Dail and Hammar's Pulmonary Pathology

Third Edition

Dail and Hammar's Pulmonary Pathology

Volume II: Neoplastic Lung Disease

Third Edition

Editor

Joseph F. Tomashefski, Jr., MD
Professor, Department of Pathology, Case Western Reserve University School of Medicine; Chairman, Department of Pathology, MetroHealth Medical Center, Cleveland, Ohio, USA

Associate Editors

Philip T. Cagle, MD
Professor, Department of Pathology, Weill Medical College of Cornell University, New York, New York; Director, Pulmonary Pathology, Department of Pathology, The Methodist Hospital, Houston, Texas, USA

Carol F. Farver, MD
Director, Pulmonary Pathology, Department of Anatomic Pathology, The Cleveland Clinic Foundation, Cleveland, Ohio, USA

Armando E. Fraire, MD
Professor, Department of Pathology, University of Massachusetts Medical School, Worcester, Massachusetts, USA

Springer

Editor:
Joseph F. Tomashefski, Jr., MD
Professor, Department of Pathology, Case Western Reserve University School of Medicine; Chairman, Department of Pathology, MetroHealth Medical Center, Cleveland, OH, USA

Associate Editors:
Philip T. Cagle, MD
Professor, Department of Pathology, Weill Medical College of Cornell University, New York, NY; Director, Pulmonary Pathology, Department of Pathology, The Methodist Hospital, Houston, TX, USA

Carol F. Farver, MD
Director, Pulmonary Pathology, Department of Anatomic Pathology, The Cleveland Clinic Foundation, Cleveland, OH, USA

Armando E. Fraire, MD
Professor, Department of Pathology, University of Massachusetts Medical School, Worcester, MA, USA

Volume II ISBN 978-1-4939-3692-2 ISBN 978-0-387-72114-9 (eBook)
DOI 10.1007/978-0-387-72114-9

Set ISBN 978-0-387-72139-2

Printed on acid-free paper.

9 8 7 6 5 4 3 2 1

springer.com

To
David H. Dail
Samuel P. Hammar

For their many contributions to pulmonary pathology, and for their conceptual and sustaining vision of this textbook

Joseph F. Tomashefski, Jr.
Philip T. Cagle
Carol F. Farver
Armando E. Fraire

To my dear wife, Cathy, and our children, Amy, Cary, David, Jessica, and Sarah

Joseph F. Tomashefski, Jr.

To my wife, Kirsten

Philip T. Cagle

To the memory of my parents, Albert and Gladys Farver

Carol F. Farver

In memory of Dr. S. Donald Greenberg, dear friend, respected colleague, and superb teacher

Armando E. Fraire

Preface

It is with a great sense of good fortune, humility, and responsibility that we, the editors, have undertaken the task of updating Dail and Hammar's *Pulmonary Pathology*, one of the great modern textbooks not only in the field of lung pathology but also in the wider arena of general pathology as well. Following the publication of its first edition, "Dail and Hammar" rapidly became the standard against which subsequent textbooks of lung pathology were measured.

First published in 1987, *Pulmonary Pathology* provided an alternative to Herbert Spencer's time-honored text, *Pathology of the Lung* which, in its fourth edition at that time, was the reigning tome on the pathology of the respiratory system. The first edition of "Dail and Hammar" was in part dedicated to Dr. Spencer, who graciously penned the foreword for that text. The first edition was also dedicated to Averill Liebow, one of the giants of pulmonary pathology, under whom Dr. Dail had served and been mentored as a fellow. Dr. Liebow's influence was notable in the first two editions, and has continued in this edition in the revised classifications and current understanding of interstitial pneumonias and lung tumors, subjects in which Dr. Liebow played such a defining role. Several of Dr. Liebow's timeless original illustrations continue to grace the pages of the third edition.

In the 13 years since the second edition there have been astounding advances in medicine and pathology. The current edition has been revised and updated to reflect these advances. As much as possible, however, we have striven to remain true to Drs. Dail and Hammar's original goals, "to present the reader with an authoritative yet readable text which hopefully answers questions that might arise in facing problem cases and to offer the reader appropriate review of particular areas within the field of pulmonary pathology." In the face of wide-reaching revisions our intent has been to maintain the unique character of *Pulmonary Pathology*, and retain continuity with previous editions. Dr. Dail and Dr. Hammar have continued to play a major role in the present text, together contributing as author or coauthor to approximately one fourth of the chapters. Nine other chapters have been updated by contributors who were also featured in the second edition. Many, if not the majority, of the illustrations in the text represent the color counterparts of previous black-and-white figures. Electron microscopy, which was emphasized in the previous two editions, continues to have a presence in the third, mainly in the volume on neoplasia, and lays the foundation for a deep understanding of the histological appearances of tumors.

The changes in the current edition, however, are significant. The previous sizable single volume text has been divided into two volumes, covering neoplastic and non-neoplastic lung diseases, to afford the reader more ready access and less strenuous effort when referencing the sections of interest. Entirely new chapters have been added on the pathology of small airways disease (Chapter 25), forensic lung pathology (Chapter 31), molecular genetics of lung and pleural neoplasms (Chapter 33), and preinvasive (neoplastic) disease (Chapter 34). The topics formerly included in the second edition chapters on AIDS and tobacco-related injury have been dispersed in the third edition, mainly throughout the sections on lung infections and lung cancer, respectively. Similarly the monumental chapters on common and uncommon lung tumors in the previous editions have been divided into seven smaller topical units housed in the second volume. Over 90 percent of the illustrations in the current edition are now presented in vivid color.

Pulmonary Pathology was one of the first pathology textbooks to emphasize the burgeoning field of immunohistochemistry and its application to diagnostic pathology, and the current edition continues to expound on the important diagnostic role of immunohistochemical stains. In this edition, however, we also embrace the molecular age with updated information on molecular pathology. In addition to extensive references to molecular aspects of lung disease, which are integrated within each of the individual chapters, the new edition includes two chapters (Chapters 33 and 34) devoted almost exclusively to molecular pathology. Chapter 33 (Molecular Genetics of Lung and Pleural Neoplasms) is essentially a text-within-a-text, serving as a compendium of information on the molecular pathology of lung tumors as well as a primer on basic molecular pathology for the uninitiated or molecularly challenged pathologist.

Within reason and to the best of our ability we have tried to maintain the reputation of *Pulmonary Pathology* as a comprehensive textbook that not only serves as a diagnostic guide to the "labyrinths of the lung," but also enables the reader to explore the etiology and pathogenesis of lung diseases. The references, both classical and modern, have been greatly increased and, as of the time that the book went to press, are relatively current. The present edition also recognizes the growing importance of electronic information sources. Relevant Internet Web sites have been included among the chapter references, and Chapter 22 on pulmonary drug toxicity is essentially constructed around Web-based resources.

There are numerous individuals to whom we owe a debt of gratitude. Most importantly, we thank the many authors who gave of their time and talent, without

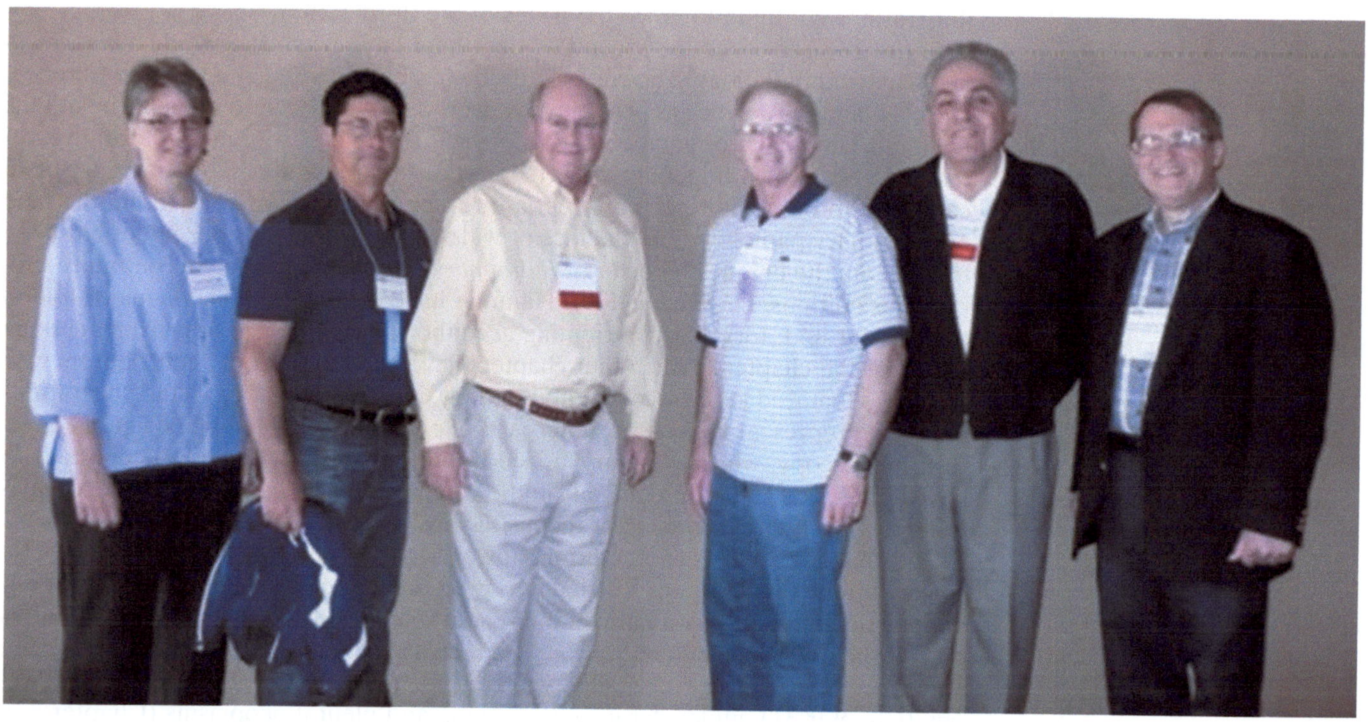

Figure 1. Members of the editorial board with Drs. Dail and Hammar. (From left to right: Carol F. Farver, Philip T. Cagle, David H. Dail, Samuel P. Hammar, Armando E. Fraire, and Joseph F. Tomashefski, Jr.)

financial compensation, to contribute to this book. Their expertise and dedication represent the soul of the work. We also appreciate their patience and understanding as both authors and editors faced the stressful implications of rapidly approaching (and receding) publication deadlines. We recognize and are especially thankful for the wonderful pulmonary pathologists under whom we have trained, who taught us the trade and served as our role models: Dr. S. Donald Greenberg (Drs. Cagle and Fraire); Dr. William Thurlbeck (Dr. Cagle); Drs. Jerome Kleinerman, John D. Reid, Merle Legg, and Lynne Reid (Dr. Tomashefski); and Drs. John Godleski and Les Kobzik (Dr. Farver). Finally, we are grateful to the Springer publishing firm, especially to our executive editor, Melissa Ramondetta and her editorial assistant, Dianne Wuori. A special thanks goes to our developmental editor, Stephanie Sakson, who kept us on track throughout the process, surmounting the hurdles of copyright permits, and the inexorable correlation of images, references, and text.

From the editors' perspective our labors now are ended (for a while at least). We leave it to you, the reader, to evaluate this text. We welcome your comments, positive or negative, which may help to direct future editions.

Joseph F. Tomashefski, Jr., MD
Philip T. Cagle, MD
Carol F. Farver, MD
Armando E. Fraire, MD

Contents

Volume II: Neoplastic Lung Disease

Volume I: Nonneoplastic Lung Disease

Contributors

Patrick A. Adegboyega, MD
Department of Pathology, University of Texas Medical Branch, Galveston, TX 77555, USA

Timothy C. Allen, MD, JD
Chairman, Department of Pathology, University of Texas Health Center at Tyler, Tyler, TX 75708, USA

Roberto Barrios, MD
Attending Pathologist, Department of Pathology, The Methodist Hospital, Houston, TX 77030, USA

Mary Beth Beasley, MD
Department of Pathology, Providence Portland Medical Center, Portland, OR 97210, USA

Kelly J. Butnor, MD
Assistant Professor, Department of Pathology, University of Vermont/Fletcher Allen Health Care, Burlington, VT 05401, USA

Philip T. Cagle, MD
Professor, Department of Pathology, Weill Medical College of Cornell University, New York; *and* Director, Pulmonary Pathology, Department of Pathology, The Methodist Hospital, Houston, TX 77030, USA

Thomas V. Colby, MD
Consultant in Pathology, Mayo Clinic Scottsdale, Scottsdale, AZ 85259, USA

Carlyne D. Cool, MD
Department of Pathology, University of Colorado Health Sciences Center, Denver, CO 80262, USA

David H. Dail, MD
Staff Pathologist, Department of Pathology, Virginia Mason Medical Center, Seattle, WA 98101, USA

Louis P. Dehner, MD
Professor and Director, Division of Anatomic Pathology, Washington University School of Medicine, St. Louis, MO 63122, USA

Ronald F. Dodson
ERI Consulting, Inc., 2026 Republic Drive, Ste A, Tyler, TX 75701, USA

Carol F. Farver, MD
Director, Pulmonary Pathology, Department of Anatomic Pathology, The Cleveland Clinic Foundation, Cleveland, OH 44195, USA

Douglas B. Flieder, MD
Chief of Surgical Pathology, Fox Chase Cancer Center, Philadelphia, PA 19111, USA

Armando E. Fraire, MD
Professor, Department of Pathology, University of Massachusetts Medical School, Worcester, MA 01655, USA

Anthony A. Gal, MD
Professor, Department of Pathology and Laboratory Medicine, Emory University Hospital, Atlanta, GA 30322, USA

Michael A. Graham, MD
Professor, St. Louis University School of Medicine; *and* Chief Medical Examiner, City of St. Louis, Division of Forensic and Environmental Pathology, St. Louis, MO 63104, USA

Steve D. Groshong, MD, PhD
Instructor, Department of Pathology, University of Colorado Health Sciences Center, Denver, CO 80262, USA

Donald G. Guinee, Jr., MD
Pathologist, Department of Pathology, Virginia Mason Medical Center, Seattle, WA 98111, USA

Samuel P. Hammar, MD
Harrison Medical Center, Pathology Associates of Kitsap County, Bremerton, WA 98310, USA

Abida K. Haque, MD
Medical Director, Department of Pathology, San Jacinto Methodist Hospital, Baytown, TX 77521, USA

Philip Hasleton, MD, FRCPath
Professor, Department of Histopathology, Clinical Sciences Block, Manchester Royal Infirmary, Manchester M13 9WL, UK

Douglas W. Henderson, MB, BS, FRCPA, FRCPath, FHKCPath (Hon)
Professor and Senior Consultant, Departments of Pathology and Anatomical Pathology, Flinders Medical Centre, Bedford Park 5042, Adelaide, South Australia

Elise R. Hoff, MD
Department of Pathology, University of Pittsburgh Medical Center—Presbyterian, Pittsburgh, PA 15213, USA

Aliya N. Husain, MB, BS
Professor, Department of Pathology, University of Chicago, Chicago, IL 60637, USA

Jaishree Jagirdar, MD
Department of Pathology, University of Texas Health Science Center at San Antonio, San Antonio, TX 78284, USA

Keith M. Kerr, BSc(Hons) MB ChB FRCPath
Consultant, Pathologist and Clinical Senior Lecturer, Department of Pathology, Aberdeen Royal Infirmary and Aberdeen University School of Medicine, Foresterhill, Aberdeen, AB25 2ZD, UK

Andras Khoor, MD
Department of Pathology, Mayo Clinic Jacksonville, Jacksonville, FL 32224, USA

Sonja Klebe, MD, PhD, FRCPA
Senior Lecturer in Anatomical Pathology, Flinders University and Consultant in Anatomical Pathology, Flinders Medical Centre, Bedford Park 5042, Adelaide, South Australia

Les Kobzik, MD
Associate Professor, Department of Environmental Health, Harvard School of Public Health, Boston, MA 02115, USA

P. Rocco LaSala, MD
Fellow, Medical Microbiology, Department of Pathology, University of Texas Medical Branch, Galveston, TX 77555, USA

Kevin O. Leslie, MD
Consultant and Professor, Mayo Clinic College of Medicine, Rochester, MN; *and* Department of Laboratory Medicine and Pathology, Mayo Clinic Scottsdale, Scottsdale, AZ 85259, USA

Aileen M. Marty, MD, FACP
Senior Scientific Advisor to the Undersecretary for Science and Technology Directorate, DHS, Department of Homeland Security, National Defense University, North Bethesda, MD 20852, USA

Michael R. McGinnis, PhD
Professor, Department of Pathology, University of Texas Medical Branch, Galveston, TX 77555, USA

William George Morice, MD, PhD
Consultant, Associate Professor of Medicine, Departments of Hematopathology and Anatomic Pathology, Mayo Clinic, Mayo Medical School, Rochester, MN 55905, USA

Andrew G. Nicholson, FRCPath DM
Professor of Respiratory Pathology, National Heart and Lung Institute Division of Imperial College School of Medicine and Consultant Histopathologist, Royal Brompton Hospital, Department of Histopathology, Sydney Street, London SW3 6NP, UK

N. Paul Ohori, MD
Medical Director of Cytopathology, Department of Pathology, University of Pittsburgh Medical Center—Presbyterian, Pittsburgh, PA 15213, USA

Christopher D. Paddock, MD, MS, MPHTM
Staff Pathologist, Department of Infectious Disease Pathology Activity, Centers for Disease Control and Prevention, Atlanta, GA 30333, USA

Helmut H. Popper, MD, Prof. Pathol.
Department of Pathology, University of Graz, Auenbruggerplatz 25, Graz A-8036, Austria

Gary W. Procop, MD, MS
Section Head, Clinical Microbiology, Division of Pathology and Laboratory Medicine, The Cleveland Clinic Foundation, 9500 Euclid Avenue, Cleveland, OH 44195

Victor L. Roggli, MD
Department of Pathology, Duke University and Durham VA Medical Centers, Durham, NC 27705, USA

Thomas A. Sporn, MD
Department of Pathology, Duke University and Durham VA Medical Centers, Durham, NC 27710, USA

J. Thomas Stocker, MD
Professor of Pathology, Uniformed Services University of the Health Sciences, 4301 Jones Bridge Road, Bethesda, MD 20814

Joseph F. Tomashefski, Jr., MD
Professor, Department of Pathology Case Western Reserve University School of Medicine; Chairman, Department of Pathology MetroHealth Medical Center Cleveland, OH 44109, USA

William D. Travis, MD
Attending Thoracic Pathologist, Department of Pathology, Memorial Sloan Kettering Cancer Center, New York, NY 10021, USA

David H. Walker, MD
Department of Pathology, University of Texas Medical Branch, Galveston, TX 77555, USA

Washington C. Winn, Jr., MD
Fletcher Allen Health Care, University of Vermont College of Medicine, Burlington, VT 05482, USA

Sherif R. Zaki, MD, PhD
Chief, Infectious Disease Pathology Activity, Department of Infectious Disease Pathology Activity, Centers for Disease Control and Prevention, Atlanta, GA 30333, USA

Dani S. Zander, MD
Professor and Chair, Department of Pathology, Penn State Milton S. Hershey Medical Center, Hershey, PA 17033, USA

32 Lymphoproliferative Diseases

William George Morice and Thomas V. Colby

Lymphoreticular diseases affecting the lung include primary and secondary lymphomas and related disorders, leukemias, and a number of lesions that are generally considered benign and hyperplastic processes. Distinguishing neoplastic disorders such as low-grade B-cell lymphomas from reactive conditions associated with prominent lymphoid infiltrates such as lymphocytic interstitial pneumonia has long been difficult for pathologists.[1–4] This difficulty is typified by the colorful history of pseudolymphoma (see below) and by lymphomatoid granulomatosis, with all its synonyms,[5–7] which has been considered by some to be a peculiar vasculitis and by others a lymphoproliferative disorder, although the weight of evidence suggests that most cases represent the latter.[8]

Classically, lymphomas involving pulmonary tissues were recognized histologically by the presence of a monomorphous population of atypical lymphoid cells and clinically by manifesting as aggressive neoplasms. However, the advent of antibody and molecular genetic reagents has allowed for a more precise definition of lymphoid malignancies as a clonal proliferation of hematolymphoid cells. This, in turn, has led to the generation of a classification scheme of these disorders based on both the cell lineage (B cell, T cell, or true histiocytic) and the putative immunologic compartment from which these neoplasms arise.[9] These tools have also enabled the recognition of a broader clinical and histologic spectrum of lymphoproliferative disorders involving the lung, including lesions that pursue a very indolent clinical course and those with a polymorphous cellular composition.

Normal Lymphoid Tissue and Lymphatic Routes of the Lung

Understanding the histology of lymphoreticular infiltrates in the lungs requires knowledge of the normal lymphatic routes and lymphoid tissue of the lung. The lymphatic routes (listed in Table 32.1) are found along the bronchovascular bundles, the pulmonary veins, and in the septa and pleura.[10,11] The lymphatics themselves are barely discernible in normal lungs but are easily recognized in pathologic states such as pulmonary edema. Lesions that tend to show a distribution along the lymphatic routes include lymphoreticular infiltrates (Fig. 32.1), lymphangitic carcinoma, sarcoidosis, and some pneumoconioses, the last reflecting lymphatic drainage of the inhaled dust.

Hilar and peribronchial lymph nodes are present in all individuals, but intrapulmonary lymph nodes are uncommon. *Intrapulmonary lymph nodes* (Fig. 32.2) are usually incidental findings encountered during computed tomography (CT) scanning of the chest, in lobectomy specimens, or at autopsy. Radiologic and pathologic studies have demonstrated that these lymph nodes most often occur singly below the level of the carina, although in some instances they may be multiple and be present in the upper lungs. Radiologically these usually appear as small (less than 2 cm), oval, smooth lesions that are either immediately subpleural or within close proximity (1 cm or less).[12] Intrapulmonary lymph nodes appear to be most commonly encountered in adult males, and an autopsy study suggested an association with smoking.[13]

TABLE 32.1. Lymphatic routes of the lung

Pleura
Interlobular septa
Bronchovascular bundles and along large intralobular veins

Note: Lymphatics are not found in alveolar septa.

On histologic examination they are usually anthracotic, and may contain or coexist with silicotic nodules.[13] The primary importance of intrapulmonary lymph nodes for the pathologist is that they may be detected during high-resolution CT scanning of the chest for cancer screening or staging. As the radiologic features of these lymph nodes are not sufficiently distinctive to reliably distinguish them from potential early malignancies, biopsy may be required for their accurate identification.[12,14]

Bienenstock et al.[15–18] and others[19] have drawn attention to a relatively extensive system of pulmonary lymphoid tissue termed bronchus-associated lymphoid tissue (BALT). BALT represents lymphoid aggregates found along airways, particularly at bifurcations, as well as those along other lymphatic routes of the lung, and is thought to be part of a more generalized immunologic compartment of mucosa-associated lymphoid tissue (MALT). MALT is specialized lymphoid tissue that is distinguished from peripheral somatic (nodal) lymphoid tissue by its ability to combat pathogens at mucosal sites through the production of immunoglobulin A (IgA) and other factors.[18,19] As might be expected from the functional role of the MALT compartment, this tissue is intimately associated with the adjacent epithelium and may even percolate between individual epithelial cells (Fig. 32.3C,D). This tropism for epithelial cells can be particularly prominent in lymphomas derived from MALT tissues, which have a proclivity to invade adjacent epithelial structures.[20–22] Lymphocytes in this system also have the ability to circulate and to "home" to other MALT organs such as the salivary glands, intestinal tract, thyroid, cervix, endometrium, and breast.[15–18,20,21,23–25]

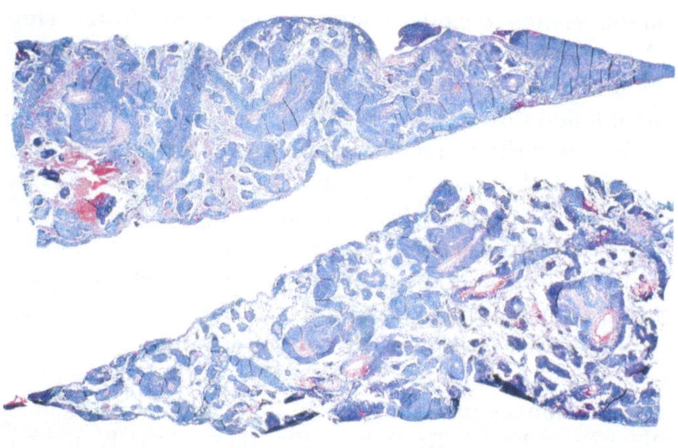

FIGURE 32.1. The lymphatic routes of the lung are illustrated in this lymphoma. The lymphomatous infiltrate is found in the pleura, septa, and along bronchovascular bundles, with relative sparing of the alveolar portions of the lung that do not have lymphatics.

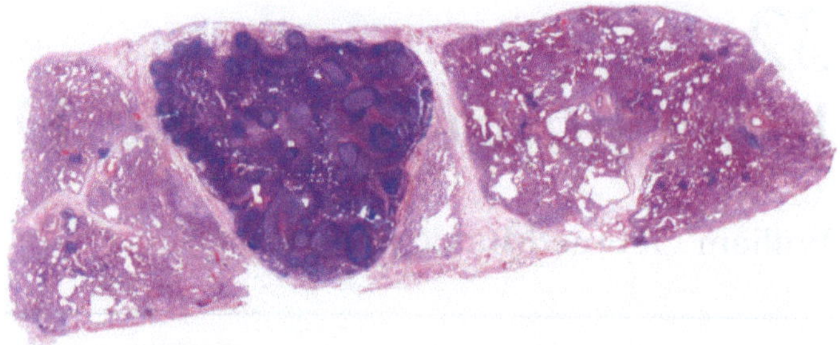

FIGURE 32.2. Intrapulmonary lymph node. This wedge biopsy shows an intrapulmonary lymph node located in an interlobular septum. Reactive follicles are apparent even at scanning power microscopy. Most intrapulmonary lymph nodes are located in or along the pleura or interlobular septa.

The radiologic manifestations of lymphoreticular infiltrates include a broad and nonspecific spectrum of changes.[26–28] The radiographic patterns of disease can often be correlated with the histologic findings: lesions that are characterized histologically by diffuse infiltrates along lymphatic routes without extensive nodular expansions produce a diffuse interstitial pattern radiologically, whereas mixed interstitial and nodular or frankly nodular patterns are associated with progressively larger nodules along the lymphatic distribution. Massive infiltration with spillover into air spaces produces a pneumonic or alveolar pattern. Combinations of these patterns are common.[26–28]

A wide variety of abnormalities may also be observed by CT examination including ground-glass opacification of pulmonary parenchyma and reticulonodular infiltrates along bronchovascular bundles. In comparison to routine chest radiology, CT scanning may be more sensitive in detecting micronodular infiltrates and peribronchovascular thickening and also may provide more detailed information regarding the character of the infiltrate, particularly in low-grade lesions. The radiologic features of lymphoreticular processes are usually not sufficiently distinctive to allow them to be distinguished from other disorders such as bronchioloalveolar carcinoma, granulomatous processes, and organizing pneumonia.[29,30] The radiologic features of specific entities are discussed in greater detail throughout the chapter.

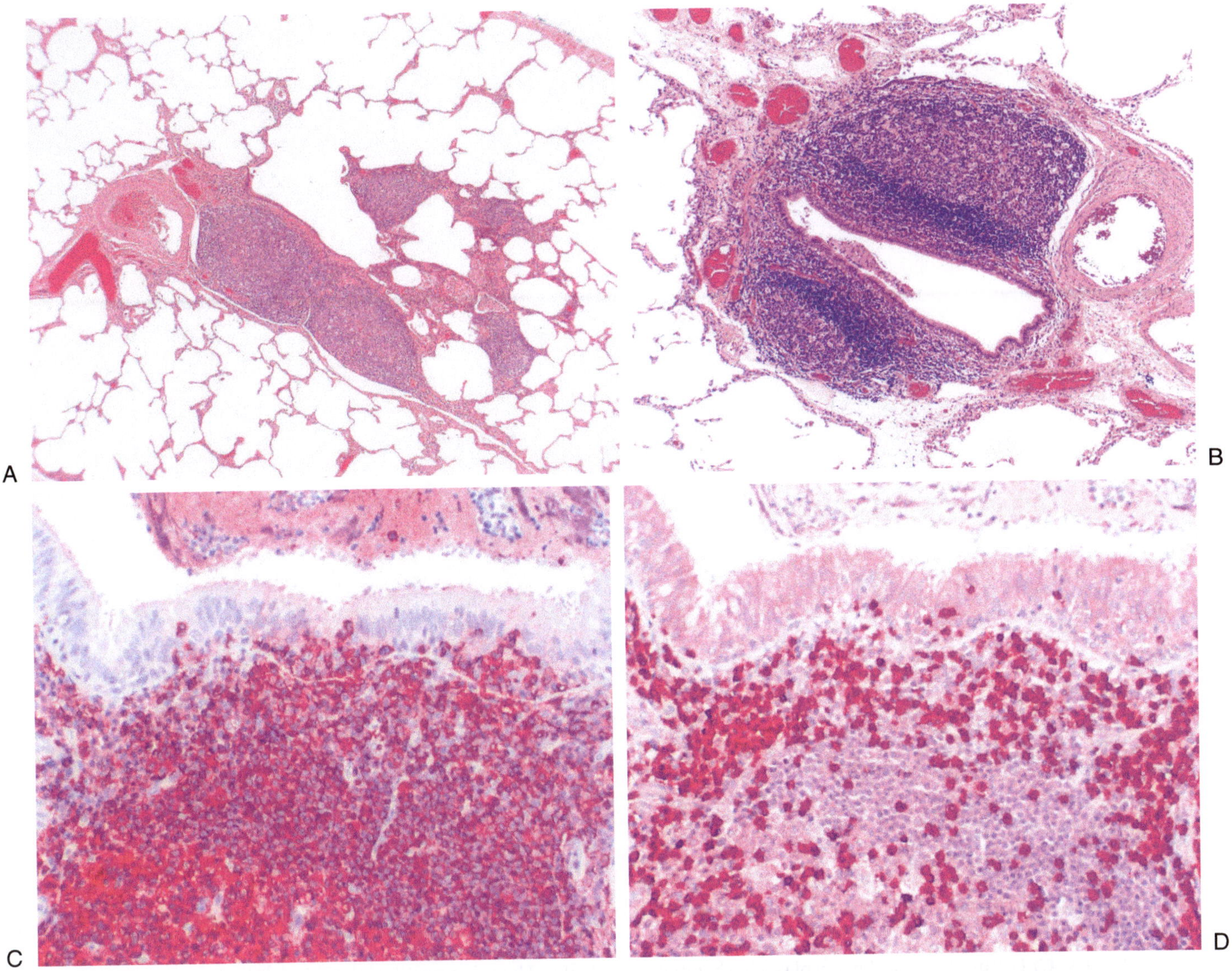

FIGURE 32.3. **(A,B)** Bronchus-associated lymphoid tissue. This case of follicular bronchiolitis shows reactive germinal centers along a small bronchiole. Immunostaining for CD20 **(C)** and CD3 **(D)** illustrates the close approximation of the lymphoid tissue to the epithelium and the extension of B cells as well as a few T cells into the epithelium.

Lymphoid Hyperplasias, Benign Lymphoid Infiltrates, and Related Lesions

Hyperplasia of lymphoid tissue in the lung is similar to lymphoid hyperplasia of other sites, with the production of germinal centers distributed along the normal locations of lymphatic tissue, specifically the pulmonary lymphatic routes. Exuberant lymphoid hyperplasia along the airways is termed follicular bronchitis or follicular bronchiolitis (Fig. 32.3), depending on the size of airway involved.[31] Lymphoid hyperplasia may also involve the septa and pleura.

In healthy children one may see a few lymphocytes and a rare germinal center in the lung. Adults generally do not have significant quantities of lymphoid tissue in parenchymal biopsy material.[19] Studies have shown the presence of small lymphoid aggregates in some bronchial biopsies from otherwise normal individuals,[32] when pulmonary lymphoid tissue is prominent; however, a pathologic condition is usually present. Hyperplasia of lymphoid tissue in the lung is most commonly a manifestation of chronic infections, chronic bronchitis, bronchiectasis, or cystic fibrosis, or is a reaction around chronic inflammatory processes such as granulomatous infections or abscesses.[33] Primary and secondary neoplasms can also have an associated lymphoid reaction including germinal

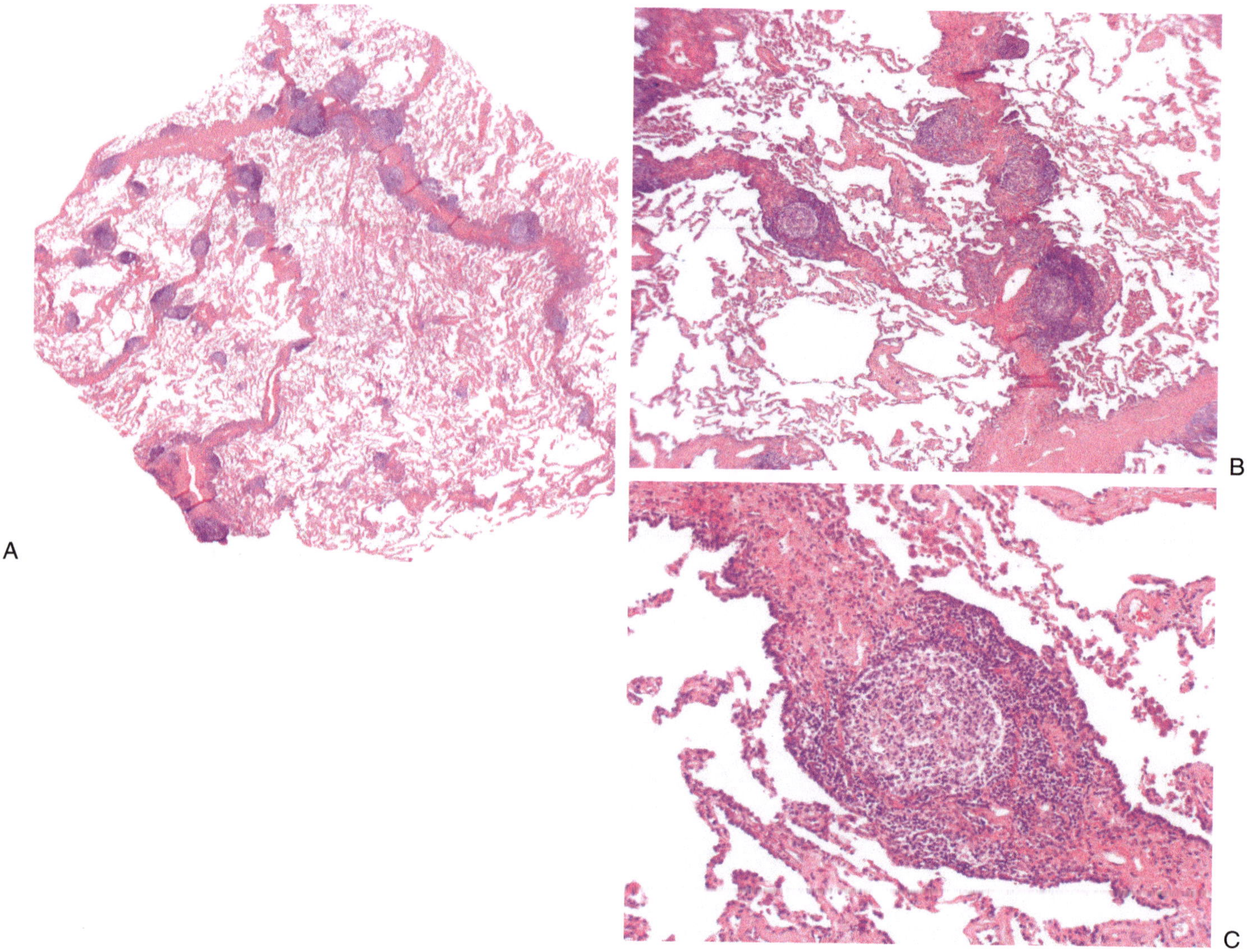

FIGURE 32.4. **(A–C)** Diffuse lymphoid hyperplasia in rheumatoid arthritis. There is a proliferation of germinal centers most prominent along interlobular septa **(A,B)**.

centers, sheets of plasma cells, or granulomas, especially in foci of obstructive pneumonia. Metastases from the lymphoepithelial variant of nasopharyngeal carcinoma and primary lymphoepithelioma-like carcinomas of the lung represent particularly florid examples.

Diffuse lymphoid hyperplasia (Fig. 32.4) producing bilateral pulmonary infiltrates on chest radiographs may sometimes be an isolated histologic finding, particularly in collagen vascular diseases (e.g., rheumatoid arthritis, Sjögren's syndrome), congenital and acquired immunodeficiency states (including HIV infection; Fig. 32.5), and systemic hypersensitivity reactions.[31,34–36] This is one of the patterns that has also been encompassed by the term *lymphocytic interstitial pneumonia* (see below). In collagen vascular diseases, this lymphoid proliferation is the lung's correlate of the exuberant lymphoid hyperplasia, which may be seen in lymph nodes in this group of disorders.[37] The lymphoid hyperplasia may at times be most prominent along airways (follicular bronchitis/bronchiolitis) and associated with clinical evidence of interstitial *or* airflow obstructive disease.[31]

When first described, *angioimmunoblastic lymphadenopathy* was thought to represent a peculiar autoimmune reaction with a syndromic clinical presentation and relatively frequent pulmonary involvement. Signs and symptoms associated with the condition included generalized lymphadenopathy, hepatosplenomegaly, Coombs-positive hemolytic anemia, skin rash, polyclonal hypergammaglobulinemia, and anemia.[38–41] While some reactive conditions with these features may occur, most cases are now recognized as being representative of a unique type of peripheral T-cell lymphoma termed angioimmunoblastic T-cell lymphoma.[42] For this reason this entity is discussed in greater detail below (see Lymphomas with Secondary Lung Involvement).

Lymphocytic Interstitial Pneumonia

Lymphocytic (lymphoid) interstitial pneumonia (LIP) (Fig. 32.6) is a chronic interstitial pneumonia characterized by a dense and diffuse polymorphous interstitial infiltrate composed of cells that are histologically benign and immunophenotypically polyclonal.[2,4,35,43,44] LIP is usually diffuse in its involvement of alveolar walls, another feature that distinguishes it from most malignant lymphomas. Lymphoid follicles are often present and there is overlap of this pattern with diffuse lymphoid hyperplasia (Fig. 32.7), although the latter is primarily related to the lymphatic routes. In the literature, both of these patterns have often been collectively referred to as lymphocytic interstitial pneumonia. However, when lymphoid follicles with germinal centers distributed along the lymphatic routes are the dominant features (Figs. 32.4 and 32.5), the term *diffuse lymphoid hyperplasia* is appropriately descriptive.[35]

With the description of the cellular pattern of nonspecific interstitial pneumonia (NSIP), many cases that might formerly have been called LIP are now called NSIP.[45] There are no precise criteria to distinguish LIP and NSIP, but most observers include as LIP only those cases with *dense* infiltrates of lymphoid cells. The following description is derived primarily from the older literature, which probably included cases that now would be called NSIP.

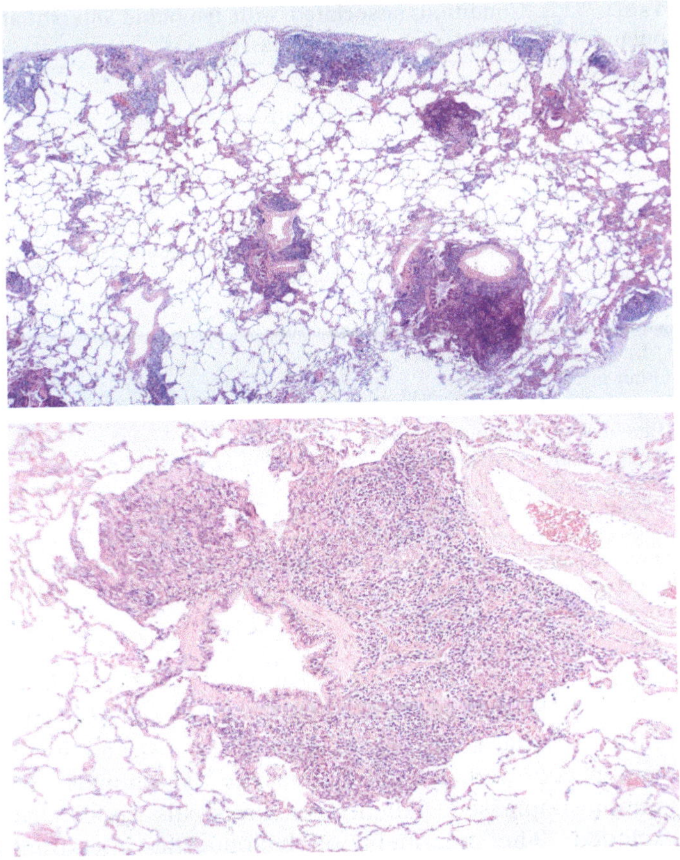

A

B

FIGURE 32.5. **(A,B)** Diffuse lymphoid hyperplasia in AIDS. Scanning power shows nodular lymphoid infiltrates along lymphatic routes, which at higher power show some features of reactive follicles **(B)**.

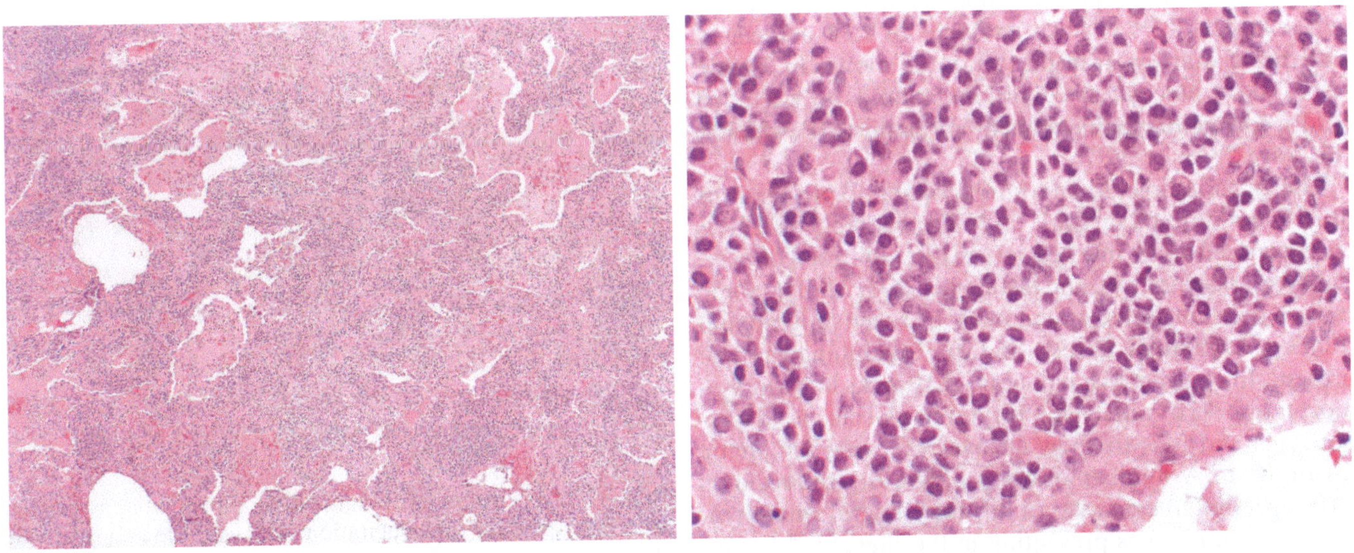

A

B

FIGURE 32.6. Lymphocytic interstitial pneumonia (LIP). There is a dense diffuse interstitial infiltrate of mononuclear cells **(A)**, which at higher power are polymorphous and include lymphocytes and plasma cells **(B)**. Immunophenotyping, including molecular studies for gene rearrangements, were negative in this case of LIP associated with Sjögren's syndrome.

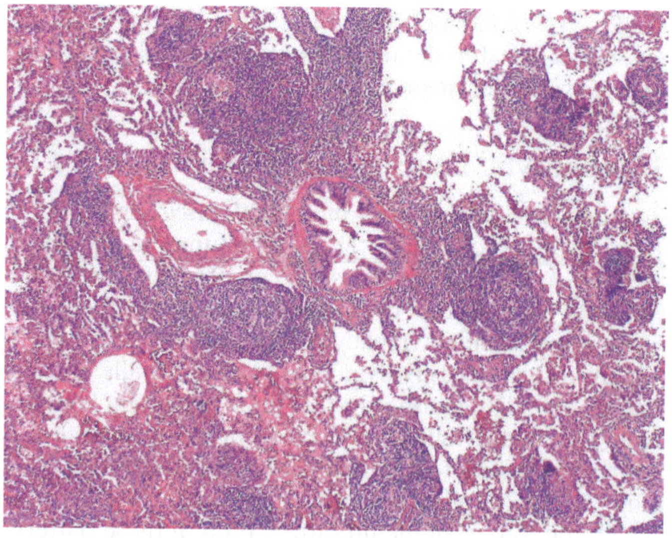

FIGURE 32.7. Diffuse lymphoid hyperplasia. There is a proliferation of germinal centers, which in this field, is predominantly along a bronchovascular structure. Diffuse lymphoid hyperplasia is one of the patterns associated with LIP. In this case there was an underlying congenital IgG deficiency.

The majority of reported cases of LIP occur in adults and have symptoms similar to other chronic interstitial pneumonias, including cough, dyspnea, weight loss, and progressive shortness of breath.[4,43,44] Children may also be affected.[46] Chest radiographs show bibasilar infiltrates. Pulmonary functions reflect infiltrative lung disease with restriction and abnormal gas exchange. Dysproteinemias are a common laboratory finding, and either hyper- or hypogammaglobulinemia may be identified. A number of conditions have been associated with LIP and diffuse lymphoid hyperplasia; they are listed in Table 32.2.[36,43,44,46–52] An example of LIP associated with bone marrow transplantation is shown in Figure 32.8. These associated conditions should be excluded before considering a diagnosis of idiopathic LIP, which is very rare.[45]

The histopathologic and immunophenotypic features of LIP are outlined in Table 32.3. The histology of LIP is characterized by a marked interstitial infiltrate of lymphocytes, plasma cells, and histiocytes (Fig. 32.6B). Some cases have giant cells, granulomas, or reactive lymphoid follicles. Interstitial fibrosis and honeycombing may be present. In contrast to lymphomas, LIP lacks large monomorphous foci of small lymphocytes or plasmacytoid lymphocytes and fails to show an overwhelming lymphatic distribution. A number of cases previously reported as LIP represented examples of diffuse bilateral small lymphocytic lymphomas presenting in the lung.[22,53,54] Immunophenotypic and molecular studies of LIP fail to show a clonal population of lymphoid cells.[43,55] T or B lymphocytes may predominate.[43,52,55]

TABLE 32.2. Conditions associated with lymphoid interstitial pneumonia/diffuse lymphoid hyperplasia

Autoimmune diseases
Sjögren's syndrome, primary biliary cirrhosis, myasthenia gravis, Hashimoto's thyroiditis, pernicious anemia/agammaglobulinemia, autoimmune hemolytic anemia, systemic lupus erythematosus, celiac disease
Immunodeficiency syndromes
Common variable immunodeficiency, acquired immunodeficiencies, unexplained childhood immunodeficiency, acquired immunodeficiency (AIDS)
Viral-associated (excluding HIV infection)
Epstein-Barr virus, chronic hepatitis
Other infections
Drug-induced
Bone marrow transplantation
Hypersensitivity pneumonitis
Miscellaneous
Familial

Modified from Colby TV, Koss MN. Travis WD. Atlas of tumor pathology. Tumors of the lower respiratory tract. Washington, DC: Armed Forces Institute of Pathology, 1994.

The differential diagnosis of LIP includes nonspecific reactive changes, extrinsic allergic alveolitis, and small lymphocytic and lymphoplasmacytic lymphomas. In immunosuppressed patients, pneumocystis should be excluded. The treatment of lymphocytic interstitial pneumonia is not resolved, but a number of patients, even those with immunodeficiency states, respond to steroids.[44,52]

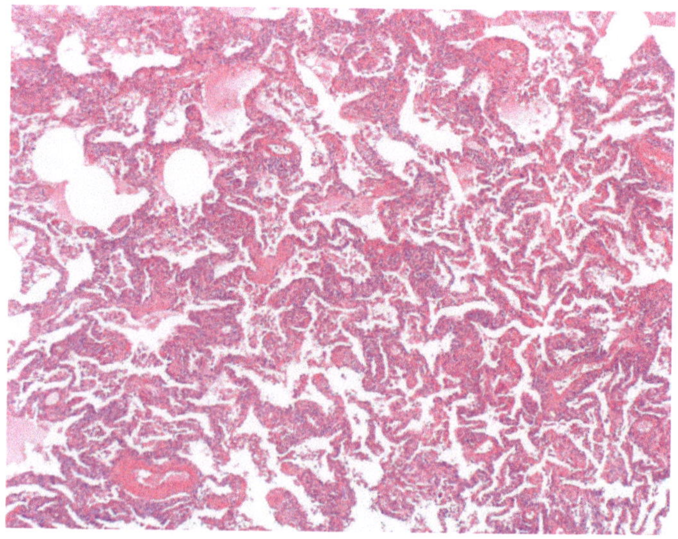

FIGURE 32.8. Lymphocytic interstitial pneumonia associated with bone marrow transplantation. This case shows a relatively dense diffuse mononuclear interstitial infiltrate. This case is right at the borderline between the degree of infiltrate expected for LIP and that expected for cellular nonspecific interstitial pneumonia (NSIP).

TABLE 32.3. Extranodal marginal zone B-cell lymphoma vs. nodular lymphoid hyperplasia and lymphocytic interstitial pneumonia

Feature	Extranodal marginal zone B-cell lymphoma	Nodular lymphoid hyperplasia	Lymphocytic interstitial pneumonia
Presentation	Single or multiple nodules consolidation, diffuse infiltrates	Localized mass/consolidation	Diffuse interstitial process
Distribution	Mass lesions with lymphatic tracking at the edges or diffuse process along lymphatic routes	Mass lesion with variable destruction of lung architecture; some lymphatic tracking of hyperplastic-appearing tissue	Diffuse proliferation of hyperplastic lymphoid tissue along lymphatic routes or dense diffuse infiltrates of interstitium
Germinal centers	Usually present with thick cuff of lymphoid tissue; colonization of germinal centers by monocytoid or centrocytic cells	Normal-appearing germinal centers present	Germinal centers are normal appearing when present
Cellular composition around germinal centers	Mixed including variable numbers of lymphocytes, monocytoid/centrocytic cells, transformed lymphocytes, plasma cells, often with Dutcher bodies	Polymorphous cellular composition, usually lymphocytes and plasma cells without Dutcher bodies	Polymorphous cellular composition, usually lymphocytes and plasma cells without Dutcher bodies
Epithelial infiltration by lymphoid cells (highlighted with cytokeratin staining)	Lymphoepithelial lesions often prominent	Lymphoepithelial lesions inconspicuous	Lymphoepithelial lesions inconspicuous
Immunophenotype	Predominant population of CD20 positive B cells (CD5, CD10, CD23 negative) with appreciable background population of CD3-positive T cells; T cells may appear predominant in some foci; plasma cells may be monotypic or polyclonal	CD20 positive B cells usually confined to follicular and immediate perifollicular regions with the remainder of the cells being predominantly T cells; polytypic plasma cells	CD20-positive B cells usually confined to follicular and immediate perifollicular regions with the remainder of the cells being predominantly T cells; polytypic plasma cells
Additional findings in some cases	Granulomas, hyaline sclerosis, amyloid deposition, crystal storing histiocytosis	Granulomas, hyaline sclerosis	Granulomas, hyaline sclerosis
Flow cytometry, molecular studies	Clonal population identified in most cases (note: these are sample dependent and false negatives may be encountered)	No clonal population identified	No clonal population identified

Note: All of the features encountered in nodular lymphoid hyperplasia and lymphocytic interstitial pneumonia may be encountered in extranodal marginal zone B-cell lymphomas and thus it is often difficult to absolutely exclude the possibility of an extranodal marginal zone B-cell lymphoma in which diagnostic tissue has not been evaluated.

Pseudolymphoma or Nodular Lymphoid Hyperplasia

Pseudolymphoma is a term that has historically been used to describe localized lymphoid proliferations in the lung presenting as a single nodule or region of consolidation confined to one lobe.[35,53,56] This moniker was coined as these lesions did not fulfill the early accepted clinical and pathologic criteria for the diagnosis of lymphoma due to lack of clinically aggressive behavior and the mixture of lymphoid elements present, respectively. The number of cases in which this descriptive category applies has dramatically diminished as most of the lesions that had been called pulmonary pseudolymphoma (synonym: nodular lymphoid hyperplasia[35]) have been reinterpreted as low-grade B-cell lymphomas.[22,53,54,56–61] Of all cases that the surgical pathologist encounters with massive accumulations of lymphocytes in the lung, roughly four of five (80%) were previously interpreted as pseudolymphomas,[62] whereas at least four of five (80%) are now interpreted as low-grade B-cell lymphomas.[56] In light of the controversy and confusion surrounding the term *pulmonary pseudolymphoma*, the term *nodular lymphoid hyperplasia* first proposed by Kradin and Mark[35] is likely a more appropriate and accurate diagnostic appellation. Regardless of whether pseudolymphoma or nodular lymphoid hyperplasia is used, this diagnosis should be restricted to those tumefactive lesions in which there is a prominent lymphoid infiltrate that by routine morphology appears reactive and that by ancillary immunophenotypic and molecular genetic analysis lacks evidence of clonality. In many cases one is left with a descriptive diagnosis (e.g., "atypical lymphoid proliferation"), since definitive characterization of a lesion may not be possible, particularly in small biopsy specimens.

Reported cases of pulmonary "pseudolymphomas" occur in adults; in a minority of cases there is a history of a prior pneumonia at the site. These lesions are most often encountered in asymptomatic patients in whom a localized mass or infiltrate is detected on routine chest radiography. Laboratory studies are generally noncontributory, but four cases in the series of Koss et al.[56] had a polyclonal hypergammaglobulinemia.

Grossly, nodular lymphoid hyperplasias are tan and well circumscribed from the surrounding tissue.[35] Fibrosis within the lesion may cause retraction of tissue toward the center of the mass. The pathologic findings in nodular lymphoid hyperplasia are described in brief in Table 32.3. A hallmark microscopic feature is the heterogeneity in cellular composition and variation from field to field. The cellular infiltrate is mixed and generally includes lymphocytes, plasma cells, and occasional histiocytes that may form nonnecrotizing granulomas; approximately one third of cases contain giant cells. Reactive germinal centers with intact mantle zones that are separated by plasma cells containing Russell bodies may be prominent, but Dutcher bodies should not be seen. There is a variable amount of scarring that may be cellular and fibroblastic or acellular and hyaline in appearance. When fibroblastic proliferation is marked, *focal* or *chronic organizing pneumonia* may be more appropriate terms.[63] Confusion with the entity *pulmonary hyalinizing granuloma* should not occur (see Chapter 21). Amyloid-like material may be present in lymphoid hyperplasias. At the edge of the lesion, one does not see prominent lymphangiitic tracking or invasion of bronchial cartilage, features that characterize lymphomas. Necrosis was found in one case reported by Koss et al.[56]

Extranodal marginal zone B-cell lymphomas of MALT involving the lung can show many similar, if not identical, histologic features to those of pseudolymphoma/nodular lymphoid hyperplasia. The pathologic features of these entities and LIP are compared in Table 32.3. For this reason the ancillary immunophenotypic and molecular genetic studies are critical in the evaluation of potential pseudolymphomas/nodular lymphoid hyperplasias. These studies should fail to reveal evidence of a clonal B-cell population in all cases in which this diagnosis is rendered.[56]

Castleman's disease (giant lymph node hyperplasia), particularly the hyaline vascular type, may involve nodes that are partially or completely intrapulmonary in location.[64]

In summary, much is made of distinguishing low-grade, indolent lymphomas from either nodular lymphoid hyperplasia or lymphocytic interstitial pneumonia. In practical terms, the distinction of nodular lymphoid hyperplasia from low-grade MALT lymphoma may be largely academic as many of these lesions may be resected for diagnosis. Solitary low-grade lymphomas managed in this way rarely recur and often lack extrapulmonary involvement, and therefore do not require further therapy.

Malignant Lymphomas Presenting in the Lung

Definitions of a primary lymphoma occurring in an extranodal site, including the lung,[65] are somewhat arbitrary, and cases that have evidence of disseminated disease are generally excluded. From a practical management point of view, it is useful to divide pulmonary lymphomas into those cases in which the lung is the major (or only) site of involvement at presentation and those in which the lung is involved in disseminated disease or is a site of relapse in a patient with a previously diagnosed lymphoma at another site.[66] Table 32.4 provides an abbreviated listing of the types of lymphoproliferative disorders that can occur as primary pulmonary disorders.

A lymphatic distribution of involvement can often be recognized histologically in pulmonary lymphomas whether they present in the lung or involve it secondarily.[53,54,66] A spectrum is encountered from diffuse infiltrates along lymphatic routes without mass formation to large necrotic masses with no discernible distribution, although in most cases with large nodules tracking of the infiltrates along lymphatic routes at the edge of the masses is often present. The lymphatic distribution is best appreciated at low power or even with naked-eye examination of the glass slide (Fig. 32.1). This distinctive distribution of lymphoreticular infiltrates has also been appreciated radiologically, particularly with high-resolution CT scanning.

Traditionally, the absence of hilar lymph node involvement has been used as evidence against a diagnosis of lymphoma when evaluating a pulmonary lesion.[62,67] Later studies emphasized that the absence of hilar lymph node involvement is a relatively frequent occurrence in primary

TABLE 32.4. Lymphomas presenting in the lung

Extranodal marginal zone B-cell lymphomas: most common (approx. 75%)
Lymphomatoid granulomatosis: next to most common
Other non-Hodgkin's lymphomas: rare
Distinct subsets: intravascular lymphomatosis, anaplastic large cell lymphoma
Hodgkin's lymphoma: rare
Lymphoproliferative disorders associated with an immunosuppressed state
Immune system dysfunction may be iatrogenic (posttransplant, methotrexate related), acquired (HIV), or congential (e.g., Wiskott-Aldrich syndrome): rare

pulmonary lymphomas and that this parameter should be considered unreliable in distinguishing benign lesions from malignant ones.[54,56,61]

If a pulmonary lymphoid lesion is suspected at the time of frozen section, the surgeon should be asked to sample hilar nodes, as they may be helpful both in establishing a diagnosis and in staging.

Practically speaking, the pathologist is often confronted with the challenge of appropriately utilizing the myriad of ancillary tests that are available to evaluate lesions composed of hematolymphoid cells. These ancillary methods are outlined and compared in Table 32.5, and they are further discussed as they pertain to specific disease entities discussed below. Many of the antibodies

TABLE 32.5. Comparison of various ancillary methods used in evaluating hematolymphoid neoplasms

Method	Reagent	Tissue required	Advantages	Shortcomings	Useful for:
Paraffin immunohistochemistry	Antibody	Paraffin embedded	Allows for optimal histopathologic correlation	Not all antigens can be detected	Evaluating all lymphoid processes
Frozen immunohistochemistry	Antibody	Frozen	Allows for some histopathologic correlation; can detect some antigens that cannot be tested in paraffin	Histology suboptimal Limited availability	Evaluating lymphoid processes composed of small lymphocytes
Flow cytometry	Fluorochrome Conjugated antibody	Fresh tissue	Allows for wide range of antigens to be detected; can examine antigen coexpression on specific cell subsets	Requires significant amounts of fresh tissue (approx. 1 cm^2) no longer available for histologic review	Evaluating lymphoid processes composed of small lymphocytes; evaluating acute leukemias and myeloid neoplasms
T-cell receptor (TCR) polymerase chain reaction (PCR)	Multiplexed PCR Primers (usually to TCR gamma chain genes)	Paraffin-embedded, fresh, or frozen	Rapid; widely available	False-positive results occur with some frequency	Evaluating potential T-cell malignancies
Immunoglobulin (Ig) PCR	Multiplexed PCR Primers (to Ig heavy and light chain genes)	Paraffin-embedded, fresh, or frozen	Rapid; widely available	False-negative results can occur, particularly in postfollicular center cell neoplasms (including mucosa-associated lymphoid tissue [MALT] lymphoma)	Evaluating potential B-cell malignancies, particularly those composed of small lymphocytes and PTLDs
TCR, Ig, and EBV Southern blot	Labeled DNA probes to TCR and Ig genes and Epstein-Barr virus (EBV) terminal repeats	Fresh or frozen	Higher specificity (TCR) and sensitivity (Ig); can confirm clonality of EBV positive processes	Labor intensive; limited availability	Evaluating potential B-cell and T-cell neoplasms; evaluating EBV-positive lymphoid disorders
In Situ Hybridization	RNA-specific DNA probes	Paraffin-embedded	Can detect RNA expression	Limited number of probes available; expensive	High sensitivity and specificity in detecting EBV positivity in lymphoid neoplasms
Fluorescence in-situ hybridization (FISH)	Fluorescently labeled DNA probes	Paraffin-embedded fresh	Detecting specific chromosomal translocations	Limited number of probes available; expensive	Evaluating for malignancies with known chromosomal translocations such as mantle cell lymphoma

used in evaluating hematolymphoid tumors are reactive in paraffin-embedded tissue.[68] Hence, obtaining well-fixed, representative paraffin blocks of the sampled tissue is of paramount importance, as paraffin immunohistochemistry may be helpful in confirming a light microscopic impression.[61] If there is sufficient tissue, some of the tumor should also be saved frozen both to allow for more detailed immunophenotyping analysis and to provide large amounts of high-quality DNA for ancillary molecular genetic studies, if needed. Flow cytometry is a powerful immunophenotyping technique. This method, however, requires the use of significant amounts of biopsy tissue that can not then be used for histologic examination; therefore, this technique should be employed only when there is an abundance of evaluable tissue.

Extranodal Marginal Zone Lymphoma of Mucosa-Associated Lymphoid Tissue

Review of this category is complicated by the evolution of both the classification of lymphomas in general and of the understanding of low-grade lymphomas in the lung in particular. As discussed above, prior to the advent of advanced immunophenotyping and molecular genetic techniques, many of these cases were inappropriately categorized as "pseudolymphomas." As most of these lesions came to be recognized as lymphomas, a variety of diagnostic labels were applied, largely reflecting the contemporaneous terminology used in lymphoma classification schemes. As such, entities in this category have been termed small (well-differentiated) lymphocytic lymphomas with or without plasmacytoid features, lymphocytic lymphomas of intermediate differentiation, and small cleaved-cell lymphomas. This confusing drift in nomenclature also reflects the historic difficulty in classifying lymphomas of MALT.[20] However, as the quintessential features of extranodal marginal zone B-cell lymphomas of the MALT type have been elucidated, it has come to be recognized that the vast majority of low-grade pulmonary lymphomas are of this type.

Multiple studies of pulmonary extranodal marginal zone B-cell lymphomas of the MALT type have revealed similar clinical, radiologic, and pathologic features. The following description is a summary of nine series.[54,56–60,69–71] Most patients are older than 20 (mean age, approximately 60 years), although patients as young as 12 have been observed. A variety of medical diseases/disorders may precede the diagnosis; most frequently described are autoimmune disorders that are present in approximately 30%. Slightly more than half are asymptomatic, with the lesion being discovered on chest radiographs. When present, the symptoms are usually relatively nonspecific and include cough, chest pain, dyspnea, hemoptysis, and fatigue. B-symptoms such as weight loss, fever, and night sweats are relatively uncommon. Pulmonary MALT lymphomas appear to occur slightly more often in females; however, the degree of female predominance varies among studies.

The abnormal laboratory findings in pulmonary MALT lymphoma, like the clinical abnormalities, are generally nonspecific. Up to one third of patients have a monoclonal serum gammopathy either at presentation or subsequently, irrespective of the presence or absence of marrow involvement. The light chain type of the monoclonal serum protein always matches that expressed by the monoclonal tumoral B cells, and is usually IgM class. The amount of serum monoclonal protein is usually low (less than 3 g/dL), in contrast to cases of lymphoplasmacytic lymphoma associated with Waldenström's macroglobulinemia, although cases of pulmonary involvement by low-grade B-cell lymphomas associated with the clinical and laboratory features of Waldenström's macroglobulinemia may occur.[72–74] Cryoglobulinemia with associated vasculitis has also been reported.[70] Pulmonary function studies are rarely recorded because the majority of patients have radiographically localized disease. In the minority of patients who have diffuse bilateral disease

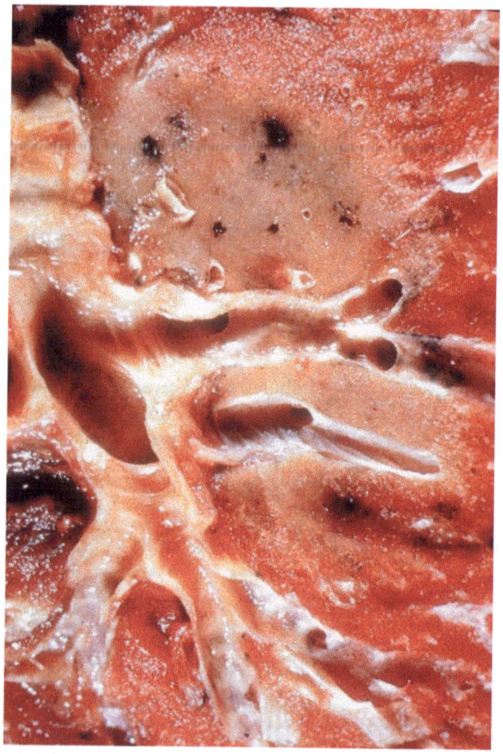

FIGURE 32.9. Low-grade extranodal marginal zone B-cell lymphoma. There is nodular consolidation without necrosis and with growth around, but not destroying, the underlying lung architecture.

radiographically, pulmonary function abnormalities of restriction and decreased diffusing capacity may be present.

The chest radiographic findings are quite variable, and any combination of the following may be seen: single or multiple nodules; unilateral or bilateral disease; localized alveolar or interstitial infiltrates; or diffuse bilateral alveolar or interstitial infiltrates. The most common presentation on routine chest radiology is a solitary, noncalcified nodule that may be 20cm or more in diameter. Air bronchograms are frequent; cavitation and hilar adenopathy are rarely observed. In a study by Wislez and colleagues,[30] the radiologic and CT features of 13 cases of primary pulmonary MALT lymphoma were compared. In this study CT examination was found to be more sensitive in detecting multiple nodules, particularly small (<7mm) nodules. The CT studies also appeared to be of greater utility in characterizing the detailed features of the infiltrates including the presence of ground-glass opacities, and a peribronchovascular growth pattern of interstitial thickening and entrapment of airways. Interestingly, dilation of the entrapped airways was seen in three cases; all lacked mucous plugging and in all the dilation resolved with treatment of the tumor.

Like other hematolymphoid neoplasms involving the lung, low-grade extranodal marginal zone lymphomas of the MALT type may form consolidative pulmonary masses (Fig. 32.9). On microscopic examination infiltration of the malignant cells along lymphatic routes can be appreciated (Fig. 32.10A,B) and these infiltrates may

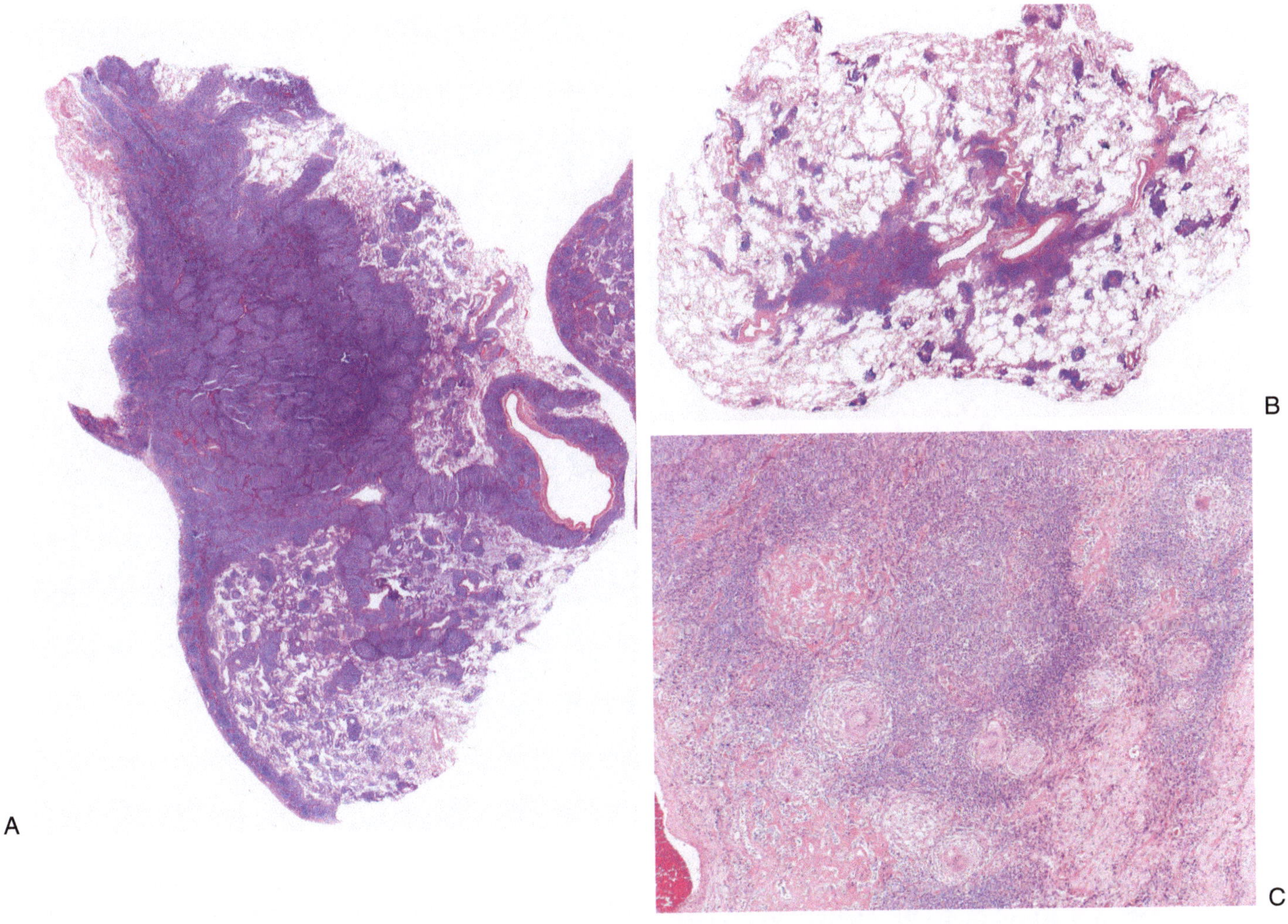

FIGURE 32.10. Low-grade of extranodal marginal zone B-cell lymphoma, low magnification features. **(A)** This whole mount illustration shows marked reactive follicular hyperplasia associated with a lesion that shows a definite tracking along perivascular and pleural lymphatic routes. **(B)** There is a nodular central zone of dense lymphoid infiltrate. There are small nodular aggregates in the surrounding lung tissue that are part of the lymphomatous process but which, in and of themselves, would be difficult to recognize as lymphoma. **(C)** This case illustrates heterogeneity with zones of sclerosis, reactive germinal centers, lymphoepithelial lesions (just below center), and granulomatous inflammation (at the 8 o'clock position).

coalesce with effacement of the normal lung architecture (Fig. 32.10B,C). The distribution may not be readily discernible in large masses, but tracking of the infiltrate along lymphatic routes may be seen at their edge, and smaller satellite lesions may be found distributed along lymphatic routes. The histopathologic findings in pulmonary MALT lymphomas are detailed in Table 32.3. Cytologically, these tumors are composed predominantly of three cell types that are present in varying proportions in each case: small lymphocytes with minimally irregular nuclear contours and sparse cytoplasm; monocytoid B cells with small irregular nuclei, abundant clear cytoplasm, and distinct cytoplasmic membranes; and cells with plasmacytoid or plasmacytic features (Fig. 32.11). When a plasma cell component is present, Dutcher bodies may be found in up to one half of cases. Interspersed among these cell populations are isolated, singly distributed "transformed" lymphocytes with large nuclei, open chromatin, and visible nucleoli.

Ideally immunologic evaluation of all suspected MALT lymphomas of the lung should be performed. In some instances this may not be possible; in such cases a diagnosis of MALT lymphoma may be proposed if morphologic features invariably associated with malignancy such as Dutcher bodies are identified. Other features such as invasion of bronchial cartilage may also suggest the diagnosis; the presence or absence of lymphoepithelial lesions does not aid in distinguishing benign and malignant processes. Given the significant histologic and radiologic overlap between MALT lymphoma and nodular lymphoid hyperplasia (the comparative features are outlined in Table 32.3), a definitive diagnosis should be deferred to immunologic and molecular evaluation unless the morphologic features are compelling. Immunophenotyp-

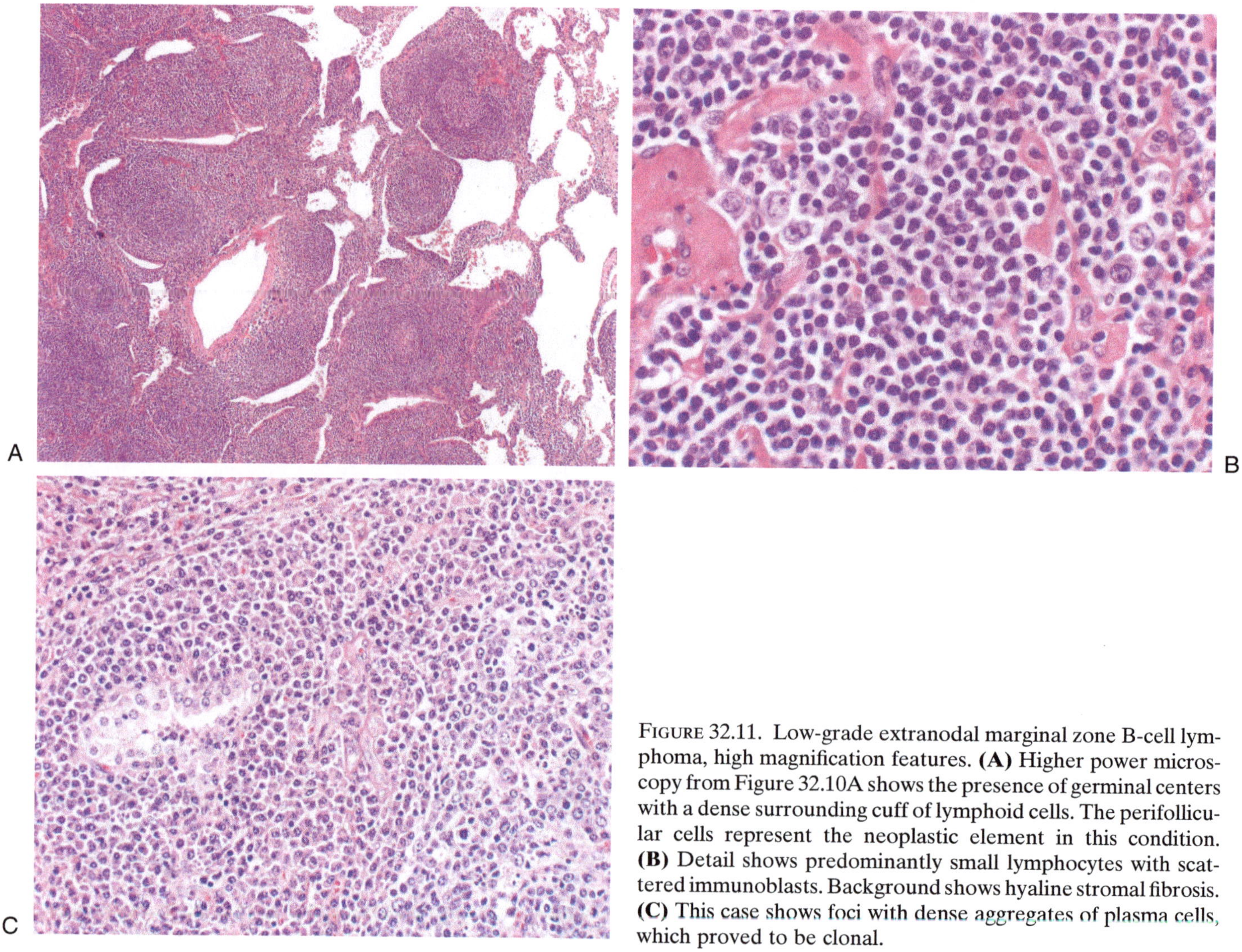

FIGURE 32.11. Low-grade extranodal marginal zone B-cell lymphoma, high magnification features. **(A)** Higher power microscopy from Figure 32.10A shows the presence of germinal centers with a dense surrounding cuff of lymphoid cells. The perifollicular cells represent the neoplastic element in this condition. **(B)** Detail shows predominantly small lymphocytes with scattered immunoblasts. Background shows hyaline stromal fibrosis. **(C)** This case shows foci with dense aggregates of plasma cells, which proved to be clonal.

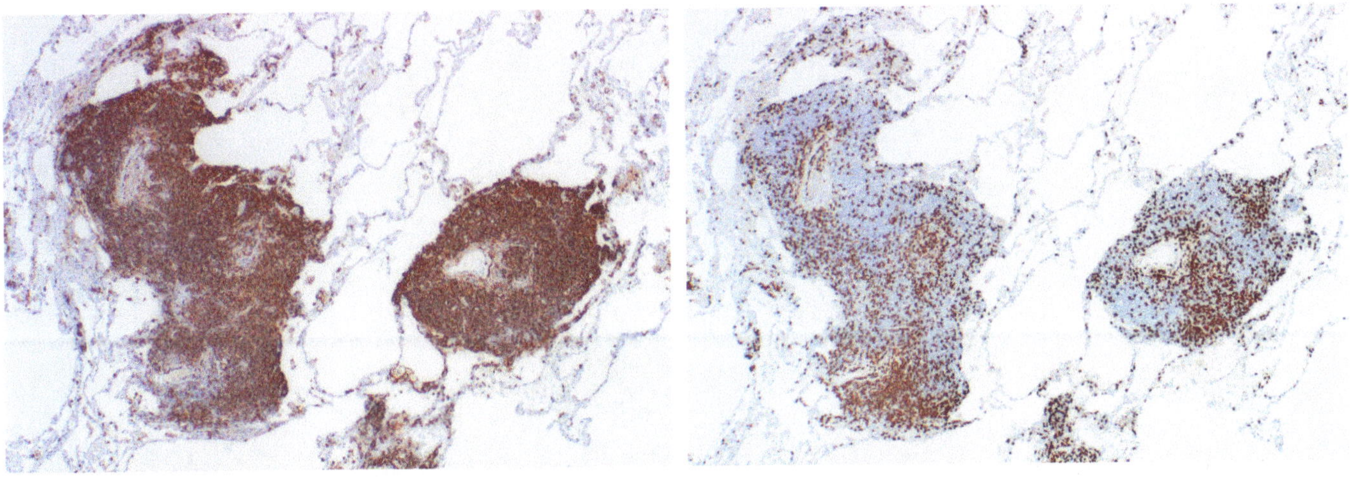

FIGURE 32.12. Low-grade extranodal marginal zone B-cell lymphoma. CD20 **(A)** and CD3 **(B)** staining shows a marked density of the B-cell infiltrate in a perivascular distribution. Although less in number, appreciable T cells are present.

ing and molecular genetic studies should demonstrate a neoplasm predominantly composed of clonal B cells (Fig. 32.12A) in all cases. T cells are also present, although they typically represent a relatively minor component of the lymphoid infiltrate (Fig. 32.12B). Immunoperoxidase staining for kappa and lambda light chains can be additionally useful in highlighting the presence of a clonal plasma cell component, which can be found in about one third of cases (Figs. 32.13 and 32.14). The presence of polyclonal plasma cells does not exclude a MALT-type lymphoma.

As in MALT lymphomas in other sites, the tumoral lesions frequently contain reactive germinal centers (Fig. 32.11A). A mixture of centrocytes and centroblasts usually populates these germinal centers, although in rare instances regressive transformation of germinal centers may be present. Colonization of these reactive germinal centers by immunoglobulin light chain restricted neoplastic plasma cells can sometimes be seen by immunoperoxidase staining.[75] Infiltration of adjacent airway and alveolar epithelium with formation of lymphoepithelial lesions is common (Fig. 32.15). The neoplastic B-cell infiltrate and the associated reactive germinal centers and lymphoepithelial lesions form an architectural unit that recapitulates the architecture seen in normal, nonneoplastic MALT tissues such as Peyer's patches. This archi-

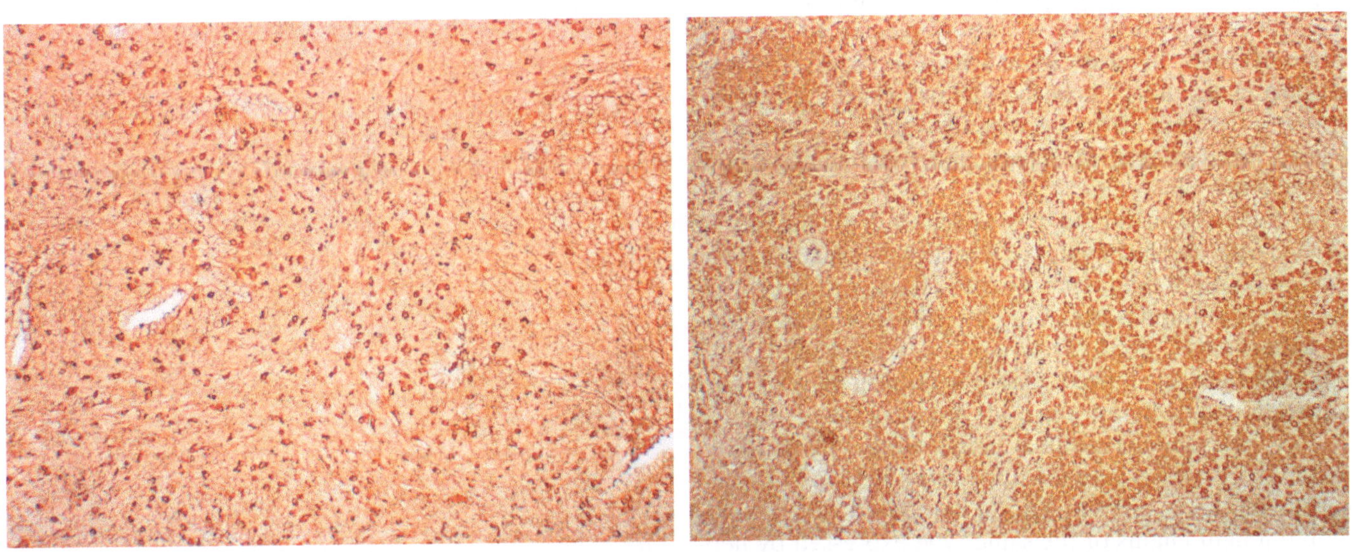

FIGURE 32.13. Low-grade extranodal marginal zone B-cell lymphoma, immunoperoxidase staining with antiimmunoglobulin light chain antibodies. Only scattered nonneoplastic kappa light chain–positive plasma cells are present **(A)**. In contrast, the neoplastic plasma cell component of the extranodal marginal zone B-cell lymphoma show strong, uniform lambda light chain restriction **(B)**.

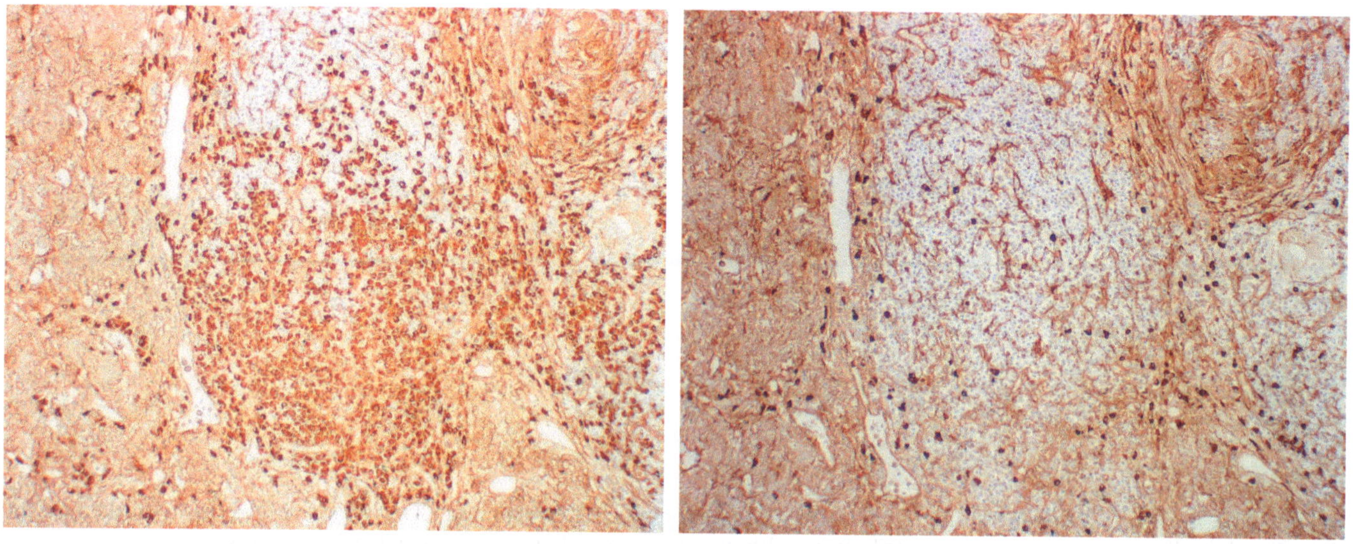

FIGURE 32.14. Low-grade extranodal marginal zone B-cell lymphoma. In some cases clonal plasma cells may be seen as focal aggregates as illustrated in this case showing kappa restriction. **(A)** Kappa. **(B)** Lambda.

tecture is characterized by subepithelial germinal centers with crescenteric accumulations of monocytoid B cells at their periphery polarized toward the overlying epithelium. When a plasma cell component is present, this also is typically polarized toward the overlying epithelium with accumulation of plasma cells in the submucosa. Accumulation of plasma cells may also be found at the periphery of small vessels if they are present within the tumor.

Some vascular infiltration (Fig. 32.16) by malignant cells, cytologically benign cells, or a mixture, is common in pulmonary MALT lymphomas. This infiltration is not typically angiodestructive and not associated with coagulative necrosis. Invasion of airways also occurs and may produce a secondary bronchiolitis or bronchiolitis obliterans with more distal obstructive changes, including foamy macrophages in alveoli and inflammatory infiltrates in alveolar walls.

At the edge of tumor masses one may find admixed plasma cells and histiocytes or a nonspecific intraalveolar accumulation of inflammatory cells. These foci may show a polyclonal immunostaining pattern for immunoglobulin light chains (Fig. 32.17). Granulomas, giant cells, dense sclerosis, and hyalinized material (which may or may not stain positively for amyloid) are sometimes seen.[76,77] A few cases mimic nodular amyloidosis. In addition, amyloid deposition with the tumor may be seen in a small subset of cases; this amyloid is composed of immunoglobulin light chains of the same type expressed by neoplastic B cells. Although this finding is not indicative of systemic amyloid deposition disease, it may be associated with an adverse prognosis. A relatively common appearance is bands of dense sclerosis surrounding islands of

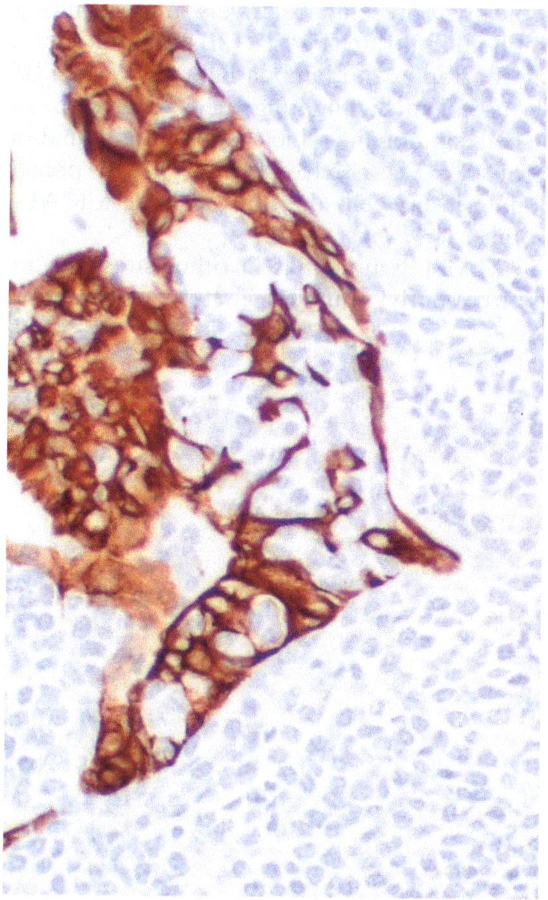

FIGURE 32.15. Low-grade extranodal marginal zone B-cell lymphoma. Lymphoepithelial lesions are highlighted with cytokeratin staining; cytokeratin-negative lymphoid cells infiltrate epithelial structures.

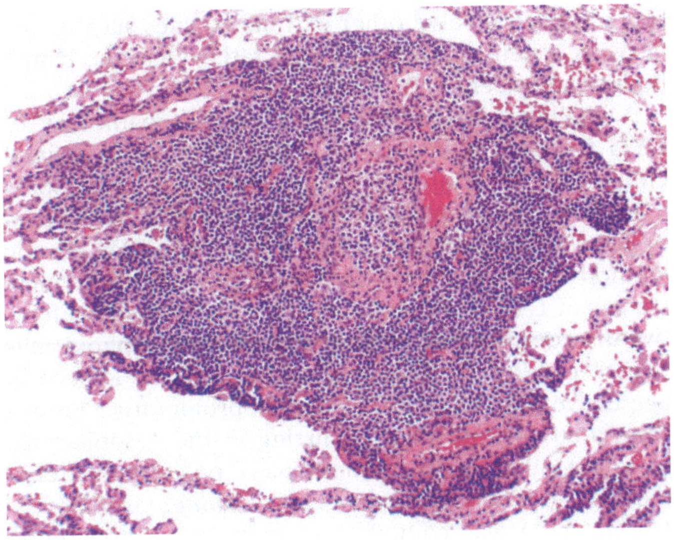

Figure 32.16. Low-grade extranodal marginal zone B-cell lymphoma. The lymphoid infiltrate is dense and shows some vascular infiltration, although classic features of vasculitis, including necrosis and fibrinoid change, are not seen.

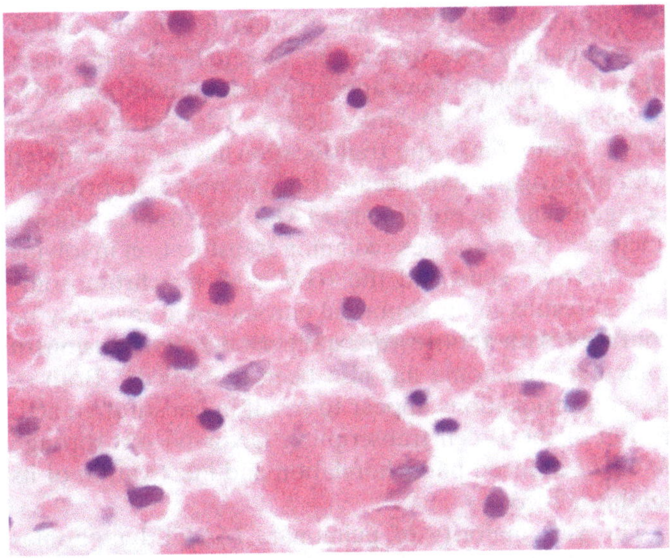

Figure 32.18. Low-grade extranodal marginal zone B-cell lymphoma with formation of immunoglobulin crystals in histiocytes.

small lymphocytes with occasional plasma cells. Immunoglobulin crystal deposition has also been described (Fig. 32.18).[78–80]

The differential diagnosis includes LIP, diffuse lymphoid hyperplasia, nodular lymphoid hyperplasia (pseudolymphoma), and other systemic low-grade lymphomas that may involve the lung, including follicular lymphoma and B-cell small lymphocytic lymphoma.

Cytogenetic abnormalities are often present in MALT lymphomas of the lung and other tissues; these abnormalities include aneuploidy and structural anomalies.[81–83] The most frequent aneuploidy in pulmonary MALT lymphomas are trisomies of chromosomes 3 and 18, which may occur singly or in combination. Trisomy of chromosome 12 may also occur, although less often.[84] Structural chromosomal abnormalities have been described. The most common structural abnormality in primary pulmonary MALT lymphoma is a reciprocal translocation involving the *API2* gene on chromosome 11q21 and the *MALT1* gene on chromosome 18q21

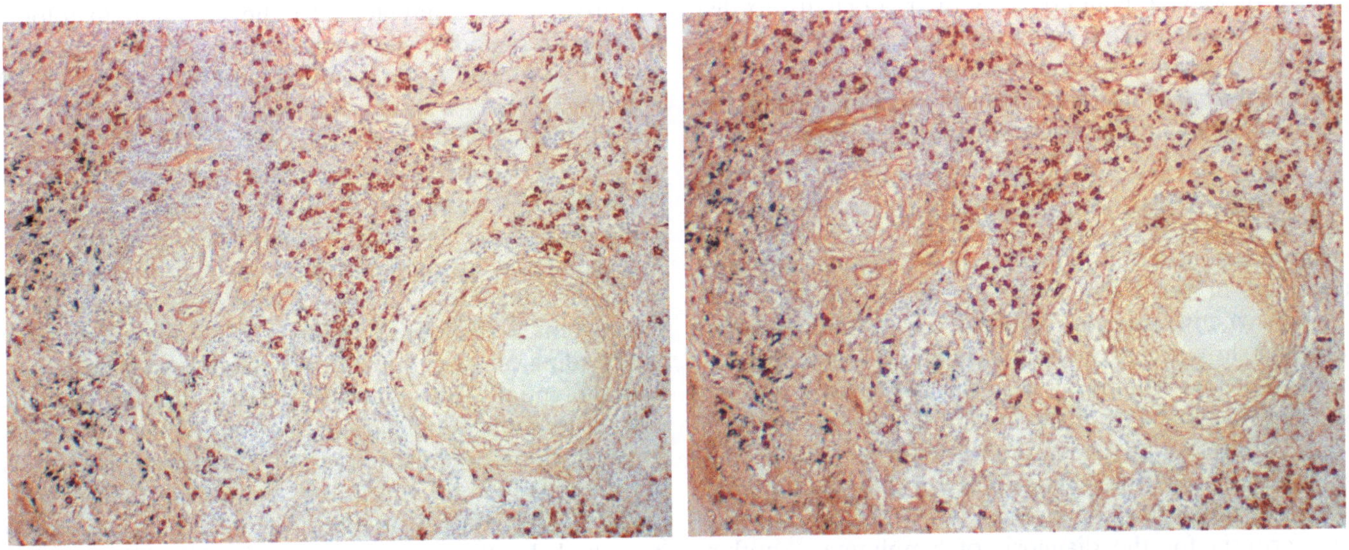

Figure 32.17. Low-grade extranodal marginal zone B-cell lymphoma. In some proven cases kappa **(A)** and lambda **(B)** staining shows that the plasma cells are polyclonal.

[t(11;18)(q21;q21)].[85,86] This abnormality is present in approximately one quarter to one half of pulmonary MALT lymphomas and appears to be mutually exclusive of aneuploidy.[87,88] In larger series of low-grade gastric MALT lymphomas, this translocation has been associated with more aggressive disease traits; however, its prognostic significance in pulmonary MALT lymphomas remains unclear.[89] A second, less common translocation involving the *MALT1* gene and the *IGH* gene on chromosome 14q32, results in an abnormal chromosome that may be confused with t(14;18)(q32;q21). *BCL2–IGH* fusion of follicular lymphoma has also been described.[90] Both of these translocations appear to result in constitutive activation of the B-cell transcription factor NF-κB through *MALT1*-induced phosphorylation and inactivation of its inhibitor I-κB.[91]

The vast majority of pulmonary MALT lymphomas are indolent and may be cured by surgery alone if they are localized.[21,23,24,54,56–60,69,71] Those that recur may do so within months or up to decades after initial recognition. At presentation, a minority, probably less than one fourth, are found to have evidence of extrapulmonary lymphoma.[54] Transformation into a large-cell lymphoma, may occur.[53,57,71] This transformation is characterized histologically by sheet-like accumulation of large transformed cells either in a biopsy also containing a low-grade MALT lymphoma or in a separate biopsy from a patient in whom a diagnosis of low-grade pulmonary MALT lymphoma has been biopsy proven either contemporaneously or previously.

Therapy and staging procedures should be tempered by the indolent nature of these lesions and the fact that resection alone may cure a significant number of patients. The indolent behavior of these lymphomas is thought to reflect lymphomas of MALT in general.[21,92] A distinctive feature of MALT lymphomas is their proclivity to disseminate to other MALT sites such as the gastrointestinal tract, thyroid, salivary glands, and lacrimal glands. For this reason, particular attention should be paid to these areas during clinical and radiologic staging procedures.[92]

Lymphomatoid Granulomatosis

Lymphomatoid granulomatosis (LYG) was originally described in the early 1970s as an angiocentric and angiodestructive process composed of "lymphoreticular" cells that showed a propensity to infiltrate blood vessels.[3] It was not clear whether it was primarily a disease of the lymphoid system, a peculiar vasculitis, or a hybrid.[3] Much of the controversy regarding the nature of LYG was related to the polymorphous nature of the inflammatory infiltrate, which did not meet widely accepted morphologic criteria for the diagnosis of lymphoma. Another confounding feature of LYG as compared to lymphomas recognized at the time of its initial description was its propensity to involve other extranodal sites such as the nervous system, kidney, and skin rather than the lymph nodes and spleen.

A challenge in understanding the histopathology of LYG is that it is in essence a morphologically defined entity that therefore may be expected to encompass a number of lymphoproliferative diseases as defined by ancillary immunophenotyping and molecular genetic methods. Early frozen-section immunohistochemical studies of LYG indicated that it was a lymphoproliferative disorder in which the majority of the lymphoid cells were T cells.[93,94] This finding was similar to that seen in aggressive angiodestructive lymphoproliferative lesions associated with necrosis occurring in the nasopharynx, so-called lethal midline granuloma or polymorphic reticulosis, and the term *angiocentric immunoproliferative lesion* (AIL) was coined to describe these apparently related diseases.[5,6] However, seminal studies using paraffin-based immunohistochemical and in-situ hybridization methods revealed fundamental differences between these two groups of cases. The majority of LYG cases were demonstrated to contain variable numbers of large Epstein-Barr virus (EBV)-positive B cells that often could be proven to be clonal, in a background of reactive small CD3 positive T cells.[95,96] In contrast, while the lesions occurring in the head and neck also contained EBV-positive atypical cells, in these cases the neoplastic cells were not B cells but rather cytotoxic lymphocytes (most often natural killer [NK] cells).[97] Hence, in the most recent World Health Organization (WHO) classification of tumors of hematopoietic and lymphoid tissues these lesions are now recognized as distinct entities called lymphomatoid granulomatosis and extranodal NK/T-cell lymphoma, nasal type, respectively.[9] Interestingly, the presence of EBV infection in these distinct lymphoproliferative lesions may lead to the common histologic findings of angiodestruction and necrosis in part through the EBV-induced elaboration of cytokines such as IP-10 and Mig.[98]

The relative biologic homogeneity of the morphologically defined entity LYG speaks to the perspicacity of the authors by whom it was initially described. However, some pathologic variability remains even within cases that fulfill the histologic criteria for the diagnosis and in which alternative diagnoses have been excluded. In the current WHO classification, LYG is included under the heading of "B-cell proliferations of uncertain malignant potential" as a disorder of EBV-positive B cells that varies in histologic grade and clinical aggressiveness in proportion to the number of EBV-positive B cells present.[9] However, rare cases in which there is no evidence of EBV positivity in the B cells have been described. Furthermore, in a small subset of cases the cytologically atypical cells are CD3–positive T cells, and B cells are virtually absent.[95] In these latter cases the

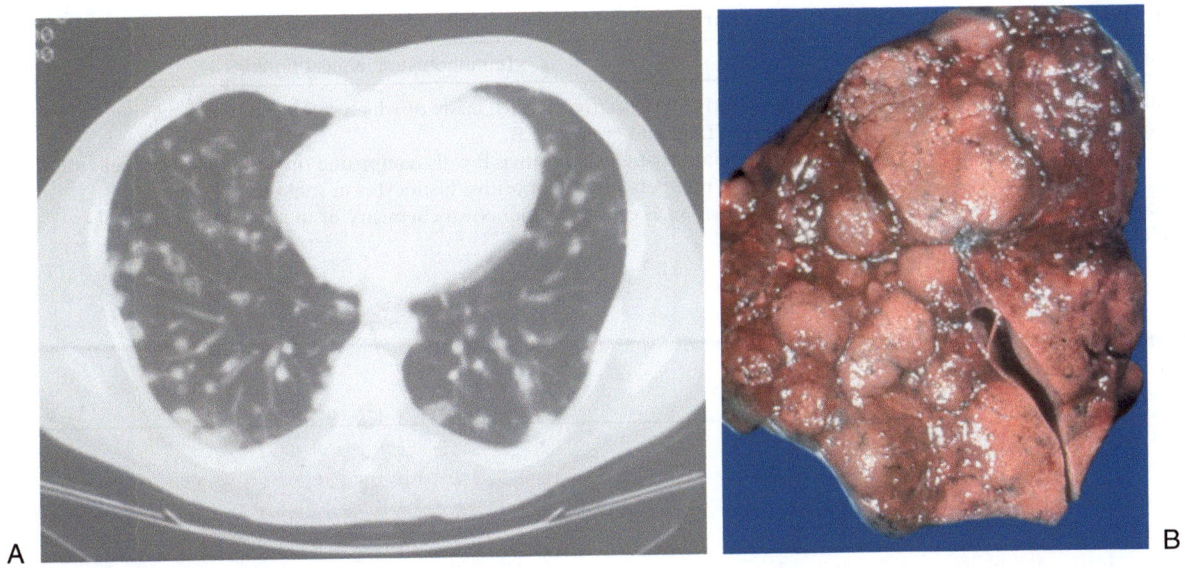

FIGURE 32.19. Lymphomatoid granulomatosis. **(A)** Typical radiologic findings with nodules, some showing cavitation. **(B)** Gross appearance with bulging, fish flesh–like nodules replacing much of the lung parenchyma. Necrosis is not prominent in this case.

atypical T cells are negative for EBV and cytotoxic granule proteins such as TIA-1 and granzyme B, features that distinguish them from extranodal NK/T-cell lymphomas of the nasal type.[99] Some contend that these "T-cell LYG" cases may be undersampled typical LYG cases, and indeed the detection of EBV-positive B cells in LYG may require studying multiple tissue blocks. However, rare cases with histologic features of LYG and the unusual attributes noted above do occur. The relationship of these cases to the entity LYG as now recognized by the WHO is unclear.

Since the initial description of lymphomatoid granulomatosis, several sizable series have been published.[100–103] Lymphomatoid granulomatosis most commonly occurs in adults with a slight male predominance. Cases have been reported in all age groups, however, including children.[104,105] Young patients affected by LYG usually have an underlying immune deficiency such as Wiskott-Aldrich syndrome, which is discussed in greater detail below. Lymphomatoid granulomatosis most commonly involves the lungs; cough as well as generalized systemic complaints such as fever and weight loss are the most common presenting symptoms. Other disease-associated clinical features in LYG are attributable to its propensity to involve other organ systems. In particular, global or localized neurologic symptoms due to involvement of the central and peripheral nervous system and rash secondary to skin involvement often occur, as these are the more frequent extrapulmonary sites of disease.[8] Although renal involvement is not uncommon, it usually is not clinically evident.[100] The laboratory findings in LYG are generally nonspecific, although patients frequently show serologic evidence of acute or prior EBV infection.[106]

Chest radiographs in LYG typically reveal both multiple nodules and/or masses, often involving both lungs, as well as linear reticulonodular infiltrates.[107,108] The nodules or masses have ill-defined borders; cavitation is infrequent and is usually found only in larger mass lesions. Multiple, bilateral pulmonary nodules can be detected along the bronchovascular structures and interlobular septa by CT and magnetic resonance imaging (MRI) scans.[109] These methods appear to be more sensitive in detecting central cavitation in smaller nodular lesions (Fig. 32.19A). CT and MRI scanning may also detect coarse linear abnormalities along bronchovascular bundles, involvement of larger bronchovascular structures in the hilum and mediastinum, and cystic lesions in the pulmonary parenchyma.[109] As would be expected from the pattern of LYG spread, mediastinal adenopathy is not commonly detected.

The gross features parallel the radiologic findings with multiple fish-flesh–like masses having varying amounts of central necrosis, which is usually more prominent in larger masses (Fig. 32.19B). The histologic features (summarized in Table 32.6 and reviewed by Jaffe and Wilson[8]) of lymphomatoid granulomatosis are distinctive (Fig. 32.20). Typically there are polymorphous nodular lymphohistiocytic infiltrates that, when small, are seen to center on or be adjacent to vascular structures (Fig. 32.20B). Less often diffuse infiltrates along vascular structures and within septa are present. Vascular infiltration by the lymphoid infiltrate with luminal narrowing is a

TABLE 32.6. Lymphomatoid granulomatosis: summary

Histologic findings	Immunohistochemical findings
Nodular infiltrates with central necrosis	Predominantly CD3-positive T cells, many of which show additional staining for cytotoxic granule proteins TIA-1 and granzyme B
Prominent vascular infiltration	Lesser population of CD20-positive B cells comprising the immunoblastic cells
Heterogeneous cell population	Appreciable numbers of CD68-positive histiocytes in some cases
Variable numbers of immunoblasts	EBV identified in B cells by immunohistochemistry or in-situ hybridization
Lack of sarcoid-like granulomas	
Lack of multinucleated giant cells	
Lack of significant numbers of neutrophils	
Lack of eosinophils	
Lack of lymphoepithelial lesions	
Lack of hyaline sclerosis	
Lack of amyloid production	
No or inconspicuous germinal centers	

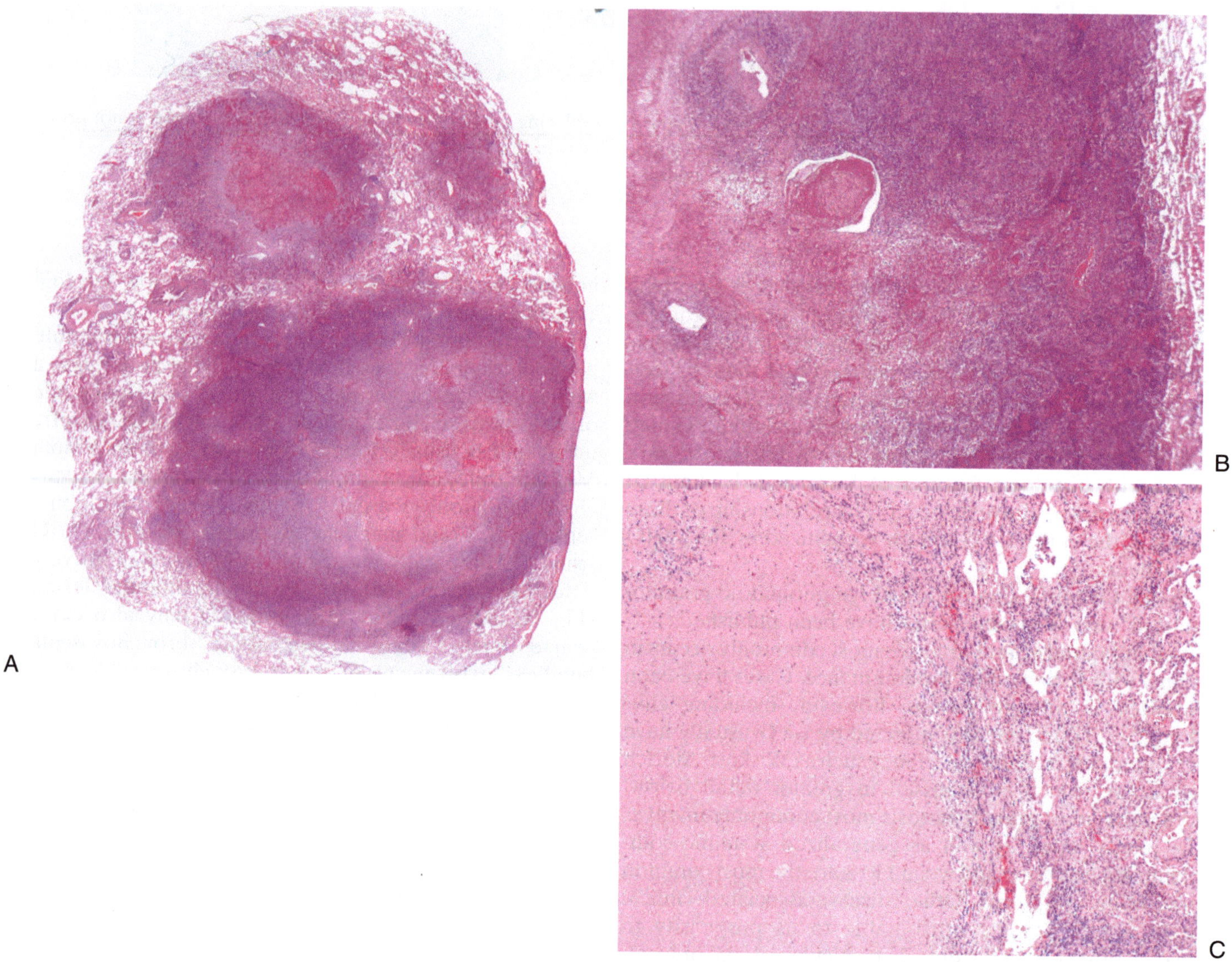

FIGURE 32.20. Lymphomatoid granulomatosis. **(A)** There are nodular infiltrates with central necrosis. The necrosis is "tumor like" and in the centers of the nodules rather than wedge-shaped as seen in infarcts. **(B)** There is a heterogeneous lymphoid infiltrate at the periphery of the necrotic nodules. Vascular infiltration may be present in the necrosis or in the viable regions (at the 11 o'clock position). **(C)** This case had some necrotic nodules in which no B cells were identified in the viable lymphoid infiltrate at the edge. Many of the necrotic cells (left) showed CD20 positive staining suggesting that the B cells had become necrotic.

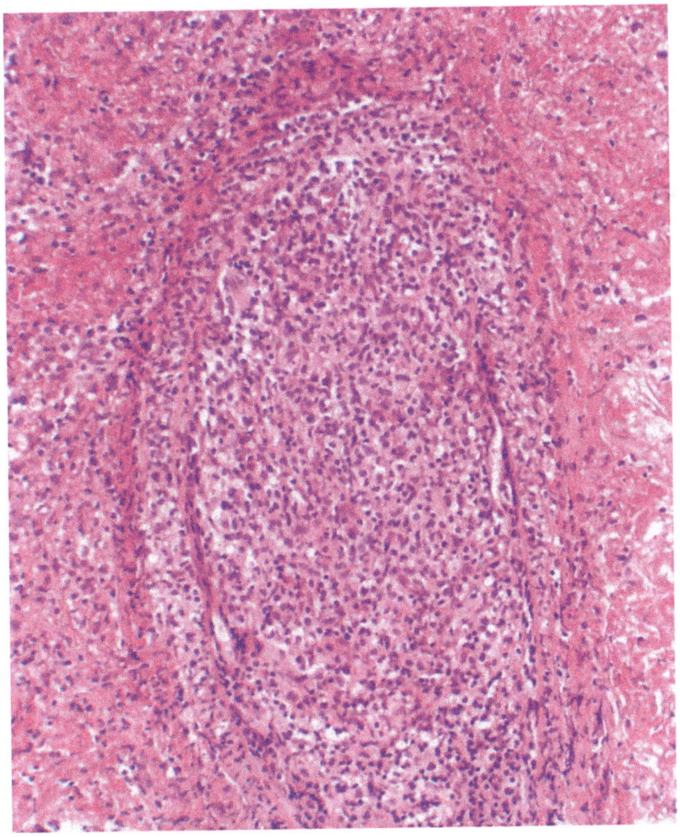

FIGURE 32.21. Lymphomatoid granulomatosis. There is vascular infiltration adjacent to the necrosis (top). Classic features of vasculitis including acute inflammatory necrosis of the vessel wall and fibrinoid change are not prominent.

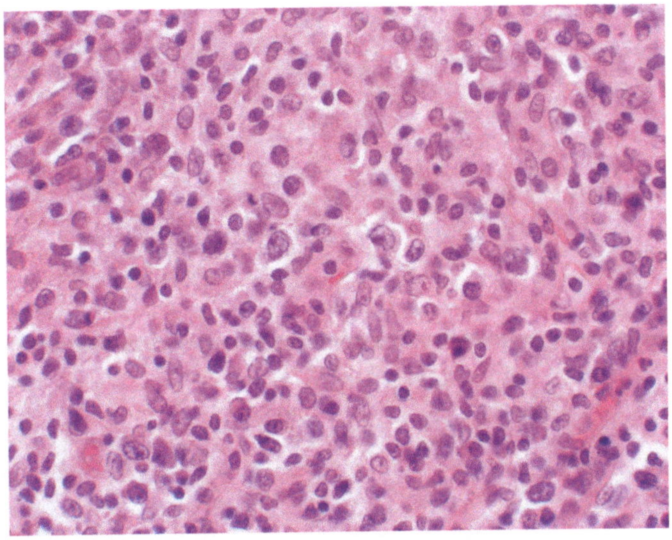

FIGURE 32.22. Lymphomatoid granulomatosis. This case shows a polymorphic cellular background including occasional immunoblasts and a mixed population of lymphocytes, plasma cells, and histiocytes.

quintessential feature (Fig. 32.21), but is not seen in all sites of involvement and may not involve all vessels. The vascular infiltration may be by cytologically benign cells, cytologically malignant cells, or a mixture of the two. The nodular lesions may vary in size, and as they enlarge there is a central fibrinous exudation into air spaces (Fig. 32.20A) and eventually central necrosis with a rim of viable tissue (Fig. 32.20B). Extremely large nodules can develop. These lymphohistiocytic infiltrates are composed of a mixture of lymphocytes, histiocytes that may form small epithelioid clusters, plasma cells, and rarely giant cells. Associated secondary changes in the air spaces including accumulation of pulmonary alveolar macrophages that may be foamy, and prominent type II cells are typical.

The lymphoid component of LYG is composed of a mixture of cells with small to intermediate-sized, angulated nuclei and variable numbers of cells with large vesicular nuclei and visible nucleoli (Fig. 32.22). The cytologic atypia in the large cells may be pronounced and in some instances they may resemble the Reed-Sternberg cells of Hodgkin's lymphoma. The number of large atypical cells varies from field to field (Fig. 32.20C), and one should search out the most atypical field in order to classify a given case. Not uncommonly, biopsies that show several nodules may reveal monomorphous foci of atypical large cells in only one of the nodules (Fig. 32.23). The large cells are often most readily detected in larger nodules and bordering areas of coagulative necrosis.

In the vast majority of LYG cases ancillary immunoperoxidase and in-situ hybridization studies reveal

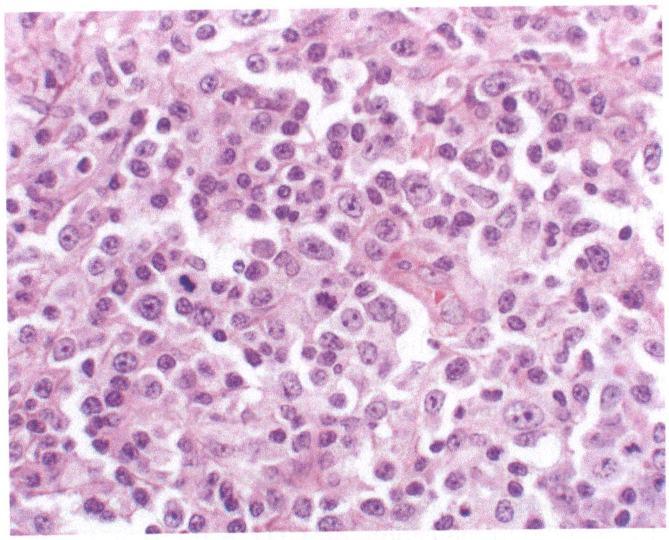

FIGURE 32.23. Lymphomatoid granulomatosis. This case shows larger numbers of immunoblasts with readily recognizable mitotic figures (center).

A B C

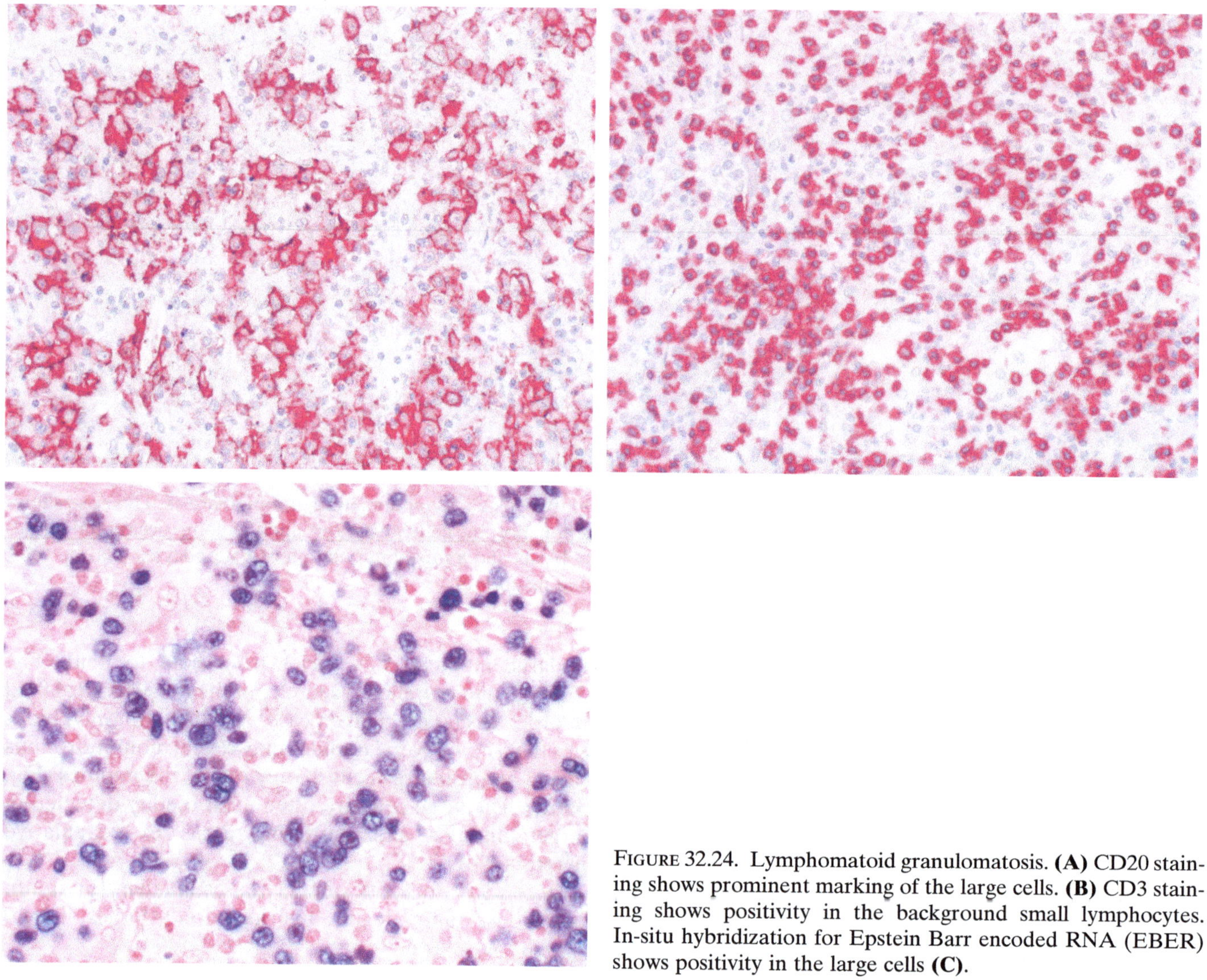

FIGURE 32.24. Lymphomatoid granulomatosis. **(A)** CD20 staining shows prominent marking of the large cells. **(B)** CD3 staining shows positivity in the background small lymphocytes. In-situ hybridization for Epstein Barr encoded RNA (EBER) shows positivity in the large cells **(C)**.

the large atypical lymphoid cells to be CD20–positive, EBV-positive B cells (Fig. 32.24A,B).[95,96] CD3–positive T-cells constitute most of the small lymphocytes (Fig. 32.24B). The results of early studies suggested that most of these T cells coexpressed CD4.[5] Subsequent analysis using a more extensive panel of immunohistochemical reagents revealed a high proportion of the small lymphocytes to express the cytotoxic granule protein TIA-1 with lesser numbers of cells positive for granzyme B, a cytotoxic granule protein expressed in T cells after cellular activation.[99] These findings are similar to those observed in large B-cell lymphomas with a prominent reactive T-cell component.[110] The results of the earlier studies suggesting a predominance of CD4 positive T cells may be attributable to detection of CD4 expression by the admixed histiocytes. Clonality can frequently be detected by EBV terminal repeat Southern blot analysis.[111] Clonal immunoglobulin gene rearrangements can often be detected by polymerase chain reaction (PCR) analysis, whereas these same studies performed using Southern blot methods are usually negative. This disparity is presumably due to the differing sensitivities of these methods.[8,112] Clonal T-cell receptor gene rearrangements are not typical in LYG, and if present, one must strongly consider the possibility of pulmonary involvement by a T-cell lineage lymphoproliferative disorder with overlapping histologic features such as extranodal NK/T-cell lymphoma of the nasal type.

When the term *angiocentric immunoproliferative lesion* was promulgated as a unifying category for what were thought to be related lymphoproliferative disorders, a three-tiered grading system was proposed.[5] In this system, the grade of the lesion increased with increasing numbers of large, cytologically atypical cells and with increased atypia in the background small lymphocytes. The complexity of this grading scheme was likely increased by the inclusion of extranodal NK/T-cell lymphomas of nasal type. If one considers as LYG the WHO-accepted lesion, a two-grade system with low-grade and high-grade categories based on the number of large B cells has proved most practical. At the low-grade end, one has difficulty believing that a neoplastic lymphoproliferative process is present. Because perivascular infiltrates are common in many conditions, a key feature is the density and mass-like character of the process; expansile nodules, central necrosis, and vascular infiltration are less common in benign lesions. At the high-grade end of the spectrum, recognition of the lymphomatous process is easy. This grading system remains relevant as it has practical implications for the treatment of these disorders. Low-grade lesions may spontaneously resolve or may respond to immunomodulatory regimens with relatively minimal cytotoxicity such as interferon-α_{2b}.[106] In contrast, high-grade lesions should in most instances be clinically approached as diffuse large B-cell lymphomas.[8] Early series of lymphomatoid granulomatosis suggested a poor prognosis despite chemotherapy,[3,100] with less than half of the patients living 2 years. Later studies suggested a more favorable prognosis with aggressive chemotherapy for high-grade lesions, with more than 50% long-term remissions.[5]

Posttransplant Lymphoproliferative Disorders

Lymphoproliferative disorders that occur following organ transplantation are, by definition, considered posttransplant lymphoproliferative disorders (PTLDs). In the case of solid organ transplantation, the frequency of these disorders varies with the type of organ transplant and the type of immunosuppressive therapy employed.[113] Increased degrees of immunosuppression are thought to incur increased risk for the development of a PTLD, as these neoplasms likely arise due to decreased T cell mediated immune surveillance. The vast majority of PTLDs are EBV-associated B-cell lineage lymphoproliferative processes that may be either polyclonal or monoclonal in nature. Monoclonality in PTLD may be demonstrated either through documentation of B-cell immunoglobulin light chain restriction or EBV Southern blot analysis.[111,114] The monoclonal PTLDs are further subdivided histologically into polymorphous and monomorphous types with the polymorphous type containing a mixture of plasmacytoid cells, smaller lymphocytes, and large transformed lymphocytes, and the monomorphic types containing a histologically malignant cell population with features of large cell lymphoma, Burkitt lymphoma, or plasmacytoma.[9]

There have been relatively few extensive studies of PTLD in the setting of pulmonary transplantation.[115–118] The reported frequency of PTLD following pulmonary transplantation varies, although more recent studies indicate that it is an uncommon complication of this procedure, occurring in approximately 5% or less of cases. As in other solid organ transplants, increasing age at transplantation appears to be associated with an increased risk for the development of PTLD. A seronegative EBV status in the transplant recipient prior to the procedure may also be a risk factor for the subsequent development of a PTLD.

The latency period between transplantation and the occurrence of PTLD in pulmonary transplants is relatively short, with many cases occurring within the first year after the procedure. These early-onset PTLDs most often occur in the allografted organ. Other sites including the gastrointestinal (GI) tract and skin may be involved in addition to, or instead of, the engrafted lung, particularly in cases that arise after the first year posttransplant.[115,116] The proclivity of early-occurring PTLDs to arise in the allografted organ raises the possibility that they may actually be derived from donor, rather than recipient, lymphocytes.[119,120] However, some pulmonary PTLDs involving the allografted organ are of host origin.[121] Most patients are either asymptomatic or have nonspecific systemic complaints.

The PTLDs typically present radiologically as single or multiple nodules, usually in the transplanted lung. Although these lesions may be detected by routine chest radiography, features seen by CT scanning such as the presence of an invasive rather than a smooth-walled border may help distinguish these lesions from other nonneoplastic causes of pulmonary nodules in transplanted lungs such as invasive pulmonary aspergillosis.[122] Definitive characterization of these lesions, however, requires tissue sampling.[123]

Pathologic studies of pulmonary PTLD suggest that the vast majority are disorders of EBV-infected B cells (Fig. 32.25). The histologic subtype varies with both polymorphous (Fig. 32.26) and monomorphous (Fig. 32.27) types described. Epstein-Barr virus–associated lesions with histopathologic features of lymphomatoid granulomatosis may also be found in this setting.[124] In most of the monomorphous PTLDs arising after transplantation, the morphologic features are those of diffuse large B-cell lymphoma.[118] However, one monomorphous PTLD arising in the colon after pulmonary transplantation was composed of atypical plasma cells and therefore was considered a plasmacytoma-like lesion. In those cases of both polymorphous and monomorphous pulmonary PTLD in which there was sufficient material for molecular genetic studies, evidence of B-cell clonality was detected by PCR or Southern blot analysis of immunoglobulin gene rearrangements.[118]

The treatment approaches to PTLD vary and may include one or more of the following: reduction of immunosuppression, surgical resection, radiation, and

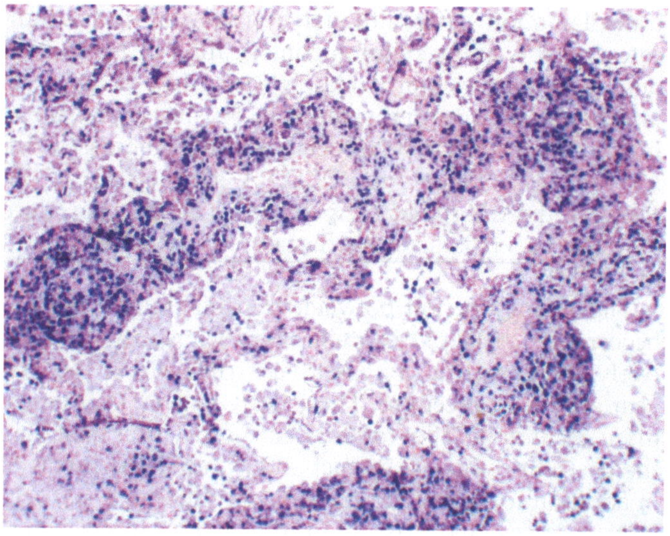

FIGURE 32.25. Primary pulmonary posttransplant lymphoproliferative disorder (PTLD). In-situ hybridization for EBER shows prominent positive staining of the lymphoid cells infiltrating a septum.

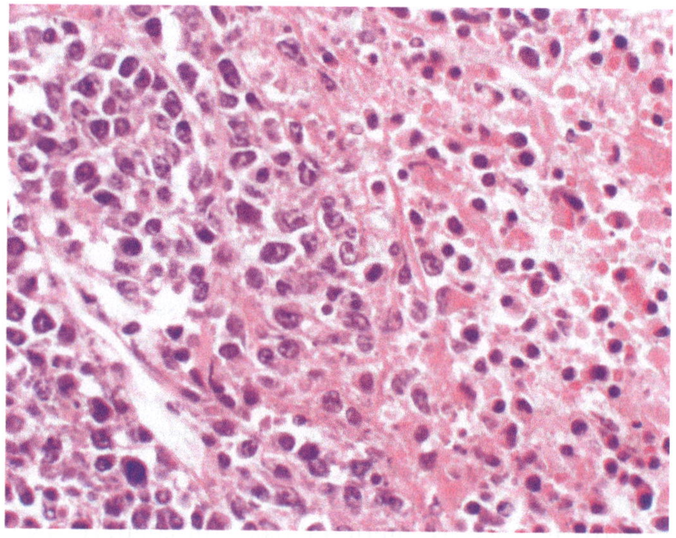

FIGURE 32.27. Primary pulmonary PTLD. This case shows features indistinguishable from large-cell lymphoma with viable lymphoid cells on the left and an area of necrosis on the right.

chemotherapy. In some cases even clonal PTLDs may regress with the lessening of immunosuppression; however, this may not be a practical approach due to the risk of allograft rejection. Some reports suggest a dire prognosis in pulmonary PTLD as compared to PTLD occurring in other settings, with a median survival time of less than 1 year.[118] Patients in whom PTLD arises in the first year after treatment tend to have disease confined to the allografted lung and may show a better response to treatment.[115,116] Also, some evidence suggests that anti-CD20 monoclonal antibody immunotherapy may be effective in treating B-cell lineage pulmonary PTLD.[117] (See also discussion in Chapter 23).

Lymphoproliferative Disorders in the Setting of Human Immunodeficiency Virus Infection and Acquired Immune Deficiency Syndrome

Acquired immunodeficiency due to HIV infection is associated with increased risk for the development of

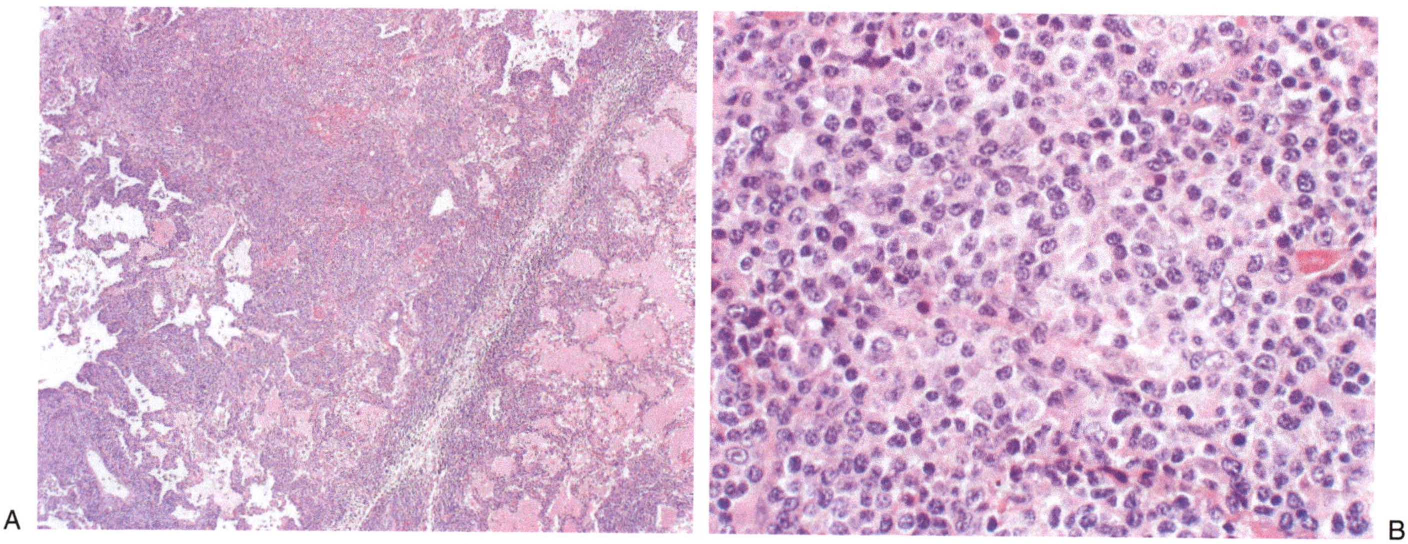

FIGURE 32.26. Primary pulmonary PTLD. There is a dense lymphoid infiltrate that shows some predilection for lymphatic routes, particularly involving a septum **(A)**; cytologically there is a polymorphic process with lymphocytes, plasma cells, and occasional immunoblasts **(B)**.

lymphoproliferative disorders. As in lymphomas arising in the setting of iatrogenic immune suppression, decreased T-cell function is thought to play a central role in the development of these disorders. Inappropriately exuberant and prolonged immune responses may also play a role in the development of lymphomas in these patients.[125]

A variety of lymphoproliferative disorders have been described as arising with increased frequency in HIV-positive patients; overall about 5% to 10% develop malignant lymphoma at some point in the disease course. Approximately 5% of HIV patients with systemic lymphoma develop clinically evident pulmonary involvement. Some studies suggest, however, that the advent of more effective highly active antiretroviral therapies (HAARTs) may have increased the proportion of lymphoma cases among HIV-positive patients referred to pulmonologists for evaluation of respiratory complications.[126] The incidence of pulmonary involvement by systemic lymphoma in HIV appears to be higher in autopsy studies, with reported frequencies as high as 70%.[127] Human immunodeficiency virus–associated primary pulmonary lymphomas are rare, occurring in less than 1% of patients.[128] Both primary and secondary pulmonary lymphomas tend to occur in advanced-stage disease in patients with low CD4 counts.

Human immunodeficiency virus–positive patients with pulmonary involvement by lymphoma tend to have nonspecific systemic and respiratory signs and symptoms including fever, cough, dyspnea, and tachypnea.[127] A variety of radiologic patterns of lung involvement may be seen in cases of systemic lymphoma with pulmonary involvement, including consolidating lobar infiltrates, nodules, and masses.[129] Multiple pulmonary nodules, usually in the lower lobes, appear to be the most common radiologic pattern in primary pulmonary lymphoma.[130,131] Hilar or mediastinal adenopathy may be observed in lymphomas with secondary lung involvement, whereas these are, by definition, absent in primary pulmonary lymphomas. Pleural effusions also may be present more often in secondary, as opposed to primary, pulmonary lymphomas in HIV patients.

Despite the variety of Hodgkin's and non-Hodgkin's lymphomas that have been described in HIV-positive patients, the vast majority of primary and secondary pulmonary lymphomas appear to be EBV-associated B-cell lymphomas of large cell or high-grade Burkitt or Burkitt-like types.[128] Lymphomatoid granulomatosis has also been described in this setting.[132] Apart from the latter, these lymphomas can usually be readily recognized as malignant processes on histologic grounds, and limited sampling procedures such as transbronchial or transthoracic needle biopsies may be sufficient for establishing the diagnosis.[128] Both primary pulmonary lymphomas and widespread systemic lymphomas with pulmonary involvement in HIV-positive patients have a poor prognosis, with many patients surviving less than 1 year after the diagnosis despite multiagent chemotherapy.[125,127,128]

Primary Effusion Lymphoma

In addition to these patterns of parenchymal lung involvement by HIV-associated lymphoma a rare type of lymphoma with preferential involvement of the pleural, pericardial, and peritoneal spaces has also been described as occurring almost exclusively in this population. This disease has been termed *primary effusion lymphoma* or body cavity–based lymphoma, as this disease usually involves only one of the sites mentioned above and rarely forms tumefactive tissue masses. Primary effusion lymphoma is a rare disorder, even in HIV-positive patients.

As one may surmise from the name given to this lymphoma, most patients present with unexplained isolated pleural, pericardial, or peritoneal effusions. The pathologic features of primary effusion lymphoma are similar, regardless of the body cavity involved.

Cytologic evaluation reveals the presence of malignant-appearing cells with large nuclei and prominent nucleoli; anaplastic nuclear features may be present. These cells often have dense, vacuolated cytoplasm and a perinuclear clearing or hof. These cells may also be identified in pleural biopsies adherent to the pleural surface with associated fibrin deposition. Leukocyte common antigen (CD45) is invariably expressed; these cells often also express the activation-associated antigens CD30 and CD38 as well as the plasma cell–associated antigen CD138.[133,134] These cells usually lack B-cell– and T-cell–associated antigens, and therefore lineage assignment can be problematic. Molecular genetic studies, however, usually reveal clonally rearranged immunoglobulin genes that when analyzed in detail are found to have undergone the somatic hypermutation process that occurs while B cells are responding to antigen in the environment of the lymphoid follicle.[135] On this basis, as well as the expression of CD138, primary effusion lymphomas are generally regarded as B-cell lymphomas derived from postfollicular center B cells. In some instances, T-cell receptor gene rearrangement may also be seen.[134,136]

In all cases of primary effusion lymphoma the neoplastic cells are positive for the human herpes virus-8/Kaposi sarcoma herpes virus (HHV-8/KSHV).[137,138] In most cases the neoplastic cells are co-infected by and therefore positive for EBV.[134,136] HHV-8/KSHV is also associated with Kaposi's sarcoma and multicentric Castleman's disease, and quite often the former and rarely the latter may also be present.[139] Primary effusion lymphomas may also be found in HIV-negative patient populations in whom other HHV-8–associated neoplasms have been described, including elderly Mediterranean men.[138] Primary effusion lymphomas arising in this setting tend to be EBV negative.[140]

The prognosis in primary effusion lymphoma is poor, with most patients dying within a year of the diagnosis, regardless of the therapeutic intervention employed.

As mentioned above, HIV infection is also associated with chronic B-cell stimulation. This may account for the prominent reactive pulmonary lymphoid proliferations associated with acquired immunodeficiency syndrome (AIDS); there is also evidence to suggest that the altered T-cell immune system may play a role in allowing these proliferations to occur.[141,142] Lymphocytic interstitial pneumonia (Fig. 32.5) may be encountered either as diffuse dense infiltration of alveolar septa by a mixed population of inflammatory cells or diffuse lymphoid hyperplasia. Lymphocytic interstitial pneumonia in AIDS is more common in children than in adults.[36,50] In isolated cases the B cells in these lesions have been proven to be clonal by immunoperoxidase staining and by molecular genetic analysis, and on this basis the lesions were categorized as MALT lymphomas. The few described cases of HIV-associated pulmonary MALT lymphoma have mostly been in pediatric patients,[143] although an instance of pulmonary MALT lymphoma with an associated *Aspergillus* fungal ball in an HIV-positive man has been described.[144]

It is important to note that some of the pulmonary lymphoid infiltrates encountered in AIDS patients are very difficult to classify into recognized disease categories. This likely reflects the varying cytology of EBV associated lymphoproliferative diseases, as detailed in the section on PTLD. In some instances these cases may be categorized as HIV-associated polymorphic B-cell lymphoma (PTLD-like) by the WHO criteria, and in other cases it is best to consider the lesions unclassifiable and to reflect this in the diagnosis. One must always bear in mind that immunoblastic reactions, some of which may be EBV associated, can occur in the setting of HIV. Given this, and the poor prognosis associated with higher grade lymphomas in AIDS patients, it is critical that ancillary immunoperoxidase and molecular genetic studies be performed to confirm a diagnosis of lymphoma and exclude a florid reactive process in cases where there is any uncertainty regarding the histologic diagnosis. Kaposi's sarcoma of the lung is sometimes an associated lesion (see Chapter 40).

Lymphoproliferative Disorders Associated with Primary Immunodeficiency States

Numerous primary immunodeficiency syndromes caused by defects in humoral and cellular immune responses have been described.[145] In many of these disorders there are increased rates of pulmonary infection, and changes secondary to chronic infection such as bronchiectasis, may be found (see Chapter 5).[146,147] In addition, in some forms of primary immunodeficiency, especially ataxia telangiectasia and Wiskott-Aldrich syndrome, the affected individuals are at increased risk for the development of malignant lymphoma.[148,149] A variety of lymphoproliferative diseases have been described in these disorders including diffuse large B-cell lymphoma. Although the rarity of these immunodeficiency states precludes systematic study of large numbers of patients, the literature suggests that pulmonary involvement by lymphoproliferative diseases may be particularly associated with Wiskott-Aldrich syndrome (WAS),[104] which is an X-linked disease characterized by eczema, recurrent infections, and thrombocytopenia with small platelets, leading to complications secondary to a bleeding diathesis.[146] This disorder, which is due to abnormalities in the gene on the X-chromosome that encodes the Wiskott-Aldrich syndrome protein (WASP),[150] has been associated with the development of EBV-associated B-cell lymphomatoid granulomatosis-like lesions in the lung and skin.[104] Florid reactive lymphoproliferations/LIP may also be encountered in these patients as well as in patients with common variable immunodeficiency, an autosomal recessive disease of various underlying genetic abnormalities that leads to abnormalities in humoral immunity.[52] As most of these disorders become manifest early in life, in cases of HIV-negative pediatric patients with massive accumulations of small lymphocytes in the lung the possibility of primary immunodeficiency should be considered and clinically excluded. Furthermore, caution must be exercised in overinterpreting these lesions as MALT lymphomas in this setting, as in some cases of primary immunodeficiency states self-limited clonal B-cell expansions have been described, albeit in the gastrointestinal tract.[151]

Hodgkin's Lymphoma Presenting in the Lung

Hodgkin's lymphoma (formerly Hodgkin's disease) is broadly categorized into the classic type containing neoplastic Hodgkin cells and Reed-Sternberg cells and the lymphocyte predominant type containing lymphocytic and histiocytic (L&H) Reed-Sternberg cell variants. The vast majority of Hodgkin's lymphomas involving the lung are of classical type and therefore the discussion focuses on this entity.

Classic Hodgkin's lymphoma is characterized by the presence of large mononucleated Hodgkin cells and multinucleated Reed-Sternberg cells in a polymorphous background containing variable proportions of small lymphocytes, plasma cells, histiocytes, and eosinophils.[9] Hodgkin and Reed-Sternberg (HRS) cells lack most B-cell– and T-cell–associated antigens and rather express

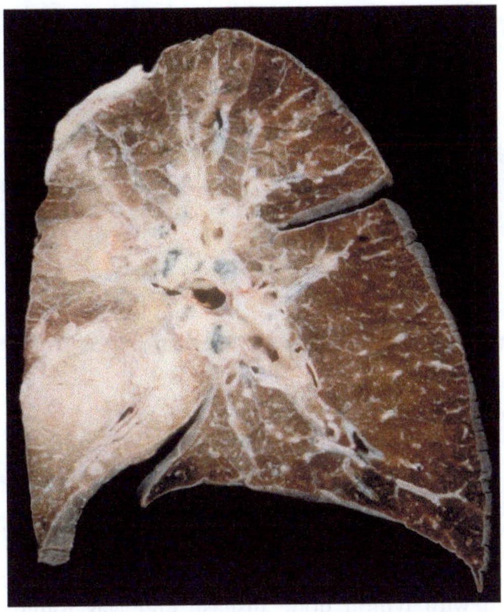

FIGURE 32.28. Pulmonary Hodgkin's lymphoma. There are nodular and linear infiltrates including some plaque-like involvement of the pleura. There is a predilection for lymphatic routes and the infiltrates extend along bronchovascular bundles from the hilum. Hilar lymph nodes are involved. This is from an autopsy in a patient who had initially presented with lymph node disease.

antigens not often expressed by lymphocytes such as CD15 and the activation-associated antigen CD30. For this reason the cellular origin of these cells was unclear. Detailed molecular genetic and immunophenotypic analyses have revealed that in most cases of classic Hodgkin's lymphoma (>95%) the HRS cells are derived from post-germinal center B cells, and in the remainder they are derived from T cells. Gene expression profiling data indicate that HRS cells are all closely related, however, regardless of their cellular origin. A unifying feature of HRS cells is their ability to "turn off" the expression of lineage-specific genes such as productively rearranged immunoglobulin genes in the B-cell type. The mechanism by which this occurs is unknown; however, in normal B cells this would be a lethal event inducing apoptosis (programmed cell death). The HRS cells, in contrast, do not undergo apoptosis in response to these abnormalities, possibly due to the expression of antiapoptotic proteins such as cFLIP and cIAP2 (reviewed by Diehl et al.[152]).

Systemic classic Hodgkin's lymphoma (not the lymphocyte predominance type) frequently involves the lung or pleura. This is especially with relapsed systemic disease where the lung is involved in approximately 40% of cases.[153] In contrast, primary pulmonary Hodgkin's lymphoma is considered rare, and some have disputed its existence. Nevertheless, case reports and small series of primary pulmonary Hodgkin's lymphoma have appeared for many years,[154–156] and 61 cases in the literature were reviewed.[157]

Primary pulmonary Hodgkin's lymphoma occurs more frequently in women (2:1), and patients are older than those with primary nodal disease; the average age is 33 years for men and 51 years for women.[91] The majority were symptomatic, and the symptoms were (in decreasing order of frequency) cough, fever, weight loss, dyspnea, fatigue, anorexia, chest pain, and pruritis.[156] Radiographically, reticulonodular infiltrates and single or multiple nodules are described.[155,156] Cavitation is not uncommon. These findings are similar to those in systemic Hodgkin's lymphoma with pulmonary involvement, where poorly marginated nodules and parenchymal infiltrates have been described.[158] Cavitation, however, is not often encountered in this setting. In Hodgkin's lymphoma, CT appears to be superior to standard radiology in both detecting and characterizing the pulmonary nodules.[158,159]

The gross findings parallel the radiologic findings (Fig. 32.28). The histologic findings of pulmonary Hodgkin's lymphoma are identical to those in lymph nodes (Figs. 32.29 to 32.32): diagnostic Reed–Sternberg cells with large multilobate nuclei with inclusion-like macronucleoli are present in the appropriate polymorphous cellular milieu composed of varying proportions of small lymphocytes, eosinophils, plasma cells, and histiocytes (Fig. 32.32B). It is worthwhile to bear in mind that many cases of primary (and secondary) pulmonary Hodgkin's lymphoma are the nodular sclerosis subtype, and therefore the majority of the Reed-Sternberg cells are lacunar variants, and the classic bilobed Reed-Sternberg cells may be few in number. The diagnosis of

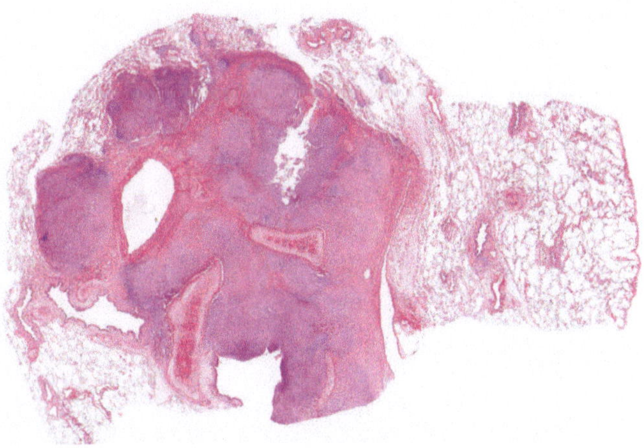

FIGURE 32.29. Primary pulmonary Hodgkin's lymphoma. In this case there is a nodular infiltrate involving a segmental bronchus. Even at scanning power magnification the nodular and sclerotic character of the process typical of the nodular sclerosing variant is apparent.

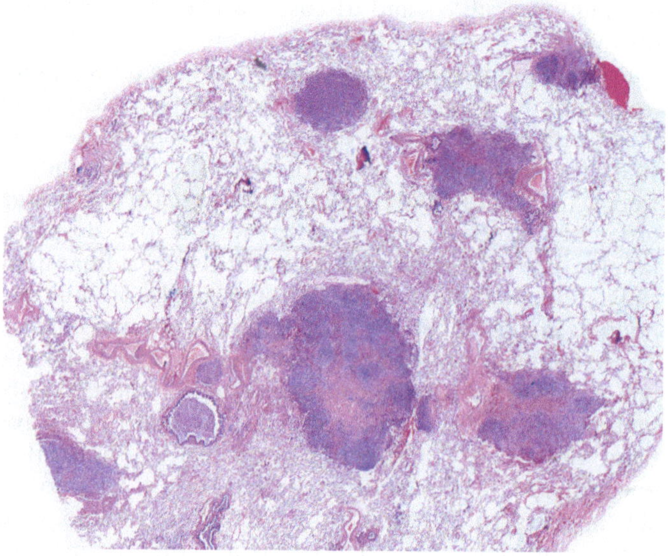

FIGURE 32.30. Primary pulmonary Hodgkin's lymphoma. This case presented as multiple small nodules, which, in most instances, can be traced to lymphatic routes in their distribution.

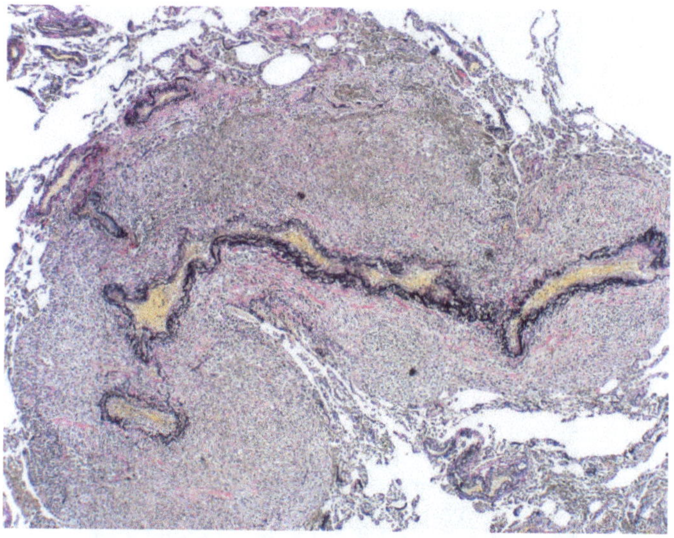

FIGURE 32.31. Pulmonary Hodgkin's lymphoma. This patient presented with lymph node disease and was found to have concurrent pulmonary infiltrates, which were confirmed to represent Hodgkin's lymphoma. The predilection for the process to infiltrate along and sometimes into vessels is apparent on elastic tissue staining.

Hodgkin's lymphoma is usually confirmed by demonstrating the appropriate immunophenotype (CD30 and CD15 positive, CD45 negative) in the Reed-Sternberg cells and variants. In small nodules and diffuse infiltrates, a lymphatic distribution of infiltration can be discerned; vascular infiltration occurs. Other patterns include a pneumonic growth pattern (in which the infiltrate fills alveoli in a consolidative fashion), endobronchial lesions, and extensive subpleural or pleural involvement.[155,156,160] Some cases may show a dramatic sarcoid-like granulomatous reaction.[161]

The patients in Yousem et al.'s[156] series were treated with conventional chemotherapeutic protocols for Hodgkin's disease. Approximately half showed a favorable

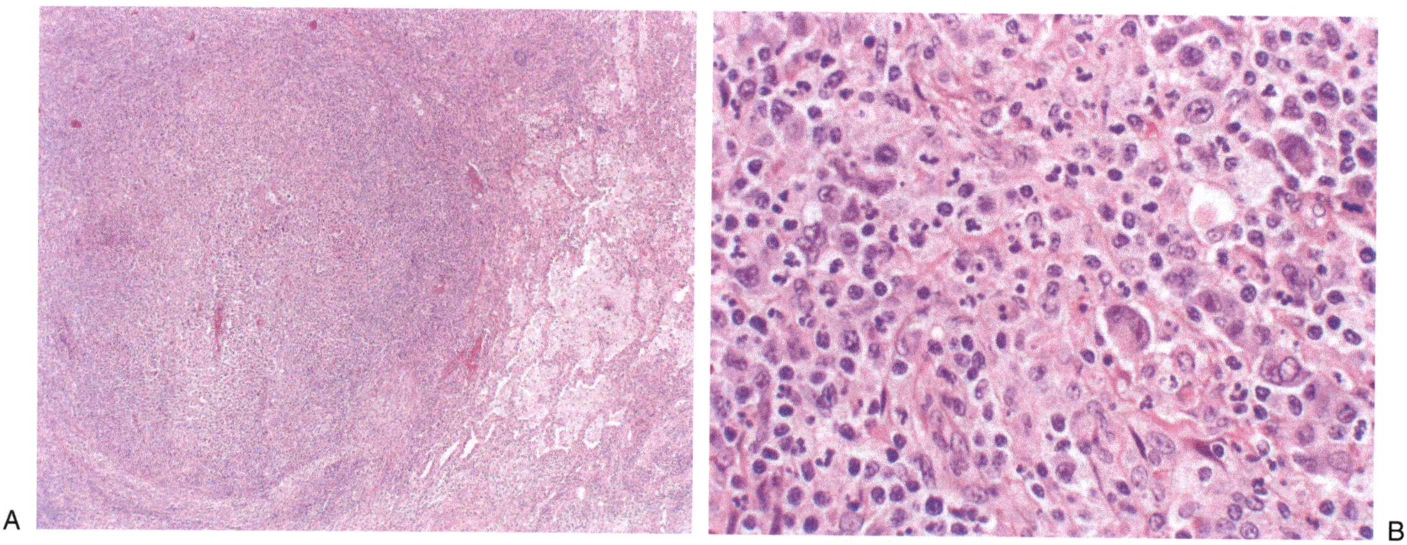

FIGURE 32.32. Primary pulmonary Hodgkin's lymphoma. The cytologic features of primary pulmonary Hodgkin's lymphoma are identical to those in lymph nodes. There are nodular infiltrates in the lung parenchyma **(A)**, which show cytologic features identical to Hodgkin's lymphoma presenting in lymph nodes **(B)**. A Reed-Sternberg cell **(B)** is apparent at the 4 o'clock position.

response to combination chemotherapy with long-term remissions. Unfavorable prognosis was linked to B-symptoms, age greater than 60 years, and bilateral disease.

Anaplastic Large Cell Lymphoma Presenting in the Lung

Anaplastic large cell lymphoma (ALCL) is a lymphoproliferative disorder with both morphologic and immunophenotypic features that overlap with those of classic Hodgkin's lymphoma. This entity has been given various names over time, with early names revolving around "histiocytoid" cytology of the neoplastic cells and more recent ones reflecting the uniform strong expression of the activation-associated antigen CD30 by the malignant cells. For a time, B-cell, T-cell and "null"-cell types of CD30–positive ALCL were accepted. However, studies in the 1990s elucidated that a cytogenetic translocation involving the anaplastic large cell lymphoma tyrosine kinase *(ALK)* gene on the short arm of chromosome 2 and the nucleophosmin gene on chromosome 5 was present in a significant subset of the CD30–positive large cell lymphoma cases of T-cell or "null"-cell types (reviewed by Stein et al.[162] and Morris et al.[163]). This translocation, which is associated with a relatively favorable prognosis, was not found in large B-cell lymphomas with CD30 expression, and furthermore this latter group exhibited a behavior more akin to diffuse large B-cell lymphoma.[164] Therefore, in the most recent WHO classification, the T-cell and "null"-cell types of ALCL are recognized and the phrase *CD30-positive* has been dropped from the name.[9] Cases of CD30–positive large B-cell lymphoma are now merely considered large B-cell lymphoma with an activated immunophenotype. It is noteworthy, however, that rare cases of large B-cell lymphoma express the *ALK* gene product through a mechanism distinct from the 2;5 chromosomal translocation of ALCL.[165,166]

When ALCL is encountered in the lung, it is most often a manifestation of widespread systemic disease[167]; however, sporadic cases of primary pulmonary ALCL have been described. A series of five cases of primary pulmonary ALCL was reported by Rush and colleagues.[168] The patients had nonspecific systemic symptoms; four of the five cases presented with isolated pulmonary nodules, one of which formed an endobronchial mass and another of which was hilar with tracheal invasion and spread into the mainstem bronchi. Histologically, these cases were all characterized by destructive infiltrates, some of which spilled into alveolar spaces, composed of large neoplastic cells with variable degrees of nuclear polymorphism (Fig. 32.33). The neoplastic cells showed strong, uniform CD30–positivity, were negative for CD15, and showed variable positivity for CD45 (leucocyte common antigen [LCA]) quintessential immunophenotypic features of ALCL. Three of the cases expressed T-cell–associated antigens; the remainder had a null cell phenotype. None of the tested cases showed evidence of the 2;5 chromosomal translocation by reverse-transcriptase (RT)-PCR analysis.

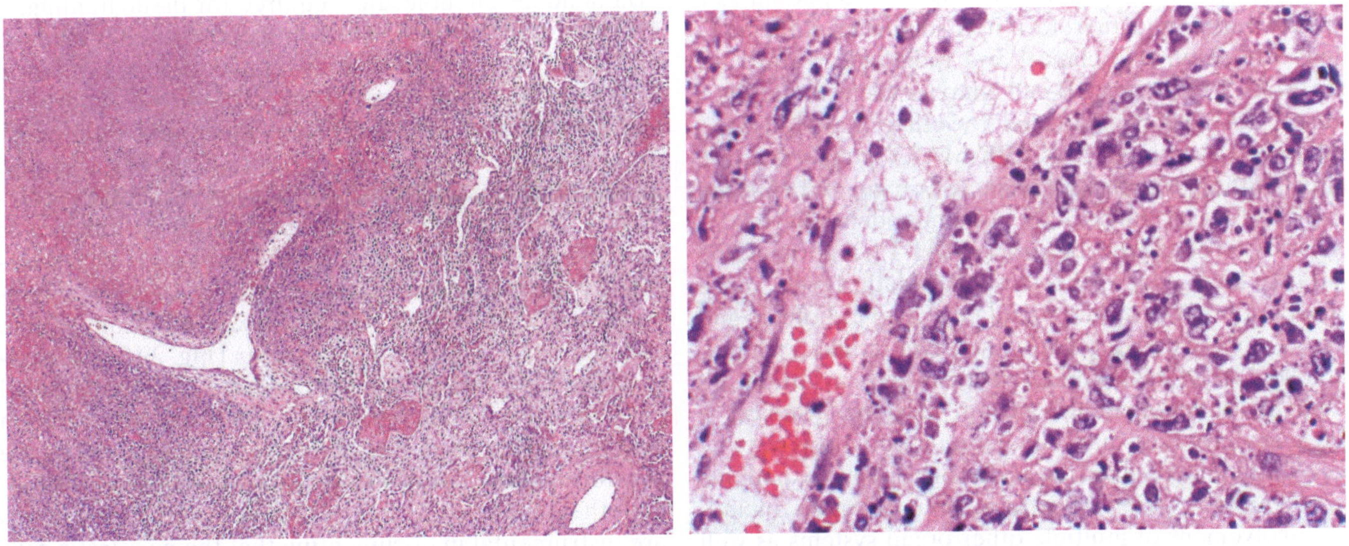

FIGURE 32.33. Primary pulmonary anaplastic large cell lymphoma. **(A)** This case presented as a single large nodule with necrosis and extensive vascular infiltration at the edge of the necrosis evident on low magnification (center left). **(B)** On higher magnification there are atypical large lymphoid cells with cytologic typical features of anaplastic large cell lymphoma. Immunophenotypically these were CD3-positive T cells, which also expressed CD30 and CD45 and were negative for CD20 and Epstein-Barr virus (EBV) (not shown).

A single case in the series of Rush et al. occurred in an HIV-positive individual. Interestingly, a review of the literature reveals other isolated instances of primary pulmonary ALCL arising in immunosuppressed patients, including one case as a PTLD following pulmonary transplantation[117] and two other cases arising in association with HIV.[128,167] This may be in keeping with the propensity for HIV-associated T-cell lymphomas to present with extranodal disease.[169] In a comparative analysis of CD30 positive and CD30 negative non-Hodgkin's lymphomas in HIV-positive patients, Nosari and colleagues[170] found a greater frequency of primary pulmonary involvement in CD30-positive cases. Lymphomas with anaplastic cytologic features occurring in AIDS patients tend to be associated with HHV-8 positivity.[171] It is difficult to glean outcome data from the literature given the rarity of primary pulmonary ALCL. However, cases occurring in immunocompromised individuals were universally associated with a poor outcome.

Other Lymphomas Presenting in the Lung

Pulmonary MALT lymphomas, lymphomatoid granulomatosis, and the other entities discussed above account for the vast majority of lymphomas that present in the lung. Once these disorders are excluded, what remains are a heterogeneous group that includes large cell B-cell lymphomas and other unclassifiable B-cell lymphomas. Follicular lymphomas, high-grade B-cell lymphomas, ALCL, and lymphoblastic lymphomas rarely involve the lung.

Most large descriptive series of pulmonary lymphoma cases predate the recognition of MALT lymphoma as a distinct entity, and therefore it is somewhat difficult to glean the distinctive clinical and radiologic features of non-MALT pulmonary B-cell lymphomas from the literature. Most patients affected by other non-Hodgkin's pulmonary lymphomas, as with MALT lymphoma, are adults, although there is a wide age range, and children may be affected, particularly in immunodeficiency states as discussed above. In contrast to MALT lymphomas, the majority have cough, shortness of breath, fever, and a variety of other systemic complaints. The radiologic and gross pathologic features vary; however, unlike with pulmonary MALT lymphomas, necrosis and cavitation are relatively common in this group. In some instances a single cavitary lung mass simulating tuberculosis may be seen. Either at presentation or during the course, patients may develop a variety of extrapulmonary lesions, including involvement of multiple other organ systems as well as paraneoplastic syndromes.

The presence of pulmonary lymphoma can be histologically obscured by a variety of factors. Like lymphomas presenting at other extranodal sites, lymphomas presenting in the lung may have an associated cytologically benign infiltrate. This infiltrate is usually at the periphery of the mass and can be remarkably extensive as compared to the foci recognizable as lymphoma.[172,173] An intraalveolar exudate and hyperplasia of type II pneumocytes is also common in the parenchyma adjacent to lymphomatous infiltrates. Reactive granulomatous inflammation and vasculitis, changes suggesting Wegener's granulomatosis, have also been described. Furthermore, extensively necrotic lesions often have a rim of viable cytologically benign cells, and one may need to search several blocks to find foci of recognizable lymphoma.

The majority of primary pulmonary lymphomas in this "wastebasket" category are large B-cell lymphomas. Histologically, these lymphomas are recognized by tumefactive lesions composed of sheets of lymphoid cells with large, atypical nuclei; however, the reactive changes described above may obfuscate the presence of lymphoma. Owing to the cytologic atypia of the neoplastic cells the differential diagnosis in the cases usually revolves around distinguishing it from other nonlymphoid malignancies such as carcinoma. The diagnosis of large B-cell lymphoma is usually confirmed by immunoperoxidase stains, which demonstrate the neoplastic cells to react with antibodies to B-cell–associated antigens such as CD20 and CD79a.

Intravascular large B-cell lymphoma is a unique subtype of large B-cell lymphoma in which the neoplastic cells are exclusively confined to the lumina of small vessels.[174–177] The neoplastic cells in this disease may remain in vascular structures due to the lack of expression of adhesion molecules required for tissue homing.[178] This unusual distribution of lymphomatous cells leads to protean clinical manifestations related to impaired blood flow such as mental status changes, nephrotic syndrome, and shortness of breath. Diffuse interstitial pulmonary infiltrates may be present on chest radiographs, and this, in combination with the presence of respiratory complaints, can lead to lung biopsy as an initial diagnostic procedure.[179,180] Histologically, this disease is characterized by the presence of large, cytologically atypical lymphoid cells within vessels, which, at low-power examination, may mimic an interstitial pneumonia (Fig. 32.34). Distinguishing these neoplastic lymphocytes from endothelial cells or intravascular infiltration by carcinoma cells on histologic grounds alone is difficult, a fact reflected by the previously used descriptive diagnosis of malignant angioendotheliomatosis. As a result, immunoperoxidase stains are instrumental in documenting that the neoplastic cells are B lymphocytes (Fig. 32.34C). Caution should be exercised, however, in rendering this diagnosis, as prominent intravascular infiltration can be seen in disseminated large B-cell lymphomas distinct from intravascular

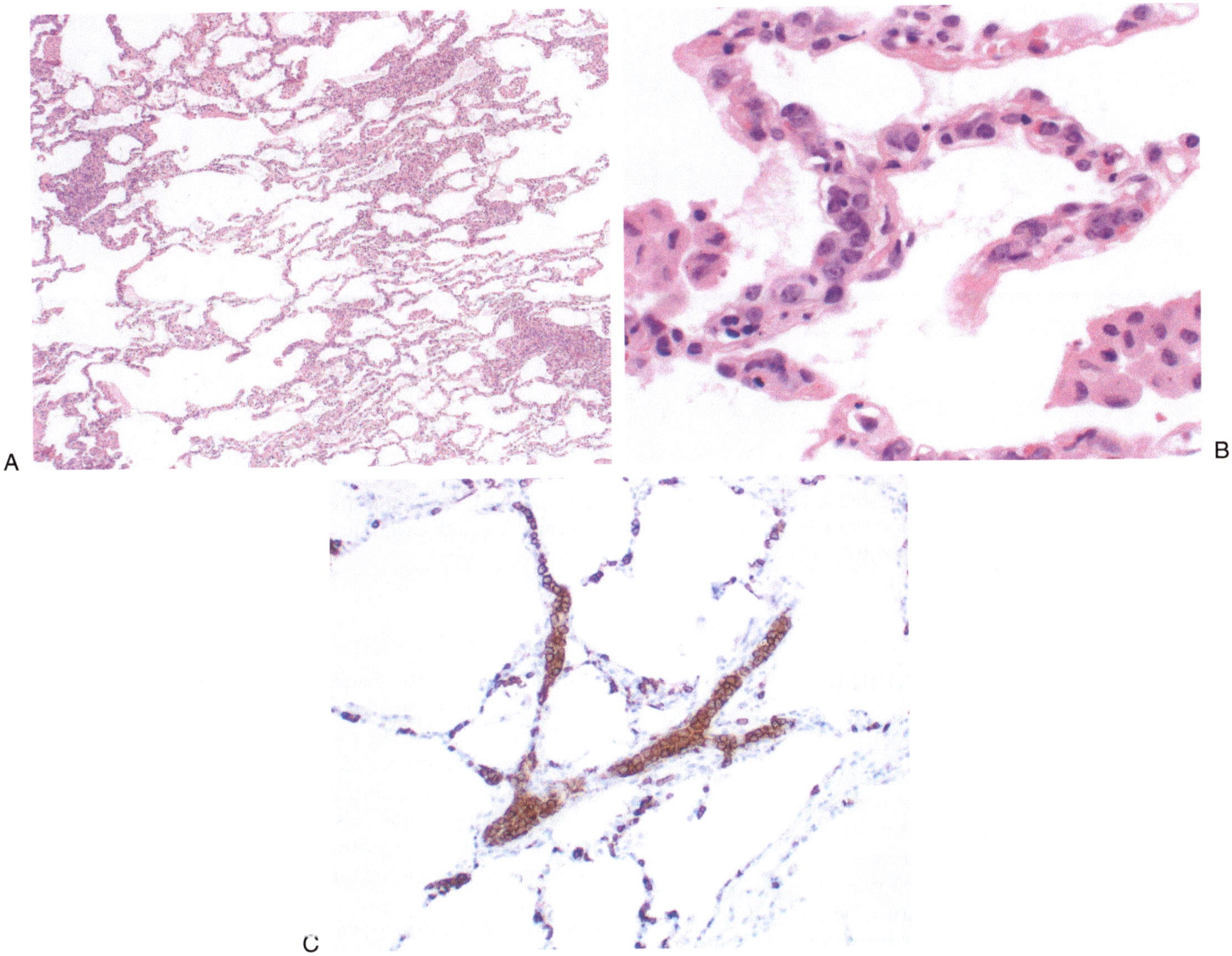

FIGURE 32.34. Intravascular lymphomatosis. Intermediate power microscopy shows some resemblance to an interstitial pneumonia **(A)**, but cytologic evaluation of the cellular areas shows atypical large lymphoid cells within capillaries in the alveolar wall **(B)**. These were confirmed as CD20-positive B cells **(C)**.

large B-cell lymphomas.[181] The latter diagnosis should only be rendered in cases in which the clinical features are typical, and clinical and radiologic examination fail to reveal evidence of lymph node, splenic, or other tissue involvement.

The remaining cases of lymphomas presenting in the lung not encompassed by the preceding discussion are few and poorly described. They are largely composed of B-cell lymphomas that cannot be further subclassified and a few T-cell lymphomas (Fig. 32.35). In cases that present as diffuse infiltrates along lymphatic routes without mass formation, the cellular heterogeneity may be so great that one is extremely reluctant to make a diagnosis of lymphoma. In such cases, cytologic atypia should be sought in infiltrates along pulmonary veins and in plaques of tumor in the pleura, because the peribronchial and peribronchiolar infiltrates tend to be the most polymorphous. The diagnosis of lymphoma should be confirmed by ancillary immunophenotyping and (when necessary) molecular genetic studies.

As with low-grade MALT lymphomas, a localized lymphoma in this group that is entirely resected may be cured.[59,182] However, the majority of patients have extensive bilateral disease, are clinically ill, and require aggressive chemotherapy that may result in either temporary or long-term remissions.[61,66,183]

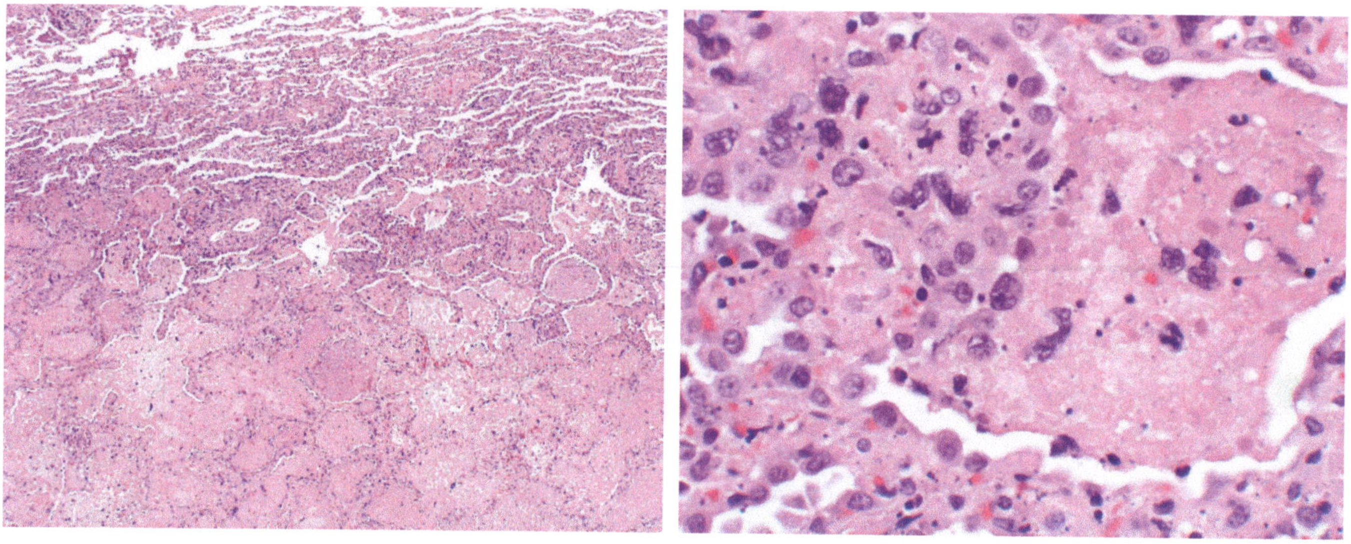

A B

FIGURE 32.35. Primary pulmonary T-cell lymphoma. This case showed nodules with extensive necrosis **(A)** resembling lymphomatoid granulomatosis with obvious cytologic features of lymphoma **(B)**. Immunohistochemistry and molecular studies confirmed T-cell lineage. The EBV studies were negative.

Lymphomas with Secondary Lung Involvement

The lung and pleura are commonly involved by a number of systemic lymphoproliferative disorders, and a detailed description of all possible entities would include a litany of most known diseases in this category. Instead, we will focus on those entities in which pulmonary involvement is a common or distinctive feature. Many of the features of secondary lung involvement by malignant lymphomas such as Hodgkin's lymphoma have been discussed comparatively with their primary pulmonary counterpart above.

Mature B-Cell Lymphoproliferative Disorders

Histologically, secondary pulmonary lymphomas in the lung cannot be distinguished from those presenting in the lung.[53,66] The knowledge of prior lymphoma is therefore critical in making the proper diagnosis. This is particularly important when confronted with a low-grade B-cell lineage malignant lymphoma, as primary pulmonary MALT lymphoma bears histologic similarity to a number of systemic lymphomas that one may encounter on pulmonary biopsies, including B-cell small lymphocytic lymphoma, mantle cell lymphoma, and follicular lymphoma. Distinguishing primary pulmonary MALT lymphoma from these other diseases is important given the propensity of MALT lymphomas to involve other MALT sites. Also, some of these disorders, particularly mantle cell lymphoma, are typically more aggressive than MALT lymphoma.[184] As when evaluating any potential recurrence of a malignant neoplasm, comparison with the cytologic features of the initial lesion is of great utility. In malignant lymphomas this bears the additional importance of assessing for potential transformation of a low-grade neoplasm to a higher-grade process.

B-cell Small Lymphocytic Lymphoma/Chronic Lymphocytic Leukemia

B-cell small lymphocytic lymphoma (Fig. 32.36) is histologically characterized by a tumefactive mass of small lymphocytes with scattered proliferation centers containing large prolymphocytes and paraimmunoblasts. Immunophenotypically B-cell small lymphocytic lymphoma is typified by aberrant coexpression of CD5 and CD23 by the neoplastic cells.[185] When proliferation centers are lacking, B-cell small lymphocytic lymphoma may resemble a MALT lymphoma. In these cases one may be forced to rely on the specific immunophenotype of B-cell small lymphocytic lymphoma, which may be detected in paraffin-embedded tissues, to establish the diagnosis.[68]

Mantle Cell Lymphoma

Mantle cell lymphoma has some similarities to B-cell small lymphocytic lymphoma in that it is typically a lymphoma composed of small B lymphocytes that aberrantly express CD5. In contrast to B-cell small lympho-

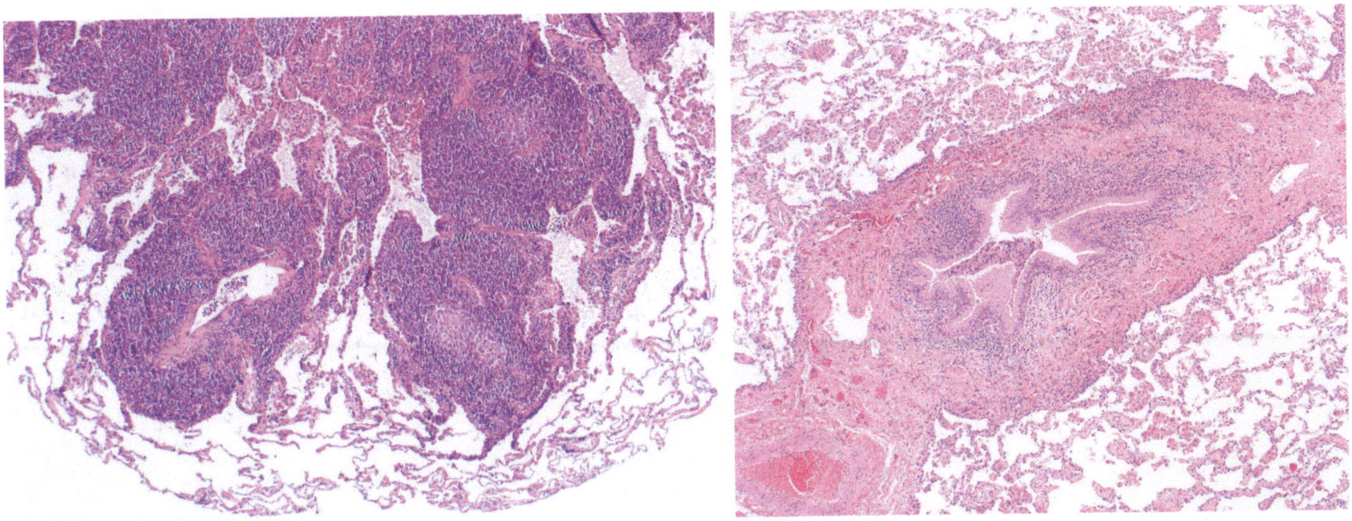

FIGURE 32.36. Pulmonary involvement in B-cell chronic lymphocytic leukemia. **(A)** There are dense perivascular infiltrates and small lymphocytes with some pseudofollicle formation (right). **(B)** This patient presented with wheezing and airflow obstruction, and the infiltrates showed a predilection for bronchioles with associated luminal narrowing, which led to the presenting symptoms. The patient was known to have chronic lymphocytic leukemia (CLL) and the bronchiolar infiltrate in this case was confirmed as CD20 positive with CD5 and CD23 coexpression.

cytic lymphoma, proliferation centers are absent and the neoplastic cells of mantle cell lymphoma usually have more nuclear irregularity and lack expression of CD23.[186] The absence of proliferation centers and the propensity of mantle cell lymphoma to encircle reactive follicles (from which the lymphoma derives its name) may lead one to entertain a diagnosis of MALT lymphoma when this process involves a MALT organ such as the lung or GI tract.[187] The quintessential feature of mantle cell lymphoma, however, is the aberrant expression of the cell cycle regulatory protein cyclin D1 resulting from the disease-specific chromosomal translocation, which juxtaposes the cyclin D1 gene on chromosome 11q23 with the immunoglobulin heavy chain gene on chromosome 14q32.[188] Cyclin D1 expression can be detected in paraffin-embedded tissues by immunoperoxidase staining, and the cyclin D1;IgH fusion can be detected by fluorescence in-situ hybridization (FISH) analysis, which can also be performed on paraffin-embedded specimens.[189,190] As mantle cell lymphoma tends to behave in a more aggressive manner than other cytologically low-grade B-cell lymphomas, performing these ancillary studies to assess for dysregulation of the cyclin D1 gene should be considered whenever this diagnosis is in question.[184]

Follicular Lymphoma

As many MALT lymphomas were probably misclassified as follicular lymphomas prior to the description of the former entity, it is difficult to accurately ascertain the frequency with which true follicular lymphomas occur in these organs.[191] The histologic resemblance between the two entities derives from the presence of reactive follicles as part of the architectural composition of MALT lymphomas. When these reactive follicles are colonized by clonal, neoplastic B cells, they can become quite prominent and mimic follicular lymphoma in appearance. For this reason one should be cautious in rendering a diagnosis of a new diagnosis of follicular lymphoma in a MALT site. Immunohistochemical stains performed on paraffin-embedded tissues can be quite helpful in revealing clusters of immunoglobulin light chain restricted BCL-2–positive plasmacytoid B cells in follicles primarily containing BCL-2–negative reactive follicular center B cells in these instances.[75,192] Bona fide follicular lymphomas should be characterized by a dense nodular growth pattern in which the nodules are populated by varying proportions of small cleaved cells, large cleaved cells, and centroblasts (Fig. 32.37). The diagnosis can be confirmed in many instances by demonstrating uniform strong BCL-2 staining in the neoplastic follicles by immunohistochemistry or the presence of *BCL-2:IgH* gene fusion by molecular genetic studies (FISH or RT-PCR).[9,193] It should be noted, however, that there can be considerable overlap between these two entities and that coincident, clonally related, localized MALT lymphomas and systemic follicular lymphomas have been described.[193]

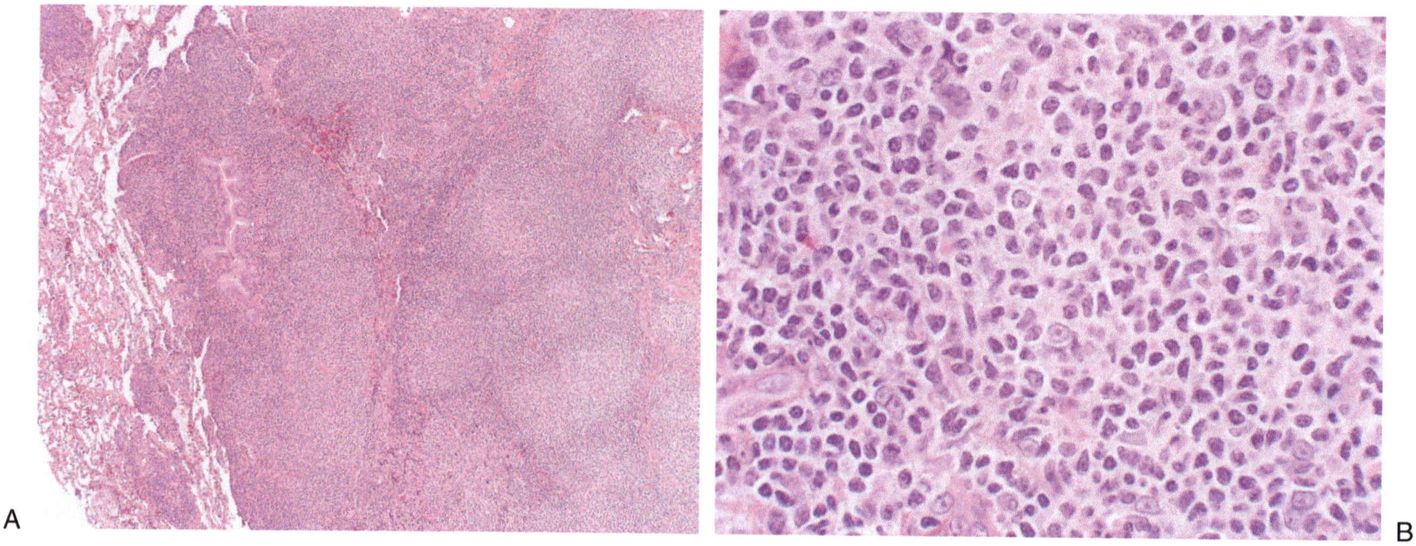

FIGURE 32.37. Primary follicular lymphoma of the lung. **(A)** The lymphoid mass shows a vague follicular architecture. **(B)** Cytologically the follicles showed typical features of follicular lymphoma, grade 1.

Mature T-Cell Lymphoproliferative Disorders

The vast majority of lymphomas are of B-cell lineage, with T-cell lymphomas representing a minor fraction of all lymphoma cases.[9] Furthermore, the features of one of the more common of these uncommon entities, ALCL of T-cell type, were discussed above. Of the remaining T-cell lymphomas, those that are most often encountered in pulmonary tissues are angioimmunoblastic T cell lymphoma and cutaneous T-cell lymphoma (Sézary syndrome and mycosis fungoides).

Angioimmunoblastic T-cell lymphoma is a nodal lymphoma that is associated with a syndromic clinical presentation that usually includes generalized lymphadenopathy, hepatosplenomegaly, Coombs-positive hemolytic anemia, skin rash, polyclonal hypergammaglobulinemia, and polyarthritis.[38] Pulmonary involvement by this lymphoma is common, occurring in up to 40% of cases. In involved lymph nodes, there is usually partial or complete architectural effacement by a polymorphous lymphoid infiltrate containing collections of neoplastic lymphoid cells with pale-staining to clear cytoplasm and variably sized, elongate, irregular nuclei. These cells are present in a background composed of a mixture of eosinophils, plasma cells, follicular dendritic cells, and venules with prominent endothelium (reviewed by Dogan et al.[42]). The groups of abnormal clear lymphoma cells may obscured by the prominent background cellular population or may even be absent in up to one half of cases, making histologic recognition difficult. Ancillary immunoperoxidase stains can be of great utility in establishing the diagnosis by highlighting the presence of cytologically atypical CD3–positive T cells, which aberrantly express the follicular center B-cell–associated antigen CD10.[194] The abnormal expression of CD10 by the T cells is a disease-specific feature that can be detected in pulmonary biopsy specimens.[195] Even in extranodal sites one should consider ancillary PCR or Southern blot studies to assess for the presence of clonal T-cell receptor gene rearrangements, which are present in most cases and help to confirm the diagnosis. The prognosis in this disease is regrettably poor, with a median survival of less than 2 years.

After lymph nodes, the lung is the second most frequent site of extracutaneous involvement by cutaneous T-cell lymphoma (Fig. 32.38).[196,197] Localized, diffuse, or sometimes nodular radiographic infiltrates are seen. The infiltrates are distributed along lymphatic routes, and the cytologic spectrum is similar to that seen in mycosis fungoides at other sites. Vascular infiltration and necrosis may be present. If symptoms requiring therapeutic intervention are required, whole-lung irradiation may be an effective treatment.[198]

Histiocytic Disorders

The early pulmonary pathology literature included descriptions of "malignant histiocytoses."[199–201] Many of these cases have now come to be recognized as T-cell lymphomas with most representing ALCLs.[202] True malignancies of histiocytic lineage are extraordinarily rare[9]; the occurrence of such neoplasms in the lung is questionable and is vastly outnumbered by benign causes of histiocytic pulmonary infiltrates such as infection and sarcoidosis.

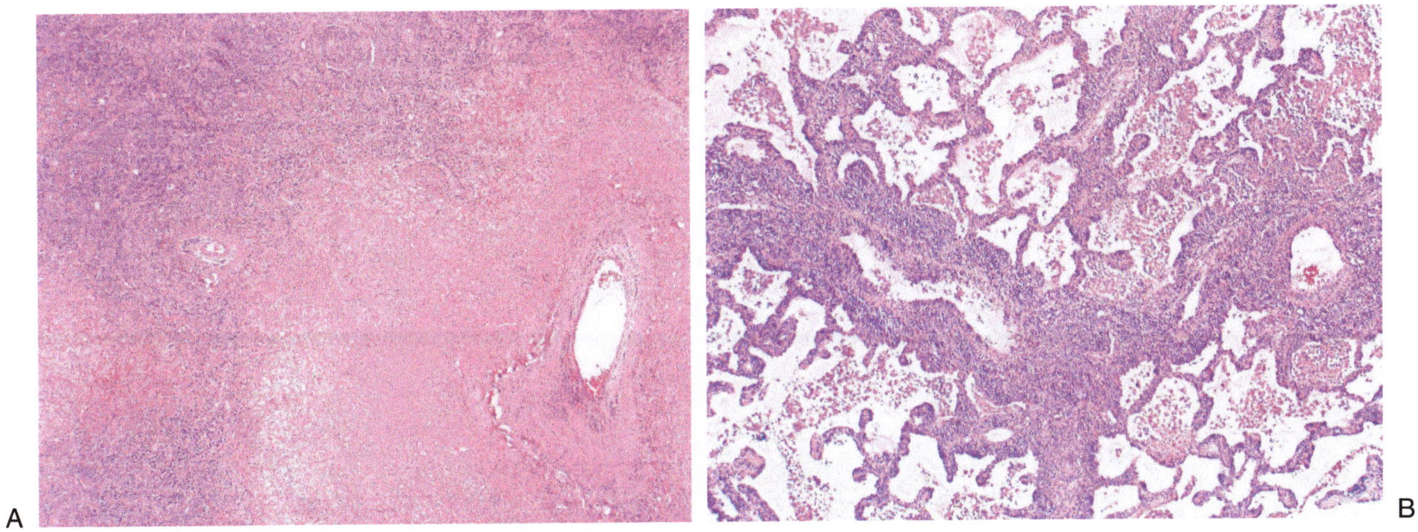

FIGURE 32.38. Secondary pulmonary involvement by cutaneous T-cell lymphoma. Some secondary lymphomas present as nodules with central necrosis similar to lymphomatoid granulomatosis **(A)**, whereas others show more diffuse involvement in which predilection for lymphatic routes is apparent along a septum and around veins **(B)**.

Despite the early misappropriation of many lymphomas as "malignant histiocytosis," there are a few well-recognized entities of histiocytic lineage that involve the lung. These pulmonary histiocytic disorders include Langerhans cell histiocytosis, which may involve the lung as a part of the disseminated disease (most often in children) or as a predominantly pulmonary disorder encountered in adult smokers called pulmonary Langerhans cell histiocytosis (PLCH; synonyms: pulmonary histiocytosis X and pulmonary eosinophilic granuloma). These disorders are discussed more extensively in Chapter 16 on histiocytic and storage diseases. Although both are rare, Erdheim-Chester disease and Rosai-Dorfman disease are well-recognized histiocytic disorders that can be encountered in the lung, which bear further discussion here (see also the discussion in Chapter 16).

Erdheim-Chester Disease

Erdheim-Chester disease is a rare non–Langerhans cell histiocytic disorder characterized by symmetric osteosclerosis of the metaphyseal and diaphyseal regions of the long bones due to bone infiltration and varied extraskeletal manifestations including pulmonary involvement.[203] Extraskeletal manifestations are present in around one half of cases, and the sites of involvement also include the skin, orbit, hypothalamus/pituitary, and retroperitoneum; these sites may be more often involved than the lung. However, lung infiltration by this disorder, when present, is symptomatic, which may lead to lung biopsy as an initial diagnostic procedure and may cause significant disease-associated morbidity and mortality.[204] Therefore, it is important for pulmonologists and pulmonary pathologists to be aware of this disease entity.

Erdheim-Chester disease typically affects middle-aged adults; cases in young adults (20 to 30 years of age) have been described, but this disease does not typically occur in children, a distinguishing feature from Langerhans cell histiocytosis. Bony disease is universal and bone pain is a common clinical manifestation.[203] Pulmonary involvement is present in approximately one quarter to one third of patients and usually presents as dyspnea of insidious onset or nonproductive cough. Pulmonary function abnormalities including decreased diffusing capacity are frequently present in this setting.[204] In selected instances, pulmonary Erdheim-Chester disease can present with acute respiratory failure. Other clinical features are directly attributable to infiltration of other organs by this process and include diabetes insipidus secondary to hypothalamic lesions and renal failure due to retroperitoneal disease.[203]

Many of the reported cases of pulmonary Erdheim-Chester have been isolated case reports, which is not unexpected given the rarity of this condition. The following discussion is largely summarized from two series of cases reported by Egan and colleagues[205] and Rush and colleagues[206] respectively. Plain film chest radiography reveals diffuse interstitial infiltrates, often with an upper lobe predominance. The CT findings in pulmonary Erdheim-Chester are characteristic and are typified by diffuse thickening of the interlobular septa and pleura associated with centrilobular opacification; these changes are more pronounced in the upper lobes.[207]

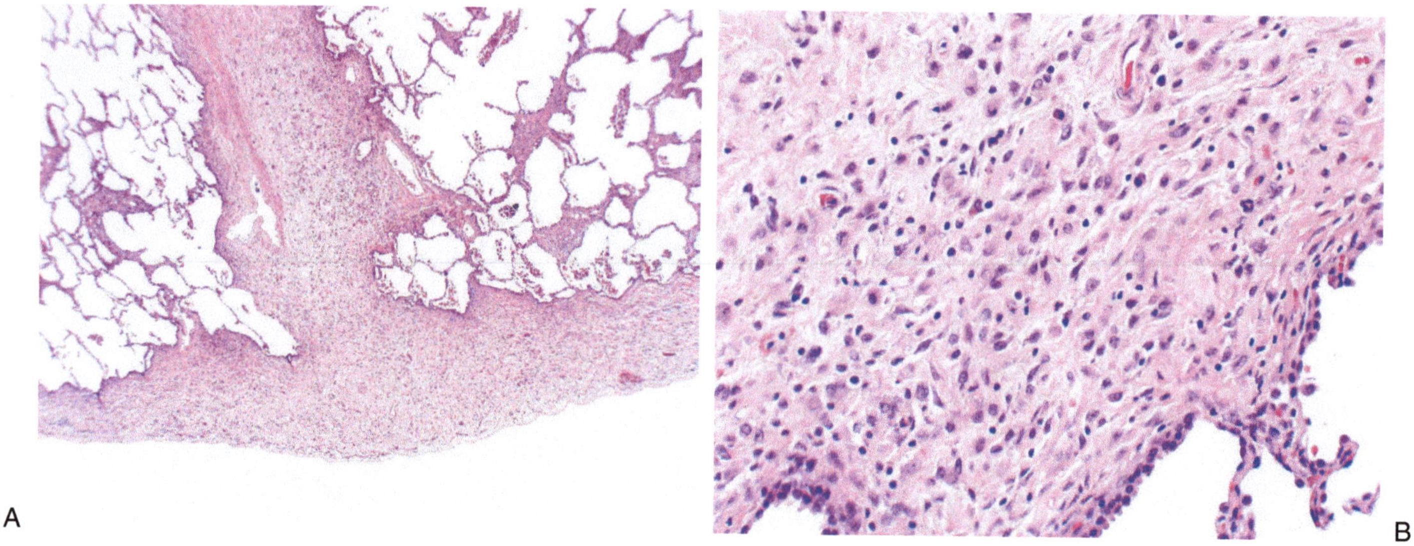

FIGURE 32.39. Pulmonary Erdheim-Chester disease. **(A)** There is a paucicellular pleural and septal thickening with relatively sparing of the alveoli. **(B)** Cytologically the infiltrate includes relatively numerous histiocytes with a background of fibroblasts and a few mixed inflammatory cells.

The low-power appearance of Erdheim-Chester in pulmonary-wedge biopsy or autopsy specimens is characterized by diffuse interstitial thickening, which follows the lymphangitic distribution of the CT abnormalities (Fig. 32.39A). Detailed cytologic evaluation reveals this thickening to be caused by a mixed infiltrate of small lymphocytes, plasma cells, and histiocytes in a background of fine, acellular fibrotic tissue (Fig. 32.39B). The histiocytes have abundant granular or vacuolated cytoplasm and lack the nuclear folding and irregularity of Langerhans-type cells. The cells are uniformly CD68 positive by immunohistochemical analysis; S-100 is expressed in a subset of cases (see Chapter 16, Figs. 16.58, 16.60). The cells lack expression of CD1a and also do not contain Birbeck granules on ultrastructural analysis—additional features that distinguish these cells from Langerhans cells.

The clinical course in Erdheim-Chester is variable, with some patients having relatively stable involvement of the lung and other sites. However, in some instances the disease pursues an unremitting course, leading to death due either to pulmonary or retroperitoneal disease.

Rosai-Dorfman Disease

Rosai-Dorfman disease, originally described in lymph nodes as sinus histiocytosis with massive lymphadenopathy (SHML), is another rare, non–Langerhans cell histiocytic disorder.[208] This usually presents as massive bilateral cervical lymphadenopathy, although a number of extranodal sites may be involved including the skin, meninges, and kidneys.[209,210] The term *Rosai-Dorfman disease* is preferred by many clinicians since lymph nodes are not always affected in individual cases. Histologically, Rosai-Dorfman disease is characterized by infiltration by large histiocytes with ovoid nuclei and abundant eosinophilic cytoplasm, which often contains entrapped small lymphocytes (emperipolesis) (see Chapter 16, Fig. 16.62). Fibrosis and infiltrates of lymphocytes, plasma cells, and occasionally neutrophils are also common, particularly in extranodal sites (Fig. 32.40A). Nasal involvement is well known.[211,212] Lower respiratory tract involvement is very rare, and when present it is usually typified by mass lesions that are centered on the large airways and hilum.[213] Some cases demonstrate a lymphatic distribution. This distribution of disease, the cytologic features of the histiocytes and their positivity for S-100 (Fig. 32.40B), and the presence of emperipolesis distinguish SHML from Erdheim-Chester disease. The number of lung cases described is too small to address prognosis. In general, SHML pursues a relatively benign course (although there are exceptions).

Leukemic Infiltrates in the Lung

Clinically significant leukemic pulmonary infiltrates recognized during life are quite rare, and infections, hemorrhage, heart failure, the effects of chemotherapy or radiotherapy, alveolar proteinosis, and opportunistic neoplasms should first be excluded.[214–216] Even when an unequivocal leukemic infiltrate is histologically identified in the lung (Fig. 32.41), it may be incidental (although still significant) to a coexisting lesion, especially infection, that is the cause of the patient's immediate lung problem. The incidence of leukemic infiltration of the lung found

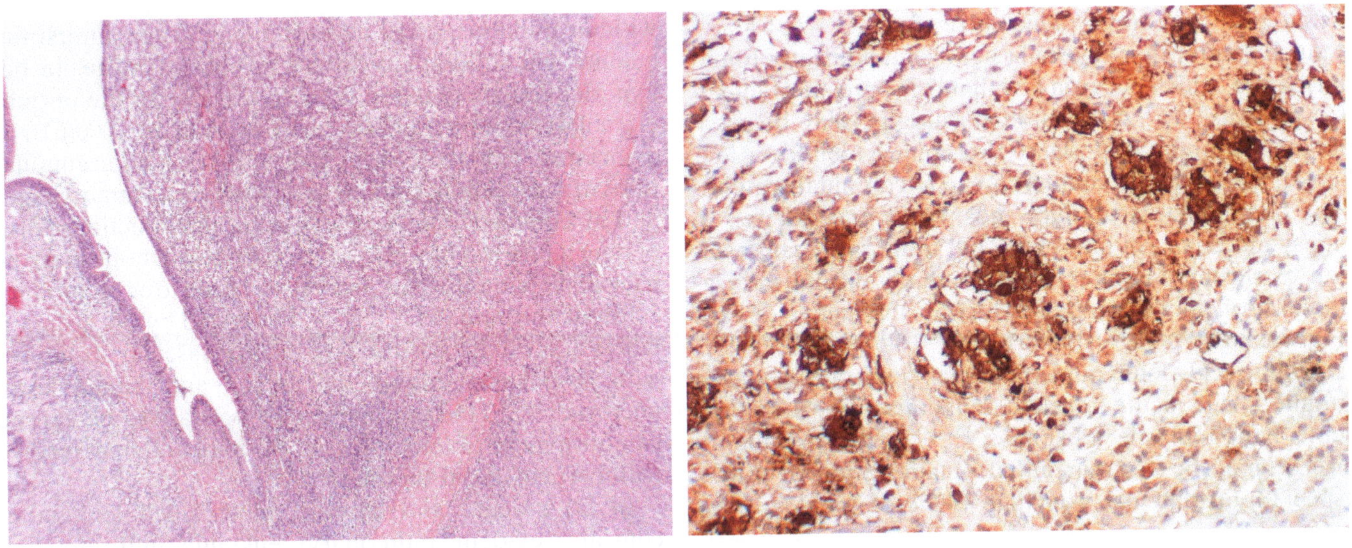

A B

FIGURE 32.40. Primary pulmonary Rosai-Dorfman disease. This case presented as a mass lesion that infiltrated and destroyed lung parenchyma including a large bronchus **(A)**. The pale histiocytic cells characteristic of Rosai-Dorfman disease are apparent at low power **(A)** and were confirmed as being S-100 positive **(B)**.

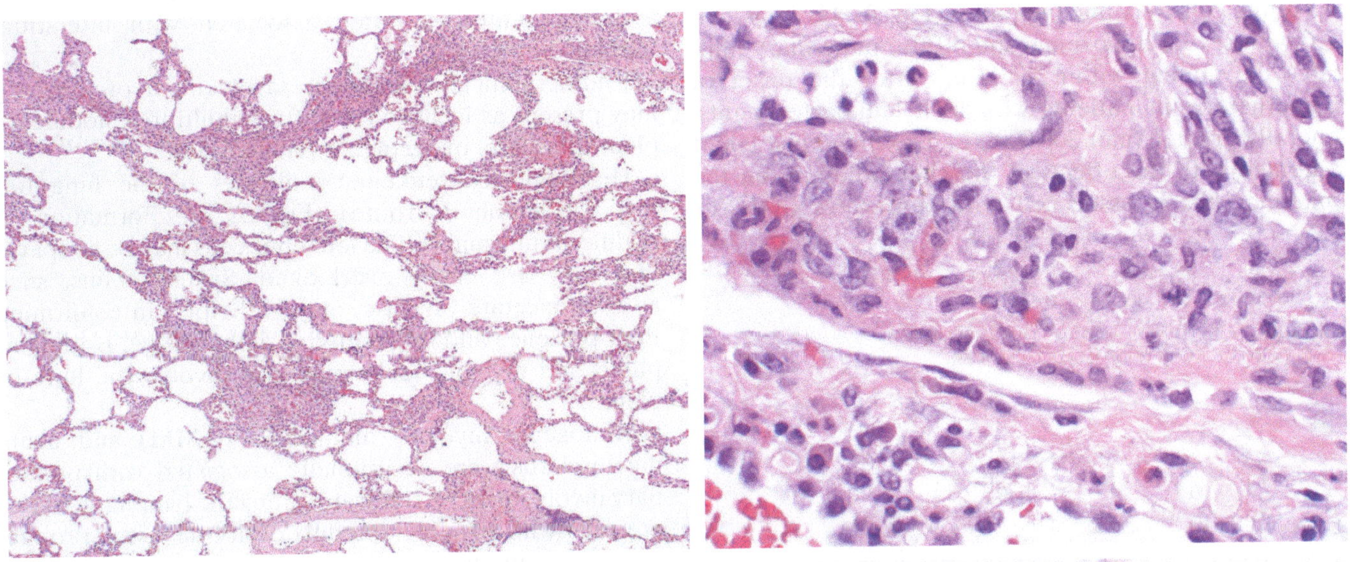

A B

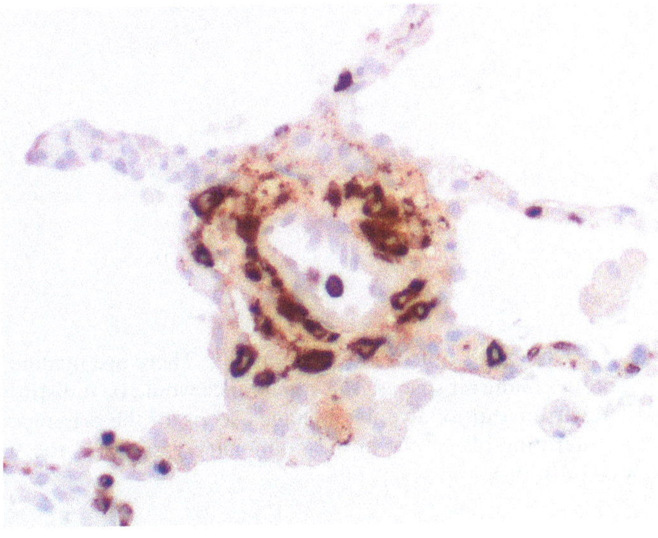

C

FIGURE 32.41. Pulmonary involvement in chronic myelomonocytic leukemia. **(A)** There is a cellular infiltrate at medium power that mimics an interstitial pneumonia. **(B)** Cytologically this infiltrate includes atypical monocytoid cells with occasional mitotic figures (at the 3 o'clock position). **(C)** The atypical cells were positive for myeloperoxidase. The patient had a history of chronic myelomonocytic leukemia.

histologically at autopsy, which varies from 25% to 64%,[215] is much greater than clinically significant infiltrates found during life, which occur in less than 7% percent of leukemic patients.[215–217] Any histologic subtype may be seen, but in the authors' experience B-chronic lymphocytic leukemia, the leukemic counterpart to B-cell small lymphocytic lymphoma, is the type most often encountered in biopsy material. An interesting but quite rare manifestation of chronic lymphocytic leukemia is diffuse infiltration of bronchioles, producing airway obstructive disease (Fig. 32.36B).[218]

Among acute leukemias, pulmonary infiltration is more common with acute myeloid leukemias (AMLs) than acute lymphoblastic leukemias.[215,219] Severe pulmonary disease may be a major initial manifestation of AML, especially in patients with high (40% or greater) blast counts.[215]

Three unusual reactions that appear unique to leukemia are leukostasis, leukemic cell lysis pneumopathy, and hyperleukocytic reaction.[216,220,221] In leukostasis, there is vascular occlusion by aggregates of blasts in patients with peripheral leukocyte counts greater than 200,000/μL. Leukemic cell lysis pneumopathy (Fig. 32.42) is associated with severe hypoxemia and diffuse pulmonary infiltrates developing within 48 hours after the onset of chemotherapy in patients with high leukocyte counts, generally greater than 200,000/μL. The high blast count combined with the effects of the chemotherapy on the leukemic cells is associated with aggregates of blasts within capillaries, small infarcts, hemorrhage, interstitial edema, and subsequent diffuse alveolar damage. In the hyperleukocytic reaction, a rapid increase in the peripheral blast count (generally greater than 245,000/μL) is associated with acute respiratory distress and accumulations of blast cells in small vessels with microhemorrhages and alveolar edema. A rare, unique noninfectious form of lung injury has recently been described in bone marrow transplant patients. This process, referred to as pulmonary cytolytic thrombi (PCT), is characterized by the accumulation of acellular basophilic debris in vascular structures with associated endothelial injury and hemorrhagic necrosis.[222–225] This vascular injury appears to be caused by entrapment of leukocytes in thrombi and may resolve with corticosteroid therapy.

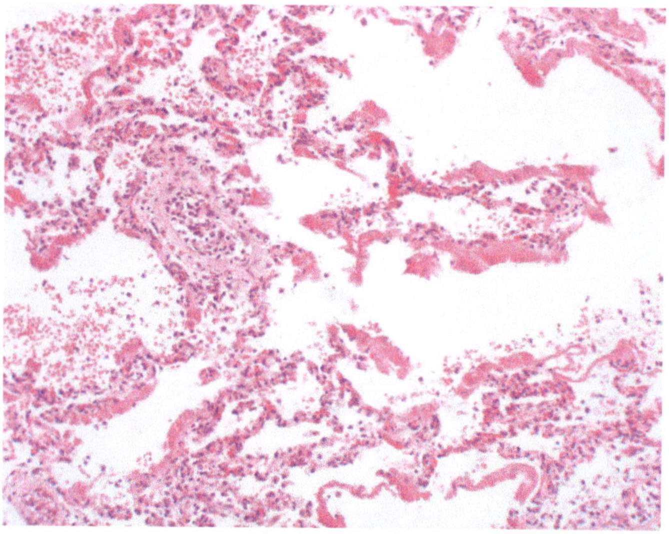

FIGURE 32.42. Leukemic lysis pneumopathy. There are hyaline membranes lining air spaces. The appearance would be indistinguishable from diffuse alveolar damage except for the presence of degenerating blast cells in the pulmonary vessels (at the 9 o'clock position).

In both acute and chronic adult T-cell leukemias, clinically evident pulmonary leukemic infiltrates appear to be relatively common and were seen in 13 of 29 patients reported by Yoshioka et al.[226] In six of the 13 cases, a diagnosis of chronic lung disease had been carried for 2 to 6 years before this diagnosis of leukemia, and four of the six were histologically confirmed as having leukemic infiltrates, often associated with interstitial fibrosis.

Radiographically, leukemic involvement of the lung may present as localized or diffuse infiltrates, nodule(s), pleural disease, or recurrent pneumonias.[216–218,227–231]

Histologically, leukemic infiltrates of the lung follow the lymphatic routes (Fig. 32.41). Formation of nodules is unusual.[227] The leukemic cells may be so sparse that they are easily overlooked. Special stains, such as chloroacetate esterase, may be helpful in confirming their presence and in identifying a phenotype. Both lymphoid and myeloid leukemias may involve the lung or pleura.[218,227,228]

Agnogenic myeloid metaplasia (AMM) and acute myelosclerosis are occasionally associated with pulmonary involvement.[232] Infiltrates along the lymphatic routes are seen with variable amounts of fibrous tissue production. The amount of fibrous tissue may overshadow the hematopoietic cells. Death from progressive restrictive disease secondary to the fibrosis associated with AMM has been reported.[233] Primary pulmonary hypertension is another uncommon pulmonary manifestation of chronic myeloproliferative disorders in general and AMM in particular.[234] The etiology of the pulmonary hypertension is unclear, although deposition of circulating megakaryocytes in the pulmonary microvasculature has been proposed. The notion that the pulmonary hypertension is caused by ectopic hematopoietic elements, which are highly radiosensitive, is supported by a report by Steensma et al.,[235] which documented dramatic improvement of AMM-associated pulmonary hypertension with a single low dose of ionizing radiation delivered to the lungs.

Plasma Cell Tumors and Multiple Myeloma

True pulmonary plasmacytomas must be distinguished from other lesions with numerous plasma cells that are more often encountered in the lung including MALT lymphomas and reactive plasma cell granulomas. When these latter entities are excluded, pulmonary neoplasms composed exclusively of plasma cells are rare, with a smattering of isolated case reports and small series in the literature.[236,237] Most of these reports describe isolated pulmonary masses formed by sheets of immunoglobulin light chain restricted plasma cells with varying degrees of cytologic atypia. Amyloid may be present, associated with the tumoral mass, and a single case with diffuse pulmonary involvement has been reported.[238] Given the rarity of primary pulmonary plasmacytomas, it is difficult to make any firm statements about their behavior. A review of the literature reveals that some patients may develop progressive disease with systemic dissemination, whereas others may experience late local recurrence or no recurrence whatsoever.[237,239,240] Although the number of bona fide cases with information regarding treatment is small, it appears that surgical excision and radiation therapy are equally efficacious in the treatment of localized pulmonary disease.

Pulmonary involvement in patients with multiple myeloma is more frequent than is primary pulmonary plasmacytoma, although it still is not common. Most of the patients have clinically obvious disseminated myeloma, and pulmonary involvement is part of the systemic disease.[241,242] Pulmonary presentation with infiltrates resembling pneumonia has also been described.[243] Multiple nodules are more frequent than diffuse infiltrates.[243] Also in this setting diffuse alveolar septal amyloid deposition or other forms of amyloidosis secondary to the myeloma may also be a cause of lung disease.[243] Kijner and Yousem[244] reported a case of systemic light chain disease presenting as bilateral nodular infiltrates on chest radiographs. Light chain deposition was distinguished from amyloid by electron microscopy.

Pleural Lymphoma and Leukemia

Pleural involvement by lymphomas and leukemias is not unexpected, because the pleura represents one of the lymphatic routes that these lesions generally affect. Indeed, identifying extrapleural infiltrative plaques is a helpful feature in distinguishing low-grade lymphomas from benign processes.[56] Elastic tissue stains may be necessary to identify the exact location of the visceral pleura in the case of massive infiltrates. Lymphomas, including lymphoplasmacytic lymphoma, rarely present as pleural disease. In these cases, the extensive and predominately visceral pleural infiltration is out of proportion to the relatively scant infiltration of the underlying pulmonary parenchyma.

Pleural effusions found at presentation in patients with Hodgkin's lymphoma and (less commonly) non-Hodgkin's lymphomas are usually caused by lymphomatous involvement of mediastinal lymph nodes and secondary lymphatic obstruction.[245] Flow cytometric immunophenotyping studies may be helpful in revealing the presence of clonal cell populations and thereby aid in establishing a diagnosis of lymphoma. This is particularly true in low-grade lymphomas in which the cytologic features may not be sufficiently distinctive to allow an unequivocal morphologic diagnosis. In cases that require biopsy, the visceral pleura should be biopsied in preference to the parietal pleura, as the extent of infiltrate is usually much more severe in the visceral pleura. Widespread myeloma may cause pleural effusions.[241,242] (See also discussion in Chapter 43).

Miscellaneous Hematolymphoid Disorders

Systemic Mast Cell Disease

Symptomatic asthma occurs frequently in systemic mast cell disease patients. In most instances this is attributed to the secretion of mediators such as histamine and leukotrienes into the circulation by the abnormal mast cells.[246] However, rare cases of systemic mastocytosis associated with infiltration of the lung parenchyma by the abnormal mast cells have been described.[247,248] Pulmonary infiltration by mast cell disease appears to be associated with increased dyspnea and abnormal pulmonary function tests, findings that may not distinguish direct organ involvement from the remote affects of mediator release. Radiographic features of parenchymal lung involvement include reticulonodular interstitial infiltrates and interstitial fibrosis; osteosclerotic and osteolytic lesions in the vertebrae due to marrow infiltration may also be noted. Computed tomography scanning reveals uniformly distributed pulmonary nodules and cysts, and mediastinal adenopathy is sometimes present. Mast cell infiltrates with associated lymphocytes and fibrosis are seen on tissue biopsy. The presence of mast cells in tissues is highlighted and confirmed through the use of immunohistochemical stains to the mast cell–associated antigens tryptase and c-kit, and these can be helpful in establishing the diagnosis given the varying cytologic features of abnormal mast cells and the polymorphous nature of the mast cell infiltrates.[249] There is currently no curative treatment for systemic mast cell disease; however, resolution of clinical and radiologic abnormalities with interferon-α therapy in a case with pulmonary involvement has been described.[248]

Immune Accessory Cell Neoplasms

Relatively recently, neoplasms that are derived from nonhistiocyte immune accessory cells have been recognized. Although some of these are derived from mesenchymal stem cells, they are generally regarded as tumors related to the hematopoietic system. As a whole these are extraordinarily rare diseases; however, they can involve the lung and are usually composed of spindled cells and therefore are considered in the differential of spindle cell neoplasms.

Follicular Dendritic Cell Tumors

Follicular dendritic cells are mesenchymal-derived cells that present antigens to B cells and thereby form an integral part of lymphoid follicles. Neoplasms derived from these cells, termed follicular dendritic cell sarcoma/tumor, can involve lymph nodes and a variety of extranodal sites including the oropharynx and GI tract.[250] Lung involvement, although not a common feature in the published reports, has been described both as a primary site of tumor and as a site of recurrence.[250,251] Some follicular dendritic cell tumors arise in association with, or are preceded by, the hyaline vascular type of Castleman's disease and this may represent a precursor lesion. In the lung and elsewhere these tumors form mass lesions with marginated, rather than infiltrative, borders that histologically are composed of spindled cells with a storiform or fascicular growth pattern. Small lymphocytes are usually intermingled. The nuclear atypia of the spindled cells varies between cases with some exhibiting striking pleomorphism; coagulative necrosis may also be present.

Based on these histologic features a number of entities may be considered in the differential diagnosis, including metaplastic carcinoma.[251] The diagnosis of follicular dendritic cell tumor is usually confirmed by immunoperoxidase stains, which reveal the neoplastic cells to be positive for CD21, CD35, and clusterin, and to be negative for a number of other antigens including CD1a, S-100 protein, and cytokeratin.[252] Given the rarity of this diagnosis, it is difficult to make conclusive statements regarding treatment, although in most cases surgical excision is described. Follicular dendritic cell tumors most often behave in an indolent fashion with local recurrences common; however, a subset of cases (approximately one quarter) behave in an aggressive fashion with lethal metastatic disease.[250]

Interdigitating Dendritic Cell Tumors

Interdigitating dendritic cell tumors/sarcomas are neoplasms derived from cells of the same name that are normally found in the lymph node paracortex where they are function in presenting antigens to T cells. These tumors appear to be even rarer than follicular dendritic cell tumors, a single case with pulmonary involvement by interdigitating dendritic cell sarcoma has been reported.[253] Like follicular dendritic cell tumors, interdigitating dendritic cell tumors are characterized histologically by storiform spindled cells, and these two types of neoplasms may be indistinguishable by morphology. Unlike follicular dendritic cells, interdigitating dendritic cells are bone marrow derived and therefore are CD45 positive. These cells are ontologically related to Langerhans cells and, like the latter are usually S-100 positive; interdigitating dendritic cells are distinguished from Langerhans cells by the lack of uniform CD1a expression and the lack of Birbeck granules by ultrastructural analysis. Interdigitating dendritic cells are also negative for the follicular dendritic cell–associated antigens CD21, CD35, and clusterin.[252,254] The behavior of these tumors is variable with both localized recurrences and widespread, fatal disease described.

References

1. Greenberg SD, Heisler JG, Gyorkey F, Jenkins DE. Pulmonary lymphoma versus pseudolymphoma: a perplexing problem. South Med J1972;65:775–784.
2. Julsrud PR, Brown LR, Li CY, Rosenow EC 3rd, Crowe JK. Pulmonary processes of mature-appearing lymphocytes: pseudolymphoma, well-differentiated lymphocytic lymphoma, and lymphocytic interstitial pneumonitis. Radiology 1978;127:289–296.
3. Liebow AA, Carrington CR, Friedman PJ. Lymphomatoid granulomatosis. Hum Pathol 1972;3:457–558.
4. Liebow AA, Carrington CB. Diffuse pulmonary lymphoreticular infiltrations associated with dysproteinemia. Med Clin North Am 1973;57:809–843.
5. Lipford EH Jr, Margolick JB, Longo DL, Fauci AS, Jaffe ES. Angiocentric immunoproliferative lesions: a clinicopathologic spectrum of post-thymic T-cell proliferations. Blood 1988;72:1674–1681.
6. DeRemee RA, Weiland LH, McDonald TJ. Polymorphic reticulosis, lymphomatoid granulomatosis. Two diseases or one? Mayo Clin Proc 1978;53:634–640.
7. Saldana MJ, Patchefsky AS, Israel HI, Atkinson GW. Pulmonary angiitis and granulomatosis. The relationship between histological features, organ involvement, and response to treatment. Hum Pathol 1977;8:391–409.
8. Jaffe ES, Wilson WH. Lymphomatoid granulomatosis: pathogenesis, pathology and clinical implications. Cancer Surv 1997;30:233–248.
9. Jaffe ES, Harris NL, Stein H, Vardiman JW. World Health Organization classification of tumours. In: Kleihues P, Sobin L, eds. Pathology and genetics of tumours of haemotopoietic and lymphoid tissues. Lyon: IARC Press, 2001.
10. Okada Y. Lymphatic system of the human lung. Kyoto: Kinpodo, 1989.
11. Nagaishi C. Functional anatomy and histology of the lung. Baltimore: University Park, 1972.

12. Sykes AM, Swensen SJ, Tazelaar HD, Jung SH. Computed tomography of benign intrapulmonary lymph nodes: retrospective comparison with sarcoma metastases. Mayo Clin Proc 2002;77:329–333.
13. Kradin RL, Spirn PW, Mark EJ. Intrapulmonary lymph nodes. Clinical, radiologic, and pathologic features. Chest 1985;87:662–667.
14. Swensen SJ, Jett JR, Hartman TE, et al. Lung cancer screening with CT: Mayo Clinic experience [see comment]. Radiology 2003;226:756–761.
15. Bienenstock J, Johnston N, Perey DY. Bronchial lymphoid tissue. I. Morphologic characteristics. Lab Invest 1973;28:686–692.
16. Bienenstock J, Johnston N, Perey DY. Bronchial lymphoid tissue. II. Functional characteristics. Lab Invest 1973;28:693–698.
17. Bienenstock J. The lung as an immunologic organ. Annu Rev Med 1984;35:49–62.
18. Bienenstock J, Befus D. Gut- and bronchus-associated lymphoid tissue. Am J Anat 1984;170:437–445.
19. Pabst R, Gehrke I. Is the bronchus-associated lymphoid tissue (BALT) an integral structure of the lung in normal mammals, including humans? Am J Respir Cell Mol Biol 1990;3:131–135.
20. Harris NL. Extranodal lymphoid infiltrates and mucosa-associated lymphoid tissue (MALT). A unifying concept. [see comment]. Am J Surg Pathol 1991;15:879–884.
21. Isaacson PG, Spencer J. Malignant lymphoma of mucosa-associated lymphoid tissue. Histopathology 1987;11:445–462.
22. Addis BJ, Hyjek E, Isaacson PG. Primary pulmonary lymphoma: a re-appraisal of its histogenesis and its relationship to pseudolymphoma and lymphoid interstitial pneumonia. Histopathology 1988;13:1–17.
23. Isaacson P, Wright DH. Extranodal malignant lymphoma arising from mucosa-associated lymphoid tissue. Cancer 1984;53:2515–2524.
24. Hernandez JA, Sheehan WW. Lymphomas of the mucosa-associated lymphoid tissue. Signet ring cell lymphomas presenting in mucosal lymphoid organs. Cancer 1985;55:592–597.
25. Morris H, Edwards J, Tiltman A, Emms M. Endometrial lymphoid tissue: an immunohistological study. J Clin Pathol 1985;38:644–652.
26. Balikian JP, Herman PG. Non-Hodgkin lymphoma of the lungs. Radiology 1979;132:569–576.
27. Bragg DG. The clinical, pathologic and radiographic spectrum of the intrathoracic lymphomas. Invest Radiol 1978;13:2–11.
28. Blank N, Castellino RA. The intrathoracic manifestations of the malignant lymphomas and the leukemias. Semin Roentgenol 1980;15:227–245.
29. Lee KS, Kim Y, Primack SL. Imaging of pulmonary lymphomas. AJR Am J Roentgenol 1997;168:339–345.
30. Wislez M, Cadranel J, Antoine M, et al. Lymphoma of pulmonary mucosa-associated lymphoid tissue: CT scan findings and pathological correlations. Eur Respir J 1999;14:423–429.
31. Yousem SA, Colby TV, Carrington CB. Follicular bronchitis/bronchiolitis. Hum Pathol 1985;16:700–706.
32. Sue-Chu M, Karjalainen EM, Altraja A, et al. Lymphoid aggregates in endobronchial biopsies from young elite cross-country skiers. Am J Respir Crit Care Med 1998;158:597–601.
33. Meuwissen HJ, Hussain M. Bronchus-associated lymphoid tissue in human lung: correlation of hyperplasia with chronic pulmonary disease. Clin Immunol Immunopathol 1982;23:548–561.
34. Yousem SA, Colby TV, Carrington CB. Lung biopsy in rheumatoid arthritis. Am Rev Respir Dis 1985;131:770–777.
35. Kradin RL, Mark EJ. Benign lymphoid disorders of the lung, with a theory regarding their development. Hum Pathol 1983;14:857–867.
36. Grieco MH, Chinoy-Acharya P. Lymphocytic interstitial pneumonia associated with the acquired immune deficiency syndrome. Am Rev Respir Dis 1985;131:952–955.
37. Dorfman RF, Warnke R. Lymphadenopathy simulating the malignant lymphomas. Hum Pathol 1974;5:519–550.
38. Frizzera G, Moran EM, Rappaport H. Angio-immunoblastic lymphadenopathy. Diagnosis and clinical course. Am J Med 1975;59:803–818.
39. Iseman MD, Schwarz MI, Stanford RE. Interstitial pneumonia in angio-immunoblastic lymphadenopathy with dysproteinemia. A case report with special histopathologic studies. Ann Intern Med 1976;85:752–755.
40. Zylak CJ, Banerjee R, Galbraith PA, McCarthy DS. Lung involvement in angioimmunoblastic lymphadenopathy (ail). Radiology 1976;121:513–519.
41. Weisenburger D, Armitage J, Dick F. Immunoblastic lymphadenopathy with pulmonary infiltrates, hypocomplementemia and vasculitis. A hyperimmune syndrome. Am J Med 1977;63:849–854.
42. Dogan A, Attygalle AD, Kyriakou C. Angioimmunoblastic T-cell lymphoma. Br J Haematol 2003;121:681–691.
43. Koss MN, Hochholzer L, Langloss JM, Wehunt WD, Lazarus AA. Lymphoid interstitial pneumonia: clinicopathological and immunopathological findings in 18 cases. Pathology 1987;19:178–185.
44. Strimlan CV, Rosenow EC 3rd, Weiland LH, Brown LR. Lymphocytic interstitial pneumonitis. Review of 13 cases. Ann Intern Med 1978;88:616–621.
45. American Thoracic Society/European Respiratory Society International Multidisciplinary Consensus Classification of the Idiopathic Interstitial Pneumonias. This joint statement of the American Thoracic Society (ATS), and the European Respiratory Society (ERS) was adopted by the ATS board of directors, June 2001 and by the ERS Executive Committee, June 2001. Am J Respir Crit Care Med 2002;165:277–304.
46. Church JA, Isaacs H, Saxon A, Keens TG, Richards W. Lymphoid interstitial pneumonitis and hypogammaglobulinemia in children. Am Rev Respir Dis 1981;124:491–496.
47. Perreault C, Cousineau S, D'Angelo G, et al. Lymphoid interstitial pneumonia after allogeneic bone marrow transplantation. A possible manifestation of chronic graft-versus-host disease. Cancer 1985;55:1–9.
48. Yoshizawa Y, Ohdama S, Ikeda A, Ohtsuka M, Masuda S, Tanaka M. Lymphoid interstitial pneumonia associated

with depressed cellular immunity and polyclonal gammopathy. Am Rev Respir Dis 1984;130:507–509.
49. Dukes RJ, Rosenow EC 3rd, Hermans PE. Pulmonary manifestations of hypogammaglobulinaemia. Thorax 1978; 33:603–607.
50. Solal-Celigny P, Couderc LJ, Herman D, et al. Lymphoid interstitial pneumonitis in acquired immunodeficiency syndrome-related complex. Am Rev Respir Dis 1985;131: 956–960.
51. Khardori R, Eagleton LE, Soler NG, McConnachie PR. Lymphocytic interstitial pneumonitis in autoimmune thyroid disease. Am J Med 1991;90:649–652.
52. Kohler PF, Cook RD, Brown WR, Manguso RL. Common variable hypogammaglobulinemia with T-cell nodular lymphoid interstitial pneumonitis and B-cell nodular lymphoid hyperplasia: different lymphocyte populations with a similar response to prednisone therapy. J Allerg Clin Immunol 1982;70:299–305.
53. Colby TV, Carrington CB. Lymphoreticular tumors and infiltrates of the lung. Pathol Annu 1983;18(pt 1): 27–70.
54. Turner RR, Colby TV, Doggett RS. Well-differentiated lymphocytic lymphoma. A study of 47 patients with primary manifestation in the lung. Cancer 1984;54:2088–2096.
55. Nicholson AG, Wotherspoon AC, Diss TC, et al. Reactive pulmonary lymphoid disorders. Histopathology 1995;26: 405–412.
56. Koss MN, Hochholzer L, Nichols PW, Wehunt WD, Lazarus AA. Primary non-Hodgkin's lymphoma and pseudolymphoma of lung: a study of 161 patients. Hum Pathol 1983;14:1024–1038.
57. Li G, Hansmann ML, Zwingers T, Lennert K. Primary lymphomas of the lung: morphological, immunohistochemical and clinical features. Histopathology 1990;16: 519 531.
58. L'Hoste RJ Jr, Filippa DA, Lieberman PH, Bretsky S. Primary pulmonary lymphomas. A clinicopathologic analysis of 36 cases. Cancer 1984;54:1397–1406.
59. Kennedy JL, Nathwani BN, Burke JS, Hill LR, Rappaport H. Pulmonary lymphomas and other pulmonary lymphoid lesions. A clinicopathologic and immunologic study of 64 patients. Cancer 1985;56:539–552.
60. Herbert A, Wright DH, Isaacson PG, Smith JL. Primary malignant lymphoma of the lung: histopathologic and immunologic evaluation of nine cases. Hum Pathol 1984; 15:415–422.
61. Weiss LM, Yousem SA, Warnke RA. Non-Hodgkin's lymphomas of the lung. A study of 19 cases emphasizing the utility of frozen section immunologic studies in differential diagnosis. Am J Surg Pathol 1985;9:480–390.
62. Saltzstein S. Pulmonary malignant lymphomas and pseudolymphomas: Classification, therapy, and prognosis. Cancer 1963;16:928–955.
63. Colby TV, Lombard C, Yousem SA, Kitaichi M. Atlas of pulmonary surgical pathology. Philadelphia: WB Saunders, 1991.
64. Keller AR, Hochholzer L, Castleman B. Hyaline-vascular and plasma-cell types of giant lymph node hyperplasia of the mediastinum and other locations. Cancer 1972;29: 670–683.
65. Papaioannou AN, Watson WL. Primary lymphoma of the lung: an appraisal of its natural history and a comparison with other localized lymphoma. J Thorac Cardiovasc Surg 1965;49:373–387.
66. Colby TV, Carrington CB. Pulmonary lymphomas simulating lymphomatoid granulomatosis. Am J Surg Pathol 1982; 6:19–32.
67. Saltzstein S. Extranodal malignant lymphomas and pseudolymphomas. Pathol Annu 1969;4:159–184.
68. Kurtin PJ, Hobday KS, Ziesmer S, Caron BL. Demonstration of distinct antigenic profiles of small B-cell lymphomas by paraffin section immunohistochemistry. Am J Clin Pathol 1999;112:319–329.
69. Fiche M, Caprons F, Berger F, et al. Primary pulmonary non-Hodgkin's lymphomas. Histopathology 1995;26:529–537.
70. Cordier JF, Chailleux E, Lauque D, et al. Primary pulmonary lymphomas. A clinical study of 70 cases in nonimmunocompromised patients. Chest 1993;103:201–208.
71. Kurtin PJ, Myers JL, Adlakha H, et al. Pathologic and clinical features of primary pulmonary extranodal marginal zone B-cell lymphoma of MALT type. Am J Surg Pathol 2001;25:997–1008.
72. Winterbauer RH, Riggins RC, Griesman FA, Bauermeister DE. Pleuropulmonary manifestations of Waldenstrom's macroglobulinemia. Chest 1974;66:368–375.
73. Essig LJ, Timms ES, Hancock DE, Sharp GC. Plasma cell interstitial pneumonia and macroglobulinemia. A response to corticosteroid and cyclophosphamide therapy. Am J Med 1974;56:398–405.
74. Case records of the Massachusetts General Hospital, Case 43–1982. N Engl J Med 1982;307:1065–1073.
75. Isaacson PG, Wotherspoon AC, Diss T, Pan LX. Follicular colonization in B-cell lymphoma of mucosa-associated lymphoid tissue. Am J Surg Pathol 1991;15:819–828.
76. Khoor A, Myers JL, Tazelaar HD, Kurtin PJ. Amyloid-like pulmonary nodules, including localized light-chain deposition: clinicopathologic analysis of three cases. Am J Clin Pathol 2004;121:200–204.
77. Lim JK, Lacy MQ, Kurtin PJ, Kyle RA, Gertz MA. Pulmonary marginal zone lymphoma of MALT type as a cause of localised pulmonary amyloidosis. J Clin Pathol 2001; 54:642–646.
78. Sun Y, Tawfiqul B, Valderrama E, Kline G, Kahn LB. Pulmonary crystal-storing histiocytosis and extranodal marginal zone B-cell lymphoma associated with a fibroleiomyomatous hamartoma. Ann Diagn Pathol 2003;7: 47–53.
79. Suarez P, el-Naggar AK, Batsakis JG. Intracellular crystalline deposits in lymphoplasmacellular disorders. Ann Otol Rhinol Laryngol 1997;106:170–172.
80. Fend F, Gabl C, Hittmair A, Greil R, Feichtinger H. Gastric malt lymphoma with crystalline immunoglobulin inclusions and secondary immunoblastic lymphoma in a cervical lymph node.[see comment]. Pathol Res Pract 1995;191: 1053–1058.
81. Murga Penas EM, Hinz K, Roser K, et al. Translocations t(11;18)(q21;q21) and t(14;18)(q32;q21) are the main chromosomal abnormalities involving MLT/MALT1 in MALT lymphomas. Leukemia 2003;17:2225–2229.

82. Cavalli F, Isaacson PG, Gascoyne RD, Zucca E. MALT Lymphomas. Hematology 2001:241–258.
83. Wotherspoon AC, Finn TM, Isaacson PG. Trisomy 3 in low-grade B-cell lymphomas of mucosa-associated lymphoid tissue. Blood 1995;85:2000–2004.
84. Remstein ED, Kurtin PJ, James CD, Wang XY, Meyer RG, Dewald GW. Mucosa-associated lymphoid tissue lymphomas with t(11;18)(q21;q21) and mucosa-associated lymphoid tissue lymphomas with aneuploidy develop along different pathogenetic pathways. Am J Pathol 2002;161: 63–71.
85. Ott G, Katzenberger T, Greiner A, et al. The t(11;18) (q21;q21) chromosome translocation is a frequent and specific aberration in low-grade but not high-grade malignant non-Hodgkin's lymphomas of the mucosa-associated lymphoid tissue (MALT-) type. Cancer Res 1997;57:3944–3948.
86. Auer IA, Gascoyne RD, Connors JM, et al. t(11;18) (q21;q21) is the most common translocation in MALT lymphomas. Ann Oncol 1997;8:979–985.
87. Remstein ED, Kurtin PJ, Einerson RR, Paternoster SF, Dewald GW. Primary pulmonary MALT lymphomas show frequent and heterogeneous cytogenetic abnormalities, including aneuploidy and translocations involving API2 and MALT1 and IGH and MALT1. Leukemia 2004;18: 156–160.
88. Okabe M, Inagaki H, Ohshima K, et al. API2–MALT1 fusion defines a distinctive clinicopathologic subtype in pulmonary extranodal marginal zone B-cell lymphoma of mucosa-associated lymphoid tissue. Am J Pathol 2003; 162:1113–1122.
89. Liu H, Ye H, Dogan A, et al. T(11;18)(q21;q21) is associated with advanced mucosa-associated lymphoid tissue lymphoma that expresses nuclear BCL10. Blood 2001; 98:1182–1187.
90. Streubel B, Lamprecht A, Dierlamm J, et al. T(14;18)(q32;q21) involving IGH and MALT1 is a frequent chromosomal aberration in MALT lymphoma. Blood 2003;101:2335–2339.
91. Lucas PC, Yonezumi M, Inohara N, et al. Bcl10 and MALT1, independent targets of chromosomal translocation in malt lymphoma, cooperate in a novel NF-kappa B signaling pathway. J Biol Chem 2001;276:19012–19019.
92. Malek SN, Hatfield AJ, Flinn IW. MALT lymphomas. Curr Treat Opt Oncol 2003;4:269–279.
93. Nichols PW, Koss M, Levine AM, Lukes RJ. Lymphomatoid granulomatosis: a T-cell disorder? Am J Med 1982; 72:467–471.
94. Jaffe ES. Pathologic and clinical spectrum of post-thymic T-cell malignancies. Cancer Invest 1984;2:413–426.
95. Myers JL, Kurtin PJ, Katzenstein AL, et al. Lymphomatoid granulomatosis. Evidence of immunophenotypic diversity and relationship to Epstein-Barr virus infection. Am J Surg Pathol 1995;19:1300–1312.
96. Guinee D Jr, Jaffe E, Kingma D, et al. Pulmonary lymphomatoid granulomatosis. Evidence for a proliferation of Epstein-Barr virus infected B-lymphocytes with a prominent T-cell component and vasculitis. Am J Surg Pathol 1994;18:753–764.
97. Jaffe ES, Chan JK, Su IJ, et al. Report of the Workshop on Nasal and Related Extranodal Angiocentric T/Natural Killer Cell Lymphomas. Definitions, differential diagnosis, and epidemiology. Am J Surg Pathol 1996;20:103–111.
98. Teruya-Feldstein J, Jaffe ES, Burd PR, et al. The role of Mig, the monokine induced by interferon-gamma, and IP-10, the interferon-gamma-inducible protein-10, in tissue necrosis and vascular damage associated with Epstein-Barr virus-positive lymphoproliferative disease. Blood 1997;90:4099–4105.
99. Morice WG, Kurtin PJ, Myers JL. Expression of cytolytic lymphocyte-associated antigens in pulmonary lymphomatoid granulomatosis. Am J Clin Pathol 2002;118:391–398.
100. Katzenstein AL, Carrington CB, Liebow AA. Lymphomatoid granulomatosis: a clinicopathologic study of 152 cases. Cancer 1979;43:360–373.
101. Koss MN, Hochholzer L, Langloss JM, Wehunt WD, Lazarus AA, Nichols PW. Lymphomatoid granulomatosis: a clinicopathologic study of 42 patients. Pathology 1986;18: 283–288.
102. Fauci AS, Haynes BF, Costa J, Katz P, Wolff SM. Lymphomatoid granulomatosis. Prospective clinical and therapeutic experience over 10 years. N Engl J Med 1982;306: 68–74.
103. Sordillo PP, Epremian B, Koziner B, Lacher M, Lieberman P. Lymphomatoid granulomatosis: an analysis of clinical and immunologic characteristics. Cancer 1982;49:2070–2076.
104. Ilowite NT, Fligner CL, Ochs HD, et al. Pulmonary angiitis with atypical lymphoreticular infiltrates in Wiskott-Aldrich syndrome: possible relationship of lymphomatoid granulomatosis and EBV infection. Clin Immunol Immunopathol 1986;41:479–484.
105. Mazzie JP, Price AP, Khullar P, et al. Lymphomatoid granulomatosis in a pediatric patient. Clin Imaging 2004;28: 209–213.
106. Wilson WH, Kingma DW, Raffeld M, Wittes RE, Jaffe ES. Association of lymphomatoid granulomatosis with Epstein-Barr viral infection of B lymphocytes and response to interferon-alpha 2b. Blood 1996;87:4531–4537.
107. Dee PM, Arora NS, Innes DJ Jr. The pulmonary manifestations of lymphomatoid granulomatosis. Radiology 1982; 143:613–618.
108. Hicken P, Dobie JC, Frew E. The radiology of lymphomatoid granulomatosis in the lung. Clin Radiol 1979;30: 661–664.
109. Lee JS, Tuder R, Lynch DA. Lymphomatoid granulomatosis: radiologic features and pathologic correlations. AJR Am J Roentgenol 2000;175:1335–1339.
110. Felgar RE, Steward KR, Cousar JB, Macon WR. T-cell-rich large-B-cell lymphomas contain non-activated CD8+ cytolytic T cells, show increased tumor cell apoptosis, and have lower Bcl-2 expression than diffuse large-B-cell lymphomas. Am J Pathol 1998;153:1707–1715.
111. Cleary ML, Nalesnik MA, Shearer WT, Sklar J. Clonal analysis of transplant-associated lymphoproliferations based on the structure of the genomic termini of the Epstein-Barr virus. Blood 1988;72:349–352.
112. Lust JA. Molecular genetics and lymphoproliferative disorders. J Clin Lab Anal 1996;10:359–367.
113. Harris NL, Swerdlow S, Frizzera G, Knowles DM. Post-transplant lymphoproliferative disorders. In: Jaffe ES,

Harris NL, Stein H, Vardiman JW, eds. World Health Organization classification of tumours. Pathology and genetics of tumours of haemotopoietic and lymphoid tissues. Lyon: IARC Press, 2001:264–269.
114. Kaplan MA, Ferry JA, Harris NL, Jacobson JO. Clonal analysis of posttransplant lymphoproliferative disorders, using both episomal Epstein-Barr virus and immunoglobulin genes as markers. Am J Clin Pathol 1994;101: 590–596.
115. Paranjothi S, Yusen RD, Kraus MD, Lynch JP, Patterson GA, Trulock EP. Lymphoproliferative disease after lung transplantation: comparison of presentation and outcome of early and late cases. J Heart Lung Transplant 2001;20: 1054–1063.
116. Armitage JM, Kormos RL, Stuart RS, et al. Posttransplant lymphoproliferative disease in thoracic organ transplant patients: ten years of cyclosporine-based immunosuppression. J Heart Lung Transplant 1991;10:877–886; discussion 886–887.
117. Reams BD, McAdams HP, Howell DN, Steele MP, Davis RD, Palmer SM. Posttransplant lymphoproliferative disorder: incidence, presentation, and response to treatment in lung transplant recipients. Chest 2003;124:1242–1249.
118. Ramalingam P, Rybicki L, Smith MD, et al. Posttransplant lymphoproliferative disorders in lung transplant patients: the Cleveland Clinic experience. Mod Pathol 2002;15: 647–656.
119. Spiro IJ, Yandell DW, Li C, et al. Brief report: lymphoma of donor origin occurring in the porta hepatis of a transplanted liver. N Engl J Med 1993;329:27–29.
120. Armes JE, Angus P, Southey MC, et al. Lymphoproliferative disease of donor origin arising in patients after orthotopic liver transplantation. Cancer 1994;74:2436–2441.
121. Randhawa PS, Yousem SA. Epstein-Barr virus-associated lymphoproliferative disease in a heart lung allograft. Demonstration of host origin by restriction fragment-length polymorphism analysis. Transplantation 1990;49: 126–130.
122. Collins J, Muller NL, Leung AN, et al. Epstein-Barr-virus-associated lymphoproliferative disease of the lung: CT and histologic findings. Radiology 1998;208:749–759.
123. Lee P, Minai OA, Mehta AC, DeCamp MM, Murthy S. Pulmonary nodules in lung transplant recipients: etiology and outcome. Chest 2004;125:165–172.
124. Saxena A, Dyker KM, Angel S, Moshynska O, Dharampaul S, Cockroft DW. Posttransplant diffuse large B-cell lymphoma of "lymphomatoid granulomatosis" type. Virchows Arch 2002;441:622–628.
125. Diebold J, Raphael M, Prevot S, Audouin J. Lymphomas associated with HIV infection. Cancer Surv 1997;30:263–293.
126. Wolff AJ, O'Donnell AE. Pulmonary manifestations of HIV infection in the era of highly active antiretroviral therapy. Chest 2001;120:1888–1893.
127. Eisner MD, Kaplan LD, Herndier B, Stulbarg MS. The pulmonary manifestations of AIDS-related non-Hodgkin's lymphoma. Chest 1996;110:729–736.
128. Ray P, Antoine M, Mary-Krause M, et al. AIDS-related primary pulmonary lymphoma. Am J Respir Crit Care Med 1998;158:1221–1229.
129. Sider L, Weiss AJ, Smith MD, VonRoenn JH, Glassroth J. Varied appearance of AIDS-related lymphoma in the chest. Radiology 1989;171:629–632.
130. Carignan S, Staples CA, Muller NL. Intrathoracic lymphoproliferative disorders in the immunocompromised patient: CT findings. Radiology 1995;197:53–58.
131. Bazot M, Cadranel J, Benayoun S, Tassart M, Bigot JM, Carette MF. Primary pulmonary AIDS-related lymphoma: radiographic and CT findings. Chest 1999;116: 1282–1286.
132. Haque AK, Myers JL, Hudnall SD, et al. Pulmonary lymphomatoid granulomatosis in acquired immunodeficiency syndrome: lesions with Epstein-Barr virus infection. Mod Pathol 1998;11:347–356.
133. Nador RG, Cesarman E, Chadburn A, et al. Primary effusion lymphoma: a distinct clinicopathologic entity associated with the Kaposi's sarcoma-associated herpes virus. Blood 1996;88:645–656.
134. Ansari MQ, Dawson DB, Nador R, et al. Primary body cavity-based AIDS-related lymphomas. Am J Clin Pathol 1996;105:221–229.
135. Matolcsy A, Nador RG, Cesarman E, Knowles DM. Immunoglobulin VH gene mutational analysis suggests that primary effusion lymphomas derive from different stages of B cell maturation.[see comment]. Am J Pathol 1998;153: 1609–1614.
136. Horenstein MG, Nador RG, Chadburn A, et al. Epstein-Barr virus latent gene expression in primary effusion lymphomas containing Kaposi's sarcoma-associated herpesvirus/human herpesvirus-8. Blood 1997;90:1186–1191.
137. Cesarman E, Chang Y, Moore PS, Said JW, Knowles DM. Kaposi's sarcoma-associated herpesvirus-like DNA sequences in AIDS-related body-cavity-based lymphomas. [see comment]. N Engl J Med 1995;332:1186–1191.
138. Cesarman E, Nador RG, Aozasa K, Delsol G, Said JW, Knowles DM. Kaposi's sarcoma-associated herpesvirus in non-AIDS related lymphomas occurring in body cavities. Am J Pathol 1996;149:53–57.
139. Hengge UR, Ruzicka T, Tyring SK, et al. Update on Kaposi's sarcoma and other HHV8 associated diseases. Part 2: pathogenesis, Castleman's disease, and pleural effusion lymphoma. Lancet Infect Dis 2002;2:344–352.
140. Cobo F, Hernandez S, Hernandez L, et al. Expression of potentially oncogenic HHV-8 genes in an EBV-negative primary effusion lymphoma occurring in an HIV-seronegative patient. J Pathol 1999;189:288–293.
141. Kurosu K, Yumoto N, Rom WN, et al. Oligoclonal T cell expansions in pulmonary lymphoproliferative disorders: demonstration of the frequent occurrence of oligoclonal T cells in human immunodeficiency virus-related lymphoid interstitial pneumonia. Am J Respir Crit Care Med 2002; 165:254–259.
142. Heitzman ER. Pulmonary neoplastic and lymphoproliferative disease in AIDS: a review. Radiology 1990;177: 347–351.
143. Teruya-Feldstein J, Temeck BK, Sloas MM, et al. Pulmonary malignant lymphoma of mucosa-associated lymphoid tissue (MALT) arising in a pediatric HIV-positive patient. Am J Surg Pathol 1995;19:357–363.

144. Mhawech P, Krishnan B, Shahab I. Primary pulmonary mucosa-associated lymphoid tissue lymphoma with associated fungal ball in a patient with human immunodeficiency virus infection. Arch Pathol Lab Med 2000;124:1506–1509.
145. Buckley RH. Primary immunodeficiency diseases: dissectors of the immune system. Immunol Rev 2002;185:206–219.
146. Buckley RH. Pulmonary complications of primary immunodeficiencies. Paediatr Respir Rev 2004;5(suppl A):S225–S233.
147. Yin EZ, Frush DP, Donnelly LF, Buckley RH. Primary immunodeficiency disorders in pediatric patients: clinical features and imaging findings. AJR Am J Roentgenol 2001;176:1541–1552.
148. Shackleford MD, McAlister WH. Primary immunodeficiency diseases and malignancy. AJR Radium Ther Nucl Med 1975;123:144–153.
149. Canioni D, Jabado N, MacIntyre E, Patey N, Emile JF, Brousse N. Lymphoproliferative disorders in children with primary immunodeficiencies: immunological status may be more predictive of the outcome than other criteria. Histopathology 2001;38:146–159.
150. Derry JM, Ochs HD, Francke U. Isolation of a novel gene mutated in Wiskott-Aldrich syndrome. Cell 1994;78:635–644.
151. Laszewski MJ, Kemp JD, Goeken JA, Mitros FA, Platz CE, Dick FR. Clonal immunoglobulin gene rearrangement in nodular lymphoid hyperplasia of the gastrointestinal tract associated with common variable immunodeficiency. Am J Clin Pathol 1990;94:338–343.
152. Diehl V, Stein H, Hummel M, Zollinger R, Connors JM. Hodgkin's lymphoma: biology and treatment strategies for primary, refractory, and relapsed disease. Hematology (Am Soc Hematol Educ Program) 2003:225–247.
153. Diehl LF, Hopper KD, Giguere J, Granger E, Lesar M. The pattern of intrathoracic Hodgkin's disease assessed by computed tomography. J Clin Oncol 1991;9:438–443.
154. Boshnakova T, Michailova V, Koss, Georgiev C, Todorov T, Sarbinova M. Primary pulmonary Hodgkin's disease—report of two cases. Respir Med 2000;94:830–831.
155. Kern WH, Crepeau AG, Jones JC. Primary Hodgkin's disease of the lung. Report of 4 cases and review of the literature. Cancer 1961;14:1151–1165.
156. Yousem SA, Weiss LM, Colby TV. Primary pulmonary Hodgkin's disease. A clinicopathologic study of 15 cases. Cancer 1986;57:1217–1224.
157. Radin AI. Primary pulmonary Hodgkin's disease. Cancer 1990;65:550–563.
158. Diederich S, Link TM, Zuhlsdorf H, Steinmeyer E, Wormanns D, Heindel W. Pulmonary manifestations of Hodgkin's disease: radiographic and CT findings. Eur Radiol 2001;11:2295–2305.
159. Lewis ER, Caskey CI, Fishman EK. Lymphoma of the lung: CT findings in 31 patients. AJR Am J Roentgenol 1991;156:711–714.
160. Harper PG, Fisher C, McLennan K, Souhami RL. Presentation of Hodgkin's disease as an endobronchial lesion. Cancer 1984;53:147–150.
161. Daly PA, O'Briain DS, Robinson I, Guckian M, Prichard JS. Hodgkin's disease with a granulomatous pulmonary presentation mimicking sarcoidosis. Thorax 1988;43:407–409.
162. Stein H, Foss HD, Durkop H, et al. CD30(+) anaplastic large cell lymphoma: a review of its histopathologic, genetic, and clinical features. Blood 2000;96:3681–3695.
163. Morris SW, Xue L, Ma Z, Kinney MC. Alk+ CD30+ lymphomas: a distinct molecular genetic subtype of non-Hodgkin's lymphoma. Br J Haematol 2001;113:275–295.
164. Haralambieva E, Pulford KA, Lamant L, et al. Anaplastic large-cell lymphomas of B-cell phenotype are anaplastic lymphoma kinase (ALK) negative and belong to the spectrum of diffuse large B-cell lymphomas. Br J Haematol 2000;109:584–591.
165. Gascoyne RD, Lamant L, Martin-Subero JI, et al. ALK-positive diffuse large B-cell lymphoma is associated with Clathrin-ALK rearrangements: report of 6 cases. Blood 2003;102:2568–2573.
166. Onciu M, Behm FG, Downing JR, et al. ALK-positive plasmablastic B-cell lymphoma with expression of the NPM-ALK fusion transcript: report of 2 cases. Blood 2003;102:2642–2644.
167. Chott A, Kaserer K, Augustin I, et al. Ki-1–positive large cell lymphoma. A clinicopathologic study of 41 cases. Am J Surg Pathol 1990;14:439–448.
168. Rush WL, Andriko JA, Taubenberger JK, et al. Primary anaplastic large cell lymphoma of the lung: a clinicopathologic study of five patients. Mod Pathol 2000;13:1285–1292.
169. Arzoo KK, Bu X, Espina BM, Seneviratne L, Nathwani B, Levine AM. T-cell lymphoma in HIV-infected patients. J Acquir Immune Defic Syndr 2004;36:1020–1027.
170. Nosari A, Cantoni S, Oreste P, et al. Anaplastic large cell (CD30/Ki-1+) lymphoma in HIV+ patients: clinical and pathological findings in a group of ten patients. Br J Haematol 1996;95:508–512.
171. Katano H, Suda T, Morishita Y, et al. Human herpesvirus 8–associated solid lymphomas that occur in AIDS patients take anaplastic large cell morphology. Mod Pathol 2000;13:77–85.
172. Lewin KJ, Ranchod M, Dorfman RF. Lymphomas of the gastrointestinal tract: a study of 117 cases presenting with gastrointestinal disease. Cancer 1978;42:693–707.
173. Colby TV, Dorfman RF. Malignant lymphomas involving the salivary glands. Pathol Annu 1979;14(pt 2):307–324.
174. Demirer T, Dail DH, Aboulafia DM. Four varied cases of intravascular lymphomatosis and a literature review. Cancer 1994;73:1738–1745.
175. DiGiuseppe JA, Nelson WG, Seifter EJ, Boitnott JK, Mann RB. Intravascular lymphomatosis: a clinicopathologic study of 10 cases and assessment of response to chemotherapy. J Clin Oncol 1994;12:2573–2579.
176. Stroup RM, Sheibani K, Moncada A, Purdy LJ, Battifora H. Angiotropic (intravascular) large cell lymphoma. A clinicopathologic study of seven cases with unique clinical presentations. Cancer 1990;66:1781–1788.
177. Wick MR, Mills SE. Intravascular lymphomatosis: clinicopathologic features and differential diagnosis. Semin Diagn Pathol 1991;8:91–101.

178. Ponzoni M, Arrigoni G, Gould VE, et al. Lack of CD 29 (beta1 integrin) and CD 54 (ICAM-1) adhesion molecules in intravascular lymphomatosis. Hum Pathol 2000;31: 220–226.
179. Yousem SA, Colby TV. Intravascular lymphomatosis presenting in the lung. Cancer 1990;65:349–353.
180. Tan TB, Spaander PJ, Blaisse M, Gerritzen FM. Angiotropic large cell lymphoma presenting as interstitial lung disease. Thorax 1988;43:578–579.
181. Morice WG, Rodriguez FJ, Hoyer JD, Kurtin PJ. Diffuse large B-cell lymphoma with distinctive patterns of splenic and bone marrow involvement: clinicopathologic features of two cases. Mod Pathol 2005;18:495–502.
182. Koss MN. Pulmonary lymphoid disorders. Semin Diagn Pathol 1995;12:158–171.
183. Cadranel J, Wislez M, Antoine M. Primary pulmonary lymphoma. Eur Respir J 2002;20:750–762.
184. Densmore JJ, Williams ME. Mantle cell lymphoma. Curr Treat Opt Oncol 2000;1:281–285.
185. Muller-Hermelink HK, Montserrat E, Catovsky D, Harris NL. Chronic lymphocytic leukemia/small lymphocytic lymphoma. In: Jaffe ES, Harris NL, Stein H, Vardiman JW, eds. World Health Organization classification of tumours. Pathology and genetics of tumours of haemotopoietic and lymphoid tissues. Lyon: IARC Press, 2001:127–130.
186. Campo E, Raffeld M, Jaffe ES. Mantle-cell lymphoma. Semin Hematol 1999;36:115–127.
187. Shibata K, Shimamoto Y, Nakano S, Miyahara M, Nakano H, Yamaguchi M. Mantle cell lymphoma with the features of mucosa-associated lymphoid tissue (MALT) lymphoma in an HTLV-I-seropositive patient. Ann Hematol 1995;70: 47–51.
188. Kurtin PJ. Mantle cell lymphoma. Adv Anat Pathol 1998;5:376–398.
189. Remstein ED, Kurtin PJ, Buno I, et al. Diagnostic utility of fluorescence in situ hybridization in mantle-cell lymphoma. Br J Haematol 2000;110:856–862.
190. Belaud-Rotureau MA, Parrens M, Dubus P, Garroste JC, de Mascarel A, Merlio JP. A comparative analysis of FISH, RT-PCR, PCR, and immunohistochemistry for the diagnosis of mantle cell lymphomas. Mod Pathol 2002; 15:517–525.
191. Isaacson PG. Lymphomas of mucosa-associated lymphoid tissue (MALT). Histopathology 1990;16:617–619.
192. Nathwani B, Piris MA, Harris NL, et al. Follicular lymphoma. In: Jaffe ES, Harris NL, Stein H, Vardiman JW, eds. World Health Organization classification of tumours. Pathology and genetics of tumours of haemotopoietic and lymphoid tissues. Lyon: IARC Press, 2001:162–167.
193. Aiello A, Du MQ, Diss TC, et al. Simultaneous phenotypically distinct but clonally identical mucosa-associated lymphoid tissue and follicular lymphoma in a patient with Sjogren's syndrome. Blood 1999;94:2247–2251.
194. Attygalle A, Al-Jehani R, Diss TC, et al. Neoplastic T cells in angioimmunoblastic T-cell lymphoma express CD10. Blood 2002;99:627–633.
195. Attygalle AD, Diss TC, Munson P, Isaacson PG, Du MQ, Dogan A. CD10 expression in extranodal dissemination of angioimmunoblastic T-cell lymphoma. Am J Surg Pathol 2004;28:54–61.
196. Wolfe JD, Trevor ED, Kjeldsberg CR. Pulmonary manifestations of mycosis fungoides. Cancer 1980;46: 2648–2653.
197. Marglin SI, Soulen RL, Blank N, Castellino RA. Mycosis fungoides. Radiographic manifestations of extracutaneous intrathoracic involvement. Radiology 1979;130:35–37.
198. Patel DJ, Griem ML, Vijayakumar S, Griem SF. Treatment of pulmonary mycosis fungoides with whole-lung radiation therapy. J Surg Oncol 1988;38:118–120.
199. van Heerde P, Feltkamp CA, Hart AA, Somers R, van Unnik JA, Vroom TM. Malignant histiocytosis and related tumors. A clinicopathologic study of 42 cases using cytological, histochemical and ultrastructural parameters. Hematol Oncol 1984;2:13–32.
200. Wongchaowart B, Kennealy JA, Crissman J, Hawkins H. Respiratory failure in malignant histiocytosis. Am Rev Respir Dis 1981;124:640–642.
201. Aozasa K, Tsujimoto M, Inoue A. Malignant histiocytosis. Report of twenty-five cases with pulmonary, renal and/or gastro-intestinal involvement. Histopathology 1985;9:39–49.
202. Delsol G, Al Saati T, Gatter KC, et al. Coexpression of epithelial membrane antigen (EMA), Ki-1, and interleukin-2 receptor by anaplastic large cell lymphomas. Diagnostic value in so-called malignant histiocytosis. Am J Pathol 1988;130:59–70.
203. Veyssier-Belot C, Cacoub P, Caparros-Lefebvre D, et al. Erdheim-Chester disease. Clinical and radiologic characteristics of 59 cases. Medicine (Baltimore) 1996;75:157–169.
204. Shamburek RD, Brewer HB Jr, Gochuico BR. Erdheim-Chester disease: a rare multisystem histiocytic disorder associated with interstitial lung disease. Am J Med Sci 2001;321:66–75.
205. Egan AJ, Boardman LA, Tazelaar HD, et al. Erdheim-Chester disease: clinical, radiologic, and histopathologic findings in five patients with interstitial lung disease. Am J Surg Pathol 1999;23:17–26.
206. Rush WL, Andriko JA, Galateau-Salle F, et al. Pulmonary pathology of Erdheim-Chester disease. Mod Pathol 2000;13:747–754.
207. Wittenberg KH, Swensen SJ, Myers JL. Pulmonary involvement with Erdheim-Chester disease: radiographic and CT findings. AJR Am J Roentgenol 2000;174:1327–1331.
208. Rosai J, Dorfman RF. Sinus histiocytosis with massive lymphadenopathy. A newly recognized benign clinicopathological entity. Arch Pathol Lab Med 1969;87:63–70.
209. Rosai J, Dorfman RF. Sinus histiocytosis with massive lymphadenopathy: a pseudolymphomatous benign disorder. Analysis of 34 cases. Cancer 1972;30:1174–1188.
210. Foucar E, Rosai J, Dorfman R. Sinus histiocytosis with massive lymphadenopathy (Rosai-Dorfman disease): review of the entity. Semin Diagn Pathol 1990;7:19–73.
211. Wright DH, Richards DB. Sinus histiocytosis with massive lymphadenopathy (Rosai-Dorfman disease): report of a case with widespread nodal and extra nodal dissemination. Histopathology 1981;5:697–709.
212. Carbone A, Passannante A, Gloghini A, Devaney KO, Rinaldo A, Ferlito A. Review of sinus histiocytosis with massive lymphadenopathy (Rosai-Dorfman disease) of

head and neck. Ann Otol Rhinol Laryngol 1999;108: 1095–1104.
213. Carpenter RJ 3rd, Banks PM, McDonald TJ, Sanderson DR. Sinus histiocytosis with massive lymphadenopathy (Rosai-Dorfman disease): Report of a case with respiratory tract involvement. Laryngoscope 1978;88: 1963–1969.
214. Rossi GA, Balbi B, Risso M, Repetto M, Ravazzoni C. Acute myelomonocytic leukemia. Demonstration of pulmonary involvement by bronchoalveolar lavage. Chest 1985;87:259–260.
215. Rosenow EC 3rd, Wilson WR, Cockerill FR 3rd. Pulmonary disease in the immunocompromised host. 1. Mayo Clin Proc 1985;60:473–487.
216. Hildebrand FL Jr, Rosenow EC 3rd, Habermann TM, Tazelaar HD. Pulmonary complications of leukemia. Chest 1990;98:1233–1239.
217. Green RA, Nichols NJ. Pulmonary involvement in leukemia. Am Rev Respir Dis 1959;80:833–844.
218. Palosaari DE, Colby TV. Bronchiolocentric chronic lymphocytic leukemia. Cancer 1986;58:1695–1698.
219. McCabe RE, Brooks RG, Mark JB, Remington JS. Open lung biopsy in patients with acute leukemia. Am J Med 1985;78:609–616.
220. Myers TJ, Cole SR, Klatsky AU, Hild DH. Respiratory failure due to pulmonary leukostasis following chemotherapy of acute nonlymphocytic leukemia. Cancer 1983; 51:1808–1813.
221. Lester TJ, Johnson JW, Cuttner J. Pulmonary leukostasis as the single worst prognostic factor in patients with acute myelocytic leukemia and hyperleukocytosis. Am J Med 1985;79:43–48.
222. Woodard JP, Gulbahce E, Shreve M, et al. Pulmonary cytolytic thrombi: a newly recognized complication of stem cell transplantation. Bone Marrow Transplant 2000;25: 293–300.
223. Castellano-Sanchez AA, Poppiti RJ. Pulmonary cytolytic thrombi (PCT). A previously unrecognized complication of bone marrow transplantation (BMT).[comment]. Am J Surg Pathol 2001;25:829–831.
224. Morales IJ, Anderson PM, Tazelaar HD, Wylam ME. Pulmonary cytolytic thrombi: unusual complication of hematopoietic stem cell transplantation. J Pediatr Hematol Oncol 2003;25:89–92.
225. Gulbahce HE, Manivel JC, Jessurun J. Pulmonary cytolytic thrombi: a previously unrecognized complication of bone marrow transplantation.[see comment]. Am J Surg Pathol 2000;24:1147–1152.
226. Yoshioka R, Yamaguchi K, Yoshinaga T, Takatsuki K. Pulmonary complications in patients with adult T-cell leukemia. Cancer 1985;55:2491–2494.
227. Callahan M, Wall S, Askin F, Delaney D, Koller C, Orringer EP. Granulocytic sarcoma presenting as pulmonary nodules and lymphadenopathy. Cancer 1987;60:1902–1904.
228. Hicklin GA, Drevyanko TF. Primary granulocytic sarcoma presenting with pleural and pulmonary involvement. Chest 1988;94:655–656.
229. Klatte EC, Yardley J, Smith EB, Rohn R, Campbell JA. The pulmonary manifestations and complications of leukemia. AJR Radium Ther Nucl Med 1963;89:598–609.
230. Desjardins A, Ostiguy G, Cousineau S, Gyger M. Recurrent localised pneumonia due to bronchial infiltration in a patient with chronic lymphocytic leukaemia. Thorax 1990; 45:570.
231. Kovalski R, Hansen-Flaschen J, Lodato RF, Pietra GG. Localized leukemic pulmonary infiltrates. Diagnosis by bronchoscopy and resolution with therapy. Chest 1990;97: 674–678.
232. Beckman EN, Oehrle JS. Fibrous hematopoietic tumors arising in agnogenic myeloid metaplasia. Hum Pathol 1982;13:804–810.
233. Asakura S, Colby TV. Agnogenic myeloid metaplasia with extramedullary hematopoiesis and fibrosis in the lung. Report of two cases. Chest 1994;105:1866–1868.
234. Dingli D, Utz JP, Krowka MJ, Oberg AL, Tefferi A. Unexplained pulmonary hypertension in chronic myeloproliferative disorders. Chest 2001;120:801–808.
235. Steensma DP, Hook CC, Stafford SL, Tefferi A. Low-dose, single-fraction, whole-lung radiotherapy for pulmonary hypertension associated with myelofibrosis with myeloid metaplasia. Br J Haematol 2002;118:813–816.
236. Joseph G, Pandit M, Korfhage L. Primary pulmonary plasmacytoma. Cancer 1993;71:721–724.
237. Koss MN, Hochholzer L, Moran CA, Frizzera G. Pulmonary plasmacytomas: a clinicopathologic and immunohistochemical study of five cases. Ann Diagn Pathol 1998; 2:1–11.
238. Horiuchi T, Hirokawa M, Oyama Y, et al. Diffuse pulmonary infiltrates as a roentgenographic manifestation of primary pulmonary plasmacytoma. Am J Med 1998;105:72–74.
239. Amin R. Extramedullary plasmacytoma of the lung. Cancer 1985;56:152–156.
240. Roikjaer O, Thomsen JK. Plasmacytoma of the lung. A case report describing two tumors of different immunologic type in a single patient. Cancer 1986;58:2671–2674.
241. Garewal H, Durie BG. Aggressive phase of multiple myeloma with pulmonary cell infiltrates. JAMA 1982;248: 1875–1876.
242. Case records of the Massachusetts General Hospital, Case 17–1984. N Engl J Med 1984;310:1103–1112.
243. Gabriel S. Multiple myeloma presenting as pulmonary infiltration. Dis Chest 1965;47:123–126.
244. Kijner CH, Yousem SA. Systemic light chain deposition disease presenting as multiple pulmonary nodules. A case report and review of the literature. Am J Surg Pathol 1988;12:405–413.
245. Kaplan HS. Hodgkin's disease. Cambridge: Harvard, 1972.
246. Valent P, Horny HP, Escribano L, et al. Diagnostic criteria and classification of mastocytosis: a consensus proposal. Leuk Res 2001;25:603–625.
247. Kelly AM, Kazerooni EA. HRCT appearance of systemic mastocytosis involving the lungs. J Thorac Imaging 2004; 19:52–55.
248. Schmidt M, Dercken C, Loke O, et al. Pulmonary manifestation of systemic mast cell disease. Eur Respir J 2000;15: 623–625.
249. Li CY. Diagnosis of mastocytosis: value of cytochemistry and immunohistochemistry. Leuk Res 2001;25: 537–541.

250. Chan JK, Fletcher CD, Nayler SJ, Cooper K. Follicular dendritic cell sarcoma. Clinicopathologic analysis of 17 cases suggesting a malignant potential higher than currently recognized. Cancer 1997;79:294–313.
251. Shah RN, Ozden O, Yeldandi A, Peterson L, Rao S, Laskin WB. Follicular dendritic cell tumor presenting in the lung: a case report. Hum Pathol 2001;32:745–749.
252. Pileri SA, Grogan TM, Harris NL, et al. Tumours of histiocytes and accessory dendritic cells: an immunohistochemical approach to classification from the International Lymphoma Study Group based on 61 cases. Histopathology 2002;41:1–29.
253. Gaertner EM, Tsokos M, Derringer GA, et al. Interdigitating dendritic cell sarcoma. A report of four cases and review of the literature. Am J Clin Pathol 2001;15:589–597.
254. Grogg KL, Lae ME, Kurtin PJ, Macon WR. Clusterin expression distinguishes follicular dendritic cell tumors from other dendritic cell neoplasms: report of a novel follicular dendritic cell marker and clinicopathologic data on 12 additional follicular dendritic cell tumors and 6 additional interdigitating dendritic cell tumors. Am J Surg Pathol 2004;28:988–998.

33
Molecular Genetics of Lung and Pleural Neoplasms

Philip T. Cagle, Jaishree Jagirdar, and Helmut H. Popper

Basic Concepts and Terminology

Molecular pathology involves study of nucleic acids, genes, and gene products.[1–9] The development and progression of human cancers are linked to genetic instability and the accumulation of multiple genetic mutations, which can be investigated with the tools of molecular pathology.[10–25] Molecular pathology provides a basis for understanding the biology of lung cancer,[26–36] including its pathogenetic relationship to tobacco smoking,[37–57] and increasingly is providing targets for therapeutic intervention.[58–78] In this section, we briefly review the basic terminology and concepts, as an introduction or refresher to subsequent sections of this chapter, and we discuss nucleic acids, genes, and gene products; replication, translation, and transcription; posttranslational modifications of gene products and protein degradation; transcription factors, cell surface receptors and signaling pathways, the cell cycle, apoptosis, cell survival and DNA damage repair; mutations; and microRNAs and siRNAs.

Nucleic Acids, Genes, and Gene Products

The two nucleic acids of primary interest to molecular pathology are deoxyribonucleic acid (DNA) and ribonucleic acid (RNA). Nucleic acids are composed of a series or chain of chemically joined nucleotides, which are basic compounds with a sugar-phosphate backbone and a nitrogenous base. Sequentially arranged nucleotides are the building blocks of nucleic acids just as sequentially arranged amino acids are the building blocks of proteins. As described below, the bits of heritable genetic information or genes are composed of DNA, which is said to contain the genetic code. DNA is composed of four different nucleotides: two purines and two pyrimidines. The two purines are adenine, abbreviated as A, and guanine, abbreviated as G. The two pyrimidines are thymine, abbreviated as T, and cytosine, abbreviated as C.

Genes are composed of DNA molecules and code for proteins that form the structural and metabolic basis of living tissues. The DNA molecules in genes are arranged in a double-stranded right-handed helix in the cell nucleus with matching nucleotides or base pairs. The nucleotides or bases in the DNA helix are paired so that A always binds with T and G always binds with C. Therefore, the sequence of nucleotides in one strand of DNA within a double helix is a "mirror image" of the other strand resulting in complementary strands of DNA composed of complementary base pairs; that is, a strand of DNA composed of the nucleotides ATC-GAT would have as its complementary strand DNA composed of the nucleotides TAG-CTA. In order for the DNA to fit in the nucleus, the DNA is arranged in nucleosomes with groups of DNA base pairs wrapped around small proteins called histones. Chromosomes, which are ordinarily indistinct in the nuclear chromatin but which are discrete during mitosis or cell division, consist of DNA packaged with histone and nonhistone proteins. Each gene is located at a specific site or locus on a specific chromosome.[79–83]

The entirety of an organism's DNA sequence or chromosomes or "complete genetic complement," including that of a human, is known as that organism's genome. Genomics is the sequencing and study of genomes, and cytogenetics is the study of chromosomes, traditionally through visualization of the karyotype or set of chromosomes of an organism. The somatic cells are diploid with a pair of each of the chromosomes (23 pairs of 46 chromosomes in humans). Therefore, a somatic cell would have two copies (alleles) of each gene, with one of the alleles at the same locus on each one of the paired chromosomes. The gametes are haploid, or have only one set of each of the chromosomes, with one copy (allele) of each gene. After fertilization, the number of chromosomes and alleles is restored to the diploid number in the fertilized egg.

The two alleles of a gene may be the same in an individual (homozygous) or different (heterozygous).

Genotype is the actual genetic information in an individual's DNA, whereas phenotype is the manifestation of the individual's genotype. When the alleles are heterozygous and one allele is manifested preferentially over the other allele, the allele that is manifested is dominant and the other allele is recessive. The features coded for by the dominant allele typically mask the features coded for by the recessive allele.

Polymorphisms are differences in DNA between individuals. The simplest polymorphism is the single nucleotide polymorphism (SNP, pronounced "snip"). A SNP is an inherited, naturally occurring difference in one base between the DNA sequences in a gene in two individuals. SNPs are responsible for most of the genetic variation between individuals. Alleles or SNPs that are in close proximity on a chromosome are often inherited together as a haplotype.

Replication is the synthesis of new DNA from an existing strand of DNA prior to cell division. Transcription is the synthesis of RNA, including messenger RNA (mRNA), from a DNA template. In order for DNA to be duplicated in replication or mRNA to be transcribed from DNA, the double-stranded helix of DNA must be unraveled and separated into single strands of DNA. Topoisomerases start the process of DNA unwinding by "nicking" or breaking a DNA strand, releasing the tension holding the helix in its coiled form. Topoisomerase I induces transient DNA single-strand breaks and topoisomerase II induces transient DNA double-strand breaks. The DNA strand that serves as the template for the mRNA is referred to as antisense, whereas sense refers to the complementary DNA strand that has the identical sequence of bases as the mRNA (except that uracil (U) replaces T).[84–99]

In transcription, a strand of RNA is formed by matching base pairs with a strand of DNA so that the RNA is a "mirror image" of the DNA template. Uracil replaces thymine as the pyrimidine base in the RNA that matches with adenosine in the DNA template, so that a strand of DNA with a sequence of nucleotides ATC-GAT results in a strand of mRNA with a sequence of matched nucleotides UAG-CUA. RNA is typically single stranded. Heterochromatin is condensed, inactive DNA at the periphery of the nucleus, and euchromatin is less condensed DNA that is available for transcription and generally in the central nucleus.

The gene product is the end molecule for which the gene codes that generates the effect of the gene. Most gene products are proteins, including those with enzymatic and structural roles. A codon is a three base pair sequence of DNA that codes for an amino acid. A sequence of base pair codons codes for a sequence of amino acids, resulting in the synthesis of the protein product through the process of translation. In translation, the mRNA template derived from the DNA template is used as a blueprint for assembling a protein molecule in association with ribosomes, which in part are made up of ribosomal RNA (rRNA). Transfer RNA (tRNA) adds amino acids to the protein molecule. Each tRNA has a specific acceptor arm for a specific amino acid, and each tRNA has a specific anticodon that binds to the corresponding specific codon in the mRNA. The amino acid is added to the protein molecule in the correct sequence determined by the mRNA, which, in turn, is derived from the sequence in the original DNA template—the gene. The end result is a specific sequence of amino acids to build a specific protein based on the original DNA template of the gene for that protein product. This manufacture of the gene product via mRNA is referred to as expression of the gene, and most control of gene expression occurs at the level of transcription.[100–102]

Genes are composed of exons and introns. Exons are segments of DNA that are eventually translated into the gene product, whereas introns are intervening segments of DNA that are spliced out of the sequence at the mRNA level. Introns are believed to play a "punctuation" or regulatory role in the gene. The splice junction is the site between an exon and an intron where splicing occurs.[103–105] A short tandem repeat (STR) consists of a sequence of two to five nucleotides that are repeated in tandem, often dozens of times, in introns.[106] Microsatellite DNA is composed of these STRs and is of interest because of its natural instability.[107–123]

Polymerases are enzymes that synthesize a target substrate: DNA polymerase synthesizes DNA using single-stranded DNA as a substrate. DNA polymerase requires a small segment of double-stranded DNA to initiate new DNA synthesis (in the polymerase chain reaction [PCR] procedure described in the next section, primers or short DNA segments of a defined length are added to serve this purpose and initiate new DNA synthesis). RNA polymerase synthesizes an RNA transcript from a DNA template by first binding to a segment of bases called the transcription initiation site (TIS) or promoter upstream of the gene that is being transcribed.[124–129] RNA polymerase I transcribes genes encoding for rRNAs, RNA polymerase II transcribes genes encoding for mRNAs, and RNA polymerase III transcribes genes encoding for tRNAs.

Certain specialized polymerases are also important to molecular pathology. Reverse transcriptase is a nucleic acid polymerase found in retroviruses that synthesizes DNA from an RNA template (the virus genome is composed of RNA), which is the reverse of normal transcription where RNA is synthesized from a DNA template. The DNA that is synthesized from an RNA template by reverse transcriptase is called complementary DNA (cDNA). This cDNA can be used for procedures to study gene expression. The cDNAs derived from RNA isolated from a particular type of tumor can be used to construct

DNA libraries that can be screened to identify cDNAs corresponding to genes that are expressed by that type of tumor.[130,131]

Telomerase is a specialized DNA polymerase that imparts immortality to cancer cells. The end regions or telomeres of the chromosomes consist of the nucleotide sequence TTAGGG repeated hundreds of times, and telomere sequences are lost each time that a cell replicates until the cell loses its ability to divide as part of the aging process. Telomerase replaces the DNA sequences at the telomeres of the chromosomes allowing cells to divide indefinitely.[132–147]

Posttranslational Modifications of Gene Products and Protein Degradation

The polypeptide chain translated from an mRNA template has a certain sequence of amino acids as noted above. The physicochemical properties of this sequence of amino acids give rise to a three-dimensional folding of the polypeptide chain into a tertiary structure that gives the protein its three-dimensional functional form. The tertiary structure of a protein typically consists of units called domains, which are compact, spherical regions of the three-dimensional form.[1–9]

Proteins may also bind to other proteins that can enhance or inhibit their function. Binding of two proteins together is dimerization. Dimers composed of identical proteins are called homodimers, whereas binding of different proteins are called heterodimers. Trimers, tetramers, and other combinations may occur.[1–9]

Gene expression does not necessarily mean gene function. Many proteins present in a given cell are inert and become functional only when activated by posttranslational modifications such as proteolytic cleavage or phosphorylation. Therefore, study of the transcriptome from RNA expression provides limited information, and study of the proteome (proteomics) provides information linking gene expression and function. Posttranslational modifications of proteins play crucial roles in control of the cell cycle, of signaling pathways, and of transcription factors (see below).

Phosphorylation and Acetylation

The activity of many proteins, including those in cell cycle control and in signaling pathways, including transcription factors, is stimulated or inhibited by phosphorylation and dephosphorylation. Phosphorylation is the addition of a phosphate group to a protein, and dephosphorylation is removal of a phosphate group from a protein. Phosphorylation and dephosphorylation causes these proteins to become active (activation) or inactive. Enzymes that catalyze phosphorylation are called kinases. Enzymes that catalyze dephosphorylation are called phosphatases. Phosphorylation may produce differing effects in a transcription factor, depending on the domain that is phosphorylated. Phosphorylation of DNA-binding domains may inhibit binding of proteins to DNA, induce transactivation of genes, or induce translocation or passage of a protein from the cytosol into the nucleus.[148–152]

The activity of other proteins is stimulated or inhibited by acetylation and deacetylation, the addition and removal of acetyl groups to the protein. Acetylation is catalyzed by acetyltransferases and deacetylation is catalyzed by deacetylases.[153]

Protein Degradation and Ubiquitinylation

Proteins must be degraded to control signaling proteins, recycle amino acids and to remove damaged or abnormal proteins. Most nuclear and cystolic proteins requiring rapid degradation are degraded by reversible cross-linkage to a polypeptide called ubiquitin in a process called ubiquitinylation or polyubiquitinylation or the ubiquitin-proteasome pathway. In the initial step, ubiquitin is activated by E1 or ubiquitin-activating enzyme. Activated ubiquitin is transferred to a ubiquitin-conjugating enzyme (E2) and then transfer of the activated ubiquitin to the specific target protein by ubiquitin ligase (E3). Multiple ubiquitins are added and the polyubiquinated proteins are degraded by a large protease complex called the proteasome. The ubiquitin is released during this process and recycled to participate in more cycles of ubiquitinylation. Ubiquitinylation is important in removal of cell cycle regulators and signaling proteins, including those involved in cell survival and cell death (apoptosis).[154]

Transcription Factors

Primary control of gene expression occurs principally at the level of initiation of transcription. Transcription requires adjusting the chromatin to make the DNA template available for transcription and is further controlled by proteins that bind to specific DNA regulatory sequences and modify RNA polymerase activity.

The tight binding of histones to DNA blocks accessibility of that DNA to gene-activating proteins. Histone acetylation by histone acetyltransferases allows binding of the gene-activating proteins to the DNA. Histone deacetylases can block this process and silence gene transcription. The transcriptional unit is the DNA unit that begins with 5′ regulatory sequences and ends with the 3′ terminator signal of the gene.[155–165]

Transcription factors are proteins that bind to DNA and directly affect gene expression by regulating the activity of RNA polymerase. Transcription factors are also known as trans-acting factors or transactivators. Transcription factors regulate gene expression by induction or activation of the gene or by silencing or inhibition of the gene, the latter via reduction in transcription levels of the gene.[166–173]

Transcriptional activators are those transcription factors that stimulate transcription or the synthesis of an RNA molecule from a DNA template. Generally, transcriptional activators consist of two domains: a DNA binding domain that recognizes and binds to a specific DNA sequence, and a transactivation domain that interacts with components of the transcriptional machinery to stimulate transcription. The DNA binding domains of different transcription factors may be related and, therefore, transcription factors can be categorized according to their DNA binding domains. Examples of families of transcription factor DNA binding domains are zinc finger, leucine zipper, copper fist, basic helix-loop-helix, helix-turn-helix, and bZIP.[174–180]

Trans-acting DNA sequences encode for diffusible transcription factors. Diffusible transcription factors bind to distant cis-acting DNA regulatory sequences (or to other proteins that subsequently bind to DNA or the transcription machinery). Diffusible transcription factors that bind to DNA are divided into two groups: (1) General transcription factors directly interact with the RNA polymerase complex and are part of the basic transcription machinery. (2) Regulatory transcription factors determine when a specific gene is activated or inactivated. The cis-acting DNA regulatory sequences include promoters and enhancers. Promoters are cis-acting DNA sequences that bind general transcription factors and operate in all genes. Enhancers are cis-acting DNA sequences that bind regulatory transcription factors, which induce specific genes.[174–180]

General transcription factors are required for the initiation of transcription by RNA polymerase. The promoters of many genes contain a TATA box (a cis-acting DNA regulatory sequence that contains adenine-thymidine–rich nucleotide sequences), and the initiation of transcription involves the binding of the TATA-binding protein (TBP) and TBP-associated factors to form the general transcription factor TFIID, which, together with other general transcription factors TFIIB, TFIIF, TFIIE, and TFIIH, bind RNA polymerase II to the promoter and initiate transcription. Binding of the transcriptional preinitiation complex to a specific sequence of nucleotides and separation or melting of the duplex DNA in association with histone acetylation creates a transcription bubble. The transcribing enzyme then separates from the preinitiation complex and moves down the DNA template along the reading frame. The transcription bubble moves down the DNA template in a 5′ to 3′ direction during transcription elongation. After transcription termination, the mRNA is released, processed and actively transported into the cytoplasm, where it enters the ribosome for translation of the protein product.[181–193]

Enhancers may be located a distance from the transcription initiation sites but are able to interact with general transcription factors or RNA polymerase complexes at the promoter because loops in the DNA bring them into proximity. Enhancers stimulate gene transcription above the otherwise low basal level.

An example of transcription factors is the Myc/Max/Mad network of transcription factors that regulate cell growth and death. The Myc family includes N-myc, c-myc, and L-myc. The Mad family includes Mad1, Mxi1, Mad3, Mad4, Mnt, and Mga. The Mad family functions in part as antagonists of the Myc family. These proteins form heterodimers that determine their effect. Myc-Max heterodimers activate transcription causing cell growth, proliferation, and death. Mad-Max heterodimers competitively inhibit the Myc-Max induced transcription causing differentiation, cell survival, and inhibition of growth and proliferation.[194–204]

Cell Surface Receptors and Signal Transduction

Ligands are extracellular messenger molecules such as growth factors, inflammatory cytokines, and hormones that bind to cell surface receptors, that is, growth factor receptors, cytokine receptors, and hormone receptors, respectively. The binding of ligands to surface receptors causes molecular "switches" to be turned on or off immediately downstream of the cell surface receptors (signaling enzyme effectors). This is followed by activation of second messengers in the cytosol and finally activation of nuclear transcription factors that regulate gene expression in order to produce the specific protein in response to the original "extracellular message" provided by the ligand. This process of passing the "message" from the cell surface receptors internally through proteins in the cytosol to the transcription factors in the nucleus is called signal transduction. The series of steps of protein activation/inactivation between the cell surface receptor activation and the transcription factor activation is called the signal transduction pathway or signaling pathway. The activation or inactivation of a protein during the steps of a signal transduction pathway generally occurs by reversible phosphorylation of an amino acid (tyrosine, serine, or threonine) and the phosphates are usually transferred from adenosine triphosphate (ATP) or guanosine triphosphate (GTP). Therefore, tyrosine kinases and serine/threonine kinases, which catalyze phosphorylation, have a prominent role in signaling pathways. Tyrosine kinases are more frequently encountered in signaling pathways than serine/threonine kinases.[205–215]

Growth factor receptors play a significant role in many cancers, including lung cancer. Most polypeptide growth factors such as epidermal growth factor (EGF) bind to cell surface receptor protein-tyrosine kinases. Binding of the ligand (growth factor) to the receptor protein-tyrosine kinase activates the receptor by dimerization of the receptor, causing autophosphorylation. The activated receptor then binds other proteins within the cell promoting their phosphorylation and stimulating their enzyme activity as a first step in the intracellular transmission of the signal. The type I growth factor receptor tyrosine kinase family consists of ErbB1 or epidermal growth factor receptor (EGFR), ErbB2, ErbB3, and ErbB4; EGFR has multiple ligands in addition to EGF, including transforming growth factor-α (TGF-α).[216–222]

A number of signaling pathways are well established and have roles in carcinogenesis and tumor progression. Several of these are briefly reviewed in the following paragraphs. These signaling pathways not only are important to our understanding of carcinogenesis, but also are potential targets of molecular therapy for cancer.

Ras/Raf-1/Mitogen-Activated Protein Kinase Pathway

A well-studied and significant signaling pathway important to carcinogenesis is the Ras/Raf-1/mitogen-activated protein kinase (MAPK) pathway. The Ras family consists of H-Ras, K-Ras, and N-Ras, and these are members of a class of small GTP-binding proteins that are downstream targets of receptor tyrosine kinases. Growth factor receptor activation causes Ras, located at the plasma membrane inner surface, to convert from the inactive GDP-bound state to the active GTP-bound state. Activated Ras interacts with the Raf protein-serine/threonine kinase and recruits Raf from the cytosol to the plasma membrane, where it is activated by kinases. Activated Raf causes activation of ERK, a member of the MAPK family, via MAP/ERK kinase (MEK). Activated ERK phosphorylates and activates multiple other genes including other protein kinases and translocates to the nucleus, where it phosphorylates and activates transcription factors including Elk-1, an important transcription factor in the immediate-early gene family. Guanosine triphosphatase (GTPase)-activating proteins (GAPs) end Ras activity by GTP hydrolysis. This is not the only pathway that the Ras genes are involved in. Epithelial cell proliferation is but one of several possible effects of Ras activation.[223–238]

The MAPK family is involved in numerous pathways that impact cell growth, differentiation, and apoptosis. The MAPK family includes ERK1 and ERK2 (extracellular stress regulated kinase); JNK1, JNK2, and JNK3 (c-jun NH2 terminal kinase), and p38 (p38 MAP kinases α, β, γ, and δ). Growth factors, oxidative stress, inflammatory cytokines, and UV radiation activate the MAP kinase kinase kinases (MKKK), which subsequently activate the MAP kinase kinases (MKK) that, in turn, activate the MAP kinases. Examples of MKKK include Raf-1, TGF-β–activated kinase (TAK), apoptosis signal regulating kinase 1 (ASK1), MAP/ERK kinase kinases (MEKK) germinal center kinase (GCK), and p21-activated kinase (PAK). ERK is antiapoptotic and also is involved in cell proliferation and differentiation and cell cycle progression. About 160 substrates have been described for the ERKs reflecting their involvement in many cellular processes. JNK and p38 are primarily proapoptotic, but have various complex effects on different cells and on the cell cycle.[239–251]

JAK Family

In contrast to growth factor receptors, cytokine receptors act through associated nonreceptor protein-tyrosine kinases that are members of the Janus kinase (JAK) family. When cytokine receptors are stimulated, the signal transducers and activators of transcription (STAT) proteins associate with the activated receptors and are phosphorylated by the JAK nonreceptor protein tyrosine kinases. The STAT proteins then undergo dimerization and they translocate to the nucleus, where they act as transcription factors for their target genes. This is known as the JAK/STAT pathway. STAT proteins may also be activated as part of growth factor receptor pathways.[252–261]

Transforming Growth Factor-β Superfamily

The TGF-β superfamily of cytokines inhibits the growth of many types of epithelial cells through formation of complexes of TGF-β type I and type II serine/threonine kinase receptors (TβRI and TβRII). TGF-β 1 binds as a ligand to TβRII, which phosphorylates and activates TβRI. TβRI phosphorylates the receptor-regulated Smads (R-Smads), Smad2 and Smad3. Activated Smad2/3 and Smad4 (Co-Smad) form a complex, translocate into the nucleus, and function as transcriptional modulators of TGF-β 1–regulated genes. The inhibitory Smads, Smad6 and Smad7, bind to Smad4, preventing association with Smad2/3 or bind to TβRI, preventing phosphorylation of Smad2 and Smad3. In both processes, the inhibitory Smads block TβRI signaling.[262–271]

Wnt/B-Catenin Pathway

In the Wnt/B-catenin pathway, Wnt (from "Wingless" in fruit-fly research) polypeptides bind to G-protein–coupled cell surface receptors that are members of the Frizzled family. In the classic or canonical Wnt pathway, signaling from Frizzled causes phosphorylation of Dishevelled, which causes inhibition of the protein kinase glycogen synthase kinase-3 (GSK-3). Ordinarily the amount of free β-catenin in the cytosol is limited when β-catenin is phosphorylated by GSK-3 and the phosphorylated β-catenin forms a complex with the adenomatous polyposis coli (APC) protein and the axin protein. Dishevelled inhibits

GSK-3 from phosphorylating β-catenin, allowing β-catenin to be stabilized and releasing free dephosphorylated β-catenin from the APC/axin complex. Although it also has roles in cell adhesion, in the Wnt pathway β-catenin complexes with the Tcf/LEF transcription factors, converting them from gene repressors to gene activators. After translocation into the nucleus, β-catenin binds to the transcription factor TCF4, which induces Myc.[272–299]

PI3K/Akt/mTOR Pathway

The PI3K/Akt/mTOR pathway plays a key role in regulating cell survival. Akt is a protein serine/threonine kinase. Inositol 1,4,5-triphosphate (PIP_3) is derived when phosphatidylinositol 4,5-biphosphate in the cell membrane is phosphorylated by phosphatidylinositol 3-kinase (PI3K). PIP_3 binds to Akt and recruits it to the inner surface of the cell membrane where Akt is phosphorylated. The activated Akt phosphorylates proteins that are direct regulators of cell survival, transcription factors, and other protein kinases.[300–315]

Hedgehog-Patched-Smoothened Signaling Pathway

In the Hedgehog-Patched-Smoothened signaling pathway, Sonic Hedgehog (Shh) polypeptide is modified by attachment of a lipid and binds to Patched on the cell surface. This stops inhibition of Smoothened (Smo) by Patched, and Smo, a G-protein–coupled receptor, activates the serine/threonine kinase Fused and the zinc finger transcription factor Gli (first detected as a mutation in gliomas). Gli induces Wnt signaling.[316–320]

Notch

Notch is a receptor for direct cell-to-cell signaling. Binding of Delta to Notch causes proteolytic cleavage of Notched and the intracellular domain of Notch is released, translocates to the nucleus, and interacts with a transcription factor.[329–337]

These are but a few of the signaling pathways identified so far, and the schemes briefly outlined here are abbreviated and simplified. Most pathways have many more complex interconnections and crosstalk. Disruption of these complicated signaling pathways at any of their many steps is common in the development and progression of cancer.

DNA Damage Repair

DNA damage occurs frequently within cells due to endogenous factors (oxygen radicals), extracellular factors (chemicals, radiation, ultraviolet [UV] light), or errors in replication, including stalled replication forks.[338] These injurious factors cause depurination, deamination, hydrolysis, and nonenzymatic methylation (alkylation), which add chemical groups called adducts to the DNA strands. Most types of DNA damage repair involve excision of the damaged DNA followed by filling of the resultant gap by newly synthesized DNA using the undamaged complementary DNA strand as a template. DNA repair occurs by several pathways including base excision repair (BER) and nucleotide excision repair (NER). Removal of intrastrand adducts from ultraviolet damage requires NER, and repair of oxidative damage from reactive oxygen species requires NER or BER, the latter initiated by DNA glycosylases.

The BER pathway repairs smaller lesions such as oxidized or reduced single bases and fragmented or nonbulky adducts. In the BER pathway, an individual damaged base (for example, oxidized 8-oxoguanine) is excised by base-specific DNA glycosylases (for example, 8-oxoguanine DNA glycosylase or OGG1). Bifunctional glycosylases have an apurinic/apyrimidinic lyase activity to incise the phosphodiester bond of the intact apurinic/apyrimidinic site, whereas monofunctional glycosylases require an apurinic/apyrimidinic endonuclease (APE1/APEX1) to incise the apurinic/apyrimidinic site. These steps create a single nucleotide gap that is filled by DNA polymerase β.[339–350] The nick is subsequently sealed by a DNA ligase III/x-ray repair cross-complementing group 1 (XRCC1) complex. This completes the repair process, generating a single nucleotide repair patch (short-patch base excision repair) and is known as the major pathway. In some cases when the terminal sugar-phosphate residue is resistant to cleavage by the apurinic/apyrimidinic lyase activity of polymerase β, the long-patch base excision repair subpathway may be necessary, involving extra steps in which additional nucleotides are added, creating a "flap" that is then removed by flap endonuclease 1 (FEN1) and proliferating cell nuclear antigen (PCNA).[351–359]

The NER pathway removes damaged bases as part of an oligonucleotide. The NER pathway repairs larger (bulky) lesions that distort the structure of DNA including pyrimidine dimers and other ultraviolet damage, bulkier chemical adducts, and cross-links. The NER pathway involves the xeroderma pigmentosum (XP) proteins. DNA damage by bulky adducts causes distortion of the DNA helical structure. This helical distortion is recognized by a protein complex including xeroderma pigmentosum group C protein (XPC) and hHR23B. Transcription factor IIH (TFIIH), xeroderma pigmentosum group A protein (XPA), and replication protein A (RPA) arrive at the site of the damage, followed by unwinding of the DNA by the TFIIH complex. TFIIH consists of nine protein subunits: p62, p52, p44, p34, cdk7, cyclin H, MAT1, and the DNA helicases XPB and XPD. XPD (xeroderma pigmentosum group D protein) is also known as ERCC2 (excision repair cross-complementation group 2) and XPB (xeroderma pigmentosum group B protein) is also known as ERCC3 (excision repair cross-complementation group 3). The XPD and XPB helicases open the DNA double helix allowing the damaged segment of DNA to be excised and removed. The damaged single-stranded fragment (usually about 27 to 30 base pairs [bp]) is excised by proteins including an excision repair cross-complementation group 1 (ERCC1) and xeroderma pigmentosum group F protein (XPF) complex. The repair process is completed by synthesis involving DNA polymerases.[360–366]

Another excision repair pathway scans newly replicated DNA for mismatched base pairs. DNA damage may cause nucleotide mismatching, for example, deamination of a nucleotide into a different nucleotide. Mismatch repair genes (MMR) form heterodimers that participate in DNA damage repair, causing cell cycle arrest. Members of the MMR family of genes include MLH1, MSH2, PMS1, and PMS2.[367–388]

Alkylating compounds in tobacco smoke form O6-methylguanine (O6-meG) in DNA, which may mispair with thymine during replication. In the direct damage reversal (DR) pathway, O6-meG–DNA methyltransferase (MGMT/AGT) repairs O6-meG and other alkylated bases.[389–403]

A particularly important type of DNA damage is the double-strand break (DSB), which causes a cascade of events referred to as the DNA damage response or DSB-repair (DSB-R) pathway (or during the S-phase checkpoint mentioned below, also known as the DNA replication stress response pathway), which includes sensing of the DNA damage, transduction of the damage signal to multiple pathways, including cell cycle checkpoints (described below), DNA repair, responses to telomere maintenance, and apoptosis (also described below).[404] Numerous genes and pathways are involved in the DNA repair process, including the MRE11/RAD50/NBS1 complex (MRN); x-ray repair cross-complementing (XRCC); the PI3K-like protein kinases (PIKKs): DNA-PKcs, ATM (mutated in ataxia telangiectasia), and ATR (ATM-Rad3–related); and ATM substrates: NBS1 (Nijmegen breakage syndrome protein 1), SMC1 (structural maintenance of chromosomes 1), CHK1, CHK2, MRE11, p53, MDM2, BRCA1 (BReast CAncer protein 1), BRCA2/FANCD1 (BReast CAncer protein 2/Fanconi anemia protein D1), and FANCD2 (Fanconi anemia protein D2). The ATM pathway responds to DSBs during all phases of the cell cycle and activates many of the downstream components of the ATR pathway. The ATR pathway responds to DSBs, but more slowly than ATM, and responds to agents that interfere with the function of replication forks. Members of the CHK kinase family are activated by PIKK family members ATM and ATR in response to replication stress. In response to damaging stimuli, ATM phosphorylates CHK2, which subsequently phosphorylates p53 and and Cdc25A, the latter causing inhibition of Cdk2 (see below).[405–430]

The Cell Cycle

Cell proliferation is a complex process primarily controlled by a series of sequential, tightly regulated steps of the cell cycle (Fig. 33.1). The steps or phases of the cell cycle are G_0 (cell at rest), G_1 (preparation for DNA synthesis), S (DNA synthesis or replication), G_2, and M (mitosis with nuclear and cellular division). The cell cycle is tightly governed by activation and inactivation of proteins through phosphorylation by cyclin-dependent kinases complexed with proteins called cyclins. Certain proteins described below act as specific "brakes" on the progression of the cell cycle. During replication or synthesis of DNA, the replication is initiated at specific points called origins of replication. The initiation of DNA replication causes a Y-shaped replication fork where the parental DNA duplex splits into two daughter DNA duplexes. Prior to DNA replication in the S phase, a pre-replicative complex is assembled consisting of the mini-chromosome maintenance protein complex (MCM), the origin recognition complex (ORC), and Cdc6/cdc18. At the onset of the S phase, S phase kinases Cdc7 and Cdk (cyclin-dependent kinase) activate the pre-replicative complex to form an initiation complex at the origin that includes binding of Cdc45 to MCM. Subsequently, the duplex DNA is unwound and various replication pro-

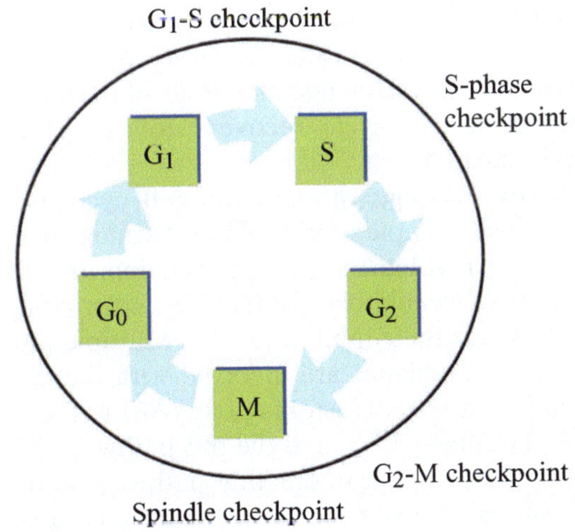

FIGURE 33.1. The cell cycle phases and its checkpoints. Phases of the cell cycle (green boxes) are G_0 (cell at rest), G_1 (preparation for DNA synthesis), S (DNA synthesis or replication), G_2, and M (mitosis with nuclear and cellular division). The checkpoints for DNA damage repair are indicated outside the circle. The G_1-S checkpoint is the restriction point at which commitment to the cell cycle occurs.

teins, including DNA polymerases, are recruited onto the unwound DNA.[431–476] Control of passage through the phases of the cell cycle is not a linear process, but involves multiple positive and negative feedback loops and interacting pathways.

There are checkpoints at specific times in the cell cycle that temporarily stop or arrest the cell cycle to permit repair of damaged DNA or, if the damage is too severe for repair, then programmed cell death or apoptosis occurs to eliminate passing on of the damaged DNA. Therefore, either by cell cycle arrest for DNA repair or by apoptosis, these checkpoints ordinarily prevent the passage of damaged DNA to daughter cells. For this reason, abnormalities of the checkpoints are of particular importance to the development of cancer since these abnormalities permit the passing on of mutations to preneoplastic and neoplastic cells. The G_1-S checkpoint prevents DNA replication when DNA damage that has not been repaired is present and the S phase checkpoint is an additional DNA damage checkpoint. Unless DNA damage repair and replication are complete, the G2–M checkpoint blocks entrance into mitosis.[477–507]

At the checkpoints, damage sensor proteins, such as the Rad9-Rad1-Hus1 heterotrimer complex (9-1-1 complex) and the Rad17-RFC complex detect DNA damage, and the 9-1-1 complex is loaded around DNA by the Rad17-RFC complex. This results in ATR-mediated and ATM-mediated phosphorylation and activation of Chk1 and Chk2. ATM and Chk2 phosphorylate and stabilize p53. The regulation of Cdc25, Wee1, and p53 inactivates cyclin-dependent kinases (cdks), which inhibit cell-cycle progression (cell cycle arrest). DNA damage repair occurs using pathways discussed above.[508–514] Subsequent to DNA damage repair, the DNA damage checkpoint is silenced, and a process called *recovery* occurs in which the cell cycle progression resumes. Polo-like kinase (Plk1) is involved in cell cycle recovery following a DNA damage-induced arrest.[515,516]

Ordinarily, passage through the cell cycle is tightly supervised by a complex series of intertwining checks and balances that involve the phosphorylation and dephosphorylation of regulatory proteins by cdks complexed with cyclins and their inhibitors.[517–525] Multiple pathways of regulatory molecules are involved with the cell cycle and include the retinoblastoma gene *(Rb)* pathway,[526–544] the TGF-β pathway,[545–555] and the p53 pathway.[556–573] Proteins in these complex interacting pathways activate or repress various steps in the cell cycle and often regulate other genes.

The major checkpoint in the cell cycle is the restriction point when commitment to the cell cycle occurs in G_1 and preparation for DNA synthesis begins (Fig. 33.2). Prior to the restriction point, growth factors initiate and maintain the transition through the G_1 phase. The restriction point is the point at which commitment to the cell cycle

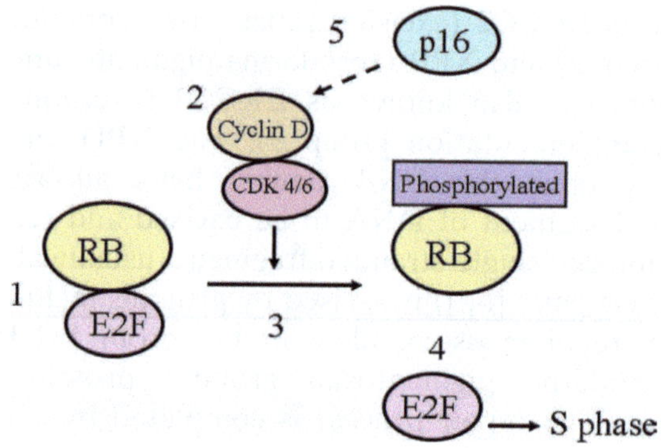

FIGURE 33.2. The restriction point: (1) Binding of unphosphorylated pRb to E2F blocks entry into the cell cycle. (2) Cyclin D complexes with cdk4 and cdk6, and (3) these complexes phosphorylate pRb during G_1. (4) Phosphorylation of pRb during G_1 results in inactivation of pRb, which initiates the S phase with release of E2F transcription factors. (5) p16 inhibits CDK4/6 kinase, which in turn prevents inactivation of pRb by phosphorylation.

occurs and the cell no longer requires growth factors to complete the cell cycle. As noted below, passage through the restriction point is determined by phosphorylation of pRb.

The RB product, pRb, manages the progression past the restriction point during the cell cycle and controls the expression of genes involved in DNA synthesis. Cyclin D activity is required for progression of the cell cycle.[574–594] In response to stimuli for mitosis, cyclin D complexes with cdk4 and cdk6 and these complexes phosphorylate pRb during G_1. Cyclin E-cdk2 complexes also phosphorylate pRb just prior to the S phase. Control of these cyclin-cdk complexes is through the activity of families of cdk inhibitors (the INK4 family including $p16^{INK4}$ and the $p21^{WAF1/Cip1}/p27^{Kip1}/p57^{Kip2}$ family).[595–609] Phosphorylation of pRb during G_1 results in inactivation of pRb, which initiates the S phase with release of E2F transcription factors[610–625] that activate transcription of numerous genes involved in DNA replication such as c-*myc*.[626–633] Cyclin A complexes with cdks and functions in both G_1/S phase transition and in mitosis, whereas cyclin B complexes with cdks and is involved in the entry into mitosis.[634, 635]

The *CDKN2A* gene encodes for two completely unrelated protein products, $p16^{INK4A}$ (mentioned above)[636–644] and $p14^{ARF}$,[645–650] which are transcribed from different exons of the *CDKN2A* gene and are active in the pRb and p53 arms of the cell cycle. As mentioned previously, p16 is a cdk inhibitor. Specifically, p16 inhibits CDK4/6 kinase, which in turn prevents inactivation of pRb by phosphorylation. Therefore, loss of p16 function would cause loss of pRb function, resulting in inappropriate cell cycling. The p14 product destabilizes the MDM2 protein (Fig. 33.3). MDM2 protein binds to and degrades p53, which, as noted previously, causes cell cycle arrest or

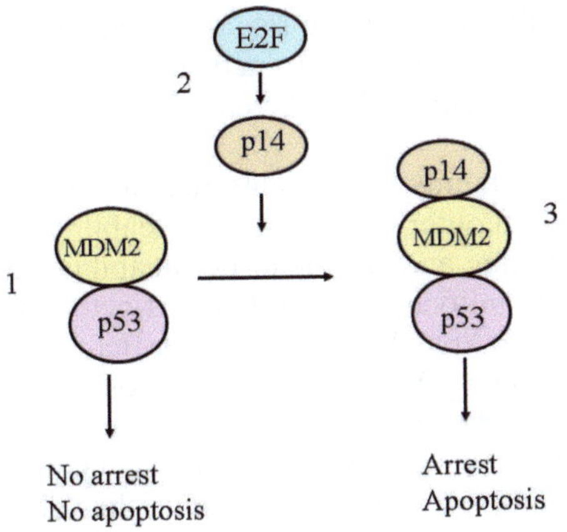

FIGURE 33.3. Control of cell cycle arrest and apoptosis: (1) MDM2 protein binds to and degrades p53, preventing p53–induced cell cycle arrest or apoptosis when DNA is damaged. (2) Release of E2F by inactivation of Rb induces p14. (3) p14 product destabilizes the MDM2 protein, allowing p53–mediated cell cycle arrest or apoptosis.

apoptosis when DNA is damaged. Loss of p53 function allows inappropriate cell cycling and interferes with apoptosis. Loss of p14 function permits excessive levels of MDM2, which results in excessive destruction of p53 and loss of p53 function. Therefore, mutations, hypermethylation, or other abnormalities of genes and their products in the pRb and p53 pathways can produce the same loss of control on the cell cycle as mutations or other abnormalities of the *RB* and *p53* genes themselve. Abnormalities of CDKN2A, p16, p14, and MDM2 are only parts of the many possibilities involving genes and their products upstream or downstream of pRb and p53 that can produce loss of control of the cell cycle.

Therefore, one of the primary roles of p53 is cell cycle regulation through the *arrest* of the cell cycle, particularly in response to DNA damage. Part of this response is mediated through activation of $p21^{WAF1}$, which inhibits cyclin-cdk complexes required for cell cycle progression.[651–662] In addition to cell cycle arrest, which permits repair of damaged DNA, p53 also induces apoptosis to destroy cells when DNA damage is beyond repair. Due to these functions, p53 has been referred to as the guardian of the genome. TGF-β is a member of a large family (superfamily) of cytokines and TGF-β1 is involved in inhibition of cell cycle progression.[663,664]

Cell Death and Survival

There is a delicate balance between cell growth and cell death in the normal growth, development, and function of various tissues. Cells that are not actively progressing through the cell cycle are either differentiated (postmitotic) or surviving (premitotic). Ordinarily, cells regulate their own death through apoptosis. Survival factors such as EGF or insulin-like growth factor-I (IGF-I) can activate survival pathways.

Apoptosis

Necrosis is a process of cell death in response to an injury by which the cytoplasm swells and bursts, spilling contents into the extracellular space, which typically invokes an inflammatory response. Apoptosis is programmed cell death that occurs during normal embryonic development, during normal tissue homeostasis and cyclical tissue processes (such as growth, death, and regeneration of hair follicles or proliferation and migration of intestinal epithelium), and when cells become aged. When DNA damage is too severe to repair, cells with DNA damage may undergo apoptosis.

Apoptosis is highly regulated by apoptotic proteins, and under normal circumstances there is a balance between proteins that promote apoptosis and proteins that inhibit apoptosis. When apoptosis occurs, there is cytoplasmic shrinkage and chromatin condensation with formation of subcellular vesicles called apoptotic bodies observable under the light microscope and breakup of DNA into 200–bp oligonucleosome-size fragments. The apoptotic bodies are removed by phagocytosis.[665–672] Similar to failure of normal DNA repair mechanisms and failure of cell cycle control, failure of normal mechanisms of apoptosis is another means by which proliferation may go unchecked during carcinogenesis, and DNA abnormalities can be passed on to daughter cells. Prominent proteins involved in the regulation of apoptosis include p53 and the Bcl-2 family of proteins. Apoptosis may be induced by p53 through activation of other proteins or may occur independent of p53 as further described below.[673–679] The Bcl-2 family of proteins includes inhibitors of apoptosis: Bcl-2, long isoform ($Bcl\text{-}X_L$), and induced myeloid leukemia cell differentiation protein (Mcl-1). It also includes promoters of apoptosis Bcl-2 associated X protein (Bax), Bcl-2 antagonistic killer 1 (Bak), Bcl-2 interacting domain (Bid), $Bcl\text{-}X_L$/Bcl-2 associated death promoter (Bad), and Bcl-2 interacting killer (Bik).[680–691]

Apoptosis involves activation of cysteine aspartate proteases (caspases) through death receptor–mediated pathways, induced by external signals and activated by p53 or JNK pathways, or through mitochondria-mediated pathways, induced by internal signals and controlled by the Bcl-2 family of proteins.[692–700] Caspases are ultimately responsible for the proteolysis of cellular substrates in apoptosis and are heterotetramers that act in a caspase cascade. Caspases 8 and 9 are initiator caspases and caspases 3, 6, and 7 are effector caspases. The formation of an apoptosome complex consisting of cytochrome c, apoptotic protease-activating factor 1 (Apaf-1), procaspase 9, and ATP is initiated by release of cytochrome c from the mitochondria into the cytosol. Procaspase 9 then undergoes autoactivation in a caspase cascade. Activated caspase 9 activates caspase 3, and caspase 3 cleaves caspase-activated deoxyribonuclease inhibitor (ICAD), causing activation of caspase-activated deoxyribonuclease (CAD). Activation of CAD is thought to cause DNA degradation resulting in the oligonucleosome-size DNA fragments characteristic of apoptosis. Caspase 3 also degrades DNA-dependent protein kinase (DNA-PK), which is a DNA repair enzyme.[701–713]

Fibroblast-associated (Fas) and tumor necrosis factor receptor (TNF-R) are the two best characterized death receptors. In the death receptor–mediated pathways, binding of ligands to the death receptors Fas, TNF-R, and TNF-related apoptosis-inducing ligand receptor (TRAIL-R) initiates apoptotic signals through death domains (DDs), death effector domains (DEDs), and caspase recruitment domains (CARDs). DDs are found in proteins such as Fas, TNF-R1, TRAIL-R1, TRAIL-R2, Fas-associated protein with death domain (FADD), TNF receptor–associated protein with death domain (TRADD), and receptor-interacting protein (RIP). DED-containing adaptor molecules, DED-containing caspase 8, and DD form the death-inducing signaling complex (DISC), which initiates the caspase cascade by binding to procaspase 8. Inhibitors of apoptosis (IAPs) inhibit caspases and IAPs are bound and inhibited by mitochondria-derived activator of caspase (SMAC/DIABLO) and HtrA2.[714–725]

Tumor necrosis factors are the best studied and most potent apoptotic ligands. Tumor necrosis factors include TNF-α and TNF-β. TNF-α is secreted by macrophages and binds to TNF-R1, which has DDs and can induce apoptosis through a signaling pathway that causes caspase activation. TNF-β is secreted by T lymphocytes and binds to TNF-R2, causing apoptosis by a different signaling pathway. Other members of the TNF superfamily may also induce apoptosis, including lymphotoxin (LT), fibroblast associated ligand (FasL), TNF-related apoptosis-inducing ligand (TRAIL), death receptor 3 ligand (DR3L), or weak homologue of TNF (TWEAK) and TNF homologue that activates apoptosis, nuclear factor (NF)-κB and JNK (THANK).[726–733]

In the mitochondria-mediated pathways, the Bcl-2 homology domains 3-only (BH3-only) proteins send signals to the mitochondria for the assembly of proapoptotic Bax and Bak, causing release of various apoptotic factors. BH3-only proteins include Bid, Bad, PMA-induced protein (Noxa), and p53 upregulated modulator of apoptosis (PUMA).[734–740]

p53 induces expression of proteins in both the death receptor–mediated pathways and the mitochondrial-mediated pathways. In the death receptor–mediated pathways, p53 activates death receptors like Fas.[741–743] In the mitochondrial-mediated pathways, p53 induces Bax, Noxa, and PUMA to cause release of cytochrome c from the mitochondria, leading to activation of caspase 9 and subsequently caspase 3 in the caspase cascade described above.[744–755]

The Bcl-2 family of proteins function by controlling mitochondrial outer membrane permeability and by controlling opening and closing of permeability pores. Bcl-2 functions by mitochondrial release of cytochrome c and interaction of Apaf-1 with caspase 9. Bcl-2 also binds to Bax and blocks c-Myc–induced apoptosis, as do Bcl-X_L and Mcl-1.[756–766]

As with previous discussions of signal transduction pathways and cell cycle regulation, this discussion of apoptosis is simplified and abbreviated. There are many interactions with other signaling pathways not described here and the complex interactions of the proteins described here have not yet been fully elucidated. In addition, apoptosis pathways interact with so-called survival pathways.

Survival Pathways

The PI3K/Akt/mTOR pathway plays a key role in regulating cell survival and was discussed above.[300–315] The NF-κB transcription factor and NF-κB signaling pathway regulate many proteins of the immune system as well as proteins that inhibit apoptosis and promote cell survival and proliferation. NF-κB includes various dimers of the Rel protein family including Rel (c-Rel), Rel A (p65), RelB, NF-κB1 (p50 and its precursor p105), and NF-κB2 (p52 and its precursor p100). The p50–p65 dimer is the most common. In most cases, binding of NF-κB complexes to promoters assists transcription but homodimer complexes of p50 or p52 can repress transcription. NF-κB proteins associate with members of the inhibitory IκB family such as IκB-α, IκB-β, and IκB-ε, which retain them in the cytoplasm in resting cells.[767–781]

Activation of NF-κB requires degradation of IκB. The degradation of IκB first requires phosphorylation of IκB by IκB kinases (IKKs). IKKs are activated by MAPKKK or by ligands for Toll-like receptors (TLRs), interleukin-1 and -18 (IL-1/IL-18) receptors, the TNF receptor superfamily, and B- and T-cell receptors. Phosphorylation of IκB by IKKs is followed by binding of $E3^{I\kappa B}$ ubiquitin ligase complex β-TrCP-SCF. $E3^{I\kappa B}$ ubiquitin ligase complex β-TrCP-SCF ubiquinylates IκB and targets it for degradation by 26S proteasome. The freed NF-κB complex translocates into the nucleus and binds to specific κB sites on DNA. The NF-κB complex is a transcription factor regulating expression of numerous inflammatory and immune proteins including proinflammatory cytokines, chemokines, adhesion molecules, cyclooxygenase-2, inducible nitric oxide synthase, major histocompatibility complex, IL-2, IL-12, and interferon-γ as well as antiapoptotic and apoptotic genes.[782–791]

Most factors that activate apoptosis also activate NF-κB. NF-κB can block TNF-induced apoptosis and chemotherapy-induced apoptosis through upregulation of antiapoptotic genes and downregulation of apoptotic genes. However, the role of NF-κB in apoptosis is very complex and, in addition to suppressing apoptosis in most cases, NF-κB may also sometimes be proapoptotic or have no role in apoptosis.

Mutations

Errors in DNA are referred to as mutations. Mutations often result in errors of the genetic code and gene product, often causing a change in the cell or tissue in which the mutation has occurred. Mutations may be silent (no effect). Mutations may cause a beneficial effect, a deleterious effect (including the death of the cell or organism), or both.[792]

Mutations are a key component in the development of cancer from normal cells. The development and progression of cancer often involves mutations in the regulatory proteins of the cell cycle, DNA damage repair, and apoptosis, resulting in uncontrolled proliferation of tumor cells. The loss of the normal controls of cell proliferation, repair, differentiation, and death is both a cause and effect of the transformation of a normal cell to a cancer cell. Disruptions in the normal cell cycle allow for the accrual of additional mutations. Development and progression of cancer is a multistep process involving accumulation of multiple mutations. Initiation of cancer is caused by an irreversible mutation, and promotion of the cancer results from proliferation of the cancer cells due to continued stimuli. In the case of cancer, the mutations confer a survival advantage to the cancer cells, allowing them to grow and proliferate unchecked. Transforming mutations generally involve three categories of genes, many of which are regulatory genes involved in the cell cycle and related normal functions: oncogenes, tumor-suppressor genes, and DNA repair genes.[793–802]

Proto-oncogenes are normal genes that code for protein kinases, growth factors, growth factor receptors, and membrane signal transducers to promote normal cell growth and differentiation. Mutation of proto-oncogenes results in oncogenes that promote unchecked cell cycle progression and cell proliferation. Tumor-suppressor genes normally encode for proteins that act as inhibitors or breaks on the cell cycle and cell growth and proliferation. Mutations causing loss of their function permits unchecked cell proliferation. Oncogenes are usually considered dominant genes, and tumor-suppressor genes are usually considered recessive genes.[803–812]

Mutations are classified according to type. *Frameshift mutations* are caused by the introduction of bases into the gene so that the shift in bases causes essentially new codons, which code for an aberrant protein. Frameshift mutations can be caused by insertion of one or more base pairs into the gene or by deletion of one or more base pairs from the gene. A *point mutation* involves substitution, insertion, or deletion of a single base pair in a gene. *Nonsense mutations* involve introduction of a stop codon in an inappropriate location in a gene, which produces a truncated protein. *Missense mutations* result from alteration of a codon so that an aberrant protein is produced. Mismatch occurs when base pairs do not match appropriately in what should be complementary DNA strands.[813–819]

In chromosomal translocations, two distinct chromosomes segments break off at a breakpoint from their respective chromosomes and join together. The translocated segments can come from two different chromosomes or from within the same chromosome (inversion). The result can be relocation of a proto-oncogene near a strong promoter, causing overexpression or activation of the oncogene product. Translocation may also cause the fusion of the proto-oncogene to another gene creating a hybrid fusion gene, which codes for an abnormal hybrid protein or chimeric protein with abnormal function.[820–831]

Oncogenes may be activated through amplification in which a gene or part of a gene is reduplicated, sometimes as much as 100- to 1000–fold. An amplified oncogene is transcribed at a higher than normal level, resulting in overexpression of its protein product. Amplified gene segments can be identified cytogenetically as homogeneously staining regions (HSRs) in a chromosome or as extrachromosomal double minutes (DMs). Oncogenes may also be activated through point mutations.[832–844]

Changes in gene expression that are heritable but do not involve alterations in base pair sequence are epigenetic changes. An example is methylation. Methylation regulates gene expression by addition of a methyl (-CH_3) group to specific sites on DNA or RNA. In humans, methylation occurs only when C is followed by G, referred to as CpG dinucleotides. CpG dinucleotides have a propensity to spontaneous mutations. Some regions of DNA have retained CpG dinucleotides called CpG islands. CpG islands are often found in association with promoters. Methylation of a promoter CpG island silences the corresponding gene, and transcription of that gene does not occur. Abnormal methylation of CpG islands associated with tumor-suppressor genes frequently occurs in cancer and contributes to cancer development.[845–853]

In some human cancers, a heterozygous situation exists in which a recessive allele that leads to cancer is masked by a normal dominant allele. If there is a mutation in the dominant allele, its protective effect is lost. The recessive cancer allele is unmasked and becomes manifest. This process in which the recessive cancer gene is unmasked when the normal dominant gene undergoes mutation is called loss of heterozygosity (LOH) and is responsible for several types of human cancer.[854–856]

MicroRNAs and siRNAs

Regulation of gene expression involves control of translation and mRNA degradation. Small RNA molecules participate in the control of gene expression and include micro RNAs (miRNAs) and short interfering RNAs (siRNAs). The miRNAs are small, regulatory, noncoding RNAs that are derived from large RNA precursors (pre-miRNAs) and are involved in the control of many critical processes during development; miRNAs help control gene expression by binding to mRNA transcripts, causing degradation or translational block. miRNA expression is altered in many cancers, and miRNAs may represent a new class of genes involved in carcinogenesis.[857–871]

Molecular Procedures

Advances in molecular procedures occur regularly. Some standard techniques, both old and new, are described here, and are mentioned in subsequent sections of this chapter.

General Principles and Techniques

For many molecular studies, the DNA or RNA must be *isolated* or *extracted* from the cells in a sample and separated and purified from other cell constituents such as proteins and lipids. DNA or RNA *isolation* for study from tissue specimens including lung cancer specimens is cell *lysis*. The initial step in *extraction* of nucleic acids from fresh or frozen tissue is homogenization of the tissue in a buffer. Extraction of nucleic acids from formalin-fixed paraffin-embedded tissue first requires removing the paraffin with an organic solvent like xylene and rehydration through alcohols. Heated protease digestion of the proteins from the lysed specimen is performed. Heated protease digestion of tissue that was formalin-fixed paraffin-embedded is prolonged to reverse formalin cross-linking between proteins (histones) and nucleic acids. Even so, DNA extracted from formalin-fixed paraffin-embedded tissue is typically no longer than the amount contained in a nucleosome. Phenol extraction is used to separate nucleic acids from other cellular constituents. Extracted nucleic acids are then precipitated in a concentrated ethanol and salt solution. Nucleic acids can also be extracted and purified by selective adsorption of nucleic acids to glass or silica columns in chaotropic salt solutions with purification by a series of washing steps with sodium azide.[871–879]

Isolation and storage of DNA from tissue samples is comparatively easy compared to RNA because cellular levels of DNA are more stable and *deoxyribonucleases* (DNAses) that normally break down DNA are easily denatured by heating. Cellular levels of RNA vary due to changing levels of transcription and rapid breakdown by *ribonucleases* (RNases) that are ubiquitous and highly stable. Therefore, additional steps must be taken to protect RNA from RNases in the cellular constituents and the laboratory environment, including prompt isolation, rigorously clean laboratory technique, wearing of gloves, agents to denature or inhibit RNases, and storage at –80°C.[880–884]

When specific quantities of nucleic acids are needed for a test, the concentration of extracted nucleic acid can be determined by measuring wavelength absorbance with ultraviolet spectrophotometry. Estimates of DNA quantity and quality can be obtained by staining sample DNA with an intercalating dye such as ethidium bromide, SYBR green, or methylene blue in an electrophoresis gel and comparing it to controls in adjacent lanes for quantity and observing distinctiveness of the band for quality.

After isolation and purification, many procedures require the use of fragments of DNA that are obtained by digesting the DNA with *restriction endonucleases*.[885–890] Restriction endonucleases are naturally occurring enzymes found in bacteria that cleave DNA at unique segments of bases called *recognition sites*. The resulting DNA *restriction fragments* of differing molecular weights are then separated using electrophoresis. Since the exact locations of restriction endonuclease recognition sites may vary between two individuals, the restriction fragments that result from digestion of DNA samples from these two individuals may be of different lengths. These are referred to as *restriction fragment length polymorphisms* (RFLPs).[891–894]

Study of the fragments of DNA obtained from restriction endonuclease digestion requires their separation from each other. *Electrophoresis* is the application of an electric field to cause migration of charged molecules (DNA is negatively charged) toward an electric pole.[895–900] When performed in a gel with microscopic pores of various sizes, DNA fragments travel through the gel primarily according to their molecular size—smaller, lighter fragments traveling faster than larger, heavier ones so that, when the current is stopped, the groups of fragments of the same size have separated out in the gel according to their molecular size as well as a few other features mentioned below. Traditionally, *polyacrylamide gels* and *agarose gels* have been used for the separation of DNA fragments by electrophoresis. DNA fragments sort themselves into groups of fragments based on their molecular size, conformation and charge, and temperature and pore size of the gel. DNA is detected by ethidium bromide staining with visualization by ultraviolet light. Since the DNA fragments are put into a rectangular well at the start of the electrophoretic separation, they retain this rectangular shape, and when visualized these separate rectangles are referred to as *bands*. *Capillary electrophoresis* is now widely used for separation of DNA fragments because it is faster, automated and more consistent than traditional gel electrophoresis and requires smaller sample volumes.[901–907] In capillary electrophoresis, DNA fragments are separated in a glass (silica) capillary tube with a polymer as electrolyte solution. The DNA fragments separate by size through the capillary and are detected by a detection system.

For most procedures, DNA must be *denatured* from a double strand (dsDNA) to single strands (ssDNA) by heating or treatment with alkali.[908–911] *Oligonucleotides* are short sequences of a few nucleotides artificially synthesized for use as probes and primers in molecular pathology procedures.[912, 913] Labeled probes are used to detect a defined segment of DNA by *hybridization*, the forming of bonds between the oligonucleotides of the probe and the complementary segment of the target DNA under study. Primers are added to initiate or prime DNA synthesis by DNA polymerase in the *polymerase chain reaction* (PCR). To apply PCR to RNA, it is necessary to create a DNA copy of the RNA known as *complementary DNA* (cDNA) using reverse transcriptase. The cDNA is then used in the PCR procedure. When synthesizing DNA segments in a procedure such as DNA sequencing, PCR, and others, the building blocks of DNA, *deoxynucleotide triphosphates* (dNTPs), must be added to the reaction.[914–917]

Bacteria have small circular pieces of extrachromosomal DNA called *plasmids*. A new DNA segment can be inserted into a plasmid where it is known as *recombinant DNA* and replicated many times when the plasmid is reintroduced to a bacterium.

To create primers and probes for the various procedures that are described below as well as for direct studies of genes, it is first necessary to identify the sequence of nucleotides in a gene or other segment of DNA of interest. The procedure by which the specific sequence of nucleotides in a piece of DNA is identified is called *DNA sequencing*.[918–921] The Sanger method of DNA sequencing using gel electrophoresis was originally developed in 1977.[922] In this procedure linear amplification of the DNA strands using sequence specific complementary primers, DNA polymerase and *dideoxynucleoside triphosphates* (ddNTPs) in addition to dNTPs are used to synthesize DNA segments of varying length complementary to the template DNA. The length of the synthesized DNA segments is determined by the point at which ddNTP was incorporated into the segment, which inhibits further extension of the DNA segment. By using different nucleoside inhibitors (ddGTP, ddATP, ddTTP, and araCTP [cytarabine triphosphate]), the segments of DNA from the same template are inhibited at different points in the DNA, and the lengths of the segments indicate the location of the nucleoside inhibitors. The lengths of the segments are determined by separation with electrophoresis; segments of different length travel at different rates. The DNA segments can be separated using gels or capillary electrophoresis. Detection of the segments can be with radioactive labeling, but currently detection is primarily by fluorescent labeling. In *dye-terminator labeling*, each ddNTP is labeled with a different fluorophore, and nucleotide sequence is determined by both the size of the DNA segment and the fluorescent colors of the segment in an automated sequencer. In capillary electrophoresis, the DNA segments are injected into a thin capillary tube and detected by laser-induced florescence. Detection software then generates an electropherogram of the DNA sequence by correlating fluorescent intensity of each dye (representing a specific ddNTP) versus the migration time.[923]

In some types of procedures, the DNA, RNA, or gene product under study is not extracted from the tissue but rather remains in tissue sections. A common example of this type of procedure is immunohistochemistry for gene protein products in which an antibody to the protein product is applied to a tissue section, washed, and, if the protein product is present and the antibody has attached to it, detected by a chromogenic reaction using an enzyme attached to the antibody directly or through a secondary antibody. This type of technique allows direct visualization by the pathologist of the location of the protein product within the tissue, which is reassuring that one is looking at, for example, expression of a protein in cancer cells and not in adjacent noncancerous tissue or necrosis. These techniques can often be applied to routine formalin-fixed, paraffin-embedded tissues, so that no special collection, storage, or other procedures are required and studies can be performed on routinely archived tissues.[924–927]

Specific Procedures

Southern Blot

Southern blots were one of the first widely used procedures developed for DNA analysis, allowing for detection of specific genes, mutations, and RFLPs.[928–931] Although no longer as widely used for clinical work as newer procedures, the Southern blot provides the basis for understanding the evolution of more current techniques. Southern blots are slow, laborious procedures compared to PCR procedures and do not involve amplification of the DNA under study. Since there is no amplification, a large amount of high-quality, intact, high molecular weight DNA is required to perform a Southern blot. Degradation of the DNA sample must be scrupulously avoided since it can produce both false-negative and false-positive results. The isolated DNA is digested into fragments by restriction endonucleases and the fragments separated by gel electrophoresis. The separated fragments of DNA are transferred from the gel onto a solid membrane, for example nylon, by capillary transfer, automated vacuum transfer, or electrotransfer. The transferred DNA fragments retain their same separated positions on the membrane that they had on the gel. This transfer procedure is referred to as blotting, and the membrane containing the transferred DNA fragments is referred to as the blot. The blotted DNA fragments are denatured with alkali and the DNA fragments are permanently fixed to the membrane by drying the blot in an oven or exposure to UV radiation. The blot is immersed in a prehybridization buffer to block nonspecific binding, and a labeled DNA probe is added to the blot. The probe hybridizes with corresponding blot DNA and, after stringent washing, only labeled probe hybridized to cDNA in the blot will remain. Visualization of the hybridized labeled probes can be visualized according to the type of label used: radioactive, chemiluminescent, or biotinylated. Visualization indicates the position of the hybridized bands relative to known control bands and it can be determined if the same specific band as a specific control band is present in the DNA under analysis. A band that is located in a position different from its corresponding control band may indicate a difference in the nucleotide sequence consistent with a mutation.

Dot Blots and Slot Blots

Similar to Southern blots, dot blots and slot blots use the same principle of hybridization of a probe to DNA undergoing investigation.[932,933] However, the DNA is applied to a spot or slot and is not digested with restriction endonucleases or electrophoresed. These procedures test for the presence or absence of the cDNA sequence to the labeled probe, which should hybridize if present. In reverse dot blots, the probe is fixed to the membrane, amplified DNA from the specimen is added, and the presence or absence of hybridization is detected by visualization.

Northern Blots and Western Blots

Northern blotting uses principles similar to Southern blotting but is used to investigate RNA expression rather than DNA.[934,935] Western blotting is used to investigate proteins using similar principles and with detection of proteins by labeled antibodies.[936–938]

Polymerase Chain Reaction

Polymerase chain reaction (PCR) is used to exponentially amplify (make multiple copies) specific DNA sequences using DNA polymerase and has been essential in the development of current molecular pathology.[939–944] PCR technology is popular for molecular pathology in the clinical laboratory because it provides high specificity and sensitivity, rapid turnaround, requires less preparation of the specimen, and is suited for the high numbers of tests required in a clinical laboratory.

The objective of the PCR technique is to amplify (make many copies) of a specific DNA sequence such as an oncogene from a DNA sample. If, for example, the oncogene is present in the DNA sample, PCR allows the investigator to make many extra copies of the oncogene from the sample to study. To perform PCR, one must know the DNA sequence to be studied from the sample DNA and make specific primers for that DNA sequence, sometimes referred to as the *target DNA*.

Primers are nucleotides that are synthesized for the target DNA that is to be amplified, and the specificity of the PCR reaction derives from the specificity of the primers for the target DNA. The primers are complementary to DNA that brackets, or sometimes overlaps, the target DNA sequence to be amplified. The three steps in the PCR cycle are *denaturation*, *annealing*, and *extension*. The target DNA is denatured from dsDNA to ssDNA by heating to about 95°C. This is followed by annealing (hybridization) between oligonucleotide primers, and complementary regions of the denatured target DNA at 30° to 65°C. Annealing forms double-stranded foci composed of oligonucleotides hybridized to the target DNA as primers for DNA polymerase. During extension at 65° to 75°C a special DNA polymerase binds to the primers and synthesizes a complementary sequence of DNA using dNTPs added to the reaction mixture with the target DNA as template. The DNA polymerase used in extension is from the hot-spring bacteria *Thermophilus aquaticus* or *Taq polymerase*. Unlike other polymerases, Taq polymerase does not denature at the high temperatures of the PCR cycle.

The PCR cycle is repeated over and over again in a thermal cycler, an instrument that holds tubes of the reagents (primers, target DNA template, Taq polymerase, and dNTPs) and cycles among the different steps (denaturation, annealing, and extension) of the PCR cycle. With each PCR cycle, the amount of DNA doubles and the DNA formed at the end of one cycle furnishes the template for the next cycle in chain reaction fashion, resulting in an exponential increase in DNA over many repeated cycles. Therefore, if one starts with a single dsDNA, there are two dsDNA after one cycle, four dsDNA after two cycles, eight dsDNA after three cycles, 16 after four cycles, 32 after five cycles, and so on, until after 32 cycles, there is a billion-fold increase over the amount of starting DNA. In the later cycles, the actual increase is not perfectly exponential due to limiting factors such as the amount of reagents like dNTPs and efficiency of the Taq polymerase and a plateau occurs.

An *amplicon* is a replicated DNA molecule produced by PCR. A *unit length amplicon* is an amplicon whose ends are defined by the primers. The exponential amplification of the target DNA sequence makes PCR much more sensitive than Southern blot. Validation of the specificity of the PCR product is necessary and verification may be done by Southern blot or sequencing.

Multiplex PCR refers to using multiple primers in one reaction in order to amplify multiple different regions of DNA at the same time.[945–949] However, it is difficult to ensure equal amplification of all regions using this technique.

Hot Start PCR

Hot start PCR refers to holding at least one of the reagents, usually *Taq*, from the reaction mixture until the reaction tube temperature has reached 60° to 80°C. This prevents *Taq* from extending primer dimers or primers that have annealed nonspecifically prior to reaching the proper reaction temperature. This approach improves sensitivity, specificity, and yield of PCR.[950–952]

Whole Genome Amplification and Multiple Displacement Amplification

The PCR techniques have been used to generate large amounts of DNA by whole genome amplification (WGA) often from tiny specimens.[953,954] Multiple displacement amplification (MDA) allows for improved reproduction of genomic DNA by using a novel DNA polymerase.[955–957]

Polymerase Chain Reaction–Restriction Fragment Length Polymorphism (PCR-RFLP)

In PCR-RFLP, the PCR products are digested by one or more restriction endonucleases and then electrophoresed to detect restriction length polymorphisms.[958,959]

Nested PCR

In nested PCR, a pair of primers is initially used to amplify a target DNA sequence. A dilution of the product is then amplified with two pairs of nested primers with one set internal to the other (nested), creating a second product that is shorter than the first one. This approach decreases the likelihood of a nonspecific amplification since there are two pairs of primers so that nested PCR increases both specificity and sensitivity. However, there is a high risk of amplicon contamination.

Reverse Transcription–Polymerase Chain Reaction (RT-PCR)

In RT-PCR, cDNA is first synthesized from an mRNA template using reverse transcriptase. As noted previously, RNA is relatively unstable due to ubiquitous RNases, but cDNA synthesized from an mRNA template is far more stable than its mRNA template. The cDNA is then used as the target DNA in PCR, providing a reliable method to study gene expression.[960–967]

Real-Time PCR

Real-time PCR allows simultaneous amplification of target DNA and detection of amplicons in real time rather than as separate steps.[968–972] Real-time PCR requires a reporter molecule that is detected by fluorescence using a detector called a fluorimeter. A fluorescent signal is generated during the log-linear phase of the PCR cycle when there is exponential amplification of target DNA. The signal detected by the built-in fluorimeter indicates the amount of PCR product synthesized during this exponential amplification phase. This approach allows for quantitation (fluorescence is proportional to initial amount of target DNA), greater accuracy and reproducibility, rapid turnaround of results, and eliminates time and costs for postamplification processing, electrophoresis, and analysis. Real-time PCR can be used for melting curve analysis, which verifies specificity and can be potentially used in the detection of unknown sequence variants.

DNA Methylation and Methylation Sensitive PCR

Sodium bisulfite treatment of DNA converts unmethylated C to U but leaves methylated C intact. C can be differentiated from U in DNA by methylation-specific PCR (MSP) using restriction endonuclease digestion with methylation-sensitive enzymes or by DNA sequencing. Primer pairs in MSP hybridize to CpG sites and identify either methylated DNA or unmethylated DNA. The presence or absence of amplicon in each PCR reaction is detected by gel electrophoresis to determine the presence or absence of methylated and unmethylated DNA. MSP is used to investigate aberrant methylated CpG islands in cancer. MSP can be combined with real-time PCR to distinguish the high amounts of CpG methylation that occur in cancer from lower amounts of methylation that sometimes occur in nonneoplastic conditions such as metaplasia.[973–978]

PCR Techniques for Unknown Sequence Variants

Most of the above techniques are used to screen for sequence variants (both mutations and polymorphisms) based on previous knowledge of the variant; that is, the sequence of the variant is either known or defined by the experimental conditions. By contrast, there is an evolving interest in both research and clinical molecular pathology to identify sequence variants by scanning without prior knowledge of their existence; that is, the sequence of the variant is unknown. Sequencing is the ultimate screening technique, but is costly and labor-intensive. The goal of the scanning techniques described below (DDGE, TGGE, HA, SSCP, DHPLC, PTT) is to identify specimens with possible variant sequences, thereby reducing costs relative to sequencing. Should an unknown variant be detected, usually by a shift in the mobility of the PCR product on a gel or capillary, the PCR product with altered mobility can be isolated and sequenced. Melting temperature analysis in real-time PCR can also be used to identify unknown sequence variants.

Denaturing Gradient Gel Electrophoresis and Temperature Gradient Gel Electrophoresis

Denaturation of dsDNA into ssDNA gradually occurs stepwise as heating increases or the concentration of a denaturing chemical increases. Regions of DNA with the most A and T content denature first and regions with highest G and C concentration denature last. Thus, a gradient of temperature or chemicals in a gel should produce increasing amounts of DNA denaturation as the DNA encounters the increasing gradient. Partially denatured DNA fragments migrate more slowly through a gel. The region within the dsDNA that denaturation occurs is called the melting domain, and the point at which the melting domain begins to denature is called the melting temperature (T_m). This terminology applies no matter whether the denature is due to heat or chemicals.

Denaturing gradient gel electrophoresis (DGGE) and temperature gradient gel electrophoresis (TGGE) are similar techniques used to identify specimens with possible mutations or polymorphisms, and are cheaper and faster screening methods than DNA sequencing. In both techniques, DNA fragments with comparatively similar lengths and with different sequences are separated by electrophoresis in a gradient of increasing ability to denature the DNA. In DGGE the gradient is a chemical denaturant composed of a mixture of urea and formamide.[979–982] In TGGE the gradient is a temperature gradient created by a combination of water baths and a cooling plate under the gel.[983–984]

The DNA fragments that melt early in the gel gradient become separated from those that melt later due to the decreased mobility caused by denaturation. The denaturing conditions and the time of electrophoresis are optimized so that normal DNA sequences migrate to an intermediate position in the gel by the end of electrophoresis and variant DNA sequences variants with a higher or lower T_m are separated from the normal sequences. After electrophoresis, specific bands can be isolated from the gel and sequenced.

Heteroduplex Analysis

In heteroduplex analysis (HA), denatured DNA fragments from a control (wild-type) sample and a test DNA sample under investigation are mixed and allowed to reanneal. This can result in homoduplexes of wild-type allele to wild-type allele, or test allele to test allele. It can also result in heteroduplexes of wild-type allele to test allele. The heteroduplexes form partially open dsDNA sequences due to their mismatched base pairs that migrate slower in electrophoresis than the completely dsDNA homoduplexes. Two types of heteroduplexes can be formed depending on the type of mutation present: insertion or deletion mutations cause bulge heteroduplexes that are easily detected, and point mutations cause bubble heteroduplexes that typically requires enhancement for detection.[985–989]

Single-Strand Conformation Polymorphism

The secondary structure or conformation of ssDNA is influenced by its nucleotide sequence. For the single-strand conformation polymorphism (SSCP) procedure, the DNA region under investigation is first amplified. The amplicons are then denatured, and ssDNA amplicons with different nucleotide sequences will have different conformations. The different conformations result in different mobility with gel or capillary electrophoresis, with mutant ssDNA migrated to different locations than wild-type ssDNA. Sequencing of the mutant DNA can subsequently be performed. Since sensitivity is decreased with longer fragments, restriction endonucleases may be used to create shorter fragments, referred to as restriction endonuclease fingerprinting–single-strand conformation polymorphism (REF-SSCP).[990–992]

Bioinformatics and Omics

Great advances have been made in recent years of our understanding of the molecular genetic basis of disease by the use of *bioiniformatics* and *omics* (*genomics*, *transcriptomics*, and *proteomics*).[993–1012] *Bioinformatics* is the use of computers and statistics to perform extensive omics-related research by searching biologic databases and comparing sequences and protein typically on a vast scale to identify sequences or proteins that are different between diseased and healthy tissues, between different biologic behaviors of the same disease, and so on.[1013–1020]

Genomics[1021–1025] studies genomes and their genes by investigating *single nucleotide polymorphisms* (SNPs) and mutations using *high-throughput* genome sequencing techniques such as high-density *DNA microarrays/DNA* (*oligonucleotide*) *chips*.[1026,1027] The base sequence of the genes of the human mitochondrial genome was completed in 1981,[1028] and the base sequence of the genes of the entire human genome was completed in 2003.[1029,1030] Tools for mining of the human genomic sequence data from the International Human Genome Sequencing

Consortium are publicly available.[1031] In addition, there are public databases that can be mined for SNPs, other human DNA polymorphic markers, and the human mitochondrial genome.[1032–1037]

Transcriptomics (also known as *functional genomics*) analyzes gene expression (mRNA) and correlates patterns of expression with biologic function.[1038–1047] Techniques used to study gene expression include serial analysis of gene expression (SAGE), suppression subtractive hybridization (SSH), differential display (DD) analysis, RNA arbitrarily primer-PCR (RAP-PCR), restriction endonucleolytic analysis of differentially expressed sequences (READS), amplified restriction fragment length polymorphism (AFLP), total gene expression analysis (TOGA), and use of internal standard competitive template primers in a quantitative multiplex RT-PCR method [StaRT-(PCR)], high-density cDNA filter hybridization analysis (HDFCA), differential screening (DS), and gene expression microarrays.[1048–1050]

Proteomics studies the structural, functional, and regulatory roles of proteins in the cell and in pathways, including how and where they are expressed.[1051–1069] Since it is the proteins transcribed from the genes and mRNA that ultimately carry out the function of the gene, proteomics is necessary to understand the actual ultimate functioning (or not) of a gene or pathway. Proteomics can be performed on surgically excised tissues, biopsies, including needle biopsies, cytology specimens, serum, and other fluids. Techniques used in proteomics to initially fractionate the groups of proteins in a specimen include two-dimensional gel electrophoresis (two-dimensional polyacrylamide gel electrophoresis [2D-PAGE]) and mass spectrometry. Proteins in a given fraction of sample can then be identified using fingerprinting or sequence tag techniques.

Metabolomics (also known as *metabonomics*) involves study of metabolic profiles by investigating the compounds in a process.[1070–1073] Techniques used in metabolomics include nuclear magnetic resonance and mass spectrometry.

The techniques used in omics are called *high-throughput* because they involve analysis of very large numbers of genes, gene expression, or proteins in one procedure or a combination of procedures. The vast amounts of data generated by these high-throughput studies typically require computers for analysis and comparison of differences between diseased and physiologic cells and tissues, a key feature of bioinformatics. Omics and bioinformatics are used not only for the study of the genes and signaling pathways involved in human diseases, but also for identifying potential targets of therapy and the design of therapeutic drugs. Several of the more common specific technologies used in omics are discussed below.

DNA Microarrays, DNA Chips, and Gene Expression Chips

DNA microarrays are used to simultaneously screen for the presence or expression of large numbers of different genes. Numerous, perhaps thousands, of different microscopic oligonucleotide probes are arranged systematically on a solid support such as glass or silicon, which is called a *DNA chip* or *oligonucleotide chip*.[1074–1076] Sample DNA under investigation is labeled with fluorescent dye, denatured, and then hybridized with the oligonucleotide probes on the chip. The chip is then scanned, and hybridization of the sample DNA to various oligonucleotide probes is detected by fluorescence and analyzed by computer.[1077–1079]

Gene expression chips bind sample mRNA to probes, often numbering thousands of different probes per chip, for analysis of patterns of gene expression compared to normal control tissues.[1080,1081]

Suppression Subtractive Hybridization

Suppression subtractive hybridization (SSH) selectively amplifies target cDNA fragments (differentially expressed genes) and suppresses nontarget DNA.[1082,1083] Total cellular RNA is isolated from two sources of tissue, for example diseased tissue and healthy tissue. The RNA is reverse-transcribed to generate cDNA, and the cDNA is digested with a restriction enzyme to generate small DNA fragments. Specially designed long terminal repeats are attached to the cDNA under investigation, followed by hybridization and PCR. During PCR, the long inverted terminal repeats attached to the DNA fragments selectively suppress amplification of unwanted DNA sequences. This achieves enrichment of the differentially expressed DNA.

Serial Analysis of Gene Expression

Serial analysis of gene expression (SAGE) is used for global analysis of gene expression and provides a comprehensive qualitative and the quantitative expression profile of virtually every gene in a cell population or tissue. SAGE isolates short (9- to 13-bp) sequences, called SAGE tags, from the expressed genes, which are linked together for efficient sequencing. The resulting sequencing data are analyzed to identify each gene and its level of expression expressed in the cells under study. The frequency of each SAGE tag directly reflects the amount of a specific transcript that is present. This technique allows new genes to be discovered since knowledge of the genes in a sample is not required prior to running the procedure. SAGE libraries from different cells and tissues have been created.[1084–1101]

Two-Dimensional Gel Electrophoresis and Mass Spectrometry

In two-dimensional polyacrylamide gel electrophoresis (2D-PAGE; also known as 2D gel electrophoresis), proteins in a sample are separated in a gel based initially on differences in isoelectric points and subsequently based on differences in molecular weight. Proteins with the same isoelectric point and molecular weight are found in the same spot in the gel. The spots of proteins in the gel are visualized with stains, most commonly silver or Coomassie brilliant blue. The spots of proteins in the gel are then excised and digested with trypsin, cyanogens bromide, or other agents. After fractionation, excision, and digestion of the proteins from a sample, several types of mass spectrometry technology are available for the subsequent further identification of specific proteins. *Mass fingerprinting* matches molecular masses of the peptides digested from the fractionated proteins in the sample to known peptide molecular masses in a database to identify proteins from the sample. The *sequence tag* method of identifying a protein involves fragmenting a peptide into a unique spectrum of derived ions in a collision chamber, and the spectra of the peptides are compared to a protein sequence in a database.[1051–1069]

Tissue Microarrays

Tissue microarrays (TMAs) are built by taking punches of cores of tissue from multiple paraffin blocks (donor blocks) and putting these core punches into another paraffin block (recipient block). The end result is a recipient block containing rows and columns of core punches representing tissue from multiple different blocks. Building a TMA requires a special instrument from Beecher Instruments (Sun Prairie, WI), and different-sized cores can be obtained from the donor blocks using needles of various sizes ranging from 0.6 to 2 mm. The recipient paraffin block is processed, and sections are cut for procedures such as immunohistochemistry, allowing the examination of dozens or hundreds of different specimens on only one or a few slides. For example, cores from 100 different lung cancer specimens can be obtained from the original tumor blocks and put into one recipient block. An immunostain for antibody X can be performed on all 100 specimens simply by cutting one section and immunostaining that one section. This saves tissue and time, and reduces technical variation as compared to sectioning, immunostaining, and examining 100 whole tissue sections on separate slides from the same 100 lung cancers.[1102–1105]

Molecular Cytogenetics

Routine cytogenetics with karyotype analyses continues to be popular. Molecular cytogenetics allows investigations that are beyond the abilities of routine cytogenetics. Molecular cytogenetic techniques include fluorescence in-situ hybridization (FISH) and its variants, comparative genomic hybridization, and array comparative genomic hybridization.[1106–1111]

Fluorescence In-Situ Hybridization

DNA or RNA probes with fluorescent tags can be hybridized to DNA within tissue sections, including formalin-fixed, paraffin-embedded tissue sections, or to chromosomes in cytogenetics. A fluorescent-tagged probe complementary to the gene under study is applied to tissue sections or karyotypes on slides. The slides are incubated so that denaturation takes place, and if DNA complementary to the probe is present, hybridization takes place. After washing away excess probe, the slide is examined with fluorescent microscopy that indicates hybridized probe. The application of FISH to formalin-fixed, paraffin-embedded tissue sections allows the pathologist to observe binding of the probes within particular cell types and allows use of archived tissue.[1112,1113]

Fluorescence in-situ hybridization increases detection of chromosomal abnormalities in karyotypes. Conventional chromosome FISH uses a single probe on metaphase spreads and fluorescent spots indicate where the probe has bound to the chromatid. In chromosome painting an entire chromosome fluoresces when multiple different probes bind to many different loci spanning the length of the chromosome.[1114] Multiplex FISH (M-FISH) uses digital imaging to visualize all of the chromosomes simultaneously using all 24 human whole chromosome painting probes. M-FISH is an example of multicolor FISH (mFISH).[1115,1116] Spectral karyotyping (SKY) is another example of mFISH that is also a 24-color, whole chromosome painting assay, allowing the visualization of each chromosome using spectral imaging.[1117–1119] Gold enhanced autometallographic in-situ hybridization (GOLDFISH) is a FISH technique that permits visualization by bright-field microscopy.[1120,1121] A variety of other modifications of FISH have been developed, including comparative genomic hybridization (CGH) (discussed below), PNA-FISH, Q-FISH, and others.[1122]

Chromogenic In-Situ Hybridization

Chromogenic in-situ hybridization (CISH) is based on the same principles as FISH and is useful to identify amplifications and chromosomal translocations. The two procedures are similar, but CISH allows for examination of formalin-fixed, paraffin-embedded tissue sections by bright-field microscopy using digoxigenin-labeled DNA probes and colorization with peroxidase and diaminobenzidine or other chromogen reactions.[1123–1126]

Comparative Genomic Hybridization

Comparative genomic hybridization uses the same principle as FISH to compare genes between two or more different populations.[1127–1131] DNA under investigation is labeled with a fluorochrome and compared to normal or control DNA that is labeled with a different fluorochrome. The ratio between the two determines relative gains or losses of genes. Comparative genomic hybridization may also be microarray-based (A-CGH).[1132–1134]

Genetic Susceptibility to Lung Cancer

Risk of Developing Lung Cancer

The risk of developing lung cancer is strongly associated with exposure to tobacco smoke, which is known to contain numerous carcinogens, procarcinogens, and suspected carcinogens including polycyclic aromatic hydrocarbons (PAHs), aromatic amines, nitrosamines, and free radical species. Other environmental exposures have been implicated in lung cancer, but their influence on the risk of developing lung cancer is small compared to the risk associated with tobacco smoking. However, not everyone with the same or similar tobacco exposure develops lung cancer. Only 10% to 20% of tobacco smokers develop lung cancer. This naturally leads to the question of why some smokers develop lung cancer and other smokers, with equivalent exposures, do not. On the other hand, about 10% to 15% of lung cancers occur in never-smokers. These individuals may have had exposure to identified or unidentified environmental carcinogens or procarcinogens, although many are classified as "idiopathic," but, since many more individuals have had these same environmental exposures and not developed lung cancer, the question again comes up as to what distinguishes those who develop lung cancer from environmental exposures or "spontaneously" as opposed to those with the same exposures who do not.

A widely held view is that individuals have differing susceptibility to the risk factors for cancer, including lung cancer.[1135–1153] This differing susceptibility would explain why some individuals with an exposure to a risk factor get cancer and others with an equivalent exposure do not. It would also help explain why some individuals get cancer with minimal risk-factor exposures or at a younger age compared to the average cancer patient. The observation that differing susceptibility appears to be inherited based on aggregation of cancers within families suggests that there is a genetic basis for this susceptibility.[1154–1181] An inherited susceptibility would help explain special categories of patients, such as those who develop lung cancer with minimal or no exposure to tobacco,[1182–1188] often in association with family histories of cancer,[1189–1193] or those who succumb to exposure at a notably earlier age than average.[1194–1197] This genetic susceptibility to cancer has a potential basis in inherited polymorphisms of genes whose products impact the individual's ability to repair DNA damage from exposures to carcinogens or whose products metabolize carcinogens to more potent forms or detoxify carcinogens. These inherited polymorphisms do not cause cancer themselves, but rather influence the effect of an exposure and the individual's response to the exposure.

Familial Risk of Lung Cancer

Multiple studies have shown an increased incidence of lung cancer and other cancers among relatives and family members of patients with lung cancer.[1154–1181] Since family members often share common environments as well as common genetics, this familial increase might potentially also be due to common exposures among family members living in the same environment or sharing common lifestyles. Therefore, potentially confounding factors such as shared smoking habits, second-hand smoke, and mutual occupational exposures should be taken into consideration before a familial cluster of cancer can be attributed to genetics. Several studies have taken these confounding factors into account and found statistically significant increased risk of lung cancer among relatives of lung cancer patients compared to controls.[1156,1160–1170,1174–1181] In particular, studies of families of nonsmokers and of younger patients with lung cancer have found an increased familial risk, which is additional evidence that genetic susceptibility is a factor in the development of lung cancer.[1163,1165,1175,1182–1197]

Presumably, at least some of the familial risk of lung cancer is likely due to inherited polymorphisms in the DNA repair genes (discussed previously) and xenobiotic-metabolizing enzyme genes discussed below. Current techniques allow investigation of potential chromosomal loci for lung cancer susceptibility in families. For example, a lung cancer susceptibility locus has been mapped to chromosome 6q23–25 in a study of multigenerational families with lung, throat, and laryngeal cancer.[1172]

Gender and Risk of Lung Cancer

Many investigators have examined potential gender differences in lung cancer susceptibility.[1198–1205] Some authors have argued that women smokers have an increased risk of developing lung cancer compared to men smokers with equivalent smoking histories,[1206–1208] while others have concluded that there are no differences.[1209,1210] A study of 7498 women and 9427 men by the International Early Lung Cancer Action Program Investigators concluded that women appear to have an increased susceptibility to tobacco carcinogens.[1205] On the other hand, an analysis of smoking and lung cancers from the Nurses'

Health Study of over 60,000 women and the Health Professionals Follow-Up Study of over 25,000 men failed to find convincing evidence of an increased lung cancer risk among women.[1210]

Several reasons for reported differences in gender-associated lung cancer susceptibility have been proposed. Hormonal influences and environmental factors may play a role. However, differences in xenobiotic-metabolizing enzymes between the sexes have also been proposed as influences on susceptibility to lung cancer.[1211,1212]

Xenobiotic-Metabolizing Enzymes

Exogenous chemicals that enter the body such as drugs, toxins, poisons, and solvents are known as xenobiotics. Xenobiotics are altered by xenobiotic-metabolizing enzymes. The xenobiotics may induce xenobiotic-metabolizing enzymes by various methods: they may act as substrate-ligands that bind receptors and activate the xenobiotic enzymes by transcription or they may stabilize the protein product. Phase I xenobiotic-metabolizing enzymes metabolize the xenobiotic chemicals into other compounds. Ironically, the phase I enzymes may cause metabolic bioactivation of xenobiotic substrates, converting them into active or more potent toxins or carcinogens known as reactive intermediates. Phase II enzymes detoxify these reactive intermediates and convert them into compounds that can be removed from the body. The cytochrome P-450s (CYPs) are an important class of phase I xenobiotic-metabolizing enzymes, and the glutathione-S-transferases GST(s) are an important class of phase II enzymes. Phase III transporters are involved in xenobiotic transport and excretion and include P-glycoprotein (P-gp), multidrug resistance-associated proteins (MRPs), and organic anion transporting polypeptide 2 (OATP2).[1213–1223]

The primary activity of the phase I enzyme CYPs is to catalyze oxidation of xenobiotics, although they may also sometimes catalyze reduction reactions (CYPs are also involved in other processes such as biosynthesis of steroid hormones and prostaglandins).[1224–1235] These reactions occur predominantly in the liver, but also take place in other tissues including the lungs.[1236–1240] CYP-dependent metabolism often produces intermediate compounds (reactive intermediates) that may be more potent as carcinogens than the parent compounds and that may bind covalently to DNA to form adducts. DNA adduct formation is considered an important step in carcinogenesis. These intermediate compounds are also the targets for phase II enzyme-dependent conjugation reactions that convert them to more soluble, inactive products that can be excreted or compartmentalized. Thus, CYP metabolism is potentially a double-edged sword, leading to production of reactive intermediates that are more carcinogenic than the original compounds but also more readily detoxified and removed than the original compounds. Nearly 60 active human P-450 genes are known and the majority are polymorphic. The CYP allele home page can be found at http://www.imm.ki.se/cypalleles. CYP enzymes and genes are designated by family number (an Arabic number), subfamily letter (A, B, C, etc.), and individual members of a subfamily (also an Arabic number). Class I polymorphic CYP enzymes metabolize procarcinogens and include *CYP1A1*, *CYP1A2*, *CYP1B1*, *CYP2A6*, *CYP2E1*, and *CYP3A4*. In particular, *CYP1A1* and *CYP1B1* are involved in the metabolism of polycyclic aromatic hydrocarbons (PAHs) from tobacco smoke, whereas *CYP2A6* and *CYP2E1* are involved in the metabolism of nitrosamines from tobacco smoke.[1224–1235]

Several CYPs are induced by the aryl hydrocarbon receptor (AhR), which dimerizes with the AhR nuclear translocator (Arnt) and induces expression of *CYP1A1* and *CYP1B1*, which encode aryl hydrocarbon hydroxylases, as well as *CYP1A2*. Ligands for AhR include PAHs and other xenobiotics, which are also substrates for the activated CYP enzymes. AhR may have low affinity or high affinity for its ligands producing low or high inducibility of CYP1 enzymes. After binding its ligand, AhR translocates into the nucleus and dimerizes with Arnt protein. The AhR/Arnt dimer binds to xenobiotic responsive elements (XREs) of the *CYP1A1* gene, activating its transcription.[1241–1244]

Benzo(a)pyrene is a PAH in tobacco smoke that has been extensively studied. When benzo(a)pyrene enters the lungs, it binds to AhR resulting in the induction of *CYP1A1* and *CYP1B1*. The benzo(a)pyrene is metabolically activated to benzo[*a*]pyrene-7,8-diol-9,10-epoxide (BPDE) by the CYP enzymes. BPDE is a carcinogen that damages DNA by covalently bonding to the DNA, forming bulky chemical adducts, for example by binding to guanine nucleobases in codons 157, 248, and 273 of *p53*, identified as mutational "hotspots" in smoking-related lung cancers.[1245–1252] In addition to PAHs, tobacco smoke also contains *N*-nitrosamines including 4-(methylnitrosoamino)-1-(3-pyridyl)-1-butanone (NNK), *N*-dimethylnitrosoamine (NDMA), *N*-diethylnitrosoamine (NDEA), *N*-nitrosophenylmethyl-amine (NMPhA), and *N*-nitrosonornicotine (NNN). The inhaled *N*-nitrosamines are metabolically activated by *CYP2A6* and *CYP2E1* to compounds that form chemical adducts with DNA.[1253–1258]

The primary activity of the phase II enzymes GSTs is to catalyze the conjugation of glutathione (GSH) to xenobiotics containing an electrophilic center, forming more soluble, nontoxic peptides that can be excreted or compartmentalized by other enzymes (phase III enzymes). The GST superfamily consists of enzymes that catalyze the conjunction of glutathione to xenobiotics and is divided into three subfamilies, each composed of multigene families: soluble or cytosolic (canonical) GSTs, microsomal or MAPEG (membrane-associated proteins involved in eicosanoid and glutathione metabolism) GSTs, and the plasmid-encoded bacterial fosfomycin-resistance GSTs. The cytosolic GSTs are polymorphic and are divided into seven classes: alpha, mu, and pi are considered specific, and sigma, omega, theta, and zeta are considered common. Of particular interest among the cytosolic GSTs in the metabolism of tobacco-derived carcinogens; GSTM1, GSTM3 and GSTP1 detoxify reactive intermediates of PAHs such as benzo(a)pyrene, and GSTT1 detoxifies reactive oxidants such as ethylene oxide.[1259–1263]

Other phase II enzymes include *N*-acetyltransferases (NAT), sulfotransferases (ST), UDP-glucuronosyltransferases (UGT), and NAD(P)H:quinone oxidoreductase (NQO1). Microsomal epoxide hydrolase (mEH) is a phase II enzyme that can also act as a phase I enzyme. mEH catalyzes the *trans*-addition of water to xenobiotics such as PAHs, including benzo(a)pyrene, producing dihydrodiol reactive intermediates involved in PAH-initiated carcinogenesis.[1264–1268]

DNA Adducts and Lung Cancer

DNA adducts from metabolically activated intermediates of compounds in tobacco smoking are considered mutagenic and carcinogenic.[1269–1272] Bulky DNA adducts can be detected by 32P-postlabeling of tumor tissues, peripheral blood lymphocytes and other tissues, immunoassays and immunohistochemistry, high-performance liquid chromatography (HPLC)-electrochemical detection, mass spectrometry, fluorescence, and phosphorescence spectroscopy.[1273] PAH-DNA adducts can be recognized by BPDE-DNA immunoassays such as the BPDE-DNA chemiluminescence immunoassay (BPDE-DNA CIA).[1274]

Increased levels of DNA adducts have been reported in lung tissues and other tissues in smokers. DNA adducts are more numerous in patients with smoking-related cancers such as lung cancer than in patients without cancer.[1275–1281] A meta-analysis in 2003 by Veglia et al.[1279] included data on 691 cancer patients and 632 controls from six studies (five studies involved lung cancer, one study oral cancer and one study bladder cancer). In this meta-analysis, current smokers with smoking-related cancers showed a statistically significant 83% higher level of adducts than controls. In a study of 85 lung cancer patients (47 smokers, 23 long-term former smokers, 15 never smokers), Gyorffy et al.[1280] found elevated levels of DNA adducts in smokers' lungs as compared to nonsmokers'/never-smokers' lungs.

Based on these studies and studies demonstrating the carcinogenicity of DNA adducts from tobacco smoke, one would expect a link between the number of DNA adducts and the development of lung cancer. In retrospective case-control studies, it is not possible to entirely exclude that levels of adducts could be a result of the disease rather than the cause of the disease. Prospective studies in which adducts were measured in blood samples collected years before the onset of cancer strongly support that adducts are a cause of cancer rather than an effect of cancer. In a 2001 nested case-control study using blood samples collected from subjects enrolled in the prospective Physicians' Health Study, Tang et al.[1276] compared samples from 89 subjects who developed primary lung cancers to 173 controls. They observed that disease-free current smokers with elevated levels of DNA adducts in blood leukocytes were three times more likely to be diagnosed with lung cancer 1 to 13 years later than current smokers with lower DNA adduct levels.

In a 2005 nested case-control study of subjects from France, Denmark, Germany, Greece, Italy, the Netherlands, Norway, Spain, Sweden, and United Kingdom in the European Prospective Investigation into Cancer and Nutrition (EPIC) investigation, Peluso et al.[1281] also measured the levels of DNA adducts in blood samples collected several years before the onset of cancer. Levels of leukocyte DNA adducts were associated with the subsequent risk of lung cancer. The association with lung cancer was stronger in never-smokers (whose sources would be environmental such as air pollution and second-hand tobacco smoke) and in younger patients. These prospective studies indicate a relationship between adduct levels and risk of lung cancer, and suggest that individuals have different susceptibilities to carcinogen exposures, highlighted by the risks observed in those with fewer years of exposure (younger patients) and those with lesser levels of exposure (never smokers).

Polymorphisms and Adduct Levels

Differences in DNA-adduct levels are related not only to levels of exposure but also to the activity levels of xenobiotic enzymes.[1282–1288] Some alleles of specific xenobiotic enzymes are more active than others. A highly active variant of a phase I enzyme (extensive metabolizer) might produce a greater number of reactive intermediates and, therefore, more DNA-adducts than a less active variant of the same phase I enzyme (poor metabolizer). A less active variant of a phase II enzyme might detoxify reactive intermediates at a slower rate than a more active variant, resulting in a greater accumulation of reactive intermediates and, hence, creating the potential for more DNA-adducts. Therefore, polymorphisms of xenobiotic enzymes have the prospect of contributing to differing adduct levels in individuals, which could cause differing susceptibilities to lung cancer among individuals. A similar principle holds when less active variants of DNA repair genes repair damage from adducts (or other sources) at a reduced rate.

Studies have shown that differing DNA adduct levels may occur in association with different variants of xenobiotic enzymes.[1282–1288] Individuals lacking the GSTM1 enzyme have higher DNA adduct levels compared to GSTM1-positive individuals. GPX1 is a phase II enzyme that conjugates polycyclic aromatic hydrocarbon-diols to glutathione. In GPX1, the *Pro198Leu* allelic variant has a lower enzyme activity, resulting in less detoxification and hence higher adduct levels compared with wild-type individuals. mEH functions as a phase II enzyme and the slow allelic variant *mEH*2* results in increased epoxide intermediates and hence higher DNA adduct levels.[1288]

Investigations of Specific Polymorphisms and Lung Cancer Susceptibility

As described further below, studies of polymorphisms of xenobiotic-metabolizing genes and DNA repair genes have identified potential allelic variants associated with greater or lesser risk of lung cancer.[1289–1292] The concept that polymorphisms of xenobiotic metabolizing enzymes and DNA repair enzymes is very attractive, but, overall, investigations that correlate single-locus alleles with lung cancer risk have produced apparently conflicting results. There are several likely reasons for this. Numbers of cases in some studies may be too few to reliably assess any moderate effects on the risk of lung cancer. The polymorphisms studied may vary. Different ethnic groups have widely differing frequencies of some polymorphisms, which impacts the results according to the ethnic group studied. The metabolism, detoxification, and repair processes involving DNA adducts are complex and it is very unlikely that one single polymorphism accounts for differences in DNA adduct levels. Studies that analyze many polymorphisms simultaneously in a single population are more likely to produce more comprehensive and consistent results. Newer technologies that permit study of SNPs and haplotypes increase statistical sensitivity.[1292] Linkage disequilibrium (LD)-based strategies are likely to improve detection of the alleles that contribute to common diseases like lung cancer.[1289–1292]

Xenobiotic Metabolizing Genes

CYP Polymorphisms and Susceptibility to Lung Cancer

In 1984, Ayesh et al.[1293] proposed an association between a polymorphism of *CYP* (debrisoquine 4–hydroxylase or *CYP2D6*), and lung cancer risk. In 1990, Kawajiri et al.[1294] suggested that polymorphisms of *CYP1A1* might impact on lung cancer risk. Subsequent studies of *CYP2D6* polymorphisms have produced mixed results.[1295–1300] Several *CYP1A1* alleles have attracted great interest.

The *CYP1A1 m1* allele, also known as *Msp*I, has a T to C transition in the 3′ noncoding flanking region and has increased enzyme activity. In 1991, Hayashi et al.[1301] were the first to describe a transition of adenine to guanine at position 2455 in exon 7 of *CYP1A1*, resulting in an isoleucine to valine amino acid substitution at codon 462 (Ile462Val). Similar to the *MspI* allele, the valine allele or *CYP1A1 m2* allele (also known as *CYP1A1*2C)* has increased enzymatic activity (extensive metabolizer), believed to result in greater carcinogenic adduct production and higher risk of tobacco smoke–related lung cancer. The *CYP1A1 m3* allele, with a mutation in intron 7, appears to be specific to African-Americans, whereas the *CYP1A1 m4* allele has a transition in exon 7 that results in a Thr for Asn substitution.[1301–1313]

Numerous studies have examined the potential association between *CYP1A1* polymorphisms and the risk of lung cancer in various ethnic populations.[1314–1354] *CYP1A1 m1* and *m2* polymorphisms are strongly correlated with the risk of lung cancer in multiple studies from Japan, particularly in regard to tobacco smokers and squamous cell carcinomas.[1314,1317,1319,1320,1325,1327,1335] In a 2001 study of 217 lung cancer cases and 404 controls from China, Song et al.[1345] reported an increased risk for squamous cell carcinoma of the lung in subjects having at least one *CYP1A1 m1* allele or at least one *CYP1A1 m2* allele, similar to findings by Lin et al.[1341] Persson et al.[1337] failed to note an association between *CYP1A1* polymorphisms and a Chinese population that consisted largely of women with adenocarcinomas.

The prevalence of the *CYP1A1 m1* and *m2* alleles is very low in Caucasians and, therefore, past studies have shown mixed results in regard to these polymorphisms and the risk of lung cancer in Caucasians.[1318,1321,1322,1331,1333,1334] A pooled analysis of data on Caucasians from 11 studies with 1153 lung cancer cases and 1449 controls in 2003 by Le Marchand et al.[1346] reported an increased risk of lung cancer, especially squamous cell carcinoma, in association with the *CYP1A1 m2* allele. A 2005 study of 1050 lung cancers and 581 controls Larsen et al.[1351] found an association between the *CYP1A1 m2* allele and lung cancer risk, particularly among women, younger individuals, and those with lesser smoking histories. Studies of American populations of mixed ethnicity have also found an increased risk of lung cancer associated with the *CYP1A1 m1* allele.[1331,1333,1334] An increased risk of lung cancer in association with the *CYP1A1 m2* allele has been reported in studies from Brazil.[1324,1328] An increased risk for adenocarcinoma of the lung, but not all types of lung cancer, has been reported among African Americans in association with the *CYP1A1 m3* allele.[1323,1326,1329,1336]

CYP2A6

CYP2A6 metabolically bioactivates *N*-nitrosamines in tobacco smoke. Several alleles of *CYP2A6* have been identified—*CYP2A6*4C*, *CYP2A6*7*, *CYP2A6*9*, and *CYP2A6*10*—which have decreased enzyme activity or decreased expression of *CYP2A6*. Consistent with the decreased metabolic bioactivation of *N*-nitrosamines, these variant alleles are associated with a decreased risk of lung cancer, particularly in regard to squamous cell carcinoma and small cell carcinoma and in heavy smokers compared to light smokers and nonsmokers.[1355–1368]

Other CYP *Alleles*

A number of other *CYP* gene alleles have undergone investigation as potential markers of lung cancer susceptibility including *CYP2A13*,[1369,1370] *CYP2E*,[1371,1372] and *CYP3A*,[1373] but data are limited.

Aryl Hydrocarbon Receptor

The aryl hydrocarbon receptor alleles have undergone limited investigation as markers of lung cancer susceptibility and, so far, no association with increased lung cancer risk has been found.[1374,1375]

Microsomal Epoxide Hydrolase

Several studies have reported that microsomal epoxide hydrolase (mEH) alleles with high activity have been associated with higher risk of smoking-related lung cancers compared to those with low activity.[1376–1381]

Glutathione-S-Transferases and Susceptibility to Lung Cancer

Variants of GST have been investigated in regard to lung cancer risk, producing mixed results.[1382–1410] GST polymorphisms may also influence cell type of lung cancers.[1411–1413] These alleles occur in the GSTM1, GSTT1, GSTP1, and GSTM3 *genes and are associated with the reduced activity or deletion (with loss of all activity) of these phase II enzymes.* These include the GSTM1*0 (GSTM1 null) allele, which is a deletion of the *GSTM1* gene; the GSTT1*0 (GSTT1 null) allele, which is a deletion of the GSTT1 gene; the GSTP1 Ile105Val variant (I105V) due to an A to G transition; the *GSTP1* Ala-114Val variant (A114V) due to a C to T transition; and the GSTM3 intron 6 polymorphism, a 3-bp deletion in intron 6.

In a 2002 nested case-control study of 89 lung cancer cases and 173 controls within the prospective Physicians' Health Study, Perera et al.,[1400] after controlling for level of smoking, concluded that adducts were significant predictors of lung cancer risk, the combined *GSTM1* null/*GSTP1* Val genotype was associated with lung cancer overall and especially among former smokers, and adducts were significantly higher among current or former smokers with lung cancer who had the *GSTM1* non-null/*GSTP1* Ile genotype.

In 2006, Ye et al.[1410] published a meta-analysis with data from 130 studies, with 23,452 lung cancer cases and 30,397 controls. They concluded that there was a weak association of the GSTM1 null and GSTT1 null polymorphisms with lung cancer risk, with possibly weaker associations in studies of individuals of European descent, whereas the *GSTP1105V*, *GSTP1114V*, and the GSTM3 intron 6 polymorphisms had no significant overall associations with lung cancer.

Other Phase II Xenobiotic Enzymes

Studies of *NQO1* alleles have produced mixed results in regard to an association with lung cancer risk.[1414–1418] *NQO1* variant allele associated with reduced activity was associated with increased risk of lung cancer in younger individuals, women, and never-smokers in a recent study by Saldivar et al.[1418]

Conflicting conclusions have been reached in studies of *NAT1* alleles and lung cancer risk.[1419–1423] In a recent study, Habalova et al.[1423] found that a slow acetylation variant (*NAT2*5B/*6*) was associated with risk of squamous cell carcinoma in younger patients, non-smokers and women.

Wang et al.[1424] reported an increased risk of lung cancer in association with the *SULT1A1*2* allele (variant A-allele), which codes for a *SULT1A1* sulfotransferase enzyme with decreased activity.

Multiple Xenobiotic Metabolizing Enzymes

Since the metabolism of xenobiotics is a complex process involving multiple enzymes, an accurate understanding of lung cancer susceptibility requires information on the interactions of multiple genes and effects of multiple enzymes. Some studies have looked at the combined effects of two or more xenobiotic enzymes.[1425–1433]

Hung et al.[1428] performed a pooled analysis of data from 14 case–control studies on 302 lung cancer cases and 1631 controls in Caucasian nonsmokers from the International Collaborative Study on Genetic Susceptibility to Environmental Carcinogens, published in 2003. They reported an increased lung cancer risk with the combined *CYP1A1 Ile462Val* variant and *GSTM1* null genotype compared with the *CYP1A1* wild-type and *GSTM1* non-null genotype.

In 2005 Raimondi et al.[1433] published a meta-analysis of data from 21 case-control studies for a total of 2764 Caucasians (555 lung cancer cases and 2209 controls) and 383 Asians (113 lung cancer cases and 270 controls) who had never smoked on a regular basis from the International Collaborative Study on Genetic Susceptibility to

Environmental Carcinogens. In their analysis of multiple xenobiotic metabolizing enzymes, they concluded that there is a significant association between lung cancer and *CYP1A1Ile462Val* polymorphism in Caucasians, *GSTT1* deletion is a risk factor for lung cancer in Caucasian nonsmokers only in studies including healthy controls, and that the combination of *CYP1A1 wild-type*, *GSTM1 null*, and *GSTT1 non-null* genotypes was associated with a decreased risk of lung cancer. None of the polymorphisms that they examined was associated with lung cancer in Asian nonsmokers.

DNA Repair Gene Polymorphisms and Susceptibility to Lung Cancer

Genes and their products involved in DNA damage repair were discussed earlier (see DNA Damage Repair). DNA repair capacity (DRC) can be measured in cultured lymphocytes using the host-cell reactivation assay and a reporter gene damaged by the activated tobacco carcinogen BPDE. In the general population, a fivefold variation in DRC has been observed. Decreased DRC has been associated with an increased risk of lung cancer.[1434–1438]

Polymorphisms in DNA repair genes may be associated with differences in efficiency of DNA repair. Decreased or increased ability to repair DNA damage is expected to influence the accumulation of significant genetic abnormalities necessary for the development of cancer. This has led to investigation of inherited polymorphisms of the DNA repair genes as factors in lung cancer susceptibility.

Nucleotide Excision Repair Pathway Polymorphisms

As discussed previously, the NER pathway removes bulky PAH-DNA adducts, and thus has been a key area of study in regard to lung cancer susceptibility. Subsequent to recognition of DNA damage such as bulky adducts by the XPC-hHR23B complex, the helicase activities of XPD (also known as ERCC2) and XPB permit opening of the DNA double helix, allowing the damaged segment of DNA to be excised and removed. The XPD protein is a necessary component of the NER pathway. Point mutations in *XPD* result in DNA repair-deficiency diseases including xeroderma pigmentosum, trichothiodystrophy, and Cockayne syndrome. Patients with xeroderma pigmentosum have a very high predilection for cancers, highlighting the association between DNA repair efficiency and the risk of cancer (see above).

Prevalence of *XPD* alleles and genotypes varies markedly according to ethnicity. Polymorphisms in codons 156, 312, 711, and 751 of the *XPD* gene are common (allele frequency >20%). Polymorphisms of codon G23592A (Asp312Asn) of exon 10 and codon A35931C (Lys751Gln) of exon 23 cause amino acid changes in the XPD protein and have been investigated in regard to susceptibility to lung cancer.[1439–1459] Some studies have looked at the levels of DNA adducts associated with these polymorphisms as an indication of the efficiency of the different alleles at DNA repair. Presumably a higher level of adducts suggests less efficiency of the allele at excising DNA adducts. In regard to codon 312 polymorphisms, most studies report a higher level of DNA adducts in association with the *Asn* allele than with the *Asp* allele. In regard to the 751 polymorphism, most studies indicate a higher level of DNA adducts in association with the *Gln* allele. Therefore, most studies seem to indicate that there is a difference in DNA repair efficiency between these specific *XPD* alleles.[1439–1459]

In a meta-analysis published in 2004 of data from nine case-control studies with 3725 lung cancer cases and 4152, Hu et al.[1454] concluded that individuals with the *XPD 751CC* genotype have a 21% higher risk of lung cancer versus those with the *XPD 751AA* genotype, and those with the *XPD 312AA* genotype have a 27% higher risk of lung cancer compared to those with the *XPD 312GG* genotype. In 2005, Benhamou and Sarasin[1456] performed a meta-analysis derived from the same studies as Hu et al., but provided a different approach and conclusions. In a meta-analysis that included 2886 cases and 3085 controls for the *XPD*-312 polymorphism from six studies, and 3374 cases and 3880 controls for the *XPD*-751 polymorphism from seven studies, Benhamou and Sarasin felt that there was no conclusive proof from these data that one or the other of these polymorphisms was associated with an increased risk of lung cancer.

Noting the results of these two meta-analyses, Hu et al.[1458] performed a case-control study of 1010 lung cancer cases and 1011 age- and sex-matched cancer-free controls in a Chinese population and examined eight SNPs/DIPs (deletion/insertion polymorphisms) of *XPD/ERCC2* and *XPB/ERCC3*. None of the eight polymorphisms was individually associated with risk of lung cancer, but the authors found that combination of genetic variants in *ERCC2* and *ERCC3* contributed to lung cancer risk in a dose-response manner.

Other studies have indicated an increased risk of lung cancer with combinations of XPD polymorphisms and polymorphisms of other DNA repair genes. Zhou et al.[1453] reported significantly increased lung cancer risk in individuals with five or six variant alleles of *XPD Asp*312*Asn*, *XPD Lys*751*Gln*, and *XRCC1 Arg*399*Gln* polymorphisms in comparison with persons with no variant alleles. Chen et al.[1444] reported that individuals with variant alleles for both *XPD Lys*751*Gln* and *XRCC1 Arg*194*Trp* polymorphisms have a higher lung cancer risk than individuals with only one variant allele in a Chinese population.

Other DNA Repair Genes

Other DNA repair gene polymorphisms have undergone limited study in regard to lung cancer susceptibility, typically with conflicting or unconfirmed results, including *XPA*,[1460–1462] *XPC*,[1463,1464] *XPG*,[1465] *XRCC1*,[1466–1472] *XRCC3*,[1473] *MMH/OGG1*, the BER pathway,[1474–1479] and *MGMT*.[1480–1482] In a study of *ATM* genotypes in 616 lung cancer patients and 616 cancer-free controls, Kim et al.[1483] found that the A allele at the site (IVS62 + 60G → A) was associated with a higher lung cancer risk than the G allele. Individuals with the ATTA haplotype showed significantly increased risk of lung cancer compared to those with the common GCCA haplotype, and individuals with the (NN)TA haplotype showed an increased lung cancer risk compared with those without the (NN)TA haplotype.

Multiple DNA Repair Genes

In a 2006 study of 44 SNPs in 20 DNA repair genes in 343 non–small-cell carcinomas and 413 controls form the Norwegian general population, Zienolddiny et al.[1484] reported the following results: (1) for the NER pathway, *ERCC1* (Asn118Asn, C → T), *ERCC1* (C15310G) and *ERCC2* (Lys751Gln) variants were associated with increased lung cancer risk, and *XPA*, *G23A*, and *ERCC5/XPG* (His46His) variants were associated with decreased lung cancer risk; (2) for the BER pathway, *OGG1* (Ser-326Cys) and *PCNA* (A1876G) variants were associated with increased lung cancer risk, the *APE1/APEX* (Ile64Val) variant was associated with decreased lung cancer risk, and the variant T allele of PCNA2352 SNP had a marginal effect on cancer risk; (3) for the DSB-R pathway, the *XRCC2* (Arg188His) variant was associated with increased lung cancer risk and *XRCC9* (Thr297Ile) and *ATR* (Thr211Met) variants were associated with decreased lung cancer risk; (4) for the DR pathway, the *MGMT/AGT* (Leu84Phe) variant in exon 3 showed a slight trend toward a higher lung cancer risk.

Other Markers of Lung Cancer Susceptibility

A large number of potential markers of lung cancer susceptibility have been examined in addition to those discussed above. Most of these have been investigated only once or a few times, and therefore conclusions have not been confirmed. These markers include common fragile sites (nonstaining gaps and breaks in specific points of chromosomes that are inducible by various clastogenic agents),[1485–1489] mutagen sensitivity (measured by the frequency of bleomycin-induced breaks in an in vitro lymphocyte assay),[1490–1492] and alleles or polymorphisms of the following: germline p53,[1493–1496] vascular endothelial growth factor (VEGF),[1497] hMLH1,[1498] human leukocyte antigen (HLA)-DRB1–related alleles,[1499] HRAS1 VNTR,[1500–1502] K-Ras,[1503] promoter of receptor for advanced glycosylation end products (RAGE),[1504] matrix metalloproteinase promoters,[1505–1509] myeloperoxidase,[1510–1514] L-*myc*,[1515,1516] surfactant genes,[1517,1518] *D19S246* locus,[1519] cyclin D1,[1520] IL-1β,[1521,1522] IL-10 promoter,[1523] methylenetetrahydrofolate reductase,[1524] *p73*,[1525] combined *p73* and *p53*,[1526] DNMT3B,[1527] cyclooxygenase-2 (prostaglandin synthase 2),[1528–1530] Semaphorin 3B (SEMA3B) T4151,[1531] folate metabolic genes,[1532] FAS and FASL,[1533] SDF-1,[1534] α_1-antitrypsin,[1535] MDM2 promoter,[1536–1538] EGFR,[1539] MBD1,[1540] MBD4,[1541] TGF,[1542] PDCD,[1543] leptin,[1544] caspase 9 promoter,[1545] and GH-IGF.[1546]

Molecular Pathology of Lung Cancer

Carcinogenesis

Carcinogenesis is a complex, multistep process in which normal cells gradually give rise to cancer cells over a period of months and years. The development of cancer from a normal cell requires the accumulation of multiple genetic and epigenetic abnormalities that result in loss of control of the cell cycle, abnormal expression and function of receptors and signaling pathways, impaired repair of DNA damage, impaired apoptosis, and other abnormalities that cause unrestricted proliferation of cells. The accumulated genetic and epigenetic abnormalities are inherited by daughter cells that continue to accumulate more abnormalities and pass them on to the next generation of cells, forming clones of cells with genetic abnormalities. Progressive cytologic and histopathologic changes accompany the accumulation of these genetic and epigenetic abnormalities and a transition from normal cells to preneoplastic cells to noninvasive cancer cells to invasive cancer cells. The accumulating genetic abnormalities provide malignant cells with distinctive means for cell survival, nutrition, resistance to host immunity, proliferation, and metastasis.

Researchers initially focused primarily on sets of functionally related genes in their studies of carcinogenesis,[1547] but focusing only on genomic alterations or RNA expression does not provide a complete understanding of cancer biology. Even in cases of gene amplification, the expression of mRNA can be inhibited by small inhibitory RNAs (siRNA), sometimes residing on introns close to the amplified gene.[1548] Also, highly expressed mRNAs may not be translated into proteins. It is now recognized that an integrated approach including investigations at the DNA, RNA, and protein levels is necessary to understand carcinogenesis.[1547]

As already noted, the development and progression of cancer from normal tissues occurs in a stepwise manner. In the early stages of cancer development, loss of cell cycle regulation by regulatory genes appears to play a major role, facilitating the proliferation of preneoplastic cells within the epithelium.[1549–1552] In this early stage, recognizable phenotypic changes may not be present and preneoplastic cells may appear histologically similar to neighboring normal cells.[1553] This is particularly evident in peripheral pulmonary carcinogenesis, where neoplastic cells develop along similar lines as reactive proliferation or regeneration of nonneoplastic cells, phenotypically simulating Clara-type secretory cylindrical cells, and cuboidal type II pneumocytes. Therefore, the preneoplastic lesions that have so far been identified either extend along the bronchiolar epithelium (bronchiolar columnar cell dysplasia[1554]), the alveolar epithelium (atypical adenomatous hyperplasia[1555]), or both (atypical goblet cell hyperplasia[1556]). Extension of these lesions most probably also includes growth within the epithelium.[1557,1558]

Preinvasive lesions may eventually become invasive. In order for invasion to occur, expression of enzymes such as collagenases, proteinases, and elastases is necessary to dissolve the basement membrane proteins, producing gaps for the cancer cells to penetrate.[1548,1559–1562] In addition, interaction of the cancer cells with host stromal cells and immune competent cells allows the invading cells to avoid host reactions.[1563] Invasive carcinoma cells have to adapt to the new environment, which involves anchorage independent growth[1564–1566] and movement of cancer cells along matrix proteins by upregulation of integrin molecules.[1567–1569] This is most often facilitated by the expression of specific adhesion molecules or downregulation of others, which correspond to the respective ligands of matrix proteins.[1570–1572] Invasion by carcinoma cells also induces a desmoplastic stroma reaction in the host, a process that currently is poorly understood, but which may have conflicting consequences. The stromal reaction results in remodeling, which is believed to enhance invasion by the cancer cells in some instances.[1562,1573–1575] However, in other cases, a desmoplastic stroma may inhibit invasion of carcinoma cells, unless the carcinoma cells undergo an epithelial-mesenchymal transition, converting into a spindle cell phenotype.[1576–1578] In addition, invasion might also stimulate a host immune response (see below).

The process of remodeling is especially important in peripheral lung because a loss of alveolar architecture is accompanied by a loss of function.[1579] Possibly because bronchioloalveolar carcinomas (BACs) fail to induce remodeling of the lung architecture, they are able to avoid stromal cell interaction.

Following tissue invasion, malignant cells may progress to lymphatic or blood vessel invasion. For vascular invasion, enzyme expression is required to dissolve the basal lamina of the respective vessels, similar to the enzymatic processes required for tissue invasion. In most instances, lung cancer cells invade and travel in the lymphatics, spreading to regional lymph nodes. In the lymph nodes, survival of malignant cells requires that they avoid detection and subsequent activation of dendritic cells and recruitment of immune cells. Malignant cells may express various receptors that cause lymphocyte adherence and activate apoptotic signaling in the adhering lymphocytes.[1580] Other defense mechanisms that may protect cancer cells from host response are production of antibodies against tumor-associated proteins,[1581,1582] activation of regulatory lymphocytes,[1583–1585] and secretion of molecules, which either cause downregulation of the immune system[1586–1589] or induce apoptosis of stromal and immune cells.[1590–1592]

Once established in lymph nodes, cancer cells proliferate, populate the lymph nodes, and finally enter the blood circulation. Some carcinomas, such as small cell lung carcinoma (SCLC), more frequently directly invade the systemic circulation, whereas adenocarcinoma (AC) and squamous cell carcinoma (SCC) more often initially invade lymphatics.

Present data indicate that most cancer cells die in the blood vessels entrapped within coagulative proteins that obstruct their nutrient and oxygen supply. Those cells that escape the coagulative proteins probably do so by expression of fibrinolytic enzymes.[1593]

Cancer cells in the circulation travel with express selectins or homing molecules. These molecules direct the cancer cells to specific sites, which could explain why pulmonary carcinoma cells prefer to metastasize to organs such as the brain, adrenal glands, and bone marrow.[1566,1594–1599] After exiting the circulation, cancer cells communicate with stromal cells and facilitate neovascularization within the new environment. Signaling of capillary sprouting, for example by vascular endothelial growth factor (VEGF), may not be as simple at the metastatic site as in the "home" organ, the lung. Multiple signaling cascades may be required for neovascularization in the metastatic site.[1559,1594,1600,1601] Presumably, only those metastatic cancer cells that are able to induce a proliferation of endothelial cells (and thus ensure nutrient and oxygen supply for their growth) will form metastatic nodules. The majority of cancer cells that arrive at the metastatic site will not grow further.[1559,1602–1606] However, they may become the source of a latent cancer cell pool.

Pulmonary Carcinogens and Their Impact on Genes

Although the majority of pulmonary carcinogens are derived from tobacco smoke, there are others, in part present within the environment (metals, asbestos, radon, etc.) and in part man-made (mineral fibers, polyaromatic hydrocarbons, aniline dyes, etc).

One of the well-known mechanisms by which carcinogens cause cancer is oxygen radical damage causing DNA strand breaks. Oxygen radicals can be formed by many tobacco carcinogens.[1607,1608] Various oxygen radicals, free or bound to aromatic hydrocarbons and glycolipids, interact with DNA, although only when the DNA is uncoiled.[1609–1615] Uncoiled DNA is most often found in dividing cells (i.e., reserve and stem cells), which therefore are the most sensitive to oxygen radical–induced DNA damage.[1616] Oxygen radicals oxidize DNA nucleotides, change their configuration, and thus inhibit pairing with their nucleotide counterparts on the complementary DNA strand. Guanine seems to be most sensitive to oxygen radical damage, which might explain why CG pairs are so often mutated.[1617]

Coiling and uncoiling of the DNA is regulated by several mechanisms that are under the control of methylating/demethylating and acetylating/deacetylating enzymes discussed previously. Under the control of histone acetyltransferases (HATs), which act with other proteins such as NF-κB, various STATs, C-amp response element binding protein (CREB), and AP1 proteins, the DNA is uncoiled and acetylated, histones are methylated, and transcription is facilitated. The histone deacetylases (HDACs), in contrast, cause coiling of the DNA by deacetylation. MeCP2 acts with HDACs to cause demethylation of methylated DNA. HDAC-SIN3 and associated proteins facilitate repression of transcription.[1618,1619] Interestingly, HDACs are sensitive to oxygen radicals, and HDACs have been found to be impaired in many non–small-cell lung carcinomas.[1620–1622]

Other mechanisms of DNA damage are chemical reactions with nucleotides that change their structure or electron configuration, or introduce $-NH_x$ or $-O-C_nH_n$ side chains. Many organic substances, sometimes with the help of metals as catalyzing agents, can cause this type of damage and metals can cause this type of damage independently.[1623,1624]

Field Cancerization

The lung, as most other organs, is compartmentalized. There are substructured areas, ill defined, but with a common regulatory system. It is now accepted that carcinogens alter one or multiple different stem cells within this area. Either one or several modified stem cells are involved in this primary event. These cells form a patch of clonally expanding preneoplastic cells and populate the area.[1625] Other genetic alterations have to take place, until cancer clones are formed, which again form small aggregates, either locally or multifocal. One consequence of this field cancerization is that after removal of a carcinoma, several clones of preneoplastic cells and cancer cells remain within the field, from which a recurrence of cancer can arise.[1625,1626]

Prevention of Damage and Repair Mechanisms

DNA damage involving xenobiotic metabolizing enzymes and DNA damage repair were discussed earlier (see sections Genetic Susceptibility to Lung Cancer and DNA Damage Repair). Detoxifying enzymes are expressed from the nasal mucosa to the alveolar region. These comprise enzymes responsible for preventing oxygen radical damage by increasing the intracellular glutathione pool, accepting or transferring oxygen radicals and thus inactivating them, or degrading toxic substances by coupling them to nontoxic substrates.[1627–1638] Phase I xenobiotic metabolizing enzymes are also present.[1639–1641] However, as previously noted, bioactivation by phase I enzymes can result in reactive intermediates that are more potent carcinogens.[1642–1648] There are, however, species specific differences in the enzyme systems, the human system being the least well equipped.[1649–1654] As previously noted, within the human population there are polymorphisms that are suspected of making some people less susceptible to the effects of tobacco carcinogens than others.[1647,1655,1656] In addition, the distribution of the enzymes is uneven within the respiratory system; high levels are present in the nasal mucosa and the bronchioloalveolar region, but lower levels are present in the trachea and main bronchi.[1657,1658]

Cell cycle checkpoints were discussed earlier (see DNA Damage Repair). Among the genes involved are the restriction point tumor suppressor genes *TP53* and *RB* and DNA repair genes, such as *MDM*, *ATR/ATM*, *MLHs*, and *MSHs*.[1659–1663] These also select the type of repair process based on the extent of damage: sanitation of the dNTPs pools, exchange of single mismatched nucleotides (point mutation), nucleotide excision repair of DNA single strands (larger pieces of DNA strands resulting in either mismatch pairing, or DNA loop formation), nucleotide incision repair, or repair of mutated/damaged segments of DNA double helix.[1662,1664–1666] In BER, a DNA glycosylase excises the mismatched base by hydrolysis of the glycoside bond between the nucleotide and the deoxyribose and generates a free base and the nucleotide is repaired.[1638,1662] In nucleotide incision repair, the mutated base is cut from both 3′ and 5′ ends and replaced.[1667] Mechanisms for repair of DNA double-strand breaks includes nonhomologous end-joining (NHEJ), in which the two ends of the DNA are joined. This usually results in mismatch of the base pair, which subsequently is repaired by one of the mechanisms described above. Homologous recombination (HR) is another mechanism that can result in repair of double-strand breaks.[1638,1668] Proteins involved in these processes, such as DNA protein kinase, the recruiting proteins Ku70 and Ku80, as well as XRCC4, Rad50, and Sir proteins, are often altered in carcinomas.[1666]

When DNA damage is irreparable, apoptosis occurs; apoptotic pathways were discussed earlier.[1664,1665,1669,1670] In some cancer types an inherited microsatellite instability results in an insufficient repair system, where many damaged cells escape repair, and mutations accumulate over time.[1670] However, this seems to play no major role in pulmonary carcinogenesis.

Nuclear Structure in Cancer Cells

During the progressive steps of carcinogenesis, chromosomes may break, parts of chromosomes are lost, and residual parts of chromosomes are rearranged, sometimes in reverse order or translocated in other cases. As a result, the structure and spatial organization of chromosomes in the interphase nucleus is changed. These chromosomal abnormalities and related abnormalities can be observed in cancer cell nuclei by light microscopy as crush artifact, grooves and clefts, aggregates of heterochromatin, asymmetric aggregates, and enlarged nucleoli. Within normal cells, various regions of the DNA are differently organized: GC-rich and highly acetylated histone H4–rich regions are active in interphase, replicate early in the S phase, and are more concentrated internally. AT-rich regions are located more peripherally. These peripheral AT-rich regions replicate later in the S phase. In cancer cells this organization of the DNA is disturbed.[1671] This disorganization might cause accumulation of losses and gains of genes during carcinogenesis and also cause altered interactions of genes that are normally spatially intimate but are separated in the disorganized nuclei.

Translocations may result in spatial shifts of genes that are normally separated into closer physical proximity, where the expression of one gene may alter the expression pattern of the other translocated gene. This effect has been observed for several oncogenes, such as *myc* and *abl*. Spatial dislocation of chromosomes can also result in a similar phenomenon: genes that are normally separated are brought into proximity where they influence each other's expression. This dislocation may be induced by a change in the histone-binding proteins, which are part of the structure fixing the chromosomes along the nuclear membrane.[1671]

Another feature of cancer cells is disruption or mislocalization of the promyelocytic leukemia body (PMLB) that harbors many suppressor genes and is involved in DNA repair processes, genomic stability, growth suppression, and cellular senescence.[1671] The PMLBs also play a role in the spatial organization of the interphase chromosomes. They are not only affected in leukemia, but also in many solid tumors, for example, PMLBs are lost in small cell lung carcinoma (SCLC).[1672] Loss of PMLBs can cause disorganization of interphase chromosomes, bringing normally distal genes into close proximity, the consequences of which are not fully explored yet.

Chromosomal Abnormalities Found in Carcinoma Cells

Different types of chromosomal abnormalities can be found in carcinoma cells, including balanced and unbalanced aberrations. The unbalanced aberrations include losses and gains of chromosomal/DNA material. The losses predominantly occur at chromosomal breakpoints (Fig. 33.4). A good example is the breakpoint on chromosome 3p, at the site of FHIT, which is frequently lost in many types of cancer. It is not known whether these breakpoints are incidental, are determined by specifically structured DNA sequences, or result from specific unique packing with histones. An example of a gain is the gain on chromosome 17q at the site of EGF receptor 2. In some cases, a gain results in an amplification of genes. However, gains are not identical to amplifications.

Unbalanced aberrations can result in translocations and inversions. When a chromosomal segment is lost, the residual chromosome material can connect to a different chromosome (translocation). This can result in an upregulation of the translocated gene when the translocated gene becomes associated with a promoter and a gene that is always active. Well-known examples are the translocation of *myc* and *abl*. Inversions are reversals of chromosome segments that happen frequently after chromosomal losses and breaks. The residual chromosome segment that broke from the original chromosome reunites with the original chromosome in a reverse orientation. It is not clear yet if this results in similar disturbances of gene interactions as in translocation.

Small Cell Lung Carcinoma

Small cell lung carcinoma (SCLC) represents one of the most aggressive types of lung cancer. No precursor lesion has yet been identified for SCLC. It is characterized by multiple balanced and unbalanced alterations involving virtually all of the chromosomes. The most common deletions are on chromosomes 3p, 5q, 9, 10, 13, 16, and 17p, whereas gains are usually found on chromosomes 1, 3q, 5p, 6p, 17q, 18, 19, and 20 (Fig. 33.5). Numerous complex chromosomal rearrangements have been reported by M-FISH, such as translocations between chromosomes 5 and 14, 5 and 11, and 1 and 6. Chromosomes 4, 5, 8, 11, 12, and 19 were most frequently involved in interchromosomal translocations.[1673]

Some of these aberrations have been investigated intensively such as 3p14 deletions resulting in the detection of tumor suppressor genes, such as *FHIT*, *FRA3B*,[1674] and *RBSP3*, a tumor suppressor gene on 3p21,[1675] or alternatively promoter hypermethylation for *RASSF1A* on 3p21.[1676] Another frequently deleted gene is the *RAF1* locus on 3p25.[1677] The function of most of these genes is largely unknown. Multiple fragile sites on different

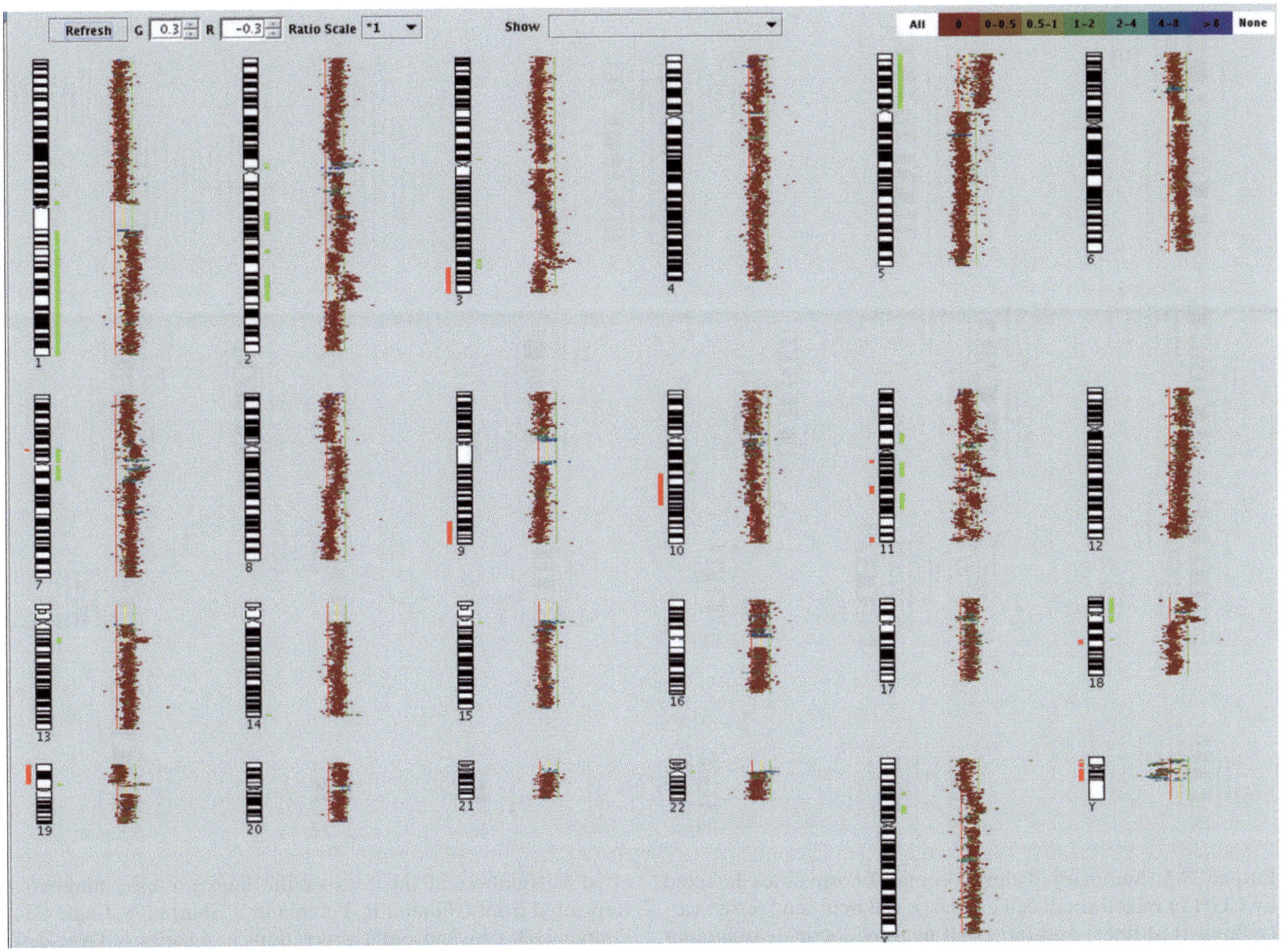

FIGURE 33.4. Complex chromosomal aberrations as detected by array comparative genomic hybridization (CGH) in a pulmonary adenocarcinoma. (Courtesy of Dr. R. Ullmann, from Popper HH, Ullmann R, Halbwedl I, et al. Complex chromosomal aberrations in pulmonary adenocarcinomas detected by array-CGH. Modern Pathol 2005;18(suppl 1):316A.)

chromosomes have been identified, but it is largely unclear why these locations are so vulnerable to breakage.

RASSF1A induces stabilization of mitotic cyclins and mitotic arrest at prometaphase. It interacts with Cdc20, an activator of the anaphase-promoting complex, resulting in the inhibition of APC activity. It was found that depletion of *RASSF1A* by RNA interference accelerated mitotic cyclin degradation and mitotic progression and caused a cell division defect characterized by centrosome abnormalities and multipolar spindles.[1678]

Neuroendocrine cells from normal tissues were found to be positive for PMLB, indicating that the absence of the PML protein found in SCLC is associated with the tumorigenic phenotype. The decreased PML expression may play an important role in SCLC development.[1672]

Another genetic pathway frequently deregulated in SCLC, as well as in non–small-cell lung carcinoma (NSCLC), is the phosphoinositol-3-kinase Akt-kinase pathway. It is frequently expressed in SCLC, but not correlated to prognosis.[1679] Expression of Akt by itself induces resistance to etoposide-mediated apoptosis. PI3K-Akt signaling promotes SCLC growth, survival, and chemotherapy resistance. Therefore, selective inhibitors of PI3K or Akt could potentially be useful as novel therapeutic agents in the treatment of SCLC.[1680]

Closely related to the PI3K-Akt and the EGFR1 mediated growth signaling is c-Met. c-Met is involved in the promotion of tumor cell growth in SCLC in cooperation with upregulated src kinase and the STAT3/5 molecules.[1681] There is no apparent correlation of c-Met expression with presence or absence of mutations. However, mutations in the juxtamembrane (JM) domain of c-met increase cell motility and migration. The JM mutations also alter c-Met receptor tyrosine kinase signaling, resulting in preferentially increased tyrosine phos-

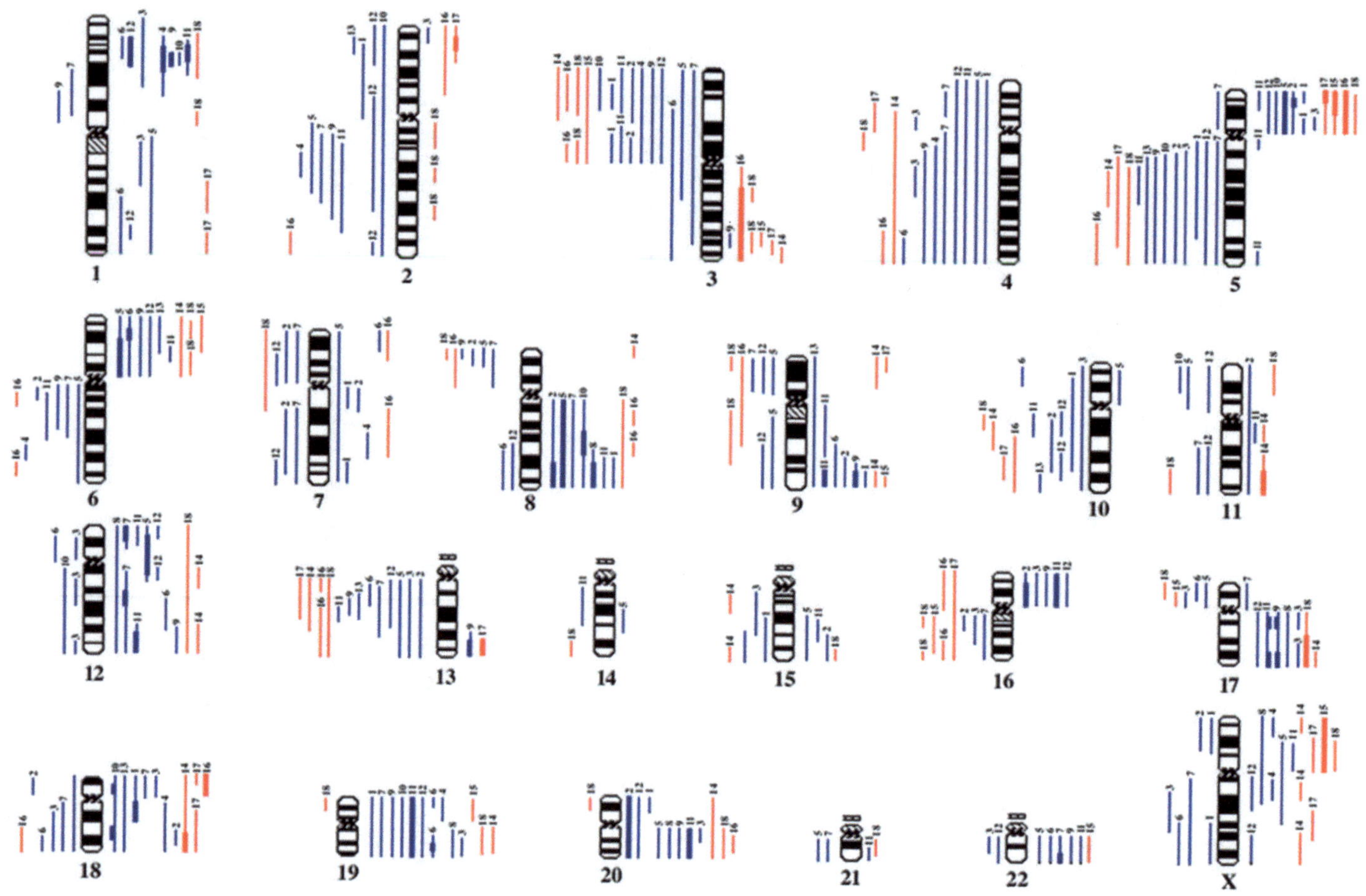

FIGURE 33.5. Summary of chromosomal abnormalities detected by CGH in mixed small cell and large cell neuroendocrine carcinomas (red lines) and large cell neuroendocrine carcinomas (blue lines). Losses are indicated by vertical lines on the left side of each ideogram and gains are indicated by vertical lines on the right side of each ideogram. Thick lines indicate a ratio of >1.5. Numbers at the tops of the lines are case numbers. Reprinted from Ullmann R, Petzmann S, Sharma A, Cagle PT, Popper HH. Chromosomal aberrations in a series of large-cell neuroendocrine carcinomas: unexpected divergence from small-cell carcinoma of the lung. Human Pathology 2001;32:1059–63, copyright Elsevier.

phorylation of various cellular proteins, including the key focal adhesion protein paxillin, correlating with increased motility. These results suggest a novel and unique role of the JM domain in c-Met signaling in SCLC with significant implications in cytoskeletal functions and metastatic potential. These somatic mutations may be associated with a more aggressive phenotype.[1682]

c-Met and hepatocyte growth factor/scatter factor (HGF/SF) are rarely coexpressed in SCLC, thus excluding an autocrine regulatory pathway, whereas the frequent coexpression of c-kit and its ligand stem cell factor (SCF) indicates that this receptor/ligand system may have an autocrine function in SCLC.[1683] c-Met is functional in SCLC and thus a possible target for therapy.[1684]

Lck (a Src-related tyrosine kinase) and, possibly, Yes are downstream of Kit in a signal transduction pathway. The inhibition of SCF-mediated proliferation and inhibition of apoptosis suggests that Src family kinases are intermediates in the signaling pathways that regulate these processes.[1685]

Gastrin-releasing peptide (GRP) and its receptor is recognized as an autocrine growth factor in SCLC. GRP now has been established as an autocrine growth factor for cancer cells in a subgroup of SCLC patients through, at least in part, upregulation of GRP receptor expression.[1686]

A marked decrease in Fas expression may be part of lung tumorigenesis, allowing tumor cells to escape from apoptosis. FasL overexpression in the context of Fas downregulation in SCLC predicts the ability of SCLC cells to induce paracrine killing of Fas-expressing cytotoxic T cells. Fas restoration may represent a key step in therapeutic strategies to reconstitute the ability of tumor cells to undergo apoptosis.[1687]

Marked reduction of *LOST1* expression was detected in SCLC. *LOST1* is a novel gene, cooperating with *14-3-3*$^{\varepsilon}$

and CRK. A significant DNA hypermethylation was found at the 5′ end of the *LOST1* gene, which might be responsible for the negligible expression of *LOST1* and 14-3-3.[1688]

A dense promoter hypermethylation of 14-3-3 sigma was seen in SCLC, but also in typical and atypical carcinoids and large cell neuroendocrine carcinomas, resulting in decreased expression.[1689] 14-3-3 functions within the apoptosis cascade by acting synergistically with IXAP proteins, and in concert and downstream of Akt kinases. It inhibits release of cytochrome c and thus acts in an antiapoptotic fashion. However, many other actions have been described such as transcription, interaction with cytoskeletal proteins, and possibly as a tumor suppressor. 14-3-3 binding can alter the localization, stability, phosphorylation state, activity, or molecular interactions of a target protein. Recent studies now indicate that the serine/threonine protein phosphatases PP1 and PP2A are important regulators of 14-3-3 binding interactions, and demonstrate a role for 14-3-3 in controlling the translocation of certain proteins from the cytoplasmic and endoplasmic reticulum to the plasma membrane.[1689–1695]

Other genes such as *PTEN*, involved in growth suppression and apoptosis, do not play a major role in SCLC or in adenocarcinomas and squamous cell carcinomas.[1696] The retinoblastoma gene *(RB)* is also not predominantly involved in SCLC carcinogenesis, whereas *p53* is mutated in almost all cases.[1697] The *ret* proto-oncogene shows an allelic loss in SCLC and thus might be involved in tumorigenesis.[1698] NCAM (neural cell adhesion molecule) is now frequently used for confirmation of the SCLC diagnosis. It is associated with neuroendocrine phenotype regardless of the histologic type of lung cancer. NCAM expression is associated with cell-to-cell adhesion and lack of substrate adhesion in cell culture, seen as floating clusters of cells. In SCLC a mutated form or splice variant occurs.[1699]

Adenocarcinoma

Currently adenocarcinoma is the most frequent cell type of lung carcinoma. In many industrialized countries it currently comprises up to 42% of all lung carcinomas.[1557] It is speculated that the relative increase in adenocarcinomas in recent years may be related to changes in smoking behavior, the lowering of the nicotine levels in cigarettes, and the invention of efficient cigarette filters 20 to 30 years ago. The lowering in the nicotine content provokes smokers to inhale more often and deeper. The filter has changed the composition of the carcinogens from particle-bound benzo-a-pyrene types to predominantly gaseous nitrosamine and polyaromatic hydrocarbon types.[1700] These result in lesions predominantly at the bronchioloalveolar border. Although the process of carcinogenesis is not fully understood, it seems that stem cells in this location already have undergone a cylindrical cell differentiation, thus paving the way for atypical adenomatous hyperplasia (AAH), bronchiolar columnar cell dysplasia (BCCD), and adenocarcinoma development.[1554,1557,1701–1704] Some early changes of adenocarcinoma development have been found, such as promoter methylation causing tumor suppressor gene silencing, or translocation of oncogenes, but other genes involved and residing on affected chromosomes and their function await detection and clarification.[1549,1552,1673,1674,1676,1679,1701,1705–1717]

In regard to molecular genetics of adenocarcinomas, it is necessary to take into account that adenocarcinomas are divided into histologic subtypes, such as tubular, papillary, bronchioloalveolar, mucinous, and so on, and that smoking-related adenocarcinomas should be differentiated from those not related to smoking, predominantly affecting women, and adenocarcinomas in children associated with congenital cystic adenomatoid malformation (Fig. 33.6).[1556,1718–1721] These various forms of pulmonary adenocarcinoma present with differing chromosomal aberrations. To complicate the picture further, when adenocarcinomas are analyzed by array CGH, the types of aberrations are even more variable. There are adenocarcinomas with "simple" aberrations, but also some with complex aberrations (Fig. 33.7). Several precursors to pulmonary adenocarcinoma have been identified including AAH,[1555] BCCD,[1554] and atypical goblet cell hyperplasia (AGCH),[1556] but other precursors are presumably still waiting to be discovered (see Chapter 34). The genetic events that facilitate the transition from the preinvasive lesion into invasive adenocarcinoma are still unknown. Recently, prognostic markers have been identified in adenocarcinomas. Positive immunohistochemical staining for cathepsin E and a negative reaction for heat shock protein 105 identified a subset of adenocarcinomas with favorable prognosis.[1590] Other factors negatively influencing the outcome of adenocarcinomas are lymphatic invasion,[1590,1722] PCNA and cyclin D expression,[1723,1724] downregulation of PTEN and nm23,[1596] upregulation of caveolin,[1725] and downregulation of TSCL1.[1726] Further discussion of this topic is found in the section Molecular Biomarkers of Lung Cancer Prognosis, below.

For many years, K-*ras* mutation has been known to occur in adenocarcinomas.[1727] More recently, a correlation between K-*ras* mutation and the activation of the PI3K/Akt kinase pathway has been established, and the function of this mutation correlated to an increase in cell movement.[1565,1728,1729] Another mechanism by which K-*ras* mutation is involved in carcinogenesis is inhibition of apoptosis.[1565] Whether or not K-*ras* mutation is definitely an early event in pulmonary adenocarcinoma genesis cannot be answered yet.

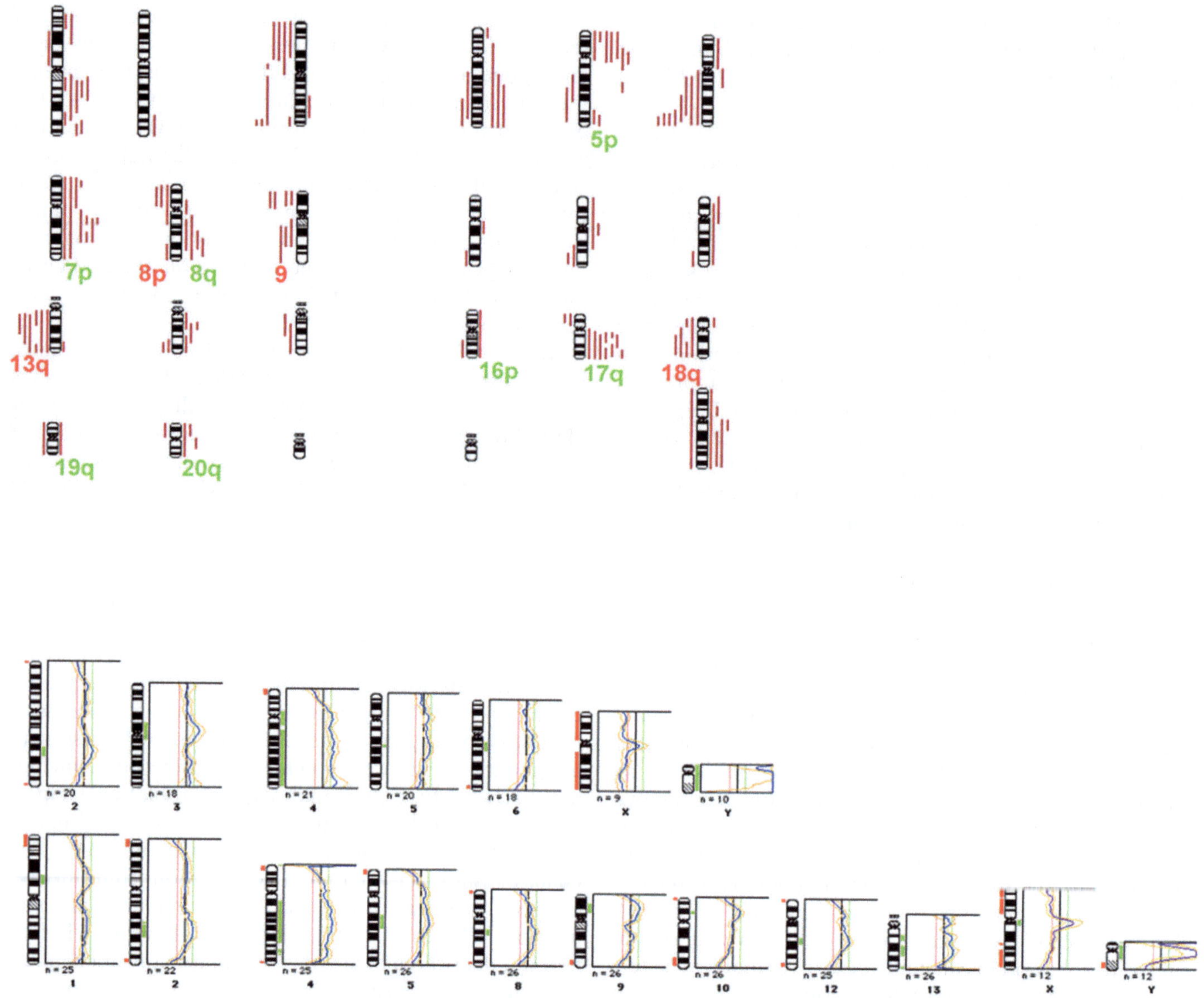

FIGURE 33.6. Comparison of chromosomal CGH in pulmonary adenocarcinomas. Upper panel CGH is from adenocarcinomas in adult smokers and never smokers. Lower panel CGH is from childhood adenocarcinomas. Losses are indicated by vertical lines on the left side of each ideogram, and gains are indicated by vertical lines on the right side of each ideogram.

Squamous Cell Carcinoma

Squamous cell carcinoma (SCC) is no longer the most common type of pulmonary carcinoma, most probably due to the changes in the composition of carcinogens in tobacco smoke due to cigarette filters and the reduction of nicotine content, resulting in deeper inhalation. Filters protect the larger airways from particle deposition and therefore carcinogen exposure. The predominant repair process in large bronchi starts with goblet cell hyperplasia and progresses to squamous metaplasia. If squamous metaplasia progresses into dysplasia, there is the potential for progression to SCC.

Chromosome gains in SCC are frequently detected at 3q, 5p, 8q, 12p, and Xq and losses at 16p, 4q, 5q, 3p, 17p, and 16q. DNA amplifications are observed at 12 regions: 3q26.1–27, 8q13–23.1, 12p12.3-pter, 12q15, 2p14–16, 4q28–31.2, 5p13.1-pter, 6q21–22.3, 7p11.2–13, 13q21.2–32, 18p11.2-pter, and 20p11.2-pter. An increased copy number at 3q may contribute to the development of SCC of the lung.[184,1730] Comparative genomic hybridization findings in NSCLC described +2 p11.2-p13, +3q25-q29, +9q13-q34, +12p, +12q12-q15, and +17q21. The CGH studies also found that −8p was preferentially associated with SCC pathogenesis, whereas the t(8;12) translocation was exclusively found in AC.[1717] Of interest, the pattern

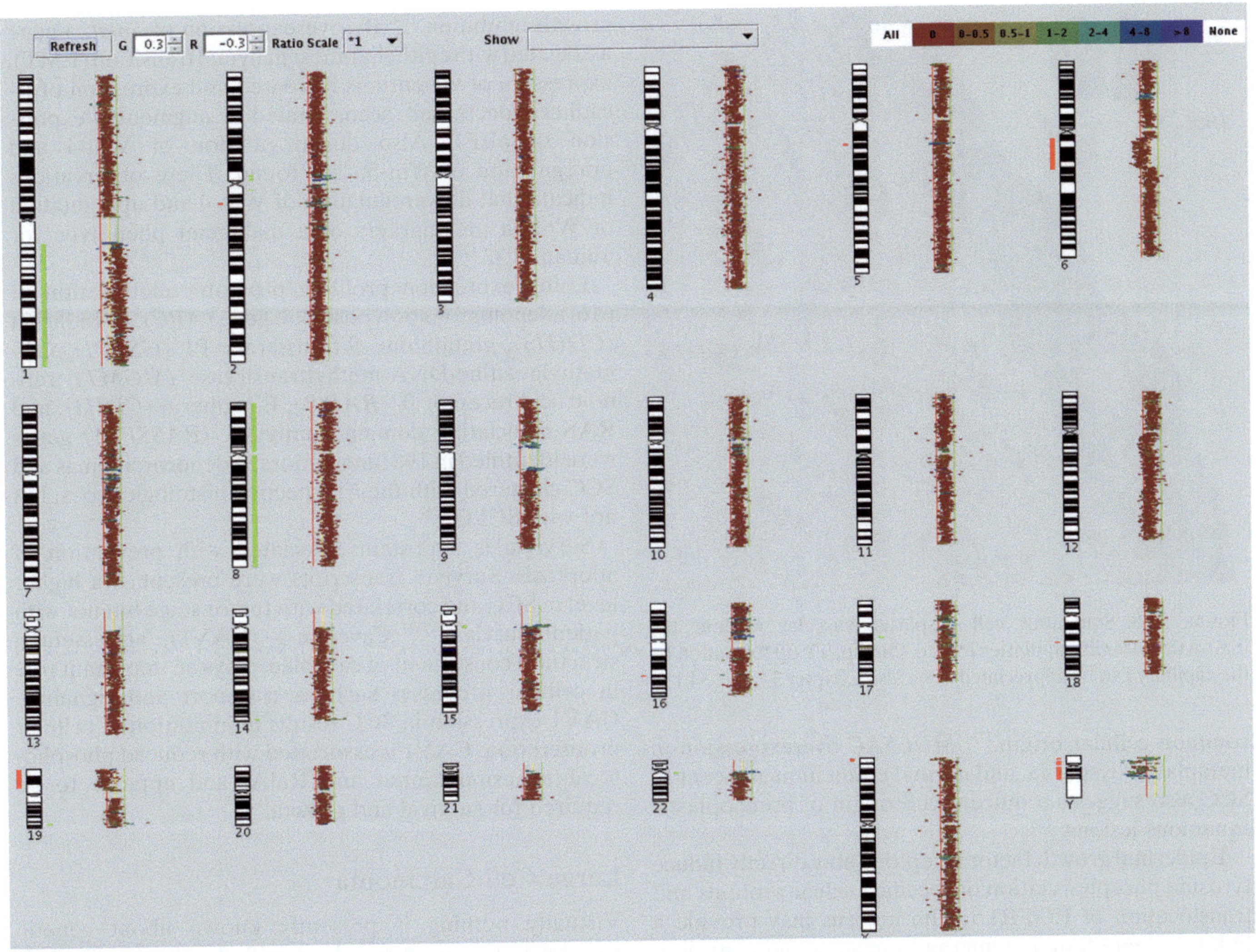

FIGURE 33.7. Array CGH of pulmonary adenocarcinoma with simple aberrations. (Courtesy of Dr. R. Ullmann, from Popper HH, Ullmann R, Halbwedl I, et al. Complex chromosomal aberrations in pulmonary adenocarcinomas detected by array-CGH. Modern Pathol 2005;18(suppl 1):316A.)

of deletions in SCC was not random: 8p21–23 allelic losses detected by LOH was always followed by 3p deletions and usually followed 9p deletions.[1731] The earliest and most frequent regions of allelic loss occurred at 3p21, 3p22–24, 3p25, and 9p21. TP53 allelic loss was present in many histologically advanced lesions (dysplasia and carcinoma-in-situ).[1553]

Recently a new precursor lesion was proposed for SCC, named angiogenic squamous dysplasia (ASD), characterized by intramucosal capillary loops (see also Chapter 34). This report suggests that an aberrant pattern of microvascularization may occur at an early stage of bronchial carcinogenesis[1732] and determine a subgroup with higher risk of progression (Fig. 33.8).

Maspin on chromosome 18q21.3 is a member of the serpin family of protease inhibitors that has tumor suppressor activity and is an angiogenesis inhibitor. Maspin has been shown to suppress motility and invasion in SCCs. Intense, uniform expression was correlated with increased survival and longer remission duration.[1709] Maspin seems to be expressed in association with cells from the proximal airways and is expressed in basal and reserve cells. An analysis of methylation status in positive and negative portions of individual tumors demonstrated intratumor diversity associated with promoter DNA methylation.[1715]

MUC genes have been identified as differentiation and cell growth associated genes. *MUC2* and *MUC5AC* are two target genes of EGFR ligands. Upregulation of these two genes results in concomitant activation of the EGFR/Ras/Raf/extracellular signal–regulated kinase-signaling pathway and Sp1 binding to their promoters.[1733] Reduced expression of *MUC4*, *MUC5AC*, and *MUC8* was observed in NSCLCs, regardless of their histologic subtype. Squamous cell carcinoma and AC display a similar pattern of mucin gene expression, supporting the concept of a

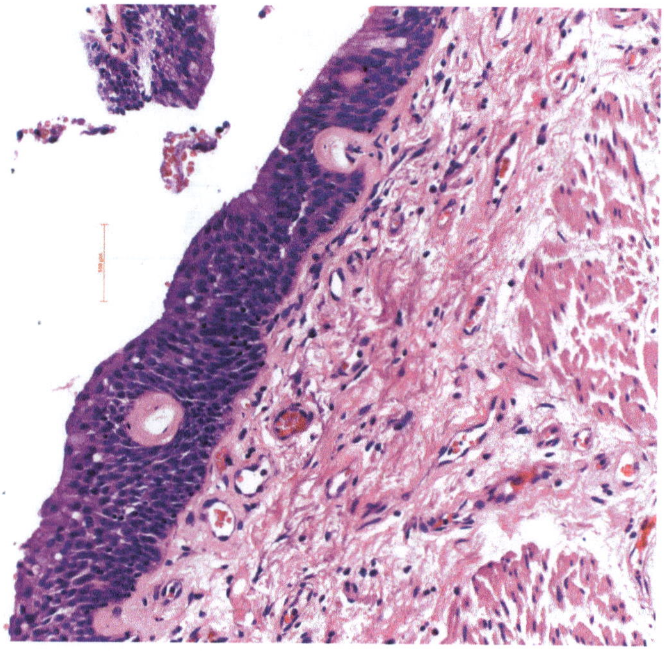

FIGURE 33.8. Squamous cell dysplasia, vascular variant; the ingrowth of fragile capillaries is seen. On top, a loop formation by the capillary can be appreciated. (See also Chapter 34, Fig. 34.15).

common cellular origin.[1734] *MUC5AC* overexpression in metaplasia, dysplasia, and normal epithelium adjacent to SCC also suggests a mucous cell origin of preneoplastic squamous lesions.[1735]

Epidermal growth factor receptor 1 may directly induce tyrosine phosphorylation of specific nuclear proteins and translocation of EGFR1 to the nucleus may provide a link between plasma membrane signaling and gene activation.[1736] Thus phosphorylation, but not overexpression, of EGFR may be the important predictor for clinical outcome of NSCLCs.[1737]

Another gene frequently involved in SCC is *FHIT*. Hypermethylation of the *FHIT* gene does not have a prognostic significance in early-stage NSCLCs. *FHIT* methylation is associated with p16 methylation and smoking in SCC, suggesting that *FHIT* may interact with p16 to contribute to the development of SCC in individuals exposed to tobacco smoke.[1738]

Many other genes such as *E2F3*, *MYBL2*, *HDAC2*, *CDK4*, and *PCNA* are expressed in the nucleus of SCC and are associated with the cell cycle and proliferation.[1702] 18q21–18qter contains the putative tumor suppressor gene *DCC* and two MAD-related genes, *DPC4* and *MADR2*, which are both components in a TGF-β–like signaling pathway that seems to be important in the progression of SCC.[1739]

The Wnt pathway is activated through Dishevelled (Dvl) overexpression in NSCLC. Dvl-3, a critical mediator of Wnt signaling, is overexpressed in SCC. Suppression decreases Dvl and β-catenin expression, resulting in growth inhibition.[1740] By overexpression of *Snail*, a gene associated with epithelial-mesenchymal transition (EMT), expression of vimentin is increased and expression of E-cadherin decreased, accompanied by augmented expression of δEF1. Also downregulation of Wnt-4 and upregulation of Wnt-5a are found. These observations indicate that downregulation of Wnt-4 and upregulation of Wnt-5a are markers of a malignant phenotype for human SCC.[1741]

Using expression profiling promoter methylation of p16, adenomatous polyposis coli gene *(APC)*, H-cadherin *(CDH13)*, glutathione S-transferase P1 *(GSTP1)*, O6–methylguanine-DNA-methyltransferase *(MGMT)*, retinoic acid receptor β_2 *(RAR-β)*, E-cadherin *(CDH1)*, and RAS association domain family 1A *(RASSF1A)* genes were identified in 198 lung tumors. Adenocarcinomas and SCC clustered with their respective histologic types, but not with SCLC.[1742]

Survivin is a protein associated with prevention of apoptosis. Survivin transcripts were present at a higher level in SCC and correlated with tumor stage but not with patient survival.[1743] Caveolin-1 (CAV1), an essential structural constituent of caveolae, plays an important role in cellular processes such as transport and signaling. CAV1 expression in SCC results in inhibition of cellular proliferation. CAV1 is associated with reduced phospho-focal adhesion kinase and RalA, and appears to be required for survival and growth.[1744]

Large Cell Carcinoma

Virtually nothing is presently known about genetic changes in tumors currently classified as large cell carcinoma, although limited data are available for one large cell carcinoma variant—large cell neuroendocrine carcinomas (LCNEC), which represents a high-grade neuroendocrine carcinoma, characterized by high mitotic counts, rapid growth, and large areas of necrosis.[1745] LCNEC has many aberrations similar to SCLC, and also some unique alterations.[1746] Especially, in contrast to SCLC, there is no gain of chromosome 3q (Fig. 33.5).

The transcription factor achaete-scute homolog-1 (hASH1) is present in LCNEC and is associated with neuroendocrine differentiation.[1747] NCAM is expressed more strongly in high-grade neuroendocrine (NE) carcinomas (SCLC and LCNEC), compared to low grade (carcinoids).[1748] Sialylated-NCAM, as found in both types of high-grade neuroendocrine carcinomas, inhibits cell adherence and thus might be responsible for the aggressive and invasive phenotype associated with these tumors.[1749] Similar to atypical carcinoids, genetic aberrations of chromosome 11q13 at, but also more distal to, the menin-gene locus are frequently found in LCNEC, as well as *p53* mutation. The loss of 5q21 is correlated with an aggressive behavior.[1750]

Molecular Biomarkers of Lung Cancer Prognosis

Approximately half of the patients with early-stage NSCLC who theoretically should be cured by surgical resection nevertheless die from their lung cancer. The ability to predict which cancers are likely to recur or progress despite apparent curative surgery has several implications. This type of information would allow patients to be categorized according to those who are likely to benefit from aggressive additional therapy and those who are unlikely to need such adjuvant therapy. In addition, it is important to know which patients are likely to do well on their own anyway versus which are likely to die of disease when evaluating the effects of new therapeutic agents. Identification of specific genes or gene products that impact on survival might also provide targets for molecular therapy.

As discussed in previous sections, lung cancer development and progression, including rate of proliferation, cell survival, resistance to apoptosis, metastatic potential, and other factors, are the result of expression of the genes of the cell cycle, signaling pathways, apoptotic pathways, cell adhesion, angiogenesis, and so on. Investigators have suspected that expression of one or more of these specific genes, especially abnormal expressions, in tumor tissue samples might predict clinical outcome and survival, probability of metastatic disease, and response to adjuvant therapy, and thus divide lung cancers into categories of better or worse prognosis.[1751–1774]

Over the past 15 years, many investigations have focused on the expression of individual genes and their potential relationship to patient survival. Some of these studies have examined point mutations, RFLPs, or other specific abnormalities of genes, but most studies have focused on immunohistochemistry to examine gene product proteins within histologic sections of tumors. Prominent among these studies have been investigations of the genes and gene products of oncogenes such as *Ras*[1775–1793] and *myc* (particularly RFLPs of L-*myc*),[1794–1800] tumor suppressor genes such as *p53*,[1801–1843] *MDM2*,[1844–1847] *RB*[1848, 1849] and *p16*,[1850–1856] cyclins such as cyclin D1,[1857–1865] apoptosis factors such as Bcl2,[1866–1880] and receptors such as ErbB2[1881–1895] and ErB3.[1896] Other genes or gene products that have been examined include *FHIT*,[1897–1900] *p21*,[1901–1905] β-catenin,[1906] p27KIP1,[1907–1909] E-cadherin,[1910] Fas,[1911] hypermethylation,[1912–1915] HIF-1,[1916] carbonic anhydrase-9,[1917] TTF-1,[1918, 1919] COX-2,[1920–1922] Skp2,[1923] E2F,[1924] *CYP1A1* and GST,[1925] chromosomes 2p and 3p,[1926,1927] chromosome 9p,[1928] EGF,[1929] metallothionein,[1930,1931] VEGF,[1932–1934] thioredoxin,[1935] Ape1/ref-1,[1936] caspase 3,[1937] nm23,[1938] BRG1/BRM,[1939,1940] telomerase,[1941,1942] p63,[1943,1944] YB-1,[1945] phospho-Akt,[1946,1947] p73,[1948] maspin,[1949] TSLC-1,[1950] p53R2,[1951] HLJ1,[1952] NF-κB,[1953] BNIP3,[1954] and Bcl-X_L.[1955] Many other studies have looked at combinations of two or more of these potential biomarkers, as well as other biomarkers, in various groupings in relation to patient survival.[1956–2028]

Overall, the data for these individual biomarkers, alone or in combination with other biomarkers, has so far produced inconsistent and conflicting results. There are several reasons for these apparent inconsistencies among studies. On a biologic level, as we have seen, signaling pathways and pathways involving the cell cycle, apoptosis, and cell survival are very complex and intertwined with many redundancies, checks and balances, and feedback loops. Examination of only one, two, or a few genes or gene products in a pathway, or conceivably of only one pathway, may be insufficient to encompass all influences on a given pathway that might affect tumor prognosis. In addition, use of different techniques and criteria to identify biomarkers, inclusion of differing populations or inadequate numbers of cases, and variable definitions of end points mean that studies of the same biomarker may not be comparable. Despite these confounding factors, the majority of studies of some biomarkers produce similar results more often than not, even with univariate analysis as an independent prognostic biomarker, for example, *p53* abnormalities as a negative prognostic biomarker.

Meta-analyses of prospective biomarkers of lung cancer prognosis have sometimes suggested that potential statistical significance does exist for some biomarkers as predictors of prognosis. A meta-analysis of 829 NSCLC cases from eight studies by Huncharek et al.[2029] yielded a relative risk of 1.52 favoring a negative prognosis associated with *p53* mutations; the authors questioned the validity of these results because of the potential of multiple sources of bias. Mitsudomi et al.[2030] performed meta-analysis on data from 43 published articles, including studies of *p53* overexpression in 3579 cases and of *p53* DNA mutations in 1031 cases, and concluded that *p53* alterations were a significant marker of poor prognosis in patients with adenocarcinoma of the lung. In a meta-analysis of data from 74 eligible articles, Steels et al.[2031] found *p53* abnormalities were associated with poorer survival in each subgroup of stage and cell type of NSCLC that they examined.

After meta-analysis of 881 NSCLC cases from eight published studies, Huncharek et al.[2032] found a relative risk of 2.35 favoring negative prognosis when K-*ras* mutations were present, but indicated that adjustments for other factors might alter these results. Mascaux et al.[2033] concluded that *ras* abnormalities including *KRAS2* mutations and *p21* overexpression were a negative prognostic factor for NSCLCs, especially for adenocarcinomas, based on a meta-analysis of data from 28 studies.

In a meta-analysis of L-*myc* EcoRI polymorphism in 3563 patients of various types of cancer from 36 studies,

Spinola et al.[2034] suggested that the S/S genotype was significantly associated with lymph node metastases, distant metastases, and stage in lung cancer patients. Based on data on 3370 patients from 25 trials, meta-analysis by Martin et al.[2035] indicated that Bcl-2 expression was associated with a better prognosis in patients with NSCLC. A meta-analysis using data on 2185 patients from 11 studies by Meert et al.[2036] concluded that EGFR expression was not a significant prognostic factor for NSCLC, but that in the studies using immunohistochemistry there was a statistical significance favoring poor prognosis, although the impact was small and possibly influenced by publication bias.

Even if a single biomarker or combination of biomarkers can be demonstrated to be a statistically significant predictor of prognosis when examining large groups of patients, the application of a single biomarker or a few biomarkers to the outcome of the individual patient is problematic. This is because of the multiple complex pathways involved in the progression of lung cancer and their many interactions, redundancies, checks and balances, and feedback loops. Therefore, in predicting the specific prognosis of the individual patient, it is logical that multiple biomarkers, that is, a molecular profile, is more likely to provide much more accurate forecast. This concept has been under investigation for a number of years, and pilot studies have shown the potential utility of neural networks or other approaches to molecular profiles to predict the unique outcomes of individual patients.[2037–2052] The availability of omics and bioinformatics now makes this type of approach much more promising than in the past.

Another area of investigation has been the detection of molecular markers of lung cancer prognosis in patient serum rather than from tumor tissue. This approach has the hypothetical advantage of providing updated information by the relatively easy technique of obtaining a blood sample. So far, studies are limited and have not been validated by additional investigations.[2053–2056]

Molecular Pathology and Therapy

Response to Conventional Therapies (Customized Therapy)

In conventional chemotherapy, platinum-based drugs are frequently used in the treatment of lung cancer, as are paclitaxel and docetaxel, drugs that bind tightly to β-tubulin and disrupt microtubule dynamics. Specific genes are involved in the response of individual lung cancers to chemotherapy by their impact on apoptosis or other signaling pathways or by their ability to repair DNA damage caused by chemotherapeutic agents. Variations in expression of these genes are believed to modulate the effectiveness of chemotherapeutic agents and resistance of tumors to chemotherapy. Therefore, it is proposed that these genes might be evaluated to tailor conventional therapy to individual patients based on their predicted responsiveness to specific conventional chemotherapeutic agents. This approach is referred to as customized therapy.[2057–2062]

Thioredoxin-1

Antioxidant enzymes and thiol proteins that regulate the cellular redox state are the major cellular protection against oxidants associated with carcinogenesis and cancer progression. Important examples of these enzymes include superoxide dismutases, glutamate cysteine ligase, catalase, thioredoxins, and peroxiredoxins. These enzymes are expressed in lung cancers that have an impact on resistance of lung cancer cells to chemotherapy and radiation in addition to influencing tumor progression.[2063–2069]

Thioredoxin-1 (TRX-1), thioredoxin reductase, and reduced nicotinamide adenine dinucleotide phosphate (NADPH) make up the thioredoxin redox system. Hypoxia causes accumulation of hypoxia-inducible factor-1 (HIF-1) and overexpression of TRX-1 activates HIF-1. Activated HIF-1 induces cyclooxygenase-2 (COX-2) expression and VEGF expression in lung cancer cells.

Thioredoxin-1 participates in reduction of bonds that regulate the ability of transcription factors AP-1 (Jun/Fos), NF-κB, and p53 to bind to DNA. Dysregulation of the TGF-β signaling pathway increases expression of TRX-1, which in turn inhibits apoptosis signal-regulating kinase 1 and activates NF-κB. Both of these effects protect the cancer cells from apoptosis caused by chemotherapeutic agents, including cisplatin.

Excision Repair Cross-Complementing Group I (ERCC1)

Genes and their products involved in DNA damage repair were discussed earlier (see DNA Damage Repair). The cytotoxicity of platinum-based drugs such as cisplatin is the result of formation of bulky platinum DNA adducts in the cancer cells, and the repair of DNA adducts is likely to decrease the effectiveness of platinum drugs.[2070–2079] In the NER pathway, ERCC1 and XPD (also known as ERCC2) are necessary for the repair of DNA adducts caused by cisplatin. DNA repair capacity (DRC) was discussed earlier (see Genetic Susceptibility to Lung Cancer). The individual response to cisplatin depends on the individual DRC since greater DRC provides greater repair of cisplatin DNA adducts in the cancer and, hence, lesser response to therapy and vice versa. For example, the XRCC3 241 MetMet allele is proposed to be an independent predictor of survival in lung cancer patients treated with cisplatin/gemcitabine.

Several studies have shown that overexpression of ERCC1 mRNA is associated with poor response to cisplatin, and low ERCC1 mRNA levels are associated with significantly better response to cisplatin in lung cancer patients. Among the DNA damage repair enzymes, ERCC1 appears to be the more important predictor of response to cisplatin therapy in lung cancer patients. In a study of 109 NSCLC patients treated with cisplatin combination chemotherapy, no effect of XPD codon 751 or 312 polymorphisms on patient survival were noted.[2074]

However, low ERCC1 activity also leads to less repair of damaged DNA in normal tissues in patients treated with chemotherapy, possibly causing greater toxicity. In one report, lung cancer patients carrying at least one ERCC1 allele with altered activity who were treated with platinum drugs had an increased incidence of grade 3 or 4 gastrointestinal toxicity.[2079]

BRCA1

As previously mentioned, BRCA1 (BReast CAncer protein 1) is a member of the ATM (mutated in ataxia telangiectasia) pathway for DNA damage repair during the cell cycle. BRCA1 causes G_2–M arrest and resistance to a range of DNA-damaging drugs and increases sensitivity to antimicrotubule chemotherapeutic agents. BRCA1 functions as a differential regulator of chemotherapy-induced apoptosis, and its impact on the response to these drugs occurs through the inhibition or induction of apoptosis.[2080–2083] BRCA1 also appears to induce 14-3-3σ by DNA damage and act synergistically with p53 to activate 14-3-3σ expression. In 2004, Taron et al.[2083] reported that patients with locally advanced NSCLC and the lowest BRCA1 mRNA expression obtained maximum benefit from neoadjuvant gemcitabine-plus-cisplatin chemotherapy and those with the highest BRCA1 mRNA expression had the poorest survival.

14-3-3 Proteins

Members of the 14-3-3 superfamily of proteins bind numerous functionally diverse signaling proteins involved in many processes, including cell-cycle control and apoptosis. 14-3-3σ is involved in cell cycle arrest at the G_2 cell cycle checkpoint in response to DNA damage. Methylation of 14-3-3σ has been proposed to be an independent prognostic factor for survival in NSCLC patients receiving platinum-based chemotherapy.[2084–2095]

Targeted Therapies

Although there has been improvement in first-line therapy for lung cancer over the past decade, the great majority of lung cancer patients, including many with apparently early stage that should be curable by resection, die from their disease. New knowledge in molecular genetics has led to the concept of targeted molecular therapy, primarily as a second-line therapy or in combination with conventional therapies. In targeted molecular therapy, specific receptors or signaling pathway proteins are targeted in a specific manner to enhance tumor specificity and sensitivity to the therapy and minimize therapy side effects.[2096–2113]

Epidermal Growth Factor Receptor Targeted Therapies

Anti-EGFR therapies include tyrosine kinase inhibitors (TKIs) and monoclonal antibodies.[2114–2124] The TKIs, such as Gefitinib (Iressa) and Erlotinib (Tarceva), act as EGFR antagonists by binding to the intracellular domain of EGFR, inhibiting downstream signaling.[2125–2154] Cetuximab (Erbitux) is a chimeric human-mouse monoclonal immunoglobulin G (IgG) antibody that binds to the extracellular domain of EGFR, which prevents ligand binding and functional activation of EGFR.[2155–2159]

Both types of anti-EGFR therapy have shown some efficacy in treating lung cancer, both as individual agents and in combination with conventional therapies, including cetuximab[2160–2165] and TKIs,[2166–2168] but results have not always been favorable. It is now apparent that some patients are more likely to respond to anti-EGFR therapy than others, and markers for those patients likely to respond have been identified. Two mutations in the tyrosine kinase domain of EGFR (a deletion at exon 19 and a missense mutation L858R at exon 21) predict improved response to EGFR TKIs. These mutations are more frequent in never-smokers, adenocarcinoma, females, and Asian patients.[2125–2154] Amplification of the EGFR gene also appears to be predictive of response.[2151]

C-Kit Antagonist Imatinib Mesylate

Imatinib mesylate (Gleevec) inhibits the ligand dependent tyrosine kinase activity of c-Kit (the receptor for stem cell factor) in some tumors (for example, gastrointestinal stromal cell tumors) that overexpress c-Kit and also inhibits other tyrosine kinases such as Abl in leukemia. There was early interest in imatinib mesylate therapy of small cell lung cancer based on tumor expression of c-Kit, but, overall, imatinib mesylate has not been found to be effective in SCLC in vivo.[2169–2188]

ErbB2/HER2/Herceptin (Trastuzumab) and ERbB2/HER2/Pertuzumab

Trastuzumab is a monoclonal antibody to the ErB2 receptor (also known as HER-2) and has proven to be an effective treatment in some women with breast carcinomas that overexpress HER-2, as demonstrated by immunohistochemistry or FISH. Trastuzumab has not proven effective in the treatment of lung cancer.[2189–2208] Pertuzumab (Omnitarg) is a HER2–specific, recombinant, humanized monoclonal antibody that prevents heterodimerization of HER2 with other HERs that is expected to undergo future clinical trials.[2209,2210]

Antiangiogenesis Therapy

Anti-VEGF therapies include monoclonal antibodies that prevent VEGF receptor (VEGFR) binding and TKIs that inhibit VEGFR activation.[2211–2220] Bevacizumab (Avastin) is a recombinant humanized monoclonal antibody that binds VEGFR. Several small-molecule receptor TKIs that inhibit VEGFR tyrosine kinase activity have been developed including ZD6474 (Zactima), sorafenib, sunitinib malate, and AG-013736. Due to structural similarities of different receptor TKIs, these receptor TKIs inhibit several receptors in addition to the VEGFR including EGFR. The VEGF Trap is a high-affinity molecule with specificity to the VEGF molecule generated as a fusion molecule of the VEGFR extracellular domain and the Fc portion of IgG1. Bevacizumab (Avastin) is usually well tolerated by patients, and several studies report improved survival of patients with metastatic lung cancer with bevacizumab in combination with chemotherapy and in combination with other targeted molecular therapies.[2221–2232]

Farnesyl Transferase Inhibitors

The ras protein undergoes posttranslational modification by the covalent addition of a nonpolar farnesyl group to the COOH-terminal by the enzyme farnesyl transferase. Farnesylation enables the ras protein to translocate from the cytoplasm to the cell membrane, and allows it to participate in signaling for increased proliferation and inhibition of apoptosis.

Farnesyl transferase inhibitors (FTIs) block farnesylation, which prevents ras signaling. Multiple agents that inhibit farnesylation have been developed. In preclinical studies, FTIs inhibited the growth of human lung cancer cell lines in vitro and in xenograft models. Farnesyl transferase inhibitors including R115777 (tipifarnib, Zarnestra) L-778,123, and lonafarnib have been studied in early clinical trials, alone or in combination with conventional treatments in lung cancer patients with relapse or refractoriness to conventional treatments. Effectiveness of these agents has been limited in these early clinical trials.[2233–2254]

The FTI SCH66336, in combination with receptor TKIs, inhibits the growth of NSCLC cells. SCH66336 appears to inhibit angiogenesis by decreasing HIF-1α expression and inhibiting VEGF production by blocking HIF-1α and Hsp90 interaction, causing degradation of HIF-1α.[2255]

Epigenetic Therapy General

Epigenetic changes such as methylation and acetylation cause alterations in gene expression without changes in the DNA coding sequence. These changes may cause significant abnormalities in carcinogenesis and tumor progression, such as silencing of tumor suppressor genes, and are passed on through cell division. Inactivation of several important genes by methylation, including *p16*, occurs frequently in lung cancer. Epigenetic changes, in contrast to genetic changes, are potentially reversible, and DNA demethylating agents have been used successfully for hematologic malignancies.[2256–2259]

Methylation Inhibitors Decitabine and 5–Azacytidine

Azanucleosides, such as decitabine and its ribonucleoside analogue 5–azacytidine, are methylation inhibitors. Demethylating agents at low doses can reactivate tumor suppressor genes in vitro. Lung cancer development has been slowed in mouse models using demethylating agents, an effect that is enhanced when combined with histone deacetylase inhibitors.[2260–2269]

Histone Deacetylase Inhibitors

DNA is wrapped around octamers of histone proteins. Histones undergo posttranslational modification by the addition of acetyl groups. Histone acetyltransferases add acetyl groups to histones and histone deacetylases (HDACs) remove acetyl groups from histones. The HDAC inhibitors (HDACIs), including suberoylanilide hydroxamic acid (SAHA), have displayed antitumor activity in preclinical models and in early clinical trials in NSCLC and other cancers. Since HDACIs also activate NF-κB antiapoptotic pathways, inhibition of NF-κB with combination therapy with bortezomib or PI3K/Akt pathway inhibition has been studied as a possible method to enhance the effects of HDACIs.[2270–2288]

Gene Therapy

In contrast to targeted molecular therapies, the hypothesis behind gene therapy for lung cancer involves replacing tumor suppressor genes using viral vectors as delivery systems. Preclinical trials indicate that this technology can inhibit cancers, and direct injection of tumor suppressor genes carried by viral vectors into tumors has caused regression of tumors locally, but delivery to a disease that is typically systemic like lung cancer remains problematic. Some studies have shown an enhanced effect of conventional DNA damaging therapies like chemotherapy and radiation therapy when combined with the tumor gene transfer therapy by restoring sensitivity to apoptosis induction.[2289–2295]

Molecular Pathology of Other Lung Tumors

Uncommon Carcinomas of the Lung

Pleomorphic Carcinomas (See Also Chapter 37)

Only one study has looked for genetic changes in pleomorphic carcinomas of the lung.[2296] Several gene products involved in cell differentiation, such as cytokeratins, epithelial membrane antigen, carcinoembryonic antigen, vimentin, S-100 protein, smooth muscle actin, and desmin, were investigated, as were the cell cycle control and apoptosis gene products *p53*, *p21Waf1*, *p27Kip1*, *FHIT*, tumor growth (proliferative fraction, assessed by Ki-67 antigen, and microvascular density, assessed by CD34 immunostaining), and tumor cell motility (fascin). It was found that the epithelial component was significantly more immunoreactive for cytokeratins, epithelial membrane antigen, carcinoembryonic antigen, cell cycle inhibitors p21Waf1 and p27Kip1, and tumor suppressor gene *FHIT*, whereas the sarcomatoid component, independent of tumor stage and size, was more immunoreactive for vimentin, fascin, and microvascular density. Accordingly, a model of tumorigenesis was suggested whereby the mesenchymal phenotype of pleomorphic cells is likely induced by the selective activation and segregation of several molecules involved in cell differentiation, cell cycle control, and tumor cell growth and motility. Whether pleomorphic carcinomas of the lung are tumors with a more dismal prognosis than NSCLCs still remains an unsettled issue. In one series, however, stage I pleomorphic carcinomas have the same clinical behavior as ordinary NSCLC, and only a high proliferative index (Ki-67 labeling index >35%) was associated with a worse prognosis.[2296] Recently, pleomorphic carcinomas were cytogenetically analyzed. They all showed common genetic aberrations, predominantly gains on chromosomes 8q, 7, 1q, 3q, and 19. Similar aberrations were also found in a carcinosarcoma. (See Chapter 37 for a further discussion of pleomorphic carcinoma.)

Carcinoids (See Also Chapter 36)

Carcinoids comprise a group of locally invasive carcinomas with either low or intermediate malignant potential. They are subclassified into typical carcinoids (TCs) and atypical carcinoids (ATCs).[2297] Both are capable of metastasizing to regional lymph nodes and distant sites, although this is more common in atypical carcinoids.[2298–2301] Most often metastases do occur late, in the experience of one of us (H.H.P.), usually at least 7 years after removal of the primary tumor.[2300,2302] Counting of mitoses is a first step toward predicting the biologic behavior, since mitoses ≥5/2 mm^2 predict worse outcome and metastasis in the majority of atypical carcinoids.[2302,2303]

The chromosome most frequently affected in pulmonary carcinoids is 11q. In contrast to carcinoids from other organ sites[2304,2305] in nearly all atypical carcinoids there is LOH of at least one locus, and by array CGH many segments of 11q are found to be lost. In those cases having lost more than one focus, the retrospective analysis of behavior showed an intermediate malignant phenotype.[2306] However, not all ATC presenting with worse biologic behavior can be identified by genetic analysis.

Understanding of the genes probably involved in carcinogenesis of carcinoids is in its infancy. *NCAM* is one of the genes; others are *nexin*, and a zinc-finger protein. The sequence and structure of *NCAM* is similar to that of the tumor suppressor gene *DCC* (deleted in colorectal carcinoma), which is associated with tumor progression of gastric carcinoma. Both *NCAM* and *DCC* are important adhesion molecules that function as tumor suppressor genes, too.[2306] The alteration of the *menin* gene is found in a minority of pulmonary sporadic carcinoids, but alterations distal to the *menin* locus are frequent in atypical carcinoids.[2304,2305] Therefore, it is speculated that genes distal to but near the *menin* locus might play a role in pulmonary carcinoids. One of these could be the *Int2* gene residing on chromosome 11q13. *Int2* was shown to be involved in an early event in the genesis of atypical pulmonary carcinoids.[2307]

In contrast to SCLC, *hASH1* gene expression is low in TC, higher in ATC, and most pronounced in the high-grade carcinomas.[2292] The interpretation of these findings is not possible at the moment, because of a lack of knowledge about *hASH1* function, other than the induction of a neuroendocrine phenotype.

Neuroendocrine hyperplasia and tumorlets are most probably the precursors of carcinoids. Genetic aberrations in these proposed precursors might tell us about progression to carcinoids. *Int2* allelic imbalance was significantly associated with carcinoid tumor formation, predicting progression from tumorlet to carcinoid.[2307]

Benign Lung Tumors

Papilloma (See Also Chapters 7, 34, and 35)

Pulmonary papillomas are most often squamous cell papillomas, although transitional and glandular papillomas do occur. In the experience of one author (H.H.P.), about 7% of SCCs show remnants of a papilloma, and most probably arose from this precursor lesion. Human papilloma virus (HPV) has been demonstrated in squamous cell papillomas.[2308] Malignant progression is associated with oncogenic types such as HPV 16 and 18. However, mutation in the *E2* gene in HPV 11 can cause malignant transformation.[2309,2310] Some aspects of oncogenic signaling have been uncovered for HPV genes; both the E6 and E7 region bind with RB and TP53 coded proteins, causing a prolonged half-life of the proteins. Both regions act as antiapoptotic molecules and inhibit cell cycle stop and repair mechanisms.[2311]

Hamartoma (See Also Chapter 40)

Hamartomas are the most common benign tumors detected in the lung, incidentally, and appear like discrete nodules with "popcorn calcifications" on radiographs. The majority of the lesions are peripheral, with 10% being endobronchial. Cytogenetic analyses have identified at least two subgroups of hamartomas characterized by either 6p21 or 12q14~q15 abnormalities.[2312–2315] The majority of 6p21 abnormalities are *translocations*, whereas 60% of the 12q14~q15 aberrations are translocations. The remaining 40% of 12q14~q15 abnormalities are inversions, insertions, and, rarely, deletions.[2315] Chromosome 14 is the preferred translocation partner for both the 12q14~q15 and the 6p21 rearrangements in the breakpoint 14q24 region. Besides these changes, other cytogenetic anomalies such as t(3;12), t(12;17), and various inversions of chromosome 12 have been found in these tumors.[2313, 2315–2319]

Chromosomal aberrations involving the breakpoint region 12q14 ~ q15 are frequently seen in a variety of human mesenchymal tumors, including uterine leiomyomas, lipomas, endometrial polyps, pleomorphic adenomas of the salivary gland, myxoid liposarcomas, and pulmonary chondroid hamartomas.[2320,2321] The 12q15 region harbors the *HMGI-C* gene and the 6p21 harbors the *HMGI(Y)* genes, members of the high-mobility-group fa mily.[2315,2316,2321,2322] The high-motility genes act as architectural transcription factors and are commonly expressed in embryonal cells,[2323] in transformed cells with a malignant phenotype,[2324] and in a variety of human cancers.[2325] Tallini et al.[2321] demonstrated that protein expression (by immunohistochemistry) of HMGI-C or HMGI(Y) is a common occurrence in lipomas, hamartomas, leiomyomata, and endometrial polyps, and it correlates with 12q15 and 6p21 chromosomal alterations. In Carney's syndrome, hamartomas and leiomyomas occur together, implying a common cytogenetic link such as a defect in either 12q15 or 6p21. However, the other tumor that occurs in this syndrome, extraadrenal paraganglioma, has not been associated with the above cytogenetic abnormality so far.

Solitary Fibrous Tumor (See Also Chapters 39 and 43)

Solitary fibrous tumors (SFTs) may occur in the pleura, pericardium, mediastinum, and retroperitoneum, but sometimes also in tissues far away from serous membranes, such as the pancreas, paranasal sinuses, and soft tissues. The molecular pathology of SFTs is largely unknown. According to one study, using CGH, 58% of the SFTs do not show any chromosomal imbalances. There appears to be no characteristic cytogenetic abnormalities in the ones that have some abnormalities. The most frequent defects are losses on chromosome arms 13q (33%) and 4q and 21q (17% each). Significant gains are seen at chromosome 8 and at 15q. There is no correlation between tumor size and molecular pathology findings, according to one study.[2326] Solitary fibrous tumors and hemangiopericytomas (HPCs) presenting at various soft tissue sites share many histologic and immunohistochemical features such as the staghorn pattern of vessels and CD34 positivity. This raises the questions of whether these tumors are related.

Miettinen et al.[2327] analyzed 15 SFTs and 11 HPCs by CGH, using DNA from formaldehyde-fixed and paraffin-embedded tissue and found that seven of eight SFTs larger than 10 cm (including four tumors with more than four mitoses per 10 high power fields) showed mostly chromosomal gains in 5q 7, 8, 12, and 18. Four cases in their study showed losses, two in chromosome 13 and two in 20q. The most common change was that of gain of the entire chromosome 8, similar to that previously described in other fibrous tumors, such as desmoids and infantile fibrosarcoma. In contrast, HPCs, including large and mitotically active tumors, showed no DNA copy number changes on CGH. Their study suggested that HPCs are genetically different from SFTs. In addition, SFTs, are strongly and diffusely positive for bcl-2 on immunohistochemical staining, whereas hemangiopericytomas, mesotheliomas, and most sarcomas are not. The specificity of immunodetection of bcl-2 in SFT has been confirmed by immunoblot analysis.[2328] *p53* gene mutations are extremely rare in SFT. A rare point mutation at codon 161 in exon 5 has been observed in one of the 13 cases analyzed.[2329]

Mixed Epithelial/Mesenchymal Cancers and Sarcomas of the Lung

Pulmonary Blastoma (See Also Chapters 37 and 42)

Pulmonary blastomas are rare lung tumors in which the glands and the mesenchymal elements are primitive or embryonal and resemble fetal lung between 10 to 16 weeks of gestation. If the tumor is biphasic with both primitive epithelial and mesenchymal elements, it is termed a *biphasic blastoma* and occurs predominantly in adults. When only the primitive *mesenchymal* component is present it is termed a *pleuropulmonary blastoma* (PPB) and constitutes a distinct clinicopathologic entity and occurs predominantly in children under 5 years of age. Pleuropulmonary blastoma presents as pulmonary and/or pleural-based tumors with cystic, solid, or combined cystic and solid features and generally has an unfavorable clinical outcome. Its primitive, sarcomatous features are analogous to those of other dysembryonic tumors, such as Wilms' tumor, hepatoblastoma, neuroblastoma, and embryonal rhabdomyosarcoma. However, abnormalities of the Wilms' tumor suppressor gene *(WT1)*, and the putative second genetic locus for Wilms' tumor *(WT2)* are not found in preliminary investigations.[2330] Approximately 25% of PPBs are associated with other lesions such as pulmonary cysts, cystic nephromas, sarcomas, medulloblastomas, thyroid dysplasias and neoplasias, malignant germ cell tumors, Hodgkin's disease, leukemia, and Langerhans cell histiocytosis. Hence, PPB should be considered as a marker of familial disease.[2330]

The β-catenin gene is one of the essential components for specification of timing and development of peripheral airways, as has been shown in a mouse model.[2331] Normally, the β-catenin protein is localized in the membrane. Gene mutation of β-catenin with subsequent nuclear/cytoplasmic (N/C) overaccumulation of the protein plays an important role in tumorigenesis of various organs including biphasic pulmonary blastoma. In the biphasic lesions, both the sarcomatous elements and the epithelial elements, aberrantly, express the β-catenin in the nucleus. Carcinosarcoma with high-grade fetal type/clear cells (so-called blastomatoid variant of carcinosarcoma) appears not to have the nuclear localization like the classic biphasic pulmonary blastomas. Mutational analysis of exon 3 of the β-catenin gene reveals that biphasic pulmonary blastomas harbor missense mutations.[2332]

p53 point mutations are variable (14–43%) in classic biphasic pulmonary blastomas.[2333,2334] However, in these lesions, *p53* may be demonstrated on immunohistochemistry without gene mutations.[2333,2335] There is better concordance of immunohistochemistry with gene mutations for spindle cell carcinomas and carcinosarcoma.[2333] The MDM2 protein gene product, believed to be significant in the pathogenesis of bronchogenic carcinoma, is present in 83% of classic biphasic pulmonary blastomas.[2335] No K-*ras* mutations are detected in classic pulmonary blastoma, and its mimics including spindle cell carcinoma and carcinosarcoma, according to one study.[2333] Monoclonal histogenesis from a single totipotential cell in a subset of these neoplasms is supported by the finding of *p53* overexpression and identical *p53* mutational genotype in both the epithelial and spindle elements of the tumors.[2333]

Comparative genomic hybridization study performed on PPB is characterized by several chromosomal imbalances. Gains observed affected regions 1q12-q23, 3q23-qter, 8pter-q24.1, 9p13–q21, 17p12–p11, 17q11–q22, 17q23–q25, 19pter-p11, and 19q11-q13.3. *Whole chromosome gains are detected on chromosomes 2 and 7.* Loss of genetic material is found at regions 6q13-qter, 10pter-p13, 10q22-qter, and 20p13. Whole chromosome gains have been confirmed by other cytogenetic studies describing gains of chromosomes 2 and 8 as recurrent abnormalities in this type of tumor, suggesting that a gene or genes of putative relevance in PPB pathogenesis are mapped at 8p11–p12. The CGH profile of PPB resembles that observed in embryonal rhabdomyosarcomas, in which gains of 2 or 2q, 7 or 7q, and 8 or 8p and loss of 10q22-qter are consistently found, implying that the two may be closely related.[2336–2338]

Synovial Sarcoma, Leiomyosarcoma, Malignant Fibrous Histiocytoma, and Malignant Peripheral Nerve Sheath Tumor (See Also Chapters 39 to 41)

Primary synovial sarcoma (SS) of the lung is rare. The tumor occurs in men and women at a median age of 50 years and ranges in size from 2 to 15.5 cm. Monophasic synovial sarcoma is far more common than biphasic synovial sarcoma in the lung. Some tumors have less than one mitosis per high power field, while others have up to five per high power field. Most are negative for e-cadherin. The aberrant expression of β-catenin within cytoplasm or nuclei is observed in two thirds of the cases. The presence of a tumor-specific SYT-SSX fusion gene as in soft tissue tumors is confirmatory. SYT-SSX1 fusion transcript is more common than the SSX2 as in soft tissue tumors. The SYT-SSX fusion gene is very valuable in diagnosing synovial sarcoma in odd locations like the lung, where it occurs rarely.[2339]

Primary leiomyosarcomas are rare in the lung. Genetic studies are not available. Kawai et al.[2340] reported the first case of renin producing leiomyosarcoma of the lung, in a 54 year old woman with parapancreatic metastases.

Malignant fibrous histiocytoma (MFH) is the most common soft tissue sarcoma in adults. However, primary MFH and primary nerve sheath tumors of the lung are rare, with only a few cases reported in the literature. Molecular genetic studies are not available.

Tarkkanen et al.[2341] compared genetic aberrations in primary sarcomas and their pulmonary metastases to explore the pathways associated with disease spreading. The primary tumor and its subsequent pulmonary metastasis of 22 patients were analyzed by comparative genomic hybridization. The mean total number of aberrations per tumor was 7.6 (range, 0–17) in primary tumors and 7.5 (range, 0–19) in metastases. The frequencies of the most common aberrations were relatively similar in primary tumors and metastases. The most frequent gain affected 1q (minimal common regions 1q21–q23 in 36% of primary tumors and 1q21 in 45% of metastases). The most frequent losses were detected at 9p. *No aberrations specific to metastases were detected.* An increase in the total number of changes during progression was a predominant feature in a majority of the cases.[2341]

Diffuse Malignant Mesothelioma (See Also Chapter 43)

Diffuse malignant mesothelioma (DMM) has a unique molecular pathogenesis compared to most cancers.[2342] Of the numerous chromosomal defects found in individual DMM tumors by karyotype, DNA cytometry, and CGH, no single cytogenetic abnormality is specific for DMM, but a typical pattern of genomic defects can be found. A DNA cytometry and CGH study of 90 cases of DMM found an average of 6.2 chromosomal imbalances per case with common losses reported in chromosomal regions 9p21, 22q, 4q31–32, 4p12–13, 14q12–24, 1p21, 13q13–14, 3p21, 6q22, 10p13-pter, and 17p12-pter, and common gains on 8q22–23, 1q23/1q32, 7p14–15, and 15q22–25.[2343] Molecular genetic analysis of 14 cases of DMM using CGH, LOH, and quantitative microsatellite analysis (QuMA) indicated at least three tumor suppressor genes mapped to chromosome 6q are commonly involved in the pathogenesis of DMM.[2344]

New genomic tools are likely to assist in understanding the molecular pathogenesis of DMM.[2345,2346] Mutations of the important tumor suppressor genes *Rb* and *p53* are distinctly rare in DMM. However, the mutations that have been most consistently described so far in DMM involve p16, p14ARF and NF2 which impact on *Rb* and *p53* expression and may cause the same final effect as direct mutations of *Rb* and *p53* as described earlier (see Molecular Procedures). Abnormalities of *p16* have been described in 31% of diffuse malignant mesotheliomas with inactivation of p16INK4a by DNA hypermethylation reported in 19% of tumors and cell lines.[2347–2349] Mutations of the Wilms' tumor gene *(WT1)* occur only in a small minority of mesotheliomas, even though *WT1* expression is a diagnostic marker of DMM.[2350] Expression of the antiapoptotic protein Bcl-xl in DMM cell lines has been proposed to be a target for antisense oligonucleotides to augment response of DMM to chemotherapy.[2351,2352] Other genes and gene products that have recently been proposed to be of potential interest in DMM pathogenesis or treatment, primarily from studies of cell lines and tissue microarrays, include SCF/c-*Kit*/Slug,[2353] DEL-1,[2354] matriptase,[2355] IGF system,[2356] c-FLIP,[2357] and several cell adhesion proteins.[2358] A microarray study of amplified mRNA from DMM cells isolated by laser capture microdissection showed overexpression of BF, FTL, IGFBP7, RARRES1, RARRES2, RBP1, SAT, and TXN, and underexpression of ALOX5AP, CLNS1A, EIF4A2, ELK3, REQ, and SYPL.[2359]

Theories about the molecular genetic pathogenesis of DMM have included hypotheses involving the oncogenic polyomavirus simian virus 40 (SV40) for more than a decade. Immortalization of human mesothelial cells by transfection with SV40 had been used to create in vitro models for the study of asbestos-induced mesothelioma.[2360] In 1993, SV40 was reported to induce DMM in hamsters,[2361] and a year later SV40-like DNA sequences were reported in 60% of 48 human DMM with SV40 large T-antigen expression in 13 of 16 specimens.[2362] Subsequently, for more than a decade, SV40 large T antigen (Tag) has been reported in human DMM from many laboratories in North America, Europe, and elsewhere by PCR amplification of frozen and paraffin-embedded tissues, sequencing, immunohistochemistry, primed in situ, and detection of SV40 Tag-specific cytotoxic T lymphocytes.[2363–2380] Other investigators have disputed a role for SV40 in the development of human DMM primarily on the basis of studies that fail to show an increase in DMM related to the inoculation of populations with polio or other vaccines contaminated with SV40, lack of serologic evidence, and failure to find evidence of SV40 in human DMM tissue samples in their studies.[2381–2395]

As noted above, tumor suppressor gene mutations in *p53* and *RB* are characteristic of many cancers, but are rare in DMM. Reports of SV40 Tag in many human mesotheliomas has led to a hypothesis that the Tag protein binds p53 or RB products in DMM, inhibiting them without causing mutation, or that SV40 Tag has effects on other gene products in interacting signaling pathways.[2396–2417] Therefore, similar to p16 and p14, SV40 Tag may impair the cell cycle control by *RB* and *p53* even when mutations of *RB* and *p53* are not present. These hypotheses have not only been considered possible explanations of how SV40 may act as an etiologic agent or cofactor (with asbestos) for DMM, but also have been considered possible targets for molecular therapy of DMM. The SV40 virus has also been reported to induce telomerase activity in human mesothelial cells.[2418]

References

1. Coleman WB, Tsongalis GJ, eds. The molecular basis of human cancer. Totowa, NJ: Humana Press, 2002.
2. Watson JD, Baker TA, Bell SP, Gann A, Levine M, Losick R, eds. Molecular biology of the gene. 5th ed. Menlo Park, CA: Benjamin Cummings, 2003.
3. Epstein RJ, ed. Human molecular biology: an introduction to the molecular basis of health and disease. Cambridge: Cambridge University Press, 2003.
4. Strachan T, Read A, eds. Human molecular genetics. 3rd ed. New York: Garland Science/Taylor and Francis Group, 2003.
5. Swansbury J, ed. Cancer cytogenetics: methods and protocols. Totowa, NJ: Humana Press, 2003.
6. Cooper GM, Hausman RE, eds. The cell: a molecular approach. 3rd ed. Washington, DC: ASM Press; Sunderland, MA: Sinauer Associates, 2004.
7. Farkas DH, ed. DNA from A to Z. Washington: AACC Press, 2004.
8. Killeen AA, ed. Principles of molecular pathology. Totowa, NJ: Humana Press, 2004.

9. Leonard DGB, ed. Molecular pathology in clinical practice. New York: Springer, 2007.
10. Fisher JC, Hollomon JH. A hypothesis for the origin of cancer foci. Cancer 1951;4:916–918.
11. Fisher JC. Multiple-mutation theory of carcinogenesis. Nature 1958;181:651–652.
12. Nowell PC. The clonal evolution of tumor cell populations. Science 1976;194:23–28.
13. Croce CM. Chromosome translocations and human cancer. Cancer Res 1986;46:6019–6023.
14. Knudson AG, Jr. Genetics of human cancer. Annu Rev Genet 1986;20:231–251.
15. Weinberg RA. Oncogenes, antioncogenes, and the molecular bases of multistep carcinogenesis. Cancer Res 1989;49:3713–3721.
16. Bishop JM. Molecular themes in oncogenesis. Cell 1991;64:235–248.
17. Ames BN, Shigenaga MK, Gold LS. DNA lesions, inducible DNA repair, and cell division: three key factors in mutagenesis and carcinogenesis. Environ Health Perspect 1993;101(suppl 5):35–44.
18. Cheng KC, Loeb LA. Genomic instability and tumor progression: mechanistic considerations. Adv Cancer Res 1993;60:121–156.
19. Renan MJ. How many mutations are required for tumorigenesis? Implications from human cancer data. Mol Carcinog 1993;7:139–146.
20. Coleman WB, Tsongalis GJ. Multiple mechanisms account for genomic instability and molecular mutation in neoplastic transformation. Clin Chem 1995;41:644–657.
21. Cairns J. Mutation and cancer: the antecedents to our studies of adaptive mutation. Genetics 1998;148:1433–1440.
22. Jackson AL, Loeb LA. The mutation rate and cancer. Genetics 1998;148:1483–1490.
23. Lengauer C, Kinzler KW, Vogelstein B. Genetic instabilities in human cancers. Nature 1998;396:643–649.
24. Coleman WB, Tsongalis GJ. The role of genomic instability in human carcinogenesis. Anticancer Res 1999;19: 4645–4664.
25. Schmutte C, Fishel R. Genomic instability: first step to carcinogenesis. Anticancer Res 1999;19:4665–4696.
26. Cagle PT. The cytogenetics and molecular genetics of lung cancer: implications for pathologists. In: Rosen PP, Fechner RE, eds. Pathology annual. East Norwalk, CT: Appleton and Lange, 1990:317–329.
27. Harris CC, Reddel R, Pfeifer A, et al. Role of oncogenes and tumour suppressor genes in human lung carcinogenesis. In: O'Neill IK, Chen J, Barsch H, eds. Relevance to human cancer of N-nitroso compounds, tobacco smoke and mycotoxins. Lyon: IARC, 1991:294–304.
28. Iman DS, Harris CC. Oncogenes and tumor suppressor genes in human lung carcinogenesis. Crit Rev Oncogen 1991;2:161–171.
29. Sozzi G, Miozzo M, Tagliabue E, et al. Cytogenetic abnormalities and overexpression of receptors for growth factors in normal bronchial epithelial and tumor samples of lung cancer patients. Cancer Res 1991;51:400–404.
30. Gazdar AF. Molecular markers for the diagnosis and prognosis of lung cancer. Cancer 1992;69:1592–1599.
31. Cagle PT. Molecular pathology of lung cancer and its clinical relevance. In: Katzenstein A-L, Churg A, eds. Current topics in pulmonary pathology. Baltimore: Williams and Wilkins, 1993.
32. Cagle PT. Lung cancer. In: Kurzrock R, Talpaz M, eds. Molecular biology in cancer medicine. London: Martin Dunitz, 1999:367–378.
33. Hanahan D, Weinberg RA. The hallmarks of cancer. Cell 2000;100:57–70.
34. Fong KM, Sekido Y, Minna J. The molecular basis of lung carcinogenesis. In: Coleman WB, Tsongalis GJ, eds. The molecular basis of human cancer. Totowa, NJ: Humana Press, 2002:379–405.
35. Fong KM, Sekido Y, Gazdar AF, Minna JD. Lung cancer. 9: Molecular biology of lung cancer: clinical implications. Thorax 2003;58:892–900.
36. Sekido Y, Fong KM, Minna JD. Molecular genetics of lung cancer. Annu Rev Med 2003;54:73–87.
37. Rodenhuis S, van de Wetering ML, Mooi WJ, Evers SG, van Zanwijk N, Bos JL. Mutational activation of the K-ras oncogene: a possible pathogenetic factor in adenocarcinoma of the lung. N Engl J Med 1987;317:929–935.
38. Belinsky SA, Devereux TR, Stoner GD, Anderson MW. Activation of the k-ras protooncogene in lung tumors from mice treated with 4-(N-methyl-N-nitrosamino)-1-(3–pyridyl)-1-butanone (NNK) or nitrosodimethylamine (NDMA). Proc AACR 1988;29:139.
39. Philips DH, Hewer A, Martin CN, Garner RC, King MM. Correlation of DNA adduct level in human lung with cigarette smoking. Nature 1988;336:790–792.
40. Rodenhuis S, Slebos RJC, Boot AJM, et al. Incidence and possible clinical significance of K-ras oncogene activation in adenocarcinoma of the human lung. Cancer Res 1988; 48:5738–5741.
41. Belinsky SA, Devereux TR, Maronpot RR, Stone G, Anderson MW. Relationship between the formation of promutagenic adducts and the activation of the K-ras protooncogene in lung tumors from A/J mice treated with nitrosamines. Cancer Res 1989;49:5305–5311.
42. Randerath R, Miller RH, Mittal D, Avitts TA, Dunsford HA, Randerath K. Covalent DNA damage in tissues of cigarette smoking as determined by 32p-postlabeling assay. J Natl Cancer Inst. 1989; 81:341–347.
43. You M, Candrian U, Maronpot R, Stoner G, Anderson M. Activation of the K-ras protooncogene in spontaneously occurring and chemically induced lung tumors of the strain A mouse. Proc Natl Acad Sci USA 1989;86: 3070–3074.
44. Chiba I, Takahashi T, Nau MM, et al. Mutations in the p53 gene are frequent in primary non-small cell lung cancer. Oncogene 1990;5:1603–1610.
45. Goodrow T, Reynolds S, Maronpot R, Anderson M. Activation of K-ras by codon 13 mutations in C57BL/6 X $C3HAF_1$ mouse tumors induced by exposure to 1,3–butadiene. Cancer Res 1990;50:4818–4823.
46. Takahashi T, D'Amico D, Chiba I, Buchhagen DL, Minna JD. Identification of intronic point mutations as an alternative mechanism for p53 inactivation in lung cancer. J Clin Invest 1990;86:363–369.

47. Brandt-Rauf PW. Advances in cancer biomarkers as applied to chemical exposures: the ras oncogene and p21 protein and pulmonary carcinogenesis. J Occup Med 1991;33:951–955.
48. Hall PA, Ray A, Lemoine NR, Midgley CA, Krauz T, Lane DP. p53 immunostaining as a marker of malignant disease in diagnostic cytopathology. Lancet 1991; 338:513.
49. Hollstein M, Sidransky D, Vogelstein B, Harris CC. p53 mutations in human cancers. Science 1991;253:49–52.
50. Lehman TA, Bennett WP, Metcalf RA, et al. p53 mutations, ras mutations, and p53–heat shock 70 protein complexes in human lung carcinoma cell lines. Cancer Res 1991;51:4090–4096.
51. Reynolds SH, Anderson MW. Activation of proto-oncogenes in human and mouse lung tumors. Environ Health Perspect 1991;93:145–148.
52. Slebos RJC, Hruban RH, Dalesio O, Mooi WJ, Offerhaus JA, Rodenhuis S. Relationship between K-ras oncogene activation and smoking in adenocarcinoma of the human lung. J Natl Cancer Inst 1991;83:1024–1027.
53. Sundaresan V, Reeve JG, Wilson B, Bleehen NM, Watson JV. Flow cytometric and immunohistochemical analysis of $p62_{c\text{-}myc}$ oncoprotein in the bronchial epithelium of lung cancer patients. Anticancer Res 1991;11:2111–2116.
54. Vahakangas KH, Samet JM, Metcalf RA, et al. Mutations of p53 and ras genes in radon-associated lung cancer from uranium miners. Lancet 1992;339:576–580.
55. Westra WH, Offerhaus JA, Goodman SN, et al. Overexpression of the p53 tumor suppressor gene product in primary lung adenocarcinomas is associated with cigarette smoking. Am J Surg Pathol 1993;17:213–220.
56. Denissenko MF, Pao A, Tang M, et al. Preferential formation of benzo[a]pyrene adducts at lung cancer mutational hotspots in P53. Science 1996;274:430–432.
57. Tammemagi MC, McLaughlin JR, Bull SB. Meta-analyses of p53 tumor suppressor gene alterations and clinicopathological features in resected lung cancers. Cancer Epidemiol Biomarkers Prev 1999;8:625–634.
58. Gautam A, Densmore CL, Waldrep JC. Inhibition of experimental lung metastasis by aerosol delivery of PEI-p53 complexes. Mol Ther 2000;2:318–323.
59. Sirotnak FM, Zakowski MF, Miller VA, Scher HI, Kris MG. Efficacy of cytotoxic agents against human tumor xenografts is markedly enhanced by coadministration of ZD1839 (Iressa), an inhibitor of EGFR tyrosine kinase. Clin Cancer Res 2000;6:4885–4892.
60. Arteaga CL, Johnson DH. Tyrosine kinase inhibitors-ZD1839 (Iressa). Curr Opin Oncol 2001;13:491–498.
61. Ramesh R, Saeki T, Templeton NS, et al. Successful treatment of primary and disseminated human lung cancers by systemic delivery of tumor suppressor genes using an improved liposome vector. Mol Ther 2001;3:337–350.
62. Kaliberov SA, Buchsbaum DJ, Gillespie GY, et al. Adenovirus-mediated transfer of BAX driven by the vascular endothelial growth factor promoter induces apoptosis in lung cancer cells. Mol Ther 2002;6:190–198.
63. Kawabe S, Nishikawa T, Munshi A, Roth JA, Chada S, Meyn RE. Adenovirus-mediated mda-7 gene expression radiosensitizes non-small cell lung cancer cells via TP53-independent mechanisms. Mol Ther 2002;6:637–644.
64. Raben D, Helfrich BA, Chan D, Johnson G, Bunn PA Jr. ZD1839, a selective epidermal growth factor receptor tyrosine kinase inhibitor, alone and in combination with radiation and chemotherapy as a new therapeutic strategy in non-small cell lung cancer. Semin Oncol 2002; 29(1 suppl 4):37–46.
65. Ranson M, Hammond LA, Ferry D, et al. Related ZD1839, a selective oral epidermal growth factor receptor-tyrosine kinase inhibitor, is well tolerated and active in patients with solid, malignant tumors: results of a phase I trial. J Clin Oncol 2002;20:2240–2250.
66. Ito I, Began G, Mohiuddin I, et al. Increased uptake of liposomal-DNA complexes by lung metastases following intravenous administration. Mol Ther 2003;7:409–418.
67. Mhashilkar AM, Stewart AL, Sieger K, et al. MDA-7 negatively regulates the beta-catenin and PI3K signaling pathways in breast and lung tumor cells. Mol Ther 2003;8:207–219.
68. Janmaat ML, Giaccone G. The epidermal growth factor receptor pathway and its inhibition as anticancer therapy. Drugs Today (Barc) 2003;n39(suppl C):61–80.
69. Rossi G, Cavazza A, Marchioni A, et al. Kit expression in small cell carcinomas of the lung: effects of chemotherapy. Mod Pathol 2003;16:1041–1047.
70. Brattstrom D, Wester K, Bergqvist M, et al. HER-2, EGFR, COX-2 expression status correlated to microvessel density and survival in resected non-small cell lung cancer. Acta Oncol 2004;43:80–86.
71. Butnor KJ, Burchette JL, Sporn TA, Hammar SP, Roggli VL. The spectrum of Kit (CD117) immunoreactivity in lung and pleural tumors: a study of 96 cases using a single-source antibody with a review of the literature. Arch Pathol Lab Med 2004;128:538–543.
72. Lynch TJ, Bell DW, Sordella R, et al. Activating mutations in the epidermal growth factor receptor underlying responsiveness of non-small-cell lung cancer to gefitinib. N Engl J Med 2004;350:2129–2139.
73. Pelosi G, Barisella M, Pasini F, et al. CD117 immunoreactivity in stage I adenocarcinoma and squamous cell carcinoma of the lung: relevance to prognosis in a subset of adenocarcinoma patients. Mod Pathol 2004;17: 711–721.
74. Onn A, Herbst RS. Molecular targeted therapy for lung cancer. Lancet 2005;366:1507–1508.
75. Ramalingam S, Belani CP. Molecularly-targeted therapies for non-small cell lung cancer. Expert Opin Pharmacother 2005;6:2667–2679.
76. Silvestri GA, Rivera MP. Targeted therapy for the treatment of advanced non-small cell lung cancer: a review of the epidermal growth factor receptor antagonists. Chest 2005;128:3975–3984.
77. Nemunaitis J, Meyers T, Senzer N, et al. Phase I trial of sequential administration of recombinant DNA and adenovirus expressing L523S protein in early stage non-small-cell lung cancer. Mol Ther 2006;13:1185–1191.
78. Sato M, Vaughan MB, Girard L, et al. Multiple oncogenic changes (K-RAS(V12), p53 knockdown, mutant EGFRs,

p16 bypass, telomerase) are not sufficient to confer a full malignant phenotype on human bronchial epithelial cells. Cancer Res 2006;66:2116–2128.
79. Watson JD, Crick FH. Molecular structure of nucleic acids; a structure for deoxyribose nucleic acid. Nature 1953;171:737–738.
80. Thoma F, Koller T. Influence of histone H1 on chromatin structure. Cell 1977;12:101–107.
81. Varshavsky AJ, Bakayev VV, Nedospasov SA, Georgiev GP. On the structure of eukaryotic, prokaryotic, and viral chromatin. Cold Spring Harb Symp Quant Biol 1978; 42(pt 1):457–473.
82. Tyler-Smith C, Willard HF. Mammalian chromosome structure. Curr Opin Genet Dev 1993;3:390–397.
83. Lamond AI, Earnshaw WC. Structure and function in the nucleus. Science 1998;280:547–553.
84. Goldberg S, Schwartz H, Darnell JE Jr. Evidence from UV transcription mapping in HeLa cells that heterogeneous nuclear RNA is the messenger RNA precursor. Proc Natl Acad Sci USA 1977;74:4520–4523.
85. Hoffmann-Berling H. DNA unwinding enzymes. Prog Clin Biol Res 1982;102(pt C):89–98.
86. Wang JC. DNA topoisomerases: why so many? J Biol Chem 1991;266:6659–6662.
87. Anderson HJ, Roberge M. DNA topoisomerase II: a review of its involvement in chromosome structure, DNA replication, transcription and mitosis. Cell Biol Int Rep 1992;16:717–724.
88. Gasser SM, Walter R, Dang Q, Cardenas ME. Topoisomerase II: its functions and phosphorylation. Antonie Van Leeuwenhoek 1992;62:15–24.
89. D'Incalci M. DNA-topoisomerase inhibitors. Curr Opin Oncol 1993;5:1023–1028.
90. Ferguson LR, Baguley BC. Topoisomerase II enzymes and mutagenicity. Environ Mol Mutagen 1994;24: 245–261.
91. Larsen AK, Skladanowski A, Bojanowski K. The roles of DNA topoisomerase II during the cell cycle. Prog Cell Cycle Res 1996;2:229–239.
92. Kato S, Kikuchi A. DNA topoisomerase: the key enzyme that regulates DNA super structure. Nagoya J Med Sci 1998;61:11–26.
93. Wang JC. Cellular roles of DNA topoisomerases: a molecular perspective. Nat Rev Mol Cell Biol 2002;3: 430–440.
94. Gimenez-Abian JF, Clarke DJ. Replication-coupled topoisomerase II templates the mitotic chromosome scaffold? Cell Cycle 2003;2:230–232.
95. Leppard JB, Champoux JJ. Human DNA topoisomerase I: relaxation, roles, and damage control. Chromosoma 2005;114:75–85.
96. Sharp PA. RNA splicing and genes. JAMA 1988;260: 3035–3041.
97. Gorlach M, Burd CG, Dreyfuss G. The mRNA poly(A)-binding protein: localization, abundance, and RNA-binding specificity. Exp Cell Res 1994;211:400–407.
98. Fotedar R, Fotedar A. Cell cycle control of DNA replication. Prog Cell Cycle Res 1995;1:73–89.
99. Auerbach AD, Verlander PC. Disorders of DNA replication and repair. Curr Opin Pediatr 1997;9:600–616.
100. Sharp SJ, Schaack J, Cooley L, Burke DJ, Soll D. Structure and transcription of eukaryotic tRNA genes. CRC Crit Rev Biochem 1985;19:107–144.
101. Persson BC. Modification of tRNA as a regulatory device. Mol Microbiol 1993;8:1011–1016.
102. Green R, Noller HF. Ribosomes and translation. Annu Rev Biochem 1997;66:679–716.
103. Cech TR. Self-splicing of group I introns. Annu Rev Biochem 1990;59:543–568.
104. Jacquier A. Self-splicing group II and nuclear pre-mRNA introns: how similar are they? Trends Biochem Sci 1990; 15:351–354.
105. Balvay L, Libri D, Fiszman MY. Pre-mRNA secondary structure and the regulation of splicing. Bioessays 1993;15:165–169.
106. Sutherland GR, Richards RI. Simple tandem DNA repeats and human genetic disease. Proc Natl Acad Sci USA 1995;92:3636–3641.
107. Horii A, Han HJ, Shimada M, et al. Frequent replication errors at microsatellite loci in tumors of patients with multiple primary cancers. Cancer Res 1994;54:3373–3375.
108. Loeb LA. Microsatellite instability: marker of a mutator phenotype in cancer. Cancer Res 1994;54:5059–5063.
109. Mao L, Lee DJ, Tockman MS, Erozan YS, Askin F, Sidransky D. Microsatellite alterations as clonal markers for the detection of human cancer. Proc Natl Acad Sci USA 1994;91:9871–9875.
110. Merlo A, Mabry M, Gabrielson E, Vollmer R, Baylin SB, Sidransky D. Frequent microsatellite instability in primary small cell lung cancer. Cancer Res 1994;54:2098–2101.
111. Wooster R, Cleton-Jansen AM, Collins N, et al. Instability of short tandem repeats (microsatellites) in human cancers. Nat Genet 1994;6:152–156.
112. Fong KM, Zimmerman PV, Smith PJ. Microsatellite instability and other molecular abnormalities in non-small cell lung cancer. Cancer Res 1995;55:28–30.
113. Miozzo M, Sozzi G, Musso K, et al. Microsatellite alterations in bronchial and sputum specimens of lung cancer patients. Cancer Res 1996;56:2285–2288.
114. Bocker T, Diermann J, Friedl W, et al. Microsatellite instability analysis: a multicenter study for reliability and quality control. Cancer Res 1997;57:4739–4743.
115. Dietmaier W, Wallinger S, Bocker T, Kullmann F, Fishel R, Ruschoff J. Diagnostic microsatellite instability: definition and correlation with mismatch repair protein expression. Cancer Res 1997;57:4749–4756.
116. Lothe RA. Microsatellite instability in human solid tumors. Mol Med Today 1997;3:61–68.
117. Arzimanoglou, II, Gilbert F, Barber HR. Microsatellite instability in human solid tumors. Cancer 1998;82: 1808–1820.
118. Boland CR, Thibodeau SN, Hamilton SR, et al. A National Cancer Institute Workshop on Microsatellite Instability for cancer detection and familial predisposition: development of international criteria for the determination of microsatellite instability in colorectal cancer. Cancer Res 1998;58:5248–5257.
119. Boyer JC, Farber RA. Mutation rate of a microsatellite sequence in normal human fibroblasts. Cancer Res 1998; 58:3946–3949.

120. Hanford MG, Rushton BC, Gowen LC, Farber RA. Microsatellite mutation rates in cancer cell lines deficient or proficient in mismatch repair. Oncogene 1998;16:2389–2393.
121. Jackson AL, Chen R, Loeb LA. Induction of microsatellite instability by oxidative DNA damage. Proc Natl Acad Sci USA 1998;95:12468–12473.
122. Johannsdottir JT, Jonasson JG, Bergthorsson JT, et al. The effect of mismatch repair deficiency on tumourigenesis; microsatellite instability affecting genes containing short repeated sequences. Int J Oncol 2000;16:133–139.
123. Kim WS, Park C, Hong SK, Park BK, Kim HS, Park K. Microsatellite instability(MSI) in non-small cell lung cancer(NSCLC) is highly associated with transforming growth factor-beta type II receptor(TGF-beta RII) frameshift mutation. Anticancer Res 2000;20:1499–1502.
124. Krieg PA, Melton DA. In vitro RNA synthesis with SP6 RNA polymerase. Methods Enzymol 1987; 155:397–415.
125. Lawyer FC, Stoffel S, Saiki RK, Myambo K, Drummond R, Gelfand DH. Isolation, characterization, and expression in Escherichia coli of the DNA polymerase gene from Thermus aquaticus. J Biol Chem 1989;264: 6427–6437.
126. Studier FW, Rosenberg AH, Dunn JJ, Dubendorff JW. Use of T7 RNA polymerase to direct expression of cloned genes. Methods Enzymol 1990;185:60–89.
127. Kollmar R, Farnham PJ. Site-specific initiation of transcription by RNA polymerase II. Proc Soc Exp Biol Med 1993;203:127–139.
128. Chou KC, Kezdy FJ, Reusser F. Kinetics of processive nucleic acid polymerases and nucleases. Anal Biochem 1994;221:217–230.
129. Tabor S, Richardson CC. A single residue in DNA polymerases of the Escherichia coli DNA polymerase I family is critical for distinguishing between deoxy- and dideoxyribonucleotides. Proc Natl Acad Sci USA 1995;92: 6339–6343.
130. Lai CJ, Markoff LJ, Zimmerman S, Cohen B, Berndt JA, Chanock RM. Cloning DNA sequences from influenza viral RNA segments. Proc Natl Acad Sci USA 1980; 77:210–214.
131. Kotewicz ML, D'Alessio JM, Driftmier KM, Blodgett KP, Gerard GF. Cloning and overexpression of Moloney murine leukemia virus reverse transcriptase in Escherichia coli. Gene 1985;35:249–258.
132. Biessmann H, Mason JM. Telomeric repeat sequences. Chromosoma 1994;103:154–161.
133. Feng J, Funk WD, Wang SS, et al. The RNA component of human telomerase. Science 1995;269:1236–1241.
134. Counter CM. The roles of telomeres and telomerase in cell life span. Mutat Res 1996;366:45–63.
135. Wellinger RJ, Sen D. The DNA structures at the ends of eukaryotic chromosomes. Eur J Cancer 1997;33:735–749.
136. Chakhparonian M, Wellinger RJ. Telomere maintenance and DNA replication: how closely are these two connected? Trends Genet 2003;19:439–446.
137. Bayne S, Liu JP. Hormones and growth factors regulate telomerase activity in ageing and cancer. Mol Cell Endocrinol 2005;240:11–22.
138. Blackburn EH. Telomeres and telomerase: their mechanisms of action and the effects of altering their functions. FEBS Lett 2005;579:859–862.
139. Blasco MA. Telomeres and human disease: ageing, cancer and beyond. Nat Rev Genet 2005;6:611–622.
140. Boukamp P, Popp S, Krunic D. Telomere-dependent chromosomal instability. J Investig Dermatol Symp Proc 2005;10:89–94.
141. Brunori M, Luciano P, Gilson E, Geli V.The telomerase cycle: normal and pathological aspects. J Mol Med 2005; 83:244–257.
142. Dong CK, Masutomi K, Hahn WC. Telomerase: regulation, function and transformation. Crit Rev Oncol Hematol 2005;54:85–93.
143. Jacobs JJ, de Lange T. p16INK4a as a second effector of the telomere damage pathway. Cell Cycle 2005;4: 1364–1368.
144. Opitz OG. Telomeres, telomerase and malignant transformation. Curr Mol Med 2005;5:219–226.
145. Viscardi V, Clerici M, Cartagena-Lirola H, Longhese MP. Telomeres and DNA damage checkpoints. Biochimie 2005;87:613–624.
146. Autexier C, Lue NF. The Structure and Function of Telomerase Reverse Transcriptase. Annu Rev Biochem 2006;75:493–517.
147. Bhattacharyya MK, Lustig AJ. Telomere dynamics in genome stability. Trends Biochem Sci 2006;31:114–122.
148. Pallen CJ, Tan YH, Guy GR. Protein phosphatases in cell signalling. Curr Opin Cell Biol 1992;4:1000–1007.
149. Boulikas T. Control of DNA replication by protein phosphorylation. Anticancer Res 1994;14:2465–2472.
150. Berndt N. Protein dephosphorylation and the intracellular control of the cell number. Front Biosci 1999;4: D22–D42.
151. Appella E, Anderson CW. Post-translational modifications and activation of p53 by genotoxic stresses. Eur J Biochem 2001;268:2764–2772.
152. Fu M, Wang C, Wang J, Zafonte BT, Lisanti MP, Pestell RG. Acetylation in hormone signaling and the cell cycle. Cytokine Growth Factor Rev 2002;13:259–276.
153. Obaya AJ, Sedivy JM. Regulation of cyclin-Cdk activity in mammalian cells. Cell Mol Life Sci 2002;59:126–142.
154. Haglund K, Dikic I. Ubiquitylation and cell signaling. EMBO J 2005;24:3353–3359.
155. Legube G, Trouche D. Regulating histone acetyltransferases and deacetylases. EMBO Rep 2003;4:944–947.
156. Marmorstein R. Structural and chemical basis of histone acetylation. Novartis Found Symp 2004;259:78–98.
157. Moore JD, Krebs JE. Histone modifications and DNA double-strand break repair. Biochem Cell Biol 2004;82: 446–452.
158. Peterson CL, Laniel MA. Histones and histone modifications. Curr Biol 2004;14:R546–R551.
159. Quivy V, Calomme C, Dekoninck A, et al. Gene activation and gene silencing: a subtle equilibrium. Cloning Stem Cells 2004;6:140–149.

160. Wang Y, Fischle W, Cheung W, Jacobs S, Khorasanizadeh S, Allis CD. Beyond the double helix: writing and reading the histone code. Novartis Found Symp 2004;259:3–17.
161. Fraga MF, Esteller M. Towards the human cancer epigenome: a first draft of histone modifications. Cell Cycle 2005;4:1377–1381.
162. Khan AU, Krishnamurthy S. Histone modifications as key regulators of transcription. Front Biosci 2005;10: 866–872.
163. Verdone L, Caserta M, Di Mauro E. Role of histone acetylation in the control of gene expression. Biochem Cell Biol 2005;83:344–353.
164. Yu Y, Waters R. Histone acetylation, chromatin remodelling and nucleotide excision repair: hint from the study on MFA2 in Saccharomyces cerevisiae. Cell Cycle 2005; 4:1043–1045.
165. Verdone L, Agricola E, Caserta M, Di Mauro E. Histone acetylation in gene regulation. Brief Funct Genomic Proteomic 2006;5:209–221.
166. Haura EB, Turkson J, Jove R. Mechanisms of disease: insights into the emerging role of signal transducers and activators of transcription in cancer. Nat Clin Pract Oncol 2005;2:315–324.
167. Wang JC. Finding primary targets of transcriptional regulators. Cell Cycle 2005;4:356–358.
168. Wittenberg C, Reed SI. Cell cycle-dependent transcription in yeast: promoters, transcription factors, and transcriptomes. Oncogene 2005;24:2746–2755.
169. Zaidi SK, Young DW, Choi JY, et al. The dynamic organization of gene-regulatory machinery in nuclear microenvironments. EMBO Rep 2005;6:128–133.
170. Barrera LO, Ren B. The transcriptional regulatory code of eukaryotic cells—insights from genome-wide analysis of chromatin organization and transcription factor binding. Curr Opin Cell Biol 2006;18:291–298.
171. Dillon N. Gene regulation and large-scale chromatin organization in the nucleus. Chromosome Res 2006;14: 117–126.
172. Maston GA, Evans SK, Green MR. Transcriptional Regulatory Elements in the Human Genome. Annu Rev Genomics Hum Genet 2006;7:29–59.
173. Thomas MC, Chiang CM. The general transcription machinery and general cofactors. Crit Rev Biochem Mol Biol 2006;41:105–178.
174. Engelkamp D, van Heyningen V. Transcription factors in disease. Curr Opin Genet Dev 1996;6:334–342.
175. Tamura T, Konishi Y, Makino Y, Mikoshiba K. Mechanisms of transcriptional regulation and neural gene expression. Neurochem Int 1996;29:573–581.
176. Bieker JJ, Ouyang L, Chen X. Transcriptional factors for specific globin genes. Ann NY Acad Sci 1998;850: 64–69.
177. Hertel KJ, Lynch KW, Maniatis T. Common themes in the function of transcription and splicing enhancers. Curr Opin Cell Biol 1997;9:350–357.
178. Arnosti DN. Analysis and function of transcriptional regulatory elements: insights from Drosophila. Annu Rev Entomol 2003;48:579–602.
179. Scannell DR, Wolfe K. Rewiring the transcriptional regulatory circuits of cells. Genome Biol 2004;5:206.
180. Villard J. Transcription regulation and human diseases. Swiss Med Wkly 2004;134:571–579.
181. Hampsey M. Molecular genetics of the RNA polymerase II general transcriptional machinery. Microbiol Mol Biol Rev 1998;62:465–503.
182. Berk AJ. Activation of RNA polymerase II transcription. Curr Opin Cell Biol 1999;11:330–335.
183. Berk AJ. TBP-like factors come into focus. Cell 2000; 103:5–8.
184. Green MR. TBP-associated factors (TAFIIs): multiple, selective transcriptional mediators in common complexes. Trends Biochem Sci 2000;25:59–63.
185. Pugh BF. Control of gene expression through regulation of the TATA-binding protein. Gene 2000;255:1–14.
186. Burley SK, Kamada K. Transcription factor complexes. Curr Opin Struct Biol 2002;12:225–230.
187. Featherstone M. Coactivators in transcription initiation: here are your orders. Curr Opin Genet Dev 2002;12: 149–155.
188. Davidson I. The genetics of TBP and TBP-related factors. Trends Biochem Sci 2003;28:391–398.
189. Hochheimer A, Tjian R. Diversified transcription initiation complexes expand promoter selectivity and tissue-specific gene expression. Genes Dev 2003;17:1309–1320.
190. Asturias FJ. RNA polymerase II structure, and organization of the preinitiation complex. Curr Opin Struct Biol 2004;14:121–129.
191. Matangkasombut O, Auty R, Buratowski S. Structure and function of the TFIID complex. Adv Protein Chem 2004;67:67–92.
192. Brady J, Kashanchi F. Tat gets the "green" light on transcription initiation. Retrovirology 2005;2:69.
193. Thomas MC, Chiang CM. The general transcription machinery and general cofactors. Crit Rev Biochem Mol Biol 2006;41:105–178.
194. Dang CV, Resar LM, Emison E, et al. Function of the c-Myc oncogenic transcription factor. Exp Cell Res 1999;253:63–77.
195. Kuramoto N, Ogita K, Yoneda Y. Gene transcription through Myc family members in eukaryotic cells. Jpn J Pharmacol 1999;80:103–109.
196. Grandori C, Cowley SM, James LP, Eisenman RN. The Myc/Max/Mad network and the transcriptional control of cell behavior. Annu Rev Cell Dev Biol 2000;16:653–699.
197. Baudino TA, Cleveland JL. The Max network gone mad. Mol Cell Biol 2001;21:691–702.
198. Eisenman RN. The Max network: coordinated transcriptional regulation of cell growth and proliferation. Harvey Lect 2000–2001;96:1–32.
199. Luscher B. Function and regulation of the transcription factors of the Myc/Max/Mad network. Gene 2001;277:1–14.
200. Zhou ZQ, Hurlin PJ. The interplay between Mad and Myc in proliferation and differentiation. Trends Cell Biol 2001;11:S10–S14.
201. Lee LA, Dang CV. Myc target transcriptomes. Curr Top Microbiol Immunol 2006;302:145–167.
202. Nair SK, Burley SK. Structural aspects of interactions within the Myc/Max/Mad network. Curr Top Microbiol Immunol 2006;302:123–143.

203. Pirity M, Blanck JK, Schreiber-Agus N. Lessons learned from Myc/Max/Mad knockout mice. Curr Top Microbiol Immunol 2006;302:205–234.
204. Rottmann S, Luscher B. The Mad side of the Max network: antagonizing the function of Myc and more. Curr Top Microbiol Immunol 2006;302:63–122.
205. Williams LT, Escobedo JA, Fantl WJ, Turck CW, Klippel A. Interactions of growth factor receptors with cytoplasmic signaling molecules. Cold Spring Harb Symp Quant Biol 1991;56:243–250.
206. Fantl WJ, Escobedo JA, Martin GA, et al. Distinct phosphotyrosines on a growth factor receptor bind to specific molecules that mediate different signaling pathways. Cell 1992;69:413–423.
207. Hunter T, Lindberg RA, Middlemas DS, Tracy S, van der Geer P. Receptor protein tyrosine kinases and phosphatases. Cold Spring Harb Symp Quant Biol 1992;57: 25–41.
208. Fantl WJ, Johnson DE, Williams LT. Signalling by receptor tyrosine kinases. Annu Rev Biochem 1993;62: 453–481.
209. Johnson GL, Vaillancourt RR. Sequential protein kinase reactions controlling cell growth and differentiation. Curr Opin Cell Biol 1994;6:230–238.
210. van der Geer P, Hunter T, Lindberg RA. Receptor protein-tyrosine kinases and their signal transduction pathways. Annu Rev Cell Biol 1994;10:251–337.
211. Schlessinger J. Cell signaling by receptor tyrosine kinases. Cell 2000;103:211–225.
212. Medinger M, Drevs J. Receptor tyrosine kinases and anticancer therapy. Curr Pharm Des 2005;11:1139–1149.
213. Gavi S, Shumay E, Wang HY, Malbon CC. G-protein-coupled receptors and tyrosine kinases: crossroads in cell signaling and regulation. Trends Endocrinol Metab 2006; 17:48–54.
214. Li E, Hristova K. Role of receptor tyrosine kinase transmembrane domains in cell signaling and human pathologies. Biochemistry 2006;45:6241–6251.
215. Perona R. Cell signalling: growth factors and tyrosine kinase receptors. Clin Transl Oncol 2006;8:77–82.
216. Tiganis T. Protein tyrosine phosphatases: dephosphorylating the epidermal growth factor receptor. IUBMB Life 2002;53:3–14.
217. Jorissen RN, Walker F, Pouliot N, Garrett TP, Ward CW, Burgess AW. Epidermal growth factor receptor: mechanisms of activation and signalling. Exp Cell Res 2003; 284:31–53.
218. Bazley LA, Gullick WJ. The epidermal growth factor receptor family. Endocr Relat Cancer 2005;12(suppl 1): S17–S27.
219. Normanno N, Bianco C, Strizzi L, et al. The ErbB receptors and their ligands in cancer: an overview. Curr Drug Targets 2005;6:243–257.
220. Zaczek A, Brandt B, Bielawski KP. The diverse signaling network of EGFR, HER2, HER3 and HER4 tyrosine kinase receptors and the consequences for therapeutic approaches. Histol Histopathol 2005;20: 1005–1015.
221. Edwin F, Wiepz GJ, Singh R, Peet CR, Chaturvedi D, Bertics PJ, Patel TB. A historical perspective of the EGF receptor and related systems. Methods Mol Biol 2006;327:1–24.
222. Warren CM, Landgraf R. Signaling through ERBB receptors: multiple layers of diversity and control. Cell Signal 2006;18:923–933.
223. Magnuson NS, Beck T, Vahidi H, Hahn H, Smola U, Rapp UR. The Raf-1 serine/threonine protein kinase. Semin Cancer Biol 1994;5:247–253.
224. Williams NG, Roberts TM. Signal transduction pathways involving the Raf proto-oncogene. Cancer Metastasis Rev 1994;13:105–116.
225. Burgering BM, Bos JL. Regulation of Ras-mediated signalling: more than one way to skin a cat. Trends Biochem Sci 1995;20:18–22.
226. Morrison DK. Mechanisms regulating Raf-1 activity in signal transduction pathways. Mol Reprod Dev 1995; 42:507–514.
227. Morrison DK, Cutler RE. The complexity of Raf-1 regulation. Curr Opin Cell Biol 1997;9:174–179.
228. Dhillon AS, Kolch W. Untying the regulation of the Raf-1 kinase. Arch Biochem Biophys 2002;404:3–9.
229. Bernards A, Settleman J. GAP control: regulating the regulators of small GTPases. Trends Cell Biol 2004; 14:377–385.
230. Bernards A, Settleman J. GAPs in growth factor signalling. Growth Factors 2005;23:143–149.
231. Chan A. Teaching resources. Ras-MAPK pathways. Sci STKE 2005;2005(271):tr5.
232. Hancock JF, Parton RG. Ras plasma membrane signalling platforms. Biochem J 2005;389(pt 1):1–11.
233. Kranenburg O. The KRAS oncogene: past, present, and future. Biochim Biophys Acta 2005;1756:81–82.
234. McCudden CR, Hains MD, Kimple RJ, Siderovski DP, Willard FS. G-protein signaling: back to the future. Cell Mol Life Sci 2005;62:551–577.
235. Mitin N, Rossman KL, Der CJ. Signaling interplay in Ras superfamily function. Curr Biol 2005;15:R563–R574.
236. Philips MR. Compartmentalized signalling of Ras. Biochem Soc Trans 2005;33(pt 4):657–661.
237. Wennerberg K, Rossman KL, Der CJ. The Ras superfamily at a glance. J Cell Sci 2005;118(pt 5):843–846.
238. Mor A, Philips MR. Compartmentalized Ras/MAPK signaling. Annu Rev Immunol 2006;24:771–800.
239. Bagrodia S, Derijard B, Davis RJ, Cerione RA. Cdc42 and PAK mediated signaling leads to Jun kinase and p38 mitogen-activated protein kinase activation. J Biol Chem 1995;270:27995–27998.
240. Pombo CM, Kehrl JH, Sanchez I, et al. Activation of the SAPK pathway by the human STE20 homologue germinal centre kinase. Nature 1995;377:750–754.
241. Xia Z, Dickens M, Raingeaud J, Davis RJ, Greenberg ME. Opposing effects of ERK and JNK p38 MAP kinases on apoptosis. Science 1995;270:1326–1331.
242. Brown JL, Stowers L, Baer M, Trejo J, Coughlin S, Chant J. Human Ste20 homologue hPAK1 links GTPases to the JNK MAP kinase pathway. Curr Biol 1996;6:598–605.
243. Ichijo H, Nishida E, Irie K, et al. Induction of apoptosis by ASK1, a mammalian MAPKKK that activates SAPK/JNK and p38 signaling pathways. Science 1997;275: 90–94.

244. Wilkinson MG, Millar JB. SAPKs and transcription factors do the nucleocytoplasmic tango. Genes Dev 1998;12:1391–1397.
245. Davis RJ. Signal transduction by the JNK group of MAP kinases. Cell 2000;103:239–252.
246. Wada T, Penninger JM. Mitogen activated protein kinases in apoptosis regulation. Oncogene 2004;23:2838–2849.
247. Bradham C, McClay DR. p38 MAPK in Development and Cancer. Cell Cycle 2006;5:824–828.
248. Gaestel M. MAPKAP kinases—MKs—two's company, three's a crowd. Nat Rev Mol Cell Biol 2006;7:120–130.
249. MacCorkle RA, Tan TH. Mitogen-activated protein kinases in cell-cycle control. Cell Biochem Biophys 2005;43:451–461.
250. Shimada K, Nakamura M, Ishida E, Konishi N. Molecular roles of MAP kinases and FADD phosphorylation in prostate cancer. Histol Histopathol 2006;21:415–422.
251. Yoon S, Seger R. The extracellular signal-regulated kinase: multiple substrates regulate diverse cellular functions. Growth Factors 2006;24:21–44.
252. Pellegrini S, Dusanter-Fourt I. The structure, regulation and function of the Janus kinases (JAKs) and the signal transducers and activators of transcription (STATs). Eur J Biochem 1997;248:615–633.
253. Liu KD, Gaffen SL, Goldsmith MA. JAK/STAT signaling by cytokine receptors. Curr Opin Immunol 1998;10: 271–278.
254. Shuai K. The STAT family of proteins in cytokine signaling. Prog Biophys Mol Biol 1999;71:405–422.
255. Boudny V, Kovarik J. JAK/STAT signaling pathways and cancer. Janus kinases/signal transducers and activators of transcription. Neoplasma 2002;49:349–355.
256. Kisseleva T, Bhattacharya S, Braunstein J, Schindler CW. Signaling through the JAK/STAT pathway, recent advances and future challenges. Gene 2002;285:1–24.
257. O'Shea JJ, Gadina M, Schreiber RD. Cytokine signaling in 2002: new surprises in the Jak/Stat pathway. Cell 2002;109(suppl):S121–S131.
258. Agaisse H, Perrimon N. The roles of JAK/STAT signaling in Drosophila immune responses. Immunol Rev 2004; 198:72–82.
259. Rawlings JS, Rosler KM, Harrison DA. The JAK/STAT signaling pathway. J Cell Sci 2004;117(pt 8):1281–1283.
260. Hebenstreit D, Horejs-Hoeck J, Duschl A. JAK/STAT-dependent gene regulation by cytokines. Drug News Perspect 2005;18:243–249.
261. Arbouzova NI, Zeidler MP. JAK/STAT signalling in Drosophila: insights into conserved regulatory and cellular functions. Development 2006;133:2605–2616.
262. Lutz M, Knaus P. Integration of the TGF-beta pathway into the cellular signalling network. Cell Signal 2002;14:977–988.
263. Mehra A, Wrana JL. TGF-beta and the Smad signal transduction pathway. Biochem Cell Biol 2002;80:605–622.
264. Cohen MM Jr. TGF beta/Smad signaling system and its pathologic correlates. Am J Med Genet A 2003;116: 1–10.
265. Derynck R, Zhang YE. Smad-dependent and Smad-independent pathways in TGF-beta family signalling. Nature 2003;425:577–584.
266. Chin D, Boyle GM, Parsons PG, Coman WB. What is transforming growth factor-beta (TGF-beta)? Br J Plast Surg 2004;57:215–221.
267. ten Dijke P, Hill CS. New insights into TGF-beta-Smad signalling. Trends Biochem Sci 2004;29:265–273.
268. Feng XH, Derynck R. Specificity and versatility in tgf-beta signaling through Smads. Annu Rev Cell Dev Biol 2005;21:659–693.
269. Park SH. Fine tuning and cross-talking of TGF-beta signal by inhibitory Smads. J Biochem Mol Biol 2005; 38:9–16.
270. Massague J, Seoane J, Wotton D. Smad transcription factors. Genes Dev 2005;19:2783–2810.
271. Massague J, Gomis RR. The logic of TGFbeta signaling. FEBS Lett 2006;580:2811–2820.
272. Gumbiner BM. Signal transduction of beta-catenin. Curr Opin Cell Biol 1995; 7:634–640.
273. Cadigan KM, Nusse R. Wnt signaling: a common theme in animal development. Genes Dev 1997;11:3286–3305.
274. Shimizu H, Julius MA, Giarre M, Zheng Z, Brown AM, Kitajewski J. Transformation by Wnt family proteins correlates with regulation of beta-catenin. Cell Growth Differ 1997;8:1349–1358.
275. Boutros M, Mlodzik M. Dishevelled: at the crossroads of divergent intracellular signaling pathways. Mech Dev 1999;83:27–37.
276. Miller JR, Hocking AM, Brown JD, Moon RT. Mechanism and function of signal transduction by the Wnt/ beta-catenin and Wnt/Ca2+ pathways. Oncogene 1999;18: 7860–7872.
277. Hinoi T, Yamamoto H, Kishida M, Takada S, Kishida S, Kikuchi A. Complex formation of adenomatous polyposis coli gene product and axin facilitates glycogen synthase kinase-3 beta-dependent phosphorylation of beta-catenin and downregulates beta-catenin. J Biol Chem 2000;275:34399–34406.
278. Polakis P. Wnt signaling and cancer. Genes Dev 2000;14: 1837–1851.
279. Civenni G, Holbro T, Hynes NE. Wnt1 and Wnt5a induce cyclin D1 expression through ErbB1 transactivation in HC11 mammary epithelial cells. EMBO Rep 2003;4: 166–171.
280. Doble BW, Woodgett JR. GSK-3: tricks of the trade for a multi-tasking kinase. J Cell Sci 2003;116:1175–1186.
281. Lee E, Salic A, Kruger R, Heinrich R, Kirschner MW. The roles of APC and Axin derived from experimental and theoretical analysis of the Wnt pathway. PLoS Biol 2003;1:E10.
282. Malliri A, Collard JG. Role of Rho-family proteins in cell adhesion and cancer. Curr Opin Cell Biol 2003;15: 583–589.
283. van Es JH, Barker N, Clevers H. You Wnt some, you lose some: oncogenes in the Wnt signaling pathway. Curr Opin Genet Dev 2003;13:28–33.
284. Veeman MT, Axelrod JD, Moon RT. A second canon. Functions and mechanisms of beta-catenin-independent Wnt signaling. Dev Cell 2003;5:367–377.
285. Cong F, Schweizer L, Varmus H. Wnt signals across the plasma membrane to activate the beta-catenin pathway

by forming oligomers containing its receptors, Frizzled and LRP. Development 2004;131:5103–5115.
286. Logan CY, Nusse R. The Wnt signaling pathway in development and disease. Annu Rev Cell Dev Biol 2004;20: 781–810.
287. Malbon CC. Frizzleds: new members of the superfamily of G-protein-coupled receptors. Front Biosci 2004;9: 1048–1058.
288. Nelson WJ, Nusse R. Convergence of Wnt, beta-catenin, and cadherin pathways. Science 2004;303:1483–1487.
289. Tolwinski NS, Wieschaus E. Rethinking WNT signaling. Trends Genet 2004;20:177–181.
290. Bejsovec A. Wnt pathway activation: new relations and locations. Cell 2005;120:11–14.
291. Gregorieff A, Clevers H. Wnt signaling in the intestinal epithelium: from endoderm to cancer. Genes Dev 2005; 19:877–890.
292. Malbon CC. Beta-catenin, cancer, and G proteins: not just for frizzleds anymore. Sci STKE 2005;2005(292): pe35.
293. Senda T, Shimomura A, Iizuka-Kogo A. Adenomatous polyposis coli (Apc) tumor suppressor gene as a multifunctional gene. Anat Sci Int 2005;80:121–131.
294. Takada R, Hijikata H, Kondoh H, Takada S. Analysis of combinatorial effects of Wnts and Frizzleds on beta-catenin/armadillo stabilization and Dishevelled phosphorylation. Genes Cells 2005;10:919–928.
295. Cadigan KM, Liu YI. Wnt signaling: complexity at the surface. J Cell Sci 2006;119:395–402.
296. Kikuchi A, Kishida S, Yamamoto H. Regulation of Wnt signaling by protein-protein interaction and post-translational modifications. Exp Mol Med 2006;38:1–10.
297. Malbon CC, Wang HY. Dishevelled: a mobile scaffold catalyzing development. Curr Top Dev Biol 2006;72: 153–166.
298. Pongracz JE, Stockley RA. Wnt signalling in lung development and diseases. Respir Res 2006;7:15.
299. Tian Q. Proteomic exploration of the Wnt/beta-catenin pathway. Curr Opin Mol Ther 2006;8:191–197.
300. Franke TF, Kaplan DR, Cantley LC. PI3K: downstream AKTion blocks apoptosis. Cell 1997;88:435–437.
301. Wymann MP, Pirola L. Structure and function of phosphoinositide 3–kinases. Biochim Biophys Acta 1998; 1436:127–150.
302. Krasilnikov MA. Phosphatidylinositol-3 kinase dependent pathways: the role in control of cell growth, survival, and malignant transformation. Biochemistry (Mosc) 2000;65:59–67.
303. Cantley LC. The phosphoinositide 3–kinase pathway. Science 2002;296:1655–1657.
304. Chang F, Lee JT, Navolanic PM, et al. Involvement of PI3K/Akt pathway in cell cycle progression, apoptosis, and neoplastic transformation: a target for cancer chemotherapy. Leukemia 2003;17:590–603.
305. Franke TF, Hornik CP, Segev L, Shostak GA, Sugimoto C. PI3K/Akt and apoptosis: size matters. Oncogene 2003;22: 8983–8998.
306. Liang J, Slingerland JM. Multiple roles of the PI3K/PKB (Akt) pathway in cell cycle progression. Cell Cycle 2003; 2:339–345.
307. Asnaghi L, Bruno P, Priulla M, Nicolin A. mTOR: a protein kinase switching between life and death. Pharmacol Res 2004;50:545–549.
308. Brader S, Eccles SA. Phosphoinositide 3-kinase signalling pathways in tumor progression, invasion and angiogenesis. Tumori 2004;90:2–8.
309. Fresno Vara JA, Casado E, de Castro J, Cejas P, Belda-Iniesta C, Gonzalez-Baron M. PI3K/Akt signalling pathway and cancer. Cancer Treat Rev 2004;30:193–204.
310. Osaki M, Oshimura M, Ito H. PI3K-Akt pathway: its functions and alterations in human cancer. Apoptosis 2004;9:667–676.
311. Chen YL, Law PY, Loh HH. Inhibition of PI3K/Akt signaling: an emerging paradigm for targeted cancer therapy. Curr Med Chem Anticancer Agents 2005;5:575–589.
312. Hay N. The Akt-mTOR tango and its relevance to cancer. Cancer Cell 2005;8:179–183.
313. Kim D, Cheng GZ, Lindsley CW, Yang H, Cheng JQ. Targeting the phosphatidylinositol-3 kinase/Akt pathway for the treatment of cancer. Curr Opin Invest Drugs 2005;6:1250–1258.
314. Morgensztern D, McLeod HL. PI3K/Akt/mTOR pathway as a target for cancer therapy. Anticancer Drugs 2005; 16:797–803.
315. Henson ES, Gibson SB. Surviving cell death through epidermal growth factor (EGF) signal transduction pathways: implications for cancer therapy. Cell Signal 2006;18:2089–2097.
316. Kalderon D. Similarities between the Hedgehog and Wnt signaling pathways. Trends Cell Biol 2002;12:523–531.
317. King RW. Roughing up Smoothened: chemical modulators of hedgehog signaling. J Biol 2002;1:8.
318. Mullor JL, Sanchez P, Altaba AR. Pathways and consequences: hedgehog signaling in human disease. Trends Cell Biol 2002;12:562–569.
319. Cohen MM Jr. The hedgehog signaling network. Am J Med Genet A 2003;123:5–28.
320. McMahon AP, Ingham PW, Tabin CJ. Developmental roles and clinical significance of hedgehog signaling. Curr Top Dev Biol 2003;53:1–114.
321. Nusse R. Wnts and Hedgehogs: lipid-modified proteins and similarities in signaling mechanisms at the cell surface. Development 2003;130:5297–5305.
322. Wetmore C. Sonic hedgehog in normal and neoplastic proliferation: insight gained from human tumors and animal models. Curr Opin Genet Dev 2003;13:34–42.
323. Lum L, Beachy PA. The Hedgehog response network: sensors, switches, and routers. Science 2004;304:1755–1759.
324. Ogden SK, Ascano M Jr, Stegman MA, Robbins DJ. Regulation of Hedgehog signaling: a complex story. Biochem Pharmacol 2004;67:805–814.
325. Yu TC, Miller SJ. The hedgehog pathway: revisited. Dermatol Surg 2004;30:583–584.
326. Hooper JE, Scott MP. Communicating with Hedgehogs. Nat Rev Mol Cell Biol 2005;6:306–317.
327. Neumann CJ. Hedgehogs as negative regulators of the cell cycle. Cell Cycle 2005;4:1139–1140.
328. Nieuwenhuis E, Hui CC. Hedgehog signaling and congenital malformations. Clin Genet 2005;67:193–208.

329. Allenspach EJ, Maillard I, Aster JC, Pear WS. Notch signaling in cancer. Cancer Biol Ther 2002;1:466–476.
330. Baron M, Aslam H, Flasza M, et al. Multiple levels of Notch signal regulation (review). Mol Membr Biol 2002; 19:27–38.
331. Baron M. An overview of the Notch signalling pathway. Semin Cell Dev Biol 2003;14:113–119.
332. Collins BJ, Kleeberger W, Ball DW. Notch in lung development and lung cancer. Semin Cancer Biol 2004;14: 357–364.
333. Hansson EM, Lendahl U, Chapman G. Notch signaling in development and disease. Semin Cancer Biol 2004;14: 320–328.
334. Kadesch T. Notch signaling: the demise of elegant simplicity. Curr Opin Genet Dev 2004;14:506–512.
335. Sjolund J, Manetopoulos C, Stockhausen MT, Axelson H. The Notch pathway in cancer: differentiation gone awry. Eur J Cancer 2005;41:2620–2629.
336. Bianchi S, Dotti MT, Federico A. Physiology and pathology of notch signalling system. J Cell Physiol 2006;207: 300–308.
337. Wilson A, Radtke F. Multiple functions of Notch signaling in self-renewing organs and cancer. FEBS Lett 2006; 580:2860–2868.
338. Abraham RT. Cell cycle checkpoint signaling through the ATM and ATR kinases. Genes Dev 2001;15:2177–2196.
339. Laval J, Jurado J, Saparbaev M, Sidorkina O. Antimutagenic role of base-excision repair enzymes upon free radical-induced DNA damage. Mutat Res 1998;402: 93–102.
340. Boiteux S, Radicella JP. Base excision repair of 8–hydroxyguanine protects DNA from endogenous oxidative stress. Biochimie 1999;81:59–67.
341. Boiteux S, Radicella JP. The human OGG1 gene: structure, functions, and its implication in the process of carcinogenesis. Arch Biochem Biophys 2000;377. 1–8.
342. Boiteux S, le Page F. Repair of 8-oxoguanine and Ogg1–incised apurinic sites in a CHO cell line. Prog Nucleic Acid Res Mol Biol 2001;68:95–105.
343. Hazra TK, Hill JW, Izumi T, Mitra S. Multiple DNA glycosylases for repair of 8-oxoguanine and their potential in vivo functions. Prog Nucleic Acid Res Mol Biol 2001; 68:193–205.
344. Ide H. DNA substrates containing defined oxidative base lesions and their application to study substrate specificities of base excision repair enzymes. Prog Nucleic Acid Res Mol Biol 2001;68:207–221.
345. Nakabeppu Y. Regulation of intracellular localization of human MTH1, OGG1, and MYH proteins for repair of oxidative DNA damage. Prog Nucleic Acid Res Mol Biol 2001;68:75–94.
346. Nishimura S. Mammalian Ogg1/Mmh gene plays a major role in repair of the 8-hydroxyguanine lesion in DNA. Prog Nucleic Acid Res Mol Biol 2001;68:107–123.
347. Shinmura K, Yokota J. The OGG1 gene encodes a repair enzyme for oxidatively damaged DNA and is involved in human carcinogenesis. Antioxid Redox Signal 2001;3: 597–609.
348. Nishimura S. Involvement of mammalian OGG1(MMH) in excision of the 8–hydroxyguanine residue in DNA. Free Radic Biol Med 2002;32:813–821.
349. Fortini P, Pascucci B, Parlanti E, D'Errico M, Simonelli V, Dogliotti E. 8-Oxoguanine DNA damage: at the crossroad of alternative repair pathways. Mutat Res 2003; 531:127–139.
350. Nakabeppu Y, Tsuchimoto D, Furuichi M, Sakumi K. The defense mechanisms in mammalian cells against oxidative damage in nucleic acids and their involvement in the suppression of mutagenesis and cell death. Free Radic Res 2004;38:423–429.
351. Thompson LH. Properties and applications of human DNA repair genes. Mutat Res 1991;247:213–219.
352. Tomkinson AE, Levin DS. Mammalian DNA ligases. Bioessays 1997;19:893–901.
353. Tomkinson AE, Mackey ZB. Structure and function of mammalian DNA ligases. Mutat Res 1998;407:1–9.
354. Thompson LH, West MG. XRCC1 keeps DNA from getting stranded. Mutat Res 2000;459:1–18.
355. Tomkinson AE, Chen L, Dong Z, et al. Completion of base excision repair by mammalian DNA ligases. Prog Nucleic Acid Res Mol Biol 2001;68:151–164.
356. Caldecott KW. XRCC1 and DNA strand break repair. DNA Repair (Amst) 2003;2:955–969.
357. Dianov GL, Sleeth KM, Dianova II, Allinson SL. Repair of abasic sites in DNA. Mutat Res 2003;531:157–163.
358. Malanga M, Althaus FR. The role of poly(ADP-ribose) in the DNA damage signaling network. Biochem Cell Biol 2005;83:354–364.
359. Williams RS, Bernstein N, Lee MS, et al. Structural basis for phosphorylation-dependent signaling in the DNA-damage response. Biochem Cell Biol 2005;83:721–727.
360. Johnson RT, Squires S. The XPD complementation group. Insights into xeroderma pigmentosum, Cockayne's syndrome and trichothiodystrophy. Mutat Res 1992; 273:97–118.
361. Wood RD. DNA damage recognition during nucleotide excision repair in mammalian cells. Biochimie 1999; 81:39–44.
362. van Brabant AJ, Stan R, Ellis NA. DNA helicases, genomic instability, and human genetic disease. Annu Rev Genomics Hum Genet 2000;1:409–459.
363. Berneburg M, Lehmann AR. Xeroderma pigmentosum and related disorders: defects in DNA repair and transcription. Adv Genet 2001;43:71–102.
364. Bernstein C, Bernstein H, Payne CM, Garewal H. DNA repair/pro-apoptotic dual-role proteins in five major DNA repair pathways: fail-safe protection against carcinogenesis. Mutat Res 2002;511:145–178.
365. Chen J, Suter B. Xpd, a structural bridge and a functional link. Cell Cycle 2003;2:503–506.
366. Lehmann AR. DNA repair-deficient diseases, xeroderma pigmentosum, Cockayne syndrome and trichothiodystrophy. Biochimie 2003;85:1101–1111.
367. Eshleman JR, Markowitz SD. Mismatch repair defects in human carcinogenesis. Hum Mol Genet 1996;5(spec. No.):1489–1494.
368. MacPhee DG. Mismatch repair as a source of mutations in non-dividing cells. Genetica 1996;97:183–195.

369. Arnheim N, Shibata D. DNA mismatch repair in mammals: role in disease and meiosis. Curr Opin Genet Dev 1997; 7:364–370.
370. Peltomaki P. DNA mismatch repair gene mutations in human cancer. Environ Health Perspect 1997;105 (suppl 4):775–780.
371. Prolla TA. DNA mismatch repair and cancer. Curr Opin Cell Biol 1998;10:311–316.
372. Kirkpatrick DT. Roles of the DNA mismatch repair and nucleotide excision repair proteins during meiosis. Cell Mol Life Sci 1999;55:437–449.
373. Kolodner RD, Marsischky GT. Eukaryotic DNA mismatch repair. Curr Opin Genet Dev 1999;9:89–96.
374. Harfe BD, Jinks-Robertson S. Mismatch repair proteins and mitotic genome stability. Mutat Res 2000;451: 151–167.
375. Harfe BD, Jinks-Robertson S. DNA mismatch repair and genetic instability. Annu Rev Genet 2000;34:359–399.
376. Taverna P, Liu L, Hanson AJ, Monks A, Gerson SL. Characterization of MLH1 and MSH2 DNA mismatch repair proteins in cell lines of the NCI anticancer drug screen. Cancer Chemother Pharmacol 2000;46:507–516.
377. Aquilina G, Bignami M. Mismatch repair in correction of replication errors and processing of DNA damage. J Cell Physiol 2001;187:145–154.
378. Bellacosa A. Functional interactions and signaling properties of mammalian DNA mismatch repair proteins. Cell Death Differ 2001;8:1076–1092.
379. Hsieh P. Molecular mechanisms of DNA mismatch repair. Mutat Res 2001;486:71–87.
380. Marti TM, Kunz C, Fleck O. DNA mismatch repair and mutation avoidance pathways. J Cell Physiol 2002; 191:28–41.
381. Schofield MJ, Hsieh P. DNA mismatch repair: molecular mechanisms and biological function. Annu Rev Microbiol 2003;57:579–608.
382. Isaacs RJ, Spielmann HP. A model for initial DNA lesion recognition by NER and MMR based on local conformational flexibility. DNA Repair (Amst) 2004;3:455–464.
383. Stojic L, Brun R, Jiricny J. Mismatch repair and DNA damage signalling. DNA Repair (Amst) 2004;3: 1091–1101.
384. Surtees JA, Argueso JL, Alani E. Mismatch repair proteins: key regulators of genetic recombination. Cytogenet Genome Res 2004;107:146–159.
385. Kunkel TA, Erie DA. DNA mismatch repair. Annu Rev Biochem 2005;74:681–710.
386. Skinner AM, Turker MS. Oxidative mutagenesis, mismatch repair, and aging. Sci Aging Knowledge Environ 2005;2005(9):re3.
387. Jiricny J. The multifaceted mismatch-repair system. Nat Rev Mol Cell Biol 2006;7:335–346.
388. Jun SH, Kim TG, Ban C. DNA mismatch repair system. Classical and fresh roles. FEBS J 2006;273:1609–1619.
389. Montesano R, Becker R, Hall J, et al. Repair of DNA alkylation adducts in mammalian cells. Biochimie 1985; 67:919–928.
390. D'Incalci M, Citti L, Taverna P, Catapano CV. Importance of the DNA repair enzyme O6–alkyl guanine alkyltransferase (AT) in cancer chemotherapy. Cancer Treat Rev 1988;15:279–292.
391. Pegg AE. Mammalian O6-alkylguanine-DNA alkyltransferase: regulation and importance in response to alkylating carcinogenic and therapeutic agents. Cancer Res 1990;50:6119–6129.
392. Erickson LC. The role of O-6 methylguanine DNA methyltransferase (MGMT) in drug resistance and strategies for its inhibition. Semin Cancer Biol 1991;2: 257–265.
393. Pegg AE, Byers TL. Repair of DNA containing O6-alkylguanine. FASEB J 1992;6:2302–2310.
394. Koc ON, Phillips WP Jr, Lee K, et al. Role of DNA repair in resistance to drugs that alkylate O6 of guanine.Cancer Treat Res 1996;87:123–146.
395. Sekiguchi M, Nakabeppu Y, Sakumi K, Tuzuki T. DNA-repair methyltransferase as a molecular device for preventing mutation and cancer. J Cancer Res Clin Oncol 1996;122:199–206.
396. Pieper RO. Understanding and manipulating O6-methylguanine-DNA methyltransferase expression. Pharmacol Ther 1997;74:285–297.
397. Sekiguchi M, Sakumi K. Roles of DNA repair methyltransferase in mutagenesis and carcinogenesis. Jpn J Hum Genet 1997;42:389–399.
398. Yu Z, Chen J, Ford BN, Brackley ME, Glickman BW. Human DNA repair systems: an overview. Environ Mol Mutagen 1999;33:3–20.
399. Kaina B, Ochs K, Grosch S, et al. BER, MGMT, and MMR in defense against alkylation-induced genotoxicity and apoptosis. Prog Nucleic Acid Res Mol Biol 2001; 68:41–54.
400. Gerson SL. Clinical relevance of MGMT in the treatment of cancer. J Clin Oncol 2002;20:2388–2399.
401. Margison GP, Santibanez-Koref MF. O6-alkylguanine-DNA alkyltransferase: role in carcinogenesis and chemotherapy. Bioessays 2002;24:255–266.
402. Drablos F, Feyzi E, Aas PA, et al. Alkylation damage in DNA and RNA—repair mechanisms and medical significance. DNA Repair (Amst) 2004;3:1389–1407.
403. Gerson SL. MGMT: its role in cancer aetiology and cancer therapeutics. Nat Rev Cancer 2004;4:296–307.
404. Gollin SM. Mechanisms leading to chromosomal instability. Semin Cancer Biol 2005;15:33–42.
405. Varon R, Vissinga C, Platzer M, et al. Nibrin, a novel DNA double-strand break repair protein, is mutated in Nijmegen breakage syndrome. Cell 1998;93:467–476.
406. Dasika GK, Lin SC, Zhao S, et al. DNA damage-induced cell cycle checkpoints and DNA strand break repair in development and tumorigenesis. Oncogene 1999;18: 7883–7899.
407. Lim DS, Kim ST, Xu B, et al. ATM phosphorylates p95/NBS1 in an S-phase checkpoint pathway. Nature 2000;404:613–617.
408. Buscemi G, Savio C, Zannini L, et al. CHK2 activation dependence on NBS1 after DNA damage. Mol Cell Biol 2001;21:5214–5222.
409. Falck J, Mailand N, Syljuasen RG, et al. The ATM-CHK2–CDC25a checkpoint pathway guards against radioresistant DNA synthesis. Nature 2001;410:842–847.

410. Xu B, Kim S, Kastan MB. Involvement of BRCA1 in S-phase and G(2)-phase checkpoints after ionizing irradiation. Mol Cell Biol 2001;21:3445–3450.
411. D'Amours D, Jackson SP. The MRE11 complex: at the crossroads of DNA repair and checkpoint signalling. Nat Rev Mol Cell Biol 2002;3:317–327.
412. Girard PM, Riballo E, Begg AC, et al. NBS1 promotes ATM dependent phosphorylation events including those required for G1/S arrest. Oncogene 2002;21:4191–4199.
413. Huang J, Dynan WS. Reconstitution of the mammalian DNA double-strand break end-joining reaction reveals a requirement for an MRE11/RAD50/NBS1–containing fraction. Nucleic Acids Res 2002;30:667–674.
414. Nakanishi K, Taniguchi T, Ranganathan V, et al. Interaction of FANCD2 and NBS1 in the DNA damage response. Nat Cell Biol 2002;4:913–920.
415. Osborn AJ, Elledge SJ, Zou L. Checking on the fork: the DNA-replication stress-response pathway. Trends Cell Biol 2002;12:509–516.
416. Tauchi H, Kobayashi J, Morishima K, et al. NBS1 is essential for DNA repair by homologous recombination in higher vertebrate cells. Nature 2002;420:93–98.
417. Tauchi H, Matsuura S, Kobayashi J, et al. Nijmegen breakage syndrome gene, NBS1, and molecular links to factors for genome stability. Oncogene 2002;21:8967–8980.
418. Yazdi PT, Wang Y, Zhao S, et al. SMC1 is a downstream effector in the ATM/NBS1 branch of the human S-phase checkpoint. Genes Dev 2002;16:571–582.
419. Carson CT, Schwartz RA, Stracker TH, et al. The MRE11 complex is required for ATM activation and the G2/M checkpoint. Embo J 2003;22:6610–6620.
420. Goodarzi AA, Block WD, Lees-Miller SP. The role of ATM and ATR in DNA damage-induced cell cycle control. Prog Cell Cycle Res 2003;5:393–411.
421. Shiloh Y. ATM and related protein kinases: safeguarding genome integrity. Nat Rev Cancer 2003;3:155–168.
422. Shiloh Y. ATM: ready, set, go. Cell Cycle 2003;2:116–117.
423. Uziel T, Lerenthal Y, Moyal L, et al. Requirement of the MRN complex for ATM activation by DNA damage. Embo J 2003;22:5612–5621.
424. Abraham RT. PI 3–kinase related kinases: "big" players in stress-induced signaling pathways. DNA Repair (Amst) 2004;3:883–887.
425. Lee JH, Paull TT. Direct activation of the ATM protein kinase by the MRE11/RAD50/NBS1 complex. Science 2004;304:93–96.
426. Matsuura S, Kobayashi J, Tauchi H, Komatsu K. Nijmegen breakage syndrome and DNA double strand break repair by NBS1 complex. Adv Biophys 2004;38:65–80.
427. Lavin MF, Birrell G, Chen P, et al. ATM signaling and genomic stability in response to DNA damage. Mutat Res 2005;569:123–132.
428. Lee JH, Paull TT. ATM activation by DNA double-strand breaks through the MRE11–RAD50–NBS1 complex. Science 2005;308:551–554.
429. O'Driscoll M, Jeggo PA. The role of double-strand break repair—insights from human genetics. Nat Rev Genet 2006;7:45–54.
430. Zhang Y, Zhou J, Lim CU. The role of NBS1 in DNA double strand break repair, telomere stability, and cell cycle checkpoint control. Cell Res 2006;16:45–54.
431. Blow JJ, Laskey RA. A role for the nuclear envelope in controlling DNA replication within the cell cycle. Nature 1988;332:546–548.
432. Nishitani H, Nurse P. p65cdc18 plays a major role controlling the initiation of DNA replication in fission yeast. Cell 1995;83:397–405.
433. Cocker JH, Piatti S, Santocanale C, Nasmyth K, Diffley JF. An essential role for the Cdc6 protein in forming the pre-replicative complexes of budding yeast. Nature 1996;379:180–182.
434. Coleman TR, Carpenter PB, Dunphy WG. The Xenopus Cdc6 protein is essential for the initiation of a single round of DNA replication in cell-free extracts. Cell 1996;87:53–63.
435. Muzi Falconi M, Brown GW, Kelly TJ. cdc18+ regulates initiation of DNA replication in Schizosaccharomyces pombe. Proc Natl Acad Sci USA 1996;93:1566–1570.
436. Owens JC, Detweiler CS, Li JJ. CDC45 is required in conjunction with CDC7/DBF4 to trigger the initiation of DNA replication. Proc Natl Acad Sci 1997;94:12521–12526.
437. Tanaka T, Knapp D, Nasmyth K. Loading of an Mcm protein onto DNA replication origins is regulated by Cdc6p and CDKs. Cell 1997;90:649–660.
438. Williams RS, Shohet RV, Stillman B. A human protein related to yeast Cdc6p. Proc Natl Acad Sci USA 1997;94:142–147.
439. Hateboer G, Wobst A, Petersen BO, et al. Cell cycle-regulated expression of mammalian CDC6 is dependent on E2F. Mol Cell Biol 1998;18:6679–6697.
440. Hua XH, Newport J. Identification of a preinitiation step in DNA replication that is independent of origin recognition complex and cdc6, but dependent on cdk2. J Cell Biol 1998;140:271 281.
441. Leatherwood J. Emerging mechanisms of eukaryotic DNA replication initiation. Curr Opin Cell Biol 1998;10:742–748.
442. McGarry TJ, Kirschner MW. Geminin, an inhibitor of DNA replication, is degraded during mitosis. Cell 1998;93:1043–1053.
443. Mimura S, Takisawa H. Xenopus Cdc45–dependent loading of DNA polymerase onto chromatin under the control of S-phase Cdk. EMBO J 1998;17:5699–5707.
444. Saha P, Chen J, Thome KC, et al. Human CDC6/Cdc18 associates with Orc1 and cyclin-cdk and is selectively eliminated from the nucleus at the onset of S phase. Mol Cell Biol 1998;18:2758–27567.
445. Williams GH, Romanowski P, Morris L, et al. Improved cervical smear assessment using antibodies against proteins that regulate DNA replication. Proc Natl Acad Sci USA1998;95:14932–14937.
446. Yan Z, DeGregori J, Shohet R, et al. Cdc6 is regulated by E2F and is essential for DNA replication in mammalian cells. Proc Natl Acad Sci USA 1998;95:3603–3608.
447. Zou L, Stillman B. Formation of a preinitiation complex by S-phase cyclin CDK-dependent loading of Cdc45p onto chromatin. Science 1998;280:593–596.

448. Donaldson AD, Blow JJ. The regulation of replication origin activation. Curr Opin Genet Dev 1999;9:62–68.
449. Fujita M, Yamada C, Goto H, et al. Cell cycle regulation of human CDC6 protein. Intracellular localization, interaction with the human mcm complex, and CDC2 kinase-mediated hyperphosphorylation. J Biol Chem 1999;274: 25927–25932.
450. Masai H, Sato N, Takeda T, Arai K. CDC7 kinase complex as a molecular switch for DNA replication. Front Biosci 1999;4:D834–D840.
451. Petersen BO, Lukas J, Sorensen CS, Bartek J, Helin K. Phosphorylation of mammalian CDC6 by cyclin A/CDK2 regulates its subcellular localization. EMBO J 1999; 18:396–410.
452. Coverley D, Pelizon C, Trewick S, Laskey RA. Chromatin-bound Cdc6 persists in S and G2 phases in human cells, while soluble Cdc6 is destroyed in a cyclin A-cdk2 dependent process. J Cell Sci 2000;113:1929–1938.
453. Homesley L, Lei M, Kawasaki Y, Sawyer S, Christensen T, Tye BK. Mcm10 and the MCM2–7 complex interact to initiate DNA synthesis and to release replication factors from origins. Genes Dev 2000;14:913–926.
454. Maiorano D, Moreau J, Mechali M. XCDT1 is required for the assembly of pre-replicative complexes in Xenopus laevis. Nature 2000;404:622–625.
455. Nishitani H, Lygerou Z, Nishimoto T, Nurse P. The Cdt1 protein is required to license DNA for replication in fission yeast. Nature 2000;404:625–628.
456. Petersen BO, Wagener C, Marinoni F, et al. Cell cycle- and cell growth-regulated proteolysis of mammalian CDC6 is dependent on APC-CDH1. Genes Dev 2000;14: 2330–2343.
457. Takisawa H, Mimura S, Kubota Y. Eukaryotic DNA replication: from pre-replication complex to initiation complex. Curr Opin Cell Biol 2000;12:690–696.
458. Whittaker AJ, Royzman I, Orr-Weaver TL. Drosophila double parked: a conserved, essential replication protein that colocalizes with the origin recognition complex and links DNA replication with mitosis and the down-regulation of S phase transcripts. Genes Dev 2000;14: 1765–1776.
459. Wohlschlegel JA, Dwyer BT, Dhar SK, Cvetic C, Walter JC, Dutta A. Inhibition of eukaryotic DNA replication by geminin binding to Cdt1. Science 2000;290:2309–2312.
460. Diffley JF. DNA replication: building the perfect switch. Curr Biol 2001;11:R367–R370.
461. Lei M, Tye BK. Initiating DNA synthesis: from recruiting to activating the MCM complex. J Cell Sci 2001;114: 1447–1454.
462. Nishitani H, Taraviras S, Lygerou Z, Nishimoto T. The human licensing factor for DNA replication Cdt1 accumulates in G1 and is destabilized after initiation of S-phase. J Biol Chem 2001;276:44905–44911.
463. Tada S, Li A, Maiorano D, Mechali M, Blow JJ. Repression of origin assembly in metaphase depends on inhibition of RLF-B/Cdt1 by geminin. Nat Cell Biol 2001; 3:107–113.
464. Yanow SK, Lygerou Z, Nurse P. Expression of Cdc18/Cdc6 and Cdt1 during G2 phase induces initiation of DNA replication. EMBO J 2001;20:4648–4656.
465. Arentson E, Faloon P, Seo J, et al. Oncogenic potential of the DNA replication licensing protein CDT1. Oncogene 2002;21:1150–1158.
466. Bell SP, Dutta A. DNA replication in eukaryotic cells. Annu Rev Biochem 2002;71:333–374.
467. Bermejo R, Vilaboa N, Cales C. Regulation of CDC6, geminin, and CDT1 in human cells that undergo polyploidization. Mol Biol Cell 2002;13:3989–4000.
468. Bonds L, Baker P, Gup C, Shroyer KR. Immunohistochemical localization of cdc6 in squamous and glandular neoplasia of the uterine cervix. Arch Pathol Lab Med 2002;26:1164–1168.
469. Mihaylov IS, Kondo T, Jones L, et al. Control of DNA replication and chromosome ploidy by geminin and cyclin A. Mol Cell Biol 2002;22:1868–1880.
470. Nishitani H, Lygerou Z. Control of DNA replication licensing in a cell cycle. Genes Cells 2002;7:523–534.
471. Robles LD, Frost AR, Davila M, Hutson AD, Grizzle WE, Chakrabarti R. Down-regulation of Cdc6, a cell cycle regulatory gene, in prostate cancer. J Biol Chem 2002; 277:25431–25438.
472. Shreeram S, Sparks A, Lane DP, Blow JJ. Cell type-specific responses of human cells to inhibition of replication licensing. Oncogene 2002;21:6624–6632.
473. Wohlschlegel JA, Kutok JL, Weng AP, Dutta A. Expression of geminin as a marker of cell proliferation in normal tissues and malignancies. Am J Pathol 2002;161:267–273.
474. Li X, Zhao Q, Liao R, Sun P, Wu X. The SCF(Skp2) ubiquitin ligase complex interacts with the human replication licensing factor Cdt1 and regulates Cdt1 degradation. J Biol Chem 2003;278:30854–30858.
475. Vaziri C, Saxena S, Jeon Y, et al. A p53–dependent checkpoint pathway prevents rereplication. Mol Cell 2003; 11:997–1008.
476. Yoshida K, Inoue I. Regulation of Geminin and Cdt1 expression by E2F transcription factors. Oncogene 2004;23:3802–3812.
477. Hartwell LH, Weinert TA. Checkpoints: controls that ensure the order of cell cycle events. Science 1989; 246:629–634.
478. Pardee AB. G1 events and regulation of cell proliferation. Science 1989;246:603–608.
479. Kastan MB, Kuerbitz SJ. Control of G1 arrest after DNA damage. Environ Health Perspect 1993;101(suppl 5): 55–58.
480. Sherr CJ. G1 phase progression: cycling on cue. Cell 1994;79:551–555.
481. Elledge SJ. Cell cycle checkpoints: preventing an identity crisis. Science 1996;274:1664–1672.
482. Rudner AD, Murray AW. The spindle assembly checkpoint. Curr Opin Cell Biol 1996;8:773–780.
483. Sanchez I, Dynlacht BD. Transcriptional control of the cell cycle. Curr Opin Cell Biol 1996;8:318–324.
484. Sherr CJ. Cancer cell cycles. Science 1996;274: 1672–1677.
485. O'Connor PM. Mammalian G1 and G2 phase checkpoints. Cancer Surv 1997;29:151–182.
486. Paulovich AG, Toczyski DP, Hartwell LH. When checkpoints fail. Cell 1997;88:315–321

487. Lengauer C, Kinzler KW, Vogelstein B. Genetic instabilities in human cancers. Nature 1998;396:643–649.
488. Mercer WE. Checking on the cell cycle. J Cell Biochem Suppl 1998;30–31:50–54.
489. Salgia R, Skarin AT. Molecular abnormalitities in lung cancer. J Clin Oncol 1998;16:1207–1217.
490. Weinert T. DNA damage checkpoints update: getting molecular. Curr Opin Genet Dev 1998;8:185–193.
491. Johnson DG, Walker CL. Cyclins and cell cycle checkpoints. Annu Rev Pharmacol Toxicol 1999;39:295–312.
492. Clarke DJ, Gimenez-Abian JF. Checkpoints controlling mitosis. Bioessays 2000;22:351–363.
493. Nyberg KA, Michelson RJ, Putnam CW, Weinert TA. Toward maintaining the genome: DNA damage and replication checkpoints. Annu Rev Genet 2002;36:617–656.
494. Shreeram S, Blow JJ. The role of the replication licensing system in cell proliferation and cancer. Prog Cell Cycle Res 2003;5:287–293.
495. Dash BC, El-Deiry WS. Cell cycle checkpoint control mechanisms that can be disrupted in cancer. Methods Mol Biol 2004;280:99–161.
496. Esposito V, Baldi A, Tonini G, et al. Analysis of cell cycle regulator proteins in non-small cell lung cancer. J Clin Pathol 2004;57:58–63.
497. Lisby M, Rothstein R. DNA damage checkpoint and repair centers. Curr Opin Cell Biol 2004;16:328–334.
498. Lukas J, Lukas C, Bartek J. Mammalian cell cycle checkpoints: signalling pathways and their organization in space and time. DNA Repair (Amst) 2004;3:997–1007.
499. Stark GR, Taylor WR. Analyzing the G2/M checkpoint. Methods Mol Biol 2004;280:51–82.
500. Swanton C. Cell-cycle targeted therapies. Lancet Oncol 2004;5:27–36.
501. Branzei D, Foiani M. The DNA damage response during DNA replication. Curr Opin Cell Biol 2005;17:568–575.
502. Hall A. Rho GTPases and the control of cell behaviour. Biochem Soc Trans 2005;33:891–895.
503. Macaluso M, Montanari M, Cinti C, Giordano A. Modulation of cell cycle components by epigenetic and genetic events. Semin Oncol 2005;32:452–457.
504. MacCorkle RA, Tan TH. Mitogen-activated protein kinases in cell-cycle control. Cell Biochem Biophys 2005;43:451–461.
505. Gaestel M. MAPKAP kinases—MKs—two's company, three's a crowd. Nat Rev Mol Cell Biol 2006;7:120–130.
506. Musgrove EA. Cyclins: roles in mitogenic signaling and oncogenic transformation. Growth Factors 2006;24:13–19.
507. Niida H, Nakanishi M. DNA damage checkpoints in mammals. Mutagenesis 2006;21:3–9.
508. Burtelow MA, Roos-Mattjus PM, Rauen M, Babendure JR, Karnitz LM. Reconstitution and molecular analysis of the hRad9–hHus1–hRad1 (9–1–1) DNA damage responsive checkpoint complex. J Biol Chem 2001;276:25903–25909.
509. Lindsey-Boltz LA, Bermudez VP, Hurwitz J, Sancar A. Purification and characterization of human DNA damage checkpoint Rad complexes. Proc Natl Acad Sci USA 2001;98:11236–11241.
510. Bao S, Lu T, Wang X, et al. Disruption of the Rad9/Rad1/Hus1 (9–1–1) complex leads to checkpoint signaling and replication defects. Oncogene 2004;23:5586–5593.
511. Parrilla-Castellar ER, Arlander SJ, Karnitz L. Dial 9–1–1 for DNA damage: the Rad9–Hus1–Rad1 (9–1–1) clamp complex. DNA Repair (Amst) 2004;3:1009–1014.
512. Majka J, Burgers PM. Function of Rad17/Mec3/Ddc1 and its partial complexes in the DNA damage checkpoint. DNA Repair (Amst) 2005;4:1189–1194.
513. Brandt PD, Helt CE, Keng PC, Bambara RA. The Rad9 protein enhances survival and promotes DNA repair following exposure to ionizing radiation. Biochem Biophys Res Commun 2006;347:232–237.
514. Niida H, Nakanishi M. DNA damage checkpoints in mammals. Mutagenesis 2006;21:3–9.
515. van Vugt MA, Medema RH. Checkpoint adaptation and recovery: back with Polo after the break. Cell Cycle 2004;3:1383–1386.
516. van Vugt MA, Bras A, Medema RH. Restarting the cell cycle when the checkpoint comes to a halt. Cancer Res 2005;65:7037–7040.
517. Chen PL, Scully P, Shew JY, Wang JY, Lee WH. Phosphorylation of the retinoblastoma gene product is modulated during the cell cycle and cellular differentiation. Cell 1989;58:1193–1198.
518. Hoppe-Seyler F, Butz K. Tumor suppressor genes in molecular medicine. Clin Investig. 1994; 72:619–630.
519. Toyoshima H, Hunter T. p27, a novel inhibitor of G1 cyclin-Cdk protein kinase activity, is related to p21. Cell 1994;78:67–74.
520. Harper JW, Elledge SJ, Keyomarsi K, et al. Inhibition of cyclin-dependent kinases by p21. Mol Biol Cell 1995; 6:387–400.
521. Sherr CJ, Roberts JM. Inhibitors of mammalian G1 cyclin-dependent kinases. Genes Dev 1995;9:1149–1163.
522. Steegenga WT, van der Eb AJ, Jochemsen AG. How phosphorylation regulates the activity of p53. J Mol Biol 1996;263:103–113.
523. Martinez JD, Craven MT, Joseloff E, Milczarek G, Bowden GT. Regulation of DNA binding and transactivation in p53 by nuclear localization and phosphorylation. Oncogene 1997;14:2511–2520.
524. Takemura M, Kitagawa T, Izuta S, et al. Phosphorylated retinoblastoma protein stimulates DNA polymerase alpha. Oncogene 1997;15:2483–2492.
525. Banin S, Moyal L, Shieh S, et al. Enhanced phosphorylation of p53 by ATM in response to DNA damage. Science 1998;281:1674–1677.
526. Dryja TP, Cavenee W, White R, et al. Homozygosity of chromosome 13 in retinoblastoma. N Engl J Med 1984; 310:550–553.
527. Lee WH, Bookstein R, Hong F, Young LJ, Shew JY, Lee EY. Human retinoblastoma susceptibility gene: cloning, identification, and sequence. Science 1987;235:1394–1399.
528. Dunn JM, Phillips RA, Becker AJ, Gallie BL. Identification of germline and somatic mutations affecting the retinoblastoma gene. Science 1988;241:1797–1800.
529. Huang HJ, Yee JK, Shew JY, et al. Suppression of the neoplastic phenotype by replacement of the RB gene in human cancer cells. Science 1988;242:1563–1566.

530. Horowitz JM, Yandell DW, Park SH, et al. Point mutational inactivation of the retinoblastoma antioncogene. Science 1989;243:937–940.
531. Bookstein R, Lee WH. Molecular genetics of the retinoblastoma suppressor gene. Crit Rev Oncog 1991;2:211–227.
532. Goodrich DW, Wang NP, Qian YW, Lee EY, Lee WH. The retinoblastoma gene product regulates progression through the G1 phase of the cell cycle. Cell 1991;67:293–302.
533. Goodrich DW, Lee WH. Molecular characterization of the retinoblastoma susceptibility gene. Biochim Biophys Acta 1993;1155:43–61.
534. Hollingsworth RE, Hensey CE, Lee W-H. Retinoblastoma protein and cell cycle. Curr Opin Genet 1993;3:55–62.
535. Wiman KG. The retinoblastoma gene: role in cell cycle control and cell differentiation. FASEB J 1993;7:841–845.
536. Riley DJ, Lee EY, Lee WH. The retinoblastoma protein: more than a tumor suppressor. Annu Rev Cell Biol 1994;10:1–29.
537. Wang JY, Knudsen ES, Welch PJ. The retinoblastoma tumor suppressor protein. Adv Cancer Res 1994;64:25–85.150.
538. Herwig S, Strauss M. The retinoblastoma protein: a master regulator of cell cycle, differentiation and apoptosis. Eur J Biochem 1997;246:581–601.
539. Weinberg RA. The retinoblastoma protein and cell cycle control. Cell 1995;81:323–330.
540. Beijersbergen RL, Bernards R. Cell cycle regulation by the retinoblastoma family of growth inhibitory proteins. Biochim Biophys Acta 1996;1287:103–120.
541. Herwig S, Strauss M. The retinoblastoma protein: a master regulator of cell cycle, differentiation and apoptosis. Eur J Biochem 1997;246:581–601.
542. Stiegler P, Kasten M, Giordano A. The RB family of cell cycle regulatory factors. J Cell Biochem Suppl 1998;30–31:30–36.
543. Stiegler P, Giordano A. The family of retinoblastoma proteins. Crit Rev Eukaryot Gene Expr 2001;11:59–76.
544. Yamasaki L. Role of the RB tumor suppressor in cancer. Cancer Treat Res 2003;115:209–239.
545. Massague J. The transforming growth factor-beta family. Annu Rev Cell Biol 1990;6:597–641.
546. Moses HL, Yang EY, Pietenpol JA. TGF-beta stimulation and inhibition of cell proliferation: new mechanistic insights. Cell 1990;63:245–247.
547. Fynan TM, Reiss M. Resistance to inhibition of cell growth by transforming growth factor-beta and its role in oncogenesis. Crit Rev Oncog 1993;4:493–540.
548. Alexandrow MG, Moses HL. Transforming growth factor beta and cell cycle regulation. Cancer Res 1995;55:1452–1457.
549. Polyak K. Negative regulation of cell growth by TGF-B. Biochim Biophys Acta 1996;1241:185–199.
550. Derynck R, Feng XH. TGF-beta receptor signaling. Biochim Biophys Acta 1997;1333:F105–F150.
551. Hartsough MT, Mulder KM. Transforming growth factor-beta signaling in epithelial cells. Pharmacol Ther 1997;75:21–41.
552. Ravitz MJ, Wenner CE. Cyclin-dependent kinase regulation during G1 phase and cell cycle regulation by TGF-beta. Adv Cancer Res 1997;71:165–207.
553. Lee KY, Bae SC. TGF-beta-dependent cell growth arrest and apoptosis. J Biochem Mol Biol 2002;35:47–53.
554. Ten Dijke P, Hill CS. New insights into TGF-beta-Smad signalling. Trends Biochem Sci 2004;29:265–273.
555. Elliott RL, Blobe GC. Role of transforming growth factor Beta in human cancer. J Clin Oncol 2005;23:2078–2093.
556. Diller L, Kassel J, Nelson CE, et al. p53 functions as a cell cycle control protein in osteosarcomas. Mol Cell Biol 1990;10:5772–5781.
557. Raycroft L, Wu H, Lozano G. Transcriptional activation by wild-type but not transforming mutants of the p53 anti-oncogene. Science 1990;249:1049–1051.
558. Kastan MB, Onyekwere O, Sidransky D, Vogelstein B, Craig RW. Participation of p53 protein in the cellular response to DNA damage. Cancer Res 1991;51:6304–6311.
559. Martinez J, Georgoff I, Levine AJ. Cellular localization and cell cycle regulation by a temperature-sensitive p53 protein. Genes Dev 1991;5:151–159.
560. Yin Y, Tainsky MA, Bischoff FZ, Strong LC, Wahl GM. Wild-type p53 restores cell cycle control and inhibits gene amplification in cells with mutant p53 alleles. Cell 1992;70:937–948.
561. Greenblatt MS, Bennett WP, Hollstein M, Harris CC. Mutations in the p53 tumor suppressor gene: clues to cancer etiology and molecular pathogenesis. Cancer Res 1994;54:4855–4878
562. Meek DW. Post-translational modification of p53. Semin Cancer Biol 1994;5:203–210.
563. Agarwal ML, Agarwal A, Taylor WR, Stark GR. p53 controls both the G2/M and the G1 cell cycle checkpoints and mediates reversible growth arrest in human fibro blasts. Proc Natl Acad Sci USA 1995;92:8493–8497.
564. Guillouf C, Rosselli F, Krishnaraju K, Moustacchi E, Hoffman B, Liebermann DA. p53 involvement in control of G2 exit of the cell cycle: role in DNA damage-induced apoptosis. Oncogene 1995;10:2263–2270.
565. Moll UM, Ostermeyer AG, Haladay R, Winkfield B, Frazier M, Zambetti G. Cytoplasmic sequestration of wild-type p53 protein impairs the G1 checkpoint after DNA damage. Mol Cell Biol 1996;16:1126–1137.
566. Almog N, Rotter V. Involvement of p53 in cell differentiation and development. Biochim Biophys Acta 1997;1333:F1–F27.
567. Levine AJ. p53, the cellular gatekeeper for growth and division. Cell 1997;88:323–331.
568. Prives C, Hall PA. The p53 pathway. J Pathol 1999;187:112–126.
569. Brooks CL, Gu W. Dynamics in the p53–Mdm2 ubiquitination pathway. Cell Cycle 2004;3:895–899.
570. Meek DW. The p53 response to DNA damage. DNA Repair (Amst) 2004;3:1049–1056.
571. Bond GL, Hu W, Levine AJ. MDM2 is a central node in the p53 pathway: 12 years and counting. Curr Cancer Drug Targets 2005;5:3–8.
572. Harris SL, Levine AJ. The p53 pathway: positive and negative feedback loops. Oncogene 2005;24:2899–2908.

573. Wang YC, Lin RK, Tan YH, Chen JT, Chen CY, Wang YC. Wild-type p53 overexpression and its correlation with MDM2 and p14ARF alterations: an alternative pathway to non-small-cell lung cancer. J Clin Oncol 2005;23:154–164.
574. Pardee AB. A restriction point for control of normal animal cell proliferation. Proc Natl Acad Sci USA 1974;71:1286–1290.
575. Campisi J, Medrano EE, Morro G, Pardee AB. Restriction point control of cell growth by a labile protein: Evidence for increased stability in transformed cells. Proc Natl Acad Sci USA 1982;79:436–440.
576. Kato J. Induction of S phase by G1 regulatory factors. Front Biosci 1999;4:D787–D792.
577. Blagosklonny MV, Pardee AB. The restriction point of the cell cycle. Cell Cycle 2002;1:103–110.
578. Boonstra J. Progression through the G1–phase of the ongoing cell cycle. J Cell Biochem 2003;90:244–252.
579. Hinds PW, Mittnacht S, Dulic V, Arnold A, Reed SI, Weinberg RA. Regulation of retinoblastoma protein functions by ectopic expression of human cyclins. Cell 1992;70:993–1006.
580. Xiong Y, Zhang H, Beach D. D type cyclins associate with multiple protein kinases and the DNA replication and repair factor PCNA. Cell 1992;71:505–514.
581. Baldin V, Lukas J, Marcote MJ, Pagano M, Draetta G. Cyclin D1 is a nuclear protein required for cell cycle progression in G1. Genes Dev 1993;7:812–821.
582. Dowdy SF, Hinds PW, Louie K, Reed SI, Arnold A, Weinberg RA. Physical interaction of the retinoblastoma protein with human D cyclins. Cell 1993;73:499–511.
583. Kato J, Matsushime H, Hiebert SW, Ewen ME, Sherr CJ. Direct binding of cyclin D to the retinoblastoma gene product (pRb) and pRb phosphorylation by the cyclin D-dependent kinase CDK4. Genes Dev 1993;7:331–342.
584. Quelle DE, Ashmun RA, Shurtleff SA, et al. Overexpression of mouse D-type cyclins accelerates G_1 phase in rodent fibroblasts. Genes Dev 1993;7:1559–1571.
585. Sewing A, Burger C, Brusselbach S, Schalk C, Lucibello FC, Muller R. Human cyclin D1 encodes a labile nuclear protein whose synthesis is directly induced by growth factors and suppressed by cyclic AMP. J Cell Sci 1993;104:545–555.
586. Lukas J, Muller H, Bartkova J, et al. DNA tumor virus oncoproteins and retinoblastoma gene mutations share the ability to relieve the cell's requirement for cyclin D1 function in G1. J Cell Biol 1994;125:625–638.
587. Pagano M, Theodoras AM, Tam SW, Draetta GF. Cyclin D1–mediated inhibition of repair and replicative DNA synthesis in human fibroblasts. Genes Dev 1994;8:1627–1639.
588. Schauer IE, Siriwardana S, Langan TA, Sclafani RA. Cyclin D1 overexpression vs. retinoblastoma inactivation: implications for growth control evasion in non-small cell and small cell lung cancer. Proc Natl Acad Sci USA 1994;91:7827–7831.
589. Bartkova J, Lukas J, Strauss M, Bartek J. Cyclin D1 oncoprotein aberrantly accumulates in malignancies of diverse histogenesis. Oncogene 1995;10:775–778.
590. Han EK, Sgambato A, Jiang W, et al. Stable overexpression of cyclin D1 in a human mammary epithelial cell line prolongs the S-phase and inhibits growth. Oncogene 1995;10:953–961.
591. Ko TC, Sheng HM, Reisman D, Thompson EA, Beauchamp RD. Transforming growth factor-beta 1 inhibits cyclin D1 expression in intestinal epithelial cells. Oncogene 1995;10:177–184.
592. Xiao ZX, Ginsberg D, Ewen M, Livingston DM. Regulation of the retinoblastoma protein-related protein p107 by G_1 cyclin-associated kinases. Proc Natl Acad Sci USA 1996;93:4633–4637.
593. Hosokawa Y, Arnold A. Mechanism of cyclin D1 (CCND1, PRAD1) overexpression in human cancer cells: analysis of allele-specific expression. Genes Chromosomes Cancer 1998;22:66–71.
594. Ortega S, Malumbres M, Barbacid M. Cyclin D-dependent kinases, INK4 inhibitors and cancer. Biochim Biophys Acta 2002;1602:73–87.
595. El-Deiry WS, Tokino T, Velculescu VE, et al. WAF1, a potential mediator of p53 tumor suppression. Cell 1993;75:817–825.
596. Polyak K, Kato JY, Solomon MJ, et al. p27Kip1, a cyclin-Cdk inhibitor, links transforming growth factor-beta and contact inhibition to cell cycle arrest. Genes Dev 1994;8:9–22.
597. Biggs JR, Kraft AS. Inhibitors of cyclin-dependent kinase and cancer. J Mol Med 1995;73:509–514.
598. Datto MB, Li Y, Panus JF, Howe DJ, Xiong Y, Wang XF. Transforming growth factor beta induces the cyclin-dependent kinase inhibitor p21 through a p53–independent mechanism. Proc Natl Acad Sci USA 1995;92:5545–5549.
599. Datto MB, Yu Y, Wang XF. Functional analysis of the transforming growth factor beta responsive elements in the WAF1/Cip1/p21 promoter. J Biol Chem 1995;270:28623–28628.
600. Deng C, Zhang P, Harper JW, Elledge SJ, Leder P. Mice lacking p21CIP1/WAF1 undergo normal development, but are defective in G1 checkpoint control. Cell 1995;82:675–684.
601. Quelle DE, Zindy F, Ashmun RA, Sherr CJ. Alternative reading frames of the INK4a tumor suppressor gene encode two unrelated proteins capable of inducing cell cycle arrest. Cell 1995;83:993–1000.
602. Yeudall WA, Jakus J. Cyclin kinase inhibitors add a new dimension to cell cycle control. Eur J Cancer B Oral Oncol 1995;31B:291–298.
603. Serrano M, Lee H, Chin L, Cordon-Cardo C, Beach D, DePinho RA. Role of the INK4a locus in tumor suppression and cell mortality. Cell 1996;85:27–37.
604. Yan Y, Frisen J, Lee MH, Massague J, Barbacid M. Ablation of the CDK inhibitor p57Kip2 results in increased apoptosis and delayed differentiation during mouse development. Genes Dev 1997;11:973–983.
605. Craig C, Kim M, Ohri E, et al. Effects of adenovirus-mediated p16INK4A expression on cell cycle arrest are determined by endogenous p16 and Rb status in human cancer cells. Oncogene 1998;16:265–272.

606. Niculescu AB 3rd, Chen X, Smeets M, Hengst L, Prives C, Reed SI. Effects of p21(Cip1/Waf1) at both the G1/S and the G2/M cell cycle transitions: pRb is a critical determinant in blocking DNA replication and in preventing endoreduplication. Mol Cell Biol 1998;18: 629–643.
607. Liggett WH Jr, Sidransky D. Role of the p16 tumor suppressor gene in cancer. J Clin Oncol 1998;16:1197–1206.
608. Sherr CJ, Roberts JM. CDK inhibitors: positive and negative regulators of G1-phase progression. Genes Dev 1999;13:1501–1512.
609. Ohtani N, Yamakoshi K, Takahashi A, Hara E. The p16INK4a-RB pathway: molecular link between cellular senescence and tumor suppression. J Med Invest 2004; 51:146–153.
610. Shan B, Zhu X, Chen PL, et al. Molecular cloning of cellular genes encoding retinoblastoma-associated proteins: identification of a gene with properties of the transcription factor E2F. Mol Cell Biol 1992;12:5620–5631.
611. Chellapan SP. The E2F transcription factor: role in cell cycle regulation and differentiation. Mol Cell Diff 1994; 2:201–220.
612. Martin K, Trouche D, Hagemeier C, Kouzarides T. Regulation of transcription by E2F1/DP1. J Cell Sci Suppl 1995;19:91–94.
613. Schwarz JK, Bassing CH, Kovesdi I, et al. Expression of the E2F1 transcription factor overcomes type beta transforming growth factor-mediated growth suppression. Proc Natl Acad Sci USA 1995;92:483–487.
614. Hurford RK Jr, Cobrinik D, Lee MH, Dyson N. pRB and p107/p130 are required for the regulated expression of different sets of E2F responsive genes. Genes Dev 1997;11:1447–1463.
615. Sellers WR, Novitch BG, Miyake S, et al. Stable binding to E2F is not required for the retinoblastoma protein to activate transcription, promote differentiation, and suppress tumor cell growth. Genes Dev 1998;12:95–106.
616. Yamaskai L, Bronson R, Williams BO, Dyson NJ, Harlow E, Jacks T. Loss of E2F-1 reduces tumorigenesis and extends the lifespan of Rb1 (+/–) mice. Nature Genet 1998;18:360–363.
617. Ohtani K. Implication of transcription factor E2F in regulation of DNA replication. Front Biosci 1999;4: D793–D804.
618. Humbert PO, Verona R, Trimarchi JM, Rogers C, Dandapani S, Lees JA. E2f3 is critical for normal cellular proliferation. Genes Dev 2000;14:690–703.
619. Ren B, Cam H, Takahashi Y, Volkert T, Terragni J, Young RA, Dynlacht BD. E2F integrates cell cycle progression with DNA repair, replication, and G(2)/M checkpoints. Genes Dev 2002;16:245–256.
620. Schlisio S, Halperin T, Vidal M, Nevins JR. Interaction of YY1 with E2Fs, mediated by RYBP, provides a mechanism for specificity of E2F function. EMBO J 2002;21:5775–5786.
621. Stevaux O, Dyson NJ. A revised picture of the E2F transcriptional network and RB function. Curr Opin Cell Biol 2002;14:684–691.
622. Mundle SD, Saberwal G. Evolving intricacies and implications of E2F-1 regulation. EMBO J 2003;17:569–574.
623. Karakaidos P, Taraviras S, Vassiliou LV, et al. Overexpression of the replication licensing regulators hCdt1 and hCdc6 characterizes a subset of non-small-cell lung carcinomas: synergistic effect with mutant p53 on tumor growth and chromosomal instability—evidence of E2F-1 transcriptional control over hCdt1. Am J Pathol 2004; 165:1351–1365.
624. Rogoff HA, Kowalik TF. Life, death and E2F: linking proliferation control and DNA damage signaling via E2F1. Cell Cycle 2004;3:845–846.
625. Korenjak M, Brehm A. E2F-Rb complexes regulating transcription of genes important for differentiation and development. Curr Opin Genet Dev 2005;15: 520–527.
626. Goodrich DW, Lee WH. Abrogation by c-myc of G1 phase arrest induced by RB protein but not by p53. Nature 1992;360:177–179.
627. Lukas J, Parry D, Aagaard L, et al. Retinoblastoma-protein-dependent cell-cycle inhibition by the tumour suppressor p16. Nature 1995;375:503–506.
628. Henriksson M, Luscher B. Proteins of the Myc network: essential regulators of cell growth and differentiation. Adv Cancer Res 1996;68:109–182.
629. Schmidt EV. MYC family ties. Nature Genet 1996; 14:8–10.
630. Alexandrow MG, Moses HL. Kips off to Myc: implications for TGF beta signaling. J Cell Biochem 1997;66: 427–432.
631. Amati B, Alevizopoulos K, Vlach J. Myc and the cell cycle. Front Biosci 1998;3:d250–d268.
632. Burgin A, Bouchard C, Eilers M. Control of cell proliferation by Myc proteins. Results Probl Cell Differ 1998; 22:181–197.
633. Matsumura I, Tanaka H, Kanakura Y. E2F1 and c-Myc in cell growth and death. Cell Cycle 2003;2:333–338.
634. Yam CH, Fung TK, Poon RY. Cyclin A in cell cycle control and cancer. Cell Mol Life Sci 2002;59:1317–1326.
635. Porter LA, Donoghue DJ. Cyclin B1 and CDK1: nuclear localization and upstream regulators. Prog Cell Cycle Res 2003;5:335–347.
636. Smith-Sorensen B, Hovig E. CDKN2A (p16INK4A) somatic and germline mutations. Hum Mutat 1996;7: 294–303.
637. Foulkes WD, Flanders TY, Pollock PM, Hayward NK. The CDKN2A (p16) gene and human cancer. Mol Med 1997;3:5–20.
638. Serrano M. The tumor suppressor protein p16INK4a. Exp Cell Res 1997;237:7–13.
639. Carnero A, Hannon GJ. The INK4 family of CDK inhibitors. Curr Top Microbiol Immunol 1998;227:43–55.
640. Liggett WH Jr, Sidransky D. Role of the p16 tumor suppressor gene in cancer. J Clin Oncol 1998;16:1197–1206.
641. Huschtscha LI, Reddel RR. p16(INK4a) and the control of cellular proliferative life span. Carcinogenesis 1999; 20:921–926.
642. Roussel MF. The INK4 family of cell cycle inhibitors in cancer. Oncogene 1999;18:5311–5317.
643. Shapiro GI, Edwards CD, Rollins BJ. The physiology of p16(INK4A)-mediated G1 proliferative arrest. Cell Biochem Biophys 2000;33:189–197.

644. Ohtani N, Yamakoshi K, Takahashi A, Hara E. The p16INK4a-RB pathway: molecular link between cellular senescence and tumor suppression. J Med Invest 2004; 51:146–153.
645. Larsen CJ. Contribution of the dual coding capacity of the p16INK4a/MTS1/CDKN2 locus to human malignancies. Prog Cell Cycle Res 1997;3:109–124.
646. Chin L, Pomerantz J, DePinho RA. The INK4a/ARF tumor suppressor: one gene—two products—two pathways. Trends Biochem Sci 1998;23:291–296.
647. Stott FJ, Bates S, James MC, et al. The alternative product from the human CDKN2A locus, p14(ARF), participates in a regulatory feedback loop with p53 and MDM2. EMBO J 1998;17:5001–5014.
648. James MC, Peters G. Alternative product of the p16/CKDN2A locus connects the Rb and p53 tumor suppressors. Prog Cell Cycle Res 2000;4:71–81.
649. Weber HO, Samuel T, Rauch P, Funk JO. Human p14(ARF)-mediated cell cycle arrest strictly depends on intact p53 signaling pathways. Oncogene 2002;21: 3207–3212.
650. Satyanarayana A, Rudolph KL. p16 and ARF: activation of teenage proteins in old age. J Clin Invest 2004;114: 1237–1240.
651. Livingstone LR, White A, Sprouse J, Livanos E, Jacks T, Tlsty TD. Altered cell cycle arrest and gene amplification potential accompany loss of wild-type p53. Cell 1992;70: 923–935.
652. Harper JW, Adami GR, Wei N, Keyomarsi K, Elledge SJ. The p21 cdk-interacting protein Cip1 is a potent inhibitor of G_1 cyclin-dependent kinases. Cell 1993;75:805–816.
653. Xiong Y, Hannon GJ, Zhang H, Casso D, Kobayashi R, Beach D. p21 is a universal inhibitor of cyclin kinases. Nature 1993;366:701–704.
654. Chen CY, Oliner JD, Zhan Q, Fornace AJ Jr, Vogelstein B, Kastan MB. Interactions between p53 and MDM2 in a mammalian cell cycle checkpoint pathway. Proc Natl Acad Sci USA 1994;91:2684–2688.
655. El-Deiry WS, Harper JW, O'Connor PM, et al. WAF1/CIP1 is induced in p53–mediated G_1 arrest and apoptosis. Cancer Res 1994;54:1169–1174.
656. Waga S, Hannon GJ, Beach D, Stillman B. The p21 inhibitor of cyclin-dependent kinases controls DNA replication by interaction with PCNA. Nature 1994;369:574–578.
657. Canman CE, Gilmer TM, Coutts SB, Kastan MB. Growth factor modulation of p53–mediated growth arrest versus apoptosis. Genes Dev 1995;9:600–611.
658. Chen X, Bargonetti J, Prives C. p53, through p21 (WAF1/CIP1), induces cyclin D1 synthesis. Cancer Res 1995;55: 4257–4263.
659. Del Sal G, Murphy M, Ruaro E, Lazarevic D, Levine AJ, Schneider C. Cyclin D1 and p21/waf1 are both involved in p53 growth suppression. Oncogene 1996;12:177–185.
660. Polyak K, Waldman T, He TC, Kinzler KW, Vogelstein B. Genetic determinants of p53–induced apoptosis and growth arrest. Genes Dev 1996;10:1945–1952.
661. Linke SP, Clarkin KC, Wahl GM. p53 mediates permanent arrest over multiple cell cycles in response to gamma-irradiation. Cancer Res 1997;57:1171–1179.
662. Cayrol C, Knibiehler M, Ducommun B. p21 binding to PCNA causes G1 and G2 cell cycle arrest in p53–deficient cells. Oncogene 1998;16:311–320.
663. Laiho M, DeCaprio JA, Ludlow JW, Livingston DM, Massague J. Growth inhibition by TGF-beta linked to suppression of retinoblastoma protein phosphorylation. Cell 1990;62:175–185.
664. Ewen ME, Sluss HK, Whitehouse LL, Livingston DM. TGF beta inhibition of Cdk4 synthesis is linked to cell cycle arrest. Cell 1993;74:1009–1020.
665. Williams GT. Programmed cell death: apoptosis and oncogenesis. Cell 1991;65:1097–1098.
666. Saraste A, Pulkki K. Morphologic and biochemical hallmarks of apoptosis. Cardiovasc Res 2000;45:528–537.
667. Martelli AM, Zweyer M, Ochs RL, et al. Nuclear apoptotic changes: an overview. J Cell Biochem 2001;82: 634–646.
668. Van Cruchten S, Van Den Broeck W. Morphological and biochemical aspects of apoptosis, oncosis and necrosis. Anat Histol Embryol 2002;31:214–223.
669. Alenzi FQ, Warrens AN. Cellular and molecular themes in apoptosis. Wien Klin Wochenschr 2003;115:563–574.
670. Schultz DR, Harrington WJ Jr. Apoptosis: programmed cell death at a molecular level. Semin Arthritis Rheum 2003;32:345–369.
671. Edinger AL, Thompson CB. Death by design: apoptosis, necrosis and autophagy. Curr Opin Cell Biol 2004;16: 663–669.
672. Jin Z, El-Deiry WS. Overview of cell death signaling pathways. Cancer Biol Ther 2005;4:139–163.
673. Yonish-Rouach E, Grunwald D, Wilder S, et al. p53–mediated cell death: relationship to cell cycle control. Mol Cell Biol 1993;13:1415–1423.
674. Oren M. Relationship of p53 to the control of apoptotic cell death. Semin Cancer Biol 1994;5:221–227.
675. Bond J, Haughton M, Blaydes J, Gire V, Wynford-Thomas D, Wyllie F. Evidence that transcriptional activation by p53 plays a direct role in the induction of cellular senescence. Oncogene 1996;13:2097–2104.
676. Chen X, Ko LJ, Jayaraman L, Prives C. p53 levels, functional domains, and DNA damage determine the extent of the apoptotic response of tumor cells. Genes Dev 1996;10:2438–2451.
677. Kagawa S, Fujiwara T, Hizuta A, et al. p53 expression overcomes p21WAF1/CIP1–mediated G1 arrest and induces apoptosis in human cancer cells. Oncogene 1997; 15:1903–1909.
678. Polyak K, Xia Y, Zweier JL, Kinzler KW, Vogelstein B. A model for p53–induced apoptosis. Nature 1997;389: 300–305.
679. Sandig V, Brand K, Herwig S, Lukas J, Bartek J, Strauss M. Adenovirally transferred p16INK4/CDKN2 and p53 genes cooperate to induce apoptotic tumor cell death. Nat Med 1997;3:313–319.
680. Hockenbery DM. The bcl-2 oncogene and apoptosis. Semin Immunol 1992;4:413–420.
681. Oltvai ZN, Milliman CL, Korsmeyer SJ. Bcl-2 heterodimerizes in vivo with a conserved homolog, Bax, that accelerates programmed cell death. Cell 1993;74:609–619.

682. Chiou SK, Rao L, White E. Bcl-2 blocks p53–dependent apoptosis. Mol Cell Biol 1994;14:2556–2563.
683. Miyashita T, Krajewski S, Krajewska M, et al. Tumor suppressor p53 is a regulator of bcl-2 and bax gene expression in vitro and in vivo. Oncogene 1994;9:1799–1805.
684. Selvakumaran M, Lin HK, Miyashita T, et al. Immediate early up-regulation of bax expression by p53 but not TGF beta 1: a paradigm for distinct apoptotic pathways. Oncogene 1994;9:1791–1798.
685. Miyashita T, Reed JC. Tumor suppressor p53 is a direct transcriptional activator of the human bax gene. Cell 1995;80:293–299.
686. Brown R. The bcl-2 family of proteins. Br Med Bull 1997; 53:466–477.
687. Jacobson MD. Apoptosis: Bcl-2–related proteins get connected. Curr Biol 1997;7:R277–R281.214.
688. Kroemer G. The proto-oncogene Bcl-2 and its role in regulating apoptosis. Nat Med 1997;3:614–620.
689. Yin C, Knudson CM, Korsmeyer SJ, Van Dyke T. Bax suppresses tumorigenesis and stimulates apoptosis in vivo. Nature 1997;385:637–640.
690. Adams JM, Cory S. The Bcl-2 protein family: arbiters of cell survival. Science 1998;281(5381):1322–1326.
691. Cory S, Adams JM. The Bcl2 family: regulators of the cellular life-or-death switch. Nat Rev Cancer 2002;2(9): 647–656.
692. Kiechle FL, Zhang X. Apoptosis: biochemical aspects and clinical implications. Clin Chim Acta 2002;326(1–2): 27–45.
693. Alenzi FQ, Warrens AN. Cellular and molecular themes in apoptosis. Wien Klin Wochenschr 2003;115(15–16): 563–574.
694. Harada H, Grant S. Apoptosis regulators. Rev Clin Exp Hematol 2003;7(2):117–138.
695. Kaina B. DNA damage-triggered apoptosis: critical role of DNA repair, double-strand breaks, cell proliferation and signaling. Biochem Pharmacol 2003;66(8):1547–1554.
696. Liston P, Fong WG, Komeluk RG. The inhibitors of apoptosis: there is more to life than Bcl2. Oncogene 2003; 22(53):8568–8580.
697. Willis S, Day CL, Hinds MG, Huang DC. The Bcl-2–regulated apoptotic pathway. J Cell Sci 2003;116(pt 20): 4053–4056.
698. Piro LD. Apoptosis, Bcl-2 antisense, and cancer therapy. Oncology (Williston Park) 2004;18(13 suppl 10):5–10.
699. Shabnam MS, Srinivasan R, Wali A, Majumdar S, Joshi K, Behera D. Expression of p53 protein and the apoptotic regulatory molecules Bcl-2, Bcl-XL, and Bax in locally advanced squamous cell carcinoma of the lung. Lung Cancer 2004;45(2):181–188.
700. Thomadaki H, Scorilas A, Hindmarsh JT. BCL2 family of apoptosis-related genes: functions and clinical implications in cancer. Crit Rev Clin Lab Sci 2006;43(1):1–67.
701. Kumar S. Mechanisms mediating caspase activation in cell death. Cell Death Differ 1999;6:1060–1066.
702. Kolenko VM, Uzzo RG, Bukowski R, Finke JH. Caspase-dependent and -independent death pathways in cancer therapy. Apoptosis 2000;5:17–20.
703. Kuida K. Caspase-9. Int J Biochem Cell Biol 2000; 32:121–124.
704. Creagh EM, Martin SJ. Caspases: cellular demolition experts. Biochem Soc Trans 2001;29:696–702.
705. Zimmermann KC, Bonzon C, Green DR. The machinery of programmed cell death. Pharmacol Ther 2001;92: 57–70.
706. Adams JM, Cory S. Apoptosomes: engines for caspase activation. Curr Opin Cell Biol 2002;14:715–720.
707. Chen M, Wang J. Initiator caspases in apoptosis signaling pathways. Apoptosis 2002;7:313–319.
708. Cho SG, Choi EJ. Apoptotic signaling pathways: caspases and stress-activated protein kinases. J Biochem Mol Biol 2002;35:24–27.
709. Gupta S. Molecular signaling in death receptor and mitochondrial pathways of apoptosis (Review). Int J Oncol 2003;22:15–20.
710. Hajra KM, Liu JR. Apoptosome dysfunction in human cancer. Apoptosis 2004;9:691–704.
711. Shi Y. Caspase activation, inhibition, and reactivation: a mechanistic view. Protein Sci 2004;13:1979–1987.
712. Fan TJ, Han LH, Cong RS, Liang J. Caspase family proteases and apoptosis. Acta Biochim Biophys Sin (Shanghai) 2005;37:719–727.
713. Kim R, Emi M, Tanabe K. Caspase-dependent and -independent cell death pathways after DNA damage (Review). Oncol Rep 2005;14:595–599.
714. Curtin JF, Cotter TG. Live and let die: regulatory mechanisms in Fas-mediated apoptosis. Cell Signal 2003;15: 983–992.
715. Dempsey PW, Doyle SE, He JQ, Cheng G. The signaling adaptors and pathways activated by TNF superfamily. Cytokine Growth Factor Rev 2003;14:193–209.
716. Gaur U, Aggarwal BB. Regulation of proliferation, survival and apoptosis by members of the TNF superfamily. Biochem Pharmacol 2003;66:1403–1408.
717. MacFarlane M. TRAIL-induced signalling and apoptosis. Toxicol Lett 2003;139:89–97.
718. Ozoren N, El-Deiry WS. Cell surface Death Receptor signaling in normal and cancer cells. Semin Cancer Biol 2003;13:135–147.
719. Tibbetts MD, Zheng L, Lenardo MJ. The death effector domain protein family: regulators of cellular homeostasis. Nat Immunol 2003;4:404–409.
720. Wajant H. Death receptors. Essays Biochem 2003;39: 53–71.
721. Thorburn A. Death receptor-induced cell killing. Cell Signal 2004;16:139–144.
722. Zhang J, Zhang D, Hua Z. FADD and its phosphorylation. IUBMB Life 2004;56:395–401.
723. de Thonel A, Eriksson JE. Regulation of death receptors-Relevance in cancer therapies. Toxicol Appl Pharmacol 2005;207(2 suppl):123–132.
724. Shakibaei M, Schulze-Tanzil G, Takada Y, Aggarwal BB. Redox regulation of apoptosis by members of the TNF superfamily. Antioxid Redox Signal 2005;7:482–496.
725. Fas SC, Fritzsching B, Suri-Payer E, Krammer PH. Death receptor signaling and its function in the immune system. Curr Dir Autoimmun 2006;9:1–17.

726. Cleveland JL, Ihle JN. Contenders in FasL/TNF death signaling. Cell 1995;81:479–482.
727. Mukhopadhyay A, Ni J, Zhai Y, Yu GL, Aggarwal BB. Identification and characterization of a novel cytokine, THANK, a TNF homologue that activates apoptosis, nuclear factor-kappaB, and c-Jun NH2–terminal kinase. J Biol Chem 1999;274:15978–15981.
728. Nakayama M, Ishidoh K, Kayagaki N, et al. Multiple pathways of TWEAK-induced cell death. J Immunol 2002;168:734–743.
729. Reichmann E. The biological role of the Fas/FasL system during tumor formation and progression. Semin Cancer Biol 2002;12:309–315.
730. Han S, Yoon K, Lee K, et al. TNF-related weak inducer of apoptosis receptor, a TNF receptor superfamily member, activates NF-kappa B through TNF receptor-associated factors. Biochem Biophys Res Commun 2003;305:789–796.
731. Wiley SR, Winkles JA. TWEAK, a member of the TNF superfamily, is a multifunctional cytokine that binds the TweakR/Fn14 receptor. Cytokine Growth Factor Rev 2003;14:241–249.
732. Campbell S, Michaelson J, Burkly L, Putterman C. The role of TWEAK/Fn14 IN the pathogenesis of inflammation and systemic autoimmunity. Front Biosci 2004; 9:2273–2284.
733. Winkles JA, Tran NL, Berens ME. TWEAK and Fn14: new molecular targets for cancer therapy? Cancer Lett 2006;235:11–17.
734. Huang DC, Strasser A. BH3–Only proteins-essential initiators of apoptotic cell death. Cell 2000;103:839–842.
735. Lutz RJ. Role of the BH3 (Bcl-2 homology 3) domain in the regulation of apoptosis and Bcl-2–related proteins. Biochem Soc Trans 2000;28:51–56.
736. Bouillet P, Strasser A. BH3–only proteins—evolutionarily conserved proapoptotic Bcl-2 family members essential for initiating programmed cell death. J Cell Sci 2002;115:1567–1574.
737. Fleischer A, Rebollo A, Ayllon V. BH3-only proteins: the lords of death. Arch Immunol Ther Exp (Warsz) 2003;51:9–17.
738. Willis SN, Adams JM. Life in the balance: how BH3–only proteins induce apoptosis. Curr Opin Cell Biol 2005; 17:617–625.
739. Shibue T, Taniguchi T. BH3–only proteins: integrated control point of apoptosis. Int J Cancer 2006;119: 2036–2043.
740. Yin XM. Bid, a BH3–only multi-functional molecule, is at the cross road of life and death. Gene 2006;369:7–19.
741. Sheikh MS, Fornace AJ Jr. Death and decoy receptors and p53–mediated apoptosis. Leukemia 2000;14:1509–1513.
742. Cappello F, Bellafiore M, Palma A, Bucchieri F. Defective apoptosis and tumorigenesis: role of p53 mutation and Fas/FasL system dysregulation. Eur J Histochem 2002;46: 199–208
743. Haupt S, Berger M, Goldberg Z, Haupt Y. Apoptosis—the p53 network. J Cell Sci 2003;116:4077–4085.
744. Oda E, Ohki R, Murasawa H, et al. Noxa, a BH3–only member of the Bcl-2 family and candidate mediator of p53–induced apoptosis. Science 2000;288:1053–1058.
745. Schuler M, Green DR. Mechanisms of p53–dependent apoptosis. Biochem Soc Trans 2001;29:684–688.
746. Wu X, Deng Y. Bax and BH3–domain-only proteins in p53–mediated apoptosis. Front Biosci 2002;7:d151–d156.
747. Jeffers JR, Parganas E, Lee Y, et al. Puma is an essential mediator of p53–dependent and -independent apoptotic pathways. Cancer Cell 2003;4:321–328.
748. Seo YW, Shin JN, Ko KH, et al. The molecular mechanism of Noxa-induced mitochondrial dysfunction in p53–mediated cell death. J Biol Chem 2003;278:48292–48299.
749. Shibue T, Takeda K, Oda E, et al. Integral role of Noxa in p53–mediated apoptotic response. Genes Dev 2003; 17:2233–2238.
750. Villunger A, Michalak EM, Coultas L, et al. p53– and drug-induced apoptotic responses mediated by BH3–only proteins puma and noxa. Science 2003;302:1036–1038.
751. Hemann MT, Zilfou JT, Zhao Z, Burgess DJ, Hannon GJ, Lowe SW. Suppression of tumorigenesis by the p53 target PUMA. Proc Natl Acad Sci U S A 2004;101:9333–9338.
752. Chipuk JE, Bouchier-Hayes L, Kuwana T, Newmeyer DD, Green DR. PUMA couples the nuclear and cytoplasmic proapoptotic function of p53. Science 2005;309: 1732–1735.
753. Tobiume K. Involvement of Bcl-2 family proteins in p53–induced apoptosis. J Nippon Med Sch 2005;72:192–193.
754. Vousden KH. Apoptosis. p53 and PUMA: a deadly duo. Science 2005;309:1685–1686.
755. Yu J, Zhang L. The transcriptional targets of p53 in apoptosis control. Biochem Biophys Res Commun 2005;331:851–858.
756. Allen RT, Cluck MW, Agrawal DK. Mechanisms controlling cellular suicide: role of Bcl-2 and caspases. Cell Mol Life Sci 1998;54:427–445.
757. Hu Y, Benedict MA, Wu D, Inohara N, Nunez G. Bcl XL interacts with Apaf-1 and inhibits Apaf-1–dependent caspase-9 activation. Proc Natl Acad Sci USA 1998; 95:4386–4391.
758. Mignotte B, Vayssiere JL. Mitochondria and apoptosis. Eur J Biochem 1998;252:1–15.
759. Pan G, O'Rourke K, Dixit VM. Caspase-9, Bcl-XL, and Apaf-1 form a ternary complex. J Biol Chem 1998;273: 5841–5845.
760. Bossy-Wetzel E, Green DR. Apoptosis: checkpoint at the mitochondrial frontier. Mutat Res 1999;434:243–251.
761. Cosulich SC, Savory PJ, Clarke PR. Bcl-2 regulates amplification of caspase activation by cytochrome c. Curr Biol 1999;9:147–150.
762. Eskes R, Desagher S, Antonsson B, Martinou JC. Bid induces the oligomerization and insertion of Bax into the outer mitochondrial membrane. Mol Cell Biol 2000;20: 929–935.
763. Haraguchi M, Torii S, Matsuzawa S, et al. Apoptotic protease activating factor 1 (Apaf-1)-independent cell death suppression by Bcl-2. J Exp Med 2000;191:1709–1720.
764. Hausmann G, O'Reilly LA, van Driel R, et al. Proapoptotic apoptosis protease-activating factor 1 (Apaf-1)

has a cytoplasmic localization distinct from Bcl-2 or Bcl-x(L). J Cell Biol 2000;149:623–634.
765. Newmeyer DD, Bossy-Wetzel E, Kluck RM, Wolf BB, Beere HM, Green DR. Bcl-xL does not inhibit the function of Apaf-1. Cell Death Differ 2000;7:402–407.
766. Cheng EH, Wei MC, Weiler S, et al. BCL-2, BCL-X(L) sequester BH3 domain-only molecules preventing BAX- and BAK-mediated mitochondrial apoptosis. Mol Cell 2001;8:705–711.
767. Liang Y, Zhou Y, Shen P. NF-kappaB and its regulation on the immune system. Cell Mol Immunol 2004;1: 343–350.
768. Xiao W. Advances in NF-kappaB signaling transduction and transcription. Cell Mol Immunol 2004;1:425–435.
769. Courtois G. The NF-kappaB signaling pathway in human genetic diseases. Cell Mol Life Sci 2005;62:1682–1691.
770. Dobrovolskaia MA, Kozlov SV. Inflammation and cancer: when NF-kappaB amalgamates the perilous partnership. Curr Cancer Drug Targets 2005;5:325–344.
771. Karin M, Greten FR. NF-kappaB: linking inflammation and immunity to cancer development and progression. Nat Rev Immunol 2005;5:749–759.
772. Luo JL, Kamata H, Karin M. IKK/NF-kappaB signaling: balancing life and death—a new approach to cancer therapy. J Clin Invest 2005;115:2625–2632.
773. Moynagh PN. The NF-kappaB pathway. J Cell Sci 2005; 118(pt 20):4589–4592.
774. Zingarelli B. Nuclear factor-kappaB. Crit Care Med 2005;33(12 suppl):S414–S416.
775. Bubici C, Papa S, Pham CG, Zazzeroni F, Franzoso G. The NF-kappaB-mediated control of ROS and JNK signaling. Histol Histopathol 2006;21:69–80.
776. Campbell KJ, Perkins ND. Regulation of NF-kappaB function. Biochem Soc Symp 2006;(73):165–180.
777. Hoffmann A, Baltimore D. Circuitry of nuclear factor kappaB signaling. Immunol Rev 2006;210:171–186.
778. Karin M. Nuclear factor-kappaB in cancer development and progression. Nature 2006;441:431–436.
779. Kovalenko A, Wallach D. If the prophet does not come to the mountain: dynamics of signaling complexes in NF-kappaB activation. Mol Cell 2006;22:433–436.
780. Piva R, Belardo G, Santoro MG. NF-kappaB: a stress-regulated switch for cell survival. Antioxid Redox Signal 2006;8:478–486.
781. Vermeulen L, Vanden Berghe W, Haegeman G. Regulation of NF-kappaB transcriptional activity. Cancer Treat Res 2006;130:89–102.
782. O'Neill LA, Greene C. Signal transduction pathways activated by the IL-1 receptor family: ancient signaling machinery in mammals, insects, and plants. J Leukoc Biol 1998;63(6):650–657.
783. Karin M. The beginning of the end: IkappaB kinase (IKK) and NF-kappaB activation. J Biol Chem 1999;274: 27339–27342.
784. Karin M. How NF-kappaB is activated: the role of the IkappaB kinase (IKK) complex. Oncogene 1999;18: 6867–6874.
785. Rothwarf DM, Karin M. The NF-kappa B activation pathway: a paradigm in information transfer from membrane to nucleus. Sci STKE 1999;1999:RE1.
786. Senftleben U, Karin M. The IKK/NF-kappa B pathway. Crit Care Med 2002;30(1 suppl):S18–S26.
787. Hayden MS, Ghosh S. Signaling to NF-kappaB. Genes Dev 2004;18:2195–2224.
788. Chen ZJ. Ubiquitin signalling in the NF-kappaB pathway. Nat Cell Biol 2005;7:758–765.
789. Hu MC, Hung MC. Role of IkappaB kinase in tumorigenesis. Future Oncol 2005;1:67–78.
790. Viatour P, Merville MP, Bours V, Chariot A. Phosphorylation of NF-kappaB and IkappaB proteins: implications in cancer and inflammation. Trends Biochem Sci 2005; 30:43–52.
791. Gloire G, Dejardin E, Piette J. Extending the nuclear roles of IkappaB kinase subunits. Biochem Pharmacol 2006;72:1081–1089.
792. Crow JF. The high spontaneous mutation rate: is it a health risk? Proc Natl Acad Sci USA 1997;94:8380–8386.
793. Hollstein M, Sidransky D, Vogelstein B, Harris CC. p53 mutations in human cancers. Science 1991;253:49–53.
794. Hartwell L. Defects in a cell cycle checkpoint may be responsible for the genomic instability of cancer cells. Cell 1992;71:543–546.
795. Zambetti GP, Levine AJ. A comparison of the biological activities of wild-type and mutant p53. Faseb J 1993; 7:855–865.
796. Hartwell LH, Kastan MB. Cell cycle control and cancer. Science 1994;266:1821–1828.
797. Foulkes WD, Flanders TY, Pollock PM, Hayward NK. The CDKN2 (p16) gene and human cancer. Mol Med 1996;3:5–20.
798. Gottlieb TM, Oren M. p53 in growth control and neoplasia. Biochim Biophys Acta 1996;1287:77–102.
799. Gao HG, Chen JK, Stewart J, et al. Distribution of p53 and K-ras mutations in human lung cancer tissues. Carcinogenesis 1997;18:473–478.
800. Peltomaki P. DNA mismatch repair gene mutations in human cancer. Environ Health Perspect 1997;105(suppl 4):775–780.
801. Cahill DP, Lengauer C, Yu J, et al. Mutations of mitotic checkpoint genes in human cancers. Nature 1998;392: 300–303.
802. Massague J, Blain SW, Lo RS. TGFbeta signaling in growth control, cancer, and heritable disorders. Cell 2000;103:295–309.
803. Chen PL, Chen YM, Bookstein R, Lee WH. Genetic mechanisms of tumor suppression by the human p53 gene. Science 1990;250:1576–1580.
804. Weinberg RA. Tumor suppressor genes. Science 1991; 254:1138–1146.
805. Levine AJ. The tumor suppressor genes. Annu Rev Biochem 1993;62:623–651.
806. Yamamoto T. Molecular basis of cancer: oncogenes and tumor suppressor genes. Microbiol Immunol 1993;37: 11–22.
807. Greenblatt MS, Bennett WP, Hollstein M, Harris CC. Mutations in the p53 tumor suppressor gene: clues to cancer etiology and molecular pathogenesis. Cancer Res 1994;54:4855–4878.
808. Ponz de Leon M. Oncogenes and tumor suppressor genes. Recent Results Cancer Res 1994;136:35–47.

809. Weinberg RA. The molecular basis of oncogenes and tumor suppressor genes. Ann NY Acad Sci 1995;758: 331–338.
810. Markowitz SD, Roberts AB. Tumor suppressor activity of the TGF-beta pathway in human cancers. Cytokine Growth Factor Rev 1996;7:93–102.
811. Shapiro GI, Rollins BJ. p16INK4A as a human tumor suppressor. Biochim Biophys Acta 1996;1242:165–169.
812. Smith-Sorensen B, Hovig E. CDKN2A (p16INK4A) somatic and germline mutations. Hum Mutat 1996;7: 294–303.
813. Eshleman JR, Markowitz SD. Mismatch repair defects in human carcinogenesis. Hum Mol Genet 1996;5 Spec No:1489–1494.
814. Malkhosyan S, Rampino N, Yamamoto H, Perucho M. Frameshift mutator mutations. Nature 1996;382:499–500.
815. Pihan G. Doxsey SJ. Mutations and aneuploidy: co-conspirators in cancer? Cancer Cell 2003;4:89–94.
816. Sarasin A. An overview of the mechanisms of mutagenesis and carcinogenesis. Mutat Res 2003;544:99–106.
817. Frank SA, Nowak MA. Problems of somatic mutation and cancer. Bioessays 2004;26:291–299.
818. Weir B, Zhao X, Meyerson M. Somatic alterations in the human cancer genome. Cancer Cell 2004;6:433–438.
819. Miller JH. Perspective on mutagenesis and repair: the standard model and alternate modes of mutagenesis. Crit Rev Biochem Mol Biol 2005;40:155–179.
820. de Klein A, van Kessel AG, Grosveld G, et al. A cellular oncogene is translocated to the Philadelphia chromosome in chronic myelocytic leukaemia. Nature 1982;300: 765–767.
821. Cory S. Activation of cellular oncogenes in hemopoietic cells by chromosome translocation. Adv Cancer Res 1986;47:189–234.
822. Cagle PT, Taylor LD, Schwartz MR, Ramzy I, Elder F. Cytogenetic abnormalities common to adenocarcinoma metastatic to the pleura. Cancer Genet Cytogenet 1989; 39:219–225.
823. Solomon E, Borrow J, Goddard AD. Chromosome aberrations and cancer. Science 1991;254:1153–60.
824. Rabbitts TH. Chromosomal translocations in human cancer. Nature 1994;372:143–149.
825. Abeysinghe SS, Stenson PD, Krawczak M, Cooper DN. Gross Rearrangement Breakpoint Database (GRaBD). Hum Mutat 2004;23:219–221.
826. Bystritskiy AA, Razin SV. Breakpoint clusters: reason or consequence? Crit Rev Eukaryot Gene Expr 2004;14: 65–77.
827. Knuutila S. Cytogenetics and molecular pathology in cancer diagnostics. Ann Med 2004;36:162–171.
828. Aplan PD. Causes of oncogenic chromosomal translocation. Trends Genet 2006;22:46–55.
829. Jefford CE, Irminger-Finger I. Mechanisms of chromosome instability in cancers. Crit Rev Oncol Hematol 2006;59:1–14.
830. Raptis S, Bapat B. Genetic instability in human tumors. EXS 2006;(96):303–320.
831. Taki T, Taniwaki M. Chromosomal translocations in cancer and their relevance for therapy. Curr Opin Oncol 2006;18:62–68.
832. Barker PE. Double minutes in human tumor cells. Cancer Genet Cytogenet 1982; 5:81–94.
833. Cowell JK. Double minutes and homogeneously staining regions: gene amplification in mammalian cells. Annu Rev Genet 1982;16:21–59.
834. Tabin CJ, Bradley SM, Bargmann CI, et al. Mechanism of activation of a human oncogene. Nature 1982;300: 143–149.
835. Alitalo K, Schwab M. Oncogene amplification in tumor cells. Adv Cancer Res 1986;47:235–281.
836. Benner SE, Wahl GM, Von Hoff DD. Double minute chromosomes and homogeneously staining regions in tumors taken directly from patients versus in human tumor cell lines. Anticancer Drugs 1991;2:11–25.
837. Hamlin JL, Leu TH, Vaughn JP, Ma C, Dijkwel PA. Amplification of DNA sequences in mammalian cells. Prog Nucleic Acid Res Mol Biol 1991;41:203–239.
838. Hahn PJ. Molecular biology of double-minute chromosomes. Bioessays 1993;15:477–484.
839. Schwab M. Amplification of oncogenes in human cancer cells. Bioessays 1998;20:473–479.
840. Schwab M. Oncogene amplification in solid tumors. Semin Cancer Biol. 1999;9:319–325.
841. Todd R, Wong DT. Oncogenes. Anticancer Res 1999;19: 4729–4746.
842. Savelyeva L. Schwab M. Amplification of oncogenes revisited: from expression profiling to clinical application. Cancer Lett 2001;167:115–123.
843. Rieger PT. The biology of cancer genetics. Semin Oncol Nurs 2004;20:145–154.
844. Gebhart E. Double minutes, cytogenetic equivalents of gene amplification, in human neoplasia—a review. Clin Transl Oncol 2005;7:477–485.
845. Wajed SA, Laird PW, DeMeester TR. DNA methylation: an alternative pathway to cancer. Ann Surg 2001;234: 10–20.
846. Fruhwald MC. DNA methylation patterns in cancer: novel prognostic indicators? Am J Pharmacogenomics 2003;3:245–260.
847. Feinberg AP. The epigenetics of cancer etiology. Semin Cancer Biol 2004;14:427–432.
848. Baylin SB. DNA methylation and gene silencing in cancer. Nat Clin Pract Oncol 2005;2(suppl 1):S4–S11.
849. Santos ES, Raez LE, DeDesare T, Singal R. DNA methylation: its role in lung carcinogenesis and therapeutic implications. Expert Rev Anticancer Ther 2005;5: 667–679.
850. Toyota M, Issa JP. Epigenetic changes in solid and hematopoietic tumors. Semin Oncol 2005;32:521–530.
851. Holmes R, Soloway PD. Regulation of imprinted DNA methylation. Cytogenet Genome Res 2006;113:122–129.
852. Klose RJ, Bird AP. Genomic DNA methylation: the mark and its mediators. Trends Biochem Sci 2006;31:89–97.
853. Pfeifer GP. Mutagenesis at methylated CpG sequences. Curr Top Microbiol Immunol 2006;301:259–281.
854. Gray JW, Collins C. Genome changes and gene expression in human solid tumors. Carcinogenesis 2000;21: 443–452.
855. Payne SR, Kemp CJ. Tumor suppressor genetics. Carcinogenesis 2005;26:2031–2045.

856. Zheng HT, Peng ZH, Li S, He L. Loss of heterozygosity analyzed by single nucleotide polymorphism array in cancer. World J Gastroenterol 2005;11:6740–6744.
857. McManus MT. MicroRNAs and cancer. Semin Cancer Biol 2003;13:253–258.
858. Ambros V. The functions of animal microRNAs. Nature 2004;431:350–355.
859. Bartel DP. MicroRNAs: genomics, biogenesis, mechanism, and function. *Cell* 2004;116:281–297.
860. Calin GA, Liu CG, Sevignani C, et al. MicroRNA profiling reveals distinct signatures in B cell chronic lymphocytic leukemias. Proc Natl Acad Sci USA 2004;101: 11755–11760.
861. Calin GA, Sevignani C, Dumitru CD, et al. Human microRNA genes are frequently located at fragile sites and genomic regions involved in cancers Proc Natl Acad Sci USA 2004;101:2999–3004.
862. Chen C-Z, Li L, Lodish HF, Bartel DP. MicroRNAs modulate hematopoietic lineage differentiation. Science 2004;303:83–87.
863. He L, Hannon GJ. MicroRNAs: small RNAs with a big role in gene regulation. Nature Rev Genet 2004;5: 522–531.
864. Du T, Zamore PD. microPrimer: the biogenesis and function of microRNA. Development 2005;132:4645–4652.
865. Hammond SM. MicroRNAs as oncogenes. Curr Opin Genet Dev 2005;16:4–9.
866. Lu J, Getz G, Miska EA, et al. MicroRNA expression profiles classify human cancers. Nature 2005;435: 834–838.
867. Zhao Y, Samal E, Srivastava D. Serum response factor regulates a muscle-specific microRNA that targets Hand2 during cardiogenesis. Nature 2005;436:214–220.
868. Davis S, Lollo B, Freier S, Esau C. Improved targeting of miRNA with antisense oligonucleotides. Nucleic Acids Res 2006;34:2294–2304.
869. Pasquinelli AE. Demystifying small RNA pathways. Dev Cell 2006;10:419–424.
870. Valencia-Sanchez MA, Liu J, Hannon GJ, Parker R. Control of translation and mRNA degradation by miRNAs and siRNAs. Genes Dev 2006;20:515–524.
871. Esch RK. Basic nucleic acid procedures. In: Coleman WB, Tsongalis GJ, eds. Molecular diagnostics for the clinical laboratorian. Totowa, NJ: Humana Press, 1997: 55–58.
872. Smith MJ, Pulliam JF, Farkas DH. Molecular pathology methodologies. In: Leonard DGB, ed. Molecular pathology in clinical practice. New York: Springer-Verlag, 2007.
873. Mardis ER, Roe BA. Automated methods for single-stranded DNA isolation and dideoxynucleotide DNA sequencing reactions on a robotic workstation. Biotechniques 1989;7:840–850.
874. Mies C. Molecular biological analysis of paraffin-embedded tissues. Hum Pathol 1994;25:555–560.
875. Poljak M, Seme K, Gale N. Rapid extraction of DNA from archival clinical specimens: our experiences. Pflugers Arch 2000;439(3 suppl):R42–R44.
876. El-Naggar AK. Methods in molecular surgical pathology. Semin Diagn Pathol 2002;19:56–71.
877. Kessler HH, Muhlbauer G, Stelzl E, Daghofer E, Santner BI, Marth E. Fully automated nucleic acid extraction: MagNA Pure LC. Clin Chem 2001;47:1124–1126.
878. Fiebelkorn KR, Lee BG, Hill CE, Caliendo AM, Nolte FS. Clinical Evaluation of an Automated Nucleic Acid Isolation System. Clin Chem 2002;48:1613–1615.
879. Williams SM, Meadows CA, Lyon E. Automated DNA Extraction for Real-Time PCR. Clin Chem 2002;48: 1629–1630.
880. Chomczynski P, Sacchi N. Single-step method of RNA isolation by acid guanidinium thiocyanate-phenol-chloroform extraction. Anal Biochem 1987;162:156–159.
881. Foss RD, Guha-Thakurta N, Conran RM, Gutman P. Effects of fixative and fixation time on the extraction and polymerase chain reaction amplification of RNA from paraffin-embedded tissue. Comparison of two housekeeping gene mRNA controls. Diagn Mol Pathol 1994; 3:148–155.
882. Krafft AE, Duncan BW, Bijwaard KE, Taubenberger JK, Lichy JH. Optimization of the isolation and amplification of RNA from formalin-fixed, paraffin-embedded tissue: the Armed Forces Institute of Pathology experience and literature review. Mol Diagn 1997;2:217–230.
883. Ramalho AS, Beck S, Farinha CM, et al. Methods for RNA extraction, cDNA preparation and analysis of CFTR transcripts. J Cyst Fibros 2004;3(suppl 2):11–15.
884. Ginsberg SD. RNA amplification strategies for small sample populations. Methods 2005;37:229–237.
885. Arber W, Linn S. DNA modification and restriction. Annu Rev Biochem 1969;38:467–500.
886. Smith HO, Wilcox KW. A restriction enzyme from Hemophilus influenzae: I. Purification and general properties. J Mol Biol 1970;51:379–391.
887. Danna K, Nathans D. Specific cleavage of simian virus 40 DNA by restriction endonuclease of Hemophilus influenzae. Proc Natl Acad Sci USA 1971;68:2913–2917.
888. Williams PJ. Restriction endonucleases: classification, properties, and applications. Mol Biotechnol 2003;23: 225–443.
889. Pingoud A, Fuxreiter M, Pingoud V, Wende W. Type II restriction endonucleases: structure and mechanism. Cell Mol Life Sci 2005;62:685–707.
890. Csako G. Present and future of rapid and/or high-throughput methods for nucleic acid testing. Clin Chim Acta 2006;363:6–31.
891. Botstein D, White RL, Skolnick M, Davis RW. Construction of a genetic linkage map in man using restriction fragment length polymorphisms. Am J Hum Genet 1980;32:314–331.
892. Pena SD, Prado VF, Epplen JT. DNA diagnosis of human genetic individuality. J Mol Med 1995;73:555–564.
893. Cullis CA. The use of DNA polymorphisms in genetic mapping. Genet Eng (NY) 2002;24:179–189.
894. Rose CM, Marsh S, Ameyaw MM, McLeod HL. Pharmacogenetic analysis of clinically relevant genetic polymorphisms. Methods Mol Med 2003;85:225–237.
895. Takahashi M, Ogino T, Baba K. Estimation of relative molecular length of DNA by electrophoresis in agarose gel. Biochim Biophys Acta 1969;174:183–187.

896. Carle GF, Frank M, Olson MV. Electrophoretic separations of large DNA molecules by periodic inversion of the electric field. Science 1986;232:65–68.
897. Olson MV. Separation of large DNA molecules by pulsed-field gel electrophoresis: a review of the basic phenomenology. J. Chromatogr 1989;470:377–383.
898. Upcroft P, Upcroft JA. Comparison of properties of agarose for electrophoresis of DNA. J Chromatogr 1993;618:79–93.
899. Borst P. Ethidium DNA agarose gel electrophoresis: how it started. IUBMB Life 2005;57:745–747.
900. Godde R, Akkad DA, Arning L, et al. Electrophoresis of DNA in human genetic diagnostics—state-of-the-art, alternatives and future prospects. Electrophoresis. 2006; 27:939–946.
901. Smith CL. Separation and analysis of DNA by electrophoresis. Curr Opin Biotechnol 1991;2:86–91.
902. Righetti PG, Gelfi C. Capillary electrophoresis of DNA for molecular diagnostics. Electrophoresis 1997;18: 1709–1714.
903. Guttman A, Ulfelder KJ. Separation of DNA by capillary electrophoresis. Adv Chromatogr 1998;38:301–340.
904. Altria KD. Overview of capillary electrophoresis and capillary electrochromatography. J Chromatogr A 1999;856: 443–463.
905. Mitchelson KR. The use of capillary electrophoresis for DNA polymorphism analysis, Mol Biotechnol 2003;24: 41–68.
906. Kan CW, Fredlake CP, Doherty EA, Barron AE. DNA sequencing and genotyping in miniaturized electrophoresis systems. Electrophoresis 2004;25:3564–3588.
907. Babu CVS, Song EJ, Babar SM, Wi MH, Yoo YS. Capillary electrophoresis at the omics level: towards systems biology. Electrophoresis 2006;27:97–110.
908. Lai CJ, Markoff LJ, Zimmerman S, Cohen B, Berndt JA, Chanock RM. Cloning DNA sequences from influenza viral RNA segments. Proc Natl Acad Sci USA 1980;77: 210–214.
909. Hoffmann-Berling H. DNA unwinding enzymes. Prog Clin Biol Res 1982;102 pt C:89–98.
910. Mullis KB, Faloona FA. Specific synthesis of DNA in vitro via a polymerase-catalyzed chain reaction. Methods Enzymol 1987;155:335–350.
911. Thomas R. The denaturation of DNA. Gene 1993;135: 77–79.
912. Kaguni JM, Kaguni LS. Enzyme-labeled probes for nucleic acid hybridization. Methods Biochem Anal 1992;36:115–127.
913. Isaac PG, Stacey J, Clee CM. Nonradioactive probes. Mol Biotechnol 1995;3:259–265.
914. Collins J. Gene cloning with small plasmids. Curr Top Microbiol Immunol 1977;78:122–170.
915. Hamer DH, Thomas CA Jr. Molecular cloning. Adv Pathobiol 1977;(6):306–319.
916. Helsinki DR. Plasmids as vectors for gene cloning. Basic Life Sci 1977;9:19–49.
917. Sinsheimer RL. Recombinant DNA. Annu Rev Biochem 1977;46:415–438.
918. Maxam AM, Gilbert W. A new method for sequencing DNA. Proc Natl Acad Sci USA 1977;74:560–564.
919. Franca LT, Carrilho E, Kist TB. A review of DNA sequencing techniques. Q Rev Biophys 2002;35:169–200.
920. Chan EY. Advances in sequencing technology. Mutat Res 2005;573:13–40.
921. Metzker ML. Emerging technologies in DNA sequencing. Genome Res 2005;15:1767–1776.
922. Sanger F, Nicklen S, Coulson AR. DNA sequencing with chain-terminating inhibitors. PNAS 1977;74:5463–5467.
923. Zimmermann J, Voss H, Schwager C, Stegemann J, Ansorge W. Automated Sanger dideoxy sequencing reaction protocol. FEBS Lett 1988;233:432–436.
924. Guesdon JL, Temynck T, Avrameas S. The use of avidin-biotin interaction in immunoenzymatic techniques. J Histochem Cytochem 1979;27:1131–1139.
925. Hsu SM. Clinical applications of immunoperoxidase technique. R I Med J 1979;62:447–452.
926. Hsu SM, Ree HJ. Self-sandwich method. An improved immunoperoxidase technic for the detection of small amounts of antigens. Am J Clin Pathol 1980;74:32–40.
927. Hsu SM, Raine L, Fanger H. Use of avidin-biotin-peroxidase complex (ABC) in immunoperoxidase techniques: a comparison between ABC and unlabeled antibody (PAP) procedures. J Histochem Cytochem 1981;29:577–580.
928. Southern EM. Detection of specific sequences among DNA fragments separated by gel electrophoresis. J Mol Biol 1975;98:503–517.
929. Cariani E, Brechot C. Detection of DNA sequences by Southern blot. Ric Clin Lab 1988;18:161–170.
930. Farkas DH. Specimen procurement, processing, tracking, and testing by the Southern blot. In: Farkas DH, ed. Molecular biology and pathology: a guidebook for quality control. San Diego: Academic Press, 1993:51–75.
931. Rose MG, Degar BA, Berliner N. Molecular diagnostics of malignant disorders. Clin Adv Hematol Oncol 2004; 2:650–660.
932. Kafatos FC, Jones CW, Efstratiadis A. Determination of nucleic acid sequence homologies and relative concentrations by a dot hybridization procedure. Nucleic Acids Res 1979;7:1541–1552.
933. Sawchuk WS. Validation of hybridization assays: correlation of filter in situ, dot blot and PCR with Southern blot. IARC Sci Publ 1992;(119):169–179.
934. Alwine JC, Kemp DJ, Stark GR. Method for detection of specific RNAs in agarose gels by transfer to diazobenzyloxymethyl-paper and hybridization with DNA probes. Proc Natl Acad Sci USA 1977;74:5350–5354.
935. Thomas PS. Hybridization of denatured RNA and small DNA fragments transferred to nitrocellulose. Proc Natl Acad Sci USA 1980;77:5201–5205.
936. Towbin H, Staehelin T, Gordon J. Electrophoretic transfer of proteins from polyacrylamide gels to nitrocellulose sheets: procedure and some applications Proc Natl Acad Sci USA 1979;76:4350–4354.
937. Burnette WN. "Western blotting": electrophoretic transfer of proteins from sodium dodecyl sulfate-polyacrylamide gels to unmodified nitrocellulose and radiographic detection with antibody and radioiodinated protein A. Anal Biochem 1981;112:195–203.

938. Kurien BT, Scofield RH. Western blotting. Methods 2006; 38:283–293.
939. Lawyer FC, Stoffel S, Saiki RK, Myambo K, Drummond R, Gelfand DH. Isolation, characterization, and expression in Escherichia coli of the DNA polymerase gene from Thermus aquaticus. J Biol Chem 1989;264:6427–6437.
940. Schutzbank TE, Stern HJ. Principles and applications of the polymerase chain reaction. J Int Fed Clin Chem 1993;5:96–105.
941. Taylor GR, Logan WP. The polymerase chain reaction: new variations on an old theme. Curr Opin Biotechnol 1995;6:24–29.
942. Kermekchiev MB, Tzekov A, Barnes WM. Cold-sensitive mutants of Taq DNA polymerase provide a hot start for PCR. Nucleic Acids Res 2003;31:6139–6147.
943. Pavlov AR, Pavlova NV, Kozyavkin SA, Slesarev AI. Recent developments in the optimization of thermostable DNA polymerases for efficient applications. Trends Biotechnol 2004;22:253–260.
944. Moore P. PCR: replicating success.Nature 2005;435: 235–238.
945. Edwards MC, Gibbs RA. Multiplex PCR: advantages, development, and applications. PCR Methods Appl 1994;3:S65–S75.
946. Elnifro EM, Ashshi AM, Cooper RJ, Klapper PE. Multiplex PCR: optimization and application in diagnostic virology. Clin Microbiol Rev 2000;13:559–570.
947. Wittwer CT, Herrmann MG, Gundry CN, Elenitoba-Johnson KS. Real-time multiplex PCR assays. Methods 2001;25:430–442.
948. Markoulatos P, Siafakas N, Moncany M. Multiplex polymerase chain reaction: a practical approach. J Clin Lab Anal 2002;16:47–51.
949. Rooney PH. Multiplex quantitative real-time PCR of laser microdissected tissue. Methods Mol Biol 2005;293:27–37.
950. Chou Q, Russell M, Birch DE, Raymond J, Bloch W. Prevention of pre-PCR mis-priming and primer dimerization improves low-copy-number amplifications, Nucleic Acids Res 1992;2:1717–1723.
951. Ailenberg M, Silverman M. Controlled hot start and improved specificity in carrying out PCR utilizing touch-up and loop incorporated primers (TULIPS). Biotechniques 2000;29:1018–1020, 1022–1024.
952. Kaboev OK, Luchkina LA, Tret'iakov AN, Bahrmand AR. PCR hot start using primers with the structure of molecular beacons (hairpin-like structure). Nucleic Acids Res 2000;28:E94.
953. Kinzler KW, Vogelstein B. Whole genome PCR: application to the identification of sequences bound by gene regulatory proteins. Nucleic Acids Res 1989;17:3645–3653.
954. Lasken RS, Egholm M. Whole genome amplification: abundant supplies of DNA from precious samples or clinical specimens, Trends Biotechnol 2003;21:531–535.
955. Blanco L, Bernad A, Lazaro JM, Martin G, Garmendia C, Salas M. Highly efficient DNA synthesis by the phage phi29 DNA polymerase. Symmetrical mode of DNA replication. J Biol Chem 1989;264:8935–8940.
956. Dean FB, Hosono S, Fang L, et al. Comprehensive human genome amplification using multiple displacement amplification. Proc Natl Acad Sci USA 2002;99:5261–5266.
957. Hawkins TL, Detter JC, Richardson PM. Whole genome amplification—applications and advances. Curr Opin Biotechnol 2002;13:65–67.
958. Kwok PY. Approaches to allele frequency determination. Pharmacogenomics 2000;1:231–235.
959. Feuilhade de Chauvin M. New diagnostic techniques. J Eur Acad Dermatol Venereol 2005;19(suppl 1):20–24.
960. Baltimore D. Viral RNA-dependent DNA polymerase. Nature 1970;226:1209–1211.
961. Myers TW, Gelfand DH. Reverse transcription and DNA amplification by a Thermus thermophilus DNA polymerase, Biochemistry 1991;30:7661–7666.
962. Gerard GF, Fox DK, Nathan M, D'Alessio JM. Reverse transcriptase. The use of cloned Moloney murine leukemia virus reverse transcriptase to synthesize DNA from RNA, Mol Biotechnol 1997;8:61–77.
963. Sellner LN, Turbett GR. Comparison of three RT-PCR methods. Biotechniques 1998;25:230–234.
964. Bustin SA. Absolute quantification of mRNA using real-time reverse transcription polymerase chain reaction assays. J Mol Endocrinol 2000;25:169–193.
965. Gerard GF, Potter RJ, Smith MD, et al. The role of template-primer in protection of reverse transcriptase from thermal inactivation. Nucleic Acids Res 2002;30: 3118–3129.
966. Kitabayashi M, Esaka M. Improvement of reverse transcription PCR by RNase H, Biosci Biotechnol Biochem 2003;67:2474–2476.
967. Bustin SA, Mueller R. Real-time reverse transcription PCR (qRT-PCR) and its potential use in clinical diagnosis. Clin Sci (Lond) 2005;109:365–379.
968. Lehmann U, Kreipe H. Real-time PCR analysis of DNA and RNA extracted from formalin-fixed and paraffin-embedded biopsies. Methods 2001;25:409–418.
969. Wilhelm J, Pingoud A. Real-time polymerase chain reaction. Chembiochem 2003;4:1120–1128.
970. Arya M, Shergill IS, Williamson M, Gommersall L, Arya N, Patel HR. Basic principles of real-time quantitative PCR. Expert Rev Mol Diagn 2005;5:209–219.
971. Bustin SA, Benes V, Nolan T, Pfaffl MW. Quantitative real-time RT-PCR—a perspective. J Mol Endocrinol 2005;34:597–601.
972. Kaltenboeck B, Wang C. Advances in real-time PCR: application to clinical laboratory diagnostics. Adv Clin Chem 2005;40:219–259.
973. Herman JG, Graff JR, Myöhänen S, Nelkin BD, Baylin SB. Methylation-specific PCR: a novel PCR assay for methylation status of CpG islands. Proc Natl Acad Sci USA 1996;93: 9821–9826.
974. Gonzalgo ML, Liang G, Spruck CH, Zingg JM, Rideout WM, Jones PA. Identification and characterization of differentially methylated regions of genomic DNA by methylationsensitive arbitrarily primed PCR. Cancer Res 1997;57: 594–599.
975. Oakeley EJ. DNA methylation analysis: a review of current methodologies. Pharmacol Ther 1999;84: 389–400.
976. Li LC, Dahiya R. MethPrimer: designing primers for methylation PCRs. Bioinformatics 2002;18:1427–1431.
977. Dahl C, Guldberg P. DNA methylation analysis techniques. Biogerontology 2003;4:233–250.

978. Liu ZJ, Maekawa M. Polymerase chain reaction-based methods of DNA methylation analysis. Anal Biochem 2003;317:259–265.
979. Lerman LS, Silverstein K. Computational simulation of DNA melting and its application to denaturing gradient gel electrophoresis. Methods Enzymol 1987;155: 482–501.
980. Abrams ES, Stanton VP. Use of denaturing gradient gel electrophoresis to study conformational transitions in nucleic acids. Methods Enzymol 1992;212:71–104.
981. Fodde R, Losekoot M. Mutation detection by denaturing gradient gel electrophoresis (DGGE). Hum Mutat 1994;3:83–94.
982. Lerman LS, Beldjord C. Comprehensive mutation detection with denaturing gradient gel electrophoresis. In: Cotton RGH, Edkins E, Forrest S, eds. Mutation detection: a practical approach. Oxford: Oxford University Press, 1998:35–59.
983. Rosenbaum V, Riesner D. Temperature-gradient gel electrophoresis. Thermodynamic analysis of nucleic acids and proteins in purified form and in cellular extracts. Biophys Chem 1987;26:235–246.
984. Riesner D, Henco K, Steger G. Temperature-gradient gel electrophoresis: a method for the analysis of conformational transitions and mutations in nucleic acids and proteins. Advances in Electrophoresis 1991;4:169–250.
985. Nagamine CM, Chan K, Lau YF. A PCR artifact: generation of heteroduplexes. Am J Hum Genet 1989;45: 337–339.
986. Keen J, Lester D, Inglehearn C, Curtis A, Bhattacharya S. Rapid detection of single base mismatches as heteroduplexes on Hydrolink gels. Trends Genet 1991;7:5.
987. Glavac D, Dean M. Applications of heteroduplex analysis for mutation detection in disease genes. Hum Mutat 1995;6:281–287.
988. Nataraj AJ, Olivos Glander I, Kusukawa N, Highsmith WE Jr. Single-strand conformation polymorphism and heteroduplex analysis for gel-based mutation detection. Electrophoresis 1999;20:1177–1185.
989. Taylor CF, Taylor GR. Current and emerging techniques for diagnostic mutation detection: an overview of methods for mutation detection. Methods Mol Med 2004;92:9–44.
990. Orita M, Iwahana H, Kanazawa H, Hayashi K, Sekiya T. Detection of polymorphisms of human DNA by gel electrophoresis as single-strand conformation polymorphisms. Proc Natl Acad Sci USA 1989;86:2766–2770.
991. Hayashi, K. PCR-SSCP: a simple and sensitive method for detection of mutations in the genomic DNA. PCR Methods Appl 1991;1:34–38.
992. Andersen PS, Jespersgaard C, Vuust J, Christiansen M, Larsen LA. Capillary electrophoresis-based single strand DNA conformation analysis in high-throughput mutation screening, Hum Mutat 2003;21:455–465.
993. Debouck C, Metcalf B. The impact of genomics on drug discovery. Annu Rev Pharmacol Toxicol 2000;40:193–207.
994. Ghosh D. High throughput and global approaches to gene expression. Comb Chem High Throughput Screen 2000;3:411–420.
995. Hanke J. Genomics and new technologies as catalysts for change in the drug discovery paradigm. J Law Med Ethics 2000;28(4 suppl):15–22.
996. Harris T. Genetics, genomics, and drug discovery. Med Res Rev 2000;20:203–211.
997. Rudert F. Genomics and proteomics tools for the clinic. Curr Opin Mol Ther 2000;2:633–642.
998. Merrick BA, Bruno ME. Genomic and proteomic profiling for biomarkers and signature profiles of toxicity. Curr Opin Mol Ther 2004;6:600–607.
999. Chalkley RJ, Hansen KC, Baldwin MA. Bioinformatic methods to exploit mass spectrometric data for proteomic applications. Methods Enzymol 2005;402:289–312.
1000. Dennis JL, Oien KA. Hunting the primary: novel strategies for defining the origin of tumours. J Pathol 2005; 205:236–247.
1001. Englbrecht CC, Facius A. Bioinformatics challenges in proteomics. Comb Chem High Throughput Screen 2005;8:705–715.
1002. Fung ET, Weinberger SR, Gavin E, Zhang F. Bioinformatics approaches in clinical proteomics. Expert Rev Proteomics 2005;2:847–862.
1003. Kremer A, Schneider R, Terstappen GC. A bioinformatics perspective on proteomics: data storage, analysis, and integration. Biosci Rep 2005;25:95–106.
1004. Mount DW, Pandey R. Using bioinformatics and genome analysis for new therapeutic interventions. Mol Cancer Ther 2005;4:1636–1643.
1005. Nishio K, Arao T, Shimoyama T, Fujiwara Y, Tamura T, Saijo N. Translational studies for target-based drugs. Cancer Chemother Pharmacol 2005;56(suppl 1):90–93.
1006. Redfern O, Grant A, Maibaum M, Orengo C. Survey of current protein family databases and their application in comparative, structural and functional genomics. J Chromatogr B Analyt Technol Biomed Life Sci 2005;815: 97–107.
1007. Iqbal O, Fareed J. Clinical applications of bioinformatics, genomics, and pharmacogenomics. Methods Mol Biol 2006;316:159–177.
1008. Katoh M, Katoh M. Bioinformatics for cancer management in the post-genome era. Technol Cancer Res Treat 2006;5:169–175.
1009. Miles AK, Matharoo-Ball B, Li G, Ahmad M, Rees RC. The identification of human tumour antigens: current status and future developments. Cancer Immunol Immunother 2006;55:996–1003.
1010. Quackenbush J. Microarray analysis and tumor classification. N Engl J Med 2006;354:2463–2472.
1011. Reeves GA, Thornton JM, BioSapiens Network of Excellence. Integrating biological data through the genome. Hum Mol Genet. 2006;15 Spec No 1:R81–R87.
1012. Waggoner A. Fluorescent labels for proteomics and genomics. Curr Opin Chem Biol 2006;10:62–66.
1013. Goodman N. Biological data becomes computer literate: new advances in bioinformatics. Curr Opin Biotechnol 2002;13:68–71.
1014. Ritchie MD. Bioinformatics approaches for detecting gene-gene and gene-environment interactions in studies of human disease. Neurosurg Focus 2005;19:E2.

1015. Hanai T, Hamada H, Okamoto M. Application of bioinformatics for DNA microarray data to bioscience, bioengineering and medical fields. J Biosci Bioeng 2006; 101:377–384.
1016. Haoudi A, Bensmail H. Bioinformatics and data mining in proteomics. Expert Rev Proteomics 2006;3:333–343.
1017. Ivanov AS, Veselovsky AV, Dubanov AV, Skvortsov VS. Bioinformatics platform development: from gene to lead compound. Methods Mol Biol 2006;316:389–431.
1018. Ness SA. Basic microarray analysis: strategies for successful experiments. Methods Mol Biol 2006;316:13–33.
1019. Perco P, Rapberger R, Siehs C, et al. Transforming omics data into context: bioinformatics on genomics and proteomics raw data. Electrophoresis 2006;27:2659–2675.
1020. Teufel A, Krupp M, Weinmann A, Galle PR. Current bioinformatics tools in genomic biomedical research (Review). Int J Mol Med 2006;17:967–973.
1021. Regnstrom K, Burgess DJ. Pharmacogenomics and its potential impact on drug and formulation development. Crit Rev Ther Drug Carrier Syst 2005;22:465–492.
1022. Thomas DC, Haile RW, Duggan D. Recent developments in genomewide association scans: a workshop summary and review. Am J Hum Genet 2005;77:337–345.
1023. Willard HF, Angrist M, Ginsburg GS. Genomic medicine: genetic variation and its impact on the future of health care. Philos Trans R Soc Lond B Biol Sci 2005;360: 1543–1550.
1024. Garraway LA, Seller WR. From integrated genomics to tumor lineage dependency. Cancer Res 2006;66:2506–2508.
1025. McDunn JE, Chung TP, Laramie JM, Townsend RR, Cobb JP. Physiologic genomics. Surgery 2006;139: 133–139.
1026. Tost J, Gut IG. Genotyping single nucleotide polymor phisms by mass spectrometry. Mass Spectrom Rev 2002; 21:388–418.
1027. Bernig T, Chanock SJ. Challenges of SNP genotyping and genetic variation: its future role in diagnosis and treatment of cancer. Expert Rev Mol Diagn 2006;6:319–331.
1028. Anderson S, Bankier AT, Barrell BG, et al. Sequence and organization of the human mitochondrial genome. Nature 1981;290:457–465.
1029. Mundy C. The human genome project: a historical perspective. Pharmacogenomics 2001;2:37–49.
1030. International Human Genome Sequencing Consortium. Finishing the euchromatic sequence of the human genome. Nature 2004;431:931–945.
1031. Baxevanis AD. Using genomic databases for sequence-based biological discovery. Mol Med 2003;9:185–192.
1032. The International HapMap Consortium. The International HapMap Project. Nature 2003;426:789–796.
1033. Thorisson GA, Stein LD. The SNP Consortium website: past, present and future, Nucleic Acids Res 2003;31: 124–127.
1034. Liu T, Johnson JA, Casella G, Wu R. Sequencing complex diseases with HapMap. Genetics 2004;168:503–511.
1035. Riva A, Kohane IS. A SNP-centric database for the investigation of the human genome, BMC Bioinformatics 2004;5:33.
1036. Kong X, Matise TC. MAP-O-MAT: internet-based linkage mapping. Bioinformatics 2005;21:557–559.
1037. Brandon MC, Lott MT, Nguyen KC, et al. MITOMAP: a human mitochondrial genome database—2004 update. Nucleic Acids Res 2005;33:D611–D613.
1038. Carulli JP, Artinger M, Swain PM, et al. High throughput analysis of differential gene expression. J Cell Biochem Suppl 1998;30–31:286–296.
1039. Scheel J, Von Brevern MC, Horlein A, Fischer A, Schneider A, Bach A. Yellow pages to the transcriptome. Pharmacogenomics 2002;3:791–807.
1040. Storck T, von Brevern MC, Behrens CK, Scheel J, Bach A. Transcriptomics in predictive toxicology. Curr Opin Drug Discov Devel 2002;5:90–97.
1041. Hedge PS, White IR, Debouck C. Interplay of transcriptomics and proteomics. Curr Opin Biotechnol 2003; 14:647–651.
1042. Jansen BJ, Schalkwijk J. Transcriptomics and proteomics of human skin. Brief Funct Genomic Proteomic 2003; 1:326–341.
1043. Suzuki M, Hayashizaki Y. Mouse-centric comparative transcriptomics of protein coding and non-coding RNAs. Bioessays 2004;26:833–843.
1044. Breitling R, Herzyk P. Biological master games: using biologists' reasoning to guide algorithm development for integrated functional genomics. OMICS 2005;9:225–232.
1045. Hu YF, Kaplow J, He Y. From traditional biomarkers to transcriptome analysis in drug development. Curr Mol Med 2005;5:29–38.
1046. Kralj M, Kraljevic S, Sedic M, Kurjak A, Pavelic K. Global approach to perinatal medicine: functional genomics and proteomics. J Perinat Med 2005;33:5–16.
1047. Morgan KT, Jayyosi Z, Hower MA, et al. The hepatic transcriptome as a window on whole-body physiology and pathophysiology. Toxicol Pathol 2005;33:136–145.
1048. Liang P, Zhu W, Zhang X, et al. Differential display using one-base anchored oligo-dT primers. Nucleic Acids Res 1994;22:5763–5764.
1049. Ahmed FE. Molecular techniques for studying gene expression in carcinogenesis. J Environ Sci Health C Environ Carcinog Ecotoxicol Rev 2002;20:77–116.
1050. Muller-Hagen G, Beinert T, Sommer A. Aspects of lung cancer gene expression profiling. Curr Opin Drug Discov Devel 2004;7:290–303.
1051. Anderson JS, Mann M. Functional genomics by mass spectrometry. FEBS Lett 2000;480:25–31
1052. Hanash S. Disease proteomics. Nature 2003;422:226–232.
1053. Liotta LA, Petricoin EF 3rd. The promise of proteomics. Clin Adv Hematol Oncol 2003;1:460–462.
1054. Jain KK. Role of oncoproteomics in the personalized management of cancer. Expert Rev Proteomics 2004;1: 49–55.
1055. Waldburg N, Kahne T, Reisenauer A, Rocken C, Welte T, Buhling F. Clinical proteomics in lung diseases. Pathol Res Pract 2004;200:147–154.
1056. Baggerman G, Vierstraete E, De Loof A, Schoofs L. Gel-based versus gel-free proteomics: a review. Comb Chem High Throughput Screen 2005;8:669–677.

1057. Brown RE. Morphoproteomics: exposing protein circuitries in tumors to identify potential therapeutic targets in cancer patients. Expert Rev Proteomics 2005;2:337–348.
1058. Calvo KR, Liotta LA, Petricoin EF. Clinical proteomics: from biomarker discovery and cell signaling profiles to individualized personal therapy. Biosci Rep 2005; 25: 107–125.
1059. Clarke W, Chan DW. ProteinChips: the essential tools for proteomic biomarker discovery and future clinical diagnostics. Clin Chem Lab Med 2005; 43:1279–1280.
1060. Kalia A, Gupta RP. Proteomics: a paradigm shift. Crit Rev Biotechnol 2005;25:173–198.
1061. Kolch w, Mischak H, Pitt AR. The molecular make-up of a tumour: proteomics in cancer research. Clin Sci (Lond) 2005;108:369–383.
1062. Patel PS, Telang SD, Rawal RM, Shah MH. A review of proteomics in cancer research. Asian Pac J Cancer Prev 2005;6:113–117.
1063. Roboz J. Mass spectrometry in diagnostic oncoproteomics. Cancer Invest 2005;23:465–478.
1064. Scaros O, Fisler R. Biomarker technology roundup: from discovery to clinical applications, a broad set of tools is required to translate from the lab to the clinic. Biotechniques 2005;suppl:30–32.
1065. Stroncek DF, Burns C, Martin BM, Rossi L, Marincola FM, Panelli MC. Advancing cancer biotherapy with proteomics. J Immunother 2005;28:183–192.
1066. Domon B, Aebersold R. Mass spectrometry and protein analysis. Science 2006;312:212–217.
1067. Fleming K, Kelley LA, Islam SA, et al. The proteome: structure, function and evolution. Philos Trans R Soc Lond B Biol Sci 2006;361:441–451.
1068. Gulmann C, Sheehan KM, Kay EW, Liotta LA, Petricoin EF 3rd. Array-based proteomics: mapping of protein circuitries for diagnostics, prognostics, and therapy guidance in cancer. J Pathol 2006;208:595–606.
1069. Kingsmore SF. Multiplexed protein measurement: technologies and applications of protein and antibody arrays. Nat Rev Drug Discov 2006;5:310–320.
1070. Davis CD, Milner J. Frontiers in nutrigenomics, proteomics, metabolomics and cancer prevention. Mutat Res 2004;551:51–64.
1071. Griffin JL, Bollard ME. Metabonomics: its potential as a tool in toxicology for safety assessment and data integration. Curr Drug Metab 2004;5:389–398.
1072. Rochfort S. Metabolomics reviewed: a new "omics" platform technology for systems biology and implications for natural products research. J Nat Prod 2005;68: 1813–1820.
1073. Griffin JL. The Cinderella story of metabolic profiling: does metabolomics get to go to the functional genomics ball? Philos Trans R Soc Lond B Biol Sci 2006;361: 147–161.
1074. Ramsay G. DNA chips: State-of-the art. Nature Biotechnol 1997;16:40–44.
1075. Duggan DJ, Bittner M, Chen Y, Meltzer P, Trent JM. Expression profiling using cDNA microarrays. Nat Genet. 1999; 21(1 suppl):10–14.
1076. Chen I, Ren J. High-throughput DNA analysis by microchip electrophoresis. Comb Chem High Throughput Screen 2004;7:29–43.
1077. Heller MJ. DNA microarray technology: devices, systems, and applications. Annu Rev Biomed Eng 2002;4: 129–153.
1078. Obeid PJ, Christopoulos TK. Microfabricated systems for nucleic acid analysis. Crit Rev Clin Lab Sci 2004;41: 429–465.
1079. Shi L, Tong W, Goodsaid F, et al. QA/QC: challenges and pitfalls facing the microarray community and regulatory agencies. Expert Rev Mol Diagn 2004;4:761–777.
1080. Zhumabayeva B, Chenchik A, Siebert PD, Herrler M. Disease profiling arrays: reverse format cDNA arrays complimentary to microarrays. Adv Biochem Eng Biotechnol 2004;86:191–213.
1081. Brentani RR, Carraro DM, Verjovski-Almeida S, et al. Gene expression arrays in cancer research: methods and applications. Crit Rev Oncol Hematol 2005;54:95–105.
1082. Diatchenko L, Lau YF, Campbell AP, et al. Suppression subtractive hybridization: a method for generating differentially regulated or tissue-specific cDNA probes and libraries. Proc Natl Acad Sci USA 1996;93:6025–6030.
1083. Wang X, Feuerstein GZ. Suppression subtractive hybridisation: application in the discovery of novel pharmacological targets. Pharmacogenomics 2000;1:101–108
1084. Velculescu VE, Vogelstein B, Kinzler KW. Analysing uncharted transcriptomes with SAGE. Trends Genet 2000;16:423–425.
1085. Polyak K, Riggins GJ. Gene discovery using the serial analysis of gene expression technique: implications for cancer research. J Clin Oncol 2001;19:2948–2958.
1086. Riggins GJ. Using Serial Analysis of Gene Expression to identify tumor markers and antigens. Dis Markers 2001;17:41 48.
1087. Scott HS, Chrast R. Global transcript expression profiling by Serial Analysis of Gene Expression (SAGE). Genet Eng (NY) 2001;23:201–219.
1088. Yamamoto M, Wakatsuki T, hada A, Ryo A. Use of serial analysis of gene expression (SAGE) technology. J Immunol Methods 2001;250:45–66
1089. Ruijter JM, Van Kampen AH, Baas F. Statistical evaluation of SAGE libraries: consequences for experimental design. Physiol Genomics 2002;11:37–44.
1090. Ye SQ, Usher DC, Zhang LO. Gene expression profiling of human diseases by serial analysis of gene expression. J Biomed Sci 2002;9:384–394.
1091. Boheler KR, Stern MD. The new role of SAGE in gene discovery. Trends Biotechnol 2003;21:55–57.
1092. Porter D, Polyak K. Cancer target discovery using SAGE. Expert Opin Ther Targets 2003;7:759–769.
1093. Cekan SZ. Methods to find out the expression of activated genes. Reprod Biol Endocrinol 2004;2:68.
1094. Liu ET. Expression genomics and cancer biology. Pharmacogenomics 2004;5:1117–1128.
1095. Tuteja R, Tuteja N. Serial analysis of gene expression (SAGE): application in cancer research. Med Sci Monit 2004;10:RA132–RA140.

1096. Tuteja R, Tuteja N. Serial analysis of gene expression: applications in human studies. J Biomed Biotechnol 2004; 2004:113–120.
1097. Tuteja R, Tuteja N. Serial analysis of gene expression (SAGE): unraveling the bioinformatics tools. Bioessays 2004;26:916–922.
1098. Matsumura H, Ito A, Saitoh H, et al. SuperSAGE. Cell Microbiol 2005;7:11–18.
1099. Romkes M, Buch SC. Strategies for measurement of biotransformation enzyme gene expression. Methods Mol Biol 2005;291:387–398.
1100. Weeraratna AT. Discovering causes and cures for cancer from gene expression analysis. Ageing Res Rev 2005;4:548–563.
1101. Porter D, Yao J, Polyak K. SAGE and related approaches for cancer target identification. Drug Discov Today 2006; 11:110–118.
1102. Wan WH, Fortuna MB, Furmanski P. A rapid and efficient method for testing immunohistochemical reactivity of monoclonal antibodies against multiple tissue samples simultaneously. J Immunol Methods 1987;103:121–129.
1103. Kononen J, Bubendorf L, Kallioniemi A, et al. Tissue microarrays for high-throughput molecular profiling of tumor specimens. Nat Med 1998;4:844–847.
1104. von Wasielewski R, Mengel M, Wiese B, Rudiger T, Muller-Hermelink HK, Kreipe H. Tissue array technology for testing interlaboratory and interobserver reproducibility of immunohistochemical estrogen receptor analysis in a large multicenter trial. Am J Clin Pathol 2002;118:675–682.
1105. Hsu FD, Nielsen TO, Alkushi A, et al. Tissue microarrays are an effective quality assurance tool for diagnostic immunohistochemistry. Modern Pathology 2002;15:1374–1380.
1106. Chang SS, Mark HF. Emerging molecular cytogenetic technologies. Cytobios 1997;90:7–22.
1107. Ried T, Liyanage M, du Manoir S, et al. Tumor cytogenetics revisited: comparative genomic hybridization and spectral karyotyping. J Mol Med 1997;75:801–814.
1108. Schrock E, Padilla-Nash H. Spectral karyotyping and multicolor fluorescence in situ hybridization reveal new tumor-specific chromosomal aberrations. Semin Hematol 2000;37:334–347.
1109. Dorritie K, Montagna C, Difilippantonio MJ, Ried T. Advanced molecular cytogenetics in human and mouse. Expert Rev Mol Diagn 2004;4:663–676.
1110. Salman M, Jhanwar SC, Ostrer H. Will the new cytogenetics replace the old cytogenetics? Clin Genet 2004;66: 265–275.
1111. Speicher MR, Carter NP. The new cytogenetics: blurring the boundaries with molecular biology. Nat Rev Genet 2005;6:782–792.
1112. Dyanov HM, Dzitoeva SG. Method for attachment of microscopic preparations on glass for in situ hybridization, PRINS, and in situ PCR studies. Biotechniques 1995;18:823–826.
1113. Hara M, Yamada S, Hirata K. Nonradioactive in situ hybridization: recent techniques and applications. Endocr Pathol 1998;9:21–29.
1114. Guan X-Y, Zhang H, Bittner M, Jiang Y, Meltzer P, Trent J. Chromosome arm painting probes. Nature Genet 1996; 12:10–11.
1115. Lee C, Lemyre E, Miron PM, Morton CC. Multicolor fluorescence in situ hybridization in clinical cytogenetic diagnostics. Curr Opin Pediatr 2001;13:550–555.
1116. Liehr T, Starke H, Weise A, Lehrer H, Claussen U. Multicolor FISH probe sets and their applications. Histol Histopathol 2004;19:229–237.
1117. Bayani J, Squire JA. Advances in the detection of chromosomal aberrations using spectral karyotyping. Clin Genet 2001;59:65–73.
1118. Bayani JM, Squire JA. Applications of SKY in cancer cytogenetics. Cancer Invest 2002;20:373–386.
1119. Jain KK. Current status of fluorescent in-situ hybridisation. Med Device Technol 2004;15:14–17.
1120. Tubbs R, Skacel M, Pettay J, et al. Interobserver interpretative reproducibility of GOLDFISH, a first generation gold-facilitated autometallographic bright field in situ hybridization assay for HER-2/neu amplification in invasive mammary carcinoma. Am J Surg Pathol 2002;26: 908–913.
1121. Tubbs R, Pettay J, Skacel M, et al. Gold-facilitated in situ hybridization: a bright-field autometallographic alternative to fluorescence in situ hybridization for detection of Her-2/neu gene amplification. Am J Pathol 2002;160: 1589–1595.
1122. Lambros MB, Simpson PT, Jones C, et al. Unlocking pathology archives for molecular genetic studies: a reliable method to generate probes for chromogenic and fluorescent in situ hybridization. Lab Invest 2006;86: 398–408.
1123. Isola J, Tanner M. Chromogenic in situ hybridization in tumor pathology. Methods Mol Med 2004;97:133–144.
1124. Hsi BL, Xiao S, Fletcher JA. Chromogenic in situ hybridization and FISH in pathology. Methods Mol Biol 2002; 204:343–351.
1125. Tanner M, Gancberg D, DiLeo A, et al. Chromogenic in situ hybridization: a practical alternative for fluorescence in situ hybridization to detect HER-2/neu oncogene amplification in archival breast cancer samples. Am J Pathol 2000;157:1467–1472.
1126. Tsukamoto T, Kusakabe M, Saga Y. In situ hybridization with non-radioactive digoxigenin-11–UTP-labeled cRNA probes: localization of developmentally regulated mouse tenascin mRNAs. Int J Dev Biol 1991;35:25–32.
1127. Mullink H, Walboomers JM, Tadema TM, Jansen DJ, Meijer CJ. Combined immuno- and non-radioactive hybridocytochemistry on cells and tissue sections: influence of fixation, enzyme pre-treatment, and choice of chromogen on detection of antigen and DNA sequences. J Histochem Cytochem 1989;37:603–609.
1128. Kallioniemi A, Kallioniemi OP, Sudar D, et al. Comparative genomic hybridization for molecular cytogenetic analysis of solid tumors. Science 1992;258:818–821.
1129. du Manoir S, Speicher MR, Joos S, et al. Detection of complete and partial chromosome gains and losses by comparative genomic in situ hybridization. Hum Genet 1993;90:590–610.

1130. Kallioniemi OP, Kallioniemi A, Piper J, et al. Optimizing comparative genomic hybridization for analysis of DNA sequence copy number changes in solid tumors. Genes Chromosomes Cancer 1994;10:231–243.
1131. Knuutila S, Bjorkqvist AM, Autio K, et al. DNA copy number amplifications in human neoplasms: review of comparative genomic hybridization studies. Am J Pathol 1998;152:1107–1123.
1132. Inazawa J, Inoue J, Imoto I. Comparative genomic hybridization (CGH)-arrays pave the way for identification of novel cancer-related genes. Cancer Sci 2004;95:559–563.
1133. Cheung SW, Shaw CA, Yu W, et al. Development and validation of a CGH microarray for clinical cytogenetic diagnosis. Genet Med 2005;7:422–432.
1134. Picard F, Robin S, Lavielle M, Vaisse C, Daudin JJ. A statistical approach for array CGH data analysis. BMC Bioinformatics 2005;6:27.
1135. Caporaso NE, Landi MT. Molecular epidemiology: a new perspective for the study of toxic exposures in man. A consideration of the influence of genetic susceptibility factors on risk in different lung cancer histologies. Med Lav 1994;85:68–77.
1136. Ikawa S, Uematsu F, Watanabe K, et al. Assessment of cancer susceptibility in humans by use of genetic polymorphisms in carcinogen metabolism. Pharmacogenetics 1995;5 Spec No:S154–S160.
1137. el-Zein R, Conforti-Froes N, Au WW. Interactions between genetic predisposition and environmental toxicants for development of lung cancer. Environ Mol Mutagen 1997;30:196–204.
1138. Mooney LA, Bell DA, Santella RM, et al. Contribution of genetic and nutritional factors to DNA damage in heavy smokers. Carcinogenesis 1997;18:503–509.
1139. Amos CI, Xu W, Spitz MR. Is there a genetic basis for lung cancer susceptibility? Recent Results Cancer Res 1999;151:3–12.
1140. Fryer AA, Jones PW. Interactions between detoxifying enzyme polymorphisms and susceptibility to cancer. IARC Sci Publ 1999;(148):303–322.
1141. Kaminsky LS, Spivack SD. Cytochromes P450 and cancer. Mol Aspects Med 1999;20:70–84, 137.
1142. Hirvonen A. Polymorphic NATs and cancer predisposition. IARC Sci Publ 1999;(148):251–270.
1143. Spitz MR, Wei Q, Li G, Wu X. Genetic susceptibility to tobacco carcinogenesis. Cancer Invest 1999;17:645–659.
1144. Bartsch H, Nair U, Risch A, Rojas M, Wikman H, Alexandrov K. Genetic polymorphism of CYP genes, alone or in combination, as a risk modifier of tobacco-related cancers. Cancer Epidemiol Biomarkers Prev 2000;9:3–28.
1145. Houlston RS. CYP1A1 polymorphisms and lung cancer risk: a meta-analysis. Pharmacogenetics 2000;10:105–114.
1146. Bouchardy C, Benhamou S, Jourenkova N, Dayer P, Hirvonen A. Metabolic genetic polymorphisms and susceptibility to lung cancer. Lung Cancer 2001;32:109–112.
1147. Goode EL, Ulrich CM, Potter JD. Polymorphisms in DNA repair genes and associations with cancer risk. Cancer Epidemiol Biomarkers Prev 2002;11:1513–1530.
1148. Kiyohara C, Otsu A, Shirakawa T, Fukuda S, Hopkin JM. Genetic polymorphisms and lung cancer susceptibility: a review. Lung Cancer 2002;37:241–256.
1149. Gorlova OY, Amos C, Henschke C, et al. Genetic susceptibility for lung cancer: interactions with gender and smoking history and impact on early detection policies. Hum Hered 2003;56:139–145.
1150. Schwartz AG. Genetic predisposition to lung cancer. Chest 2004;125(5 suppl):86S-9S.
1151. Kiyohara C, Yoshimasu K, Shirakawa T, Hopkin JM. Genetic polymorphisms and environmental risk of lung cancer: a review. Rev Environ Health 2004;19:15–38.
1152. Miller YE, Fain P. Genetic susceptibility to lung cancer. Semin Respir Crit Care Med 2003;24:197–204.
1153. Christiani DC. Genetic susceptibility to lung cancer. J Clin Oncol 2006;24:1651–1652.
1154. Anderson D. Familial susceptibility to cancer. CA Cancer J Clin 1976;26:143–149.
1155. Ooi WL, Elston RC, Chen VW, Bailey-Wilson JE, Rothschild H. Increased familial risk for lung cancer. J Natl Cancer Inst 1986;76:217–222.
1156. Ooi WL, Elston RC, Chen VW, Bailey-Wilson JE, Rothschild H. Familial lung cancer—correcting an error in calculation. J Natl Cancer Inst 1986;77:990.
1157. Sellers TA, Ooi WL, Elston RC, Chen VW, Bailey-Wilson JE, Rothschild H. Increased familial risk for non-lung cancer among relatives of lung cancer patients. Am J Epidemiol 1987;126:237–246.
1158. McDuffie HH. Clustering of cancer in families of patients with primary lung cancer. J Clin Epidemiol 1991;44:69–76.
1159. Ambrosone CB, Rao U, Michalek AM, Cummings KM, Mettlin CJ. Lung cancer histologic types and family history of cancer. Analysis of histologic subtypes of 872 patients with primary lung cancer. Cancer 1993;72:1192–1198.
1160. Sellers TA, Chen PL, Potter JD, Bailey-Wilson JE, Rothschild H, Elston RC. Segregation analysis of smoking-associated malignancies: evidence for Mendelian inheritance. Am J Med Genet 1994;52:308–314.
1161. Dragani TA, Manenti G, Pierotti MA. Polygenic inheritance of predisposition to lung cancer. Ann Ist Super Sanita 1996;32:145–150
1162. Ahlbom A, Lichtenstein P, Malmstrom H, Feychting M, Hemminki K, Pedersen NL. Cancer in twins: genetic and nongenetic familial risk factors. J Natl Cancer Inst 1997;89:287–293.
1163. Li H, Yang P, Schwartz AG. Analysis of age of onset data from case-control family studies. Biometrics 1998;54:1030–109.
1164. Suzuki K, Ogura T, Yokose T, et al. Microsatellite instability in female non-small-cell lung cancer patients with familial clustering of malignancy. Br J Cancer 1998;77:1003–1008.
1165. Hemminki K, Vaittinen P. Familial cancers in a nationwide family cancer database: age distribution and prevalence. Eur J Cancer 1999;35:1109–1117.
1166. Bromen K, Pohlabeln H, Jahn I, Ahrens W, Jockel KH. Aggregation of lung cancer in families: results from a population-based case-control study in Germany. Am J Epidemiol 2000;152:497–505.

1167. Gupta D, Aggarwal AN, Vikrant S, Jindal SK. Familial aggregation of cancer in patients with bronchogenic carcinoma. Indian J Cancer 2000;37:43–49.
1168. Wunsch-Filho V, Boffetta P, Colin D, Moncau JE. Familial cancer aggregation and the risk of lung cancer. Sao Paulo Med J 2002;120:38–44.
1169. Etzel CJ, Amos CI, Spitz MR. Risk for smoking-related cancer among relatives of lung cancer patients. Cancer Res 2003;63:8531–8535.
1170. Li X, Hemminki K. Familial and second lung cancers: a nation-wide epidemiologic study from Sweden. Lung Cancer 2003;39:255–263.
1171. Rooney A. Family history reveals lung-cancer risk. Lancet Oncol 2003;4:267.
1172. Bailey-Wilson JE, Amos CI, Pinney SM, et al. A major lung cancer susceptibility locus maps to chromosome 6q23–25. Am J Hum Genet 2004;75:460–474.
1173. Hemminki K, Li X, Czene K. Familial risk of cancer: data for clinical counseling and cancer genetics. Int J Cancer 2004;108:109–114.
1174. Jonsson S, Thorsteinsdottir U, Gudbjartsson DF, et al. Familial risk of lung carcinoma in the Icelandic population. JAMA 2004;292:2977–2983.
1175. Hemminki K, Li X. Familial risk for lung cancer by histology and age of onset: evidence for recessive inheritance. Exp Lung Res 2005;31:205–215.
1176. Jin YT, Xu YC, Yang RD, Huang CF, Xu CW, He XZ. Familial aggregation of lung cancer in a high incidence area in China. Br J Cancer 2005;92:1321–1325.
1177. Jin Y, Xu Y, Xu M, Xue S. Increased risk of cancer among relatives of patients with lung cancer in China. BMC Cancer 2005;5:146.
1178. Keith RL, Miller YE. Lung cancer: genetics of risk and advances in chemoprevention. Curr Opin Pulm Med 2005;11:265–271.
1179. Li X, Hemminki K. Familial multiple primary lung cancers: a population-based analysis from Sweden. Lung Cancer 2005;47:301–307.
1180. Matakidou A, Eisen T, Houlston RS. Systematic review of the relationship between family history and lung cancer risk. Br J Cancer 2005;93:825–833.
1181. Schwartz AG, Ruckdeschel JC. Familial lung cancer: genetic susceptibility and relationship to chronic obstructive pulmonary disease. Am J Respir Crit Care Med 2006;173:16–22.
1182. Bennett WP, Alavanja MC, Blomeke B, et al. Environmental tobacco smoke, genetic susceptibility, and risk of lung cancer in never-smoking women. J Natl Cancer Inst 1999;91:2009–2014.
1183. Yang P, Yokomizo A, Tazelaar HD, et al. Genetic determinants of lung cancer short-term survival: the role of glutathione-related genes. Lung Cancer 2002;35:221–229.
1184. Kiyohara C, Wakai K, Mikami H, Sido K, Ando M, Ohno Y. Risk modification by CYP1A1 and GSTM1 polymorphisms in the association of environmental tobacco smoke and lung cancer: a case-control study in Japanese nonsmoking women. Int J Cancer 2003;107:139–144.
1185. Cohet C, Borel S, Nyberg F, et al. Exon 5 polymorphisms in the O6–alkylguanine DNA alkyltransferase gene and lung cancer risk in non-smokers exposed to second-hand smoke. Cancer Epidemiol Biomarkers Prev 2004;13: 320–323.
1186. Wenzlaff AS, Cote ML, Bock CH, et al. CYP1A1 and CYP1B1 polymorphisms and risk of lung cancer among never smokers: a population-based study. Carcinogenesis 2005;26:2207–2212.
1187. Wenzlaff AS, Cote ML, Bock CH, Land SJ, Schwartz AG. GSTM1, GSTT1 and GSTP1 polymorphisms, environmental tobacco smoke exposure and risk of lung cancer among never smokers: a population-based study. Carcinogenesis 2005;26:395–401.
1188. Gorlova OY, Zhang Y, Schabath MB, et al. Never smokers and lung cancer risk: a case-control study of epidemiological factors. Int J Cancer 2006;118:1798–1804.
1189. Schwartz AG, Yang P, Swanson GM. Familial risk of lung cancer among nonsmokers and their relatives. Am J Epidemiol 1996;144:554–562.
1190. Yang P, Schwartz AG, McAllister AE, Aston CE, Swanson GM. Genetic analysis of families with nonsmoking lung cancer probands. Genet Epidemiol 1997;14:181–197.
1191. Mayne ST, Buenconsejo J, Janerich DT. Familial cancer history and lung cancer risk in United States nonsmoking men and women. Cancer Epidemiol Biomarkers Prev 1999;8:1065–1069.
1192. Schwartz AG, Rothrock M, Yang P, Swanson GM. Increased cancer risk among relatives of nonsmoking lung cancer cases. Genet Epidemiol 1999;17:1–15.
1193. Yang P, Schwartz AG, McAllister AE, Swanson GM, Aston CE. Lung cancer risk in families of nonsmoking probands: heterogeneity by age at diagnosis. Genet Epidemiol 1999;17:253–273.
1194. Kreuzer M, Kreienbrock L, Gerken M, et al. Risk factors for lung cancer in young adults. Am J Epidemiol 1998; 147:1028–1037.
1195. Gauderman WJ, Morrison JL. Evidence for age-specific genetic relative risks in lung cancer. Am J Epidemiol 2000;151:41–49.
1196. Li X, Hemminki K. Inherited predisposition to early onset lung cancer according to histological type. Int J Cancer 2004;112:451–457.
1197. Cote ML, Kardia SL, Wenzlaff AS, Land SJ, Schwartz AG. Combinations of glutathione S-transferase genotypes and risk of early-onset lung cancer in Caucasians and African Americans: a population-based study. Carcinogenesis 2005;26:811–819.
1198. Dresler CM, Fratelli C, Babb J, Everley L, Evans AA, Clapper ML. Gender differences in genetic susceptibility for lung cancer. Lung Cancer 2000;30:153–160.
1199. Kreuzer M, Wichmann HE. Lung cancer in young females. Eur Respir J 2001;17:1333–1334.
1200. Haugen A. Women who smoke: are women more susceptible to tobacco-induced lung cancer? Carcinogenesis 2002;23:227–229.
1201. Stabile LP, Siegfried JM. Sex and gender differences in lung cancer. J Gend Specif Med 2003;6:37–48.
1202. Pauk N, Kubik A, Zatloukal P, Krepela E. Lung cancer in women. Lung Cancer 2005;48:1–9.

1203. Matakidou A, Eisen T, Bridle H, O'Brien M, Mutch R, Houlston RS. Case-control study of familial lung cancer risks in UK women. Int J Cancer 2005;116:445–450.
1204. Patel JD. Lung cancer in women. J Clin Oncol 2005;23: 3212–3218.
1205. International Early Lung Cancer Action Program Investigators, Henschke CI, Yip R, Miettinen OS. Women's susceptibility to tobacco carcinogens and survival after diagnosis of lung cancer. JAMA 2006;296:180–184.
1206. Risch HA, Howe GR, Jain M, et al. Are female smokers at higher risk for lung cancer than male smokers? A case-control analysis by histologic type. Am J Epidemiol 1993;138:281–293.
1207. Zang EA, Wynder EL. Differences in lung cancer risk between men and women: Examination of the evidence. J Natl Cancer Inst 1996;88:183–192.
1208. Henschke CI, Miettinen O. Women's susceptibility to tobacco carcinogens. Lung Cancer 2004;43:1–5.
1209. Bach PB, Kattan MW, Thornquist MD, et al. Variations in lung cancer risk among smokers. J Natl Cancer Inst 2003;95:470–478.
1210. Bain C, Feskanich D, Speizer FE, et al. Lung cancer rates in men and women with comparable histories of smoking. J Natl Cancer Inst 2004;96:826–834.
1211. Ng DP, Tan KW, Zhao B, Seow A. CYP1A1 polymorphisms and risk of lung cancer in non-smoking Chinese women: influence of environmental tobacco smoke exposure and GSTM1/T1 genetic variation. Cancer Causes Control 2005;16:399–405.
1212. Mollerup S, Berge G, Baera R, et al. Sex differences in risk of lung cancer: Expression of genes in the PAH bioactivation pathway in relation to smoking and bulky DNA adducts. Int J Cancer 2006;119:741–744.
1213. Bond JA. Metabolism and elimination of inhaled drugs and airborne chemicals from the lungs. Pharmacol Toxicol 1993;72(suppl 3):36–47.
1214. Raunio H, Husgafvel-Pursiainen K, Anttila S, Hietanen E, Hirvonen A, Pelkonen O. Diagnosis of polymorphisms in carcinogen-activating and inactivating enzymes and cancer susceptibility—a review. Gene 1995;159:113–121.
1215. Wormhoudt LW, Commandeur JN, Vermeulen NP. Genetic polymorphisms of human N-acetyltransferase, cytochrome P450, glutathione-S-transferase, and epoxide hydrolase enzymes: relevance to xenobiotic metabolism and toxicity. Crit Rev Toxicol 1999;29:59–124.
1216. Nakajima T, Aoyama T. Polymorphism of drug-metabolizing enzymes in relation to individual susceptibility to industrial chemicals. Ind Health 2000;38: 143–152.
1217. Miller MC 3rd, Mohrenweiser HW, Bell DA. Genetic variability in susceptibility and response to toxicants. Toxicol Lett 2001;120:269–280.
1218. Rushmore TH, Kong AN. Pharmacogenomics, regulation and signaling pathways of phase I and II drug metabolizing enzymes. Curr Drug Metab 2002;3:481–490.
1219. Daly AK. Pharmacogenetics of the major polymorphic metabolizing enzymes. Fundam Clin Pharmacol 2003; 17:27–41.
1220. Sheweita SA, Tilmisany AK. Cancer and phase II drug-metabolizing enzymes. Curr Drug Metab 2003;4:45–58.
1221. Xu C, Li CY, Kong AN. Induction of phase I, II and III drug metabolism/transport by xenobiotics. Arch Pharm Res 2005;28:249–268.
1222. Nishikawa A, Mori Y, Lee IS, Tanaka T, Hirose M. Cigarette smoking, metabolic activation and carcinogenesis. Curr Drug Metab 2004;5:363–373.
1223. Cascorbi I. Genetic basis of toxic reactions to drugs and chemicals. Toxicol Lett 2006;162:16–28.
1224. Raunio H, Husgafvel-Pursiainen K, Anttila S, Hietanen E, Hirvonen A, Pelkonen O. Diagnosis of polymorphisms in carcinogen-activating and inactivating enzymes and cancer susceptibility—a review. Gene 1995;159:113–121.
1225. Kerremans AL. Cytochrome P450 isoenzymes—importance for the internist. Neth J Med 1996;48:237–243.
1226. Dogra SC, Whitelaw ML, May BK. Transcriptional activation of cytochrome P450 genes by different classes of chemical inducers. Clin Exp Pharmacol Physiol 1998; 25:1–9.
1227. Lewis DF, Watson E, Lake BG. Evolution of the cytochrome P450 superfamily: sequence alignments and pharmacogenetics. Mutat Res 1998;410:245–270.
1228. McKinnon RA, Nebert DW. Cytochrome P450 knockout mice: new toxicological models. Clin Exp Pharmacol Physiol 1998;25:783–787.
1229. Ingelman-Sundberg M. Genetic susceptibility to adverse effects of drugs and environmental toxicants. The role of the CYP family of enzymes. Mutat Res 2001;482:11–19.
1230. Ingelman-Sundberg M. Polymorphism of cytochrome P450 and xenobiotic toxicity. Toxicology 2002;181–182: 447–452.
1231. Lewis DF. Human cytochromes P450 associated with the phase 1 metabolism of drugs and other xenobiotics: a compilation of substrates and inhibitors of the CYP1, CYP2 and CYP3 families. Curr Med Chem 2003;10: 1955–1972.
1232. Shimada T, Fujii-Kuriyama Y. Metabolic activation of polycyclic aromatic hydrocarbons to carcinogens by cyto chromes P450 1A1 and 1B1. Cancer Sci 2004;95:1–6.
1233. Lewis DF. 57 varieties: the human cytochromes P450. Pharmacogenomics 2004;5:305–318.
1234. Rodriguez-Antona C, Ingelman-Sundberg M. Cytochrome P450 pharmacogenetics and cancer. Oncogene 2006;25:1679–1691.
1235. Sim SC, Ingelman-Sundberg M. The human cytochrome P450 Allele Nomenclature Committee Web site: submission criteria, procedures, and objectives. Methods Mol Biol 2006;320:183–191.
1236. Raunio H, Hakkola J, Hukkanen J, et al. Expression of xenobiotic-metabolizing CYPs in human pulmonary tissue. Exp Toxicol Pathol 1999;51:412–417.
1237. Hukkanen J, Pelkonen O, Raunio H. Expression of xenobiotic-metabolizing enzymes in human pulmonary tissue: possible role in susceptibility for ILD. Eur Respir J Suppl 2001;32:122s–126s.
1238. Hukkanen J, Pelkonen O, Hakkola J, Raunio H. Expression and regulation of xenobiotic-metabolizing cytochrome P450 (CYP) enzymes in human lung. Crit Rev Toxicol 2002;32:391–411.
1239. Ding X, Kaminsky LS. Human extrahepatic cytochromes P450: function in xenobiotic metabolism and tissue-

selective chemical toxicity in the respiratory and gastrointestinal tracts. Annu Rev Pharmacol Toxicol 2003;43: 149–173.

1240. Castell JV, Donato MT, Gomez-Lechon MJ. Metabolism and bioactivation of toxicants in the lung. The in vitro cellular approach. Exp Toxicol Pathol 2005;57(suppl 1): 189–204.

1241. Fujii-Kuriyama Y, Ema M, Mimura J, Matsushita N, Sogawa K. Polymorphic forms of the Ah receptor and induction of the CYP1A1 gene. Pharmacogenetics 1995;5 Spec No:S149–S153.

1242. Denison MS, Nagy SR. Activation of the aryl hydrocarbon receptor by structurally diverse exogenous and endogenous chemicals. Annu Rev Pharmacol Toxicol 2003;43:309–334.

1243. Fujii-Kuriyama Y, Mimura J. Molecular mechanisms of AhR functions in the regulation of cytochrome P450 genes. Biochem Biophys Res Commun 2005;338:311–317.

1244. Hankinson O. Role of coactivators in transcriptional activation by the aryl hydrocarbon receptor. Arch Biochem Biophys 2005;433:379–386.

1245. Gelboin HV. Benzo(a)pyrene metabolism, activation, and carcinogenesis. role and regulation of mixed function oxidases and related enzymes. Physiol Rev 1980;60: 1107–1166.

1246. Phillips DH. Fifty years of benzo(a)pyrene. Nature (Lond.) 1983;303:468–472.

1247. Jeffrey AM. DNA modification by chemical carcinogens. Pharmacol Ther 1985;28:237–272.

1248. Graslund A, Jernstrom B. DNA-carcinogen interaction: covalent DNA-adducts of benzo(a)pyrene 7,8–dihydrodiol 9,10–epoxides studied by biochemical and biophysical techniques. Q Rev Biophys 1989;22:1–37.

1249. Denissenko MF, Pao A, Tang M S, Pfeifer GP. Preferential formation of benzo[a]pyrene adducts at lung cancer mutational hotspots in p53. Science 1996;274:430–432.

1250. Kozack R, Seo KY, Jelinsky SA, Loechler EL. Toward an understanding of the role of DNA adduct conformation in defining mutagenic mechanism based on studies of the major adduct (formed at N(2)-dG) of the potent environmental carcinogen, benzo[a]pyrene. Mutat Res 2000; 450:41–59.

1251. Pfeifer GP, Denissenko MF, Olivier M, Tretyakova N, Hecht SS, Hainaut P. Tobacco smoke carcinogens, DNA damage and p53 mutations in smoking-associated cancers. Oncogene 2002;21:7435–7451.

1252. Baird WM, Hooven LA, Mahadevan B. Carcinogenic polycyclic aromatic hydrocarbon-DNA adducts and mechanism of action. Environ Mol Mutagen 2005;45: 106–114.

1253. Hoffmann D, Brunnemann KD, Adams JD, Hecht SS. Formation and analysis of N-nitrosamines in tobacco products and their endogenous formation in consumers. IARC Sci Publ 1984;57:743–762.

1254. Brunnemann KD, Hoffmann D. Analytical studies on tobacco-specific N-nitrosamines in tobacco and tobacco smoke. Crit Rev Toxicol 1991;21:235–240.

1255. Amin S, Desai D, Hecht SS, Hoffmann D. Synthesis of tobacco-specific N-nitrosamines and their metabolites and results of related bioassays. Crit Rev Toxicol 1996; 26:139–147.

1256. Brunnemann KD, Prokopczyk B, Djordjevic MV, Hoffmann D. Formation and analysis of tobacco-specific N-nitrosamines. Crit Rev Toxicol 1996;26:121–137.

1257. Hecht SS, Biochemistry, biology, and carcinogenicity of tabacco-specific N-nitrosamines. Chem Res Toxicol 1998;11:559–603.

1258. Hecht SS. DNA adduct formation from tobacco-specific N-nitrosamines. Mutat Res 1999;424:127–142.

1259. Vos RM, Van Bladeren PJ. Glutathione S-transferases in relation to their role in the biotransformation of xenobiotics. Chem Biol Interact 1990;75:241–265.

1260. Daniel V. Glutathione S-transferases: gene structure and regulation of expression. Crit Rev Biochem Mol Biol 1993;28:173–207.

1261. Hayes JD, Pulford DJ. The glutathione S-transferase supergene family: regulation of GST and the contribution of the isoenzymes to cancer chemoprotection and drug resistance. Crit Rev Biochem Mol Biol 1995;30:445–600.

1262. Rahman Q, Abidi P, Afaq F, et al. Glutathione redox system in oxidative lung injury. Crit Rev Toxicol 1999; 29:543–568.

1263. Salinas AE, Wong MG. Glutathione S-transferases—a review. Curr Med Chem 1999;6:279–309.

1264. Baron J, Voigt JM. Localization, distribution, and induction of xenobiotic-metabolizing enzymes and aryl hydrocarbon hydroxylase activity within lung. Pharmacol Ther 1990;47:419–445.

1265. Seidegard J, Ekstrom G. The role of human glutathione transferases and epoxide hydrolases in the metabolism of xenobiotics. Environ Health Perspect 1997;105(suppl 4): 791–799.

1266. Omiecinski CJ, Hassett C, Hosagrahara V. Epoxide hydrolase polymorphism and role in toxicology. Toxicol Lett 2000;112–113:365–370.

1267. Fretland AJ, Omiecinski CJ. Epoxide hydrolases: biochemistry and molecular biology. Chem Biol Interact 2000;129:41–59.

1268. Arand M, Cronin A, Adamska M, Oesch F. Epoxide hydrolases: structure, function, mechanism, and assay. Methods Enzymol 2005;400:569–588.

1269. Miller EC, Miller JA. Searches for ultimate chemical carcinogens and their reaction with cellular macromolecules. Cancer 1981;47:2327–2345.

1270. Pelkonen O, Nebert DW. Metabolism of polycyclic aromatic hydrocarbons: etiologic role in carcinogenesis. Pharmacol Rev 1982;34:189–222.

1271. Poirier MC, Beland FA. DNA adduct measurement and tumor incidence during chronic carcinogen exposure in animal models: implications for DNA adduct-based human cancer risk assessment. Chem Res Toxicol 1992; 5:749–755.

1272. Bartsch H, Rojas M, Nair U, Nair J, Alexandrov K. Genetic cancer susceptibility and DNA adducts: studies in smokers, tobacco chewers, and coke oven workers. Cancer Detect Prev 1999;23:445–453.

1273. Poirier MC, Santella RM, Weston A. Carcinogen macromolecular adducts and their measurement. Carcinogenesis 2000;21:353–359.

1274. Weston A, Manchester DK, Poirier MC, et al. Derivative fluorescence spectral analysis of polycyclic aromatic hydrocarbon-DNA adducts in human placenta. Chem Res Toxicol 1989;2:104–108.
1275. Vulimiri SV, Wu X, Baer-Dubowska W, et al. Analysis of aromatic DNA adducts and 7,8–dihydro-8–oxo- 2′-deoxyguanosine in lymphocyte DNA from a case-control study of lung cancer involving minority populations. Mol Carcinog 2000;27:34–46.
1276. Tang D, Phillips DH, Stampfer M, et al. Association between carcinogen DNA adducts in white blood cells and lung cancer risk in the Physicians Health Study. Cancer Res 2001;61:6708–6712.
1277. Phillips DH. Smoking-related DNA and protein adducts in human tissues. Carcinogenesis 2002;23:1979–2004.
1278. Wiencke JD. DNA adduct burden and tobacco carcinogenesis. Oncogene 2002;21:7376–7391.
1279. Veglia F, Matullo G, Vineis P. Bulky DNA adducts and risk of cancer: a meta-analysis. Cancer Epidemiol Biomarkers Prev 2003;12:157–160.
1280. Gyorffy E, Anna L, Gyori Z, et al. DNA adducts in tumour, normal peripheral lung and bronchus, and peripheral blood lymphocytes from smoking and non-smoking lung cancer patients: correlations between tissues and detection by 32P-postlabelling and immunoassay. Carcinogenesis 2004;25:1201–1209.
1281. Peluso M, Munnia A, Hoek G, et al. DNA adducts and lung cancer risk: a prospective study. Cancer Res 2005; 65:8042–8048.
1282. Hassett C, Robinson KB, Beck NB, Omiecinski CJ. The human microsomal epoxide hydrolase gene (EPHX1): complete nucleotide sequence and structural characterization. Genomics 1994;23:433–442.
1283. Kato S, Bowman ED, Harrington AM, Blomeke B, Shields PG. Human lung carcinogen-DNA adduct levels mediated by genetic polymorphisms in vivo. J Natl Cancer Inst 1995;87:902–907.
1284. Butkiewicz D, Grzybowska E, Hemminki K, et al. Modulation of DNA adduct levels in human mononuclear white blood cells and granulocytes by CYP1A1 CYP2D6 and GSTM1 genetic polymorphisms. Mutat Res 1998;415:97–108.
1285. Rojas M, Alexandrov K, Cascorbi I, et al. High benzo[a]pyrene diol-epoxide DNA adduct levels in lung and blood cells from individuals with combined CYP1A1 MspI/Msp-GSTM1*0/*0 genotypes. Pharmacogenetics 1998;8:109–118.
1286. Ratnasinghe D, Tangrea JA, Andersen MR, et al. Glutathione peroxidase codon 198 polymorphism variant increases lung cancer risk. Cancer Res 2000;60: 6381–6383.
1287. Godschalk RW, Dallinga JW, Wikman H, et al. Modulation of DNA and protein adducts in smokers by genetic polymorphisms in GSTM1, GSTT1, NAT1 and NAT2. Pharmacogenetics 2001;11:389–398.
1288. Ketelslegers HB, Gottschalk RW, Godschalk RW, et al. Interindividual variations in DNA adduct levels assessed by analysis of multiple genetic polymorphisms in smokers. Cancer Epidemiol Biomarkers Prev 2006;15: 624–629.
1289. Kawajiri K, Watanabe J, Eguchi H, Hayashi S. Genetic polymorphisms of drug-metabolizing enzymes and lung cancer susceptibility. Pharmacogenetics. 1995;5 Spec No: S70–S73.
1290. Watanabe M. Polymorphic CYP genes and disease predisposition—what have the studies shown so far? Toxicol Lett 1998;102–103:167–171.
1291. Smith GB, Harper PA, Wong JM, et al. Human lung microsomal cytochrome P4501A1 (CYP1A1) activities: impact of smoking status and CYP1A1, aryl hydrocarbon receptor, and glutathione S-transferase M1 genetic polymorphisms. Cancer Epidemiol Biomarkers Prev. 2001;10:839–853.
1292. Liang G, Pu Y, Yin L. Rapid detection of single nucleotide polymorphisms related with lung cancer susceptibility of Chinese population. Cancer Lett 2005;223:265–274.
1293. Ayesh R, Idle JR, Ritchie JC, Crothers MJ, Hetzel MR. Metabolic oxidation phenotypes as markers for susceptibility to lung cancer. Nature 1984;312:169–170.
1294. Kawajiri K, Nakachi K, Imai K, Yoshii A, Shinoda N, Watanabe J. Identification of genetically high risk individuals to lung cancer by DNA polymorphisms of the cytochrome P450IA1 gene. FEBS Lett 1990;263: 131–133.
1295. Caporaso N, Pickle LW, Bale S, Ayesh R, Hetzel M, Idle J. The distribution of debrisoquine metabolic phenotypes and implications for the suggested association with lung cancer risk. Genet Epidemiol 1989;6:517–524.
1296. Nebert DW. Polymorphism of human CYP2D genes involved in drug metabolism: possible relationship to individual cancer risk. Cancer Cells 1991;3:93–96.
1297. Puchetti V, Faccini GB, Micciolo R, Ghimenton F, Bertrand C, Zatti N. Dextromethorphan test for evaluation of congenital predisposition to lung cancer. Chest 1994;105:449–453.
1298. Caporaso N, DeBaun MR, Rothman N. Lung cancer and CYP2D6 (the debrisoquine polymorphism): sources of heterogeneity in the proposed association. Pharmacogenetics 1995;5:S129–S134.
1299. Gao Y, Zhang Q. Polymorphisms of the GSTM1 and CYP2D6 genes associated with susceptibility to lung cancer in Chinese. Mutat Res 1999;444:441–449.
1300. Laforest L, Wikman H, Benhamou S, et al. CYP2D6 gene polymorphism in caucasian smokers: lung cancer susceptibility and phenotype-genotype relationships. Eur J Cancer 2000;36:1825–1832.
1301. Hayashi S, Watanabe J, Nakachi K, Kawajiri K Genetic linkage of lung cancer-associated MspI polymorphisms with amino acid replacement in the heme binding region of the human cytochrome P450IA1 gene. J Biochem (Tokyo) 1991;110:407–411.
1302. Petersen DD, Mckinney CE, Ikeya K, et al. Human CYP1A1 gene: cosegregation of the enzyme inducibility phenotype and an RFLP. Am J Hum Genet 1991;48: 720–725.
1303. Ingelman-Sundberg M, Johansson I, Persson I, et al. Genetic polymorphism of cytochromes P450: interethnic differences and relationship to incidence of lung cancer. Pharmacogenetics 1992;2:264–2671.

1304. Cosma G, Crofts F, Taioli E, Toniolo P, Garte S. Relationship between genotype and function of the human CYP1A1 gene. J Toxicol Environ Health 1993;40:309–316.
1305. Crofts F, Cosma GN, Taioli E, Currie DC, Toniolo PT, Garte SJ. A novel CYP1A1 gene polymorphism in African-Americans. Carcinogenesis 1993;14:1729–1731.
1306. Kawajiri K, Nakachi K, Imai K, Watanabe J, Hayashi S. The CYP1A1 gene and cancer susceptibility. Crit Rev Oncol Hematol 1993;14:77–87.
1307. Crofts F, Taioli E, Trachman J, et al. Functional significance of di erent human CYP1A1 genotypes. Carcinogenesis 1994;15:2961–2963.
1308. Drakoulis N, Cascorbi I, Brockmoller J, Gross CR, Roots I. Polymorphisms in the human CYP1A1 gene as susceptibility factors for lung cancer: exon-7 mutation (4889 A to G), and a T to C mutation in the 3′-flanking region. Clin Invest 1994;72:240–248.
1309. Landi MT, Bertazzi PA, Shields PG, et al. Association between CYP1A1 genotype, mRNA expression and enzymatic activity in humans. Pharmacogenetics 1994;4:242–246.
1310. Nakachi K, Hayashi S, Kawajiri K, Imai K. Association of cigarette smoking and CYP1A1 polymorphisms with adenocarcinoma of the lung by grades of differentiation. Carcinogenesis 1995;16:2209–2213.
1311. Kawajiri K, Eguchi H, Nakachi K, Sekiya T, Yamamoto M. Association of CYP1A1 germ line polymorphisms with mutations of the p53 gene in lung cancer. Cancer Res 1996;56:72–76.
1312. Kiyohara C, Hirohata T, Inutsuka S. The relationship between aryl hydrocarbon hydroxylase and polymorphisms of the CYP1A1 gene. Jpn J Cancer Res 1996;87:18–24.
1313. Kiyohara C, Nakanishi Y, Inutsuka S, et al. The relationship between CYP1A1 aryl hydrocarbon hydroxylase activity and lung cancer in a Japanese population. Pharmacogenetics 1998;8:315–323.
1314. Kawajiri K, Nakachi K, Imai K, Hayashi S, Watanabe J. Individual differences in lung cancer susceptibility in relation to polymorphisms of P-450IA1 gene and cigarette dose. Princess Takamatsu Symp 1990;21:55–61.
1315. Nakachi K, Imai K, Hayashi S, Watanabe J, Kawajiri K. Genetic susceptibility to squamous cell carcinoma of the lung in relation to cigarette smoking dose. Cancer Res 1991;51:5177–5180.
1316. Uematsu F, Kikuchi H, Motomiya M, et al. Association between restriction fragment length polymorphism of the human cytochrome P450IIE1 gene and susceptibility to lung cancer. Jpn J Cancer Res 1991;82:254–256.
1317. Hayashi S, Watanabe J, Kawajiri K. High susceptibility to lung cancer analyzed in term of combined genotypes of CYP1A1 and Mu-class glutathione S-transferase genes. Jpn J Cancer Res 1992;83:866–870.
1318. Hirvonen A, Husgafvel-Pursiainen K, Karjalainen A, Anttila S, Vainio H. Point-mutational MspI and Ile-Val polymorphisms closely linked in the CYP1A1 gene: lack of association with susceptibility to lung cancer in a Finnish study population. Cancer Epidemiol Biomarkers Prev 1992;1:485–489.
1319. Kawajiri K, Nakachi K, Imai K, Watanabe J, Hayashi S. The CYP1A1 gene and cancer susceptibility. Crit Rev Oncol Hematol 1993;14:77–87.
1320. Nakachi K, Imai K, Hayashi S, Kawajiri K. Polymorphisms of the CYP1A1 and glutathione S-transferase genes associated with susceptibility to lung cancer in relation to cigarette dose in a Japanese population. Cancer Res 1993;53:2994–2999.
1321. Shields PG, Caporaso NE, Falk RT, et al. Lung cancer, race, and a CYP1A1 genetic polymorphism. Cancer Epidemiol Biomarkers Prev 1993;2:481–485.
1322. Alexandrie AK, Sundberg MI, Seidegard J, Tornling G, Rannug A. Genetic susceptibility to lung cancer with special emphasis to CYP1A1 and GSTM1: a study on host factors in relation to age at onset, gender and histological cancer types. Carcinogenesis 1994;15:1785–1790.
1323. Kelsey KT, Wiencke JK, Spitz MR. A race-specific genetic polymorphism in the CYP1A1 gene is not associated with lung cancer in African-Americans. Carcinogenesis 1994;15:1121–1124.
1324. Hamada GS, Sugimura H, Suzuki I, et al. The heme-binding region polymorphism of cytochrome P450IA1 (CypIA1), rather than the RsaI polymorphism of IIE1 (CypIIE1), is associated with lung cancer in Rio de Janeiro. Cancer Epidemiol Biomarkers Prev 1995;4:63–67.
1325. Kihara M, Kihara M, Noda K. Risk of smoking for squamous and small cell carcinomas of the lung modulated by combinations of CYP1A1 and GSTM1 gene polymorphisms in a Japanese population. Carcinogenesis 1995;16:2331–2336.
1326. London SJ, Daly AK, Fairbrother KS, et al. Lung cancer risk in African-Americans in relation to a race-specific polymorphism. Cancer Res 1995;55:6035–6037.
1327. Nakachi K, Hayashi S, Kawajiri K, Imai K. Association of cigarette smoking and CYP1A1 polymorphisms with adenocarcinoma of the lung by grades of differentiation. Carcinogenesis 1995;16:2209–2213.
1328. Sugimura H, Hamada GS, Suzuki I, et al. CYP1A1 and CYP2E1 polymorphism and lung cancer, case-control study in Rio de Janeiro, Brazil. Pharmacogenetics 1995;5 (Special Issue):145–148.
1329. Taioli E, Crofts F, Demopoulos R, Trachman J, Toniolo P, Garte MSJ. An African American specific CYP1A1 polymorphism is associated with adenocarcinoma of the lung. Cancer Res 1995;55:472–473.
1330. Cascorbi I, Brockmoller J, Roots I. A C4887A polymorphism in exon 7 of human CYP1A1: population frequency, mutation linkages, and impact on lung cancer susceptibility. Cancer Res 1996;56:4965–4969.
1331. Xu X, Kelsey KT, Wiencke JK, Wain JC, Christiani DC. Cytochrome P450 CYP1A1 MspI polymorphism and lung cancer susceptibility. Cancer Epidemiol Biomarkers Prev 1996;5:687–692.
1332. Bouchardy C, Wikman H, Benhamou S, Hirvonen A, Dayer P, Husgafvel-Pursianinen K. CYP1A1 genetic polymorphisms, tobacco smoking and lung cancer risk in a French Caucasian population. Biomarkers 1997;2:131–134.

1333. Garcia Closas M, Kelsey KT, et al. A case-control study of cytochrome P450 1A1, glutathione S-transferase M1, cigarette smoking and lung cancer susceptibility (Massachusetts, United States). Cancer Causes Control 1997;8:544–553.
1334. Le Marchand L, Sivaraman L, Pierce L, et al. Association of CYP1A1, GSTM1, and CYP2E1 polymorphisms with lung cancer suggest cell type specificities to tobacco carcinogens. Cancer Res 1998;58:4858–4863.
1335. Sugimura H, Wakai K, Genka K, et al. Association of Ile462Val (Exon 7) polymorphism of cytochrome P450 IA1 with lung cancer in the Asian population: further evidence from a case-control study in Okinawa. Cancer Epidemiol Biomarkers Prev 1998;7: 413–417.
1336. Taioli E, Fordd J, Li Y, Demopoulos R, Garte S. Lung cancer risk and CYP1A1 genotype in African Americans. Carcinogenesis 1998;19:813–817.
1337. Persson I, Johansson I, Lou Y-C, et al. Genetic polymorphism of xenobiotic metabolizing enzymes among Chinese lung cancer patients. Int J Cancer 1999;81: 325–329.
1338. Quinones L, Berthou F, Varela N, Simon B, Gil L, Lucas D. Ethnic susceptibility to lung cancer: differences in CYP2E1, CYP1A1 and GSTM1 genetic polymorphisms between French Caucasian and Chilean populations. Cancer Lett 1999;141:167–171.
1339. Dolzan V, Rudolf Z, Breskvar K. Genetic polymorphism of xenobiotic metabolising enzymes in Slovenian lung cancer patients. Pflugers Arch 2000;439(3 suppl): R29–R30.
1340. Han XM, Zhou HH. Polymorphism of CYP450 and cancer susceptibility. Acta Pharmacol Sin 2000;21: 673–679.
1341. Lin P, Wang S-L, Wang H-J, et al. Association of CYP1A1 and microsomal epoxide hydrolase polymorphisms with lung squamous cell carcinoma. Br J Cancer 2000;82: 852–857.
1342. Chen S, Xue K, Xu L, Ma G, Wu J. Polymorphisms of the CYP1A1 and GSTM1 genes in relation to individual susceptibility to lung carcinoma in Chinese population. Mutat Res 2001;458:41–47.
1343. Gsur A, Haidinger G, Hollaus P, et al. Genetic polymorphisms of CYP1A1 and GSTM1 and lung cancer risk. Anticancer Res 2001;21:2237–2242.
1344. Quinones L, Lucas D, Godoy J, et al. CYP1A1, CYP2E1 and GSTM1 genetic polymorphisms. The effect of single and combined genotypes on lung cancer susceptibility in Chilean people. Cancer Lett 2001;174:35–44.
1345. Song N, Tan W, Xing D, Lin D. CYP 1A1 polymorphism and risk of lung cancer in relation to tobacco smoking: a case-control study in China. Carcinogenesis 2001;22: 11–16.
1346. Le Marchand L, Guo C, Benhamou S, et al. Pooled analysis of the CYP1A1 exon 7 polymorphism and lung cancer (United States). Cancer Causes Control 2003;14:339–346.
1347. Vineis P, Veglia F, Benhamou S, et al. CYP1A1 T3801 C polymorphism and lung cancer: a pooled analysis of 2451 cases and 3358 controls. Int J Cancer 2003;104:650–657.
1348. Wang J, Deng Y, Li L, et al. Association of GSTM1, CYP1A1 and CYP2E1 genetic polymorphisms with susceptibility to lung adenocarcinoma: a case-control study in Chinese population. Cancer Sci 2003;94:448–452.
1349. Sobti RC, Sharma S, Joshi A, Jindal SK, Janmeja A. Genetic polymorphism of the CYP1A1, CYP2E1, GSTM1 and GSTT1 genes and lung cancer susceptibility in a north indian population. Mol Cell Biochem 2004;266:1–9.
1350. Demir A, Altin S, Demir I, Koksal V, Cetincelik U, Dincer I. The role of CYP1A1 Msp1 gene polymorphisms on lung cancer development in Turkey. Tuberk Toraks 2005;53:5–9.
1351. Larsen JE, Colosimo ML, Yang IA, Bowman R, Zimmerman PV, Fong KM. Risk of non-small cell lung cancer and the cytochrome P4501A1 Ile462Val polymorphism. Cancer Causes Control 2005;16:579–585.
1352. Sreeja L, Syamala V, Hariharan S, Madhavan J, Devan SC, Ankathil R. Possible risk modification by CYP1A1, GSTM1 and GSTT1 gene polymorphisms in lung cancer susceptibility in a South Indian population. J Hum Genet 2005;50:618–627.
1353. Larsen JE, Colosimo ML, Yang IA, Bowman R, Zimmerman PV, Fong KM. CYP1A1 Ile462Val and MPO G-463A interact to increase risk of adenocarcinoma but not squamous cell carcinoma of the lung. Carcinogenesis 2006;27:525–532.
1354. Pisani P, Srivatanakul P, Randerson-Moor J, et al. GSTM1 and CYP1A1 polymorphisms, tobacco, air pollution, and lung cancer: a study in rural Thailand. Cancer Epidemiol Biomarkers Prev 2006;15:667–674.
1355. Kamataki T, Nunoya K, Sakai Y, Kushida H, Fujita K. Genetic polymorphism of CYP2A6 in relation to cancer. Mutat Res 1999;428:125–130.
1356. Miyamoto M, Umetsu Y, Dosaka-Akita H, et al. CYP2A6 gene deletion reduces susceptibility to lung cancer. Biochem Biophys Res Commun 1999;261:658–660.
1357. Nunoya KI, Yokoi T, Kimura K, et al. A new CYP2A6 gene deletion responsible for the in vivo polymorphic metabolism of (+)-cis-3,5-dimethyl-2-(3-pyridyl)thiazolidin-4-one hydrochloride in humans. J Pharmacol Exp Ther 1999;289:437–442.
1358. Nunoya K, Yokoi T, Takahashi Y, Kimura K, Kinoshita M, Kamataki T. Homologous unequal cross-over within the human CYP2A gene cluster as a mechanism for the deletion of the entire CYP2A6 gene associated with the poor metabolizer phenotype. J Biochem (Tokyo) 1999;126: 402–407.
1359. Ariyoshi N, Takahashi Y, Miyamoto M, et al. Structural characterization of a new variant of the CYP2A6 gene (CYP2A6*1B) apparently diagnosed as heterozygotes of CYP2A6*1A and CYP2A6*4C. Pharmacogenetics 2000;10:687–693.
1360. Kushida H, Fujita K, Suzuki A, Yamada M, Nohmi T, Kamataki T. Development of a Salmonella tester strain sensitive to promutagenic N-nitrosamines: expression of recombinant CYP2A6 and human NADPH-cytochrome P450 reductase in S. typhimurium YG7108. Mutat Res 2000;471:135–143.
1361. Ariyoshi N, Sawamura Y, Kamataki T. A novel single nucleotide polymorphism altering stability and activity of

CYP2A6. Biochem. Biophys. Res. Commun 2001;281: 810–814.
1362. Loriot MA, Rebuissou S, Oscarson M, et al. Genetic polymorphisms of cytochrome P450 2A6 in a case-control study on lung cancer in a French population. Pharmacogenetics 2001;11:39–44.
1363. Pitarque M, von Richter O, Oke B, Berkkan H, Oscarson M, Ingelman-Sundberg M. Identification of a single nucleotide polymorphism in the TATA box of the CYP2A6 gene: impairment of its promoter activity. Biochem Biophys Res Commun 2001;284:455–460.
1364. Tan W, Chen GF, Xing DY, Song CY, Kadlubar FF, Lin DX. Frequency of CYP2A6 gene deletion and its relation to risk of lung and esophageal cancer in the Chinese population. Int J Cancer 2001;95:96–101.
1365. Xu C, Rao YS, Xu B, et al. An in vivo pilot study characterizing the new CYP2A6*7, 8, and 10 alleles. Biochem Biophys Res Commun 2002;290:318–324.
1366. Kiyotani K, Yamazaki H, Fujieda M, et al. Decreased coumarin 7–hydroxylase activities and CYP2A6 expression levels in humans caused by genetic polymorphism in CYP2A6 promoter region (CYP2A6*9). Pharmacogenetics 2003;13:689–695.
1367. Fujieda M, Yamazaki H, Saito T, et al. Evaluation of CYP2A6 genetic polymorphisms as determinants of smoking behavior and tobacco-related lung cancer risk in male Japanese smokers. Carcinogenesis 2004; 25:2451–2458.
1368. Kamataki T, Fujieda M, Kiyotani K, Iwano S, Kunitoh H. Genetic polymorphism of CYP2A6 as one of the potential determinants of tobacco-related cancer risk. Biochem Biophys Res Commun 2005;338:306–310.
1369. Wang H, Tan W, Hao B, et al. Substantial reduction in risk of lung adenocarcinoma associated with genetic polymorphism in CYP2A13, the most active cytochrome P450 for the metabolic activation of tobacco-specific carcinogen NNK. Cancer Res 2003;63:8057–8061.
1370. Cauffiez C, Lo-Guidice JM, Quaranta S, et al. Genetic polymorphism of the human cytochrome CYP2A13 in a French population: implication in lung cancer susceptibility. Biochem Biophys Res Commun 2004;317:662–669.
1371. Itoga S, Nomura F, Makino Y, et al. Tandem repeat polymorphism of the CYP2E1 gene: an association study with esophageal cancer and lung cancer. Alcohol Clin Exp Res 2002;26(8 suppl):15S-19S.
1372. Iizasa T, Baba M, Saitoh Y, et al. A polymorphism in the 5′-flanking region of the CYP2E1 gene and elevated lung adenocarcinoma risk in a Japanese population. Oncol Rep 2005;14:919–923.
1373. Dally H, Edler L, Jager B, et al. The CYP3A4*1B allele increases risk for small cell lung cancer: effect of gender and smoking dose. Pharmacogenetics 2003;13:607–618.
1374. Cauchi S, Stucker I, Solas C, et al. Polymorphisms of human aryl hydrocarbon receptor (AhR) gene in a French population: relationship with CYP1A1 inducibility and lung cancer. Carcinogenesis 2001;22:1819–1824.
1375. Cauchi S, Stucker I, Cenee S, Kremers P, Beaune P, Massaad-Massade L. Structure and polymorphisms of human aryl hydrocarbon receptor repressor (AhRR) gene in a French population: relationship with CYP1A1 inducibility and lung cancer. Pharmacogenetics 2003;13: 339–347.
1376. Persson I, Johansson I, Lou YC, et al. Genetic polymorphism of xenobiotic metabolizing enzymes among Chinese lung cancer patients. Int J Cancer 1999;81: 325–329.
1377. London SJ, Smart J, Daly AK. Lung cancer risk in relation to genetic polymorphisms of microsomal epoxide hydrolase among African-Americans and Caucasians in Los Angeles County. Lung Cancer 2000;28:147–155.
1378. Wu X, Gwyn K, Amos CI, Makan N, Hong WK, Spitz MR. The association of microsomal epoxide hydrolase polymorphisms and lung cancer risk in African-Americans and Mexican-Americans. Carcinogenesis 2001;22:923–928.
1379. To-Figueras J, Gene M, Gomez-Catalan J, Pique E, Borrego N, Corbella J. Lung cancer susceptibility in relation to combined polymorphisms of microsomal epoxide hydrolase and glutathione S-transferase P1. Cancer Lett 2001;173:155–162.
1380. Cajas-Salazar N, Au WW, Zwischenberger JB, et al. Effect of epoxide hydrolase polymorphisms on chromosome aberrations and risk for lung cancer. Cancer Genet Cytogenet 2003;145:97–102.
1381. Park JY, Chen L, Elahi A, Lazarus P, Tockman MS. Genetic analysis of microsomal epoxide hydrolase gene and its association with lung cancer risk. Eur J Cancer Prev 2005;14:223–230.
1382. Seidegard J, Pero RW, Markowitz MM, Roush G, Miller DG, Beattie EJ. Isoenzyme(s) of glutathione transferase (class Mu) as a marker for the susceptibility to lung cancer: a follow up study. Carcinogenesis 1990;11:33–36.
1383. Zhong S, Howie AF, Ketterer B, et al. Glutathione S-transferase mu locus: use of genotyping and phenotyping assays to assess association with lung cancer susceptibility. Carcinogenesis 1991;12:1533–1537.
1384. Hirvonen A, Husgafvel-Pursiainen K, Anttila S, Vainio H. The GSTM1 null genotype as a potential risk modifier for squamous cell carcinoma of the lung. Carcinogenesis 1993;14:1479–1481.
1385. Kihara M, Kihara M, Noda K, Okamoto N. Increased risk of lung cancer in Japanese smokers with class mu glutathione S-transferase gene deficiency. Cancer Lett 1993; 71:151–155.
1386. Nazar-Stewart V, Motulsky AG, Eaton DL, et al. The glutathione S-transferase mu polymorphism as a marker for susceptibility to lung carcinoma. Cancer Res 1993;53(10 suppl):2313–2318.
1387. Deakin M, Elder J, Hendrickse C, et al. Glutathione S-transferase GSTT1 genotypes and susceptibility to cancer: studies of interactions with GSTM1 in lung, oral, gastric and colorectal cancers. Carcinogenesis 1996;17:881–884.
1388. To-Figueras J, Gene M, Gomez-Catalan J, et al. Glutathione-S-Transferase M1 and codon 72 p53 polymorphisms in a northwestern Mediterranean population and their relation to lung cancer susceptibility. Cancer Epidemiol Biomarkers Prev 1996;5:337–342.
1389. Kelsey KT, Spitz MR, Zuo ZF, Wiencke JK. Polymorphisms in the glutathione S-transferase class mu and theta genes interact and increase susceptibility to lung

cancer in minority populations (Texas, United States). Cancer Causes Control 1997;8:554–559.
1390. Sun GF, Shimojo N, Pi JB, Lee S, Kumagai Y. Gene deficiency of glutathione S-transferase mu isoform associated with susceptibility to lung cancer in a Chinese population. Cancer Lett 1997;113:169–172.
1391. Jourenkova-Mironova N, Wikman H, Bouchardy C, et al. Role of glutathione S-transferase GSTM1, GSTM3, GSTP1 and GSTT1 genotypes in modulating susceptibility to smoking-related lung cancer. Pharmacogenetics 1998;8:495–502.
1392. Stucker I, de Waziers I, Cenee S, et al. GSTM1, smoking and lung cancer: a case-control study. Int J Epidemiol 1999;28:829–835.
1393. To-Figueras J, Gene M, Gomez-Catalan J, et al. Genetic polymorphism of glutathione S-transferase P1 gene and lung cancer risk. Cancer Causes Control 1999;10:65–70.
1394. Belogubova EV, Togo AV, Kondratieva TV, Lemehov VG, Hanson KP, Imyanitov EN. GSTM1 genotypes in elderly tumour-free smokers and non-smokers. Lung Cancer 2000;29:189–195.
1395. Reszka E, Wasowicz W. Significance of genetic polymorphisms in glutathione S-transferase multigene family and lung cancer risk. Int J Occup Med Environ Health 2001;14:99–113.
1396. Benhamou S, Lee WJ, Alexandrie AK, et al. Meta- and pooled analyses of the effects of glutathione S-transferase M1 polymorphisms and smoking on lung cancer risk. Carcinogenesis 2002;23:1343–1350.
1397. Cerrahoglu K, Kunter E, Isitmangil T, et al. Can't lung cancer patients detoxify procarcinogens? Allerg Immunol (Paris) 2002;34:51–55.
1398. Lewis SJ, Cherry NM, Niven RM, Barber PV, Povey AC. GSTM1, GSTT1 and GSTP1 polymorphisms and lung cancer risk. Cancer Lett 2002;180:165–171.
1399. Liloglou T, Walters M, Maloney P, Youngson J, Field JK. A T2517C polymorphism in the GSTM4 gene is associated with risk of developing lung cancer. Lung Cancer 2002;37:143–146.
1400. Perera FP, Mooney LA, Stampfer M, et al.; Physicians' Health Cohort Study. Associations between carcinogen-DNA damage, glutathione S-transferase genotypes, and risk of lung cancer in the prospective Physicians' Health Cohort Study. Carcinogenesis 2002;23:1641–1646.
1401. Stucker I, Hirvonen A, de Waziers I, et al. Genetic polymorphisms of glutathione S-transferases as modulators of lung cancer susceptibility. Carcinogenesis 2002;23: 1475–1481.
1402. Nazar-Stewart V, Vaughan TL, Stapleton P, Van Loo J, Nicol-Blades B, Eaton DL. A population-based study of glutathione S-transferase M1, T1 and P1 genotypes and risk for lung cancer. Lung Cancer 2003;40:247–258.
1403. Mohr LC, Rodgers JK, Silvestri GA. Glutathione S-transferase M1 polymorphism and the risk of lung cancer. Anticancer Res 2003;23:2111–2124.
1404. Pinarbasi H, Silig Y, Cetinkaya O, Seyfikli Z, Pinarbasi E. Strong association between the GSTM1–null genotype and lung cancer in a Turkish population. Cancer Genet Cytogenet 2003;146:125–129.
1405. Wang J, Deng Y, Cheng J, Ding J, Tokudome S. GST genetic polymorphisms and lung adenocarcinoma susceptibility in a Chinese population. Cancer Lett 2003;201: 185–193.
1406. Reszka E, Wasowicz W, Rydzynski K, Szeszenia-Dabrowska N, Szymczak W. Glutathione S-transferase M1 and P1 metabolic polymorphism and lung cancer predisposition. Neoplasma 2003;50:357–362.
1407. Schneider J, Bernges U, Philipp M, Woitowitz HJ. GSTM1, GSTT1, and GSTP1 polymorphism and lung cancer risk in relation to tobacco smoking. Cancer Lett 2004;208: 65–74.
1408. Yang P, Bamlet WR, Ebbert JO, Taylor WR, de Andrade M. Glutathione pathway genes and lung cancer risk in young and old populations. Carcinogenesis 2004;25: 1935–1944.
1409. Chan-Yeung M, Tan-Un KC, Ip MS, et al. Lung cancer susceptibility and polymorphisms of glutathione-S-transferase genes in Hong Kong. Lung Cancer 2004;45: 155–160.
1410. Ye Z, Song H, Higgins JP, Pharoah P, Danesh J. Five glutathione s-transferase gene variants in 23,452 cases of lung cancer and 30,397 controls: meta-analysis of 130 studies. PLoS Med 2006;3:e91.
1411. Le Marchand L, Sivaraman L, Pierce L, et al. Associations of CYP1A1, GSTM1, and CYP2E1 polymorphisms with lung cancer suggest cell type specificities to tobacco carcinogens. Cancer Res 1998;58:4858–4863.
1412. Liu G, Miller DP, Zhou W, et al. Differential association of the codon 72 p53 and GSTM1 polymorphisms on histological subtype of non-small cell lung carcinoma. Cancer Res 2001;61:8718–8722.
1413. Risch A, Wikman H, Thiel S, et al. Glutathione-S-transferase M1, M3, T1 and P1 polymorphisms and susceptibility to non-small-cell lung cancer subtypes and hamartomas. Pharmacogenetics 2001;11:757–764.
1414. Rosvold EA, McGlynn KA, Lustbader ED, Buetow KH. Identification of an NAD(P)H: quinone oxidoreductase polymorphism and its association with lung cancer and smoking. Pharmacogenetics 1995;5:199–206.
1415. Wiencke JK, Spitz MR, McMillan A, Kelsey KT. Lung cancer in Mexican-Americans and African-Americans is associated with the wild-type genotype of the NAD(P)H: quinone oxidoreductase polymorphism. Cancer Epidemiol Biomarkers Prev 1997;6:87–92.
1416. Xu LL, Wain JC, Miller DP, et al. The NAD(P)H: quinone oxidoreductase 1 gene polymorphism and lung cancer: differential susceptibility based on smoking behavior. Cancer Epidemiol Biomarkers Prev 2001;10:303–309.
1417. Lawson KA, Woodson K, Virtamo J, Albanes D. Association of the NAD(P)H: quinone oxidoreductase (NQO1) 609C- >T polymorphism with lung cancer risk among male smokers. Cancer Epidemiol Biomarkers Prev 2005; 14:2275–2276.
1418. Saldivar SJ, Wang Y, Zhao H, et al. An association between a NQO1 genetic polymorphism and risk of lung cancer. Mutat Res 2005;582:71–78.
1419. Abdel-Rahman SZ, El-Zein RA, Zwischenberger JB, Au WW. Association of the NAT1*10 genotype with increased

chromosome aberrations and higher lung cancer risk in cigarette smokers. Mutat Res 1998;398:43–54.
1420. Seow A, Zhao B, Poh WT, et al. NAT2 slow acetylator genotype is associated with increased risk of lung cancer among non-smoking Chinese women in Singapore. Carcinogenesis 1999;20:1877–1881.
1421. Wikman H, Thiel S, Jager B, et al. Relevance of N-acetyltransferase 1 and 2 (NAT1, NAT2) genetic polymorphisms in non-small cell lung cancer susceptibility. Pharmacogenetics 2001;11:157–168.
1422. Belogubova EV, Kuligina ESh, Togo AV, et al. "Comparison of extremes" approach provides evidence against the modifying role of NAT2 polymorphism in lung cancer susceptibility. Cancer Lett 2005;221:177–183.
1423. Habalova V, Salagovic J, Kalina I, Stubna J. A pilot study testing the genetic polymorphism of N-acetyltransferase 2 as a risk factor in lung cancer. Neoplasma 2005;52: 364–368.
1424. Wang Y, Spitz MR, Tsou AM, Zhang K, Makan N, Wu X. Sulfotransferase (SULT) 1A1 polymorphism as a predisposition factor for lung cancer: a case-control analysis. Lung Cancer 2002;35:137–142.
1425. Roots I, Brockmoller J, Drakoulis N, Loddenkemper R. Mutant genes of cytochrome P-450IID6, glutathione S-transferase class Mu, and arylamine N-acetyltransferase in lung cancer patients. Clin Investig 1992;70:307–319.
1426. Miller DP, Liu G, De Vivo I, et al. Combinations of the variant genotypes of GSTP1, GSTM1, and p53 are associated with an increased lung cancer risk. Cancer Res 2002;62:2819–2823.
1427. Sunaga N, Kohno T, Yanagitani N, et al. Contribution of the NQO1 and GSTT1 polymorphisms to lung adenocarcinoma susceptibility. Cancer Epidemiol Biomarkers Prev 2002;11:730–738.
1428. Hung RJ, Boffetta P, Brockmoller J, et al. CYP1A1 and GSTM1 genetic polymorphisms and lung cancer risk in Caucasian non-smokers: a pooled analysis. Carcinogenesis 2003;24:875–882.
1429. Cajas-Salazar N, Sierra-Torres CH, Salama SA, Zwischenberger JB, Au WW. Combined effect of MPO, GSTM1 and GSTT1 polymorphisms on chromosome aberrations and lung cancer risk. Int J Hyg Environ Health 2003;206:473–483.
1430. Lin P, Hsueh YM, Ko JL, Liang YF, Tsai KJ, Chen CY. Analysis of NQO1, GSTP1, and MnSOD genetic polymorphisms on lung cancer risk in Taiwan. Lung Cancer 2003;40:123–129.
1431. Alexandrie AK, Nyberg F, Warholm M, Rannug A. Influence of CYP1A1, GSTM1, GSTT1, and NQO1 genotypes and cumulative smoking dose on lung cancer risk in a Swedish population. Cancer Epidemiol Biomarkers Prev 2004;13:908–914.
1432. Liu G, Zhou W, Park S, et al. The SOD2 Val/Val genotype enhances the risk of nonsmall cell lung carcinoma by p53 and XRCC1 polymorphisms. Cancer 2004;101:2802–2808.
1433. Raimondi S, Boffetta P, Anttila S, et al. Metabolic gene polymorphisms and lung cancer risk in non-smokers An update of the GSEC study. Mutat Res 2005;592:45–57.
1434. Wei Q, Cheng L, Hong WK, Spitz MR. Reduced DNA repair capacity in lung cancer patients. Cancer Res 1996;56:4103–4107.
1435. Wei Q, Spitz MR. The role of DNA repair capacity in susceptibility to lung cancer: a review. Cancer Metastasis Rev 1997;16:295–307.
1436. Wei Q, Cheng L, Amos CI, et al. Repair of tobacco carcinogen-induced DNA adducts and lung cancer risk: a molecular epidemiologic study. J Natl Cancer Inst 2000;92:1764–1772.
1437. Shen H, Spitz MR, Qiao Y, et al. Smoking, DNA repair capacity and risk of nonsmall cell lung cancer. Int J Cancer 2003;107:84–88.
1438. Spitz MR, Wei Q, Dong Q, Amos CI, Wu X. Genetic susceptibility to lung cancer: the role of DNA damage and repair. Cancer Epidemiol Biomarkers Prev. 2003;12:689–698.
1439. Duell EJ, Wiencke JK, Cheng TJ, et al. Polymorphisms in the DNA repair genes XRCC1 and ERCC2 and biomarkers of DNA damage in human blood mononuclear cells. Carcinogenesis 2000;21:965–971.
1440. Butkiewicz D, Rusin M, Enewold L, et al. Genetic polymorphisms in DNA repair genes and risk of lung cancer. Carcinogenesis 2001;22:593–597.
1441. David-Beabes GL, Lunn RM, London SJ. No association between the XPD (Lys751Gln) polymorphism or the XRCC3 (Thr241Met) polymorphism and lung cancer risk. Cancer Epidemiol Biomarkers Prev 2001;10: 911–912.
1442. Palli D, Russo A, Masala G, et al. DNA adduct levels and DNA repair polymorphisms in traffic-exposed workers and a general population sample. Int J Cancer 2001; 94:121–127.
1443. Spitz MR, Wu X, Wang Y, et al. Modulation of nucleotide excision repair capacity by XPD polymorphisms in lung cancer patients. Cancer Res 2001;61:1354–1357.
1444. Chen S, Tang D, Xue K, et al. DNA repair gene XRCC1 and XPD polymorphisms and risk of lung cancer in a Chinese population. Carcinogenesis 2002;23:1321–1325.
1445. Hou SM, Falt S, Angelini S, et al. The XPD variant alleles are associated with increased aromatic DNA adduct level and lung cancer risk. Carcinogenesis 2002;23:599–603.
1446. Qiao Y, Spitz MR, Guo Z, et al. Rapid assessment of repair of ultraviolet DNA damage with a modified host-cell reactivation assay using a luciferase reporter gene and correlation with polymorphisms of DNA repair genes in normal human lymphocytes. Mutat Res 2002;509: 165–174.
1447. Park JY, Lee SY, Jeon HS, et al. Lys751Gln polymorphism in the DNA repair gene XPD and risk of primary lung cancer. (Letter). Lung Cancer 2002;36:15–16.
1448. Tang D, Cho S, Rundle A, et al. Polymorphisms in the DNA repair enzyme XPD are associated with increased levels of PAH–DNA adducts in a case-control study of breast cancer. Breast Cancer Res Treat 2002;75:159–166.
1449. Xing D, Tan W, Wei Q, Lin D. Polymorphisms of the DNA repair gene XPD and risk of lung cancer in a Chinese population. Lung Cancer 2002;38:123–129.

1450. Liang G, Xing D, Miao X, et al. Sequence variations in the DNA repair gene XPD and risk of lung cancer in a Chinese population. Int J Cancer 2003;105:669–673.
1451. Matullo G, Peluso M, Polidoro S, et al. Combination of DNA repair gene single nucleotide polymorphisms and increased levels of DNA adducts in a population-based study. Cancer Epidemiol Biomarkers Prev 2003;12:674–677.
1452. Misra RR, Ratnasinghe D, Tangrea JA, et al. Polymorphisms in the DNA repair genes XPD, XRCC1, XRCC3, and APE/ref-1, and the risk of lung cancer among male smokers in Finland. Cancer Lett 2003;191:171–178.
1453. Zhou W, Liu G, Miller DP, et al. Polymorphisms in the DNA repair genes XRCC1 and ERCC2, smoking, and lung cancer risk. Cancer Epidemiol Biomarkers Prev 2003;12:359–365.
1454. Hu Z, Wei Q, Wang X, Shen H. DNA repair gene XPD polymorphism and lung cancer risk: a meta-analysis. Lung Cancer 2004;46:1–10.
1455. Vogel U, Laros I, Jacobsen NR, et al. Two regions in chromosome 19q13.2–3 are associated with risk of lung cancer. Mutat Res 2004;546:65–74.
1456. Benhamou S, Sarasin A. ERCC2 /XPD gene polymorphisms and lung cancer: a HuGE review. Am J Epidemiol 2005;161:1–14.
1457. Yin J, Li J, Ma Y, Guo L, Wang H, Vogel U. The DNA repair gene ERCC2/XPD polymorphism Arg 156Arg (A22541C) and risk of lung cancer in a Chinese population. Cancer Lett 2005;223:219–226.
1458. Hu Z, Xu L, Shao M, et al. Polymorphisms in the Two Helicases ERCC2/XPD and ERCC3/XPB of the Transcription Factor IIH Complex and Risk of Lung Cancer: A Case-Control Analysis in a Chinese Population. Cancer Epidemiol. Biomarkers Prev 2006;15:1336–1340.
1459. Yin J, Vogel U, Ma Y, Guo L, Wang H, Qi R. Polymorphism of the DNA repair gene ERCC2 Lys751Gln and risk of lung cancer in a northeastern Chinese population. Cancer Genet Cytogenet 2006;169:27–32.
1460. Park JY, Park SH, Choi JE, et al. Polymorphisms of the DNA repair gene xeroderma pigmentosum group A and risk of primary lung cancer. Cancer Epidemiol Biomarkers Prev 2002;11:993–997.
1461. Butkiewicz D, Popanda O, Risch A, et al. Association between the risk for lung adenocarcinoma and a (-4) G-to-A polymorphism in the XPA gene. Cancer Epidemiol Biomarkers Prev 2004;13:2242–2246.
1462. Vogel U, Overvad K, Wallin H, Tjonneland A, Nexo BA, Raaschou-Nielsen O. Combinations of polymorphisms in XPD, XPC and XPA in relation to risk of lung cancer. Cancer Lett 2005;222:67–74.
1463. Hu Z, Wang Y, Wang X, et al. DNA repair gene XPC genotypes/haplotypes and risk of lung cancer in a Chinese population. Int J Cancer 2005;115:478–483.
1464. Lee GY, Jang JS, Lee SY, et al. XPC polymorphisms and lung cancer risk. Int J Cancer 2005;115:807–813.
1465. Jeon HS, Kim KM, Park SH, et al. Relationship between XPG codon 1104 polymorphism and risk of primary lung cancer. Carcinogenesis 2003;24:1677–1681.
1466. David-Beabes GL, London SJ. Genetic polymorphism of XRCC1 and lung cancer risk among African-Americans and Caucasians. Lung Cancer 2001;34:333–339.
1467. Divine KK, Gilliland FD, Crowell RE, et al. The XRCC1 399 glutamine allele is a risk factor for adenocarcinoma of the lung. Mutat Res 2001;461:273–278.
1468. Ito H, Matsuo K, Hamajima N, et al. Gene-environment interactions between the smoking habit and polymorphisms in the DNA repair genes, APE1 Asp148Glu and XRCC1 Arg399Gln, in Japanese lung cancer risk. Carcinogenesis 2004;25:1395–1401.
1469. Vogel U, Nexo BA, Wallin H, Overvad K, Tjonneland A, Raaschou-Nielsen O. No association between base excision repair gene polymorphisms and risk of lung cancer. Biochem Genet 2004;42:453–460.
1470. Schneider J, Classen V, Bernges U, Philipp M. XRCC1 polymorphism and lung cancer risk in relation to tobacco smoking. Int J Mol Med 2005;16:709–716.
1471. Zhang X, Miao X, Liang G, et al. Polymorphisms in DNA base excision repair genes ADPRT and XRCC1 and risk of lung cancer. Cancer Res 2005;65:722–726.
1472. Yin J, Vogel U, Guo L, Ma Y, Wang H. Lack of association between DNA repair gene ERCC1 polymorphism and risk of lung cancer in a Chinese population. Cancer Genet Cytogenet 2006;164:66–70.
1473. Jacobsen NR, Raaschou-Nielsen O, Nexo B, et al. XRCC3 polymorphisms and risk of lung cancer. Cancer Lett 2004;213:67–72.
1474. Ishida T, Takashima R, Fukayama M, et al. New DNA polymorphisms of human MMH/OGG1 gene: prevalence of one polymorphism among lung-adenocarcinoma patients in Japanese. Int J Cancer 1999;80:18–21.
1475. Sugimura H, Kohno T, Wakai K, et al. hOGG1 Ser326Cys polymorphism and lung cancer susceptibility. Cancer Epidemiol Biomarkers Prev 1999;8:669–674.
1476. Wikman H, Risch A, Klimek F, et al. hOGG1 polymorphism and loss of heterozygosity (LOH): significance for lung cancer susceptibility in a caucasian population. Int J Cancer 2000;88:932–937.
1477. Ito H, Hamajima N, Takezaki T, et al. A limited association of OGG1 Ser326Cys polymorphism for adenocarcinoma of the lung. J Epidemiol 2002;12:258–265.
1478. Hu YC, Ahrendt SA. hOGG1 Ser326Cys polymorphism and G:C-to-T:A mutations: no evidence for a role in tobacco-related non small cell lung cancer. Int J Cancer 2005;114:387–393.
1479. Kohno T, Kunitoh H, Toyama K, et al. Association of the OGG1-Ser326Cys polymorphism with lung adenocarcinoma risk. Cancer Sci 2006;97:724–728.
1480. Gackowski D, Speina E, Zielinska M, et al. Products of oxidative DNA damage and repair as possible biomarkers of susceptibility to lung cancer. Cancer Res 2003;63:4899–4902.
1481. Yang M, Coles BF, Caporaso NE, Choi Y, Lang NP, Kadlubar FF. Lack of association between Caucasian lung cancer risk and O6-methylguanine-DNA methyltransferase-codon 178 genetic polymorphism. Lung Cancer 2004;44:281–286.

1482. Chae MH, Jang JS, Kang HG, et al. O6–alkylguanine-DNA alkyltransferase gene polymorphisms and the risk of primary lung cancer. Mol Carcinog 2006;45:239–249.
1483. Kim JH, Kim H, Lee KY, et al. Genetic polymorphisms of ataxia telangiectasia mutated affect lung cancer risk. Hum Mol Genet 2006;15(7):1181–1186
1484. Zienolddiny S, Campa D, Lind H, et al. Polymorphisms of DNA repair genes and risk of non-small cell lung cancer. Carcinogenesis 2006;27:560–567.
1485. Liu CX, Wang GH, Li P. The expression frequency of common fragile sites and genetic susceptibility to lung cancers. Cancer Genet Cytogenet 1989;42:107–114.
1486. Egeli U, Karadag M, Tunca B, Ozyardimci N. The expression of common fragile sites and genetic predisposition to squamous cell lung cancers. Cancer Genet Cytogenet 1997;95:153–158.
1487. Karadag M, Tunca B, Cecener G, et al. Chromosomal fragile sites and relationship between genetic predisposition to small cell lung cancer. Teratog Carcinog Mutagen 2002;22:31–40.
1488. Tunca B, Cecener G, Gebitekin C, Egeli U, Ediz B, Ercan I. Investigation of genetic susceptibility to non-small cell lung cancer by fragile site expression. Teratog Carcinog Mutagen 2002;22:205–215.
1489. Dhillon VS, Husain SA, Ray GN. Expression of aphidicolin-induced fragile sites and their relationship between genetic susceptibility in breast cancer, ovarian cancer, and non-small-cell lung cancer patients. Teratog Carcinog Mutagen 2003;(suppl 1):35–45.
1490. Spitz MR, Hsu TC, Wu X, Fueger JJ, Amos CI, Roth JA. Mutagen sensitivity as a biological marker of lung cancer risk in African Americans. Cancer Epidemiol Biomarkers Prev 1995;4:99–103.
1491. Strom SS, Wu S, Sigurdson AJ, et al. Lung cancer, smoking patterns, and mutagen sensitivity in Mexican-Americans. J Natl Cancer Inst Monogr 1995;(18):29–33.
1492. Spitz MR, Wu X, Jiang H, Hsu TC. Mutagen sensitivity as a marker of cancer susceptibility. J Cell Biochem Suppl 1996;25:80–84.
1493. Kawajiri K, Nakachi K, Imai K, Watanabe J, Hayashi S. Germ line polymorphisms of p53 and CYP1A1 genes involved in human lung cancer. Carcinogenesis 1993;14:1085–1089.
1494. Wang YC, Chen CY, Chen SK, Chang YY, Lin P. p53 codon 72 polymorphism in Taiwanese lung cancer patients: association with lung cancer susceptibility and prognosis. Clin Cancer Res 1999; 5:129–134.
1495. Biros E, Kalina I, Kohut A, Stubna J, Salagovic J. Germ line polymorphisms of the tumor suppressor gene p53 and lung cancer. Lung Cancer 2001;31:157–162.
1496. Hwang SJ, Cheng LS, Lozano G, Amos CI, Gu X, Strong LC. Lung cancer risk in germline p53 mutation carriers: association between an inherited cancer predisposition, cigarette smoking, and cancer risk. Hum Genet 2003;113:238–243.
1497. Lee SJ, Lee SY, Jeon HS, et al. Vascular endothelial growth factor gene polymorphisms and risk of primary lung cancer. Cancer Epidemiol Biomarkers Prev 2005;14:571–575.
1498. Park SH, Lee GY, Jeon HS, et al. –93G → A polymorphism of hMLH1 and risk of primary lung cancer. Int J Cancer 2004;112:678–682.
1499. Tokumoto H. Analysis of HLA-DRB1–related alleles in Japanese patients with lung cancer—relationship to genetic susceptibility and resistance to lung cancer. J Cancer Res Clin Oncol 1998;124:511–516.
1500. Lindstedt BA, Ryberg D, Zienolddiny S, Khan H, Haugen A. Hras1 VNTR alleles as susceptibility markers for lung cancer: relationship to microsatellite instability in tumors. Anticancer Res 1999;19:5523–5527.
1501. Rosell R, Calvo R, Sanchez JJ, et al. Genetic susceptibility associated with rare HRAS1 variable number of tandem repeats alleles in Spanish non-small cell lung cancer patients. Clin Cancer Res 1999;5:1849–1854.
1502. Pierce LM, Sivaraman L, Chang W, et al. Relationships of TP53 codon 72 and HRAS1 polymorphisms with lung cancer risk in an ethnically diverse population. Cancer Epidemiol Biomarkers Prev 2000;9:1199–1204.
1503. Wang M, Wang Y, You M. Identification of genetic polymorphisms through comparative DNA sequence analysis on the K-ras gene: implications for lung tumor susceptibility. Exp Lung Res 2005;31:165–177.
1504. Schenk S, Schraml P, Bendik I, Ludwig CU. A novel polymorphism in the promoter of the RAGE gene is associated with non-small cell lung cancer. Lung Cancer 2001;32:7–12.
1505. Zhu Y, Spitz MR, Lei L, Mills GB, Wu X. A single nucleotide polymorphism in the matrix metalloproteinase-1 promoter enhances lung cancer susceptibility. Cancer Res 2001;61:7825–7829.
1506. Yu C, Pan K, Xing D, et al. Correlation between a single nucleotide polymorphism in the matrix metalloproteinase-2 promoter and risk of lung cancer. Cancer Res 2002,62.6430–6433.
1507. Hu Z, Huo X, Lu D, et al. Functional polymorphisms of matrix metalloproteinase-9 are associated with risk of occurrence and metastasis of lung cancer. Clin Cancer Res 2005;11:5433–5439.
1508. Zhang J, Jin X, Fang S, et al. The functional polymorphism in the matrix metalloproteinase-7 promoter increases susceptibility to esophageal squamous cell carcinoma, gastric cardiac adenocarcinoma and non-small cell lung carcinoma. Carcinogenesis 2005;26:1748–1753.
1509. Zhou Y, Yu C, Miao X, et al. Functional haplotypes in the promoter of matrix metalloproteinase-2 and lung cancer susceptibility. Carcinogenesis 2005;26:1117–1121.
1510. Feyler A, Voho A, Bouchardy C, et al. Point: myeloperoxidase –463G → a polymorphism and lung cancer risk. Cancer Epidemiol Biomarkers Prev 2002;11:1550–1554.
1511. Kantarci OH, Lesnick TG, Yang P, et al. Myeloperoxidase –463 (G → A) polymorphism associated with lower risk of lung cancer. Mayo Clin Proc 2002;77:17–22.
1512. Schabath MB, Spitz MR, Hong WK, et al. A myeloperoxidase polymorphism associated with reduced risk of lung cancer. Lung Cancer 2002;37:35–40.
1513. Xu LL, Liu G, Miller DP, et al. Counterpoint: the myeloperoxidase –463G → a polymorphism does not decrease lung cancer susceptibility in Caucasians. Cancer Epidemiol Biomarkers Prev 2002;11:1555–1559.

1514. Liu G, Zhou W, Wang LI, et al. MPO and SOD2 polymorphisms, gender, and the risk of non-small cell lung carcinoma. Cancer Lett 2004;214:69–79.
1515. Kumimoto H, Hamajima N, Nishimoto Y, et al. L-myc genotype is associated with different susceptibility to lung cancer in smokers. Jpn J Cancer Res 2002;93:1–5.
1516. Shih CM, Kuo YY, Wang YC, et al. Association of L-myc polymorphism with lung cancer susceptibility and prognosis in relation to age-selected controls and stratified cases. Lung Cancer 2002;36:125–132.
1517. Seifart C, Seifart U, Plagens A, Wolf M, von Wichert P. Surfactant protein B gene variations enhance susceptibility to squamous cell carcinoma of the lung in German patients. Br J Cancer 2002;87:212–217.
1518. Seifart C, Lin HM, Seifart U, et al. Rare SP-A alleles and the SP-A1–6A(4) allele associate with risk for lung carcinoma. Clin Genet 2005;68:128–136.
1519. Yanagitani N, Kohno T, Kim JG, et al. Identification of D19S246 as a novel lung adenocarcinoma susceptibility locus by genome survey with 10–cM resolution micro satellite markers. Cancer Epidemiol Biomarkers Prev 2003;12:366–371.
1520. Qiuling S, Yuxin Z, Suhua Z, Cheng X, Shuguang L, Fengsheng H. Cyclin D1 gene polymorphism and susceptibility to lung cancer in a Chinese population. Carcinogenesis 2003;24:1499–1503.
1521. Zienolddiny S, Ryberg D, Maggini V, Skaug V, Canzian F, Haugen A. Polymorphisms of the interleukin-1 beta gene are associated with increased risk of non-small cell lung cancer. Int J Cancer 2004;109:353–356.
1522. Lind H, Zienolddiny S, Ryberg D, Skaug V, Phillips DH, Haugen A. Interleukin 1 receptor antagonist gene polymorphism and risk of lung cancer: a possible interaction with polymorphisms in the interleukin 1 beta gene. Lung Cancer 2005;50:285–290.
1523. Shih CM, Lee YL, Chiou HL, et al. The involvement of genetic polymorphism of IL-10 promoter in non-small cell lung cancer. Lung Cancer 2005;50:291–297.
1524. Jeng YL, Wu MH, Huang HB, et al. The methylenetetrahydrofolate reductase 677C → T polymorphism and lung cancer risk in a Chinese population. Anticancer Res 2003;23:5149–5152.
1525. Li G, Wang LE, Chamberlain RM, Amos CI, Spitz MR, Wei Q. p73 G4C14–to-A4T14 polymorphism and risk of lung cancer. Cancer Res 2004;64:6863–6866.
1526. Schabath MB, Wu X, Wei Q, Li G, Gu J, Spitz MR. Combined effects of the p53 and p73 polymorphisms on lung cancer risk. Cancer Epidemiol Biomarkers Prev 2006; 15:158–161.
1527. Lee SJ, Jeon HS, Jang JS, et al. DNMT3B polymorphisms and risk of primary lung cancer. Carcinogenesis 2005;26:403–409.
1528. Hu Z, Miao X, Ma H, et al. A common polymorphism in the 3′UTR of cyclooxygenase 2/prostaglandin synthase 2 gene and risk of lung cancer in a Chinese population. Lung Cancer 2005;48:11–17.
1529. Sorensen M, Autrup H, Tjonneland A, Overvad K, Raaschou-Nielsen O. A genetic polymorphism in prostaglandin synthase 2 (8473, T → C) and the risk of lung cancer. Cancer Lett 2005;226:49–54.
1530. Park JM, Choi JE, Chae MH, et al. Relationship between cyclooxygenase 8473T > C polymorphism and the risk of lung cancer: a case-control study. BMC Cancer 2006;6: 70.
1531. Marsit CJ, Wiencke JK, Liu M, Kelsey KT. The race associated allele of Semaphorin 3B (SEMA3B) T415I and its role in lung cancer in African-Americans and Latino-Americans. Carcinogenesis 2005;26:1446–1449.
1532. Shen M, Rothman N, Berndt SI, et al. Polymorphisms in folate metabolic genes and lung cancer risk in Xuan Wei, China. Lung Cancer 2005;49:299–309.
1533. Zhang X, Miao X, Sun T, et al. Functional polymorphisms in cell death pathway genes FAS and FASL contribute to risk of lung cancer. J Med Genet 2005;42:479–484.
1534. Razmkhah M, Doroudchi M, Ghayumi SM, Erfani N, Ghaderi A. Stromal cell-derived factor-1 (SDF-1) gene and susceptibility of Iranian patients with lung cancer. Lung Cancer 2005;49:311–315.
1535. Yang P, Bamlet WR, Sun Z, et al. Alpha1–antitrypsin and neutrophil elastase imbalance and lung cancer risk. Chest 2005;128:445–452.
1536. Hu Z, Ma H, Lu D, et al. Genetic variants in the MDM2 promoter and lung cancer risk in a Chinese population. Int J Cancer 2006;118:1275–1278.
1537. Li G, Zhai X, Zhang Z, Chamberlain RM, Spitz MR, Wei Q. MDM2 gene promoter polymorphisms and risk of lung cancer: a case-control analysis. Carcinogenesis 2006;27:2028–2033.
1538. Lind H, Zienolddiny S, Ekstrom PO, Skaug V, Haugen A. Association of a functional polymorphism in the promoter of the MDM2 gene with risk of nonsmall cell lung cancer. Int J Cancer 2006;119:718–721.
1539. Bell DW, Gore I, Okimoto RA, et al. Inherited susceptibility to lung cancer may be associated with the T790M drug resistance mutation in EGFR. Nat Genet 2005; 37:1315–1316.
1540. Jang JS, Lee SJ, Choi JE, et al. Methyl-CpG binding domain 1 gene polymorphisms and risk of primary lung cancer. Cancer Epidemiol Biomarkers Prev 2005;14: 2474–2480.
1541. Shin MC, Lee SJ, Choi JE, et al. Glu346lys Polymorphism in the Methyl-Cpg Binding Domain 4 Gene and the Risk of Primary Lung Cancer. Jpn J Clin Oncol 2006;36:483–488.
1542. Kang HG, Chae MH, Park JM, et al. Polymorphisms in TGF-beta1 gene and the risk of lung cancer. Lung Cancer 2006;52:1–7.
1543. Spinola M, Meyer P, Kammerer S, et al. Association of the PDCD5 locus with lung cancer risk and prognosis in smokers. J Clin Oncol 2006;24:1672–1678.
1544. Ribeiro R, Araujo AP, Coelho A, et al. A functional polymorphism in the promoter region of leptin gene increases susceptibility for non-small cell lung cancer. Eur J Cancer 2006;42:1188–1193.
1545. Park JY, Park JM, Jang JS, et al. Caspase 9 promoter polymorphisms and risk of primary lung cancer. Hum Mol Genet 2006;15:1963–1971.
1546. Rudd MF, Webb EL, Matakidou A, et al. GELCAPS Consortium. Variants in the GH-IGF axis confer susceptibility to lung cancer. Genome Res 2006;16:693–701.

1547. Hanash S. Integrated global profiling of cancer. Nature Reviews Cancer 2004;4:638–643.

1548. Liu LT, Chang HC, Chiang LC, Hung WC. Histone deacetylase inhibitor up-regulates RECK to inhibit MMP-2 activation and cancer cell invasion. Cancer Res 2003;63:3069–3072.

1549. Hayashi H, Miyamoto H, Ito T, et al. Analysis of p21Waf1/Cip1 expression in normal, premalignant, and malignant cells during the development of human lung adenocarcinoma. Am J Pathol 1997;151:461–470.

1550. Kim S, Jung Y, Kim D, Koh H, Chung J. Extracellular zinc activates p70 S6 kinase through the phosphatidylinositol 3–kinase signaling pathway. J Biol Chem 2000;275: 25979–25984.

1551. Moore SM, Rintoul RC, Walker TR, Chilvers ER, Haslett C, Sethi T. The presence of a constitutively active phosphoinositide 3–kinase in small cell lung cancer cells mediates anchorage-independent proliferation via a protein kinase B and p70s6k-dependent pathway. Cancer Res 1998;58:5239–5247.

1552. Singhal S, Amin KM, Kruklitis R, et al. Alterations in cell cycle genes in early stage lung adenocarcinoma identified by expression profiling. Cancer Biol Ther 2003;2:291–298.

1553. Wistuba, II, Behrens C, Milchgrub S, et al. Sequential molecular abnormalities are involved in the multistage development of squamous cell lung carcinoma. Oncogene 1999;18:643–650.

1554. Ullmann R, Bongiovanni M, Halbwedl I, et al. Bronchiolar columnar cell dysplasia—genetic analysis of a novel preneoplastic lesion of peripheral lung. Virchows Arch 2003;442:429–436.

1555. Miller RR. Alveolar atypical hyperplasia in association with primary pulmonary adenocarcinoma: a clinicopathological study of 10 cases. Thorax 1993;48:679–680.

1556. Stacher E, Ullmann R, Halbwedl I, et al. Atypical goblet cell hyperplasia in congenital cystic adenomatoid malformation as a possible preneoplasia for pulmonary adenocarcinoma in childhood: a genetic analysis. Hum Pathol 2004;35:565–570.

1557. Ullmann R, Bongiovanni M, Halbwedl I, et al. Is high-grade adenomatous hyperplasia an early bronchioloalveolar adenocarcinoma? J Pathol 2003;201:371–376.

1558. Simon R, Eltze E, Schafer KL, et al. Cytogenetic analysis of multifocal bladder cancer supports a monoclonal origin and intraepithelial spread of tumor cells. Cancer Res 2001;61:355–362.

1559. Brader S, Eccles SA. Phosphoinositide 3-kinase signalling pathways in tumor progression, invasion and angiogenesis. Tumori 2004;90:2–8.

1560. Kumaki F, Matsui K, Kawai T, et al. Expression of matrix metalloproteinases in invasive pulmonary adenocarcinoma with bronchioloalveolar component and atypical adenomatous hyperplasia. Am J Pathol 2001;159:2125–2135.

1561. Park BK, Zeng X, Glazer RI. Akt1 induces extracellular matrix invasion and matrix metalloproteinase-2 activity in mouse mammary epithelial cells. Cancer Res 2001; 61:7647–7653.

1562. Masuya D, Huang C, Liu D, et al. The tumour-stromal interaction between intratumoral c-Met and stromal hepatocyte growth factor associated with tumour growth and prognosis in non-small-cell lung cancer patients. Br J Cancer 2004;90:1555–1562.

1563. Brabek J, Constancio SS, Shin NY, Pozzi A, Weaver AM, Hanks SK. CAS promotes invasiveness of Src-transformed cells. Oncogene 2004;23:7406–7415.

1564. Cheng CH, Yu KC, Chen HL, et al. Blockade of v-Src-stimulated tumor formation by the Src homology 3 domain of Crk-associated substrate (Cas). FEBS Lett 2004;557:221–227.

1565. Guerrero S, Casanova I, Farre L, Mazo A, Capella G, Mangues R. K-ras codon 12 mutation induces higher level of resistance to apoptosis and predisposition to anchorage-independent growth than codon 13 mutation or proto-oncogene overexpression. Cancer Res 2000;60: 6750–6756.

1566. Yokota J, Nishioka M, Tani M, Kohno T. Genetic alterations responsible for metastatic phenotypes of lung cancer cells. Clin Exp Metastasis 2003;20:189–193.

1567. Altun-Gultekin ZF, Chandriani S, Bougeret C, et al. Activation of Rho-dependent cell spreading and focal adhesion biogenesis by the v-Crk adaptor protein. Mol Cell Biol 1998;18:3044–3058.

1568. Harte MT, Hildebrand JD, Burnham MR, Bouton AH, Parsons JT. p130Cas, a substrate associated with v-Src and v-Crk, localizes to focal adhesions and binds to focal adhesion kinase. J Biol Chem 1996;271:13649–13655.

1569. Wang KK, Liu N, Radulovich N, et al. Novel candidate tumor marker genes for lung adenocarcinoma. Oncogene 2002;21:7598–7604.

1570. Burger M, Glodek A, Hartmann T, et al. Functional expression of CXCR4 (CD184) on small-cell lung cancer cells mediates migration, integrin activation, and adhesion to stromal cells. Oncogene 2003;22:8093–8101.

1571. Fujikawa K, de Aos Scherpenseel I, Jain SK, Presman E, Christensen RA, Varticovski L. Role of PI 3–kinase in angiopoietin-1–mediated migration and attachment-dependent survival of endothelial cells. Exp Cell Res 1999;253:663–672.

1572. Shelly C, Herrera R. Activation of SGK1 by HGF, Rac1 and integrin-mediated cell adhesion in MDCK cells: PI-3K-dependent and -independent pathways. J Cell Sci 2002;115:1985–1993.

1573. Allinen M, Beroukhim R, Cai L, et al. Molecular characterization of the tumor microenvironment in breast cancer. Cancer Cell 2004;6:17–32.

1574. Kurose K, Gilley K, Matsumoto S, et al. Frequent somatic mutations in PTEN and TP53 are mutually exclusive in the stroma of breast carcinomas. Nat Genet 2002; 32:355–357.

1575. Tuhkanen H, Anttila M, Kosma VM, et al. Genetic alterations in the peritumoral stromal cells of malignant and borderline epithelial ovarian tumors as indicated by allelic imbalance on chromosome 3p. Int J Cancer 2004;109:247–252.

1576. Barbera MJ, Puig I, Dominguez D, et al. Regulation of Snail transcription during epithelial to mesenchymal transition of tumor cells. Oncogene 2004;23:7345–7354.

1577. Xue C, Plieth D, Venkov C, Xu C, Neilson EG. The gatekeeper effect of epithelial-mesenchymal transition regu-

lates the frequency of breast cancer metastasis. Cancer Res 2003;63:3386–3394.
1578. Zavadil J, Cermak L, Soto-Nieves N, Bottinger EP. Integration of TGF-beta/Smad and Jagged1/Notch signalling in epithelial-to-mesenchymal transition. Embo J 2004;23:1155–1165.
1579. Garantziotis S, Steele MP, Schwartz DA. Pulmonary fibrosis: thinking outside of the lung. J Clin Invest 2004;114:319–321.
1580. Hallermalm K, De Geer A, Kiessling R, Levitsky V, Levitskaya J. Autocrine secretion of Fas ligand shields tumor cells from Fas-mediated killing by cytotoxic lymphocytes. Cancer Res 2004;64:6775–6782.
1581. Brandlein S, Pohle T, Ruoff N, Wozniak E, Muller-Hermelink HK, Vollmers HP. Natural IgM antibodies and immunosurveillance mechanisms against epithelial cancer cells in humans. Cancer Res 2003;63:7995–8005.
1582. Bergqvist M, Brattstrom D, Lamberg K, et al. The presence of anti-p53 antibodies in sera prior to thoracic surgery in non small cell lung cancer patients: its implications on tumor volume, nodal involvement, and survival. Neoplasia 2003;5:283–287.
1583. Casares N, Arribillaga L, Sarobe P, et al. CD4+/CD25+ regulatory cells inhibit activation of tumor-primed CD4+ T cells with IFN-gamma-dependent antiangiogenic activity, as well as long-lasting tumor immunity elicited by peptide vaccination. J Immunol 2003;171:5931–5939.
1584. Turk MJ, Guevara-Patino JA, Rizzuto GA, Engelhorn ME, Houghton AN. Concomitant tumor immunity to a poorly immunogenic melanoma is prevented by regulatory T cells. J Exp Med 2004;200:771–782.
1585. Wang HY, Lee DA, Peng G, et al. Tumor-specific human CD4+ regulatory T cells and their ligands: implications for immunotherapy. Immunity 2004;20:107–118.
1586. Aoudjit F, Guo W, Gagnon-Houde JV, et al. HLA-DR signaling inhibits Fas mediated apoptosis in A375 mela noma cells. Exp Cell Res 2004;299:79–90.
1587. Atkins D, Ferrone S, Schmahl GE, Storkel S, Seliger B. Down-regulation of HLA class I antigen processing molecules: an immune escape mechanism of renal cell carcinoma? J Urol 2004;171:885–889.
1588. Makarenkova VP, Shurin GV, Tourkova IL, et al. Lung cancer-derived bombesin-like peptides down-regulate the generation and function of human dendritic cells. J Neuroimmunol 2003;145:55–67.
1589. Ohshima K, Hamasaki M, Makimoto Y, et al. Differential chemokine, chemokine receptor, cytokine and cytokine receptor expression in pulmonary adenocarcinoma: diffuse down-regulation is associated with immune evasion and brain metastasis. Int J Oncol 2003;23:965–973.
1590. Ullmann R, Morbini P, Halbwedl I, et al. Protein expression profiles in adenocarcinomas and squamous cell carcinomas of the lung generated using tissue microarrays. J Pathol 2004;203:798–807.
1591. Sugita J, Ohtani H, Mizoi T, et al. Close association between Fas ligand (FasL; CD95L)-positive tumor-associated macrophages and apoptotic cancer cells along invasive margin of colorectal carcinoma: a proposal on tumor-host interactions. Jpn J Cancer Res 2002;93:320–328.
1592. Zusman I, Gurevich P, Gurevich E, Ben-Hur H. The immune system, apoptosis and apoptosis-related proteins in human ovarian tumors (a review). Int J Oncol 2001;18:965–972.
1593. Hataji O, Taguchi O, Gabazza EC, et al. Increased circulating levels of thrombin-activatable fibrinolysis inhibitor in lung cancer patients. Am J Hematol 2004;76:214–219.
1594. Cha HJ, Jeong MJ, Kleinman HK. Role of thymosin beta4 in tumor metastasis and angiogenesis. J Natl Cancer Inst 2003;95:1674–1680.
1595. Diederichs S, Bulk E, Steffen B, et al. S100 family members and trypsinogens are predictors of distant metastasis and survival in early-stage non-small cell lung cancer. Cancer Res 2004;64:5564–5569.
1596. Goncharuk VN, del-Rosario A, Kren L, et al. Co-downregulation of PTEN, KAI-1, and nm23-H1 tumor/metastasis suppressor proteins in non-small cell lung cancer. Ann Diagn Pathol 2004;8:6–16.
1597. Ji P, Diederichs S, Wang W, et al. MALAT-1, a novel non-coding RNA, and thymosin beta4 predict metastasis and survival in early-stage non-small cell lung cancer. Oncogene 2003;22:8031–8041.
1598. Kikuchi T, Daigo Y, Katagiri T, et al. Expression profiles of non-small cell lung cancers on cDNA microarrays: identification of genes for prediction of lymph-node metastasis and sensitivity to anti-cancer drugs. Oncogene 2003;22:2192–2205.
1599. Yang J, Mani SA, Donaher JL, et al. Twist, a master regulator of morphogenesis, plays an essential role in tumor metastasis. Cell 2004;117:927–939.
1600. Natori T, Sata M, Washida M, Hirata Y, Nagai R, Makuuchi M. Nicotine enhances neovascularization and promotes tumor growth. Mol Cells 2003;16:143–146.
1601. Yen L, You XL, Al Moustafa AE, et al. Heregulin selectively upregulates vascular endothelial growth factor secretion in cancer cells and stimulates angiogenesis. Oncogene 2000;19:3460–3469.
1602. Su JL, Shih JY, Yen ML, et al. Cyclooxygenase-2 induces EP1- and HER-2/Neu-dependent vascular endothelial growth factor-C up-regulation: a novel mechanism of lymphangiogenesis in lung adenocarcinoma. Cancer Res 2004;64:554–564.
1603. Arinaga M, Noguchi T, Takeno S, et al. Clinical significance of vascular endothelial growth factor C and vascular endothelial growth factor receptor 3 in patients with nonsmall cell lung carcinoma. Cancer 2003;97:457–464.
1604. Bartoli M, Platt D, Lemtalsi T, et al. VEGF differentially activates STAT3 in microvascular endothelial cells. Faseb J 2003;17:1562–1564.
1605. Cooke JP, Bitterman H. Nicotine and angiogenesis: a new paradigm for tobacco-related diseases. Ann Med 2004;36:33–40.
1606. Philp D, Huff T, Gho YS, Hannappel E, Kleinman HK. The actin binding site on thymosin beta4 promotes angiogenesis. Faseb J 2003;17:2103–2105. Epub 2003 Sep 2118.
1607. Shields PG. Epidemiology of tobacco carcinogenesis. Curr Oncol Rep 2000;2:257–262.

1608. Shimada T, Sugie A, Shindo M, et al. Tissue-specific induction of cytochromes P450 1A1 and 1B1 by polycyclic aromatic hydrocarbons and polychlorinated biphenyls in engineered C57BL/6J mice of arylhydrocarbon receptor gene. Toxicol Appl Pharmacol 2003;187:1–10.
1609. Blair IA. Lipid hydroperoxide-mediated DNA damage. Exp Gerontol 2001;36:1473–1481.
1610. Box HC, Dawidzik JB, Budzinski EE. Free radical-induced double lesions in DNA. Free Radic Biol Med 2001;31:856–868.
1611. Cadet J, Delatour T, Douki T, et al. Hydroxyl radicals and DNA base damage. Mutat Res 1999;424:9–21.
1612. Leonard SS, Bower JJ, Shi X. Metal-induced toxicity, carcinogenesis, mechanisms and cellular responses. Mol Cell Biochem 2004;255:3–10.
1613. Martinez GR, Loureiro AP, Marques SA, et al. Oxidative and alkylating damage in DNA. Mutat Res 2003;544:115–127.
1614. Pryor WA. Cigarette smoke radicals and the role of free radicals in chemical carcinogenicity. Environ Health Perspect 1997;105(suppl 4):875–882.
1615. Shackelford RE, Kaufmann WK, Paules RS. Oxidative stress and cell cycle checkpoint function. Free Radic Biol Med 2000;28:1387–1404.
1616. Lopez-Larraza DM, Bianchi NO. DNA response to bleomycin in mammalian cells with variable degrees of chromatin condensation. Environ Mol Mutagen 1993;21:258–264.
1617. Cloutier JF, Drouin R, Weinfeld M, O'Connor TR, Castonguay A. Characterization and mapping of DNA damage induced by reactive metabolites of 4–(methylnitrosamino)-1–(3-pyridyl)-1–butanone (NNK) at nucleotide resolution in human genomic DNA. J Mol Biol 2001;313:539–557.
1618. Insinga A, Monestiroli S, Ronzoni S, et al. Inhibitors of histone deacetylases induce tumor-selective apoptosis through activation of the death receptor pathway. Nat Med 2005;11:71–76.
1619. Zhu P, Huber E, Kiefer F, Gottlicher M. Specific and redundant functions of histone deacetylases in regulation of cell cycle and apoptosis. Cell Cycle 2004;3:1240–1242.
1620. Mayo MW, Denlinger CE, Broad RM, et al. Ineffectiveness of histone deacetylase inhibitors to induce apoptosis involves the transcriptional activation of NF-kappa B through the Akt pathway. J Biol Chem 2003;278:18980–18989.
1621. Osada H, Tatematsu Y, Saito H, Yatabe Y, Mitsudomi T, Takahashi T. Reduced expression of class II histone deacetylase genes is associated with poor prognosis in lung cancer patients. Int J Cancer 2004;112:26–32.
1622. Sasaki H, Moriyama S, Nakashima Y, et al. Histone deacetylase 1 mRNA expression in lung cancer. Lung Cancer 2004;46:171–178.
1623. Kasprzak KS, Sunderman FW Jr, Salnikow K. Nickel carcinogenesis. Mutat Res 2003;533:67–97.
1624. Waalkes MP. Cadmium carcinogenesis. Mutat Res 2003;533:107–120.
1625. Braakhuis BJ, Tabor MP, Kummer JA, Leemans CR, Brakenhoff RH. A genetic explanation of Slaughter's concept of field cancerization: evidence and clinical implications. Cancer Res 2003;63:1727–1730.
1626. Hafner C, Knuechel R, Zanardo L, et al. Evidence for oligoclonality and tumor spread by intraluminal seeding in multifocal urothelial carcinomas of the upper and lower urinary tract. Oncogene 2001;20:4910–4915.
1627. Hayes JD, Flanagan JU, Jowsey IR. Glutathione transferases. Annu Rev Pharmacol Toxicol 2005;45:51–88.
1628. Lewis SJ, Cherry NM, Niven RM, Barber PV, Povey AC. Associations between smoking, GST genotypes and N7–methylguanine levels in DNA extracted from bronchial lavage cells. Mutat Res 2004;559:11–18.
1629. Mohr LC, Rodgers JK, Silvestri GA. Glutathione S-transferase M1 polymorphism and the risk of lung cancer. Anticancer Res 2003;23:2111–2124.
1630. Nazar-Stewart V, Vaughan TL, Stapleton P, Van Loo J, Nicol-Blades B, Eaton DL. A population-based study of glutathione S-transferase M1, T1 and P1 genotypes and risk for lung cancer. Lung Cancer 2003;40:247–258.
1631. Pinarbasi H, Silig Y, Cetinkaya O, Seyfikli Z, Pinarbasi E. Strong association between the GSTM1–null genotype and lung cancer in a Turkish population. Cancer Genet Cytogenet 2003;146:125–129.
1632. Reszka E, Wasowicz W, Rydzynski K, Szeszenia-Dabrowska N, Szymczak W. Glutathione S-transferase M1 and P1 metabolic polymorphism and lung cancer predisposition. Neoplasma 2003;50:357–362.
1633. Schneider J, Bernges U, Philipp M, Woitowitz HJ. GSTM1, GSTT1, and GSTP1 polymorphism and lung cancer risk in relation to tobacco smoking. Cancer Lett 2004;208:65–74.
1634. Sgambato A, Campisi B, Zupa A, et al. Glutathione S-transferase (GST) polymorphisms as risk factors for cancer in a highly homogeneous population from southern Italy. Anticancer Res 2002;22:3647–3652.
1635. Stucker I, Hirvonen A, de Waziers I, et al. Genetic polymorphisms of glutathione S-transferases as modulators of lung cancer susceptibility. Carcinogenesis 2002;23:1475–1481.
1636. Wang Y, Spitz MR, Schabath MB, Ali-Osman F, Mata H, Wu X. Association between glutathione S-transferase p1 polymorphisms and lung cancer risk in Caucasians: a case-control study. Lung Cancer 2003;40:25–32.
1637. Svensson R, Pamedytyte V, Juodaityte J, Makuska R, Morgenstern R. Characterisation of polymeric surfactants that are glutathione transferase mimics. Toxicology 2001;168:251–258.
1638. Slupphaug G, Kavli B, Krokan HE. The interacting pathways for prevention and repair of oxidative DNA damage. Mutat Res 2003;531:231–251.
1639. Kim SY, Adachi H, Koo JS, Jetten AM. Induction of the cytochrome P450 gene CYP26 during mucous cell differentiation of normal human tracheobronchial epithelial cells. Mol Pharmacol 2000;58:483–490.
1640. Knaapen AM, Borm PJ, Albrecht C, Schins RP. Inhaled particles and lung cancer. Part A: Mechanisms. Int J Cancer 2004;109:799–809.
1641. Ueng TH, Wang HW, Hung CC, Chang HL. Effects of motorcycle exhaust inhalation exposure on cytochrome P-450 2B1, antioxidant enzymes, and lipid peroxidation

in rat liver and lung. J Toxicol Environ Health A 2004; 67:875–888.
1642. O'Brien TJ, Ceryak S, Patierno SR. Complexities of chromium carcinogenesis: role of cellular response, repair and recovery mechanisms. Mutat Res 2003;533:3–36.
1643. Andrew AS, Warren AJ, Barchowsky A, et al. Genomic and proteomic profiling of responses to toxic metals in human lung cells. Environ Health Perspect 2003;111: 825–835.
1644. Baldwin RM, Shultz MA, Buckpitt AR. Bioactivation of the Pulmonary Toxicants Naphthalene and 1-Nitronaphthalene by Rat Cytochrome CYP2F4. J Pharmacol Exp Ther 2005;312:857–865.
1645. Baulig A, Garlatti M, Bonvallot V, et al. Involvement of reactive oxygen species in the metabolic pathways triggered by diesel exhaust particles in human airway epithelial cells. Am J Physiol Lung Cell Mol Physiol 2003;285: L671–L679.
1646. Buckpitt A, Boland B, Isbell M, et al. Naphthalene-induced respiratory tract toxicity: metabolic mechanisms of toxicity. Drug Metab Rev 2002;34:791–820.
1647. Le Marchand L, Guo C, Benhamou S, et al. Pooled analysis of the CYP1A1 exon 7 polymorphism and lung cancer (United States). Cancer Causes Control 2003;14:339–346.
1648. Rengasamy A, Barger MW, Kane E, Ma JK, Castranova V, Ma JY. Diesel exhaust particle-induced alterations of pulmonary phase I and phase II enzymes of rats. J Toxicol Environ Health A 2003;66:153–167.
1649. Collins AR. Molecular epidemiology in cancer research. Mol Aspects Med 1998;19:359–432.
1650. Godin DV, Garnett ME. Species-related variations in tissue antioxidant status—I. Differences in antioxidant enzyme profiles. Comp Biochem Physiol B 1992;103: 737–742.
1651. Stagsted J, Young JF. Large differences in erythrocyte stability between species reflect different antioxidative defense mechanisms. Free Radic Res 2002;36:779–789.
1652. Dorger M, Allmeling AM, Neuber A, Behr J, Rambeck W, Krombach F. Interspecies comparison of rat and hamster alveolar macrophage antioxidative and oxidative capacity. Environ Health Perspect 1997;105(suppl 5): 1309–1312.
1653. Hissink AM, Oudshoorn MJ, Van Ommen B, Van Bladeren PJ. Species and strain differences in the hepatic cytochrome P450–mediated biotransformation of 1,4–dichlorobenzene. Toxicol Appl Pharmacol 1997;145:1–9.
1654. Bryan CL, Jenkinson SG. Species variation in lung antioxidant enzyme activities. J Appl Physiol 1987;63: 597–602.
1655. Pitarque M, von Richter O, Rodriguez-Antona C, Wang J, Oscarson M, Ingelman-Sundberg M. A nicotine C-oxidase gene (CYP2A6) polymorphism important for promoter activity. Hum Mutat 2004;23:258–266.
1656. Wang H, Tan W, Hao B, et al. Substantial reduction in risk of lung adenocarcinoma associated with genetic polymorphism in CYP2A13, the most active cytochrome P450 for the metabolic activation of tobacco-specific carcinogen NNK. Cancer Res 2003;63:8057–8061.
1657. Serabjit-Singh CJ, Nishio SJ, Philpot RM, Plopper CG. The distribution of cytochrome P-450 monooxygenase in cells of the rabbit lung: an ultrastructural immunocytochemical characterization. Mol Pharmacol 1988;33: 279–289.
1658. Sipal Z, Ahlenius T, Bergstrand A, Rodriquez L, Jakobsson SW. Oxidative biotransformation of benzo(a) pyrene by human lung microsomal fractions prepared from surgical specimens. Xenobiotica 1979;9:633–645.
1659. Dash BC, El-Deiry WS. Cell cycle checkpoint control mechanisms that can be disrupted in cancer. Methods Mol Biol 2004;280:99–161.
1660. Kolas NK, Cohen PE. Novel and diverse functions of the DNA mismatch repair family in mammalian meiosis and recombination. Cytogenet Genome Res 2004;107: 216–231.
1661. Koundrioukoff S, Polo S, Almouzni G. Interplay between chromatin and cell cycle checkpoints in the context of ATR/ATM-dependent checkpoints, DNA Repair (Amst) 2004;3:969–978.
1662. Sancar A, Lindsey-Boltz LA, Unsal-Kacmaz K, Linn S. Molecular mechanisms of mammalian DNA repair and the DNA damage checkpoints. Annu Rev Biochem 2004;73:39–85.
1663. Surtees JA, Argueso JL, Alani E. Mismatch repair proteins: key regulators of genetic recombination. Cytogenet Genome Res 2004;107:146–159.
1664. Ljungman M, Lane DP. Transcription—guarding the genome by sensing DNA damage. Nat Rev Cancer 2004;4:727–737.
1665. Norbury CJ, Zhivotovsky B. DNA damage-induced apoptosis. Oncogene 2004;23:2797–2808.
1666. Pastwa E, Blasiak J. Non-homologous DNA end joining. Acta Biochim Pol 2003;50:891–908.
1667. Mone MJ, Bernas T, Dinant C, et al. In vivo dynamics of chromatin-associated complex formation in mammalian nucleotide excision repair. Proc Natl Acad Sci USA 2004;101:15933–15937.
1668. Tauchi H, Kobayashi J, Morishima K, et al. Nbs1 is essential for DNA repair by homologous recombination in higher vertebrate cells. Nature 2002;420:93–98.
1669. Berardi P, Russell M, El-Osta A, Riabowol K. Functional links between transcription, DNA repair and apoptosis. Cell Mol Life Sci 2004;61:2173–2180.
1670. Zhivotovsky B, Kroemer G. Apoptosis and genomic instability. Nat Rev Mol Cell Biol 2004;5:752–762.
1671. Zink D, Fische AH, Nickerson JA. Nuclear structure in cancer cells. Nat Rev Cancer 2004;4:677–687.
1672. Zhang P, Chin W, Chow LT, et al. Lack of expression for the suppressor PML in human small cell lung carcinoma. Int J Cancer 2000;85:599–605.
1673. Berrieman HK, Ashman JN, Cowen ME, Greenman J, Lind MJ, Cawkwell L. Chromosomal analysis of non-small-cell lung cancer by multicolour fluorescent in situ hybridization. Br J Cancer 2004;90:900–905.
1674. Fong KM, Biesterveld EJ, Virmani A, et al. FHIT and FRA3B 3p14.2 allele loss are common in lung cancer and preneoplastic bronchial lesions and are associated with cancer-related FHIT cDNA splicing aberrations. Cancer Res 1997;57:2256–2267.

1675. Kashuba VI, Li J, Wang F, et al. RBSP3 (HYA22) is a tumor suppressor gene implicated in major epithelial malignancies. Proc Natl Acad Sci USA 2004;101:4906–4911.
1676. Burbee DG, Forgacs E, Zochbauer-Muller S, et al. Epigenetic inactivation of RASSF1A in lung and breast cancers and malignant phenotype suppression. J Natl Cancer Inst 2001;93:691–699.
1677. Graziano SL, Pfeifer AM, Testa JR, et al. Involvement of the RAF1 locus, at band 3p25, in the 3p deletion of small-cell lung cancer. Am J Pathol 1991;139:317–325.
1678. Song MS, Song SJ, Ayad NG, et al. The tumour suppressor RASSF1A regulates mitosis by inhibiting the APC-Cdc20 complex. Nat Cell Biol 2004;6:129–137.
1679. Massion PP, Taflan PM, Shyr Y, et al. Early involvement of the phosphatidylinositol 3–kinase/Akt pathway in lung cancer progression. Am J Respir Crit Care Med 2004;170: 1088–1094.
1680. Krystal GW, Sulanke G, Litz J. Inhibition of phosphatidylinositol 3–kinase-Akt signaling blocks growth, promotes apoptosis, and enhances sensitivity of small cell lung cancer cells to chemotherapy. Mol Cancer Ther 2002;1:913–922.
1681. Boccaccio C, Ando M, Tamagnone L, et al. Induction of epithelial tubules by growth factor HGF depends on the STAT pathway. Nature 1998;391:285–288.
1682. Ma PC, Kijima T, Maulik G, et al. c-MET mutational analysis in small cell lung cancer: novel juxtamembrane domain mutations regulating cytoskeletal functions. Cancer Res 2003;63:6272–6281.
1683. Rygaard K, Nakamura T, Spang-Thomsen M. Expression of the proto-oncogenes c-met and c-kit and their ligands, hepatocyte growth factor/scatter factor and stem cell factor, in SCLC cell lines and xenografts. Br J Cancer 1993;67:37–46.
1684. Maulik G, Kijima T, Ma PC, et al. Modulation of the c-Met/hepatocyte growth factor pathway in small cell lung cancer. Clin Cancer Res 2002;8:620–627.
1685. Krystal GW, DeBerry CS, Linnekin D, Litz J. Lck associates with and is activated by Kit in a small cell lung cancer cell line: inhibition of SCF-mediated growth by the Src family kinase inhibitor PP1. Cancer Res 1998;58:4660–4666.
1686. Uchida K, Kojima A, Morokawa N, et al. Expression of progastrin-releasing peptide and gastrin-releasing peptide receptor mRNA transcripts in tumor cells of patients with small cell lung cancer. J Cancer Res Clin Oncol 2002; 128:633–640.
1687. Senderowicz AM, Viard-Leveugle I, Veyrenc S, French LE, Brambilla C, Brambilla E. Small-molecule cyclin-dependent kinase modulators: Frequent loss of Fas expression and function in human lung tumours with overexpression of FasL in small cell lung carcinoma. Oncogene 2003;22:6609–6620.
1688. Konishi H, Sugiyama M, Mizuno K, et al. Detailed characterization of a homozygously deleted region corresponding to a candidate tumor suppressor locus at distal 17p13.3 in human lung cancer. Oncogene 2003;22:1892–1905.
1689. Yatabe Y, Osada H, Tatematsu Y, Mitsudomi T, Takahashi T. Decreased expression of 14-3-3sigma in neuroendocrine tumors is independent of origin and malignant potential. Oncogene 2002;21:8310–8319.
1690. Dougherty MK, Morrison DK. Unlocking the code of 14-3-3, J Cell Sci 2004;117:1875–1884.
1691. Hermeking H. The 14-3-3 cancer connection. Nat Rev Cancer 2003;3:931–943.
1692. Kovacina KS, Park GY, Bae SS, et al. Identification of a proline-rich Akt substrate as a 14-3-3 binding partner. J Biol Chem 2003;278:10189–10194.
1693. Masters SC, Subramanian RR, Truong A, et al. Survival-promoting functions of 14-3-3 proteins. Biochem Soc Trans 2002;30:360–365.
1694. Nomura M, Shimizu S, Sugiyama T, et al. 14-3-3 Interacts directly with and negatively regulates pro-apoptotic Bax. J Biol Chem 2003;278:2058–2065.
1695. Qi W, Liu X, Qiao D, Martinez JD. Isoform-specific expression of 14-3-3 proteins in human lung cancer tissues. Int J Cancer 2005;113:359–363.
1696. Forgacs E, Biesterveld EJ, Sekido Y, et al. Mutation analysis of the PTEN/MMAC1 gene in lung cancer. Oncogene 1998;17:1557–1565.
1697. Harbour JW, Lai SL, Whang-Peng J, Gazdar AF, Minna JD, Kaye FJ. Abnormalities in structure and expression of the human retinoblastoma gene in SCLC. Science 1988;241:353–357.
1698. Futami H, Egawa S, Takasaki K, Tsukada T, Shiraishi M, Yamaguchi K. Allelic loss of DNA locus of the RET proto-oncogene in small cell lung cancer. Cancer Lett 2003;195:59–65.
1699. Carbone DP, Koros AM, Linnoila RI, Jewett P, Gazdar AF. Neural cell adhesion molecule expression and messenger RNA splicing patterns in lung cancer cell lines are correlated with neuroendocrine phenotype and growth morphology. Cancer Res 1991;51:6142–6149.
1700. Popper HH. Bronchiolitis, an update. Virchows Arch 2000;437:471–481.
1701. Aoyagi Y, Yokose T, Minami Y, et al. Accumulation of losses of heterozygosity and multistep carcinogenesis in pulmonary adenocarcinoma. Cancer Res 2001;61: 7950–7954.
1702. Borczuk AC, Gorenstein L, Walter KL, Assaad AA, Wang L, Powell CA. Non-small-cell lung cancer molecular signatures recapitulate lung developmental pathways. Am J Pathol 2003;163:1949–1960.
1703. Copin MC, Buisine MP, Devisme L, et al. Normal respiratory mucosa, precursor lesions and lung carcinomas: differential expression of human mucin genes. Front Biosci 2001;6:D1264–1275.
1704. Mori M, Rao SK, Popper HH, Cagle PT, Fraire AE. Atypical adenomatous hyperplasia of the lung: a probable forerunner in the development of adenocarcinoma of the lung. Mod Pathol 2001;14:72–84.
1705. Kishimoto Y, Sugio K, Hung JY, et al. Allele-specific loss in chromosome 9p loci in preneoplastic lesions accompanying non-small-cell lung cancers. J Natl Cancer Inst 1995;87:1224–1229.
1706. Massion PP, Taflan PM, Jamshedur Rahman SM, et al. Significance of p63 amplification and overexpression in lung cancer development and prognosis. Cancer Res 2003;63:7113–7121.

1707. Park IW, Wistuba II, Maitra A, et al. Multiple clonal abnormalities in the bronchial epithelium of patients with lung cancer. J Natl Cancer Inst 1999;91:1863–1868.
1708. Singhal S, Amin KM, Kruklitis R, et al. Differentially expressed apoptotic genes in early stage lung adenocarcinoma predicted by expression profiling. Cancer Biol Ther 2003;2:566–571.
1709. Smith SL, Watson SG, Ratschiller D, Gugger M, Betticher DC, Heighway J. Maspin—the most commonly-expressed gene of the 18q21.3 serpin cluster in lung cancer—is strongly expressed in preneoplastic bronchial lesions. Oncogene 2003;22:8677–8687.
1710. Takamochi K, Ogura T, Suzuki K, et al. Loss of heterozygosity on chromosomes 9q and 16p in atypical adenomatous hyperplasia concomitant with adenocarcinoma of the lung. Am J Pathol 2001;159:1941–1948.
1711. Yamasaki M, Takeshima Y, Fujii S, et al. Correlation between genetic alterations and histopathological subtypes in bronchiolo-alveolar carcinoma and atypical adenomatous hyperplasia of the lung. Pathol Int 2000;50: 778–785.
1712. He B, You L, Uematsu K, et al. SOCS-3 is frequently silenced by hypermethylation and suppresses cell growth in human lung cancer. Proc Natl Acad Sci USA 2003; 100:14133–14138.
1713. Lamy A, Sesboue R, Bourguignon J, et al. Aberrant methylation of the CDKN2a/p16INK4a gene promoter region in preinvasive bronchial lesions: a prospective study in high-risk patients without invasive cancer. Int J Cancer 2002;100:189–193.
1714. Maruyama R, Sugio K, Yoshino I, Maehara Y, Gazdar AF. Hypermethylation of FHIT as a prognostic marker in nonsmall cell lung carcinoma. Cancer 2004;100:1472–1477.
1715. Yatabe Y, Mitsudomi T, Takahashi T. Maspin expression in normal lung and non-small-cell lung cancers: cellular property-associated expression under the control of promoter DNA methylation. Oncogene 2004;23:4041–4049.
1716. Dang TP, Gazdar AF, Virmani AK, et al. Chromosome 19 translocation, overexpression of Notch3, and human lung cancer. J Natl Cancer Inst 2000;92:1355–1357.
1717. Sy SM, Wong N, Lee TW, et al. Distinct patterns of genetic alterations in adenocarcinoma and squamous cell carcinoma of the lung. Eur J Cancer 2004;40:1082–1094.
1718. Hashimoto T, Tokuchi Y, Hayashi M, et al. Different subtypes of human lung adenocarcinoma caused by different etiological factors. Evidence from p53 mutational spectra. Am J Pathol 2000;157:2133–2141.
1719. Powell CA, Spira A, Derti A, et al. Gene expression in lung adenocarcinomas of smokers and nonsmokers. Am J Respir Cell Mol Biol 2003;29:157–162.
1720. Sanchez-Cespedes M, Ahrendt SA, Piantadosi S, et al. Chromosomal alterations in lung adenocarcinoma from smokers and nonsmokers. Cancer Res 2001;61:1309–1313.
1721. Wong MP, Fung LF, Wang E, et al. Chromosomal aberrations of primary lung adenocarcinomas in nonsmokers. Cancer 2003;97:1263–1270.
1722. Okada M, Nishio W, Sakamoto T, et al. Correlation between computed tomographic findings, bronchioloalveolar carcinoma component, and biologic behavior of small-sized lung adenocarcinomas. J Thorac Cardiovasc Surg 2004;127:857–861.
1723. Caputi M, Esposito V, Groger AM, et al. Prognostic role of proliferating cell nuclear antigen in lung cancer: an immunohistochemical analysis. In Vivo 1998;12:85–88.
1724. Caputi M, Groeger AM, Esposito V, et al. Prognostic role of cyclin D1 in lung cancer. Relationship to proliferating cell nuclear antigen. Am J Respir Cell Mol Biol 1999; 20:746–750.
1725. Ho CC, Huang PH, Huang HY, Chen YH, Yang PC, Hsu SM. Up-regulated caveolin-1 accentuates the metastasis capability of lung adenocarcinoma by inducing filopodia formation. Am J Pathol 2002;161:1647–1656.
1726. Uchino K, Ito A, Wakayama T, et al. Clinical implication and prognostic significance of the tumor suppressor TSLC1 gene detected in adenocarcinoma of the lung. Cancer 2003;98:1002–1007.
1727. Li ZH, Zheng J, Weiss LM, Shibata D. c-k-ras and p53 mutations occur very early in adenocarcinoma of the lung. Am J Pathol 1994;144:303–309.
1728. Chong H, Vikis HG, Guan KL. Mechanisms of regulating the Raf kinase family. Cell Signal 2003;15:463–469.
1729. Devereux TR, Holliday W, Anna C, Ress N, Roycroft J, Sills RC. Map kinase activation correlates with K-ras mutation and loss of heterozygosity on chromosome 6 in alveolar bronchiolar carcinomas from B6C3F1 mice exposed to vanadium pentoxide for 2 years. Carcinogenesis 2002;23:1737–1743.
1730. Chujo M, Noguchi T, Miura T, Arinaga M, Uchida Y, Tagawa Y. Comparative genomic hybridization analysis detected frequent overrepresentation of chromosome 3q in squamous cell carcinoma of the lung. Lung Cancer 2002;38:23–29.
1731. Wistuba II, Behrens C, Virmani AK, et al. Allelic losses at chromosome 8p21–23 are early and frequent events in the pathogenesis of lung cancer. Cancer Res 1999;59:1973–1979.
1732. Keith RL, Miller YE, Gemmill RM, et al. Angiogenic squamous dysplasia in bronchi of individuals at high risk for lung cancer. Clin Cancer Res 2000;6:1616–1625.
1733. Perrais M, Pigny P, Copin MC, Aubert JP, Van Seuningen I. Induction of MUC2 and MUC5AC mucins by factors of the epidermal growth factor (EGF) family is mediated by EGF receptor/Ras/Raf/extracellular signal-regulated kinase cascade and Sp1. J Biol Chem 2002;277:32258–32267.
1734. Lopez-Ferrer A, Curull V, Barranco C, et al. Mucins as differentiation markers in bronchial epithelium. Squamous cell carcinoma and adenocarcinoma display similar expression patterns. Am J Respir Cell Mol Biol 2001; 24:22–29.
1735. Copin MC, Devisme L, Buisine MP, et al. From normal respiratory mucosa to epidermoid carcinoma: expression of human mucin genes. Int J Cancer 2000;86:162–168.
1736. Holt SJ, Alexander P, Inman CB, Davies DE. Epidermal growth factor induced tyrosine phosphorylation of nuclear proteins associated with translocation of epidermal growth factor receptor into the nucleus. Biochem Pharmacol 1994;47:117–126.

1737. Kanematsu T, Yano S, Uehara H, Bando Y, Sone S. Phosphorylation, but not overexpression, of epidermal growth factor receptor is associated with poor prognosis of non-small cell lung cancer patients. Oncol Res 2003;13:289–298.
1738. Kim JS, Kim H, Shim YM, Han J, Park J, Kim DH. Aberrant methylation of the FHIT gene in chronic smokers with early stage squamous cell carcinoma of the lung. Carcinogenesis 2004;25:2165–2171.
1739. Frank CJ, McClatchey KD, Devaney KO, Carey TE. Evidence that loss of chromosome 18q is associated with tumor progression. Cancer Res 1997;57:824–827.
1740. Uematsu K, He B, You L, Xu Z, McCormick F, Jablons DM. Activation of the Wnt pathway in non small cell lung cancer: evidence of dishevelled overexpression. Oncogene 2003;22:7218–7221.
1741. Taki M, Kamata N, Yokoyama K, Fujimoto R, Tsutsumi S, Nagayama M. Down-regulation of Wnt-4 and up-regulation of Wnt-5a expression by epithelial-mesenchymal transition in human squamous carcinoma cells. Cancer Sci 2003;94:593–597.
1742. Toyooka S, Toyooka KO, Maruyama R, et al. DNA methylation profiles of lung tumors. Mol Cancer Ther 2001;1:61–67.
1743. Falleni M, Pellegrini C, Marchetti A, et al. Survivin gene expression in early-stage non-small cell lung cancer. J Pathol 2003;200:620–626.
1744. Sunaga N, Miyajima K, Suzuki M, et al. Different roles for caveolin-1 in the development of non-small cell lung cancer versus small cell lung cancer. Cancer Res 2004;64:4277–4285.
1745. Travis WD, Gal AA, Colby TV, Klimstra DS, Falk R, Koss MN. Neuroendocrine tumors of the lung with proposed criteria for large-cell neuroendocrine carcinoma. An ultrastructural, immunohistochemical, and flow cytometric study of 35 cases. Hum Pathol 1998;29:272–279.
1746. Ullmann R, Schwendel A, Klemen H, Wolf G, Petersen I, Popper HH. Unbalanced chromosomal aberrations in neuroendocrine lung tumors as detected by comparative genomic hybridization. Hum Pathol 1998;29:1145–1149.
1747. Jiang SX, Kameya T, Asamura H, et al. hASH1 expression is closely correlated with endocrine phenotype and differentiation extent in pulmonary neuroendocrine tumors. Mod Pathol 2004;17:222–229.
1748. Lantuejoul S, Moro D, Michalides RJ, Brambilla C, Brambilla E. Neural cell adhesion molecules (NCAM) and NCAM-PSA expression in neuroendocrine lung tumors. Am J Surg Pathol 1998;22:1267–1276.
1749. Patriarca C, Pruneri G, Alfano RM, et al. Polysialylated N-CAM, chromogranin A and B, and secretogranin II in neuroendocrine tumours of the lung. Virchows Arch 1997;430:455–460.
1750. Onuki N, Wistuba II, Travis WD, et al. Genetic changes in the spectrum of neuroendocrine lung tumors. Cancer 1999;85:600–607.
1751. Schwab M, Amler LC. Amplification of cellular oncogenes: a predictor of clinical outcome in human cancer. Genes Chromosomes Cancer 1990;1:181–193.
1752. Stahel RA. Antigens, receptors and dominant oncogenes and the prognosis of non-small cell lung cancer. Lung Cancer 1994;11(suppl 3):S31–S38.
1753. Johnson BE. Biologic and molecular prognostic factors—impact on treatment of patients with non-small cell lung cancer. Chest 1995;107(6 suppl):287S-290S.
1754. Kanters SD, Lammers JW, Voest EE. Molecular and biological factors in the prognosis of non-small cell lung cancer. Eur Respir J 1995;8:1389–1397.
1755. Mountain CF. New prognostic factors in lung cancer. Biologic prophets of cancer cell aggression. Chest 1995;108:246–254.
1756. Scagliotti GV, Masiero P, Pozzi E. Biological prognostic factors in non-small cell lung cancer. Lung Cancer 1995;12(suppl 1):S13–S25.
1757. van Zandwijk N, Mooi WJ, Rodenhuis S. Prognostic factors in NSCLC. Recent experiences. Lung Cancer 1995;12(suppl 1):S27–S33.
1758. Smit EF, Groen HJ, Splinter TA, Ebels T, Postmus PE. New prognostic factors in resectable non-small cell lung cancer. Thorax 1996;51:638–646.
1759. Tockman MS. Clinical detection of lung cancer progression markers. J Cell Biochem Suppl 1996;25:177–184.
1760. Graziano SL. Non-small cell lung cancer: clinical value of new biological predictors. Lung Cancer 1997;17(suppl 1): S37–S58.
1761. Lucchi M, Fontanini G, Mussi A, et al. Tumor angiogenesis and biologic markers in resected stage I NSCLC. Eur J Cardiothorac Surg 1997;12:535–541.
1762. Rosell R, Pifarre A, Monzo M, et al. Reduced survival in patients with stage-I non-small-cell lung cancer associated with DNA-replication errors. Int J Cancer 1997;74:330–334.
1763. de Juan C, Iniesta P, Vega FJ, et al. Prognostic value of genomic damage in non-small-cell lung cancer. Br J Cancer 1998;77:1971–1977.
1764. Greatens TM, Niehans GA, Rubins JB, et al. Do molecular markers predict survival in non-small-cell lung cancer? Am J Respir Crit Care Med 1998;157:1093–1097.
1765. Komaki R, Milas L, Ro JY, et al. Prognostic biomarker study in pathologically staged N1 non-small cell lung cancer. Int J Radiat Oncol Biol Phys 1998;40:787–796.
1766. Fu XL, Zhu XZ, Shi DR, et al. Study of prognostic predictors for non-small cell lung cancer. Lung Cancer 1999; 23:143–152.
1767. Lavezzi AM, Santambrogio L, Bellaviti N, et al. Prognostic significance of different biomarkers in non-small cell lung cancer. Oncol Rep 1999;6:819–825.
1768. Cagini L, Monacelli M, Giustozzi G, et al. Biological prognostic factors for early stage completely resected non-small cell lung cancer. J Surg Oncol 2000;74:53–60.
1769. Moldvay J, Scheid P, Wild P, et al. Predictive survival markers in patients with surgically resected non-small cell lung carcinoma. Clin Cancer Res 2000;6:1125–1134.
1770. Stevens CW, Lee JS, Cox J, Komaki R. Novel approaches to locally advanced unresectable non-small cell lung cancer. Radiother Oncol 2000;55:11–8.
1771. Junker K. Prognostic factors in stage I/II non-small cell lung cancer. Lung Cancer 2001;33(suppl 1):S17–S24.

1772. Niklinski J, Niklinska W, Laudanski J, Chyczewska E, Chyczewski L. Prognostic molecular markers in non-small cell lung cancer. Lung Cancer 2001;34(suppl 2): S53–S58.
1773. Osaki T, Oyama T, Inoue M, et al. Molecular biological markers and micrometastasis in resected non-small-cell lung cancer. Prognostic implications. Jpn J Thorac Cardiovasc Surg 2001;49:545–551.
1774. Baksh FK, Dacic S, Finkelstein SD, et al. Widespread molecular alterations present in stage I non-small cell lung carcinoma fail to predict tumor recurrence. Mod Pathol 2003;16:28–34.
1775. Slebos RJ, Kibbelaar RE, Dalesio O, et al. K-ras oncogene activation as a prognostic marker in adenocarcinoma of the lung. N Engl J Med 1990;323:561–565.
1776. Mitsudomi T, Steinberg SM, Oie HK, et al. ras gene mutations in non-small cell lung cancers are associated with shortened survival irrespective of treatment intent. Cancer Res 1991;51:4999–5002.
1777. Miyamoto H, Harada M, Isobe H, et al. Prognostic value of nuclear DNA content and expression of the ras oncogene product in lung cancer. Cancer Res 1991;51: 6346–6350.
1778. Harada M, Dosaka-Akita H, Miyamoto H, Kuzumaki N, Kawakami Y. Prognostic significance of the expression of ras oncogene product in non-small cell lung cancer. Cancer 1992;69:72–77.
1779. Rodenhuis S, Slebos RJ. Clinical significance of ras oncogene activation in human lung cancer. Cancer Res 1992;52(9 suppl):2665s–2669s.
1780. Sugio K, Ishida T, Yokoyama H, Inoue T, Sugimachi K, Sasazuki T. ras gene mutations as a prognostic marker in adenocarcinoma of the human lung without lymph node metastasis. Cancer Res 1992;52:2903–2906.
1781. Rosell R, Li S, Skacel Z, et al. Prognostic impact of mutated K-ras gene in surgically resected non-small cell lung cancer patients. Oncogene 1993;8:2407–2412.
1782. Silini EM, Bosi F, Pellegata NS, et al. K-ras gene mutations: an unfavorable prognostic marker in stage I lung adenocarcinoma. Virchows Arch 1994;424:367–373.
1783. Rosell R, Monzo M, Molina F, et al. K-ras genotypes and prognosis in non-small-cell lung cancer. Ann Oncol 1995;6(suppl 3):S15–S20.
1784. Keohavong P, DeMichele MA, Melacrinos AC, Landreneau RJ, Weyant RJ, Siegfried JM. Detection of K-ras mutations in lung carcinomas: relationship to prognosis. Clin Cancer Res 1996;2:411–418.
1785. Cho JY, Kim JH, Lee YH, et al. Correlation between K-ras gene mutation and prognosis of patients with nonsmall cell lung carcinoma. Cancer 1997;79:462–467.
1786. Siegfried JM, Gillespie AT, Mera R, et al. Prognostic value of specific KRAS mutations in lung adenocarcinomas. Cancer Epidemiol Biomarkers Prev 1997;6:841–847.
1787. De Gregorio L, Manenti G, Incarbone M, et al. Prognostic value of loss of heterozygosity and KRAS2 mutations in lung adenocarcinoma. Int J Cancer 1998;79:269–272.
1788. Graziano SL, Gamble GP, Newman NB, et al. Prognostic significance of K-ras codon 12 mutations in patients with resected stage I and II non-small-cell lung cancer. J Clin Oncol 1999;17:668–675.
1789. Nelson HH, Christiani DC, Mark EJ, Wiencke JK, Wain JC, Kelsey KT. Implications and prognostic value of K-ras mutation for early-stage lung cancer in women. J Natl Cancer Inst 1999;91:2032–2038.
1790. Wang YC, Lee HS, Chen SK, Yang SC, Chen CY. Analysis of K-ras gene mutations in lung carcinomas: correlation with gender, histological subtypes, and clinical outcome. J Cancer Res Clin Oncol 1998;124:517–522.
1791. Tomizawa Y, Kohno T, Kondo H, et al. Clinicopathological significance of epigenetic inactivation of RASSF1A at 3p21.3 in stage I lung adenocarcinoma. Clin Cancer Res 2002;8:2362–2368.
1792. Kim DH, Kim JS, Ji YI, et al. Hypermethylation of RASSF1A promoter is associated with the age at starting smoking and a poor prognosis in primary non-small cell lung cancer. Cancer Res 2003;63:3743–3746.
1793. Pulling LC, Divine KK, Klinge DM, et al. Promoter hypermethylation of the O6–methylguanine-DNA methyltransferase gene: more common in lung adenocarcinomas from never-smokers than smokers and associated with tumor progression. Cancer Res 2003;63:4842–4848.
1794. Funa K, Steinholtz L, Nou E, Bergh J. Increased expression of N-myc in human small cell lung cancer biopsies predicts lack of response to chemotherapy and poor prognosis. Am J Clin Pathol 1987;88:216–220.
1795. Johnson BE, Ihde DC, Makuch RW, et al. myc family oncogene amplification in tumor cell lines established from small cell lung cancer patients and its relationship to clinical status and course. J Clin Invest 1987;79: 1629–1634.
1796. Kawashima K, Shikama H, Imoto K, et al. Close correlation between restriction fragment length polymorphism of the L-MYC gene and metastasis of human lung cancer to the lymph nodes and other organs. Proc Natl Acad Sci USA 1988;85:2353–2356.
1797. Kawashima K, Nomura S, Hirai H, et al. Correlation of L-myc RFLP with metastasis, prognosis and multiple cancer in lung-cancer patients. Int J Cancer 1992;50: 557–561.
1798. Shih CM, Kuo YY, Wang YC, et al. Association of L-myc polymorphism with lung cancer susceptibility and prognosis in relation to age-selected controls and stratified cases. Lung Cancer 2002;36:125–132.
1799. Yaylim I, Isbir T, Ozturk O, et al. Is there any correlation between restriction fragment length polymorphism of the L-MYC gene and metastasis of human nonsmall cell lung cancer? Cancer Genet Cytogenet 2002;134:118–122.
1800. Spinola M, Conti B, Ravagnani F, et al. A new polymorphism (Ser362Thr) of the L-myc gene is not associated with lung adenocarcinoma risk and prognosis. Eur J Cancer Prev 2004;13:87–89.
1801. Horio Y, Takahashi T, Kuroishi T, et al. Prognostic significance of p53 mutations and 3p deletions in primary resected non-small cell lung cancer. Cancer Res 1993; 53:1–4.
1802. Mitsudomi T, Oyama T, Kusano T, Osaki T, Nakanishi R, Shirakusa T. Mutations of the p53 gene as a predictor of

poor prognosis in patients with non-small-cell lung cancer. J Natl Cancer Inst 1993;85:2018–2023.
1803. Morkve O, Halvorsen OJ, Skjaerven R, Stangeland L, Gulsvik A, Laerum OD. Prognostic significance of p53 protein expression and DNA ploidy in surgically treated non-small cell lung carcinomas. Anticancer Res 1993; 13:571–578.
1804. Carbone DP, Mitsudomi T, Chiba I, et al. p53 immunostaining positivity is associated with reduced survival and is imperfectly correlated with gene mutations in resected non-small cell lung cancer. A preliminary report of LCSG 871. Chest 1994;106(6 suppl):377S–381S.
1805. Sauter ER, Gwin JL, Mandel J, Keller SM. p53 and disease progression in patients with non-small cell lung cancer. Surg Oncol 1995;4:157–161.
1806. Langendijk JA, Thunnissen FB, Lamers RJ, de Jong JM, ten Velde GP, Wouters EF. The prognostic significance of accumulation of p53 protein in stage III non-small cell lung cancer treated by radiotherapy. Radiother Oncol 1995;36:218–224.
1807. Lee JS, Yoon A, Kalapurakal SK, et al. Expression of p53 oncoprotein in non-small-cell lung cancer: a favorable prognostic factor. J Clin Oncol 1995;13:1893–1903.
1808. Passlick B, Izbicki JR, Haussinger K, Thetter O, Pantel K. Immunohistochemical detection of P53 protein is not associated with a poor prognosis in non-small-cell lung cancer. J Thorac Cardiovasc Surg 1995;109:1205–1211.
1809. Tormanen U, Eerola AK, Rainio P, et al. Enhanced apoptosis predicts shortened survival in non-small cell lung carcinoma. Cancer Res 1995;55:5595–5602.
1810. Dalquen P, Sauter G, Torhorst J, et al. Nuclear p53 overexpression is an independent prognostic parameter in node-negative non-small cell lung carcinoma. J Pathol 1996;178:53–58.
1811. Nishio M, Koshikawa T, Kuroishi T, et al. Prognostic significance of abnormal p53 accumulation in primary, resected non-small-cell lung cancers. J Clin Oncol 1996; 14:497–502.
1812. Pappot H, Francis D, Brunner N, Grondahl-Hansen J, Osterlind K. p53 protein in non-small cell lung cancer as quantitated by enzyme-linked immunosorbent assay: relation to prognosis. Clin Cancer Res 1996;2:155–160.
1813. Dalquen P, Moch H, Feichter G, et al. DNA aneuploidy, S-phase fraction, nuclear p53 positivity, and survival in non-small-cell lung carcinoma. Virchows Arch 1997; 431:173–179.
1814. de Anta JM, Jassem E, Rosell R, et al. TP53 mutational pattern in Spanish and Polish non-small cell lung cancer patients: null mutations are associated with poor prognosis. Oncogene 1997;15:2951–2958.
1815. Dobashi K, Sugio K, Osaki T, Oka T, Yasumoto K. Micrometastatic P53–positive cells in the lymph nodes of non-small-cell lung cancer: prognostic significance. J Thorac Cardiovasc Surg 1997;114:339–346.
1816. Fontanini G, Vignati S, Lucchi M, et al. Neoangiogenesis and p53 protein in lung cancer: their prognostic role and their relation with vascular endothelial growth factor (VEGF) expression. Br J Cancer 1997;75:1295–1301.
1817. Guang SG, Ogura T, Sekine I, et al. Association between p53 mutation and clinicopathological features of non-small cell lung cancer. Jpn J Clin Oncol 1997;27:211–215.
1818. Quantin X, Pujol JL, Lehmann M, Simony J, Serre I, Michel FB. Immunohistochemical detection of p53 protein and prognosis of surgically resected non-small-cell lung cancer. Cancer Detect Prev 1997;21: 418–425.
1819. Vega FJ, Iniesta P, Caldes T, et al. p53 exon 5 mutations as a prognostic indicator of shortened survival in non-small-cell lung cancer. Br J Cancer 1997;76:44–51.
1820. Hayakawa K, Mitsuhashi N, Hasegawa M, et al. The prognostic significance of immunohistochemically detected p53 protein expression in non-small cell lung cancer treated with radiation therapy. Anticancer Res 1998; 18:3685–3688.
1821. Huang C, Taki T, Adachi M, Konishi T, Higashiyama M, Miyake M. Mutations in exon 7 and 8 of p53 as poor prognostic factors in patients with non-small cell lung cancer. Oncogene 1998;16:2469–2477.
1822. Levesque MA, D'Costa M, Spratt EH, Yaman MM, Diamandis EP. Quantitative analysis of p53 protein in non-small cell lung cancer and its prognostic value. Int J Cancer 1998;79:494–501.
1823. Sanchez-Pernaute A, Torres A, Iniesta P, et al. Prognostic significance of p53 gene mutations in squamous cell carcinoma of the lung. Oncol Rep 1998;5:1129–1133.
1824. Tagawa M, Murata M, Kimura H. Prognostic value of mutations and a germ line polymorphism of the p53 gene in non-small cell lung carcinoma: association with clinicopathological features. Cancer Lett 1998;128:93–99.
1825. Dursun BA, Memis L, Dursun A, Bayiz H, Ozkul M. Clinical importance of correlations between p53 immunoreactivity and clinicopathological parameters in lung carcinoma. Pathol Oncol Res 1999;5:285–290.
1826. Hashimoto T, Tokuchi Y, Hayashi M, et al. p53 null mutations undetected by immunohistochemical staining predict a poor outcome with early-stage non-small cell lung carcinomas. Cancer Res 1999;59:5572–5577.
1827. Komiya T, Hirashima T, Kawase I. Clinical significance of p53 in non-small-cell lung cancer. Oncol Rep 1999;6: 19–28.
1828. Tomizawa Y, Kohno T, Fujita T, et al. Correlation between the status of the p53 gene and survival in patients with stage I non-small cell lung carcinoma. Oncogene 1999; 18:1007–1014.
1829. Wang YC, Chen CY, Wang HJ, Chen SK, Chang YY, Lin P. Influence of polymorphism at p53, CYP1A1 and GSTM1 loci on p53 mutation and association of p53 mutation with prognosis in lung cancer. Zhonghua Yi Xue Za Zhi (Taipei) 1999;62:402–410.
1830. Wang YC, Lee HS, Chen SK, Chang YY, Chen CY. Prognostic significance of p53 codon 72 polymorphism in lung carcinomas. Eur J Cancer 1999;35:226–230.
1831. Hashimoto T, Kobayashi Y, Ishikawa Y, et al. Prognostic value of genetically diagnosed lymph node micrometastasis in non-small cell lung carcinoma cases. Cancer Res 2000;60:6472–6478.
1832. Murakami I, Hiyama K, Ishioka S, Yamakido M, Kasagi F, Yokosaki Y. p53 gene mutations are associated with shortened survival in patients with advanced non-small

cell lung cancer: an analysis of medically managed patients. Clin Cancer Res 2000;6:526–530.
1833. Sioris T, Husgafvel-Pursiainen K, Karjalainen A, et al. Survival in operable non-small-cell lung cancer: role of p53 mutations, tobacco smoking and asbestos exposure. Int J Cancer 2000;86:590–594.
1834. Skaug V, Ryberg D, Kure EH, et al. p53 mutations in defined structural and functional domains are related to poor clinical outcome in non-small cell lung cancer patients. Clin Cancer Res 2000;6:1031–1037.
1835. Tanaka F, Yanagihara K, Otake Y, et al. Prognostic factors in patients with resected pathologic (p-) T1–2N1M0 non-small cell lung cancer (NSCLC). Eur J Cardiothorac Surg 2001;19:555–561.
1836. Gajra A, Tatum AH, Newman N, et al. The predictive value of neuroendocrine markers and p53 for response to chemotherapy and survival in patients with advanced non-small cell lung cancer. Lung Cancer 2002;36: 159–165.
1837. Hanaoka N, Tanaka F, Wada H. Prognostic significance of p53 status in non-small cell lung cancer in correlation with postoperative adjuvant therapy. Thorac Cardiovasc Surg 2002;50:355–359.
1838. Ahrendt SA, Hu Y, Buta M, et al. p53 mutations and survival in stage I non-small-cell lung cancer: results of a prospective study. J Natl Cancer Inst 2003;95:961–970.
1839. Campling BG, El-Deiry WS. Clinical implication of p53 mutation in lung cancer. Mol Biotechnol 2003;24: 141–156.
1840. Tan DF, Li Q, Rammath N, et al. Prognostic significance of expression of p53 oncoprotein in primary (stage I-IIIa) non-small cell lung cancer. Anticancer Res 2003;23: 1665–1672.
1841. Haque AK, Au W, Cajas-Salazar N, et al. CYP2E1 polymorphism, cigarette smoking, p53 expression, and survival in non-small cell lung cancer: a long term follow-up study. Appl Immunohistochem Mol Morphol 2004;12: 315–322.
1842. Tanaka F, Yanagihara K, Otake Y, et al. Prognostic factors in resected pathologic (p-) stage IIIA-N2, non-small-cell lung cancer. Ann Surg Oncol 2004;11:612–618.
1843. Berghmans T, Mascaux C, Martin B, Ninane V, Sculier JP. Prognostic role of p53 in stage III non-small cell lung cancer. Anticancer Res 2005;25:2385–2389.
1844. Higashiyama M, Doi O, Kodama K, et al. MDM2 gene amplification and expression in non-small-cell lung cancer: immunohistochemical expression of its protein is a favourable prognostic marker in patients without p53 protein accumulation. Br J Cancer 1997;75:1302–1308.
1845. Aikawa H, Sato M, Fujimura S, et al. MDM2 expression is associated with progress of disease and WAF1 expression in resected lung cancer. Int J Mol Med 2000;5:631–633.
1846. Ko JL, Cheng YW, Chang SL, Su JM, Chen CY, Lee H. MDM2 mRNA expression is a favorable prognostic factor in non-small-cell lung cancer. Int J Cancer 2000;89: 265–270.
1847. Dworakowska D, Jassem E, Jassem J, et al. MDM2 gene amplification: a new independent factor of adverse prognosis in non-small cell lung cancer (NSCLC). Lung Cancer 2004;43:285–295.
1848. Xu HJ, Quinlan DC, Davidson AG, et al. Altered retinoblastoma protein expression and prognosis in early-stage non-small-cell lung carcinoma. J Natl Cancer Inst 1994;86:695–699.
1849. Caputi M, Groeger AM, Esposito V, et al. Loss of pRb2/p130 expression is associated with unfavorable clinical outcome in lung cancer. Clin Cancer Res 2002;8: 3850–3856.
1850. Taga S, Osaki T, Ohgami A, et al. Prognostic value of the immunohistochemical detection of p16INK4 expression in nonsmall cell lung carcinoma. Cancer 1997;80: 389–395.
1851. Volm M, Koomagi R, Mattern J. Prognostic value of p16INK4A expression in lung adenocarcinoma. Anticancer Res 1998;18:2309–2312.
1852. Groeger AM, Caputi M, Esposito V, et al. Independent prognostic role of p16 expression in lung cancer. J Thorac Cardiovasc Surg 1999;118:529–535.
1853. Kawabuchi B, Moriyama S, Hironaka M, et al. p16 inactivation in small-sized lung adenocarcinoma: its association with poor prognosis. Int J Cancer 1999;84:49–53.
1854. Huang CI, Taki T, Higashiyama M, Kohno N, Miyake M. p16 protein expression is associated with a poor prognosis in squamous cell carcinoma of the lung. Br J Cancer 2000;82:374–380.
1855. Ng CS, Zhang J, Wan S, et al. Tumor p16M is a possible marker of advanced stage in non-small cell lung cancer. J Surg Oncol 2002;79:101–106.
1856. Tanaka R, Wang D, Morishita Y, et al. Loss of function of p16 gene and prognosis of pulmonary adenocarcinoma. Cancer 2005;103:608–615.
1857. Betticher DC, Heighway J, Hasleton PS, et al. Prognostic significance of CCND1 (cyclin D1) overexpression in primary resected non-small-cell lung cancer. Br J Cancer 1996;73:294–300.
1858. Kwa HB, Michalides RJ, Dijkman JH, Mooi WJ. The prognostic value of NCAM, p53 and cyclin D1 in resected non-small cell lung cancer. Lung Cancer 1996;14: 207–217.
1859. Caputi M, De Luca L, Papaccio G, et al. Prognostic role of cyclin D1 in non small cell lung cancer: an immunohistochemical analysis. Eur J Histochem 1997;41:133–138.
1860. Caputi M, Groeger AM, Esposito V, et al. Prognostic role of cyclin D1 in lung cancer. Relationship to proliferating cell nuclear antigen. Am J Respir Cell Mol Biol 1999; 20:746–750.
1861. Keum JS, Kong G, Yang SC, et al. Cyclin D1 overexpression is an indicator of poor prognosis in resectable non-small cell lung cancer. Br J Cancer 1999;81:127–132.
1862. Mishina T, Dosaka-Akita H, Kinoshita I, et al. Cyclin D1 expression in non-small-cell lung cancers: its association with altered p53 expression, cell proliferation and clinical outcome. Br J Cancer 1999;80:1289–1295.
1863. Anton RC, Coffey DM, Gondo MM, Stephenson MA, Brown RW, Cagle PT. The expression of cyclins D1 and E in predicting short-term survival in squamous cell carcinoma of the lung. Mod Pathol 2000;13:1167–1172.

1864. Ikehara M, Oshita F, Ito H, et al. Expression of cyclin D1 but not of cyclin E is an indicator of poor prognosis in small adenocarcinomas of the lung. Oncol Rep 2003;10: 137–139.
1865. Dobashi Y, Goto A, Fukayama M, Abe A, Ooi A. Overexpression of cdk4/cyclin D1, a possible mediator of apoptosis and an indicator of prognosis in human primary lung carcinoma. Int J Cancer 2004;110:532–541.
1866. Gaffney EF, O'Neil AJ, Staunton MJ. bcl-2 and prognosis in non-small-cell lung carcinoma. N Engl J Med 1994; 330:1757–1758.
1867. Fontanini G, Vignati S, Bigini D, et al. Bcl-2 protein: a prognostic factor inversely correlated to p53 in non-small-cell lung cancer. Br J Cancer 1995;71:1003–1007.
1868. Ritter JH, Dresler CM, Wick MR. Expression of bcl-2 protein in stage T1N0M0 non-small cell lung carcinoma. Hum Pathol 1995;26:1227–1232.
1869. Higashiyama M, Doi O, Kodama K, Yokouchi H, Nakamori S, Tateishi R. bcl-2 oncoprotein in surgically resected non-small cell lung cancer: possibly favorable prognostic factor in association with low incidence of distant metastasis. J Surg Oncol 1997;64:48–54.
1870. Anton RC, Brown RW, Younes M, Gondo MM, Stephenson MA, Cagle PT. Absence of prognostic significance of bcl-2 immunopositivity in non-small cell lung cancer: analysis of 427 cases. Hum Pathol 1997;28:1079–1082.
1871. Silvestrini R, Costa A, Lequaglie C, et al. Bcl-2 protein and prognosis in patients with potentially curable non-small-cell lung cancer. Virchows Arch 1998;432:441–444.
1872. Eerola AK, Ruokolainen H, Soini Y, Raunio H, Paakko P. Accelerated apoptosis and low bcl-2 expression associated with neuroendocrine differentiation predict shortened survival in operated large cell carcinoma of the lung. Pathol Oncol Res 1999;5:179–186.
1873. Laudanski J, Chyczewski L, Niklinska WE, et al. Expression of bcl-2 protein in non-small cell lung cancer: correlation with clinicopathology and patient survival. Neoplasma 1999;46:25–30.
1874. Cox G, Walker RA, Muller S, Abrams KR, Steward WP, O'Byrne KJ. Does immunointensity account for the differences in prognostic significance of Bcl-2 expression in non-small cell lung cancer? Pathol Oncol Res 2000;6: 87–92.
1875. Cox G, Louise Jones J, Andi A, Abrams KR, O'Byrne KJ. Bcl-2 is an independent prognostic factor and adds to a biological model for predicting outcome in operable non-small cell lung cancer. Lung Cancer 2001;34:417–426.
1876. Hwang JH, Lim SC, Kim YC, Park KO, Ahn SJ, Chung WK. Apoptosis and bcl-2 expression as predictors of survival in radiation-treated non-small-cell lung cancer. Int J Radiat Oncol Biol Phys 2001;50:13–18.
1877. Huang CI, Neuberg D, Johnson BE, Wei JY, Christiani DC. Expression of bcl-2 protein is associated with shorter survival in nonsmall cell lung carcinoma. Cancer 2003; 98:135–143.
1878. Tomita M, Matsuzaki Y, Edagawa M, Shimizu T, Hara M, Onitsuka T. Prognostic significance of bcl-2 expression in resected pN2 non-small cell lung cancer. Eur J Surg Oncol 2003;29:654–657.
1879. Shibata Y, Hidaka S, Tagawa Y, Nagayasu T. Bcl-2 protein expression correlates with better prognosis in patients with advanced non-small cell lung cancer. Anticancer Res 2004;24:1925–1928.
1880. Yilmaz A, Savas I, Dizbay Sak S, et al. Distribution of Bcl-2 gene expression and its prognostic value in non-small cell lung cancer. Tuberk Toraks 2005;53:323–329.
1881. Kern JA, Schwartz DA, Nordberg JE, et al. p185neu expression in human lung adenocarcinomas predicts shortened survival. Cancer Res 1990;50:5184–5187.
1882. Tateishi M, Ishida T, Mitsudomi T, Kaneko S, Sugimachi K. Prognostic value of c-erbB-2 protein expression in human lung adenocarcinoma and squamous cell carcinoma. Eur J Cancer 1991;27:1372–1375.
1883. Giatromanolaki A, Koukourakis MI, O'Byrne K, et al. Non-small cell lung cancer: c-erbB-2 overexpression correlates with low angiogenesis and poor prognosis. Anticancer Res 1996;16:3819–3825.
1884. Hsieh CC, Chow KC, Fahn HJ, et al. Prognostic significance of HER-2/neu overexpression in stage I adenocarcinoma of lung. Ann Thorac Surg 1998;66:1159–1163.
1885. Cantero R, Torres AJ, Maestro ML, et al. Prognostic value of the quantified expression of p185 in non-small cell lung cancer. J Thorac Cardiovasc Surg 2000;119:1119–1125.
1886. Micke P, Hengstler JG, Ros R, et al. c-erbB-2 expression in small-cell lung cancer is associated with poor prognosis. Int J Cancer 2001;92:474–479.
1887. Bakir K, Ucak R, Tuncozgur B, Elbeyli L. Prognostic factors and c-erbB-2 expression in non-small-cell lung carcinoma (c-erbB-2 in non-small cell lung carcinoma). Thorac Cardiovasc Surg 2002;50:55–58.
1888. Selvaggi G, Scagliotti GV, Torri V, et al. HER-2/neu overexpression in patients with radically resected nonsmall cell lung carcinoma. Impact on long-term survival. Cancer 2002;94:2669–2674.
1889. Meert AP, Martin B, Paesmans M, et al. The role of HER-2/neu expression on the survival of patients with lung cancer: a systematic review of the literature. Br J Cancer 2003;89:959–965.
1890. Nakamura H, Saji H, Ogata A, et al. Correlation between encoded protein overexpression and copy number of the HER2 gene with survival in non-small cell lung cancer. Int J Cancer 2003;103:61–66.
1891. Turken O, Kunter E, Cermik H, et al. Prevalence and prognostic value of c-erbB2 expression in non-small cell lung cancer (NSCLC). Neoplasma 2003;50:257–261.
1892. Nakamura H, Kawasaki N, Taguchi M, Kabasawa K. Association of HER-2 overexpression with prognosis in nonsmall cell lung carcinoma: a metaanalysis. Cancer 2005;103:1865–1873.
1893. Pelosi G, Del Curto B, Dell'Orto P, et al. Lack of prognostic implications of HER-2/neu abnormalities in 345 stage I non-small cell carcinomas (NSCLC) and 207 stage I-III neuroendocrine tumours (NET) of the lung. Int J Cancer 2005;113:101–108.
1894. Vallbohmer D, Brabender J, Yang DY, et al. Sex differences in the predictive power of the molecular prognostic factor HER2/neu in patients with non-small-cell lung cancer. Clin Lung Cancer 2006;7:332–337.

1895. Brandt B, Vogt U, Schlotter CM, et al. Prognostic relevance of aberrations in the erbB oncogenes from breast, ovarian, oral and lung cancers: double-differential polymerase chain reaction (ddPCR) for clinical diagnosis. Gene 1995;159:35–42.
1896. Yi ES, Harclerode D, Gondo M, et al. High c-erbB-3 protein expression is associated with shorter survival in advanced non-small cell lung carcinomas. Mod Pathol 1997;10:142–148.
1897. Burke L, Khan MA, Freedman AN, et al. Allelic deletion analysis of the FHIT gene predicts poor survival in non-small cell lung cancer. Cancer Res 1998;58:2533–2536.
1898. Geradts J, Fong KM, Zimmerman PV, Minna JD. Loss of Fhit expression in non-small-cell lung cancer: correlation with molecular genetic abnormalities and clinicopathological features. Br J Cancer 2000;82:1191–1197.
1899. Maruyama R, Sugio K, Yoshino I, Maehara Y, Gazdar AF. Hypermethylation of FHIT as a prognostic marker in nonsmall cell lung carcinoma. Cancer 2004;100: 1472–1477.
1900. Toledo G, Sola JJ, Lozano MD, Soria E, Pardo J. Loss of FHIT protein expression is related to high proliferation, low apoptosis and worse prognosis in non-small-cell lung cancer. Mod Pathol 2004;17:440–448.
1901. Komiya T, Hosono Y, Hirashima T, et al. p21 expression as a predictor for favorable prognosis in squamous cell carcinoma of the lung. Clin Cancer Res 1997;3:1831–1835.
1902. Levesque MA, D'Costa M, Diamandis EP. p21WAF1 protein expression determined by quantitative immunoassay in relation to non-small-cell lung cancer aggressiveness. J Cancer Res Clin Oncol 2000;126:48–52.
1903. Shih CM, Lin PT, Wang HC, Huang WC, Wang YC. Lack of evidence of association of p21WAF1/CIP1 polymorphism with lung cancer susceptibility and prognosis in Taiwan. Jpn J Cancer Res 2000;91:9–15.
1904. Shoji T, Tanaka F, Takata T, et al. Clinical significance of p21 expression in non-small-cell lung cancer. J Clin Oncol 2002;20:3865–3871.
1905. Dworakowska D, Jassem E, Jassem J, et al. Absence of prognostic significance of p21(WAF1/CIP1) protein expression in non-small cell lung cancer. Acta Oncol 2005;44:75–79.
1906. Hommura F, Furuuchi K, Yamazaki K, et al. Increased expression of beta-catenin predicts better prognosis in nonsmall cell lung carcinomas. Cancer 2002;94:752–758.
1907. Catzavelos C, Tsao MS, DeBoer G, Bhattacharya N, Shepherd FA, Slingerland JM. Reduced expression of the cell cycle inhibitor p27Kip1 in non-small cell lung carcinoma: a prognostic factor independent of Ras. Cancer Res 1999;59:684–688.
1908. Hommura F, Dosaka-Akita H, Mishina T, et al. Prognostic significance of p27KIP1 protein and ki-67 growth fraction in non-small cell lung cancers. Clin Cancer Res 2000; 6:4073–4081.
1909. Hirabayashi H, Ohta M, Tanaka H, et al. Prognostic significance of p27KIP1 expression in resected non-small cell lung cancers: analysis in combination with expressions of p16INK4A, pRB, and p53. J Surg Oncol 2002; 81:177–184.
1910. Shimamoto T, Ohyashiki JH, Hirano T, Kato H, Ohyashiki K. Hypermethylation of E-cadherin gene is frequent and independent of p16INK4A methylation in non-small cell lung cancer: potential prognostic implication. Oncol Rep 2004;12:389–395.
1911. Uramoto H, Osaki T, Inoue M, et al. Fas expression in non-small cell lung cancer: its prognostic effect in completely resected stage III patients. Eur J Cancer 1999;35:1462–1465.
1912. Kim YT, Park SJ, Lee SH, et al. Prognostic implication of aberrant promoter hypermethylation of CpG islands in adenocarcinoma of the lung. J Thorac Cardiovasc Surg 2005;130:1378.
1913. Safar AM, Spencer H 3rd, Su X, et al. Methylation profiling of archived non-small cell lung cancer: a promising prognostic system. Clin Cancer Res 2005;11:4400–4405.
1914. Kim JS, Kim JW, Han J, Shim YM, Park J, Kim DH. Cohypermethylation of p16 and FHIT promoters as a prognostic factor of recurrence in surgically resected stage I non-small cell lung cancer. Cancer Res 2006;66: 4049–4054.
1915. Nakata S, Sugio K, Uramoto H, et al. The methylation status and protein expression of CDH1, p16(INK4A), and fragile histidine triad in nonsmall cell lung carcinoma: epigenetic silencing, clinical features, and prognostic significance. Cancer 2006;106:2190–2199.
1916. Giatromanolaki A, Koukourakis MI, Sivridis E, et al. Relation of hypoxia inducible factor 1 alpha and 2 alpha in operable non-small cell lung cancer to angiogenic/molecular profile of tumours and survival. Br J Cancer 2001;85:881–890.
1917. Giatromanolaki A, Koukourakis MI, Sivridis E, et al. Expression of hypoxia-inducible carbonic anhydrase-9 relates to angiogenic pathways and independently to poor outcome in non-small cell lung cancer. Cancer Res 2001;61:7992–7998.
1918. Haque AK, Syed S, Lele SM, Freeman DH, Adegboyega PA. Immunohistochemical study of thyroid transcription factor-1 and HER2/neu in non-small cell lung cancer: strong thyroid transcription factor-1 expression predicts better survival. Appl Immunohistochem Mol Morphol 2002;10:103–109.
1919. Myong NH. Thyroid transcription factor-1 (TTF-1) expression in human lung carcinomas: its prognostic implication and relationship with wxpressions of p53 and Ki-67 proteins. J Korean Med Sci 2003;18:494–500.
1920. Khuri FR, Wu H, Lee JJ, et al. Cyclooxygenase-2 over-expression is a marker of poor prognosis in stage I non-small cell lung cancer. Clin Cancer Res 2001;7:861–867.
1921. Laga AC, Zander DS, Cagle PT. Prognostic significance of cyclooxygenase 2 expression in 259 cases of non-small cell lung cancer. Arch Pathol Lab Med 2005;129: 1113–1117.
1922. Mascaux C, Martin B, Paesmans M, et al. Has Cox-2 a prognostic role in non-small-cell lung cancer? A systematic review of the literature with meta-analysis of the survival results. Br J Cancer 2006;95:139–145.
1923. Zhu CQ, Blackhall FH, Pintilie M, et al. Skp2 gene copy number aberrations are common in non-small cell lung

carcinoma, and its overexpression in tumors with ras mutation is a poor prognostic marker. Clin Cancer Res 2004;10:1984–1991.

1924. Gorgoulis VG, Zacharatos P, Mariatos G, et al. Transcription factor E2F-1 acts as a growth-promoting factor and is associated with adverse prognosis in non-small cell lung carcinomas. J Pathol 2002;198:142–156.

1925. Goto I, Yoneda S, Yamamoto M, Kawajiri K. Prognostic significance of germ line polymorphisms of the CYP1A1 and glutathione S-transferase genes in patients with non-small cell lung cancer. Cancer Res 1996;56:3725–3730.

1926. Pifarre A, Rosell R, Monzo M, et al. Prognostic value of replication errors on chromosomes 2p and 3p in non-small-cell lung cancer. Br J Cancer 1997;75:184–189.

1927. Marsit CJ, Hasegawa M, Hirao T, et al. Loss of heterozygosity of chromosome 3p21 is associated with mutant TP53 and better patient survival in non-small-cell lung cancer. Cancer Res 2004;64:8702–8707.

1928. Tomizawa Y, Adachi J, Kohno T, et al. Prognostic significance of allelic imbalances on chromosome 9p in stage I non-small cell lung carcinoma. Clin Cancer Res 1999;5: 1139–1146.

1929. Ohsaki Y, Tanno S, Fujita Y, et al. Epidermal growth factor receptor expression correlates with poor prognosis in non-small cell lung cancer patients with p53 overexpression. Oncol Rep 2000;7:603–607.

1930. Joseph MG, Banerjee D, Kocha W, Feld R, Stitt LW, Cherian MG. Metallothionein expression in patients with small cell carcinoma of the lung: correlation with other molecular markers and clinical outcome. Cancer 2001;92: 836–842.

1931. Pinto CA, Carvalho PE, Antonangelo L, et al. Morphometric evaluation of tumor matrix metalloproteinase 9 predicts survival after surgical resection of adenocarcinoma of the lung. Clin Cancer Res 2003;9:3098–3104.

1932. Liao M, Wang H, Lin Z, Feng J, Zhu D. Vascular endothelial growth factor and other biological predictors related to the postoperative survival rate on non-small cell lung cancer. Lung Cancer 2001;33:125–132.

1933. Niklinska W, Burzykowski T, Chyczewski L, Niklinski J. Expression of vascular endothelial growth factor (VEGF) in non-small cell lung cancer (NSCLC): association with p53 gene mutation and prognosis. Lung Cancer 2001;34(suppl 2):S59–S64.

1934. Fontanini G, Faviana P, Lucchi M, et al. A high vascular count and overexpression of vascular endothelial growth factor are associated with unfavourable prognosis in operated small cell lung carcinoma. Br J Cancer 2002;86:558–563.

1935. Kakolyris S, Giatromanolaki A, Koukourakis M, et al. Thioredoxin expression is associated with lymph node status and prognosis in early operable non-small cell lung cancer. Clin Cancer Res 2001;7:3087–3091.

1936. Puglisi F, Aprile G, Minisini AM, et al. Prognostic significance of Apel/ref-1 subcellular localization in non-small cell lung carcinomas. Anticancer Res 2001;21:4041–4049.

1937. Takata T, Tanaka F, Yamada T, et al. Clinical significance of caspase-3 expression in pathologic-stage I, nonsmall-cell lung cancer. Int J Cancer 2001;96(suppl):54–60.

1938. Katakura H, Tanaka F, Oyanagi H, et al. Clinical significance of nm23 expression in resected pathologic-stage I, non-small cell lung cancer. Ann Thorac Surg 2002;73: 1060–1064.

1939. Reisman DN, Sciarrotta J, Wang W, Funkhouser WK, Weissman BE. Loss of BRG1/BRM in human lung cancer cell lines and primary lung cancers: correlation with poor prognosis. Cancer Res 2003;63:560–566.

1940. Fukuoka J, Fujii T, Shih JH, et al. Chromatin remodeling factors and BRM/BRG1 expression as prognostic indicators in non-small cell lung cancer. Clin Cancer Res 2004;10:4314–4324.

1941. Wang J, Liu X, Jiang W, Liang L. Telomerase activity and expression of the telomerase catalytic subunit gene in non-small cell lung cancer: correlation with decreased apoptosis and clinical prognosis. Chin Med J (Engl) 2000;113:985–990.

1942. Wu TC, Lin P, Hsu CP, et al. Loss of telomerase activity may be a potential favorable prognostic marker in lung carcinomas. Lung Cancer 2003;41:163–169.

1943. Massion PP, Taflan PM, Jamshedur Rahman SM, et al. Significance of p63 amplification and overexpression in lung cancer development and prognosis. Cancer Res 2003;63:7113–7121.

1944. Iwata T, Uramoto H, Sugio K, et al. A lack of prognostic significance regarding DeltaNp63 immunoreactivity in lung cancer. Lung Cancer 2005;50:67–73.

1945. Gessner C, Woischwill C, Schumacher A, et al. Nuclear YB-1 expression as a negative prognostic marker in non-small cell lung cancer. Eur Respir J 2004;23:14–19.

1946. David O, LeBeau H, Brody AR, Friedman M, Jett J. Phospho-Akt overexpression in non-small cell lung cancer confers significant stage-independent survival disadvantage. Chest 2004;125(5 suppl):152S.

1947. David O, Jett J, LeBeau H, et al. Phospho-Akt overexpression in non-small cell lung cancer confers significant stage-independent survival disadvantage. Clin Cancer Res 2004;10:6865–6871.

1948. Uramoto H, Sugio K, Oyama T, et al. Expression of deltaNp73 predicts poor prognosis in lung cancer. Clin Cancer Res 2004;10:6905–6911.

1949. Hirai K, Koizumi K, Haraguchi S, et al. Prognostic significance of the tumor suppressor gene maspin in non-small cell lung cancer. Ann Thorac Surg 2005;79:248–253.

1950. Goto A, Niki T, Chi-Pin L, et al. Loss of TSLC1 expression in lung adenocarcinoma: relationships with histological subtypes, sex and prognostic significance. Cancer Sci 2005;96:480–486.

1951. Uramoto H, Sugio K, Oyama T, Hanagiri T, Yasumoto K. P53R2, p53 inducible ribonucleotide reductase gene, correlated with tumor progression of non-small cell lung cancer. Anticancer Res 2006;26:983–988.

1952. Tsai MF, Wang CC, et al. A new tumor suppressor DnaJ-like heat shock protein, HLJ1, and survival of patients with non-small-cell lung carcinoma. J Natl Cancer Inst 2006;98:825–838.

1953. Zhang Z, Ma J, Li N, Sun N, Wang C. Expression of nuclear factor-kappaB and its clinical significance in nonsmall-cell lung cancer. Ann Thorac Surg 2006;82:243–248.

1954. Giatromanolaki A, Koukourakis MI, Sowter HM, et al. BNIP3 expression is linked with hypoxia-regulated protein expression and with poor prognosis in non-small cell lung cancer. Clin Cancer Res 2004;10:5566–5571.
1955. Karczmarek-Borowska B, Filip A, Wojcierowski J, et al. Estimation of prognostic value of Bcl-xL gene expression in non-small cell lung cancer. Lung Cancer 2006;51: 61–69.
1956. Volm M, Efferth T, Mattern J. Oncoprotein (c-myc, c-erbB1, c-erbB2, c-fos) and suppressor gene product (p53) expression in squamous cell carcinomas of the lung. Clinical and biological correlations. Anticancer Res 1992;12:11–20.
1957. Weston A, Caporaso NE, Perrin LS, et al. Relationship of H-ras-1, L-myc, and p53 polymorphisms with lung cancer risk and prognosis. Environ Health Perspect 1992;8: 61–67.
1958. Volm M, Drings P, Wodrich W. Prognostic significance of the expression of c-fos, c-jun and c-erbB-1 oncogene products in human squamous cell lung carcinomas. J Cancer Res Clin Oncol 1993;119:507–510.
1959. Ebina M, Steinberg SM, Mulshine JL, Linnoila RI. Relationship of p53 overexpression and up-regulation of proliferating cell nuclear antigen with the clinical course of non-small cell lung cancer. Cancer Res 1994; 54:2496–2503.
1960. Isobe T, Hiyama K, Yoshida Y, Fujiwara Y, Yamakido M. Prognostic significance of p53 and ras gene abnormalities in lung adenocarcinoma patients with stage I disease after curative resection. Jpn J Cancer Res 1994;85:1240–1246.
1961. Kern JA, Slebos RJ, Top B, et al. C-erbB-2 expression and codon 12 K-ras mutations both predict shortened survival for patients with pulmonary adenocarcinomas. J Clin Invest 1994;93:516–520.
1962. Tateishi M, Ishida T, Kohdono S, Hamatake M, Fukuyama Y, Sugimachi K. Prognostic influence of the co-expression of epidermal growth factor receptor and c-erbB-2 protein in human lung adenocarcinoma. Surg Oncol 1994;3: 109–113.
1963. Fujino M, Dosaka-Akita H, Harada M, et al. Prognostic significance of p53 and ras p21 expression in nonsmall cell lung cancer. Cancer 1995;76:2457–2463.
1964. Kratzke RA, Greatens TM, Rubins JB, et al. Rb and p16INK4a expression in resected non-small cell lung tumors. Cancer Res 1996;56:3415–3420.
1965. Kwa HB, Michalides RJ, Dijkman JH, Mooi WJ. The prognostic value of NCAM, p53 and cyclin D1 in resected non-small cell lung cancer. Lung Cancer 1996; 14:207–217.
1966. Ohsaki Y, Toyoshima E, Fujiuchi S, et al. bcl-2 and p53 protein expression in non-small cell lung cancers: correlation with survival time. Clin Cancer Res 1996;2:915–920.
1967. Pfeiffer P, Clausen PP, Andersen K, Rose C. Lack of prognostic significance of epidermal growth factor receptor and the oncoprotein p185HER-2 in patients with systemically untreated non-small-cell lung cancer: an immunohistochemical study on cryosections. Br J Cancer 1996;74: 86–91.
1968. Xu HJ, Cagle PT, Hu SX, Li J, Benedict WF. Altered retinoblastoma and p53 protein status in non-small cell carcinoma of the lung: potential synergistic effects on prognosis. Clin Cancer Res 1996;2:1169–76.
1969. Apolinario RM, van der Valk P, de Jong JS, et al. Prognostic value of the expression of p53, bcl-2, and bax oncoproteins, and neovascularization in patients with radically resected non-small-cell lung cancer. J Clin Oncol 1997; 15:2456–2466.
1970. Dosaka-Akita H, Hu SX, Fujino M, et al. Altered retinoblastoma protein expression in nonsmall cell lung cancer: its synergistic effects with altered ras and p53 protein status on prognosis. Cancer 1997;79:1329–1337.
1971. Fukuyama Y, Mitsudomi T, Sugio K, Ishida T, Akazawa K, Sugimachi K. K-ras and p53 mutations are an independent unfavourable prognostic indicator in patients with non-small-cell lung cancer. Br J Cancer 1997;75:1125–1130.
1972. Ishida H, Irie K, Itoh T, Furukawa T, Tokunaga O. The prognostic significance of p53 and bcl-2 expression in lung adenocarcinoma and its correlation with Ki-67 growth fraction. Cancer 1997;80:1034–1045.
1973. MacKinnon M, Kerr KM, King G, Kennedy MM, Cockburn JS, Jeffrey RR. p53, c-erbB-2 and nm23 expression have no prognostic significance in primary pulmonary adenocarcinoma. Eur J Cardiothorac Surg 1997; 11:838–842.
1974. Nishio M, Koshikawa T, Yatabe Y, et al. Prognostic significance of cyclin D1 and retinoblastoma expression in combination with p53 abnormalities in primary, resected non-small cell lung cancers. Clin Cancer Res 1997;3: 1051–1058.
1975. Pastorino U, Andreola S, Tagliabue E, et al. Immunocytochemical markers in stage I lung cancer: relevance to prognosis. J Clin Oncol 1997;15:2858–2865.
1976. Sanchez-Cespedes M, Rosell R, Pifarre A, et al. Microsatellite alterations at 5q21, 11p13, and 11p15.5 do not predict survival in non-small cell lung cancer. Clin Cancer Res 1997;3:1229–1235.
1977. Bennett WP, el-Deiry WS, Rush WL, et al. p21waf1/cip1 and transforming growth factor beta 1 protein expression correlate with survival in non-small cell lung cancer. Clin Cancer Res 1998;4:1499–1506.
1978. Huang CL, Taki T, Adachi M, et al. Mutations of p53 and K-ras genes as prognostic factors for non-small cell lung cancer. Int J Oncol 1998;12:553–563.
1979. Kim YC, Park KO, Kern JA, et al. The interactive effect of Ras, HER2, P53 and Bcl-2 expression in predicting the survival of non-small cell lung cancer patients. Lung Cancer 1998;22:181–190.
1980. Nemunaitis J, Klemow S, Tong A, et al. Prognostic value of K-ras mutations, ras oncoprotein, and c-erb B-2 oncoprotein expression in adenocarcinoma of the lung. Am J Clin Oncol 1998;21:155–160.
1981. Volm M, Rittgen W, Drings P. Prognostic value of ERBB-1, VEGF, cyclin A, FOS, JUN and MYC in patients with squamous cell lung carcinomas. Br J Cancer 1998;77: 663–669.
1982. Brambilla E, Moro D, Gazzeri S, Brambilla C. Alterations of expression of Rb, p16(INK4A) and cyclin D1 in non-small cell lung carcinoma and their clinical significance. J Pathol 1999;188:351–360.

1983. Cantero R, Torres AJ, Maestro M, et al. Use of possible synergistic expression of p53 and p185 as a prognostic tool for stage I non-small-cell lung cancer. World J Surg 1999;23:1294–1299.
1984. Hommura F, Dosaka-Akita H, Kinoshita I, et al. Predictive value of expression of p16INK4A, retinoblastoma and p53 proteins for the prognosis of non-small-cell lung cancers. Br J Cancer 1999;81:696–701.
1985. Boldrini L, Calcinai A, Samaritani E, et al. Tumour necrosis factor-alpha and transforming growth factor-beta are significantly associated with better prognosis in non-small cell lung carcinoma: putative relation with BCL-2–mediated neovascularization. Br J Cancer 2000;83:480–486.
1986. Carvalho PE, Antonangelo L, Bernardi FD, Leao LE, Rodrigues OR, Capelozzi VL. Useful prognostic panel markers to express the biological tumor status in resected lung adenocarcinomas. Jpn J Clin Oncol 2000;30: 478–486.
1987. Demarchi LM, Reis MM, Palomino SA, et al. Prognostic values of stromal proportion and PCNA, Ki-67, and p53 proteins in patients with resected adenocarcinoma of the lung. Mod Pathol 2000;13:511–520.
1988. Moldvay J, Scheid P, Wild P, et al. Predictive survival markers in patients with surgically resected non-small cell lung carcinoma. Clin Cancer Res 2000;6:1125–1134.
1989. Nguyen VN, Mirejovsky P, Mirejovsky T, Melinova L, Mandys V. Expression of cyclin D1, Ki-67 and PCNA in non-small cell lung cancer: prognostic significance and comparison with p53 and bcl-2. Acta Histochem 2000; 102:323–338.
1990. Volm M, Koomagi R. Prognostic relevance of c-Myc and caspase-3 for patients with non-small cell lung cancer. Oncol Rep 2000;7:95–98.
1991. Brabender J, Danenberg KD, Metzger R, et al. Epidermal growth factor receptor and HER2-neu mRNA expression in non-small cell lung cancer Is correlated with survival. Clin Cancer Res 2001;7:1850–1855.
1992. Chen JT, Chen YC, Chen CY, Wang YC. Loss of p16 and/or pRb protein expression in NSCLC. An immunohistochemical and prognostic study. Lung Cancer 2001; 31:163–170.
1993. Dosaka-Akita H, Hommura F, Mishina T, et al. A risk-stratification model of non-small cell lung cancers using cyclin E, Ki-67, and ras p21: different roles of G1 cyclins in cell proliferation and prognosis. Cancer Res 2001;61:2500–2504.
1994. Jin M, Inoue S, Umemura T, et al. Cyclin D1, p16 and retinoblastoma gene product expression as a predictor for prognosis in non-small cell lung cancer at stages I and II. Lung Cancer 2001;34:207–218.
1995. Laudanski J, Niklinska W, Burzykowski T, Chyczewski L, Niklinski J. Prognostic significance of p53 and bcl-2 abnormalities in operable nonsmall cell lung cancer. Eur Respir J 2001;17:660–666.
1996. Saitoh G, Sugio K, Ishida T, Sugimachi K. Prognostic significance of p21waf1, cyclin D1 and retinoblastoma expression detected by immunohistochemistry in non-small cell lung cancer. Oncol Rep 2001;8:737–743.
1997. Schiller JH, Adak S, Feins RH, et al. Lack of prognostic significance of p53 and K-ras mutations in primary resected non-small-cell lung cancer on E4592: a Laboratory Ancillary Study on an Eastern Cooperative Oncology Group Prospective Randomized Trial of Postoperative Adjuvant Therapy. J Clin Oncol. 2001; 19:448–457.
1998. Sugio K, Tsukamoto S, Ushijima C, et al. Clinical significance of the Rb expression in adenocarcinoma of the lung. Anticancer Res 2001;21:1931–1935.
1999. Dworakowska D, Gozdz S, Jassem E, et al. Prognostic relevance of proliferating cell nuclear antigen and p53 expression in non-small cell lung cancer. Lung Cancer 2002;35:35–41.
2000. Gessner C, Liebers U, Kuhn H, et al. BAX and p16INK4A are independent positive prognostic markers for advanced tumour stage of nonsmall cell lung cancer. Eur Respir J 2002;19:134–140.
2001. Gonzalez-Quevedo R, Iniesta P, Moran A, et al. Cooperative role of telomerase activity and p16 expression in the prognosis of non-small-cell lung cancer. J Clin Oncol 2002;20:254–262.
2002. Han H, Landreneau RJ, Santucci TS, et al. Prognostic value of immunohistochemical expressions of p53, HER-2/neu, and bcl-2 in stage I non-small-cell lung cancer. Hum Pathol 2002;33:105–110.
2003. Lai RS, Wang JS, Hsu HK, Chang HC, Lin CH, Lin MH. Prognostic evaluation of the expression of p53 and bcl-2 oncoproteins in patients with surgically resected non-small cell lung cancer. Jpn J Clin Oncol 2002;32: 393–397.
2004. Minami K, Saito Y, Imamura H, Okamura A. Prognostic significance of p53, Ki-67, VEGF and Glut-1 in resected stage I adenocarcinoma of the lung. Lung Cancer 2002; 38:51–67.
2005. Cheng YL, Lee SC, Harn HJ, et al. Prognostic prediction of the immunohistochemical expression of p53 and p16 in resected non-small cell lung cancer. Eur J Cardiothorac Surg 2003;23:221–228.
2006. Grossi F, Loprevite M, Chiaramondia M, et al. Prognostic significance of K-ras, p53, bcl-2, PCNA, CD34 in radically resected non-small cell lung cancers. Eur J Cancer 2003;39:1242–1250.
2007. Hilbe W, Dirnhofer S, Oberwasserlechner F, et al. Immunohistochemical typing of non-small cell lung cancer on cryostat sections: correlation with clinical parameters and prognosis. J Clin Pathol 2003;56:736–741.
2008. Miyatake K, Gemba K, Ueoka H, et al. Prognostic significance of mutant p53 protein, P-glycoprotein and glutathione S-transferase-pi in patients with unresectable non-small cell lung cancer. Anticancer Res 2003; 23:2829–2836.
2009. Pollan M, Varela G, Torres A, et al. Clinical value of p53, c-erbB-2, CEA and CA125 regarding relapse, metastasis and death in resectable non-small cell lung cancer. Int J Cancer 2003;107:781–790.
2010. Zereu M, Vinholes JJ, Zettler CG. p53 and Bcl-2 protein expression and its relationship with prognosis in small-cell lung cancer. Clin Lung Cancer 2003;4:298–302.
2011. Brattstrom D, Wester K, Bergqvist M, et al. HER-2, EGFR, COX-2 expression status correlated to micro vessel density and survival in resected non-small cell lung cancer. Acta Oncol 2004;43:80–86.

2012. Dworakowska D, Jassem E, Jassem J, et al. Prognostic relevance of altered pRb and p53 protein expression in surgically treated non-small cell lung cancer patients. Oncology 2004;67:60–66.
2013. Esposito V, Baldi A, Tonini G, et al. Analysis of cell cycle regulator proteins in non-small cell lung cancer. J Clin Pathol 2004;57:58–63.
2014. Groeger AM, Esposito V, De Luca A, et al. Prognostic value of immunohistochemical expression of p53, bax, Bcl-2 and Bcl-xL in resected non-small-cell lung cancers. Histopathology 2004;44:54–63.
2015. Onn A, Correa AM, Gilcrease M, et al. Synchronous overexpression of epidermal growth factor receptor and HER2–neu protein is a predictor of poor outcome in patients with stage I non-small cell lung cancer. Clin Cancer Res 2004;10:136–143.
2016. Oshita F, Ito H, Ikehara M, et al. Prognostic impact of survivin, cyclin D1, integrin beta1, and VEGF in patients with small adenocarcinoma of stage I lung cancer. Am J Clin Oncol 2004;27:425–428.
2017. Saad RS, Liu Y, Han H, Landreneau RJ, Silverman JF. Prognostic significance of HER2/neu, p53, and vascular endothelial growth factor expression in early stage conventional adenocarcinoma and bronchioloalveolar carcinoma of the lung. Mod Pathol 2004;17:1235–1242.
2018. Szelachowska J, Jelen M. Laminin, Her2/neu and Ki-67 as prognostic factors in non-small cell lung cancer. Rocz Akad Med Bialymst 2004;49:256–261.
2019. Wang J, Lee JJ, Wang L, et al. Value of p16INK4a and RASSF1A promoter hypermethylation in prognosis of patients with resectable non-small cell lung cancer. Clin Cancer Res 2004;10:6119–6125.
2020. Abdulkader I, Sanchez L, Cameselle-Teijeiro J, et al. Cell-cycle-associated markers and clinical outcome in human epithelial cancers: a tissue microarray study. Oncol Rep 2005;14:1527–1531.
2021. Bozcuk H, Gumus A, Ozbilim G, et al. Cluster analysis of p-glycoprotein, c-erb-B2 and P53 in relation to tumor histology strongly indicates prognosis in patients with operable non-small cell lung cancer. Med Sci Monit 2005;11:HY11–HY20.
2022. Burke L, Flieder DB, Guinee DG, et al. Prognostic implications of molecular and immunohistochemical profiles of the Rb and p53 cell cycle regulatory pathways in primary non-small cell lung carcinoma. Clin Cancer Res 2005;11:232–241.
2023. Dworakowska D, Jassem E, Jassem J, et al. Prognostic value of cyclin D1 overexpression in correlation with pRb and p53 status in non-small cell lung cancer (NSCLC). J Cancer Res Clin Oncol 2005;131:479–485.
2024. Esposito V, Baldi A, De Luca A, et al. Cell cycle related proteins as prognostic parameters in radically resected non-small cell lung cancer. J Clin Pathol 2005;58:734–739.
2025. Ghazizadeh M, Jin E, Shimizu H, et al. Role of cdk4, p16INK4, and Rb expression in the prognosis of bronchioloalveolar carcinomas. Respiration 2005;72:68–73.
2026. Maddau C, Confortini M, Bisanzi S, et al. Prognostic significance of p53 and Ki-67 antigen expression in surgically treated non-small cell lung cancer: immunocytochemical detection with imprint cytology. Am J Clin Pathol 2006;125:425–431.
2027. Paik KH, Park YH, Ryoo BY, et al. Prognostic value of immunohistochemical staining of p53, bcl-2, and Ki-67 in small cell lung cancer. J Korean Med Sci 2006;21:35–39.
2028. Yaren A, Oztop I, Kargi A, et al. Bax, bcl-2 and c-kit expression in non-small-cell lung cancer and their effects on prognosis. Int J Clin Pract 2006;60:675–682.
2029. Huncharek M, Kupelnick B, Geschwind JF, Caubet JF. Prognostic significance of p53 mutations in non-small cell lung cancer: a meta-analysis of 829 cases from eight published studies. Cancer Lett 2000;153:219–226.
2030. Mitsudomi T, Hamajima N, Ogawa M, Takahashi T. Prognostic significance of p53 alterations in patients with non-small cell lung cancer: a meta-analysis. Clin Cancer Res 2000;6:4055–4063.
2031. Steels E, Paesmans M, Berghmans T, et al. Role of p53 as a prognostic factor for survival in lung cancer: a systematic review of the literature with a meta-analysis. Eur Respir J 2001;18:705–719.
2032. Huncharek M, Muscat J, Geschwind JF. K-ras oncogene mutation as a prognostic marker in non-small cell lung cancer: a combined analysis of 881 cases. Carcinogenesis 1999;20:1507–1510.
2033. Mascaux C, Iannino N, Martin B, et al. The role of RAS oncogene in survival of patients with lung cancer: a systematic review of the literature with meta-analysis. Br J Cancer 2005;92:131–139.
2034. Spinola M, Pedotti P, Dragani TA, Taioli E. Meta-analysis suggests association of L-myc EcoRI polymorphism with cancer prognosis. Clin Cancer Res 2004;10:4769–4775.
2035. Martin B, Paesmans M, Berghmans T, et al. Role of Bcl-2 as a prognostic factor for survival in lung cancer: a systematic review of the literature with meta-analysis. Br J Cancer 2003;89:55–64.
2036. Meert AP, Martin B, Delmotte P, et al. The role of EGF-R expression on patient survival in lung cancer: a systematic review with meta-analysis. Eur Respir J 2002;20:975–981.
2037. Harpole DH Jr, Herndon JE 2nd, Wolfe WG, Iglehart JD, Marks JR. A prognostic model of recurrence and death in stage I non-small cell lung cancer utilizing presentation, histopathology, and oncoprotein expression. Cancer Res 1995;55:51–56.
2038. Fontanini G, Vignati S, Bigini D, et al. Recurrence and death in non-small cell lung carcinomas: a prognostic model using pathological parameters, microvessel count, and gene protein products. Clin Cancer Res 1996;2:1067–1075.
2039. Zborovskaya I, Gasparian A, Kitaeva M, et al. Simultaneous detection of genetic and immunological markers in non-small cell lung cancer: prediction of metastatic potential of tumor. Clin Exp Metastasis 1996;14:490–500.
2040. Bellotti M, Elsner B, Paez De Lima A, Esteva H, Marchevsky AM. Neural networks as a prognostic tool for patients with non-small cell carcinoma of the lung. Mod Pathol 1997;10:1221–1227.
2041. Kwiatkowski DJ, Harpole DH Jr, Godleski J, et al. Molecular pathologic substaging in 244 stage I non-small-cell

lung cancer patients: clinical implications. J Clin Oncol 1998;16:2468–2477.
2042. Marchevsky AM, Patel S, Wiley KJ, et al. Artificial neural networks and logistic regression as tools for prediction of survival in patients with Stages I and II non-small cell lung cancer. Mod Pathol 1998;11:618–625.
2043. Miyake M, Adachi M, Huang C, Higashiyama M, Kodama K, Taki T. A novel molecular staging protocol for non-small cell lung cancer. Oncogene 1999;18:2397–2404.
2044. Schneider PM, Praeuer HW, Stoeltzing O, et al. Multiple molecular marker testing (p53, C-Ki-ras, c-erbB-2) improves estimation of prognosis in potentially curative resected non-small cell lung cancer. Br J Cancer 2000;83: 473–479.
2045. O'Byrne KJ, Cox G, Swinson D, et al. Towards a biological staging model for operable non-small cell lung cancer. Lung Cancer 2001;34(suppl 2):S83–S89.
2046. Gandara DR, Lara PN, Lau DH, Mack P, Gumerlock PH. Molecular-clinical correlative studies in non-small cell lung cancer: application of a three-tiered approach. Lung Cancer 2001;34(suppl 3):S75–S80.
2047. Dosaka-Akita H, Hommura F, Mishina T, et al. A risk-stratification model of non-small cell lung cancers using cyclin E, Ki-67, and ras p21: different roles of G1 cyclins in cell proliferation and prognosis. Cancer Res 2001; 61:2500–2504.
2048. Volm M, Koomagi R, Mattern J, Efferth T. Expression profile of genes in non-small cell lung carcinomas from long-term surviving patients. Clin Cancer Res 2002; 8:1843–1848.
2049. Hanai T, Yatabe Y, Nakayama Y, et al. Prognostic models in patients with non-small-cell lung cancer using artificial neural networks in comparison with logistic regression. Cancer Sci 2003;94:473–477.
2050. Au NH, Cheang M, Huntsman DG, et al. Evaluation of immunohistochemical markers in non-small cell lung cancer by unsupervised hierarchical clustering analysis: a tissue microarray study of 284 cases and 18 markers. J Pathol 2004;204:101–109.
2051. Lu C, Soria JC, Tang X, et al. Prognostic factors in resected stage I non-small-cell lung cancer: a multivariate analysis of six molecular markers. J Clin Oncol 2004;22: 4575–4583.
2052. Berrar D, Sturgeon B, Bradbury I, Downes CS, Dubitzky W. Survival trees for analyzing clinical outcome in lung adenocarcinomas based on gene expression profiles: identification of neogenin and diacylglycerol kinase alpha expression as critical factors. J Comput Biol 2005;12: 534–544.
2053. Komiya T, Hirashima T, Takada M, et al. Prognostic significance of serum p53 antibodies in squamous cell carcinoma of the lung. Anticancer Res 1997;17:3721–3724.
2054. Gonzalez R, Silva JM, Sanchez A, et al. Microsatellite alterations and TP53 mutations in plasma DNA of small-cell lung cancer patients: follow-up study and prognostic significance. Ann Oncol 2000;11:1097–1104.
2055. Jacot W, Pujol JL, Boher JM, Lamy PJ. Serum EGF-receptor and HER-2 extracellular domains and prognosis of non-small-cell lung cancer. Br J Cancer 2004;91: 430–433.
2056. Camps C, Sirera R, Bremnes R, et al. Is there a prognostic role of K-ras point mutations in the serum of patients with advanced non-small cell lung cancer? Lung Cancer 2005;50:339–346.
2057. Rosell R, Fossella F, Milas L; Spanish Lung Cancer Group. Molecular markers and targeted therapy with novel agents: prospects in the treatment of non-small cell lung cancer. Lung Cancer 2002;38(suppl 4):43–49.
2058. Rosell R, Taron M, Ariza A, et al. Molecular predictors of response to chemotherapy in lung cancer. Semin Oncol 2004;31(1 suppl 1):20–27.
2059. Fanucchi M, Khuri FR. Taxanes in the treatment of non-small cell lung cancer. Treat Respir Med 2006;5:181–191.
2060. Rosell R, Cecere F, Santarpia M, Reguart N, Taron M. Predicting the outcome of chemotherapy for lung cancer. Curr Opin Pharmacol 2006;6:323–331.
2061. Rosell R, Cuello M, Cecere F, et al. Treatment of non-small-cell lung cancer and pharmacogenomics: where we are and where we are going. Curr Opin Oncol 2006;18: 135–143.
2062. Santarpia M, Altavilla G, Salazar F, Taron M, Rosell R. From the bench to the bed: individualizing treatment in non-small-cell lung cancer. Clin Transl Oncol 2006;8: 71–76.
2063. Heppell-Parton A, Cahn A, Bench A, et al. Thioredoxin, a mediator of growth inhibition, maps to 9q31. Genomics 1995;26:379–381.
2064. Kakolyris S, Giatromanolaki A, Koukourakis M, et al. Thioredoxin expression is associated with lymph node status and prognosis in early operable non-small cell lung cancer. Clin Cancer Res 2001;7:3087–3091.
2065. Soini Y, Kahlos K, Napankangas U, et al. Widespread expression of thioredoxin and thioredoxin reductase in non small cell lung carcinoma. Clin Cancer Res 2001, 7:1750–1757.
2066. Kim HJ, Chae HZ, Kim YJ, et al. Preferential elevation of Prx I and Trx expression in lung cancer cells following hypoxia and in human lung cancer tissues. Cell Biol Toxicol 2003;19:285–298.
2067. Arnold NB, Ketterer K, Kleeff J, Friess H, Buchler MW, Korc M. Thioredoxin is downstream of Smad7 in a pathway that promotes growth and suppresses cisplatin-induced apoptosis in pancreatic cancer. Cancer Res 2004;64:3599–3606.
2068. Kinnula VL, Paakko P, Soini Y. Antioxidant enzymes and redox regulating thiol proteins in malignancies of human lung. FEBS Lett 2004;569:1–6.
2069. Csiki I, Yanagisawa K, Haruki N, et al. Thioredoxin-1 modulates transcription of cyclooxygenase-2 via hypoxia-inducible factor-1{alpha} in non-small cell lung cancer. Cancer Res 2006;66:143–150.
2070. Rosell R, Lord RV, Taron M, Reguart N. DNA repair and cisplatin resistance in non-small-cell lung cancer. Lung Cancer 2002;38:217–227.
2071. Camps C, Sarries C, Roig B, et al. Assessment of nucleotide excision repair XPD polymorphisms in the peripheral blood of gemcitabine/cisplatin-treated advanced non-small-cell lung cancer patients. Clin Lung Cancer 2003;4:237–241.

2072. Rosell R, Taron M, Barnadas A, Scagliotti G, Sarries C, Roig B. Nucleotide excision repair pathways involved in Cisplatin resistance in non-small-cell lung cancer. Cancer Control 2003;10:297–305.
2073. Isla D, Sarries C, Rosell R, et al. Single nucleotide polymorphisms and outcome in docetaxel-cisplatin-treated advanced non-small-cell lung cancer. Ann Oncol 2004; 15:1194–1203.
2074. Ryu JS, Hong YC, Han HS, et al. Association between polymorphisms of ERCC1 and XPD and survival in non-small-cell lung cancer patients treated with cisplatin combination chemotherapy. Lung Cancer 2004;44:311–316.
2075. Zhou W, Gurubhagavatula S, Liu G, et al. Excision repair cross-complementation group 1 polymorphism predicts overall survival in advanced non-small cell lung cancer patients treated with platinum-based chemotherapy. Clin Cancer Res 2004;10:4939–4943.
2076. Garcia-Campelo R, Alonso-Curbera G, Anton Aparicio LM, Rosell R. Pharmacogenomics in lung cancer: an analysis of DNA repair gene expression in patients treated with platinum-based chemotherapy. Expert Opin Pharmacother 2005;6:2015–2026.
2077. Rosell R, Cobo M, Isla D, et al. Applications of genomics in NSCLC. Lung Cancer 2005;50(suppl 2):S33–S40.
2078. Seve P, Dumontet C. Chemoresistance in non-small cell lung cancer. Curr Med Chem Anticancer Agents 2005; 5:73–88.
2079. Simon GR, Sharma S, Cantor A, Smith P, Bepler G. Polymorphisms in ERCC1 and grade 3 or 4 toxicity in non-small cell lung cancer patients. Clin Cancer Res 2005;11:1534–1538.
2080. Wachters FM, Wong LS, Timens W, Kampinga HH, Groen HJ. ERCC1, hRad51, and BRCA1 protein expression in relation to tumour response and survival of stage III/IV NSCLC patients treated with chemotherapy. Lung Cancer 2005;50:211–219.
2081. Aprelikova O, Pace AJ, Fang B, et al. BRCA1 is a selective co-activator of 14-3-3 sigma gene transcription in mouse embryonic stem cells. J Biol Chem 2001;276:25647–25650.
2082. Quinn JE, Kennedy RD, Mullan PB, et al. BRCA1 functions as a differential modulator of chemotherapy-induced apoptosis. Cancer Res 2003;63:6221–6228.
2083. Taron M, Rosell R, Felip E, et al. BRCA1 mRNA expression levels as an indicator of chemoresistance in lung cancer. Hum Mol Genet 2004;13:2443–2449.
2084. Hermeking H, Lengauer C, Polyak K, et al. 14–3–3κ is a p53–regulated inhibitor of G2/M progression. Mol Cell 1997;1:3–11.
2085. Chan TA, Hermeking H, Lengauer C, et al. 14–3–3σ is required to prevent mitotic catastrophe after DNA damage. Nature 1999;401:616–620.
2086. Ferguson AT, Evron E, Umbricht CB, et al. High frequency of hypermethylation at the 14–3–3 sigma locus leads to gene silencing in breast cancer. Proc Natl Acad Sci USA 2000;97:6049–6054.
2087. Fu H, Subramanian RR, Masters SC. 14–3–3 proteins: structure, function, and regulation, Annu Rev Pharmacol Toxicol 2000;40:617–647.
2088. Suzuki H, Itoh F, Toyota M, et al. Inactivation of the 14–3–3 sigma gene is associated with 5′ CpG island hypermethylation in human cancers. Cancer Res 2000;60: 4353–4357.
2089. Masters SC, Fu H. 14–3–3 proteins mediate an essential anti-apoptotic signal. J Biol Chem 2001;276:45193–45200.
2090. Umbricht CB, Evron E, Gabrielson E, et al. Hypermethylation of 14–3–3σ (stratifin) is an early event in breast cancer. Oncogene 2001;20:3348–3353.
2091. Vercoutter-Edouart AS, Lemoine J, Le Bourhis X, et al. Proteomic analysis reveals that 14–3–3σ is downregulated in human breast cancer cells. Cancer Res 2001;61:76–80.
2092. Osada H, Tatematsu Y, Yatabe Y, et al. Frequent and histogical type-specific inactivation of 14–3–3σ in human lung cancers. Oncogene 2002;21:2418–2424.
2093. Hermeking H. The 14–3–3 cancer connection. Nature Rev Cancer 2003;3:931–943.
2094. Bhatia K, Siraj AK, Hussain A, et al. The tumor suppressor gene 14–3–3 sigma is commonly methylated in normal and malignant lymphoid cells. Cancer Epidemiol Biomarkers Prev 2004;12:165–169.
2095. Ramirez JL, Rosell R, Taron M, et al. 14–3–3s methylation in pretreatment serum circulating DNA of cisplatin-plus-gemcitabine-treated advanced non-small-cell lung cancer patients predicts survival: the spanish lung cancer group. J Clin Oncol 2005;23:9105–9112.
2096. Herbst RS. Targeted therapy in non-small-cell lung cancer. Oncology (Williston Park) 2002;16(9 suppl 9):19–24.
2097. Rosell R, Fossella F, Milas L; Spanish Lung Cancer Group. Molecular markers and targeted therapy with novel agents: prospects in the treatment of non-small cell lung cancer. Lung Cancer 2002;38(suppl 4):43–49.
2098. Stephenson J. Cancer studies explore targeted therapy, researchers seek new prevention strategies. JAMA 2002;287:3063–3067.
2099. Dancey JE. Recent advances of molecular targeted agents: opportunities for imaging. Cancer Biol Ther 2003;2:601–609.
2100. Johnson DH. Targeted therapy in non-small cell lung cancer: myth or reality. Lung Cancer 2003;41(suppl 1): S3–S8.
2101. Levitzki A. Protein kinase inhibitors as a therapeutic modality. Acc Chem Res 2003;36:462–469.
2102. Vlahovic G, Crawford J. Activation of tyrosine kinases in cancer. Oncologist 2003;8:531–538.
2103. Kim R, Toge T. Changes in therapy for solid tumors: potential for overcoming drug resistance in vivo with molecular targeting agents. Surg Today 2004;34:293–303.
2104. Murray N, Salgia R, Fossella FV. Targeted molecules in small cell lung cancer. Semin Oncol 2004;31(1 suppl 1): 106–111.
2105. Ross JS, Schenkein DP, Pietrusko R, et al. Targeted therapies for cancer 2004. Am J Clin Pathol 2004;122:598–609.
2106. Adams GP, Weiner LM. Monoclonal antibody therapy of cancer. Nat Biotechnol 2005;23:1147–1157.
2107. Blackhall F, Papakotoulas PI, Danson S, Thatcher N. Perspectives on novel therapies for bronchial carcinoma. Expert Opin Pharmacother 2005;6:1157–1167.

2108. Caponigro F, Basile M, de Rosa V, Normanno N. New drugs in cancer therapy, National Tumor Institute, Naples, 17–18 June 2004. Anticancer Drugs 2005;16:211–221.
2109. Lynch T Jr, Kim E. Optimizing chemotherapy and targeted agent combinations in NSCLC. Lung Cancer 2005;50(suppl 2):S25–S32.
2110. Ramalingam S, Belani CP. Molecularly-targeted therapies for non-small cell lung cancer. Expert Opin Pharmacother 2005;6:2667–2679.
2111. Maione P, Gridelli C, Troiani T, Ciardiello F. Combining targeted therapies and drugs with multiple targets in the treatment of NSCLC. Oncologist 2006;11:274–284.
2112. Massarelli E, Herbst RS. Use of novel second-line targeted therapies in non-small cell lung cancer. Semin Oncol 2006;33(1 suppl 1):S9–S16.
2113. Stinchcombe TE, Lee CB, Socinski MA. Current approaches to advanced-stage non-small-cell lung cancer: first-line therapy in patients with a good functional status. Clin Lung Cancer 2006;7(suppl 4):S111–S117.
2114. Ciardiello F, De Vita F, Orditura M, De Placido S, Tortora G. Epidermal growth factor receptor tyrosine kinase inhibitors in late stage clinical trials. Expert Opin Emerg Drugs 2003;8:501–514.
2115. Gatzemeier U. Targeting the HER1/EGFR receptor to improve outcomes in non-small-cell lung cancer. Oncology (Williston Park) 2003;17(11 suppl 12):7–10.
2116. Khalil MY, Grandis JR, Shin DM. Targeting epidermal growth factor receptor: novel therapeutics in the management of cancer. Expert Rev Anticancer Ther 2003;3:367–380.
2117. Seymour L. Epidermal growth factor receptor inhibitors: an update on their development as cancer therapeutics. Curr Opin Investig Drugs 2003;4:658–666.
2118. Sridhar SS, Seymour L, Shepherd FA. Inhibitors of epidermal-growth-factor receptors: a review of clinical research with a focus on non-small-cell lung cancer. Lancet Oncol 2003;4:397–406.
2119. Byrne BJ, Garst J. Epidermal growth factor receptor inhibitors and their role in non-small-cell lung cancer. Curr Oncol Rep 2005;7:241–247.
2120. Giaccone G. Epidermal growth factor receptor inhibitors in the treatment of non-small-cell lung cancer. J Clin Oncol 2005;23:3235–3242.
2121. Silvestri GA, Rivera MP. Targeted therapy for the treatment of advanced non-small cell lung cancer: a review of the epidermal growth factor receptor antagonists. Chest 2005;128:3975–3984.
2122. Ho C, Davies AM, Lara PN Jr, Gandara DR. Second-line treatment for advanced-stage non-small-cell lung cancer: current and future options. Clin Lung Cancer 2006;7(suppl 4):S118–S125.
2123. Ji H, Li D, Chen L, et al. The impact of human EGFR kinase domain mutations on lung tumorigenesis and in vivo sensitivity to EGFR-targeted therapies. Cancer Cell 2006;9:485–495.
2124. Vokes EE, Chu E. Anti-EGFR therapies: clinical experience in colorectal, lung, and head and neck cancers. Oncology (Williston Park) 2006;20(5 suppl 2):15–25.
2125. Schiller JH, Harrington D, Belani CP, et al. Comparison of four chemotherapy regimens for advanced non-small-cell lung cancer. N Engl J Med 2002;346:92–98.
2126. Kris MG, Natale RB, Herbst RS, et al. Efficacy of gefitinib, an inhibitor of the epidermal growth factor receptor tyrosine kinase, in symptomatic patients with non-small cell lung cancer: a randomized trial. JAMA 2003;290:2149–2158.
2127. Amador ML, Oppenheimer D, Perea S, et al. An epidermal growth factor receptor intron 1 polymorphism mediates response to epidermal growth factor receptor inhibitors. Cancer Res 2004;64:9139–9143.
2128. Calvo E, Rowinsky EK. Effect of epidermal growth factor receptor mutations on the response to epidermal growth factor receptor tyrosine kinase inhibitors: target-based populations for target-based drugs. Clin Lung Cancer 2004;6(suppl 1):S35–S42.
2129. Huang SF, Liu HP, Li LH, et al. High frequency of epidermal growth factor receptor mutations with complex patterns in non-small cell lung cancers related to gefitinib responsiveness in Taiwan. Clin Cancer Res 2004;10:8195–8203.
2130. Janne PA, Gurubhagavatula S, Yeap BY, et al. Outcomes of patients with advanced non-small cell lung cancer treated with gefitinib (ZD1839, "Iressa") on an expanded access study. Lung Cancer 2004;44:221–230.
2131. Miller VA, Kris MG, Shah N, et al. Bronchioloalveolar pathologic subtype and smoking history predict sensitivity to gefitinib in advanced non-small-cell lung cancer. J Clin Oncol 2004;22:1103–1109.
2132. Paez JG, Janne PA, Lee JC, et al. EGFR mutations in lung cancer: correlation with clinical response to gefitinib therapy. Science 2004;304:1497–1500.
2133. Pao W, Miller V, Zakowski M, et al. EGF receptor gene mutations are common in lung cancers from "never smokers" and are associated with sensitivity of tumors to gefitinib and erlotinib. Proc Natl Acad Sci USA 2004;101:13306–13311.
2134. Sordella R, Bell DW, Haber DA, Settleman J. Gefitinib-sensitizing EGFR mutations in lung cancer activate anti-apoptotic pathways. Science 2004;305:1163–1167.
2135. Vastag B. Research unveils the "who" and "why" of gefitinib. J Natl Cancer Inst 2004;96:1352–1354.
2136. Amann J, Kalyankrishna S, Massion PP, et al. Aberrant epidermal growth factor receptor signaling and enhanced sensitivity to EGFR inhibitors in lung cancer. Cancer Res 2005;65:226–235.
2137. Bell DW, Lynch TJ, Haserlat SM, et al. Epidermal growth factor receptor mutations and gene amplification in non-small-cell lung cancer: molecular analysis of the IDEAL/INTACT gefitinib trials. J Clin Oncol 2005;23:8081–8092.
2138. Cortes-Funes H, Gomez C, Rosell R, et al. Epidermal growth factor receptor activating mutations in Spanish gefitinib-treated non-small-cell lung cancer patients. Ann Oncol 2005;16:1081–1086.
2139. Han SW, Kim TY, Hwang PG, et al. Predictive and prognostic impact of epidermal growth factor receptor mutation in non-small-cell lung cancer patients treated with gefitinib. J Clin Oncol 2005;23:2493–2501.

2140. Kobayashi S, Boggon TJ, Dayaram T, et al. EGFR mutation and resistance of non-small-cell lung cancer to gefitinib. N Engl J Med 2005;352:786–792.
2141. Kwak EL, Sordella R, Bell DW, et al. Irreversible inhibitors of the EGF receptor may circumvent acquired resistance to gefitinib. Proc Natl Acad Sci USA 2005;102: 7665–7670.
2142. Lee DH, Han JY, Lee HG, et al. Gefitinib as a first-line therapy of advanced or metastatic adenocarcinoma of the lung in never-smokers. Clin Cancer Res 2005;11:3032–3037.
2143. Lynch TJ. Predictive tests for EGFR inhibitors. Clin Adv Hematol Oncol 2005;3:678–679.
2144. Mitsudomi T, Kosaka T, Endoh H, et al. Mutations of the epidermal growth factor receptor gene predict prolonged survival after gefitinib treatment in patients with non-small-cell lung cancer with postoperative recurrence. J Clin Oncol 2005;23:2513–2520.
2145. Mukohara T, Engelman JA, Hanna NH, et al. Differential effects of gefitinib and cetuximab on non-small-cell lung cancers bearing epidermal growth factor receptor mutations. J Natl Cancer Inst 2005;97:1185–1194.
2146. Pan Q, Pao W, Ladanyi M. Rapid polymerase chain reaction-based detection of epidermal growth factor receptor gene mutations in lung adenocarcinomas. J Mol Diagn 2005;7:396–403.
2147. Pao W, Miller VA, Politi KA, Riely GJ, Somwar R, Zakowski MF. Acquired resistance of lung adenocarcinomas to gefitinib or erlotinib is associated with a second mutation in the EGFR kinase domain. PLoS Med 2005; 2:e73.
2148. Sequist LV, Haber DA, Lynch TJ. Epidermal growth factor receptor mutations in non-small cell lung cancer: predicting clinical response to kinase inhibitors. Clin Cancer Res 2005;11:5668–5670.
2149. Shigematsu H, Lin L, Takahashi T, et al. Clinical and biological features associated with epidermal growth factor receptor gene mutations in lung cancers. J Natl Cancer Inst 2005;97:339–346.
2150. Speake G, Holloway B, Costello G. Recent developments related to the EGFR as a target for cancer chemotherapy. Curr Opin Pharmacol 2005;5:343–349.
2151. Takano T, Ohe Y, Sakamoto H, et al. Epidermal growth factor receptor gene mutations and increased copy numbers predict gefitinib sensitivity in patients with recurrent non-small-cell lung cancer. J Clin Oncol 2005;23: 6829–6837.
2152. Taron M, Ichinose Y, Rosell R, et al. Activating mutations in the tyrosine kinase domain of the epidermal growth factor receptor are associated with improved survival in gefitinib-treated chemorefractory lung adenocarcinomas. Clin Cancer Res 2005;11:5878–5885.
2153. Thomson S, Buck E, Petti F, et al. Epithelial to mesenchymal transition is a determinant of sensitivity of non-small-cell lung carcinoma cell lines and xenografts to epidermal growth factor receptor inhibition, Cancer Res 2005;65: 9455–9462.
2154. Yauch RL, Januario T, Eberhard DA, et al. Epithelial versus mesenchymal phenotype determines in vitro sensitivity and predicts clinical activity of erlotinib in lung cancer patients. Clin Cancer Res 2005;11:8686–8698.
2155. Govindan R. Cetuximab in advanced non-small cell lung cancer. Clin Cancer Res 2004;10(12 pt 2):4241s–4244s.
2156. Humblet Y. Cetuximab: an IgG(1) monoclonal antibody for the treatment of epidermal growth factor receptor-expressing tumours. Expert Opin Pharmacother 2004;5: 1621–1633.
2157. Kim ES. Cetuximab as a single agent or in combination with chemotherapy in lung cancer. Clin Lung Cancer 2004;6(suppl 2):S80–S84.
2158. Kim ES, Vokes EE, Kies MS. Cetuximab in cancers of the lung and head & neck. Semin Oncol 2004;31(1 suppl 1): 61–67.
2159. Harding J, Burtness B. Cetuximab: an epidermal growth factor receptor chemeric human-murine monoclonal antibody. Drugs Today (Barc) 2005;41:107–127.
2160. Mukohara T, Engelman JA, Hanna NH, et al. Differential effects of gefitinib and cetuximab on non-small-cell lung cancers bearing epidermal growth factor receptor mutations. J Natl Cancer Inst 2005;97:1185–1194.
2161. Raben D, Helfrich B, Chan DC, et al. The effects of cetuximab alone and in combination with radiation and/or chemotherapy in lung cancer. Clin Cancer Res 2005; 11(2 pt 1):795–805.
2162. Robert F, Blumenschein G, Herbst RS, et al. Phase I/IIa study of cetuximab with gemcitabine plus carboplatin in patients with chemotherapy-naive advanced non-small-cell lung cancer. J Clin Oncol 2005;23:9089–9096.
2163. Thienelt CD, Bunn PA Jr, Hanna N, et al. Multicenter phase I/II study of cetuximab with paclitaxel and carboplatin in untreated patients with stage IV non-small-cell lung cancer. J Clin Oncol 2005;23:8786–8793.
2164. Bogart JA, Govindan R. A randomized phase II study of radiation therapy, pemetrexed, and carboplatin with or without cetuximab in stage III non-small cell lung cancer. Clin Lung Cancer 2006;7:285–287.
2165. Jensen AD, Munter MW, Bischoff H, et al. Treatment of non-small cell lung cancer with intensity-modulated radiation therapy in combination with cetuximab: the NEAR protocol (NCT00115518). BMC Cancer 2006;6:122.
2166. Herbst RS, Giaccone G, Schiller JH, et al. Gefitinib in combination with paclitaxel and carboplatin in advanced non-small-cell lung cancer: a phase III trial—INTACT 2. J Clin Oncol 2004;22:785–794.
2167. Giaccone G, Herbst RS, Manegold C, et al. Gefitinib in combination with gemcitabine and cisplatin in advanced non-small-cell lung cancer: a phase III trial—INTACT 1. J Clin Oncol 2004;22:777–784.
2168. Herbst RS, Giaccone G, Schiller JH, et al. Gefitinib in combination with paclitaxel and carboplatin in advanced non-small-cell lung cancer: a phase III trial—INTACT 2. J Clin Oncol 2004;22:785–794.
2169. Krystal GW, Honsawek S, Litz J, Buchdunger E. The selective tyrosine kinase inhibitor STI571 inhibits small cell lung cancer growth. Clin Cancer Res 2000;6: 3319–3326.
2170. Wang WL, Healy ME, Sattler M, et al. Growth inhibition and modulation of kinase pathways of small cell lung

cancer cell lines by the novel tyrosine kinase inhibitor STI 571. Oncogene 2000;19:3521–3528.
2171. Buchdunger E, O'Reilly T, Wood J. Pharmacology of imatinib (STI571). Eur J Cancer 2002;38(suppl 5):S28–S36.
2172. Kijima T, Maulik G, Ma PC, et al. Regulation of cellular proliferation, cytoskeletal function, and signal transduction through CXCR4 and c-Kit in small cell lung cancer cells. Cancer Res 2002;62:6304–6311.
2173. Radford IR. Imatinib. Novartis. Curr Opin Investig Drugs 2002;3:492–499.
2174. Abrams TJ, Lee LB, Murray LJ, Pryer NK, Cherrington JM. SU11248 inhibits KIT and platelet-derived growth factor receptor beta in preclinical models of human small cell lung cancer. Mol Cancer Ther 2003;2:471–478.
2175. Heinrich MC. Is KIT an important therapeutic target in small cell lung cancer? Clin Cancer Res 2003;9(16 pt 1):5825–5828.
2176. Johnson BE, Fischer T, Fischer B, et al. Phase II study of imatinib in patients with small cell lung cancer. Clin Cancer Res 2003;9:5880–5887.
2177. Soria JC, Johnson BE, Chevalier TL. Imatinib in small cell lung cancer. Lung Cancer 2003;41(suppl 1):S49–S53.
2178. Zhang P, Gao WY, Turner S, Ducatman BS. Gleevec (STI-571) inhibits lung cancer cell growth (A549) and potentiates the cisplatin effect in vitro. Mol Cancer 2003; 2:1.
2179. Johnson BE. Imatinib for small cell lung cancer, aiming for a target in vivo. Clin Cancer Res 2004;10:3235–3236.
2180. Maulik G, Bharti A, Khan E, Broderick RJ, Kijima T, Salgia R. Modulation of c-Kit/SCF pathway leads to alterations in topoisomerase-I activity in small cell lung cancer. J Environ Pathol Toxicol Oncol 2004;23:237–251.
2181. Micke P, Hengstler JG, Albrecht H, et al. c-kit expression in adenocarcinomas of the lung. Tumour Biol 2004;25: 235–242.
2182. Wolff NC, Randle DE, Egorin MJ, Minna JD, Ilaria RL Jr. Imatinib mesylate efficiently achieves therapeutic intratumor concentrations in vivo but has limited activity in a xenograft model of small cell lung cancer. Clin Cancer Res 2004;10:3528–3534.
2183. Altundag O, Altundag K, Boruban C, Silay YS, Turen S. Imatinib mesylate lacks activity in small cell lung carcinoma expressing c-kit protein: a Phase II clinical trial. Cancer 2005;104:2033–2034.
2184. Decaudin D, de Cremoux P, Sastre X, et al. In vivo efficacy of STI571 in xenografted human small cell lung cancer alone or combined with chemotherapy. Int J Cancer 2005;113:849–856.
2185. Dy GK, Miller AA, Mandrekar SJ, et al. A phase II trial of imatinib (ST1571) in patients with c-kit expressing relapsed small-cell lung cancer: a CALGB and NCCTG study. Ann Oncol 2005;16:1811–1816.
2186. Krug LM, Crapanzano JP, Azzoli CG, et al. Imatinib mesylate lacks activity in small cell lung carcinoma expressing c-kit protein: a phase II clinical trial. Cancer 2005;103:2128–2131.
2187. Yokoyama T, Miyazawa K, Yoshida T, Ohyashiki K. Combination of vitamin K2 plus imatinib mesylate enhances induction of apoptosis in small cell lung cancer cell lines. Int J Oncol 2005;26:33–40.
2188. Johnson FM, Krug LM, Tran HT, et al. Phase I studies of imatinib mesylate combined with cisplatin and irinotecan in patients with small cell lung carcinoma. Cancer 2006; 106:366–374.
2189. Hirsch FR, Franklin WA, Bunn PA. What is the role of HER-2/neu and trastuzumab (Herceptin) in lung cancer? Lung Cancer 2002;36:263–264.
2190. Zinner RG, Kim J, Herbst RS. Non-small cell lung cancer clinical trials with trastuzumab: their foundation and preliminary results. Lung Cancer 2002;37:17–27.
2191. Ferrone M, Motl SE. Trastuzumab for the treatment of non-small-cell lung cancer. Ann Pharmacother 2003;37: 1904–1908.
2192. Heinmoller P, Gross C, Beyser K, et al. HER2 status in non-small cell lung cancer: results from patient screening for enrollment to a phase II study of herceptin. Clin Cancer Res 2003;9:5238–5243.
2193. Krawczyk P, Chocholska S, Milanowski J. Anti-HER therapeutic agents in the treatment of non-small-cell lung cancer. Ann Univ Mariae Curie Sklodowska [Med] 2003;58:113–117.
2194. Andre F, Le Chevalier T, Soria JC. Her2–neu: a target in lung cancer? Ann Oncol 2004;15:3–4.
2195. Gatzemeier U, Groth G, Butts C, et al. Randomized phase II trial of gemcitabine-cisplatin with or without trastuzumab in HER2–positive non-small-cell lung cancer. Ann Oncol 2004;15:19–27.
2196. Hirsch FR, Langer CJ. The role of HER2/neu expression and trastuzumab in non-small cell lung cancer. Semin Oncol 2004;31(1 suppl 1):75–82.
2197. Langer CJ, Stephenson P, Thor A, Vangel M, Johnson DH; Eastern Cooperative Oncology Group Study 2598. Trastuzumab in the treatment of advanced non small cell lung cancer: is there a role? Focus on Eastern Cooperative Oncology Group study 2598. J Clin Oncol 2004;22: 1180–1187.
2198. Lara PN Jr, Laptalo L, Longmate J, et al.; California Cancer Consortium. Trastuzumab plus docetaxel in HER2/neu-positive non-small-cell lung cancer: a California Cancer Consortium screening and phase II trial. Clin Lung Cancer 2004;5:231–236.
2199. Rousel R. Toward customized trastuzumab in HER-2/ neu-overexpressing non-small-cell lung cancers. J Clin Oncol 2004;22:1171–1173.
2200. Zinner RG, Glisson BS, Fossella FV, et al. Trastuzumab in combination with cisplatin and gemcitabine in patients with Her2–overexpressing, untreated, advanced non-small cell lung cancer: report of a phase II trial and findings regarding optimal identification of patients with Her2–overexpressing disease. Lung Cancer 2004;44:99–110.
2201. Altundag K, Altundag O, Morandi P, Gunduz M. Targeted therapy for targeted patients: trastuzumab in adjuvant treatment of non-small-cell lung cancer. J Clin Oncol 2005;23:1325.
2202. Altundag O, Altundag K, Ozcakar B, Silay YS. HER2/neu intragenic kinase domain mutations may be major determinant of response to trastuzumab or specific kinase

inhibitors in non-small cell lung cancer patients. Lung Cancer 2005;49:279–280.
2203. Clamon G, Herndon J, Kern J, Govindan R, Garst J, Watson D, Green M; Cancer and Leukemia Group B. Lack of trastuzumab activity in nonsmall cell lung carcinoma with overexpression of erb-B2: 39810: a phase II trial of Cancer and Leukemia Group B. Cancer 2005; 103:1670–1675.
2204. Kalemkerian G. Trastuzumab in the treatment of advanced non-small-cell lung cancer: is there a role? J Clin Oncol 2005;23:1325–1326.
2205. Krug LM, Miller VA, Patel J, et al. Randomized phase II study of weekly docetaxel plus trastuzumab versus weekly paclitaxel plus trastuzumab in patients with previously untreated advanced nonsmall cell lung carcinoma. Cancer 2005;104:2149–2155.
2206. Lee JW, Soung YH, Kim SY, et al. Absence of the ERBB2 kinase domain mutation in lung adenocarcinomas in Korean patients. Int J Cancer 2005;116:652–653.
2207. Nakamura H, Takamori S, Fujii T, et al. Cooperative cell-growth inhibition by combination treatment with ZD1839 (Iressa) and trastuzumab (Herceptin) in non-small-cell lung cancer. Cancer Lett 2005;230:33–46.
2208. Cappuzzo F, Bemis L, Varella-Garcia M. HER2 mutation and response to trastuzumab therapy in non-small-cell lung cancer. N Engl J Med 2006;354:2619–2621.
2209. Friess T, Scheuer W, Hasmann M. Combination treatment with erlotinib and pertuzumab against human tumor xenografts is superior to monotherapy. Clin Cancer Res 2005;11:5300–5309.
2210. Bianco AR. Targeting c-erbB2 and other receptors of the c-erbB family: rationale and clinical applications. J Chemother 2004;16(suppl 4):52–54.
2211. Langer CJ, Natalie RB. The emerging role of vascular endothelial growth factor receptor tyrosine kinase inhibitors. Semin Oncol 2005;32(6 suppl 10):S23–S29.
2212. Rhee J, Hoff PM. Angiogenesis inhibitors in the treatment of cancer. Expert Opin Pharmacother 2005;6: 1701–1711.
2213. Wakelee HA, Schiller JH. Targeting angiogenesis with vascular endothelial growth factor receptor small-molecule inhibitors: novel agents with potential in lung cancer. Clin Lung Cancer 2005;7(suppl 1):S31–S38.
2214. Cascone T, Troiani T, Morelli MP, Gridelli C, Ciardiello F. Antiangiogenic drugs in non-small cell lung cancer treatment. Curr Opin Oncol 2006;18:151–155.
2215. de Castro Junior G, Puglisi F, de Azambuja E, El Saghir NS, Awada A. Angiogenesis and cancer: A cross-talk between basic science and clinical trials (the "do ut des" paradigm). Crit Rev Oncol Hematol 2006;59:40–50.
2216. Ellis LM, Rosen L, Gordon MS. Overview of anti-VEGF therapy and angiogenesis. Part 1: Angiogenesis inhibition in solid tumor malignancies. Clin Adv Hematol Oncol 2006;4:suppl 1–10.
2217. Jain RK, Duda DG, Clark JW, Loeffler JS. Lessons from phase III clinical trials on anti-VEGF therapy for cancer. Nat Clin Pract Oncol 2006;3:24–40.
2218. Lee D, Heymach JV. Emerging antiangiogenic agents in lung cancer. Clin Lung Cancer 2006;7:304–308.
2219. Morgensztern D, Govindan R. Clinical trials of antiangiogenic therapy in non-small cell lung cancer: focus on bevacizumab and ZD6474. Expert Rev Anticancer Ther 2006;6:545–551.
2220. Yano S, Matsumori Y, Ikuta K, Ogino H, Doljinsuren T, Sone S. Current status and perspective of angiogenesis and antivascular therapeutic strategy: non-small cell lung cancer. Int J Clin Oncol 2006;11:73–81.
2221. Herbst RS, Sandler AB. Non-small cell lung cancer and antiangiogenic therapy: what can be expected of bevacizumab? Oncologist 2004;9(suppl 1):19–26.
2222. Johnson DH, Fehrenbacher L, Novotny WF, et al. Randomized phase II trial comparing bevacizumab plus carboplatin and paclitaxel with carboplatin and paclitaxel alone in previously untreated locally advanced or metastatic non-small-cell lung cancer. J Clin Oncol 2004; 22:2184–2191.
2223. Sandler AB, Johnson DH, Herbst RS. Anti-vascular endothelial growth factor monoclonals in non-small cell lung cancer. Clin Cancer Res 2004;10:4258s-4262s.
2224. Belani CP, Ramalingam S. Bevacizumab extends survival for patients with nonsquamous non-small-cell lung cancer. Clin Lung Cancer 2005;6:267–268.
2225. Culy C. Bevacizumab: antiangiogenic cancer therapy. Drugs Today (Barc) 2005;41:23–36.
2226. Herbst RS, Johnson DH, Mininberg E, et al. Phase I/II trial evaluating the anti-vascular endothelial growth factor monoclonal antibody bevacizumab in combination with the HER-1/epidermal growth factor receptor tyrosine kinase inhibitor erlotinib for patients with recurrent non-small-cell lung cancer. J Clin Oncol 2005;23:2544–2555.
2227. Kerr C. Bevacizumab and chemotherapy improves survival in NSCLC. Lancet Oncol 2005;6:266.
2228. Midgley R, Kerr D. Bevacizumab—current status and future directions. Ann Oncol 2005;16:999–1004.
2229. Tyagi P. Bevacizumab, when added to paclitaxel/carboplatin, prolongs survival in previously untreated patients with advanced non-small-cell lung cancer: preliminary results from the ECOG 4599 trial. Clin Lung Cancer 2005;6:276–278.
2230. Bozec A, Fischel JL, Milano G. Epidermal growth factor receptor/angiogenesis dual targeting: preclinical experience. Curr Opin Oncol 2006;18:330–334.
2231. Dy GK, Adjei AA. Angiogenesis inhibitors in lung cancer: a promise fulfilled. Clin Lung Cancer 2006;7(suppl 4): S145–S149.
2232. Lyseng-Williamson KA, Robinson DM. Spotlight on bevacizumab in advanced colorectal cancer, breast cancer, and non-small cell lung cancer. BioDrugs 2006;20: 193–195.
2233. Nagasu T, Yoshimatsu K, Rowell C, Lewis MD, Garcia AM. Inhibition of human tumor xenograft growth by treatment with the farnesyl transferase inhibitor B956. Cancer Res 1995;55:5310–5314.
2234. Sepp-Lorenzino L, Ma Z, Rands E, et al. A peptidomimetic inhibitor of farnesyl:protein transferase blocks the anchorage-dependent and -independent growth of human tumor cell lines. Cancer Res 1995;55:5302–5309.

2235. Liu M, Bryant MS, Chen J, et al. Antitumor activity of SCH 66336, an orally bioavailable tricyclic inhibitor of farnesyl protein transferase, in human tumor xenograft models and wap-ras transgenic mice. Cancer Res 1998; 58:4947–4956.
2236. Adjei AA, Erlichman C, Davis JN, et al. A Phase I trial of the farnesyl transferase inhibitor SCH66336: evidence for biological and clinical activity. Cancer Res 2000;60: 1871–1877.
2237. Adjei AA, Davis JN, Bruzek LM, Erlichman C, Kaufmann SH. Synergy of the protein farnesyltransferase inhibitor SCH66336 and cisplatin in human cancer cell lines. Clin Cancer Res 2001;7:1438–1445.
2238. Britten CD, Rowinsky EK, Soignet S, et al. A Phase I and pharmacological study of the farnesyl protein transferase inhibitor L-778,123 in patients with solid malignancies. Clin Cancer Res 2001;7:3894–3903.
2239. Crul M, de Klerk GJ, Beijnen JH, Schellens JH. Ras biochemistry and farnesyl transferase inhibitors: a literature survey. Anticancer Drugs 2001;12:163–184.
2240. End DW, Smets G, Todd AV, et al. Characterization of the antitumor effects of the selective farnesyl protein transferase inhibitor R115777 in vivo and in vitro. Cancer Res 2001;61:131–137.
2241. Dy GK, Adjei AA. The role of farnesyltransferase inhibitors in lung cancer therapy. Clin Lung Cancer 2002; 4:57–62.
2242. Evans TL, Fidias P, Skarin A, et al. Phase II study of efficacy and tolerability of the farnesl-protein transferase inhibitor L-778,123 as first-line therapy in patients with advanced non-small cell lung cancer (NSCLC). Proc Am Soc Clin Oncol 2002;2:13.
2243. Ghobrial IM, Adjei AA. Inhibitors of the ras oncogene as therapeutic targets. Hematol Oncol Clin N Am 2002; 16:1065 1088.
2244. Heymach JV, De Porre PM, DeVore RF, et al. Phase II study of the farnesyl transferase inhibitor (FTI) R115777 (Zarnestra) in patients with relapsed small cell lung cancer (SCLC). Proc Am Soc Clin Oncol 2002;21: 319.
2245. Kim ES, Kies MS, Fossella FV, et al. A Phase I/II study of the farnesyl transferase inhibitor (FTI) SCH66336 (lonafarnib) with paclitaxel in taxane-refractory patients with non-small cell lung cancer (NSCLC): final report. Proc Am Assoc Cancer Res 2002;43:550.
2246. Marangolo M. Targeted biological treatments in NSCLC. Farnesyl transferase inhibitors. Suppl Tumori 2002;1: S49.
2247. Adjei AA. Farnesyltransferase inhibitors. Cancer Chemother Biol Response Modif 2003;21:127–144.
2248. Adjei AA. An overview of farnesyltransferase inhibitors and their role in lung cancer therapy. Lung Cancer 2003;41(suppl 1):S55–S62.
2249. Adjei AA, Mauer A, Bruzek L, et al. Phase II study of the farnesyl transferase inhibitor R115777 in patients with advanced non-small cell lung cancer. J Clin Oncol 2003;21:1760–1766.
2250. Brunner TB, Gupta AK, Shi Y, et al. Farnesyltransferase inhibitors as radiation sensitizers. Int J Radiat Biol 2003;79:569–576.
2251. Johnson BE, Heymach JV. Farnesyl transferase inhibitors for patients with lung cancer. Clin Cancer Res 2004;10: 4254s–4257s.
2252. Heymach JV, Johnson DH, Khuri FR, et al. Phase II study of the farnesyl transferase inhibitor R115777 in patients with sensitive relapse small-cell lung cancer. Ann Oncol 2004;15:1187–1193.
2253. Sebti SM, Adjei AA. Farnesyltransferase inhibitors. Semin Oncol 2004;31(1 suppl 1):28–39.
2254. Adjei AA. Farnesyltransferase inhibitors. Cancer Chemother Biol Response Modif 2005;22:123–133.
2255. Han JY, Oh SH, Morgillo F, et al. Hypoxia-inducible factor 1alpha and antiangiogenic activity of farnesyltransferase inhibitor SCH66336 in human aerodigestive tract cancer. J Natl Cancer Inst 2005;97:1272–1286.
2256. Kopelovich L, Crowell JA, Fay JR. The epigenome as a target for cancer chemoprevention. J Natl Cancer Inst 2003;95:1747–1757.
2257. Digel W, Lubbert M. DNA methylation disturbances as novel therapeutic target in lung cancer: preclinical and clinical results. Crit Rev Oncol Hematol 2005;55:1–11.
2258. Miyamoto K, Ushijima T. Diagnostic and therapeutic applications of epigenetics. Jpn J Clin Oncol 2005; 35:293–301.
2259. Schrump DS, Nguyen DM. Targeting the epigenome for the treatment and prevention of lung cancer. Semin Oncol 2005;32:488–502.
2260. Otterson GA, Khleif SN, Chen W, Coxon AB, Kaye FJ. CDKN2 gene silencing in lung cancer by DNA hypermethylation and kinetics of p16INK4 protein induction by 5–aza 2′deoxycytidine. Oncogene 1995;11:1211–1216.
2261. Momparler RL, Bouffard DY, Momparler LF, Dionne J, Belanger K, Ayoub J. Pilot phase I-II study on 5–aza-2′-deoxycytidine (Decitabine) in patients with metastatic lung cancer. Anticancer Drugs 1997;8:358–368.
2262. Lantry LE, Zhang Z, Crist KA, et al. 5-Aza-2′-deoxycytidine is chemopreventive in a 4-(methyl-nitrosamino)-1-(3-pyridyl)-1-butanone-induced primary mouse lung tumor model. Carcinogenesis 1999;20:343–346.
2263. Momparler RL, Eliopoulos N, Ayoub J. Evaluation of an inhibitor of DNA methylation, 5–aza-2′-deoxycytidine, for the treatment of lung cancer and the future role of gene therapy. Adv Exp Med Biol 2000;465:433–446.
2264. Schwartsmann G, Schunemann H, Gorini CN, et al. A phase I trial of cisplatin plus decitabine, a new DNA-hypomethylating agent, in patients with advanced solid tumors and a follow-up early phase II evaluation in patients with inoperable non-small cell lung cancer. Invest New Drugs 2000;18:83–91.
2265. Momparler RL, Ayoub J. Potential of 5–aza-2′-deoxycytidine (Decitabine) a potent inhibitor of DNA methylation for therapy of advanced non-small cell lung cancer. Lung Cancer 2001;34(suppl 4):S111–S115.
2266. Boivin AJ, Momparler LF, Hurtubise A, Momparler RL. Antineoplastic action of 5–aza-2′-deoxycytidine and phenylbutyrate on human lung carcinoma cells. Anticancer Drugs 2002;13:869–874.
2267. Belinsky SA, Klinge DM, Stidley CA, et al. Inhibition of DNA methylation and histone deacetylation prevents murine lung cancer. Cancer Res 2003;63:7089–7093.

2268. Hurtubise A, Momparler RL. Evaluation of antineoplastic action of 5–aza-2′-deoxycytidine (Dacogen) and docetaxel (Taxotere) on human breast, lung and prostate carcinoma cell lines. Anticancer Drugs 2004;15:161–167.
2269. Momparler RL. Epigenetic therapy of cancer with 5–aza-2′-deoxycytidine (decitabine). Semin Oncol 2005;32: 443–451.
2270. Ardizzoni A, Loprevite M. Histone deacetylation inhibitors. Suppl Tumori 2002;1:S52–S54.
2271. Belinsky SA, Klinge DM, Stidley CA, et al. Inhibition of DNA methylation and histone deacetylation prevents murine lung cancer. Cancer Res 2003;63:7089–7093.
2272. Liu LT, Chang HC, Chiang LC, Hung WC. Histone deacetylase inhibitor up-regulates RECK to inhibit MMP-2 activation and cancer cell invasion. Cancer Res 2003;63:3069–3072.
2273. Mie Lee Y, Kim SH, Kim HS, et al. Inhibition of hypoxia-induced angiogenesis by FK228, a specific histone deacetylase inhibitor, via suppression of HIF-1alpha activity. Biochem Biophys Res Commun 2003;300:241–246.
2274. Sasakawa Y, Naoe Y, Inoue T, et al. Effects of FK228, a novel histone deacetylase inhibitor, on tumor growth and expression of p21 and c-myc genes in vivo. Cancer Lett 2003;195:161–168.
2275. Denlinger CE, Keller MD, Mayo MW, Broad RM, Jones DR. Combined proteasome and histone deacetylase inhibition in non-small cell lung cancer. J Thorac Cardiovasc Surg 2004;127:1078–1086.
2276. Denlinger CE, Rundall BK, Jones DR. Modulation of antiapoptotic cell signaling pathways in non-small cell lung cancer: the role of NF-kappaB. Semin Thorac Cardiovasc Surg 2004;16:28–39.
2277. Marks PA, Richon VM, Kelly WK, Chiao JH, Miller T. Histone deacetylase inhibitors: development as cancer therapy. Novartis Found Symp. 2004;259:269–281.
2278. Rundall BK, Denlinger CE, Jones DR. Combined histone deacetylase and NF-kappaB inhibition sensitizes non-small cell lung cancer to cell death. Surgery 2004;136: 416–425.
2279. Denlinger CE, Rundall BK, Jones DR. Inhibition of phosphatidylinositol 3–kinase/Akt and histone deacetylase activity induces apoptosis in non-small cell lung cancer in vitro and in vivo. J Thorac Cardiovasc Surg 2005;130:1422–1429.
2280. Kristeleit R, Fong P, Aherne GW, de Bono J. Histone deacetylase inhibitors: emerging anticancer therapeutic agents? Clin Lung Cancer 2005;7(suppl 1):S19–S30.
2281. Maxhimer JB, Reddy RM, Zuo J, Cole GW, Schrump DS, Nguyen DM. Induction of apoptosis of lung and esophageal cancer cells treated with the combination of histone deacetylase inhibitor (trichostatin A) and protein kinase C inhibitor (calphostin C). J Thorac Cardiovasc Surg 2005;129:53–63.
2282. Mitic T, McKay JS. Immunohistochemical analysis of acetylation, proliferation, mitosis, and apoptosis in tumor xenografts following administration of a histone deacetylase inhibitor—a pilot study. Toxicol Pathol 2005;33: 792–799.
2283. Sonnemann J, Gange J, Kumar KS, Muller C, Bader P, Beck JF. Histone deacetylase inhibitors interact synergistically with tumor necrosis factor-related apoptosis-inducing ligand (TRAIL) to induce apoptosis in carcinoma cell lines. Invest New Drugs 2005; 23:99–109.
2284. Aparicio A. The potential of histone deacetylase inhibitors in lung cancer. Clin Lung Cancer 2006;7:309–312.
2285. Komatsu N, Kawamata N, Takeuchi S, et al. SAHA, a HDAC inhibitor, has profound anti-growth activity against non-small cell lung cancer cells. Oncol Rep 2006;15:187–191.
2286. Ota H, Tokunaga E, Chang K, et al. Sirt1 inhibitor, Sirtinol, induces senescence-like growth arrest with attenuated Ras-MAPK signaling in human cancer cells. Oncogene 2006;25:176–185.
2287. Sonnemann J, Hartwig M, Plath A, Saravana Kumar K, Muller C, Beck JF. Histone deacetylase inhibitors require caspase activity to induce apoptosis in lung and prostate carcinoma cells. Cancer Lett 2006;232:148–160.
2288. Watanabe T, Hioki M, Fujiwara T, et al. Histone deacetylase inhibitor FR901228 enhances the antitumor effect of telomerase-specific replication-selective adenoviral agent OBP-301 in human lung cancer cells. Exp Cell Res 2006;312:256–265.
2289. Nguyen DM, Spitz FR, Yen N, et al. Gene therapy for lung cancer: enhancement of tumor suppression by a combination of sequential systemic cisplatin and adenovirus-mediated p53 gene transfer. J Thorac Cardiovasc Surg 1996;112:1372–1377.
2290. Roth JA, Nguyen D, Lawrence DD, et al. Retrovirus-mediated wild-type p53 gene transfer to tumors of patients with lung cancer. Nat Med 1996;2:985–991.
2291. Roth JA. Clinical protocol: modification of mutant K-ras gene expression in non-small cell lung cancer (NSCLC). Hum Gene Ther 1996;7:875–889.
2292. Roth JA. Clinical protocol: modification of tumor suppressor gene expression and induction of apoptosis in non-small cell lung cancer (NSCLC) with an adenovirus vector expressing wildtype p53 and cisplatin. Hum Gene Ther 1996;7:1013–1030.
2293. Swisher SG, Roth JA, Nemunaitis J, et al. Adenovirus-mediated p53 gene transfer in advanced non-small cell lung cancer. J Natl Cancer Inst 1999;91:763–771.
2294. Nemunaitis J, Swisher SG, Timmons T, et al. Adenovirus-mediated p53 gene transfer in sequence with cisplatin to tumors of patients with non-small-cell lung cancer. J Clin Oncol 2000;18(3):609–622.
2295. Schuler M, Herrmann R, De Greve JL, et al. Adenovirus-mediated wild-type p53 gene transfer in patients receiving chemotherapy for advanced non-small-cell lung cancer: results of a multicenter phase II study. J Clin Oncol 2001;19:1750–1758.
2296. Pelosi G, Fraggetta F, Nappi O, et al. Pleomorphic carcinomas of the lung show a selective distribution of gene products involved in cell differentiation, cell cycle control, tumor growth, and tumor cell motility: a clinicopathologic and immunohistochemical study of 31 cases. Am J Surg Pathol 2003;27:1203–1215.
2297. Travis W, Colby TV, Corrin B, et al., eds. Histological typing of lung and pleura tumours. Berlin: Spinger; 1999:1–156.

2298. Cardillo G, Sera F, Di Martino M, et al. Bronchial carcinoid tumors: nodal status and long-term survival after resection. Ann Thorac Surg 2004;77:1781–1785.
2299. Filosso PL, Rena O, Donati G, et al. Bronchial carcinoid tumors: surgical management and long-term outcome. J Thorac Cardiovasc Surg 2002;123:303–309.
2300. Smolle-Juttner FM, Popper H, Klemen H, et al. Clinical features and therapy of "typical" and "atypical" bronchial carcinoid tumors (grade 1 and grade 2 neuroendocrine carcinoma). Eur J Cardiothorac Surg 1993;7:121–124; discussion 125.
2301. Thomas CF Jr, Tazelaar HD, Jett JR. Typical and atypical pulmonary carcinoids: outcome in patients presenting with regional lymph node involvement. Chest 2001; 119:1143–1150.
2302. Klemen H S-JF, Popper HH. Morphological and Immunohistochemical study of typical and atypical carcinoids of the lung, on the bases of 55 cases with clinico-pathological correlation and proposal of a new classification. Endocrine-related Cancer 1994;1:53–62.
2303. Beasley MB, Thunnissen FB, Brambilla E, et al. Pulmonary atypical carcinoid: predictors of survival in 106 cases. Hum Pathol 2000;31:1255–1265.
2304. Debelenko LV, Brambilla E, Agarwal SK, et al. Identification of MEN1 gene mutations in sporadic carcinoid tumors of the lung. Hum Mol Genet 1997;6:2285–2290.
2305. Petzmann S, Ullmann R, Klemen H, Renner H, Popper HH. Loss of heterozygosity on chromosome arm 11q in lung carcinoids. Hum Pathol 2001;32:333–338.
2306. Petzmann S, Ullmann R, Halbwedl I, Popper HH. Analysis of chromosome-11 aberrations in pulmonary and gastrointestinal carcinoids: an array comparative genomic hybridization-based study. Virchows Arch 2004; 445:151–159.
2307. Finkelstein SD, Hasegawa T, Colby T, Yousem SA. 11q13 allelic imbalance discriminates pulmonary carcinoids from tumorlets. A microdissection-based genotyping approach useful in clinical practice. Am J Pathol 1999; 155:633–640.
2308. Popper HH, el-Shabrawi Y, Wockel W, et al. Prognostic importance of human papilloma virus typing in squamous cell papilloma of the bronchus: comparison of in situ hybridization and the polymerase chain reaction. Hum Pathol 1994;25:1191–1197.
2309. Lin BY, Makhov AM, Griffith JD, Broker TR, Chow LT. Chaperone proteins abrogate inhibition of the human papillomavirus (HPV) E1 replicative helicase by the HPV E2 protein. Mol Cell Biol 2002;22:6592–6604.
2310. Zobel T, Iftner T, Stubenrauch F. The papillomavirus E8–E2C protein represses DNA replication from extrachromosomal origins. Mol Cell Biol 2003;23:8352–8362.
2311. Munger K, Baldwin A, Edwards KM, et al. Mechanisms of human papillomavirus-induced oncogenesis. J Virol 2004;78:11451–11460.
2312. Johansson M, Heim S, Mandahl N, Johansson L, Hambraeus G, Mitelman F. t(3;6;14)(p21;p21;q24) as the sole clonal chromosome abnormality in a hamartoma of the lung. Cancer Genet Cytogenet 1992;60:219–220.
2313. Johansson M, Dietrich C, Mandahl N, et al. Recombinations of chromosomal bands 6p21 and 14q24 characterize pulmonary hamartomas. Br J Cancer 1993;67:1236–1241.
2314. Fletcher JA, Longtine J, Wallace K, Mentzer SJ, Sugarbaker DJ. Cytogenetic and histologic findings in 17 pulmonary chondroid hamartomas: evidence for a pathogenic relationship with lipomas and leiomyomas. Genes Chromosomes Cancer 1995;12:220–223.
2315. Kazmierczak B, Meyer-Bolte K, Tran KH, et al. A high frequency of tumors with rearrangements of genes of the HMGI(Y) family in a series of 191 pulmonary chondroid hamartomas. Genes Chromosomes Cancer 1999;26: 125–133.
2316. Dal-Cin P, Kools P, De Jonge I, Moerman P, Van de Ven W, Van den Berghe H. Rearrangement of 12q14–15 in pulmonary chondroid hamartoma. Genes Chromosomes Cancer 1993;8:131–133.
2317. Kazmierczak B, Rosigkeit J, Wanschura S, et al. HMGI-C rearrangements as the molecular basis for the majority of pulmonary chondroid hamartomas: a survey of 30 tumors. Oncogene 1996;12:515–521.
2318. Wanschura S, Dal-Cin P, Kazmierczak B, Bartnitzke S, Van Den Berghe H, Bullerdiek J. Hidden paracentric inversions of chromosome arm 12q affecting the HMGIC gene. Genes Chromosomes Cancer 1997;18: 322–323.
2319. Rogalla P, Lemke I, Kazmierczak B, Bullerdiek J. An identical HMGIC-LPP fusion transcript is consistently expressed in pulmonary chondroid hamartomas with t(3;12)(q27–28;q14–15). Genes Chromosomes Cancer 2000;4:363–366.
2320. Mitelman F. Catalog of chromosomal aberrations in cancer. New York: Wiley Liss; 1998.
2321. Tallini G, Vanni R, Manfioletti G, et al. HMGI-C and HMGI(Y) immunoreactivity correlates with cytogenetic abnormalities in lipomas, pulmonary chondroid hamartomas, endometrial polyps, and uterine leiomyomas and is compatible with rearrangement of the HMGI-C and HMGI(Y) genes. Lab Invest 2000;80:359–369.
2322. Wanschura S, Kazmierczak B, Schoenmakers EFPM, et al. Regional fine mapping of the multiple aberration region involved in uterine leiomyomas, lipomas and pleomorphic adenomas of the salivary gland to 12q15. Genes Chromosomes Cancer 1995;14:68–70.
2323. Chiappetta G, Avantaggiato V, Visconti R, et al. High level expression of the HMGI (Y) gene during embryonic development. Oncogene 1996; 13:2439–2446.
2324. Berlingieri MT, Manfioletti G, Santoro M, et al. Inhibition of HMGI-C protein synthesis suppresses retrovirally induced neoplastic transformation of rat thyroid cells. Mol Cell Biol 1995;15:1545–1553.
2325. Bandiera A, Bonifacio D, Manfioletti G, et al. Expression of HMGI(Y) proteins in squamous intraepithelial and invasive lesions of the uterine cervix. Cancer Res 1998; 58:426–431.
2326. Krismann M, Adams H, Jaworska Klaus-Michael Müller M, Johnen G. Patterns of chromosomal imbalances in benign solitary fibrous tumours of the pleura. Virchows Archiv 2000;437:248–255.
2327. Miettinen MM, el-Rifai W, Sarlomo-Rikala M, Andersson LC, Knuutila S. Tumor size-related DNA copy number

changes occur in solitary fibrous tumors but not in hemangiopericytomas. Mod Pathol 1997;10:1194–200.
2328. Chilosi M, Facchettti F, Dei Tos AP, et al. bcl-2 expression in pleural and extrapleural solitary fibrous tumours. J Pathol 1997;181:362–367.
2329. Morimitsu Y, Nakajima M, Hisaoka M, Hashimoto H. Extrapleural solitary fibrous tumor: clinicopathologic study of 17 cases and molecular analysis of the p53 pathway. APMIS 2000;108:617–625.
2330. Priest JR, Watterson J, Strong L, et al. Pleuropulmonary blastoma: a marker for familial disease. J Pediatr 1996; 28:220–224.
2331. Mucenski ML, Wert SE, Nation JM, et al. beta-Catenin is required for specification of proximal/distal cell fate during lung morphogenesis. J Biol Chem 2003;278:40231–40238.
2332. Nakatani Y, Miyagi Y, Takemura T, et al. Aberrant nuclear/cytoplasmic localization and gene mutation of beta-catenin in classic pulmonary blastoma: beta-catenin immunostaining is useful for distinguishing between classic pulmonary blastoma and a blastomatoid variant of carcinosarcoma. Am J Surg Pathol 2004;28:921–927.
2333. Holst VA, Finkelstein S, Colby TV, Myers JL, Yousem SA. p53 and K-ras mutational genotyping in pulmonary carcinosarcoma, spindle cell carcinoma, and pulmonary blastoma: implications for histogenesis. Am J Surg Pathol 1997;21:801–811.
2334. Bodner SM, Koss MN. Mutations in the p53 gene in pulmonary blastomas: immunohistochemical and molecular studies. Hum Pathol 1996;27:1117–1123.
2335. Pacinda SJ, Ledet SC, Gondo MM, et al. p53 and MDM2 immunostaining in pulmonary blastomas and bronchogenic carcinomas Hum Pathol 1996;27:542–546.
2336. Roque L, Rodrigues R, Martins C, et al. Comparative genomic hybridization analysis of a pleuropulmonary blastoma. Cancer Genet Cytogenet 2004;149:58–62.
2337. Hong B, Chen Z, Coffin CM, et al. Molecular cytogenetic analysis of a pleuropulmonary blastoma. Cancer Genet Cytogenet 2003;142:65–69.
2338. Barnard M, Bayani J, Grant R, Teshima I, Thorner P, Squire J. Use of multicolor spectral karyotyping in genetic analysis of pleuropulmonary blastoma. Pediatr Dev Pathol 2000;3:479–486.
2339. Okamoto S, Hisaoka M, Daa T, Hatakeyama K, Iwamasa T, Hashimoto H. Primary pulmonary synovial sarcoma: a clinicopathologic, immunohistochemical, and molecular study of 11 cases. Hum Pathol 2004;35:850–856.
2340. Kawai K, Fukamizu A, Kawakami Y, et al. A case of renin producing leiomyosarcoma originating in the lung. Endocrinol Jpn 1991;38:603–609.
2341. Tarkkanen M, Huuhtanen R, Virolainen M, et al. Comparison of genetic changes in primary sarcomas and their pulmonary metastases. Genes Chromosomes Cancer 1999;25:323–331.
2342. Carbone M, Kratzke RA, Testa JR. The pathogenesis of mesothelioma. Semin Oncol 2002;29:2–17.
2343. Krismann M, Muller KM, Jaworska M, Johnen G. Molecular cytogenetic differences between histological subtypes of malignant mesotheliomas: DNA cytometry and comparative genomic hybridization of 90 cases. J Pathol 2002;197:363–371.
2344. Jensen RH, Tiirikainen M, You L, et al. Genomic alterations in human mesothelioma including high resolution mapping of common regions of DNA loss in chromosome arm 6q. Anticancer Res 2003;23(3B):2281–2289.
2345. Bueno R, Gordon GJ. Genetics of malignant pleural mesothelioma: molecular markers and biologic targets. Thorac Surg Clin 2004;14(4):461–468.
2346. Krismann M, Muller KM, Jaworska M, Johnen G. Pathological anatomy and molecular pathology. Lung Cancer 2004;45(suppl 1):S29–S33.
2347. Dopp E, Poser I, Papp T. Interphase fish analysis of cell cycle genes in asbestos-treated human mesothelial cells (HMC), SV40–transformed HMC (MeT-5A) and mesothelioma cells (COLO). Cell Mol Biol (Noisy-le-grand) 2002;48:OL271–OL277.
2348. Hirao T, Bueno R, Chen C-J, Gordon GJ, Heilig E, Kelsey KT. Alterations of the p16^{INK4} locus in human malignant mesothelial tumors. Carcinogenesis 2002;23:1127–1130.
2349. Wong L, Zhou J, Anderson D, Kratzke RA. Inactivation of p16INK4a expression in malignant mesothelioma by methylation. Lung Cancer 2002;38(2):131–136.
2350. Scharnhorst V, van der Eb AJ, Jochemsen AG. WT1 proteins: functions in growth and differentiation. Gene 2001;273:141–161.
2351. Smythe WR, Mohuiddin I, Ozveran M, Cao XX. Antisense therapy for malignant mesothelioma with oligonucleotides targeting the bcl-xl gene product. J Thorac Cardiovasc Surg 2002;123(6):1191–1198.
2352. Ozvaran MK, Cao XX, Miller SD, Monia BA, Hong WK, Smythe WR. Antisense oligonucleotides directed at the bcl-xl gene product augment chemotherapy response in mesothelioma. Mol Cancer Ther 2004;3(5):545–550.
2353. Catalano A, Rodilossi S, Rippo MR, Caprari P, Procopio A. Induction of stem cell factor/c-Kit/slug signal transduction in multidrug-resistant malignant mesothelioma cells. J Biol Chem 2004;279(45):46706–46714.
2354. Hegmans JP, Bard MP, Hemmes A, et al. Proteomic analysis of exosomes secreted by human mesothelioma cells. Am J Pathol 2004;164(5):1807–1815.
2355. Hoang CD, D'Cunha J, Kratzke MG, et al. Gene expression profiling identifies matriptase overexpression in malignant mesothelioma. Chest 2004;125(5):1843–1852.
2356. Hoang CD, Zhang X, Scott PD, et al. Selective activation of insulin receptor substrate-1 and -2 in pleural mesothelioma cells: association with distinct malignant phenotypes. Cancer Res 2004;64(20):7479–7485.
2357. Rippo MR, Moretti S, Vescovi S, et al. FLIP overexpression inhibits death receptor-induced apoptosis in malignant mesothelial cells. Oncogene 2004;23(47):7753–7760.
2358. Kettunen E, Nicholson AG, Nagy B, et al. L1CAM, INP10, P-cadherin, tPA and ITGB4 over-expression in malignant pleural mesotheliomas revealed by combined use of cDNA and tissue microarray. Carcinogenesis 2005;26(1): 17–25.
2359. Mohr S, Bottin MC, Lannes B, et al. Microdissection, mRNA amplification and microarray: a study of pleural

mesothelial and malignant mesothelioma cells. Biochimie 2004;86(1):13–9.
2360. Ke Y, Reddel RR, Gerwin BI, et al. Establishment of a human in vitro mesothelial cell model system for investigating mechanisms of asbestos-induced mesothelioma. Am J Pathol 1989;134(5):979–991.
2361. Cicala C, Pompetti F, Carbone M. SV40 induces mesotheliomas in hamsters. Am J Pathol 1993;142(5):1524–1533.
2362. Carbone M, Pass HI, Rizzo P, et al. Simian virus 40–like DNA sequences in human pleural mesothelioma. Oncogene 1994;9(6):1781–1790.
2363. Pepper C, Jasani B, Navabi H, Wynford-Thomas D, Gibbs AR. Simian virus 40 large T antigen (SV40LTAg) primer specific DNA amplification in human pleural mesothelioma tissue. Thorax 1996;51(11):1074–1076.
2364. Galateau-Salle F, Bidet P, Iwatsubo Y, et al. SV40–like DNA sequences in pleural mesothelioma, bronchopulmonary carcinoma, and non-malignant pulmonary diseases. J Pathol 1998;184(3):252–257.
2365. Gibbs AR, Jasani B, Pepper C, Navabi H, Wynford-Thomas D. SV40 DNA sequences in mesotheliomas. Dev Biol Stand 1998;94:41–45.
2366. Galateau-Salle F, Bidet P, Iwatsubo Y, et al. Detection of SV40–like DNA sequences in pleural mesothelioma, bronchopulmonary carcinoma and other pulmonary diseases. Dev Biol Stand 1998;94:147–152.
2367. Testa JR, Carbone M, Hirvonen A, et al. A multi-institutional study confirms the presence and expression of simian virus 40 in human malignant mesotheliomas. Cancer Res 1998;58(20):4505–4509.
2368. Shivapurkar N, Wiethege T, Wistuba II, et al. Presence of simian virus 40 sequences in malignant mesotheliomas and mesothelial cell proliferations. J Cell Biochem 1999; 76(2):181–188.
2369. Ramael M, Nagels J, Heylen H, et al. Detection of SV40 like viral DNA and viral antigens in malignant pleural mesothelioma. Eur Respir J 1999;14(6):1381–1386.
2370. Cristaudo A, Powers A, Vivaldi A, et al. SV40 can be reproducibly detected in paraffin-embedded mesothelioma samples. Anticancer Res 2000;20(2A):895–898.
2371. Procopio A, Strizzi L, Vianale G, et al. Simian virus-40 sequences are a negative prognostic cofactor in patients with malignant pleural mesothelioma. Genes Chromosomes Cancer 2000;29(2):173–179.
2372. McLaren BR, Haenel T, Stevenson S, Mukherjee S, Robinson BW, Lake RA. Simian virus (SV) 40 like sequences in cell lines and tumour biopsies from Australian malignant mesotheliomas. Aust NZ J Med 2000;30(4):450–456.
2373. Jasani B, Jones CJ, Radu C, et al. Simian virus 40 detection in human mesothelioma: reliability and significance of the available molecular evidence. Front Biosci 2001;6: E12–E22.
2374. De Rienzo A, Tor M, Sterman DH, Aksoy F, Albelda SM, Testa JR. Detection of SV40 DNA sequences in malignant mesothelioma specimens from the United States, but not from Turkey. J Cell Biochem 2002;84(3):455–459.
2375. Bright RK, Kimchi ET, Shearer MH, Kennedy RC, Pass HI. SV40 Tag-specific cytotoxic T lymphocytes generated from the peripheral blood of malignant pleural mesothelioma patients. Cancer Immunol Immunother 2002; 50(12):682–690.
2376. Cerrano PG, Jasani B, Filiberti R, et al. Simian virus 40 and malignant mesothelioma (review). Int J Oncol 2003; 22(1):187–194.
2377. Vilchez RA, Kozinetz CA, Arrington AS, Madden CR, Butel JS. Simian virus 40 in human cancers. Am J Med 2003;114(8):675–684.
2378. Gazdar AF, Carbone M. Molecular pathogenesis of malignant mesothelioma and its relationship to simian virus 40. Clin Lung Cancer 2003;5(3):177–181.
2379. Jin M, Sawa H, Suzuki T, et al. Investigation of simian virus 40 large T antigen in 18 autopsied malignant mesothelioma patients in Japan. J Med Virol 2004;74(4): 668–676.
2380. Vilchez RA, Butel JS. Emergent human pathogen simian virus 40 and its role in cancer. Clin Microbiol Rev 2004;17(3):495–508.
2381. Strickler HD, Rosenberg PS, Devesa SS, Hertel J, Fraumeni JF Jr, Goedert JJ. Contamination of poliovirus vaccines with simian virus 40 (1955–1963) and subsequent cancer rates. JAMA 1998;279(4):292–295.
2382. Shah KV. Search for SV40 in human mesotheliomas. Dev Biol Stand 1998;94:67–68.
2383. Griffiths DJ, Nicholson AG, Weiss RA. Detection of SV40 sequences in human mesothelioma. Dev Biol Stand 1998;94:127–136.
2384. Olin P, Giesecke J. Potential exposure to SV40 in polio vaccines used in Sweden during 1957: no impact on cancer incidence rates 1960 to 1993. Dev Biol Stand 1998;94: 227–233.
2385. Mulatero C, Surentheran T, Breuer J, Rudd RM. Simian virus 40 and human pleural mesothelioma. Thorax 1999; 54(1):60–61.
2386. Strizzi L, Vianale G, Giuliano M, et al. SV40, JC and BK expression in tissue, urine and blood samples from patients with malignant and nonmalignant pleural disease. Anticancer Res 2000;20(2A):885–889.
2387. Pilatte Y, Vivo C, Renier A, Kheuang L, Greffard A, Jaurand MC. Absence of SV40 large T-antigen expression in human mesothelioma cell lines. Am J Respir Cell Mol Biol 2000;23(6):788–793.
2388. Strickler HD; International SV40 Working Group. A multicenter evaluation of assays for detection of SV40 DNA and results in masked mesothelioma specimens. Cancer Epidemiol Biomarkers Prev 2001;10(5):523–532.
2389. Strickler HD, Goedert JJ, Devesa SS, Lahey J, Fraumeni JF Jr, Rosenberg PS. Trends in U.S. pleural mesothelioma incidence rates following simian virus 40 contamination of early poliovirus vaccines. J Natl Cancer Inst 2003;95(1): 38–45.
2390. Engels EA, Katki HA, Nielsen NM, et al. Cancer incidence in Denmark following exposure to poliovirus vaccine contaminated with simian virus 40. J Natl Cancer Inst 2003;95(7):532–539.
2391. Mayall F, Barratt K, Shanks J. The detection of Simian virus 40 in mesotheliomas from New Zealand and England using real time FRET probe PCR protocols. J Clin Pathol 2003;56(10):728–730.

2392. Shah KV, Galloway DA, Knowles WA, Viscidi RP. Simian virus 40 (SV40) and human cancer: a review of the serological data. Rev Med Virol 2004;14(4):231–239.
2393. Rollison DE, Page WF, Crawford H, et al. Case-control study of cancer among US Army veterans exposed to simian virus 40–contaminated adenovirus vaccine. Am J Epidemiol. 2004;160(4):317–324.
2394. Lopez-Rios F, Illei PB, Rusch V, Ladanyi M Evidence against a role for SV40 infection in human mesotheliomas and high risk of false-positive PCR results owing to presence of SV40 sequences in common laboratory plasmids. Lancet 2004;364(9440):1157–1166.
2395. Shah KV. Causality of mesothelioma: SV40 question. Thorac Surg Clin 2004;14(4):497–504.
2396. Carbone M, Rizzo P, Grimley PM, et al. Simian virus-40 large-T antigen binds p53 in human mesotheliomas. Nat Med 1997;3(8):908–912.
2397. De Luca A, Baldi A, Esposito V, et al. The retinoblastoma gene family pRb/p105, p107, pRb2/p130 and simian virus-40 large T-antigen in human mesotheliomas. Nat Med 1997;3(8):913–916.
2398. Lechner JF, Tesfaigzi J, Gerwin BI. Oncogenes and Tumor-Suppressor Genes in Mesothelioma—Asynopsis Environ Health Perspect 1997;105S(suppl 5):1061–1067.
2399. Levresse V, Moritz S, Renier A, et al. Effect of simian virus large T antigen expression on cell cycle control and apoptosis in rat pleural mesothelial cells exposed to DNA damaging agents. Oncogene 1998;16(8):1041–1053.
2400. Matker CM, Rizzo P, Pass HI, et al. The biological activities of simian virus 40 large-T antigen and its possible oncogenic effects in humans. Monaldi Arch Chest Dis 1998;53(2):193–197.
2401. Mutti L, Carbone M, Giordano GG, Giordano A. Simian virus 40 and human cancer. Monaldi Arch Chest Dis 1998;53(2):198–201.
2402. Procopio A, Strizzi L, Giuffrida A, et al. Human malignant mesothelioma of the pleura: new perspectives for diagnosis and therapy. Monaldi Arch Chest Dis 1998; 53(2):241–243.
2403. Mutti L, De Luca A, Claudio PP, Convertino G, Carbone M, Giordano A. Simian virus 40–like DNA sequences and large-T antigen-retinoblastoma family protein pRb2/p130 interaction in human mesothelioma. Dev Biol Stand 1998;94:47–53.
2404. Murthy SS, Testa JR. Asbestos, chromosomal deletions, and tumor suppressor gene alterations in human malignant mesothelioma. J Cell Physiol 1999;180(2): 150–157.
2405. Mayall FG, Jacobson G, Wilkins R. Mutations of p53 gene and SV40 sequences in asbestos associated and non-asbestos-associated mesotheliomas. J Clin Pathol 1999;52(4):291–293.
2406. Emri S, Kocagoz T, Olut A, Gungen Y, Mutti L, Baris YI. Simian virus 40 is not a cofactor in the pathogenesis of environmentally induced malignant pleural mesothelioma in Turkey. Anticancer Res 2000;20(2A):891–894.
2407. Modi S, Kubo A, Oie H, Coxon AB, Rehmatulla A, Kaye FJ. Protein expression of the RB-related gene family and SV40 large T antigen in mesothelioma and lung cancer. Oncogene 2000;19(40):4632–4639.
2408. De Rienzo A, Testa JR. Recent advances in the molecular analysis of human malignant mesothelioma. Clin Ter 2000;151(6):433–438.
2409. Schrump DS, Waheed I. Strategies to circumvent SV40 oncoprotein expression in malignant pleural mesotheliomas. Semin Cancer Biol 2001;11(1):73–80.
2410. Toyooka S, Pass HI, Shivapurkar N, et al. Aberrant methylation and simian virus 40 tag sequences in malignant mesothelioma. Cancer Res 2001;61(15):5727–5730.
2411. Cacciotti P, Libener R, Betta P, et al. SV40 replication in human mesothelial cells induces HGF/Met receptor activation: a model for viral-related carcinogenesis of human malignant mesothelioma. Proc Natl Acad Sci USA 2001;98(21):12032–12037.
2412. Cacciotti P, Strizzi L, Vianale G, et al. The presence of simian-virus 40 sequences in mesothelioma and mesothelial cells is associated with high levels of vascular endothelial growth factor. Am J Respir Cell Mol Biol 2002; 26(2):189–193.
2413. Baldi A, Groeger AM, Esposito V, et al. Expression of p21 in SV40 large T antigen positive human pleural mesothelioma: relationship with survival. Thorax 2002;57(4): 353–356.
2414. Carbone M, Rudzinski J, Bocchetta M. High throughput testing of the SV40 Large T antigen binding to cellular p53 identifies putative drugs for the treatment of SV40–related cancers. Virology 2003;315(2):409–414.
2415. Barbanti-Brodano G, Sabbioni S, Martini F, Negrini M, Corallini A, Tognon M. Simian virus 40 infection in humans and association with human diseases: results and hypotheses. Virology 2004;318(1):1–9.
2416. Jaurand MC, Fleury-Feith J. Pathogenesis of malignant pleural mesothelioma. Respirology 2005;10(1):2–8.
2417. Wali A, Morin PJ, Hough CD, Lonardo F, Seya T, Carbone M, Pass HI. Identification of intelectin overexpression in malignant pleural mesothelioma by serial analysis of gene expression (SAGE). Lung Cancer 2005;48(1):19–29.
2418. Foddis R, De Rienzo A, Broccoli D, et al. SV40 infection induces telomerase activity in human mesothelial cells. Oncogene 2002;221:1434–1442.

34 Preinvasive Disease

Keith M. Kerr and Armando E. Fraire

Primary lung cancer is the most frequent cause of death from malignant disease worldwide. In many Western countries the overall incidence of lung cancer shows signs of decreasing, yet the explosion in tobacco consumption in many Asian countries in particular suggests this disease will remain a major worldwide health problem for the foreseeable future. Despite a decline in lung cancer incidence in Western male populations, and, coincident with this, a fall in rates of squamous cell carcinoma, many of these same Western countries are witnessing a continued rise in lung cancer cases in females. At the same time, and probably not entirely unrelated to this change in sex demography, primary adenocarcinoma of the lung is on the increase, although there is evidence of this tumor type also rising in males.

Although lung cancer is a common disease, its overall prognosis is dismal. Only about 15% of patients can be offered potentially curative treatment, and only half of them will actually be cured. As a general rule, symptomatic lung cancer is fatal. Recent technological advances in diagnostic imaging and molecular biology have rekindled interest in screening for lung cancer, and thus renewed attention has been focused on early lung cancer and the lesions that may precede invasion. Unless there is some dramatic development in our ability to cure advanced (invasive) lung cancer, progress in reducing lung cancer mortality will clearly depend on improving detection of those early or preinvasive lesions before they become incurable.

The World Health Organization (WHO) classification of lung cancer[1] recognizes three preinvasive diseases that are thought to be precursors of malignant lung tumors. These are squamous dysplasia/carcinoma in situ (SD/CIS), atypical adenomatous hyperplasia (AAH), and diffuse idiopathic pulmonary neuroendocrine cell hyperplasia (DIPNECH). Before considering these morphologically distinctive precursors of lung malignancy, this chapter discusses a number of other diseases or changes in the lung that are variably associated with the development of lung cancer. The relevance of pulmonary preinvasive disease to current developments in lung cancer screening is also discussed.

Preexisting Lung Disease and Lung Cancer

There are several pulmonary diseases or pathologic processes that appear to carry a risk of the development of primary lung cancer or other malignancy. Principal among these is lung fibrosis, either localized or diffuse. Diffuse fibrosis may be idiopathic or occur in the context of connective tissue disease or pneumoconiosis. Lesions such as cystic adenomatoid malformations (CAMs), human papilloma virus (HPV)-associated papillomatosis, and other cystic, inflammatory, and congenital lesions must also be considered.

Localized Lung Fibrosis: The "Scar Cancer" Hypothesis

The frequent finding of a hyalinized central scar surrounded by tumor led to the belief that the scar predated the cancer and may have been in some way responsible for the tumor's development: the *Narbenkrebs* or "scar cancer" hypothesis first proposed by Rossle[2] in 1943, some 4 years after the first description of an association between adenocarcinoma and pulmonary fibrosis by Freidrich.[3,4] The fact that these scars are often bereft of tumor cells and show anthracotic pigmentation reinforced the belief in their preexistence to the tumor[5] (Fig. 34.1). In an autopsy study of such tumors, which included squamous cell carcinomas and carcinoid tumorlets as well as adenocarcinomas,[6] areas of atypical alveolar epithelium were noted in close proximity to the scars, and this was considered of significance both in terms of development of the tumors and the differential diagnosis of reactive

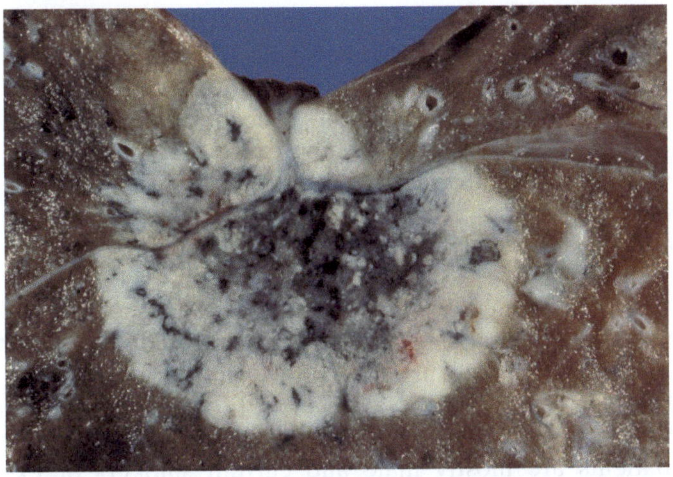

FIGURE 34.1. Peripheral adenocarcinoma with central anthracotic scar.

hyperplasia and malignancy. Further support for this hypothesis was presented in a study of 82 scar cancers, derived from a larger group of 1186 lung carcinomas.[7] About half of these study cases were peripheral, 72% were adenocarcinomas, 18% were squamous cell carcinomas, and 10% were large cell undifferentiated carcinomas. These scar cancers were predominantly upper lobe tumors and were not associated with smoking, in contrast to the remainder of the tumors in the rest of the study group. These authors considered pulmonary infarction to be the most likely cause of the scar that led to the cancer, differing from many earlier reports in which tuberculosis was considered the dominant precursor disease.

In practice it is extremely difficult to say in an individual case whether or not the localized central scar in a peripheral tumor pre- or postdates the development of the cancer.[8,9] The body of evidence now largely refutes the scar cancer hypothesis and suggests the central scar is a product rather than a cause of tumor development. The fact that Auerbach et al.[7] described an apparent increase in the incidence of scar cancers, predominantly adenocarcinomas, over a 20-year period in nonsmokers is entirely consistent with what we now know about the development of peripheral adenocarcinoma of the lung (see below). Shimosato et al.[10,11] and others[12] have led the way in refuting the scar cancer hypothesis by making the following pathologic and radiologic observations:

- Adenocarcinoma is common in scar-free lung.
- The relative sizes of the central scar and the overall tumor are generally proportionate.
- Both metastatic tumors *to* lung and extrapulmonary metastases *from* lung adenocarcinomas frequently show central scars.
- The presence of psammoma bodies in some scars suggests the preexistence of papillary tumor at that site.
- Retrospective examination of chest radiographs rarely shows a scar.
- Repeated radiologic observations of tumors in development may show shrinkage of the tumor shadow, convergence of adjacent vessels and airways on the tumor mass, and increasing central radiodensity, all implying contraction of a central scar *after* the tumor first appears. These findings are more recently supported by observations made by spiral computed tomography (CT) scanning of peripheral lung nodules in lung cancer screening programs (see below)
- In tumors less than 3 cm in diameter, the presence of a central scar carries a worse prognosis and implies that such tumors may be more likely to have metastasized because they are older lesions.[10] This point is supported by another study of 22 scar cancers, 19 of which were adenocarcinoma, followed-up over 10 years.[13]

Others have described the tendency for lymph node metastases from peripheral lung adenocarcinoma to undergo central scarring.[14] Kolin and Koutoulakis[15] suggested that, in both primary tumors and metastases, central ischemic tumor cell necrosis due to vascular obliteration by tumor may be the cause of central scarring, while others have proposed that small airway obstruction by expanding tumor may lead to collapse of the alveolar elastin network prior to the development of the central scar, pointing out that in such peripheral sites collateral drift is poor, making alveolar collapse more likely.[16]

Studies of the cell content and collagen type in the fibrous tissue in scar cancers further supports the suggestion that the scar postdates the tumor. Myofibroblasts are readily found in the central scars of tumors, but are less frequent in mature apical pulmonary scars unassociated with malignancy.[17] Fibrosis in scar cancer shows abundant collagen type III, typical of recent fibroplasia, while in old, mature pulmonary scars collagen types I and V predominate.[14,17,18] The presence of histoplasma organisms within the central scars in some Clara cell–type adenocarcinomas, however, was held to support the suggestion that these particular tumors may have developed from preexisting histoplasma foci,[19] albeit that these patients were from a state (Kentucky) where histoplasmosis is endemic.

In summary, the term *scar cancer* may be a reasonable description of a tumor with a central area of fibrosis, but for the vast majority of lesions, this scar almost certainly develops with or is caused by the tumor. However, there may be rare exceptions where the tumor does arise in association with a preexisting localized scar.

Diffuse Lung Fibrosis and Lung Cancer

While the suggestions that localized pulmonary scars may give rise to lung cancer have been effectively rejected, there is good evidence that diffuse pulmonary fibrosis occurring in a number of different circumstances does increase the risk of pulmonary malignancy.

Historically, both Bell[20] and Geevers et al.[21] speculated that regenerative hyperplasia of alveolar epithelium, as seen after an inflammatory process, may be atypical, that such epithelial hyperplasia "may give rise to localized or diffuse adenomatous growth which may form metastases,"[20] and that "alveolar cell tumors of the lung may result from such atypical pulmonary inflammatory reactions."[21] Even earlier reports following the 1918 influenza pandemic predicted that the prevalence of lung cancer would rise as a result of the postinflammatory changes that were widespread in the population surviving infection,[22] and even described cases of early epidermoid carcinoma found at autopsy in patients dying during the pandemic. It seems much more likely, however, that the squamous epithelium described in these few cases represents the common atypical squamous metaplasia seen in the epithelial proliferative/reparative phase of diffuse alveolar damage (DAD) syndrome, a frequent complication in fatal influenza; indeed, the predicted rise in lung cancer was never convincingly demonstrated.[23]

Idiopathic Pulmonary Fibrosis

Meyer and Liebow[23] gave one of the earliest detailed accounts of the association between diffuse pulmonary fibrosis and honeycombing and lung cancer, pointing out that the epithelium in areas of honeycomb lung is often atypical. They found that 22% of a series of 153 resected lung cancers were associated with honeycomb lung and atypical alveolar cell hyperplasia, while 21% of their 19 autopsy cases with honeycomb lung also had lung cancer. Fraire and Greenberg[24] reported three cases of lung cancer found in 16 autopsied patients who had diffuse interstitial fibrosis, a prevalence of 19%. The risk of developing lung cancer was reported to be increased 14-fold and sevenfold, respectively, in male and female patients with cryptogenic fibrosing alveolitis compared with controls matched for sex, age, and smoking habit.[25]

More recent reports give a wide range of figures for the proportion of patients with idiopathic pulmonary fibrosis (IPF) who develop lung cancer. Ma et al.[26] reviewed this issue and stated that, while rates as low as 4.8% are reported from the United States, and similar relatively low figures of 5.2%[27] and 9.7%[25] have been found in United Kingdom patients, much higher rates seem to be reported from Japan. Matsushita et al.[28] reported an autopsy study of 83 patients with usual interstitial pneumonia (UIP) of whom 40 (48.2%) also had lung cancer compared with 9.1% of their control cases without UIP, while in a very similar study Qunn et al.[29] reported a cancer rate of 42% in 72 IPF autopsies versus 8.1% in the control cases. Mizushima et al.[30] reviewed the literature on Japanese patients with IPF and lung cancer and found 154 reported cases; 23 of these patients (15%) had multiple synchronous lung cancers, a more frequent occurrence than is seen in lung cancer patients without fibrosis. There are reports finding no link between IPF and lung cancer,[31] but these were based on data taken from death certificates, a questionable source of medical histories.

Wherever these cases are found, several characteristics seem to be consistent: the tumors, including those of squamous cell type, are most often found within or at the margins of the peripheral zones of honeycombing (ipso facto predominantly in the lower lobes) (Fig. 34.2), and patients are mostly male and current smokers or ex-smokers.[28,30,32,33] Exposure to metal dust may also increase the likelihood of cancer developing in IPF.[26,31] The association with smoking is of interest since it is a potential confounder of the link between IPF and lung cancer, given that there is evidence that IPF, as well as lung cancer, may be smoking related.[34] In a substantial study of 890 patients with IPF and 5884 controls, Hubbard et al.[35] showed that the risk of developing lung cancer was increased sevenfold in IPF, independent of the effect of cigarette smoking.

There is controversy over whether or not adenocarcinoma is the predominant cell type in IPF-associated lung cancer. In their review, Ma and colleagues[26] declared adenocarcinoma was the most frequent cell type, which Mizushima et al.[30] also found in a review of female

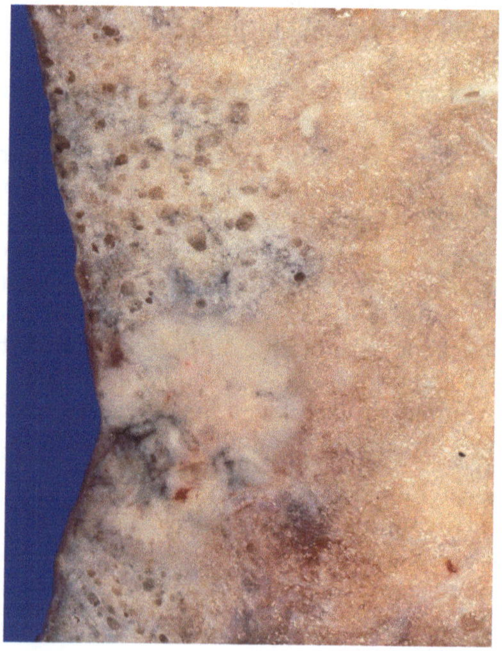

FIGURE 34.2. Peripheral adenocarcinoma that has arisen in a subpleural zone of honeycombing.

Japanese patients (64% adenocarcinoma vs. 31% squamous cell carcinoma), while male Japanese patients showed an excess of squamous cell cancers (47%) over adenocarcinoma (31%). Even fewer adenocarcinomas (19%) were reported by Sakai et al.,[33] who noted that 66% of the tumors were squamous cell and 27% were small cell lung cancers, while Aubry et al.[36] showed 66% of the tumors in their study to be squamous cell. Meyer and Liebow[23] reported a 31% incidence of adenocarcinoma in their cases, higher than the frequency of adenocarcinoma in the general lung cancer population of the time. Turner-Warwick et al.[25] found 27% were adenocarcinomas, although one quarter of their cases were not histologically proven. On balance, there does appear to be an excess of adenocarcinoma in IPF-associated lung cancer.

It is not clear why IPF would predispose a patient to lung cancer. The issue of a common etiology with cancer, especially smoking tobacco, has been mentioned above. Inflammatory changes and, in particular, cytokine production has been implicated in the process.[37] Epithelial hyperproliferation is a forerunner or predisposing factor in the development of many epithelial tumors. Meyer and Liebow[23] drew attention to the presence of proliferation and atypia in the (bronchiolo)alveolar epithelium in fibrotic, honeycomb lung, and this fits intuitively with the potential for adenocarcinoma development, while others have described more squamous metaplasia in carcinoma–associated UIP when compared to those without tumors.[32] However, in this study the degree of atypia was not increased in the metaplastic squamous or glandular epithelium in the UIP of those with malignancy, and both p53 expression and proliferative index (Ki-67) were also no different.

Qunn et al.[29] reported that the hyperplastic epithelium in IPF showed DNA aneuploidy in eight of 12 cases examined, that hyperplastic epithelium overexpressed p53, and, in those patients with IPF-associated lung cancer, the hyperplastic foci were more prominent than in those without cancer. Overexpression of p53 protein and mutation of the *P53* gene were also found in another study of hyperplastic/metaplastic epithelial changes in IPF associated with cancer.[38] Squamous metaplasia with and without atypia showed overexpression of p53 protein in 60% and 54% of lesions, and *P53* mutation in 4% and 23% of lesions, respectively. Mutation of *P53* and *KRAS* was also found by Takahashi et al.[39] in hyperplastic epithelium in IPF, but the case numbers examined were very small. These authors also found significantly higher expression of K-ras protein in type II pneumocytes in IPF in those with cancer (75% of cases), when compared to those IPF patients without cancer (40%). In a search for genomic instability in sputum cells from IPF patients, loss of heterozygosity (LOH) was demonstrated in lung cancer–associated loci including sites corresponding to the *MYCL1*, *FHIT*, *SPARC*, *P16*^{INK4}, and *P53* genes.[40] Loss of heterozygosity at the *FHIT* locus on chromosome 3p, together with commensurate loss of demonstrable DNA by fluorescence in-situ hybridization (FISH) analysis and loss of stainable Fhit protein by immunohistochemistry, was found to be more frequent in cancer-associated IPF epithelial metaplasia than in those cases that were not cancer associated.[41]

It seems very likely that the epithelial proliferation and metaplasia occurring in association with IPF provides a background upon which further genetic alterations, perhaps caused by tobacco smoke carcinogens, or metal or mineral exposure (see below), may occur, leading to lung cancer development. In addition, there is evidence that radiation-induced pulmonary fibrosis also carries an increased risk, in particular, of adenocarcinoma.[42] The data so far available suggest that the genetic alterations occurring during malignant transformation in the IPF setting are the same as those occurring in central bronchial and peripheral bronchioloalveolar epithelia during usual lung carcinogenesis.

Connective Tissue Disease

Lung cancer may also be seen in the setting of connective tissue diseases, usually complicated by diffuse pulmonary fibrosis. One report found that 12% of patients with connective tissue disease developed lung cancer.[43] Most of the available literature is in the form of case reports, but this subject was comprehensively reviewed by Yang et al.,[44] who found 153 reported cases in the world literature since 1944. There was a slight preponderance in females (82 cases versus 71 in males), and the mean age of 58 is rather young when compared to an average group of lung cancer patients. Adenocarcinoma was the clearly predominant cell type with 85 cases (56%) reported, of which just over half were described as bronchioloalveolar carcinoma (BAC). It seems unlikely, however, that many of this latter group would be BAC as currently defined, that is to say, with no evidence of stromal invasion. Twenty-eight cases (18%) were squamous cell carcinomas, while a similar number of small cell cancers were found.

Ninety-six cases, about two thirds of the total, in the review by Yang et al.[44] were found in patients with progressive systemic sclerosis (PSS; scleroderma), the majority of whom were female; slightly less than half were smokers and virtually all had pulmonary fibrosis. Two thirds of these 96 tumors were described as either BAC (36 cases) or adenocarcinoma (26 cases) and these BACs accounted for the vast majority of tumors of this type found with any connective tissue disease. Peters-Golden et al.[45] calculated that the relative risk ratio for lung cancer in PSS is 16.5.

Twenty-seven cases of lung cancer arising in patients with rheumatoid arthritis (RA) were also reviewed.[44] Most patients were male smokers, but again most patients had pulmonary fibrosis. Bronchioloalveolar carcinoma was rare in this group, with squamous cell, small cell, and adenocarcinomas each accounting for 21% to 25% of cases.

In patients with polymyositis/dermatomyositis (PM/DM), there were 24 tumors again seen predominantly in male smokers, but only half the patients had pulmonary fibrosis.[44] Small cell carcinoma was the most frequent cell type, followed by squamous cell; adenocarcinoma and BAC were uncommon. Relatively speaking, reports of lung cancer in patients with systemic lupus erythematosus and Sjögren's syndrome are rare.

The association between PSS and adenocarcinoma, particularly with a BAC component, is striking. One report found that 77% of the tumors in PSS patients were BAC.[46] This and the association with pulmonary fibrosis suggest a similar pathogenesis to that discussed above with respect to IPF. In contrast, there appears to be a strong association with smoking and cancer in both RA and PM/DM patients, and, in the latter group at least, tumor development is not necessarily associated with lung fibrosis. This appears to be reflected in the tumor types that predominate in these diseases. Apart from speculation about the possible effect of inflammatory mediators on lung epithelium, some have raised the possibility that immunosuppressant drugs may increase the risk of neoplasia in some patients.[47] With PM/DM in particular, the possibility remains that in some way the connective tissue disorder may be caused by, rather than be a cause of, the tumor. Nonetheless a range of connective tissue disorders, but in particular PSS, do appear to carry an increased risk for the development of lung cancer, with the associated pulmonary fibrosis implicated as the preneoplastic lesion in many instances.

Mineral Pneumoconiosis

Asbestosis certainly confers an increased risk for the development of primary lung cancer, but the literature shows that the issue is far from being clear-cut.[48–50] There are a few points that can be regarded as consistent findings:

- Lung cancer is more likely to occur when asbestosis (fibrosis) is present.
- Lung cancer is increased in those with asbestos exposure but without fibrosis. Thus there is a dose-response curve; low levels of exposure appear to confer an increased risk, but there is a minimum level below which no excess risk appears to exist.[51]
- Lung cancer in asbestosis is most frequent in the fibrotic lower lobes.

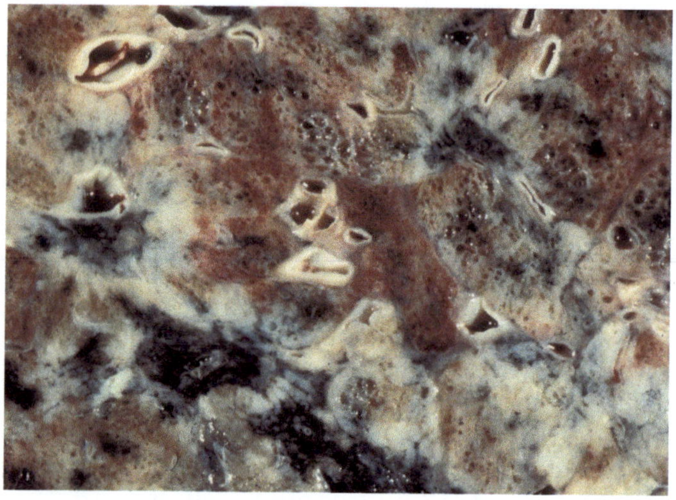

FIGURE 34.3. This patient with silicosis (the gray/black nodules) also developed adenocarcinoma (the cream/white tissue), which was multifocal and of mixed pattern histologically, including bronchioloalveolar carcinoma.

- Contrary to earlier studies suggesting there was an excess of adenocarcinomas in this setting, all types of lung cancer appear increased, and occur in the same proportions as they do in smokers in the general population,[52] commensurate with the fact that there is synergism between asbestos and cigarette smoking. The effect is independent of the mechanisms giving rise to fibrosis and much, perhaps most, of the carcinogenicity of asbestos may be through its enhancement of the mutagenicity of tobacco carcinogens.[53]

Other forms of pneumoconiosis not associated with asbestos appear to be associated with lung cancer. Katabami et al.[54] found that peripheral squamous cell carcinoma was associated with the presence of diffuse fibrosis caused by pneumoconiosis. Silica is now recognized as a human carcinogen,[49] and evidence suggests that silicosis carries a higher risk for lung cancer development than silica exposure without fibrosis[55–57] (Fig. 34.3).

Other Lung Lesions and Lung Cancer

Cystic Adenomatoid Malformation

Type I congenital cystic adenomatoid malformation appears to carry a risk of developing mucinous bronchioloalveolar carcinoma (MBAC).[58] Tumors have been reported in children as young as 11 years,[59] as well as in adulthood,[60] and may occur in the lung years after resection of the CAM from an infant or neonate.[61,62] Sheffield et al.[63] speculated that groups of sometimes atypical mucous cells, characteristic of the cyst lining but also found in the adjacent alveolar walls, may be the origin of MBAC in these cases. Such cells in lung adjacent to the cyst are not necessarily removed at cystectomy and may explain why MBAC has arisen many years after resection of the CAM. MacSweeney et al.[58] found microscopic foci of MBAC in five of 16 type I CAMs, further examples of adjacent mucous cell hyperplasia and, in two patients, foci of atypical adenomatous hyperplasia (see below). Using comparative genomic hybridization, gains in chromosomes 2 and 4 were demonstrated by Stacher et al.[64] in two examples of goblet cell hyperplasia associated with type I CAM. Immunocytochemistry was used to show nuclear translocation of interleukin (IL)-4Rα and upregulation of *Muc2*, reflecting aberrant goblet cell differentiation. Cystic adenomatoid malformation may be associated with rhabdomyosarcoma,[59] while type IV CAM may carry a risk of transformation into pleuropulmonary blastoma.[58]

Juvenile Tracheobronchial Squamous Papillomatosis

Radiation therapy and tobacco smoking increase the risk of malignant transformation in this condition.[65] Simma et al.,[66] however, reported a case of squamous cell carcinoma arising in the lungs of a 16-year-old who had presented at 1 year of age with HPV-associated tracheobronchial squamous papillomatosis. The child had not been irradiated, and the authors found 11 similar cases in a literature review. HPV11[65] and HPV6a DNA[67] have been found in cancers arising in such patients who have not been irradiated, and it has also been suggested that papillomas positive for HPV16 or -18 may be at high risk of malignant change.[68]

Cysts, Sequestration, and Bronchiectasis

Lung cancer has been reported in association with peripheral lung cysts,[69] bronchogenic cyst,[70] bronchopulmonary sequestration,[71] and bronchiectasis.[72,73] While the tumors arising in the cysts were both described as MBAC, the tumor arising in the sequestration and most of those seen in bronchiectasis were squamous cell carcinomas. One of us has also seen examples of peripheral squamous cell carcinoma apparently arising in the wall of cystic cavities, almost certainly bronchiectatic in origin, and partly lined by metaplastic squamous epithelium. Care would always have to be taken in the case of a tumor apparently arising within bronchiectasis that the bronchiectasis predated the tumor rather than it being the result of airway obstruction by tumor. Sawada et al.[74] demonstrated allelic loss of 9p21 (see below) in the metaplastic squamous epithelium of a lung cyst, which was found in a resection specimen removed for an intercurrent but noncontiguous squamous cell carcinoma.

From the foregoing it is clear that there are a variety of preexisting lung diseases or lesions that are entities in their own right as opposed to being primarily preinvasive hyperplastic/dysplastic changes in lung epithelium and that appear to confer on the sufferer an increased risk for developing lung cancer. With regard to asbestos, this risk appears to be more about potentiating the carcinogenic effects of tobacco smoke rather than by causing fibrosis. Nonetheless, diffuse pulmonary fibrosis of a variety of causes, tracheobronchial papillomatosis and type I CAM in particular, probably by creating abnormally proliferating epithelial cell populations, may be considered preneoplastic lesions in the lung.

Preinvasive Lesions in the World Health Organization Classification

The third edition of the WHO classification of lung tumors[1] contained a new section that identified three preinvasive lesions: squamous dysplasia/carcinoma in situ (SD/CIS), atypical adenomatous hyperplasia (AAH), and diffuse idiopathic pulmonary neuroendocrine cell hyperplasia (DIPNECH). Each is associated with a variety of different pulmonary neoplasms, and there is evidence that these preinvasive lesions are the precursors that may progress to invasive neoplasia. This last point raises a number of fundamental issues relating to matters of definition and the exact nature of the lesions under discussion. Rupert Willis[75] defined a neoplasm as "an abnormal mass of tissue, the growth of which exceeds and is uncoordinated with that of the normal tissues, and persists in the same excessive manner after cessation of the stimuli which evoked the change." Although some of the lesions we are about to discuss appear to have, at least in some patients, sufficient autonomy of growth control to fulfill this definition of neoplasia, yet are not invasive, a discussion of preinvasive lesions in the lung should also include lesions that are preneoplastic, that is, not yet capable of independent growth. Sometimes we can be reasonably clear about whether we consider a lesion to be hyperplastic or neoplastic; in some circumstances this distinction is anything but clear.

Much of the evidence described below suggests that epithelial hyperplasia is one of the earliest recognizable alterations of the lung epithelia associated with tumor development. A hyperproliferating epithelium is a frequent, if not necessarily obligatory, precursor of tumor development following current theories of multistep carcinogenesis. Some genetic alterations such as chromosomal loss, translocation, or gene mutation are mechanistically dependent on mitosis. The preinvasive stage of tumor development thus encompasses both hyperplastic and neoplastic lesions.

Squamous Dysplasia/Carcinoma-in-Situ and Other Bronchial Preinvasive Lesions

This group of lesions, which occur in tracheobronchial, and to a lesser extent in bronchiolar, epithelium, is the best known of the preinvasive lung lesions and the archetypal progenitor for what might be called bronchogenic carcinoma. It is likely that most bronchogenic squamous cell carcinomas, but also many small cell lung cancers and possibly other tumor types arising in the central airways, develop from such alterations in the airway epithelium. As well as considering SD/CIS in detail, it is appropriate to discuss the other, possibly earlier changes believed to occur in the bronchial epithelium prior to the development of SD/CIS.

Basal Cell Hyperplasia

Basal cell hyperplasia (BCH), also known as reserve cell hyperplasia, is defined by the presence of three or more layers of basal cells in otherwise normal respiratory epithelium[76] (Fig. 34.4). Assessment of possible BCH can be hampered by cross-cutting of the epithelium, making the basal layer (but also the basement membrane) appear thicker than it really is. Occasionally basal cells may replace the entire epithelium and care must be taken not to confuse this with severe dysplasia or CIS[77] (Fig. 34.5). Within a strict definition of BCH, these cells do not ordinarily show evidence of keratinization or intercellular bridge formation and atypia is lacking. Not infrequently, however, the expanded basal layer does show intercellular bridges, yet differentiated columnar epithelial cells remain on the epithelial surface (Fig. 34.6). Such lesions have also been termed immature squamous metaplasia, though this is not recognized in the WHO classification.

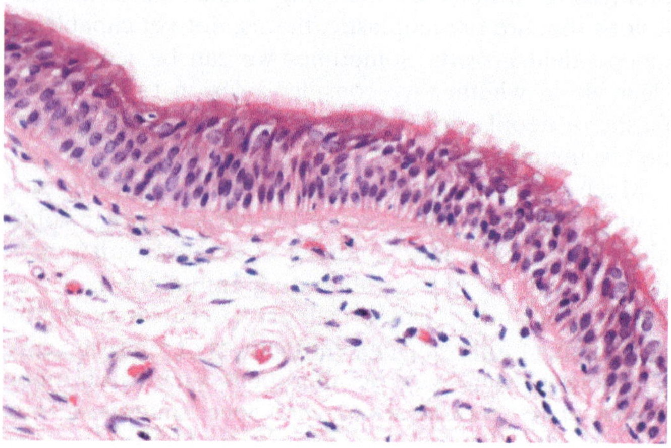

FIGURE 34.4. Basal cell hyperplasia. The zone of basal cells is expanded to a three- to four-cell thickness.

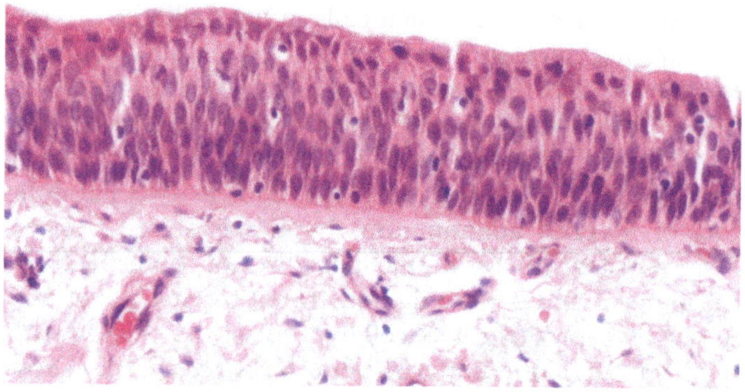

FIGURE 34.5. Basal cell hyperplasia. In this example the basal cell zone occupies most of the epithelium. Columnar cells remain on the surface. There is no atypia.

This immature squamous cell population may develop atypia (see below).

Goblet Cell Hyperplasia

Airways from patients with chronic bronchitis and asthma frequently show excess numbers of mucus-secreting goblet cells in the respiratory epithelium. There may be ciliated cells admixed with the goblet cells or short runs of only goblet cells may be present (Fig. 34.7), sometimes with a slightly papillary or tufted appearance. These cells lack atypia, and while their presence in increased numbers is a recognized reactive response to chronic irritation, such as from tobacco smoke,[78] any relationship with the development of cancer is uncertain. While most consider goblet cell hyperplasia to be a reactive change sharing a common etiology with SD/CIS, but not a progenitor lesion of preinvasive neoplasia in the airways, others have challenged this view (see below).[79]

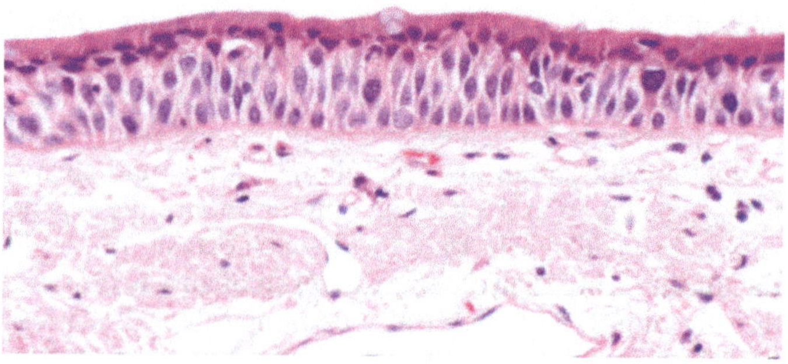

FIGURE 34.6. Basal cell hyperplasia that shows squamous differentiation. Intercellular bridges are evident in the basal cell zone.

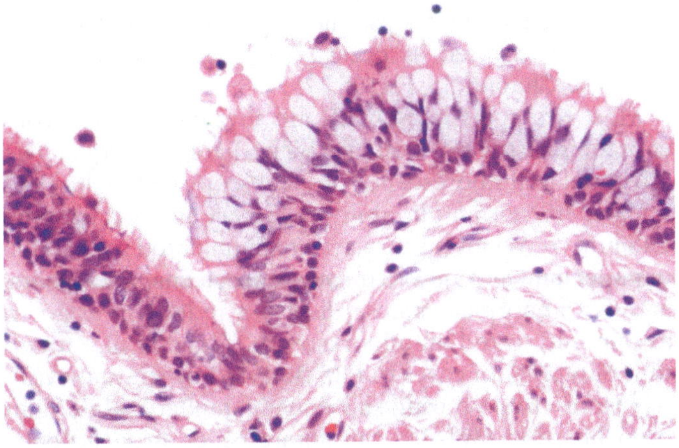

FIGURE 34.7. Goblet cell hyperplasia. Excess numbers of mucin-secreting goblet cells occupy the respiratory epithelium. Typically this is a focal epithelial change but may be diffuse throughout the bronchial epithelium.

Squamous Metaplasia

In squamous metaplasia the full thickness of the pseudostratified respiratory epithelium is replaced by a population of squamous cells showing intercellular bridges in an intermediate zone lying above the basal cell layer and below a superficial zone of cell maturation, flattening, and keratinization (Fig. 34.8). More frequently, however, keratinization is minimal and in squamous metaplasia the cells are not atypical. While there is a strong association between squamous metaplasia and cigarette smoking,[76,80,81] other factors such as exposure to irradiation,[82] air pollution,[83] smoking marijuana,[84] vitamin A deficiency,[85] and chronic lung diseases such as bronchiectasis, tuberculosis, and pneumoconiosis[86] may also be responsible. Squamous metaplasia may be seen in airways draining chronic suppurative lesions and around the site of tracheostomy or other points of bronchial trauma, and may be found overlying a typical carcinoid or a variety of benign bronchial tumors (Fig. 34.9). Basal cell hyperplasia, loss of ciliated cells, and squamous metaplasia may be seen in association with pneumonia, but atypia is not seen.[87] In most of these scenarios it is clear that chronic irritation is the factor that induces this adaptive change to an epithelium better able to deal with the prevailing environment. In vitamin A deficiency both hyperplasia and squamous metaplasia of the tracheobronchial epithelium occur.[88] Since many of the dysplasias and carcinomas-in-situ that occur in the human airway have squamous features, squamous metaplasia is often assumed to be the precursor of squamous dysplasia and CIS. This may not always be the case.[89] The presence of squamous metaplasia indicates a response to airway mucosal injury, but it does not necessarily mean that atypical changes will follow.

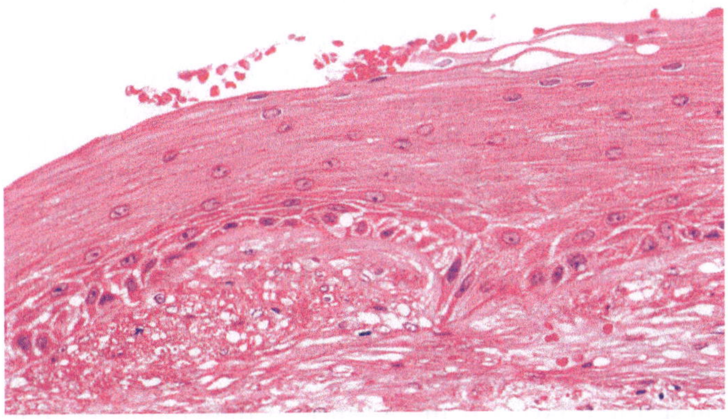

FIGURE 34.8. Squamous metaplasia. Full-thickness squamous epithelium may occur with or without a surface layer of keratinized squamous cells.

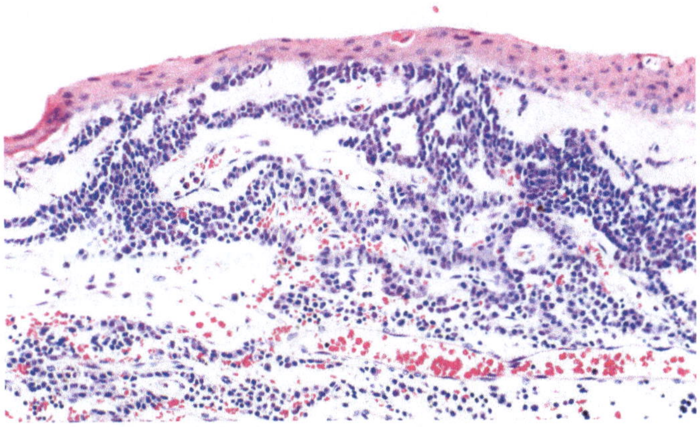

FIGURE 34.9. Squamous metaplasia overlying a typical bronchial carcinoid tumour.

Sqaumous Dysplasia and Carcinoma-in-Situ

Until the recent publication of criteria for the diagnosis and grading of dysplasia in tracheobronchial epithelium,[1] few descriptions were available and many authors simply referred to criteria applied to squamous epithelial dysplasia in other sites, such as the cervix, or described complex systems that were difficult to apply.[80,90] The published WHO classification is still relatively complex and has four categories: mild, moderate, and severe dysplasia, and carcinoma in situ. In classifications of epithelial dysplasia in other sites, such as cervix and esophagus, there has been a recent trend toward more simplified systems of low- and high-grade dysplasia, and some recent publications concerning bronchial epithelial dysplasia have followed this trend, referring to moderate/severe dysplasia and CIS as high-grade disease.[91]

Gross Features

On examination of airways in surgical specimens or at autopsy, the gross features of SD/CIS, if apparent at all, may be subtle. Foci of CIS are most often found at bronchial bifurcations, often on the spur of the carina.[92,93] These foci may appear pale compared to the surrounding mucosa, with a vague nodular or granular character, and the mucosa loses its transparent appearance. The fine ridges and rugae of the mucosa are lost, as are the pitted openings of bronchial gland ducts.[89] Nonetheless, even in surgical resection specimens where lesions were actively sought, having been previously diagnosed by bronchial biopsy/cytology, up to 39% of CIS lesions and even 17% of invasive carcinomas caused no grossly visible abnormality.[94] In this study the mean diameter of the CIS lesions was 9mm (range 2 to 17mm); most lesions were 2 to 4mm in thickness, with focal broadening up to 7mm. In a series of 19 cases of isolated CIS[93] identified by sputum cytology and bronchial biopsy in the context of a lung cancer screening program, the maximum lesion size was 12mm while four lesions were 4mm or less. Rarely a lesion may be circumferential, resulting in loss of mucociliary function and impaired clearance of the distal lung. Thus CIS can lead to distal collapse and retention pneumonia. Uncommonly an exophytic polypoid or papillary CIS lesion may occur, without evidence of stromal invasion (Fig. 34.10). Spencer et al.[95] described four such cases, two of which occurred in conjunction with invasive squamous cell carcinoma in another airway, but two were isolated lesions. In the WHO classification of squamous cell carcinoma, however, the papillary variant is accepted as occasionally being noninvasive.[1] (See also Chapter 35, Fig. 35.37).

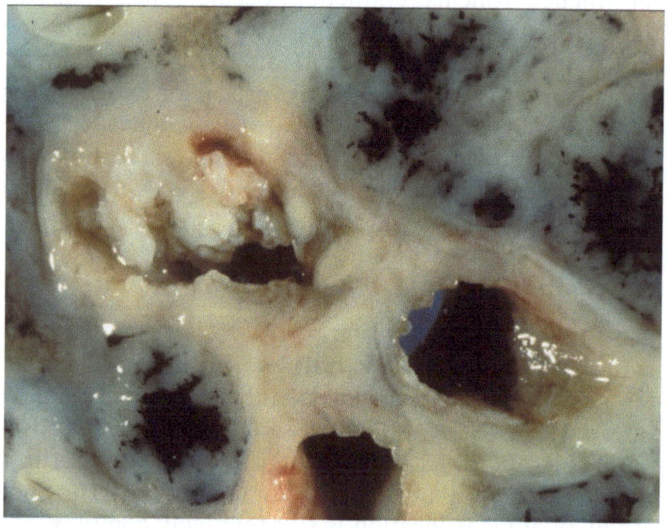

Figure 34.10. This papillary endobronchial tumor was associated with obstructive pneumonia and reactive lymphadenopathy, but there was no evidence of invasive disease.

Most examples of SD/CIS are invisible to the bronchoscopist using the standard white-light technique. The advent of autofluorescence bronchoscopy (AFB) has had a major impact on our ability to detect and localize SD/CIS in vivo. When the airways are illuminated with a blue or violet light and viewed through special imaging sensors, areas of abnormal mucosa display a reduction in green as opposed to red autofluorescence.[96] Lam et al.[97] found that only 29% of cases of CIS detected by sputum cytology were visible during subsequent standard white-light bronchoscopy (WLB). Autofluorescence bronchoscopy had a 6.3-fold greater sensitivity than WLB for detecting moderate/severe dysplasia, and CIS and was even better, by a factor of 2.7, at detecting invasive carcinoma. In the same study, however, nearly half of the AFB-abnormal areas that were biopsied were histologically normal, while a further third showed reactive inflammatory, hyperplastic, or metaplastic changes. Hirsch et al.[91] also found AFB had better sensitivity than WLB (68.8 vs. 21.9%) for detecting high-grade dysplasia. It is worth noting, however, that this group also noted that 31% of their severe dysplasias were not localized at AFB.

Measurement of a small series of AFB-detected SD/CIS lesions revealed that 45% were between 1.6 and 4mm in maximum dimension, while 55% measured 1.5mm or less.[98] Obviously patient selection, experience with the technique, and biopsy policy influence the findings when using AFB, which remains a highly sensitive but less specific technique for detecting bronchial preinvasive lesions in vivo.

Microscopic Diagnosis and Grading

The criteria for microscopic diagnosis and grading of SD/CIS assume a full-thickness squamous-type epithelium. Although four categories are described, it is recognized that these changes represent a biologic continuum, and the divisions are artificial. Furthermore, the degree of atypia as defined in these criteria may vary considerably between adjacent high-power microscopic fields, and a "full house" of features of the assigned category will not always be present in any given lesion. The tabulation of criteria published by WHO[99] is shown in Table 34.1. Following the practice applied in other squamous epithelia, the epithelium is divided into lower, middle, and upper thirds, and the distribution of certain features within these three layers is the essence of the grading system. Epithelial thickness, cell size, changes in maturation and orientation, and nuclear features will inevitably be assessed somewhat subjectively. In some cases cell matu-

TABLE 34.1. Histologic features of bronchial squamous dysplasia and carcinoma in situ

	Mild dysplasia	Moderate dysplasia	Severe dysplasia	Carcinoma in situ
Epithelial thickness	Mild increase	Moderate increase	Marked increase	Variable. Ranges from greatly increased to thinner than normal
Cell size	Mild increase Minimal variation and pleomorphism	Mild increase in cell size; cells often small Moderate variation and pleomorphism	Marked increase May be marked variation and pleomorphism	Marked increase May be marked variation and pleomorphism
Cell maturation and orientation	• Continuous progression of maturation from base to luminal surface • Basilar zone expanded with cellular crowding in *lower third* • Distinct intermediate (prickle cell) zone often present • Superficial flattening of epithelial cells	• Partial progression of maturation from base to luminal surface • Basilar zone expanded with cellular crowding in *lower two thirds* of epithelium • Intermediate zone confined to upper third of epithelium • Superficial flattening of epithelial cells	• Little progression of maturation from base to luminal surface • Basilar zone expanded with cellular crowding *well into upper third* • Intermediate zone greatly attenuated • Superficial flattening of epithelial cells	• No progression of maturation from base to luminal surface; *epithelium could be inverted with little change in appearance* • Basilar zone expanded with cellular crowding *throughout epithelium* • Intermediate zone absent • Surface flattening confined to the most superficial cells
Nuclear features	• Mild variation of N/C ratio • Finely granular chromatin • Minimal angulation • Nucleoli inconspicuous or absent • Nuclei vertically oriented in lower third • Mitoses *absent* or very rare	• Moderate variation of N/C ratio • Finely granular chromatin • Angulations, grooves and lobulations present • Nucleoli inconspicuous or absent • Nuclei vertically oriented in lower two thirds • Mitotic figures present in *lower third*	• N/C ratio often high and variable • Chromatin uneven and coarse • Nuclear angulations and folding prominent • Nucleoli frequently present and conspicuous • Nuclei vertically oriented in lower two thirds • Mitotic figures present in *lower two thirds*	• N/C ratio often high and variable • Chromatin uneven and coarse • Nuclear angulations and folding prominent • Nucleoli may be present or inconspicuous • No consistent orientation of nuclei in relation to epithelial surface • Mitotic figures present *throughout epithelium*

N/C, nuclear to cytoplasmic ratio.
Modified from Franklin et al.[99]

ration is complete, resulting in keratinization, while in others a more basaloid phenotype is retained.

The key feature in allowing a diagnosis of *mild dysplasia* is expansion of the basilar zone of cells into, but not beyond, the lower third of the epithelium (Fig. 34.11). Atypia and pleomorphism are minimal, but the crowded cells in the lower third have vertically orientated nuclei with few irregular features. Mitoses are absent or very rare.

In *moderate dysplasia* the crowded population of basal cells with vertically orientated nuclei extends into, but not above, the middle third of what is still clearly recognizable as squamous epithelium (Fig. 34.12). Epithelial thickness is increased, cell size is increased, though not markedly so, and nuclear contours may be irregular. Mitotic figures may be present anywhere in the lower third of the epithelium.

Severe dysplasia is characterized by a marked increase in cell size, pleomorphism, and nuclear variability. Nucleoli may be seen. As well as the crowded basilar zone of cells clearly extending into the upper third of the epithelium, both mitoses and vertically orientated nuclei may be found in the lower two thirds of the epithelium (Fig. 34.13). There remains evidence of flattening of epithelial cells on the surface.

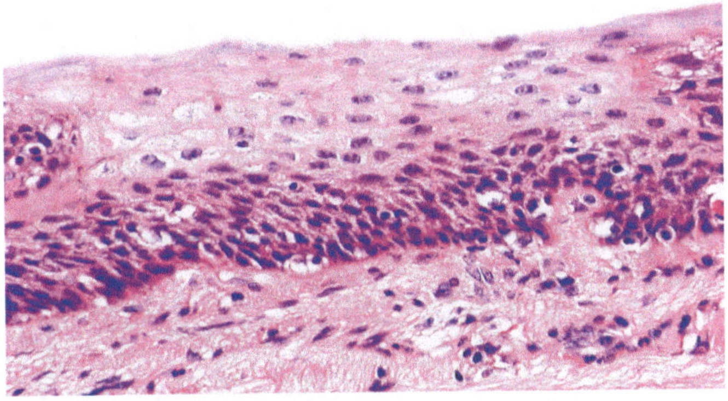

FIGURE 34.11. Mild squamous dysplasia. This example occurred in an epithelium exhibiting obvious squamous differentiation.

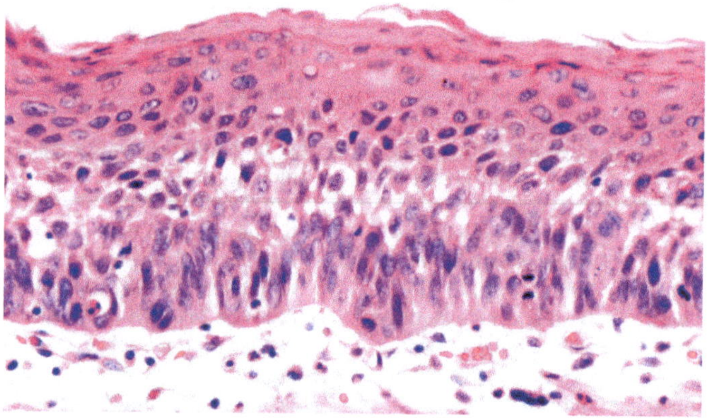

FIGURE 34.12. Moderate squamous dysplasia. Mitotic figures are clearly seen in the lower third of the epithelium.

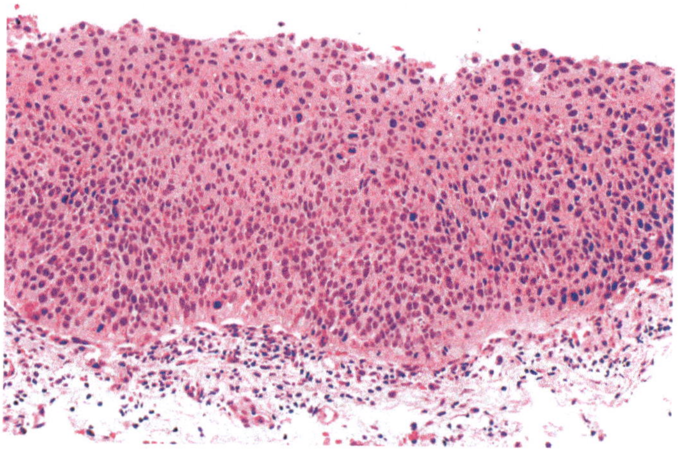

FIGURE 34.14. Carcinoma in situ (CIS). Chaotic epithelium with no obvious maturation and mitoses throughout. This is a rather thick example of CIS, photographed at half the magnification of Figures 34.11 to 34.13.

The key feature in the recognition of CIS is a completely haphazard orientation of markedly enlarged and pleomorphic cells that look like malignant cells (Fig. 34.14). There is usually no evidence of cell maturation such that if the epithelium were inverted it would look the same. Mitotic figures may be found at any level. Paradoxically, although CIS may be associated with considerable increase in epithelial thickness, it may also be present as a thinned epithelium.

As atypia develops in this squamous-type epithelium, the basement membrane may also thicken.[80] Nuorva et al.[100] described occasional disruptions of the basement membrane beneath moderate to severe dysplasia, but not in association with mild dysplasia. The disintegration of basement membrane as dysplasia increases in severity is also described by Fisseler-Eckhoff et al.,[101] who also noted that, in severe dysplasia and CIS, increased deposition of laminin and type III collagen is accompanied by neoangiogenesis.

Possibly related to this phenomenon is a lesion described by Keith et al.[102] as *angiogenic squamous dysplasia* (ASD). Here, capillary vessels project upward into the metaplastic or dysplastic squamous epithelium, resulting in a micropapillary architecture (Fig. 34.15; see also Chapter 33, Fig. 33.8). Serial sections confirmed that these lesions were indeed tufts of capillary loops gathered

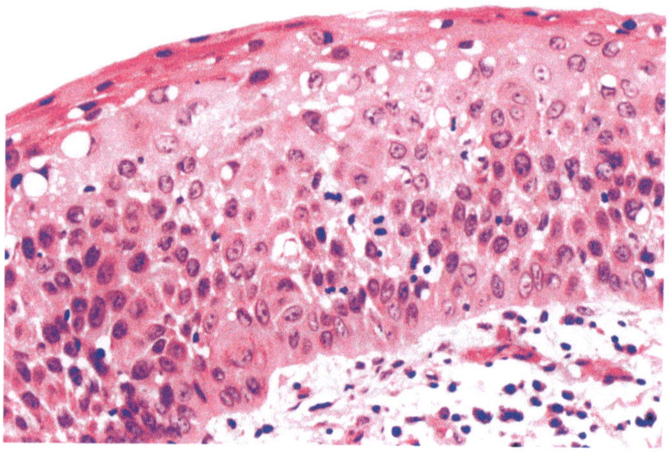

FIGURE 34.13. Severe squamous dysplasia. Nuclear atypia present throughout most of the epithelium. Mitotic figures in the mid-zone.

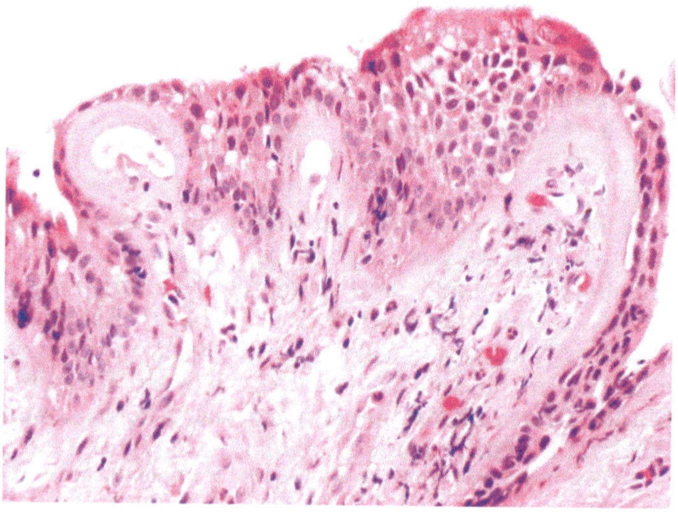

FIGURE 34.15. Angiogenic squamous dysplasia in a bronchial biopsy specimen. This example shows mild atypia.

beneath the intact basement membrane, which was surmounted by a thinned and often dysplastic squamous epithelium. Microvessel density was significantly increased in these areas. Such lesions were detected at AFB in 34% of a group of heavy cigarette smokers without cancer, but never found in the nonsmoking control group. Angiogenic squamous dysplasia was also found in 60% of patients with squamous cell carcinoma. The mechanisms of neoangiogenesis in this setting are unknown, but its association with patients at high risk of developing lung cancer and with preinvasive epithelial changes tempts speculation about a possible role for ASD in the evolution of invasive disease. These morphologic changes have been previously described by the term *micropapillomatosis*[103,104] and may be more efficiently detected in vivo utilizing high magnification bronchovideoscopy and narrow band filter imaging.[105]

Cytologic Diagnosis of Bronchial Squamous Atypia

Exfoliative cytology may be used to examine sputum or bronchial washings and brushings for atypical squamous cells, and these have been related to histopathologic findings to create classification systems for bronchial squamous atypia[104,106,107] and CIS.[108] As would be predicted, these classifications are based on the recognition of metaplastic squamous cells in flat sheets, clusters, and individually. They are larger than basal cells but smaller than the oral squames that are found in sputum samples, have usually basophilic or orangeophilic cytoplasm, and regular round to oval nuclei. Dysplasias are characterized by increasingly severe cellular aberration. Variability in cell size and nuclear/cytoplasmic ratio are the key features, and increasing cytoplasmic acidophilia (orangeophilia) is seen. The chromatin pattern changes from a fine powdery and even distribution to become increasingly coarse with perinuclear membrane clumping. In the more severe atypias, nucleoli appear and nuclear outlines become increasingly irregular. In CIS, cellular cannibalism and multinucleation may be seen. Clearly a range of atypical appearances may be found in exfoliated airway cells, which at least have the potential to reflect the degrees of dysplasia present. How reliably these atypias may be accurately graded depends, as ever, on the experience of the cytopathologist. While criteria for distinguishing between CIS and invasive carcinoma have been published,[108] the consensus view is that these cannot be reliably distinguished (see Chapter 45).

It is difficult to say what proportion of preinvasive lesions would be expected to be found using sputum cytology, but the overall figure is probably low, since in screening studies for cancer where tumors on average are less advanced than in the symptomatic population, 40% of detected squamous cell carcinomas were advanced enough to be seen on chest radiography yet were not identified on sputum cytology.[109] Woolner et al.,[110] however, found sputum cytology had a sensitivity of 78% for CIS and invasive carcinoma combined, while a more recent study has shown that in 79 patients with a normal chest radiograph but moderate sputum atypia, combined white light and AFB examination revealed early squamous cell carcinoma in 4%, CIS in 3%, and severe dysplasia in 9% of subjects.[111]

Historical Perspective

Animal Models

Many of the ideas surrounding the evolution of SD/CIS and the development of invasive disease have come from animal models, a topic extensively reviewed elsewhere.[104,112] Although caution must be exercised in drawing too many conclusions about human disease from these studies,[112] useful insights are provided by this work, particularly since it is clearly impossible to repeat it in human subjects. Becci et al.[113] described a sequence of changes in the hamster tracheobronchial epithelium after regular carcinogen exposure. The earliest changes were mucous cell hyperplasia, followed by expansion of the basal cell layer and squamous metaplasia, and, much later, focal severe atypia and CIS. Mucous cells were retained in the surface layer (see below). Nettesheim et al.[112] describe three phases in the morphogenesis of experimental carcinogen-induced neoplasia in rodent airway mucosa: an acute toxic phase, a subacute or preneoplastic phase, and a neoplastic phase. In the first phase there is evidence of acute cellular damage (toxicity) and hyperplasia of both mucous and basal cells. Soon after the mucous cell and BCH develops, stratified squamous metaplasia appears in places. These hyperplastic/metaplastic changes are considered to be a nonspecific toxic reaction to injury, which may occur in other circumstances without the presence of carcinogens and are generally rapidly reversible when the inducing chemicals are removed. In some airways, however, damage persists in the form of an atrophic squamous epithelium. Where the initial carcinogenic insult was severe, some animals develop foci of stratified squamous metaplasia months later (the subacute phase). Unlike the metaplasia seen in the acute phase, these are focal, discrete lesions showing an orderly structure, orthokeratinization, an absence of mucous cells, and lacking inflammatory cells. Gradually, many of these lesions develop increasing cytologic atypia and may be classified as dysplastic. The neoplastic phase begins with lesions classified as CIS, upon which invasion supervenes.

Nasiell et al.[104] have described a similar sequence of events in the airways of dogs treated with carcinogens. These changes, including those considered CIS, appeared to be reversible when carcinogen treatment was withdrawn.[114] While most of these studies involved the administration of quite high concentrations of pure carcinogenic agents to animals that developed preinvasive and invasive disease remarkably quickly, Hammond et al.[115] found that, in the infamous smoking beagle model, while the sequence of changes was the same, namely BCH followed by squamous metaplasia, atypia only developed in a few squamous metaplastic lesions after years of exposure, and few of these lesions subsequently progressed to invasive disease.

Human Studies

Although the conventional belief is that a progression of changes, similar to those seen in experimental animals, occurs in the human airway, viz. BCH evolving into squamous metaplastic epithelium, which in turn is the background for the development of dysplasia and CIS,[104] this idea has been challenged. Melamed and Zaman[89] proposed that in the human tracheobronchial epithelium, in response to both the nonspecific irritant effect and the specific carcinogenic effects of tobacco smoke, BCH and squamous metaplasia may occur independently of each other in different parts of the airway and that each of these lesions may develop atypia (dysplasia) and CIS. These authors also proposed that CIS can arise de novo in otherwise normal respiratory mucosa without any preceding lesion. It is certainly true that some SD/CIS lesions have distinctive squamous differentiation, as in Figures 34.11 to 34.14, while others have a more basal cell morphology (Fig. 34.16). It is not known whether these variations in SD/CIS reflect a different exposure to carcinogens or are more likely to give rise to different types of invasive tumor (see later). In our experience, a patient will have SD/CIS with more or less keratinization (and thus a more basaloid morphology), but not both patterns. When full maturation to keratinization is absent, columnar epithelial cells appear to persist on the surface, making grading difficult (see below). Trump et al.[79] have also challenged the conventional view that BCH is the precursor of squamous metaplasia, suggesting that goblet cells may convert into keratinizing squamous cells either directly or via an intermediate form of mucous cell.

Some of the earliest and best-known work on preinvasive lesions in the human tracheobronchial tree and their relationship with invasive cancer and tobacco smoking was published by Auerbach and colleagues.[76,80,87,90,116] In an extensive autopsy-based study of 402 white males in which the entire tracheobronchial tree from each patient was removed and sectioned, Auerbach et al. found changes from BCH and squamous metaplasia to the presence of atypical cells and lesions they regarded as CIS. These lesions were found throughout the tracheobronchial tree, although atypia and CIS were less frequent in the trachea than elsewhere. Lesions were more frequent, more extensive, and more atypical with increasing exposure to tobacco smoke.[76,90] The authors concluded that bronchogenic carcinoma developed on a background of BCH and loss of ciliated epithelium, with a concurrent increase in cytologic atypia, and that this process was potentially reversible at any point in the proposed continuum, should smoking cease. Progression of disease appeared to occur over many years.[80,116]

In a study of 210 males who had died of primary lung cancer, some of whom were uranium miners, Auerbach

A

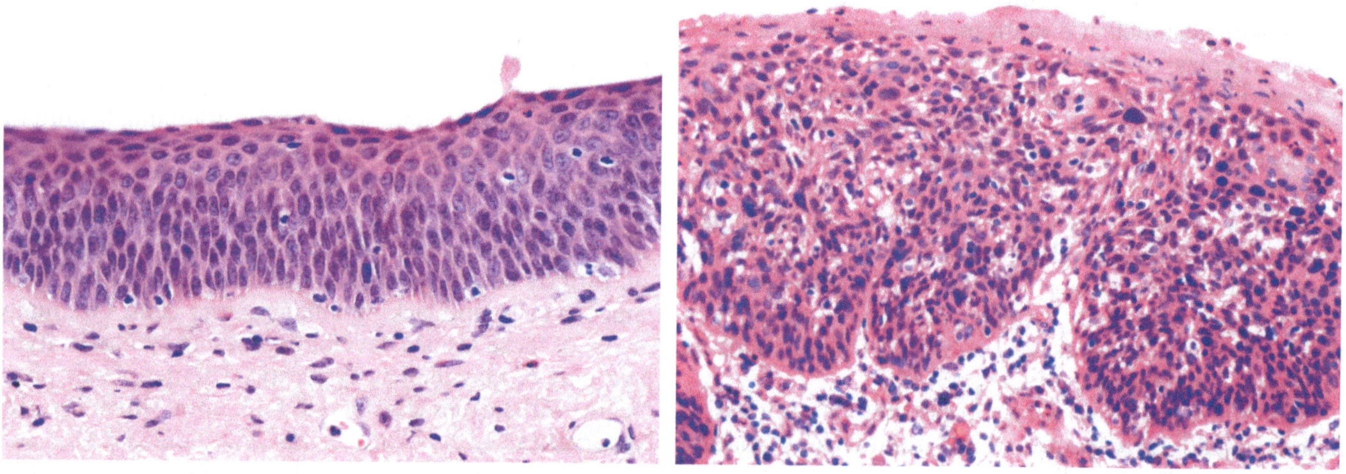

B

FIGURE 34.16. These examples of squamous dysplasia (SD)/CIS show the basaloid pattern with keratinization and intercellular bridges less evident. **(A)** Moderate dysplasia showing crowding of cells with vertically orientated nuclei in the lower two thirds of the epithelium. **(B)** Carcinoma in situ. No evidence of maturation in this pleomorphic epithelium covered in fibrinous coagulum.

et al.[117] found CIS in the residual tracheobronchial tree in 96% of the miners and 92% of the nonminers, and found that high-grade dysplasia was more widespread in the respiratory mucosa of the miners when compared with the nonminers. Peters et al.,[81] who studied 106 heavy cigarette smokers and multiple biopsy specimens taken at fiberoptic bronchoscopy, found that squamous metaplasia was more frequent and extensive, and that the mitotic index in these lesions was higher in those with increased exposure to tobacco smoke. Their data also suggested that the intensity of exposure was more important than chronicity in developing squamous metaplasia. Auerbach at al.[80] found that SD/CIS was present in up to 40% of those who were heavy smokers, but did not have invasive carcinoma. While BCH and squamous dysplasia are frequent in smokers without cancer, and dysplasia and CIS are increased in heavy smokers, these high-grade changes are even more frequent in lungs that have already developed carcinoma.[116] High-grade dysplasia and CIS are more often found in male rather than female heavy smokers, both in autopsy studies[87] and in patients screened by cytology and AFB.[118]

Dysplasia may also be detected by sputum cytology, especially in high-risk populations such as heavy tobacco smokers, particularly those with chronic obstructive pulmonary disease (COPD) and those exposed to radiation.[91,106,119] Hirsch et al.[91] reported finding mild dysplasia in 48% and moderate/severe dysplasia in 26% of a sputum cytology–screened high-risk population, while Frost at al.,[119] whose study population was perhaps less at risk, found a similar frequency of low-grade abnormalities, but found high-grade dysplasia in only 3.5% of their subjects.

Squamous dysplasia/CIS and the changes that precede it are frequent in the airways of smokers, as well as in other at-risk groups, with evidence of a positive correlation between smoking exposure and degree of atypia. While hyperplasia and metaplasia as a result of air pollution are recognized, an association between SD/CIS and urban pollution independent of tobacco smoke has not been demonstrated.[120,121]

Issues in the Diagnosis of Preinvasive Bronchial Lesions

There are considerable benefits in having an agreed set of criteria that may be applied to the difficult job of diagnosing and grading bronchial SD/CIS. Although there have been major advances in our understanding of the biology of SD/CIS, much remains to be learned. It is essential that there is consistency in reporting SD/CIS so that correct conclusions are drawn and data can be compared between centers. This issue has been raised by Venmans et al.,[122] who speculated that misclassification of SD/CIS has probably influenced the findings of AFB screening studies. A report suggested that it was possible to achieve reasonable consistency in applying the WHO classification,[123] but more studies of this type are required.

Relatively few pathologists have extensive experience of SD/CIS in small bronchial biopsy specimens, and most pulmonary pathologists have difficulties with this area of diagnosis. Most SD/CIS is invisible at standard bronchoscopy and so is an incidental finding in the usual surgical pathology setting. The situation is rather different in a screening program (see below). The WHO criteria can be quite difficult to apply since there may be partial loss of surface epithelial cells and orientation of the tissue sections on the slide is all-important. As in the cervix, distinction between BCH and mild dysplasia may be almost impossible (Fig. 34.17). Application of the "thirds" rule can be problematic, even in an intact squamous epithelium, which is frequently quite thin. As previously mentioned, squamous change may occur only in the lower part of the respiratory epithelium, in the zone of BCH, and differentiated columnar cells may persist over metaplastic or dysplastic squamous epithelium (Fig. 34.18). In such a case it may be best to ignore the overlying residual columnar cells and take a pragmatic approach by attempting to classify the lesion as low or high grade based on the cytologic features.

If CIS is found in a bronchial biopsy specimen, careful examination of multiple levels should be made to rule out mucosal invasion. Not infrequently, such samples contain cytologically malignant squamous epithelium without any underlying stroma. Caution must be exercised in

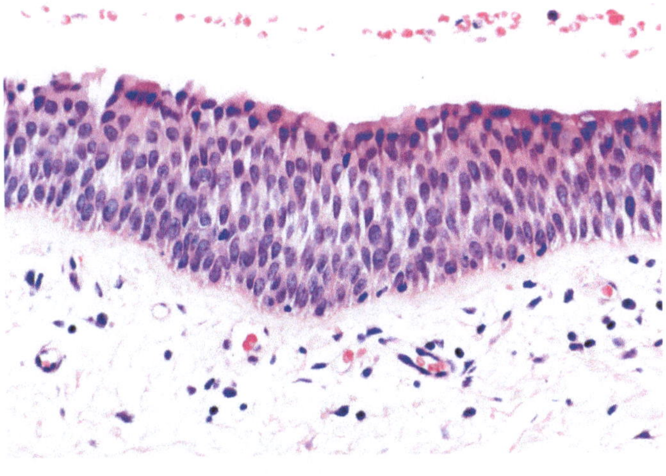

FIGURE 34.17. Basal cell hyperplasia with squamous differentiation (intermediate zone present) and persistent columnar cells superficially. There is more nuclear variation and irregularity in this lesion compared to that in Figure 34.5. A classification of mild dysplasia is acceptable in this case, but this field highlights some of the difficulties encountered with these lesions.

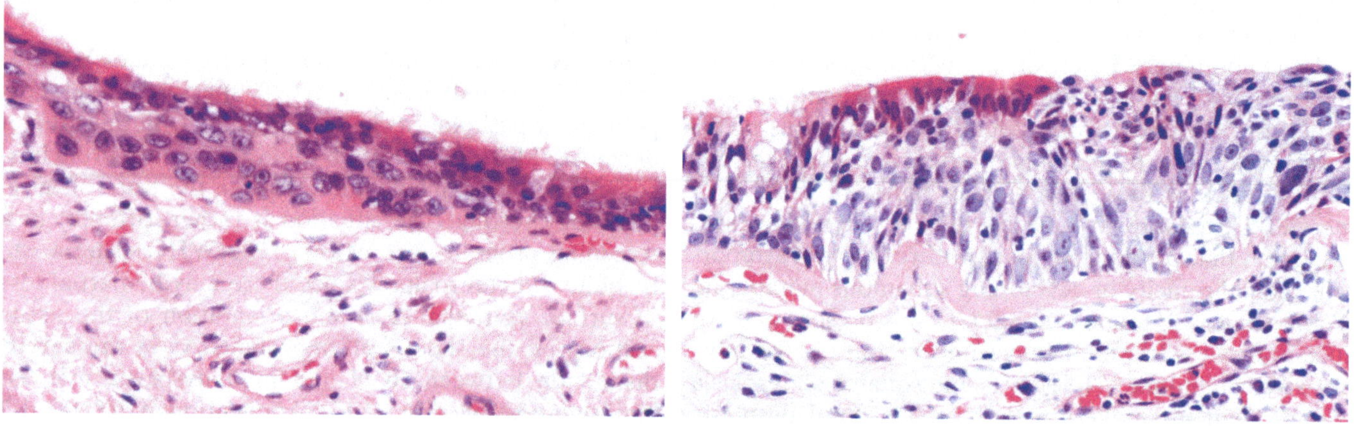

FIGURE 34.18. **(A)** A thin layer of dysplastic squamous cells covered by ciliated epithelium. Do such lesions develop from such as is illustrated in Figure 34.6? **(B)** Carcinoma in situ partially covered by respiratory epithelium. Transformation of incomplete squamous epithelium or lateral extension of CIS undermining nonneoplastic epithelium?

diagnosing invasive disease in the absence of definite evidence of such; the phrase "at least carcinoma in situ" is useful, and correlation with bronchoscopic and radiologic findings often leads to the correct diagnosis. Dysplasia and CIS may extend from the surface of the bronchus, down the bronchial gland ducts, and replace the bronchial glands. This is still CIS, but the unwary pathologist may make an erroneous diagnosis of invasive carcinoma if the lobular architecture of the aberrant squamous epithelium replacing the clustered bronchial gland acini is not appreciated (Fig. 34.19).

Squamous metaplasia not infrequently occurs when there is long-standing inflammation of airways, bronchial mucosal ulceration, or in diffuse lung diseases such as UIP/IPF and organizing DAD (Fig. 34.20). Atypical cells may occur in such epithelia, and this reactive atypia can be misdiagnosed as dysplasia if the context is not appreciated or allowance is not made for any coexistent inflammation. Viral infection may lead to atypia whether or not the bronchial epithelium is squamous, and both

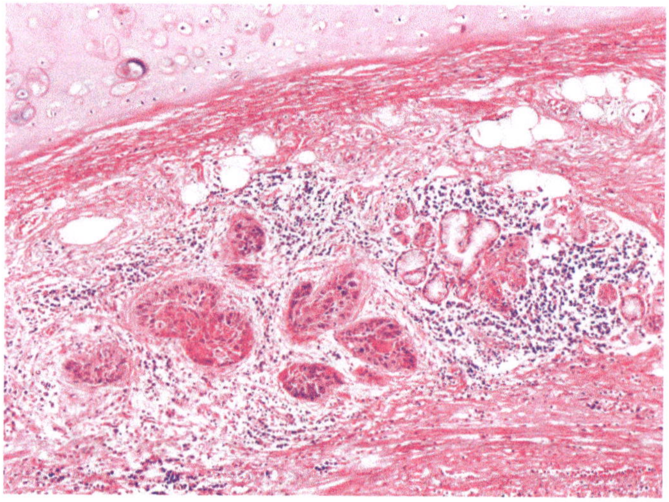

FIGURE 34.19. Carcinoma in situ involving bronchial submucous gland acini and ducts. This does not represent invasive disease.

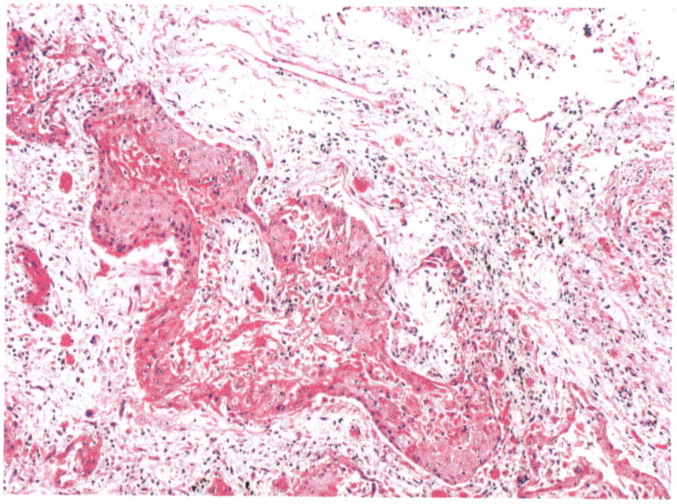

FIGURE 34.20. Squamous metaplasia with evidence of nuclear atypia. This patient had organizing-phase diffuse alveolar damage (DAD). The squamous metaplasia occurs in the regenerating alveolar epithelium rather than in bronchial epithelium.

chemo- and radiotherapy may also give quite marked cytologic atypia in both bronchial surface epithelium and seromucous glands. Although atypia may be present in these circumstances, the abnormal epithelial architecture of SD/CIS is absent.

The identification of CIS in an airway may raise the possibility of invasive disease elsewhere in the tracheobronchial tree. This will have implications for patient follow-up and, possibly, may indicate chemopreventive therapy (see below). Carcinoma in situ in association with invasive carcinoma is good evidence that the cancer is primary in the bronchus. In a tumor with an epidermoid and a glandular component, any CIS would favor a diagnosis of adenosquamous carcinoma over one of high-grade mucoepidermoid carcinoma.[124] Carcinoma in situ may be quite extensive in surgical specimens resected for invasive carcinoma and may be present at the bronchial resection margin in the absence of invasive disease at this level. In a series of cases of resected lung cancer with CIS at the bronchial resection margin, no difference in outcome was observed with stage-matched controls with normal resection margins.[125] While this has been confirmed by more recent studies, others have found an adverse outcome in those patients with CIS at bronchial resection margins, especially if it extends into bronchial glands.[126] In a large retrospective study of surgically resected non–small-cell lung cancers (NSCLCs), CIS found in the vicinity of the tumor in 8.5% of 1501 cases had no influence on patient survival.[127]

Progression of Squamous Dysplasia/Carcinoma in Situ to Invasive Disease

Morphologic studies and the coexistence of SD/CIS with invasive disease provide strong circumstantial evidence that SD/CIS is a precursor of invasive cancer. While the animal models facilitate direct longitudinal observation of tumor development, similar studies are clearly not possible in human subjects. Instead we must rely on subjects who are, voluntarily or otherwise, exposed to factors that increase their chances of developing lung cancer, seek evidence of preinvasive disease, and, with the passage of time, identify cases of invasive carcinoma. As a scientific experiment, this methodology has many problems, but it is the only practical approach available. Bronchial preinvasive lesions are invisible on the plain chest radiograph, and for many years the only way to detect SD/CIS (or early invasive disease) was by sputum cytology.

Suprun et al.[128] found, on follow-up of patients who had squamous metaplasia and dysplasia detectable on sputum cytology, that 17% and 33%, respectively, went on to develop carcinoma. Over a period of 17 years Saccomanno and colleagues[106] collected over 50,000 sputum samples from approximately 6000 uranium miners, ex-miners, and nonminers. As would be expected in both the mining and nonmining groups, those who smoked had a much lower prevalence of normal sputum cytology than those who did not. In those subjects who developed sputum atypia, the mean age at which each successive stage or degree of atypia appeared also increased. Patients who developed CIS in their sputum during the study did so after anywhere between a few months and 10 years of examination, but the degree of disease on entry to the study varies, making interpretation of the data difficult. Average times to develop invasive squamous cell carcinoma from stages of moderate atypia, severe atypia, and CIS in sputum were 4.8, 2.9 and 2.5 years, respectively. Frost et al.[119] reported on a series of cases detected during the Johns Hopkins Lung Project. Of those who had marked sputum atypia, follow-up over 9 years showed 42.6% developed invasive carcinoma. Over the same period 10.6% of those with moderate atypia, but 4% of those with lesser atypia or normal sputum, developed lung cancer. Follow-up over 2 to 8 years of 46 patients with a sputum cytology diagnosis of severe dysplasia found that 21 patients (46%) developed invasive disease.[129]

Studies using sputum cytology to observe progression of this disease are prone to sampling error, and as always the possibility of diagnostic inaccuracy is present; there is thus doubt as to how representative of the bronchial disease the sputum sample is. Nonetheless, these studies provide valuable data on the predictive value of sputum cytology and do suggest that severe degrees of sputum atypia carry a substantial risk of lung cancer development.

Satoh et al.[130] found that in four chromate workers with biopsy-proven dysplasia, three with severe dysplasia developed invasive squamous cell carcinoma within 7 to 13 months, while the fourth who had only mild dysplasia developed invasive disease after 82 months. Increasing use of AFB has improved detection rates for SD/CIS and also allows localization, and therefore repeated observation, of the diseased airway, something not possible with sputum cytology. An early AFB study, in which 18 SD/CIS lesions of varying grade were followed for between 3 months and 2 years, found that one CIS lesion became invasive.[131] Worthy of note is the fact that some high-grade lesions reverted to a lower grade or showed BCH at follow-up biopsy.

Venmans et al.[132] found that, during a follow-up period of 6 to 60 months, two of six patients with biopsy-proven CIS and all three patients with severe dysplasia went on to develop invasive disease. Of the four patients who had CIS and did not develop invasive disease, three reverted to normal histology on repeat bronchoscopy. However, extended follow-up of these four patients over up to 6 more years has shown that all four have subsequently developed invasive carcinoma.[133,134] In the largest study of its kind so far published, Bota et al.[135] studied 104 patients over a 2-year period. Each patient received up to four AFB examinations, and in total over 1000 biopsy samples were taken. Most of those lesions that were normal or inflammatory after biopsy remained so, though 17% progressed to severe dysplasia. Of those lesions that were originally found to be hyperplastic, metaplastic, or dysplastic (any grade), about one third were stable at 2 years, between one and two thirds regressed to a lower grade lesion or became normal, while evidence of disease progression was variable. Of the hyperplastic and metaplastic lesions, 30% became mild or moderate dysplasia, 2% became CIS, and one lesion became invasive squamous cell carcinoma over 2 years. Over the same time period only 3.5% of mild/moderate dysplasias progressed no further than severe dysplasia. Most CIS lesions were stable, none progressed to invasion, and a few regressed to normal.

Banerjee et al.[96] reported five of 17 patients with CIS progressing to invasive disease over 6 to 48 months' follow-up, while the remaining 12 patients have remained stable. Ponticiello et al.[136] also found that, over a 4-year follow-up period, 25%, 50%, and 75%, respectively, of mild, moderate, and severe dysplasia progressed to invasive squamous cell carcinoma, but the case numbers were small, and statistically significant differences could not be demonstrated. Moro-Sibilot et al.[137] prospectively studied 27 patients with severe dysplasia or CIS and found progression to cancer in 17% at 1 year and 63% at 3 years. Persistence of smoking in the presence of a high-grade lesion did not seem to alter outcome, nor did the number of biopsies performed on the patient.

The data from bronchoscopy studies are difficult to interpret for a number of reasons. In many of these studies, high-grade lesions were treated, though in some a wait-and-see policy was followed. Biopsy at subsequent bronchoscopy may miss the crucial area, giving a false impression of disease regression. Biopsy of the lesion may remove it (many of these lesions are small [see above] and potentially resectable by forceps biopsy) or alter the lesion such that the behavior of the residual disease may be modified. It is theoretically possible that progression (through growth stimulation) or regression (via biopsy-induced inflammation) could result. The possibility of misclassification of disease on biopsy specimens may also affect the results and explain some examples of disease regression.[122]

Despite these caveats it seems likely that the following assertions are true:

- Progression of disease takes years rather than months.
- Each stage of disease can last a considerable period of time but the rate of progression increases as disease advances.
- Progression of disease is not inevitable: lesions may wax and wane or regress completely, especially after smoking cessation.
- As disease becomes more advanced, regression is less likely and progression more likely.
- It is difficult to generate hard data on this topic!

Recently there has been considerable interest in the use of molecular biology to predict progression of SD/CIS. This will be considered in the next section.

Cell and Molecular Biology of Squamous Dysplasia/Carcinoma in Situ

Developments in immunohistochemistry, molecular biology, and genetics have led to considerable advances in our knowledge of the molecular events, which occur during the progression of preinvasive disease in the bronchial epithelium. It must be emphasized that the widely held stepwise progression from the so-called reactive stages of hyperplasia/metaplasia, through increasing SD/CIS, to invasive disease is still to some extent speculative, though supported by a large body of circumstantial evidence. Until the advent of AFB, it was impossible to perform directly observational longitudinal studies of SD/CIS (accepting that the cytologic studies of Saccomanno et al.[82,106] do not fall into this category). A large number of studies have shown that there is progression in the patterns of protein expression and genetic alteration in step with the morphologic progression of disease, and it is almost intuitive that at least some of the elements within the increasingly altered genotype determine the altered phenotype; however, it is not known which alterations these are. Furthermore there is evidence that certain genetic or epigenetic changes may help predict which SD/CIS lesions will progress and which will not, something that has enormous potential utility in the assessment of this disease (see below).

Altered Cell Proliferation

As would be expected, there is evidence that the earliest precursors, as well as SD/CIS, demonstrate various degrees of hyperproliferation. This is implicit, given that the presence of increased numbers of often abnormally located mitotic figures is part of the definition of SD/CIS. Using anti–proliferating cell nuclear antigen (PCNA) antibodies, Hirano et al.[138] demonstrated that, while the proliferating compartment of normal mucosa was confined to the lowest 25% of the respiratory epithelial cells, that compartment expanded to 35% to 40% of the epithelium in low- and high-grade dysplasia, while in invasive disease, 85% to 90% of cells were "cycling." Others have found similar results, with PCNA-positive nuclei co-located to the expanded basal layer found in bronchial dysplasia[139] or by using anti-MIB1 antibodies.[140,141] In one study the MIB1 labeling index in squamous metaplasia/

dysplasia could not predict those patients who also had carcinoma.[140]

Khuri et al.[142] also found increasing PCNA expression in the progression from normal, through hyperplasia and metaplasia, to dysplasia in an extensive study of 706 bronchial biopsies taken from 86 patients. Furthermore, they found that smoking cessation saw a fall in PCNA expression commensurate with a reversal in the presence of metaplasia, and this change was promoted by 13-cis-retinoic acid treatment. By detection of Ki-67, the same authors also showed that there is a dose-related proliferative response in bronchial epithelium of active smokers, an effect that may persist for up to 20 years after smoking cessation.[143] One other study, using anti-PCNA antibodies to measure proliferative activity in preinvasive bronchial lesions, also showed that there is increased apoptotic activity in these lesions (threefold above normal in squamous metaplasia and a fourfold increase in dysplasia), which parallels the increase in proliferative activity. The authors found no relationship between apoptotic activity and related oncogene and tumor suppressor gene (TSG) expression (*p53, bcl2, BAX*; see below).[144] Tan et al.[145] showed, in a relatively small number of cases, that use of minichromosome maintenance protein MCM2 as a surrogate marker of cell cycling activity in bronchial metaplasia, dysplasia, and CIS may provide a more sensitive method to detect the proliferative compartment in preinvasive bronchial lesions. They found that on average the MCM2 count in any lesion was two to three times higher that that found using anti–Ki-67 antibodies and concluded that MCM2 could be a useful marker in screening sputum for premalignancy.

Neovascularization

Evidence for increased vascular density in the stroma immediately deep to the basement membrane underpinning various preinvasive bronchial lesions was found by Fisseler-Eckhoff et al.,[101] who described vascularity increased by 1.5, 2.5, and 3.0 times, respectively, in squamous metaplasia, dysplasia, and CIS. Interestingly, they also described the concentration of new vessels closer to the basement membrane as dysplasia increased, in association with intraepithelial sprouts of endothelial cells. Similar associations between disease progression and microvascular density were reported by Fontanini et al.,[146] who found a significant rise in subepithelial vessel count when comparing hyperplasia/metaplasia, moderate squamous dysplasia, and CIS. They also found an increasing expression of vascular endothelial growth factor (VEGF) and p53 protein, though between dysplasia and CIS the difference in VEGF expression was not significant.

These findings tempt speculation that molecular events in the evolving SD/CIS lesion stimulate angiogenesis in preparation for tissue invasion and that, in some cases, this leads to the development of ASD. Lantuejoul et al.[147] also found significant elevations of VEGF expression from hyperplasia, through increasing atypia to severe SD/CIS, but found no particular excess of VEGF expression in those lesion that were classified as ASD,[102] a lesion that might have been expected to demonstrate abundant angiogenic signals and that possibly is one morphologic expression of the so-called angiogenic switch in bronchial carcinogenesis.[148] This angiogenic switch in bronchial preinvasive lesions may thus not be (solely) dependent on VEGF and, given the relative lack of p53 mutations in this setting, high p53 protein is also an unlikely candidate.[102] Merrick et al.[149] recently confirmed the progressive increase in microvascular density and VEGF expression as SD/CIS develops, noting that BCH did not demonstrate this alteration. This study also demonstrated elevation in VEGF messenger RNA (mRNA) levels commensurate with the change in VEGF protein expression in SD/CIS epithelial cells, showed that there was a switch from VEGF165 to VEGF121 isoform during SD/CIS development, and that VEGF receptors KDR, flt1, and neuropilin 1 were increasingly expressed. These authors found a trend toward the most angiogenic expression profile in ASD.

Class 3 semaphorins may compete with VEGF for binding the transmembrane VEGF co-receptors neuropilin 1 and 2 (NP1 and NP2). Thus semaphorins such as SEMA3F may act as tumor suppressors by competitive inhibition of the tumor promoting effects of VEGF.[147] It is thus of interest that loss of SEMA3F expression was found early in bronchial carcinogenesis,[147] entirely consistent with the observation that the relevant allele(s) may well be lost in the common and early loss of semaphorin gene loci at 3p21.3 in bronchial carcinogenesis,[150] a loss also described in ASD.[102] Lantuejoul et al.[147] also showed that NP1 and NP2 expression increased with increasing grade of preinvasive bronchial lesion.

It is clear that several factors of potential importance in enabling the angiogenic switch in bronchial carcinogenesis are increasingly dysregulated as the morphologic progression of disease unfolds. The precise molecular changes that are key to this event remain to be determined.

Adhesion Molecules, Cytokeratins, and Matrix Alterations

CD44v6 is a cell adhesion molecule that is consistently expressed in bronchial epithelial basal cells and also in squamous metaplasia.[151] Wimmel et al.[152] reported CD44s and CD44v6 expression confined to the base of normal respiratory epithelium, but CD44v6 was found increasingly expressed throughout all layers in SD/CIS.

In one study, disease progression was associated with decrease in expression of CK4 and CK17, while CK10 was not seen until invasion occurred.[153] Conversely, others found that CK10 was expressed in dysplastic, though not in normal, bronchial epithelium and also described loss of CK6 and the appearance of CK14 in association with disease progression.[154]

While matrix metalloproteinase 2 (MMP-2) and metalloproteinase tissue inhibitor 1 (TIMP-1) show no change in expression throughout the spectrum of preinvasive bronchial lesions, there appears to be a reciprocal expression of MMP-9 and MMP-1, MMP-9 increasing as disease progresses from BCH to CIS, while MMP-1 expression shows the reverse.[155] Bolon et al.[156] found little expression of either MMP-1 or MMP-7 in any grade of lesion, MMP-3 expression in 31% of lesions of all types, and MMP-11 present in dysplasia and CIS but not in invasive disease. The transcription factor c-Ets-1, which regulates MMP-1 and MMP-3 expression, was not dysregulated in any lesion.

These studies demonstrate altered expression of various proteins that reflect altered differentiation and potential changes in the interaction of cells with their neighbors and their surrounding matrix commensurate with evolving neoplasia.

Human Papilloma Virus Genome

While one of six squamous metaplastic lesions was found to have HPV6 DNA, Bejui-Thivolet et al.[157] found DNA of HPV18 in three cases, and HPV16, -11, and -6 in one case each of invasive squamous carcinoma. Other studies have failed to find any HPV DNA,[158] and the role of this factor in bronchial carcinogenesis remains uncertain.

P53

The TSG *P53* is located at 17p13, and its protein product p53 functions as a tumor suppressor in response to carcinogen-induced DNA damage, principally as a transcription factor for a number of genes that promote G_1 cell-cycle arrest and either DNA repair or apoptosis.[159] Inactivation of wild-type p53 protein is one of the most common changes seen in human carcinogenesis, with p53 alterations detectable in about half of squamous cell lung cancers and most small cell lung carcinomas. Loss of heterozygosity at 17p may lead to allelic deletion of one copy of the *P53* gene, while loss of functional p53 in the cell may be completed by mutation of the other allele. Most of the somatic *P53* mutations that occur are missense. This stabilizes the normally labile wild-type p53, leading to intranuclear accumulation of protein, rendering it detectable by immunohistochemistry. A minority of mutations do not lead to elevated p53 levels. Other changes, either genetic or epigenetic, may alter p53 metabolism and lead to accumulation.[160] Most of the antibodies used to identify p53 protein bind wild-type and mutated forms.

The earliest studies of p53 in lung carcinogenesis demonstrated *P53* gene mutations in radon-induced squamous cell carcinoma,[161] and both LOH within the *P53* gene and elevated p53 levels in both invasive squamous carcinoma and associated CIS[162] and in severe dysplasia.[163] These studies involved small numbers of cases, but confirmed that relatively advanced preinvasive bronchial lesions showed both deletion within the *P53* gene and gene mutation.

Since then a large amount of data on p53 immunohistochemistry has accumulated. The findings of comparable studies for increased p53 expression at various stages in the stepwise progression of preinvasive bronchial squamous lesions are shown in Table 34.2. Direct comparisons are difficult to make since authors used different antibodies to p53, different detection systems, and scored lesions as positive using different criteria. There is clear evidence, however, that stainable p53 protein becomes more abundant as lesions become morphologically more advanced, and in lesser grades of dysplasia, positive nuclei are found in the basal parts of the epithelium.

While most have found that stainable p53 is absent in morphologically normal bronchial epithelium, there are caveats to this generality. Walker et al.[165] described infrequent solitary p53-positive cells, predominantly in the basal layer of morphologically normal bronchial epithelium. This was rarely seen in patients without cancer, but was present in 53% of bronchial resection margins in cases of surgically resected lung cancer. However, it has been suggested that overexpression of p53 of this magnitude may reflect alteration of cellular metabolism and protein turnover rather than point mutation of the *P53* gene.[160,166] Martin et al.[170] counted the number of positive cells in normal epithelium and preinvasive lesions detected at AFB in patients without lung cancer, but who were at increased risk due to a previous history of head/neck cancer or heavy smoking habit. In this population, almost one third of patients with histologically normal bronchial epithelium had more than 1% of cells with stainable p53.

In those studies where p53 expression was compared in the preinvasive lesions and squamous cell carcinoma in the same patient, a high degree of concordance is found. In a small number of cases Satoh et al.[130] found 100% concordance between the p53 status of SD/CIS and that of the squamous cell carcinoma each patient later developed after years of follow-up (see above).

Nuorva et al.[100] found that all of the p53-positive SD/CIS were associated with p53-positive carcinomas, while only three of eight p53-negative SD/CIS lesions were associated with a p53-positive tumor. Walker et al.[165] again found that most SD/CIS coexisting with resected squamous cell carcinoma showed the same p53 status as

TABLE 34.2. Published data on p53 immunohistochemistry in bronchial preinvasive lesions

Reference	Normal bronchial epithelium	Basal cell hyperplasia	Squamous metaplasia	Mild dysplasia	Moderate dysplasia	Severe dysplasia	Carcinoma in situ
Nuorva et al.[100]				20	0	78	50
Bennett et al.[164]	0		7	30	27	60	59
Hirano et al.[138]	0			0		6*	
Walker et al.[165]	0			14	25	59	
Fontanini et al.[166]	0	0	0				76
Katabami et al.[167]	0	0	0	11	27	50	
Brambilla et al.[168]		0	0	19	36		59**
Lonardo et al.[169]	0		0	0	50***		53**
Martin et al.[170] #	0.9	3.4	9.1	20.5		50.2	34.7

All data except # presented as % of cases described as positive for p53 protein.
*Data for high-grade dysplasia, that is, moderate and severe dysplasia.
**Data for severe dysplasia and CIS.
***One of two cases examined showed very weak positive staining (see text).
#Data shown is mean percentage of cells positive for p53 in each lesion type.

the invasive tumor, but 25% of their cases did not. Brambilla et al.[168] found that, while all patients with p53-negative cancer also has p53-negative SD/CIS, 62% of those with p53-positive carcinoma had concurrent p53-positive CIS. These authors also showed that SD/CIS adjacent to invasive carcinoma was more likely to be p53-positive than SD/CIS distant to a cancer. These findings support the concept of field cancerization in the airway, although p53 alteration may not be an obligatory part of this process.

Although Bennett et al.[164] found that p53 positivity rates in SD/CIS were no different between patients with and without concurrent cancer, most authors have found p53 more likely to be expressed in preinvasive lesions in cancer bearers or those at increased risk than in those without cancer. In a study of the relationships among SD/CIS, lung cancer, and pneumoconiosis, Katabami et al.[167] found that while bronchial dysplasia showed p53-positivity rates of 21% and 27% in those with and without pneumoconiosis respectively, p53-positivity was more common in *bronchiolar* squamous dysplasia in pneumoconiotics (56%) than in nonpneumoconiotics (18%), an interesting observation given that in pneumoconiosis squamous cell carcinomas tend to arise in more peripheral small airways.

P21[waf1/cip1] is a downstream target of p53, which inhibits cyclin/cyclin-dependent kinases. Although this protein was found more often and in haphazard distribution in preinvasive lesions when compared to normal epithelium, there was no consistent relationship between expression and grade of lesion.[168]

In a study of 51 patients who had squamous metaplasia or dysplasia diagnosed after bronchial biopsy, 31 of whom had synchronous or metachronous carcinoma, a positive p53 stain and high grade of dysplasia had a positive predictive value for carcinoma of 91% and 80%, respectively.[140] In another study the association of p53-positive SD/CIS with concurrent or previous cancer and the absence of p53-positivity in SD/CIS in those with no cancer history also support the suggestion that p53 positivity in SD/CIS may have predictive value for the development of invasive disease.[168] Over a period of 4 years, Ponticiello et al.[136] followed-up 22 heavy smokers in whom SD/CIS had been diagnosed at bronchoscopy. Nine of their patients (41%) had p53-positive SD/CIS and seven of these (78%) went on to develop invasive squamous cell carcinoma; these seven SD/CIS lesions had particularly high expression of p53. Of the 13 patients with p53-negative SD/CIS, only three (23%) developed invasive carcinoma, and two of these tumors were adenocarcinoma, possibly unrelated to the SD/CIS. Jeanmart et al.[171] however, were unable to demonstrate significant predictive value for p53 status in SD/CIS found in at-risk patients after at least 18 months' follow-up. However, these authors also assessed levels of cyclin D1, cyclin E, Bax, and Bcl2 (see below), and found that, if more than two of the markers studied were aberrantly expressed, progression to CIS or invasive carcinoma was more likely.

Mutation of the *P53* gene has also been directly demonstrated, albeit in only a few preinvasive bronchial lesions,[161–163] and this appears to be associated with relatively high-grade disease. While Kohno et al.[172] found no evidence of *P53* mutation in squamous metaplasia, two of 22 (9%) dysplasias showed mutation and 17p LOH, alterations they shared with their concurrent squamous cell carcinomas. In this study, a further two dysplasias showed 17p LOH, but no *P53* mutation. The presence of a single identical point mutation of *P53* found in multiple metaplastic and dysplastic lesions from throughout the tracheobronchial tree of an at-risk, but cancer-free, subject was interpreted as evidence of a single clone of premalignant cells that had expanded to populate extensive areas of the airway epithelium.[173] This finding reinforced the suggestion of clonal evolution made in an earlier study,[174] which is also notable for the demonstration that an area of dysplasia with one mutated *P53* allele in a patient without cancer evolved into a lesion homozygous for the mutation 9 months later. This mechanism of field cancerization, however, has been challenged by the finding of different patterns of genetic alteration, particularly in *P53* in synchronous neoplastic lesions in the bronchi.[175–177] This issue is further discussed below. A detailed study of multiple preinvasive lesions in two patients over a 4-year period, during which various SD/CIS lesions progressed and regressed, but invasive carcinoma developed, concluded that LOH in *FHIT* (see below) and *P53* mutations were associated with progression of disease.[178]

P63

The p63 protein is a member of the p53 family, a p53 homologue that transactivates *P53* genes and induces apoptosis in cells expressing one of the six splice variants. Massion et al.[179] found that the *P63* gene at 3q27 is amplified in most squamous cell carcinomas and the splice variant expressed was ΔNp63α. Increase in gene copy number was also found in severe dysplasia and CIS, but not in lower grade lesions, and this correlated with an increase in stainable p63 protein in the expanded basal cell layers.

The Fragile Histidine Triad (FHIT)

The *FHIT* gene located at 3p14.2 spans the *FRA3B* common fragile site and is a putative TSG with possible functions related to apoptosis and control of cell proliferation. It is frequently lost in many human tumors including lung cancer.[180] Allelic losses and homozygous deletions have been described at the *FHIT* locus, but the relative rarity of mutations of this gene has questioned its role in tumor suppression, suggesting instead that the frequent losses are simply a by-product of the location in a fragile site.

Loss of immunohistochemically detectable Fhit protein was found in 93% of preinvasive bronchial lesions overall (in 60% of moderate dysplasias and all severe dysplasia and CIS), and may be an important and early change in squamous cell carcinogenesis,[181] a suggestion supported by Geradts et al.[182]

In one study, LOH at 3p14.2 appeared relatively late in CIS, but not in lesser degrees of dysplasia,[183] but others have found losses at this locus much earlier in hyperplasia and metaplasia and in bronchial biopsies from smokers with no evidence of lung cancer.[184–186] Curiously, Tseng et al.[185] did not show the expected strong association between *FHIT* LOH and lack of Fhit expression, suggesting Fhit inactivation may be a complex process. These authors also showed that loss of Fhit expression was associated with active smoking.

Epidermal Growth Factor Receptor and Other Tyrosine Kinases

The epidermal growth factor receptor (EGFR) ERBB1, one of the ERBB family of transmembrane receptor tyrosine kinases, has epidermal growth factor (EGF) and transforming growth factor-α (TGF-α) as ligands, and regulates epithelial cell proliferation and differentiation. EGFR is frequently overexpressed in NSCLC, particularly squamous cell carcinoma, as opposed to small cell lung cancer (SCLC),[159] and has been studied in bronchial preinvasive lesions.

Rusch et al.[187] found excess EGFR detectable by immunocytochemistry in SD/CIS, but also in squamous metaplasia, and concluded this overexpression was an early event. Their findings for TGF-α were inconclusive. Khuri et al.[142] found that EGFR expression was positively correlated with proliferative activity (PCNA expression) in preinvasive lesions and that EGFR expression reversed with smoking cessation. Both EGFR and TGF-α have been found overexpressed in normal and hyperplastic bronchial epithelium of cancer bearers when compared to those without lung cancer,[188] but are more often found in dysplasia in which, in the small number of lesions examined, membrane expression was greater than that in the cytoplasm, suggesting a switch from cytoplasmic to membrane expression as SD/CIS develops and progresses. These authors also found that erbB-2, another ERBB family member with growth promoting function, was more highly expressed in normal and hyperplastic mucosa of cancer-bearers when compared to controls, but otherwise the place of erbB-2 in the development of SD/CIS is not clear from this study. Another study failed to detect c-erbB2 expression at any stage in the development of bronchial SD/CIS.[189] Franklin et al.[190] also highlighted how EFGR is consistently overexpressed even at the earliest stage of BCH and persists through all stages to CIS and invasive disease; they also showed how coexpression of this and other members of the ERBB family could determine the response of preinvasive lesions to inhibitors of receptor tyrosine kinases in chemoprevention trials (see below).

Phosphorylated AKT (Protein Kinase B)

The serine/threonine kinase Akt is a downstream effector of the phosphatidylinositol 3-kinase (PI3K) pathway, the activation of which may cause malignant transformation in mouse models of human cancer. *AKT* may be activated in respiratory epithelial cells by components of tobacco smoke.[191] Immunohistochemical detection of activated p-AKT Ser[473] was found in 27% of normal bronchial epithelia, 44% of hyperplasias, and 88% of dysplasias, but in only 33% of invasive NSCLCs.[192] Expression in invasive disease was not related to tumor histology, and the authors concluded that p-AKT activation is an early event in bronchial carcinogenesis.

K-*ras* Mutations

Although K-*ras* mutation is described in around 20% of NSCLCs, the vast majority of these are adenocarcinomas.[193] Given what we now believe regarding the genesis of most adenocarcinomas of the lung (see below), it is probably not surprising that the K-*ras* mutation has not been convincingly demonstrated with any regularity in SD/CIS. Sugio et al.[194] found no evidence of mutation in any bronchial or bronchiolar dysplasia examined. Although one of their study patients had a squamous cell carcinoma with K-*ras* mutation and is described as also showing mutation in noninvasive carcinoma, it is not clear if this really refers to bronchial squamous cell CIS. None of the normal or hyperplastic epithelium showed mutation. Accepting that the relatively unusual form of central bronchial-type adenocarcinoma may arise from transformation of the bronchial epithelium, these types of adenocarcinoma do not show K-*ras* mutation, unlike their peripheral counterparts.[195]

$p16^{INK4A}$-Cyclin D1-CDK4-RB Pathway

The $p16^{INK4A}$-cyclin D1-CDK4-*RB* pathway has a central role in controlling progression from the G_1 to S phase of the cell cycle. This pathway is altered in many lung cancers and may be disrupted if any component is dysfunctional. While *RB* alteration is a common event (90%) in SCLC development (see below), it is seen relatively infrequently (15–30%) in NSCLCs.[159] Abnormalities of the other components, however, are common in NSCLC.[196,197] Cyclin D1 inhibits Rb function by stimulation of Rb phosphorylation through complexing with cyclin-dependent kinase 4 (CDK4). CDK4 function is inhibited by p16. Thus Rb function may be lost by modification of the gene itself or by hyperphosphorylation through loss of p16 function or upregulation of cyclin D1. Both hypophosphorylated Rb protein and p16 protein act as tumor suppressors by promoting G1 arrest.

In an immunohistochemical study of this pathway in SD/CIS, Brambilla et al.[198] found that Rb was consistently expressed in all grades of preinvasive lesion, but that 12% of moderate dysplasias and 30% of CIS lesions showed loss of p16 expression. Cyclin D1 overexpression was seen in 6% of hyperplastic/metaplastic lesions, 17% of mild dysplasias, 46% of moderate dysplasias, and 38% of CIS lesions, suggesting this may be an earlier alteration that p16 loss. These authors also showed that p16 loss, and, to a lesser extent, cyclin D1 overexpression may be associated with a greater likelihood of SD/CIS progression to invasion. Lonardo et al.[169] made similar observations, finding Rb loss was absent in preinvasive lesions and present in only 6% of squamous cell carcinomas. Cyclin D1 was increasingly overexpressed, being undetectable in normal epithelium, but overexpressed in 7% of squamous metaplasias, 18% of low-grade dysplasia, and 47% of high-grade SD/CIS. These authors also found that cyclin E, another cell-cycle regulator active at the G_1-S transition, was overexpressed in 33% of high grade SD/CIS, but rarely expressed in lesions of a lesser grade. Betticher et al.,[199] however, did detect diminished Rb expression in some preinvasive lesions present at bronchial resection margins of cancer-bearing lungs. Jeanmart et al.[171] also studied cyclins D1 and E in squamous metaplasia and all grades of SD/CIS and found, in contrast to others,[169] overexpression of cyclin E in low-grade dysplasia and also significant increases in expression of both in high-grade versus low-grade dysplasia.

The bulk of the evidence, therefore, would suggest that, in the evolution of bronchogenic NSCLC, this pathway is disrupted through overexpression of cyclin D1 and reduced expression of p16, rather than loss of Rb expression.

The *CDKN2A/p16*^{INK4a} gene is located at 9p21. Gene function may be lost through mutation or deletion (LOH) or through epigenetic inactivation via promoter hypermethylation, the latter event sometimes occurring in one allele while the other is deleted.

Loss of heterozygosity at 9p was detected in none of the hyperplastic/metaplastic lesions, 31% of dysplasias, and 83% of CIS lesions studied by Thiberville et al.[131] Similar findings were reported by Kishimoto et al.,[200] though they did report LOH in hyperplasia. Wistuba et al.[184] found evidence of even earlier 9p LOH, reporting losses in 15% of morphologically normal epithelia, 20% of hyperplastic/metaplastic lesions, 35% of dysplasias, and 80% of CIS lesions. Boyle et al.[177] reported 9p LOH in 75% of dysplasias that were informative. Allelic loss of 9p21 has also been detected in the squamous metaplastic epithelium lining a lung cyst in a patient with resected squamous cell carcinoma.[74]

CDKN2A promoter hypermethylation was found in 75% of CIS lesions occurring adjacent to invasive squamous cell carcinoma, which also showed hypermethylation.[201] These authors also demonstrated an increasing frequency of *CDNK2A* promoter hypermethylation in earlier lesions, finding 17% of BCHs, 24% of squamous metaplasias, and 50% of all CIS lesions so affected. Increasingly frequent hypermethylation was also detected in a range of preinvasive lesions found at fluorescence bronchoscopy in patients without cancer.[202] In the latter study, 5% of normal epithelia, 21% of metaplastic/mild-moderate dysplastic lesions, and 50% of severe dysplasia/CIS lesions showed this epigenetic change, which correlated closely with p16 immunohistochemistry.

CDKN2A methylation did not help predict outcome in these patients, but appeared to be a relatively early event in bronchogenic carcinogenesis that persisted years after smoking cessation,[202] and there is evidence that gene methylation is associated with tobacco smoking.[203]

Another smaller study found loss of p16 protein expression in only two of 20 preinvasive lesions examined (one severe dysplasia and one CIS lesion), attributed this p16 loss to gene hypermethylation in the CIS lesion only, and postulated a further epigenetic mechanism for loss of p16 function; the authors demonstrated downregulation of *P16*, due to overexpression of the polycomb-group gene *BMI-1*, in around half the samples studied, though this excess of bmi-1 protein was seen in normal and hyperplastic, as well as dysplastic, epithelium.[204]

Bcl2 and Related Proteins

Bcl2 protects cells from apoptosis and is negatively regulated by p53. Bcl2 may become overexpressed in tumor cells as a mechanism to avoid apoptosis.[205] The *BAX* gene is a downstream transcription target for p53, and the bax protein appears to promote apoptosis and act as a tumor suppressor.[206] Bax complexes with bcl2, and the bcl2/bax ratio may determine the apoptotic susceptibility of a cell.

Bcl2 tends to be confined to the basal cell layer in normal respiratory epithelium, but in SD/CIS there is increased expression of bcl2, mirroring the distribution of morphologically atypical cells.[207] While Boers et al.[140] could not demonstrate overexpression of bcl2 in squamous metaplasia, Katabami et al.[167] found excess bcl2 in BCH, and squamous metaplasia and squamous dysplasia in around 30% to 50% of cases, with no significant difference in expression between different grades of lesion. Similar findings for bcl2 overexpression were reported by Brambilla et al.,[168] who also showed a more consistent relationship between loss of bax expression and disease progression, an observation maintained with the onset of invasion, unlike the inconsistent relationship with bcl2 overexpression. Thus the bcl2/bax ratio was consistently low in normal or hyperplastic epithelium, but ratios greater than 1 (bcl2 expression > bax expression) were seen with increasing frequency across the spectrum from squamous metaplasia to CIS. A high bcl2/bax ratio was more common in SD/CIS adjacent to invasive cancer, and the authors suggested this ratio may indicate a more unstable lesion, although it is apparently not an independent predictor of disease progression.[171] There seems to be no relationship between p53 and bcl2 or bax expression in bronchial preinvasive lesions.[168,207]

Retinoic Acid Receptors (RARs)

It is known that retinoid deficiency may induce squamous metaplasia and therefore could be related to the genesis of bronchial carcinoma. A functional loss of retinoid activity may be induced through loss of *RAR* genes at 3p during bronchial carcinogenesis, and *RAR*-β has been proposed as a TSG. Losses in 3p and therefore corresponding loss of expression of RAR-β protein has been shown in SD/CIS, more so in higher-grade than low-grade lesions.[208]

Heterologous Nuclear Ribonucleoprotein (hnRNP) B1

hnRNP B1 is an RNA-binding protein required for mRNA precursor maturation, and has been found in the majority of squamous cell lung cancers.[209] It was also expressed in bronchial epithelium in cancer-bearing lungs,[209] and was found in 63% of SD/CIS lesions.[210] It has thus been proposed as a candidate biomarker for bronchial lung cancer detection and diagnosis, but more work is needed, given that at least one of these studies also found it expressed in alveolar macrophages.[209]

Telomerase

Telomerase is inactive in most adult cells. Activated telomerase ribonucleoprotein complex may prevent progressive telomere shortening after cell division, and after p53/Rb inactivation, thus preventing cell senescence. Activated telomerase, which is found in most human tumors after activation at some stage during carcinogenesis, may therefore confer immortality on cancer cell populations.

Yashima et al.[211] found that both hyperplastic and dysplastic bronchial epithelia showed frequent strong human telomerase RNA component (hTERC) expression in 70% to 80% of cases, while normal epithelium showed weak reactions in 20% of cases and CIS and invasive disease in 95% to 100% of cases. Human telomerase reverse transcriptase (hTERT) enzyme activity, however, showed only a fourfold increase from normal in all preinvasive lesions, including CIS, while in invasive disease the difference was forty times greater. Quantitative increase in hTERT mRNA levels during SD/CIS development has also been reported,[212] and has even been suggested as a predictive marker, in nondysplastic mucosa, of future CIS development.[213] Lantuejoul et al.[214] found the same progressive increase in telomerase activity from normal, through squamous metaplasia and dysplasia to CIS as well as a significant correlation with p53 expression, bcl2/bax ratio, and cell proliferation, suggesting telomerase reactivation occurs in tandem with increased cell cycle activity and resistance to apoptosis. The same group also demonstrated that the marked telomere shortening seen in squamous metaplasia was reversed as dysplasia supervened, presumably a function of increased telomerase activity.

Telomerase dysregulation and reactivation would appear to be a key factor in bronchial carcinogenesis.

Cellular DNA and Genomic Studies

Among the factors that allow a diagnosis of squamous dysplasia in the airway epithelium is the identification of abnormalities in nuclear size, shape, and tinctorial characteristics, which, at least in part, reflect alteration in nuclear DNA content. These changes reflect genomic instability, which has been demonstrated in preinvasive bronchial lesions by nuclear DNA ploidy analysis both in animal and human studies.[104,138] Hirano et al.[138] showed that, while normal bronchial epithelium showed no aneuploidy, 8% of low-grade dysplasias, 33% of high-grade dysplasias, and 100% of invasive squamous cell carcinomas showed DNA aneuploidy. These authors also showed that the development of aneuploidy, which is clearly a relatively early event in the evolution of bronchogenic carcinoma, depended on the presence of hyperproliferation of the epithelium. Smith et al.[215] also demonstrated aneuploidy in multifocal preinvasive lesions and confirmed the increasing frequency of aneuploidy with increasing grade of lesion.

Fluorescence in-situ hybridization was used to determine that, in one case of squamous metaplasia adjacent to invasive squamous carcinoma, the aneuploidy rate was 21% and chromosome 7 showed a mean copy number of 3.3.[216] Comparative genomic hybridization (CGH) detected numerical changes in chromosome 3 in preinvasive bronchial lesions detected using AFB,[217] while high-resolution CGH was used to demonstrate amplification of both 8q21 (*MYC*) and 8q22 in bronchial CIS.[218]

Technological advances in tissue microdissection and DNA analysis have increased our knowledge of the genetic events that occur in the bronchial epithelium during central bronchial carcinogenesis. Some of these findings have already been discussed in earlier sections concerned with specific genes, pathways, or processes.

Genomic alterations and, in particular, evidence of LOH at various loci appear to be associated with tobacco smoking, may be found in morphologically normal respiratory epithelium in smokers, and may persist in the epithelium after smoking cessation and for years after any morphologically recognizable preinvasive lesion has resolved.[219,220] These areas or clones of genetically abnormal yet morphologically normal or minimally abnormal bronchial epithelial cells number in the thousands, are small, and are estimated to contain approximately 90,000 cells,[176] which would occupy roughly 1 to 2 mm^2 of mucosa. Individual losses of genetic material are smaller and less frequent in preinvasive lesions when compared to invasive carcinoma.[184,221] As the morphologic changes of preinvasive lesions evolved in the proposed stepwise fashion, so the number and degree of allele specific molecular alterations increases, apparently as clonally independent foci.[184]

Losses in chromosome 3p are among the earliest changes to occur. Loci at 3p21.3 (*RASSF1A* and *SEMA3B*), 3p22–24 (*BAP-1*), and 3p25, and less frequently 3p14.2 (*FHIT*) (see above) and 3p14.21, occur in normal and hyperplastic epithelium in 31% and 42% of cases, respectively.[184] Losses at 9p21 ($P16^{INK4}$) are also found at this stage (see above). Hung et al.[222] found LOH somewhere in 3p in 76% of hyperplasias, 86% of dysplasias, and 100% of CIS lesions. Wistuba et al.[150] also reported allelic losses in 3p in 78% of preinvasive lesions, by which stage losses were frequently multiple, and found that 95% of squamous cell carcinomas demonstrated losses of large segments of 3p. The previously mentioned loci were involved, together with 3p12 (*DUTT1*), wherein losses appear in dysplasia, but not earlier.[184] In addition, between 78% and 88% of cases the preinvasive lesions showed the same allelic losses as the patient's concurrent squamous cell carcinoma,[150,222] a parallel with the data on *P53* mutations described above. Deletions at 8p21–23 also appear relatively early, at the hyperplasia/metaplasia stage in cancer-bearers and in smokers without cancer,[223] although this tended to follow 3p and, usually, 9p deletions.

Loss of heterozygosity at 17p13 (*P53*) has also been described at the hyperplasia/metaplasia stage, but is more frequent in more advanced lesions.[184] Losses at 13q14 (*RB*) and 5q (*APC-MCC*) also appear at the dysplasia stage, are more frequent in CIS and invasive squamous cell carcinoma, but are less frequent at any stage than the other losses already described.[184] Thiberville et al.,[131] however, described 5q21 LOH in 11% of hyperplastic lesions detected at autofluorescence bronchoscopy. As mentioned above, the K-*ras* mutation is a late and infrequent event in central bronchial carcinogenesis, and *P53* mutations occur at variable times,[194,224] while $P16^{INK4}$ promoter hypermethylation is a relatively early event. None of these changes appears to predict the likelihood of disease progression, despite the accumulation of changes being associated with higher-grade disease. As well as in $P16^{INK4}$, abnormal promoter hypermethylation of *RARβ*, *H-cadherin*, *FHIT*, and *RASSF1A* is also seen in bronchial epithelial cells in heavy smokers.[224]

Using complementary DNA (cDNA) microanalysis data to identify differential gene expression, which is important in lung squamous cell tumorigenesis, Smith et al.[225,226] found maspin, a protein product of the serpin gene cluster on 18q21.3, and S100A2 protein, a potential TSG, to be overexpressed in bronchial epithelial basal cells and increasingly so in preinvasive lesions.

Multiple genomic alterations thus occur in the morphologic progression of SD/CIS and appear in some semblance of order rather than at random. It is not known for sure how the earliest changes may influence later alterations, yet a degree of interdependence may be inferred from the above and certainly fits with current concepts of "multi-hit" carcinogenesis. Early dysregulation of cell cycle regulators may lead to hyperproliferation. This, in turn, increases the likelihood of genetic accidents during mitosis, further genomic losses, mutations, aberrant gene expression, and overall genomic instability. The large amount of evidence reviewed above indicates that the proposed morphologic progression runs in parallel with increasing genomic changes and altered gene expression, and it is intuitive to suppose that some of these genetic changes drive the process and orchestrate the morphologic evolution of SD/CIS. There is experimental evidence that correction of even a single genetic abnormality may reverse the malignant phenotype.[227] Jeanmart et al.[171] provided evidence that in this progression the molecular findings in moderate dysplasia are closer to those found in severe rather than mild dysplasia, supporting the tendency to consider moderate and severe dysplasia together as high-grade disease.

The presence of both concordant and discordant alterations in tumors, preinvasive lesions, and even morphologically normal epithelium suggests there may well be multiple potential pathways, at least at a genomic level, for the development of bronchogenic carcinoma.[177] This may account for the observation that while some tumors appear to develop through the proposed series of steps, at a morphologic and also at a genetic level (the so-called sequential theory of lung cancer development), others apparently jump stages, at least in terms of the morphologic evolution of disease, or appear to arise de novo without a morphologically recognizable preinvasive stage (the parallel theory).[224] The latter scenario may particularly apply in the development of SCLC (see below).

This section has reviewed the morphology, development, diagnosis, and molecular and cell biology of bronchial preinvasive lesions. Squamous dysplasia/CIS is the archetypal precursor lesion for invasive squamous cell carcinoma. This lesion is also seen in association with small cell undifferentiated carcinoma, but whether it serves as a true precursor or coexists due to a common etiology is unclear. The role of SD/CIS in the genesis of other bronchogenic cancers is uncertain. Bronchial-type adenocarcinomas occur and may arise from bronchial glands or surface epithelium, but their precursor is essentially unknown. Around 25% of basaloid carcinomas are associated with CIS, which is rich in basaloid cells,[228] an interesting observation given that the basaloid immunophenotype, as identified by staining with the 34βE12 antibody (cytokeratins 1, 5, 10, and 14), is also strongly associated with this tumor type.[229] This lends further support both to the idea that SD/CIS may be the precursor to more than just squamous cell carcinoma and to the suggestion that malignant transformation may occur not only within fully differentiated keratinizing squamous epithelium (squamous metaplasia), but also in BCH, which becomes atypical without keratinization/maturation.[89]

Atypical Adenomatous Hyperplasia

The previous section dealt in some detail with bronchial SD/CIS in a discussion of how this group of lesions shows all the hallmarks of preinvasive malignancy and comprises the likely precursors of bronchial squamous cell carcinoma and probably some other bronchogenic NSCLCs. There is also evidence that SD/CIS could be related to the development of bronchial SCLC (see below). Leaving aside those rare bronchial adenocarcinomas about whose origin we know little, it is a fact that most adenocarcinomas do not have a bronchial origin, arising instead in the peripheral parenchymal compartment of the lung. This poses the question, How do these adenocarcinomas arise? This is all the more pertinent given that this form of lung cancer is now the dominant type worldwide; this has been so in Japan, Hong Kong, and probably in many Asian countries for decades, and in the United States for some time,[230] and there is evidence that this rise in adenocarcinoma has occurred in at least some European countries.[231] For many years the answer to this question was unknown or thought to relate in some way to pulmonary scars or fibrosis (see above). More recently, however, the lesion now called atypical adenomatous hyperplasia (AAH) was recognized and now appears in the WHO classification as a putative precursor of invasive adenocarcinoma.

This section describes the morphology of AAH, its association with invasive pulmonary adenocarcinoma, and the cell and molecular biologic evidence that underpins the place of AAH as a pulmonary preinvasive lesion. By necessity this discussion also considers the relationship between AAH and localized nonmucinous bronchioloalveolar carcinoma (LNMBAC) and how the latter, as currently defined in the WHO classification as a noninvasive tumor, may well represent the stage between AAH and invasive adenocarcinoma in the stepwise development of peripheral lung adenocarcinoma. Although therefore conceptually a preinvasive lesion in the lung, LNMBAC will be considered in more detail in Chapter 35, section on Bronchioloalveolar Carcinoma. To discuss published studies on AAH, however, it is relevant and helpful to consider their findings in conjunction with data on LNMBAC and, indeed, on invasive adenocarcinoma.

Some early literature refers to "atypical regenerative hyperplasia"[6] and "atypical epithelial proliferation"[23] of the alveolar epithelium in the context of lung tumor development, but these descriptions appear to be related to the bronchioloalveolar cell proliferation seen in association with pulmonary fibrosis, as previously discussed. Most peripheral pulmonary adenocarcinomas arise in the lung, which is devoid of preexisting scars, diffuse fibrosis,

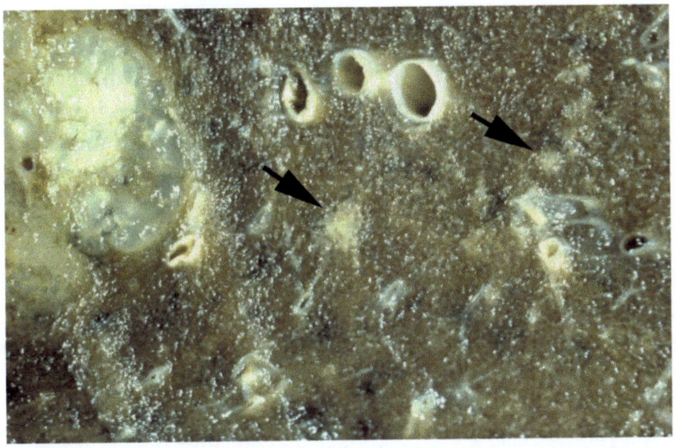

FIGURE 34.21. Two foci of atypical adenomatous hyperplasia (AAH) on the cut surface of resected lung previously inflated with 10% formalin before slicing. Associated mucinous adenocarcinoma is seen on the left.

or honeycombing. From a series of 1015 surgically resected lung cancers, Shimosato et al.[11] identified five patients in whom an incidental atypical hyperplastic lesion of the alveolated lung, measuring between 1.5 and 13 mm, was found in the routine pathologic sections taken from each resection specimen. These authors described these lesions as atypical alveolar cuboidal cell hyperplasia and concluded that "one can assume that some peripheral adenocarcinomas arise without any association with preexisting scar tissue as an in-situ carcinoma from almost normal appearing bronchioloalveoli. However, it is not certain whether or not cancer develops through a stage of atypical hyperplasia." In 1988 Miller et al.[232] described another five patients, from a series of 57 with primary adenocarcinoma of the lung, whose resected lung showed multiple foci of "bronchioloalveolar cell atypia or dysplasia." Due to these lesions' similarity to BAC and their association with adenocarcinoma in particular, these authors proposed the analogy between this and the adenoma-carcinoma sequence seen in colon cancer development.

Since then a number of other descriptions have been published, using a variety of terms, such as alveolar epithelial hyperplasia,[233] atypical alveolar hyperplasia,[234] atypical bronchioloalveolar cell hyperplasia,[235] atypical adenomatous hyperplasia,[236,237] and bronchioloalveolar adenoma.[238] The term *atypical adenomatous hyperplasia* has emerged as the preferred one.

Morphology of Atypical Adenomatous Hyperplasia

Gross Features

While the vast majority of AAH lesions are incidental microscopic findings, occasional lesions may be detected on gross examination of the cut surface of the lung. Lesions are small, a few millimeters in diameter, and may be visible as discrete, rather ill-defined, grayish, tan, or yellowish foci (Fig. 34.21). Occasionally a lesion may be large and distinct enough to allow appreciation of the alveolar architecture by the presence of a stippled pattern of depressions or holes on its cut surface (Fig. 34.22). The AAH lesions are most often found close to the pleura[233] and in the upper lobes.[239]

For all practical purposes it is not possible to localize AAH lesions macroscopically unless the lung tissue has previously been subject to inflation-fixation and the lung slices are examined carefully under a good light. Miller[238] advocated the use of Bouin's fluid to inflate the specimens, since the enhanced yellow color of the lesions made them easier to detect. This is a particularly toxic fixative, however, and it is not conducive to subsequent DNA and immunohistochemical analysis of the tissues. One of us uses 10% neutral-buffered formalin to inflate per-bronchially fresh surgical resection specimens received from the operating room within minutes of removal. Lungs are cut, after 24 hours' fixation, into 1-cm-thick parasagittal slices using a purpose-built board. The slices are examined under a bright light while keeping the slices flooded with running water, which partially reexpands the parenchyma and washes away obscuring blood and secretions. Although many foci so identified prove not to be AAH, this technique has been successful in identifying many lesions.[240] Nonetheless, most of these authors' AAH lesions are still incidental findings in random parenchymal blocks. As suggested above, AAH is most often found in the most lateral parasagittal slices, consistent with a subpleural concentration of lesions. While this may reflect the true distribution of the lesions, macroscopic identification is easiest in peripheral lung uncluttered by large vessels and airways. Coexistent lung

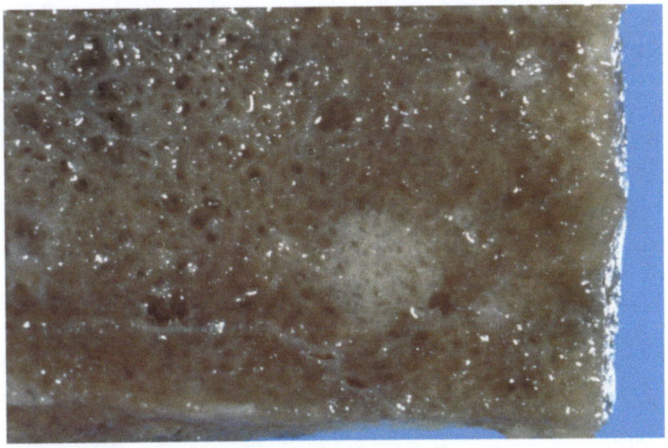

FIGURE 34.22. Close-up gross view of AAH in a sampled tissue block. The holes pitting the surface of the pale 2-mm lesion represent alveolar spaces.

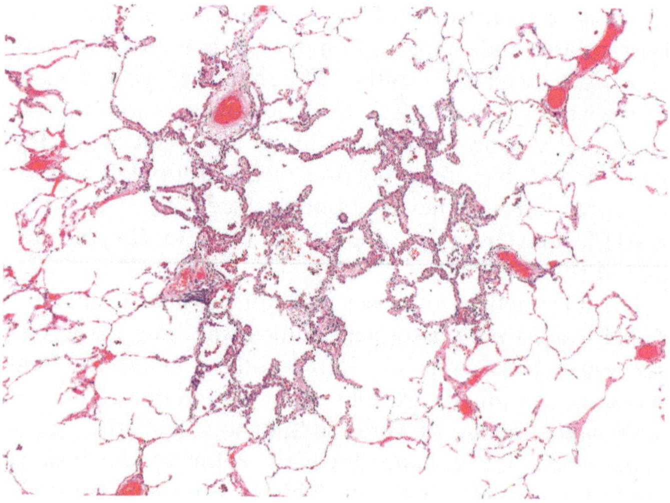

FIGURE 34.23. Atypical adenomatous hyperplasia. Low-power view of a small lesion. Slight thickening of alveolar walls and prominent alveolar lining cells can be seen.

disease such as emphysema, fibrosis, or pneumonia, particularly of the retention-type related to carcinoma, renders AAH impossible to identify.

Microscopic Features

In the latest WHO classification, AAH is defined as "a localized proliferation of mild to moderately atypical cells lining involved alveoli and, sometimes, respiratory bronchioles, resulting in focal lesions in peripheral alveolated lung, usually less than 5 mm in diameter and generally in the absence of underlying interstitial inflammation and fibrosis"[241] (Fig. 34.23).

One of the most striking characteristics of AAH is the cytologic and, to a lesser extent, architectural heterogeneity that may be seen. The cells lining the involved alveoli may be cuboidal, low columnar, or round in shape, and are frequently admixed with "peg" cells showing apical snouts. Cell size and shape usually vary, sometimes markedly so, and the population of cells forms an interrupted, intermittent layer, with little or no stratification, and with small gaps between the cells or admixed with apparently normal flat type I pneumocytes (Fig. 34.24). Nuclei are round or oval, with regular outlines, the chromatin pattern is homogeneous, sometimes quite hyperchromatic, and nuclear inclusions are quite common, seen in at least 25% of cells.[233] Double nuclei, particularly in large round cells, are not infrequent. Mitotic figures are extremely uncommon. Some of these cells have both light microscopic and ultrastructural features of either type II pneumocytes, showing cytoplasmic lamellar bodies and nuclear branching microtubules,[238,242–245] or Clara cells with typical electron-dense granules.[238,242,244,245] The immunohistochemical findings are discussed below. This cytology is consistent with an origin from the bronchioloalveolar lining, perhaps from progenitor cells capable of differentiating into type II pneumocytes or Clara cells. Ciliated or mucous cells are not seen in AAH.

Typically the alveolar walls are slightly thickened due to an increase in interstitial collagen and occasional fibroblasts. There may also be an excess of lymphocytes, occasionally in small aggregates, and occasional lesions show quite marked fibrosis. It is not unusual to find moderate aggregates of alveolar macrophages within the alveolar airspaces. Elastosis was noted in 34 of 38 lesions studied

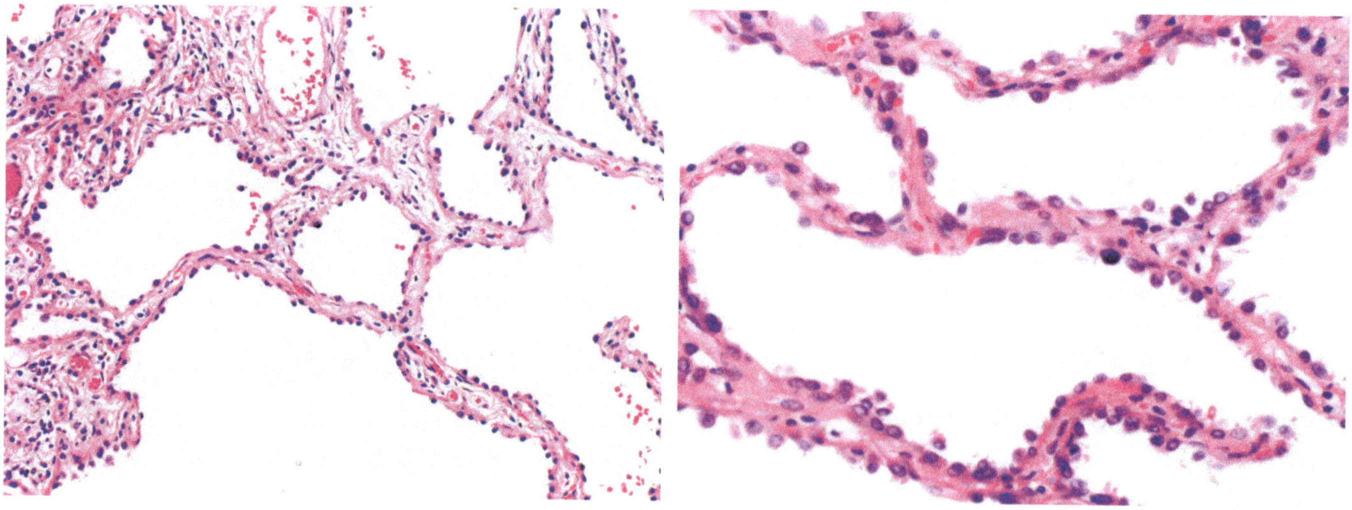

A B

FIGURE 34.24. Atypical adenomatous hyperplasia. **(A,B)** Thickened alveolar walls lined by an interrupted single layer of rounded or cuboidal cells of variable appearance.

by Weng et al.,[235] who also reported significant fibrosis in 14 of the larger lesions in their study group. Miller[238] described moderate inflammation and fibrosis in about one fifth of lesions.

Characteristically these lesions are discrete localized foci, particularly when viewed at low magnification. There is some blending with the normal alveolar lining at the edges of the lesion, especially in less cellular examples where the cell population is more discontinuous. Sometimes, if an associated respiratory bronchiole is present in the section, atypical columnar or "peg" cells can be seen lining the airway. In some lesions, especially those with more alveolar wall fibrosis, the alveolar spaces appear to be reduced in size, while in other larger examples some alveolar spaces may be increased in size, giving a microcystic appearance.

When AAH was first included in the WHO classification of preinvasive lung lesions, it was defined as a lesion less than 5 mm and, indeed, Miller[238] considered any lesion over 5 mm a carcinoma. It is clear, however, that there are some lesions measuring over 5 mm, which are AAH-like and lack sufficient features to be classified as LNMBAC. Weng et al.[235] found that 25% of the lesions in their study measured less than 1 mm, 55% from 1 mm up to 3 mm, 10% greater than 3 mm up to 5 mm, while 10% measure greater than 5 mm up to 10 mm. The largest AAH lesion described by Nakanishi[233] measured 24 mm. Chapman and Kerr found that 64% of lesions measured less than 3 mm, 17% from 3 mm up to 5 mm, 9% measured greater than 5 mm up to 10 mm, while 10% measured over 10 mm, the largest being 19 mm (unpublished data).

There is some variation in the range of cellularity and atypia seen in AAH, both within a single lesion and between multiple foci occurring in the same lung.[236] Some authors have made reference to low-grade and high-grade AAH,[246–248] noting that some lesions are more cellular, with a tendency to have more continuous runs of cells lining alveoli, a predominance of "peg" or columnar cells, and moderate nuclear atypia (Fig. 34.25). Consequently more cell-cell contact is evident. Such lesions tend to be larger, and occasional small tufts or pseudopapillae may be seen. In one study, any lesion with mild atypia and a simple intermittent layer of cuboidal cells on slightly thickened alveolar walls was considered grade I, while grade II lesions were those with thicker alveolar walls and a continuous lining of columnar cells with occasional evidence of stratification or papilla formation.[235] Of the 67 lesions in this study 72% were grade I and 28% were grade II. Miller[238] noted a tendency for larger lesions to be more atypical, 76% of her series of lesions under 3 mm showing mild atypia while 67% of those over 4 mm showed moderate or severe atypia. Kitamura et al.[249] found the same trend and made a distinction between high- and low-grade AAH. While Koga et al.[250] found 91% of 119 AAH lesions were low grade, they found no difference in size between low- and high-grade lesions. Kerr[251] found that 18 of 111 (16%) measured AAH lesions were considered high grade and 67% of these measured over 5 mm.

It should be emphasized, however, that the practice of grading the degree of atypia in AAH is not currently recommended in the WHO classification, since this practice has, as yet, no known clinical significance and reproducibility is untested. The distinction between AAH and BAC is discussed below.

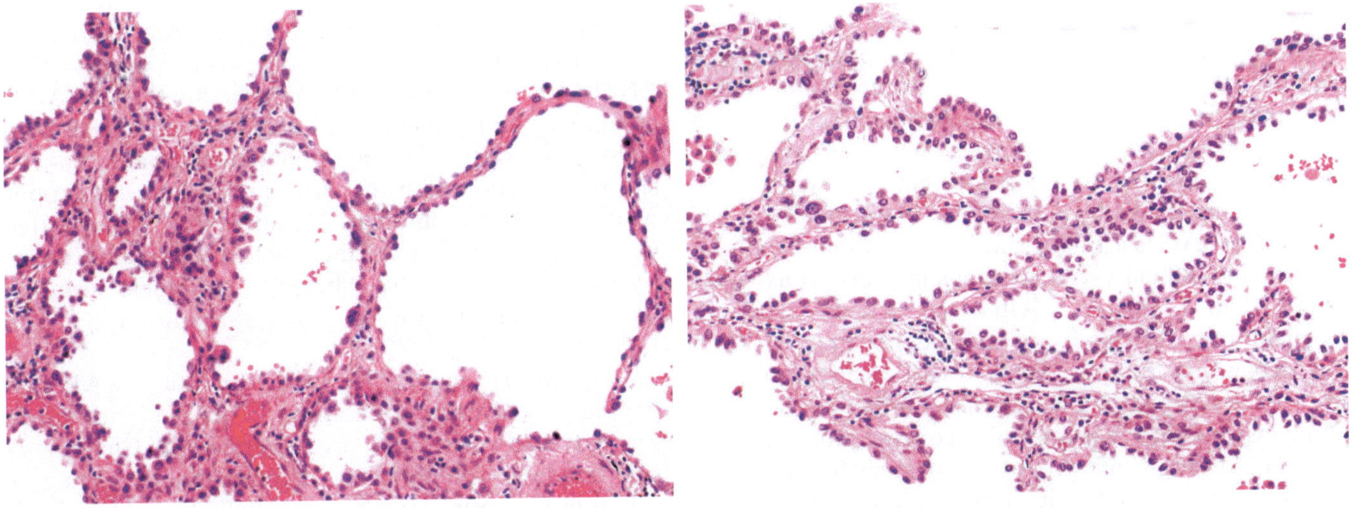

A B

Figure 34.25. Two examples of atypical adenomatous hyperplasia that are rather more cellular and atypical. **(A)** Lesion demonstrates considerable cellular heterogeneity. **(B)** The cell population is more crowded but remains a single layer.

Differential Diagnosis

There are two major distinctions to be made in diagnosing AAH while a number of other less common lesions must also be considered.

In the distinction between AAH and reactive pneumocyte hyperplasia, common sense must prevail. Epithelial hyperplasia, which may be quite atypical, is part of the picture in IPF/UIP, honeycomb lung, DAD, radiation pneumonitis, and virtually every other situation where there has been injury to the alveolar epithelium. This is the reason for the relevant caveat in the current WHO definition that AAH cannot ever be diagnosed in the presence of the above; indeed, the frequent presence of emphysema may also make identification of AAH difficult. Atypical adenomatous hyperplasia is a discrete, localized lesion whose distinction relies, at least in part, on the contrast with adjacent surrounding normal alveoli. That said, it is equally wrong to dismiss a diagnosis of AAH if there is fibrosis or chronic inflammation *within* the lesion; a mild degree of fibrosis or inflammation is the rule, and sometimes these features may be marked. Occasionally lymphoid follicles may be seen. In the original description of AAH, Shimosato et al.[11] described sclerosis and partial alveolar collapse, and it is likely that some AAH lesions may regress or sclerose rather than progress.[252] Fibrosis and inflammation of alveolar walls within the lesion is thus acceptable, but if these changes extend significantly beyond the limits of the lesion as defined by the epithelial cell population, then one should be most cautious in diagnosing AAH. Similarly, where there is any degree of obstructive pneumonitis/retention pneumonia, a diagnosis of AAH should be made with great care. Many AAH lesions can be appreciated as centriacinar in location and should not be confused with the subpleural and paraseptal alveolar cuboidal cell hyperplasia relatively common distal to tumors.

The hypothesis surrounding the concept of AAH as a precursor lesion of pulmonary adenocarcinoma places this lesion at the beginning of a biologic continuum in which AAH becomes LNMBAC, wherein invasion subsequently develops and adenocarcinoma supervenes. Thus the line drawn by pathologists to distinguish AAH from LNMBAC is artificial and has led to some pathologists having difficulty in accepting some lesions as AAH rather than LNMBAC. After the seminal work of Noguchi et al.[253] in classifying small adenocarcinomas and the recognition that pure BAC has an excellent prognosis,[10,254] the refining of a narrower definition of BAC as a noninvasive lesion[1] has made this concept more tangible (Fig. 34.26). Noguchi[255] proposed a strategy for allocating problematic lesions to either the AAH or LNMBAC category, and this has been incorporated in the latest WHO classification.[256] If a lesion fulfills three or more of

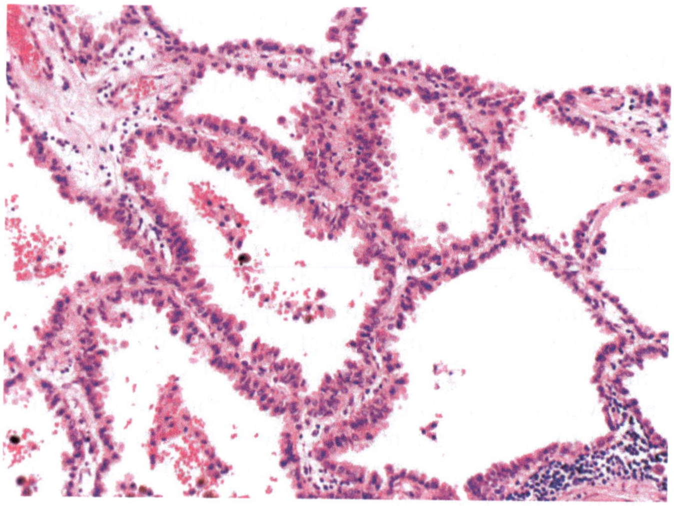

FIGURE 34.26. Bronchioloalveolar carcinoma. This field from a localized nonmucinous bronchioloalveolar carcinoma (LNMBAC) shows marked crowding and overlapping of atypical columnar cells. These features are unacceptable as AAH. Compare with Figure 34.25.

the following five histologic criteria, a diagnosis of LNMBAC (de facto adenocarcinoma in situ) is appropriate. In general, AAH would not show more than one of these features:

- Marked cell stratification
- High cell density with marked overlapping of nuclei
- Coarse nuclear chromatin and prominent nucleoli
- True papillae or cells growing in a "picket-fence"–type arrangement
- Tumor cell height is increased and tends to exceed that of the columnar cells in surrounding terminal bronchioles

Those lesions that fulfill criteria for LNMBAC are generally larger than AAH, certainly over 5 mm, and most over 15 mm in size. The cell population in LNMBAC is much more homogeneous than in AAH, comprising more compacted columnar cells with close cell-cell apposition.[248] This population usually makes a sharp distinction with the surrounding lung. In support of the pathologic findings, Nomori et al.[257] found that, in spiral CT studies in the context of a lung cancer screening program (see below), radiologic size was not a useful criteria for distinguishing AAH from LNMBAC.

The unwary may be tempted to confuse AAH with papillary or alveolar adenomas.[258,259] These latter lesions are extremely rare and are described in Chapter 41. Micronodular pneumocyte hyperplasia occurring in tuberous sclerosis may also potentially be confused with AAH,[260,261] and clearly the clinical context is important in the differential diagnosis (see Chapter 39, Fig. 39.28).

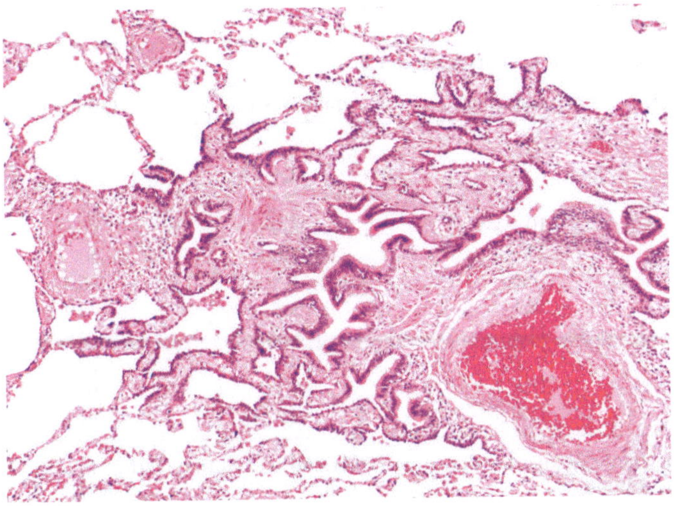

FIGURE 34.27. Bronchiolar epithelial hyperplasia (bronchiolar metaplasia or lambertosis). Reactive proliferation of bronchiolar epithelium lining centriacinar alveoli associated with some fibrosis.

Bronchioloalveolar carcinoma–like lesions have been described in adolescent cancer patients.[262] A more common lesion is so-called bronchiolar epithelial hyperplasia or bronchiolization of alveoli (lambertosis), a localized centriacinar proliferation of bronchiolar columnar epithelium distinct from AAH, which shows ciliated cells among the respiratory-type epithelium that lines centriacinar alveoli, often in association with scarring and distortion of the bronchioles (Fig. 34.27).

Associations and Prevalence of Atypical Adenomatous Hyperplasia

The prevalence of AAH in the general population is not known. These lesions cannot be detected in vivo with any reliability, even using advanced spiral CT scanning techniques in the context of a lung cancer screening program. To date their detection has been the preserve of pathologists, either through serendipity or more likely by actively seeking them in surgical lung specimens or autopsy material. Success will be improved by taking many tissue blocks, both of any suspicious foci and at random from the subpleural parenchyma in particular.

Some authors have sought AAH lesions in autopsy lungs. Yanagisawa[263] reported finding lesions considered by Weng et al.[235] to be AAH in 3.6% of 140 autopsies. In a series of 100 consecutive autopsies, from which any patient with primary or metastatic lung cancer was excluded, Sterner et al.[264] found two patients with AAH. Both these patients were ex-smokers. Yokose et al.[265] sought AAH in a population of 241 patients over 60 years of age and found lesions in 3.4% of patients without concurrent malignancy of any sort, but in 10.2% of patients who had a malignant tumor at autopsy. The same pathologists, working with different colleagues in a different hospital, repeated their study on a group of 179 patients ranging from 0 to 90 years old. Five patients (2.8%), all men between 52 and 63 years of age, had AAH, and one of them had a malignant (nonpulmonary) tumor.[266] While Sterner et al. averaged three to five tissue blocks per case, Yokose and co-workers[265,266] averaged seven blocks. Most of these patients had only one AAH, occasionally two were found. Given that intercurrent lung pathology is very frequent in autopsy cases, any search for AAH in this setting is particularly challenging, and this, together with the relatively low tissue block numbers studied, suggests that the prevalence of AAH is likely to be underestimated.

The vast majority of AAH lesions reported have been found in surgical resection specimens, in most instances removed for primary malignancy. Given that lung resection for disease other than primary cancer is relatively unusual and that success in finding AAH is in part dependent on the lack of any intercurrent diffuse disease, the collective experience of AAH in lungs without primary cancer is limited, which introduces a degree of bias. Nonetheless, there is good evidence that AAH is more common in lungs bearing a primary carcinoma than in those without, and in particular in lungs with adenocarcinoma (Tables 34.3 and 34.4).

The data in Table 34.3 give an average prevalence of 18% for AAH in lungs bearing a primary cancer, though it must be emphasized that these studies are by no means comparable. Some data[267,268] are reproduced from a secondary source,[235] and some are not true prospective studies.[233,269] Nonetheless, the average prevalence from

TABLE 34.3. Prevalence of atypical adenomatous hyperplasia (AAH) in primary cancer-bearing surgical lung resections

Reference	No. of lungs examined	Cases showing AAH (%)
Morinaga and Shimosato 1987[267]	203	13.9
Kodama et al. 1988[268]	131	12.2
Miller 1990*[238]	247	9.3
Nakanishi 1990[233]	70	21.4
Weng et al. 1992*[235]	165	16.4
Noguchi and Shimosato 1994[269]	2098	5.1
Chapman and Kerr 2000*[240]	554	12.1
Nakahara et al. 2001*[239]	508	23.2
Koga et al. 2002*[250]	61	49
Total; average (%)	4037	18
Total; average of five prospective studies*(%)	1535	22

The enormous variation in reported figures probably reflects differences in methodology for detecting AAH and makes the average figures of limited value.

TABLE 34.4. Prevalence of AAH in resections bearing different primary lung cancer types

	Cell type of primary lung cancer			
Reference	Adenocarcinoma (%)	Large cell (%)	Squamous (%)	Others (%)
Morinaga and Shimosato 1987[267]	18.8		5.9	
Kodama et al. 1988[268]	19.2		11.1	
Miller 1990*[238]	15.6		3	
Nakanishi 1990[233]	34.5	10	6.9	
Weng et al. 1992*[235]	17	23	11.6	20
Noguchi and Shimosato 1994[269]	7.8	6.6	1	6.5
Chapman and Kerr 2000*[240]	23.2	12.5	3.3	5.4
Nakahara et al. 2001*[239]	29.3	11.8	9.8	19.5
Koga et al. 2002*[250]	57		30	29
Average%	24.7	12.8	9.1	16
Average of five prospective studies*%	28.4	15.8	11.5	18.4

The enormous variation in reported figures probably reflects differences in methodology for detecting AAH and makes the average figures of limited value. It may be more valid to compare within rather than between studies.

those five studies that were essentially prospective is 22%.[235,238–240,250] Notable are the findings of Koga et al.,[250] whose figures are by far the highest for AAH prevalence (Tables 34.3 and 34.4). These authors sliced formalin-inflated lungs in 4-mm slices and averaged 60 tissue blocks per specimen. In resections for metastatic disease, prevalences of 9.6% and 4.4% have been reported where, at least in the later study, reasonable numbers of cases were studied.[235,267]

When the prevalence of AAH is compared with the cell type of the associated primary lung cancer, a consistent and statistically significant association with adenocarcinoma is found (Table 34.4). Koga et al.[250] reported a particular association with the BAC subtype and a tendency for AAH to be more atypical in these cases.

Clearly these data again vary, and it may be more meaningful to compare figures within each study. Atypical adenomatous hyperplasia is much more frequently seen in association with adenocarcinoma than with squamous cell carcinoma. Although obstructive pneumonitis is more common with bronchogenic squamous cell carcinomas and makes detection of AAH harder, this difference is real. The figures for large cell carcinoma may seem relatively high, but many large cell carcinomas may well be terminally differentiated adenocarcinomas, and up to 80% of large cell carcinomas show ultrastructural evidence of glandular differentiation. The "others" category contains a large proportion of adenosquamous carcinomas, though whether they fulfill the current criteria for this diagnosis is debatable. In those patients who have AAH, the proportion of these with adenocarcinoma is high and remarkably consistent in five prospective studies at between 72% and 81%.[235,238–240,250]

The number of lesions varies between patients and is clearly in part a function of the volume of lung examined and the methods used for their detection. Atypical adenomatous hyperplasia is likely to be multifocal in each case. While most early reports described patients with mostly single lesions, the more comprehensive studies have found more AAH and show further interesting associations. Between 40% and 66% (mean 48%) of resections with AAH show multiple lesions.[233,235,238–240] Most of these cases have between two and six AAH lesions detected, but there are reports of some very large numbers of AAHs found in even single lobectomy specimens. Weng et al.,[235] who averaged 51 blocks per resection, had one case with 14 AAHs. Chapman and Kerr,[240] who made more careful gross examination, sampled suspicious foci and took up to six random blocks, found four patients with 12, 19, 34, and 42 AAHs, respectively, and since this report have another patient with 125 lesions. Miller,[238] who also paid attention to gross examination, described five patients whose lungs were studded with multiple AAH lesions. In one exceptional case report, Anami et al.[270] reported a left upper lobectomy with 161 AAH lesions.

Almost without exception, patients with large numbers of AAH lesions have concurrent BAC or invasive adenocarcinoma. Furthermore, there is a clear association between large numbers of AAH lesions and multiple synchronous primary adenocarcinomas (Table 34.5). Chapman and Kerr[240] found that 10 of their 70 AAH patients had multiple synchronous primary adenocarcinomas. Nakahara et al.[239] reported that while 21% of patients with a single lung tumor had AAH (64% of which were single), 46% of those with multiple cancers had AAH (63% of which were multiple).

The prevalence of AAH between the sexes varies between studies (Table 34.6), and conclusions are difficult to draw. One of us favors the view that AAH is commoner in females, at least in a Caucasian

TABLE 34.5. Reported cases of multiple synchronous primary adenocarcinoma and multiple AAH in surgical resections

Reference	No. of AAH lesions	No. of synchronous carcinomas
Anami et al. 1998[270]	161	2 (left upper lobe)
Suzuki et al. 1998[271]	12	2 (bilateral)
Chapman and Kerr 2000[240]	42	6
	34	3
	19	3
	8	4
Dohmoto et al. 2000[272]	2	4 (bilateral)
Takamochi et al. 2001[273]	6	3
	3	4
	2	4
Koga et al. 2002[250]	3	2 (bilateral)

(Scottish) population studied, especially those with adenocarcinoma. The Japanese data do not allow a clear conclusion.

Data from autopsy studies described above suggested an association between AAH and concurrent or previous malignancy at any site, not only in the lung.[265] This is supported by three other studies in Japanese subjects,[239,274,275] but not in a Western case study.[276] The reverse findings were reported with respect to AAH and a family history of malignancy; an association was found in the Scottish patients,[276] but not for the Japanese.[239,274] Once more this is a confusing picture that may be confounded by ethnic differences.

Evidence in Support of Atypical Adenomatous Hyperplasia as a Preinvasive Lesion: Morphology, Morphometry, and Cytofluorimetry

That AAH is found most frequently in association with adenocarcinoma of the lung, exhibits minor degrees of cytologic atypia, and has an architecture reminiscent of the earliest stages of lung adenocarcinoma (localized nonmucinous bronchioloalveolar carcinoma) is fairly persuasive that AAH is a precursor lesion of LNMBAC and therefore invasive adenocarcinoma. Some of the earliest reports of AAH seem to refer to a lesion that was contiguous with an established adenocarcinoma, rather than a discrete focal lesion as described above. This led to confusion and discredited the case for AAH as an adenocarcinoma precursor in some minds. The confusion is understandable, but the presence of an AAH-like zone at the periphery of an established tumor not only is supportive of the hypothesis, but also is more or less expected, once one accepts that a diagnosis of AAH is not necessary limited to a focus of less than 5 mm in diameter. One of us has seen several examples of lesions that show invasive adenocarcinoma, a peripheral BAC component, and marginal zones where the histologic features differ from the BAC component of the tumor and are identical to those seen in discrete AAH. The temptation to compare this with the residual adenoma at the margin of some colorectal carcinomas is too great to resist, especially since, as one might expect, such AAH-like zones are more frequent in smaller peripheral-type adenocarcinomas.[254]

Studies of cell and nuclear size and nuclear DNA content in AAH and adenocarcinomas also reflect both the differences and the continuity between these lesions and confirm the observation that some lesions have both adenocarcinoma and AAH-like areas. Kodama et al.[246] demonstrated that AAH lesions had a significantly lower mean nuclear area (MNA; 50 μm^2 or less) than LNMBACs, in which the MNA was always over 50 μm^2. They also found several lesions with two distinct cell populations defined by MNA, corresponding to AAH and LNMBAC. Nakanishi[233] and Yokozaki et al.[277] reported almost identical results on MNA, while Kitamura et al.[249] favored a value of 40 μm^2, in combination with a lesion diameter of 5 mm, as a cutoff between AAH and BAC. In a more detailed morphometric study, Mori et al.[278] measured 12 different parameters of cell and nuclear morphology and subjected the data to cluster analysis. Lesions considered AAH clearly segregated into one group and Clara cell type adenocarcinomas (BACs) into another. A third group contained both lesions considered type II pneumocyte type adenocarcinoma (BACs) and AAHs. On review these latter AAHs were more atypical than those that segregated into a group by themselves.

Using cytofluorimetry[237] and image cytometry,[277] the mean cell DNA content in AAH has been shown to be higher than in reactive pneumocyte hyperplasia, but lower than that found in small adenocarcinomas. Both these studies showed that some lesions clearly designated AAH or adenocarcinoma shared nuclear characteristics.

TABLE 34.6. Prevalence of AAH in males and females

Reference	Males with lung cancer (%)	Males with adenocarcinoma (%)	Females with lung cancer (%)	Females with adenocarcinoma (%)
Weng et al. 1992[235]	20	26	9	8.3
Nakahara et al. 2001[239]	21	No data	28	No data
Chapman and Kerr 2000[240]	9.2	18.8	19	30.2

Aneuploidy was noted in 77% to 85% of the adenocarcinomas, but also in 36% to 54% of the AAH lesions. Nakanishi et al.[279] found less aneuploidy (absent in low-grade AAH but present in 25% of high-grade AAHs and 35% of BACs) and described an increase in argyrophilic nucleolar-organizer region (AgNOR) counts across the spectrum of lesions.

These objective measurements of the nuclear and cytologic characteristics of AAH and LNMBAC reflect the subjective assessments of the same characteristics made on microscopy of hematoxylin and eosin (H&E)-stained sections. There is a range of cytologic features found in AAH that corresponds to our assessment of atypia, and at the most atypical end of the spectrum there is overlap with lesions regarded as LNMBAC. These data and the existence of combined lesions strongly support the place of AAH as a precursor of adenocarcinoma.

Evidence in Support of Atypical Adenomatous Hyperplasia as a Preinvasive Lesion: Cell and Molecular Biology

There is an increasing amount of evidence that AAH exhibits a variety of changes in protein expression and numerous genetic alterations that are associated with neoplastic transformation in cell populations. In addition, in some studies, there is evidence of molecular as well as morphologic progression of abnormality as AAH becomes more atypical and develops into LNMBAC. In many instances, however, relatively few AAH lesions have been studied, making the significance of the findings difficult to ascertain. Certainly this aspect of the literature on AAH is much less voluminous when compared to that available from the study of bronchial SD/CIS.

Altered Cell Proliferation

A few studies have measured proliferative (cycle cell) activity in AAH. Both Carey et al.[234] and Kitaguchi et al.[280] observed that the Ki-67 index was higher in AAH than in surrounding normal alveoli. Kitamura et al.[247] reported a Ki-67 index (percent of positive cells) of 0.59% for low-grade AAH, 2.05% for high-grade AAH, while AAH-like carcinomas (pure LNMBAC) had an average Ki-67 index of 6.08%, and in some well-differentiated adenocarcinoma it was 15.6%. Kurasono et al.[281] found similar results: low-grade AAH (0.73%), high-grade AAH (1.53%), 3.7% in early adenocarcinoma, and 12.10% in overt adenocarcinoma. These authors infer that these adenocarcinomas are probably LNMBAC. Similarly, Mori et al.[244] found a mean Ki-67 index of 1.8% in AAH, while their adenocarcinomas (almost certainly LNMBAC) recorded 3.5%. Koga et al.[250] reported a Ki-67 index of 1.4% in low-grade AAH and 3.5% in high-grade lesions, and Yamasaki et al.[282] reported a similar progression in Ki-67 index from 2.2% in AAH to 5% in LNMBAC and 12% in sclerosing forms of BAC. Using MCM2, which probably identifies more cycling cells than Ki-67, Kerr et al.[283] reported a mean proliferative index of 0.87% for low-grade AAH, 2.56% for high-grade AAH, 11.5% for LNMBAC, 49.5% for the BAC component of mixed adenocarcinoma, and 65.5% for invasive adenocarcinoma. In this latter study the range of values for the BAC component of mixed adenocarcinoma ranged from 20% to 80%. The overlap with data for pure LNMBAC raises the possibility that the BAC component of a mixed adenocarcinoma may be heterogeneous biologically, consisting of invasive (lepidic) adenocarcinoma and true BAC, that is, adenocarcinoma in situ, a concept already raised by the morphometric data discussed above.

Carcinoembryonic Antigen

While Carey et al.[234] found quite frequent staining of AAH for carcinoembryonic antigen (CEA), Rao and Fraire[284] found CEA infrequently expressed. Kitamura et al.[249] demonstrated increasing CEA staining as atypia increased such that 25% of low-grade AAH, 35% of high-grade AAH, 67% of LNMBAC, and 77% of adenocarcinomas were positive, while Nakanishi[233] and Mori et al.[285] showed a similar trend.

Blood Group Antigens

Nakanishi[233] described decreasing frequency of staining for A, B, and H blood group antigens as AAH lesions became more atypical.

Markers of Peripheral Airway Cells

Mori et al.[285] stained a range of lesions, previously characterized using morphometry,[278] for surfactant apoprotein A (SPA; a type 2 pneumocyte marker) and urine protein 1 (UP1; a Clara cell marker). While many AAH lesions expressed SPA, relatively few stained for UP1. Kitamura et al.[242] also used these markers and similarly found that from low-grade AAH to invasive adenocarcinoma, SPA expression became progressively weaker and more infrequent, whereas UP1 was not found in AAH but was seen in 20% of LNMBAC and in 70% of adenocarcinomas. To some extent these findings reflect the H&E morphology and ultrastructural studies of AAH (see above). Thyroid transcription factor-1 (TTF-1) has been suggested as a lineage marker for lesions derived from peripheral airways epithelium and as such is expressed in all AAH lesions and LNMBACs.[286]

Cytochrome P-450

The cytochrome P-450 (CYP) enzymes metabolize xenobiotics and as such are probably important in activating some tobacco carcinogens. Intense staining for CYP1A1–

2, CYP2B1–2, and CYP2E1 was found in AAH and adenocarcinoma, while normal alveoli stained less, the differences being most marked with CYP1A1–2 and least with CYP2B1–2.[285]

Matrix Metalloproteinases and Related Stromal Factors

In AAH, MMP-2 expression was found to be strong in 30% to 40% of cases by some,[287,288] but absent by others.[289] The tissue inhibitor of this enzyme, TIMP-2, has been found in about 40% of cases.[287,288] MT1-MMP was not found in AAH, although its inhibitor (TIMP-1) was present in all AAHs studied.[287] These authors and Kitamura et al.[289] also report variable staining of AAH for MMP-3, -7, and -9 and an intact basement membrane, as assessed by collagen type IV staining, in AAH and BAC, but not in invasive disease. MMP-2 and TIMP-2 appear to be upregulated in LNMBAC.[287,288] Iijima et al.[290] have further refined this observation by noting that MMP-2, but not MMP-9, is more highly expressed in LNMBAC with central fibroblastic scarring (a change in BAC that probably heralds the onset of invasion), when compared to LNMBAC without central fibrosis, that is, true adenocarcinoma in situ. While Kumaki et al.[287] demonstrated preservation and increased MMP-2/TIMP-2 expression in invasive disease, others have demonstrated a diminution of expression in invasive tumor.[288,289] There is evidence that the vascularity of AAH is increased when compared to normal lung.[291]

Cell Adhesion Molecules

While high-level expression of CD44v6, one of the CD44 family particularly expressed in lung epithelium, was relatively frequent in AAH (64% of cases) and less so (24%) in invasive adenocarcinoma, expression of both E-cadherin and β-catenin was high in only a third of AAHs and high in 60% to 80% of LNMBACs and invasive adenocarcinomas.[288] While these losses in CD44v6 expression may reflect an invasive phenotype developing, the E-cadherin/β-catenin changes appeared to mirror the degree of cell-cell contact within the lesions examined. Another study, however, reported that over 90% of AAH lesions and over 70% of LNMBACs expressed both E-cadherin and β-catenin, but much less staining in invasive tumors.[292] Definitions of positivity differ between these studies. Galectins 1, 1b, 3b, and 7b were shown to be overexpressed in AAH when compared to normal lung.[291]

Mucins

Awaya and coworkers[293] found a significant decrease in MUC1 expression but significantly increased expression of MUC2, MUC5AC, MUC6, and depolarized MUC1 in the progression from AAH through LNMBAC to adenocarcinoma.

Oncogenes

A number of oncogenes and tumor suppressor genes, together with related chromosome regions have been studied in AAH. Their relevance and importance to carcinogenesis is described in the relevant section on the cell and molecular biology of SD/CIS.

Fragile Histidine Triad (FHIT)

The protein product (Fhit) of this putative TSG is extensively expressed in both AAH and LNMBAC, but is lost as invasion develops in adenocarcinomas.[288] Mixed adenocarcinomas show differential staining of their BAC and invasive solid and acinar components. The potential of Fhit loss as a marker of invasion is yet to be explored.

Commensurate with this finding, LOH at 3p14.2 was not found in any AAHs examined.[282]

$p16^{INK4A}$-Cyclin D1-CDK4-RB Pathway

The proteins involved in this pathway were studied by Kurasono et al.,[281] who found relatively high expression of cyclin D1 in AAH, but a decrease in expression in both LNMBAC and adenocarcinoma. They also found that loss of Rb expression was rare in AAH and LNMBAC and infrequent in adenocarcinoma, as was loss of p16 expression. They suggest that overexpression of cyclin D1 may be important at the early stages of adenocarcinogenesis (AAH), but less important in the later stages.

Analysis of chromosome 9p has shown evidence of LOH at selected loci in up to one third of AAHs examined. Kitaguchi et al.[280] reported 9p LOH in 13% of cases, while Kohno et al.[172] found 5% of AAHs had LOH. Both report that the lesions with LOH were moderate to severely atypical and that LOH was more frequent in concurrent adenocarcinoma. Yamasaki et al.[282] studied AAH and LNMBAC with and without central scarring. In AAH LOH at *D9S144* (9p) and *IFNA* (9p21) was found in 7% and 33%, respectively. The frequency of LOH of these microsatellite markers was the same in the BACs studied. LOH at 13q (*D13S176 RB*) was found in three out of nine AAH studied (see below).

It is difficult to draw conclusions on the basis of such limited data. There is evidence for alterations of genes and gene expression for this pathway that is all consistent with neoplasia. The importance of these alterations in adenocarcinogenesis remains uncertain, however, and we await data on hypermethylation of *P16* in AAH, given that this mechanism of gene inactivation seems so important in central bronchial carcinogenesis.

Tyrosine Kinases: HER-2/neu and EGFR

Given that overexpression of membrane-bound c-erbB-2, the product of the *HER2/Neu* oncogene, is found in up to 70% of lung adenocarcinomas, its expression in AAH is clearly of interest. While low-grade AAH did not express c-erbB-2, some high-grade AAHs were positive, representing 7% of all AAH studied.[294] This implies that this factor may be upregulated relatively late in adenocarcinogenesis. Mori et al.[244] also demonstrated some c-erbB-2 protein in AAH and rather more in BAC, but actual figures are not given.

There has been considerable recent interest in *EGFR* mutations in adenocarcinomas due to their apparent association with tumor sensitivity to tyrosine kinase inhibitors. This literature is now considerable and beyond the scope of this chapter. However, Yatabe et al.,[295] as well as reporting that *EGFR* mutation was strongly associated with peripheral-type pulmonary adenocarcinoma, also found mutations in two of five AAH lesions studied. Yoshida et al.[296] found *EGFR* mutation in only one of 35 (3%) AAH lesions, in 11% of LNMBACs, and in 42% of invasive adenocarcinomas. A consistent finding is the apparent mutual exclusivity of *EGFR* and K-*ras* mutations in particular lesions, though in patients with multiple lung lesions either mutation may be found.[296] This subject is now a major growth area in lung cancer research

Cyclooxygenase-2 (COX-2)

Cyclooxygenases catalyze the synthesis of prostaglandins and other eicosanoids and play a role in carcinogenesis. They are upregulated in many tumors, including lung cancer and adenocarcinoma in particular.[297] While one study showed COX-2 expressed in only 22% of AAH,[298] Hosomi et al.[299] found, as with BAC and invasive adenocarcinomas, over 80% of AAH lesions showed upregulation of COX-2. This may explain the apparent success of long-term aspirin therapy as a chemopreventive agent for lung cancer.[300]

Eukaryotic Initiation Factor 4E (eIF4E)

This factor is a key regulator of protein synthesis and is overexpressed in many lung cancers. Expression of eIF4E is above normal background levels in AAH and increases through BAC to invasive adenocarcinoma.[301]

Telomerase

Nakanishi et al.[302] studied hTERC and hTERT mRNA using in-situ hybridization in formalin-fixed paraffin-embedded AAH and LNMBAC. Expression of both was found in 27% of low-grade AAH, around 75% of high-grade AAH, and 98% of LNMBAC. These data support the neoplastic progression of low-grade AAH through a higher-grade lesion to LNMBAC.

Apoptosis-Related Factors

Nakanishi et al.[303] found bcl-2 overexpressed in no low-grade AAH, 28% of high-grade AAH, and 48% of BAC. These authors also found survivin overexpressed in 9% of low-grade AAH, but in 89% and 100%, respectively, of high-grade AAH and LNMBAC. Although Kayser et al.[291] reported overexpression of bcl-2 in 70% of AAH lesions, one of us has found that bcl-2 is infrequently overexpressed in AAH (unpublished observations). Nonetheless, there is evidence that antiapoptotic mechanisms are upregulated during adenocarcinogenesis, although Mori et al.[244] described less expression of bcl2 in LNMBAC, when compared to AAH.

P27

Another tumor suppressor gene, *P27*, functions as an inhibitor of cyclin-dependent kinase 2, and loss of this protein promotes oncogenesis. This protein is conserved in AAH when associated with p27-positive adenocarcinoma, but is consistently low in AAH found with p27-negative adenocarcinomas.[304] Jab-1, a P27 degradation pathway protein was found in 36% of AAH lesions, was absent in normal lung epithelia, and showed reciprocal expression with p27 protein.[305]

P53

Abnormalities of the *P53* gene and altered expression of p53 protein rank among the commonest changes seen in human tumors. Several studies using immunohistochemistry to detect p53 protein in AAH are published, but comparison is very difficult due to different scoring systems and staining methods. Kerr et al.[294] reported altered expression of p53 protein in AAH. Strong nuclear staining of 5% to 70% of nuclei was reported in 28% of AAH cases, while a further 30% showed only weak focal staining of <5% of the cells (58% overall positivity). High p53 expression was associated with greater cellular pleomorphism and crowding (high-grade AAH). One group found less staining of both low- and high-grade AAH, but published two different sets of data with overall positivity rates in all AAH of 19%[247] and 9%.[249] Other studies have reported variable rates of p53 positivity in AAH, namely 3%,[306] 17%,[303] and 35%.[280,307] Katabami et al.[167] found stainable p53 in 25% of AAH lesions in patients without pneumoconiosis, but 36% of AAHs from patients with pneumoconiosis were p53-positive.

It is likely that technical differences explain these wide discrepancies. Although lesion classification could also play a part, frequent review of case material has ensured that LNMBAC has not been underdiagnosed in at least some of the published work.[294] It does seem clear from all the published data, however, that higher levels are more likely to be seen in more atypical higher-grade lesions, with higher levels still in LNMBAC and invasive disease.

Expression of the p53-inducible cyclin-dependent kinase inhibitor p21$^{waf1/cip1}$ was compared with p53 expression and, while reactive lesions demonstrated low levels of both proteins, elevated levels of p21 were seen in some AAH lesions. There was no relationship between p21 level and grade of lesion or p53 status.[308]

It has been suggested that relatively low levels of p53 protein, possibly detected by some systems and not by others, may be the result of stabilization of wild-type p53, but that higher levels may correlate with gene mutation and mutant protein. Mutations of *P53*, however, have been difficult to detect, not least because of the technical challenges of dealing with such small lesions. Hayashi et al.,[308] Slebos et al.,[306] and Yamasaki et al.[282] were unable to find any mutation in one, three, and 20 AAHs, respectively, although Slebos et al. reported a missense mutation in exon 7 of *P53* in an AAH-like carcinoma (high-grade AAH or LNMBAC). Kohno et al.,[172] however, found a *P53* exon 8 mutation in one of 20 AAHs (5%). Unspecified mutations of *P53* were found in 23% of adenocarcinomas associated with AAH[172] and in 16% and 33%, respectively, of nonsclerosing and sclerosing LNMBACs.[282]

Hayashi et al.[308] reported LOH in exon 4 of *P53* in one of seven AAH lesions examined. The LOH in 17p was reported in 6% of AAH and 17% of adenocarcinomas in one study[280] and in 6% of AAH, 11% of nonsclerosing LNMBAC, and in 36% of sclerosing LNMBAC in another.[282] Alveolar collapse and fibrosis/sclerosis probably represent malignant progression within LNMBAC,[253] and Aoyagi et al.[309] also demonstrated an increasing frequency on 17p LOH (and LOH at other sites; see below) in this progression.

Abnormalities of *P53* and its protein product are clearly present in the early stages of adenocarcinogenesis. While stainable p53 protein appears to accumulate at an early stage, even at high levels, this is not, insofar as the limited data may be interpreted, apparently associated with frequent *P53* mutation or LOH, events that appear later at the BAC (adenocarcinoma in situ) stage.

P63

This p53 protein homologue, which transactivates the *P53* gene and may induce apoptosis, is found in reserve cells in bronchiolar epithelium. As well as being expressed more or less uniformly in reactive peripheral lung epithelia, it was found strongly expressed in two of five AAH lesions and in only one of 33 adenocarcinomas.[310]

K-*ras* Mutations

Point mutation of *ras* proto-oncogenes, especially K-*ras* codons 12, 13, or 61, is described in around 20% of NSCLCs, the vast majority of these being adenocarcinomas with codon 12 the most frequently mutated.[159,193] The nature of these mutations suggests they result from DNA damage by tobacco carcinogens. There is experimental evidence that activation of the RAS signaling pathway of kinases is associated with cell transformation and tumor progression,[159] and in particular, activation of K-*ras* in the mouse may lead to adenocarcinoma via an adenomatous lesion.[311,312] Thus the status of K-*ras* in AAH is of considerable interest.

The earliest reports of K-*ras* codon 12 point mutation in AAH were made by Ohshima et al.[313] and Sugio et al.,[194] who each examined six AAHs and found mutation in two and one case respectively. Sagawa et al.,[314] on the other hand, found no mutation in five AAHs examined. A key piece of work in this area was reported by Westra et al.,[315] who found codon 12 mutations in 16 of 41 AAHs examined (39%) as well as in 42% of the associated adenocarcinomas. Furthermore, they showed that the type of mutation most frequent in AAH is a G-T transversion at position 1 or 2, the type that is also most frequently found in adenocarcinomas. They also showed that the base change at codon 12 present in the adenocarcinoma was not necessarily the same as that in concurrent AAH, and indeed cases with multiple AAHs may show different mutations. This is very strong evidence, not only for the neoplastic nature of AAH, but that AAHs represent independent foci of neoplastic development within a field undergoing transformation. Cooper et al.[195] found a lower frequency of the same mutation in AAH (15%) and peripheral type adenocarcinomas (35%), the type most likely derived from AAH, but never in bronchial type adenocarcinomas.

Cellular DNA and Genomic Studies

The clonality of AAH was first demonstrated by Nakayama et al.[237] using cytofluorimetry. Clonal analysis based on polymorphism of the X-linked human androgen receptor gene *(HUMARA)* has also demonstrated that AAH is a clonal proliferation.[316] The independent origin of multiple AAHs in the same patient, alluded to in the K-*ras* work, is supported by the presence of different polymorphisms in multiple AAHs in one patient. Also of interest is the finding of the same polymorphism in adenocarcinoma and contiguous AAH, supporting observations made in morphometric and cell cycle studies.

Chromosomal studies have been carried out on a few AAH lesions. Zojer et al.[216] used interphase FISH with probes for chromosomes 7, 8, 9, and 18, and demonstrated an aneuploidy rate of 11% in chromosome 7 in one of two AAHs studied. Two areas considered AAH in continuity with adenocarcinoma both showed similar gains in chromosome 7, and, in one lesion, gains in chromosome. Using comparative genomic hybridization, Ullmann et al.[317] found occasional gains or losses in four low-grade AAHs, but more frequent changes in 13 high-grade AAHs of a degree similar to that in the two LNMBACs in the study. These authors concluded that this similarity between high-grade AAH and LNMBAC meant these lesions are one and the same. They also noted that the pattern of changes in high-grade AAH and concurrent BAC or adenocarcinoma showed some similarities (there were also differences), and regarded this as evidence that AAH may be metastatic spread from the associated adenocarcinoma. This appears to contradict the conclusions drawn from all the other morphologic, immunocytochemical, and genetic studies described above, and cannot account for AAH that occurs in the absence of adenocarcinoma.

Studies that have shown LOH at 17p (*P53*) and 9p (*P16 CDKN2A/p16*^{INK4a}) in AAH have been described above in the relevant section.

Loss of heterozygosity in 3p, seen so frequently and early in central bronchial carcinogenesis, has been found in between 10% and 18% of AAHs, depending on which microsatellite marker is examined.[172,280,282] As with other markers, 3p LOH was only found in the most atypical lesions. One study found LOH in both 3p and 17p in one lesion,[280] while Yamasaki et al.[282] reported no LOH at *D3S1234* (3p14.2 *FHIT*), but 25% of AAHs showed LOH at *D3S1300*, a finding repeated in LNMBAC with and without central fibrosis. The LOH at 3p14.2 has been described in 43% of BACs[318] although other studies failed to find 3p LOH.[319]

Takamochi et al.[273] described 9q LOH in 39% of AAHs (in particular 25% had LOH at 9q34 in the region of the tuberous sclerosis *TSC1* gene) and 16p LOH in 22% (with 6% showing LOH at 16p13.3 in the region of *TSC2*). Interestingly, LOH was just as frequent in low-grade as in high-grade lesions. Commensurate rates of LOH were higher and allelic losses more extensive in associated adenocarcinomas. The same group had earlier shown that adenocarcinomas with these genetic abnormalities were more likely to occur in association with multiple AAH when compared to those without these regions of LOH.[320] In another study, LOH at 9q (*D9S51*) was found in one of six AAH lesions, all from the same patient.[270]

The *TSC1* gene at 9q34, or some gene very close to this region, is therefore a candidate TSG of possible importance in adenocarcinogenesis. The occurrence of micronodular pneumocyte hyperplasia (MPH), a lesion morphologically very similar to AAH, in tuberous sclerosis (TS) is thus a tantalizing parallel, but MPH is rare in TS, case material is extremely limited, and it may be that the real TSG in AAH is not *TSC1* but rather an unknown gene in the immediate vicinity.[273] Recently, Takamochi et al.[321] raised a further possibility, that TSC-1 is a TSG but is silenced by hypermethylation rather than by LOH or mutation.

As well as showing 9q LOH, Anami et al.[270] showed LOH at 17q (*D17S791*) in two of six AAHs in the same patient, in whom the concurrent two adenocarcinomas also showed the same LOH. Another AAH showed microsatellite instability at this locus. Nomori et al.[322] examined nine AAH lesions from the same patient and found that, as well as CEA, c-erbB-2 and p53 were detected immunohistochemically in four, one, and three lesions, respectively, with the largest (10mm) lesion expressing all three proteins; one third of the AAH lesions, excluding the largest lesion, showed LOH at 13q (*RB*) while LOH at 3p (*FHIT*), 5q (*APC*), 9p (*P16*), 17p (*P53*), and 22q (BandM) was absent. The importance of these two studies is that considerable genetic heterogeneity is again demonstrated within a group of AAHs occurring in the same patient, supporting their place as independent neoplastic foci in a cancerization field.

In a detailed study of LNMBACs with or without evidence of evolving tissue invasion, Aoyagi et al.[309] examined eight key regions for possible LOH and concluded the following: deletions of 5q (*APC*), 9p (*P16*), 11q (*Int-2*), and 13q (*RB*) were relatively early events and implicated inactivation of the associated genes in pulmonary adenocarcinogenesis; deletion of 3p, 17p, 18q (Smad4), and 22q (BandM) increased significantly during malignant progression of LNMBAC and tumor cells within the central fibrotic zones of more advanced LNMBAC exhibited more genetic abnormalities than those lining alveolar walls at the lesions periphery.

Thus there is evidence, albeit in a limited number of cases, that AAH (and LNMBAC) shows the genetic characteristics that would be expected of a putative precursor of a malignant tumor. Which genetic alterations are the important ones and which are background noise, resulting from the genomic instability inherent in the carcinogen-damaged genome, are less clear, though some of the candidates are beginning to emerge from the fog.

Atypical Adenomatous Hyperplasia: Possible Etiologic Factors

There are little or no data to support the role of any particular etiologic agent in the development of AAH. Tobacco smoke is an obvious suspect, but the data that exist do not allow a clear conclusion. While most of the patients with AAH studied by one of us have been cigarette smokers,[234,240] Nakahara et al.[239] found no association between smoking history and prevalence of AAH. Kitagawa et al.[275] made similar findings in a small group of Japanese patients, but suggested that smoking may be associated with multiple synchronous primary adenocarcinomas arising with AAH.

There may be something to be learned from animal studies, but, again, data are few. Alveolar hyperplasia occurs in dogs exposed to tobacco smoke,[323] while exposure of rats to asbestos causes adenomatosis and invasive adenocarcinoma. These lesions are similar to AAH, LNMBAC, and invasive adenocarcinoma occurring in humans, and the sheep disease jaagsiekte (ovine pulmonary adenomatosis) has similarities to multifocal BAC in humans.

Although Kayser et al.[291] showed an excess asbestos fiber burden in AAH-bearing lungs, no control data were given. There is no tendency for those with AAH to have occupations more at risk of asbestos exposure than those without AAH,[324] and AAH is not more prevalent at necropsy where there is evidence of asbestos exposure.[325] Studies of human BAC have generally failed to demonstrate jaagsiekte sheep retrovirus.[326] Animal models of adenocarcinogenesis[312,327] may give insight into the molecular mechanisms, and perhaps the etiology, of this disease, but apart from a possible role for tobacco smoke, etiologic factors in humans are not well characterized.

The possibility of a genetic predisposition to AAH is fascinating, but there are no hard data, only a few hints. Various studies have found an association with AAH, particularly multiple lesions, and a (previous) history of cancer in the patient or close relatives (see above), but a definite conclusion on this subject is lacking. The finding of one AAH lesion and three synchronous primary adenocarcinomas in a patient with Li-Fraumeni syndrome is interesting, but singular.[328] Takamochi et al.[273] speculated about a constitutive inherited loss of *TSC1* in some patients with AAH. Given the greater prevalence of adenocarcinoma in women, the finding of a relative excess of AAH in females, at least in one study,[276] is interesting. Furthermore, women appear to be more susceptible than men to the carcinogenic effects of tobacco smoke, and current trends indicate still rising incidences of both smoking and adenocarcinoma in females.[329,330] Perhaps changes in cigarette manufacture have altered smoking habits and put the lung periphery more at risk; perhaps the response to this exposure is AAH, which results in a rising incidence of adenocarcinoma, particularly in a more susceptible and increasingly smoking female population. This scenario does not, however, explain the relatively high frequency of adenocarcinoma in nonsmoking Asiatic women, some of whom have AAH, although other possible toxic exposures, such as cooking oil, have been implicated. Given that the majority of the AAH literature concerns Japanese patients, one could speculate that oriental genes may also have a role to play in this complex picture.

Atypical Adenomatous Hyperplasia: Risk of Progression and Prognostic Implication

The rate or risk of progression of AAH is unknown, with no formal longitudinal studies to inform us. Until recently, such a study would have been impossible since AAH is so difficult to detect, even in pathologic material and far more so in vivo. Leading-edge spiral CT scanning, usually deployed in the context of a lung cancer screening program (see below) means, however, that lesions such as AAH and BAC can now be detected,[331,332] and we can anticipate data on longitudinal observations with interest. There is a report, in the Japanese literature, of a patient with multiple AAH diagnosed 10 years after resection for adenocarcinoma[322] and one of us has seen two patients who have survived resection of lung cancer associated with AAH, only to present 2 and 5 years later, respectively, with a second primary adenocarcinoma. Until some hard data are available, it is probably prudent to advise follow-up, should a diagnosis of AAH be made in the absence of concurrent disease that would demand treatment.

Several studies have been published in which patients with AAH, diagnosed in lung tissue resected for primary carcinoma, have been followed, and their postoperative survival compared with comparable patients without AAH.[240,250,274,333,334] In these studies an assumption is made, not unreasonably, that further AAH will remain in the unresected lung. While Takigawa et al.[274] showed a tendency for patients with AAH to have a better survival, the difference was not significant, possibly due to small case numbers. Other studies have failed to show any difference in survival between those with and without AAH.[240,250,333,334] For many patients the outcome will be determined by the cancer for which they had surgery, before any AAH may have had a chance to progress, but even if only patients with stage I disease are considered, for whom cure rates will be high, there is still no difference in survival.[240]

Peripheral Lung Adenocarcinogenesis: An Adenoma-Carcinoma Sequence

As with SD/CIS, there is now a considerable amount of morphologic, morphometric, cytofluorometric, immunohistochemical, and genetic data on AAH and LNMBAC, presented above and reviewed elsewhere,[243,252,335,336] which supports the following conclusions:

- AAH is a monoclonal proliferative lesion exhibiting genetic and epigenetic features commensurate with neoplasia.
- Multiple lesions in the same patient are heterogeneous, supporting their independent origin within a field of cancerization.
- The morphologic progression of AAH is paralleled by progression in gene alteration and protein expression.
- AAH is similar to but distinct from LNMBAC, a lesion that probably develops from AAH.
- LNMBAC is now defined as a lesion lacking stromal invasion, and as such may be considered adenocarci-

noma in situ. This is supported by the observation that such lesions as currently defined, and without central fibrosis (see below), have a 5-year survival of 100%.[253]

Thus a parallel is made between AAH/BAC and SD/CIS, although much more is known about the molecular biology and risk and rates of progression of the latter. Nonetheless, there is now excellent evidence to support the concept of pulmonary alveolar intraepithelial neoplasia (PAIN) as the precursor of many and perhaps most peripheral adenocarcinomas of the lung.

The work of Noguchi and others[253] proposes that the pure LNMBAC with an intact alveolar architecture may also be referred to as type A carcinoma. Gradually such lesions show collapse and compression of the alveolar architecture centrally (a type B carcinoma), but these lesions still have excellent prognosis (100% 5-year survival). The process of collapse is then superseded by active fibroblastic proliferation, new collagen synthesis, and evidence of biochemical and physical alteration in basement membranes, a process that is seen even at the stage of alveolar collapse.[253,337] Such lesions are referred to by Noguchi et al.[253] as type C carcinoma, are the equivalent of lesions formerly classified as sclerosing BAC, and demonstrate further progression of disease at a genetic level (see above). These changes herald the onset of early stromal invasion and the development of what would be classified as mixed-type adenocarcinoma (BAC plus other components classified by the histologic patterns seen in the stromally invasive parts of the tumor) in the WHO classification. Overall type C carcinomas have a 5-year survival of 80%, reflecting the presence of invasion in some lesions and thus the potential for metastasis. Interestingly, those lesions that have a central fibrotic focus of less than 5-mm diameter still have a 5-year survival of 100%.[338]

Some concerns have been justifiably raised over the concept of AAH, its distinction from reactive lesions, and the differential diagnosis of AAH and LNMBAC.[77,339] While some authors have been less than clear in some of the terms used, for example, AAH-like carcinoma, and referred in some cases to AAH in continuity with what is otherwise obvious adenocarcinoma, concepts have evolved and been clarified. As already discussed, it is entirely in keeping with the overall hypothesis that some established adenocarcinomas may retain an area that morphologically resembles AAH at a margin. The criteria given above for distinguishing AAH from LNMBAC are helpful and provide a usable approach to the problem. We share the view, expressed by Ritter,[339] that there are (still) no reliable immunohistochemical solutions to making this distinction. As pathologists we are, as with the classification of SD/CIS, attempting to "draw a line in the sand" to distinguish between stages of what is, in fact, a biologic continuum, and all the evidence suggests that at a molecular level there is heterogeneity of the alterations found in lesions that are morphologically similar. It would be wrong to expect to be able to confidently classify every lesion, but this approach should allow most to be diagnosed. Given that the prognosis for pure LNMBAC is so good, it may be less of an issue to distinguish between AAH and LNMBAC and more important to identify invasion.[248] Although we do not yet know how quickly, if at all, AAH may progress, it is still worth noting its existence in cancer resections. High-resolution spiral CT scanning may detect other lesions in residual lung that may either warrant immediate intervention or close follow-up, especially given that radiologic features of prognostic value are beginning to emerge.

We have no idea of how many adenocarcinomas arise via this pathway. In the lung periphery it is likely that a majority evolve through stages of AAH and LNMBAC, but we cannot discount the possibility of tumors arising de novo from peripheral lung epithelium. Bronchiolar columnar cell dysplasia has been described,[340] but until this lesion is more widely recognized it is impossible to draw a conclusion about its role. A small proportion of adenocarcinomas, which are morphologically different from most peripheral tumors, appear to arise within larger bronchi. Most of these tumors, however, are large and advanced at presentation, and progression and differentiation mean that the appearance at this stage may give no clue about how the tumor began. Small, malignant papillary endobronchial adenocarcinomas occur and are rare, but their precursor is unknown. Similar tumors also occur very occasionally in the periphery, perhaps from bronchiolar epithelium but are also very uncommon. Prospective detailed searches for small peripheral lesions by pathologists reveal foci of AAH, LNMBAC, and various reactive lesions, but millimeter-sized adenocarcinomas lacking an AAH/LNMBAC component are almost unknown in this setting.[240,250] When more data are available from various prospective high-resolution CT–based screening studies, it will be interesting to see if small, solid (millimeter-sized) invasive cancers are found. So far, very few have been reported (see below).

Multifocal nonmucinous and mucinous BACs are dealt with elsewhere in this book (see Chapter 35). These lesions sit less well with the concept of BAC as adenocarcinoma in situ, being progressive lesions that grow, spread within the lung, and may kill the patient. While this behavior is not exclusive of the concept of carcinoma in situ, we must consider the possibility that such multifocal disease, certainly the mucinous type and probably the nonmucinous and rare mixed type, are biologically distinct from LNMBAC. Clearly there is much work to be done in evolving ideas about and understanding the biology of these tumors.

Diffuse Idiopathic Pulmonary Neuroendocrine Cell Hyperplasia

Diffuse idiopathic pulmonary neuroendocrine cell hyperplasia (DIPNECH) is an exceedingly rare lesion. It is included in the WHO classification of pulmonary preinvasive lesions because some patients with this disease develop one or more peripheral-type spindle cell carcinoid tumors. The typical presentation is of a slowly progressive disease characterized by an unproductive cough and shortness of breath. Patients have ranged widely in age but are typically between 40 and 60 years old, and there is an excess of females. Reported cases were frequently initially misdiagnosed as asthma, and examination usually reveals little, but pulmonary function testing shows an obstructive or mixed obstructive/restrictive pattern and reduced pulmonary gas transfer.

Aguayo et al.[341] highlighted this condition and named it in 1992. They described six patients, four of whom, by current criteria also had typical carcinoid tumors. Since then we have been able to find reports of a further 11 cases of probable DIPNECH in the English literature.[342–346] The case of pulmonary neuroendocrine cell (PNC) hyperplasia reported by Armas et al.,[344] however, is significantly different from the others, and curious in that there were no tumorlets or carcinoids, and gas transfer was reduced, but there was neither obstructive nor restrictive disease and the hyperplastic PNCs seemed to be alveolar/interstitial rather than bronchiolar in distribution. It is possible that other reports before 1992 do refer to cases of what would now be termed DIPNECH.[347–349]

Morphology

DIPNECH is characterized by the widespread proliferation of PNCs in the form of increased numbers of single cells, small groups, and linear intraepithelial proliferations (Fig. 34.28A). Larger nodules of cells may protrude into the bronchial or bronchiolar lumen, but remain covered by respiratory epithelial cells and are contained by the basement membrane. There may be bronchiolar fibrosis associated with these more pronounced collections of cells, and the fibrosis or the nodules of PNCs themselves may cause bronchiolar obstruction (Fig. 34.28B). Consequently, there may be evidence of distal bronchiolar dilatation, while, radiologically, signs of air trapping may be seen.[346] The remainder of the alveolated lung is generally normal. These changes would be the minimum required for a diagnosis of DIPNECH, assuming that other evidence of fibrosing or inflammatory lung disease, which is known to be associated with reactive PNC proliferation, is absent.

In addition, patients with DIPNECH often show more extensive manifestations of PNC hyperplasia in the form of so-called carcinoid tumorlets. These lesions are characterized by the extension of PNCs beyond the respiratory epithelial basement membrane and not infrequently just beyond the limits of the involved bronchiole (Fig. 34.28C). These lesions are typically 2 to 3 mm, though by definition never more than 5 mm, in maximum dimension. Any lesion over 5 mm is arbitrarily considered a carcinoid tumor.[1,124] Occasionally larger tumorlets and small carcinoid tumors may be visible to the naked eye on the cut surface of the lung (see Chapter 36).

Tumorlets are accompanied by variable amounts of fibrous tissue and their development may lead to bronchiolar obliteration. It has been suggested that in DIPNECH the fibrosis that accompanies the PNC hyperplasia is a reactive phenomenon and the result of bombesin or some other paracrine substance produced by the neuroendocrine cells.[341] Although this view prevails, it has been challenged by a suggestion that inflammation causes reactive PNC hyperplasia.[343]

Only typical carcinoid tumors occurring in the peripheral lung have been reported in association with DIPNECH. Other types of pulmonary neuroendocrine tumor have not been reported in this setting. There are no published studies of the molecular genetics of the PNC lesions found in DIPNECH. High levels of expression of neutral endopeptidase have been shown in the PNCs in DIPNECH, possibly a secondary effect since PNCs are rich in bombesin-like proteins, the substrate of neutral endopeptidase.[350] Given that the diagnosis of DIPNECH, tumorlets, and carcinoid tumor, at least in the DIPNECH setting, is based on a quantitative assessment of PNCs and their distribution, the distinction between hyperplasia and neoplasia is distinctly blurred.

Pulmonary Neuroendocrine Cell Hyperplasia Without DIPNECH

The relationship among carcinoid tumors, tumorlets, and PNC hyperplasia without the context of DIPNECH is also particularly hazy. Miller and Muller[351] found, in a study of 25 patients with peripheral carcinoid tumors, that 19 patients (76%) had intercurrent PNC hyperplasia; of these, eight (32% of the total) had obliterative bronchiolitis associated with the foci of PNC hyperplasia, and two of these had asymptomatic airflow limitation that could not be explained by COPD or any other lung disease. Some of these PNC foci appear large enough to be considered tumorlets. Interestingly, the authors speculated that these cases and other examples of less prominent PNC hyperplasia, without underlying chronic lung disease, could be part of a spectrum of change with DIPNECH as the most extreme manifestation.

Pulmonary tumorlets most likely represent a localized form of PNC hyperplasia, although previously they have been considered neoplastic and even early or in-situ car-

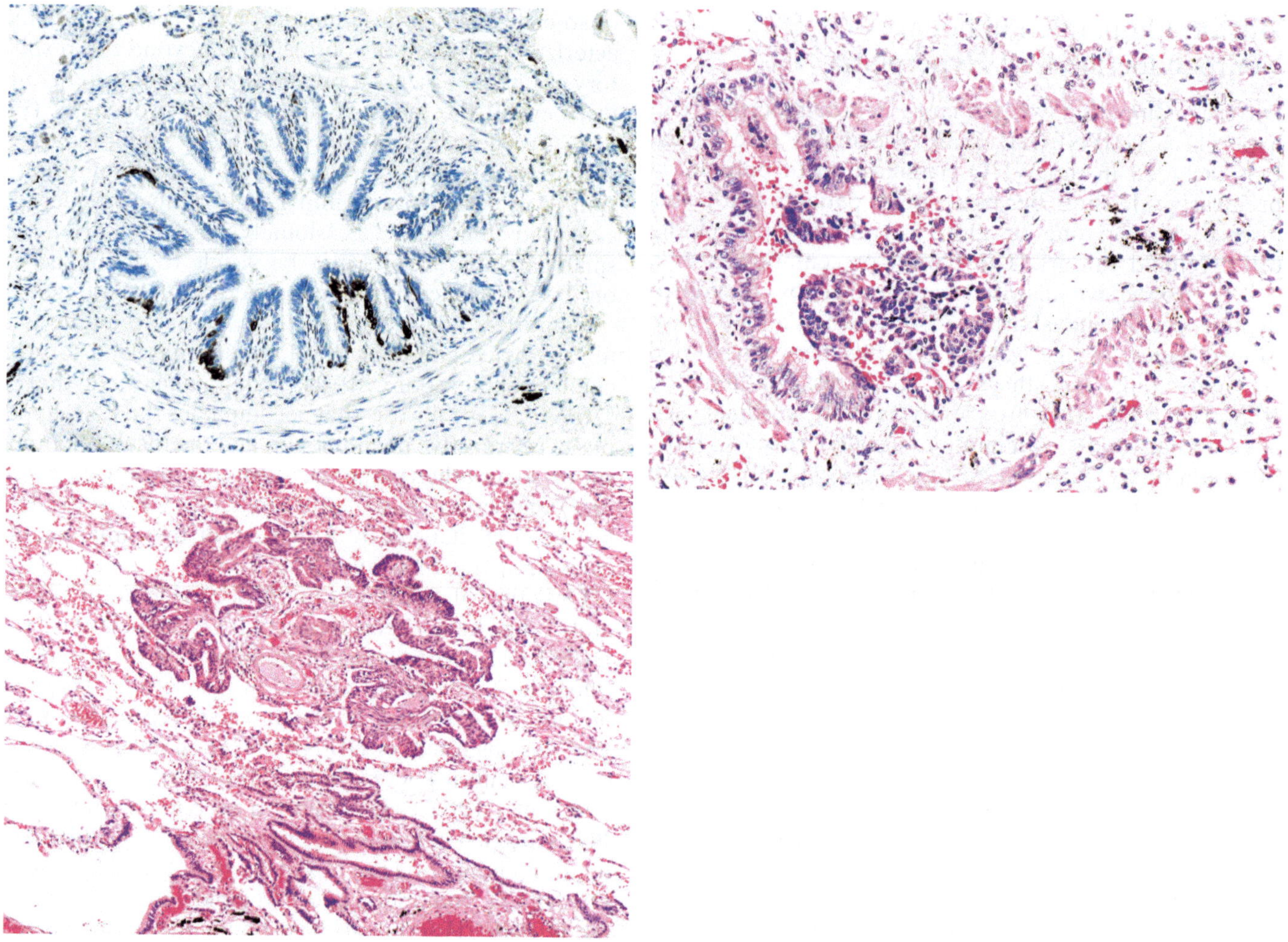

FIGURE 34.28. These images are from a patient with diffuse idiopathic pulmonary neuroendocrine cell hyperplasia (DIPNECH), who developed multiple peripheral spindle-cell carcinoid tumors. **(A)** This bronchiole shows linear proliferation of neuroendocrine cells. Antichromogranin A. **(B)** A bronchiole is obliterated by a nodular proliferation of neuroendocrine cells and fibrosis. Hematoxylin and eosin (H&E). **(C)** A distorted bronchiole with a carcinoid tumorlet. H&E.

cinoma.[352,353] Examples of tumorlets with regional lymph node metastases are reported, though in some cases we would now consider the primary lesion a carcinoid tumor on the basis of its size.[354,355] D'Agati and Perzin,[356] however, appear to have a bona fide case and report three others from the literature. Although not common, PNC hyperplasia including tumorlets is well recognized in association with a number of preexisting chronic fibrosing or inflammatory diseases, especially bronchiectasis and chronic lung abscess.[352,353,357] They have also been reported in association with a number of other conditions such as bronchopulmonary dysplasia,[358] cystic fibrosis,[359] diffuse panbronchiolitis,[360] COPD,[361] Langerhans cell histiocytosis,[362] and intralobar sequestration.[363] Whitwell[352] described 22 patients with tumorlets, of whom 36% had severe bronchiectasis. Churg and Warnock[353] found five of their 20 cases with tumorlets had bronchiectasis, while another three patients had significant localized pulmonary scarring. Nine of their patients had multiple tumorlets. These authors also pointed out that as well as sharing cytologic features with peripheral spindle cell carcinoid tumors, tumorlets, like peripheral carcinoids, may be multiple and predominate in females.

It is clear, however, that tumorlets may arise in relatively normal lung (Fig. 34.29). A case reported by Gmelich et al.[348] demonstrated no fibrosis or other underlying abnormalities in the lung, which bore multiple tumorlets and carcinoid tumors measuring from 1 to 10mm. There is insufficient detail given to know if this patient had DIPNECH, as described by Aguayo et al.[341] with altered pulmonary function, or had a forme fruste of such, as described by Miller and Muller.[351] In the case of multiple tumorlets reported by Ranchod,[364] the lung bearing them had been resected for small cell carcinoma.

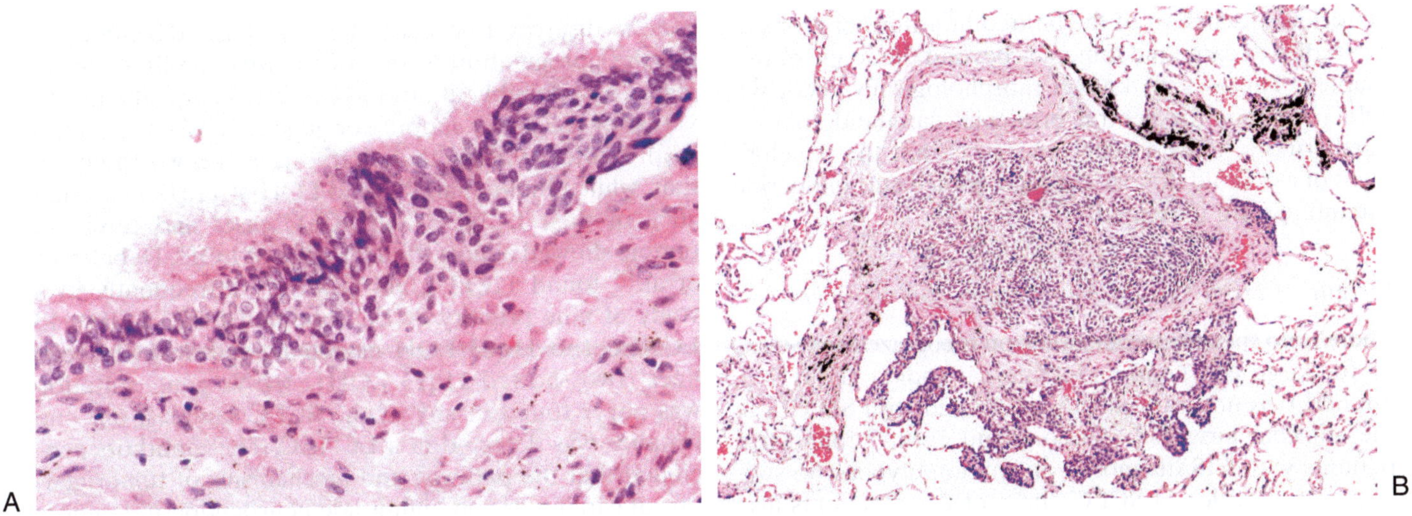

FIGURE 34.29. This patient did not have a diagnosis of DIPNECH. Her mild airflow limitation was attributed to emphysema. There was widespread evidence of PNC hyperplasia in the lobectomy specimen, removed for squamous cell carcinoma. No carcinoid tumour was found. **(A)** The bronchial epithelium shows focal nodular neuroendocrine cell hyperplasia. **(B)** Bronchioles obliterated by PNC hyperplasia and carcinoid tumorlets were readily found in the resected left upper lobe.

The author expressed surprise that as both lesions show neuroendocrine differentiation, this association was not more common. In fact, not a single case of peripheral carcinoid tumor or any other type of neuroendocrine tumor is reported in any of those patients with multiple carcinoid tumorlets that have occurred in the setting of preexisting chronic lung disease.

It seems odd that while peripheral carcinoids are seen not infrequently in the setting of DIPNECH and perhaps in a forme fruste of that disease,[351] they are not found with tumorlets in chronic scarring/bronchiectasis, especially since the latter scenario is much more common, relatively speaking. There are no data to suggest why such a difference should exist. Although it could be argued that tumorlets occurring in the setting of chronic lung inflammation reflect reactive hyperplasia and that those seen in the absence of fibrosis may have neoplastic potential, the poor distinction between hyperplasia and neoplasia in this context makes any conclusion difficult.

Apart from the coexistence of tumorlets and peripheral spindle cell type carcinoid tumors in particular, whether or not in the context of DIPNECH, the expression of TTF-1 in both these types of lesion, with much less staining seen in central-type carcinoids, supports the morphologic evidence that peripheral carcinoids derive from tumorlets but central carcinoids arise through a different mechanism. While the expression of TTF-1 was absent in one study,[365] the experience of one of us and the findings of Du et al.[366] show that TTF-1 is expressed in tumorlets and peripheral-type carcinoids. This fits with the suggestion that TTF-1 is a peripheral airway epithelial cell lineage marker that is not found in central bronchial airway cells, including neuroendocrine cells.[286,365]

While tumorlets may thus be a precursor for peripheral spindle cell carcinoids, almost nothing is known about the origin of central-type bronchial carcinoid tumors. In the past there has been speculation, but without any real evidence, that they may derive from bronchial submucous glands.[367] Pulmonary neuroendocrine cells are believed to differentiate from bronchial epithelial stem cells, and, as such, neoplasms arising in the airways may well express this form of differentiation. Sporadic typical bronchial carcinoid tumors have been shown to have both *MEN1* gene mutation in about one third of cases[368] and LOH of chromosome 11, especially in the region of 11q13, close to the site of the *MEN1* gene in 22% to 47% of tumors.[368–370] Finkelstein et al.[371] also showed allelic imbalance in the region of 11q13 (*int-2*) in 73% of typical carcinoids, while similar imbalance was found in one carcinoid tumorlet (9%), which had not coexisted with any carcinoid tumor. In four patients with carcinoid tumors and tumorlets, the latter showed no losses at 11q13, in contrast to the associated tumor. This discordance in genotype rules out the possibility that the tumorlets were some form of metastasis from the carcinoid tumor. Although two of their cases were described as peripheral spindle cell carcinoids, specific data on these cases are not given.

The presence of alterations in the 11q13 region may be of importance in the development of carcinoid tumors, but the relationship between this and tumorlet formation is unclear. In the absence of any other molecular data on tumorlets, discussion of the limited literature of molecular studies of carcinoid tumors is beyond the scope of this chapter. There is no known morphologically recognizable precursor for central bronchial carcinoid tumors. Furthermore, most evidence suggests that the development of carcinoid tumors and high-grade neuroendocrine carcinomas are unrelated.

Origin of High-Grade Neuroendocrine Tumors

There is no specific precursor lesion recognized for SCLC or for large cell neuroendocrine carcinoma (LCNEC), but SCLC is not infrequently associated with SD/CIS in the adjacent airways.[372] Saccomanno et al.[106] found five patients with CIS diagnosed on sputum atypia who subsequently developed SCLC; three of these patients also developed squamous cell carcinoma. In this study there was no significant difference in the duration of the stages of moderate and severe atypia and CIS prior to the onset of either squamous cell or small cell carcinoma. The authors thus speculated that small cell carcinoma might develop from preexisting SD/CIS, through some "sudden chromosomal change," into a very rapidly progressive invasive tumor. This may well be a remarkably prescient hypothesis, given what we now know of the genetic events involved in SCLC development.

In a murine model of lung carcinogenesis, animals with somatic inactivation of both the *P53* and *RB* genes developed tumors with very close resemblance to human SCLC.[327] These animals also developed precursor lesions consisting of nodules of cells in the airway epithelium whose immunophenotype suggested they were neuroendocrine cells derived from multipotent airway epithelial cells.[373] Despite a temptation to relate this observation to PNC hyperplasia and SCLC in humans, and recognizing the enormous potential importance that this elegant mouse model has for predicting the molecular events that determine the development of human SCLC, there is no known relationship between PNC hyperplasia, tumorlets, and human SCLC.

However, there is evidence that inactivation of Rb is a key step in the genesis of human SCLC. Shapiro et al.[374] reported that the p16^{INK4A}-cyclin D1-CDK4-RB pathway is inactivated by Rb loss in SCLC, while in NSCLC Rb is generally normal, but p16 is low or absent, a state that promotes Rb hyperphosphorylation and loss of function. Rb loss has been found in both LCNEC and SCLC, but not in typical carcinoid tumors.[375] This is one of many genetic and epigenetic alterations that precede and drive the development of SCLC[376] and that differ either qualitatively or quantitatively from NSCLC. Apart from *RB* (13q14) and 5q21–22 losses being more frequent in SCLC, the absence of a K-*ras* mutation in SCLC is another notable difference between this tumor type and NSCLC.[150,376] Other almost universal features in the genetic disarray that characterizes SCLC development are the upregulation of one of the *myc* family of oncogenes, and possibly, if not the earliest change, the inactivation of the tumor suppressor gene *RASSF1A* at 3p21.3 by promoter hypermethylation.[377] It is also worth noting that, while Onuki et al.[378] found LOH at 11q13 in around 70% of their LCNEC and SCLC cases and carcinoid tumors showed almost the same rate of LOH, Debelenko et al.[379] found 11q13 LOH relatively infrequently in a study of nine primary SCLC (one had 11q13 LOH), 13 LCNEC (no 11q13 LOH detected), and 36 SCLC cell lines (two showed 11q13 LOH). *MEN1* gene mutation was never found in any of the SCLC samples, but one instance was detected in a LCNEC. These authors concluded that the pathway and mechanisms of tumorigenesis of carcinoids and high-grade neuroendocrine tumors are different.

While it is conceivable that the various genetic and epigenetic events required to determine the small cell phenotype may occur within SD/CIS as predicted by Saccomanno et al.,[106] an alternative scenario has been proposed by Wistuba et al.[380] In their study of patients with both SCLC and NSCLC, allelic losses were up to 10 times more frequent and more extensive in histologically normal or hyperplastic bronchial epithelium from the bronchi of smokers with SCLC when compared to those with NSCLC. In particular, histologically normal epithelium from those with SCLC showed much more frequent LOH at 5q21–22 and 17p13 (*P53*), although 13q14 (*RB*) loss was not demonstrated. Thus they propose that SCLC may develop directly from histologically normal or hyperplastic bronchial epithelium without any morphologically recognizable precursor, the so-called parallel theory of lung cancer development.[224,380] (Fig. 34.30).

This is clearly a complex and poorly understood area in lung carcinogenesis and much remains to be learned. Squamous dysplasia/CIS does occur in association with SCLC, but may not be the precursor lesion. Instead it may be a case of coexistence due to a shared common etiology with SCLC—tobacco smoke. Perhaps, as predicted, certain genetic alterations occur leading to the rapid development of SCLC, but these events occur not on a background of SD/CIS but within phenotypically normal, genotypically scrambled bronchial epithelium.[376,380]

Although there are qualitative similarities, but quantitative differences, in the genetic abnormalities found in the range of neuroendocrine tumors,[378] most evidence suggests that the morphogenesis of SCLC and LCNEC is quite distinct from that of carcinoid tumors. Epidemiologically the former are seen in older smokers with a male preponderance, whereas carcinoids are not smoking-associated and predominate in younger females. Also, SCLC and LCNEC are not seen in DIPNECH. Carcinoid tumor is, in general, not seen as part of a lung cancer

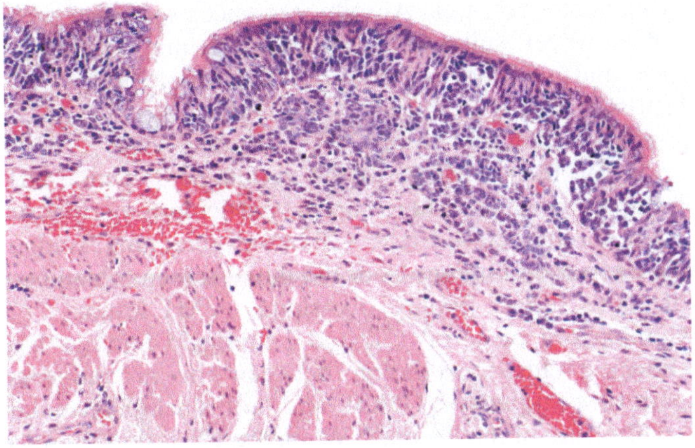

FIGURE 34.30. An example of small cell lung carcinoma developing de novo from bronchial epithelium. This tiny plaque-like lesion was found incidentally in bronchial mucosa during routine microscopic examination of a lung resected for squamous cell carcinoma.

showing mixed differentiation, while high-grade neuroendocrine tumors are seen in this setting. Sturm et al.[365] demonstrated TTF-1 expression in 85% of SCLC and 49% of LCNEC but none in PNC hyperplasia, tumorlets or carcinoid tumors providing further support for distinct pathways of development, even although these data on TTF-1 in carcinoids have been challenged.

Lung Tumor Development: Lessons from Immunocytochemistry and Genetics

The classification of preinvasive lung lesions has followed a traditional morphologic approach. Simple H&E histology is cheap, easy, and with a degree of expertise may provide a wealth of clinically useful information. There is, however, a current vogue for the molecular classification of lung cancer, seeking better prognostication of disease and the possibility of tailoring therapy according to the tumor's genetic or protein expression profile.

Studies of morphologically normal respiratory epithelium in smokers have demonstrated genetic "lesions," and Mao[381] has suggested that, in parallel with evolving SD/CIS, there are between three and 12 critical alterations needed for the malignant phenotype. The pattern of genetic change in smoking-damaged bronchial epithelium is different (and more extensive) in those with SCLC when compared to patients with NSCLC. This raises a number of questions regarding the histologic type of tumor that emerges when the full malignant phenotype develops. Ultimately the tumor is the product of a number of critical genetic alterations, which determine both the dysregulated growth and the pattern of differentiation. The type of lung cancer that develops may also depend on the particular stem cells that are transformed. Preinvasive lesions retain many of the characteristics of their progenitor cell population, presumably since their genotype is less deviant. Certain factors may determine patterns of differentiation, but the relationship between these and transforming genetic events, such as inactivation of TSGs and upregulation of other genes, is unclear. Some changes may be more deterministic of malignant transformation regardless of tumor type (*FHIT, P53*), but others are more type (differentiation) specific (K-*ras* and adenocarcinoma, *P16* in NSCLC, *RB* in SCLC, etc.). Other changes may be more likely in cells that are differentiating in a particular direction. It is difficult to know, however, what is cause and what is effect in these circumstances.

Some treated SCLC may recur as NSCLC.[382] In mixed tumors, an LCNEC component differentiates from and retains the TTF-1 status of the adenocarcinoma or squamous cell carcinoma from which it derives,[229] and many large cell undifferentiated carcinomas may be terminally differentiated adenocarcinomas. This demonstrates the potential for neoplastic clones to switch patterns of differentiation and how, by the time a tumor is advanced and symptomatic it may have progressed from a preinvasive precursor, through a stage of early cancer reflecting its origin, to a lesion that has deviated further, both morphologically and genetically, from its original form.

Preinvasive Lung Lesions: Lessons for and from Lung Cancer Screening

As already mentioned, lung cancer is a major global health problem; it is almost universally fatal if it presents symptomatically. On the other hand, populations at risk from lung cancer may be defined, the disease may be cured if treated early, and new technology has improved our ability to detect early disease. Lung cancer is thus an ideal candidate for cancer screening.[383] Although surgical resection of stage IA disease may give an 85% cure rate,[384] up to 15% of patients with tumors of 1 cm or less have metastatic disease at presentation.[385] The onset of invasion poses an immediate risk of metastases, so there is a premium on detecting preinvasive disease. If the proportion of detected cases that are still at a preinvasive stage can be increased, then improved outcomes can be expected.

In general, for a lung tumor to be visible on a plain chest x-ray film, it must be at least 1 cm in diameter and not obscured by any normal structure. Such a lesion is unlikely to be symptomatic and thus will not come to medical attention unless through screening or as an incidental finding. A solid 1-cm tumor mass contains very approximately 10^{10} cells, and assuming we start with one cell, such a mass would take approximately 30 volume doublings to appear. Doubling time (DT) varies enormously between tumors and during the natural history of a tumor, but again assuming, for the sake of this argument, that DT is 100 days,[386] then the tumor has taken over 8 years to reach a 1-cm diameter. Even if we start with a hypothetical clonal patch of 1 to 2 mm^2 in the bronchial epithelium,[176] about 4 years would be needed. Of course this makes a number of barely justifiable assumptions. Preinvasive lesions are clonal, but can we relate the lesion back to one cell? Preinvasive lesions in the lung periphery are clearly not solid. The assumed DT of 100 days may be wildly wrong, though cell proliferation studies suggest perhaps not. Constant progression is assumed when in fact there is evidence, at least with SD/CIS, that lesions may wax and wane. The essence of this argument, however, is that even allowing for some considerable errors in estimating early tumor growth kinetics, the preclinical phase of a tumor (no symptoms, undetectable by conventional means) is very long, relative to the clinical phase, assuming exponential growth. For much of this time the lesion will be in a preinvasive stage. For success in lung cancer screening, it is thus essential to shift our detection phase backward into the preclinical phase to detect preinvasive or very early invasive disease.

This chapter has described in considerable detail two completely separate pathways of lung tumor development, one in the central bronchi based on SD/CIS from which most squamous cell and possibly some small cell lung cancers develop, and one in the lung periphery based on AAH, which probably accounts for the majority of adenocarcinomas. It is essential that lung cancer screening strategies take both these pathways into account.

The plain chest radiograph views the whole lung, but cannot detect any preinvasive disease, and any visible cancer, almost by definition, is relatively advanced, particularly if centrally located. This may be part of the reason why chest radiograph-based screening programs in the 1970s were unsuccessful in reducing cancer mortality.[109] Sputum cytology is less efficient than the chest radiograph for detecting lung cancer, has an overall average sensitivity of approximately 65% (though quoted figures range from 22% to 98%), and is most successful with central tumors, squamous cell tumors, and more advanced disease, but may also detect SD/CIS.[387] Chest radiography and sputum cytology in combination detect more tumors than either alone, but preinvasive disease remains elusive. Autofluorescence bronchoscopy has provided a sensitive method of localizing preinvasive or very early, radiographically occult invasive bronchial disease, which may be detected by sputum cytology, but which is invisible at standard white-light bronchoscopy.[388] This approach has facilitated many studies of bronchial preinvasive neoplasia and is responsible, in part, for the considerable advances made in our understanding of the biology of SD/CIS by making more pathologic material available for research. Autofluorescence bronchoscopy is not, however, suitable as a practical primary screening tool and will not identify all bronchial preinvasive lesions.[91]

High-resolution spiral CT scanning has greatly improved the sensitivity of the radiologic detection and localization of early lung cancer, particularly peripheral adenocarcinoma.[389] Eight CT-based screening studies have reported findings from the initial screen,[390] and two of these report finding occasional AAH lesions.[391,392] Comparison of spiral CT and pathologic findings has shown a close correlation between the ground-glass pattern of opacity (GGO) and a bronchioloalveolar architecture in the lesion.[393] When the CT lesion shows a pure GGO pattern, 70% of these lesions are LNMBAC and 27% are AAH, but only 3% are invasive adenocarcinoma.[394] Furthermore, the presence of solid areas within a GGO is even more strongly associated with a malignant diagnosis and corresponds to the alveolar collapse and fibroblastic proliferation of type B and C tumors.[331,395] So far confirmation of diagnosis of these lesions has required surgical excision, since AAH and LNMBAC cannot be diagnosed by fine-needle aspiration cytology.[396]

Currently available technology has the capability of detecting (sputum cytology plus spiral CT) and localizing (autofluorescence bronchoscopy and spiral CT) early lung cancers and a proportion of preinvasive lesions. It remains to be seen whether newer methods such as combined CT and positron emission tomography will have anything to offer in the detection of small invasive tumors (possibly) or preinvasive disease (unlikely). Our knowledge of the molecular biology of preinvasive diseases may highlight possible marker-based approaches to refining sputum cytology detection of neoplastic cells or even suggest a potential molecular marker present in sputum or blood.[387,397,398]

Once disease is detected and localized, what next? These decisions will depend on the prevailing knowledge of the likelihood of progression of the disease, and, at least in SD/CIS, there are potential markers that may help decide. Should lung cancer screening become mainstream, pathologists will be faced with handling and diagnosing lesions that, to date, are relatively uncommon in surgical histopathologic practice. This reinforces the need for robust, repeatable criteria for lesion classification. It will also be essential that every opportunity be taken to ensure that new radiologic and molecular biologic approaches to detecting and diagnosing preinvasive or early invasive lung cancer are underpinned by adequate pathologic evidence as the gold-standard diagnosis. There is optimism that, as more is learned about preinvasive disease, better chemopreventive strategies may evolve.[399] With increased opportunity to handle more of these hitherto relatively rare lesions comes the chance to undertake research in this crucially important area, to improve our ability to detect, diagnose, and treat this most common and deadly malignancy.

Conclusion

This chapter has reviewed in some detail those lesions in the lung that are considered to be preinvasive precursors of invasive lung cancer. As well as considering the specific lesions included in the WHO classification of lung tumors, namely squamous dysplasia/carcinoma in situ, atypical adenomatous hyperplasia, and diffuse idiopathic neuroendocrine cell hyperplasia, other lung diseases that carry an additional risk of lung cancer development have been described.

Recent times have seen a considerable increase in our knowledge of the structure, cell biology, and genetics of preinvasive lung disease. While the work of Auerbach and colleagues in the late 1950s laid the foundation for our current ideas on bronchial carcinogenesis through SD/CIS, it was 30 years later that a similar basis for peripheral lung adenocarcinogenesis was proposed by Shimosato, Miller, and others. These careful morphologic studies underpinned the extensive and ever-expanding literature on the biology of these pathways of lung carcinogenesis discussed in this chapter. There are clearly different pathways of lung carcinogenesis, which in part define the type of tumor that develops, but it is possible that other pathways remain to be discovered. There is abundant evidence that genetic changes occur that drive the evolution of the lesions, but many of these changes are not consistently found or do not occur in the same order. It has been suggested that perhaps between three and 12 critical genetic alterations are required for the full malignant phenotype to evolve.[381] There is no inevitability to the progression of these lesions. Longitudinal studies are very difficult to conduct, but many lesions appear to wax and wane and, if malignancy develops, this probably takes some considerable time.

The relative inaccessibility of the lung has made it difficult to obtain material from preinvasive disease for research. The earliest work on bronchial carcinogenesis relied on detailed examination of tens of thousands of sections derived from autopsy lungs and the study of sputum cytology specimens. The more recent introduction of fiberoptic bronchoscopy, in particular utilizing autofluorescence detection methods, has been a key advance in the study of SD/CIS, allowing direct visualization and biopsy of much of the bronchial tree and improved lesion detection, and has presented the prospect of longitudinal studies of lesions' natural history. Obtaining material to study peripheral adenocarcinogenesis is even more difficult. It remains to be seen whether spiral CT scanning and limited surgical resection of screen-detected lesions will provide us with opportunities to replicate the amount of detailed genetic work that has been possible on SD/CIS. The lack of a recognized precursor lesion of small cell lung cancer has meant this pathway of lung carcinogenesis has remained largely unexplored. The possibility of a genetic lesion without a specific morphologic correlate is suggested by recent work in patients with SCLC and by an exciting new animal model.

Examination of increasingly small tissue samples in an attempt to identify or rule out precancerous changes is an increasing part of the surgical pathologist's work,[400] and lung cancer screening may add to this load. Although we have an improved classification of pulmonary preinvasive lesions, there are still many unknowns and much has still to be learned. The fact that these lesions represent only a partial evolution, from normal, of the malignant phenotype, and our classification is, to a large extent, an artificial division of a biologic continuum means that preinvasive lesions are more difficult to recognize than full-blown cancer. While some of the criticism of pathologists over our lack of diagnostic consistency may be justified,[122] these are difficult lesions to work with, and we must guard against being inappropriately confident in our diagnosis in an area littered with uncertainty.[401]

And what does our diagnosis mean for the patient? Page[402] described preinvasive disease as having "specific anatomic features with only suggested clinical implications." Indeed the core issue is one of risk, the risk of developing invasive disease. We know little about this risk in preinvasive lung disease. Even though SD/CIS has been extensively studied, there is still much debate over the likelihood of progression and therefore the need for treatment.[403] We currently have little or no idea of the relative risks posed by the other forms of preinvasive lung disease. As Foucar[401] eloquently stated, "It is important that pathologists evaluating changes in early malignancy avoid the trap of moving from prediction to prophesy."

Lung cancer remains a considerable medical problem in Europe and North America and the rise in tobacco consumption that parallels economic development elsewhere in the world means that it will be a global health problem for many years to come. This, coupled with key technological advances, has returned lung cancer screening to the health agenda. Our relative lack of success, to date, in treating symptomatic lung cancer coupled with the prospect of screening for the disease has given new relevance to and kindled renewed interest in preinvasive and early lung cancer. To improve detection and treatment of this disease at an early stage, a full understanding of its pathology and biology will be essential.

References

1. Travis WD, Colby TV, Corrin B, et al., eds. Histological typing of lung and pleural tumours. WHO International histological classification of tumours. 3rd ed. Berlin: Springer, 1999.
2. Rossle R. Die Narbenkrebse der Lungen. Schweiz Med Wochenschr 1943;73:1200–1203.
3. Friedrich G. Periphere Lungenkrebse auf dem Boden pleuranaher Narben. Virchows Arch (Pathol Anat) 1939; 304:230–247.
4. Spencer H. Lung scar cancer. In: Shimosato Y, Melamed MD, Nettesheim P, eds. Morphogenesis of lung cancer. Vol 1. Boca Raton, FL: CRC Press, 1982:111–120.
5. Carroll R. The influence of lung scars on primary lung cancer. J Path Bact 1962;83:293–297.
6. Raeburn C, Spencer H. A study of the origin and development of lung cancer. Thorax 1953;8:1–10.
7. Auerbach O, Garfinkel L, Parks VR. Scar cancer of the lung. Increase over a 21 year period. Cancer 1979; 43:636–642.
8. Bakris GL, Mulopulos GP, Korchik R, et al. Pulmonary scar carcinoma. A clinicopathological analysis. Cancer 1983;52:493–497.
9. Edwards C, Carlile A. Scar adenocarcinoma of the lung: a light and electron microscopic study. J Clin Pathol 1986;39:423–427.
10. Shimosato Y, Hashimoto T, Kodama T, et al. Prognostic implications of fibrotic focus (scar) in small peripheral lung cancers. Am J Surg Pathol 1980;4:365–373.
11. Shimosato Y, Kodama T, Kameya T. Morphogenesis of peripheral type adenocarcinoma of the lung. In: Shimosato Y, Melamed MR, Nettesheim P, eds. Morphogenesis of lung cancer. Vol 1. Boca Raton, FL: CRC Press, 1982:65–90.
12. Suzuki A. Growth characteristics of peripheral type adenocarcinoma in terms of roentgenologic findings. In: Shimosato Y, Melamed MR, Nettesheim P, eds. Morphogenesis of lung cancer. Vol 1. Boca Raton, FL: CRC Press, 1982:91–110.
13. Cagle PT, Cohle SD, Greenberg SD. Natural history of pulmonary scar cancers. Clinical and pathological implications. Cancer 1985;56:2031–2035.
14. Madri JA, Carter D. Scar cancers of the lung: origin and significance. Hum Pathol 1984;15:625–631.
15. Kolin A, Koutoulakis T. Role of arterial occlusion in pulmonary scar cancers. Hum Pathol 1988;19:1161–1167.
16. Kung ITM, Mok CK, Lui IOL, et al. Pulmonary scar cancer. A pathologic reappraisal. Am J Surg Pathol 1985; 9:391–400.
17. Barsky SH, Huang SJ, Bhuta S. The extracellular matrix of pulmonary scar carcinomas is suggestive of a desmoplastic origin. Am J Pathol 1986;124: 412–419.
18. El-Torkey M, Giltman LI, Dabbous M. Collagens in scar carcinoma of the lung. Am J Pathol 1985;121:322–326.
19. Yoneda K. Scar carcinomas of the lung in a Histoplasmosis endemic area. Cancer 1990;65:164–168.
20. Bell ET. Hyperplasia of the pulmonary alveolar epithelium in disease. Am J Pathol 1943;19:901–907.
21. Geevers EF, Neubuerger KT, Davis CL. The pulmonary alveolar lining under various pathologic conditions in man and animals. Am J Pathol 1943;19:913–937.
22. Winternitz MC, Wason IM, Mcnamara FP. The pathology of influenza. New Haven: Yale University Press, 1920.
23. Meyer EC, Liebow AA. Relationship of interstitial pneumonia honeycombing and atypical epithelial proliferation to cancer of the lung. Cancer 1965;18:322–351.
24. Fraire AE, Greenberg SD. Carcinoma and diffuse interstitial fibrosis of lung. Cancer 1973;31:1078–1086.
25. Turner-Warwick M, Lebowitz M, Burrows B, et al. Cryptogenic fibrosing alveolitis and lung cancer. Thorax 1980; 35:496–499.
26. Ma Y, Seneviratne CK, Koss M. Idiopathic pulmonary fibrosis and malignancy. Curr Opin Pulm Med 2001;7: 278–282.
27. Stack BH, Choo-Kang YF, Heard BE. The prognosis of cryptogenic fibrosing alveolitis. Thorax 1972;27:535–542.
28. Matsushita H, Tanaka S, Saiki Y, et al. Lung cancer associated with usual interstitial pneumonia. Pathol Int 1995; 45:925–932.
29. Qunn L, Takemura T, Ikushima S, et al. Hyperplastic epithelial foci in honeycomb lesions in idiopathic pulmonary fibrosis. Virchows Arch 2002;441:271–278.
30. Mizushima Y, Kobayashi M. Clinical characteristics of synchronous multiple lung cancer associated with idiopathic pulmonary fibrosis. A review of Japanese cases. Chest 1995;108:1271–1277.
31. Samet JM. Does idiopathic pulmonary fibrosis increase lung cancer risk? Am J Respir Crit Care Med 2000; 161:1–2.
32. Hironaka M, Fukayama M. Pulmonary fibrosis and lung carcinoma: a comparative study of metaplastic epithelia in honeycombed areas of usual interstitial pneumonia with or without lung carcinoma. Pathol Int 1999;49: 1060–1066.
33. Sakai S, Ono M, Nishio T, et al. Lung cancer associated with diffuse pulmonary fibrosis: CT-pathologic correlation. J Thorac Imaging 2003;18:67–71.
34. Baumgartner KB, Samet JM, Stidley CA, et al. Cigarette smoking—a risk factor for idiopathic pulmonary fibrosis. Am J Respir Crit Care Med 1997;155:242–248.
35. Hubbard R, Venn A, Lewis S, et al. Lung cancer and cryptogenic fibrosing alveolitis. A population-based cohort study. Am J Respir Crit Care Med 2000;161:5–8.
36. Aubry MC, Myers JL, Douglas WW, et al. Primary pulmonary carcinoma in patients with idiopathic pulmonary fibrosis. Mayo Clin Proc 2002;77:763–770.
37. Ardies CM. Inflammation as cause for scar cancers of the lung. Integr Cancer Ther 2003;2:238–246.
38. Kawasaki H, Ogura T, Yokose T, et al. p53 gene alteration in atypical epithelial lesions and carcinoma in patients with idiopathic pulmonary fibrosis. Hum Pathol 2001;32: 1043–1049.
39. Takahashi T, Munakata M, Ohtsuka Y, et al. Expression and alteration of ras and p53 proteins in patients with lung carcinoma accompanied by idiopathic pulmonary fibrosis. Cancer 2002;95:624–633.
40. Demopoulos K, Arvanitis DA, Vassilakis DA, et al. MYCL1, FHIT, SPARC, p16(INK4) and TP53 genes

associated to lung cancer in idiopathic pulmonary fibrosis. J Cell Mol Med 2002;6:215–222.
41. Uematsu K, Yoshimura A, Gemma A, et al. Aberrations in the fragile histidine triad (FHIT) gene in idiopathic pulmonary fibrosis. Cancer Res 2001;61:8527–8533.
42. Tokarskaya ZB, Okladnikova ND, Belyaeva ZD, et al. The influence of radiation and nonradiation factors on the lung cancer incidence among the workers of the nuclear enterprise. Mayak Health Phys 1995;69:356–366.
43. Ohno S, Oshikawa K, Kitamura S, et al. Clinicopathological analysis of interstitial pneumonia associated with collagen vascular disease in patients with lung cancer. (In Japanese. English abstract). Nihon Kyobu Shikkan Gakkai Zasshi 1997;35:1324–1329.
44. Yang Y, Fujita J, Tokuda M, et al. Lung cancer associated with several connective tissue diseases: with a review of literature. Rheumatol Int 2001;21:106–111.
45. Peters-Golden M, Wide RA, Hochberg M, et al. Incidence of lung cancer in systemic sclerosis. J Rheumatol 1985; 12:1136–1139.
46. Talbott JH, Barrocas M. Carcinoma of the lung in progressive systemic sclerosis: a tabular review of the literature and a detailed report of the roentgenographic changes in two cases. Semin Arthritis Rheum 1980;9:191–217.
47. Matteson EL, Hickey AR, Maguire L, et al. Occurrence of neoplasia in patients with rheumatoid arthritis enrolled on DMARD Registry. Rheumatoid Arthritis Azathioprine Registry Steering Committee. J Rheumatol 1991; 18:809–814.
48. Greenberg SD, Roggli VL. Carcinoma of the lung. In: Roggli VL, Greenberg SD, Pratt PC, eds. Pathology of asbestos-associated diseases. Boston: Little, Brown, 1993: 189–210.
49. Mossman BT, Churg A. Mechanisms in the pathogenesis of asbestosis and silicosis. Am J Respir Crit Care Med 1998;157:1666–1680.
50. Henderson DW, de Klerk NH, Hammar SP, et al. Asbestos and lung cancer: is it attributable to asbestosis or asbestos fibre burden? In: Corrin B, ed. Pathology of lung tumours. Edinburgh: Churchill Livingstone, 1997: 83–118.
51. Jones RN, Hughes JM, Weill H. Asbestos exposure, asbestosis and asbestos-attributable lung cancer. Thorax 1996; 51(suppl 2):S9–S15.
52. Churg A. Lung cancer cell type and asbestos exposure. JAMA 1985;253:2984–2985.
53. Nelson HH, Kelsey KT. The molecular epidemiology of asbestos and tobacco in lung cancer. Oncogene 2002; 21:7284–7288.
54. Katabami M, Dosaka-Akita H, Honma K, et al. Pneumoconiosis-related lung cancers: preferential occurrence from diffuse interstitial fibrosis-type pneumoconiosis. Am J Respir Crit Care Med 2000;162:295–300.
55. Silicosis and Silicate Disease Committee: Craighead JE (chairman). Diseases associated with exposure to silica and nonfibrous silicate minerals. Arch Pathol Lab Med 1988;112:673–720.
56. Churg A, Green FHY. Occupational lung disease. In: Thurlbeck WM, Churg AM, eds. Pathology of the lung. 2nd ed. New York: Thieme, 1995:851–929.
57. Weill H, McDonald JC. Exposure to crystalline silica and risk of lung cancer: the epidemiological evidence. Thorax 1995;51:97–102.
58. MacSweeney F, Papagiannopoulos K, Goldstraw P, et al. An assessment of the expanded classification of congenital cystic adenomatoid malformations and their relationship to malignant transformation. Am J Surg Pathol 2003; 27:1139–1146.
59. Granata C, Gambini C, Balducci T, et al. Bronchioloalveolar carcinoma arising in congenital cystic adenomatoid malformation in a child: a case report and review on malignancies originating in congenital cystic adenomatoid malformation. Pediatr Pulmonol 1998;25:62–66.
60. Ribet ME, Copin MC, Soots JG, et al. Bronchioloalveolar carcinoma and congenital cystic adenomatoid malformation. Ann Thorac Surg 1995;60:1126–1128.
61. Kaslovsky RA, Purdy S, Dangman BC, et al. Bronchioloalveolar carcinoma in a child with congenital cystic adenomatoid malformation. Chest 1997;112:548–551.
62. Benjamin DR, Cahill JL. Bronchioloalveolar carcinoma of the lung and congenital cystic adenomatoid malformation. Am J Clin Pathol 1991;95:889–892.
63. Sheffield EA, Addis BJ, Corrin B, et al. Epithelial hyperplasia and malignant change in congenital lung cysts. J Clin Pathol 1987;40:612–614.
64. Stacher E, Ullmann R, Halbwedl I, et al. Atypical goblet cell hyperplasia in congenital cystic adenomatoid malformation as a possible preneoplasia for pulmonary adenocarcinoma in childhood: A genetic analysis. Hum Pathol 2004;35:565–570.
65. Guillou L, Sahli R, Chaubert P, et al. Squamous cell carcinoma of the lung in a non-smoking, nonirradiated patient with juvenile laryngotracheal papillomatosis. Evidence of human papillomavirus-11 DNA in both carcinoma and papillomas. Am J Surg Pathol 1991;15:891–898.
66. Simma B, Burger R, Uehlinger J, et al. Squamous-cell carcinoma arising in a non-irradiated child with recurrent respiratory papillomatosis. Eur J Pediatr 1993; 152:776–778.
67. DiLorenzo TP, Tamsen A, Abramson AL, et al. Human papillomavirus type 6a DNA in the lung carcinoma of a patient with recurrent laryngeal papillomatosis is characterized by a partial duplication. J Gen Virol 1992; 73:423–428.
68. Popper HH, el-Shabrawi Y, Wockel W, et al. Prognostic importance of human papilloma virus typing in squamous cell papilloma of the bronchus: comparison of in situ hybridisation and the polymerase chain reaction. Hum Pathol 1994;25:1191–1197.
69. Prichard MG, Brown PJ, Sterrett GF. Bronchioloalveolar carcinoma arising in longstanding lung cysts. Thorax 1984;39:545–549.
70. De Perrot M, Pache JC, Spiliopoulos A. Carcinoma arising in congenital lung cysts. J Thorac Cardiovasc Surg 2001; 49:184–185.
71. Bell-Thomson J, Missier P, Sommers SC. Lung carcinoma arising in bronchopulmonary sequestration. Cancer 1979; 44:334–339.
72. Konwaler BE, Reingold IM. Carcinoma arising in bronchiectatic cavities. Cancer 1952;5:525–529.

73. Tonelli P. A morphological study of nodular lung carcinomas and their possible pathogenesis from a cluster of non-obstructive bronchiectasis. Lung Cancer 1997;17:135–145.
74. Sawada M, Inase N, Imai M, et al. Chromosome 9p deletion in squamous metaplasia in cystic lesion of the lung. Respirology 2003;8:239–242.
75. Willis RA. The pathology of tumours, fourth edition. London: Butterworths, 1967:1.
76. Auerbach O, Gere JB, Forman JB, et al. Changes in the bronchial epithelium in relation to smoking and cancer of the lung. N Engl J Med 1957;256:97–104.
77. Travis WD. Lung. In: Henson DE, Albores-Saavedra J, eds. Pathology of incipient neoplasia. New York: Oxford University Press, 2001:295–316.
78. Lamb D, Reid L. Goblet cell increases in rat bronchial epithelium after exposure to cigarette and cigar tobacco smoke. Br Med J 1969;1:33–35.
79. Trump BF, McDowell EM, Glavin F, et al. The respiratory epithelium. III Histogenesis of epidermoid metaplasia and carcinoma in situ in the human. J Natl Cancer Inst 1978; 61:563–575.
80. Auerbach O, Hammond EC, Garfinkel L. Changes in bronchial epithelium in relation to smoking, 1955–1960 vs. 1970–1977. N Engl J Med 1979;300:381–386.
81. Peters EJ, Morice R, Benner SE, et al. Squamous metaplasia of the bronchial mucosa and its relationship to smoking. Chest 1993;103:1429–1432.
82. Saccomanno G, Saunders RP, Archer VE, et al. Cancer of the lung—the cytology of sputum prior to the development of carcinoma. Acta Cytol 1965;9:413–423.
83. Calderon-Garciduenas L, Rodriguez-Alcaraz A, Villarreal-Calderon A, et al. Nasal epithelium as a sentinel for airborne environmental pollution. Toxicol Sci 1998;46:352–364.
84. Gong H Jr, Fligiel S, Tashkin DP, et al. Tracheobronchial changes in habitual, heavy smokers of marijuana with and without tobacco. Am Rev Respir Dis 1987;136:142–149.
85. Mayne ST Redlich CA, Cullen MR. Dietary vitamin A and prevalence of bronchial metaplasia in asbestos-exposed workers. Am J Clin Nutr 1998;68:630–635.
86. Valentine EH. Squamous metaplasia of the bronchus; a study of metaplastic changes occurring in the epithelium of the major bronchi in cancerous and noncancerous cases. Cancer 1957;10:272–279.
87. Auerbach O, Stout AP, Hammond EC, et al. Changes in bronchial epithelium in relation to sex, age, residence, smoking and pneumonia. N Engl J Med 1962; 267:111–119.
88. Gazdar AF, Carbone DP. The biology and molecular genetics of lung cancer. Austin, TX: RG Landes; 1994:54.
89. Melamed MR, Zaman MB. Pathogenesis of epidermoid carcinoma of lung. In: Shimosato Y, Melamed MR, Nettesheim P, eds. Morphogenesis of lung cancer. Volume 1. Boca Raton, FL: CRC Press, 1982:37–64.
90. Auerbach O, Stout AP, Hammond EC, et al. Changes in bronchial epithelium in relation to cigarette smoking and in relation to lung cancer. N Engl J Med 1961; 265:255–267.
91. Hirsch FR, Prindiville SA, Miller YE, et al. Fluorescence versus white-light bronchoscopy for detection of preneoplastic lesions: a randomised study. J Natl Cancer Inst 2001;93:1385–1391.
92. Carter D, Marsh BR, Baker RR, et al. Relationship of morphology to clinical presentation in ten cases of early squamous cell carcinoma of the lung. Cancer 1976; 37:1389–1396.
93. Nagamoto N, Saito Y, Sato M, et al. Clinicopathological analysis of 19 cases of isolated carcinoma in situ of the bronchus. Am J Surg Pathol 1993;17:1234–1243.
94. Woolner LB, Fontana RS, Cortese DA, et al. Roentgenographically occult lung cancer: pathologic findings and frequency of multicentricity during a 10-year period. Mayo Clin Proc 1984;59:453–466.
95. Spencer H, Dail DH, Arneaud J. Non-invasive bronchial epithelial papillary tumors. Cancer 1980;45:1486–1497.
96. Banerjee AK, Rabbitts PH, George J. Lung cancer 3: Fluorescence bronchoscopy: clinical dilemmas and research opportunities. Thorax 2003;58:266–271.
97. Lam S, Kennedy T, Unger M, et al. Localization of bronchial intraepithelial lesions by fluorescence bronchoscopy. Chest 1998;113:696–702.
98. Lam S, MacAulay C, LeRiche JC, et al. Detection and localization of early lung cancer by fluorescence bronchoscopy. Cancer 2000;89:2468–2473.
99. Franklin WA, Wistuba II, Geisinger KR, et al. Squamous dysplasia and carcinoma in situ. In: Travis WD, Brambilla E, Muller-Hermelink HK, et al., eds. World Health Organisation classification of tumours. Pathology and genetics of tumours of the lung, pleura, thymus and heart. Lyon: IARC Press, 2004:68–72.
100. Nuorva K, Soini Y, Kamel D, et al. Concurrent p53 expression in bronchial dysplasias and squamous cell lung carcinomas. Am J Pathol 1993;142:725–732.
101. Fisseler-Eckhoff A, Prebeg M, Voss B, et al. Extracellular matrix in preneoplastic lesions and early cancer of the lung. Pathol Res Pract 1990;186:95–101.
102. Keith RL, Miller YE, Gemmill RM, et al. Angiogenic squamous dysplasia in bronchi of individuals at high risk for lung cancer. Clin Cancer Res 2000;6:1616–1625.
103. Muller KM, Muller G. The ultrastructure of preneoplastic changes in the bronchial mucosa. Curr Top Pathol 1983; 73:233–263.
104. Nasiell M, Auer G, Kato H. Cytological studies in man and animals on development of bronchogenic carcinoma. In: McDowell EM, ed. Lung carcinomas. Edinburgh: Churchill Livingstone, 1987:207–242.
105. Shibuya K, Hoshino H, Chiyo M, et al. High magnification bronchovideoscopy combined with narrow band imaging could detect capillary loops of angiogenic squamous dysplasia in heavy smokers at high risk for lung cancer. Thorax 2003;58:989–995.
106. Saccomanno G, Archer VE, Auerbach O, et al. Development of carcinoma of the lung as reflected in exfoliated cells. Cancer 1974;33:256–270.
107. Frost JK, Erozan YS, Gupta PK. Cytopathology. In: National Cancer Institute cooperative early lung cancer group. Atlas of early lung cancer. Tokyo: Igaku-Shoin, 1983.

108. Tao LC, Chamberlain DW, Delarue NC, et al. Cytologic diagnosis of radiographically occult squamous cell carcinoma of the lung. Cancer 1982;50:1580–1586.
109. Unattributed. Early lung cancer detection: summary and conclusions. Am Rev Respir Dis 1984;130:565–570.
110. Woolner LB, David E, Fontana RS, et al. In situ and early invasive bronchogenic carcinoma. Report of 28 cases with postoperative survival data. J Thorac Cardiovasc Surg 1970;60:275–290.
111. Kennedy TC, Franklin WA, Prindiville SA, et al. High prevalence of occult endobronchial malignancy in high risk patients with moderate sputum atypia. Lung Cancer 2005;49:187–191.
112. Nettesheim P, Klein-Szanto AJP, Yarita T. Experimental models for the study of morphogenesis of lung cancer. In: Shimosato Y, Melamed MR, Nettesheim P, eds. Morphogenesis of lung cancer. Volume 2. Boca Raton, FL: CRC Press, 1982:131–166.
113. Becci PJ, McDowell EM, Trump BF. The respiratory epithelium. IV. Histogenesis of epidermoid metaplasia and carcinoma in situ in the hamster. J Natl Cancer Inst 1978;61:577–586.
114. Auer G, Ono J, Nasiell M, et al. Reversibility of bronchial cell atypia. Cancer Res 1982;42:4241–4247.
115. Hammond EC, Auerbach O, Kirman D, et al. Effects of cigarette smoking in dogs. Arch Environ Health 1970; 21:740–753.
116. Auerbach O. Pathogenesis of lung cancer. Cancer 1961; 7:11–21.
117. Auerbach O, Saccomanno G, Kuschner M, et al. Histologic findings in the tracheobronchial tree of uranium miners and non-miners with lung cancer. Cancer 1978; 42:483–489.
118. Lam S, LeRiche JC, Zheng Y, et al. Sex-related differences in bronchial epithelial changes associated with tobacco smoking. J Natl Cancer Inst 1999;91:691–696.
119. Frost JK, Ball WC, Levin ML, et al. Sputum cytopathology: use and potential in monitoring the workplace environment by screening for biological effects of exposure. J Occup Med 1986;28:692–703.
120. Agapitos E, Delsedime L, Kalandidi A, et al. Correlation with early pathological lesions in the bronchial tree with environmental exposures: study objectives and preliminary findings. IARC Sci Publ 1991;112:263–268.
121. Lam S, Hung JY, Kennedy SM, et al. Detection of dysplasia and carcinoma in situ by ratio fluorimetry. Am Rev Respir Dis 1992;146:1458–1461.
122. Venmans BJ, Van der Linden JC, Elbers JRJ, et al. Observer variability in histopathological reporting of bronchial biopsy specimens: Influence on the results of autofluorescence bronchoscopy in detection of bronchial neoplasia. J Bronchol 2000;7:210–214.
123. Nicholson AG, Perry LJ, Cury PM, et al. Reproducibility of the WHO/IASLC grading system for pre-invasive squamous lesions of the bronchus: a study of inter-observer and intra-observer variation. Histopathology 2001;38: 202–208.
124. Colby TV, Koss MN, Travis WD. Tumours of the lower respiratory tract. Atlas of tumour pathology. Washington, DC: AFIP, 1995.
125. Tan KK, Kennedy MM, Kerr KM, et al. Patient survival and bronchial resection line status in primary lung carcinoma. Thorax 1995;50:437P.
126. Pasic A, Grünberg K, Mooi W, et al. The natural history of carcinoma in situ involving bronchial resection margins. Lung Cancer 2005;49(suppl 2):S57.
127. Aubert Amoro-Sibilot D, Diab S, et al. Prognostic significance of carcinoma in situ in the vicinity of non small cell resected lung cancer in stage I to IIIA. Lung Cancer 2005;49(suppl 2):S57.
128. Suprun H, Hjerpe A, Nasiell M, et al. A correlative cytologic study of the incidence of pulmonary cancer and other lung diseases associated with squamous metaplasia of the bronchial epithelium. In: Niebergs HE, ed. Prevention and detection of cancer: Part 2, detection. New York: Marcel Dekker, 1980:1303–1320.
129. Risse EKJ, Vooijs GP, van't Hof MA. Diagnostic significance of 'severe dysplasia' in sputum cytology. Acta Cytol 1988;32:629–634.
130. Satoh Y, Ishikawa Y, Nakagawa K, et al. A follow-up study of progression from dysplasia to squamous cell carcinoma with immunohistochemical examination of p53 protein overexpression in the bronchi of ex-chromate workers. Br J Cancer 1997;75:678–683.
131. Thiberville L, Payne P, Vielkinds J, et al. Evidence of cumulative gene losses with progression of premalignant epithelial lesions to carcinoma of the bronchus. Cancer Res 1995;55:5133–5139.
132. Venmans BJ, van Boxem TJ, Smit EF, et al. Outcome of bronchial carcinoma in situ. Chest 2000;117:1572–1576.
133. Sutedja TG, Venmans BJ, Smit EF, et al. Fluorescence bronchoscopy for early detection of lung cancer. A clinical perspective. Lung Cancer 2001;34:157–168.
134. Sutedja TG, Postmus PE. Personal communication, 2004.
135. Bota S, Auliac J-B, Paris C, et al. Follow-up of bronchial precancerous lesions and carcinoma in situ using fluorescence endoscopy. Am J Crit Care Med 2001;164: 1688–1693.
136. Ponticiello A, Barra E, Giani U, et al. P53 immunohistochemistry can identify bronchial dysplastic lesions proceeding to lung cancer: a prospective study. Eur Respir J 2000;15:547–552.
137. Moro-Sibilot D, Fievet F, Jeanmart M, et al. Clinical prognostic indicators of high-grade pre-invasive bronchial lesions. Eur Respir J 2004;24:24–29.
138. Hirano T, Franzen B, Kato H, et al. Genesis of squamous cell lung carcinoma. Sequential changes of proliferation, DNA ploidy and p53 expression. Am J Pathol 1994; 144:296–302.
139. Pendelton N, Dixon GR, Burnett HE, et al. Expression of proliferating cell nuclear antigen (PCNA) in dysplasia of the bronchial epithelium. J Pathol 1993;170:169–172.
140. Boers JE, ten Velde GP, Thunnissen FB. P53 in squamous metaplasia: a marker for risk of respiratory tract carcinoma. Am J Respir Crit Care Med 1996;153:411–416.
141. Schlake G, Muller KM. Carcinogenesis in bronchial epithelium—an immunohistochemical evaluation of preneoplastic lesions. Virchows Arch 2003;443:291.
142. Khuri FR, Lee JS, Lippman SM, et al. Modulation of proliferating cell nuclear antigen in the bronchial epithe-

lium of smokers. Cancer Epidemiol Biomark Prev 2001; 10:311–318.
143. Lee JJ, Liu D, Lee JS, et al. Long-term impact of smoking on lung epithelial proliferation in current and former smokers. J Natl Cancer Inst 2001;93:1081–1088.
144. Tormanen U, Nuorva K, Soini Y, et al. Apoptotic activity is increased in parallel with the metaplasia-dysplasia-carcinoma sequence of the bronchial epithelium. Br J Cancer 1999;79:996–1002.
145. Tan D-F, Huberman JA, Hyland A, et al. MCM2—a promising marker for premalignant lesions of the lung: a cohort study. BMC Cancer 2001;1:6–14.
146. Fontanini G, Calcinai A, Boldrini L, et al. Modulation of neoangiogenesis in bronchial preneoplastic lesions. Oncol Rep 1999;6:813–817.
147. Lantuejoul S, Constantin B, Drabkin H, et al. Expression of VEGF, semaphorin SEMA3F, and their common receptors neuropilins NP1 and NP2 in preinvasive bronchial lesions, lung tumours, and cell lines. J Pathol 2003; 200:336–347.
148. Gazdar AF, Minna JD. Angiogenesis and the multistage development of lung cancers. Clin Cancer Res 2000; 6:1611–1612.
149. Merrick DT, Haney J, Petrunich S, et al. Overexpression of vascular endothelial growth factor and its receptors in bronchial dysplasia demonstrated by quantitative RT-PCR analysis. Lung Cancer 2005;48:31–45.
150. Wistuba II, Behrens C, Virmani AK, et al. High resolution chromosome 3p allelotyping of human lung cancer and preneoplastic/preinvasive bronchial epithelium reveals multiple, discontinuous sites of 3p allele loss and three regions of frequent breakpoints. Cancer Res 2000; 60:1949–1960.
151. Fasano M, Sabatini MT, Wieczorek R, et al. CD44 and its spliced variant in lung tumours. A role in histogenesis? Cancer 1997;80:34–41.
152. Wimmel A, Kogan E, Ramaswamy A, et al. Variant expression of CD44 in preneoplastic lesions of the lung. Cancer 2001;92:1231–1236.
153. Fisseler-Eckhoff A, Rothstein D, Muller KM. Neovascularisation in hyperplastic, metaplastic and potentially preneoplastic lesions of the bronchial mucosa. Virchows Arch 1996;429:95–100.
154. Pendleton N, Dixon GR, Green JA, et al. Expression of markers of differentiation in normal bronchial epithelium and bronchial dysplasia. J Pathol 1996;178:146–150.
155. Galateau-Salle FB, Luna RE, Horiba K, et al. Matrix metalloproteinases and tissue inhibitors of metalloproteinases in bronchial squamous preinvasive lesions. Hum Pathol 2000;31:296–305.
156. Bolon I, Brambilla E, Vandenbunder B, et al. Changes in the expression of matrix proteases and of the transcription factor c-Ets-1 during progression of precancerous bronchial lesions. Lab Invest 1996;75:1–13.
157. Bejui-Thivolet F, Liagre N, Chignol MC, et al. Detection of human papillomavirus DNA in squamous bronchial metaplasia and squamous cell carcinomas of the lung by in situ hybridization using biotinylated probes in paraffin-embedded specimens. Hum Pathol 1990;21: 111–116.
158. Carey FA, Salter DM, Kerr KM, et al. An investigation into the role of human papillomavirus in endobronchial papillary squamous tumours. Respir Med 1990;84: 445–447.
159. Sekido Y, Fong KM, Minna JD. Molecular genetics of lung cancer. Annu Rev Med 2003;54:73–87.
160. Hall PA, Lane DP. P53 in tumour pathology: can we trust immunohistochemistry? Revisited. J Pathol 1994; 172:1–4.
161. Vahakangas KH, Samet JM, Metcalf RA, et al. Mutations of p53 and ras genes in radon-associated lung cancer from uranium miners. Lancet 1992;339:576–580.
162. Sundaresan V, Ganly P, Hasleton PS, et al. P53 and chromosome 3 abnormalities, characteristic of malignant lung tumours, are detectable in preinvasive lesions of the bronchus. Oncogene 1992;7:1989–1997.
163. Sozzi G, Miozzo M, Donghi R, et al. Deletions of 17p and p53 mutations in preneoplastic lesions of the lung. Cancer Res 1992;52:6079–6082.
164. Bennett WP, Colby TV, Travis WD, et al. p53 protein accumulates frequently in early bronchial neoplasia. Cancer Res 1993;53:4817–4822.
165. Walker C, Robertson LJ, Myskow MW, et al. P53 expression in normal and dysplastic bronchial epithelium and in lung carcinomas. Br J Cancer 1994;70:297–303.
166. Fontanini G, Vignati S, Bigini D, et al. Human non-small cell lung cancer: p53 protein accumulation is an early event and persists during metastatic progression. J Pathol 1994;174:23–31.
167. Katabami M, Dosaka-Akita H, Honma K, et al. P53 and bcl-2 expression in pneumoconiosis-related pre-cancerous lesions and lung cancers: frequent and preferential p53 expression in pneumoconiotic bronchiolar dysplasias. Int J Cancer 1998;75:504–511.
168. Brambilla E, Gazzeri S, Lantuejoul S, et al. P53 mutant immunophenotype and deregulation of p53 transcription pathway (bcl2, bax and waf1) in precursor bronchial lesions of lung cancer. Clin Cancer Res 1998;4: 1609–1618.
169. Lonardo F, Rusch V, Langenfeld J, et al. Overexpression of cyclins D1 and E is frequent in bronchial preneoplasia and precedes squamous cell carcinoma development. Cancer Res 1999;59:2470–2476.
170. Martin B, Verdebout J-M, Mascaux C, et al. Expression of p53 in preneoplastic and early neoplastic bronchial lesions. Oncol Rep 2002;9:223–229.
171. Jeanmart M, Lantuejoul S, Fievet F, et al. Value of immunohistochemical markers in preinvasive bronchial lesions in risk assessment of lung cancer. Clin Cancer Res 2003; 9:2195–2203.
172. Kohno H, Hiroshima K, Toyozaki T, et al. p53 mutation and allelic loss of chromosome 3p, 9p of preneoplastic lesions in patients with non-small cell lung carcinoma. Cancer 1999;85:341–347.
173. Franklin WA, Gazdar AF, Haney J, et al. Widely dispersed p53 mutation in respiratory epithelium. A novel mechanism for field carcinogenesis. J Clin Invest 1997; 100:2133–2137.
174. Chung GT, Sundaresan V, Hasleton P, et al. Clonal evolution of lung tumours. Cancer Res 1996;56:1609–1614.

175. Sozzi G, Miozzo M, Pastorino U, et al. Genetic evidence for an independent origin for multiple preneoplastic and neoplastic lung lesions. Cancer Res 1995;55:135–140.
176. Park IW, Wistuba II, Maitra A, et al. Multiple clonal abnormalities in the bronchial epithelium of patients with lung cancer. J Natl Cancer Inst 1999;91:1863–1868.
177. Boyle JO, Lonardo F, Chang JH, et al. Multiple high-grade bronchial dysplasia and squamous cell carcinoma: concordant and discordant mutations. Clin Cancer Res 2001;7:259–266.
178. Sozzi G, Oggionni M, Alasio L, et al. Molecular changes track recurrence and progression of bronchial precancerous lesions. Lung Cancer 2002;37:267–270.
179. Massion PP, Taflan PM, Jamshedur Rahman SM, et al. Significance of p63 amplification and overexpression in lung cancer development and prognosis. Cancer Res 2003; 63:7113–7121.
180. Sozzi G, Tornielli S, Tagliabue E, et al. Absence of Fhit protein in primary lung tumors and cell lines with FHIT gene abnormalities. Cancer Res 1997;57: 5207–5212.
181. Sozzi G, Pastorino U, Moiraghi L, et al. Loss of FHIT function in lung cancer and preinvasive bronchial lesions. Cancer Res 1998;58:5032–5037.
182. Geradts J, Fong KM, Zimmerman PV, et al. Loss of Fhit expression in non-small-cell lung cancer: correlation with molecular genetic abnormalities and clinicopathological features. Br J Cancer 2000;82:1191–1197.
183. Fong KM, Biesterveld EJ, Virmani A, et al. FHIT and FRA3B 3p14.2 allele loss are common in lung cancer and preneoplastic bronchial lesions and are associated with cancer-related FHIT cDNA splicing aberrations. Cancer Res 1997;57:2256–2267.
184. Wistuba II, Behrens C, Milchgrub S, et al. Sequential molecular abnormalities are involved in the multistage development of squamous cell lung carcinomas. Oncogene 1999;18:643–650.
185. Tseng JE, Kemp BL, Khuri FR, et al. Loss of Fhit is frequent in stage I non-small cell lung cancer and in the lungs of chronic smokers. Cancer Res 1999;59:4798–4803.
186. Zochbauer-Muller S, Wistuba II, Minna JD, et al. Fragile histidine triad (FHIT) gene abnormalities in lung cancer. Clin Lung Cancer 2000;2:141–145.
187. Rusch V, Klimstra D, Linkov I, et al. Aberrant expression of p53 or the epidermal growth factor receptor is frequent in early bronchial neoplasia and coexpression precedes squamous cell carcinoma development. Cancer Res 1995; 55:1365–1372.
188. Piyathilake CJ, Frost AR, Manne U, et al. Differential expression of growth factors in squamous cell carcinoma and precancerous lesions of the lung. Clin Cancer Res 2002;8:734–744.
189. Meert A, Martin B, Verdebout J, et al. Is there a role of c-erb-B2 in the first steps of lung carcinogenesis? Lung Cancer 2005;49(suppl 2):S183.
190. Franklin WA, Veve R, Hirsch FR, et al. Epidermal growth factor receptor family in lung cancer and premalignancy. Semin Oncol 2002;29:3–14.
191. West KA, Brognard J, Clark AS, et al. Rapid Akt activation by nicotine and a tobacco carcinogen modulates the phenotype of normal human airway epithelial cells. J Clin Invest 2003;111:81–90.
192. Tsao AS, McDonnell T, Lam S, et al. Increased phospho-AKT (Ser^{473}) expression in bronchial dysplasia: Implications for lung cancer prevention studies. Cancer Epidemiol Biomark Prev 2003;12:660–664.
193. Rodenhuis S, Slebos RJC, Boot AJM, et al. Incidence and possible clinical significance of K-ras oncogene activation in adenocarcinoma of the human lung. Cancer Res 1988; 48:5738–5741.
194. Sugio K, Kishimoto Y, Virmani AK, et al. K-ras mutations are a relatively late event in the pathogenesis of lung carcinomas. Cancer Res 1994;54:5811–5815.
195. Cooper CA, Carey FA, Bubb VJ, et al. The pattern of K-ras mutation in pulmonary adenocarcinoma defines a new pathway of tumour development in the human lung. J Pathol 1997;181:401–404.
196. Brambilla E, Moro D, Gazzeri S, et al. Alterations of expression of Rb, p16(INK4A) and cyclin D1 in non-small cell lung carcinoma and their clinical significance. J Pathol 1999;188:351–360.
197. Fong KM, Sekido Y, Gazdar AF, et al. Molecular biology of lung cancer: clinical implications. Thorax 2003; 58:892–900.
198. Brambilla E, Gazzeri S, Moro D, et al. Alterations of Rb pathway (Rb-p16INK4–cyclin D1) in preinvasive bronchial lesions. Clin Cancer Res 1999;5:243–250.
199. Betticher DC, Heighway J, Thatcher N, et al. Abnormal expression of CCND1 and RB1 in resection margin epithelia of lung cancer patients. Br J Cancer 1997; 75:1761–1768.
200. Kishimoto Y, Sugio K, Hung JY, et al. Allele-specific loss in chromosome 9p loci in preneoplastic lesions accompanying non-small-cell lung cancers. J Natl Cancer Inst 1995; 87:1224–1229.
201. Belinsky SA, Nikula KJ, Palmisano WA, et al. Aberrant methylation of $p16^{INK4a}$ is an early event in lung cancer and a potential biomarker for early diagnosis. Proc Natl Acad Sci USA 1998;95:11891–11896.
202. Lamy A, Sesboue R, Bourguignon J, et al. Aberrant methylation of the CDKN2A/$P16^{INK4A}$ gene promoter region in preinvasive bronchial lesions: A prospective study in high-risk patients without invasive cancer. Int J Cancer 2002; 100:189–193.
203. Toyooka S, Maruyama R, Toyooka KO, et al. Smoke exposure, histologic type and geography-related differences in the methylation profiles of non-small cell lung cancer. Int J Cancer 2003;103:153–160.
204. Breuer RHJ, Snijders PJF, Sutedja GT, et al. expression of the $P16^{INK4a}$ gene product, methylation of the $p16^{INK4a}$ promoter region and expression of the polycomb-group gene BMI-1 in squamous cell carcinoma and premalignant endobronchial lesions. Lung Cancer 2005;48: 299–306.
205. Zochenbauer-Muller S, Gazdar AF, Minna JD. Molecular pathogenesis of lung cancer. Annu Rev Physiol 2002; 64:681–708.
206. Sekido Y, Fong KM, Minna JD. Progression in understanding the molecular pathogenesis of human lung cancer. Biochim Biophys Acta 1998;1378:F21–F59.

207. Walker C, Robertson L, Myskow M, et al. Expression of the bcl-2 protein in normal and dysplastic bronchial epithelium and in lung carcinomas. Br J Cancer 1995; 72:164–169.
208. Martinet N, Alla F, Farre G, et al. Retinoic acid receptor and retinoid X receptor alterations in lung cancer precursor lesions. Cancer Res 2000;60:2869–2875.
209. Snead DR, Perunovic B, Cullen N, et al. hnRNP B1 expression in benign and malignant lung disease. J Pathol 2003; 200:88–94.
210. Wu S, Sato M, Endo C, et al. hnRNP B1 protein may be a possible prognostic factor in squamous cell carcinoma of the lung. Lung Cancer 2003;41:179–186.
211. Yashima K, Litzky LA, Kaiser L, et al. Telomerase expression in respiratory epithelium during the multistage pathogenesis of lung carcinomas. Cancer Res 1997; 57:2373–2377.
212. Shibuya K, Fujisawa T, Hoshino H, et al. Increased telomerase activity and elevated hTERT mRNA expression during multistage carcinogenesis of squamous cell carcinoma of the lung. Cancer 2001;92:849–855.
213. Snijders PJ, Breuer RH, Sutedja GT, et al. Elevated hTERT mRNA levels: a potential determinant of bronchial squamous cell carcinoma (in situ). Int J Cancer 2004;109:412–417.
214. Lantuejoul S, Soria JC, Morat L, et al. Telomere shortening and telomerase reverse transcriptase expression in preinvasive bronchial lesions. Clin Cancer Res 2005;11:2074–2082.
215. Smith AL, Hung J, Walker L, et al. Extensive areas of aneuploidy are present in the respiratory epithelium of lung cancer patients. Br J Cancer 1996;73:203–209.
216. Zojer N, Dekan G, Ackermann J, et al. Aneuploidy of chromosome 7 can be detected in invasive lung cancer and associated premalignant lesions of the lung by fluorescence in situ hybridization. Lung Cancer 2000; 28:225–235.
217. Helfritzsch H, Junker K, Bartel M, et al. Differentiation of positive autofluorescence bronchoscopy findings by comparative genomic hybridisation. Oncol Rep 2002; 9:697–701.
218. Garnis C, MacAuley C, Lam S, et al. Genetic alteration on 8q distinct from MYC in bronchial carcinoma in situ lesions (letter). Lung Cancer 2004;44:403–404.
219. Mao L, Lee JS, Kurie JM, et al. Clonal genetic alterations in the lungs of current and former smokers. J Natl Cancer Inst 1997;89:857–862.
220. Wistuba II, Lam S, Behrens C, et al. Molecular damage in the bronchial epithelium of current and former smokers. J Natl Cancer Inst 1997;89:1366–1373.
221. Chung GT, Sundaresan V, Hasleton P, et al. Sequential molecular genetic changes in lung cancer development. Oncogene 1995;11:2591–2598.
222. Hung J, Kishimoto Y, Sugio K, et al. Allele-specific chromosome 3p deletions occur at an early stage in the pathogenesis of lung carcinoma. JAMA 1995;273:558–563.
223. Wistuba II, Behrens C, Virmani AK, et al. Allelic losses at chromosome 8p21–23 are early and frequent events in the pathogenesis of lung cancer. Cancer Res 1999; 59:1973–1979.
224. Wistuba II, Mao L, Gazdar AF. Smoking molecular damage in bronchial epithelium. Oncogene 2002; 21:7298–7306.
225. Smith SL, Watson SG, Ratschiller D, et al. Maspin—the most commonly-expressed gene of the 18q21.3 serpin cluster in lung cancer—is strongly expressed in preneoplastic bronchial lesions. Oncogene 2003;22:8677–8687.
226. Smith SL, Gugger M, Hoban P, et al. S100A2 is strongly expressed in airway basal cells, preneoplastic bronchial lesions and primary non-small cell carcinomas. Br J Cancer 2004;91:1515–1524.
227. Minna JD, Fong K, Zochbauer-Muller S, et al. Molecular pathogenesis of lung cancer and potential translational applications. Cancer J 2002;8(suppl 1):S41–S46.
228. Brambilla E, Moro D, Veale D, et al. Basal cell (basaloid) carcinoma of the lung. A new morphologic and phenotypic entity with separate prognostic significance. Hum Pathol 1992;23:993–1003.
229. Sturm N, Lantuejoul S, Laverriere M-H, et al. Thyroid transcription factor 1 and cytokeratins 1,5,10,14 (34ßE12) expression in basaloid and large-cell neuroendocrine carcinomas of the lung. Hum Pathol 2001;32:918–925.
230. Travis WD, Travis LB, Devesa SS. Lung cancer. Cancer 1995;75(suppl):191–202.
231. Harkness EF, Brewster DH, Kerr KM, et al. Changing trends in incidence of lung cancer by histological type in Scotland. Int J Cancer 2002;102:179–183.
232. Miller RR, Nelems B, Evans KG, et al. Glandular neoplasia of the lung. A proposed analogy to colonic tumours. Cancer 1988;61:1009–1014.
233. Nakanishi K. Alveolar epithelial hyperplasia and adenocarcinoma of the lung. Arch Pathol Lab Med 1990; 114:363–368.
234. Carey FA, Wallace WAH, Fergusson RJ, et al. Alveolar atypical hyperplasia in association with primary pulmonary adenocarcinoma: a clinicopathological study of 10 cases. Thorax 1992;47:1041–1043.
235. Weng S-Y, Tsuchiya E, Kasuga T, et al. Incidence of atypical bronchioloalveolar cell hyperplasia of the lung: relation to histological subtypes of lung cancer. Virchows Arch A Pathol Anat 1992;420:463–471.
236. Weng S, Tsuchiya E, Satoh Y, et al. Multiple atypical adenomatous hyperplasia of type II pneumocytes and bronchioloalveolar carcinoma. Histopathology 1990; 16:101–103.
237. Nakayama H, Noguchi M, Tsuchiya R, et al. Clonal growth of atypical adenomatous hyperplasia of the lung: cytofluorometric analysis of nuclear DNA content. Mod Pathol 1990;3:314–320.
238. Miller RR. Bronchioloalveolar cell adenomas. Am J Surg Pathol 1990;14:904–912.
239. Nakahara R, Yokose T, Nagai K, et al. Atypical adenomatous hyperplasia of the lung: a clinicopathological study of 118 cases including cases with multiple atypical adenomatous hyperplasia. Thorax 2001;56:302–305.
240. Chapman AD, Kerr KM. The association between atypical adenomatous hyperplasia and primary lung cancer. Br J Cancer 2000;83:632–636.
241. Kerr KM, Fraire AE, Pugatch B, et al. Atypical adenomatous hyperplasia. In: Travis WD, Brambilla E,

Muller-Hermelink HK, et al, eds. World Health Organisation classification of tumours. Pathology and genetics of tumours of the lung, pleura, thymus and heart. Lyon: IARC Press, 2004:73–75.
242. Kitamura H, Kameda Y, Ito T, et al. Cytodifferentiation of atypical adenomatous hyperplasia and bronchioloalveolar lung carcinoma: immunohistochemical and ultrastructural studies. Virchows Arch 1997;431: 415–424.
243. Kitamura H, Kameda Y, Ito T, et al. Atypical adenomatous hyperplasia of the lung. Implications for the pathogenesis of peripheral lung adenocarcinoma. Am J Clin Pathol 1999;111:610–622.
244. Mori M, Kaji M, Tezuka F, et al. Comparative ultrastructural study of atypical adenomatous hyperplasia and adenocarcinoma of the human lung. Ultrastruct Pathol 1998;22:459–466.
245. Osanai M, Igarashi T, Yoshida Y. Unique cellular features in atypical adenomatous hyperplasia of the lung: ultrastructural evidence of its cytodifferentiation. Ultrastruct Pathol 2001;25:367–373.
246. Kodama T, Biyajima S, Watanabe S, et al. Morphometric study of adenocarcinomas and hyperplastic epithelial lesions in the peripheral lung. Am J Clin Pathol 1986; 85:146–151.
247. Kitamura H, Kameda Y, Nakamura N, et al. Proliferative potential and p53 overexpression in precursor and early stage lesions of bronchioloalveolar lung carcinoma. Am J Pathol 1995;146:876–887.
248. Kerr KM. Atypical adenomatous hyperplasia versus nonmucinous bronchioloalveolar carcinoma. A spectrum of neoplasia in the lung periphery. Lung Cancer 2000;29(S2):94–95.
249. Kitamura H, Kameda Y, Nakamura N, et al. Atypical adenomatous hyperplasia and bronchoalveolar lung carcinoma. Analysis by morphometry and the expressions of p53 and carcinoembryonic antigen. Am J Surg Pathol 1996;20:553–562.
250. Koga T, Hashimoto S, Sugio K, et al. Lung adenocarcinoma with bronchioloalveolar carcinoma component is frequently associated with foci of high-grade atypical adenomatous hyperplasia. Am J Clin Pathol 2002; 117:464–70.
251. Kerr KM. Morphology and genetics of preinvasive pulmonary disease. Curr Diag Pathol 2004;10:259–268.
252. Kerr KM. Adenomatous hyperplasia and the origin of peripheral adenocarcinoma of the lung. In: Corrin B, ed. Pathology of lung tumours. Edinburgh: Churchill Livingstone, 1997:119–134.
253. Noguchi M, Morokawa A, Kawasaki M, et al. Small adenocarcinoma of the lung. Histologic characteristics and prognosis. Cancer 1995;75:2844–2852.
254. Kurokawa T, Matsuno Y, Noguchi M, et al. Surgically curable "early" adenocarcinoma in the periphery of the lung. Am J Surg Pathol 1994;18:431–438.
255. Noguchi M. Personal communication, 2003.
256. Colby TV, Noguchi M, Henschke C, et al. Adenocarcinoma. In: Travis WD, Brambilla E, Muller-Hermelink HK, et al., eds. World Health Organisation classification of tumours. Pathology and genetics of tumours of the lung, pleura, thymus and heart. Lyon: IARC Press, 2004: 35–44.
257. Nomori H, Ohtsuka T, Naruke T, et al. Differentiating between atypical adenomatous hyperplasia and bronchioloalveolar carcinoma using the computed tomography number histogram. Ann Thorac Surg 2003;76: 867–871.
258. Noguchi M, Kodama T, Shimosato Y, et al. Papillary adenoma of type 2 pneumocytes. Am J Surg Pathol 1986;10:134–139.
259. Yousem SA, Hochholzer L. Alveolar adenoma. Hum Pathol 1986;17:1066–1071.
260. Lantuejoul S, Ferretti G, Negoescu A, et al. Multifocal alveolar hyperplasia associated with lymphangioleiomyomatosis in tuberous sclerosis. Histopathology 1997; 30:570–575.
261. Muir TE, Leslie KO, Popper H, et al. Micronodular pneumocyte hyperplasia. Am J Surg Pathol 1998;22:465–472.
262. Travis WD, Linnoila RI, Horowitz M, et al. Pulmonary nodules resembling bronchioloalveolar carcinoma in adolescent cancer patients. Mod Pathol 1998;1:372–377.
263. Yanagisawa M. A histopathological study of proliferative changes of the epithelial components of the lung. A contribution to the histogenesis of pulmonary carcinoma (in Japanese). Jpn J Cancer Clin 1959;5:667–680.
264. Sterner DJ, Masuko M, Roggli VL, et al. Prevalence of pulmonary atypical alveolar cell hyperplasia in an autopsy population: a study of 100 cases. Mod Pathol 1997; 10:469–473.
265. Yokose T, Ito Y, Ochiai A. High prevalence of atypical adenomatous hyperplasia of the lung in autopsy specimens from elderly patients with malignant neoplasms. Lung Cancer 2000;29:125–130.
266. Yokose T, Doi M, Tanno K, Yamazaki K, Ochiai A. Atypical adenomatous hyperplasia of the lung in autopsy cases. Lung Cancer 2001;33:155–161.
267. Morinaga S, Shimosato Y. Microcancer of the bronchus and lung: pathology of the microadenocarcinoma in the periphery of the lung (in Japanese). Pathol Clin Med 1987;5(suppl):74–80.
268. Kodama T, Nishiyama H, Nishiwaki Y, et al. Histopathological study of adenocarcinoma and hyperplastic epithelial lesion of the lung (in Japanese, abstract in English). Haigan (Lung Cancer) 1988;28:325–333.
269. Noguchi M, Shimosato Y. The development and progression of adenocarcinoma of the lung. In: Hansen HH, ed. Lung cancer. Boston: Kluwer Academic, 1994:131–142.
270. Anami Y, Matsuno Y, Yamada T, et al. A case of double primary adenocarcinoma of the lung with multiple atypical adenomatous hyperplasia. Pathol Int 1998;48:634–640.
271. Suzuki K, Takahashi K, Yoshida J, et al. Synchronous double primary lung carcinomas associated with multiple atypical adenomatous hyperplasia. Lung Cancer 1998; 19:131–139.
272. Dohmoto K, Fujita J, Ohtsuki Y, et al. Synchronous four primary lung adenocarcinoma associated with multiple atypical adenomatous hyperplasia. Lung Cancer 2000; 27:125–130.
273. Takamochi K, Ogura T, Suzuki K. Loss of heterozygosity on chromosomes 9q and 16p in atypical adenomatous

hyperplasia concomitant with adenocarcinoma of the lung. Am J Pathol 2001;159:1941–1948.
274. Takigawa N, Segawa Y, Nakata M, et al. Clinical investigation of atypical adenomatous hyperplasia of the lung. Lung Cancer 1999;25:115–121.
275. Kitagawa H, Goto A, Niki T, et al. Lung adenocarcinoma associated with atypical adenomatous hyperplasia. A clinicopathological study with special reference to smoking and cancer multiplicity. Pathol Int 2003;53:823–827.
276. Chapman AD, Thetford D, Kerr KM. Pathological and clinical investigation of pulmonary atypical adenomatous hyperplasia and its association with primary lung adenocarcinoma Lung Cancer 2000;29(S1):215–216.
277. Yokozaki M, Kodama T, Yokose T, et al. Differentiation of atypical adenomatous hyperplasia and adenocarcinoma of the lung by use of DNA ploidy and morphometric analysis. Mod Pathol 1996;9:1156–1164.
278. Mori M, Chiba R, Takahashi T. Atypical adenomatous hyperplasia of the lung and its differentiation from adenocarcinoma. Characterisation of atypical cells by morphometry and multivariate cluster analysis. Cancer 1993; 72:2331–2340.
279. Nakanishi K, Hiroi S, Kawai T, et al. Argyrophilic nucleolar-organiser region counts and DNA status in bronchioloalveolar epithelial hyperplasia and adenocarcinoma of the lung. Hum Pathol 1998;29:235–239.
280. Kitaguchi S, Takeshima Y, Nishisaka T, et al. Proliferative activity, p53 expression and loss of heterozygosity on 3p, 9p and 17p in atypical adenomatous hyperplasia of the lung. Hiroshima J Med Sci 1998;47:17–25.
281. Kurasono Y, Ito T, Kameda Y, et al. Expression of cyclin D1, retinoblastoma gene protein and p16 MTS1 protein in atypical adenomatous hyperplasia and adenocarcinoma of the lung. An immunohistochemical analysis. Virchows Arch 1998;432:207–215.
282. Yamasaki M, Takeshima Y, Fujii S, et al. Correlation between genetic alterations and histopathological subtypes in bronchiolo-alveolar carcinoma and atypical adenomatous hyperplasia of the lung. Pathol Int 2000;50:778–785.
283. Kerr KM, Fyfe N, Chapman AD, et al. Cell cycle marker MCM2 in peripheral lung adenocarcinoma and its precursors. Lung Cancer 2003;41:S15.
284. Rao SK, Fraire AE. Alveolar cell hyperplasia in association with adenocarcinoma of lung. Mod Pathol 1995;9:99–108.
285. Mori M, Tezuka F, Chiba R, et al. Atypical adenomatous hyperplasia and adenocarcinoma of the human lung. Their heterology in form and analogy in immunohistochemical characteristics. Cancer 1996;77:665–674.
286. Stenhouse G, Fyfe N, King G, et al. Thyroid transcription factor 1 in pulmonary adenocarcinoma. J Clin Pathol 2004;57:383–387.
287. Kumaki F, Matsui K, Kawai T, et al. Expression of matrix metalloproteinases in invasive pulmonary adenocarcinoma with bronchioloalveolar component and atypical adenomatous hyperplasia. Am J Pathol 2001; 159:2125–2135.
288. Kerr KM, MacKenzie SJ, Ramasami S, et al. Expression of Fhit, cell adhesion molecules and matrix metalloproteinases in atypical adenomatous hyperplasia and pulmonary adenocarcinoma. J Pathol 2004;203:638–644.
289. Kitamura H, Oosawa Y, Kawano N, et al. Basement membrane patterns, gelatinase A and tissue inhibitor of metalloproteinase-2 expressions, and stromal fibrosis during the development of peripheral lung adenocarcinoma. Hum Pathol 1999;30:331–338.
290. Iijima T, Minami Y, Nakamura N, et al. MMP-2 activation and stepwise progression of pulmonary adenocarcinoma. Analysis of MMP-2 and MMP-9 with gelatin zymography. Pathol Int 2004;54:295–301.
291. Kayser K, Nwoye JO, Kosjerina Z, et al. Atypical adenomatous hyperplasia of lung: its incidence and analysis of clinical, glycohistochemical and structural features including newly defined growth factor regulators and vascularisation. Lung Cancer 2003;42:171–182.
292. Awaya H, Takeshima Y, Amatya VJ, et al. Loss of expression of E-cadherin and beta-catenin is associated with progression of pulmonary adenocarcinoma. Pathol Int 2005;55:14–18.
293. Awaya H, Takeshima Y, Yamasaki M, et al. Expression of MUC1, MUC2, MUC5AC, and MUC6 in atypical adenomatous hyperplasia, bronchioloalveolar carcinoma, adenocarcinoma with mixed subtypes, and mucinous bronchioloalveolar carcinoma of the lung. Am J Clin Pathol 2004;121:644–653.
294. Kerr KM, Carey FA, King G, et al. Atypical alveolar hyperplasia: relationship with pulmonary adenocarcinoma, p53 and c-erbB-2 expression. J Pathol 1994; 174:249–256.
295. Yatabe Y, Kosaka T, Takahashi T, et al. EGFR mutation is specific for terminal respiratory unit type adenocarcinoma. Am J Surg Pathol 2005;29:633–639.
296. Yoshida Y, Sibata T, Kokubu A, et al. Mutations of the epidermal growth factor receptor gene in atypical adenomatous hyperplasia and bronchioloalveolar carcinoma of the lung. Lung Cancer 2005;49(suppl 2):S76.
297. Hida T, Yatabe Y, Achiwa H, et al. Increased expression of cyclooxygenase 2 occurs frequently in human lung cancers, specifically in adenocarcinomas. Cancer Res 1998;58:3761–3764.
298. Takigawa N, Ida M, Segawa Y, et al. Expression of cyclooxygenase-2, Fas and Fas ligand in pulmonary adenocarcinoma and atypical adenomatous hyperplasia. Anticancer Res 2003;23:5069–5073.
299. Hosomi Y, Yokose T, Hirose Y, et al. Increased cyclooxygenase 2 (COX-2) expression occurs frequently in precursor lesions of human adenocarcinoma of the lung. Lung Cancer 2000;30:73–81.
300. Schreinemachers DM, Everson RB. Aspirin use and lung, colon, and breast cancer incidence in a prospective study. Epidemiology 1994;5:138–146.
301. Seki N, Takasu T, Mandai K, et al. Expression of eukaryotic initiation factor 4E in atypical adenomatous hyperplasia and adenocarcinoma of the human peripheral lung. Clin Cancer Res 2002;8:3046–3053.
302. Nakanishi K, Kawai T, Kumaki F, et al. Expression of human telomerase RNA component and telomerase reverse transcriptase mRNA in atypical adenomatous hyperplasia of the lung. Hum Pathol 2002;33:697–702.

303. Nakanishi K, Kawai T, Kumaki F, et al. Survivin expression in atypical adenomatous hyperplasia of the lung. Am J Clin Pathol 2003;120:712–719.
304. Barrios R, Khoor A, Ostrowski B, et al. Analysis of p27 expression in lung adenocarcinoma vs. adenomatous hyperplasia of the lung. Mod Pathol 2000;13:206A.
305. Goto A, Niki T, Moriyama S, et al. Immunohistochemical study of Skp2 and Jab1, two key molecules in the degradation of P27, in lung adenocarcinoma. Pathol Int 2004; 54:675–681.
306. Slebos RJC, Baas IO, Clement MJ, et al. p53 alterations in atypical alveolar hyperplasia of the human lung. Hum Pathol 1998;29:801–808.
307. Pueblitz S, Hieger LR. Expression of p53 and CEA in atypical adenomatous hyperplasia of the lung (letter). Am J Surg Pathol 1997;2:867–869.
308. Hayashi H, Miyamoto H, Ito T, et al. Analysis of p21waf1/cip1 expression in normal, premalignant and malignant cells during the development of human lung adenocarcinoma. Am J Pathol 1997;151:461–470.
309. Aoyagi Y, Yokose T, Minami Y, et al. Accumulation of losses of heterozygosity and multistep carcinogenesis in pulmonary adenocarcinoma. Cancer Res 2001;61:7950–7954.
310. Sheikh HA, Fuhrer K, Cieply K, et al. p63 expression in assessment of bronchioloalveolar proliferations of the lung. Mod Pathol 2004;17:1134–1140.
311. Johnson L, Mercer K, Greenbaum D, et al. Somatic activation of the K-ras oncogene causes early onset lung cancer in mice. Nature 2001;410:1111–1116.
312. Meuwissen R, Linn SC, van der Valk M, et al. Mouse model for lung tumorigenesis through Cre/lox controlled sporadic activation of the K-Ras oncogene. Oncogene 2001;20:6551–6558.
313. Ohshima S, Shimizu Y, Takahama M. Detection of c-Ki-ras gene mutation in paraffin sections of adenocarcinoma and atypical bronchioloalveolar cell hyperplasia of human lung. Virchows Arch 1994;424:129–134.
314. Sagawa M, Saito Y, Fujimura S, et al. K-ras point mutation occurs in the early stage of carcinogenesis in lung cancer. Br J Cancer 1998;77:720–723.
315. Westra WH, Baas IO, Hruban RH, et al. K-ras oncogene activation in atypical alveolar hyperplasias of the human lung. Cancer Res 1996;56:2224–2228.
316. Niho S, Yokose T, Suzuki K, et al. Monoclonality of atypical adenomatous hyperplasia of the lung. Am J Pathol 1999;154:249–254.
317. Ullmann R, Bongiovanni M, Halbwedl I, et al. Is high-grade adenomatous hyperplasia an early bronchioloalveolar carcinoma? J Pathol 2003;201:371–376.
318. Marchetti A, Pellegrini S, Bertacca G, et al. FHIT and p53 gene abnormalities in bronchioloalveolar carcinomas. Correlations with clinicopathological data and K-ras mutations. J Pathol 1998;184:240–246.
319. Sasatomi E, Johnson LR, Aldeeb DN et al. Genetic profile of cumulative mutational damage associated with early pulmonary adenocarcinoma: bronchioloalveolar carcinoma vs. stage I invasive adenocarcinoma. Am J Surg Pathol 2004;28:1280–1288.
320. Suzuki K, Ogura T, Yokose T, et al. Loss of heterozygosity in the tuberous sclerosis gene associated regions in adenocarcinoma of the lung accompanied by multiple atypical adenomatous hyperplasia. Int J Cancer 1998;79:384–389.
321. Takamochi K, Ogura T, Yokose T, et al. Molecular analysis of the TSC1 gene in adenocarcinoma of the lung. Lung Cancer 2004;46:271–281.
322. Nomori H, Horio H, Naruke T, et al. A case of multiple atypical adenomatous hyperplasia of the lung detected by computed tomography. Jpn J Clin Oncol 2001;31: 514–516.
323. Frasca JM, Auerbach O, Parks VR, et al. Alveolar cell hyperplasia in the lungs of smoking dogs. Exp Mol Pathol 1974;21:300–312.
324. Foster C, Kerr KM. Unpublished observations.
325. Attenoos R. Personal communication.
326. Yousem SA, Finkelstein SD, Swalsky PA, et al. Absence of jaagsiekte sheep retrovirus DNA and RNA in bronchioloalveolar and conventional human pulmonary adenocarcinoma by PCR and RT-PCR analysis. Hum Pathol 2001;32:1039–1042.
327. Meuwissen R, Lin SC, Linnoila RI, et al. Induction of small cell lung cancer by somatic inactivation of both Trp53 and Rb1 in a conditional mouse model. Cancer Cell 2003;4:181–189.
328. Nadav Y, Pastorino U, Nicholson AG. Multiple synchronous lung cancers and atypical adenomatous hyperplasia in Li-Fraumeni syndrome. Histopathology 1998;33: 52–54.
329. Gazdar AF, Minna JD. Cigarettes, sex and lung adenocarcinoma. J Natl Cancer Inst 1997;89:1563–1565.
330. Thun MJ, Lally CA, Flannery JT, et al. Cigarette smoking and changes in the histopathology of lung cancer. J Natl Cancer Inst 1997;89:1580–1586.
331. Aoki T, Nakata H, Watanabe H, et al. Evolution of peripheral lung adenocarcinomas: CT findings correlated with histology and tumour doubling time. Am J Roengenol 2000;174:763–768.
332. Asamura H, Suzuki K, Watanabe S, et al. A clinicopatho logical study of resected subcentimeter lung cancers: a favourable prognosis for ground glass opacity lesions. Ann Thorac Surg 2003;76:1016–1022.
333. Logan PM, Miller RR, Evans K, et al. Bronchogenic carcinoma and coexistent bronchioloalveolar cell adenomas. Assessment of radiologic detection and follow-up in 28 patients. Chest 1996;109:713–717.
334. Suzuki K, Nagai K, Yoshida J, et al. The prognosis of resected lung carcinoma associated with atypical adenomatous hyperplasia: a comparison of the prognosis of well-differentiated adenocarcinoma associated with atypical adenomatous hyperplasia and intrapulmonary metastasis. Cancer 1997;79:1521–1526.
335. Kerr KM. Pulmonary preinvasive neoplasia. J Clin Pathol 2001;54:257–271.
336. Mori M, Rao SK, Popper HH, et al. Atypical adenomatous hyperplasia of the lung: A probable forerunner in the development of adenocarcinoma of the lung. Mod Pathol 2001;14:72–84.
337. Nakano K, Iyama K, Mori T, et al. Loss of alveolar basement membrane type IV collagen α3, α4, α5 chains in bronchioloalveolar carcinoma of the lung. J Pathol 2001; 194:420–427.

338. Suzuki K, Yokose T, Yoshida J, et al. Prognostic significance of the size of central fibrosis in peripheral adenocarcinoma of the lung. Ann Thorac Surg 2000;69:893–897.
339. Ritter JH. Pulmonary atypical adenomatous hyperplasia. A histological lesion in search of usable criteria and clinical significance. Am J Clin Pathol 1999;111:587–589.
340. Ullman R, Bongiovanni M, Halbwedl I, et al. Bronchiolar columnar cell dysplasia—genetic analysis of a novel preneoplastic lesion of peripheral lung. Virchows Arch 2003;442:429–436.
341. Aguayo SM, Miller YE, Waldron JA, et al. Idiopathic diffuse hyperplasia of pulmonary neuroendocrine cells and airway disease. N Engl J Med 1992;327:1285–1288.
342. Sheerin N, Harrison NK, Sheppard, et al. Obliterative bronchiolitis caused by multiple tumourlets and microcarcinoids successfully treated by single lung transplantation. Thorax 1995;50:207–209.
343. Jessurun J, Manivel JC, Simpson R. Idiopathic diffuse hyperplasia of pulmonary neuroendocrine cells (IDHPNC): a consequence of diffuse bronchiolitis. Lab Invest 1994; 70:151A.
344. Armas OA, White DA, Erlandson RA. Diffuse idiopathic pulmonary neuroendocrine cell proliferation presenting as interstitial lung disease. Am J Surg Pathol 1995; 19:963–970.
345. Brown MJ, English J, Muller NL. Bronchiolitis obliterans due to neuroendocrine hyperplasia: high-resolution CT-pathologic correlation. Am J Roentgenol 1997; 168:1561–1562.
346. Lee JS, Brown KK, Cool C, et al. Diffuse pulmonary neuroendocrine cell hyperplasia: Radiologic and clinical features. J Comput Assist Tomogr 2002;26:180–184.
347. Felton WL, Liebow AA, Lindskog GF. Peripheral and multiple bronchial adenomas. Cancer 1953;6:555–567.
348. Gmelich JT, Bensch KG, Liebow AA. Cells of Kulchitsky type in bronchioles and their relation to the origin of peripheral carcinoid tumours. Lab Invest 1967; 17:88–98.
349. Miller MA, Mark GJ, Kanarek D. Multiple peripheral pulmonary carcinoids and tumourlets of carcinoid type, with restrictive and obstructive lung disease. Am J Med 1978;65:373–378.
350. Cohen AJ, King TE, Gilman LB, et al. High expression of neutral endopeptidase in idiopathic diffuse hyperplasia of pulmonary neuroendocrine cells. Am J Respir Crit Care Med 1998;158:1593–1599.
351. Miller RR, Muller NL. Neuroendocrine cell hyperplasia and obliterative bronchiolitis in patients with peripheral carcinoid tumours. Am J Surg Pathol 1995;19:653–658.
352. Whitwell F. Tumourlets of the lung. J Path Bact 1955; 70:529–541.
353. Churg A, Warnock ML. Pulmonary tumourlet. A form of peripheral carcinoid. Cancer 1976;37:1469–1477.
354. Kay S. Histologic and histogenetic observations on the peripheral adenoma of the lung. Arch Pathol 1958;65: 395–402.
355. Hausman DH, Weimann RB. Pulmonary tumourlet with hilar lymph node metastases. Cancer 1967;20:1515–1519.
356. D'Agati VD, Perzin KH. Carcinoid tumorlets of the lung with metastasis to a peribronchial lymph node. Report of a case and review of the literature. Cancer 1985; 55:2472–2476.
357. Bonikos DS, Bensch KG, Jamplis RW. Peripheral pulmonary carcinoid tumours. Cancer 1976;37:1977–1998.
358. Johnson DE, Lock JE, Elde RP, et al. Pulmonary neuroendocrine cells in hyaline membrane disease and bronchopulmonary dysplasia. Pediatr Res 1982;16:446–454.
359. Johnson DE, Wobken JD, Landrum BG. Changes in bombesin, calcitonin, and serotonin immunoreactive pulmonary neuroendocrine cells in cystic fibrosis and after prolonged mechanical ventilation. Am Rev Respir Dis 1988;137:123–131.
360. Watanabe H, Kobayashi H, Honma K, et al. Diffuse panbronchiolitis with multiple tumourlets. A quantitative study of the Kultschitzky cells and the clusters. Acta Pathol Jpn 1985;35:1221–1231.
361. Gosney JR, Sissons MC, Allibone RO, et al. Pulmonary endocrine cells in chronic bronchitis and emphysema. J Pathol 1989;157:127–133.
362. Aguayo SM, King TE Jr, Waldron JA, Jr, et al. Increased pulmonary neuroendocrine cells with bombesin-like immunoreactivity in adult patients with eosinophilic granuloma. J Clin Invest 1990;86:838–844.
363. Pelosi G, Zancanaro C, Sbabo L, et al. Development of innumerable neuroendocrine tumourlets in pulmonary lobe scarred by intralobar sequestration. Immunohistochemical and ultrastructural study of an unusual case. Arch Pathol Lab Med 1992;116:1167–1174.
364. Ranchod M. The histogenesis and development of pulmonary tumourlets. Cancer 1977;39:1135–1145.
365. Sturm N, Rossi G, Lantuejoul S, et al. Expression of thyroid transcription factor-1 in the spectrum of neuroendocrine cell lung proliferations with special interest in carcinoids. Hum Pathol 2002;33:175–182.
366. Du EZ, Goldstraw P, Zacharias J, et al. TTF-1 expression is specific for lung primary in typical and atypical carcinoids: TTF-1–positive carcinoids are predominantly in peripheral location. Hum Pathol 2004;35:825–831.
367. Salyer DC, Salyer WR, Eggleston JC. Bronchial carcinoid tumours. Cancer 1975;36:1522–1537.
368. Debelenko LV, Brambilla E, Agarwal SK, et al. Identification of MEN1 gene mutations in sporadic carcinoid tumours of the lung. Hum Mol Genet 1997;6: 2285–2290.
369. Walch AK, Zitzelsberger HF, Aubele MM, et al. Typical and atypical carcinoid tumours of the lung are characterised by 11q deletions as detected by comparative genomic hybridisation. Am J Pathol 1998;153:1089–1098.
370. Petzmann S, Ullmann R, Klemen H, et al. Loss of heterozygosity on chromosome arm 11q in lung carcinoids. Hum Pathol 2001;32:333–338.
371. Finkelstein SD, Hasegawa T, Colby T, et al. 11q13 allelic imbalance discriminates pulmonary carcinoids from tumourlets. A microdissection-based genotyping approach useful in clinical practice. Am J Pathol 1999;155:633–640.
372. Matthews MJ, Gazdar AF. Small cell carcinoma of the lung. Its morphology, behaviour and nature. In: Shimosato Y, Melamed MR, Nettesheim P, eds. Morphogenesis of lung cancer. Vol 2. Boca Raton, FL: CRC Press, 1982: 1–14.

373. Linnoila RI. Murine models for human lung neuroendocrine (NE) carcinomas: pathology and molecular determinants of differentiation. Lung Cancer 2003;41(suppl 2):3.
374. Shapiro GI, Edwards CD, Kobzik L, et al. Reciprocal Rb inactivation and p16INK4 expression in primary lung cancers and cell lines. Cancer Res 1995;55:505–509.
375. Beasley MB, Lantuejoul S, Abbondanzo S, et al. The P16/cyclin D1/Rb pathway in neuroendocrine tumors of the lung. Hum Pathol 2003;34:136–142.
376. Wistuba II, Gazdar AF, Minna JD. Molecular genetics of small cell lung carcinoma. Semin Oncol 2001;28(suppl 4):3–13.
377. Minna JD, Kurie JM, Jacks T. A big step in the study of small cell lung cancer. Cancer Cell 2003;4:163–166.
378. Onuki N, Wistuba II, Travis WD, et al. Genetic changes in the spectrum of neuroendocrine lung tumours. Cancer 1999;85:600–607.
379. Debelenko LV, Swalwell JI, Kelley MJ, et al. MEN1 gene mutation analysis of high-grade neuroendocrine lung carcinoma. Genes Chrom Cancer 2000;28:58–65.
380. Wistuba II, Berry J, Behrens C, et al. Molecular changes in the bronchial epithelium of patients with small cell lung cancer. Clin Cancer Res 2000;6:2604–2610.
381. Mao L. Molecular abnormalities in lung carcinogenesis and their potential clinical implications. Lung Cancer 2001;34:S27–S34.
382. Brambilla E, Moro D, Gazzeri S, et al. Cytotoxic chemotherapy induces cell differentiation in small cell lung carcinoma. J Clin Oncol 1991;9:50–61.
383. Mulshine JL, Smith RA. Screening and early diagnosis of lung cancer. Thorax 2002;57:1071–1078.
384. Strauss GM. Randomized population trials and screening for lung cancer. Cancer 2000;89:2399–2421.
385. Yoshida J, Nagai K, Yokose T, et al. Primary peripheral lung carcinoma smaller than 1 cm in diameter. Chest 1998;114:710–712.
386. Kerr KM, Lamb D. Actual growth rate and tumour cell proliferation in human pulmonary neoplasms. Br J Cancer 1984;50:343–349.
387. Thunnissen FBJM. Sputum examination for early detection of lung cancer. J Clin Pathol 2003;56:805–810.
388. Hirsch FR, Franklin WA, Gazdar AF, et al. Early detection of lung cancer: clinical perspectives of recent advances in biology and radiology. Clin Cancer Res 2001;7:5–22.
389. Henschke CI, McCauley DI, Yankelevitz DF, et al. Early lung cancer action project: overall design and findings from baseline screening. Lancet 1999;354:99–105.
390. Kerr KM, Noguchi M. Pathology of Screen-detected lesions. In: Hirsch FR, Bunn PA, Kato JL, et al., eds. Prevention and early detection of lung cancer. London: IASLC/Martin Dunitz, 2005.
391. Sone S, Takashima S, Li F, et al. Mass screening for lung cancer with mobile spiral computed tomography scanner. Lancet 1998;351:1242–1245.
392. Nawa T, Nakagawa T, Kusano S, et al. Lung cancer screening using low-dose spiral CT. Results of baseline and 1-year follow-up studies. Chest 2002;122:15–20.
393. Kodama K, Higashiyama M, Yokouchi H, et al. Prognostic value of ground-glass opacity found in small lung adenocarcinoma on high-resolution CT scanning. Lung Cancer 2001;33:17–25.
394. Nakata M, Sawada S, Saeki H, et al. Prospective study of thoracoscopic limited resection for ground-glass opacity selected by computed tomography. Ann Thorac Surg 2003;75:1601–1605.
395. Takashima S, Maruyama Y, Hasegawa M, et al. Prognostic significance of high-resolution CT findings in small peripheral adenocarcinoma of the lung: a retrospective study on 64 patients. Lung Cancer 2002;36:289–295.
396. Flieder DB. Recent advances in the diagnosis of adenocarcinoma: the impact of lung cancer screening on histopathologists. Curr Diag Pathol 2004;10:269–278.
397. Kennedy TC, Miller Y, Prindiville S. Screening for lung cancer revisited and the role of sputum cytology and fluorescence bronchoscopy in a high-risk group. Chest 2000;117:72S-79S.
398. McWilliams A, Mayo J, MacDonald S, et al. Lung cancer screening. A different paradigm. Am J Respir Crit Care Med 2003;168:1167–1173.
399. van Zandwijk N, Hirsch FR. Chemoprevention of lung cancer: current status and future prospects. Lung Cancer 2003;42:S71–S79.
400. Berman JJ, Henson DE. The precancers: Waiting for a classification. Hum Pathol 2003;34:833–834.
401. Foucar E. Do pathologists play dice? Uncertainty and early histopathological diagnosis of common malignancies. Histopathology 1997;31:495–502.
402. Page DL. Atypical Hyperplasia, narrowly and broadly defined. Hum Pathol 1991;22:631–632.
403. Banerjee AK, Rabbitts PH, George PJ. Preinvasive bronchial lesions. Surveillance or intervention? Chest 2004;125:95S–96S.

35 Common Non–Small-Cell Carcinomas and Their Variants

Douglas B. Flieder and Samuel P. Hammar

Lung cancer is the leading cause of cancer death in the world; over 1.2 million new cases and 1.1 million worldwide deaths were predicted for 2004.[1] These statistics are astounding given the rarity of lung cancer during the first half of the 20th century, when lung cancer had a lower incidence than liver, prostate, colon, stomach, uterine, breast, and even ovarian cancer. Only a sound understanding of the complex epidemiologic, etiologic, and clinicopathologic aspects of lung carcinoma will enable clinical and scientific progress against this deadly disease regardless of technological advances. Recent modifications in the World Health Organization (WHO) classification of non–small-cell lung cancer (NSCLC) reflect our greater understanding of lung cancer pathology. This chapter provides the necessary information for sound pathologic diagnoses by reviewing general aspects of lung carcinoma as well as the clinicopathologic features of the most common types of NSCLC, namely squamous cell carcinoma (SCC), adenocarcinoma, large cell carcinoma (LCC), and their variants.

Epidemiology

Incidence and Mortality

Lung cancer is the most common and deadliest cancer in the world. Estimated numbers of lung cancer cases worldwide increased 51% since 1985.[2] The worldwide incidence of lung carcinoma in 2002 reached an astonishing 1,352,132 cases and represented 12.4% of newly diagnosed cancer cases[1,2] (Fig. 35.1). The more than one million deaths represent almost 18% of worldwide cancer deaths[1] (Fig. 35.2). The 5-year survival rate in the United States stands at 15%, and in Europe only 10%, which is not much better than the recorded rate of 8.9% noted in developing countries[2] (Fig. 35.3).

Geographic trends in lung cancer incidence and mortality basically reflect regional differences in smoking behavior (Fig. 35.4). While developed countries had 676,681 new cases and 584,979 deaths and developing nations including China reported 672,221 new cases and 591,162 deaths in 2002, these data are misleading since the rising incidence and mortality of lung cancer will produce huge epidemics in developing countries in the decades to come.[2] Presently, the risk of dying from lung cancer is highest in North America, Australia, New Zealand, Europe (particularly Central and Eastern Europe), and South America, while the rates in China, Japan, and Southeast Asia are rising steeply. The lowest rates are observed in southern Asia and sub-Saharan Africa. Declining lung cancer rates first observed in the United Kingdom, and then in Finland, Australia, Netherlands, New Zealand, the U.S., Singapore, Denmark, Germany, Italy, and Sweden are related to the generational diminution in smoking.

Gender

In 2002, 965,241 men and 386,891 women were stricken with lung cancer and 848,132 and 330,786, respectively, died worldwide. The global lung cancer incidence rate is 35.5 per 100,000 men and 12.1 per 100,000 women, and accounts for 16% and 7.6% of new cancer cases in men and women, respectively.[1,2] The epidemic is simply less advanced in women.

Although the estimated number of lung cancer cases in men has increased by 44% since 1985, this is due to population growth and aging. In fact, there has been a 3.3% decrease in the actual age-standardized incidence (risk).[2] In the U.S., the annual percent change in the lung cancer incidence rate for men fell from 1.4% for the period 1975–1982 to –1.9% for the period 1991–2001 (Fig. 35.5). The death rate also fell from 1.8% to –1.9% during the same time periods (Fig. 35.6).[3] In the European Union, the lung cancer mortality rate per 100,000 men declined 1.6% from 1990 to 2000 despite the addition of Central and Eastern European nations with the

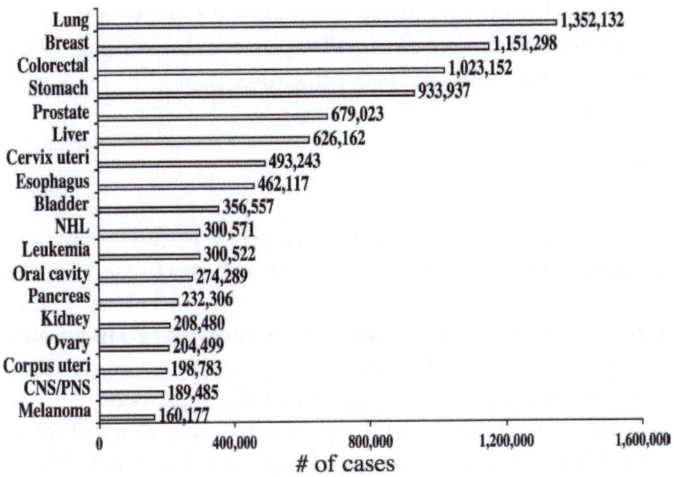

FIGURE 35.1. World cancer incidence by site, 2002. NHL, non-Hodgkin's lymphoma; CNS/PNS, central nervous system/peripheral nervous system.

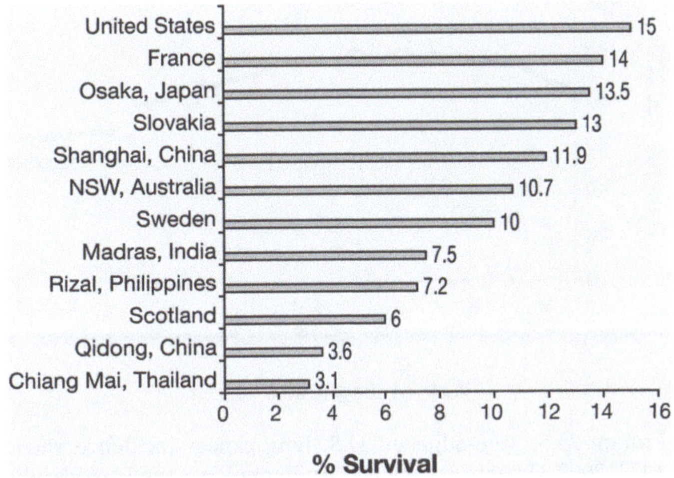

FIGURE 35.3. Five-year survival rates of lung cancer patients following diagnosis.

highest European lung cancer rates.[4–7] In 1996, tobacco smoking among Chinese men reached levels seen in the U.S. in 1950. With 300 million current male smokers, lung cancer will soon be responsible for more than two million deaths a year in Chinese men.[8,9]

In women, the estimated numbers of lung cancer cases worldwide has increased 76% since 1985.[2] While reported cases have perhaps peaked in the U.K., most Western countries show a rising incidence and mortality trend.[6,7,10] The highest incidence rates are noted in North America and North Western Europe, and the greatest rises are noted in Southern and Eastern Europe.[11]

The 600% increase in the death rate from lung cancer in American women from 1930 through 1997 corresponds to the availability and social acceptability of tobacco use among women and is now responsible for the current lung cancer epidemic in women.[12–14] While smoking prevalence in American men has decreased by nearly 50% from its peak in the 1960s and the death rate in men from lung cancer has decreased slightly, the smoking prevalence in American women has only decreased by 25% during the same period.[15] Although the annual percent change in the lung cancer incidence rate for U.S. women

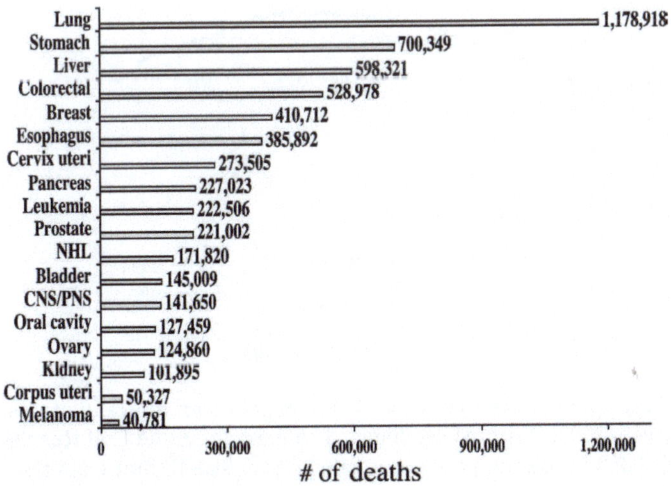

FIGURE 35.2. World cancer mortality by site, 2002. NHL, non-Hodgkin's lymphoma; CNS/PNS, central nervous system/peripheral nervous system.

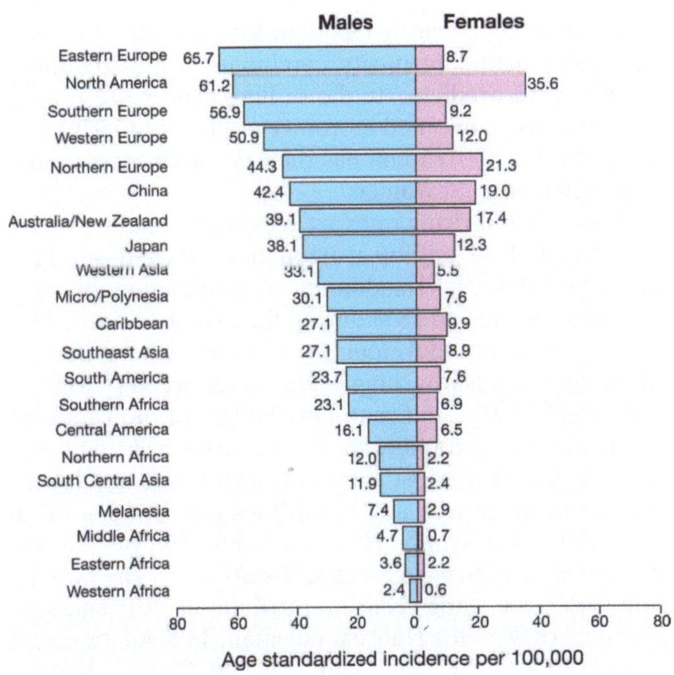

FIGURE 35.4. Age-standardized global lung cancer incidence rates. (From Parkin et al.,[2] with permission of Lippincott Williams & Wilkins.)

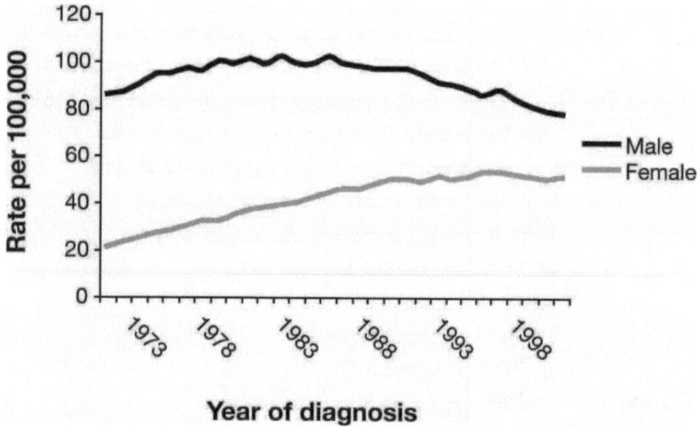

FIGURE 35.5. Age-adjusted U.S. lung cancer incidence rates, 1973–2002. (From Surveillance, Epidemiology, and End Results [SEER] Program [www.seer.cancer.gov] SEER*Stat Database: Mortality—All COD, Public-Use With State, Total U.S. [1969–2004], National Cancer Institute, DCCPS, Surveillance Research Program, Cancer Statistics Branch, released April 2007. Underlying mortality data provided by NCHS (_www.cdc.gov/nchs_ (http://www.cdc.gov/nchs)).

fell from 5.5% for the period 1975–1982 to 1.1% for the period 1991–2001, an increase is almost certain as groups of U.S. women with the highest rates of smoking will soon reach the age when lung cancer develops[16] (Fig. 35.6). In the European Union, the lung cancer mortality rate per 100,000 women rose 1.2% from 1990 to 2000 and a striking 38% in women younger than 55 years.[4]

In the U.S. it is estimated that in 2006, 47% (81,770) of newly diagnosed lung cancers are in women. While this incidence is significantly less than that attributed to breast cancer including in-situ carcinoma (212,920), more women were predicted to die of lung cancer (72,130) in 2006 than the combined mortality of breast (40,970) and colorectal (27,300) carcinoma, the next two most common carcinomas in U.S. women.[17]

Moderate but rising rates are reported in China, where an estimated 20 million women have started smoking since the 1990s.[1,18,19] In addition, smoking among women in Japan doubled to 18% during the 5-year period 1986–1991.[20] In many developing countries where female smoking remains low, lung cancer rates are very low.

A small but significant percentage of nonsmoking women also develop and die of lung cancer. Lung carcinoma is the third most common cancer among Chinese women in Singapore and constitutes almost 10% of all cancers in this group. However, only 3% of Chinese women aged 18 to 64 in Singapore smoke.[21,22] The population risk for lung cancer attributable to smoking approaches 80% for Hawaiian women, 45% for Japanese women living in Hawaii, and 15% for Chinese women living in Hawaii.[23] While the effect of cigarette smoking on lung cancer risk among Chinese females is qualitatively and quantitatively similar to its effect on lung cancer risk in women in other parts of the world, environmental tobacco smoke and other environmental carcinogens including cooking oil vapor, coal burning-devices, and perhaps genetic susceptibilities probably also play etiologic roles.[24,25]

Age

Non–small-cell lung cancer may occur in newborns and octogenarians,[26,27] but most cases are diagnosed in the sixth and seventh decades of life. Diagnoses rise exponentially and plateau at the age of 80 in men and 70 in women before decreasing. The median age of lung cancer diagnosis in the general population of the U.S. is 68 years.[28] No more than 10% of lung cancers are diagnosed in individuals under 50 years of age and less than 5% in individuals under 40 years of age.[29–36]

Whether in Asia, Europe, or North America, a larger percentage of lung cancer patients under age 40 are women as compared to older cohorts.[26,33,37–40] In the U.S., younger African Americans are also overrepresented.[29] The vast majority of cases are adenocarcinomas, and while many patients have significant smoking histories, up to 34% are never-smokers.[26,30–39,41,42] This percentage of nonsmokers does not appear to differ from that in the older populations.[42,43] Nevertheless, environmental, hormonal, and genetic factors are probably codeterminants.[29,31,33,35,38,39,42,44]

Younger patients present with more advanced stage than older cohorts, and are more likely to receive multimodality therapy for a variety of reasons, including the relative absence of comorbidities and the reluctance of physicians and patients to accept realistic therapeutic limitations. Overall survival and disease-free survival

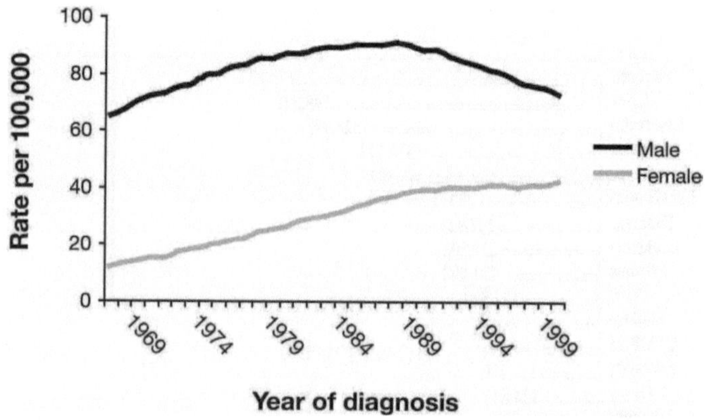

FIGURE 35.6. Age-adjusted U.S. lung cancer mortality rates, 1969–2002. (From Surveillance, Epidemiology, and End Results [SEER] Program [www.seer.cancer.gov] SEER*Stat Database: Mortality—All COD, Public-Use With State, Total U.S. [1969–2004], National Cancer Institute, DCCPS, Surveillance Research Program, Cancer Statistics Branch, released April 2007. Underlying mortality data provided by NCHS (_www.cdc.gov/nchs_ (http://www.cdc.gov/nchs)).

rates are probably not significantly different in younger populations.[29,31,33,37,42]

Non–small-cell carcinoma in children is rare. Fewer than 100 sporadic cases have been reported[45–50] (see Chapter 42). An equal sex distribution is noted, and adenocarcinomas are more common than SCC and LCC in the published series. Several cases have been reported arising in association with congenital cystic adenomatoid malformations.[51] Survival appears stage related and parallels that seen in adults.[45]

Race

Smoking-specific lung cancer mortality rates are consistently higher in British, Norwegian, Swedish, and American Caucasian male smokers than in Japanese male smokers.[52,53] Since the 1950s lung cancer rates in American Caucasian men have been two to three times higher than in Japanese men despite a lower prevalence of smoking in the U.S.[54–57] Furthermore, rates of lung cancer in Japanese migrants and their offspring in the U.S. remain below those of U.S.-born Caucasians.[58]

There is significant variation in the incidence of lung cancer among ethnic and racial groups in the U.S. Age-standardized incidence and death rates for African Americans and American Indian/Alaskan Natives vary from 117.2 and 104.1 for African-American males to 46.0 and 49.8 for American Indian/Alaskan Natives[3] (Fig. 35.7). African-American males have an almost 13% chance of developing lung cancer by age 75.[59] Black males between the ages of 40 and 54 are two to four times more likely to develop lung cancer than white males regardless

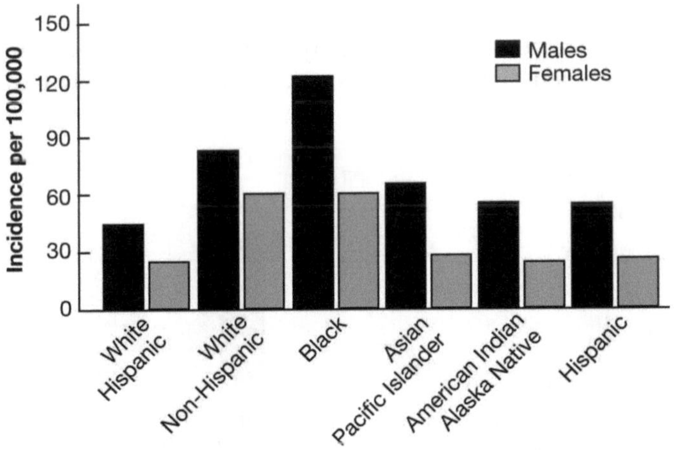

FIGURE 35.7. Age-adjusted U.S. lung cancer incidence rates by ethnicity, 1996–2000. (From Surveillance, Epidemiology, and End Results [SEER] Program [www.seer.cancer.gov] SEER*Stat Database: Mortality—All COD, Public-Use With State, Total U.S. [1969–2004], National Cancer Institute, DCCPS, Surveillance Research Program, Cancer Statistics Branch, released April 2007. Underlying mortality data provided by NCHS (_www.cdc.gov/nchs_(http://www.cdc.gov/nchs)).

of smoking habits.[60,61] And even African-American nonsmokers are eight times more likely to develop lung cancer than their white counterparts.[60] Furthermore, African Americans develop lung cancer at an earlier age than their white counterparts although they as a group begin to smoke later in life and smoke fewer cigarettes per day.[61–64] Native Hawaiians also appear more susceptible to lung cancer than whites, Japanese Americans, and Latinos.[58]

A greater racial susceptibility to lung cancer seems likely; however, cigarette formulation (more toxic with higher concentrations of tobacco-specific nitrosamines in American-manufactured cigarettes), smoking habits, occupation, and diet also play large roles.[58,62,65–67] For example, African Americans prefer menthol cigarettes, and suffer greater industrial exposure to carcinogens.[68,69] Furthermore, almost a dozen recent credible studies evaluating the role of cytochrome P-450 enzymes CYP2C9, CYP2D6, and CYP2E1 and the African-American–specific m3 mutation of *CYP1A1* in lung cancer in African Americans do not conclusively support a correlation between the genetic polymorphisms and susceptibility to lung carcinoma.[70–79] Suffice it to say, the etiologic roles of race and ethnicity are incompletely understood.

Histology

Almost 80% of lung cancers are NSCLC and about 20% are small cell lung cancer (SCLC). Worldwide, SCC is the most common lung carcinoma, but when one views the histologic breakdown according to region and gender, interesting trends are noted. Squamous cell carcinoma comprises 44% of lung cancers in men and 25% in women. Adenocarcinomas comprise 28% of cases in men and 42% in women. Only in China, Japan, the U.S., and Canada does the incidence of adenocarcinoma in men exceed that of SCC. In women, adenocarcinoma is the leading histologic type worldwide except in Poland, England, and Scotland, where SCC remains the most common histologic type.[80–82] Large cell carcinoma comprises less than 10% of NSCLC in both sexes.

In the 1950s adenocarcinoma constituted only 5% of male lung cancer in the U.S. but is now the most frequent form.[83,84] The current shift is due to both the decrease in SCC and increase in adenocarcinoma incidence rather than a drastic disappearance or surge in one of the histologic subtypes. In the U.S., SCC in men reached its maximum incidence in 1981, while the incidence of adenocarcinoma continued to rise until the early 1990s.[83,85] In contrast, both adenocarcinoma and SCC incidence rates continue to rise in American women. For this gender, the specific birth cohort values lag approximately 20 years beyond the male figures. Similar observations have been reported in Japan, the U.K., and in the Netherlands.[86–88]

These histologic differences are greatly influenced by differing smoking behavior and cigarette design in different regions of the world.[89–92] The growing numbers of ex-smokers in the population also play a large role since the decline in risk of lung cancer on smoking cessation is faster for SCC than for adenocarcinoma.[93,94] Lastly, a small component of the observed shift might be due to changes in diagnostic criteria, coding, and technological advances including fiberoptic bronchoscopy, thin-needle aspiration, and immunohistochemical stains. However, the increase in adenocarcinoma rates antedated these diagnostic innovations.[87,95]

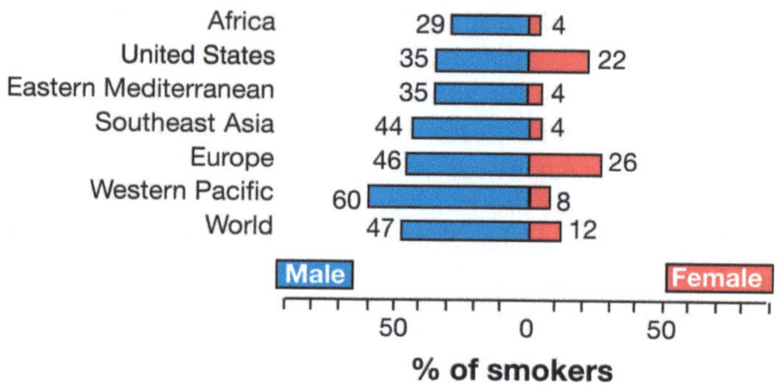

FIGURE 35.8. Estimated prevalence of adult smoking by geographic region in the early 1990s. (From Stewart and Kleihues.[926])

Etiology

Tobacco

The causal relationship between smoking and lung cancer was first suggested in 1898, and clearly established with cohort and case-controlled studies in the 1950s and 1960s.[96–104] The link is indisputable, and following the U.S. Surgeon General's 1964 report on smoking, which summarized existing evidence and declared cigarette smoking to be the major cause of lung cancer among American men, additional studies have further defined the relationship with regard to other epidemiologic factors.[105] These recent studies have great public health implications since they address the newer and purportedly lower-risk cigarettes.

The International Agency for Research on Cancer (IARC) estimated that in populations with prolonged cigarette use, the proportion of lung cancer attributable to cigarette smoking is greater than 90%.[53] According to studies conducted in Europe, Japan, and North America, 91% of all lung cancers in men and 69% in women are attributable to cigarette smoking[53,106] (Table 35.1); 90% to 95% of cases in men in Europe and North America and 85% and 74% of cases in women in North American and northern Europe are tobacco-related.[2] While cigarette consumption has decreased by half in the U.S. and several European nations, one billion men and a quarter of a billion women smoke worldwide. Sixty percent of adult men in China are estimated to smoke, representing one third of the worldwide smokers[107] (Fig. 35.8). Approximately 30 million young adults also start to smoke each year (Fig. 35.9). The worst consequences of tobacco have not yet been seen.

The risk of lung cancer in cigarette smokers depends on various aspects of smoking behavior including duration of smoking, number of cigarettes smoked, type of cigarette smoked, and inhaling pattern. Nevertheless, the relative risk for males aged 35 and older ranges from 11.4 to 22.4, and for women the mortality rate from lung cancer approaches 16 per 100,000 in women with a history of cigarette smoking versus 7 per 100,00 in never-smokers.[108,109]

TABLE 35.1. Percentage of deaths from lung cancer attributable to tobacco smoking in developed countries in 1990

	35–69 years	≥70 years
Men	93.9	90.3
Women	68.8	68.9

Source: Data from Sasco et al.[187]

Smoking causes genetic changes in cells of the lung that lead to the development of lung cancer. More than 4000 chemicals have been identified in tobacco smoke.[108] Approximately 2550 come from processed unadulterated tobacco, while the remainder are additives, pesticides, and other organic and metallic compounds.[110,111] Known or recognized carcinogens include polycyclic aromatic hydrocarbons (PAHs), *N*-nitrosamines, aromatic amines, aldehydes, organic compounds (e.g., benzene, vinyl chloride), and inorganic compounds (e.g., arsenic, chromium, radon, lead-210, polonium-210)[108,112] (Table 35.2). Polycyclic aromatic hydrocarbons and tobacco-specific nitrosamines are the most potent carcinogens in tobacco smoke.[112]

The concentrations of many of these carcinogens in mainstream (i.e., inhaled) smoke are above levels that

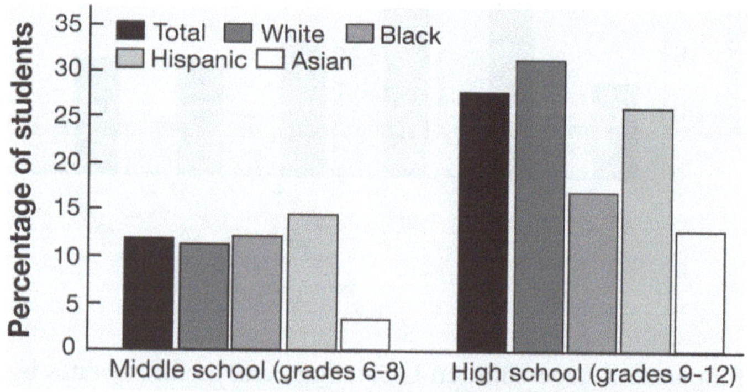

FIGURE 35.9. Active tobacco use among middle and high school students in the United States, 2004. (From Anonymous. Tobacco use, access, and exposure to tobacco in media among middle and high school students—United States 2004. MMWR 2005;54: 297–301.)

TABLE 35.2. Carcinogenic agents in tobacco smoke

Substances	Tobacco smoke (per cigarette)
Volatile aldehydes	
Formaldehyde	20–105 μg
Acetaldehyde	18–1400 μg
Crotonaldehyde	10–20 μg
N-nitrosamines	
N-nitrosodimethylamine	0.1–180 ng
N-nitrosodiethylamine	0–36 ng
N-nitrosopyrolidine	1.5–110 ng
Tobacco-specific nitrosamines	
N′-nitrosonornicotine (NNN)	3–3700 ng
4-(Methylnitrosamino)-1-(3-pyridyl)-1-butanone (NNK)	0–770 ng
4-(Methylnitrosamino)-1-(3-pyridyl)-1-butanol (NNAL)	Present
N′-nitrosoanabasine (NAB)	14–46 ng
Metals	
Nickel	0–600 ng
Cadmium	41–62 ng
Polonium 210	1–10 mBq
Arsenic	40–120 ng
Polycyclic aromatic hydrocarbons	
Benzo[*a*]pyrene	20–40 ng
Benzo[*a*]anthracene	20–70 ng
Benzo[*b*]fluoranthene	4–22 ng
Chrysene	40–60 ng
Dibenzo[*a,l*]pyrene	1.7–3.2 ng
Dibenzo[*a,h*]anthracene	Present

Source: Data from Stewart and Kleihues.[107]

would be fatal with uninterrupted exposure, but the dilution of the smoke with air and intermittency of smoke inhalation prevents cigarette smoking from being immediately lethal.[113] The 10^9 to 10^{10} particles per milliliter of cigarette smoke range from 0.1 to 1.0 μm in diameter. The size of the particles and inhalation pattern of the smoker (only subjectively studied) determine where the particles will be deposited. The deposition of particulates containing PAHs, polonium-210, or lead-210 in proximal bronchi are associated with the development of SCC, while the deeper inhalation of volatile nitrosamines results in their deposition in terminal bronchioles and alveoli and perhaps development of adenocarcinoma.[85,94,114]

Major determinants of lung cancer risk in cigarette smokers have been elucidated through epidemiologic studies. The duration of cigarette smoking is the strongest determinant of risk for both men and women.[53,115,116] For example, women smoking 20 cigarettes per day for 41 to 70 years had a mortality ratio (MR) of 25.1 compared to an MR of 13.6 for women who smoked for 21 to 30 years.[117] This determinant is responsible for the observation that an early age of onset is associated with a morbid lung cancer risk later in life.[53,118–120] An effect of age at starting to smoke independent of duration of smoking has not been demonstrated.[53,118,119] The intensity or quantity of cigarettes smoked is also significant, but not as important as the years of smoking.[115,116] The relative risk has been shown to be lesser in women, but these results probably reflect differences in duration of smoking. Remarkably, 1.5 pack per day smokers may bathe their bronchial epithelium with as much radiation as their skin receives from almost one chest x-ray per day.[121,122]

Whether low-tar cigarettes lower the risk of lung cancer remains controversial. The U.S. Surgeon General report states that "although characteristics of cigarettes have changed during the last 50 years . . . the risk of lung cancer in smokers has not declined."[123] While tar content has decreased from approximately 35 mg in the 1950s to 10 mg in the 1980s and most smokers use filtered cigarettes, deeper inhalation and increasing intensity of tobacco smoking (more cigarettes per day and more puffs per cigarette) make epidemiologic studies difficult to interpret.[53,124–134] Yet the risk of lung cancer is higher among lifetime nonfilter smokers than among lifetime filter smokers.[130,132] Furthermore, the risk of lung cancer appears no different in people who smoke medium-tar (15–21 mg), low-tar (8–14 mg), or very low tar cigarettes (≤7 mg).[135] Also, lung cancer risk from mentholated cigarettes resembles the risk from smoking nonmentholated cigarettes.[136] Interestingly, the widely advertised threefold decrease in the tar (containing PAHs) and nicotine content of American cigarettes included an increase in other carcinogens including tobacco-specific *N*-nitrosamines.[137] Lastly, studies have shown higher risk of lung cancer among deep versus slight or moderate inhalers.[109,138]

Substantial controversy surrounds the possibility that women are more susceptible than men to developing lung cancer after exposure to similar amounts of cigarette smoke.[12,139–144] Since women with lung cancer are younger than men, are two to three times more likely to have never smoked, start smoking at a later date, smoke less on average (31 vs. 52 pack-years), smoke lower tar content cigarettes, and inhale less deeply than men,[139,145] epidemiologic studies have not been precise or complete enough to conclusively argue the case for unequal risk of lung cancer for men and women with identical smoking exposure.[12,146,147] Sex-related biologic differences including gender-related nicotine clearance abilities, higher levels of DNA adducts, decreased DNA repair capacity, increased frequency of mutations in tumor suppressor genes, and the role of estrogens in smokers are not entirely understood.[148,149] At this time though, it appears that the carcinogenic effect of smoking on the lung is similar in men and women.[150]

Tobacco smoking increases the risk of both NSCLC and SCLC. The association is strongest for SCC, LCC, and SCLC, but the association between adenocarcinoma and tobacco smoking has become stronger over the past decade[151] (Fig. 35.10). Perhaps deeper and more

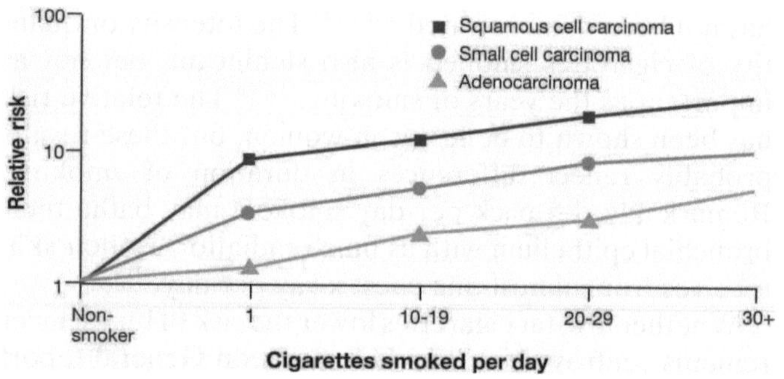

FIGURE 35.10. The relative risk of major histologic types of lung cancer according to cigarette consumption. (From Stewart and Kleihues.[927])

frequent inhalation of very low tar and nicotine cigarettes with greater deposition of carcinogens including *N*-nitrosamines are in part responsible for the inevitable ascendancy of adenocarcinoma as the most common type of lung cancer in smokers.[151–153]

Although the risk of lung cancer in former smokers remains higher than in individuals who have never smoked, the risk for former smokers decreases over time[53,123] Numerous studies have demonstrated risk reduction for men and women with all histologic types of lung cancer and for different types of tobacco smoked.[115,154] The most important modifier of risk reduction in ex-smokers is the number of years of abstinence.[155,156] The benefit of cessation becomes apparent approximately 5 years after quitting and increases as the length of abstinence lengthens (Fig. 35.11). The magnitude of risk reduction may be less for heavy smokers than for light smokers, for those who smoked for a shorter period of time, for those who quit at a younger age, or for those who inhaled less often and less deeply.[155,157–160]

While the prevalence of cigarette smoking is decreasing in many parts of the world, consumption of cigars and cigarillos is becoming increasingly popular in the U.S. and Europe, especially among teenagers.[161–166] Cigar consumption rose 75% between 1993 and 1998 in the U.S.[162,163] A similar trend is expected in Europe.[167] Since cigars are wrapped in tobacco, unlike cigarettes, mainstream cigar smoke has greater concentrations of nicotine, benzene, PAHs, hydrogen cyanide, lead nitrogen oxides, *N*-nitrosamines, ammonia, and carbon monoxide than mainstream smoke from cigarettes.[168,169] Cigar smoke also tends to have a higher pH than cigarette smoke, which not only increases the amount of free nicotine in both the particulate and vapor phases of smoke, but also facilitates the absorption of nicotine through buccal and nasal mucosa.[162,170,171]

Cigar and cigarillo smokers are at greater risk of developing lung cancer than nonsmokers, but lung cancer risk is less strongly associated with cigar than with cigarette smoking.[162,172] An American study noted a fivefold risk of lung cancer for cigar-only smoking men, and a European case-control study reported that cigar smokers were nine times more likely to develop lung cancer than nonsmokers compared to 15 times for cigarette smokers.[173] A dose-response relationship between lung cancer risk and either duration of smoking or average and cumulative consumption was seen for cigar smoking.[167,173] The proportion of SCC or SCLC was noted in one study to be higher than in cigarette-only smokers.[174] Similar findings have been reported for pipe smoking, with the additional observation that the relative risk of lung cancer for pipe smokers decreases with years since quitting.[175] Lastly, smokers who switch from cigarettes to pipes or cigars can halve their risk of dying of lung cancer but that risk still remains 50% higher than that of lifelong nonsmokers.[176] Individuals who smoke cigarettes along with either cigars or pipes have a lung cancer risk two-thirds that of pure cigarette smokers.[174] This effect is probably due to the reduction in the quantity of tobacco smoked and shallower inhalation.

Tobacco smoking with water pipes is a growing public health issue. This centuries-old practice was in decline as recently as the 1980s but its popularity, especially with adolescent Middle Easterners, is on the rise.[177,178] Perhaps 100 million people smoke water pipes daily.[179] Though mistakenly considered safer than cigarette smoking, water pipes produce high plasma concentrations of

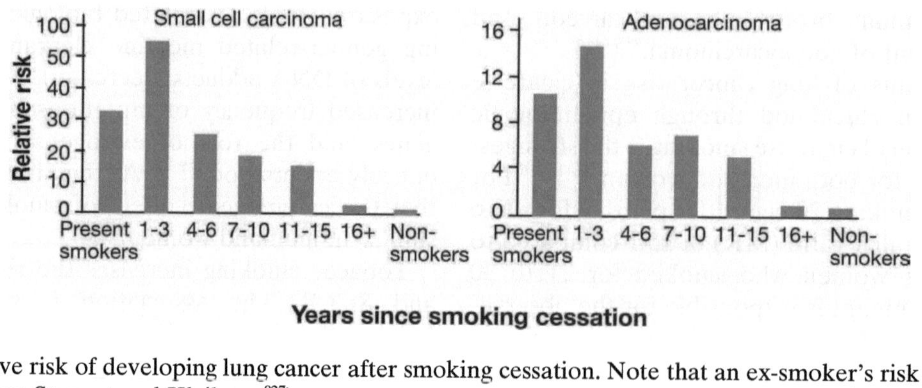

FIGURE 35.11. Relative risk of developing lung cancer after smoking cessation. Note that an ex-smoker's risk never equals that of a never-smoker. (From Stewart and Kleihues.[927])

carbon monoxide, nicotine, tar, arsenic, chromium, and lead.[180] An increased risk of lung cancer has also been reported with bidis smoked in India and water pipes in China.[53,181]

Marijuana smoking may also be a risk factor for lung cancer.[182] A marijuana cigarette deposits four times as much tar in the respiratory tract as that deposited from a single comparable sized filtered cigarette and contains many carcinogens including PAHs and phenols at concentrations higher than those found in cigarettes.[182,183] Histopathologic studies of bronchial epithelium in habitual marijuana smokers suggest that smoking marijuana exerts field cancerization effects similar to those seen in tobacco smokers.[184] Since marijuana use is becoming more prevalent, especially among adolescents, carefully designed retrospective and prospective studies are necessary to determine the exact relationship between this illicit drug and lung cancer risk.

Involuntary or passive smoking, also referred to as environmental tobacco smoke (ETS), also causes lung cancer and is estimated to be responsible for up to 3000 cases (20%) of lung cancer per year in nonsmoking American men and women.[185,186] In stark comparison to the observation that 90% of lung cancers in men are attributable to tobacco smoking, only 50% to 70% of lung cancers in women are the consequence of tobacco smoking.[150,187] Lung cancer cohorts report female never-smoker rates ranging up to 43%[188–191]; however, up to 82% of these women had histories of environmental tobacco smoke.[188] In fact, never smokers with lung cancer in one recent study had a higher exposure to ETS in childhood (13%) compared with ever smokers (5%).[188] Since accurate assessments of ETS exposure are difficult to ascertain, one cannot be entirely certain of a never smoking woman's risk of developing lung cancer.

Environmental tobacco smoke is composed of sidestream smoke released from the burning tobacco product (80%) and mainstream smoke exhaled by smokers (20%). Sidestream smoke contains higher concentrations of some carcinogens (e.g., nitrosamines, benzo[*a*]pyrene [BaP]) and other toxic compounds than measured in inhaled mainstream smoke (Table 35.3). Based on urinary and serum levels of cotinine, the metabolite of nicotine, nonsmoking spouses of "heavy" smokers may absorb the equivalent of one cigarette a day.

Large-scale studies and meta-analyses report a statistically significant and consistent association between lung cancer risk in spouses of smokers and exposure to secondhand tobacco smoke from the spouse who smokes.[192–196] In addition, workplace and social setting ETS equally increase the risk of lung cancer.[185,193] The excessive risk is of the order of 20% for women and 30% for men and increases with both the number of cigarettes smoked by the spouse and duration of the exposure.[194] This risk is equivalent to a relative risk on the order of 1.2.[197] It is uncertain whether ETS imparts a greater risk of developing SCC and SCLC than adenocarcinoma.[195,196,198–208] Unlike the persistent risk of lung cancer in ex-smokers, no increase in risk has been detected in individuals whose exposure to ETS ended more than 15 years earlier.[189,192,196,198]

TABLE 35.3. Tobacco constituents in mainstream smoke (MS) of one cigarette and environmental tobacco smoke (ETS) in polluted environments

Constituent	Amount in MS of 1 cigarette	Inhaled ETS in 1 hour
Acrolein	60–100 μg	8–72 μg
Benzo[*a*]pyrene	20–40 ng	1.7–460 ng
Carbon monoxide	10–23 mg	1.2–22 mg
Dimethylnitrosamine	10–40 ng	6–140 ng
Nicotine	1–2.5 mg	0.6–30 μg

Source: Data from U.S. Surgeon General Report.[924]

Environmental Factors

While radioactive forms including radon-222, lead-210, and polonium-210 are recognized carcinogens in tobacco smoke, inhalation of radioactive radon gas originating from the earth's core and ubiquitous in the environment is considered the second leading cause of lung cancer in the U.S. The 1998 National Academy of Science report attributes 15,000 to 20,000 annual U.S. lung cancer cases and deaths (10–15%) to residential radon exposure.[209,210] Epidemiologic studies suggest that radon may be responsible for 20% of lung cancers in Sweden, 7% in Germany, and 4% in the Netherlands.[211,212]

Radon is a naturally occurring inert radioactive decay product of radium-226, the fifth daughter of uranium-238. Both uranium-238 and radium-226 are present in most soils and rocks, although their concentrations vary. Radon rises through the earth and enters air or water and is the most important isotope of uranium-238 owing to its relatively long half-life of 3.82 days. Solid radon decay products including 218-polonium and 214-polonium, also referred to as progeny or daughters, settle on dust particles, and are inspired and retained in the lung (Fig. 35.12). These progeny emit high-energy and high-mass particles (i.e., alpha particles), which damage the respiratory epithelium.

The primary site of radon exposure for most people is the home. Radon enters the home from the soil through cracks in the foundation, loose-fitting pipe penetrations, sump openings, crawl spaces, and block walls. Lesser amounts are waterborne. Areas of the world with the highest radon levels include Scandinavia and Southern Europe (Fig. 35.13). The Reading Prong crossing through

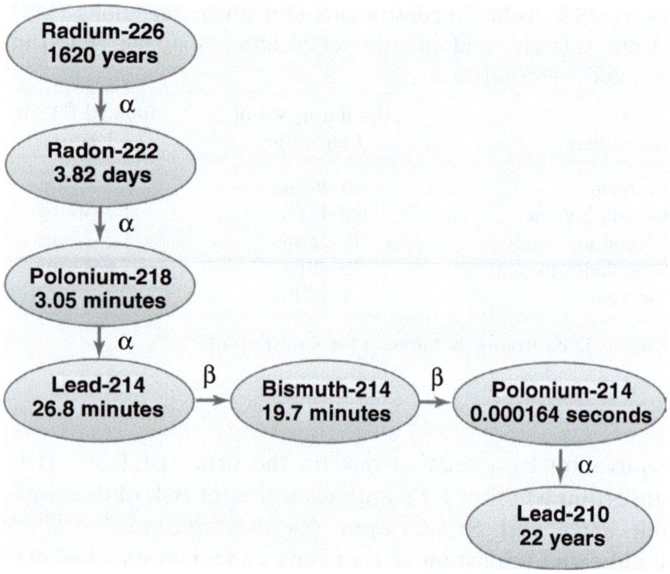

FIGURE 35.12. Decay pathway of radium-226 to lead-210.

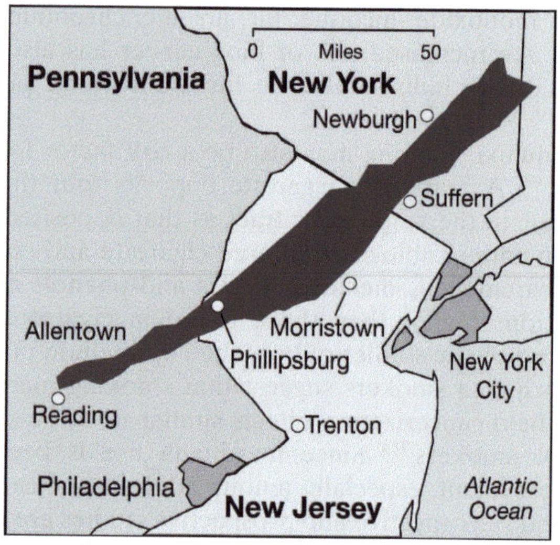

FIGURE 35.14. The Reading Prong is a thin belt of igneous and metamorphic rocks containing high concentrations of uranium-238, and thus high levels of radon.

Pennsylvania, New York, and New Jersey is a well-publicized "hot spot" in the United States (Fig. 35.14). The recognition of radon as a lung cancer risk has over the past decade spawned a large commercial industry offering home radon tests and remediation.

Radon is classified as a human carcinogen primarily on the basis of findings in miners.[213–215] Residential exposure is at much lower levels and the risk of lung cancer in this population was originally established by extrapolating data from miners.[213,215,216] While debated whether data from miners should be extrapolated to residential radon exposure where radon levels are 50- to 100-fold less than the lowest levels in uranium mines, animal and in vitro studies support the findings, and recent case-control studies and meta-analyses conclusively demonstrate an association between residential radon and lung cancer risk.[210,217–225] The interaction between radon exposure and smoking with regard to lung cancer appears more than additive but less than multiplicative.[219] The risk for SCLC is higher in residential radon-associated lung cancer.[218]

Although cigarette smoking and radon are the principle causes of lung cancer, indoor and outdoor air pollution remain public health concerns. After all, an adult

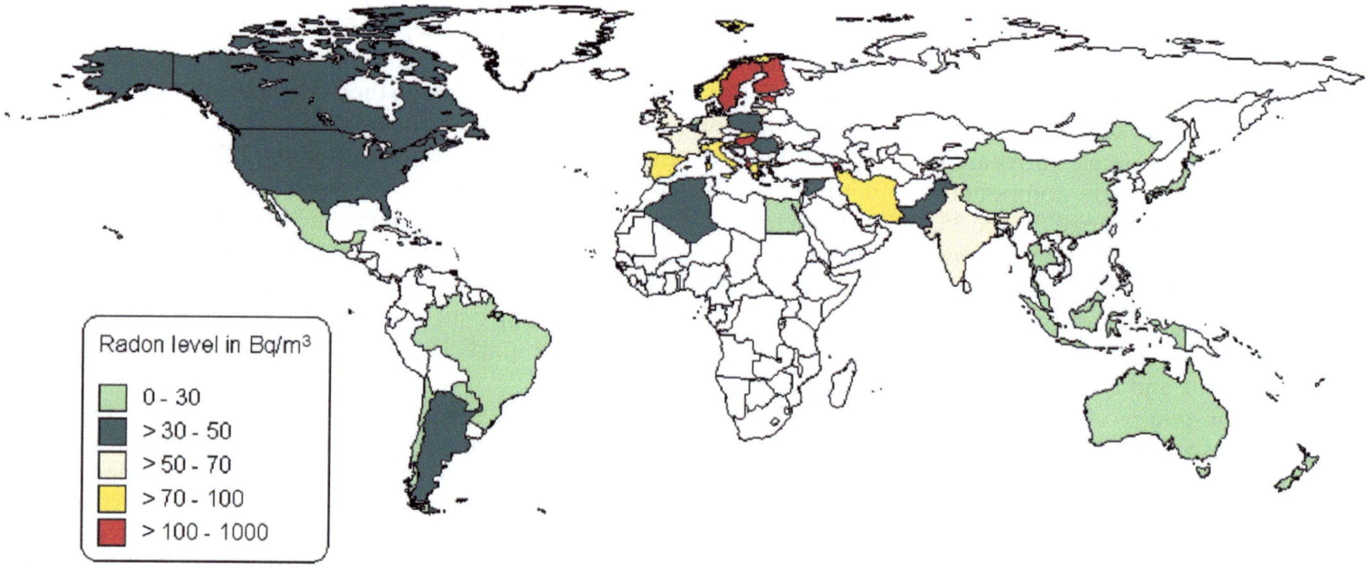

FIGURE 35.13. World radon levels. (Courtesy of Daniel Steck, Ph.D., St. John's University, MN.)

human inhales over 10,000 liters of air per day. Carcinogens emitted by industries, power plants, motor vehicles, and heating materials including wood and coal, contaminate outdoor air. Mid-20th century industries in Europe and North America spewed, and developing nations continue to release, enormous amounts of organic and inorganic substances including carcinogens such as arsenic, copper, cadmium, and sulfuric acid into the air and soil.[226,227] Fossil-fuel combustion resplendent with PAHs also contaminates ambient air across the globe and is associated with a moderate increase in lung cancer risk in the U.S.[228]

Data suggest that 1% to 2% of lung cancers are directly attributable to air pollution.[229–232] A European study noted an elevated lung cancer risk for city dwellers compared to residents of rural areas after controlling for age, smoking habits, social class, and occupation. Increased risks of SCLC, adenocarcinoma, and LCC were reported.[233] And although an American Cancer Society study noted only minimal differences in lung cancer mortality in urban or rural areas or among cities according to pollution indices, the U.S. Environmental Protection Agency estimated a median excess of 18 lifetime cancer cases (not all lung) per 100,000 people for all hazardous air pollutant concentrations.[234,235] In regions of China, arsenic from copper smelters accounts for a proportion of the excess risk of lung cancer, and similar findings were noted near a coke oven in Genoa, Italy.[236,237]

Indoor pollution is categorized into four classes: combustion products, chemicals, radon, and biologicals. Combustion sources include ETS, but of great interest in the developing world is the excessive cancer risk associated with cooking and heating stoves.[238] Across China, air pollution from coal-burning heating and cooking devices are linked to lung cancer.[237,239] In instances, measured BaP levels in poorly ventilated homes using unvented coal-burning stoves or fire pits exceeded the recommended upper limit for U.S. cities by 60 times.[237] In one region, an age–, education–, and tobacco-smoking–adjusted relative risk of 2.3 was noted.[25,240] Individuals' risks rise in proportion to duration of exposure but may also be associated with genetic factors.[241,242] In at least one province, stove improvement reduced levels of indoor air pollution by 35% and thus reduced the risk of lung cancer.[243] Whether the elevated risk of lung cancer in nonsmoking Chinese women is at least in part due to prolonged exposure to mutagenic vapors from rapeseed oil produced in wok cooking is postulated but not proven.[244–246] Epidemiologic studies do not account for the fact that while lung cancer rates are rising in this population, the use of rapeseed oil has been constant for many decades. The presence of heterocyclic amines in cooked meat and fumes generated during frying or grilling of meats may also increase the risk of lung cancer among current and ex-smokers.[247]

Occupational Factors

The distinction between occupational and environmental exposure to carcinogenic compounds is arbitrary given the presence of many substances in both the workplace and general environment. While uranium miners are exposed to high concentrations of radon, the ubiquitous nature of the radioactive material is also an environmental risk factor for lung cancer. Nonferrous metal smelting, wood preservation, glass manufacturing, and production and use of agricultural chemicals expose workers to arsenic and increase lung cancer risk, but drinking water contaminated with arsenic is also associated with an increased risk of SCC and SCLC.[248–250] The idiosyncratic nature of the evidence also complicates efforts to improve workplace environments. In some instances, such as asbestos mining, a causative agent is apparent, while in others, such as painting and welding, an excessive risk is noted but the causative agents are not known.[251] For this reason, the IARC lists occupational agents as definite, probable, or possible human carcinogens,[53] while the U.S. Department of Health and Human Services lists substances as either known to be or reasonably anticipated to be human carcinogens.[252]

Although occupational carcinogens are responsible for a significant percentage of lung cancer among exposed workers, known carcinogens are not a major cause of lung cancer (Tables 35.4 and 35.5). While an association between SCLC and radiation as well as chloromethyl ether exposure is accepted, there are no specific associations between particular occupational exposures and lung cancer cell types.[253,254]

Of the many occupational factors, more has been written about asbestos exposure and lung cancer than the other exposures. While a complete discussion of asbestos is beyond the scope of this chapter (see Chapter 27, Asbestos), the association between heavy asbestos exposure and carcinoma of the lung is universally accepted.[255] Epidemiologic studies have demonstrated a dose-response relationship between asbestos exposure and lung cancer risk and note an at least 15-year latency period between first exposure and disease.[256–259] The relative risk of lung cancer is estimated to increase 0.5% to 4% for each fiber per cubic centimeter per year (fiber-years) of cumulative exposure. Thus, a cumulative exposure of 25 fiber-years increases the risk of lung cancer at least twofold.[260]

Asbestos exposure acts synergistically with cigarette smoking.[257,261–263] An often-quoted study noted cigarette smoking increased lung cancer risk 11-fold and asbestos exposure fivefold when compared to a nonsmoking, nonexposed reference population. The lung cancer risk among cigarette-smoking asbestos insulators was 55-fold, indicating that the two effects are multiplicative rather than additive.[257] Cigarette smoking appears to increase

TABLE 35.4. Occupational agents and exposures evaluated by the International Agency for Research on Cancer (IARC) as definite human lung carcinogens

Substance or mixture	Occupation or industry
Physical agents	
Ionizing radiation including x-rays, γ-rays, and radon gas	Radiologists; technologists, nuclear workers, radium-dial painters, underground miners, plutonium workers, aircraft crew
Respirable dusts and fibers	
Asbestos	Mining and milling, by-product manufacture insulating, shipyard workers, asbestos cement industry
Silica, crystalline	Granite and stone industries, ceramic, glass, and related industries, foundries and metallurgical industries, abrasives, construction, farming
Talc containing asbestiform fibers	Manufacture of pottery, paper, paint, cosmetics
Metals and metal compounds	
Arsenic and arsenic compounds	Nonferrous metal smelting, production, packaging, and use of arsenic containing pesticides, sheep dip manufacture, wool fiber production, mining of ores containing arsenic
Beryllium	Beryllium extraction and processing, aircraft and aerospace industries, electronics and nuclear industries, jewelers
Cadmium and cadmium compounds	Cadmium-smelter workers, battery production workers, cadmium-copper alloy workers, dyes and pigment production, electroplating processes
Chromium compounds, hexavalent	Chromate production plants, dyes and pigments, plating and engraving, chromium ferro-alloy production, stainless-steel welding, in wood preservatives, leather tanning, water treatment, inks, photography, lithography, drilling muds, synthetic perfumes, pyrotechnics, corrosion resistance
Selected nickel compounds including combinations of nickel oxides and sulfides in the nickel-refining industry	Nickel refining and smelting, welding
Wood and fossil fuels and their by-products	
Coal tars and pitches	Production of refined chemicals and coal tar products (patent-fuel), coke production, coal gasification, aluminum production, foundries, road paving and construction (roofers and slaters)
Mineral oils, untreated and mildly treated	Production, used as lubricant by metal workers, machinists, engineers, printing industry (ink formulation), used in cosmetics, medicinal and pharmaceutical preparations
Soots	Chimney sweeps, heating-unit service personnel, brick masons and helpers, building demolition workers, insulators, firefighters, metallurgical workers, work involving burning or organic materials
Intermediates in plastics and rubber manufacturing	
Bis(chloromethyl) ether and chloromethyl methyl ether (technical grade)	Production, chemical intermediate, alkylating agent, laboratory reagent, plastic manufacturing, ion-exchange resins and polymers
2,3,7,8-tetrachlorodibenzo-*para*-dioxin (TCDD)	Production, use of chlorophenols and chlorophenoxy herbicides, waste incineration, PCB production, pulp and paper bleaching
Others	
Involuntary (passive) smoking	Workers in bars and restaurants, office workers
Mustard gas	Production, used in research laboratories, military personnel
Strong inorganic-acid mists containing sulfuric acid	Pickling operations, steel industry, petrochemical industry, phosphate acid fertilizer manufacturing

Source: Siemiatycki et al.,[251] with permission.

the penetration of asbestos fibers into the bronchial mucosa and may interfere with the clearance of asbestos fibers.[264–266]

The effects of asbestos fibers on bronchial epithelium are not unlike those of classic tumor promoters. Asbestos fibers can induce protein kinase C, and activate proto-oncogenes c-*fos* and c-*jun* as well as nuclear factor (NF)-κB–dependent gene expression, including interleukins, nitric oxide synthetase, and the proto-oncogene c-*myc*.[267–271] In addition, asbestos fibers adsorb and enhance the transport of carcinogens including BaP into cells and may enhance the generation of the active carcinogenic metabolites.[272]

Less than 2% of lung cancers are asbestos related, but carcinoma of the lung may develop in response to exposure to *any* type of asbestos.[273] Data suggest chrysotile is as potent a lung carcinogen as the amphiboles amosite and crocidolite.[256,258,274–277] Reported variations in lung

TABLE 35.5. Occupational agents and exposures evaluated by IARC as probable human lung carcinogens

Substance or mixture	Occupation or industry
Polyaromatic hydrocarbons	
Benz[*a*]anthracene	Work involving combustion of organic matter, foundries, steel mills, firefighters, vehicle mechanics
Benzo[*a*]pyrene	Work involving combustion of organic matter, foundries, steel mills, firefighters, vehicle mechanics
Dibenz[*a,h*]anthracene	Work involving combustion of organic matter, foundries, steel mills, firefighters, vehicle mechanics
Wood and fossil fuels and their by-products	
Diesel engine exhaust	Railroad workers, professional drivers, dock workers, mechanics
Chlorinated hydrocarbons	
α-Chlorinated toluenes	Production, dye and pesticide manufacture
Monomers	
Epichlorohydrin	Production and use of resins, glycerine, and propylene-based rubbers, used as a solvent
Pesticides	
Nonarsenical insecticides	Production, pest control and agricultural workers, flour and grain mill workers

Source: Siemiatycki et al.,[251] with permission.

cancer rates are most likely due to the concentration and duration of exposure, the size of the fibers, and concomitant tobacco use. For example, the low lung cancer rate among brake repair workers is attributable to the relatively low dust level, low proportion of asbestos in the dust, and the presence of very short chrysotile fibers in that dust.[279,280] The only indication of a greater risk for developing an asbestos-related lung carcinoma in this work group might be concomitant smoking, since cigarette smoking increases the penetration of chrysotile fibers to a greater extent than amphiboles.[265]

Nonoccupational asbestos exposure including living with an asbestos worker or residing near asbestos mines may have a small increase in lung cancer risk.[197] The assessment of this type of exposure is fraught with difficulties since exposure levels are usually low and the duration of the exposure is rarely known. Studies reported in China and South Africa find a small risk, but this has not been observed in either European or North American investigations.[240,281,282]

The clinical and pathologic features of lung carcinoma in asbestos workers are no different from those seen in individuals without asbestos exposure. There is no difference in tumor location, either central or peripheral, nor is there a particular lobar distribution associated with asbestos-related carcinoma. Although assertions correlating histologic cell type with asbestos exposure litter the medical literature, it is often stated that adenocarcinoma is the cell type most often observed in asbestos-related cancers.[283–288] Most carcinomas of the lung occurring in asbestos workers are histologically similar to those occurring in nonexposed cigarette smokers.[254,289,290] For these reasons it does not appear that any pathologic feature of a lung carcinoma is of value in deciding whether the tumor represents an asbestos-related malignancy.

Along these lines, there remains a fair bit of controversy regarding the pathologist's ability to determine whether a lung carcinoma is associated with asbestos exposure. While some experts believe that a lung cancer cannot be designated as asbestos related without a radiographic or pathologic diagnosis of asbestosis,[291–294] others believe that a sufficient asbestos dose or tissue burden (equivalent to values seen in individuals with asbestosis) is enough evidence to establish a causal link between asbestos exposure and lung carcinoma.[284,295–303] Aside from legal ramifications, if the former theory is true and lung cancer is a complication of asbestosis and not a primary consequence of exposure, then those exposed to asbestos without radiographic or pathologic evidence of asbestosis might be somewhat reassured.

Infections

The etiologic role of infectious agents in the development of lung carcinoma is an intriguing area of clinical and epidemiologic research. While strong associations, such as human papilloma viruses (HPV) and cervical SCC are not present in lung cancer, viruses, mycobacteria, bacteria, and fungi may play etiologic roles in rare cases.

Human papilloma virus is perhaps the most likely virus to play a role in lung carcinogenesis. Some HPV types are considered oncogenic and responsible for most anogenital carcinomas and also implicated in esophageal and head and neck neoplasms. Since HPV-induced lesions occur at squamocolumnar mucosal junctions, and cigarette smokers often have foci of metaplastic squamous mucosa, it is not unreasonable to postulate a role for HPV in the development of SCC. While juvenile-onset laryngeal papillomatosis with malignant transformation is a recognized HPV-associated lesion, the detection rate of HPV (mostly high-risk subtypes 16 and 18) by a variety of methods in de novo SCC ranges from 0% to 80%.[304–312] An uncritical literature review noted that almost 22% of bronchial carcinomas harbored HPV DNA.[313] Geographic, racial, and perhaps seasonal variations may also confound the findings, but reports from similar locations have shown entirely opposite results, suggesting methodologic flaws.[314–318] Human papilloma virus protein expression in blood and tumor samples from Asian women with lung adenocarcinoma also suggests a possible link between HPV and the risk of developing lung adenocarcinoma in female nonsmokers; however, few limited studies have investigated this risk.[319,320] Hematogenous spread of virus from cervical infections (subtypes 16 and 18) rather than inhaled virus (subtypes 6 and 11) is postulated, but additional studies are necessary.

Epstein-Barr virus (EBV) is associated with primary pulmonary lymphoepithelioma-like carcinoma (LELC) in Chinese, Japanese, Taiwanese, and Eskimo populations.[321–330] This EBV-associated carcinoma morphologically resembles the EBV-associated undifferentiated nasopharyngeal carcinoma and presumably represents a clonal expansion of a single EBV-infected progenitor cell.[331] The absence of EBV genome in most Western LELC suggests that EBV is not a required etiologic factor.[307,322,332,333] This pattern is analogous to that seen in Burkitt lymphoma, which has a 100% association with EBV in African patients but less than 25% association in non-Africans. Rare instances of EBV-positive NSCLC including a signet-ring cell adenocarcinoma are of uncertain significance.[325,328,333–336] In fact, in-situ hybridization staining of these tumors is heterogeneous and patchy rather than convincingly diffuse as noted in Asian lymphoepithelioma-like carcinoma.[327,328]

Lung cancer is not an acquired immunodeficiency syndrome (AIDS)-defining malignancy. Nevertheless, human immunodeficiency virus (HIV)-infected men and women appear to have a small but significant risk of developing lung cancer compared to age- and gender-matched populations.[337–343] This increase is not accounted for by smoking alone.[339,344] Recent studies evaluating malignancy-related death in HIV-infected patients treated with highly active antiretroviral therapy (HAART) indicate that lung cancer is the most common solid tumor in patients with controlled HIV infection and occurs more frequently in the post-HAART era.[338,345–348] With a mean age of diagnosis ranging from 38 to 49 years, these 30- to 60-pack-year smokers have mostly NSCLC, often adenocarcinomas, but without a statistically significant subtype association.[349–352] The majority of patients present with advanced-stage disease, and all cases are fatal. Whether the carcinomas are intrinsically more aggressive than NSCLC in HIV-negative patients is debated.[353,354] Dysregulation of immune mechanisms such as decreased natural killer cell activity and aberrant inflammatory cytokine production related to Tat protein–induced angiogenesis have been reported in HIV-infected lung cancer patients.[355,356] Perhaps this results in an unchecked proliferation of spontaneously developing tumor cells.[357] Yet the development of lung cancer may not be associated with a low CD4 cell count, thus calling into question the role of immune function in carcinogenesis.[344,358,359] Lastly, while the role of HIV is unknown, the virus might stimulate the release of aberrant growth factors resulting in oncogenesis.[360]

Statistically significant increases in lung cancer risk are also associated with particular pulmonary mycobacterial and bacterial organisms. Previous pulmonary tuberculosis appears to be an independent risk factor for lung cancer. Not surprisingly, tuberculosis is often cited as a major etiologic factor in the nonsmoking Asian women with lung cancer.[361] Among those diagnosed with tuberculosis within 20 years, the risk of lung cancer exceeded 2.5-fold in a case-control study adjusting for cigarette smoking in Shanghai, China.[362,363] This risk is apparently not related to treatment with isoniazid, prior radiation therapy, or socioeconomic status.[362,364–366] The association appears stronger with adenocarcinoma than SCC or SCLC, an unsurprising fact given that most tuberculosis-associated carcinomas are peripheral.[201,362,367,368] The chronic inflammatory process might enhance the effects of other carcinogenic exposures or stimulate cell proliferation and growth.[362] Underlying weakened host immunity may also predispose to the development of lung cancer.[369] The possibility that a very small percentage of lung carcinomas arise from tuberculosis-associated scars cannot be entirely discounted (see sections Lung Injury and Adenocarcinoma, below) (see also Chapter 9).

Prospective and retrospective epidemiologic studies have also reported an association between serologic evidence of chronic *Chlamydophila pneumoniae* infection and risk of lung cancer in male smokers.[370–375] Elevated immunoglobulin A (IgA) and immune complex levels are associated with SCC and SCLC subtypes.[370] Only a single case-control study investigated the association for women, and found a statistically significant positive association.[376] Another group did not find an association among nonsmoking Chinese women in Singapore.[377] Not unlike the organism's role in the pathogenesis of coronary artery disease, chronic inflammation resulting from persistent infection may induce production of reactive oxygen species and other inflammatory stimuli.[378,379] Chronic *C. pneumoniae* infection may also act synergistically with cigarette smoke carcinogens and either initiate or promote carcinogenesis.

Epidemiologic studies investigating high lung cancer rates among nonsmoking women in Asia and Africa raise the possibility that chronic fungal infections may play an etiologic role. In northern Thailand, for example, *Microsporum canis*, a zoophilic dermatophyte, has been suggested as a risk factor.[24,380] Whether organisms usually responsible for superficial fungal infections could initiate or promote lung carcinogenesis, however, has yet to be proven.

Lung Injury

Several noninfectious pulmonary and systemic diseases are also associated with an increased risk of developing lung cancer. Chronic obstructive pulmonary diseases (COPD) and inflammatory/fibrosing lung diseases have been studied, and while not all investigations yielded statistically significant results, the risk for lung cancer is generally elevated for patients with chronic bronchitis and emphysema as well as various chronic interstitial lung diseases.

The association between both chronic bronchitis and emphysema and lung cancer is densely clouded by the role of tobacco smoking. Since only a small percentage of smokers develop lung cancer, other local inflammatory conditions must play a role. Impaired pulmonary function, even in the absence of cigarette smoking, is associated with an increased risk for lung cancer.[381,382] Case-control and cohort studies note an association after adjusting for active smoking.[9,25,366,368,383–389] The risk increases linearly in proportion to the degree of airway obstruction. In one study individuals with a forced expiratory volume of less than 60% of predicted had an almost fivefold excess risk of lung cancer.[387,390,391] Squamous cell carcinoma and SCLC are reported more often than adenocarcinomas, but all types are seen.[25,201,367,368,383,392] While mucostasis contributing to impaired carcinogen clearance may be in part responsible for the COPD-associated increase in lung cancer,[381,386] such a theory does not account for the long latency periods of both COPD and lung cancer and would require significant obstructive disease to precede the development of carcinoma by many years.[387] Perhaps long-standing inflammation in the bronchi leads to cellular injury and repair, resulting in increased cell turnover and propagation of genetic errors.

An association between asthma and lung cancer is not certain. Evidence supporting an association exists, but the overall epidemiologic evidence is not entirely convincing.[366,368,383,389,392–394] Misclassification of chronic bronchitis or even allergies as asthma may be responsible for conflicting results.

While several chronic fibrosing lung diseases including asbestosis are unequivocally associated with the development of lung cancer, the relationship between idiopathic pulmonary fibrosis (IPF) and lung cancer is probable but not certain. Although the scientific literature is replete with studies indicating a greater incidence of lung cancer in IPF patients with relative risks of 7 to 14 manifesting as a greater than expected number of peripheral lower lobe SCC in older males, relatively limited observational evidence and conflicting findings on follow-up and death certificate–based studies question the association.[395–405] Evidence indicating that cigarette smoking is an independent risk factor for IPF may confound the vast majority of studies suggesting an IPF-lung cancer connection.[406] Nevertheless, accelerated cell proliferation in honeycomb lesions may very well hold clues for the pathogenesis of both IPF and lung cancer[407,408] (see Chapter 34).

Epidemiologic studies also note modest associations between several collagen-vascular diseases and lung cancer. Scleroderma and systemic sclerosis have been thoroughly studied and most but not all investigations note relative risks ranging from 2 to as high as 16.[409–413] The bronchioloalveolar carcinoma (BAC) subtype of adenocarcinoma may be seen with increased frequency in systemic sclerosis patients, but the data are historical and may not represent true BAC. The observation that lung cancer in these patients arises in the setting of chronic lung fibrosis again raises the possibility that inflammation-induced pulmonary fibrosis may lead to NSCLC. Both dermatomyositis and polymyositis are associated with an increased risk of NSCLC. The risk is greater for dermatomyositis with relative risks approaching 3.5.[414–416] Yet the possibility that some myositis-associated lung cancers represent paraneoplastic syndromes clouds the data[415,417] (see Chapter 34).

Diet

Much is theorized but little known about the influence of diet on lung cancer risk. The epidemiologic observation made over 30 years ago that lung cancer patients had low vitamin A levels ushered in decades of research focusing on vitamins and antioxidant micronutrients as putative preventive agents.[418] It was recently shown that individuals with low dietary folate intake have markedly diminished DNA repair capacity, and it has been hypothesized that antioxidant micronutrients might reduce lung cancer risk by protecting against oxidative damage to DNA.[419]

Case-control and cohort studies generally indicate that individuals with high dietary intake of fruits or vegetables have lower lung cancer risks that those with low fruit or vegetable intake[420–423] (Fig. 35.15). These findings may be stronger for fruits than vegetables, and stronger for women than men.[424–427] The protective effect might only apply to SCC and SCLC.[428] Smokers appear to eat fewer fruits and vegetables compared to never-smokers.[429,430] Despite the apparent inverse associations of total fruit,

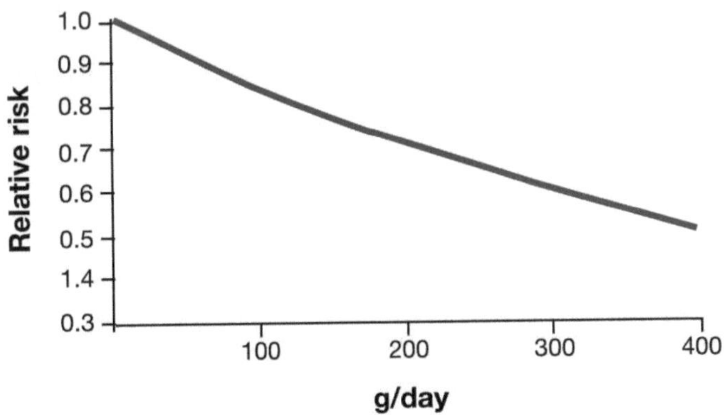

FIGURE 35.15. Relative risk of lung cancer associated with fruit consumption. Similar findings have been reported with vegetable consumption. (From Stewart and Kleihues.[927])

rosaceae fruit, cruciferae vegetables, and "other" vegetables such as corn, onions, and sweet potatoes with lung cancer risk, three large chemopreventive studies in Western populations showed no association between ß-carotene, retinoid, and α-tocopherol supplements and lung cancer risk.[431–433] In fact, in two of the three studies ß-carotene supplements were unequivocally responsible for an increased risk of lung cancer and mortality.

Thus the search continues for meaningful chemicals in fruits and vegetables. Data regarding the association between vitamin C, folate, and phytochemicals such as flavonoids and lung cancer are to date inconclusive.[422,434] Genetics–diet interactions may play a large role. Dithiolthiones, glucosinolates, indoles and sulforaphanes found in cruciferae vegetables can inhibit phase I carcinogen-acting enzymes and induce phase II carcinogen detoxification enzymes.[435–437] A decreased risk of lung cancer associated with isothiocyanates might be pronounced in individuals with a particular glutathione S-transferase (GST) M1 genotype.[438–441]

Familial and Genetic Factors

Although 70% to 90% of lung cancer cases occur in current or past tobacco smokers, the absolute lifetime risk of a smoker developing lung cancer is no greater than 20%.[154,442] Despite the wealth of known epidemiologic causal risk factors for lung cancer, determinants of host susceptibility to tobacco-induced lung cancer are not well characterized. While genetic epidemiology, metabolic phenotyping, and other research approaches support the intuitive notion that lung cancer has a genetic basis, current data do not identify those individuals at greatest risk.

Epidemiologic studies dating back to the 1960s indicate a familial susceptibility to lung cancer with a distinct early-onset component.[385,443–447] The proportion of lung cancer patients with a familial history for lung cancer ranges from 3% to 16.5%.[448,449] Most studies controlled for cigarette smoking, as this behavior also aggregates in families, and a recent report from Iceland indicates that the relative risk estimates for first-, second-, and third-degree relatives of patients with lung cancer are significantly increased (parents, 2.69; siblings, 2.02; children, 1.96) and in fact strongest for relatives of patients with lung cancer before age 61 (parents, 3.48; siblings, 3.30; children, 2.84).[446,450] A stronger genetic influence has been reported for adenocarcinoma than for SCC, LCC, and SCLC.[446]

Genetic modeling studies suggest that familial aggregation may be due to mendelian inheritance of only a few genetic factors.[451] Either a rare major autosomal dominant or codominant gene or a high-penetrant recessive gene(s) has been suggested.[448,452,453] However, the largest study of lung cancer in twins did not demonstrate a genetic basis for susceptibility.[454] Interestingly, a major lung cancer susceptibility locus was recently mapped to chromosome 6q23–25.[455] The Genetic Epidemiology of Lung Cancer Consortium plans to identify lung cancer genes though multicenter linkage studies.

The search for inherited host factors has emphasized metabolic pathways related to carcinogen detoxification, activation, and DNA repair (Fig. 35.16). Differences in susceptibility to carcinogens probably result from a delicate balance between the formation of genotoxic intermediates and detoxification. Genetically determined polymorphisms in the cytochrome P-450 system are well studied, and several phase I and phase II enzymes appear to be associated with an increased risk of lung cancer. It should be noted, however, that particular polymorphisms have a racial component and should only be viewed within the context of risk factors including tobacco use and occupational exposure.[456–458]

Phase I enzymes activate tobacco carcinogens such as PAH into reactive intermediates that can bind DNA. These adducts can lead to mutations in oncogenes or tumor suppressor genes. Two specific polymorphisms in the *CYP1A1* gene, the MspI polymorphism and a polymorphism in exon 7, are associated with increased lung cancer risk.[459,460] CYP2D6, a phase I enzyme that determines the phenotype for debrisoquine metabolism, may be involved in the metabolism of tobacco smoke carcinogens. Phenotype studies including a meta-analysis suggest that fast metabolizers are at a slightly increased risk of

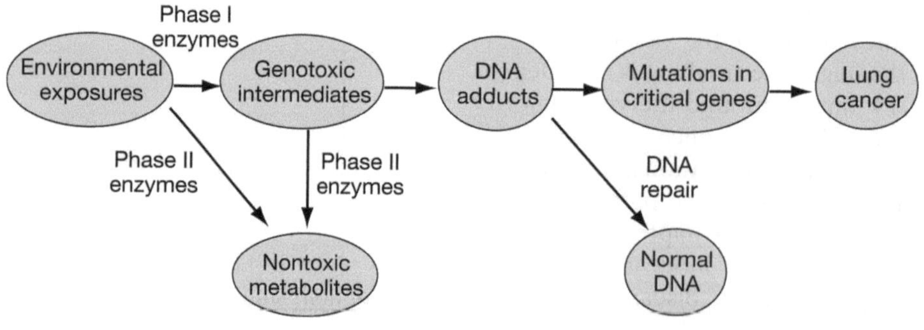

FIGURE 35.16. Postulated roles of phase I and II enzymes and DNA repair in lung cancer development.

lung cancer while slow metabolizers are at reduced risk for lung cancer.[461–463] However, genotypic analysis does not confirm the result.[464]

Glutathione S-transferase is a well-studied phase II enzyme. At least four genetically distinct classes, μ, α, π, and θ, are responsible for the detoxification of PAH reactive metabolites. While a complete discussion is beyond the scope of this chapter, a modest increased lung cancer risk is associated with the GSTM1 null genotype (50% of Caucasians) as compared to those with a GSTM1 present genotype.[465,466] Interestingly, this susceptibility is not stronger in smokers than in nonsmokers, yet this genotype may increase the risk of nonsmokers exposed to ETS.[466,467]

Interactions between phase I and II enzymes and exposure levels may be more meaningful than individual enzyme genotypes.[468] Individuals who build up phase I intermediates and are deficient in phase II metabolism seem to be at increased risk of lung cancer. Nonsmokers with *CYP1A1 Ile462Val* and *GSTTM1* null polymorphisms have a greater than fourfold increased likelihood of lung cancer compared with those with nonvariant genotypes.[469]

Variations between individuals in DNA repair capacity may be a risk factor for lung cancer. Not unlike enzyme polymorphisms, DNA repair capacity may modulate the risk of smoking-related lung cancer.[449,470–473] In fact, DNA repair capacity seems lower in lung cancer cases than in healthy controls and especially pronounced among younger patients and smokers.[474] This area of research is moving forward but only a few large population-based studies have been published. While consistent patterns of associations are still lacking, polymorphisms in DNA repair target genes including xeroderma pigmentosum complementation group D (XPD), and x-ray repair complementation groups 1 and 3 (XRCC1 and XRCC3) may affect one's risk of developing lung cancer.[474,475,476]

Molecular epidemiology has also uncovered an association between folate metabolism and increased risk of lung cancer. While a risk cannot be ascribed, individuals in Xuan Wei, China, are exposed to high levels of PAHs from smoky coal use and have a high probability of dietary folate deficiency, and it appears that single nucleotide polymorphisms in several genes involved in folate metabolism also increase the risk of lung cancer.[477] Associations among human ABO blood groups, human leukocyte antigens (HLAs), and lung cancer have also been examined. Conflicting data and weak statistical results argue against such associations.[478]

Lung Cancer Screening

Given the notable survival advantage afforded to the small percentage of patients diagnosed with early-stage disease as compared to the majority of patients with advanced-stage disease, it would seem that screening high-risk individuals might lower lung cancer mortality. Yet screening for lung cancer is not recommended on a population basis since to date there is no evidence that screening reduces mortality.[479]

Before the advent of computed tomography (CT) and laser-induced fluorescence endoscopy (LIFE), trials dating back to the 1950s examined potential benefits of chest x-ray (CXR) screening with or without sputum examination. Nonrandomized studies preceded randomized trials in the U.S. and Europe.[480–484] For example, the North London Lung Cancer Study assigned over 55,000 individuals to either a plain CXR every 6 months for 3 years or a single plain CXR at the start and end of the 3-year period. There were more lung cancers and resections in the screened group than in the control group (132 vs. 96 and 44% vs. 29%), but no difference in lung cancer mortality between the groups.[484]

Randomized trials assessed the impact of plain CXR and sputum cytology during the 1970s. Over 35,000 males enrolled in National Cancer Institute–sponsored studies at the Mayo Clinic, the Johns Hopkins Hospital, Memorial Sloan-Kettering Cancer Center, and also in Czechoslovakia.[485–488] While the screened groups had lower stage disease and increased 5-year survival (35% vs. 15%), lung cancer mortality was not affected. Additional findings were surprising. In the Johns Hopkins Lung Project, approximately 50% of the patients who developed lung cancer did so between scheduled follow-ups, suggesting that some carcinomas are very aggressive and that close surveillance and early detection do not alter the natural history of the disease. Although it was predicted that the screened group would have more patients with early-stage disease rather than advanced disease, this expected stage shift did not occur.

Unfortunately, these studies suffered from methodologic flaws including absence of true control arms and short duration of screening. For example, the Mayo Lung Project had the statistical power to detect only a 50% or larger reduction in mortality.[489] Follow-up analysis suggested that overdiagnosis of carcinoma explained the observed longer survival without mortality benefit.[490] The notion that lung carcinomas may have limited clinical relevance might appear absurd, but the identification of clinically unimportant lung cancers may have occurred. Perhaps the inclusion of seven to 14 cases of SCC in situ in the screened arm contributed to the belief in overdiagnosis[491] (see below).

The National Cancer Institute responded with the Prostate, Lung, Colorectal, and Ovarian Cancer Screening Trial (PLCO). The study enrolled more than 154,000 men and women between the ages of 55 and 74 from 1992 to 2001, and the lung cancer portion randomized smokers, but not necessarily high-risk individuals, to screening with CXR for 2 to 3 years or no screening. The study is powered to detect a 10% reduction in mortality due to lung cancer, but since participants will be followed for 13 years, final analysis is not expected until 2014. The baseline screening round noted that only 2.1% of participants with an abnormal CXR were diagnosed with cancer within 12 months, yet 44% of those carcinomas were stage I tumors.[492]

A persuasive result might not lead to enthusiastic support of CXR screening of high-risk individuals. Great technological advances in thoracic imaging late last century led lung cancer researchers to suggest that low-dose computed tomography (LDCT) was a better screening tool. Uncontrolled trials from Japan, the U.S., and Europe encompassing more than 15,000 mostly tobacco smoking men and women at least 40 years old detected over 100 carcinomas with a mean diameter of 1.5 cm.[493–501] Seventy-eight percent were stage I and only 14% were either stage III or IV. Thus, LDCT detects more cancers than CXR with a higher proportion of early-stage malignancies. These studies also narrowed the "at-risk" population to at least 60-year-old former or current smokers. However, compiled data indicate that over 50% of participants have at least one noncalcified nodule detected on screening scans. While the vast majority of these nodules are benign, all require follow-up scans and at least 30% undergo invasive procedures including fine-needle aspirates or wedge resections for benign lesions.[502]

Other issues clouding the utility of high-resolution CT (HRCT) screening include cancer risk from radiation exposure, a reported 12% incidence of SCLC in screening trials, and epidemiologic concerns inherent in mass screening programs.[501,503–508] Lead-time bias (apparent increase in survival attributable to the longer interval after a diagnosis made on the basis of a screening test as compared with one made after the onset of symptoms), length-time bias (possibility that relatively slow-growing cancers that are less likely to cause symptoms may be preferentially detected by screening suggesting that the apparently longer survival with screening may represent the indolent nature of the carcinomas detected rather than a benefit of screening), and overdiagnosis bias (detection of tumors that despite histologic evidence of malignancy do not cause the subject's death) may distort survival data.[509] In addition, the cost-effectiveness of LDCT remains unknown.

Biologic questions also dampen enthusiasm for lung cancer screening. Size is a definite determinant of outcome, with recent data even suggesting the need for subclassification of T1 carcinomas; however, the exponential model of lung cancer growth indicates that most of a tumor's life occurs prior to detection[510–514] (Fig. 35.17). Twenty doublings are required for a 10-μm cell to have a diameter of 0.1 cm (10^6 cells), 30 doublings for a diameter of 1.0 cm (10^9 cells), and 35 doublings for a diameter of 3.0 cm ($10^{10.5}$ cells). Even if growth slows as the malignancy enlarges, all these lesions occur late in the course of the disease, as death from cancer usually occurs with tumor burdens of approximately 10^{12} cells. Assuming a doubling time of 118 days for an adenocarcinoma, 22.5 years are required for that carcinoma to achieve a volume of 1 cm^3. If this tumor is detected in a 73-year-old man, then it started to grow when he was 50 years old and would not have been detectable at 65 years of age.[515–517]

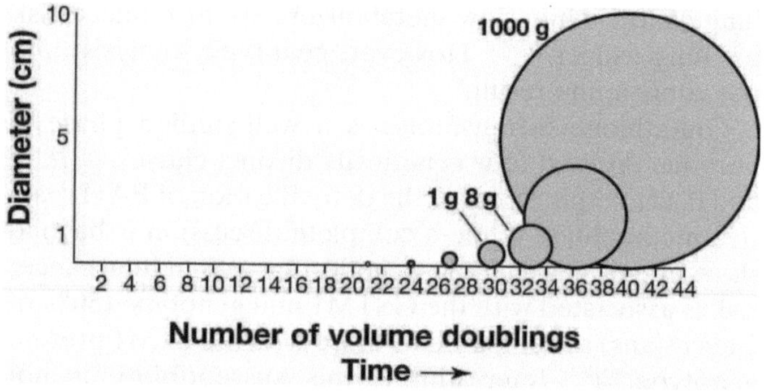

FIGURE 35.17. Life of a solid tumor. Time is expressed as volume doublings. A carcinoma with a doubling time of 1 month requires 40 months to reach 1000 g or 10 cm in diameter, while a carcinoma with a doubling time of 1 year requires 40 years.

Mortality reduction must be proven through prospective randomized controlled trials. The U.S. National Lung Screening Trial (NLST) has enrolled 50,000 high-risk men and women to screening with CT or CXR for 3 years with a 5-year follow-up period. Unfortunately, the study is only powered to detect a 50% reduction in lung cancer mortality by LDCT, and although accrual was completed in 2004, results will not be available for at least 5 years. Of interest, the pilot study preceding the NLST found only 40% of HRCT-detected carcinomas to be stage I, with an equal distribution between HRCT and CXR arms.[506] Prospective randomized controlled trials are also ongoing in France and the Netherlands.

Since LDCT images peripheral lung better than central parenchyma, the great majority of LDCT-detected carcinomas are peripheral adenocarcinomas. However, with rare exceptions in particular geographic and gender groups, central SCC is still the most common primary lung cancer. While the controlled trials of the 1970s failed to demonstrate a mortality benefit in assessing sputum cytology, recent advances may change the screening algorithm.

The development of SCC was documented in exfoliated cells over 40 years ago,[518,519] but screening sputum cytology has a sensitivity rate less than 20%. Narrowing the screened population to current and ex-smokers with airflow obstruction, a positive family history, or occupational exposures improves the sensitivity of sputum analysis.[520] Technological advances including immunostaining, polymerase chain reaction (PCR)-based

Table 35.6. Common signs and symptoms of lung cancer

Symptoms attributable to a central tumor
Cough
Hemoptysis
Wheeze and stridor
Dyspnea
Pneumonia
Symptoms attributable to a peripheral tumor
Pain
Cough
Dyspnea
Pneumonia
Symptoms related to regional spread of tumor in the thorax
Tracheal obstruction
Esophageal compression with dysphagia
Bronchopulmonary fistula
Recurrent laryngeal nerve paralysis with hoarseness
Phrenic nerve paralysis with hemidiaphragm elevation and dyspnea
Sympathetic nerve paralysis with Horner's syndrome
Eighth cervical and first thoracic nerves with ulnar pain and Pancoast syndrome
Superior vena cava syndrome from vascular obstruction
Pericardial and cardiac extension with tamponade, arrhythmia, or cardiac failure
Lymphatic obstruction with pleural effusion
Lymphangitic spread through lungs with hypoxemia and dyspnea

assays, and computer-assisted image analysis of exfoliated sputum cells may bring the noninvasive, inexpensive, and very specific (approximately 95%) test into standard use.[521,522]

Even with a sputum cytology diagnosis of dysplasia, recognition of preinvasive and early invasive bronchial SCC is difficult, as white light bronchoscopy detects less than 40% of carcinoma in situ. Autofluorescence bronchoscopy is much more sensitive, but with a high false-positive rate due to inflammation and goblet cell hyperplasia, this modality is currently better suited for clinical surveillance.[523,524] Virtual bronchoscopy and optical coherent tomography may enter the clinical realm in the next few years.

Clinical Manifestations

Signs and symptoms associated with pulmonary NSCLC depend on tumor location and extent, as well as tumor biology.[525,526] From 1995 through 2001, 16% of Americans presented with localized disease, 37% with regional disease, 39% with distant disease, and 8% were unstaged[527] (Tables 35.6 and 35.7). Probably 5% and certainly no more than 20% of patients with lung cancer are asymptomatic and diagnosed during investigation of an unrelated medical problem.[525,528,529]

Central tumors arising in larger airways usually cause cough, sputum production, wheezing, or hemoptysis.[526,529] Massive bleeding is rarely encountered. Atelectasis with subsequent pneumonia and abscess may occur. Peripheral tumors can cause cough, dyspnea, and chest pain that may be confused with angina. Chest pain is poorly understood and usually not caused by tumor invasion of nerve-rich structures such as the parietal pleura. Pneumonia and abscess may also lead to a diagnosis.

Intrathoracic spread of carcinoma can produce a myriad of clinical complaints. Pleural involvement manifests with malignant effusions and chest pain leading to dyspnea. Of note, pleural effusions associated with NSCLC may be due to pleural seeding of tumor cells, lymphatic obstruction, pulmonary venous obstruction, or mesothelial cell response to carcinoma. Apical lung carcinomas may present with Pancoast syndrome (lower brachial plexopathy, Horner's syndrome, and shoulder pain), while vascular obstruction occasionally manifests as superior vena cava syndrome. Nodal involvement or tumor extension into the posterior mediastinum can lead to partial or complete esophageal obstruction. Involvement of the left recurrent laryngeal nerve causes hoarseness, while phrenic nerve involvement leads to an elevated hemidiaphragm with or without dyspnea. Pericardial or cardiac involvement can present as tamponade.

Since lymphangitic and hematogenous dissemination are so common in lung cancer, regional and distal nodal metastases as well as visceral metastases are often responsible for initial symptoms or signs. It is not surprising that extrathoracic manifestations are the presenting symptoms in about one third of lung cancer patients.[530] Reported patterns of metastatic spread are not strikingly different[531–533] (Table 35.8). Any site can be affected, but brain, liver, bone, adrenal gland, and kidney metastases are most common. In fact, over 70% of carcinomas that present with symptomatic brain metastases are of lung origin.[534]

Constitutional symptoms including malaise, fever, anorexia, and weight loss are common yet poorly

Table 35.7. Clinical manifestations of non–small-cell lung cancer

Tumor	Effects of primary tumor	Intrathoracic spread	Distant metastases	Paraneoplastic syndromes
SCC	>50%	10–25%	<10%	<10%
Adenocarcinoma	10–25%	<10%	10–25%	<10%
LCC	up to 50%	10–25%	10–25%	<10%

SCC, squamous cell carcinoma; LCC, large cell carcinoma.
Source: Modified from Colby et al.[925]

Table 35.8. Metastatic sites of non–small-cell lung cancer

Site	Squamous cell carcinoma (%)	Adeno-carcinoma (%)	Large cell carcinoma (%)
Regional lymph nodes	83	91	89
Pleura	24	30	18
Chest wall	16	18	14
Pericardium	15	19	17
Heart	20	16	16
Esophagus	14	10	9
Distant lymph nodes	29	48	45
Brain	36	47	49
Liver	37	42	33
Spleen	6	9	9
Adrenal	20	41	35
Kidney	23	26	19
Bone	26	44	25
Skin	1	6	2

Source: Modified from Colby et al.[925]

understood presenting symptoms, while up to 25% of patients with lung cancer present with a paraneoplastic syndrome (Table 35.9). These syndromes are not specific to lung cancer but often indicate the presence of a lung carcinoma. Occasionally, lung cancer patients present with multiple synchronous or metachronous paraneoplastic syndromes.[535] Of note, certain endocrinologic derangements seen in lung cancer patients, such as hypercalcemia or syndrome of inappropriate antidiuretic hormone (SIADH) secretion can be a direct effect of bone or pituitary gland involvement, respectively, rather than a paraneoplastic syndrome. Although most paraneoplastic syndromes including virtually all neurologic syndromes such as Lambert-Eaton syndrome are found in patients with SCLC, hyperparathyroidism due to tumor secretion of a parathormone-like substance is common in patients with SCC.[536,537] Nonbacterial thrombotic endocarditis, while rare, is associated with adenocarcinoma, and both clubbing and hypertrophic osteoarthropathy are most frequently associated with SCC or adenocarcinoma.[538,539] Interestingly, rare instances of bone and joint pain improvement and radiographic resolution have been reported following treatment of the primary tumor.[540,541] Cutaneous paraneoplastic syndromes associated with NSCLC are legion, including pigmented lesions, keratoses, and erythemas.

Not all patients with elevated serum hormone levels manifest disease. For example, while up to 70% of SCLC patients have excess antidiuretic hormone production, and almost 50% have elevated serum levels of adrenocorticotrophic hormone, less than 15% have either SIADH or Cushing syndrome.[542,543] Inactive biologic forms of tumor-produced hormones are thought responsible.[544,545]

Table 35.9. Paraneoplastic, endocrinologic, and hematologic manifestations of lung cancer

Endocrine
- Hypercalcemia (parathormone-like substance)
- Hyponatremia (syndrome of inappropriate antidiuretic hormone secretion)
- Cushing's syndrome (adrenocorticotropic hormone [ACTH])
- Carcinoid syndrome (serotonin)
- Gynecomastia (gonadotropins)
- Hypercalcitonemia
- Elevated growth hormone
- Prolactinemia
- Hypoglycemia
- Hyperglycemia
- Diarrhea (vasoactive intestinal polypeptide)
- Hypertension (renin)

Neurologic
- Encephalopathy
- Subacute cerebellar degeneration
- Progressive multifocal leukoencephalopathy
- Transverse myelitis
- Peripheral neuropathy
- Polymyositis
- Autonomic neuropathy
- Myasthenic syndromes including Eaton-Lambert syndrome
- Optic neuritis

Skeletal
- Clubbing
- Hypertrophic pulmonary osteoarthropathy

Hematologic
- Anemia
- Pure red cell aplasia
- Leukemoid reactions
- Eosinophilia
- Thrombocytosis
- Thrombocytopenia
- Leukoerythroblastosis
- Disseminated intravascular coagulation
- Recurrent venous thrombosis
- Nonbacterial thrombotic (marantic) endocarditis
- Dysproteinemia
- Hypoalbuminemia
- Marrow plasmacytosis

Cutaneous
- Hyperkeratosis
- Dermatomyositis
- Acanthosis nigricans
- Hyperpigmentation
- Erythema gyratum repens
- Hypertrichosis lanuginosa acquisita

Other
- Systemic lupus erythematosus
- Dermatomyositis
- Nephrotic syndrome
- Lactic acidosis
- Hypouricemia
- Henoch-Schönlein purpura
- Amyloidosis

Lung cancer patients with a history of tobacco use successfully treated with surgical resection are at increased risk of developing a second lung cancer. The incidence of second primary lung cancer after resection of NSCLC ranges from 1% to 4%, but those with stage I carcinomas may have an incidence as high as 8.6%.[546] It is estimated that the risk is 2% per patient per year of follow-up, accumulating over time.[546] Current smokers have a higher incidence than ex-smokers, while age, sex, stage, histology, tumor location, and initial surgery do not appear to have an effect on the development of a second primary lung cancer.[546,547] In most, but not all, studies, tumors appear between 2 and 5 years after the initial surgery, and the majority of patients are asymptomatic.[546,548–551] The carcinomas are usually of the same histology as the first carcinoma. Surveillance with postoperative CT may prolong survival.[547]

Methods of Diagnosis

Patients with either symptoms or radiographic findings suggestive of lung cancer require a tissue diagnosis and disease staging before appropriate treatment. Radiographic and nuclear medicine tests including CT, 2-^{18}F-fluoro-2-deoxy-D-glucose positron emission tomography (FDG-PET), magnetic resonance imaging (MRI), and scintigraphy can indicate extent of disease, while a myriad of minimally invasive procedures can provide a tissue diagnosis depending on clinical presentation and radiographic location of the tumor[552,553] (Table 35.10). Central lung lesions can be diagnosed with sputum cytology, bronchoscopic biopsy, brushing, washing, or fine-needle aspiration (FNA), while peripheral lung lesions are usually sampled via either fluoroscopic or CT-guided percutaneous FNA. Transbronchial biopsy, brushing, or needle aspiration can also be employed. Many studies have demonstrated high accuracy rates for cytologic procedures with improved sensitivity and specificity achieved when combined with tissue biopsies.[552] Metastatic lung cancer can also be diagnosed with CT-guided FNA. Immunohistochemical studies often confirm the pulmonary nature of the metastasis.

Every histologic diagnosis of carcinoma requires clinical and radiographic correlation. Reactive processes and nonepithelial tumors including lymphomas and sarcomas should be excluded, and metastatic lesions should be considered in the differential diagnosis. Aside from poor fixation, processing, or staining, overinterpretation of crush artifact, detached strips of benign bronchial mucosa, bronchial squamous metaplasia, and reactive processes represent the most likely histologic pitfalls in the diagnosis of NSCLC.

Distinguishing SCLC from NSCLC is of paramount importance on account of different treatment options and markedly different prognoses. The distinction is usually possible with cytologic specimens such as sputum, transthoracic needle aspirate and bronchoscopic washings, brushings, and lavage cytology.[553,554] Yet a cytologic diagnosis of NSCLC is more reliable than a cytologic diagnosis of SCLC with average misclassification rates of 2% and 9%, respectively.[552] Not surprisingly, combining bronchial brushings, washings, and biopsies leads to fewer discrepancies.[555] The combination of different samples forces the pathologist to synthesize numerous cytologic and histologic features including nuclear-to-cytoplasmic ratio, nuclear chromatin, and cell shape rather than simply evaluating cell size and presence or absence of nucleoli (see Chapter 36).

Preoperative histologic classification of NSCLC is more problematic. While a definitive diagnosis may not be possible in all cases, one achieves the greatest accuracy in subtyping with the use of more than one sampling modality and strict adherence to diagnostic criteria.[555–557] Distinctions among SCC, adenocarcinoma, and LCC were until recently of no therapeutic significance. With widespread use of flexible fiberoptic bronchoscopy producing tissue fragments only 2 mm in diameter, presurgical subtyping is incorrect in up to 38% of cases.[558] Small sample size and the fact that almost 60% of lung carcinomas exhibit more than one of the major histologic types accounts for these poor results.[559–561] Variation in appearance and degree of differentiation from microscopic field to field and slide to slide has great implications for classification and perhaps treatment and prognosis. Adenocarcinoma diagnoses are the least reproducible with the lowest specificity, negative predictive value, and percent exact agreement.[562,563] As a consequence, use of the term NSCLC is encouraged.[530,557,558,564] Furthermore, BAC and LCC diagnoses can only be suggested on small samples (see sections Bronchioloalveolar Carcinoma and Large Cell Carcinoma, below).

Lastly, although more than 95% of tumors are accurately diagnosed without a thoracotomy, increasing numbers of subcentimeter lesions detected on LDCT are exceedingly difficult to diagnose with minimally invasive techniques. Intraoperative palpation and wedge resection has become a not infrequent diagnostic procedure, and frozen section diagnosis is an accurate tool for most of these pulmonary nodules.[565] A definitive diagnosis allows the surgeon to proceed with lung cancer surgery, while an uncertain interpretation aborts the surgery. The 1.5% discordance rate between frozen section and definitive diagnoses reported by the College of American Pathologists (CAP) for multiple organ frozen sections is most often due to misinterpretation of the frozen section slide, the presence of diagnostic tissue in permanent sections not present on the frozen section slide, or diagnostic tissue in the specimen not

TABLE 35.10. Radiographic findings of non-small cell lung cancer at diagnosis

Radiographic feature	Squamous cell carcinoma	Adenocarcinoma	Large cell carcinoma
Nodule ≤4 cm	14%	46%	18%
Peripheral location	29%	65%	61%
Central location	64%	5%	42%
Hilar/perihilar mass	40%	17%	32%
Cavitation	5%	3%	4%
Pleural/chest wall involvement	3%	5%	2%
Hilar adenopathy	38%	19%	32%
Mediastinal adenopathy	5%	9%	10%

Source: Colby et al.[925]

sampled at frozen section. Two thirds of the incorrect frozen section diagnoses are considered false negatives while only one third are false positives.[566,567] Particular areas of difficulty with subcentimeter lung nodules at frozen section include differentiating reactive atypia from neoplasia and atypical adenomatous hyperplasia (AAH) from BAC[565] (see Chapter 34 and below).

Individuals with clinical or radiographic evidence of extrapulmonary lung cancer rarely have their primary lung tumor sampled. Computed tomography and FDG-PET often indicate possible mediastinal lymph node metastases as well as distal metastases and aid in preventing nontherapeutic thoracotomies.[568,569] Mediastinoscopy, endoscopic ultrasonography with fine aspiration, thoracentesis, and thoracoscopy are established methods of diagnosis and staging.[570–573]

Interestingly, there is considerable debate in the surgical field about whether individuals with peripheral T1 tumors require free-standing mediastinoscopy since the likelihood of N2 disease is only 10% to 15%. A recent study reported the sensitivity, specificity, positive predictive value, negative predictive value, and accuracy of PET scan as 64%, 77%, 45%, 88%, and 74%, respectively.[574] At this time, FDG-PET should not be relied on as a sole staging modality.

Staging

Surgical resection of NSCLC offers the only chance of cure. Since surgery is a reasonable treatment option in only 20% of patients, a reproducible and meaningful system for identifying patients with potentially curable disease as well as other subgroups that may benefit from chemotherapy or radiation therapy is necessary. While the first clinical classification of cancer was formulated by the League of Nations Health Organization in 1929, the current tumor, node, metastasis (TNM) system developed from a 1945 proposal for stage grouping.[575] The recent International System for Staging Lung Cancer adopted by the American Joint Committee on Cancer (AJCC) and the Union Internationale Contre le Cancer (UICC) was introduced in 1986 and revised in 1997[576] (Table 35.11). Regional lymph node station classification was also standardized in 1997[576] (Fig. 35.18). This staging system is based on over 5000 clinically and pathologically staged patients followed for at least 5 years. The primary tumor is subdivided into four categories (T1 to T4) depending on size and location. Lymph nodes are identified according to anatomic location, and involvement is divided into bronchopulmonary (N1), ipsilateral mediastinal (N2), and contralateral mediastinal or supraclavicular disease (N3) (Table 35.11). Metastases are either present (M1) or absent (M0). Using this system, four broad stages with seven separate substages identify significant differences in 5-year survival, ranging from 67% to 23% respectively for pathologic stages IA and IIIA, and 7% to 1% for clinical stages IIIB and IV, respectively.[577] (Table 35.12) (Figs. 35.19 and 35.20). While this TNM can be applied to SCLC, most thoracic surgical, medical, and radiation oncologists use the two category limited versus extensive staging system. Generally speaking, patients with clinical stage IIIA or lower NSCLC may be surgical candidates, while stage IIIB or IV patients are usually not[578] (Fig. 35.21).

Staging of individual patients has clinical, imaging, surgical, and pathologic phases with increasingly precise data. Initial treatment is mostly based on clinical and

Table 35.11. Tumor, node, metastasis (TNM) classification of the lung

DEFINITION OF TNM

Primary Tumor (T)

TX	Primary tumor cannot be assessed, or tumor proven by the presence of malignant cells in sputum or bronchial washings but not visualized by imaging or bronchoscopy
T0	No evidence of primary tumor
Tis	Carcinoma *in situ*
T1	Tumor 3 cm or less in greatest dimension, surrounded by lung or visceral pleura, without bronchoscopic evidence of invasion more proximal than the lobar bronchus,* (i.e., not in the main bronchus)
T2	Tumor with any of the following features of size or extent: More than 3 cm in greatest dimension Involves main bronchus, 2 cm or more distal to the carina Invades the visceral pleura Associated with atelectasis or obstructive pneumonitis that extends to the hilar region but does not involve the entire lung
T3	Tumor of any size that directly invades any of the following: chest wall (including superior sulcus tumors), diaphragm, mediastinal pleura, parietal pericardium; or tumor in the main bronchus less than 2 cm distal to the carina, but without involvement of the carina; or associated atelectasis or obstructive pneumonitis of the entire lung
T4	Tumor of any size that invades any of the following: mediastinum, heart, great vessels, trachea, esophagus, vertebral body, carina; or separate tumor nodules in the same lobe; or tumor with malignant pleural effusion**

**Note:* The uncommon superficial tumor of any size with its invasive component limited to the bronchial wall, which may extend proximal to the main bronchus, is also classified T1.

***Note:* Most pleural effusions associated with lung cancer are due to tumor. However, there are a few patients in whom multiple cytopathologic examinations of pleural fluid are negative for tumor. In these cases, fluid is non-bloody and is not an exudate. Such patients may be further evaluated by videothoracoscopy (VATS) and direct pleural biopsies. When these elements and clinical judgment dictate that the effusion is not related to the tumor, the effusion should be excluded as a staging element and the patient should be staged T1, T2, or T3.

Regional Lymph Nodes (N)

NX	Regional lymph nodes cannot be assessed
N0	No regional lymph node metastasis
N1	Metastasis to ipsilateral peribronchial and/or ipsilateral hilar lymph nodes, and intrapulmonary nodes including involvement by direct extension of the primary tumor
N2	Metastasis to ipsilateral mediastinal and/or subcarinal lymph nodes(s)
N3	Metastasis to contralateral mediastinal, contralateral hilar, ipsilateral or contralateral scalene, or supraclavicular lymph nodes(s)

Distant Metastasis (M)

MX	Distant metastasis cannot be assessed
M0	No distant metastasis
M1	Distant metastasis present

Note: M1 includes separate tumor nodule(s) in a different lobe (ipsilateral or contralateral).

Source: Used with the permission of the American Joint Committee on Cancer (AJCC), Chicago, Illinois. The original source for this material is the AJCC Cancer Staging Manual, Sixth Edition (2002) published by Springer Science and Business Media, LCC, www.springer.com.

imaging data, but lymph node sampling at mediastinoscopy may be performed to assess nodal status before considering lung cancer surgery. Currently, the accuracy of clinical staging in predicting the final pathologic TNM (pTNM) is quite poor—less than 50%.[579] Obviously, the more extensive the testing, the more likely more patients will be staged with advanced rather than early disease. Survival curves reflect this fact (Fig. 35.22). Thus, each lung cancer report must include either the pTNM or information allowing for correct pathologic staging. Published practice protocols from CAP or Association of Directors of Anatomic and Surgical Pathology are available in paper and electronic versions.

Although the TNM system is relatively easy to apply, several issues require additional comments. The status of thoracic lymph nodes is the main determinant of outcome for patients with resectable lung cancer. The UICC TNM book states that pN0 requires histologic examination of at least six hilar and mediastinal lymph nodes, but adds "if the lymph nodes are negative, but the number ordinarily examined is not met, classify as pN0."[580] Whether complete mediastinal lymphadenectomy as opposed to nodal sampling becomes the recommended treatment depends on the results of an ongoing American College of Surgeons Oncology Group trial. Sentinel lymph node sampling and ancillary studies searching for isolated tumor cells or micrometastases are of uncertain clinical utility at the present time.[581–583]

Up to one third of patients with NSCLC have a pleural effusion at diagnosis. While this finding indicates a poor prognosis whether or not malignant cell are identified in the fluid, a malignant effusion is a T4 stage IIIB designation.[530] Unfortunately, cytologic examination of fluid is positive for malignant cells in no more than 65% of patients with malignant pleural effusions.[530] Closed needle pleural biopsy does not raise the

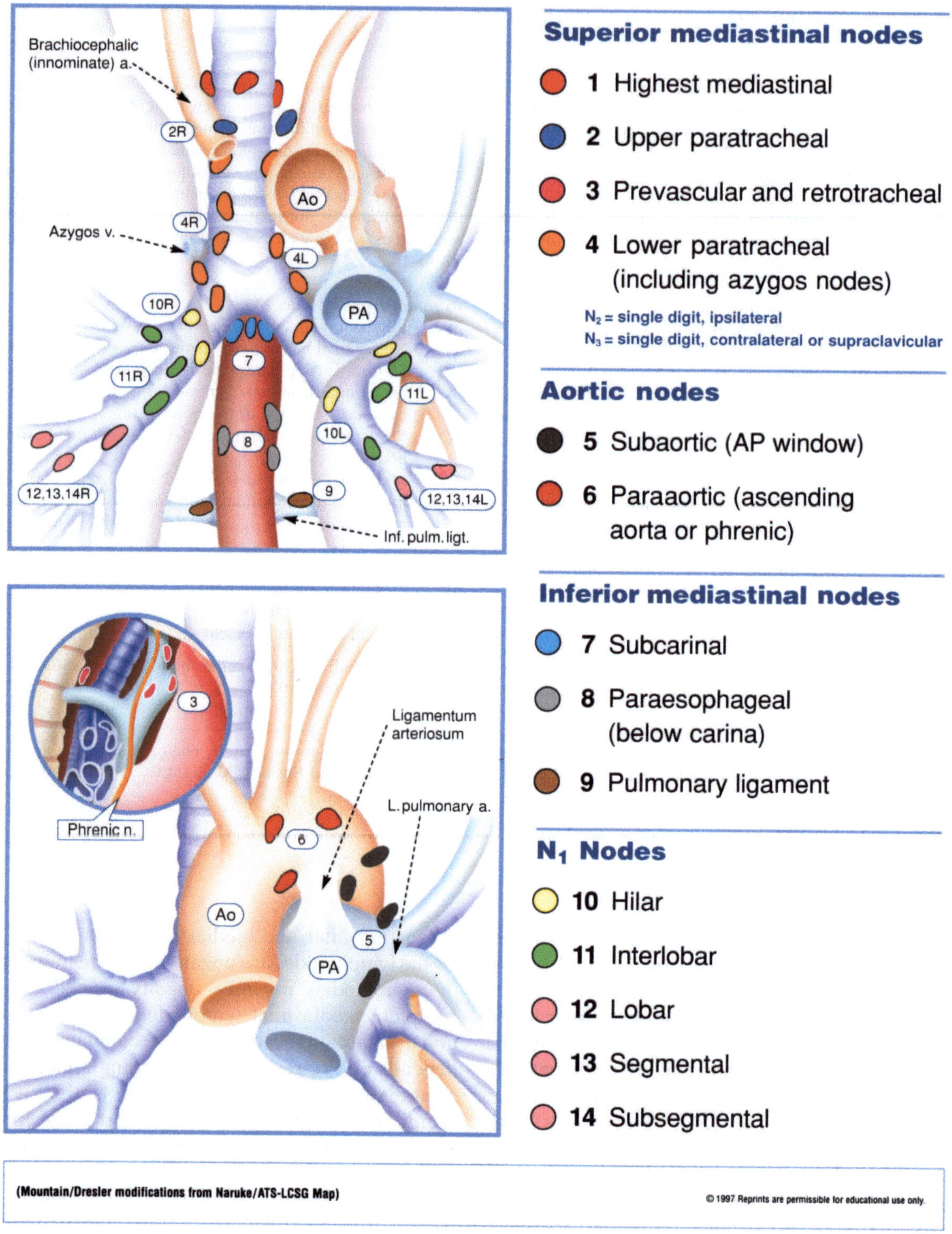

FIGURE 35.18. Regional lymph node stations for lung cancer staging. (From Mountain and Dresler CM,[576] with permission of *Chest.*)

TABLE 35.12. Stage Grouping

Occult Carcinoma	TX	N0	M0
Stage 0	Tis	N0	M0
Stage IA	T1	N0	M0
Stage IB	T2	N0	M0
Stage IIA	T1	N1	M0
Stage IIB	T2	N1	M0
	T3	N0	M0
Stage IIIA	T1	N2	M0
	T2	N2	M0
	T3	N1	M0
	T3	N2	M0
Stage IIIB	Any T	N3	M0
	T4	Any N	M0
Stage IV	Any T	Any N	M1

Source: Used with the permission of the American Joint Committee on Cancer (AJCC), Chicago, Illinois. The original source for this material is the AJCC Cancer Staging Manual, Sixth Edition (2002) published by Springer Science and Business Media, LCC, www.springer.com.

sensitivity as much as a second thoracentesis procedure.[584] Thoracoscopy confirms a diagnosis of pleural involvement in greater than 95% of patients, but is often performed at the time of the surgical resection and thus differs little from intraoperative pre-resection lavage.[585–587] 2–^{18}F-fluoro-2-deoxy-D-glucose PET may be useful in improving staging in NSCLC patients with pleural effusions.[588]

Several pathologic findings may lead to confusion in applying a pTNM designation. The prognostic value of visceral pleural invasion cannot be overemphasized. Previous editions of this text offered a classification for pleural invasion, and while the Japan Lung Cancer Society uses the system, recent studies have demonstrated that there is no prognostic difference between tumors that merely invade into visceral pleura (p1) and tumors that invade through visceral pleura with surface involvement (p2).[589–592] Carcinomas 3.0 cm or smaller with invasion into the visceral pleura require T2 stage IB or IIB designations. Pleural invasion also correlates with more extensive mediastinal lymph node involvement.[593] Full-faced histologic sections of pleural puckers are required for evaluation, and elastic tissue stains highlighting the fragmented pleural internal elastic lamina directly above lung parenchyma may aid in the evaluation.[589,594]

Bronchial involvement by carcinomas of any size ensures an at least T2 designation except for superficial spreading tumors with invasion confined to the bronchial wall (T1 status). If the tumor comes within less than 2.0 cm of the carina, a T3 designation is applied while carinal involvement necessitates a T4 assignment. Whether the invasive component of a tumor involves a main bronchus or comes within 2.0 cm of the carina requires clinical and bronchoscopic correlation. One should be aware that the right main bronchus is usually less than 2.0 cm in length, and the right upper lobe bronchus can be at the carina.

Greater confusion surrounds the pathologist's ability to stage a resection specimen containing more than one histologically similar or identical carcinoma. The staging system states that satellite tumor nodules within the primary tumor-bearing lobe necessitate a T4 designation, while tumor nodules in the ipsilateral nonprimary tumor lobe(s) are classified M1. While the historical literature estimates that no more than 2% of lung cancer patients harbor synchronous tumors, pathologic findings from a large LDCT screening study report 25% of patients with adenocarcinomas had additional tumors, most of which were not clinically detected.[595,596] Whether such cases warrant either stage IIIB or IV status is uncertain but unlikely given the up to 60% 5-year survival rates for individuals with stage-suggested rates of no greater than 7%.[597–600] Furthermore, the surgical pathologist cannot differentiate synchronous SCC or adenocarcinoma primaries from intrapulmonary metastases in many instances on the basis of published morphologic criteria or molecular studies.[601,602]

Histogenesis of Common Lung Neoplasms

While our understanding of the histogenesis of NSCLCs is incomplete, great strides have been made over the past 20 years. Mid- to late 20th century observational studies noted the heterogeneity of lung cancers and considered that SCC, adenocarcinoma, and LCC arose from undifferentiated SCLC.[603–605] It is probably an oversimplification to believe that these common lung cancers arise from a single cell, but not unreasonable to suppose that all epithelial neoplasms develop from progressive transformation of normal epithelial cells into atypical cells that eventually become neoplastic.[606–608] The process of multistep carcinogenesis suggests that SCC arises from metaplastic/dysplastic respiratory epithelium and that peripheral adenocarcinoma arises from Clara cells, bronchiolar cells, mucin-producing cells, or pneumocytes (see Chapter 34). While many genetic changes occur in all histologic types, the frequency and timing of the changes differ in SCLC and NSCLC.[609] In addition, particular genetic and epigenetic differences are noted between SCC and adenocarcinoma[610] (see Chapter 33, which discusses genetic alteration in lung tumors). At the very least, this knowledge confirms the surgical pathologist's belief that morphologic diversity suggests molecular diversity. Cancer stem cell research also suggests that particular lung stem cells may be precursors to airway and airspace-derived carcinomas.[611–613] On the basis of this work, therapeutic interventions including chemoprevention may become commonplace.

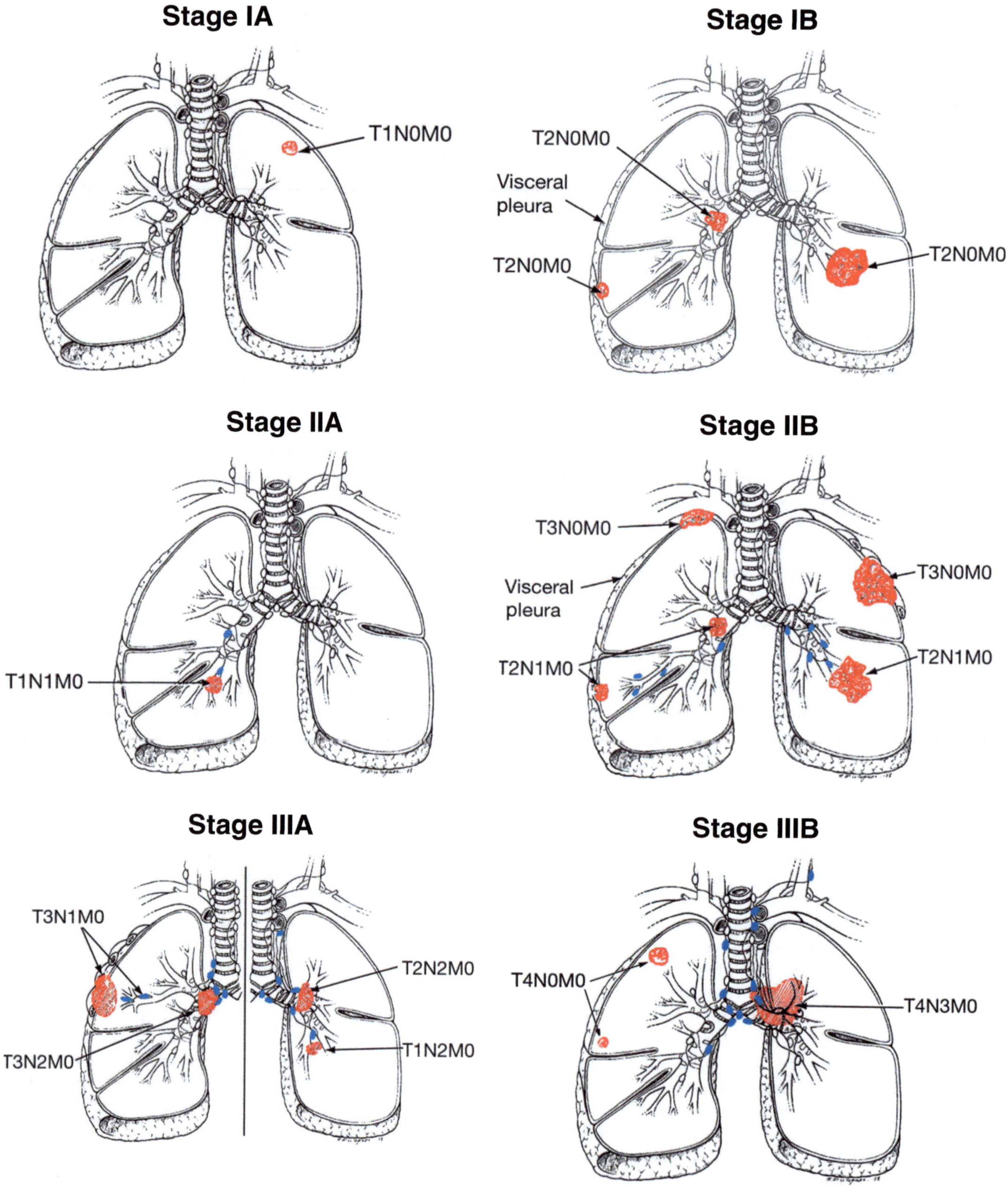

FIGURES 35.19. Stage IA through stage IV lung cancer staging. See Table 35.12 for details. (From Mountain CF. The international system for staging lung cancer. Semin Surg Oncol 2000;18:106–115, with permission of John Wiley & Sons.)

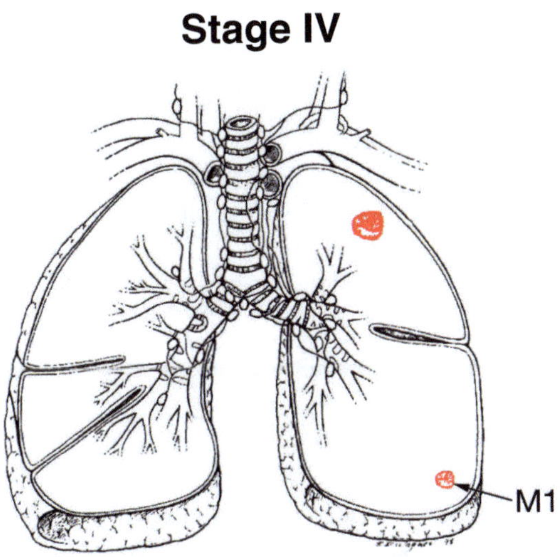

FIGURES 35.19. (*Continued*)

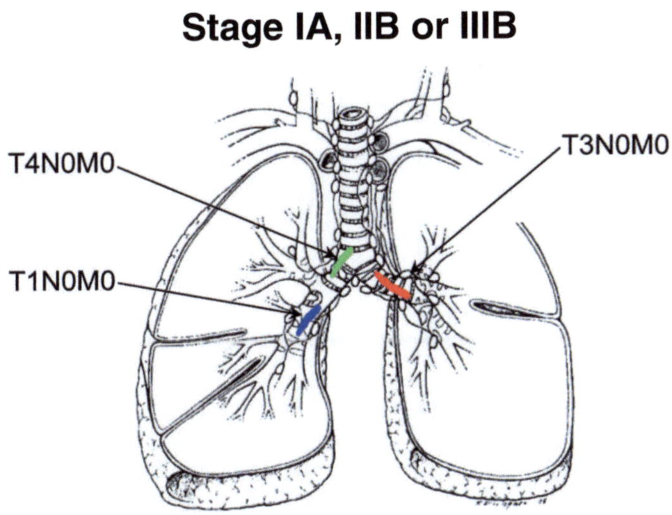

FIGURE 35.20. Staging of superficial spreading carcinomas. Carcinomas confined to the bronchial wall are staged based on their location. Tumors greater than 2.0 cm from the carina are T1N0M0 (stage IA), those within 2.0 cm of the carina are T3N0M0 (stage IIB), and those involving the carina are T4N0M0 (stage IIIB).

Histologic Classification of Lung Cancer

A standard international system of tumor classification is necessary to maintain consistency in patient diagnoses, treatment, and prognosis as well as to provide for comparative clinical, epidemiologic, and biologic studies. The Manual of Tumor Nomenclature and Coding was introduced in 1951 and eventually evolved into the International Classification of Diseases (ICD), while the Systematized Nomenclature of Pathology (SNOP) was

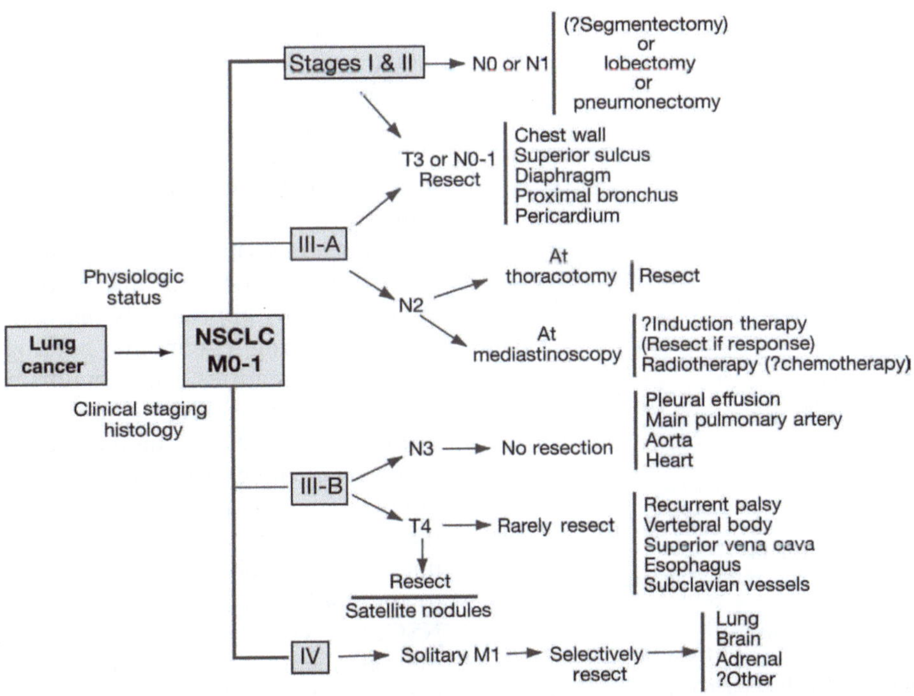

FIGURE 35.21. General algorithm for considering surgical treatment of non–small-cell lung cancer (NSCLC). The decision to undertake surgical resection depends on accurate pre- or intraoperative staging.

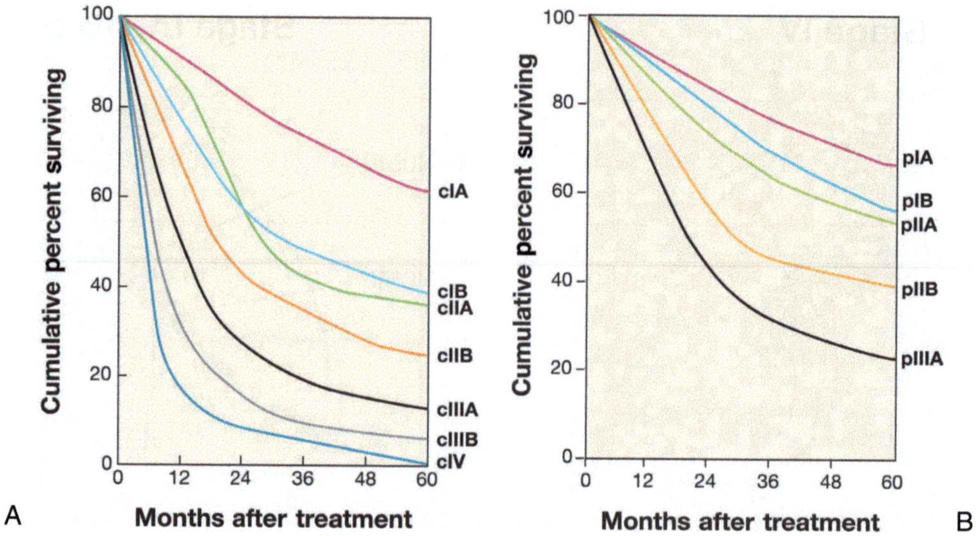

FIGURE 35.22. Cumulative proportions of patients with NSCLC surviving after treatment according to clinical **(A)** or surgical-pathologic **(B)** stage. (From Mountain CF. The international system for staging lung cancer. Semin Surg Oncol 2000;18:106–115, with permission of John Wiley & Sons.)

TABLE 35.13. World Health Organization histologic classification of common pulmonary non–small-cell carcinomas

Squamous cell carcinoma
Variants
Papillary
Clear cell
Small cell
Basaloid
Adenocarcinoma
Adenocarcinoma, mixed subtype
Acinar adenocarcinoma
Papillary adenocarcinoma
Bronchioloalveolar carcinoma
Nonmucinous
Mucinous
Mixed nonmucinous and mucinous or indeterminate
Solid adenocarcinoma with mucin production
Variants:
Fetal adenocarcinoma
Mucinous ("colloid") carcinoma
Mucinous cystadenocarcinoma
Signet ring adenocarcinoma
Clear cell adenocarcinoma
Large cell carcinoma
Variants:
Large cell neuroendocrine carcinoma
Combined large cell neuroendocrine carcinoma
Basaloid carcinoma
Lymphoepithelioma-like carcinoma
Clear cell carcinoma
Large cell carcinoma with rhabdoid phenotype
Adenosquamous carcinoma

Source: Travis.[617]

introduced in 1965 and became the Systematized Nomenclature of Medicine (SNOMED) in 1976. The first WHO International Histological Classification of Tumors was published in 1967 and major revisions in the lung tumor classification appeared in 1981 and 1999.[614–616] The current classification appearing in the WHO Classification of Tumor–Pathology and Genetics series is the globally recognized lung tumor classification scheme[617] (Table 35.13).

Pathologists involved in the formulation of the 2004 WHO classification attempted to adhere to principles of reproducibility, clinical significance, and simplicity, while minimizing the number of unclassifiable lesions. The classification is descriptive rather than histogenetic and based almost entirely on light microscopic features. A consequence of this approach is the expansion of histologic subtypes. Lung carcinoma heterogeneity necessitates combined categories, while tumors with histologic peculiarities require splitting into separate categories. For example, clear cell carcinoma is classified as a variant of LCC, yet clear cell variants of SCC and adenocarcinoma are also included in the classification scheme. While the major diagnostic categories remain fundamentally unchanged, modifications in the classification compared to the 1981 version affected many categories including NSCLC. Expanded morphologic categories and a fundamental reworking of the adenocarcinoma group figure prominently. Early genomic and proteomic profiling of lung cancer recapitulate these broad histologic subtypes.[618–621]

Squamous Cell Carcinoma

Squamous cell carcinoma (SCC) of the lung is a malignant epithelial tumor with keratinization or intercellular bridges. Squamous cell carcinoma arises from a progressive dysplasia of metaplastic squamous epithelium. While most SCC probably arise from metaplastic basal cells, columnar goblet cells may also develop into carcinoma through the metaplasia-dysplasia-carcinoma sequence.[622–625] Histologic heterogeneity is common, and although many morphologic variants have been described, the current WHO classification recognizes only papillary, clear cell, small cell, and basaloid (Table 35.13). In addition, SCC may be combined with adenocarcinoma, SCLC, and other malignancies, even in endobronchial locations[626] (see Chapters 36 and 37). Rare mucin vacuoles can be seen in otherwise typical SCC.[627] Unless an unequivocal glandular component comprises at least 10% of the tumor, a diagnosis of adenosquamous carcinoma should not be entertained (see Adenosquamous Carcinoma, below).

Most SCCs arise in main, lobar, segmental, or subsegmental bronchi, while approximately one third arise from small peripheral airways.[628–630] In general, SCCs are smaller than other lung carcinomas since obstructive symptoms manifest early in the clinical course. Tumors are white or gray with varying degrees of hemorrhage and necrosis. Large tumors are prone to central cavitation, but small tumors also cavitate. Lesions can be firm or soft depending on the amount of stromal desmoplasia, keratin production, and necrosis. Central tumors form intraluminal polypoid masses and mucosal thickening, and often infiltrate through the bronchial wall into peribronchial tissue, lung, hilar and mediastinal lymph nodes, and mediastinal structures (Fig. 35.23A). Even partial bronchial lumen obstruction can lead to

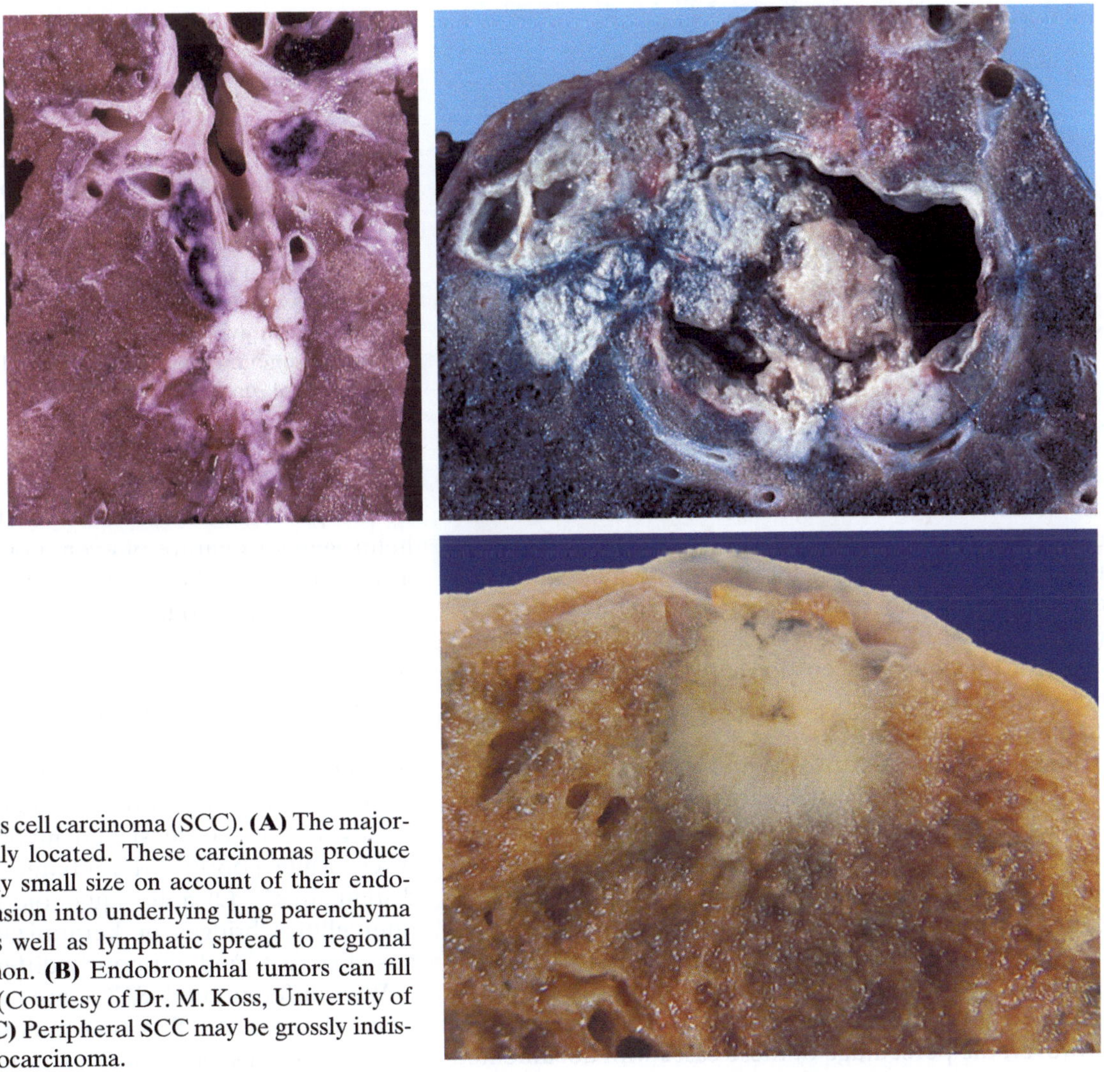
A B C

FIGURE 35.23. Squamous cell carcinoma (SCC). **(A)** The majority of SCCs are centrally located. These carcinomas produce symptoms at a relatively small size on account of their endobronchial location. Invasion into underlying lung parenchyma and direct extension as well as lymphatic spread to regional lymph nodes are common. **(B)** Endobronchial tumors can fill bronchiectatic cavities. (Courtesy of Dr. M. Koss, University of Southern California.) **(C)** Peripheral SCC may be grossly indistinguishable from adenocarcinoma.

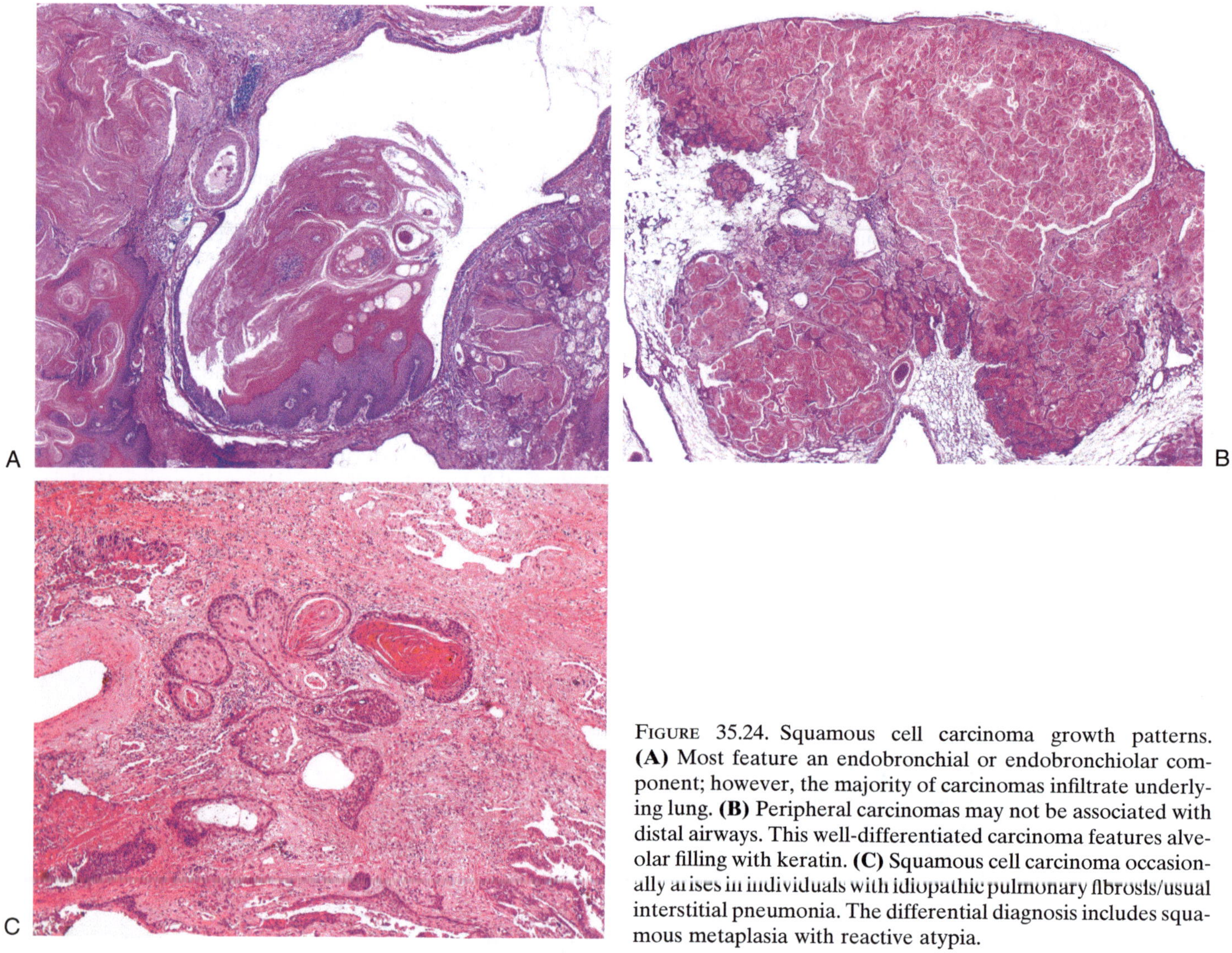

FIGURE 35.24. Squamous cell carcinoma growth patterns. **(A)** Most feature an endobronchial or endobronchiolar component; however, the majority of carcinomas infiltrate underlying lung. **(B)** Peripheral carcinomas may not be associated with distal airways. This well-differentiated carcinoma features alveolar filling with keratin. **(C)** Squamous cell carcinoma occasionally arises in individuals with idiopathic pulmonary fibrosis/usual interstitial pneumonia. The differential diagnosis includes squamous metaplasia with reactive atypia.

mucostasis with atelectasis, obstructive lipoid pneumonia, infectious pneumonia, abscess formation, and bronchiectasis (Fig. 35.23B). Peripheral tumors have an upper lobe predilection, form solid nodules, and may cause pleural puckering or chest wall involvement[628] (Fig. 35.23C). In some surgical series, SCC is the most common histology seen in superior sulcus tumors; however, less than half of superior sulcus tumors are of squamous histology.[631–635]

Since central SCCs arise in large airways, an endobronchial component is almost always observed (Fig. 35.24A). Adjacent bronchial mucosa usually features metaplasia, dysplasia, and in situ changes. Only one third of peripheral SCCs have an endobronchial/endobronchiolar component[628] (Fig. 35.24B,C). Peripheral SCCs are also less likely to invade lymphatics or spread to hilar lymph nodes.[629,630] Viral cytopathic effect suggestive of HPV infection is noted in up to 50% of all pulmonary SCCs; however, the percentage of these cases with documented HPV DNA is uncertain.[312]

Keratinization or intercellular bridges are the diagnostic morphologic features of SCC (Fig. 35.25). Given the heterogeneous nature of even a pure SCC, one may find a tumor containing areas with obvious intercellular bridges and numerous keratin pearls (well differentiated) and areas with subtle bridges or rare keratin pearls (poorly differentiated). An SCC is graded as well, moderately, or poorly differentiated according to the most poorly differentiated component. Grading is obviously subjective and of uncertain clinical utility; however, generally speaking, well-differentiated SCC tends to spread locally within the chest and involve mediastinal structures, while poorly differentiated SCC metastasizes to distant sites.[636] Of note, squamoid tumors lacking either intercellular bridges or keratinization should be diagnosed as LCC and not poorly differentiated SCC.

Well-differentiated SCCs are cohesive tumors with nests or cords of infiltrating tumor cells vaguely resembling epidermis or squamous mucosa (Fig. 35.26A,B). Tumor cells are usually separated by desmoplastic stroma

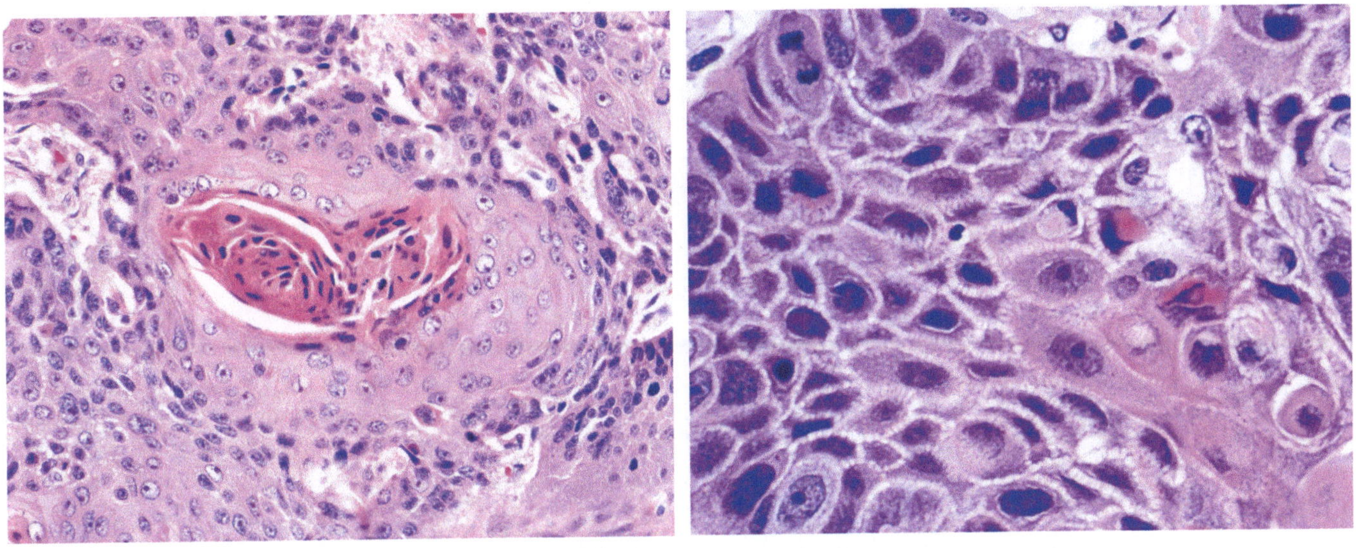

FIGURE 35.25. Squamous cell carcinoma, diagnostic features. **(A)** Extracellular keratin is commonly seen in well-differentiated carcinomas. **(B)** Intercellular bridges and intracytoplasmic keratin are diagnostic features but often focal in poorly differentiated carcinomas.

and inflammatory cells. Keratinization is most often found in the center of the nests along with loose keratin, neutrophils, and occasional multinucleated giant cells. A pseudoglandular arrangement can be seen owing to individual cell necrosis (Fig. 35.26C). The edges of infiltrating carcinomas and some peripheral SCCs feature air-space filling by tumor cells. Solid and lepidic architectural patterns can be seen with displaced pneumocytes filling the central portions of alveolar sacs (Fig. 35.26D–F). Tumor cells feature abundant eosinophilic to clear cytoplasm with large nuclei, prominent nucleoli, and chromatin condensation along the nuclear membrane. Mitoses are abundant, but atypical forms are not common. Extremely well-differentiated SCC lacking cytologic features of malignancy is diagnosed on the basis of stromal invasion alone.

Moderately and poorly differentiated carcinomas often form sheets, and individual tumor cells feature variation in size and shape. Tumor cells may be spindled or pleomorphic, and atypical mitoses are common. Necrosis can be extensive. In instances where obvious squamous features are not appreciated, one might consider sarcoma or lymphoma diagnoses.

While SCCs typically stain for both low and high molecular weight keratins (such as AE1, AE3, Cam5.2, 34ßE12, cytokeratin 5/6, and cytokeratin 14) in addition to B72.3, CEA, and p63, immunohistochemistry has a very limited role in SCC diagnosis.[637–639] No single immunohistochemical marker or panel of markers aids in differentiating a lung SCC from a nonpulmonary metastasis. For example, few pulmonary SCCs stain with thyroid transcription factor-1 (TTF-1) or cytokeratin 7.[640–642] While up to 30% of SCCs react with antibodies directed against synaptophysin, chromogranin, or CD56 antigens, this neuroendocrine differentiation does not alter the light microscopic diagnosis and is of no prognostic significance.[643–645] Up to one third of moderately and poorly differentiated SCCs also stain with trophoblastic cell markers human chorionic gonadotropin (hCG) or human placental lactogen (hPL). Yet such results do not suggest a diagnosis of choriocarcinoma, just as α-fetoprotein (AFP) expression does not a hepatoid or yolk sac tumor make.[646–648]

Ultrastructurally, SCC cells have short filopodial processes that interdigitate with processes of neighboring cells[649–652] (Fig. 35.27A). Desmosomes connect the processes to each other and correspond to the intercellular bridges seen on light microscopy. Well- to moderately differentiated SCC typically contains numerous cytoplasmic tonofilaments attached to the desmosomes (Fig. 35.27B). These tonofilaments impart an eosinophilic hue to tumor cells. Poorly differentiated SCC usually demonstrates fewer cytoplasmic tonofilaments and desmosomes and lacks filopodial processes.[650] In some cases mucin and neurosecretory-type granules may be seen, but the remainder of the cytoplasm is relatively unspecialized. Invasive tumor cells demonstrate highly variable basement membrane deposition, while tumor cell nests on the periphery of the lesion are encircled with basement membrane.[653,654] Alveolar space-filling SCCs displace pneumocytes but do not destroy the alveolar wall basement membrane.[655]

The differential diagnosis of SCC includes reactive and neoplastic processes. Squamous metaplasia of respiratory epithelium and alveolar pneumocytes associated with diffuse alveolar damage, healing infarcts, infections, and chemo- and radiation therapy can produce discrete lesions oftentimes centered on airways. Recognition of

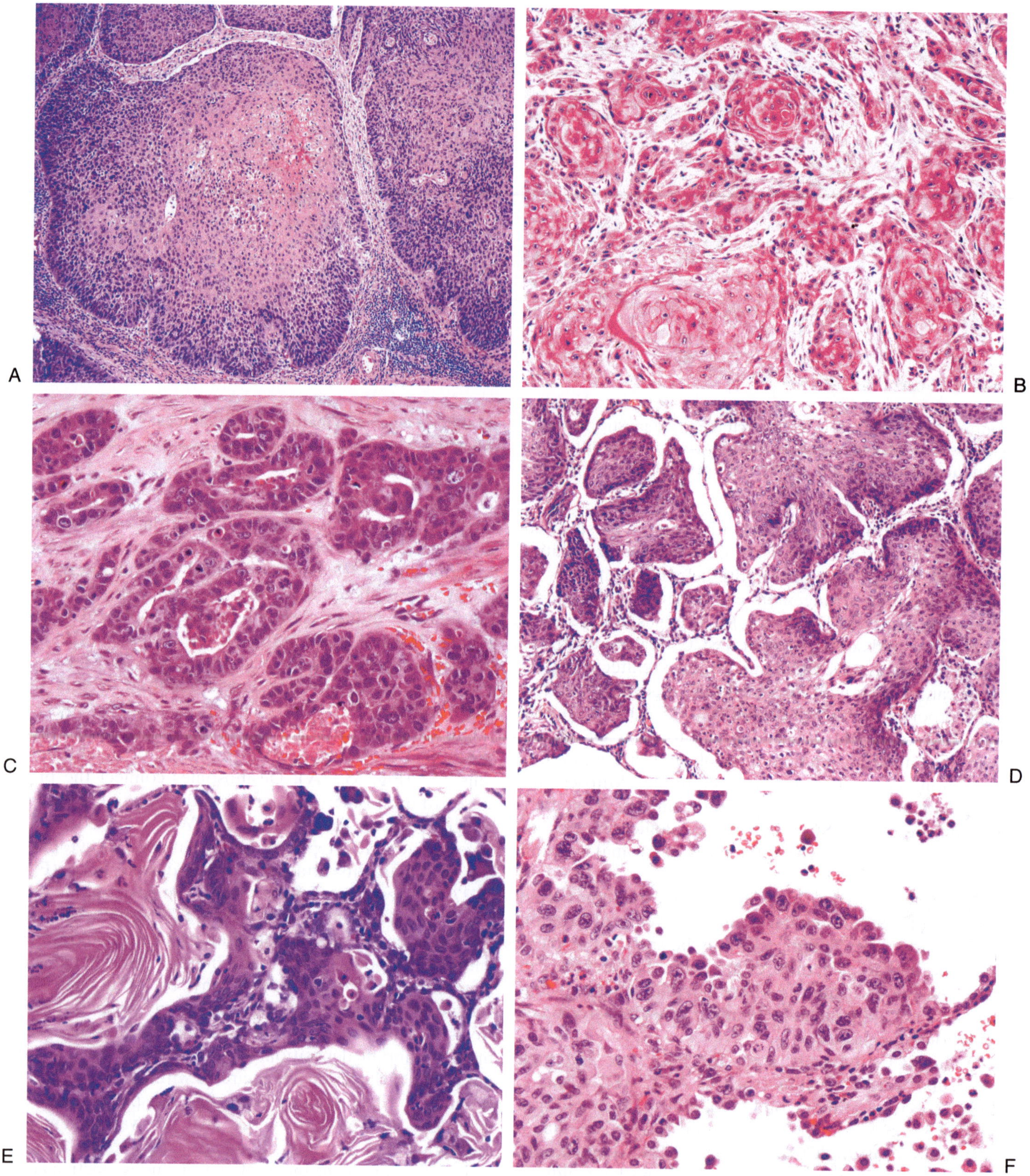

FIGURE 35.26. Squamous cell carcinoma (SCC), histologic growth patterns. **(A)** Nests of tumor cells resemble a jigsaw puzzle and feature scant intervening desmoplastic stroma and inflammatory cells. Central degeneration leads to cavitation. **(B)** Morpheaform growth is not uncommon. Desmoplasia is more pronounced in this example. **(C)** Poorly differentiated carcinomas may have a pseudoglandular growth pattern owing to individual cell necrosis and microcavitation. **(D)** Air-space filling can be seen at the edges of otherwise destructive carcinomas. **(E)** Lepidic growth may feature abundant intraalveolar keratin. **(F)** Multiple layers of nonkeratinizing SCC can overgrow alveolar septa.

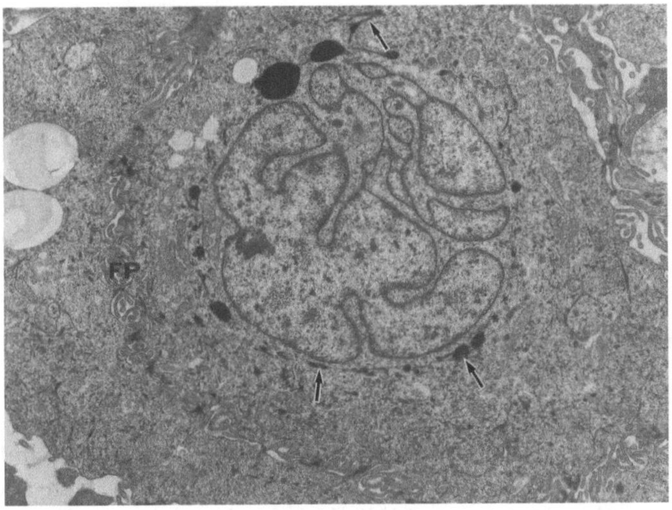

A

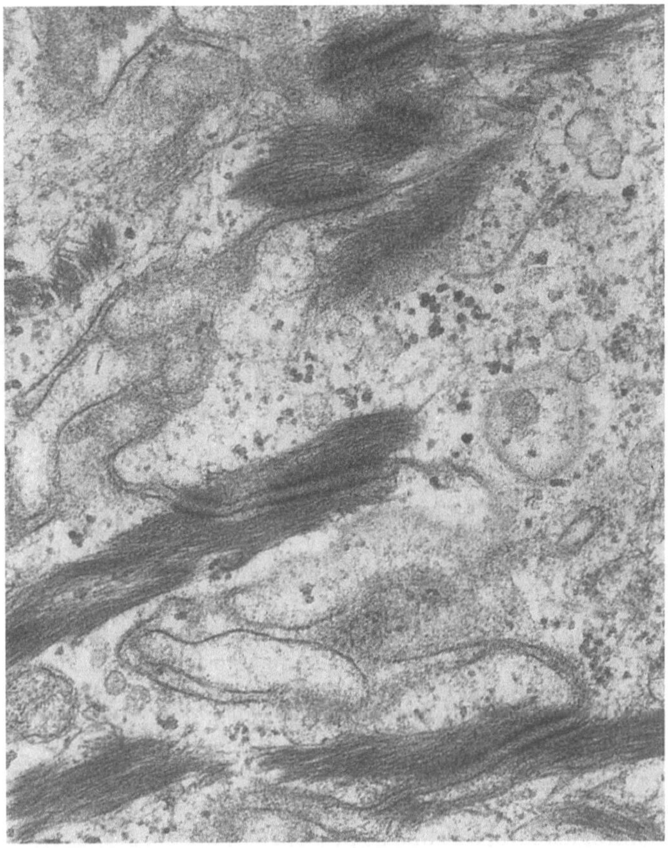

B

FIGURE 35.27. Squamous cell carcinoma, ultrastructural features. **(A)** This tumor cells features filopodial processes (FPs), numerous desmosomes, and cytoplasmic tonofilaments. Electron-dense material represents keratohyaline granules (arrows). **(B)** This greatly magnified field demonstrates filopodial processes interconnected by desmosomes. Tonofilaments insert into desmosomal plaques.

the primary pathologic process and extension of metaplastic epithelium through canals of Lambert into alveolar spaces in the absence of parenchymal destruction suggest the proper diagnosis. Biopsy fragments with metaplasia overlying unsampled malignancies can also be mistaken for SCC. Squamous cell papillomas lack frankly malignant cytology and stromal invasion, while pulmonary involvement with laryngotracheal papillomatosis, although rare, should also be differentiated from invasive carcinoma. An SCC with entrapped glandular epithelium should not be misinterpreted as adenosquamous carcinoma, while endobronchial mucoepidermoid carcinoma features intermediate and mucinous cells. Lung SCC with mediastinal extension can be distinguished from histopathologically identical primary thymic carcinoma with a CD5 stain since the former is always negative and the latter is often positive.[656–659] Differentiating a primary lung SCC from a metastasis on histologic grounds alone can be impossible. Molecular studies show great promise and appear more accurate than clinical criteria in distinguishing a de novo lung primary from a metastasis.[660,661] Metastatic malignant melanoma can also mimic SCC.

Surgery is the only therapy that offers any chance of cure to patients with resectable SCC. Superior sulcus tumors and other bulky SCC may be resected after chemotherapy or radiation treatments. For the vast majority of patients with inoperable SCC, radiation therapy can provide intermediate to long-term local control. The overall 5-year survival rate is approximately 15%, yet stage I resected SCCs have an at least 50% 5-year survival rate.[662] Adjuvant chemotherapy for resectable SCC also appears to prolong survival.[663–667]

While almost 200 individual NSCLC prognostic factors including biomarkers have been studied, stage and performance status are the only universally accepted prognostic indicators[668–670] (Fig. 35.28). Peripheral SCCs do not

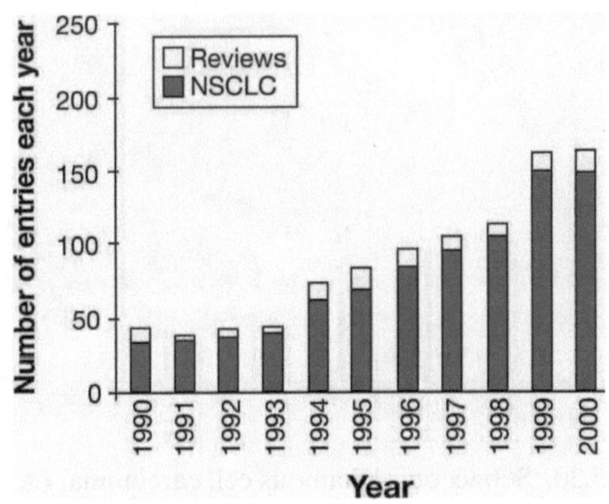

FIGURE 35.28. Indexed English-language literature pertaining to prognostic factors in non–small-cell lung cancer (NSCLC). (From Brundage et al.,[668] with permission of *Chest*.)

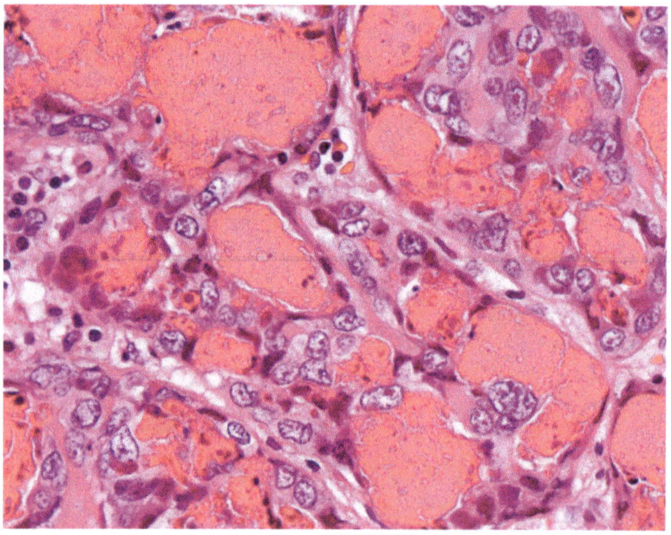

FIGURE 35.29. Pseudoangiosarcomatous/pseudovascular adenoid squamous cell carcinoma. Cuboidal and flattened malignant epithelioid tumor cells line interanastomosing sinuous blood vessel-like spaces. Immunohistochemical studies may be required to differentiate this variant from a true angiosarcoma.

have a different survival rate than central tumors, and histologic features, such as presence or absence of cavitation, may or may not indicate a more aggressive clinical course.[629,671] Although investigators have studied whether SCC survival rates are stage for stage better than adenocarcinoma, a consensus opinion is lacking.[636,672–677]

Squamous Cell Carcinoma Variants

While many morphologic variants of SCC including verrucous, oncocytic, spindle cell, giant cell, pleomorphic (see Chapter 37), pseudovascular adenoid/pseudoangiosarcomatous[678,679] (Fig. 35.29), sebaceous[680] (Fig. 35.30), and pilomatricoma-like[681] have been described, the current WHO classification includes only papillary, clear cell, small cell, and basaloid. Pure variants are rare, but many SCCs contain areas with these particular patterns.

Papillary Variant

Although many SCCs feature endobronchial polypoid growth, a rare percentage are almost completely papillary. These carcinomas are more common in men and nearly always are T1N0 lesions; however, their prognosis is not better than that of other stage IA lung carcinomas.[682–684] Histologically, tumors are well differentiated and feature polypoid or papillary growth into bronchial lumens (Fig. 35.31A). Nonkeratinizing tumor cells line fibrovascular cores and rarely exhibit more than moderate cytologic atypia (Fig. 35.31B). Adjacent bronchial mucosa is almost always metaplastic and usually dysplastic. Although most cases are invasive carcinomas, histologic findings of submucosal invasion may be subtle, and spread into submucosal glands should not be mistaken for invasion. With well-differentiated cytology, only the appreciation of cellular crowding and incomplete maturation allow for a diagnosis of carcinoma. Koilocytosis is not commonly seen,

A

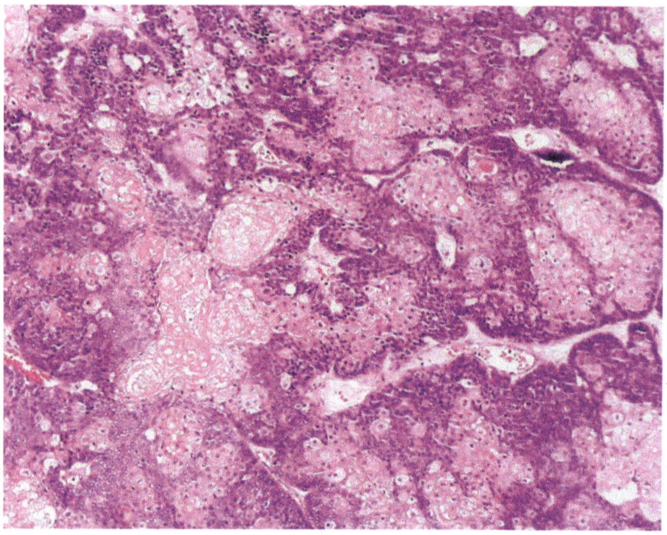

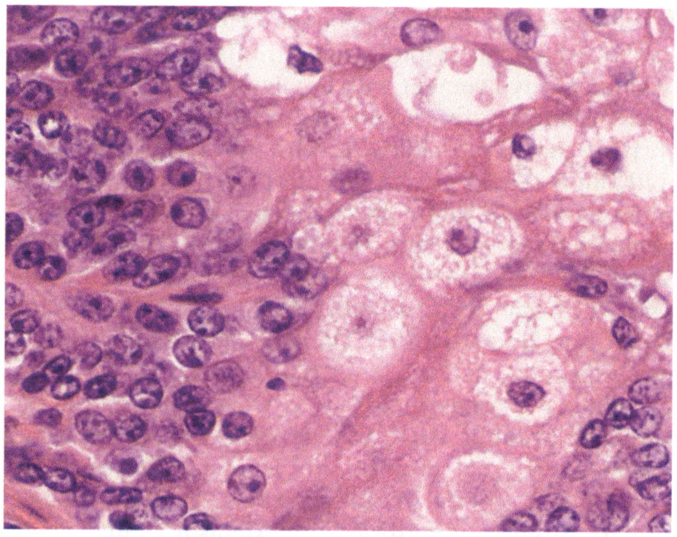

B

FIGURE 35.30. Sebaceous squamous cell carcinoma. **(A)** Tumor lobules composed of dark and light zones punctuate the low-magnification appearance of this neoplasm. **(B)** Basaloid-type cells with uniform vesicular nuclei and scant cytoplasm are intimately associated with sebaceous cells featuring abundant cytoplasm and small lipid-filled vesicles. Note the virtually identical nuclear features of both components. Other microscopic fields feature typical squamous morphology. (Courtesy of Dr. A. Borczuk, New York Presbyterian Hospital-Columbia University.)

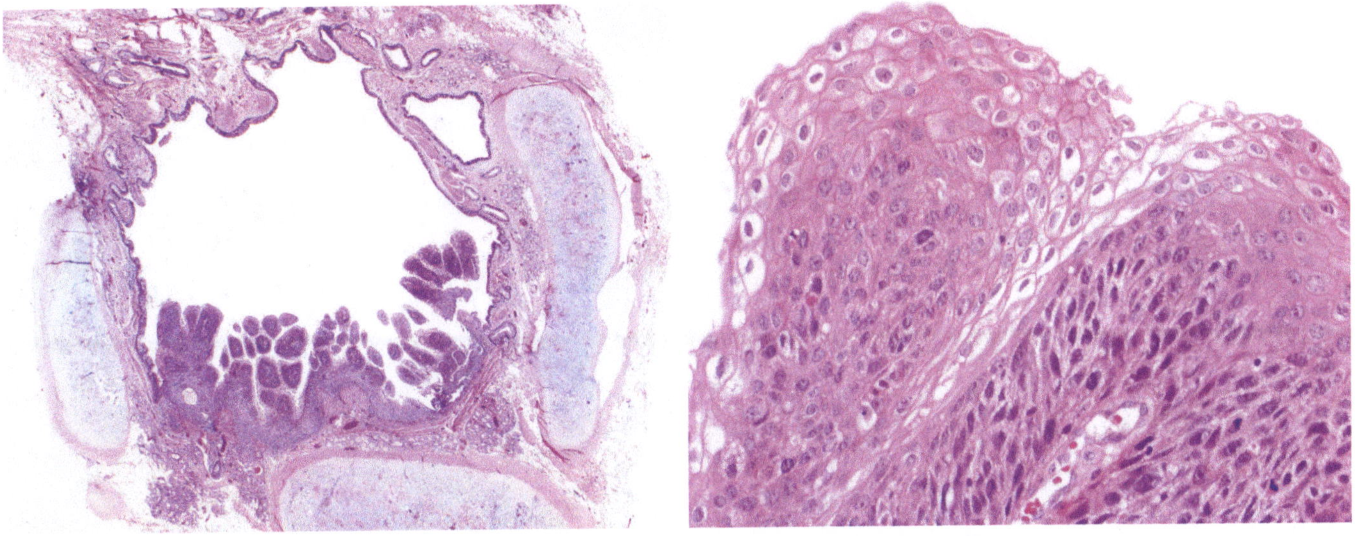

A B

FIGURE 35.31. Papillary variant of squamous cell carcinoma. **(A)** Exclusive endobronchial growth is quite rare and does not portend a more favorable outcome. **(B)** Papillary fronds are usually lined by well- or moderately differentiated tumor cells. Surface vacuolation is not diagnostic of koilocytosis. Unlike squamous cell papillomas, these carcinomas are broad based and feature uniform malignant cytology. (See also Chapter 34, Fig. 34.10).

and when present should raise the possibility of a solitary squamous cell papilloma.[685] These rare benign tumors are usually exophytic with a single fibrovascular core. Cytologic atypia may be seen, yet progression to carcinoma is infrequent. Stromal invasion is only suggested with the uncommon inverted growth pattern. Endobronchial metastases of nonpulmonary carcinomas, most notably head and neck SCC, rarely feature only papillary architecture and lack adjacent dysplastic epithelium.

Clear Cell Variant

Up to 30% of SCCs feature focal clear cell morphology, but rare tumors have almost complete clear cell histology.[686] However, these tumors must demonstrate unequivocal, albeit focal, squamous differentiation in the form of either intercellular bridges or keratinization. This poorly differentiated variant is composed of large solid nests or sheets of tumor cells with ample optically clear cytoplasm, irregularly shaped hyperchromatic nuclei, prominent nucleoli, and distinct cell borders separated by thin fibrous septa with areas of necrosis (Fig. 35.32). The periodic acid-Schiff (PAS)-positive diastase sensitive histochemical profile indicates cytoplasmic glycogen. The main differential diagnosis concerns metastatic clear cell carcinoma from nonpulmonary sites such as the kidney or salivary gland.

Small Cell Variant

This variant is of great clinical importance given its morphologic resemblance to SCLC. Although this poorly differentiated SCC features a high nuclear/cytoplasmic ratio and focal nuclear molding, architectural and cytologic features of SCC are apparent. Tumor cells form well-defined nests or cords with intervening desmoplastic stroma (Fig. 35.33A; see also Fig. 36.126 in Chapter 36). Sheets of necrosis and chromatin streaming (Azzopardi effect) are not prominent.[687] In comparison to SCLC, tumor cells have coarse to vesicular chromatin, obvious nucleoli, and distinct cell borders (Fig. 35.33B). Intercellular bridges or keratinization, though focal, are the sine qua non of diagnosis. The differential diagnosis may be impossible on small biopsy fragments, while excluding a combined SCLC on a large biopsy or excision may be equally challenging. High molecular weight keratin (34ßE12) and p63 immunohistochemical stains decorate SCC but not SCLC and thus aid in discriminating between the two entities[688,689] (see Figs. 36.127 to 36.129 in Chapter 36).

Basaloid Variant

Basaloid morphology can be seen in SCC. Nomenclature is confusing, as pure basaloid carcinoma, a subtype of LCC, can have abrupt keratin pearl formation mimicking hair follicles, although such is not considered squamous differentiation (see Large Cell Carcinoma, below). The basaloid variant of SCC requires at least focal intercellular bridges and individual cell keratinization. These poorly differentiated carcinomas can have endobronchial or peripheral locations and form solid lobules or trabecular masses with striking peripheral palisading of small cuboidal to fusiform cells with scant cytoplasm, hyper-

A 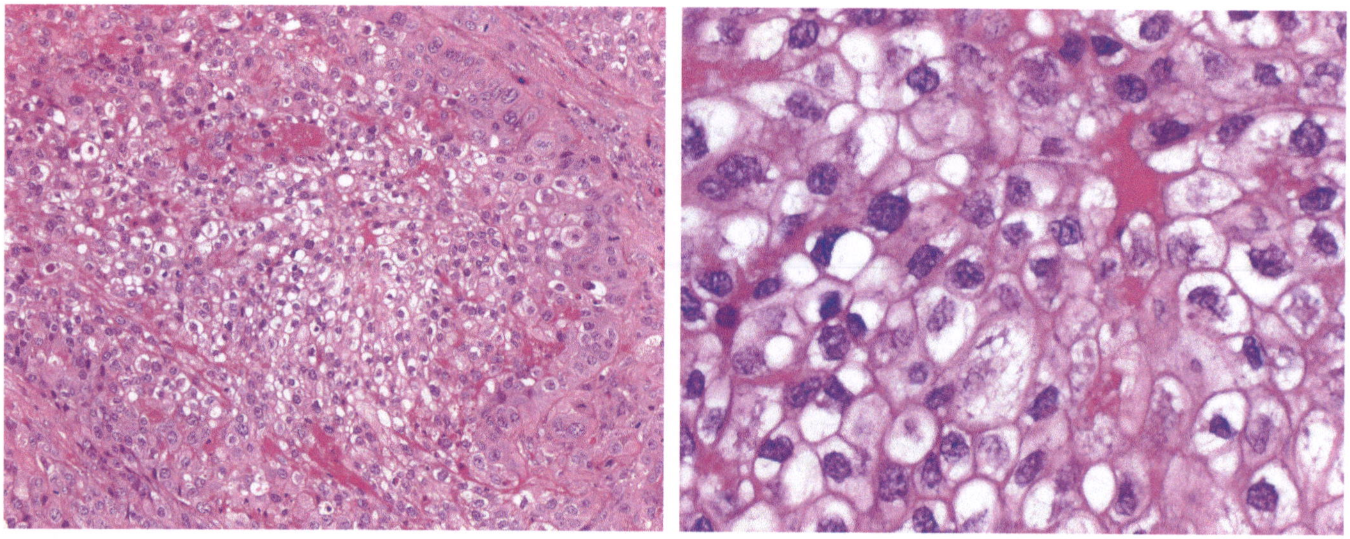 B

FIGURE 35.32. Clear cell variant of squamous cell carcinoma. **(A)** While the tumor features eosinophilic cytoplasm and individual cell keratinization along the periphery, the central area is composed of clear cells. Focal clear cell change is common, and predominant clear cell morphology is quite rare. **(B)** These glycogen-rich cells lack morphologic features of squamous cell carcinoma.

chromatic nuclei with granular chromatin, inconspicuous nucleoli, and a high mitotic rate (Fig. 35.34). Central necrosis is usually present, and hyaline stroma can be seen in up to one third of cases. Survival rates for this variant are as poor as those noted for the pure basaloid carcinoma.[690] The differential diagnosis includes adenoid cystic carcinoma, especially for central lesions (see Chapter 38).[691]

Adenocarcinoma

Adenocarcinoma of the lung is defined as a malignant epithelial tumor with glandular differentiation or mucin production. As the most common histologic subtype in some countries, in women, and in nonsmokers, much attention is focused on prevention, early diagnosis, and treatment of these morphologically heterogeneous carci-

A 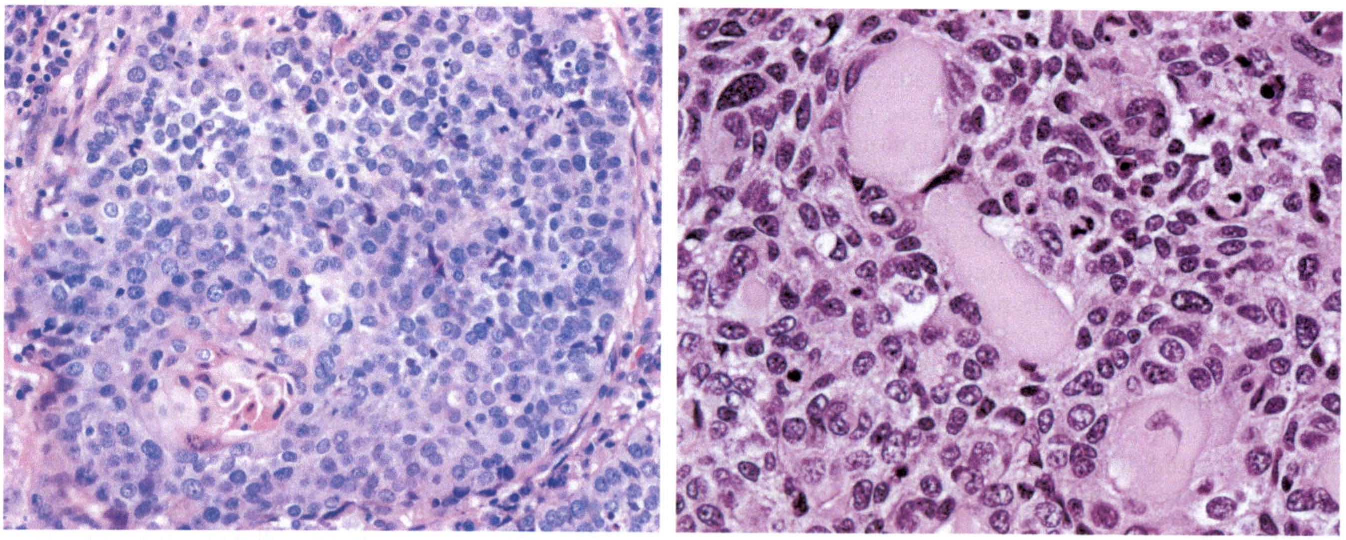 B

FIGURE 35.33. Small cell variant of squamous cell carcinoma. **(A)** Tumor nodules feature peripheral palisading and focal keratinization. Tumor cells are round with less cytoplasm than typical squamous cell carcinomas. (Courtesy of Dr. C. Moran, M.D. Anderson Cancer Center, Houston, TX.) **(B)** This example features ample cytoplasm, vesicular chromatin and nucleoli. Amyloid-like stroma is a rare light microscopic finding.

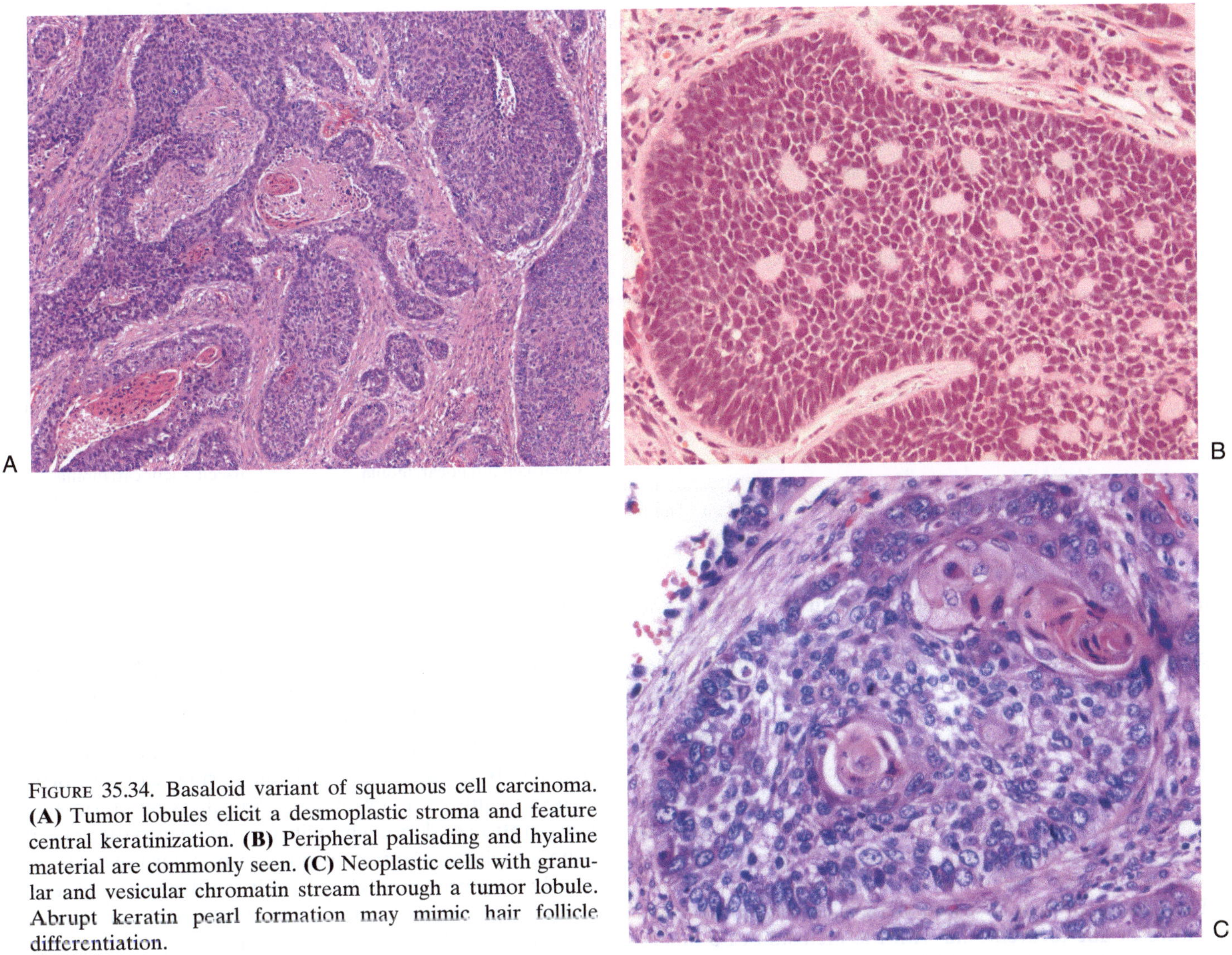

FIGURE 35.34. Basaloid variant of squamous cell carcinoma. **(A)** Tumor lobules elicit a desmoplastic stroma and feature central keratinization. **(B)** Peripheral palisading and hyaline material are commonly seen. **(C)** Neoplastic cells with granular and vesicular chromatin stream through a tumor lobule. Abrupt keratin pearl formation may mimic hair follicle differentiation.

nomas. Most adenocarcinomas are peripheral tumors and probably arise from Clara cells or type II pneumocytes, while central carcinomas develop from bronchial epithelium or bronchial gland epithelium.[606,607,619,621,692–694] Adenocarcinomas rarely arise in association with congenital cysts, congenital cystic adenomatoid malformations, and bullae including placentoid bullous lesions.[51,695–700]

Many pulmonary adenocarcinomas are associated with parenchymal scars. In the first half of the 20th century, pathologists believed that carcinomas arose from old tuberculosis, infarcts, pneumoconiosis, emphysematous blebs, and bronchiectasis from chronic inflammatory processes.[608,701–704] Suggested causes of epithelial proliferation and malignant transformation included trapping of carcinogens in fibrotic tissue or the effect of chronic inflammation.[608] Most peripheral and almost all upper lobe apical carcinomas were considered scar carcinomas as long as the tumor did not obviously arise from or involve the nearest bronchus. The 1981 WHO classification considered papillary adenocarcinoma and BAC the most frequent morphologic patterns in scar carcinomas.[615] Diffuse parenchymal scarring was extrapolated as a risk factor for the development of lung carcinoma. The etiologic role of tobacco and immunologic derangements confound this association (see sections Infections and Lung Injury, above).[397,406,705,706]

While rare cases of carcinoma arise in association with preexisting localized or diffuse pulmonary fibrosis,[707] prior radiographs from patients with scar carcinomas without scars, and psammoma bodies in the center of scars surrounded by psammoma body-rich carcinomas suggest a different course of events. Peripheral scars associated with adenocarcinoma are now considered the result of tumor factors and host response.[708–711] Vascular or airway occlusion by tumor along with increased tumor cell secretion of metalloproteinase inhibitors probably lead to alveolar collapse and fibrosis, while the large

TABLE 35.14. Historical World Health Organization (WHO) classifications of pulmonary adenocarcinoma

1967	1981	1999	2004
Bronchogenic			Adenocarcinoma, mixed subtype
Acinar	Acinar adenocarcinoma	Acinar adenocarcinoma	Acinar adenocarcinoma
Papillary	Papillary adenocarcinoma	Papillary adenocarcinoma	Papillary adenocarcinoma
Bronchioloalveolar carcinoma	Bronchioloalveolar carcinoma	Bronchioloalveolar carcinoma	Bronchioloalveolar carcinoma
		Nonmucinous	Nonmucinous
		Mucinous	Mucinous
		Mixed	Mixed or indeterminate
	Solid with mucus formation	Solid with mucin	Solid with mucin production
		Variants	Variants
		Well-differentiated fetal adenocarcinoma	Fetal adenocarcinoma
		Mucinous (colloid) adenocarcinoma	Mucinous (colloid) adenocarcinoma
		Mucinous cystadenocarcinoma	Mucinous cystadenocarcinoma
		Signet-ring adenocarcinoma	Signet-ring adenocarcinoma
		Clear-cell adenocarcinoma	Clear-cell adenocarcinoma

Source: World Health Organization Histologic Typing of Lung Tumours.[614–617]

numbers of myofibroblasts, extracellular matrix, and type III collagen in scars indicate a vigorous host desmoplastic response.[710–715] Recent investigations suggest that the quantity and quality of the scar have prognostic significance.[716]

The WHO scheme has greatly expanded over the past 40 years (Table 35.14). The current classification recognizes five major adenocarcinoma subtypes—acinar, papillary, BAC, solid with mucin production, and mixed—as well as five variants (Table 35.13). As with SCC, adenocarcinoma is often a component of combined carcinomas. This system not only acknowledges the heterogeneous nature of adenocarcinoma with the inclusion of a mixed category, but restricts BAC diagnoses to carcinomas without stromal, vascular, or lymphatic invasion.

Although critics contend that the WHO subgroups are indistinct on account of the overwhelming predominance of the mixed subtype, and the fact that adenocarcinomas have similar cytology regardless of the architectural pattern, subclassification is morphologically useful and should be undertaken in order to elucidate different responses to therapies and differences in prognosis. Since BAC differs from the other major subtypes in so many ways, clinical and histologic features of this subtype are discussed separately.

Nonbronchioloalveolar Carcinoma

Non-BAC adenocarcinomas are usually peripheral lung tumors, although up to 13% may be central.[693,717–719] Peripheral tumors can have several different growth patterns. Most are 4.0cm or smaller, solitary, firm and gritty, solid, gray-tan subpleural lesions with either lobulated or spiculated edges (Fig. 35.35A). Tumors with mucinous features may have glistening mucoid, gray cut surfaces (Fig. 35.35B). Central necrosis or hemorrhage is common. The periphery may be semifirm with preserved air spaces. These qualities can be identified on HRCT scans with varying degrees of hazy increased attenuation and preserved bronchial and vascular structures (ground-glass opacities [GGOs]).[718] Pleural puckering can be pronounced resulting in a V-shaped pleural invagination and incorporation of dense white fibrous tissue into the center of the neoplasm. Central lesions can be hilar/perihilar or entirely endobronchial (Fig. 35.35C). Obstructive pneumonia or atelectasis is often seen. Unlike SCC, cavitation is uncommon. Peripheral adenocarcinoma is the most common tumor type to invade through overlying visceral pleura and spread along the pleural surface as a thick rind or with many nodules (Fig. 35.35D). These patterns resemble malignant mesothelioma and are referred to as pseudomesotheliomatous carcinoma.[720–724] Diffuse bilateral lung disease with multiple nodules of varying sizes or prominent interstitial expansion secondary to lymphangitic spread are commonly encountered, though usually at autopsy (Fig. 35.35E). Adenocarcinoma can also mimic interstitial lung disease clinically, radiographically, and even in tissue samples.[725] Pagetoid spread of adenocarcinoma in small and large airways may complicate surgical attempts at complete resection[726,727] (Fig. 35.35F).

Regardless of the architectural pattern, adenocarcinoma cells are cuboidal, columnar, or polygonal with moderate to abundant clear, eosinophilic, or mucin-filled basophilic cytoplasm. Nuclei are large and vesicular with prominent nucleoli. Clara cell differentiation manifests as eosinophilic cytoplasm with apical bulbs; PAS stains demonstrate diastase-resistant apical stain-

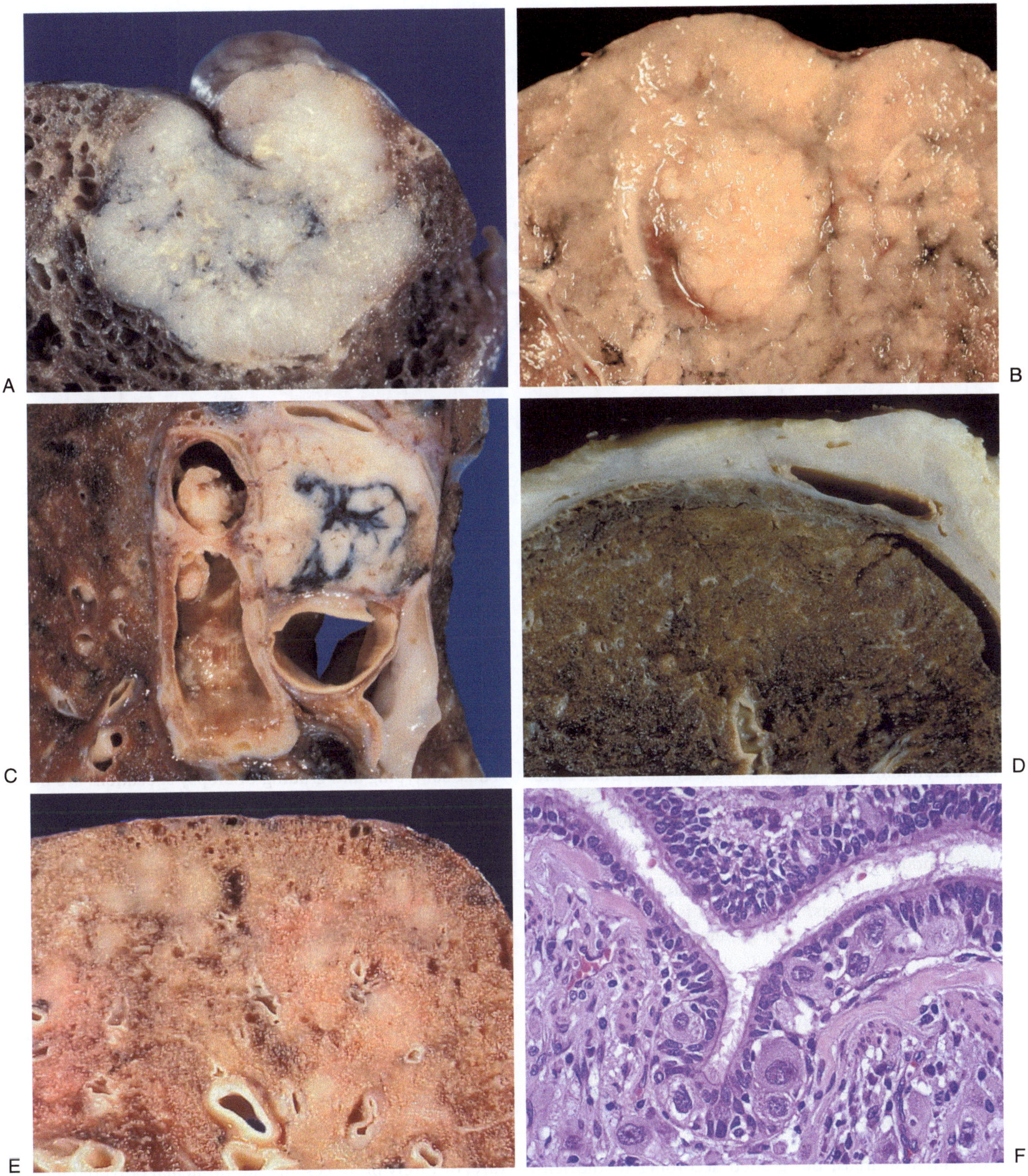

FIGURE 35.35. Invasive adenocarcinoma. **(A)** Subpleural tumors often cause pleural puckering. This well-circumscribed carcinoma has overrun anthracotic parenchyma and features punctate necrosis. **(B)** Adenocarcinomas with mucinous features have gelatinous cut surfaces. A papillary growth pattern is appreciated in this example. **(C)** Central adenocarcinomas may be indistinguishable from squamous cell carcinoma. Direct extension into peribronchial lymph nodes is not uncommon. **(D)** A thick pleural rind, while associated with malignant mesothelioma, can be the dominant pattern of lung cancer spread. The primary lung adenocarcinoma may be quite small and difficult to identify on gross specimen examination. **(E)** Multiple intraparenchymal foci of carcinoma are rarely encountered in surgical specimens. In the absence of a dominant lung mass, this radiographic pattern may suggest a nonpulmonary primary or even an infectious process. **(F)** Pagetoid spread is usually an incidental microscopic finding but may complicate attempts at complete surgical resection.

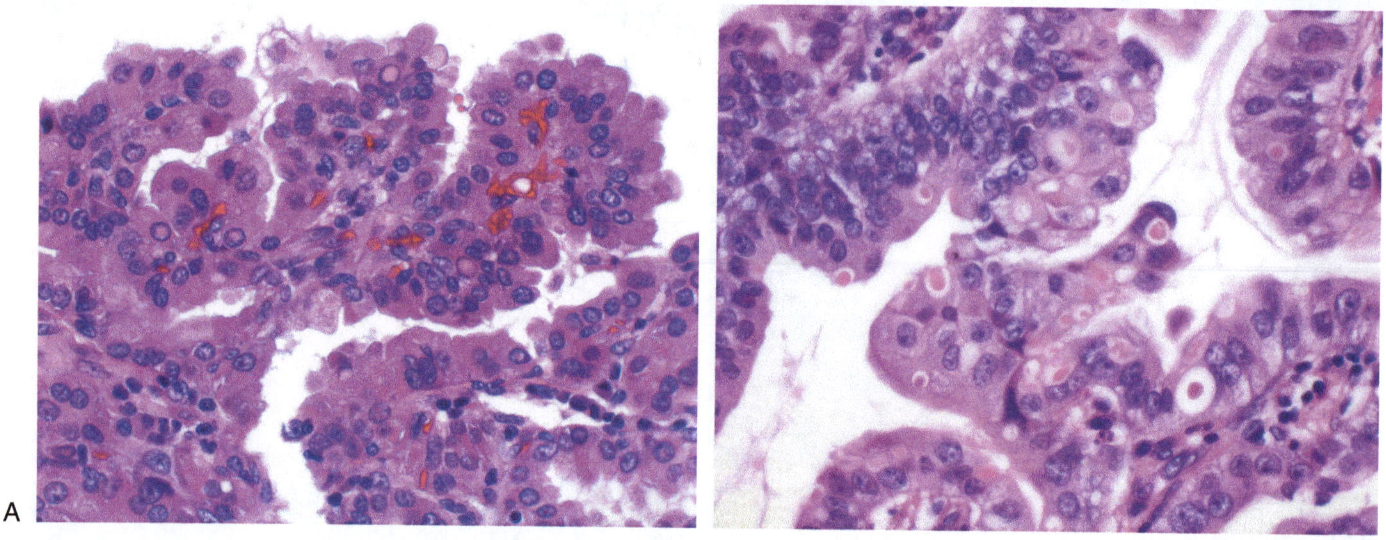

FIGURE 35.36. Adenocarcinoma morphology. **(A)** Cuboidal to columnar cells may feature both abundant eosinophilic apical cytoplasm suggestive of Clara cell differentiation as well as intranuclear pseudoinclusions suggestive of type II pneumocyte differentiation. The distinction is of no clinical importance. **(B)** Globular eosinophilic intracytoplasmic inclusions are encountered in degenerating cells, including tumors treated with chemotherapy or radiation prior to surgical excision.

ing. Intranuclear pseudoinclusions usually indicate type II pneumocyte differentiation, and globular eosinophilic intracytoplasmic inclusions may be seen, especially following induction therapy[728–730] (Fig. 35.36). Intracytoplasmic mucin can be subtle and only noted on mucin stains (mucicarmine, PAS diastase, Alcian blue) or obvious with signet-ring forms. Extracellular mucin can manifest as intraluminal wisps or extensive acellular pools. Intracellular glycogen may also be seen.

Virtually all invasive lung adenocarcinomas elicit stromal desmoplasia, varying degrees of host inflammation including eosinophilic, neutrophilic, or lymphoplasmacytic infiltrates with/without germinal center formation, parenchymal necrosis, and vasculitis. Granulomatous inflammation may be seen. Psammoma bodies, calcifications, and metaplastic bone are not uncommon.[731,732]

Adenocarcinomas are graded according to architectural and cytologic features. Tumors can be well (grade I), moderately (grade II), or poorly differentiated (grade III), depending on the extent to which the tumor resembles normal lung architecture and the degree of cytologic atypia. Poorly differentiated carcinomas are often solid with discohesive tumor cells. Given intratumoral heterogeneity, adenocarcinomas are recognized by their most differentiated areas, but graded according to the least differentiated area. Approximately 5% are well, 70% moderately, and 25% poorly differentiated. Tumoral necrosis can be seen in well-differentiated adenocarcinomas, but is usually more prominent in poorly differentiated lesions.

Adenocarcinoma, mixed subtype is listed first in the WHO classification as the most common histologic pattern. Over 80% of resected adenocarcinomas feature at least two and often three individual patterns, while less than 10% lack a BAC component[733] (Fig. 35.37). The larger the tumor, the more likely one is to identify additional architectural patterns and degrees of differentiation. Tumors usually feature solid or acinar components centrally and BAC morphology at the periphery.[734,735] Thus, subtyping and grading of biopsy specimens are not recommended.

The *acinar* pattern is the most common pure subtype, the most common pattern in mixed carcinomas, and cytologically resembles bronchial gland, bronchial lining epithelium, or Clara cells.[693,736,737] This pattern may be well, moderately, or poorly differentiated and features acini and tubules (Fig. 35.38). Cells may contain abundant cytoplasmic mucin, and extracellular mucin can be plentiful. A pseudoglandular pattern can be seen in SCC (Fig. 35.26C) and LCC with individual cell necrosis and should not be mistaken for acinar adenocarcinoma. Rhabdoid cells, usually identified in LCC, may be seen in acinar adenocarcinoma[738] (see "rhabdoid phenotype" under Large Cell Carcinoma Variants, below).

The *papillary* variant is defined as an adenocarcinoma with papillary structures that replace alveolar architecture, or rarely produces an endobronchial polypoid mass (Fig. 35.39A). This subtype represents from 3% to 10% of lung adenocarcinomas yet is a common component of mixed adenocarcinomas.[732,734,735] Architectural destruction and stromal invasion may not be obvious since secondary and tertiary papillary fronds with fibrovascular cores mimic normal alveolar parenchyma (Fig. 35.39B). Cuboidal to low columnar cells resembling Clara cells or

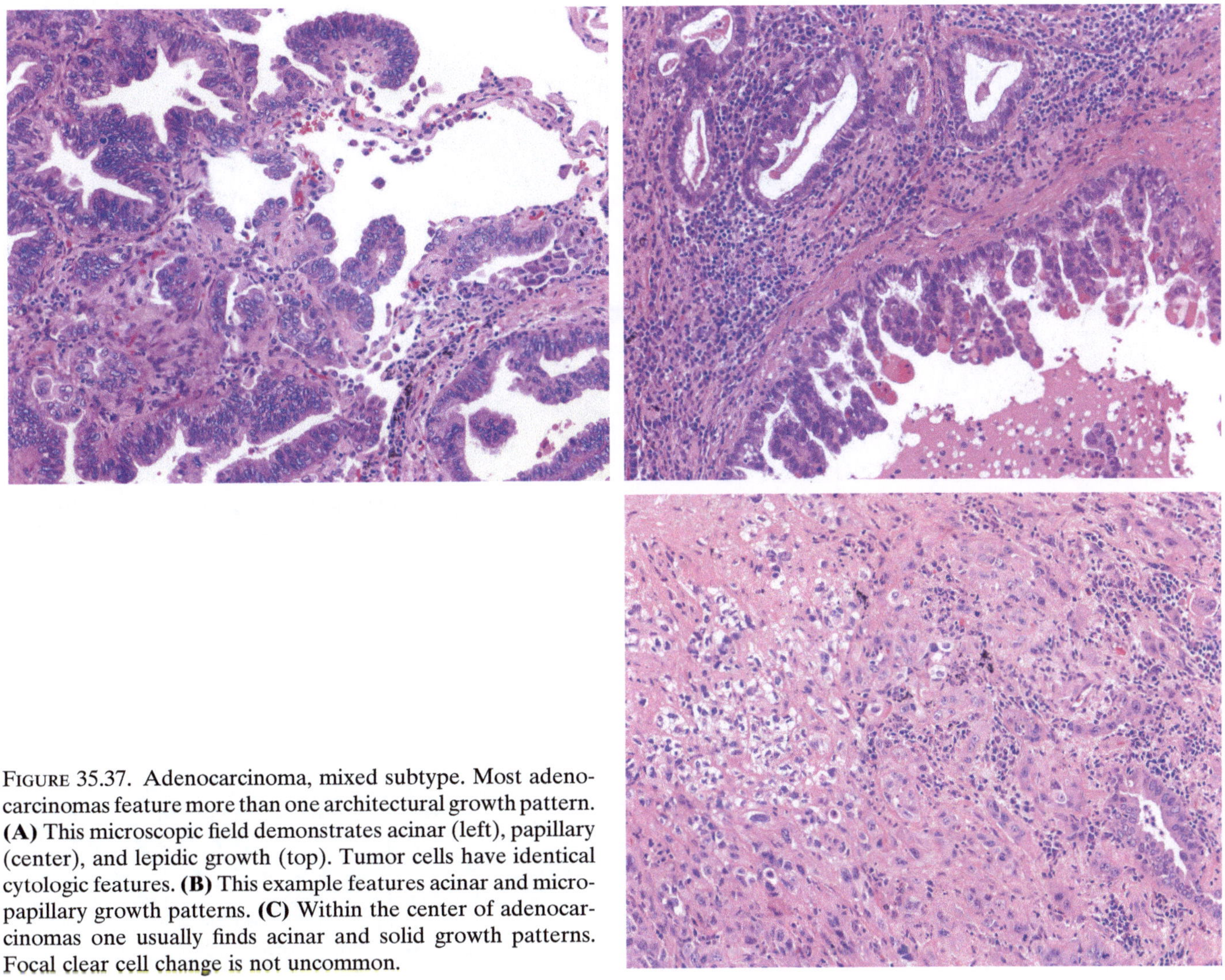

A B C

FIGURE 35.37. Adenocarcinoma, mixed subtype. Most adenocarcinomas feature more than one architectural growth pattern. **(A)** This microscopic field demonstrates acinar (left), papillary (center), and lepidic growth (top). Tumor cells have identical cytologic features. **(B)** This example features acinar and micropapillary growth patterns. **(C)** Within the center of adenocarcinomas one usually finds acinar and solid growth patterns. Focal clear cell change is not uncommon.

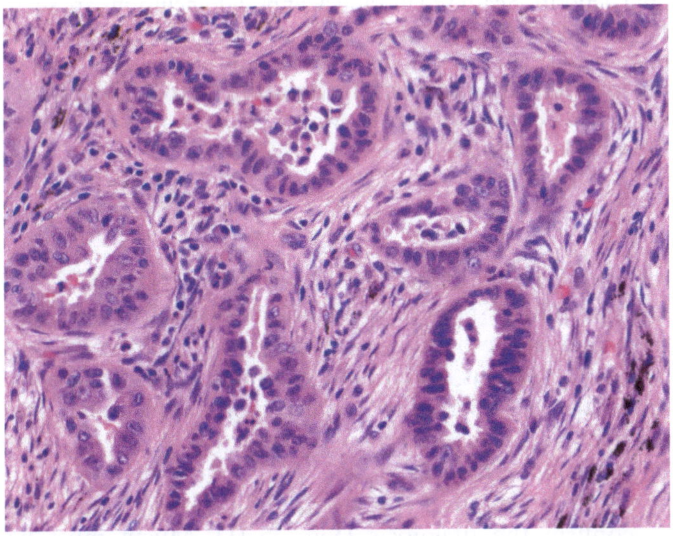

FIGURE 35.38. Adenocarcinoma, acinar subtype. Infiltrating tubules or glands elicit a desmoplastic stroma. Intraluminal mucin and inflammatory cells are commonly seen.

type II pneumocytes, or tall columnar cells line the fibrovascular cores. Mucinous differentiation is infrequent (Fig. 35.39C). Cytologic atypia is usually apparent, and rare cases contain prominent spindle cell morules[739] (Fig. 35.39D). Secondary findings include psammoma bodies and stromal lymphocytes.

The micropapillary pattern has attracted much attention of late. Characterized by small papillary tufts growing from alveolar septa or floating within alveolar spaces yet lacking fibrovascular cores, this pattern is not exclusively associated with papillary carcinoma, but is seen in a large percentage of papillary carcinomas[732,740] (Fig. 35.40A). The pattern is often observed at the periphery of mixed adenocarcinomas and is frequently the morphology of lymph node metastases.[740,741] Cells feature a high nuclear/cytoplasmic ratio with little eosinophilic cytoplasm and nuclear characteristics similar to those seen in adjacent nonmicropapillary areas (Fig. 35.40B). Recent data suggest that this morphology may be more likely to metastasize and thus indicate an

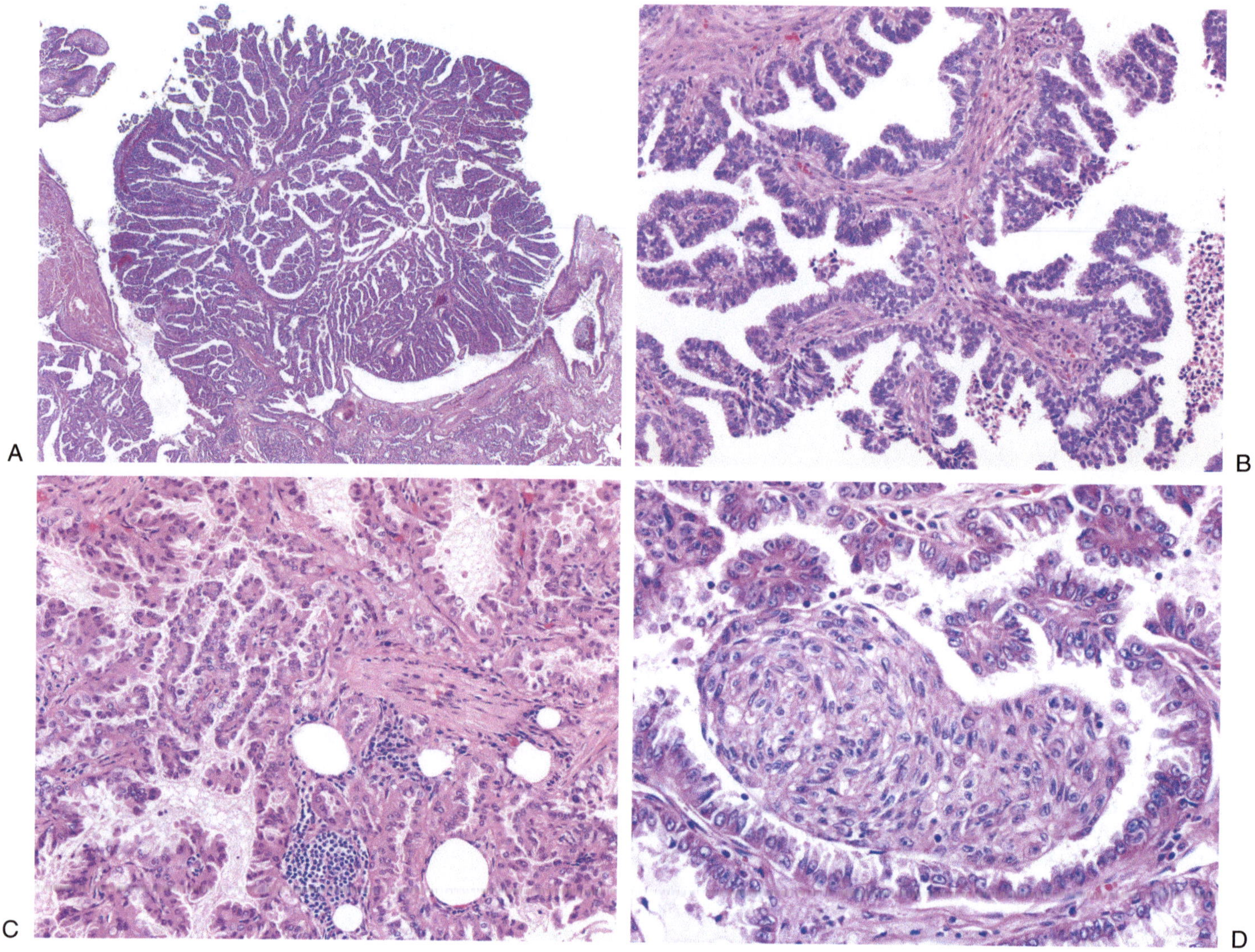

FIGURE 35.39. Adenocarcinoma, papillary subtype. **(A)** This endobronchial tumor demonstrates arborizing large central and thin peripheral fibrovascular cores. **(B)** The fibrovascular cores should not be mistaken for preserved alveolar septa. Note the micropapillary proliferations streaming from larger papillae. **(C)** This histologic field from the tumor illustrated in Figure 35.35B is from an individual with a long history of nasal spray use and exogenous lipoid pneumonia. Papillary fronds encircle lipid deposits. Scattered intranuclear pseudoinclusions are seen. **(D)** Spindle cell morules are a curious morphologic finding in this adenocarcinoma subtype. These tightly packed cells without nuclear atypia or mitotic activity stain with thyroid transcription factor-1. (Courtesy of Dr. C. Moran, M.D. Anderson Cancer Center, Houston, TX.)

unfavorable prognosis, even for patients with small (≤2.0 cm) lung adenocarcinomas.[740,742]

Papillary adenocarcinoma can be difficult to differentiate from BAC. However, nuclear atypia and dirty necrosis are usually conspicuous in papillary adenocarcinoma but not in BAC. Intranuclear pseudoinclusions, clear cell change, and intracytoplasmic eosinophilic globules are not discriminators. The distinction is of great clinical importance as papillary adenocarcinoma has a poorer stage-for-stage prognosis than BAC, yet perhaps a greater likelihood of responding to epidermal growth factor receptor tyrosine kinase inhibitors (EGFR-TKIs).[732,743,744] Differentiating papillary adenocarcinoma of the lung from metastatic papillary carcinoma of the thyroid and metastatic serous carcinoma originating in the female reproductive tract may require immunohistochemical studies.

The *solid adenocarcinoma with mucin* subtype is a poorly differentiated carcinoma requiring a mucin stain to confirm the diagnosis (Fig. 35.41). Mucin must be identified in at least five tumor cells in each of two high power (40×) fields. Although less than 15% of mixed

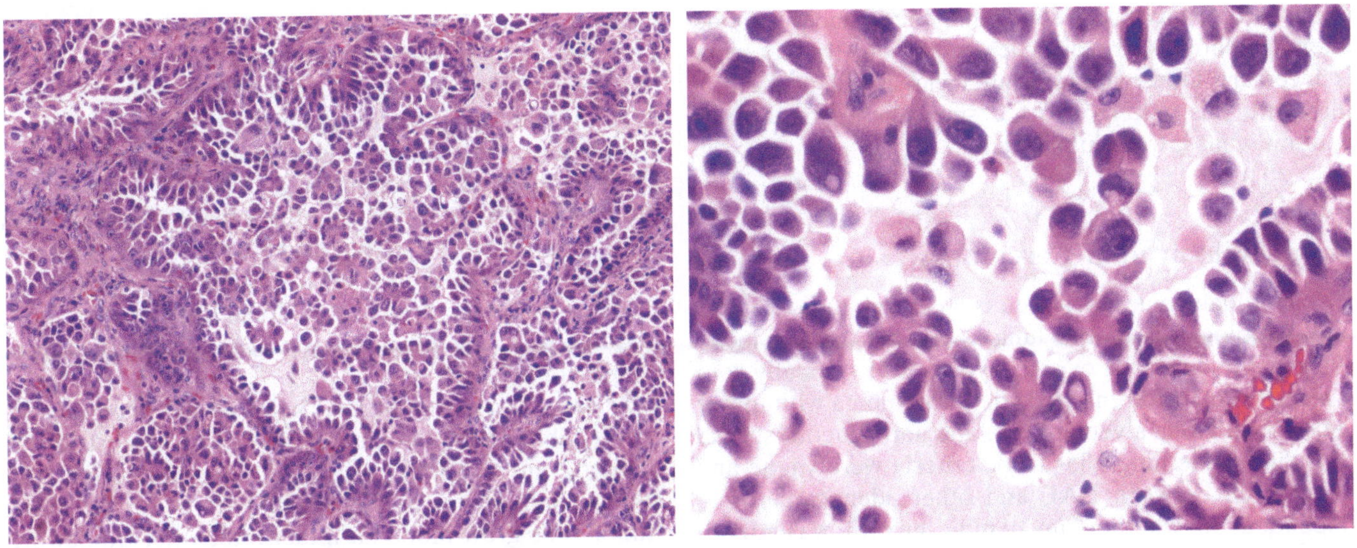

FIGURE 35.40. Adenocarcinoma, micropapillary pattern. **(A)** Small papillary tufts of tumor cells without individual fibrovascular cores float in alveolar spaces. **(B)** High-grade cytology is usually seen. This morphology might be more aggressive that other adenocarcinoma subtypes.

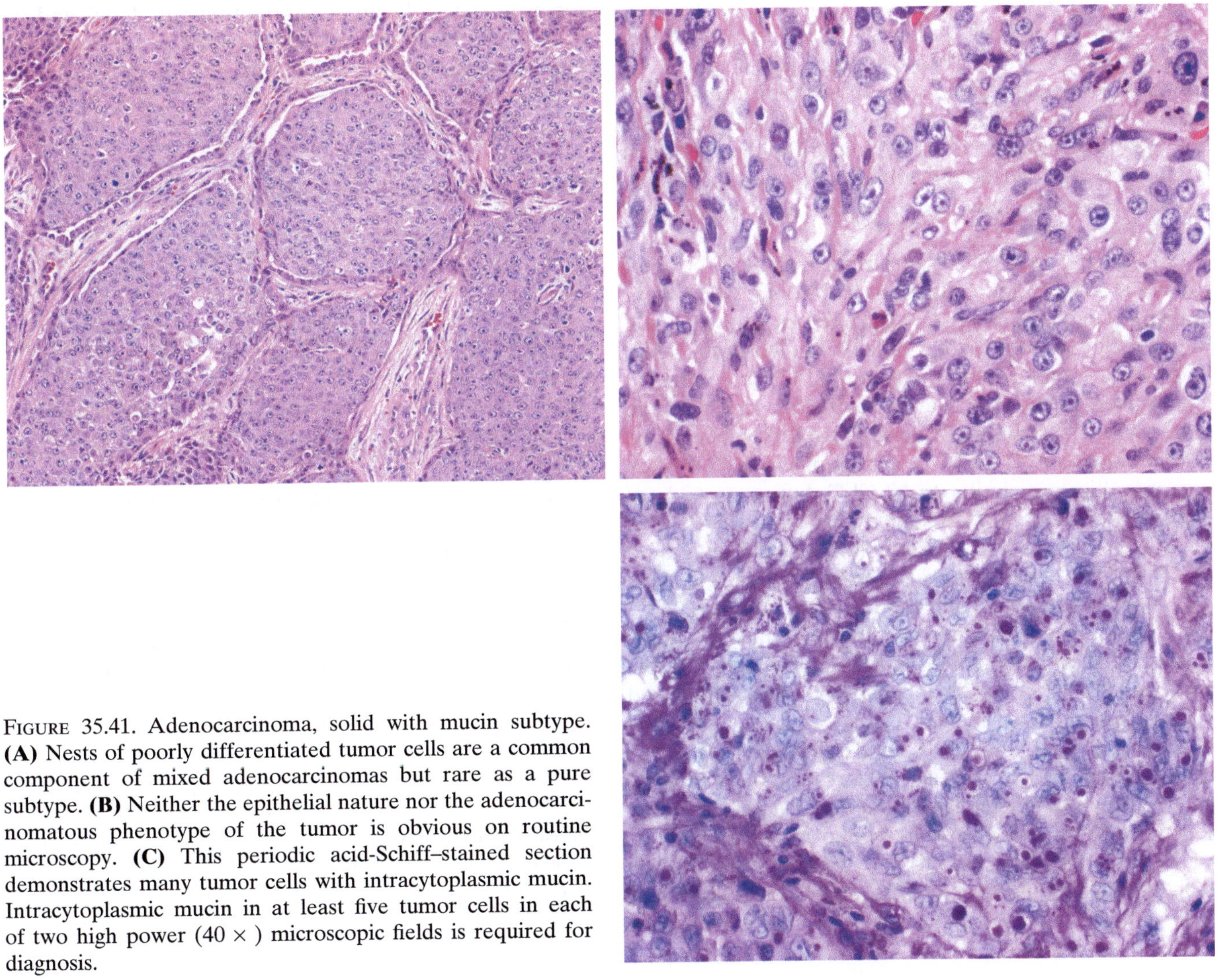

FIGURE 35.41. Adenocarcinoma, solid with mucin subtype. **(A)** Nests of poorly differentiated tumor cells are a common component of mixed adenocarcinomas but rare as a pure subtype. **(B)** Neither the epithelial nature nor the adenocarcinomatous phenotype of the tumor is obvious on routine microscopy. **(C)** This periodic acid-Schiff–stained section demonstrates many tumor cells with intracytoplasmic mucin. Intracytoplasmic mucin in at least five tumor cells in each of two high power (40 ×) microscopic fields is required for diagnosis.

adenocarcinomas have a solid component, and pure solid adenocarcinomas are even less common, the category is necessary. Otherwise, one might classify adenocarcinomas with this pattern as LCC since these tumors may contain scant intracellular mucin.

Bronchioloalveolar Carcinoma

Bronchioloalveolar carcinoma is a clinical, radiographic, and pathologically unique lung carcinoma that has interested pathologists for over 125 years.[745] Historically considered a well-differentiated adenocarcinoma with tumor cell growth along alveolar septa and aerogeneous spread throughout the lung, diagnostic criteria were vague and distinctions between BAC and other adenocarcinomas depended on whether any lepidic growth was identified.[746,747] Previous WHO classifications did not comment on the amount of this pattern required to diagnose a lung adenocarcinoma as BAC.[614,615] Clinicopathologic studies in the 1990s, however, suggested a significant survival advantage for patients with small adenocarcinomas composed entirely of BAC pattern.[735] On the basis of this work, the 1999 WHO classification required that BAC demonstrate pure lepidic growth without invasion of stroma, vessels, or pleura.[616] The 2004 classification did not alter this definition.[617] Three morphologic types of BAC are recognized: nonmucinous, mucinous, and mixed. A BAC diagnosis cannot be made on either cytologic or biopsy specimens.

Before the recent refinement in the diagnostic criteria, clinicopathologic generalizations regarding BAC were not reproducible. Though less than 10 years have passed since the definitional change, much is known about BAC, thanks in no small part to the advent of CT screening for lung cancer. Bronchioloalveolar carcinoma represents no more than 5% of lung carcinomas but 16% of resected carcinomas in a HRCT screening program.[596,748] Age demographics are similar to NSCLC, but up to 63% of patients with BAC are women and 26% of patients with BAC are nonsmokers.[748] Although it has been suggested that BAC may be more prevalent in Japan than in Europe and North America, confirmatory data are lacking.[716] Bronchioloalveolar carcinoma, often the mucinous type, is associated with congenital cystic adenomatoid malformations.[51,699,700,749] Despite morphologic similarities and weak immunohistochemical cross-reactivity between BAC and retrovirus-induced ovine pulmonary adenocarcinoma (also known as jaagsiekte or sheep pulmonary adenomatosis), molecular evidence of jaagsiekte sheep retrovirus in human adenocarcinomas is lacking.[750–753]

The majority of patients are asymptomatic, some present with cough, dyspnea, or weight loss, while less than 10% with advanced mucinous BAC have bronchorrhea producing up to 900 mL of watery sputum per day.[754] Patterns of lung involvement include solitary nodules, multiple nodules, or, rarely, lobar consolidation. Perhaps 25% of cases are multifocal and if a dominant nodule is not present, the radiographic appearance suggests metastatic carcinoma. Topographic genotyping suggests that multifocal BAC represents monoclonal disease rather than de novo tumor growth at multiple sites.[755] The consolidative pattern is difficult to distinguish radiographically or macroscopically from lobar pneumonia. Lung nodules with significant percentages of GGO may be nonmucinous BAC.[756–758]

At least two-thirds of BACs are of the nonmucinous type (Table 35.15). Nonmucinous BACs are usually ill-defined, tan, semifirm peripheral nodules ranging from several millimeters to many centimeters in size. Since tumor cells grow along an intact interstitial framework, air spaces are visible grossly (Fig. 35.42A). Central scarring and pleural fibrosis with or without puckering can be seen. Hemorrhage and necrosis are absent. Multifocality can be seen in a minority of cases. Mucinous BAC, however, is usually larger, more often multifocal, and can present as segmental or lobar consolidation. This tumor was first described as resembling "fromage de Roque-

TABLE 35.15. Pathologic features of bronchioloalveolar carcinoma

	Nonmucinous	Mucinous
Gross features		
Solitary or multifocal	Usually solitary	Usually multifocal
Pneumonic pattern	Not seen	Occasionally seen
Histologic features		
Multifocality	Occasional	Frequent
Cell morphology	Cuboidal to columnar	Tall columnar
Micropapillary formation	Common	Common
Central scar	Occasional	Rare
Cytologic atypia	At least centrally	Uniform
Degree of atypia	Mild to severe	Mild
Desquamated cells	Often	Always
Ciliated cells	Incredibly rare	Never
Apical mucin	Not present	Present
Septal fibrosis	Always	Rare
Septal inflammation	Often	Infrequent
Immunohistochemical features		
CK7	+	+/–
CK20	–	Often +
TTF-1	Usually +	Usually –
SPA	+	Usually –
Ultrastructural features		
Clara cell	Common	Never
Type II pneumocyte	Occasional	Never
Mucin cell	Never	Always

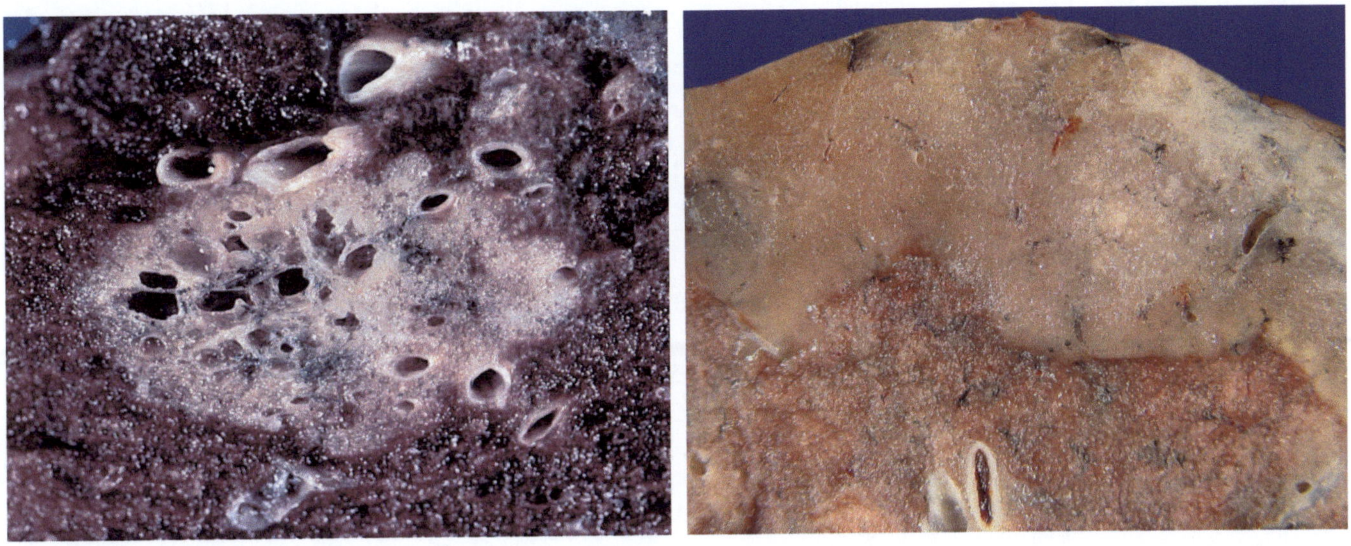

A B

FIGURE 35.42. Bronchioloalveolar carcinoma (BAC). **(A)** Both airways and air spaces are preserved in this nonmucinous BAC. A very small central scar and scattered anthracosis are appreciated. **(B)** Mucinous BAC often fills the lung with yellow gelatinous mucin. Underlying alveolar parenchyma is also intact.

fort" on the basis of its tan gray and glistening mucinous cut surface[745] (Fig. 35.42B). Parenchymal architecture may be distorted, but is not destroyed. Hemorrhage and necrosis are not seen in this type.

Nonmucinous BACs are usually well or moderately differentiated and feature uniform cuboidal to columnar epithelial cells with mild to moderate cytologic atypia without cilia proliferating along alveolar septa (Fig. 35.43A). Central areas feature cellular crowding, desquamated tumor cells in alveolar spaces, and oftentimes fibrosis (Fig. 35.43B). While cellular tufts can be seen, complex papillary structures indicate papillary carcinoma. The periphery of the tumor is poorly defined since tumor cell density, height, and cytologic atypia lessen at the edges and blend almost imperceptibly with benign or reactive pneumocytes (Fig. 35.43C). Individual tumor cells or clusters may float in alveolar spaces, and satellite nodules may be only a few millimeters in size. Nucleomegaly and prominent nucleoli are usually identified and nuclear pleomorphism can rarely be seen (Fig. 35.43D). Most tumor cells resemble Clara cells rather than type II pneumocytes, though the distinction is of no clinical import.[746] Clara cell differentiation features columnar cells with eosinophilic cytoplasm, apical granules, and sometimes apical nuclei, while type II pneumocyte-like cells are cuboidal with clear to foamy cytoplasm and eosinophilic or clear intranuclear pseudoinclusions.[728,759] These inclusions, however, are not specific for BAC. Mixed cell types are not infrequently observed, and mitotic activity is rarely brisk. Cytoplasmic mucin or glycogen may be seen in either cell type. Periodic acid-Schiff with diastase staining highlights both apical cytoplasmic granules and intranuclear inclusions. Involved alveolar septa may be slightly or significantly expanded with either fibrosis or lymphoplasmacytic infiltrates along with germinal centers. T-lymphocytes predominate.[760] Surrounding noninvolved lung may feature intraalveolar collections of histiocytes, sometimes pigmented, and scattered nonnecrotizing granulomas.

Central scars are a common finding in pulmonary adenocarcinomas and especially in tumors with BAC morphology (Fig. 35.44). In fact, three-dimensional analysis of blood vessels in BAC has shown continuous remodeling of alveolar capillaries rather than new vessel formation in central scars.[761] Tumors with angulated malignant glands embedded in fibroelastotic stroma may be entrapped or invasive foci (Fig. 35.44B,C). Whether a tumor is diagnosed as BAC or invasive adenocarcinoma, mixed subtype with a prominent BAC component, is quite challenging and requires that the entire tumor be examined histologically. Infiltrating single cells or irregular glands with stromal desmoplasia are required to diagnose invasion. While elastic tissue and type IV collagen immunohistochemical stains might highlight parenchymal destruction by tumor cells, interpretation is difficult.[762] Molecular studies may become an ancillary tool in the coming years.[763]

Mucinous BAC is a well-differentiated adenocarcinoma that features a sharp separation with nonneoplastic lung and minimal if any stromal fibrosis or inflammation (Table 35.15). Alveolar spaces fill with mucin but parenchymal destruction or fibrous demarcations are not

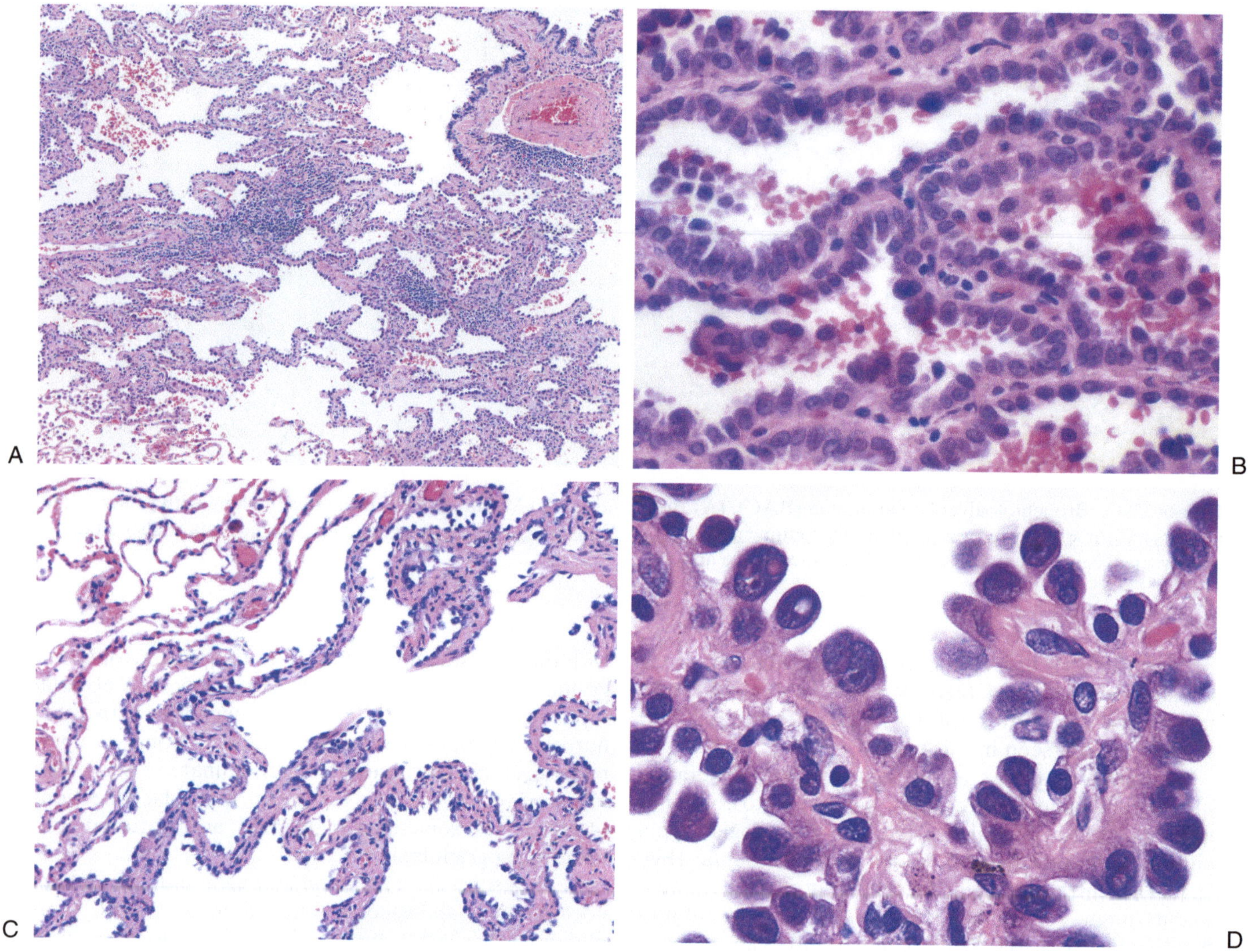

FIGURE 35.43. Bronchioloalveolar carcinoma, nonmucinous subtype. **(A)** The lepidic growth pattern differs from the destructive complex arborizing architecture seen in papillary adenocarcinomas. **(B)** Central zones are replete with malignant cells crowding alveolar septa. Air spaces may contain desquamated tumor cells or alveolar macrophages. This example features fairly well-differentiated tumor cells. **(C)** The periphery of a nonmucinous BAC is often less cellular with less cytologic atypia than the central portions of the tumor. This "zonation effect" can make frozen section diagnosis challenging. **(D)** Not all BACs are well or moderately differentiated. High-grade nuclear features may be encountered. Septal fibrosis is usually present, but oftentimes subtle. A brisk inflammatory response is not always seen.

seen (Fig. 35.45A). Tall uniform columnar cells without cilia line alveolar walls in a discontinuous fashion (Fig. 35.45B). Cells often resemble goblet cells with basal nuclei and ample clear, gray, or foamy cytoplasm (Fig. 35.45C). Vesicular chromatin and inconspicuous nucleoli are seen while significant atypia or mitotic activity is rare. Alveolar macrophages and occasional neutrophils float in air-space mucin. In comparison to the nonmucinous BAC, lymphoid infiltrates associated with this subtype are reportedly B lymphocytes.[760]

Bronchioloalveolar carcinoma with both nonmucinous and mucinous cells are rarely seen, while in some instances one cannot be certain of the cell type. The WHO classification features a "mixed nonmucinous and mucinous or indeterminate" designation for such tumors.

One cannot speak of a single lung adenocarcinoma immunohistochemical profile. While most adenocarcinomas express many epithelial markers, including various cyto-keratins, epithelial membrane antigen (EMA), carcinoembryonic antigen (CEA), CD15 (LeuM1), BER. EP4, and B72.3, staining fluctuates with tumor subtype and grade. Low molecular weight keratin and TTF-1 expression patterns differ for nonmucinous and mucinous lung tumors, while adenocarcinomas do not stain for CK5/6.[642]

Greater than 90% of nonmucinous carcinomas including virtually all nonmucinous BACs stain with CK7 while

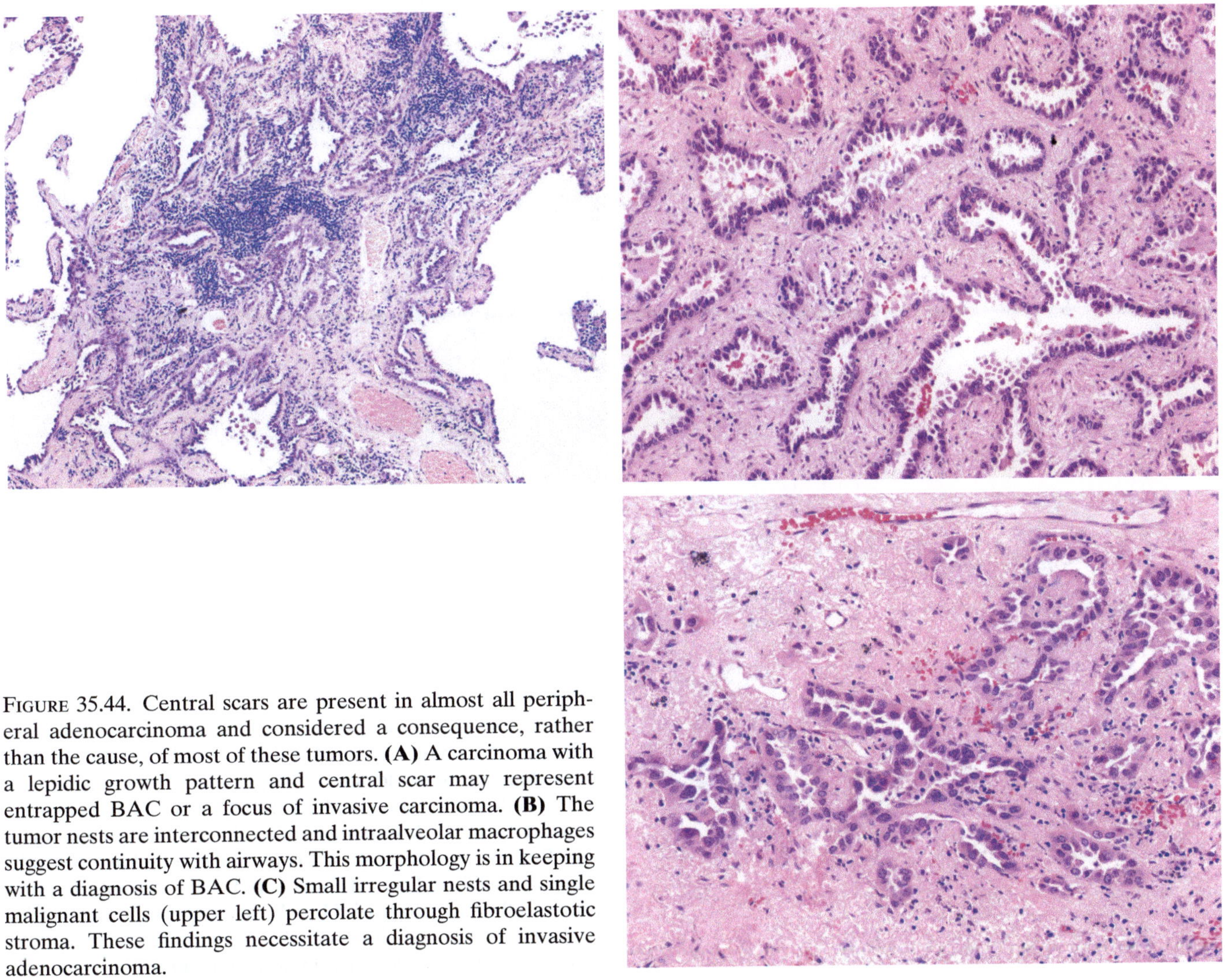

FIGURE 35.44. Central scars are present in almost all peripheral adenocarcinoma and considered a consequence, rather than the cause, of most of these tumors. **(A)** A carcinoma with a lepidic growth pattern and central scar may represent entrapped BAC or a focus of invasive carcinoma. **(B)** The tumor nests are interconnected and intraalveolar macrophages suggest continuity with airways. This morphology is in keeping with a diagnosis of BAC. **(C)** Small irregular nests and single malignant cells (upper left) percolate through fibroelastotic stroma. These findings necessitate a diagnosis of invasive adenocarcinoma.

only rare cases express CK20.[637,764–767] Approximately 75% of these tumors demonstrate nuclear staining for TTF-1. This marker is superior to surfactant proteins A and B, which stain less than 50% of tumors.[759,768,769] Thus, approximately 70% of nonmucinous adenocarcinomas demonstrate a CK7$^+$/CK20$^-$/TTF-1$^+$ profile.

Mucinous adenocarcinomas including almost all mucinous BACs stain with CK7, while tumors with goblet cell morphology including BAC express CK20 in up to 90% of cases. Thyroid transcription factor-1 marks less than 25% of these tumors.[764,770,771] Additional comments regarding staining profiles of mucinous lung tumors are discussed below (Table 35.16).

Not unlike SCC, up to 30% of adenocarcinomas without any suggestion of neuroendocrine morphology stain with chromogranin, synaptophysin, or CD56.[637,643,645] A similar percentage, especially poorly differentiated adenocarcinomas, also stain with trophoblastic cell markers hCG or hPL.[646,648] Lastly, CDX2, a reliable marker of colorectal adenocarcinoma, rarely stains lung adenocarcinomas including mucinous BAC.[772–775] A CDX2$^+$/TTF-1$^+$ profile, however, is most unlikely.[773]

Ultrastructurally, adenocarcinomas of the lung demonstrate the same morphologic heterogeneity appreciated with the light microscope, histochemical, and immunohistochemical studies.[650,776] Findings parallel the degree of differentiation. However, all adenocarcinomas feature lumina bounded by tight junctions surfaced with usually short surface microvilli.[649,777] Abundant endoplasmic reticulum and Golgi complexes, and cytoplasmic secretory granules are usually found. The microvilli with glycocalyx project into acinar spaces, while desmosomes are not as plentiful as in SCC. Free intracytoplasmic mucin or glycogen can be seen.[778]

Most adenocarcinomas demonstrate Clara cell differentiation, but type II pneumocyte or mucinous features are not uncommon.[779,780] Clara cell differentiation shows apical bulbous cytoplasm filled with abundant smooth and rough endoplasmic reticulum and electron-dense spherical granules (Fig. 35.46A). Ultrastructurally most

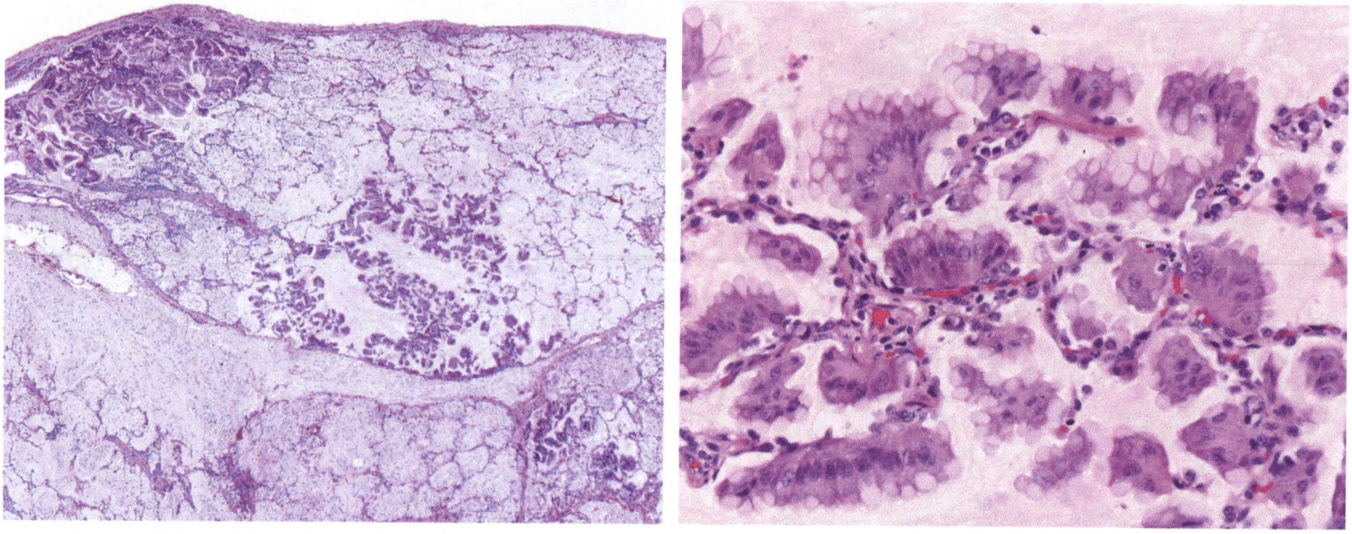

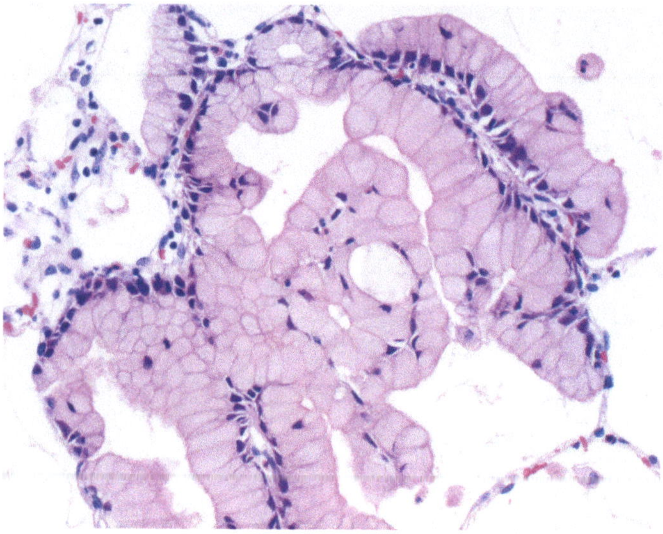

FIGURE 35.45. Bronchioloalveolar carcinoma, mucinous subtype. **(A)** These carcinomas are usually larger but less cellular than the nonmucinous subtype. Scattered collections of tumor cells line alveolar septa. Underlying lung parenchyma is intact. **(B)** Small clusters of tumor cells displace pneumocytes and float free in air spaces. Eosinophilic cells have centrally located nuclei and apical mucin. **(C)** This example features goblet cell morphology with basally located compressed nuclei. Unlike the nonmucinous BAC, alveolar septal fibrosis and lymphocytic infiltrates are not commonly encountered.

TABLE 35.16. Histologic and immunohistochemical features of mucinous/intestinal-type lung adenocarcinomas

	Mucinous BAC	Mucinous "colloid" adenocarcinoma	Mucinous cystadenocarcinoma	Signet ring adenocarcinoma	Intestinal-type adenocarcinoma
Histology	Lepidic	Goblet cell in pools of mucin No capsule	Mucinous cyst lined with goblet cells	Sheets, nests of signet ring cells	Cribriform with "dirty necrosis" stratified columnar cells
Immunohistochemistry					
CK7	Usually –	+/–	+	+	+
CK20	+	+	?	–	–
TTF-1	Usually –	+/–	?	+	+
CDX2	–	+	?	–	–
MUC1	?	?	?	+	+
MUC2	–	+	?	–	–
MUC5AC	+	–	?	+	+/–
SP-A	Usually –	+/–	?	–	?

BAC, bronchioloalveolar carcinoma.
?, uncertain or unknown.
Source: Data from Castro,[843] Gao,[836] Goldstein,[764] Kish,[846] Merchant,[847] Rossi,[829] Shah,[770] and Yousem.[831]

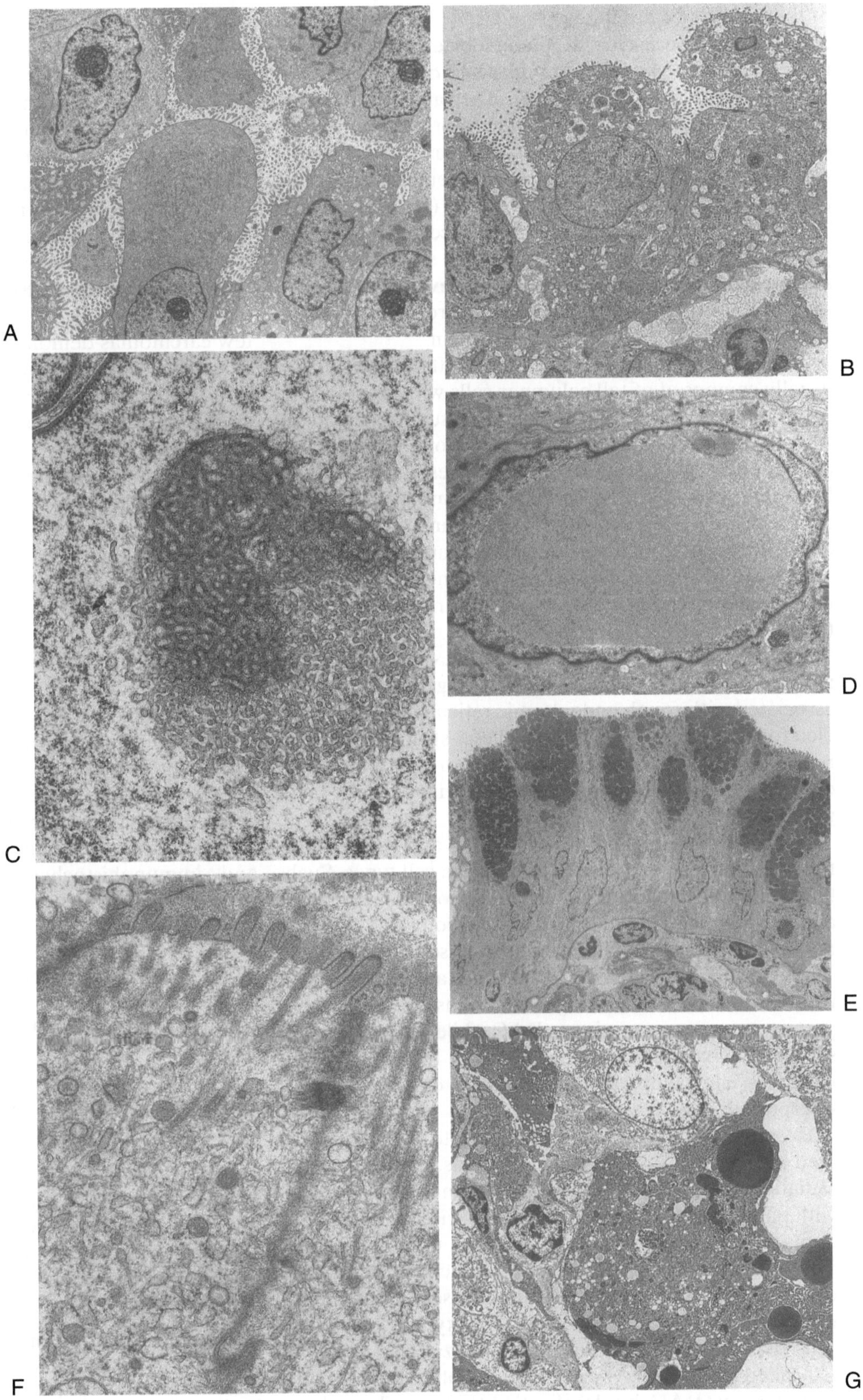

FIGURE 35.46. Adenocarcinoma, ultrastructural features. **(A)** Nonmucinous tumor cells feature short surface microvilli. Prominent apical cytoplasmic endoplasmic reticulum is consistent with Clara cell differentiation. **(B)** Cytoplasmic lamellar granules suggest type II pneumocyte differentiation. **(C)** Intranuclear inclusions stain for surfactant proteins. A tubular configuration can be seen. **(D)** Intranuclear inclusions may be amorphous and can displace much of the nuclear chromatin. (Courtesy of Drs. H. Shimazaki and S. Aida, National Defense Medical Hospital, Saitama, Japan.) **(E)** Mucinous adenocarcinomas including BAC contain abundant cytoplasmic mucous vacuoles. Nuclei are basally located. **(F)** The apical portion of a mucinous adenocarcinoma cell has short uniform microvilli covered by fuzzy glycocalyx and associated with glycocalyceal bodies. Apical cytoplasmic filaments are also numerous. **(G)** Eosinophilic bodies (see Fig. 35.36B) occur in degenerating cells and have the same electron density as red blood cells.

of these densities are finely granular.[781] Tumor cells with complete or focal type II pneumocyte differentiation have cytoplasmic lamellar granules and occasional intranuclear inclusions (Fig. 35.46B). The lamellar granules are electron dense with osmiophilic whorls that resemble surfactant granules.[746] The intranuclear inclusions are usually bounded to the inner nuclear membrane and can be either tubular or amorphous[728,730,782] (Fig. 35.46C,D). These structures are not restricted to cells with type II pneumocyte differentiation and are not specific for lung adenocarcinomas.[728,783] They are, however, most often identified in nonmucinous BAC and are immunohistochemically positive for surfactant protein.[728]

Adenocarcinomas with mucinous differentiation are usually composed of tall columnar cells with cytoplasmic mucous vacuoles. The vacuoles are usually located in apical cytoplasm and have a wide range of ultrastructural appearances suggesting to some investigators either bronchial goblet cell or bronchial gland cell origin[779] (Fig. 35.46E). Glycocalyceal bodies and microvillous dense-core rootlets with extensions into apical cytoplasm, often seen in colonic and ovarian mucinous tumors, are not uncommon in mucinous lung adenocarcinomas.[650,746,784] (Fig. 35.46F).

Eosinophilic intracytoplasmic globules in adenocarcinomas are usually encountered in degenerating cells, associated with rough endoplasmic reticulum and appear electron dense (Fig. 35.46G). These structures might represent accumulated secretory glycoprotein in injured or degenerating tumor cells or variant Clara cell granules.[729,785]

Evidence of squamous differentiation and neurosecretory granules may be found in any of the cell types. Such findings should not alter a light microscopic diagnosis of adenocarcinoma since electron microscopy findings are not included in the WHO classification scheme.

The differential diagnosis of lung adenocarcinoma includes reactive and malignant lesions. Some lesions pertain more to nonmucinous BAC while others must be separated from invasive carcinomas. In virtually all instances, clinical history is necessary to ensure a correct interpretation.

Reactive bronchiolar and pneumocyte atypia associated with acute and organizing infections, chemotherapy, radiation therapy, and chronic inflammatory processes with parenchymal fibrosis can mimic various adenocarcinoma subtypes. These reactive changes usually lack the cytologic monotony of carcinoma. Parenchymal scars and organizing pneumonia usually feature squamous metaplasia and ciliated cells admixed with atypical glandular cells. Bronchiolar scars and bronchiolization of alveoli (so-called lambertosis) bear architectural resemblance to nonmucinous BAC, but localization to the peribronchiolar compartment and obvious cilia differentiate reactive from malignant. Apical caps and honeycomb lung contain metaplastic epithelium and cytologic atypia but papillary or invasive growth and significant cytoplasmic mucin indicate malignancy. Adenocarcinoma rarely arises in emphysematous bullae but one should not confuse hyperplastic epithelium with BAC. Therapy effect is usually diffuse rather than tumoral, and cytomegaly, nuclear pleomorphism, and prominent nucleoli are associated with other inflammatory changes such as hyaline membranes or organizing pneumonia.[786,787] However, pulmonary nodules in cancer patients treated with chemotherapy can be histologically inseparable from BAC.[788] p63 may be a useful immunohistochemical tool, especially in small biopsies, since reactive bronchioloalveolar processes but few carcinomas demonstrate positive staining.[789]

Atypical adenomatous hyperplasia, a putative precursor of adenocarcinoma, has overlapping features with nonmucinous BAC (Table 35.17) (see Chapter 34). While both are proliferative pneumocyte lesions with lepidic growth, carcinomas generally measure >0.5 cm and feature more columnar morphology and cellular crowding, with micropapillary fronds and overlapping nuclei. Cytologic atypia is usually greater in BAC, which has coarser nuclear chromatin and prominent nucleoli. Atypical adenomatous hyperplasia rarely has more than one of these features.[790]

Small adenocarcinomas may be mistaken for benign tumors including sclerosing hemangioma and papillary adenoma. Despite vague resemblances to adenocarcinomas, these well-circumscribed tumors lack malignant cytologic features.

Differentiating malignant mesothelioma from adenocarcinoma is a clinicopathologic exercise in every case. Morphology may be indistinguishable, and both mucin and immunohistochemical stains are required (see

TABLE 35.17. Radiographic and morphologic features of nonmucinous bronchioloalveolar carcinoma and atypical adenomatous hyperplasia

	Nonmucinous bronchioloalveolar carcinoma	Atypical adenomatous hyperplasia
Radiographically detected	Almost always	Almost never
Size	Any size	Usually <5 mm
Location	Anywhere	Peribronchiolar
Borders	Irregular	Sharp
Growth pattern	Lepidic	Lepidic
Cellular crowding	Yes	No
Cell shape	Cuboidal to columnar	Cuboidal to low columnar
Cytoplasm	Abundant	Sparse
Nuclei	Uniform to pleomorphic	Uniform
Chromatin	Variable	Dense
Nucleoli	Present	Inconspicuous
Inclusions	Occasional	Occasional
Septal fibrosis	Usually present	Absent to minimal
Septal inflammation	Minimal to severe	Minimal

Chapter 43). The role of electron microscopy has diminished with the recent development of mesothelial cell immunohistochemical markers calretinin, CK5/6, and WT-1.

Differentiating a metastasis from a primary lung carcinoma relies heavily on clinical history and review of previous tumors, and is aided by immunohistochemistry. Metastatic adenocarcinomas can mimic lung primaries grossly and microscopically. However, endobronchial, peripheral, interstitial, or multifocal metastases with central cavitation and BAC-like growth usually lack morphologic heterogeneity common to lung adenocarcinomas and feature only a single microscopic pattern (see Chapter 44).

Since most nonmucinous and signet-ring cell lung adenocarcinomas have a $CK7^+/CK20^-/TTF\text{-}1^+$ immunophenotype, almost all sinonasal, pancreas, small intestinal, colorectal, renal, bladder, and prostatic primaries can be excluded. Additional markers including thyroglobulin, CDX2, and prostatic-specific antigen aid in identifying papillary and follicular thyroid, colorectal, and prostatic adenocarcinomas, respectively. Breast and nonmucinous endometrial and ovarian carcinomas may require additional stains, especially in instances where the carcinoma is poorly differentiated and TTF-1 negative. Caution should be exercised with estrogen receptor antibodies since expression is not predictable and particular clones, including 6F11, reportedly stain the majority of lung adenocarcinomas.[791–794]

Distinguishing a mucinous lung primary from a metastatic carcinoma arising in the bladder, pancreaticobiliary tract, colon, or ovary is rarely possible on morphologic grounds alone, especially on biopsy specimens. Lepidic growth is rarely seen with these metastases. Immunohistochemical stains may be helpful. Although mucinous lung tumors including mucinous BAC are often $CK20^+$ and $TTF\text{-}1^-$, most retain CK7 immunoreactivity. This $CK7^+/CK20^+$ profile is shared by the majority of pancreatic and ovarian mucinous carcinomas but not seen in many colorectal primaries. In addition, CDX2 is usually negative in common mucinous lung carcinomas (see "Mucinous 'Colloid' Adenocarcinoma" under Adenocarcinoma Variants, below).

As with SCC, surgery offers the only possibility of cure for patients with lung adenocarcinoma, while locally advanced tumor may be treated with neoadjuvant therapy prior to surgical resection. Individuals with multiple lung adenocarcinomas may be surgical candidates given reported 3- and 5-year survival rates of over 60%.[597,598,795] Adjuvant chemotherapy for resectable invasive adenocarcinomas also appears to prolong survival.[663–667] Radiation therapy is reserved for poor surgical candidates and is a palliative treatment.

Performance status and stage are the strongest indicators of outcome. Of note, invasive adenocarcinomas measuring ≤2.0cm also have a better 5-year survival rate than those measuring between 2.1 and 3.0cm.[510,511,764] Tumor morphology also appears to play a role, at least in small tumors. Three centimeter and smaller nonmucinous BAC have a 5-year survival rate of almost 100%.[733,735,796–802] However, difficulties in making a reproducible diagnosis of nonmucinous BAC have resulted in studies evaluating morphologic features seen in adenocarcinomas with prominent if not complete BAC morphology.[803] Studies investigating the size and quality of the central scar as well as the location and size of invasive foci within these tumors suggest that 3.0 and smaller adenocarcinomas with scars less than 0.5cm and invasion along the edge of the scar measuring less than 0.5cm have survival rates approaching that of the pure nonmucinous BAC.[733,796,797,804] The therapeutic ramifications of these findings are great. Small peripheral carcinomas with radiographic findings suggestive of nonmucinous BAC, that is, greater than 50% GGO, may be amenable to limited resection.[758,795,802,805,806] However, not all GGOs are BAC.[716]

The morphologic pattern may also indicate response to particular therapies. Recent data suggest that in addition to age, gender, and smoking history, nonmucinous BAC, mixed adenocarcinomas with a BAC component, and papillary adenocarcinomas are more likely to respond to EGFR-TKI than other lung adenocarcinomas.[743,807,808] While data are inconsistent and conflicting, neuroendocrine differentiation in typical adenocarcinomas probably does not independently influence response to chemotherapy or survival.[645,809–811]

Aside from nonmucinous BAC, pulmonary adenocarcinoma is as deadly as SCC, with a 16% 5-year survival rate.[662]

Adenocarcinoma Variants

In addition to the five common patterns, five distinctive yet rare histologic variants are included in the WHO classification, while several other histologic patterns are not included (Table 35.13). These morphologies may comprise entire tumors or may be combined with but not limited to the adenocarcinoma subtypes.

Fetal adenocarcinoma is composed of neoplastic glands resembling fetal lung tubules seen between 10 and 16 weeks' gestation. This tumor exemplifies the necessity of detailed morphologic studies in a molecular age. Light microscopic refinements in the classification of so-called blastomatous lung tumors have led to the recognition of both low- and high-grade variants of fetal adenocarcinoma and suggest a continuum with pulmonary blastoma[812,813] (Table 35.18)(see Chapter 37). This recent development necessitated a change in nomenclature from well-differentiated fetal adenocarcinoma in the 1999 classification to simply fetal adenocarcinoma in the 2004 scheme. Although *fetal adenocarcinoma* is the WHO-preferred term, the carcinoma was originally

TABLE 35.18. Clinical and pathologic features of pulmonary fetal adenocarcinomas

	Fetal adenocarcinomas	
	Low grade	High grade
Clinical		
Age (mean)	34 years	64 years
Gender	Male ≤ female	Male > female
Smoking	76%	85%
Stage at presentation	Usually early	Often advanced
>stage I	10%	37%
Prognosis	Good	Poor
Died of tumor (mean follow-up)	9.5% (70 months)	42% (24 months)
Histopathologic		
Arrangement of glands	Orderly	Disorganized
Necrosis	Spotty if present	Commonly broad
Nuclear size	Small	Large
Anisonucleosis	Mild	Obvious
Nuclear chromatin	Usually condensed	Dispersed
Nucleoli	Inconspicuous	Prominent
Morules	Common	Absent
Biotin-rich nucleus	Common	Uncommon
Stroma		
Amount	Slight to moderate	Abundant
Appearance	Loose fibromyxoid	Desmoplastic
Endocrine cells	Almost always	Common
AFP-positive cells	Occasional	Always
p53 protein overexpression	Uncommon	Common
β-catenin expression	Nuclear and cytoplasmic	Membranous

AFP, α-fetoprotein.
Source: Modified from Nakatani et al.,[813] with permission of Lippincott Williams & Wilkins.

named *pulmonary endodermal tumor resembling fetal lung*.[814] Rare cases of combined fetal adenocarcinoma with other lung cancers and with yolk sac tumor have been reported.[815]

Fetal adenocarcinomas are predominantly tumors of adults in the fourth decade of life and have not been reported in children under age 10.[813,816–819] As a group, an equal sex distribution is noted and 80% of patients are smokers. Individuals are often asymptomatic, and solitary peripheral tumors measure from 1.0 to 10 cm with a mean size of 4.5 cm.[813,818,819] An endobronchial location is rare.[818,820,821]

The carcinoma is unencapsulated white, tan, or brown, and fleshy with hemorrhage and cystic change. Histologically, the well-circumscribed mass is composed of branching tubules and scant intervening stroma (Fig. 35.47A). A cribriform pattern may be prominent (Fig. 35.47B). The tubules are lined by pseudostratified nonciliated columnar cells with frequent subnuclear or supranuclear cytoplasmic vacuoles. Cords and ribbons of cells with peripheral palisading and rosette-like structures are also seen (Fig. 35.47C). Nuclei are usually oval to round. Structures resembling squamous morules of endometrioid adenocarcinoma feature solid cell nests at the base of the glands with polygonal cells, eosinophilic finely granular cytoplasm, and occasional clear nuclei (Fig. 35.47D). The optically clear nuclei due to biotin accumulation are similar to those recognized in gestational endometrium and nonpulmonary neoplasms including pancreatoblastoma.[822–824] Mitoses are easily seen, and necrosis varies from spotty to extensive. The amount of stroma also varies from slight to moderate and is usually myxoid with spindle cells without hypercellularity, nuclear pleomorphism, or necrosis. Desmoplasia is not a stromal finding, and only scant lymphoplasmacytic infiltrates are noted. Tumor grading should be based on architectural and cytologic features alone (Table 35.18) (Fig. 35.48).

While clear cytoplasm is due to glycogen, intraluminal mucin may be seen though goblet cell morphology or cytoplasmic mucin is rare. The immunohistochemical profile may correspond to tumor grade[813,818] (Table 35.18). Tumor cells stain with cytokeratins, EMA, and CEA. Varying percentages of epithelial cells, mostly morular cells, react with antibodies directed against surfactant apoprotein, Clara cell antigen, and TTF-1.[819,825] Neuroendocrine cell differentiation is always seen in low-grade carcinomas and in approximately one third of high-grade lesions. Positive staining for chromogranin, synaptophysin, and Leu-7 are observed in a few glandular cells and in scattered morular cells. Specific amines and polypeptide hormones including calcitonin, serotonin, and somatostatin may also be identified in the morules. Interestingly, low-grade lesions feature nuclear and cytoplasmic ß-catenin staining, while high-grade tumors demonstrate a membranous pattern.[826] Similarly, AFP staining is more common in high-grade lesions. Vimentin and smooth muscle actin staining are localized to stromal cells.[818,819]

Ultrastructurally, neoplastic glands are surrounded by a distinct basal lamina and feature apical junctional complexes, occasional luminal microvilli, and glycogen-free spaces in sub- or supranuclear cytoplasm.[814,819] Morular cells are cohesive with cytoplasmic interdigitations and desmosomes, while primitive lumina with microvilli can be observed. The cytoplasm has well-developed rough endoplasmic reticulum, mitochondria, lipid droplets, electron-dense membrane-bound granules, and neuroendocrine-type granules. Optically clear nuclei represent many tightly packed 7- to 10-nm filaments. Osmiophilic lamellar bodies in the cytoplasm of cuboidal cells lining alveolus-like structures suggest type II pneumocyte differentiation. Peculiar round bodies with beaded borders are of uncertain function yet bear a resemblance to fibrous granules noted in primitive ciliated cells. Stromal cells show myofibroblastic differentiation.

One must differentiate fetal adenocarcinoma from clear cell adenocarcinoma, carcinoid tumors, as well as pulmonary blastoma and pleuropulmonary blastoma.

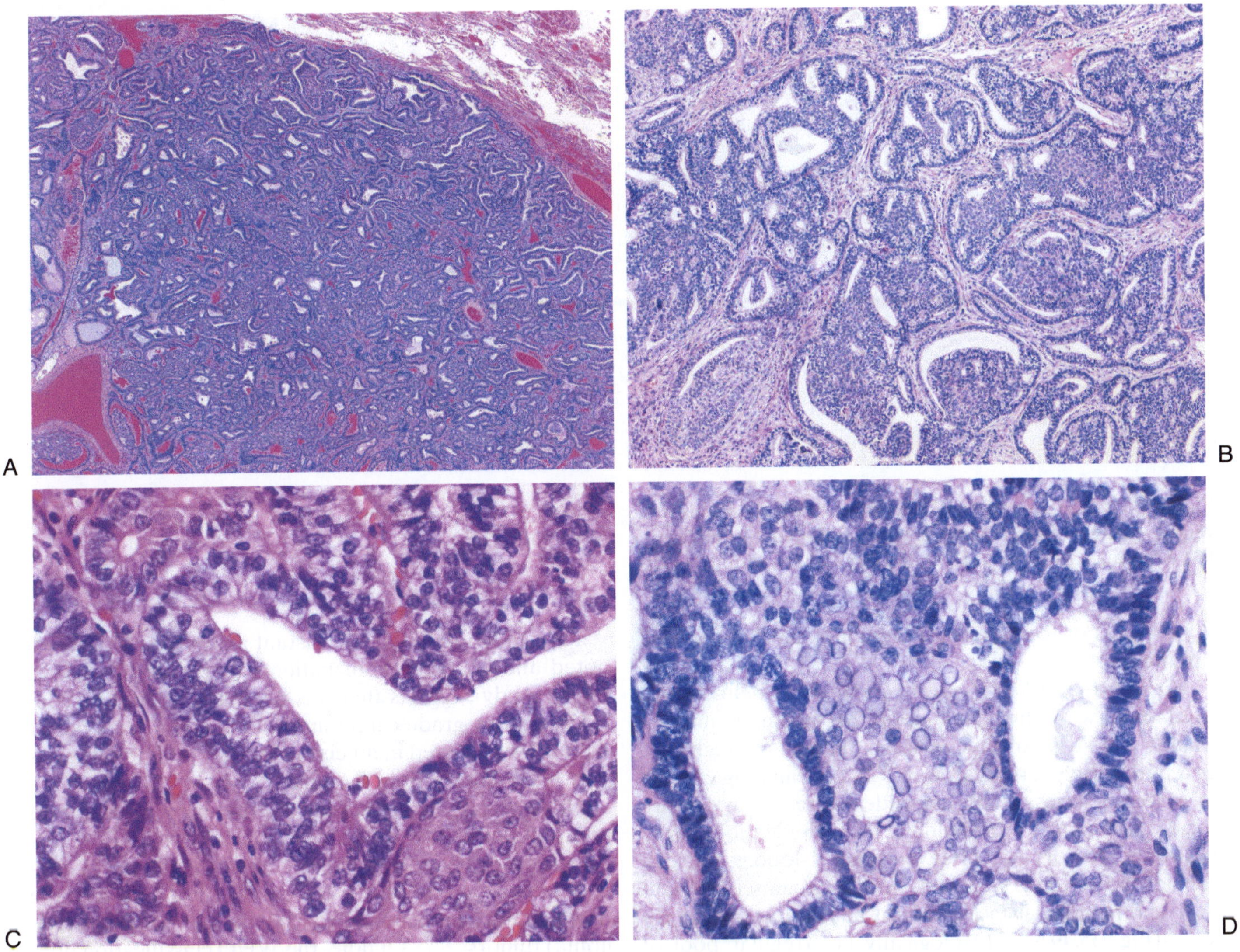

FIGURE 35.47. Fetal adenocarcinoma. **(A)** Low magnification demonstrates a well-circumscribed tumor with branching tubules and little intervening stroma. **(B)** A cribriform arrangement can be striking. **(C)** Columnar nonciliated cells with clear cytoplasm may form rosettes (upper left). Solid cell nests (i.e., morules) are usually composed of polygonal cells with eosinophilic cytoplasm. **(D)** Morular cells in low-grade lesions may have optically clear nuclei on account of biotin accumulation. This finding is not limited to this tumor type.

The endometrioid appearance with morules and lack of sarcomatous stroma distinguish the tumors. Carcinoid tumors also demonstrate diffuse neuroendocrine marker positivity.

Surgical excision is the primary treatment, while chemotherapy and/or radiation therapy may be of palliative benefit.[818,827] While clinicopathologic studies have shown a significantly better survival for patients with fetal adenocarcinoma as compared to adenocarcinomas in general, these data might reflect only clinical follow-up from patients with the low-grade subtype (Table 35.18). Thirty percent of low-grade tumors recur locally and are amenable to resection, while tumor-associated mortality is approximately 10%.[813] The high-grade tumors appear to be as aggressive as usual adenocarcinomas; however, it is difficult to generalize given the paucity of reported cases.

Three mucin-producing adenocarcinoma variants recognized by the WHO—mucinous ("colloid") adenocarcinoma, mucinous cystadenocarcinoma, and signet ring adenocarcinoma—are morphologically similar to nonpulmonary mucinous carcinomas including gastrointestinal, pancreatic, ovarian, and breast primaries (Table 35.16). While minimally invasive diagnostic procedures may yield mucin or clusters of goblet cells, surgical excision and complete histologic sampling are required for diagnosis. Diagnostic difficulties may arise when confronted with one of these tumors in a patient with

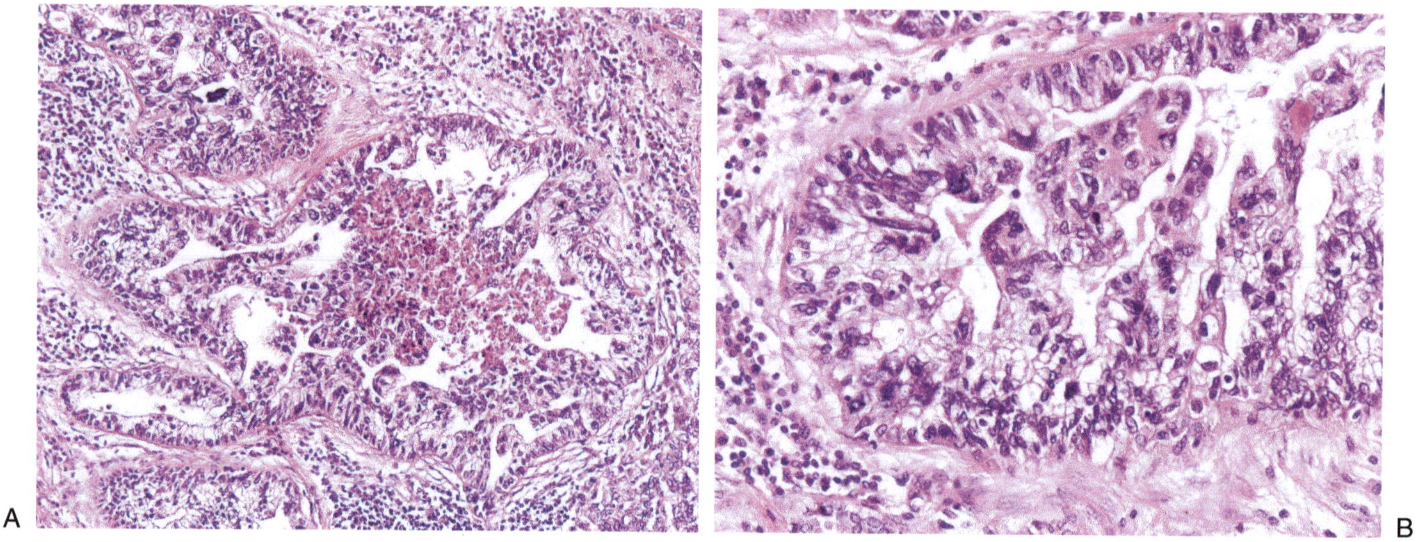

FIGURE 35.48. High-grade fetal adenocarcinoma. **(A)** This rare variant features architectural disorder and abundant necrosis. **(B)** Anisonucleosis is prominent and morules are absent. (Courtesy of Dr. W. Travis, Memorial Sloan-Kettering Cancer Center, New York, NY.)

a previous or concurrent nonpulmonary "mucinous" carcinoma.

Mucinous ("colloid") adenocarcinoma is defined as a carcinoma with dissecting pools of mucin containing islands and strips of mucinous epithelium. Though rare as a pure subtype, representing 0.24% of all lung cancers in a recent series, many lung adenocarcinomas feature focal mucinous morphology.[828,829] Epidemiologically indistinct, tumors are often peripheral lesions but can replace entire lobes with soft, poorly circumscribed tan-gray and mucoid surfaces without hemorrhage or necrosis[830] (Fig. 35.49A). Histologically an irregular pool of paucicellular mucin fills, distorts, and destroys pulmonary air spaces with minimal lymphoplasmacytic inflammation. Histiocytes and foreign body–type giant cells comprise the majority of cells and especially at low magnification neoplastic cells may be inapparent. However, small clusters of mucinous cuboidal epithelium float in the mucin, and mucinous columnar cells focally line scattered fibrotic alveoli (Fig. 35.49B). The epithelium may be extremely well differentiated but usually features at least focal crowding with nucleomegaly and hyperchromasia (Fig. 35.49C). A fibrous capsule is not present and mitoses are rare.

The neoplastic goblet cells express enteric markers CDX2 and MUC2 along with CK20 with only focal and often weak CK7 and TTF-1 expression[771,829,831,832] (Table 35.16). Thus, clinical correlation is required to diagnose this tumor as a lung primary. The differential diagnosis also includes the other mucinous lung tumors discussed below and mucinous BAC. Mucinous BAC features an overabundance of neoplastic cells lining alveolar walls and does not stain for CDX2 or MUC2.[829,831]

Though lymph node and distant metastases have been noted and almost half of patients die of the disease, a recent study suggests that this neoplasm should be considered a low-grade carcinoma with survival rates better than those reported in mucinous BAC.[828,829] Surgical excision is the appropriate therapy.

Mucinous cystadenocarcinoma belongs to the rare group of pulmonary mucinous cystic neoplasms. The histologic spectrum encompasses benign (mucinous cystadenoma), borderline (mucinous cystic tumor of borderline malignancy), and malignant (mucinous cystadenocarcinoma) tumors.[833–840] Of note, the WHO classification does not recognize the borderline category.[617]

These lesions have been reported in asymptomatic adult smokers and present as round well-demarcated masses without calcifications. Tumors can be as large as 15 cm and are unilocular glistening gray mucus-filled cysts without mural nodules. Communications with bronchi are not seen. Tumors are well circumscribed with a partial fibrous capsule lacking complex septations (Fig. 35.50A). Microscopic mucin dissection into adjacent lung tissue is frequently observed. The cyst is filled with mucus and the fibrous tissue wall or peripheral alveolar walls are lined by a discontinuous layer of low cuboidal to tall columnar cells with considerable cytoplasmic mucin. Cells may also float in mucin. The cyst wall may contain lymphoplasmacytic infiltrates, and giant cell reaction to mucin is common. Giant cells can also line the capsule wall.

Cystadenomas feature uniform basally located round or flattened nuclei with inconspicuous nucleoli and little or no cellular crowding, while mucinous cystadenocarcinomas show greater cellularity, nuclear stratification

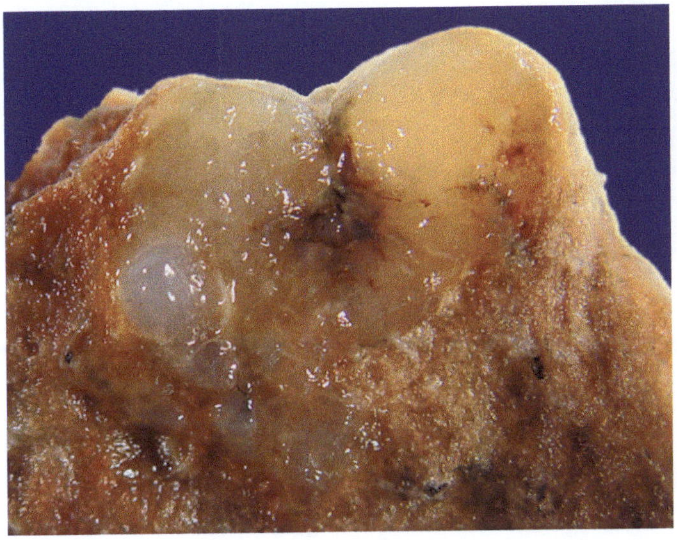

A

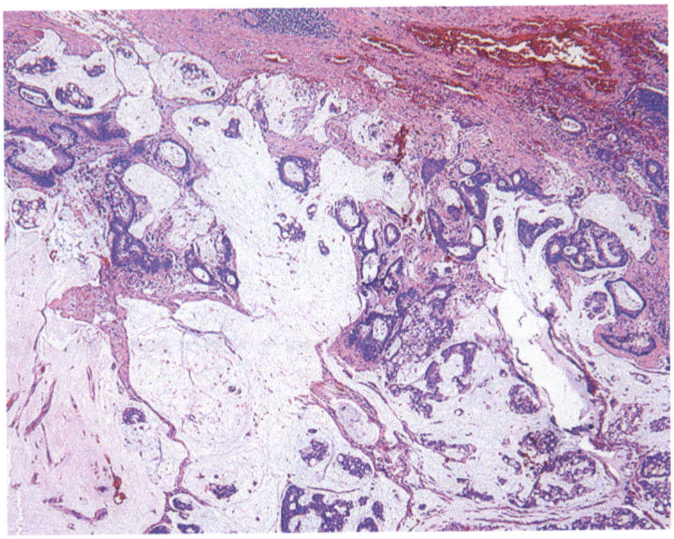

B

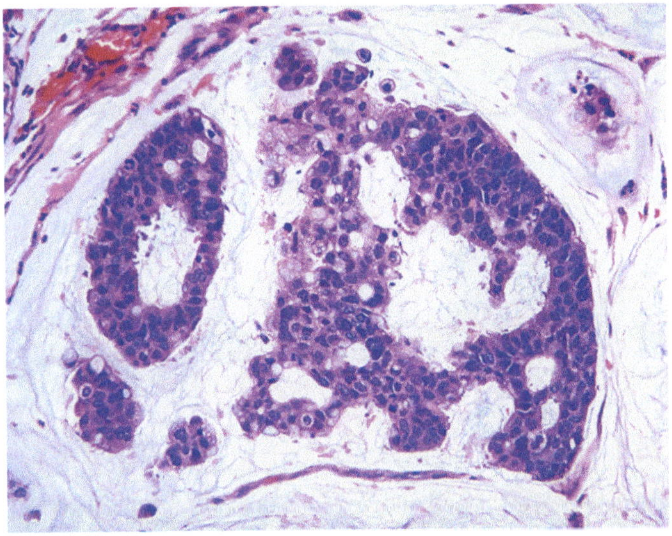

C

FIGURE 35.49. Mucinous ("colloid") adenocarcinoma. **(A)** This peripheral solitary mass is unencapsulated. **(B)** Malignant glands line and float within mucin-rich air spaces, as well as infiltrate stroma. **(C)** Cribriform arrangements of tumor cells are overtly malignant with nucleomegaly and nuclear hyperchromasia. This carcinoma may be histologically, immunohistochemically and ultrastructurally indistinguishable from a colorectal metastasis (see Fig. 35.46F).

including cribriforming, and cytologic atypia including nuclear envelope irregularities, hyperchromasia, prominent nucleoli, and not infrequent mitoses (Fig. 35.50B,D). Signet ring cells are not seen in this pure subtype. Malignant cytology may be only focal, while necrosis is absent. Microscopic invasion of surrounding lung removes the carcinoma from this category and necessitates a diagnosis of adenocarcinoma, mixed subtype. If atypical cytologic or architectural features not reaching the level of carcinoma are observed, then a designation of mucinous cystic tumor of borderline malignancy is appropriate[834,836,838,841,842] (Fig. 35.50C). However, such tumors are exceedingly rare and complete tumor sampling almost always uncovers at least focal adenocarcinoma.

The mucinous epithelium in all these lesions is cytokeratin and CK7 positive, and CEA, EMA, CK20, and TTF-1 indeterminate.[833,834,836,838,842] Tumors staining patterns with antibodies such MUC2, MUC5AC, and CDX2 are not known.

Mucinous cystadenocarcinoma should be differentiated from metastatic ovarian, breast, pancreatic, and gastrointestinal carcinomas. Helpful features include the absence of necrosis in this lung carcinoma and staining with CK7; however, clinical history and review of other tumor resections are required.

Mucinous cystic neoplasms require formal anatomic lobectomies since wedge resections with intraoperative frozen sections can be inconclusive regarding the presence of malignancy, and recurrences of both mucinous cystadenomas and carcinomas have been reported.[835,840] Lymph node metastases, or death from either mucinous cystadenocarcinomas or bona fide borderline tumors have not been reported.[838,839] Lesions with even a single microscopic focus of typical invasive adenocarcinoma behave as invasive adenocarcinomas.[836]

Signet-ring adenocarcinoma is the most aggressive mucin-producing lung tumor. Although rarely seen as a pure subtype, up to 2% of surgically resected primary

A B C D

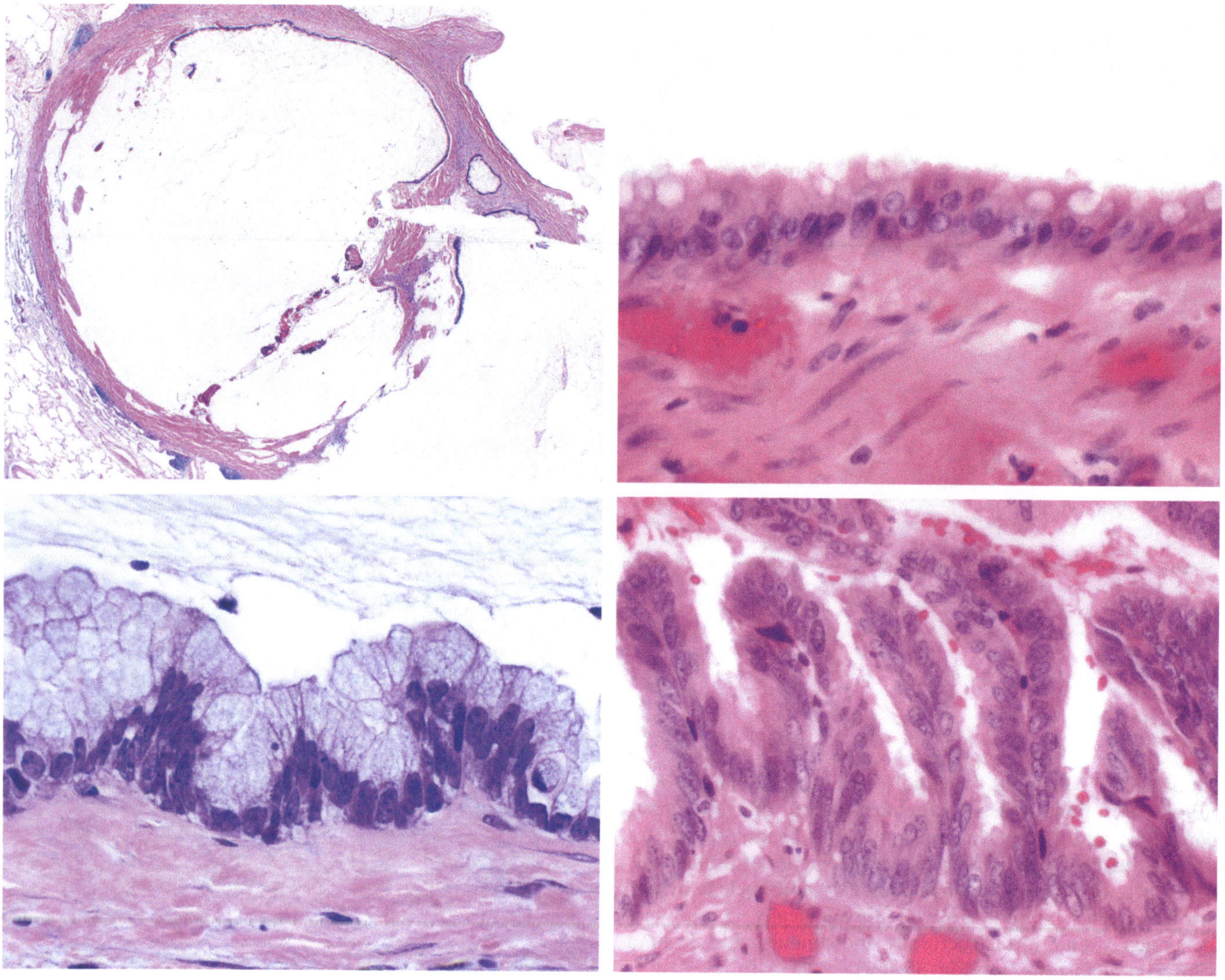

FIGURE 35.50. Mucinous cystic neoplasms. **(A)** Whether an adenoma, so-called borderline tumor, or carcinoma, these unilocular mucin-filled lesions are partially lined with neoplastic epithelium. **(B)** Basally located uniform cells are not crowded and the cuboidal nuclei are cytologically bland. This morphology is compatible with a diagnosis of cystadenoma. **(C)** Mucinous epithelium may be hyperchromatic and appear pseudostratified; however, the epithelium is not proliferative enough and the cytology does not reach the level of carcinoma. A designation of borderline malignancy is appropriate. **(D)** Papillary fronds with pseudostratification and malignant nuclear features are diagnostic of carcinoma. (Courtesy of Dr. A. Patchefsky, Fox Chase Cancer Center, Fox Chase, PA.)

lung adeno- or adenosquamous carcinomas feature a signet-ring cell component[693] (Fig. 35.51A). The average age of patients with tumors containing a predominant signet-ring cell pattern is 54 years, almost 10 years younger than the average age of lung cancer patients.[693,843,844] Most cases are peripheral lesions, but endobronchial and pseudomesotheliomatous presentations have also been reported.[693,724] Lung cancers with focal signet-ring morphology are poorly differentiated.

Unlike the common adenocarcinoma subtypes, this variant is defined according to tumor cytology. Medium-sized cells with distinct cell borders feature abundant clear to basophilic cytoplasm with peripherally displaced crescentic hyperchromatic nuclei. Tumor cells form destructive acini or sheets, or fill alveolar spaces (Fig. 35.51B). Cellular atypia, mitoses, necrosis, desmoplasia, and inflammatory response may be seen. Histochemical stains (PAS diastase, mucicarmine, and Alcian blue at pH 2.7) indicate the presence of both neutral and acid mucins.[845,846]

Immunohistochemical studies demonstrate tumor cell positivity for cytokeratin, CEA, MUC1, and MUC5AC, while indicating a $CK7^{+}/CK20^{-}$ phenotype in almost 95% of cases. Thyroid transcription factor-1 stains over

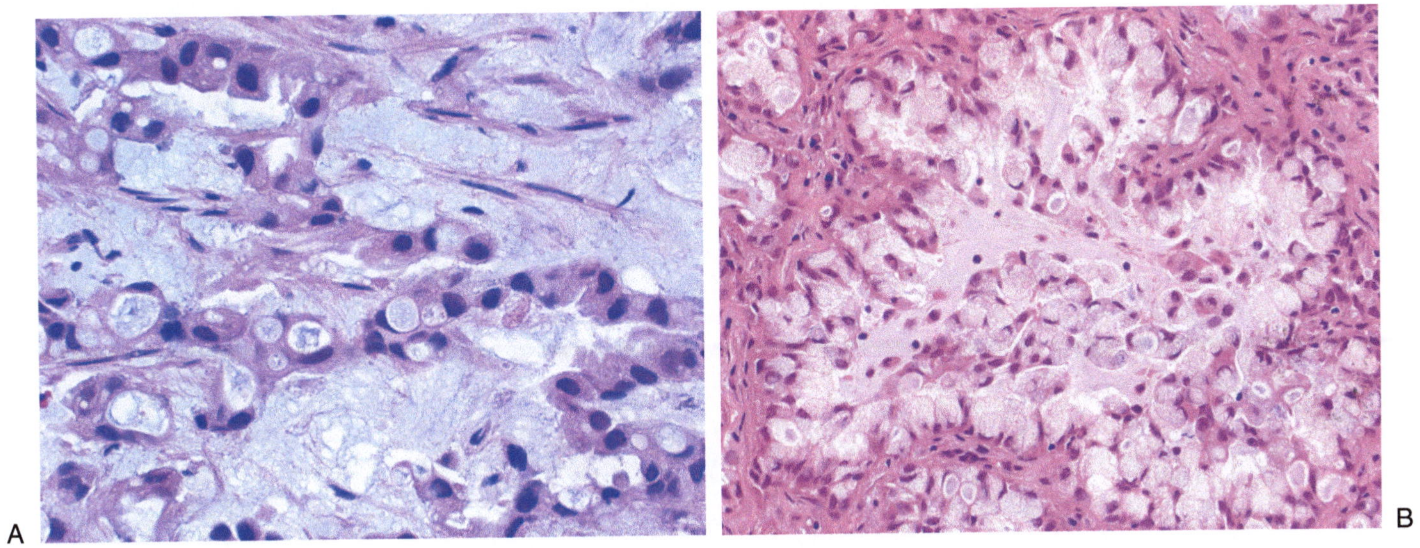

FIGURE 35.51. Signet-ring cell adenocarcinoma. **(A)** Signet-ring cell morphology is commonly identified in mixed adenocarcinomas. Cytoplasmic mucin displaces nuclei to cell edges. **(B)** The pure subtype may have an acinar growth pattern. Extracellular mucin is also apparent.

80% of tumors.[843,845–847] Neuroendocrine differentiation has been reported in two cases, and EBV has been documented in a single case.[334,848] Ultrastructurally, tumor cells contain abundant cytoplasmic mucin granules similar to those observed in goblet cells.[849]

Immunohistochemical stains discriminate this lung primary from breast, stomach, and colon metastases. Mucoepidermoid and acinic cell carcinomas are also differential considerations. Mucocytes in a mucoepidermoid carcinoma lack cytologic atypia, while acinic cell carcinomas are mucicarmine negative.[850]

A recent clinicopathologic analysis suggests that tumors composed of at least 50% signet-ring cells have higher frequency of lymph node metastases and poorer 5-year survival rate than tumors with only a minor signet-ring cell component.[844] This latter category has a typical adenocarcinoma prognosis.

Clear cell adenocarcinoma is a WHO-recognized subtype with no more than 20 reported cases in the world literature.[686,718,851,852] However, almost a third of adenocarcinomas feature focal clear cell change.[686] This rare tumor may be endobronchial or peripheral, and tumor cells form sheets with at least focal tubule formation[718] (Fig. 35.52A). Papillae may also be seen.[853] Gland formation is required for diagnosis. Sheets of polygonal cells with clear to eosinophilic cytoplasm have irregular nuclei and prominent nucleoli (Fig. 35.52B). The PAS-positive, diastase-sensitive, histochemical profile indicates cytoplasmic glycogen. Histochemical evidence of cytoplasmic mucin may be seen but is not required for diagnosis.[851] A $CK7^+/CK20^-/TTF\text{-}1^+$ immunohistochemical profile was reported in a single case.[853] Differentiating clear cell adenocarcinoma from a renal metastasis relies on clinical information, identifying a heterogeneous growth pattern along with intracytoplasmic mucin, and immunohistochemical markers specific for renal cell carcinoma.[854] The absence of morules excludes the possibility of a fetal adenocarcinoma. This poorly differentiated tumor does not have a different clinical course from other nonmucinous invasive adenocarcinomas.

Additional unusual patterns of lung adenocarcinoma may be seen in pure forms or in combination with the more common WHO recognized subtypes.

Adenocarcinomas with massive inflammatory infiltrates might be mistaken for LELC[855,856] (Fig. 35.53A) (see discussion of "lymphoepithelioma-like carcinoma" under Large Cell Carcinoma Variants, below). This morphologic pattern has been reported in older Asian individuals, mostly men, and the histology may correlate with a better outcome than predicted by stage. $CD8^+$ and $CD4^+$ T lymphocytes infiltrate tumor nests, while polyclonal B lymphocytes form follicles around the edges of the acinar and solid nonmucinous neoplastic cells[855,856] (Fig. 35.53B). Lymph node metastases feature identical morphology. While similar to LELC, this carcinoma is first and foremost an adenocarcinoma rather than a LCC. Epstein-Barr virus infection was not present in the nine studied cases.[855]

Nonmucinous pulmonary adenocarcinomas may resemble colorectal, small intestinal adenocarcinoma or high-grade sinonasal adenocarcinoma of the intestinal type.[831,857,858] Typical cribriform "gland in gland" patterns and lumina filled with necrotic debris are composed of stratified columnar cells with hyperchromatic nuclei and

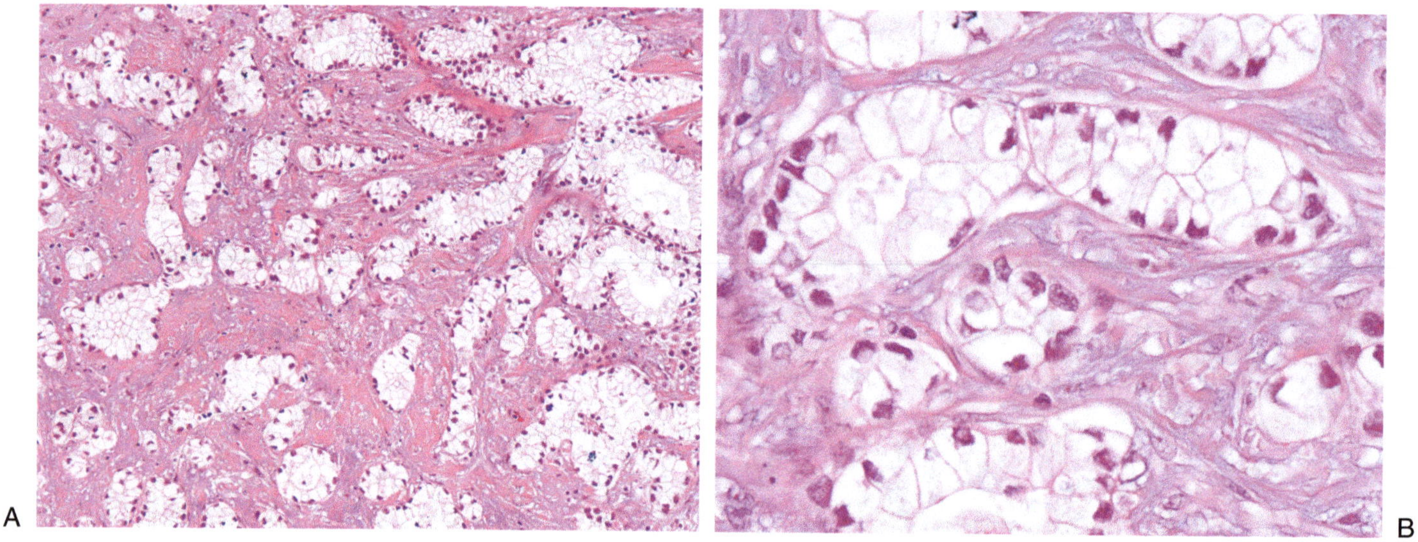

Figure 35.52. Clear cell adenocarcinoma. **(A)** This rare adenocarcinoma subtype features tubules and glands composed exclusively of clear tumor cells. **(B)** Irregularly shaped nuclei are less compressed by cytoplasmic glycogen than one finds with signet-ring cell adenocarcinomas.

apical eosinophilic cytoplasm (Fig. 35.54). Mitoses are frequent, and occasional goblet or Paneth cell differentiation can be observed. These carcinomas express CK7 and TTF-1 but not CK20 or CDX2.[775,831] Immunoreactivity for MUC1 but not MUC2 staining also distinguish these lung carcinomas from their enteric counterparts[831] (Table 35.16). This variant has no particular clinical relevance.

Hepatoid adenocarcinoma of the lung has been reported only in men, while AFP-producing tumors are not as rare or gender limited.[647,859,860] Hepatoid adenocarcinomas average 9.0 cm in size and usually feature papillary, trabecular, or sheet-like proliferation of cuboidal cells with eosinophilic cytoplasm and hyaline globules[861–863] (Fig. 35.55A). Centrally located round nuclei have vesicular chromatin and prominent nucleoli (Fig. 35.55B). These cells react with Hepar-1, AFP, polyclonal CEA in a canalicular pattern, and surfactant antibodies, while TTF-1 demonstrates cytoplasmic but not nuclear staining.[861,863] Electron microscopy indicates typical findings of hepatocellular carcinoma including paranuclear aggregations of intermediate filaments and electron dense round bodies.[861] In the absence of typical

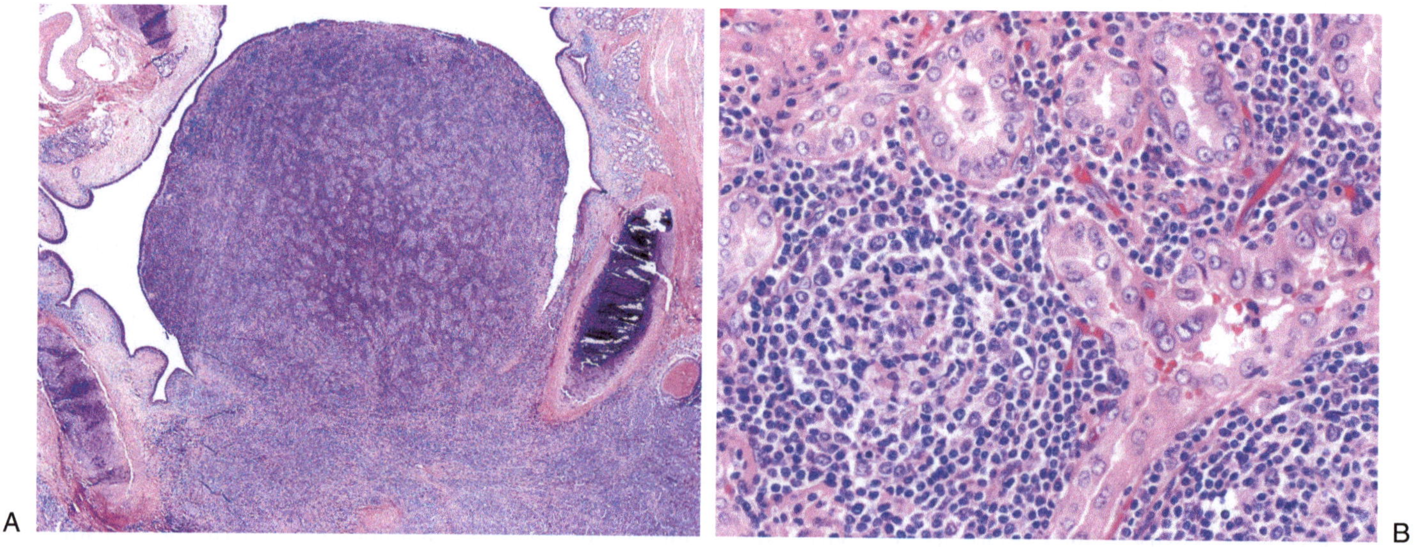

Figure 35.53. Adenocarcinoma with massive lymphoid infiltrates. **(A)** More than half of this endobronchial carcinoma is composed of benign lymphoid infiltrates. Paler cellular aggregates represent tumor cells. **(B)** Malignant glands are surrounded by benign T lymphocytes while benign B lymphocytes form a germinal center.

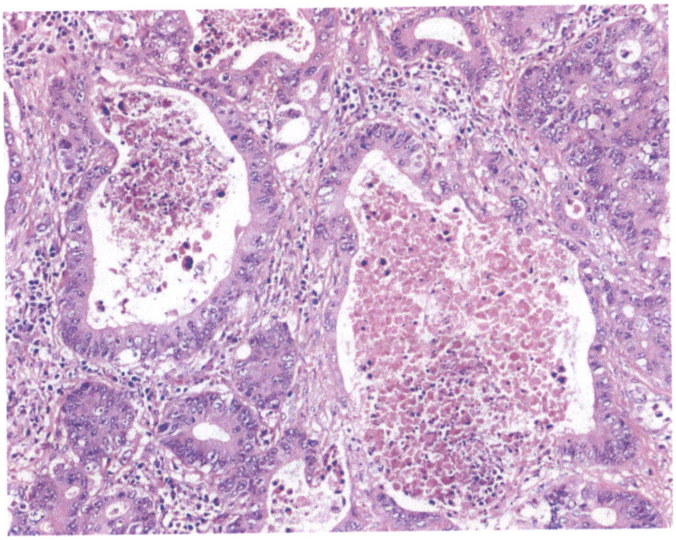

FIGURE 35.54. Nonmucinous adenocarcinoma resembling enteric-type adenocarcinoma. The cribriform architecture, cellular pseudostratification, and luminal "dirty necrosis" suggest a nonpulmonary origin. Clinical history and immunohistochemistry aid in the differential diagnosis. (Courtesy of Dr. S. Yousem, University of Pittsburgh Medical Center, Pittsburgh, PA.)

adenocarcinoma morphology, one must rely on clinical and radiographic data to diagnose this tumor as a primary lung cancer. Patients with hepatoid adenocarcinoma have a poor prognosis.[860]

Large Cell Carcinoma

The WHO classification defines pulmonary LCC as an NSCLC without light microscopic or histochemical evidence of glandular or squamous differentiation. As such, LCC is not a single tumor but rather a collection of poorly differentiated carcinomas that account for less than 10% of lung cancers.[84,617,864] However, if NSCLC were classified on the basis of either ultrastructural or expression profile analysis rather than only light microscopy and histochemistry, then probably no more than 1% of lung cancers would be bona fide LCC[618–621,650,865–867] (Table 35.19). Derived from a pluripotent epithelial cell, most cases do not demonstrate an in situ component.[617] Morphologic subtypes with unique features are recognized in the classification scheme (Table 35.13).

Large cell carcinomas are usually large peripheral tumors. Pleural and chest wall invasion are common. Tan tumors are often necrotic and hemorrhagic, but cavitation is rare (Fig. 35.56).

Tumor histopathology is varied. The neoplasm usually grows in cohesive sheets or nests, but may flood alveolar spaces or percolate through pulmonary interstitium (Fig. 35.57). Intermediate to large polygonal cells with abundant eosinophilic, clear or foamy cytoplasm, large vesicular nuclei, and prominent nucleoli are the norm (Fig. 35.58A). Nuclear pleomorphism and a brisk mitotic rate including atypical forms are common. Cell borders may be well defined, imparting a squamoid appearance, but intercellular bridges and keratinization are absent (Fig. 35.58B). Gland formation is not seen; if five or more cells

A

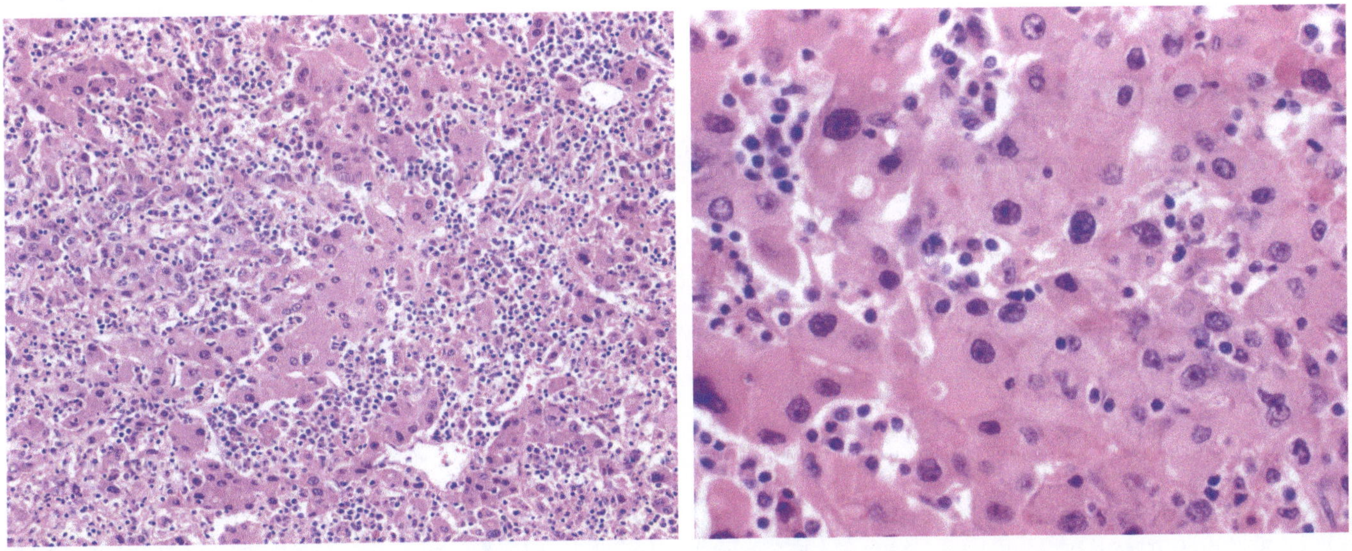

B

FIGURE 35.55. Hepatoid adenocarcinoma. **(A)** Tumor cells form trabeculae and hug thin-walled blood vessels. **(B)** Cuboidal cells have eosinophilic cytoplasm, round nuclei, and single nucleoli. In its pure form, morphology, immunohistochemistry and electron microscopy cannot distinguish this lung primary from a liver metastasis. (Courtesy of Dr. H. Cooper, Fox Chase Cancer Center, Fox Chase, PA.)

TABLE 35.19. Ultrastructural assessment of large cell carcinomas diagnosed by light microscopy

No. cases	Squamous differentiation	Adenocarcinomatous differentiation	Adenosquamous differentiation	Neuroendocrine +/– adenosquamous features	Undifferentiated
198	27 (14%)	111 (56%)	25 (12%)	16 (8%)	19 (10%)

Source: Data from Churg,[867] Carter,[877] Delmonte,[872] Dunnill,[560] Hammar,[865] Kodama,[866] Leong,[874] and Saba.[875]

in at least two high-power (40×) fields have intracytoplasmic mucin, then a diagnosis of solid adenocarcinoma with mucin production is appropriate. Focal spindle cell morphology may be seen. Large areas of coagulative tumor cell necrosis are not uncommon. Stroma may be scant to extensive and both neutrophilic and lymphoplasmacytic infiltrates can be striking. Marked tumor-associated and systemic eosinophilia have also been reported.[868]

Immunophenotyping and hierarchical clustering analysis of immunohistochemical markers in NSCLC indicate that LCC is not a pure group.[869,870] Most LCCs stain with at least one epithelial marker including cytokeratins, Cam5.2, CEA, or EMA, but discohesive tumors may be negative for epithelial markers.[866,871,872] Upward of 80% stain with CK7, while approximately 50% stain with TTF-1.[642,659,768,869] Rare tumors stain with CK5/6.[873] Vimentin is positive in less than half of the tumors. Greater than 90% of LCCs stain with hCG and more than 50% stain with hPL.[646]

Ultrastructural examination of LCC clearly demonstrates glandular or squamous differentiation in 70% of cases, and the majority are adenocarcinomatous.[865–867,872,874–877] Neurosecretory-type granules are also noted in 8% of cases excluding large cell neuroendocrine carcinoma (LCNEC).

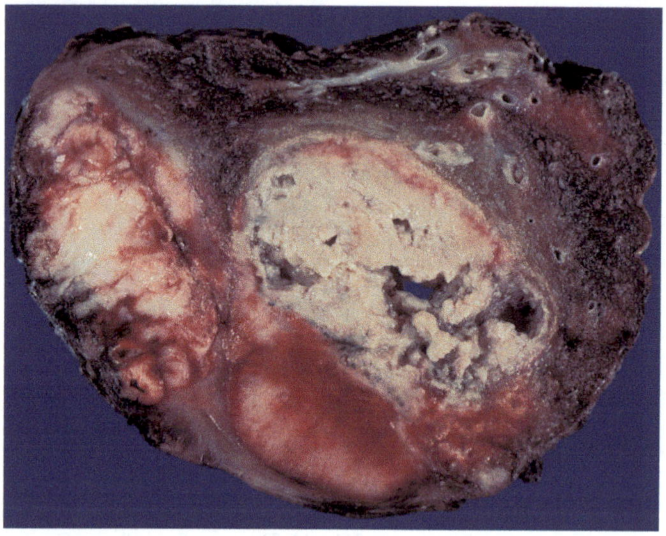

FIGURE 35.56. Large cell carcinoma. Large tan fleshy tumors may resemble sarcomas. Necrosis is common.

A diagnosis of LCC requires extensive tumor sampling and is not possible on cytologic or histologic biopsies. After excluding adenocarcinoma and SCC from consideration, one must consider sarcomas, lymphomas, and metastatic neoplasms including malignant melanoma. Large cell lymphoma and malignant melanoma can easily be mistaken for LCC, and immunohistochemical studies

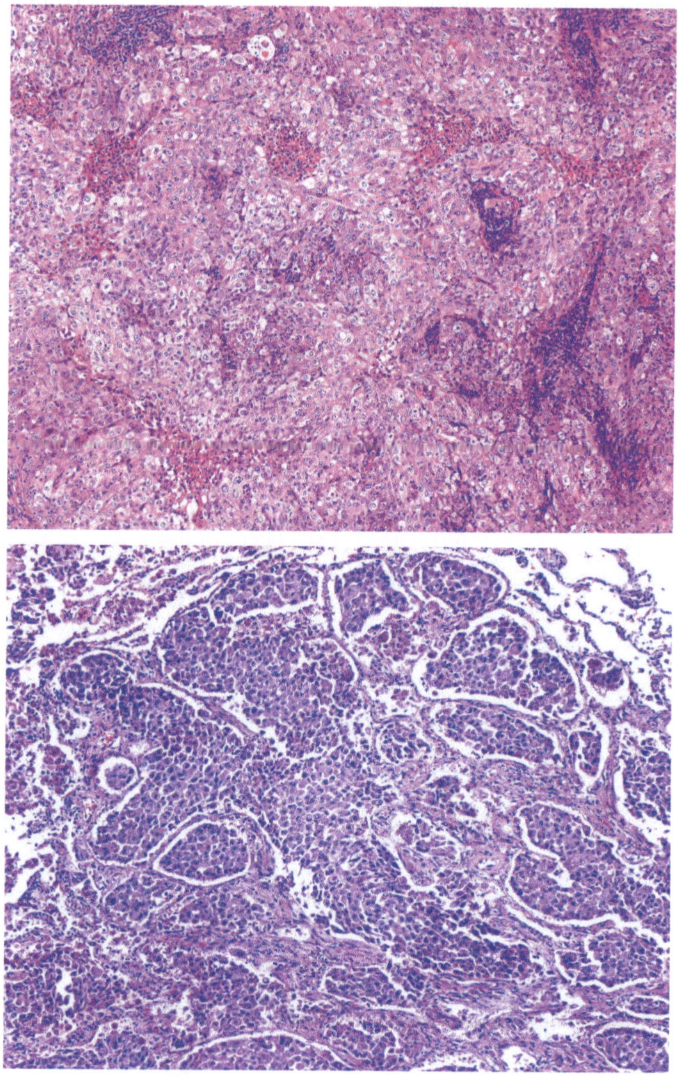

A

B

FIGURE 35.57. Large cell carcinoma growth patterns. **(A)** Destructive growth is usually seen. **(B)** Tumor may fill alveolar spaces.

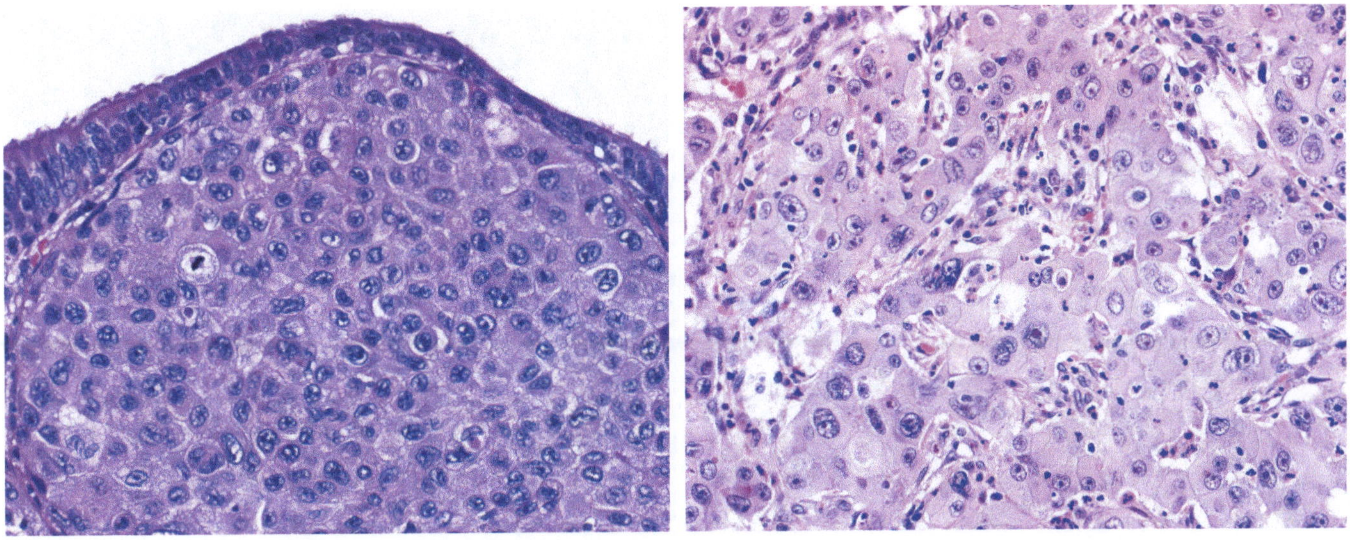

FIGURE 35.58. Large cell carcinoma, morphology. **(A)** Sheets of large cells usually feature large vesicular nuclei with nucleoli and abundant cytoplasm. **(B)** Prominent cell membranes are not indicative of squamous differentiation. Scattered neutrophils highlight tumor cell size.

are recommended for all discohesive undifferentiated neoplasms.[865] Metastatic carcinomas and sarcomas can be diagnosed or excluded on the basis of clinical history and previous tumor histology. Immunohistochemistry may be helpful depending on the clinical scenario.

Large cell carcinomas are best treated surgically. Prognosis, not unlike that reported for other NSCLC, depends on patient performance status and the pathologic tumor stage. Whether LCC histology affects outcome is uncertain; however, one can state with confidence that this collection of poorly differentiated carcinomas does not have a better 5-year survival than either SCC or adenocarcinoma.[871,878–881]

Large Cell Carcinoma Variants

Large cell carcinoma subtypes are poorly differentiated carcinomas with distinctive etiologic, clinical, or pathologic features.

Large cell neuroendocrine carcinoma is a large cell carcinoma with neuroendocrine morphology and immunohistochemical or ultrastructural evidence of neuroendocrine differentiation. *Combined LCNEC* has both LCNEC morphology and evidence of neuroendocrine (NE) differentiation along with adenocarcinoma, SCC, or pleomorphic carcinoma morphology. These are the only neoplasms in the WHO classification scheme whose diagnoses require either immunohistochemical or ultrastructural studies. Tumors featuring LCNEC and SCLC are considered combined SCLC. Although LCNEC and combined LCNEC share many features with SCLC including a very poor prognosis, neuroendocrine differentiation does not imply tumor origin from a specific neuroendocrine cell, and thus the tumors need not be classified together. Furthermore, it is uncertain whether SCLC therapy benefits patients with LCNEC. These carcinomas are discussed within the spectrum of neuroendocrine lung tumors (see Chapter 36).

Basaloid carcinoma is a recently recognized variant of LCC resembling basal cell carcinomas of the skin and anal canal.[690] Unlike other LCC, most basaloid carcinomas are exophytic endobronchial tumors with adjacent squamous dysplasia. This tumor most likely arises from either basal or suprabasal bronchial cells.[690,882]

Tumors feature solid lobular or anastomosing trabecular invasive growth patterns with well-defined borders and peripheral palisading (Fig. 35.59A,B; see also Fig. 36.132 in Chapter 36). Rosettes may be observed. Small cuboidal or fusiform cells have scant cytoplasm and hyperchromatic nuclei with finely granular chromatin without prominent nucleoli (Fig. 35.59C). The mitotic rate is between 15 and 45 per 10 high-power (40×) fields. Central necrosis is common. While pure basaloid carcinoma lacks glandular or squamous differentiation, abrupt keratin formation mimicking hair follicles is permitted. Stroma is often hyalinized or features mucoid degeneration. These tumors stain with cytokeratins and 34ßE12, but not TTF-1.[883] No more than 10% of cases feature staining with one neuroendocrine marker (chromogranin, synaptophysin, or CD56). In these instances, less than 30% of tumor cells stain.[884]

The differential diagnosis includes SCC, SCLC, and LCNEC, and a correct diagnosis on small samples may not be possible. If focal squamous differentiation is seen,

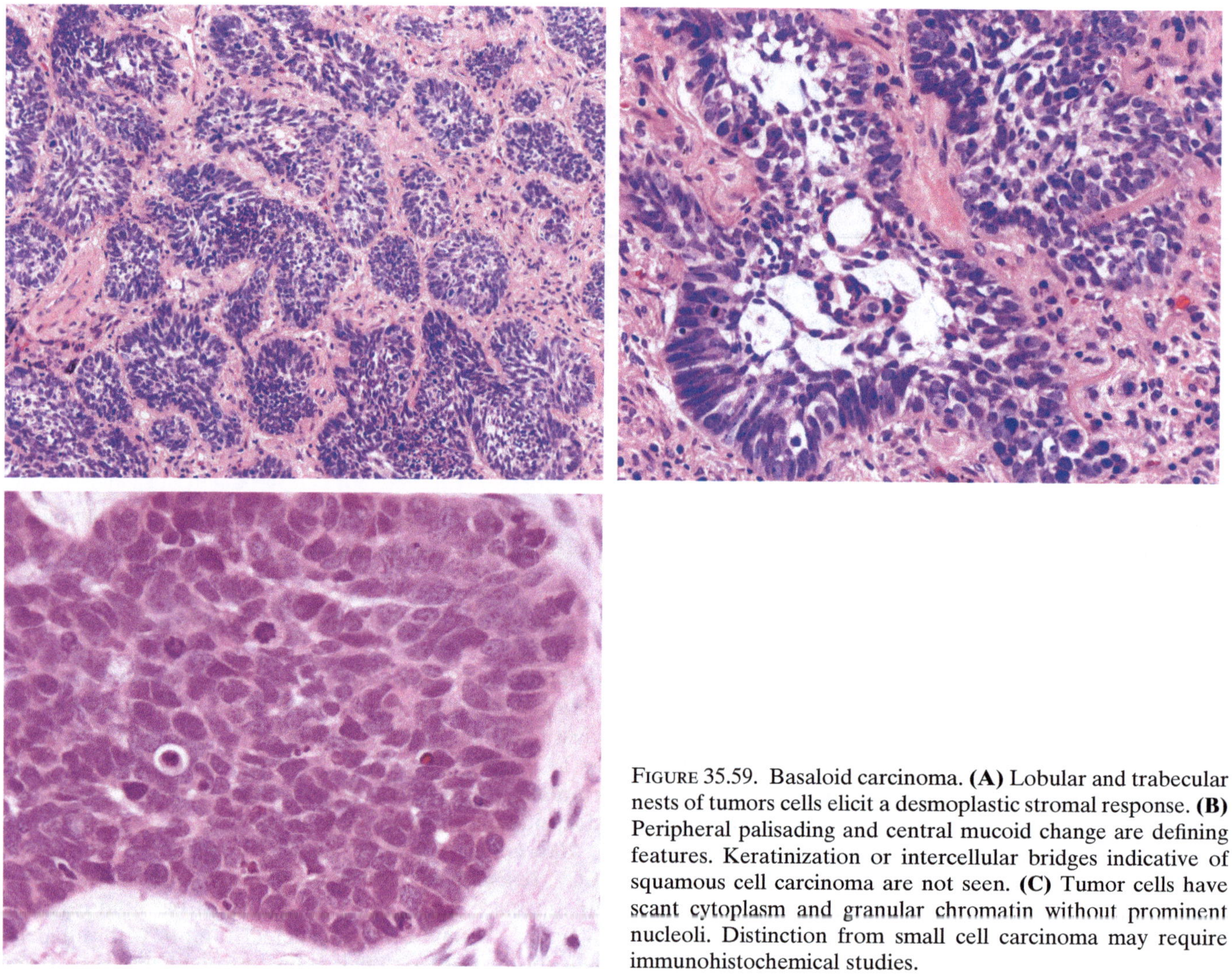

FIGURE 35.59. Basaloid carcinoma. **(A)** Lobular and trabecular nests of tumors cells elicit a desmoplastic stromal response. **(B)** Peripheral palisading and central mucoid change are defining features. Keratinization or intercellular bridges indicative of squamous cell carcinoma are not seen. **(C)** Tumor cells have scant cytoplasm and granular chromatin without prominent nucleoli. Distinction from small cell carcinoma may require immunohistochemical studies.

then one should diagnose SCC, basaloid variant. Obvious nodular growth with palisading and absence of nuclear molding differentiate basaloid carcinoma from SCLC, but the distinction may very difficult on biopsy specimens. Ninety percent of SCLCs are TTF-1 positive and only 10% are negative for chromogranin, synaptophysin, or CD56.[885,886] Large cell neuroendocrine carcinoma may be histologically indistinguishable, since both tumors feature palisading and one third of basaloid carcinomas have rosettes. A $34\beta E12^{+}/TTF\text{-}1^{-}$ immunohistochemical profile supports a diagnosis of basaloid carcinoma.[883]

This high-grade LCC might be more aggressive than SCC, but with inconsistent results among the less than 100 reported cases, prognostication is not possible.[690,887–890]

Lymphoepithelioma-like carcinoma (LELC) is a clinicopathologically distinct rare neoplasm.[322,323,327–330,333] Most cases arise in Asians, and an association with tobacco is not nearly as strong as the association with EBV in this population. Lymphoepithelioma-like carcinoma in Westerners, however, is not associated with EBV[332,333] (see Infections, above).

Tumors are most often solitary white, firm, and well circumscribed, and histologically resemble undifferentiated nasopharyngeal carcinoma. Sheets and irregularly shaped nests of large epithelial cells are surrounded and infiltrated by lymphocytes and plasma cells (Fig. 35.60A,B). The tumor has a pushing border, and malignant undifferentiated cells clump together in a so-called syncytial arrangement (Fig. 35.60C). Tumor cells feature vesicular nuclei, prominent nucleoli, and moderate amounts of cytoplasm (Fig. 35.60C). Mitoses are frequent and pagetoid spread within intact bronchioles is not uncommon. Tumoral necrosis is rare. Spindled cells are rarely seen but if glandular or squamous differentiation is present, then the carcinoma is not LELC. The inflammatory cell reaction is composed of mostly $CD8^{+}$ T lymphocytes, and germinal centers or granulomas may form.

Neutrophils and eosinophils may be seen. Stroma is focally sclerotic and amyloid has been noted.[327] Metastases feature identical morphology. Tumor cells are cytokeratin positive and most stain with bcl-2.[329] Asian patients with Epstein-Barr virus-encoded RNA-1 (EBER-1) in tumor cells usually have either elevated IgA or IgG serum titers against EBV-viral capsid antigen (EBV-VCA).[327,329] Interestingly, EBV-VCA IgG titers may correlate with tumor size and stage. Of note, latent membrane protein-1 (LMP-1) is negative in almost all cases.[329]

The differential diagnosis includes inflammatory pseudotumor, metastatic undifferentiated nasopharyngeal carcinoma, malignant lymphoma, and malignant melanoma. Although the syncytial nests of tumor cells may not be apparent at low magnification, the neoplastic nature of the process should be obvious on further study. Clinical history usually allows one to diagnose an LELC as a lung primary, but cases reported in patients 6 to 13 years after treatment for nasopharyngeal carcinoma may indicate late metastases.[335] Anaplastic large cell lymphoma and malignant melanoma can be differentiated from LELC with standard immunohistochemical stains.

Based on limited follow-up data, LELC has a variable clinical course. While many tumors are localized at diagnosis, extensive disease is not uncommon. Whether LELC has a better stage for stage survival than LCC or NSCLC is not known.[327–329,333]

Clear cell carcinoma is an exquisitely rare LCC, while clear cell morphology is observed in almost one third of NSCLCs and rarely with SCLCs.[686,891,892] Clear cell variants of both SCC and adenocarcinoma are appreciated (see sections Squamous Cell Carcinoma and Adenocarcinoma, above), and while it has been suggested that clear cell carcinoma is not a distinct entity, the WHO has not removed it from the last three classifications.[686,852] The infiltrative and ill-defined tumors are composed of large polygonal cells with abundant clear to slightly

A

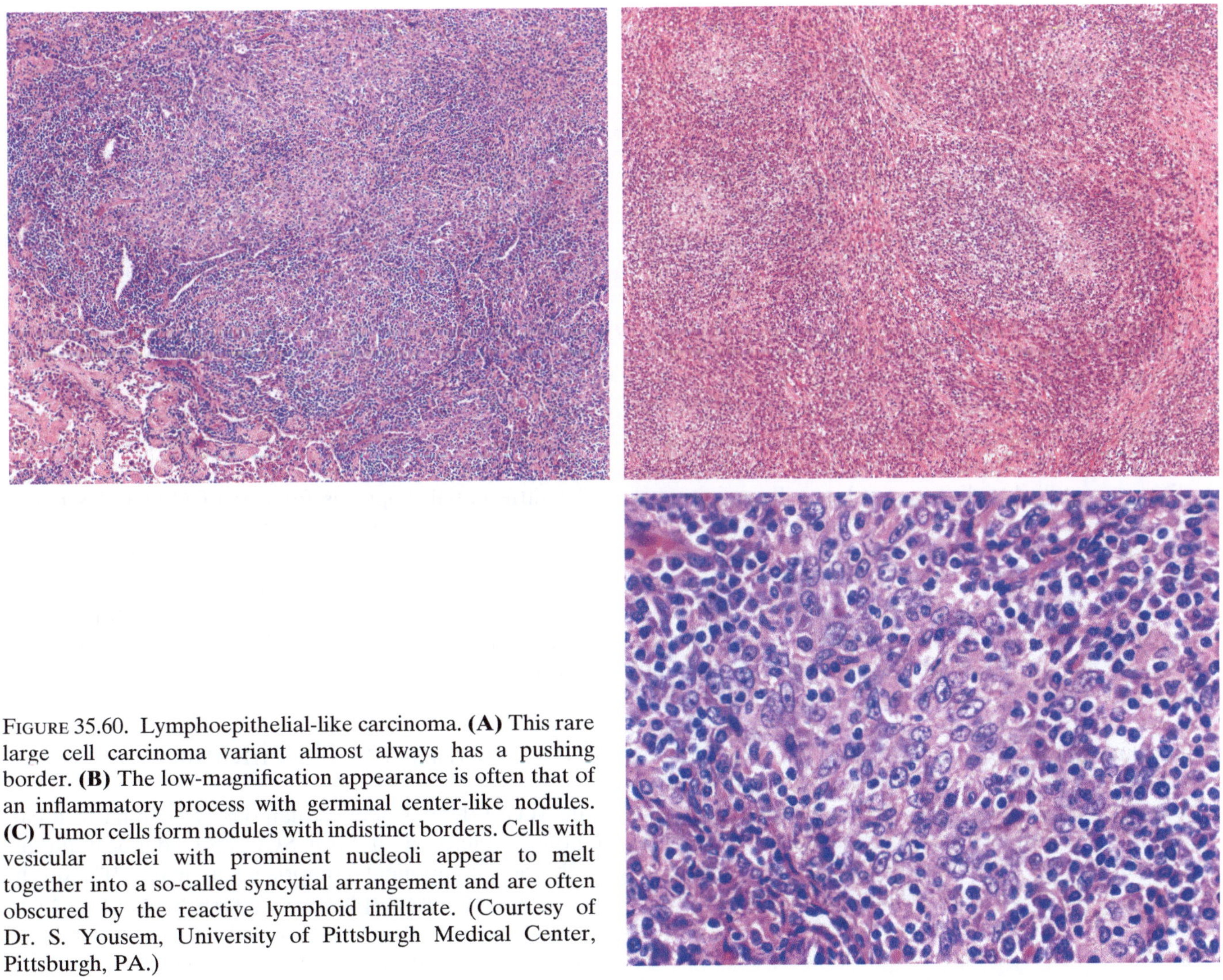

B

C

FIGURE 35.60. Lymphoepithelial-like carcinoma. **(A)** This rare large cell carcinoma variant almost always has a pushing border. **(B)** The low-magnification appearance is often that of an inflammatory process with germinal center-like nodules. **(C)** Tumor cells form nodules with indistinct borders. Cells with vesicular nuclei with prominent nucleoli appear to melt together into a so-called syncytial arrangement and are often obscured by the reactive lymphoid infiltrate. (Courtesy of Dr. S. Yousem, University of Pittsburgh Medical Center, Pittsburgh, PA.)

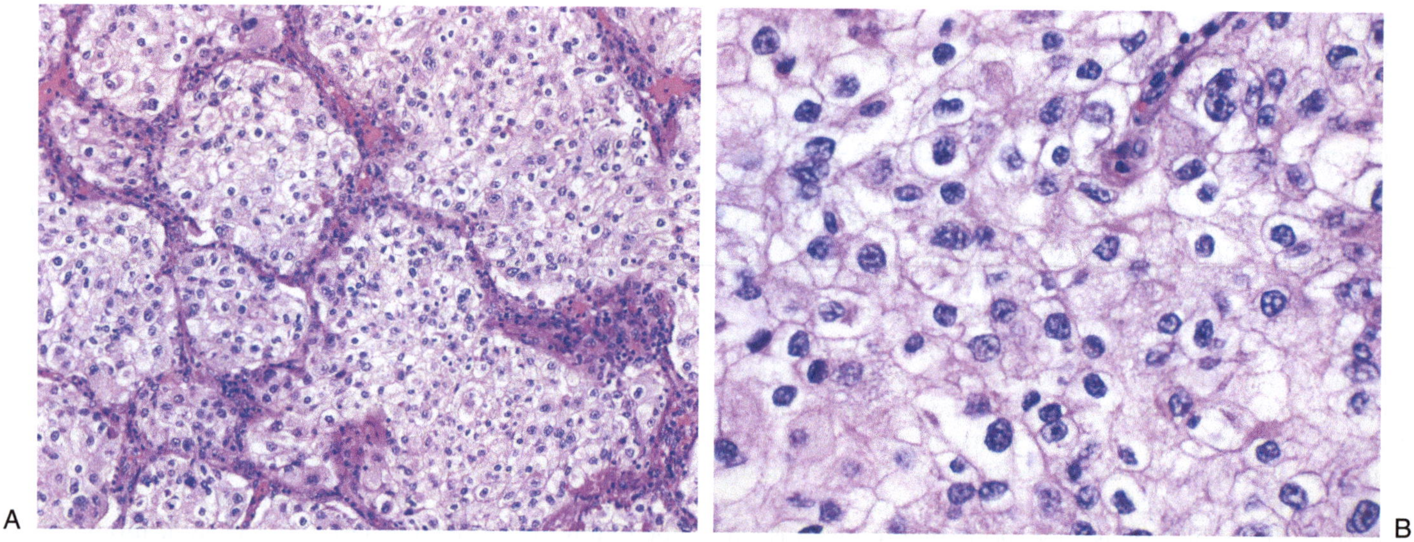

FIGURE 35.61. Clear cell carcinoma. **(A)** Sheets of tumor cells often fill alveolar spaces. Note the absence of either squamous or glandular features. **(B)** Large tumor cells are irregular with malignant cytology. Periodic acid-Schiff stains highlight abundant intracytoplasmic glycogen. As with clear cell SCC and adenocarcinoma, distinction from metastatic renal, thyroid, and salivary gland carcinomas may be difficult.

foamy cytoplasm and prominent cell borders (Fig. 35.61). Cytoplasmic glycogen is usually abundant and confirmed with a PAS diastase stain. Clear cell change in nonneoplastic bronchial epithelium adjacent to an endobronchial carcinoma may be seen, and cytokeratin AE1/AE3 and CK7 positivity but TTF-1, chromogranin, and synaptophysin negativity have been reported in a single case.[893] Ultrastructural studies may demonstrate glandular or squamous differentiation in addition to cytoplasmic glycogen.[852,894]

Clear cell carcinoma of the lung must be differentiated from metastatic carcinomas arising in the kidney, thyroid gland, and salivary glands, and clear cell carcinoid tumor and clear cell tumor of lung (so-called sugar tumor) (CCTL). Clinical history and immunohistochemical studies are required to diagnose a clear cell carcinoma as a lung primary. Clear cell carcinoid tumor lacks nuclear pleomorphism, necrosis, and mitoses, and stains for neuroendocrine markers.[895] Clear cell tumor of lung may feature focal cytologic atypia, but not diffuse malignant features. Furthermore, clear cell carcinoma is cytokeratin positive while CCTL stains with HMB-45 but not cytokeratin.[896]

Large cell carcinoma with rhabdoid phenotype is not a single clinicopathologic entity. Rhabdoid cells can be seen in many extrarenal sites and as a part of lung carcinomas including SCLC.[897–903] Lung carcinomas composed entirely of rhabdoid cells are exceedingly rare.[904,905] If more than 10% of a LCC is composed of rhabdoid cells, then a diagnosis of LCC with rhabdoid phenotype is warranted.[617,738,906,907] Tumors may be solitary or multifocal at diagnosis and grow in sheets or nests, or fill alveoli (Fig. 35.62A). Rhabdoid morphology may be apparent only at the periphery of the carcinoma. The neoplastic cells are round, polygonal, or pleomorphic with round vesicular nuclei and a large eosinophilic globular cytoplasmic inclusion (Fig. 35.62B,C). Tumor cells are diffusely positive for vimentin, and usually stain with cytokeratin and EMA. Cytokeratin positive cells often stain with CK7 but not CK20.[901] Thyroid transcription factor-1 and, of course, muscle-specific actin, desmin, and myoD are negative. Neuroendocrine differentiation, especially chromogranin positivity, is not uncommon, while Leu-7 and glial fibrillary acidic protein staining have been reported in several cases.[906,908] Ultrastructurally, the cytoplasmic inclusions are composed of whorled intermediate filaments, and dense core granules may be seen.[902,904,906] (Fig. 35.62D). The differential diagnosis for this LCC includes malignant melanoma and malignant lymphoma. Immunohistochemical studies usually reveal the epithelial nature of the tumor. Metastatic tumors with rhabdoid features can only be excluded on the basis of clinical history. These carcinomas are aggressive and few survivors have been reported.[909,910]

Adenosquamous Carcinoma

The WHO defines adenosquamous carcinoma as a carcinoma composed of both SCC and adenocarcinoma, with each component comprising at least 10% of the tumor. Given the morphologic heterogeneity of lung carcinomas, one would expect to encounter a significant number of adenosquamous carcinomas. However, its

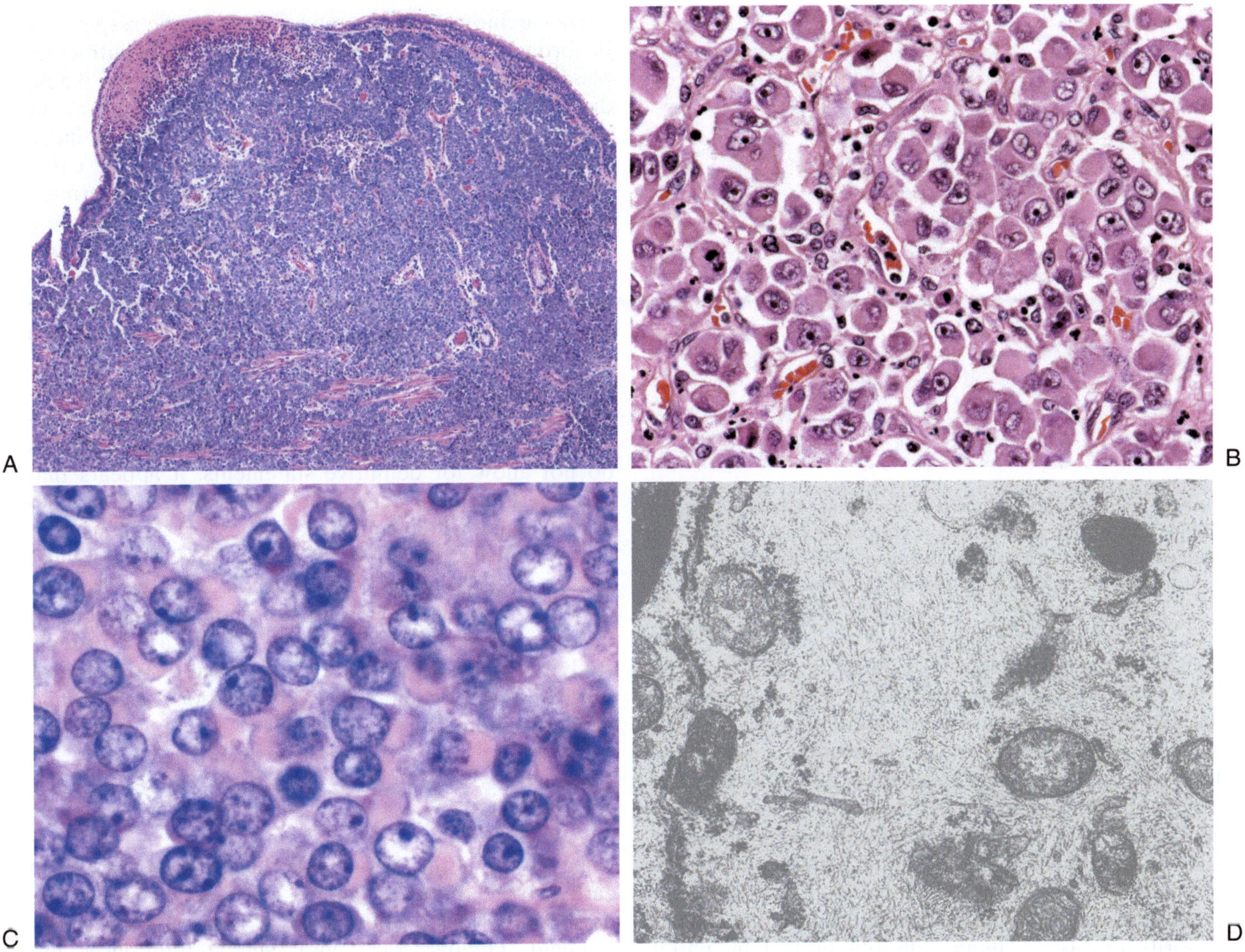

FIGURE 35.62. Large cell carcinoma with rhabdoid phenotype. **(A)** Sheets of tumor cells destroy underlying parenchyma. In this example the carcinoma infiltrates bronchial wall with surface ulceration. **(B)** The carcinoma may be partly or entirely composed of pleomorphic cells with eosinophilic cytoplasm. (Courtesy of Drs. H. Shimazaki and S. Aida, National Defense Medical Hospital, Saitama, Japan.) **(C)** This carcinoma may also resemble other small round blue cell tumors, yet the globular eosinophilic cytoplasmic inclusions suggest a rhabdoid phenotype. **(D)** Ultrastructural examination reveals abundant intracytoplasmic intermediate filaments and occasional dense core granules. (Courtesy of Drs. H. Shimazaki and S. Aida, National Defense Medical Hospital, Saitama, Japan.)

frequency based on this arbitrary definition may be no more than 2% and perhaps less than 1% of lung carcinomas.[911–915] The histogenesis is unknown, yet prevailing opinion suggests that this tumor arises from a single pluripotent bronchial reserve cell rather than representing squamous metaplasia of adenocarcinoma or a collision tumor.[913,916–918]

While detailed epidemiologic information is limited, given the rarity of the tumor and lack of diagnostic conformity in the literature, adenosquamous carcinoma has a slight male predominance, is strongly associated with tobacco use, and most often presents as a peripheral tumor with either central scarring or pleural puckering.[911–914] Gross features are not unlike those of other NSCLCs, although central or endobronchial cases are rare.

Morphologic requirements for a diagnosis of adenosquamous carcinoma require the light microscopic presence of well-defined SCC and adenocarcinoma. Thus unequivocal intracellular keratin, keratin pearls, or intercellular bridges as well as true gland formation should be identified (Fig. 35.63). Solid areas with a squamoid or "pavement" appearance do not suffice for squamous differentiation, while solid adenocarcinoma requires more

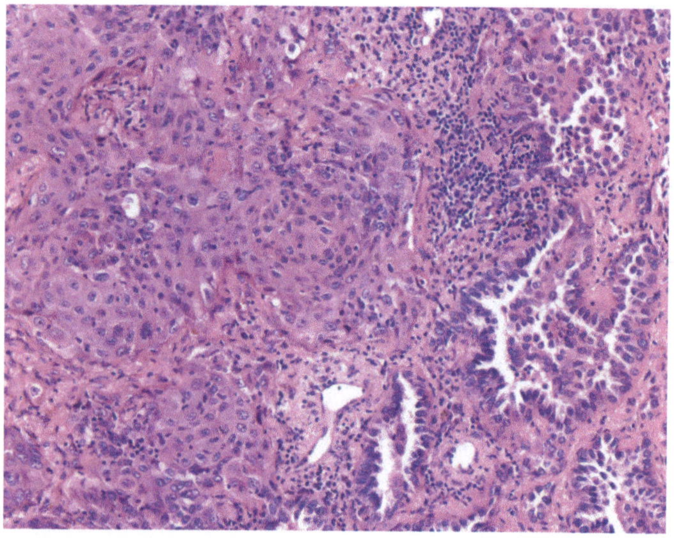

FIGURE 35.63. Adenosquamous carcinoma. Gland formation (right) and either keratinization (upper left) or intercellular bridges are necessary for this diagnosis. The minority component must constitute at least 10% of the tumor.

than five mucin droplets in each of at least two high power fields[911] (see Adenocarcinoma, above). As long as the minority component comprises 10% of the tumor, a diagnosis of adenosquamous carcinoma is warranted. The components may be intertwined or separate, and the degree of differentiation of each component is independent. Most cases are composed of either well- or moderately differentiated SCC and adenocarcinoma. Illustrated examples feature acinar and papillary patterns of adenocarcinoma. Areas of LCC morphology are also seen in a minority of cases. Tumor cells obliterate lung parenchyma and elicit a desmoplastic response. Amyloid-like stroma has been described.[919] Lymph node metastases often feature the morphology of the dominant primary tumor component and rarely feature both phenotypes.[920]

The immunohistochemical and ultrastructural findings of adenosquamous carcinoma hold no great surprises. The squamous component stains with low and high molecular weight keratins, while the glandular areas usually do not stain with high molecular weight keratin but express TTF-1 and EMA. Electron microscopy demonstrates SCC and adenocarcinoma features in the respective tumor populations. Ultrastructural evidence of adenosquamous carcinoma in the absence of light microscopy findings, reported in almost 50% of NSCLCs, is not synonymous with a diagnosis of adenosquamous carcinoma.[622,921,922]

A diagnosis of adenosquamous carcinoma on anything less than a tumor resection specimen is not possible, given the need to assess relative percentages of the different morphologies. The differential diagnosis includes adenocarcinoma with entrapped metaplastic respiratory or bronchiolar epithelium, and SCC with intracytoplasmic mucin or entrapped glandular epithelium. These distinctions are usually apparent, while central or endobronchial adenosquamous carcinoma may be indistinguishable from high-grade mucoepidermoid carcinoma. However, most high-grade mucoepidermoid carcinomas have areas of low-grade histology, feature a mixture of mucinous and squamous cells, but usually lack keratinization and keratin pearls in the squamoid areas as well as tubular and papillary growth in the glandular component. In addition, dysplasia and carcinoma in situ are not seen in overlying squamous mucosa.[923]

Adenosquamous carcinomas are treated surgically. While the rarity of the tumor combined with inconsistent diagnostic criteria used in clinicopathologic studies do not allow for definitive statements, it appears that this tumor is more aggressive than either SCC or adenocarcinoma when compared stage for stage with 5-year survival rates of 62.5% and 35% for resected localized disease and all resectable cases, respectively.[914,915] Adenosquamous morphology may be an independent prognostic factor.[912,913,916,920] Lastly, a single study did not note a difference in stage distribution or survival based on the relative proportions of SCC and adenocarcinoma.[913]

Conclusion

Lung cancer is the great public health epidemic of the early 21st century. Incidence rates are rising in the developing world, while survival rates are essentially stagnant. Gender, race, and genetic differences are acknowledged, though poorly understood. Tobacco use is mostly responsible for lung carcinoma, while occupational and environmental exposures are secondary etiologies. Sophisticated diagnostic and therapeutic tools aid in patient diagnosis, staging, and treatment. The current WHO classification of lung tumors separates most NSCLC into SCC, adenocarcinoma, and LCC categories. Squamous cell carcinoma, LCC, and adenosquamous variants are notable mostly for morphologic reasons, while particular adenocarcinoma diagnoses impact therapy and prognosis. Small nonmucinous BACs have an extremely favorable prognosis in comparison to most other invasive adenocarcinomas. As we step deeper into the molecular age of oncology, pathologic diagnoses retain great importance and are the foundation for future therapeutic successes.

References

1. Ferlay J, Bray F, Pisani P, et al. GLOBOCAN 2002: Cancer incidence, mortality and prevalence worldwide. IARC

cancer base No. 5, version 2.0, 2002. Lyon, France: IARC Press, 2004.
2. Parkin DM, Bray F, Ferlay J, et al. Global cancer statistics, 2002. CA Cancer J Clin 2005;55(2):74–108.
3. Jemal A, Murray T, Ward E, et al. Cancer statistics, 2005. CA Cancer J Clin 2005;55(1):10–30.
4. Levi F, Lucchini F, Negri E, et al. Trends in mortality from major cancers in the European Union, including acceding countries, in 2004. Cancer 2004;101(12):2843–2850.
5. Brennan P, Bray I. Recent trends and future directions for lung cancer mortality in Europe. Br J Cancer 2002;87(1): 43–48.
6. Tyczynski JE, Bray F, Parkin DM. Lung cancer in Europe in 2000: epidemiology, prevention, and early detection. Lancet Oncol 2003;4(7):396.
7. Boyle P, Ferlay J. Cancer incidence and mortality in Europe, 2004. Ann Oncol 2005;16:481–488.
8. Chen ZM, Xu Z, Collins R, et al. Early health effects of the emerging tobacco epidemic in China. A 16-year prospective study. JAMA 1997;278(18):1500–1504.
9. Liu BQ, Peto R, Chen ZM, et al. Emerging tobacco hazards in China: 1. Retrospective proportional mortality study of one million deaths. BMJ 1998;317(7170):1411–1422.
10. Bray F, Tyczynski JE, Parkin DM. Going up or coming down? The changing phases of the lung cancer epidemic from 1967 to 1999 in the 15 European Union countries. Eur J Cancer 2004;40(1):96–125.
11. Tyczynski JE, Bray F, Areleid T, et al. Lung cancer mortality patterns in selected central, eastern and southern European countries. Int J Cancer 2004;109:598–610.
12. Bain C, Feskanich D, Speizer FE, et al. Lung cancer rates in men and women with comparable histories of smoking. J Natl Cancer Inst 2004;96(11):826–834.
13. Kreuzer M, Boffetta P, Whitley E, et al. Gender differences in lung cancer risk by smoking: a multicentre case-control study in Germany and Italy. Br J Cancer 2000;82(1): 227–233.
14. U. S. Public Health Service Office of Surgeon General. Women and smoking: a report of the Surgeon General. Washington, DC: U.S. Department of Health and Human Services, Public Health Service, Office of the Surgeon General, 2001.
15. Giovino GA. Epidemiology of tobacco use in the United States. Oncogene 2002;21:7326–7340.
16. Jemal AR, Tiawari RC, Murray T, et al. Cancer statistics 2004. CA Cancer J Clin 2004;54(1):8–29.
17. Jemal A, Siegel R, Ward E, et al. Cancer statistics, 2006. CA Cancer J Clin 2006;56(2):106–130.
18. Tomlinson R. Smoking death toll shifts to Third World. BMJ 1997;3:315–565.
19. Pisani P, Parkin DM, Bray F, et al. Estimates of the worldwide mortality from 25 cancers in 1990. Int J Cancer 1999; 83:18–29.
20. Chaloupka F, Lixuthal A. Cigarette smoking in Pacific Rim countries; the impact of US trade policy: National Bureau for Economic Research. In: Program and abstracts of the WEA International 1996 Pacific Rim Allied Economic Organizations Conference. Working Paper No. 5543, 1996:10–15.
21. Tan YK, Wee TC, Koh WP, et al. Survival among Chinese women with lung cancer in Singapore: a comparison by stage, histology and smoking status. Lung Cancer 2003;40: 237–246.
22. Epidemiology and Disease Control Department of Ministry and Health Singapore. National Health Survey 1998, 1999: Epidemiology and Disease Control Department, 1998.
23. Hinds MW, Stemmermann GN, Yang HY, et al. Differences in lung cancer risk from smoking among Japanese, Chinese and Hawaiian women in Hawaii. Int J Cancer 1981;27(3):297–302.
24. Lam WK, White NW, Chan-Yeung MM. Lung cancer epidemiology and risk factors in Asia and Africa. Int J Tuberc Lung Dis 2004;8(9):1045–1057.
25. Wu-Williams AH, Dai XD, Blot W, et al. Lung cancer among women in north-east China. Br J Cancer 1990;62(6): 982–987.
26. Kuo CW, Chen YM, Chao JY, et al. Non-small cell lung cancer in very young and very old patients. Chest 2000; 117(2):354–357.
27. Port JL, Kent M, Korst RJ, et al. Surgical resection for lung cancer in the octogenarian. Chest 2004;126(3):733–738.
28. Ries LAG, Kosary CL, Hankey BF. SEER Cancer Statistics Review 1975–2000. Bethesda, MD: National Cancer Institute, 2003.
29. Ramalingam S, Pawlish K, Gadgeel S, et al. Lung cancer in young patients: analysis of a Surveillance, Epidemiology, and End Results database. J Clin Oncol 1998;16(2):651–657.
30. McDuffie HH, Klaassen DJ, Dosman JA. Characteristics of patients with primary lung cancer diagnosed at age of 50 years or younger. Chest 1989;96(6):1298–1301.
31. Skarin AT, Herbst RS, Leong TL, et al. Lung cancer in patients under age 40. Lung Cancer 2001;32(3):255–264.
32. Tian DL, Liu HX, Zhang L, et al. Surgery for young patients with lung cancer. Lung Cancer 2003;42(2):215–220.
33. Liu NS, Spitz MR, Kemp BL, et al. Adenocarcinoma of the lung in young patients. Cancer 2000;88(8):1837–1841.
34. Whooley BP, Urschel JD, Antkowiak JG, et al. Bronchogenic carcinoma in patients age 30 and younger. Ann Thorac Cardiovasc Surg 2000;6(2):86–88.
35. Mizushima Y, Yokoyama A, Ito M, et al. Lung carcinoma in patients age younger than 30 years. Cancer 1999;85(8): 1730–1733.
36. Roviaro GC, Varoli F, Zannini P, et al. Lung cancer in the young. Chest 1985;87(4):456–459.
37. Rocha MP, Fraire AE, Guntupalli KK, et al. Lung cancer in the young. Cancer Detect Prev 1994;18(5):349–355.
38. Cornere MM, Fergusson W, Kolbe J, et al. Characteristics of patients with lung cancer under the age of 45 years: a case control study. Respirology 2001;6(4):293–296.
39. Kreuzer M, Kreienbrock L, Gerken M, et al. Risk factors for lung cancer in young adults. Am J Epidemiol 1998; 147(11):1028–1037.
40. Kreuzer M, Kreienbrock L, Muller KM, et al. Histologic types of lung carcinoma and age at onset. Cancer 1999; 85(9):1958–1965.

41. Maruyama R, Yoshino I, Yohena T, et al. Lung cancer in patients younger than 40 years of age. J Surg Oncol 2001; 77:208–212.
42. Sekine I, Nishiwaki Y, Yokose T, et al. Young lung cancer patients in Japan: different characteristics between the sexes. Ann Thorac Surg 1999;67(5):1451–1455.
43. Tominaga K, Mori K, Yokoi K, et al. Lung cancer in patients under 50 years old. Jpn J Cancer Res 1999;90:490–495.
44. Lienert T, Serke M, Schonfeld N, et al. Lung cancer in young females. Eur Respir J 2000;16(5):986–990.
45. Hartman GE, Shochat SJ. Primary pulmonary neoplasms of childhood: a review. Ann Thorac Surg 1983;36(1):108–119.
46. Fontenelle LJ. Primary adenocarcinoma of lung in a child: review of the literature. Am Surg 1976;42(4):296–299.
47. Cayley CK, Caez HJ, Mersheimer W. Primary bronchogenic carcinoma of the lung in children; review of the literature; report of a case. AMA Am J Dis Child 1951;82(1): 49–60.
48. Niitu Y, Kubota H, Hasegawa S, et al. Lung cancer (squamous cell carcinoma) in adolescence. Am J Dis Child 1974;127(1):108–111.
49. La Salle AJ, Andrassy RJ, Stanford W. Bronchogenic squamous cell carcinoma in childhood; a case report. J Pediatr Surg 1977;12(4):519–521.
50. Epstein DM, Aronchick JM. Lung cancer in childhood. Med Pediatr Oncol 1989;17(6):510–513.
51. MacSweeney F, Papagiannopoulos K, Goldstraw P, et al. An assessment of the expanded classification of congenital cystic adenomatoid malformations and their relationship to malignant transformation. Am J Surg Pathol 2003;27(8): 1139–1146.
52. Hirayama T. Life-style and mortality: a large-scale census-based cohort study in Japan. In: Wahrendorf J, ed. Contributions to epidemiology and biostatistics. Vol. 6. Basel, Switzerland: Karger, 1990:41–45.
53. IARC. Tobacco smoking. In: IARC Monographs on the evaluation of carcinogenic risk of chemicals to humans. Lyon, France: IARC, 1986.
54. Stellman SD, Takezaki T, Wang L, et al. Smoking and lung cancer risk in American and Japanese men: an international case-control study. Cancer Epidemiol Biomarkers Prev 2001;10(11):1193–1199.
55. Wynder EL, Hirayama T. Comparative epidemiology of cancers of the United States and Japan. Prev Med 1977;6: 567–594.
56. Wynder EL, Fujita Y, Harris RE, et al. Comparative epidemiology of cancer between the United States and Japan-a second look. Cancer (Phila) 1991;67:746–763.
57. Parkin DM, Whelan SL, Ferlay J, et al. Incidence in five continents, VII. IARC Scientific Publication No. 143, 1997.
58. Haiman CA, Stram DO, Wilkens LR, et al. Ethnic and racial differences in the smoking-related risk of lung cancer. N Engl J Med 2006;354:333–342.
59. Devesa SS, Grauman DJ, Blot WJ, et al. Cancer surveillance series: changing geographic patterns of lung cancer mortality in the United States, 1950 through 1994. J Natl Cancer Inst 1999;91(12):1040–1050.
60. Schwartz AG, Swanson GM. Lung carcinoma in African Americans and whites. A population-based study in metropolitan Detroit, Michigan. Cancer 1997;79(1):45–52.
61. Schneiderman M, Davis DL, Wagener DK. Smokers: black and white. Science 1990;249(4966):228–229.
62. Wynder EL, Hoffmann D. Smoking and lung cancer: scientific challenges and opportunities. Cancer Res 1994; 54(20):5284–5295.
63. Fiori MC, Nootny TE, Pierce JP, et al. Trends in cigarette smoking in the United States. The changing influence of gender and race. JAMA 1989;261:49–55.
64. U. S. Department of Health and Human Services. Tobacco use among U.S. racial/ethnic minority groups—African-Americans, American-Indians and Alaska Natives, Asian-Americans and Pacific Islanders, and Hispanics: a report of the Surgeon General. Atlanta, GA: U.S. Department of Health and Human Services, Centers for Disease Control and Prevention, National Center for Chronic Disease Prevention and Health Promotion, Office on Smoking and Health, 1998.
65. Stellman SD, Resnicow K. Tobacco smoking, cancer and social class. IARC Sci Publ 1997(138):229–250.
66. Stellman SD, Chen Y, Muscat JE, et al. Lung cancer risk in white and black Americans. Ann Epidemiol 2003; 13(4):294–302.
67. Brawley OW, Freeman HP. Race and outcomes: is this the end of the beginning for minority health research? J Natl Cancer Inst 1999;91:1908–1909.
68. Swanson GM, Lin CS, Burns PB. Diversity in the association between occupation and lung cancer among black and white men. Cancer Epidemiol Biomarkers Prev 1993;2(4): 313–320.
69. Muscat JE, Stellman SD, Richie JP Jr, et al. Lung cancer risk and workplace exposures in black men and women. Environ Res 1998;76(2):78–84.
70. Wrensch MR, Miike R, Sison JD, et al. CYP1A1 variants and smoking-related lung cancer in San Francisco Bay Area Latinos and African Americans. Int J Cancer 2004;114:141–147.
71. Kelsey KT, Wiencke JK, Spitz MR. A race specific genetic polymorphism in the CYP1A1 gene is not associated with lung cancer in African Americans. Carcinogenesis 1994;15: 1121–1124.
72. Taioli E, Crofts F, Demopoulos R, et al. A specific African-American CYP1A1 polymorphism is associated with adenocarcinoma of the lung. Cancer Res 1995;55:472–473.
73. London SJ, Daly AK, Fairbrother KS, et al. Lung cancer risk in African-Americans in relation to a race specific CYP1A1 polymorphism. Cancer Res 1995;55:6035–6037.
74. Ishibe N, Wiencke JK, Zheng-fa Z, et al. Susceptibility to lung cancer in light smokers associated with CYP1A1 polymorphisms in Mexican and African-Americans. Cancer Epidemiol Biomarkers Prev 1997;6:1075–1080.
75. Taioli E, Ford J, Trachman J, et al. Lung cancer risk and CYP1A1 genotype in African Americans. Carcinogenesis 1998;19(5):813–817.
76. London SJ, Daly AK, Leathart JB, et al. Lung cancer risk in relation to the CYP2C9*1/CYP2C9*2 genetic polymorphism among African-Americans and Caucasians in Los

Angeles County, California. Pharmacogenetics 1996;6(6): 527–533.
77. London SJ, Daly AK, Cooper J, et al. Lung cancer risks in relation to Rsa I polymorphism among African-Americans and Caucasians in Los Angeles County. Pharmacogenetics 1996;6:151–158.
78. London SJ, Daly AK, Leathart JB, et al. Genetic poly-morphism of CDP2D6 and lung cancer risk in African-Americans and Caucasians in Los Angeles California. Carcinogenesis 1997;18:1203–1204.
79. Wu X, Shi H, Jiang H, et al. Associations between cytochrome P4502E1 genotype, mutagen sensitivity, cigarette smoking and susceptibility to lung cancer. Carcinogenesis 1997;18:967–973.
80. Devesa SS, Bray F, Vizcaino AP, et al. International lung cancer trends by histologic type: male:female differences diminishing and adenocarcinoma rates rising. Int J Cancer 2005.
81. Parkin DM, Whelan SL, Ferlay J, et al. Cancer incidence in five continents, vol VIII. IARC Scientific Publications No. 155. Lyon: IARC Press, 2002.
82. Ringer G, Smith JM, Engel AM, et al. Influence of sex on lung cancer histology, stage, and survival in a midwestern United States tumor registry. Clin Lung Cancer 2005;7(3): 180–182.
83. Travis WD, Lubin J, Ries L, et al. United States lung carcinoma incidence trends: declining for most histologic types among males, increasing among females. Cancer 1996;77(12):2464–2470.
84. Travis WD, Travis LB, Devesa SS. Lung cancer. Cancer 1995;75(1 suppl):191–202.
85. Devesa SS, Shaw GL, Blot WJ. Changing patterns of lung cancer incidence by histological type. Cancer Epidemiol Biomarkers Prev 1991;1(1):29–34.
86. Sobue T, Ajiki W, Tsukuma H, et al. Trends of lung cancer incidence by histologic type: a population-based study in Osaka, Japan. Jpn J Cancer Res 1999;90(1):6 15.
87. Harkness EF, Brewster DH, Kerr KM, et al. Changing trends in incidence of lung cancer by histologic type in Scotland. Int J Cancer 2002;102(2):179–183.
88. Janssen-Heijnen ML, Nab HW, van Reek J, et al. Striking changes in smoking behaviour and lung cancer incidence by histological type in south-east Netherlands, 1960–1991. Eur J Cancer 1995;31A(6):949–952.
89. Wynder EL, Muscat JE. The changing epidemiology of smoking and lung cancer histology. Environ Health Perspect 1995;103(suppl 8):143–148.
90. Sobue T, Tsukuma H, Oshima A, et al. Lung cancer incidence rates by histologic type in high- and low-risk areas; a population-based study in Osaka, Okinawa, and Saku Nagano, Japan. J Epidemiol 1999;9(3):134–142.
91. Hatcher J, Dover DC. Trends in histopathology of lung cancer in Alberta. Can J Public Health 2003;94(4):292–296.
92. Levi F, Franceschi S, La Vecchia C, et al. Lung carcinoma trends by histologic type in Vaud and Neuchatel, Switzerland, 1974–1994. Cancer 1997;79(5):906–914.
93. Jedrychowski W, Becher H, Wahrendorf J, et al. Effect of tobacco smoking on various histological types of lung cancer. J Cancer Res Clin Oncol 1992;118(4):276–282.
94. Lubin JH, Blot WJ. Assessment of lung cancer risk factors by histologic category. J Natl Cancer Inst 1984;73(2):383–389.
95. Thun MJ, Lally CA, Flannery JT, et al. Cigarette smoking and changes in the histopathology of lung cancer. J Natl Cancer Inst 1997;89(21):1580–1586.
96. Rottman H. Uber Primarere Lungencarcinoma. 1898; Inaugural dissertation. Wurzburg, Germany: Universitat Wurzburg, 1898.
97. Schrek R, Baker LA, et al. Tobacco smoking as an etiologic factor in disease; cancer. Cancer Res 1950;10(1):49–58.
98. Mills CA, Porter MM. Tobacco smoking habits and cancer of the mouth and respiratory system. Cancer Res 1950; 10(9):539–542.
99. Levin ML, Goldstein H, Gerhardt PR. Cancer and tobacco smoking. JAMA 1950;143:336–338.
100. Wynder EL, Graham EA. Tobacco smoking as a possible etiologic factor in bronchiogenic carcinoma; a study of 684 proved cases. JAMA 1950;143(4):329–336.
101. Doll R, Hill AB. Smoking and carcinoma of the lung; preliminary report. BMJ 1950;2(4682):739–748.
102. Muller FH. Tabakmissbrauch und Lungencarcinom. Z Krebsforsch 1939;49:57–85.
103. Schairer E, Schoniger E. Lungenkrebs and Tabakverbrauch. Z Krebsforsch 1943;54:261–269.
104. Wassink WE. Onstaansvoorwasrden voor Longkanker. Med Tijdschr Geneesk 1948;92:3732–3747.
105. U. S. Public Health Service. Smoking and health. Report of the advisory committee to the Surgeon General of the Public Health Service. DHEW Publication No. (PHS) 1103. Washington, DC: U.S. Government Printing Office, 1964.
106. Peto R, Lopez AD, Boreham J, et al. Mortality from smoking in developed countries 1950–2000: indirect estimates from National Vital Statistics. Oxford: Oxford University Press, 1994.
107. Tobacco. In: Stewart BW, Kleihues P, International Agency for Research on Cancer, eds. World Cancer Report. Lyon: IARC Press, 2003:22–28.
108. U. S. Department of Health and Human Services. Reducing the health consequences of smoking: 25 years of progress: a report of the Surgeon General. Publication No. (CDC) 89–8411. Washington, DC: U.S. Department of Health and Human Services U.S. Government Printing Office, 1989.
109. Hammond EC. Smoking in relation to the death rates of one million men and women. Natl Cancer Inst Monogr 1966;19:127–204.
110. Dube M, Green CR. Methods of collection of smoke for analytical purposes. Recent Adv Tobacco Sci 1984;10: 88–150.
111. Wynder EL, Hoffman D. Tobacco and tobacco smoke: studies in experimental carcinogenesis. New York: Academic Press, 1967.
112. Hecht SS. Tobacco smoke carcinogens and lung cancer. J Natl Cancer Inst 1999;91(14):1194–1210.
113. Burns DM. Tobacco smoking. In: Samet JM, ed. Epidemiology of lung cancer. New York: Marcel Dekker, 1994.

114. Schraufnagel D, Peloquin A, Pare JA, et al. Differentiating bronchioloalveolar carcinoma from adenocarcinoma. Am Rev Respir Dis 1982;125(1):74–79.
115. Doll R, Peto R. Cigarette smoking and bronchial carcinoma: dose and time relationships among regular smokers and lifelong non-smokers. J Epidemiol Community Health 1978;32(4):303–313.
116. Flanders WD, Lally CA, Zhu BP, et al. Lung cancer mortality in relation to age, duration of smoking, and daily cigarette consumption: results from Cancer Prevention Study II. Cancer Res 2003;63(19):6556–6562.
117. Garfinkel L, Stellman SD. Smoking and lung cancer in women: findings in a prospective study. Cancer Res 1988; 48(23):6951–6955.
118. U. S. Department of Health and Human Services. The health consequences of smoking: cancer. A report of the Surgeon General. Report No. (PHS) 82–50179. Washington, DC: U.S. Department of Health and Human Services, 1982.
119. Peto R, Parish SE, Gray RG. There is no such thing as aging, and cancer is not related to it. In: Likhachev A, Anisimov V, Montesano R, eds. IARC Sci Publication No. 58. Lyon: International Agency for Research on Cancer, 1985:43–53.
120. Knoke JD, Shanks TG, Vaughn JW, et al. Lung cancer mortality is related to age in addition to duration and intensity of cigarette smoking: an analysis of CPS-I data. Cancer Epidemiol Biomarkers Prev 2004;13(6):949–957.
121. Winters TH, Di Franza JR. Radioactivity in cigarette smoking. N Engl J Med 1982;306(6):364–365.
122. Martell EA. Radioactivity of tobacco trichomes and insoluble cigarette smoke particles. Nature 1974;249(454): 215–217.
123. U.S. Department of Health and Human Services. The health effects of active smoking: a report of the Surgeon General. Washington, DC: U.S. Government Printing Office, 2004.
124. Bross ID, Gibson R. Risks of lung cancer in smokers who switch to filter cigarettes. Am J Public Health Nations Health 1968;58(8):1396–1403.
125. Wynder EL, Mabuchi K, Beattie EJ Jr. The epidemiology of lung cancer. Recent trends. JAMA 1970;213(13): 2221–2228.
126. Hammond EC, Garfinkel L, Seidman H, et al. "Tar" and nicotine content of cigarette smoke in relation to death rates. Environ Res 1976;12(3):263–274.
127. Dean G, Lee PN, Todd GF, et al. Report on a second retrospective mortality study in northeast England. Part I: Factors related to mortality from lung cancer, bronchitis, heart disease and stroke in Cleveland County with particular emphasis on the relative risks associated with filter and plain cigarettes. Paper No. 14, part I. London: Tobacco Research Council, 1977.
128. Hawthorne VM, Fry JS. Smoking and health: the association between smoking behaviour, total mortality, and cardiorespiratory disease in west central Scotland. J Epidemiol Community Health 1978;32(4):260–266.
129. Rimington J. The effect of filters on the incidence of lung cancer in cigarette smokers. Environ Res 1981;24(1):162–166.
130. Lubin JH, Blot WJ, Berrino F, et al. Patterns of lung cancer risk according to type of cigarette smoked. Int J Cancer 1984;33(5):569–576.
131. Wynder EL, Kabat GC. The effect of low-yield cigarette smoking on lung cancer risk. Cancer 1988;62(6):1223–1230.
132. Pathak DR, Samet JM, Humble CG, et al. Determinants of lung cancer risk in cigarette smokers in New Mexico. J Natl Cancer Inst 1986;76(4):597–604.
133. Joly OG, Lubin JH, Caraballoso M. Dark tobacco and lung cancer in Cuba. J Natl Cancer Inst 1983;70(6): 1033–1039.
134. Wilcox HB, Schoenberg JB, Mason TJ, et al. Smoking and lung cancer: risk as a function of cigarette tar content. Prev Med 1988;17(3):263–272.
135. Harris JE, Thun MJ, Mondul AM, et al. Cigarette tar yeilds in relation to mortality from lung cancer in the cancer prevention study II prospective cohort, 1982–1988. Br Med J 2004;328:1–8.
136. Carpenter CL, Jarvik ME, Morgenstern H, et al. Mentholated cigarette smoking and lung-cancer risk. Ann Epidemiol 1999;9(2):114–120.
137. Hoffmann D, Hoffmann I. The changing cigarette, 1950–1995. J Toxicol Environ Health 1997;50(4):307–364.
138. Cederlof R, Friberg L, Hrubec Z, et al. The relationship of smoking and smoke social covariables to mortality and cancer morbidity. A ten year follow-up in a probability sample of 55000 Swedish subjects age 18 to 69, Part I and Part 2. Stockholm, Sweden: The Karolinska Institute, 1975.
139. Zang EA, Wynder EL. Differences in lung cancer risk between men and women: examination of the evidence. J Natl Cancer Inst 1996;88:183–192.
140. Perneger TV. Sex, smoking, and cancer: a reappraisal. J Natl Cancer Inst 2001;93:1600–1602.
141. Thun MJ, Henley SJ, Calle EE. Tobacco use and cancer: an epidemiologic perspective for geneticists. Oncogene 2002;21:7307–7325.
142. Khuder SA. Effect of cigarette smoking on major histological types of lung cancer: a meta-analysis. Lung Cancer 2001;31:139–148.
143. Thun MJ, Day-Lally CA, Calle EE, et al. Excess mortality among cigarette smokers: changes in a 20–year interval. Am J Public Health 1995;85(9):1223–1230.
144. Thun MJ, Myers DG, Day-Lally C, et al. Age and the exposure-response relationships between cigarette smoking and premature death in Cancer Prevention Study II. In: Burns DM, Garfinkel L, Samet J, eds. Smoking and tobacco control monograph no. 8: Changes in cigarette-related disease risks and their implication for prevention and control. Bethesda, MD: U.S. Department of Health and Human Services, Pubic Health Service, National Institutes of Health, National Cancer Institute, 1997:383–413.
145. Olak J, Colson Y. Gender differences in lung cancer: have we really come a long way, baby? J Thorac Cardiovasc Surg 2004;128(3):346–351.

146. Patel JD, Bach PB, Kris MG. Lung cancer in US women. JAMA 2004;291:1763–1768.
147. Jemal AR, Travis WD, Tarone RE, et al. Lung cancer rates convergence in young men and women in the United States: analysis by birth cohort and histologic type. Int J Cancer 2003;105:101–107.
148. Beckett AH, Gorrod JW, Jenner P. The effect of smoking on nicotine metabolism in vivo in man. J Pharm Pharmacol 1971;23:62S-7S.
149. Rivera MP, Stover DE. Gender and lung cancer. Clin Chest Med 2004;25(2):391–400.
150. Parkin JE, Tyczynski JE, Boffetta J, et al. Lung cancer epidemiology and etiology. In: Travis WD, Brambilla E, Kourad H, Muller-Hermelink HK, Harris CC, eds. Tumours of the lung, pleura, thymus and heart. Lyon, France: IARC Press, 2004.
151. Muscat JE, Joshua E, Stellman SD, et al. Cigarette smoking and large cell carcinoma of the lung. Cancer Epidemiol Biomarkers Prev 1997;7:477–480.
152. Hoffmann D, Rivenson A, Hecht SS. The biological significance of tobacco-specific N-nitrosamines: smoking and adenocarcinoma of the lung. Crit Rev Toxicol 1996;26(2): 199–211.
153. Stellman SD, Muscat JE, Thompson S, et al. Risk of squamous cell carcinoma and adenocarcinoma of the lung in relation to lifetime filter cigarette smoking. Cancer 1997; 80(3):382–388.
154. U.S. Department of Health and Human Services. The health benefits of smoking cessation. A report of the Surgeon General. Report No. (CDC) 90–8416. Washington, DC: U.S. Department of Health and Human Services, 1990.
155. Lubin JH, Blot WJ, Berrino F, et al. Modifying risk of developing lung cancer by changing habits of cigarette smoking. Br Med J 1984;288:1953–1956.
156. Brown CC, Chu KC. Use of multistage models to infer stage affected by carcinogenic exposure: example of lung cancer and cigarette smoking. J Chronic Dis 1987;40(suppl 2):171S–179S.
157. Graham S, Levin ML. Smoking withdrawal in the reduction of risk of lung cancer. Cancer 1971;27(4):865–871.
158. Doll R, Peto R, Boreham J, et al. Mortality in relation to smoking: 50 years' observations on male British doctors. BMJ 2004;328(7455):1519–1527.
159. Halpern MT, Gillespie BW, Warner KE. Patterns of absolute risk of lung cancer mortality in former smokers. J Natl Cancer Inst 1993;85(6):457–464.
160. Godtfredsen NS, Prescott E, Osler M. Effect of smoking reduction on lung cancer risk. JAMA 2005;294(12):1505–1510.
161. Nicolaides-Bowman A, Wald NJ, Forey B, et al. International smoking statistics: a collection of historical data from 22 economically developed countries. Oxford, UK: Oxford University Press, 1993.
162. U. S. Department of Health and Human Services. Cigars: health effects and trends. Bethesda, MD: National Cancer Institute U.S. Department of Health and Human Services National Institutes of Health, 1997.
163. U. S. Department of Agriculture. Tobacco situation and outlook report. Washington, DC: U.S. Department of Agriculture, 1999.
164. Anonymous. Cigar smoking among teenagers—United States, Massachusetts, and New York, 1996. MMWR 1997;46:433–440.
165. Baker F, Ainsworth SR, Dye JT, et al. Health risks associated with cigar smoking. JAMA 2000;284(6):735–740.
166. Frazier AL, Fisher L, Camargo CA, et al. Association of adolescent cigar use with other high-risk behaviors. Pediatrics 2000;106(2):E26.
167. Boffetta P, Pershagen G, Jockel KH, et al. Cigar and pipe smoking and lung cancer risk: a multicenter study from Europe. J Natl Cancer Inst 1999;91(8):697–701.
168. Appel BR, Guirguis G, Kim IS, et al. Benzene, benzo(a)pyrene, and lead in smoke from tobacco products other than cigarettes. Am J Public Health 1990;80(5): 560–564.
169. Brunnemann KD, Hoffmann D. Chemical studies on tobacco smoke. XXIV. A quantitative method for carbon monoxide and carbon dioxide in cigarette and cigar smoke. J Chromatogr Sci 1974;12(2):70–75.
170. Armitage A, Dollery C, Houseman T, et al. Absorption of nicotine from small cigars. Clin Pharmacol Ther 1978; 23(2):143–151.
171. Henningfield JE, Hariharan M, Kozlowski LT. Nicotine content and health risks of cigars. JAMA 1996;276(276): 1857.
172. Iribarren C, Tekawa IS, Sidney S, et al. Effect of cigar smoking on the risk of cardiovascular disease, chronic obstructive pulmonary disease, and cancer in men. N Engl J Med 1999;340(23):1773–1780.
173. Shapiro JA, Jacobs EJ, Thun MJ. Cigar smoking in men and risk of death from tobacco-related cancers. J Natl Cancer Inst 2000;92(4):333–337.
174. Higgins IT, Mahan CM, Wynder EL. Lung cancer among cigar and pipe smokers. Prev Med 1988;17(1):116–128.
175. Henley SJ, Thun MJ, Chao A, et al. Association between exclusive pipe smoking and mortality from cancer and other diseases. J Natl Cancer Inst 2004;96(11):853–861.
176. Wald NJ, Watt HC. Prospective study of effect of switching from cigarettes to pipes or cigars on mortality from three smoking related diseases. BMJ 1997;314(7098): 1860–1863.
177. Varsano S, Ganz I, Eldor N, et al. [Water-pipe tobacco smoking among school children in Israel: frequencies, habits, and attitudes]. Harefuah 2003;142(11):736–741, 807.
178. Maziak W, Ward KD, Afifi Soweid RA, et al. Tobacco smoking using a waterpipe: a re-emerging strain in a global epidemic. Tob Control 2004;13(4):327–333.
179. Wolfram RM, Chehne F, Oguogho A, et al. Narghile (water pipe) smoking influences platelet function and (iso-)eicosanoids. Life Sci 2003;74(1):47–53.
180. Shihadeh A. Investigation of mainstream smoke aerosol of the argileh water pipe. Food Chem Toxicol 2003;41(1): 143–152.
181. Gupta D, Boffetta P, Gaborieau V, et al. Risk factors of lung cancer in Chandigarh, India. Indian J Med Res 2001;113:142–150.
182. Wu TC, Tashkin DP, Djahed B, et al. Pulmonary hazards of smoking marijuana as compared with tobacco. N Engl J Med 1988;318(6):347–351.

183. Hoffman D, Brunneman DK, Gori GB, et al. On the carcinogenicity of marijuana smoke. Recent Adv Phytochem 1975;9:63–81.
184. Barsky SH, Roth MD, Kleerup EC, et al. Histopathologic and molecular alterations in bronchial epithelium in habitual smokers of marijuana, cocaine, and/or tobacco. J Natl Cancer Inst 1998;90(16):1198–1205.
185. IARC. Tobacco smoke and involuntary smoking. In: IARC monographs on the evaluation of carcinogenic risks to humans. Lyon, France: IARC Press, 2003.
186. Council NR. Environmental tobacco smoke. Washington, DC: National Academy Press, 1986.
187. Sasco AJ, Secretan MB, Straif K. Tobacco smoking and cancer: a brief review of recent epidemiological evidence. Lung Cancer 2004;45:s3–s9.
188. de Andrade M, Ebbert JO, Wampfler JA, et al. Environmental tobacco smoke exposure in women with lung cancer. Lung Cancer 2004;43(2):127–134.
189. Wang L, Lubin JH, Zhang SR, et al. Lung cancer and environmental tobacco smoke in a non-industrial area of China. Int J Cancer 2000;91:139–145.
190. Pandey M, Mathew A, Nair MK. Global perspective of tobacco habits and lung cancer: a lesson for third world countries. Eur J Cancer Prev 1999;8(4):271–279.
191. Shopland DR. Cigarette smoking as a cause of cancer. Cancer rates and risks. National Cancer Institutes of Health 1996;967:67–72.
192. Vineis P, Airoldi L, Veglia P, et al. Environmental tobacco smoke and risk of respiratory cancer and chronic obstructive pulmonary disease in former smokers and never smokers in the EPIC prospective study. BMJ 2005; 330(7486):277.
193. Brennan P, Buffler PA, Reynolds P, et al. Secondhand smoke exposure in adulthood and risk of lung cancer among never smokers: a pooled analysis of two large studies. Int J Cancer 2004;109(1):125–131.
194. Hackshaw AK, Law MR, Wald NJ. The accumulated evidence on lung cancer and environmental tobacco smoke. BMJ 1997;315(7114):980–988.
195. Fontham ET, Correa P, Reynolds P, et al. Environmental tobacco smoke and lung cancer in nonsmoking women. A multicenter study. JAMA 1994;271(22):1752–1759.
196. Boffetta P, Agudo A, Ahrens W, et al. Multicenter case-control study of exposure to environmental tobacco smoke and lung cancer in Europe. J Natl Cancer Inst 1998;90(19): 1440–1450.
197. Boffetta P. Epidemiology of environmental and occupational cancer. Oncogene 2004;23(38):6392–6403.
198. Boffetta P, Ahrens W, Nyberg F, et al. Exposure to environmental tobacco smoke and risk of adenocarcinoma of the lung. Int J Cancer 1999;83(5):635–639.
199. Akiba S, Kato H, Blot WJ. Passive smoking and lung cancer among Japanese women. Cancer Res 1986;46(9): 4804–4807.
200. Brownson RC, Reif JS, Keefe TJ, et al. Risk factors for adenocarcinoma of the lung. Am J Epidemiol 1987;125(1): 25–34.
201. Gao YT, Blot WJ, Zheng W, et al. Lung cancer among Chinese women. Int J Cancer 1987;40(5):604–609.
202. Stockwell HG, Goldman AL, Lyman GH, et al. Environmental tobacco smoke and lung cancer risk in nonsmoking women. J Natl Cancer Inst 1992;84(18):1417–1422.
203. Koo LC, Ho JH, Saw D, et al. Measurements of passive smoking and estimates of lung cancer risk among nonsmoking Chinese females. Int J Cancer 1987;39(2):162–169.
204. Lam TH, Kung IT, Wong CM, et al. Smoking, passive smoking and histological types in lung cancer in Hong Kong Chinese women. Br J Cancer 1987;56(5):673–678.
205. Garfinkel L, Auerbach O, Joubert L. Involuntary smoking and lung cancer: a case-control study. J Natl Cancer Inst 1985;75(3):463–469.
206. Kalandidi A, Katsouyanni K, Voropoulou N, et al. Passive smoking and diet in the etiology of lung cancer among non-smokers. Cancer Causes Control 1990;1(1): 15–21.
207. Zaridze D, Maximovitch D, Zemlyanaya G, et al. Exposure to environmental tobacco smoke and risk of lung cancer in non-smoking women from Moscow, Russia. Int J Cancer 1998;75(3):335–338.
208. Pershagen G, Hrubec Z, Svensson C. Passive smoking and lung cancer in Swedish women. Am J Epidemiol 1987;125: 17–24.
209. National Research Council. Health effects of exposure to radon (BEIR VI). Washington, DC: National Academy Press, 1999.
210. Lubin JH, Tomasek L, Edling C, et al. Estimating lung cancer mortality from residential radon using data for low exposures of miners. Radiat Res 1997;147(2):126–134.
211. Steindorf K, Lubin J, Wichmann HE, et al. Lung cancer deaths attributable to indoor radon exposure in West Germany. Int J Epidemiol 1995;24(3):485–492.
212. Leenhouts HP, Brugmans MJ. Calculation of the 1995 lung cancer incidence in The Netherlands and Sweden caused by smoking and radon: risk implications for radon. Radiat Environ Biophys 2001;40(1):11–21.
213. Samet JM. Radon and lung cancer. J Natl Cancer Inst 1989;81(10):745–757.
214. Samet JM, Pathak DR, Morgan MV, et al. Lung cancer mortality and exposure to radon progeny in a cohort of New Mexico underground uranium miners. Health Phys 1991;61(6):745–752.
215. United States National Academy of Sciences. Health risks of radon and other internally deposited alpha-emitters. Washington, DC: United States National Academy of Sciences, Committee on biological effects of ionizing radiation (BEIR IV) National Research Council, National Academy Press, 1988.
216. National Council on Radiation Protection and Measurements. Ionizing radiation exposure of the population of the United States. NCRP report No. 93. Bethesda, MD: National Council on Radiation Protection and Measurements, 1987.
217. Baysson H, Tirmarche M, Tymen G, et al. Indoor radon and lung cancer in France. Epidemiology 2004;15(6): 709–716.
218. Wichmann HE, Rosario AS, Heid IM, et al. Increased lung cancer risk due to residential radon in a pooled and

extended analysis of studies in Germany. Health Phys 2005;88(1):71–79.
219. Pershagen G, Akerblom G, Axelson O, et al. Residential radon exposure and lung cancer in Sweden. N Engl J Med 1994;330(3):159–164.
220. Lubin JH. Studies of radon and lung cancer in North America and China. Radiat Prot Dosimetry 2003;104(4): 315–319.
221. Alavanja MC, Lubin JH, Mahaffey JA, et al. Residential radon exposure and risk of lung cancer in Missouri. Am J Public Health 1999;89(7):1042–1048.
222. Darby S, Hill D, Auvinen A, et al. Radon in homes and risk of lung cancer: collaborative analysis of individual data from 13 European case-control studies. BMJ 2005;330(7485):223.
223. Krewski D, Lubin JH, Zielinski JM, et al. Residential radon and risk of lung cancer: a combined analysis of 7 North American case-control studies. Epidemiology 2005;16(2):137–145.
224. Lubin JH, Boice JD, Jr. Lung cancer risk from residential radon: meta-analysis of eight epidemiologic studies. J Natl Cancer Inst 1997;89(1):49–57.
225. Lubin JH, Wang ZY, Boice JD, et al. Risk of lung cancer and residential radon in China: pooled results of two studies. Int J Cancer 2004;109:132–137.
226. Brown LM, Pottern LM, Blot WJ. Lung cancer in relation to environmental pollutants emitted from industrial sources. Environ Res 1984;34(2):250–261.
227. Besso A, Nyberg F, Pershagen G. Air pollution and lung cancer mortality in the vicinity of a nonferrous metal smelter in Sweden. Int J Cancer 2003;107(3):448–452.
228. Pope CA, 3rd, Thun MJ, Namboodiri MM, et al. Particulate air pollution as a predictor of mortality in a prospective study of U.S. adults. Am J Respir Crit Care Med 1995;151(3 pt 1):669–674.
229. Dockery DW, Pope CA, 3rd, Xu X, et al. An association between air pollution and mortality in six U.S. cities. N Engl J Med 1993;329(24):1753–1759.
230. Nyberg F, Gustavsson P, Jarup L, et al. Urban air pollution and lung cancer in Stockholm. Epidemiology 2000; 11(5):487–495.
231. Whitrow MJ, Smith BJ, Pilotto LS, et al. Environmental exposure to carcinogens causing lung cancer: epidemiological evidence from the medical literature. Respirology 2003;8(4):513–521.
232. Boffetta P, Nyberg F. Contribution of environmental factors to cancer risk. Br Med Bull 2003;68:71–94.
233. Barbone F, Bovenzi M, Cavallieri F, et al. Air pollution and lung cancer in Trieste, Italy. Am J Epidemiol 1995; 141(12):1161–1169.
234. Hammond EC, Garfinkel L. General air pollution and cancer in the United States. Prev Med 1980;9(2):206–211.
235. Woodruff TJ, Caldwell J, Cogliano VJ, et al. Estimating cancer risk from outdoor concentrations of hazardous air pollutants in 1990. Environ Res 2000;82(3):194–206.
236. Parodi S, Stagnaro E, Casella C, et al. Lung cancer in an urban area in Northern Italy near a coke oven plant. Lung Cancer 2005;47(2):155–164.
237. Xu ZY, Blot WJ, Li G, et al. Environmental determinants of lung cancer in Shenyang, China. IARC Sci Publ 1991;(105):460–465.
238. Chen BH, Hong CJ, Pandey MR, et al. Indoor air pollution in developing countries. Lancet 1990;336(8730):1548.
239. Mumford JL, He XZ, Chapman RS, et al. Lung cancer and indoor air pollution in Xuan Wei, China. Science 1987; 235(4785):217–220.
240. Xu ZY, Blot WJ, Xiao HP, et al. Smoking, air pollution, and the high rates of lung cancer in Shenyang, China. J Natl Cancer Inst 1989;81(23):1800–1806.
241. Kleinerman RA, Wang Z, Wang L, et al. Lung cancer and indoor exposure to coal and biomass in rural China. J Occup Environ Med 2002;44(4):338–344.
242. Lan Q, Feng Z, Tian D, et al. p53 gene expression in relation to indoor exposure to unvented coal smoke in Xuan Wei, China. J Occup Environ Med 2001;43(3):226–230.
243. Lan Q, Chapman RS, Schreinemachers DM, et al. Household stove improvement and risk of lung cancer in Xuanwei, China. J Natl Cancer Inst 2002;94(11):826–835.
244. Kleinerman R, Wang Z, Lubin J, et al. Lung cancer and indoor air pollution in rural china. Ann Epidemiol 2000;10(7):469.
245. Zhou BS, Wang TJ, Guan P, et al. Indoor air pollution and pulmonary adenocarcinoma among females: a case-control study in Shenyang, China. Oncol Rep 2000;7(6):1253–1259.
246. Zhong L, Goldberg MS, Gao YT, et al. Lung cancer and indoor air pollution arising from Chinese-style cooking among nonsmoking women living in Shanghai, China. Epidemiology 1999;10(5):488–494.
247. Seow A, Poh WT, Teh M, et al. Fumes from meat cooking and lung cancer risk in Chinese women. Cancer Epidemiol Biomarkers Prev 2000;9(11):1215–1221.
248. ATSDR. Toxicological profile for arsenic. Atlanta, GA: Agency for Substances and Disease Registry, 2000.
249. Guo HR. Arsenic level in drinking water and mortality of lung cancer (Taiwan). Cancer Causes Control 2004; 15(2):171–177.
250. Chen CL, Hsu LI, Chiou HY, et al. Ingested arsenic, cigarette smoking, and lung cancer risk: a follow-up study in arseniasis-endemic areas in Taiwan. JAMA 2004; 292(24):2984–2990.
251. Siemiatycki J, Richardson L, Straif K, et al. Listing occupational carcinogens. Environ Health Perspect 2004; 112(15):1447–1459.
252. U. S. Department of Health and Human Services. The report on carcinogens. 11th ed. Washington, DC: Department for Health and Human Services, Public Health Service, National Toxicology Program, 2005.
253. Ives JC, Buffler PA, Greenberg SD. Environmental associations and histopathologic patterns of carcinoma of the lung: the challenge and dilemma in epidemiologic studies. Am Rev Respir Dis 1983;128(1):195–209.
254. Churg A. Lung cancer cell type and occupational exposure. In: Samet JM, ed. Epidemiology of lung cancer. New York: Marcel Dekker, 1994:413–436.
255. Mark EJ, Shin DH. Asbestos and the histogenesis of lung carcinoma. Semin Diagn Pathol 1992;9(2):110–116.

256. Selikoff IJ, Lee DHK. Asbestos and disease. New York: Academic Press, 1978.
257. Hammond EC, Selikoff IJ, Seidman H. Asbestos exposure, cigarette smoking and death rates. Ann NY Acad Sci 1979;330:473–490.
258. McDonald JC, McDonald AD. Epidemiology of asbestos-related lung cancer. In: Antman K, Aisner J, eds. Asbestos related malignancy. Orlando: Grune & Stratton, 1987:57–79.
259. Hughes JM, Weill H, Hammad YY. Mortality of workers employed in two asbestos cement manufacturing plants. Br J Ind Med 1987;44(3):161–174.
260. Cullen MR, Barnett MJ, Balmes JR, et al. Predictors of lung cancer among asbestos-exposed men in the beta-carotene and retinol efficacy trial. Am J Epidemiol 2005; 161(3):260–270.
261. Selikoff IJ, Hammond EC, Churg J. Asbestos exposure, smoking, and neoplasia. JAMA 1968;204(2):106–112.
262. Selikoff IJ, Hammond EC. Asbestos and smoking. JAMA 1979;242(5):458–459.
263. Selikoff IJ, Seidman H, Hammond EC. Mortality effects of cigarette smoking among amosite asbestos factory workers. J Natl Cancer Inst 1980;65(3):507–513.
264. McFadden D, Wright J, Wiggs B, et al. Cigarette smoke increases the penetration of asbestos fibers into airway walls. Am J Pathol 1986;123(1):95–99.
265. Churg A, Stevens B. Enhanced retention of asbestos fibers in the airways of human smokers. Am J Respir Crit Care Med 1995;151(5):1409–1413.
266. McFadden D, Wright JL, Wiggs B, et al. Smoking inhibits asbestos clearance. Am Rev Respir Dis 1986;133(3):372–374.
267. Mossman BT, Kamp DW, Weitzman SA. Mechanisms of carcinogenesis and clinical features of asbestos-associated cancers. Cancer Invest 1996;14(5):466–480.
268. Marsh JP, Mossman BT. Mechanisms of induction of ornithine decarboxylase activity in tracheal epithelial cells by asbestiform minerals. Cancer Res 1988;48(3):709–714.
269. Perderiset M, Marsch JP, Mossman BT. Activation of protein kinase C by crocidolite asbestos in hamster tracheal epithelial cells. Carcinogenesis 1991;12:1499–1502.
270. Heintz NH, Janssen YM, Mossman BT. Persistent induction of c-fos and c-jun expression by asbestos. Proc Natl Acad Sci U S A 1993;90(8):3299–3303.
271. Janssen YMW, Barchowsky A, Treadwell Mea. Asbestos induces nuclear factor kB (NF-kB) DNA-binding activity and NF-kB-dependent gene expression in tracheal epithelial cells. Proc Natl Acad Sci U S A 1995;92:8458–8462.
272. Reiss B, Tong C, Telang S, et al. Enhancement of benzo[a]pyrene mutagenicity by chrysotile asbestos in rat liver epithelial cells. Environ Res 1983;31:100–104.
273. Lilienfeld DE, Mandel JS, Coin P, et al. Projection of asbestos related diseases in the United States, 1985–2009. I. Cancer. Br J Ind Med 1988;45(5):283–291.
274. Acheson ED, Gardner MJ, Winter PD, et al. Cancer in a factory using amosite asbestos. Int J Epidemiol 1984;13(1): 3–10.
275. Dement JM, Harris RL Jr, Symons MJ, et al. Exposures and mortality among chrysotile asbestos workers. Part II: mortality. Am J Ind Med 1983;4(3):421–433.
276. Meurman LO, Kiviluoto R, Hakama M. Combined effect of asbestos exposure and tobacco smoking on Finnish anthophyllite miners and millers. Ann N Y Acad Sci 1979;330:491–495.
277. Roggli VL, Greenberg SD, Seitzman LH, et al. Pulmonary fibrosis, carcinoma, and ferruginous body counts in amosite asbestos workers. A study of six cases. Am J Clin Pathol 1980;73(4):496–503.
278. Rushton L, Alderson MR, Nagarajah CR. Epidemiological survey of maintenance workers in London Transport Executive bus garages and Chiswick Works. Br J Ind Med 1983;40(3):340–345.
279. Cheng VK, O'Kelly FJ. Asbestos exposure in the motor vehicle repair and servicing industry in Hong Kong. J Soc Occup Med 1986;36(3):104–106.
280. Williams RL, Muhlbaier JL. Asbestos brake emissions. Environ Res 1982;29(1):70–82.
281. Luce D, Bugel I, Goldberg P, et al. Environmental exposure to tremolite and respiratory cancer in New Caledonia: a case-control study. Am J Epidemiol 2000;151(3):259–265.
282. Mzileni O, Sitas F, Steyn K, et al. Lung cancer, tobacco, and environmental factors in the African population of the Northern Province, South Africa. Tob Control 1999;8(4):398–401.
283. Buchanan WD. Asbestosis and primary intrathoracic neoplasms. Ann NY Acad Sci 1965;132(1):507–518.
284. Karjalainen A, Anttila S, Vanhala E, et al. Asbestos exposure and the risk of lung cancer in a general urban population. Scand J Work Environ Health 1994;20(4): 243–250.
285. Whitwell F, Newhouse ML, Bennett DR. A study of the histologic cell types of lung cancer in workers suffering from asbestosis in the United Kingdom. Br J Ind Med 1974;31:298–303.
286. Hourihane DO, McCaughey WT. Pathological aspects of asbestosis. Postgrad Med J 1966;42(492):613–622.
287. Hasan FM, Nash G, Kazemi H. Asbestos exposure and related neoplasia. The 28 year experience of a major urban hospital. Am J Med 1978;65(4):649–654.
288. Johansson L, Albin M, Jakobsson K, et al. Histological type of lung carcinoma in asbestos cement workers and matched controls. Br J Ind Med 1992;49(9):626–630.
289. Craighead JE, Abraham JL, Churg A, et al. The pathology of asbestos-associated diseases of the lungs and pleural cavities: diagnostic criteria and proposed grading schema. Report of the Pneumoconiosis Committee of the College of American Pathologists and the National Institute for Occupational Safety and Health. Arch Pathol Lab Med 1982;106(11):544–596.
290. Churg A, Golden J. Current problems in the pathology of asbestos—related disease. Pathol Annu 1982;17(pt 2):33–66.
291. Hughes JM, Weill H. Asbestosis as a precursor of asbestos-related lung cancer: results of prospective mortality study. Br J Ind Med 1991;48:229–233.
292. Churg A. Asbestos, asbestosis, and lung cancer. Mod Pathol 1993;6(5):509–511.

293. Jones RN, Hughes JM, Weil H. Asbestos exposure, asbestosis and asbestos-attributable lung cancer. Thorax 1996; 51(suppl):S9–S15.
294. Weiss W. Asbestosis: a marker for the increased risk of lung cancer among workers exposed to asbestos. Chest 1999;115(2):536–549.
295. Roggli VL, Sanders LL. Asbestos content of lung tissue and carcinoma of the lung: a clinicopathologic correlation and mineral fiber analysis of 234 cases. Am Occup Hys 1999:109–117.
296. Hillerdal G. Pleural plaques and risk for bronchial carcinoma and mesothelioma. A prospective study. Chest 1994; 105(1):144–150.
297. Roggli VL, Hammar SP, Pratt PC, et al. Does asbestos or asbestosis cause carcinoma of the lung? Am J Ind Med 1994;26(6):835–838.
298. Abraham JL. Asbestos inhalation, not asbestosis, causes lung cancer. Am J Ind Med 1994;26(6):839–842.
299. Egilman D, Reinert A. Lung cancer and asbestos exposure: asbestosis is not necessary. Am J Ind Med 1996;30: 398–406.
300. Banks DE, Wang ML, Parker JE. Asbestos exposure, asbestosis, and lung cancer. Chest 1999;115(2):320–322.
301. Nelson HH, Christiani DC, Wiencke JK, et al. k-ras mutation and occupational asbestos exposure in lung adenocarcinoma: asbestos-related cancer without asbestosis. Cancer Res 1999;59(18):4570–4573.
302. Henderson DW, de Klerk NH, Hammar SP, et al. Asbestos and lung cancer: is it attributable to asbestosis or to asbestos fiber burden? In: Corrin B, ed. Lung cancer. New York: Churchill-Livingstone, 1997:83–118.
303. Henderson DW, Rodelsperger K, Woitowitz HJ, et al. After Helsinki: a multidisciplinary review of the relationship between asbestos exposure and lung cancer, with emphasis on studies published during 1997–2004. Pathology 2004:517–550.
304. Cook JR, Hill DA, Humphrey PA, et al. Squamous cell carcinoma arising in recurrent respiratory papillomatosis with pulmonary involvement: emerging common pattern of clinical features and human papillomavirus serotype association. Mod Pathol 2000;13(8):914–918.
305. Guillou L, Sahli R, Chaubert P, et al. Squamous cell carcinoma of the lung in a nonsmoking, nonirradiated patient with juvenile laryngotracheal papillomatosis. Evidence of human papillomavirus-11 DNA in both carcinoma and papillomas. Am J Surg Pathol 1991;15(9):891–898.
306. Lele SM, Pou AM, Ventura K, et al. Molecular events in the progression of recurrent respiratory papillomatosis to carcinoma. Arch Pathol Lab Med 2002;126(10):1184–1188.
307. Brouchet L, Valmary S, Dahan M, et al. Detection of oncogenic virus genomes and gene products in lung carcinoma. Br J Cancer 2005;92(4):743–746.
308. Welt A, Hummel M, Niedobitek G, et al. Human papillomavirus infection is not associated with bronchial carcinoma: evaluation by in situ hybridization and the polymerase chain reaction. J Pathol 1997;181:276–280.
309. Clavel CE, Nawrocki B, Bosseaux B, et al. Detection of human papillomavirus DNA in bronchopulmonary carcinomas by hybrid capture II: a study of 185 tumors. Cancer 2000;88(6):1347–1352.
310. Yousem SA, Ohori NP, Sonmez-Alpan E. Occurrence of human papillomavirus DNA in primary lung neoplasms. Cancer 1992;69(3):693–697.
311. Bohlmeyer T, Le TN, Shroyer AL, et al. Detection of human papillomavirus in squamous cell carcinomas of the lung by polymerase chain reaction. Am J Respir Cell Mol Biol 1998;18(2):265–269.
312. Jain N, Singh V, Hedau S, et al. Infection of human papillomavirus type 18 and p53 codon 72 polymorphism in lung cancer patients from India. Chest 2005;128(6):3999–4007.
313. Syrjanen KJ. HPV infections and lung cancer. J Clin Pathol 2002;55(12):885–891.
314. Papadopoulou K, Labropoulou V, Davaris P, et al. Detection of human papillomaviruses in squamous cell carcinomas of the lung. Virchows Arch 1998;433(1):49–54.
315. Gorgoulis VG, Zacharatos P, Kotsinas A, et al. Human papilloma virus (HPV) is possibly involved in laryngeal but not in lung carcinogenesis. Hum Pathol 1999;30(3): 274–283.
316. Tsuhako K, Nakazato I, Hirayasu T, et al. Human papillomavirus DNA in adenosquamous carcinoma of the lung. J Clin Pathol 1998;51(10):741–749.
317. Hirayasu T, Iwamasa T, Kamada Y, et al. Human papillomavirus DNA in squamous cell carcinoma of the lung. J Clin Pathol 1996;49(10):810–817.
318. Miyagi J, Tsuhako K, Kinjo T, et al. Recent striking changes in histological differentiation and rate of human papillomavirus infection in squamous cell carcinoma of the lung in Okinawa, a subtropical island in southern Japan. J Clin Pathol 2000;53(9):676–684.
319. Cheng YW, Chiou HL, Sheu GT, et al. The association of human papillomavirus 16/18 infection with lung cancer among nonsmoking Taiwanese women. Cancer Res 2001;61(7):2799–2803.
320. Chen YC, Chen JH, Richard K, et al. Lung adenocarcinoma and human papillomavirus infection. Cancer 2004; 101(6):1428–1436.
321. Han AJ, Xiong M, Zong YS. Association of Epstein-Barr virus with lymphoepithelioma-like carcinoma of the lung in southern China. Am J Clin Pathol 2000;114(2):220–226.
322. Butler AE, Colby TV, Weiss L, et al. Lymphoepithelioma-like carcinoma of the lung. Am J Surg Pathol 1989;14(7): 698.
323. Gal AA, Unger ER, Koss MN, et al. Detection of Epstein-Barr virus in lymphoepithelioma-like carcinoma of the lung. Mod Pathol 1991;4(2):264–268.
324. Pittaluga S, Wong MP, Chung LPea. Clonal Epstein-Barr virus in lymphoepithelioma-like carcinoma of the lung. Am J Surg Pathol 1993;17:678–682.
325. Kasai K, Sato Y, Kameya T, et al. Incidence of latent infection of Epstein-Barr virus in lung cancers—an analysis of EBER1 expression in lung cancers by in situ hybridization. J Pathol 1994;174(4):257–265.
326. Higashiyama M, Doi O, Kodama K, et al. Lymphoepithelioma-like carcinoma of the lung: analysis of two cases for Epstein-Barr virus infection. Hum Pathol 1995;26(11): 1278–1282.

327. Chan JK, Hui PK, Tsang WY, et al. Primary lymphoepithelioma-like carcinoma of the lung. A clinicopathologic study of 11 cases. Cancer 1995;76(3):413–422.
328. Chen F-F, Yan J-J, Lai W-W, et al. Epstein-Barr virus-associated nonsmall cell lung carcinoma. Undifferentiated "lymphoepithelioma-like" carcinoma as a distinct entity with better prognosis. Cancer 1998;82:2334–2342.
329. Chang YL, Wu CT, Shih JY, et al. New aspects in clinicopathologic and oncogene studies of 23 pulmonary lymphoepithelioma-like carcinomas. Am J Surg Pathol 2002; 26(6):715–723.
330. Begin LR, Eskandari J, Joncas J, et al. Epstein-Barr virus related lymphoepithelioma-like carcinoma of lung. J Surg Oncol 1987;36(4):280–283.
331. Anagnostopoulos I, Hummel M. Epstein-Barr virus in tumours. Histopathology 1996;29(4):297–315.
332. Weiss LM, Movahed LA, Butler AE, et al. Analysis of lymphoepithelioma and lymphoepithelioma-like carcinomas for Epstein-Barr viral genomes by in situ hybridization. Am J Surg Pathol 1989;13(8):625–631.
333. Castro CY, Ostrowski ML, Barrios R, et al. Relationship between Epstein-Barr virus and lymphoepithelioma-like carcinoma of the lung: a clinicopathologic study of 6 cases and review of the literature. Hum Pathol 2001; 32(8):863–872.
334. Huber M, Pavlova B, Muhlberger H, et al. Detection of the Epstein-Barr virus in primary adenocarcinoma of the lung with signet-ring cells. Virchows Arch 2002;441(1): 25–30.
335. Wong MP, Chung LP, Yuen ST, et al. In situ detection of Epstein-Barr virus in non-small cell lung carcinomas. J Pathol 1995;177(3):233–240.
336. Conway EJ, Hudnall SD, Lazarides A, et al. Absence of evidence for an etiologic role for Epstein-Barr virus in neoplasms of the lung and pleura. Mod Pathol 1996;9(5): 491–495.
337. Phelps RM, Smith DK, Heilig CM, et al. Cancer incidence in women with or at risk for HIV. Int J Cancer 2001; 94(5):753–757.
338. Herida M, Mary-Krause M, Kaphan R, et al. Incidence of non-AIDS-defining cancers before and during the highly active antiretroviral therapy era in a cohort of human immunodeficiency virus-infected patients. J Clin Oncol 2003;21(18):3447–3453.
339. Parker MS, Leveno DM, Campbell TJ, et al. AIDS-related bronchogenic carcinoma: fact or fiction? Chest 1998; 113(1):154–161.
340. Frisch M, Biggar RJ, Engels EA, et al. Association of cancer with AIDS-related immunosuppression in adults. JAMA 2001;285(13):1736–1745.
341. Grulich AE, Wan X, Law MG, et al. Risk of cancer in people with AIDS. AIDS 1999;13(7):839–843.
342. Gallagher B, Wang Z, Schymura MJ, et al. Cancer incidence in New York State acquired immunodeficiency syndrome patients. Am J Epidemiol 2001;154(6):544–556.
343. Serraino D, Boschini A, Carrieri Pea. Cancer risk among men with, or at risk of, HIV infection in Southern Europe. AIDS 2000;14:553–559.
344. Powles T, Nelson M, Bower M. HIV-related lung cancer—a growing concern? Int J STD AIDS 2003;14(10):647–651.
345. Bower M, Powles T, Nelson M, et al. HIV-related lung cancer in the era of highly active antiretroviral therapy. AIDS 2003;17(3):371–375.
346. Bonnet F, Lewden C, May T, et al. Malignancy-related causes of death in human immunodeficiency virus-infected patients in the era of highly active antiretroviral therapy. Cancer 2004;101(2):317–324.
347. Lewden C, Salmon D, Morlat P, et al. Causes of death among human immunodeficiency virus (HIV)-infected adults in the era of potent antiretroviral therapy: emerging role of hepatitis and cancers, persistent role of AIDS. Int J Epidemiol 2005;34(1):121–130.
348. Louie JK, Hsu LC, Osmond DH, et al. Trends in causes of death among persons with acquired immunodeficiency syndrome in the era of highly active antiretroviral therapy. J Infect Dis 2002:1023–1027.
349. Vyzula R, Remick SC. Lung cancer in patients with HIV-infection. Lung Cancer 1996;15(3):325–339.
350. Tirelli U, Spina M, Sandri S, et al. Lung carcinoma in 36 patients with human immunodeficiency virus infection. The Italian Cooperative Group on AIDS and Tumors. Cancer 2000;88(3):563–569.
351. Chiao EY, Krown SE. Update on non-acquired immunodeficiency syndrome-defining malignancies. Curr Opin Oncol 2003;15(5):389–397.
352. Lavole A, Wislez M, Antoine M, et al. Lung cancer, a new challenge in the HIV-infected population. Lung Cancer 2006;51(1):1–11.
353. Spano JP, Massiani MA, Bentata M, et al. Lung cancer in patients with HIV Infection and review of the literature. Med Oncol 2004;21(2):109–115.
354. Powles T, Thirwell C, Newsom-Davis T, et al. Does HIV adversely influence the outcome in advanced non-small-cell lung cancer in the era of HAART? Br J Cancer 2003; 89(3):457–459.
355. Wistuba II, Behrens C, Gazdar AF. Pathogenesis of non-AIDS-defining cancers: a review. AIDS Patient Care STDS 1999;13(7):415–426.
356. Wistuba, II, Behrens C, Milchgrub S, et al. Comparison of molecular changes in lung cancers in HIV-positive and HIV-indeterminate subjects. JAMA 1998;279(19):1554–1559.
357. Agostini C, Trentin L, Zambello R, et al. HIV-1 and lung. Infectivity, pathologenic mechanisms and cellular immune response taking place in the lower respiratory tract. Am Rev Respir Dis 1993;147:1038–1049.
358. Cooley TP. Non-AIDS-defining cancer in HIV-infected people. Hematol Oncol Clin North Am 2003;17(3):889–899.
359. Burke M, Furman A, Hoffman M, et al. Lung cancer in patients with HIV infection: is it AIDS-related? HIV Med 2004;5(2):110–114.
360. Semenzato G, de Rossi A, Agostini C. Human retroviruses and their aetiological link to pulmonary diseases. Eur Respir J 1993;6(7):925–929.
361. Hinds MW, Cohen HI, Kolonel LN. Tuberculosis and lung cancer risk in nonsmoking women. Am Rev Respir Dis 1982;125(6):776–778.

362. Zheng W, Blot WJ, Liao ML, et al. Lung cancer and prior tuberculosis infection in Shanghai. Br J Cancer 1987; 56(4):501–504.
363. Ko YC, Lee CH, Chen MJ, et al. Risk factors for primary lung cancer among non-smoking women in Taiwan. Int J Epidemiol 1997;26(1):24–31.
364. Howe GR, Lindsay J, Coppock E, et al. Isoniazid exposure in relation to cancer incidence and mortality in a cohort of tuberculosis patients. Int J Epidemiol 1979;8(4):305–312.
365. Campbell AH. Pulmonary tuberculosis, isoniazid and cancer. Br J Dis Chest 1970;64:141–149.
366. Brenner AV, Wang Z, Kleinerman RA, et al. Previous pulmonary diseases and risk of lung cancer in Gansu Province, China. Int J Epidemiol 2001;30(1):118–124.
367. Avalanja MCR, Brownson RC, Boice JD Jr, et al. Pre-existing lung disease and lung cancer among non-smoking women. Am J Epidemiol 1992;136:623–632.
368. Wu AH, Fontham ET, Reynolds P, et al. Previous lung disease and risk of lung cancer among lifetime nonsmoking women in the United States. Am J Epidemiol 1995;141(11):1023–1032.
369. Ohshima H, Bartsch H. Chronic infections and inflammatory processes as cancer risk factors: possible role of nitric oxide in carcinogenesis. Mutat Res 1994;305: 253–264.
370. Laurila AL, Anttila T, Laara E, et al. Serological evidence of an association between Chlamydia pneumoniae infection and lung cancer. Int J Cancer 1997;74(1):31–34.
371. Koyi H, Branden E, Gnarpe J, et al. An association between chronic infection with Chlamydia pneumoniae and lung cancer. A prospective 2-year study. APMIS 2001; 109(9):572–580.
372. Jackson LA, Wang SP, Nazar-Stewart V, et al. Association of Chlamydia pneumoniae immunoglobulin A seropositivity and risk of lung cancer. Cancer Epidemiol Biomarkers Prev 2000;9(11):1263–1266.
373. Kocazeybek B. Chronic Chlamydophila pneumoniae infection in lung cancer, a risk factor: a case-control study. J Med Microbiol 2003;52(Pt 8):721–726.
374. Littman AJ, White E, Jackson LA, et al. Chlamydia pneumoniae infection and risk of lung cancer. Cancer Epidemiol Biomarkers Prev 2004;13(10):1624–1630.
375. Littman AJ, Jackson LA, Vaughan TL. Chlamydia pneumoniae and lung cancer: epidemiologic evidence. Cancer Epidemiol Biomarkers Prev 2005;14(4):773–778.
376. Anttila T, Koskela P, Leinonen M, et al. Chlamydia pneumoniae infection and the risk of female early-onset lung cancer. Int J Cancer 2003;107(4):681–682.
377. Koh WP, Vincent TK, Chow M-CP, et al. Lack of association between chronic Chlamydophila pneumoniae infection and lung cancer among nonsmoking Chinese women in Singapore. Int J Cancer 2005;114:502–504.
378. Wong Y, Ward ME. Chlamydia pneumoniae and atherosclerosis. J Clin Pathol 1999;52(5):398–399.
379. Huittinen T, Leinonen M, Tenkanen L, et al. Synergistic effect of persistent Chlamydia pneumoniae infection, autoimmunity, and inflammation on coronary risk. Circulation 2003;107(20):2566–2570.
380. Nakachi K, Limtrakul P, Sonklin P, et al. Risk factors for lung cancer among Northern Thai women: epidemiological, nutritional, serological, and bacteriological surveys of residents in high- and low-incidence areas. Jpn J Cancer Res 1999;90(11):1187–1195.
381. Cohen BH. Chronic obstructive pulmonary disease: a challenge in genetic epidemiology. Am J Epidemiol 1980; 112(2):274–288.
382. Davis AL. Bronchogenic carcinoma in chronic obstructive pulmonary disease. JAMA 1876;235:621–622.
383. Mayne ST, Buenconsejo J, Janerich DT. Previous lung disease and risk of lung cancer among men and women nonsmokers. Am J Epidemiol 1999;149(1):13–20.
384. Shen XB, Wang GX, Huang YZ, et al. Analysis and estimates of attributable risk factors for lung cancer in Nanjing, China. Lung Cancer 1996;14(suppl 1):S107–S112.
385. Samet JM, Humble CG, Pathak DR. Personal and family history of respiratory disease and lung cancer risk. Am Rev Respir Dis 1986;134(3):466–470.
386. Skillrud DM, Offord KP, Miller RD. Higher risk of lung cancer in chronic obstructive pulmonary disease. A prospective, matched, controlled study. Ann Intern Med 1986;105(4):503–507.
387. Tockman MS, Anthonisen NR, Wright EC, et al. Airways obstruction and the risk for lung cancer. Ann Intern Med 1987;106(4):512–518.
388. Schabath MB, Delclos GL, Martynowicz MM, et al. Opposing effects of emphysema, hay fever, and select genetic variants on lung cancer risk. Am J Epidemiol 2005;161(5):412–422.
389. Alavanja MC, Brownson RC, Boice JD Jr, et al. Preexisting lung disease and lung cancer among nonsmoking women. Am J Epidemiol 1992;136(6):623–632.
390. Kuller LH, Ockene J, Meilahn E, et al. Relation of forced expiratory volume in one second (FEV1) to lung cancer mortality in the Multiple Risk Factor Intervention Trial (MRFIT). Am J Epidemiol 1990;132(2):265–274.
391. Lange P, Nyboe J, Appleyard M, et al. Ventilatory function and chronic mucus hypersecretion as predictors of death from lung cancer. Am Rev Respir Dis 1990;141(3): 613–617.
392. Littman AJ, Thornquist MD, White E, et al. Prior lung disease and risk of lung cancer in a large prospective study. Cancer Causes Control 2004;15(8):819–827.
393. Santillan AA, Camargo CA Jr, Colditz GA. A meta-analysis of asthma and risk of lung cancer (United States). Cancer Causes Control 2003;14(4):327–334.
394. Turner MC, Chen Y, Krewski D, et al. An overview of the association between allergy and cancer. Int J Cancer 2006.
395. Daniels CE, Jett JR. Does interstitial lung disease predispose to lung cancer? Curr Opin Pulm Med 2005;11: 431–437.
396. Stack BH, Choo-Kang YF, Heard BE. The prognosis of cryptogenic fibrosing alveolitis. Thorax 1972;27(5):535–542.
397. Turner-Warwick M, Lebowitz M, Burrows B, et al. Cryptogenic fibrosing alveolitis and lung cancer. Thorax 1980; 35(7):496–499.

398. Matsushita H, Tanaka S, Saiki Y, et al. Lung cancer associated with usual interstitial pneumonia. Pathol Int 1995; 45(12):925–932.
399. Hubbard R, Venn A, Lewis S, et al. Lung cancer and cryptogenic fibrosing alveolitis. A population-based cohort study. Am J Respir Crit Care Med 2000;161(1):5–8.
400. Aubry MC, Myers JL, Douglas WW, et al. Primary pulmonary carcinoma in patients with idiopathic pulmonary fibrosis. Mayo Clin Proc 2002;77(8):763–770.
401. Kawasaki H, Nagai K, Yokose T, et al. Clinicopathological characteristics of surgically resected lung cancer associated with idiopathic pulmonary fibrosis. J Surg Oncol 2001;76(1):53–57.
402. Wells C, Mannino DM. Pulmonary fibrosis and lung cancer in the United States: analysis of the multiple cause of death mortality data, 1979 through 1991. South Med J 1996;89:505–510.
403. Harris JM, Cullinan P, McDonald JC. Does cryptogenic fibrosing alveolitis carry an increased risk of death from lung cancer? J Epidemiol Community Health 1998;52(9): 602–603.
404. Samet JM. Does idiopathic pulmonary fibrosis increase lung cancer risk? Am J Respir Crit Care Med 2000;161(1): 1–2.
405. Nagai A, Chiyotani A, Nakadate T, et al. Lung cancer in patients with idiopathic pulmonary fibrosis. Tohoku J Exp Med 1992;167(3):231–237.
406. Baumgartner KB, Samet JM, Stidley CA, et al. Cigarette smoking: a risk factor for idiopathic pulmonary fibrosis. Am J Respir Crit Care Med 1997;155(1):242–248.
407. Qunn L, Takemura T, Ikushima S, et al. Hyperplastic epithelial foci in honeycomb lesions in idiopathic pulmonary fibrosis. Virchows Arch 2002;441(3):271–278.
408. Hironaka M, Fukayama M. Pulmonary fibrosis and lung carcinoma: a comparative study of metaplastic epithelia in honeycombed areas of usual interstitial pneumonia with or without lung carcinoma. Pathol Int 1999;49(12):1060–1066.
409. Peters-Golden M, Wise RA, Hochberg M, et al. Incidence of lung cancer in systemic sclerosis. J Rheumatol 1985; 12(6):1136–1139.
410. Roumm AD, Medsger TA, Jr. Cancer and systemic sclerosis. An epidemiologic study. Arthritis Rheum 1985; 28(12):1336–1340.
411. Rosenthal AK, McLaughlin JK, Gridley G, et al. Incidence of cancer among patients with systemic sclerosis. Cancer 1995;76(5):910–914.
412. Hill CL, Nguyen AM, Roder D, et al. Risk of cancer in patients with scleroderma: a population based cohort study. Ann Rheum Dis 2003;62(8):728–731.
413. Chatterjee S, Severson RK, Weiss LK, et al. Risk of malignancy in scleroderma [abstract]. Arthritis Rheum 2000; 43(suppl):S315.
414. Sigurgeirsson B, Lindelof B, Edhag O, et al. Risk of cancer in patients with dermatomyositis or polymyositis. A population-based study. N Engl J Med 1992;326(6):363–367.
415. Chow WH, Gridley G, Mellemkjaer L, et al. Cancer risk following polymyositis and dermatomyositis: a nationwide cohort study in Denmark. Cancer Causes Control 1995; 6(1):9–13.
416. Hill CL, Zhang Y, Sigurgeirsson B, et al. Frequency of specific cancer types in dermatomyositis and polymyositis: a population-based study. Lancet 2001;357(9250):96–100.
417. Buchbinder R, Hill CL. Malignancy in patients with inflammatory myopathy. Curr Rheumatol Rep 2002;4(5): 415–426.
418. Bjelke E. Dietary vitamin A and human lung cancer. Int J Cancer 1975;15(4):561–565.
419. Wei Q, Shen H, Wang LE, et al. Association between low dietary folate intake and suboptimal cellular DNA repair capacity. Cancer Epidemiol Biomarkers Prev 2003;12(10): 963–969.
420. Wright ME, Mayne ST, Swanson CA, et al. Dietary carotenoids, vegetables, and lung cancer risk in women: the Missouri women's health study (United States). Cancer Causes Control 2003;14(1):85–96.
421. Skuladottir H, Tjoenneland A, Overvad K, et al. Does insufficient adjustment for smoking explain the preventive effects of fruit and vegetables on lung cancer? Lung Cancer 2004;45(1):1–10.
422. Neuhouser ML, Patterson RE, Thornquist MD, et al. Fruits and vegetables are associated with lower lung cancer risk only in the placebo arm of the beta-carotene and retinol efficacy trial (CARET). Cancer Epidemiol Biomarkers Prev 2003;12(4):350–358.
423. Holick CN, Michaud DS, Stolzenberg-Solomon R, et al. Dietary carotenoids, serum beta-carotene, and retinol and risk of lung cancer in the alpha-tocopherol, beta-carotene cohort study. Am J Epidemiol 2002;156(6):536–547.
424. Feskanich D, Ziegler RG, Michaud DS, et al. Prospective study of fruit and vegetable consumption and risk of lung cancer among men and women. J Natl Cancer Inst 2000;92(22):1812–1823.
425. Smith Warner SA, Spiegelman D, Yaun SS, et al. Fruits, vegetables and lung cancer: a pooled analysis of cohort studies. Int J Cancer 2003;107(6):1001–1011.
426. Miller AB, Altenburg HP, Bueno-de-Mesquita B, et al. Fruits and vegetables and lung cancer: findings from the European Prospective Investigation into Cancer and Nutrition. Int J Cancer 2004;108(2):269–276.
427. Mannisto S, Smith-Warner SA, Spiegelman D, et al. Dietary carotenoids and risk of lung cancer in a pooled analysis of seven cohort studies. Cancer Epidemiol Biomarkers Prev 2004;13(1):40–48.
428. Brennan P, Fortes C, Butler J, et al. A multicenter case-control study of diet and lung cancer among non-smokers. Cancer Causes Control 2000;11(1):49–58.
429. Subar AF, Harlan LC, Mattson ME. Food and nutrient intake differences between smokers and non-smokers in the US. Am J Public Health 1990;80(11):1323–1329.
430. Thornton A, Lee P, Fry J. Differences between smokers, ex-smokers, passive smokers and non-smokers. J Clin Epidemiol 1994;47(10):1143–1162.
431. The alpha Tocopherol B Carotene Cancer Prevention Study Group. The effect of vitamin E and B carotene on the incidence of lung cancer and other cancers in male smokers. N Engl J Med 1994(330):1029–1035.
432. Omenn GS, Goodman GE, Thornquist MD, et al. Effects of a combination of beta carotene and vitamin A on lung

cancer and cardiovascular disease. N Engl J Med 1996; 334(18):1150–1155.
433. Hennekens CH, Buring JE, Manson JE, et al. Lack of effect of long-term supplementation with beta carotene on the incidence of malignant neoplasms and cardiovascular disease. N Engl J Med 1996;334(18):1145–1149.
434. Neuhouser ML. Dietary flavonoids and cancer risk: evidence from human population studies. Nutr Cancer 2004;50(1):1–7.
435. Shapiro TA, Fahey JW, Wade KL, et al. Chemoprotective glucosinolates and isothiocyanates of broccoli sprouts: metabolism and excretion in humans. Cancer Epidemiol Biomarkers Prev 2001;10(5):501–508.
436. Zhang Y, Talalay P, Cho C, et al. A major induce of anticarcinogenic protective enzymes from broccoli: isolation and elucidation of structure. Proc Natl Acad Sci 1992(89): 2399–2403.
437. Lampe JW, Chen C, Li S, et al. Modulation of human glutathione S-transferases by botanically defined vegetable diets. Cancer Epidemiol Biomarkers Prev 2000;9(8):787–793.
438. Zhao B, Seow A, Lee EJ, et al. Dietary isothiocyanates, glutathione S-transferase-M1, -T1 polymorphisms and lung cancer risk among Chinese women in Singapore. Cancer Epidemiol Biomarkers Prev 2001;10(10):1063–1067.
439. Spitz MR, Duphoma CM, Detry MA, et al. Dietary intake of isothiocyanates: Evidence of a joint effect with glutathione S-transferase polymorphisms in lung cancer risk. Cancer 2000;9:1017–1020.
440. London SJ, Yuan JM, Chung FL, et al. Isothiocyanates, glutathione S-transferase M1 and T1 polymorphisms, and lung-cancer risk: a prospective study of men in Shanghai, China. Lancet 2000;356(9231):724–729.
441. Wang LI, Giovannucci EL, Hunter D, et al. Dietary intake of Cruciferous vegetables, glutathione S-transferase (GST) polymorphisms and lung cancer risk in a Caucasian population. Cancer Causes Control 2004;15(10): 977–985.
442. Mattson ME, Pollack ES, Cullen JW. What are the odds that smoking will kill you? Am J Public Health 1987;77(4): 425–431.
443. Jin YT, Xu YC, Yang RD, et al. Familial aggregation of lung cancer in a high incidence area in China. Br J Cancer 2005;92(7):1321–1325.
444. Etzel CJ, Amos CI, Spitz MR. Risk for smoking-related cancer among relatives of lung cancer patients. Cancer Res 2003;63(23):8531–8535.
445. Tokuhata GK, Lillienfeld AM. Familial aggregation of lung cancer in humans. J Natl Cancer Inst 1963;30:289–312.
446. Jonsson S, Thorsteinsdottir U, Gudbjartsson DF, et al. Familial risk of lung carcinoma in the Icelandic population. JAMA 2004;292(24):2977–2983.
447. Li X, Hemminki K. Familial and second lung cancers: a nation-wide epidemiologic study from Sweden. Lung Cancer 2003;39(3):255–263.
448. Li X, Hemminki K. Inherited predisposition to early onset lung cancer according to histological type. Int J Cancer 2004;112(3):451–457.
449. Sellers TA, Elston RC, Atwood LD, et al. Lung cancer histologic type and family history of cancer. Cancer 1992; 69:86–91.
450. Gauderman WJ, Morrison JL. Evidence for age-specific genetic relative risks in lung cancer. Am J Epidemiol 2000;151(1):41–49.
451. Sellers TA, Chen PL, Potter JD, et al. Segregation analysis of smoking-associated malignancies: evidence for Mendelian inheritance. Am J Med Genet 1994;52(3):308–314.
452. Wu PF, Lee CH, Wang MJ, et al. Cancer aggregation and complex segregation analysis of families with female non-smoking lung cancer probands in Taiwan. Eur J Cancer 2004;40(2):260–266.
453. Sellers TA, Bailey-Wilson JE, Elston RC, et al. Evidence for mendelian inheritance in the pathogenesis of lung cancer. J Natl Cancer Inst 1990;82(15):1272–1279.
454. Braun MM, Caporaso NE, Page WF, et al. Genetic component of lung cancer: cohort study of twins. Lancet 1994; 344(8920):440–443.
455. Bailey-Wilson JE, Amos CI, Pinney SM, et al. A major lung cancer susceptibility locus maps to chromosome 6q23–25. Am J Hum Genet 2004;75(3):460–474.
456. Nakachi K, Imai K, Hayashi S, et al. Polymorphisms of the CYP1A1 and glutathione S-transferase genes associated with susceptibility to lung cancer in relation to cigarette dose in a Japanese population. Cancer Res 1993;53(13): 2994–2999.
457. Shields PG, Caporaso NE, Falk RT, et al. Lung cancer, race, and a CYP1A1 genetic polymorphism. Cancer Epidemiol Biomarkers Prev 1993;2(5):481–485.
458. Sugimura H, Suzuki I, Hamada GS, et al. Cytochrome P-450 lA1 genotype in lung cancer patients and controls in Rio de Janeiro, Brazil. Cancer Epidemiol Biomarkers Prev 1994;3(2):145–148.
459. Vineis P, Veglia F, Benhamou S, et al. CYP1A1 T3801 C polymorphism and lung cancer: a pooled analysis of 2451 cases and 3358 controls. Int J Cancer 2003;104(5):650–657.
460. Le Marchand L, Guo C, Benhamou S, et al. Pooled analysis of the CYP1A1 exon 7 polymorphism and lung cancer (United States). Cancer Causes Control 2003;14(4):339–346.
461. Amos CI. Host factors in lung cancer risk: A review of interdisciplinary studies. Cancer Epidemiol Biomarkers Prev 1 1992:505–513.
462. Shaw GL, Falk RT, Deslauriers J, et al. Debrisoquine metabolism and lung cancer risk. Cancer Epidemiol Biomarkers Prev 1995;4(1):41–48.
463. Christensen PM, Gotzsche PC, Brosen K. The sparteine/debrisoquine (CYP2D6) oxidation polymorphism and the risk of lung cancer: a meta-analysis. Eur J Clin Pharmacol 1997;51(5):389–393.
464. Rostami-Hodjegan A, Lennard MS, Woods HF, et al. Meta-analysis of studies of the CYP2D6 polymorphism in relation to lung cancer and Parkinson's disease. Pharmacogenetics 1998;8(3):227–238.
465. Houlston RS. Glutathione S-transferase M1 status and lung cancer risk: a meta-analysis. Cancer Epidemiol Biomarkers Prev 1999;8(8):675–682.

466. Benhamou S, Lee WJ, Alexandrie AK, et al. Meta- and pooled analyses of the effects of glutathione S-transferase M1 polymorphisms and smoking on lung cancer risk. Carcinogenesis 2002;23(8):1343–1350.
467. Bennett WP, Alavanja MC, Blomeke B, et al. Environmental tobacco smoke, genetic susceptibility, and risk of lung cancer in never-smoking women. J Natl Cancer Inst 1999;91(23):2009–2014.
468. Vineis P, Martone T. Genetic-environmental interactions and low-level exposure to carcinogens. Epidemiology 1995;6(4):455–457.
469. Hung RJ, Boffetta P, Brockmoller J, et al. CYP1A1 and GSTM1 genetic polymorphisms and lung cancer risk in Caucasian non-smokers: a pooled analysis. Carcinogenesis 2003;24(5):875–882.
470. Raunio H, Husgafvel-Pursiainen K, Anttila S, et al. Diagnosis of polymorphisms in carcinogen-activating and inactivating enzymes and cancer susceptibility—a review. Gene 1995;159(1):113–121.
471. Perera FP. Molecular epidemiology: insights into cancer susceptibility, risk assessment and prevention. J Natl Cancer Inst 1996;88:496–509.
472. Li D, Wang M, Cheng L, et al. In vitro induction of benzo(a)pyrene diol epoxide-DNA adducts in peripheral lymphocytes as a susceptibility marker for human lung cancer. Cancer Res 1996;56(16):3638–3641.
473. Zienolddiny S, Campa D, Lind H, et al. Polymorphisms of DNA repair genes and risk of non-small cell lung cancer. Carcinogenesis 2006;27(3):560–567.
474. Wei Q, Cheng L, Hong WK, et al. Reduced DNA repair capacity in lung cancer patients. Cancer Res 1996;56(18): 4103–4107.
475. Butkiewicz D, Rusin M, Enewold L, et al. Genetic polymorphisms in DNA repair genes and risk of lung cancer. Carcinogenesis 2001;22(4):593–597.
476. Goode EL, Ulrich CM, Potter JD. Polymorphisms in DNA repair genes and associations with cancer risk. Cancer Epidemiol Biomarkers Prev 2002;11(12):1513–1530.
477. Shen M, Rothman N, Berndt SI, et al. Polymorphisms in folate metabolic genes and lung cancer risk in Xuan Wei, China. Lung Cancer 2005;49(3):299–309.
478. Economou P, Lechner JF, Samet JM. Familial and genetic factors in the pathogenesis of lung cancer. In: Samet JM, ed. Epidemiology of lung cancer. New York: Marcel Dekker, 1994:353–396.
479. Smith RA, Cokkinides V, Eyre HJ. American Cancer Society Guidelines for the Early Detection of Cancer, 2005. CA Cancer J Clin 2005;55(1):31–44; quiz 55–56.
480. Weiss W, Boucot KR. The Philadelphia Pulmonary Neoplasm Research Project. Early roentgenographic appearance of bronchogenic carcinoma. Arch Intern Med 1974; 134(2):306–311.
481. An evaluation of radiologic and cytologic screening for the early detection of lung cancer: a cooperative pilot study of the American Cancer Society and the Veterans Administration. Cancer Res 1966;26(10):2083–2121.
482. Nash FA, Morgan JM, Tomkins JG. South London Lung Cancer Study. Br Med J 1968;2(607):715–721.
483. Wilde J. A 10 year follow-up of semi-annual screening for early detection of lung cancer in the Erfurt County, GDR. Eur Respir J 1989;2(7):656–662.
484. Brett GZ. The value of lung cancer detection by six-monthly chest radiographs. Thorax 1968;23(4):414–420.
485. Fontana RS, Sanderson DR, Taylor WF, et al. Early lung cancer detection: results of the initial (prevalence) radiologic and cytologic screening in the Mayo Clinic study. Am Rev Respir Dis 1984;130(4):561–565.
486. Frost JK, Ball WC Jr, Levin ML, et al. Early lung cancer detection: results of the initial (prevalence) radiologic and cytologic screening in the Johns Hopkins study. Am Rev Respir Dis 1984;130(4):549–554.
487. Flehinger BJ, Melamed MR, Zaman MB, et al. Early lung cancer detection: results of the initial (prevalence) radiologic and cytologic screening in the Memorial Sloan-Kettering study. Am Rev Respir Dis 1984;130(4):555–560.
488. Kubik A, Polak J. Lung cancer detection. Results of a randomized prospective study in Czechoslovakia. Cancer 1986;57(12):2427–2437.
489. Fontana RS, Sanderson DR, Woolner LB, et al. Screening for lung cancer. A critique of the Mayo Lung Project. Cancer 1991;67(4 suppl):1155–1164.
490. Marcus PM, Bergstralh EJ, Fagerstrom RM, et al. Lung cancer mortality in the Mayo Lung Project: impact of extended follow-up. J Natl Cancer Inst 2000;92(16):1308–1316.
491. Colby TV, Tazelaar HD, Travis WD, et al. Pathologic review of the Mayo Lung Project cancers [corrected]. Is there a case for misdiagnosis or overdiagnosis of lung carcinoma in the screened group? Cancer 2002;95(11): 2361–2365.
492. Oken MM, Marcus PM, Hu P, et al. Baseline chest radiograph for lung cancer detection in the randomized Prostate, Lung, Colorectal and Ovarian Cancer Screening Trial. J Natl Cancer Inst 2005;97(24):1832–1839.
493. Kaneko M, Eguchi K, Ohmatsu H, et al. Peripheral lung cancer: screening and detection with low-dose spiral CT versus radiography. Radiology 1996;201(3):798–802.
494. Sone S, Takashima S, Li F, et al. Mass screening for lung cancer with mobile spiral computed tomography scanner. Lancet 1998;351(9111):1242–1245.
495. Sobue T, Moriyama N, Kaneko M, et al. Screening for lung cancer with low-dose helical computed tomography: anti-lung cancer association project. J Clin Oncol 2002; 20(4):911–920.
496. Sone S, Li F, Yang ZG, et al. Results of three-year mass screening programme for lung cancer using mobile low-dose spiral computed tomography scanner. Br J Cancer 2001;84(1):25–32.
497. Henschke CI, McCauley DI, Yankelevitz DF, et al. Early Lung Cancer Action Project: overall design and findings from baseline screening. Lancet 1999;354(9173):99–105.
498. Henschke CI, Naidich DP, Yankelevitz DF, et al. Early lung cancer action project: initial findings on repeat screenings. Cancer 2001;92(1):153–159.
499. Swensen SJ, Jett JR, Sloan JA, et al. Screening for lung cancer with low-dose spiral computed tomography. Am J Respir Crit Care Med 2002;165(4):508–513.

500. Diederich S, Wormanns D, Semik M, et al. Screening for early lung cancer with low-dose spiral CT: prevalence in 817 asymptomatic smokers. Radiology 2002;222(3):773–781.
501. Diederich S, Thomas M, Semik M, et al. Screening for early lung cancer with low-dose spiral computed tomography: results of annual follow-up examinations in asymptomatic smokers. Eur Radiol 2004;14(4):691–702.
502. Jett JR. Limitations of screening for lung cancer with low-dose spiral computed tomography. Clin Cancer Res 2005;11(13 Pt 2):4988s-92s.
503. Diederich S, Wormanns D. Impact of low-dose CT on lung cancer screening. Lung Cancer 2004;45(suppl 2):S13–S19.
504. Brenner DJ. Radiation risks potentially associated with low-dose CT screening of adult smokers for lung cancer. Radiology 2004;231(2):440–445.
505. Berrington de Gonzalez A, Darby S. Risk of cancer from diagnostic X-rays: estimates for the UK and 14 other countries. Lancet 2004;363(9406):345–351.
506. Gohagan JK, Marcus PM, Fagerstrom RM, et al. Final results of the Lung Screening Study, a randomized feasibility study of spiral CT versus chest X-ray screening for lung cancer. Lung Cancer 2005;47(1):9–15.
507. Black WC, Welch HG. Screening for disease. AJR Am J Roentgenol 1997;168(1):3–11.
508. Hulka BS. Cancer screening. Degrees of proof and practical application. Cancer 1988;62(8 suppl):1776–1780.
509. Patz EF Jr, Goodman PC, Bepler G. Screening for lung cancer. N Engl J Med 2000;343(22):1627–1633.
510. Flieder DB, Port JL, Korst RJ, et al. Tumor size is a determinant of stage distribution in T1 non-small cell lung cancer. Chest 2005;128(4):2304–2308.
511. Mery CM, Pappas AN, Burt BM, et al. Diameter of non-small cell lung cancer correlates with long-term survival: implications for T stage. Chest 2005;128(5):3255–3260.
512. Collins VP, Loeffler RK, Tivey H. Observations on growth rates of human tumors. Am J Roentgenol Radium Ther Nucl Med 1956;76(5):988–1000.
513. Geddes DM. The natural history of lung cancer: a review based on rates of tumour growth. Br J Dis Chest 1979; 73(1):1–17.
514. Iwasaki A, Shirakusa T, Enatsu S, et al. The value of tumor volume in surgically resected non-small cell lung cancer. Thorac Cardiovasc Surg 2006;54(2):112–116.
515. Spratt JS, Meyer JS, Spratt JA. Rates of growth of human neoplasms: part II. J Surg Oncol 1996;61(1):68–83.
516. Friberg S, Mattson S. On the growth rates of human malignant tumors: implications for medical decision making. J Surg Oncol 1997;65(4):284–297.
517. Kerr KM, Lamb D. Actual growth rate and tumour cell proliferation in human pulmonary neoplasms. Br J Cancer 1984;50(3):343–349.
518. Saccomanno G, Saunders RP, Archer VE, et al. Cancer of the lung: the cytology of sputum prior to the development of carcinoma. Acta Cytol 1965;9(6):413–423.
519. Saccomanno G, Archer VE, Auerbach O, et al. Development of carcinoma of the lung as reflected in exfoliated cells. Cancer 1974;33(1):256–270.
520. Kennedy TC, Proudfoot SP, Franklin WA, et al. Cytopathological analysis of sputum in patients with airflow obstruction and significant smoking histories. Cancer Res 1996;56(20):4673–4678.
521. McWilliams A, MacAulay C, Gazdar AF, et al. Innovative molecular and imaging approaches for the detection of lung cancer and its precursor lesions. Oncogene 2002;21(45): 6949–6959.
522. Kennedy TC, Hirsch FR. Using molecular markers in sputum for the early detection of lung cancer: a review. Lung Cancer 2004;45(suppl 2):S21–S27.
523. Hirsch FR, Prindiville SA, Miller YE, et al. Fluorescence versus white-light bronchoscopy for detection of preneoplastic lesions: a randomized study. J Natl Cancer Inst 2001;93(18):1385–1391.
524. Lam S, Kennedy T, Unger M, et al. Localization of bronchial intraepithelial neoplastic lesions by fluorescence bronchoscopy. Chest 1998;113(3):696–702.
525. Chute CG, Greenberg ER, Baron J, et al. Presenting conditions of 1539 population-based lung cancer patients by cell type and stage in New Hampshire and Vermont. Cancer 1985;56(8):2107–2111.
526. Patel AM, Peters SG. Clinical manifestations of lung cancer. Mayo Clin Proc 1993;68(3):273–277.
527. SEER Stage Distribution by Sex, Lung and Bronchus Cancer, All Ages, SEER 9 Registries for 1975–79, 1985–89, 1995–2001. April 2005. www.seer.cancer.gov.
528. Tammemagi CM, Neslund-Dudas C, Simoff M, et al. Lung carcinoma symptoms—an independent predictor of survival and an important mediator of African-American disparity in survival. Cancer 2004;101(7):1655–1663.
529. Beckles MA, Spiro SG, Colice GL, et al. Initial evaluation of the patient with lung cancer: symptoms, signs, laboratory tests, and paraneoplastic syndromes. Chest 2003;123(1 suppl):97S–104S.
530. Pretreatment evaluation of non-small-cell lung cancer. The American Thoracic Society and the European Respiratory Society. Am J Respir Crit Care Med 1997;156(1):320–332.
531. Stenbygaard LE, Sorensen JB, Larsen H, et al. Metastatic pattern in non-resectable non-small cell lung cancer. Acta Oncol 1999;38(8):993–998.
532. Auerbach O, Garfinkel L, Parks VR. Histologic type of lung cancer in relation to smoking habits, year of diagnosis and sites of metastases. Chest 1975;67(4):382–387.
533. Line DH, Deeley TJ. The necropsy findings in carcinoma of the bronchus. Br J Dis Chest 1971;65(4):238–242.
534. Merchut MP. Brain metastases from undiagnosed systemic neoplasms. Arch Intern Med 1989;149(5):1076–1080.
535. Monsieur I, Meysman M, Noppen M, et al. Non-small-cell lung cancer with multiple paraneoplastic syndromes. Eur Respir J 1995;8(7):1231–1234.
536. Coggeshall J, Merrill W, Hande K, et al. Implications of hypercalcemia with respect to diagnosis and treatment of lung cancer. Am J Med 1986;80(2):325–328.
537. Martin TJ, Moseley JM, Gillespie MT. Parathyroid hormone-related protein: biochemistry and molecular biology. Crit Rev Biochem Mol Biol 1991;26(3–4):377–395.

538. Green KB, Silverstein RL. Hypercoagulability in cancer. Hematol Oncol Clin North Am 1996;10(2):499–530.
539. Sridhar KS, Lobo CF, Altman RD. Digital clubbing and lung cancer. Chest 1998;114(6):1535–1597.
540. Albrecht S, Keller A. Postchemotherapeutic reversibility of hypertrophic osteoarthropathy in a patient with bronchogenic adenocarcinoma. Clin Nucl Med 2003;28(6):463–466.
541. Hayashi M, Sekikawa A, Saijo A, et al. Successful treatment of hypertrophic osteoarthropathy by gefitinib in a case with lung adenocarcinoma. Anticancer Res 2005;25(3c):2435–2438.
542. Johnson BE, Chute JP, Rushin J, et al. A prospective study of patients with lung cancer and hyponatremia of malignancy. Am J Respir Crit Care Med 1997;156(5): 1669–1678.
543. Yalow RS, Eastridge CE, Higgins G Jr, et al. Plasma and tumor ACTH in carcinoma of the lung. Cancer 1979;44(5): 1789–1792.
544. Patel AM, Davila DG, Peters SG. Paraneoplastic syndromes associated with lung cancer. Mayo Clin Proc 1993; 68(3):278–287.
545. Hansen M, Bork E. Peptide hormones in patients with lung cancer. Recent Results Cancer Res 1985;99:180–186.
546. Rice D, Kim HW, Sabichi A, et al. The risk of second primary tumors after resection of stage I nonsmall cell lung cancer. Ann Thorac Surg 2003;76(4):1001–1007; discussion 1007–1008.
547. Kent MS, Korn P, Port JL, et al. Cost effectiveness of chest computed tomography after lung cancer resection: a decision analysis model. Ann Thorac Surg 2005;80(4):1215–1222; discussion 1222–1223.
548. Pairolero PC, Williams DE, Bergstralh EJ, et al. Postsurgical stage I bronchogenic carcinoma: morbid implications of recurrent disease. Ann Thorac Surg 1984;38(4):331–338.
549. Deschamps C, Pairolero PC, Trastek VF, et al. Multiple primary lung cancers. Results of surgical treatment. J Thorac Cardiovasc Surg 1990;99(5):769–777; discussion 777–778.
550. Martini N, Bains MS, Burt ME, et al. Incidence of local recurrence and second primary tumors in resected stage I lung cancer. J Thorac Cardiovasc Surg 1995;109(1):120–129.
551. Thomas PA Jr, Rubinstein L. Malignant disease appearing late after operation for T1 N0 non-small-cell lung cancer. The Lung Cancer Study Group. J Thorac Cardiovasc Surg 1993;106(6):1053–1058.
552. Schreiber G, McCrory DC. Performance characteristics of different modalities for diagnosis of suspected lung cancer: summary of published evidence. Chest 2003;123(1 suppl): 115S-28S.
553. Rivera MP, Detterbeck F, Mehta AC. Diagnosis of lung cancer: the guidelines. Chest 2003;123(1 suppl):129S-36S.
554. Delgado PI, Jorda M, Ganjei-Azar P. Small cell carcinoma versus other lung malignancies: diagnosis by fine-needle aspiration cytology. Cancer 2000;90(5):279–285.
555. Jones AM, Hanson IM, Armstrong GR, et al. Value and accuracy of cytology in addition to histology in the diagnosis of lung cancer at flexible bronchoscopy. Respir Med 2001;95(5):374–378.
556. Johnston WW. Fine needle aspiration biopsy versus sputum and bronchial material in the diagnosis of lung cancer. A comparative study of 168 patients. Acta Cytol 1988;32(5):641–646.
557. Cataluna JJ, Perpina M, Greses JV, et al. Cell type accuracy of bronchial biopsy specimens in primary lung cancer. Chest 1996;109(5):1199–1203.
558. Chuang MT, Marchevsky A, Teirstein AS, et al. Diagnosis of lung cancer by fibreoptic bronchoscopy: problems in the histological classification of non-small cell carcinomas. Thorax 1984;39(3):175–178.
559. Roggli VL, Vollmer RT, Greenberg SD, et al. Lung cancer heterogeneity: a blinded and randomized study of 100 consecutive cases. Hum Pathol 1985;16(6):569–579.
560. Dunnill MS, Gatter KC. Cellular heterogeneity in lung cancer. Histopathology 1986;10(5):461–475.
561. Mooi WJ, Dingemans KP, Wagenaar SS, et al. Ultrastructural heterogeneity of lung carcinomas: representativity of samples for electron microscopy in tumor classification. Hum Pathol 1990;21(12):1227–1234.
562. Field RW, Smith BJ, Platz CE, et al. Lung cancer histologic type in the surveillance, epidemiology, and end results registry versus independent review. J Natl Cancer Inst 2004;96(14):1105–1107.
563. Sorensen JB, Hirsch FR, Gazdar A, et al. Interobserver variability in histopathologic subtyping and grading of pulmonary adenocarcinoma. Cancer 1993;71(10):2971–2976.
564. Edwards SL, Roberts C, McKean ME, et al. Preoperative histological classification of primary lung cancer: accuracy of diagnosis and use of the non-small cell category. J Clin Pathol 2000;53(7):537–540.
565. Marchevsky AM, Changsri C, Gupta I, et al. Frozen section diagnoses of small pulmonary nodules: accuracy and clinical implications. Ann Thorac Surg 2004;78(5):1755–1759.
566. Novis DA, Zarbo RJ. Interinstitutional comparison of frozen section turnaround time. A College of American Pathologists Q-Probes study of 32868 frozen sections in 700 hospitals. Arch Pathol Lab Med 1997;121(6):559–567.
567. Gephardt GN, Zarbo RJ. Interinstitutional comparison of frozen section consultations. A college of American Pathologists Q-Probes study of 90,538 cases in 461 institutions. Arch Pathol Lab Med 1996;120(9):804–809.
568. Reed CE, Harpole DH, Posther KE, et al. Results of the American College of Surgeons Oncology Group Z0050 trial: the utility of positron emission tomography in staging potentially operable non-small cell lung cancer. J Thorac Cardiovasc Surg 2003;126(6):1943–1951.
569. Pozo-Rodriguez F, Martin de Nicolas JL, Sanchez-Nistal MA, et al. Accuracy of helical computed tomography and [18F] fluorodeoxyglucose positron emission tomography for identifying lymph node mediastinal metastases in potentially resectable non-small-cell lung cancer. J Clin Oncol 2005;23:8283–8285.
570. Hermens FH, Van Engelenburg TC, Visser FJ, et al. Diagnostic yield of transbronchial histology needle aspiration

in patients with mediastinal lymph node enlargement. Respiration 2003;70(6):631–635.
571. Yung RC. Tissue diagnosis of suspected lung cancer: selecting between bronchoscopy, transthoracic needle aspiration, and resectional biopsy. Respir Care Clin North Am 2003;9(1):51–76.
572. Yasufuku K, Chiyo M, Koh E, et al. Endobronchial ultrasound guided transbronchial needle aspiration for staging of lung cancer. Lung Cancer 2005;50:347–354.
573. Detterbeck FC, DeCamp MM Jr, Kohman LJ, et al. Lung cancer. Invasive staging: the guidelines. Chest 2003;123(1 suppl):167S–175S.
574. Gonzalez-Stawinski GV, Lemaire A, Merchant F, et al. A comparative analysis of positron emission tomography and mediastinoscopy in staging non-small cell lung cancer. J Thorac Cardiovasc Surg 2003;126(6):1900–1905.
575. Denoix PF. Enquete permanent dans les centres antercancereux. Bull Inst Nat Hyg 1946;1:70–75.
576. Mountain CF, Dresler CM. Regional lymph node classification for lung cancer staging. Chest 1997;111(6):1718–1723.
577. Mountain CF. Revisions in the International System for Staging Lung Cancer. Chest 1997;111(6):1710–1717.
578. Jett JR, Scott WJ, Rivera MP, et al. Guidelines on treatment of stage IIIB non-small cell lung cancer. Chest 2003;123(1 suppl):221S-5S.
579. Lopez-Encuentra A, Garcia-Lujan R, Rivas JJ, et al. Comparison between clinical and pathologic staging in 2,994 cases of lung cancer. Ann Thorac Surg 2005;79(3):974–979; discussion 979.
580. Sobin LH, Wittekind C, International Union against Cancer. TNM: classification of malignant tumours. 6th ed. New York: Wiley-Liss, 2002.
581. Tiffet O, Nicholson AG, Khaddage A, et al. Feasibility of the detection of the sentinel lymph node in peripheral non-small cell lung cancer with radio isotopic and blue dye techniques. Chest 2005;127(2):443–448.
582. Jiao X, Krasna MJ. Clinical significance of micrometastasis in lung and esophageal cancer: a new paradigm in thoracic oncology. Ann Thorac Surg 2002;74(1):278–284.
583. Goldstein NS, Mani A, Chmielewski G, et al. Immunohistochemically detected micrometastases in peribronchial and mediastinal lymph nodes from patients with T1, N0, M0 pulmonary adenocarcinomas. Am J Surg Pathol 2000;24(2):274–279.
584. Prakash UB, Reiman HM. Comparison of needle biopsy with cytologic analysis for the evaluation of pleural effusion: analysis of 414 cases. Mayo Clin Proc 1985;60(3):158–164.
585. Menzies R, Charbonneau M. Thoracoscopy for the diagnosis of pleural disease. Ann Intern Med 1991;114(4):271–276.
586. Vicidomini G, Santini M, Fiorello A, et al. Intraoperative pleural lavage: is it a valid prognostic factor in lung cancer? Ann Thorac Surg 2005;79(1):254–257; discussion 257.
587. Dresler CM, Fratelli C, Babb J. Prognostic value of positive pleural lavage in patients with lung cancer resection. Ann Thorac Surg 1999;67(5):1435–1439.
588. Erasmus JJ, McAdams HP, Rossi SE, et al. FDG PET of pleural effusions in patients with non-small cell lung cancer. AJR Am J Roentgenol 2000;175(1):245–249.
589. Bunker ML, Raab SS, Landreneau RJ, et al. The diagnosis and significance of visceral pleural invasion in lung carcinoma. Histologic predictors and the role of elastic stains. Am J Clin Pathol 1999;112(6):777–783.
590. Shimizu K, Yoshida J, Nagai K, et al. Visceral pleural invasion classification in non-small cell lung cancer: a proposal on the basis of outcome assessment. J Thorac Cardiovasc Surg 2004;127(6):1574–1578.
591. Osaki T, Nagashima A, Yoshimatsu T, et al. Visceral pleural involvement in nonsmall cell lung cancer: prognostic significance. Ann Thorac Surg 2004;77(5):1769–1773; discussion 1773.
592. Maruyama R, Shoji F, Okamoto T, et al. Prognostic value of visceral pleural invasion in resected non-small cell lung cancer diagnosed by using a jet stream of saline solution. J Thorac Cardiovasc Surg 2004;127(6):1587–1592.
593. Kang JH, Kim KD, Chung KY. Prognostic value of visceral pleura invasion in non-small cell lung cancer. Eur J Cardiothorac Surg 2003;23(6):865–869.
594. Butnor KJ, Cooper K. Visceral pleural invasion in lung cancer: recognizing histologic parameters that impact staging and prognosis. Adv Anat Pathol 2005;12(1):1–6.
595. Bewtra C. Multiple primary bronchogenic carcinomas, with a review of the literature. J Surg Oncol 1984;25(3):207–213.
596. Flieder DB, Vazquez M, Carter D, et al. Pathologic findings of lung tumors diagnosed on baseline CT screening. Am J Surg Pathol 2006;30:606–613.
597. Battafarano RJ, Meyers BF, Guthrie TJ, et al. Surgical resection of multifocal non-small cell lung cancer is associated with prolonged survival. Ann Thorac Surg 2002;74(4):988–993; discussion 993–994.
598. Roberts PF, Straznicka M, Lara PN, et al. Resection of multifocal non-small cell lung cancer when the bronchioloalveolar subtype is involved. J Thorac Cardiovasc Surg 2003;126(5):1597–1602.
599. Kamiyoshihara M, Kawashima O, Sakata S, et al. Management of ipsilateral intrapulmonary metastases in the new TNM system for non-small cell lung cancer. J Cardiovasc Surg (Torino) 2000;41(6):931–934.
600. Okada M, Tsubota N, Yoshimura M, et al. Evaluation of TMN classification for lung carcinoma with ipsilateral intrapulmonary metastasis. Ann Thorac Surg 1999;68(2):326–330; discussion 331.
601. Martini N, Melamed MR. Multiple primary lung cancers. J Thorac Cardiovasc Surg 1975;70(4):606–612.
602. Dacic S, Ionescu DN, Finkelstein S, et al. Patterns of allelic loss of synchronous adenocarcinomas of the lung. Am J Surg Pathol 2005;29(7):897–902.
603. Strauss B, Weller CV. Bronchogenic carcinoma: a statistical analysis of two hundred ninety-six cases with necropsy as to relationships between cell types and age, sex, and metastasis. AMA Arch Pathol 1957;63(6):602–611.
604. Reid JD. The classification of lung cancer. Aust N Z J Surg 1963;32:239–243.

605. Yesner R. Spectrum of lung cancer and ectopic hormones. Pathol Annu 1978;13 Pt 1:207–240.
606. Dermer GB. Autoradiography of cellular glycoproteins reveals histogenesis of bronchogenic adenocarcinomas. Cancer 1981;47(8):2000–2006.
607. Dermer GB. Origin of bronchioloalveolar carcinoma and peripheral bronchial adenocarcinoma. Cancer 1982;49(5): 881–887.
608. Auerbach O. Pathogenesis of lung cancer. Compr Ther 1981;7(12):11–21.
609. Yokota J, Kohno T. Molecular footprints of human lung cancer progression. Cancer Sci 2004;95(3):197–204.
610. Toyooka S, Maruyama R, Toyooka KO, et al. Smoke exposure, histologic type and geography-related differences in the methylation profiles of non-small cell lung cancer. Int J Cancer 2003;103(2):153–160.
611. Hong KU, Reynolds SD, Watkins S, et al. Basal cells are a multipotent progenitor capable of renewing the bronchial epithelium. Am J Pathol 2004;164(2):577–588.
612. Kim CF, Jackson EL, Woolfenden AE, et al. Identification of bronchioalveolar stem cells in normal lung and lung cancer. Cell 2005;121(6):823–835.
613. Giangreco A, Reynolds SD, Stripp BR. Terminal bronchioles harbor a unique airway stem cell population that localizes to the bronchoalveolar duct junction. Am J Pathol 2002;161(1):173–182.
614. Kreyberg L, Liebow AA, Uehlinger EA. Histological Typing of Lung Tumours. 1st ed. Geneva: World Health Organization, 1967.
615. Histological typing of lung tumours. 2nd ed. Geneva: World Health Organization, 1981.
616. Travis WD, Colby TV, Corrin B, et al. Histological typing of lung and pleural tumours. 3rd ed. Berlin: Springer-Verlag, 1999.
617. Travis WD, Brambilla E, Muller Hermelink HK, et al. Pathology and genetics of tumours of the lung, pleura, thymus and heart. Lyon: IARC Press, 2004.
618. Nacht M, Dracheva T, Gao Y, et al. Molecular characteristics of non-small cell lung cancer. Proc Natl Acad Sci USA 2001;98(26):15203–15208.
619. Garber ME, Troyanskaya OG, Schluens K, et al. Diversity of gene expression in adenocarcinoma of the lung. Proc Natl Acad Sci U S A 2001;98(24):13784–13789.
620. Virtanen C, Ishikawa Y, Honjoh D, et al. Integrated classification of lung tumors and cell lines by expression profiling. Proc Natl Acad Sci USA 2002;99(19):12357–12362.
621. Bhattacharjee A, Richards WG, Staunton J, et al. Classification of human lung carcinomas by mRNA expression profiling reveals distinct adenocarcinoma subclasses. Proc Natl Acad Sci USA 2001;98(24):13790–13795.
622. McDowell EM, McLaughlin JS, Merenyl DK, et al. The respiratory epithelium. V. Histogenesis of lung carcinomas in the human. J Natl Cancer Inst 1978;61(2):587–606.
623. Trump BF, McDowell EM, Glavin F, et al. The respiratory epithelium. III. Histogenesis of epidermoid metaplasia and carcinoma in situ in the human. J Natl Cancer Inst 1978;61(2):563–575.
624. Yamamoto M, Shimokata K, Nagura H. Immunoelectron microscopic study on the histogenesis of epidermoid metaplasia in respiratory epithelium. Am Rev Respir Dis 1987;135(3):713–718.
625. Copin MC, Devisme L, Buisine MP, et al. From normal respiratory mucosa to epidermoid carcinoma: expression of human mucin genes. Int J Cancer 2000;86(2):162–168.
626. Fukushima M, Homma K, Hashimoto T, et al. Histologically unique case of combined small cell and squamous cell carcinoma in a polypoid bronchial tumor. Pathol Int 2005;55(12):785–791.
627. Gatter KC, Dunnill MS, Heryet A, et al. Human lung tumours: does intermediate filament co-expression correlate with other morphological or immunocytochemical features? Histopathology 1987;11(7):705–714.
628. Tomashefski JF Jr, Connors AF Jr, Rosenthal ES, et al. Peripheral vs central squamous cell carcinoma of the lung. A comparison of clinical features, histopathology, and survival. Arch Pathol Lab Med 1990;114(5):468–474.
629. Funai K, Yokose T, Ishii G, et al. Clinicopathologic characteristics of peripheral squamous cell carcinoma of the lung. Am J Surg Pathol 2003;27(7):978–984.
630. Sakurai H, Asamura H, Watanabe S, et al. Clinicopathologic features of peripheral squamous cell carcinoma of the lung. Ann Thorac Surg 2004;78(1):222–227.
631. Arcasoy SM, Jett JR. Superior pulmonary sulcus tumors and Pancoast's syndrome. N Engl J Med 1997;337(19): 1370–1376.
632. Rusch VW, Parekh KR, Leon L, et al. Factors determining outcome after surgical resection of T3 and T4 lung cancers of the superior sulcus. J Thorac Cardiovasc Surg 2000; 119(6):1147–1153.
633. Goldberg M, Gupta D, Sasson AR, et al. The surgical management of superior sulcus tumors: a retrospective review with long-term follow-up. Ann Thorac Surg 2005; 79(4):1174–1179.
634. Komaki R, Roth JA, Walsh GL, et al. Outcome predictors for 143 patients with superior sulcus tumors treated by multidisciplinary approach at the University of Texas M. D. Anderson Cancer Center. Int J Radiat Oncol Biol Phys 2000;48(2):347–354.
635. Hagan MP, Choi NC, Mathisen DJ, et al. Superior sulcus lung tumors: impact of local control on survival. J Thorac Cardiovasc Surg 1999;117(6):1086–1094.
636. Ichinose Y, Yano T, Asoh H, et al. Prognostic factors obtained by a pathologic examination in completely resected non-small-cell lung cancer. An analysis in each pathologic stage. J Thorac Cardiovasc Surg 1995;110(3): 601–605.
637. Lyda MH, Weiss LM. Immunoreactivity for epithelial and neuroendocrine antibodies are useful in the differential diagnosis of lung carcinomas. Hum Pathol 2000;31(8): 980–987.
638. Chu PG, Weiss LM. Expression of cytokeratin 5/6 in epithelial neoplasms: an immunohistochemical study of 509 cases. Mod Pathol 2002;15(1):6–10.
639. Chu PG, Lyda MH, Weiss LM. Cytokeratin 14 expression in epithelial neoplasms: a survey of 435 cases with emphasis on its value in differentiating squamous cell carcinomas

from other epithelial tumours. Histopathology 2001;39(1): 9–16.
640. Tan D, Li Q, Deeb G, et al. Thyroid transcription factor-1 expression prevalence and its clinical implications in non-small cell lung cancer: a high-throughput tissue microarray and immunohistochemistry study. Hum Pathol 2003;34(6): 597–604.
641. Wang PW, Zee S, Zarbo RJ, et al. Coordinate expression of cytokeratins 7 and 20 defines unique subsets of carcinoma. Appl Immunohistochem 1995;3(2):99–107.
642. Jerome Marson V, Mazieres J, Groussard O, et al. Expression of TTF-1 and cytokeratins in primary and secondary epithelial lung tumours: correlation with histological type and grade. Histopathology 2004;45(2):125–134.
643. Visscher DW, Zarbo RJ, Trojanowski JQ, et al. Neuroendocrine differentiation in poorly differentiated lung carcinomas: a light microscopic and immunohistologic study. Mod Pathol 1990;3(4):508–512.
644. Pelosi G, Pasini F, Sonzogni A, et al. Prognostic implications of neuroendocrine differentiation and hormone production in patients with Stage I nonsmall cell lung carcinoma. Cancer 2003;97(10):2487–2497.
645. Howe MC, Chapman A, Kerr K, et al. Neuroendocrine differentiation in non-small cell lung cancer and its relation to prognosis and therapy. Histopathology 2005;46(2): 195–201.
646. Boucher LD, Yoneda K. The expression of trophoblastic cell markers by lung carcinomas. Hum Pathol 1995;26(11): 1201–1206.
647. Hiroshima K, Iyoda A, Toyozaki T, et al. Alpha-fetoprotein-producing lung carcinoma: report of three cases. Pathol Int 2002;52(1):46–53.
648. Dirnhofer S, Freund M, Rogatsch H, et al. Selective expression of trophoblastic hormones by lung carcinoma: neuroendocrine tumors exclusively produce human chorionic gonadotropin alpha-subunit (hCGalpha). Hum Pathol 2000;31(8):966–972.
649. Hammar SP, Bolen JW, Bockus D, et al. Ultrastructural and immunohistochemical features of common lung tumors: an overview. Ultrastruct Pathol 1985;9(3–4):283–318.
650. Hammar S. The use of electron microscopy and immunohistochemistry in the diagnosis and understanding of lung neoplasms. Clin Lab Med 1987;7(1):1–30.
651. Sidhu GS. The ultrastructure of malignant epithelial neoplasms of the lung. Pathol Annu 1982;17 (Pt 1):235–266.
652. Dingemans KP, Mooi WJ. Ultrastructure of squamous cell carcinoma of the lung. Pathol Annu 1984;19 Pt 1:249–273.
653. Dingemans KP, Mooi WJ. Ultrastructure of tumour invasion and desmoplastic response of bronchogenic squamous cell carcinoma. Virchows Arch A Pathol Anat Histopathol 1987;411(3):283–291.
654. Havenith MG, Dingemans KP, Cleutjens JP, et al. Basement membranes in bronchogenic squamous cell carcinoma: an immunohistochemical and ultrastructural study. Ultrastruct Pathol 1990;14(1):51–63.
655. Nakanishi K, Kawai T, Suzuki M, et al. Bronchogenic squamous cell carcinomas with invasion along alveolar walls. Histopathology 1996;29(4):363–368.
656. Kornstein MJ, Rosai J. CD5 labeling of thymic carcinomas and other nonlymphoid neoplasms. Am J Clin Pathol 1998;109(6):722–726.
657. Dorfman DM, Shahsafaei A, Chan JK. Thymic carcinomas, but not thymomas and carcinomas of other sites, show CD5 immunoreactivity. Am J Surg Pathol 1997;21(8):936–940.
658. Tateyama H, Eimoto T, Tada T, et al. Immunoreactivity of a new CD5 antibody with normal epithelium and malignant tumors including thymic carcinoma. Am J Clin Pathol 1999;111(2):235–240.
659. Pomplun S, Wotherspoon AC, Shah G, et al. Immunohistochemical markers in the differentiation of thymic and pulmonary neoplasms. Histopathology 2002;40(2):152–158.
660. Geurts TW, Nederlof PM, van den Brekel MW, et al. Pulmonary squamous cell carcinoma following head and neck squamous cell carcinoma: metastasis or second primary? Clin Cancer Res 2005;11(18):6608–6614.
661. Leong PP, Rezai B, Koch WM, et al. Distinguishing second primary tumors from lung metastases in patients with head and neck squamous cell carcinoma. J Natl Cancer Inst 1998;90(13):972–977.
662. Mountain CF. Prognostic implications of the International Staging System for Lung Cancer. Semin Oncol 1988;15(3): 236–245.
663. Kato H, Tsuboi M, Kato Y, et al. Postoperative adjuvant therapy for completely resected early-stage non-small cell lung cancer. Int J Clin Oncol 2005;10(3):157–164.
664. Visbal AL, Leighl NB, Feld R, et al. Adjuvant chemotherapy for early-stage non-small cell lung cancer. Chest 2005;128(4):2933–2943.
665. Park JH, Lee CT, Lee HW, et al. Postoperative adjuvant chemotherapy for stage I non-small cell lung cancer. Eur J Cardiothorac Surg 2005;27(6):1086–1091.
666. Park JH, Shim YM, Baek HJ, et al. Postoperative adjuvant therapy for stage II non-small-cell lung cancer. Ann Thorac Surg 1999;68(5):1821–1826.
667. Winton T, Livingston R, Johnson D, et al. Vinorelbine plus cisplatin vs. observation in resected non-small-cell lung cancer. N Engl J Med 2005;352(25):2589–2597.
668. Brundage MD, Davies D, Mackillop WJ. Prognostic factors in non-small cell lung cancer: a decade of progress. Chest 2002;122(3):1037–1057.
669. Pelletier MP, Edwardes MD, Michel RP, et al. Prognostic markers in resectable non-small cell lung cancer: a multivariate analysis. Can J Surg 2001;44(3):180–188.
670. Gomez de la Camara A, Lopez-Encuentra A, Ferrando P. Heterogeneity of prognostic profiles in non-small cell lung cancer: too many variables but a few relevant. Eur J Epidemiol 2005;20(11):907–914.
671. Gasinska A, Kolodziejski L, Niemiec J, et al. Clinical significance of biological differences between cavitated and solid form of squamous cell lung cancer. Lung Cancer 2005;49(2):171–179.
672. Harpole DH Jr, Herndon JE, 2nd, Young WG Jr, et al. Stage I nonsmall cell lung cancer. A multivariate analysis of treatment methods and patterns of recurrence. Cancer 1995;76(5):787–796.

673. Nesbitt JC, Putnam JB Jr, Walsh GL, et al. Survival in early-stage non-small cell lung cancer. Ann Thorac Surg 1995;60(2):466–472.
674. Padilla J, Calvo V, Penalver JC, et al. Surgical results and prognostic factors in early non-small cell lung cancer. Ann Thorac Surg 1997;63(2):324–326.
675. Gail MH, Eagan RT, Feld R, et al. Prognostic factors in patients with resected stage I non-small cell lung cancer. A report from the Lung Cancer Study Group. Cancer 1984;54(9):1802–1813.
676. Martini N, Burt ME, Bains MS, et al. Survival after resection of stage II non-small cell lung cancer. Ann Thorac Surg 1992;54(3):460–465; discussion 466.
677. Martini N, Flehinger BJ. The role of surgery in N2 lung cancer. Surg Clin North Am 1987;67(5):1037–1049.
678. Nappi O, Swanson PE, Wick MR. Pseudovascular adenoid squamous cell carcinoma of the lung: clinicopathologic study of three cases and comparison with true pleuropulmonary angiosarcoma. Hum Pathol 1994;25(4):373–378.
679. Banerjee SS, Eyden BP, Wells S, et al. Pseudoangiosarcomatous carcinoma: a clinicopathological study of seven cases. Histopathology 1992;21(1):13–23.
680. Borczuk AC, Sha KK, Hisler SE, et al. Sebaceous carcinoma of the lung: histologic and immunohistochemical characterization of an unusual pulmonary neoplasm: report of a case and review of the literature. Am J Surg Pathol 2002;26(6):795–798.
681. Garcia-Escudero A, Navarro-Bustos G, Jurado-Escamez P, et al. Primary squamous cell carcinoma of the lung with pilomatricoma-like features. Histopathology 2002;40(2): 201–202.
682. Sherwin RP, Laforet EG, Strieder JW. Exophytic endobronchial carcinoma. J Thorac Cardiovasc Surg 1962;43: 716 730.
683. Dulmet-Brender E, Jaubert F, Huchon G. Exophytic endobronchial epidermoid carcinoma. Cancer 1986;57(7): 1358–1364.
684. Cooper L, Hagenschneider JK, Banky S, et al. Papillary endobronchial squamous cell carcinoma. Ann Diagn Pathol 2005;9(5):284–288.
685. Flieder DB, Koss MN, Nicholson A, et al. Solitary pulmonary papillomas in adults: a clinicopathologic and in situ hybridization study of 14 cases combined with 27 cases in the literature. Am J Surg Pathol 1998;22(11):1328–1342.
686. Katzenstein AL, Prioleau PG, Askin FB. The histologic spectrum and significance of clear-cell change in lung carcinoma. Cancer 1980;45(5):943–947.
687. Churg A, Johnston WH, Stulbarg M. Small cell squamous and mixed small cell squamous—small cell anaplastic carcinomas of the lung. Am J Surg Pathol 1980;4(3):255–263.
688. Wang BY, Gil J, Kaufman D, et al. P63 in pulmonary epithelium, pulmonary squamous neoplasms, and other pulmonary tumors. Hum Pathol 2002;33(9):921–926.
689. Zhang H, Liu J, Cagle PT, et al. Distinction of pulmonary small cell carcinoma from poorly differentiated squamous cell carcinoma: an immunohistochemical approach. Mod Pathol 2005;18(1):111–118.
690. Brambilla E, Moro D, Veale D, et al. Basal cell (basaloid) carcinoma of the lung: a new morphologic and phenotypic entity with separate prognostic significance. Hum Pathol 1992;23(9):993–1003.
691. Lin O, Harkin TJ, Jagirdar J. Basaloid-squamous cell carcinoma of the bronchus. Report of a case with review of the literature. Arch Pathol Lab Med 1995;119(12):1167–1170.
692. Kitamura H, Kameda Y, Ito T, et al. Atypical adenomatous hyperplasia of the lung. Implications for the pathogenesis of peripheral lung adenocarcinoma. Am J Clin Pathol 1999;111(5):610–622.
693. Hirata H, Noguchi M, Shimosato Y, et al. Clinicopathologic and immunohistochemical characteristics of bronchial gland cell type adenocarcinoma of the lung. Am J Clin Pathol 1990;93(1):20–25.
694. Ten Have-Opbroek AA, Benfield JR, van Krieken JH, et al. The alveolar type II cell is a pluripotential stem cell in the genesis of human adenocarcinomas and squamous cell carcinomas. Histol Histopathol 1997;12(2):319–336.
695. Hano H, Cui S, Ushigome S, et al. Papillary adenocarcinoma arising in placentoid bullous lesion of the lung: report of a case with immunohistochemical study. Arch Pathol Lab Med 1998;122(10):915–919.
696. Hanaoka N, Tanaka F, Otake Y, et al. Primary lung carcinoma arising from emphysematous bullae. Lung Cancer 2002;38(2):185–191.
697. Sheffield EA, Addis BJ, Corrin B, et al. Epithelial hyperplasia and malignant change in congenital lung cysts. J Clin Pathol 1987;40(6):612–614.
698. Prichard MG, Brown PJ, Sterrett GF. Bronchioloalveolar carcinoma arising in longstanding lung cysts. Thorax 1984;39(7):545–549.
699. Granata C, Gambini C, Balducci T, et al. Bronchioloalveolar carcinoma arising in congenital cystic adenomatoid malformation in a child: a case report and review on malignancies originating in congenital cystic adenomatoid malformation. Pediatr Pulmonol 1998;25(1):62–66.
700. Sudou M, Sugi K, Murakami T. Bronchioloalveolar carcinoma arising from a congenital cystic adenomatoid malformation in an adolescent: the first case report from the orient. J Thorac Cardiovasc Surg 2003;126(3):902–903.
701. Friedrich G. Periphere Lungenkrebse auf dem Boden pleuranaher Narben. Virchows Arch Pathol Anat 1939;304: 230–247.
702. Roessle R. Die Narbenkrebse der Lungen. Schweiz Med Wochenschr 1943;73:1200–1203.
703. Yokoo H, Suckow EE. Peripheral lung cancers arising in scars. Cancer 1961;14:1205–1215.
704. Auerbach O, Garfinkel L, Parks VR. Scar cancer of the lung: increase over a 21 year period. Cancer 1979;43(2): 636–642.
705. Fraire AE, Greenberg SD. Carcinoma and diffuse interstitial fibrosis of lung. Cancer 1973;31(5):1078–1086.
706. Meyer EC, Liebow AA. Relationship of interstitial pneumonia honeycombing and atypical epithelial proliferation to cancer of the lung. Cancer 1965;18:322–351.
707. Yoneda K. Scar carcinomas of the lung in a histoplasmosis endemic area. Cancer 1990;65(1):164–168.

708. Cagle PT, Cohle SD, Greenberg SD. Natural history of pulmonary scar cancers. Clinical and pathologic implications. Cancer 1985;56(8):2031–2035.
709. Shimosato Y, Suzuki A, Hashimoto T, et al. Prognostic implications of fibrotic focus (scar) in small peripheral lung cancers. Am J Surg Pathol 1980;4(4):365–373.
710. Madri JA, Carter D. Scar cancers of the lung: origin and significance. Hum Pathol 1984;15(7):625–631.
711. Kung IT, Lui IO, Loke SL, et al. Pulmonary scar cancer. A pathologic reappraisal. Am J Surg Pathol 1985;9(6): 391–400.
712. Kumaki F, Matsui K, Kawai T, et al. Expression of matrix metalloproteinases in invasive pulmonary adenocarcinoma with bronchioloalveolar component and atypical adenomatous hyperplasia. Am J Pathol 2001;159(6):2125–2135.
713. Kolin A, Koutoulakis T. Role of arterial occlusion in pulmonary scar cancers. Hum Pathol 1988;19(10):1161–1167.
714. el-Torkey M, Giltman LI, Dabbous M. Collagens in scar carcinoma of the lung. Am J Pathol 1985;121(2):322–326.
715. Moriya Y, Niki T, Yamada T, et al. Increased expression of laminin-5 and its prognostic significance in lung adenocarcinomas of small size. An immunohistochemical analysis of 102 cases. Cancer 2001;91(6):1129–1141.
716. Travis WD, Garg K, Franklin WA, et al. Evolving concepts in the pathology and computed tomography imaging of lung adenocarcinoma and bronchioloalveolar carcinoma. J Clin Oncol 2005;23(14):3279–3287.
717. Edwards CW. Pulmonary adenocarcinoma: review of 106 cases and proposed new classification. J Clin Pathol 1987; 40(2):125–135.
718. Iyoda A, Hiroshima K, Toyozaki T, et al. Clear cell adenocarcinoma with endobronchial polypoid growth. Pathol Int 2000;50(12):979–983.
719. Kodama T, Shimosato Y, Koide T, et al. Endobronchial polypoid adenocarcinoma of the lung. Histological and ultrastructural studies of five cases. Am J Surg Pathol 1984;8(11):845–854.
720. Harwood TR, Gracey DR, Yokoo H. Pseudomesotheliomatous carcinoma of the lung. A variant of peripheral lung cancer. Am J Clin Pathol 1976;65(2):159–167.
721. Koss M, Travis W, Moran C, et al. Pseudomesotheliomatous adenocarcinoma: a reappraisal. Semin Diagn Pathol 1992;9(2):117–123.
722. Koss MN, Fleming M, Przygodzki RM, et al. Adenocarcinoma simulating mesothelioma: a clinicopathologic and immunohistochemical study of 29 cases. Ann Diagn Pathol 1998;2(2):93–102.
723. Attanoos RL, Gibbs AR. 'Pseudomesotheliomatous' carcinomas of the pleura: a 10-year analysis of cases from the Environmental Lung Disease Research Group, Cardiff. Histopathology 2003;43(5):444–452.
724. Guru PK, Phillips S, Ball MM, et al. Pseudomesotheliomatous presentation of primary signet ring cell carcinoma of lung. Indian J Chest Dis Allied Sci 2005;47(3):209–211.
725. Lantuejoul S, Colby TV, Ferretti GR, et al. Adenocarcinoma of the lung mimicking inflammatory lung disease with honeycombing. Eur Respir J 2004;24(3):502–505.
726. Kawabuchi B, Ishikawa Y, Tsuchiya S, et al. Mucosal spreading adenocarcinoma at the hilar portion of the lung. Acta Pathol Jpn 1993;43(11):690–695.
727. Higashiyama M, Doi O, Kodama K, et al. Extramammary Paget's disease of the bronchial epithelium. Arch Pathol Lab Med 1991;115(2):185–188.
728. Aida S, Shimazaki H, Sato K, et al. Prognostic significance of frequent acidophilic nuclear inclusions in adenocarcinoma of the lung with immunohistochemical and ultrastructural studies. Cancer 2001;91(10):1896–1904.
729. Scroggs MW, Roggli VL, Fraire AE, et al. Eosinophilic intracytoplasmic globules in pulmonary adenocarcinomas: a histochemical, immunohistochemical, and ultrastructural study of six cases. Hum Pathol 1989;20(9):845–849.
730. Tsumuraya M, Kodama T, Kameya T, et al. Light and electron microscopic analysis of intranuclear inclusions in papillary adenocarcinoma of the lung. Acta Cytol 1981; 25(5):523–532.
731. Hara H, Iwabuchi K, Shinada J, et al. Pulmonary adenocarcinoma with heterotopic bone formation. Pathol Int 2000;50(11):910–913.
732. Silver SA, Askin FB. True papillary carcinoma of the lung: a distinct clinicopathologic entity. Am J Surg Pathol 1997; 21(1):43–51.
733. Terasaki H, Niki T, Matsuno Y, et al. Lung adenocarcinoma with mixed bronchioloalveolar and invasive components: clinicopathological features, subclassification by extent of invasive foci, and immunohistochemical characterization. Am J Surg Pathol 2003;27(7):937–951.
734. Jian Z, Tomizawa Y, Yanagitani N, et al. Papillary adenocarcinoma of the lung is a more advanced adenocarcinoma than bronchioloalveolar carcinoma that is composed of two distinct histological subtypes. Pathol Int 2005;55(10): 619–625.
735. Noguchi M, Morikawa A, Kawasaki M, et al. Small adenocarcinoma of the lung. Histologic characteristics and prognosis. Cancer 1995;75(12):2844–2852.
736. Sorensen JB, Hirsch FR, Olsen J. The prognostic implication of histopathologic subtyping of pulmonary adenocarcinoma according to the classification of the World Health Organization. An analysis of 259 consecutive patients with advanced disease. Cancer 1988;62(2):361–367.
737. Sorensen JB, Olsen JE. Prognostic implications of histopathologic subtyping in patients with surgically treated stage I or II adenocarcinoma of the lung. J Thorac Cardiovasc Surg 1989;97(2):245–251.
738. Shimazaki H, Aida S, Sato M, et al. Lung carcinoma with rhabdoid cells: a clinicopathological study and survival analysis of 14 cases. Histopathology 2001;38(5):425–434.
739. Moran CA, Jagirdar J, Suster S. Papillary lung carcinoma with prominent "morular" component. Am J Clin Pathol 2004;122(1):106–109.
740. Amin MB, Tamboli P, Merchant SH, et al. Micropapillary component in lung adenocarcinoma: a distinctive histologic feature with possible prognostic significance. Am J Surg Pathol 2002;26(3):358–364.
741. Roh MS, Lee JI, Choi PJ, et al. Relationship between micropapillary component and micrometastasis in the

regional lymph nodes of patients with stage I lung adenocarcinoma. Histopathology 2004;45(6):580–586.
742. Makimoto Y, Nabeshima K, Iwasaki H, et al. Micropapillary pattern: a distinct pathological marker to subclassify tumours with a significantly poor prognosis within small peripheral lung adenocarcinoma (≤20mm) with mixed bronchioloalveolar and invasive subtypes (Noguchi's type C tumours). Histopathology 2005;46(6):677–684.
743. Kim YH, Ishii G, Goto K, et al. Dominant papillary subtype is a significant predictor of the response to gefitinib in adenocarcinoma of the lung. Clin Cancer Res 2004; 10(21):7311–7317.
744. Aida S, Shimazaki H, Sato K, et al. Prognostic analysis of pulmonary adenocarcinoma subclassification with special consideration of papillary and bronchioloalveolar types. Histopathology 2004;45(5):468–476.
745. Malassez L. Examen histologique d'un cas de cancer encephaloide du poumon (epithelioma). Arch Physiol Normale Pathol 1876;3:353–372.
746. Clayton F. Bronchioloalveolar carcinomas. Cell types, patterns of growth, and prognostic correlates. Cancer 1986;57(8):1555–1564.
747. Liebow AA. Bronchiolo-alveolar carcinoma. Adv Intern Med 1960;10:329–358.
748. Zell JA, Ou SH, Ziogas A, et al. Epidemiology of bronchioloalveolar carcinoma: improvement in survival after release of the 1999 WHO classification of lung tumors. J Clin Oncol 2005;23(33):8396–8405.
749. Lantuejoul S, Ferretti GR, Goldstraw P, et al. Metastases from bronchioloalveolar carcinomas associated with longstanding type 1 congenital cystic adenomatoid malformations. A report of two cases. Histopathology 2006;48(2): 204–206.
750. De las Heras M, Barsky SH, Hasleton P, et al. Evidence for a protein related immunologically to the jaagsiekte sheep retrovirus in some human lung tumours. Eur Respir J 2000;16(2):330–332.
751. Palmarini M, Fan H. Retrovirus-induced ovine pulmonary adenocarcinoma, an animal model for lung cancer. J Natl Cancer Inst 2001;93(21):1603–1614.
752. Yousem SA, Finkelstein SD, Swalsky PA, et al. Absence of jaagsiekte sheep retrovirus DNA and RNA in bronchioloalveolar and conventional human pulmonary adenocarcinoma by PCR and RT-PCR analysis. Hum Pathol 2001;32(10):1039–1042.
753. Hiatt KM, Highsmith WE. Lack of DNA evidence for jaagsiekte sheep retrovirus in human bronchioloalveolar carcinoma. Hum Pathol 2002;33(6):680.
754. Daly RC, Trastek VF, Pairolero PC, et al. Bronchoalveolar carcinoma: factors affecting survival. Ann Thorac Surg 1991;51(3):368–376; discussion 376–377.
755. Holst VA, Finkelstein S, Yousem SA. Bronchioloalveolar adenocarcinoma of lung: monoclonal origin for multifocal disease. Am J Surg Pathol 1998;22(11):1343–1350.
756. Mirtcheva RM, Vazquez M, Yankelevitz DF, et al. Bronchioloalveolar carcinoma and adenocarcinoma with bronchioloalveolar features presenting as ground-glass opacities on CT. Clin Imaging 2002;26(2):95–100.
757. Matsuguma H, Nakahara R, Anraku M, et al. Objective definition and measurement method of ground-glass opacity for planning limited resection in patients with clinical stage IA adenocarcinoma of the lung. Eur J Cardiothorac Surg 2004;25(6):1102–1106.
758. Suzuki K, Kusumoto M, Watanabe S, et al. Radiologic classification of small adenocarcinoma of the lung: radiologic-pathologic correlation and its prognostic impact. Ann Thorac Surg 2006;81(2):413–419.
759. Mizutani Y, Nakajima T, Morinaga S, et al. Immunohistochemical localization of pulmonary surfactant apoproteins in various lung tumors. Special reference to nonmucus producing lung adenocarcinomas. Cancer 1988;61(3):532–537.
760. Axiotis CA, Jennings TA. Observations on bronchioloalveolar carcinomas with special emphasis on localized lesions. A clinicopathological, ultrastructural, and immunohistochemical study of 11 cases. Am J Surg Pathol 1988; 12(12):918–931.
761. Uehara T, Honda T, Sano K, et al. A three-dimensional analysis of blood vessels in bronchioloalveolar carcinoma. Lung 2004;182(6):343–353.
762. Goto K, Yokose T, Kodama T, et al. Detection of early invasion on the basis of basement membrane destruction in small adenocarcinomas of the lung and its clinical implications. Mod Pathol 2001;14(12):1237–1245.
763. Sheikh HA, Sasatomi E, Finkelstein S, et al. Comparative mutational analysis of pulmonary scar epithelium, bronchioloalveolar carcinomas, and invasive well-differentiated pulmonary adenocarcinomas: a molecular approach to diagnostically challenging cases. Am J Surg Pathol 2005; 29(10):1267–1273.
764. Goldstein NS, Thomas M. Mucinous and nonmucinous bronchioloalveolar adenocarcinomas have distinct staining patterns with thyroid transcription factor and cytokeratin 20 antibodies. Am J Clin Pathol 2001;116(3):319–325.
765. Lau SK, Desrochers MJ, Luthringer DJ. Expression of thyroid transcription factor-1, cytokeratin 7, and cytokeratin 20 in bronchioloalveolar carcinomas: an immunohistochemical evaluation of 67 cases. Mod Pathol 2002;15(5): 538–542.
766. Chu P, Wu E, Weiss LM. Cytokeratin 7 and cytokeratin 20 expression in epithelial neoplasms: a survey of 435 cases. Mod Pathol 2000;13(9):962–972.
767. Kummar S, Fogarasi M, Canova A, et al. Cytokeratin 7 and 20 staining for the diagnosis of lung and colorectal adenocarcinoma. Br J Cancer 2002;86(12):1884–1887.
768. Kaufmann O, Dietel M. Thyroid transcription factor-1 is the superior immunohistochemical marker for pulmonary adenocarcinomas and large cell carcinomas compared to surfactant proteins A and B. Histopathology 2000;36(1):8–16.
769. Zamecnik J, Kodet R. Value of thyroid transcription factor-1 and surfactant apoprotein A in the differential diagnosis of pulmonary carcinomas: a study of 109 cases. Virchows Arch 2002;440(4):353–361.
770. Shah RN, Badve S, Papreddy K, et al. Expression of cytokeratin 20 in mucinous bronchioloalveolar carcinoma. Hum Pathol 2002;33(9):915–920.
771. Yatabe Y, Koga T, Mitsudomi T, et al. CK20 expression, CDX2 expression, K-ras mutation, and goblet cell mor-

phology in a subset of lung adenocarcinomas. J Pathol 2004;203(2):645–652.
772. Saad RS, Cho P, Silverman JF, et al. Usefulness of Cdx2 in separating mucinous bronchioloalveolar adenocarcinoma of the lung from metastatic mucinous colorectal adenocarcinoma. Am J Clin Pathol 2004;122(3):421–427.
773. Mazziotta RM, Borczuk AC, Powell CA, et al. CDX2 immunostaining as a gastrointestinal marker: expression in lung carcinomas is a potential pitfall. Appl Immunohistochem Mol Morphol 2005;13(1):55–60.
774. Barbareschi M, Murer B, Colby TV, et al. CDX-2 homeobox gene expression is a reliable marker of colorectal adenocarcinoma metastases to the lungs. Am J Surg Pathol 2003;27(2):141–149.
775. De Lott LB, Morrison C, Suster S, et al. CDX2 is a useful marker of intestinal-type differentiation: a tissue microarray-based study of 629 tumors from various sites. Arch Pathol Lab Med 2005;129(9):1100–1105.
776. Bedrossian CW, Weilbaecher DG, Bentinck DC, et al. Ultrastructure of human bronchiolo-alveolar cell carcinoma. Cancer 1975;36(4):1399–1413.
777. McGregor DH, Dixon AY, McGregor DK. Adenocarcinoma of the lung: a comparative diagnostic study using light and electron microscopy. Hum Pathol 1988;19(8): 910–913.
778. Sidhu GS, Forrester EM. Glycogen-rich Clara cell-type bronchiolo-alveolar carcinoma: light and electron microscopic study. Cancer 1977;40(5):2209–2215.
779. Kimula Y. A histochemical and ultrastructural study of adenocarcinoma of the lung. Am J Surg Pathol 1978; 2(3):253–264.
780. Herrera GA, Alexander CB, DeMoraes HP. Ultrastructural subtypes of pulmonary adenocarcinoma. A correlation with patient survival. Chest 1983;84(5):581–586.
781. Ogata T, Endo K. Clara cell granules of peripheral lung cancers. Cancer 1984;54(8):1635–1644.
782. Hiroshima K, Toyozaki T, Iyoda A, et al. Ultrastructural study of intranuclear inclusion bodies of pulmonary adenocarcinoma. Ultrastruct Pathol 1999;23(6):383–389.
783. Caruso RA. Intranuclear and intranucleolar tubular inclusions in gastric adenocarcinoma cells. Ultrastruct Pathol 1991;15(2):139–148.
784. Weidner N. Pulmonary adenocarcinoma with intestinal-type differentiation. Ultrastruct Pathol 1992;16(1–2):7–10.
785. Nakanishi K, Kawai T, Suzuki M. Large intracytoplasmic body in lung cancer compared with Clara cell granule. Am J Clin Pathol 1987;88(4):472–477.
786. Bennett DE, Million RR, Ackerman LV. Bilateral radiation pneumonitis, a complication of the radiotherapy of bronchogenic carcinoma. (Report and analysis of seven cases with autopsy.) Cancer 1969;23(5):1001–1018.
787. Flieder DB, Travis WD. Pathologic characteristics of drug-induced lung disease. Clin Chest Med 2004;25(1): 37–45.
788. Travis WD, Linnoila RI, Horowitz M, et al. Pulmonary nodules resembling bronchioloalveolar carcinoma in adolescent cancer patients. Mod Pathol 1988;1(5):372–377.
789. Sheikh HA, Fuhrer K, Cieply K, et al. p63 expression in assessment of bronchioloalveolar proliferations of the lung. Mod Pathol 2004;17(9):1134–1140.
790. Minami Y, Matsuno Y, Iijima T, et al. Prognostication of small-sized primary pulmonary adenocarcinomas by histopathological and karyometric analysis. Lung Cancer 2005;48(3):339–348.
791. Wu CT, Chang YL, Shih JY, et al. The significance of estrogen receptor beta in 301 surgically treated non-small cell lung cancers. J Thorac Cardiovasc Surg 2005;130(4): 979–986.
792. Ollayos CW, Riordan GP, Rushin JM. Estrogen receptor detection in paraffin sections of adenocarcinoma of the colon, pancreas, and lung. Arch Pathol Lab Med 1994; 118(6):630–632.
793. Vargas SO, Leslie KO, Vacek PM, et al. Estrogen-receptor-related protein p29 in primary nonsmall cell lung carcinoma: pathologic and prognostic correlations. Cancer 1998;82(8):1495–1500.
794. Dabbs DJ, Landreneau RJ, Liu Y, et al. Detection of estrogen receptor by immunohistochemistry in pulmonary adenocarcinoma. Ann Thorac Surg 2002;73(2):403–405; discussion 406.
795. Nakata M, Sawada S, Yamashita M, et al. Objective radiologic analysis of ground-glass opacity aimed at curative limited resection for small peripheral non-small cell lung cancer. J Thorac Cardiovasc Surg 2005;129(6):1226–1231.
796. Yokose T, Suzuki K, Nagai K, et al. Favorable and unfavorable morphological prognostic factors in peripheral adenocarcinoma of the lung 3 cm or less in diameter. Lung Cancer 2000;29(3):179–188.
797. Suzuki K, Yokose T, Yoshida J, et al. Prognostic significance of the size of central fibrosis in peripheral adenocarcinoma of the lung. Ann Thorac Surg 2000;69(3):893–897.
798. Maeshima AM, Niki T, Maeshima A, et al. Modified scar grade: a prognostic indicator in small peripheral lung adenocarcinoma. Cancer 2002;95(12):2546–2554.
799. Sakuragi T, Sakao Y, Fujita H, et al. Lymph node metastasis, recurrence, and prognosis in small peripheral lung adenocarcinoma. Analysis based on replacement. Jpn J Thorac Cardiovasc Surg 2002;50(10):424–429.
800. Kondo D, Yamada K, Kitayama Y, et al. Peripheral lung adenocarcinomas: 10 mm or less in diameter. Ann Thorac Surg 2003;76(2):350–355.
801. Sakurai H, Dobashi Y, Mizutani E, et al. Bronchioloalveolar carcinoma of the lung 3 centimeters or less in diameter: a prognostic assessment. Ann Thorac Surg 2004;78(5): 1728–1733.
802. Asamura H, Suzuki K, Watanabe S, et al. A clinicopathological study of resected subcentimeter lung cancers: a favorable prognosis for ground glass opacity lesions. Ann Thorac Surg 2003;76(4):1016–1022.
803. Noguchi M, Minami Y, Iijima T, et al. Reproducibility of the diagnosis of small adenocarcinoma of the lung and usefulness of an educational program for the diagnostic criteria. Pathol Int 2005;55(1):8–13.
804. Sakurai H, Maeshima A, Watanabe S, et al. Grade of stromal invasion in small adenocarcinoma of the lung: his-

topathological minimal invasion and prognosis. Am J Surg Pathol 2004;28(2):198–206.
805. Aoki T, Tomoda Y, Watanabe H, et al. Peripheral lung adenocarcinoma: correlation of thin-section CT findings with histologic prognostic factors and survival. Radiology 2001;220(3):803–809.
806. Yoshida J, Nagai K, Yokose T, et al. Limited resection trial for pulmonary ground-glass opacity nodules: fifty-case experience. J Thorac Cardiovasc Surg 2005;129(5): 991–996.
807. Miller VA, Kris MG, Shah N, et al. Bronchioloalveolar pathologic subtype and smoking history predict sensitivity to gefitinib in advanced non-small-cell lung cancer. J Clin Oncol 2004;22(6):1103–1109.
808. Hirsch FR, Varella-Garcia M, McCoy J, et al. Increased epidermal growth factor receptor gene copy number detected by fluorescence in situ hybridization associates with increased sensitivity to gefitinib in patients with bronchioloalveolar carcinoma subtypes: a Southwest Oncology Group Study. J Clin Oncol 2005;23(28):6838–6845.
809. Schleusener JT, Tazelaar HD, Jung SH, et al. Neuroendocrine differentiation is an independent prognostic factor in chemotherapy-treated nonsmall cell lung carcinoma. Cancer 1996;77(7):1284–1291.
810. Skov BG, Sorensen JB, Hirsch FR, et al. Prognostic impact of histologic demonstration of chromogranin A and neuron specific enolase in pulmonary adenocarcinoma. Ann Oncol 1991;2(5):355–360.
811. Hiroshima K, Iyoda A, Shibuya K, et al. Prognostic significance of neuroendocrine differentiation in adenocarcinoma of the lung. Ann Thorac Surg 2002;73(6):1732–1735.
812. Kodama T, Shimosato Y, Watanabe S, et al. Six cases of well-differentiated adenocarcinoma simulating fetal lung tubules in pseudoglandular stage. Comparison with pulmonary blastoma. Am J Surg Pathol 1984;8(10):735–744.
813. Nakatani Y, Kitamura H, Inayama Y, et al. Pulmonary adenocarcinomas of the fetal lung type: a clinicopathologic study indicating differences in histology, epidemiology, and natural history of low-grade and high-grade forms. Am J Surg Pathol 1998;22(4):399–411.
814. Kradin RL, Young RH, Dickersin GR, et al. Pulmonary blastoma with argyrophil cells and lacking sarcomatous features (pulmonary endodermal tumor resembling fetal lung). Am J Surg Pathol 1982;6(2):165–172.
815. Siegel RJ, Bueso-Ramos C, Cohen C, et al. Pulmonary blastoma with germ cell (yolk sac) differentiation: report of two cases. Mod Pathol 1991;4(5):566–570.
816. DiFurio MJ, Auerbach A, Kaplan KJ. Well-differentiated fetal adenocarcinoma: rare tumor in the pediatric population. Pediatr Dev Pathol 2003;6(6):564–567.
817. Singh SP, Besner GE, Schauer GM. Pulmonary endodermal tumor resembling fetal lung: report of a case in a 14-year-old girl. Pediatr Pathol Lab Med 1997;17(6):951–958.
818. Koss MN, Hochholzer L, O'Leary T. Pulmonary blastomas. Cancer 1991;67(9):2368–2381.
819. Nakatani Y, Dickersin GR, Mark EJ. Pulmonary endodermal tumor resembling fetal lung: a clinicopathologic study of five cases with immunohistochemical and ultrastructural characterization. Hum Pathol 1990;21(11):1097–1107.
820. Babycos PB, Daroca PJ, Jr. Polypoid pulmonary endodermal tumor resembling fetal lung: report of a case. Mod Pathol 1995;8(3):303–306.
821. Mardini G, Pai U, Chavez AM, et al. Endobronchial adenocarcinoma with endometrioid features and prominent neuroendocrine differentiation. A variant of fetal adenocarcinoma. Cancer 1994;73(5):1383–1389.
822. Nakatani Y, Kitamura H, Inayama Y, et al. Pulmonary endodermal tumor resembling fetal lung. The optically clear nucleus is rich in biotin. Am J Surg Pathol 1994;18(6):637–642.
823. Nakatani Y, Masudo K, Nozawa A, et al. Biotin-rich, optically clear nuclei express estrogen receptor-beta: tumors with morules may develop under the influence of estrogen and aberrant beta-catenin expression. Hum Pathol 2004; 35(7):869–874.
824. Gamachi A, Kashima K, Daa T, et al. Aberrant intranuclear localization of biotin, biotin-binding enzymes, and beta-catenin in pregnancy-related endometrium and morule-associated neoplastic lesions. Mod Pathol 2003; 16(11):1124–1131.
825. Yamazaki K. Pulmonary well-differentiated fetal adenocarcinoma expressing lineage-specific transcription factors (TTF-1 and GATA-6) to respiratory epithelial differentiation: an immunohistochemical and ultrastructural study. Virchows Arch 2003;442(4):393–399.
826. Nakatani Y, Masudo K, Miyagi Y, et al. Aberrant nuclear localization and gene mutation of beta-catenin in low-grade adenocarcinoma of fetal lung type: up-regulation of the Wnt signaling pathway may be a common denominator for the development of tumors that form morules. Mod Pathol 2002;15(6):617–624.
827. Shiojima K, Hayakawa K, Mitsuhashi N, et al. An autopsy case of pulmonary adenocarcinoma of fetal type treated with radiation therapy. Radiat Med 1994;12(1):36–38.
828. Moran CA, Hochholzer L, Fishback N, et al. Mucinous (so-called colloid) carcinomas of lung. Mod Pathol 1992; 5(6):634–638.
829. Rossi G, Murer B, Cavazza A, et al. Primary mucinous (so-called colloid) carcinomas of the lung: a clinicopathologic and immunohistochemical study with special reference to CDX-2 homeobox gene and MUC2 expression. Am J Surg Pathol 2004;28(4):442–452.
830. Brownlee NA, Mott RT, Mahar A, et al. Mucinous (colloid) adenocarcinoma of the lung. Arch Pathol Lab Med 2005;129(1):121–122.
831. Yousem SA. Pulmonary intestinal-type adenocarcinoma does not show enteric differentiation by immunohistochemical study. Mod Pathol 2005;18(6):816–821.
832. Maeshima A, Miyagi A, Hirai T, et al. Mucin-producing adenocarcinoma of the lung, with special reference to goblet cell type adenocarcinoma: immunohistochemical observation and Ki-ras gene mutation. Pathol Int 1997; 47(7):454–460.
833. Kragel PJ, Devaney KO, Meth BM, et al. Mucinous cystadenoma of the lung. A report of two cases with immu-

nohistochemical and ultrastructural analysis. Arch Pathol Lab Med 1990;114(10):1053–1056.

834. Roux FJ, Lantuejoul S, Brambilla E, et al. Mucinous cystadenoma of the lung. Cancer 1995;76(9):1540–1544.
835. Matsuo T, Yusuke Kimura N, Takamori S, et al. Recurrent pulmonary mucinous cystadenoma. Eur J Cardiothorac Surg 2005;28(1):176–177.
836. Gao ZH, Urbanski SJ. The spectrum of pulmonary mucinous cystic neoplasia: a clinicopathologic and immunohistochemical study of ten cases and review of literature. Am J Clin Pathol 2005;124(1):62–70.
837. Davison AM, Lowe JW, Da Costa P. Adenocarcinoma arising in a mucinous cystadenoma of the lung. Thorax 1992;47(2):129–130.
838. Graeme-Cook F, Mark EJ. Pulmonary mucinous cystic tumors of borderline malignancy. Hum Pathol 1991;22(2): 185–190.
839. Higashiyama M, Doi O, Kodama K, et al. Cystic mucinous adenocarcinoma of the lung. Two cases of cystic variant of mucus-producing lung adenocarcinoma. Chest 1992; 101(3):763–766.
840. Mann GN, Wilczynski SP, Sager K, et al. Recurrence of pulmonary mucinous cystic tumor of borderline malignancy. Ann Thorac Surg 2001;71(2):696–697.
841. Traub B. Mucinous cystadenoma of the lung. Arch Pathol Lab Med 1991;115(8):740–741.
842. Dixon AY, Moran JF, Wesselius LJ, et al. Pulmonary mucinous cystic tumor. Case report with review of the literature. Am J Surg Pathol 1993;17(7):722–728.
843. Castro CY, Moran CA, Flieder DG, et al. Primary signet ring cell adenocarcinomas of the lung: a clinicopathological study of 15 cases. Histopathology 2001;39(4):397–401.
844. Tsuta K, Ishii G, Yoh K, et al. Primary lung carcinoma with signet-ring cell carcinoma components: clinicopathological analysis of 39 cases. Am J Surg Pathol 2004; 28(7):868–874.
845. Hayashi H, Kitamura H, Nakatani Y, et al. Primary signet ring cell carcinoma of the lung: histochemical and immunohistochemical characterization. Hum Pathol 1999;30(4): 378–383.
846. Kish JK, Ro JY, Ayala AG, et al. Primary mucinous adenocarcinoma of the lung with signet-ring cells: a histochemical comparison with signet-ring cell carcinomas of other sites. Hum Pathol 1989;20(11):1097–1102.
847. Merchant SH, Amin MB, Tamboli P, et al. Primary signet-ring cell carcinoma of lung: immunohistochemical study and comparison with non-pulmonary signet-ring cell carcinomas. Am J Surg Pathol 2001;25(12):1515–1519.
848. Butala RM, Moscovic EA. Neuroendocrine markers in pulmonary adenocarcinomas with signet-ring cells. Hum Pathol 1990;21(10):1082.
849. Sarma DP, Hoffmann EO. Primary signet-ring cell carcinoma of the lung. Hum Pathol 1990;21(4):459–460.
850. Moran CA, Suster S, Koss MN. Acinic cell carcinoma of the lung ("Fechner tumor"). A clinicopathologic, immunohistochemical, and ultrastructural study of five cases. Am J Surg Pathol 1992;16(11):1039–1050.
851. Morgan AD, Mackenzie DH. Clear-cell carcinoma of the lung. J Pathol Bacteriol 1964;87:25–27.
852. Edwards C, Carlile A. Clear cell carcinoma of the lung. J Clin Pathol 1985;38(8):880–885.
853. Steinhauer JR, Moran CA, Suster S. "Secretory endometrioid-like" adenocarcinoma of the lung. Histopathology 2005;47(2):219–220.
854. Katzenstein AL, Purvis R Jr, Gmelich J, et al. Pulmonary resection for metastatic renal adenocarcinoma: pathologic findings and therapeutic value. Cancer 1978;41(2):712–723.
855. Tsuta K, Ishii G, Kim E, et al. Primary lung adenocarcinoma with massive lymphocyte infiltration. Am J Clin Pathol 2005;123(4):547–552.
856. Minami Y, Iijima T, Onizuka M, et al. Pulmonary adenocarcinoma with massive lymphocyte infiltration: report of three cases. Lung Cancer 2003;42(1):63–68.
857. Tsao MS, Fraser RS. Primary pulmonary adenocarcinoma with enteric differentiation. Cancer 1991;68(8):1754–1757.
858. Inamura K, Satoh Y, Okumura S, et al. Pulmonary adenocarcinomas with enteric differentiation: histologic and immunohistochemical characteristics compared with metastatic colorectal cancers and usual pulmonary adenocarcinomas. Am J Surg Pathol 2005;29(5):660–665.
859. Ishikura H, Kanda M, Ito M, et al. Hepatoid adenocarcinoma: a distinctive histological subtype of alpha-fetoprotein-producing lung carcinoma. Virchows Arch A Pathol Anat Histopathol 1990;417(1):73–80.
860. Hayashi Y, Takanashi Y, Ohsawa H, et al. Hepatoid adenocarcinoma in the lung. Lung Cancer 2002;38(2):211–214.
861. Carlinfante G, Foschini MP, Pasquinelli G, et al. Hepatoid carcinoma of the lung: a case report with immunohistochemical, ultrastructural and in-situ hybridization findings. Histopathology 2000;37(1):88–89.
862. Arnould L, Drouot F, Fargeot P, et al. Hepatoid adenocarcinoma of the lung: report of a case of an unusual alpha-fetoprotein-producing lung tumor. Am J Surg Pathol 1997;21(9):1113–1118.
863. Nasu M, Soma T, Fukushima H, et al. Hepatoid carcinoma of the lung with production of alpha-fetoprotein and abnormal prothrombin: an autopsy case report. Mod Pathol 1997;10(10):1054–1058.
864. Yesner R. Large cell carcinoma of the lung. Semin Diagn Pathol 1985;2(4):255–269.
865. Hammar S. Adenocarcinoma and large cell undifferentiated carcinoma of the lung. Ultrastruct Pathol 1987; 11(2–3):263–291.
866. Kodama T, Shimosato Y, Koide T, et al. Large cell carcinoma of the lung—ultrastructural and immunohistochemical studies. Jpn J Clin Oncol 1985;15(2):431–441.
867. Churg A. The fine structure of large cell undifferentiated carcinoma of the lung. Evidence for its relation to squamous cell carcinomas and adenocarcinomas. Hum Pathol 1978;9(2):143–156.
868. Kodama T, Takada K, Kameya T, et al. Large cell carcinoma of the lung associated with marked eosinophilia. A case report. Cancer 1984;54(10):2313–2317.
869. Johansson L. Histopathologic classification of lung cancer: Relevance of cytokeratin and TTF-1 immunophenotyping. Ann Diagn Pathol 2004;8(5):259–267.

870. Au NH, Cheang M, Huntsman DG, et al. Evaluation of immunohistochemical markers in non-small cell lung cancer by unsupervised hierarchical clustering analysis: a tissue microarray study of 284 cases and 18 markers. J Pathol 2004;204(1):101–109.
871. Ishida T, Kaneko S, Tateishi M, et al. Large cell carcinoma of the lung. Prognostic implications of histopathologic and immunohistochemical subtyping. Am J Clin Pathol 1990; 93(2):176–182.
872. Delmonte VC, Alberti O, Saldiva PH. Large cell carcinoma of the lung. Ultrastructural and immunohistochemical features. Chest 1986;90(4):524–527.
873. Ordonez NG. Value of cytokeratin 5/6 immunostaining in distinguishing epithelial mesothelioma of the pleura from lung adenocarcinoma. Am J Surg Pathol 1998;22(10): 1215–1221.
874. Leong AS. The relevance of ultrastructural examination in the classification of primary lung tumours. Pathology 1982;14(1):37–46.
875. Saba SR, Espinoza CG, Richman AV, et al. Carcinomas of the lung: an ultrastructural and immunocytochemical study. Am J Clin Pathol 1983;80(1):6–13.
876. Albain KS, True LD, Golomb HM, et al. Large cell carcinoma of the lung. Ultrastructural differentiation and clinicopathologic correlations. Cancer 1985;56(7):1618–1623.
877. Carter N, Nelson F, Gosney JR. Ultrastructural heterogeneity in undifferentiated bronchial carcinoma. J Pathol 1993;171(1):53–57.
878. Downey RS, Sewell CW, Mansour KA. Large cell carcinoma of the lung: a highly aggressive tumor with dismal prognosis. Ann Thorac Surg 1989;47(6):806–808.
879. Downey RJ, Asakura S, Deschamps C, et al. Large cell carcinoma of the lung: results of resection for a cure. J Thorac Cardiovasc Surg 1999;117(3):599–604.
880. Wertzel H, Grahmann PR, Bansbach S, et al. Results after surgery in undifferentiated large cell carcinoma of the lung: the role of neuroendocrine expression. Eur J Cardiothorac Surg 1997;12(5):698–702.
881. Martini N, Rusch VW, Bains MS, et al. Factors influencing ten-year survival in resected stages I to IIIa non-small cell lung cancer. J Thorac Cardiovasc Surg 1999;117(1):32–36; discussion 37–38.
882. McDowell EM, Barrett LA, Glavin F, et al. The respiratory epithelium. I. Human bronchus. J Natl Cancer Inst 1978;61(2):539–549.
883. Sturm N, Lantuejoul S, Laverriere MH, et al. Thyroid transcription factor 1 and cytokeratins 1, 5, 10, 14 (34betaE12) expression in basaloid and large-cell neuroendocrine carcinomas of the lung. Hum Pathol 2001;32(9):918–925.
884. Geddy PM, Gouldesbrough DR. Basal cell (basaloid) carcinoma of the lung. Hum Pathol 1993;24(4):452–453.
885. Guinee DG Jr, Fishback NF, Koss MN, et al. The spectrum of immunohistochemical staining of small-cell lung carcinoma in specimens from transbronchial and open-lung biopsies. Am J Clin Pathol 1994;102(4):406–414.
886. Folpe AL, Gown AM, Lamps LW, et al. Thyroid transcription factor-1: immunohistochemical evaluation in pulmonary neuroendocrine tumors. Mod Pathol 1999;12(1): 5–8.
887. Moro D, Brichon PY, Brambilla E, et al. Basaloid bronchial carcinoma. A histologic group with a poor prognosis. Cancer 1994;73(11):2734–2739.
888. Foroulis CN, Iliadis KH, Mauroudis PM, et al. Basaloid carcinoma, a rare primary lung neoplasm: report of a case and review of the literature. Lung Cancer 2002;35(3):335–338.
889. Ro YS, Park JH, Park CK, et al. Basaloid carcinoma of the lung presenting concurrently with cutaneous metastasis. J Am Acad Dermatol 2003;49(3):523–526.
890. Kim DJ, Kim KD, Shin DH, et al. Basaloid carcinoma of the lung: a really dismal histologic variant? Ann Thorac Surg 2003;76(6):1833–1837.
891. Inase N, Takayama S, Nakayama M, et al. Pulmonary clear cell carcinoma. J Surg Oncol 1991;48(2):145–147.
892. McNamee CJ, Simpson RH, Pagliero KM, et al. Primary clear-cell carcinoma of the lung. Respir Med 1993;87(6): 471–473.
893. Garzon JC, Lai FM, Mok TS, et al. Clear cell carcinoma of the lung revisited. J Thorac Cardiovasc Surg 2005; 130(4):1198–1199.
894. Yamamato T, Yazawa T, Ogata T, et al. Clear cell carcinoma of the lung: a case report and review of the literature. Lung Cancer 1993;10(1–2):101–106.
895. Gaffey MJ, Mills SE, Frierson HF Jr, et al. Pulmonary clear cell carcinoid tumor: another entity in the differential diagnosis of pulmonary clear cell neoplasia. Am J Surg Pathol 1998;22(8):1020–1025.
896. Gaffey MJ, Mills SE, Zarbo RJ, et al. Clear cell tumor of the lung. Immunohistochemical and ultrastructural evidence of melanogenesis. Am J Surg Pathol 1991;15(7): 644–653.
897. Parham DM, Weeks DA, Beckwith JB. The clinicopathologic spectrum of putative extrarenal rhabdoid tumors. An analysis of 42 cases studied with immunohistochemistry or electron microscopy. Am J Surg Pathol 1994;18(10):1010–1029.
898. Chetty R, Bhana B, Batitang S, et al. Lung carcinomas composed of rhabdoid cells. Eur J Surg Oncol 1997;23(5): 432–434.
899. Chetty R. Combined large cell neuroendocrine, small cell and squamous carcinomas of the lung with rhabdoid cells. Pathology 2000;32(3):209–212.
900. Attems JH, Lintner F. Pseudomesotheliomatous adenocarcinoma of the lung with rhabdoid features. Pathol Res Pract 2001;197(12):841–846.
901. Miyagi J, Tsuhako K, Kinjo T, et al. Rhabdoid tumour of the lung is a dedifferentiated phenotype of pulmonary adenocarcinoma. Histopathology 2000;37(1):37–44.
902. Hammar S, Troncoso P, Yowell R, et al. Use of electron microscopy in the diagnosis of uncommon lung tumors. Ultrastruct Pathol 1993;17(3–4):319–351.
903. Ordonez NG. Mesothelioma with rhabdoid features: an ultrastructural and immunohistochemical study of 10 cases. Mod Pathol 2006;19:373–383.
904. Hiroshima K, Shibuya K, Shimamura F, et al. Pulmonary large cell carcinoma with rhabdoid phenotype. Ultrastruct Pathol 2003;27(1):55–59.

905. Yilmazbayhan D, Ates LE, Dilege S, et al. Pulmonary large cell carcinoma with rhabdoid phenotype. Ann Diagn Pathol 2005;9(4):223–226.
906. Cavazza A, Colby TV, Tsokos M, et al. Lung tumors with a rhabdoid phenotype. Am J Clin Pathol 1996;105(2):182–188.
907. Rubenchik I, Dardick I, Auger M. Cytopathology and ultrastructure of primary rhabdoid tumor of lung. Ultrastruct Pathol 1996;20(4):355–360.
908. Colby TV, Koss MN, Travis WD. Carcinoid and other neuroendocrine tumors. In: Colby TV, Koss MN, Travis WD, eds. Tumors of the lower respiratory tract. 3rd ed. Washington, DC: Armed Forces Institute of Pathology, 1995:311–312.
909. Kaneko T, Honda T, Fukushima M, et al. Large cell carcinoma of the lung with a rhabdoid phenotype. Pathol Int 2002;52(10):643–647.
910. Tamboli P, Toprani TH, Amin MB, et al. Carcinoma of lung with rhabdoid features. Hum Pathol 2004;35(1):8–13.
911. Fitzgibbons PL, Kern WH. Adenosquamous carcinoma of the lung: a clinical and pathologic study of seven cases. Hum Pathol 1985;16(5):463–466.
912. Nakagawa K, Yasumitu T, Fukuhara K, et al. Poor prognosis after lung resection for patients with adenosquamous carcinoma of the lung. Ann Thorac Surg 2003;75(6):1740–1744.
913. Takamori S, Noguchi M, Morinaga S, et al. Clinicopathologic characteristics of adenosquamous carcinoma of the lung. Cancer 1991;67(3):649–654.
914. Ishida T, Kaneko S, Yokoyama H, et al. Adenosquamous carcinoma of the lung. Clinicopathologic and immunohistochemical features. Am J Clin Pathol 1992;97(5):678–685.
915. Gawrychowski J, Brulinski K, Malinowski E, et al. Prognosis and survival after radical resection of primary adenosquamous lung carcinoma. Eur J Cardiothorac Surg 2005;27(4):686–692.
916. Naunheim KS, Taylor JR, Skosey C, et al. Adenosquamous lung carcinoma: clinical characteristics, treatment, and prognosis. Ann Thorac Surg 1987;44(5):462–466.
917. Ichinose Y, Hara N, Takamori S, et al. DNA ploidy pattern of each carcinomatous component in adenosquamous lung carcinoma. Ann Thorac Surg 1993;55(3):593–596.
918. Steele VE, Nettesheim P. Unstable cellular differentiation in adenosquamous cell carcinoma. J Natl Cancer Inst 1981;67(1):149–154.
919. Yousem SA. Pulmonary adenosquamous carcinomas with amyloid-like stroma. Mod Pathol 1989;2(5):420–426.
920. Shimizu J, Oda M, Hayashi Y, et al. A clinicopathologic study of resected cases of adenosquamous carcinoma of the lung. Chest 1996;109(4):989–994.
921. Horie A, Ohta M. Ultrastructural features of large cell carcinoma of the lung with reference to the prognosis of patients. Hum Pathol 1981;12(5):423–432.
922. Auerbach O, Frasca JM, Parks VR, et al. A comparison of World Health Organization (WHO) classification of lung tumors by light and electron microscopy. Cancer 1982;50(10):2079–2088.
923. Yousem SA, Hochholzer L. Mucoepidermoid tumors of the lung. Cancer 1987;60(6):1346–1352.
924. Department of Health and Human Services. The health consequences of involuntary smoking. Report No. 87–8398. Washington, DC: United States Department of Health and Human Services, Centers for Disease Control, 1986.
925. Colby TV, Koss MN, Travis WD. Carcinoma of the lung: Clinical and radiographic aspects, spread, staging, management, and prognosis. In: Colby TV, Koss MN, Travis WD, eds. Tumors of the lower respiratory tract. 3rd ed. Washington, DC: Armed Forces Institute of Pathology, 1995:107–134.
926. Diet and nutrition. In: Stewart BW, Kleihues P, International Agency for Research on Cancer, eds. World cancer report. Lyon: IARC Press, 2003:62–68.

36
Neuroendocrine Tumors

Samuel P. Hammar

Neuroendocrine Neoplasms of the Lung

Of all neoplasms that occur in the body, few have been studied or written about as much as neuroendocrine lung tumors. Neuroendocrine lung neoplasms exhibit a wide variety of morphologic appearances, ranging from typical carcinoid to small cell (undifferentiated) carcinoma (small cell lung cancer [SCLC]). A conceptual understanding of these neoplasms is based on knowledge of the neuroendocrine cell system and the evolution of the amine precursor uptake and decarboxylase (APUD) concept.

There exists in many tissues and organs in the body a population of cells, initially conceptualized by Feyrter[1] in 1938, referred to as epithelial clear cells and considered to be part of a diffuse epithelial endocrine system; the cells have similar morphologic and biochemical features. These cells were designated APUD cells on the basis of their capability to take up and decarboxylate amine precursors, including 3,4-dihydroxyphenylalanine (L-dopa) and 5-hydroxytryptophan (5-HTP). Because of this property, the cells could be identified histochemically as decarboxylated amines, and they form highly fluorescent derivatives with formaldehyde vapor. Pearse[2] initially thought all these cells were of neural crest origin, although numerous studies proved this to be incorrect. Pearse and Takor[3] later suggested that neuroendocrine cells could be (1) derivatives of neural crest, which include the adrenal medulla, all paraganglia, perifollicular-C cells of the thyroid, melanocytes, and possibly Merkel cells of the skin; (2) neural tube- and ridge-derived cells, which include those in the hypophysis, and the hypothalamic neuroendocrine cells; and (3) derivatives of the neuroendocrine-programmed ectoblast, which include the neuroendocrine cells in the gastroenteropancreatic system, the bronchopulmonary tree, parathyroid chief cells, placental endocrine cells, and various other related cells. Pearse[4] introduced the term *diffuse neuroendocrine system* to refer to this group of cells.

Gould and DeLellis[5] and Gould et a1.[6,7] extensively reviewed the cellular components and neoplasms of this system and suggested the term *dispersed neuroendocrine system* to refer to these cells (Fig. 36.1). As summarized by Gould et a1.[8] in 1987,

> The dispersed neuroendocrine system, as currently understood, encompasses elements of the central and peripheral nervous systems; a number of traditional neuroendocrine organs such as the hypophysis; assemblies of endocrine cells such as the pancreatic islets and the pulmonary neuroepithelial bodies; and a large number of widely distributed single endocrine cells demonstrable in numerous organs and tissues, including the thyroid, gastrointestinal and bronchopulmonary tract, and the skin.

Not surprisingly, many of these cells have similar biochemical features and contain a variety of biogenic amines, peptide hormones, and neurotransmitters that can be identified biochemically or immunohistochemically.[9] The location of neuropeptides within the autonomic nervous system of the lung and function of these neuropeptides has been reviewed.[10]

Identification of Neuroendocrine Cells and Neuroendocrine Neoplasms

Normal neuroendocrine cells and neoplasms of neuroendocrine cells can be identified in several ways.

Histochemical Identification

Neuroendocrine Cells

Neuroendocrine cells are argyrophilic, which can be demonstrated with a Grimelius or Sevier–Munger silver nitrate stain, or they express the property of argentaffin-

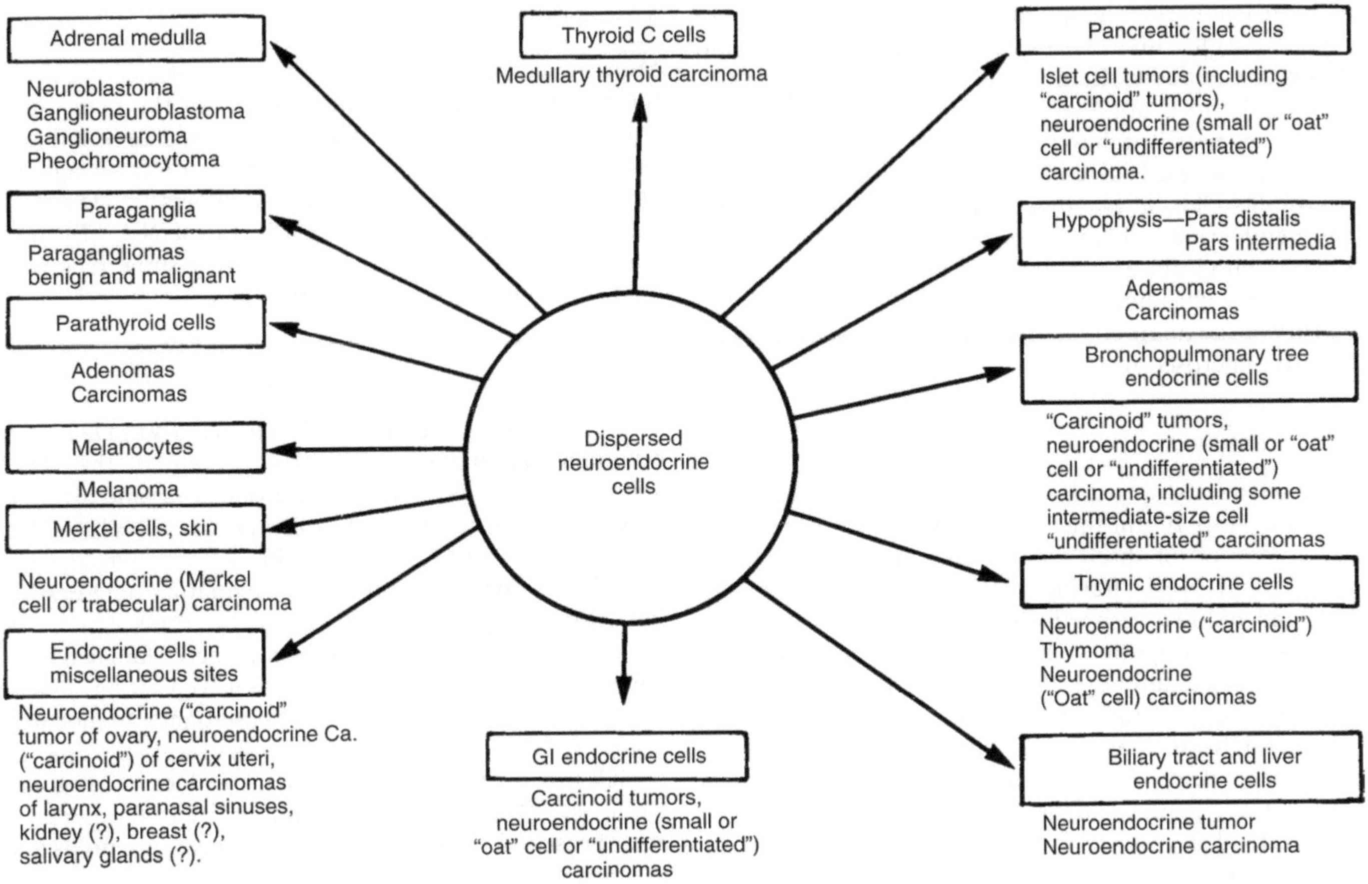

FIGURE 36.1. Diagrammatic representation of dispersed neuroendocrine system. (From Gould and DeLellis.[5] Copyright © 1983 by Churchill Livingstone, with permission.)

ity. The cells exhibit marked metachromasia with toluidine blue or coriophosphine O after acid hydrolysis.

Immunohistochemical-Biochemical Identification

Neuron-specific enolase (2-phospho-D-glycerate hydrolase) catalyzes the interconversion of 2-phosphoglycerate and phosphoenolpyruvate in the glycolytic pathway. Enolases are dimers composed of three distinct subunits—alpha, beta, and gamma. The gamma subunit is in the highest concentration in the central and peripheral nervous system as alpha–gamma and gamma-gamma dimers. Neuron-specific enolase refers to gamma enolase, which can be identified biochemically or immunohistochemically in high concentrations in neuronal and neuroendocrine cells. Neuron-specific enolase is not found exclusively in neurons or neuroendocrine cells.

Haimoto et al.[11] reported immunohistochemical localization of gamma enolase in many normal nonneural and nonneuroendocrine cells (see their Table 1) such as smooth muscle cells, renal epithelial cells, lymphocytes, myoepithelial cells, megakaryocytes, and plasma cells. Pahlman et al.[12] measured neuron-specific enolase enzymatically and by radioimmunoassay in several different tumors and cell lines and found the enzyme was present in a variety of nonneuroendocrine neoplasms and neuroendocrine tumors. Vinores et al.[13] reported similar findings, identifying neuron-specific enolase in breast carcinoma, chordoma, and renal cell carcinoma. Bergh et al.[14] reported that 14 of 21 non–small-cell lung cancers (NSCLCs) showed immunocytochemical staining for neuron-specific enolase, and Said et al.[15] found that 57% of nonneuroendocrine lung tumors showed immunostaining for the enzyme. Schmechel[16] reviewed the specificity of neuron-specific enolase and stated the gamma subunit of enolase was neither nonspecific nor neuron specific.

Chromogranins

Chromogranins are a family of acidic proteins containing high concentrations of glutamic acid and are located within the matrix of neuroendocrine granules in many normal neuroendocrine cells and in the cells of a variety of neuroendocrine neoplasms.[17–22] Chromogranins are subdivided into three classes: A, B, and C. Chromogranin-A was discovered by Banks and Helle[23] in 1965. Chromogranins B and C are also referred to as secretogranin 1 and 2. Angeletti[24] updated our knowledge on chromogranins and discussed the controversy concerning these glycoproteins. Chromogranin A has been identified in normal neuroendocrine cells of the bronchopulmonary tract.[25,26] I agree with Said et al.[15] that the intensity of immunostaining for chromogranin A usually correlates with the density of the neuroendocrine granules as determined by electron microscopy.

Neurofilaments

Neurofilaments are one of five major classes of intermediate 7- to 10-nm-thick filaments that in vertebrates are composed of three polypeptides designated NF-H, NF-M, and NF-L having molecular weights of 200, 160, and 68 kDa, respectively. Neurons and some normal and neoplastic neuroendocrine cells contain neurofilaments, although they may be difficult or impossible to demonstrate in conventional formalin-fixed processed tissue. They are often difficult to identify immunohistochemically in neuroendocrine neoplasms.[27] In a study of 112 neuroendocrine tumors, Shah et al.[28] were unable to demonstrate immunoreactivity for NF-H or NF-L in any of the neoplasms. Leoncini et al.[29] reported that the ability to demonstrate neurofilaments in neuroendocrine lung neoplasms depends on whether the neurofilament epitopes are phosphorylated. Immunoreactivity for NF-M and NF-H was much more frequent when phosphorylation of the neurofilament subunit was present. Leoncini et al. suggested the lack of phosphorylation could explain the reported low rate of neurofilament expression.

Synaptophysin

Synaptophysin is a 38-kDa glycoprotein component of presynaptic vesicles that was originally isolated from bovine neurons.[30] Using immunofluorescence microscopy on frozen sections, synaptophysin can be demonstrated in neurons and neuroendocrine cells and in a variety of neuroendocrine neoplasms, including neuroendocrine tumors of the lung.[8,31]

Leu7

Leu7, initially used as a monoclonal antibody to identify natural killer cells, was observed to immunostain neuroendocrine tumor cells, including those of small cell lung carcinoma.[32,33] Leu7 has been demonstrated to react with a 75- to 82-kDa protein within the matrix of some neuroendocrine granules.[34]

Monoclonal Antibody 735

Monoclonal antibody 735, directed against the long-chain form of polysialic acid, which is part of the neural cell adhesion molecule (NCAM), immunostains small cell carcinomas but shows minimal or no reaction against typical carcinoids and atypical carcinoids.[35,36] This and other similar antibodies directed against N-CAM antibody have also been reported to rarely show reactivity toward non–small-cell lung neoplasms.[37]

Thyroid Transcription Factor 1

Thyroid transcription factor-1 (TTF-1) is a 40-kDa homeodomain-containing transcription protein of the Nkx2 gene family that is expressed in bronchiolar and alveolar type II cells of the lung, in follicular and C cells of the thyroid, and in the developing brain.[38–40] Thyroid transcription factor-1 is important in regulating lung epithelial morphogenesis in activating the transcription of surfactant proteins A, B, and C genes, and Clara cell–specific secretory protein gene. In addition to showing nuclear immunostaining of about 70% of pulmonary adenocarcinomas, TTF-1 is also expressed in a significant percentage of SCLCs[40–46] and in large cell neuroendocrine lung carcinomas.[45,47,48] There has been variability in the percentage of cases of TTF-1 expression in typical carcinoids and atypical cardinoids.[42,45,47,49]

Sturm et al.[50] evaluated TTF-1 expression in 15 cases of neuroendocrine hyperplasia, 23 pulmonary tumorlets, 27 typical carcinoids, 23 atypical carcinoids, 64 large cell neuroendocrine carcinomas, and 55 SCLCs. No cases of neuroendocrine hyperplasia, tumorlet, typical carcinoid, or atypical carcinoid showed TTF-1 expression. In contrast, 31 of 64 (48%) large cell neuroendocrine carcinomas showed TTF-1 expression and 37 of 55 (67%) SCLCs showed TTF-1 expression. In contrast, Saqi et al.[51] found TTF-1 expression in eight of 15 (53%) typical pulmonary carcinoids but did not find TTF-1 expression in gastrointestinal (GI) tract carcinoid tumors.

CD117

CD117 (c-Kit) is a transmembrane tyrosine kinase receptor that has been immunolocalized in various neoplasms, the most noticeable of which are gastrointestinal stromal tumors and chronic granulocytic leukemia.[52] c-Kit expression has also been observed in large cell neuroendocrine carcinomas and is associated with a worse prognosis than those large cell neuroendocrine carcinomas that do not express c-Kit.[53] Butnor et al.[54] evaluated 61 carcinomas, including 11 small cell carcinomas, four large cell neuroendocrine carcinomas, 22 squamous cell carcinomas, 23 adenocarcinomas, 11 typical pulmonary carcinoid tumors, 19 pleural malignant mesotheliomas, and six localized

TABLE 36.1. Neuropeptides and neuroamines commonly found in neuroendocrine lung neoplasms

Bombesin
Calcitonin
Adrenocorticotropic hormone
Leu-enkephalin
Gastrin
Somatostatin
Vasoactive intestinal polypeptide
Neurotensin
Arginine vasopressin
Serotonin

pleural fibrous tumors using a polyclonal c-Kit antibody. c-Kit staining was observed in 82% of the SCLCs and in 25% of the large cell neuroendocrine carcinomas. Typical pulmonary carcinoids showed no reactivity with c-Kit. The authors concluded the high frequency of c-Kit immunoreactivity in SCLC could have important potential therapeutic implications.

Other Immunocytochemical Markers

Other immunocytochemical markers of neuroendocrine cells and neoplasms include various neuropeptides that can be identified in normal and neoplastic neuroendocrine cells (Table 36.1). For example, calcitonin, vasoactive intestinal polypeptide, and adrenocorticotrophic hormone can be identified in neuroendocrine tumors of the skin and lung.[6,7] These substances are not present in every tumor cell and are not specific for any given neuroendocrine neoplasm. It should also be stressed that a significant number of nonneuroendocrine lung neoplasms contain one or more of these substances.[55] Although initially controversial,[56–61] all neuroendocrine tumors of epithelial origin, such as neuroendocrine neoplasms of the lung, contain keratin[62–65] and desmoplakin proteins.[66] Funa et al.[67] reported in 1986 that small cell carcinomas of lung and some other neuroendocrine neoplasms lacked β_2-microglobulin, whereas NSCLC strongly expressed this antigen. They suggested the demonstration of β_2-microglobulin could be used to differentiate neuroendocrine lung tumors from nonneuroendocrine lung neoplasms.

Ultrastructural Identification

In 1984, Payne et al.[68] described a specific ultrastructural cytochemical stain, called the uranaffin stain, which distinguished true neuroendocrine granules from neuroendocrine-like granules found in a variety of nonneuroendocrine neoplasms. Nagle et al.[69] studied 41 neuroendocrine tumors by an avidin-biotin immunoperoxidase technique for neuron-specific enolase, bombesin, adrenocorticotrophic hormone, calcitonin, and serotonin. In addition, they studied the tumors by transmission electron microscopy and with the uranaffin stain. All tumors contained neuroendocrine granules demonstrable by electron microscopy and the uranaffin stain, but seven of 16 poorly differentiated neuroendocrine neoplasms were negative with all antisera tested. The authors suggested the uranaffin reaction and transmission electron microscopy were more specific for diagnosing poorly differentiated neuroendocrine tumors. Ultrastructurally, the most distinctive feature of all neuroendocrine lung neoplasms are dense-core, membrane-bound, neuroendocrine granules, which are occasionally referred to as neurosecretory granules. The number and size of neuroendocrine granules vary considerably from one neuroendocrine tumor to the next.[9] For example, neuroendocrine granules are numerous in most typical lung carcinoids but are usually rare in small cell neuroendocrine lung neoplasms. It should be emphasized that ultrastructurally, dense-core granules in normal neuroendocrine cells resemble neuroendocrine granules in neoplastic cells.[70,71] Another ultrastructural feature common to most neoplastic neuroendocrine cells are processes that usually contain microtubules and intermediate filaments.

Molecular Biology Techniques

The study of gene expression has been useful in identifying some neuroendocrine lung neoplasms and requires molecular biology techniques, including Northern and Southern blotting, polymerase chain reaction, and in-situ hybridization. Using chromosomal RNA (cRNA) probes and in-situ hybridization, gastrin-releasing polypeptide gene expression has been identified in most typical bronchopulmonary carcinoids but only in a few small cell and large cell neuroendocrine carcinomas.[72] Chromogranin A is identified by immunohistochemistry in approximately 25% of small cell lung carcinomas because of the relatively low concentration of neuroendocrine granules, whereas using molecular biology techniques, messenger RNA for chromogranin A can be identified in nearly all small cell lung carcinomas (see Chapter 33).[73]

Normal Neuroendocrine Cells of the Lung

In 1949, Frohlich[74] described solitary and nodular aggregates of neuroendocrine cells in the bronchi. He thought these cells had a chemoreceptive or neurosecretory function. The presence of these cells was confirmed by Feyrter,[75] who suggested bronchial carcinoids originated from them. In the mid-1960s, Bensch and colleagues[76,77]

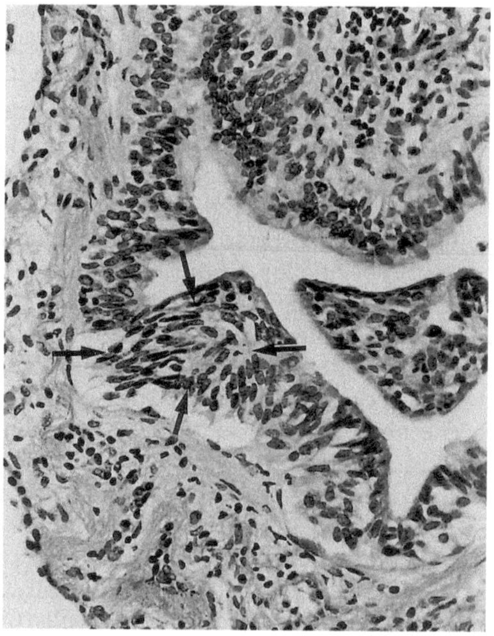

FIGURE 36.2. Portion of bronchus of 10-year-old child whose lung tissue showed diffuse interstitial fibrosis. Neuroepithelial body (*arrows*) is composed mostly of spindle-shaped cells.

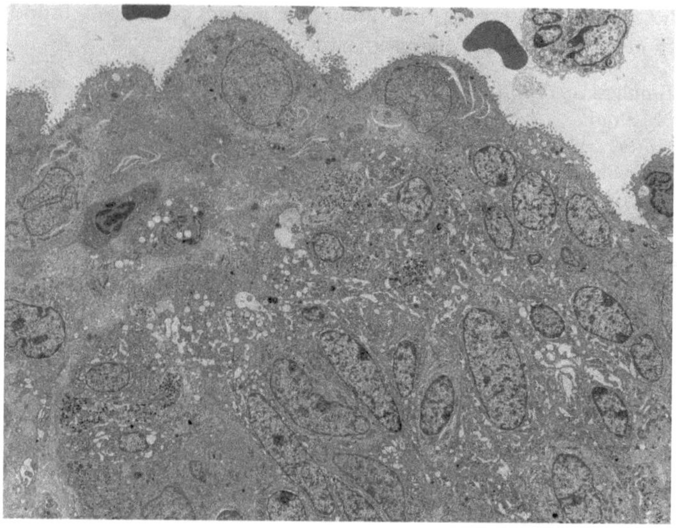

FIGURE 36.4. Ultrastructural appearance of neuroepithelial body. Note surface epithelial cells and underlying neuroendocrine cells containing cytoplasmic electron-dense granules. ×2700.

and Gmelich and Bensch[78] described the ultrastructural appearance of neuroendocrine cells and related these cells to bronchial carcinoids and to small cell lung carcinomas that were found to contain the same type of neuroendocrine granules. In 1972 and 1973, Lauweryns et al.[79] and Lauweryns and Goddeeris[80] reemphasized the morphology of neuroepithelial bodies (Figs. 36.2 and 36.3) as clusters of eosinophilic cells in hematoxylin and eosin (H&E)-stained sections that extended from basement membrane of the bronchial mucosa to the lumen, displayed argyrophilia, and contained neuroendocrine granules when examined ultrastructurally (Figs. 36.4 and 36.5). Neuroepithelial bodies appear to be innervated and are frequently found in association with vessels,

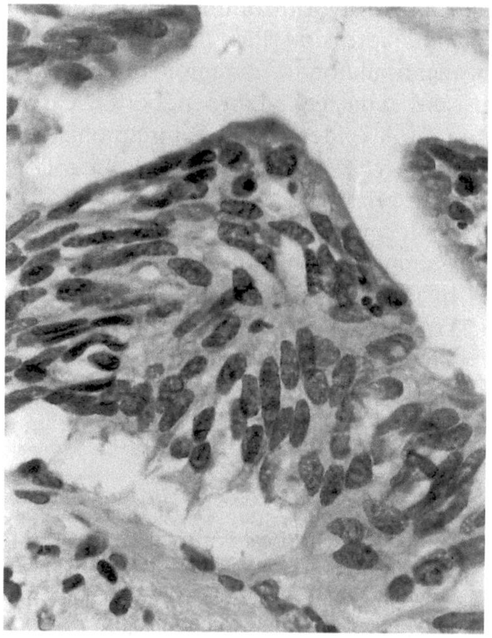

FIGURE 36.3. Neuroepithelial body at greater magnification. ×775.

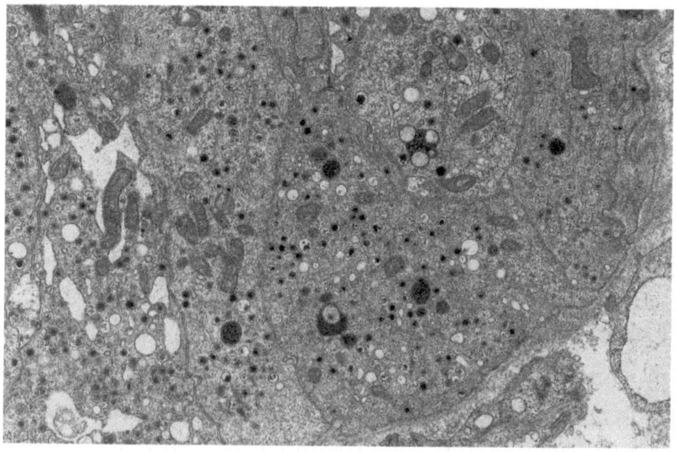

FIGURE 36.5. At greater magnification, ultrastructural features of neuroendocrine cells forming neuroepithelial bodies are better seen. Note obvious dense-core granules and prominent lysosomes (residual bodies-ceroid pigment). ×16,000.

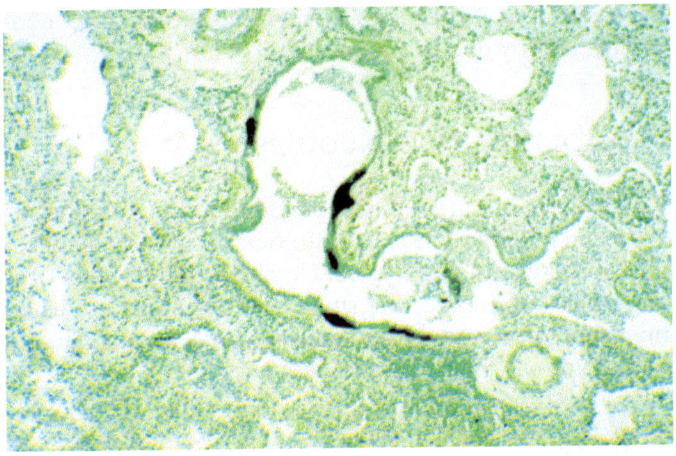

FIGURE 36.6. Lung tissue shown in Figure 36.2 immunostained for neuron-specific enolase, which highlights (*black*) neuroepithelial bodies.

which suggests they have a neurosecretory or chemoreceptive function.

Pulmonary neuroendocrine cells are increased in persons living at high altitude, and are seen in increased numbers in children with bronchopulmonary dysplasia, cystic fibrosis, and bronchiectasis.[81,82] Their prominence in fetal tissue suggested they produce growth factors such as gastrin-releasing peptide, which might contribute to the morphogenesis and maturation of the lung.[83–85] They are also increased (or possibly induced) in cigarette smoke–associated pulmonary diseases in adults.[86–88] Aguayo et al.[89] reported increased concentrations of peptides of bombesin-like immunoreactivity in bronchoalveolar lavage fluid from normal cigarette smokers, and

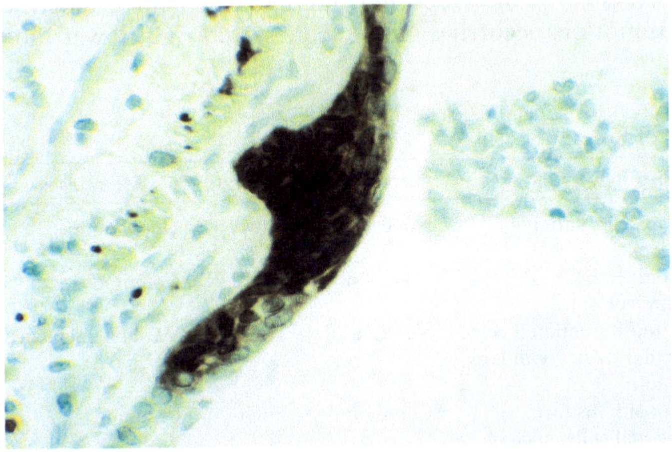

FIGURE 36.7. Neuroepithelial body in lung tissue shows intense immunostaining (*black*) for chromogranin.

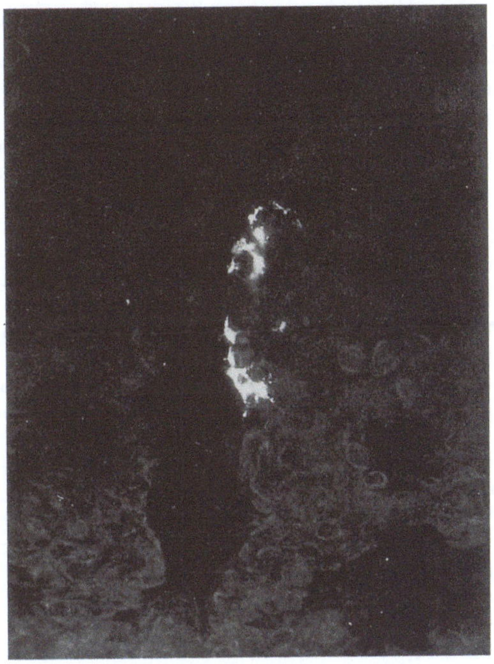

FIGURE 36.8. Neuroepithelial body also expresses synaptophysin using direct immunofluorescent technique. (Courtesy of V. E. Gould, M.D.)

Tabassian et al.[90] found that subchronic cigarette-smoke exposure caused increased pulmonary concentrations of immunoreactive calcitonin and mammalian bombesin in hamster lungs. In 1992, Aguayo et al.[91] reported hyperplasia of pulmonary neuroendocrine cells in six nonsmokers with obliteration of small airways and suggested the product(s) produced by these neuroendocrine cells, for example, bombesin, was the cause of the fibrotic airway disease (see Chapter 34). A summary of the reactions of normal neuroendocrine cells to stimuli is provided by Gould et al.[6] Neuroepithelial bodies are easily identified immunohistochemically with antibodies against neuron-specific enolase, chromogranin, or synaptophysin (Figs. 36.6 to 36.8).

Nomenclature of Neuroendocrine Neoplasms of Lung

The nomenclature of neuroendocrine lung neoplasms has undergone an evolution over the years.[92] Neuroendocrine proliferations and neoplasms are listed in Table 36.2. As discussed below, some neuroendocrine lung neoplasms have been referred to by various names, and it is important to recognize this, especially when discussing cases with clinicians.

TABLE 36.2. The spectrum of neuroendocrine proliferations and neoplasms

I. Neuroendocrine cell hyperplasia and tumorlets	A. Neuroendocrine cell hyperplasia
	(1) Neuroendocrine cell hyperplasia associated with fibrosis and/or inflammation
	(2) Neuroendocrine cell hyperplasia adjacent to carcinoid tumors
	(3) Diffuse idiopathic neuroendocrine cell hyperplasia with or without airway fibrosis/obstruction
	B. Tumorlets
II. Tumors with neuroendocrine morphology	A. Typical carcinoid
	B. Atypical carcinoid
	C. Large cell neuroendocrine carcinoma
	D. Small cell carcinoma
III. Non-small-cell carcinomas with neuroendocrine differentiation	
IV. Other tumors with neuroendocrine properties	A. Pulmonary blastoma
	B. Primitive neuroectodermal tumor
	C. Desmoplastic round cell tumor
	D. Carcinomas with rhabdoid phenotype
	E. Paraganglioma
	F. Amphicrine carcinoma

Preinvasive Lesions

The majority of neuroendocrine cell hyperplasias are secondary to airway fibrosis or inflammation. Diffuse idiopathic pulmonary neuroendocrine cell hyperplasia (DIPNECH) may be associated with airway fibrosis or obstruction, and is thought to be a precursor to the development of multiple tumorlets and typical or atypical carcinoids. A thorough discussion of neuroendocrine cell hyperplasia as a precursor to neuroendocrine lung neoplasms is provided in Chapter 34.

Neuroendocrine Neoplasms

The general features of neuroendocrine lung neoplasms are listed in Table 36.3. The histologic criteria for diagnosing typical carcinoid, atypical carcinoid, large cell neuroendocrine carcinoma, and small cell carcinoma are listed in Table 36.4 and based on the 2004 World Health Organization (WHO) classification.[93,94]

Tumorlet

Tumorlet is a term coined by Whitwell[95] in 1955, who described 24 cases of localized neuroendocrine cell proliferation in lobes resected for bronchiectasis or lung abscess. Tumorlets represent localized regions of neuroendocrine cell proliferation, usually centered on scarred small airways, often in association with pulmonary fibrosis or bronchiectasis (Fig. 36.9). However, in the Churg and Warnock[96] autopsy study of 20 tumorlets, only one third occurred in diseased lungs.

Tumorlets are often discovered incidentally at autopsy, in open biopsies that show pulmonary fibrosis, or in lobes that are resected for bronchiectasis or other chronic conditions. Ultrastructurally the cells of tumorlets closely resemble those forming neuroepithelial bodies and typical carcinoid tumors. Conceptually, tumorlets can be thought of as large neuroepithelial bodies or small typical carcinoids. An unusual case of multiple tumorlets and mature carcinoid tumors was reported in a 53-year-old woman with a 25-year history of nonproductive hacking cough and occasional traces of hemoptysis.[97] These tumors were thought to be responsible for the observed pulmonary function test abnormalities of mild restrictive and obstructive defects.

Pelosi et al.[98] reported hundreds of neuroendocrine tumorlets occurring in the sequestered right lower lobe

TABLE 36.3. General features of neuroendocrine (NE) neoplasms of lung

Type of NE neoplasm	Relative frequency	Location in lung	Histology-cytology	Necrosis	Mitotic rate	Metastases
Carcinoid	Infrequent	Central	Uniform cells; variable patterns	None	Low	Uncommon
Atypical carcinoid	Uncommon	Peripheral in 60% of cases	Organoid; cellular pleomorphism	Common	High	Common
Large cell neuroendocrine carcinoma	Uncertain	Midzone or peripheral	Large undifferentiated cells; vesicular nuclei with large nucleoli	Variable	High	Variable incidence
Small cell neuroendocrine carcinoma	Frequent; 20% of common lung neoplasms	Central	Small ovoid, fusiform, or polygonal cells; nucleoli inconspicuous	Common	High	Common

TABLE 36.4. Criteria for diagnosis of neuroendocrine tumors

Typical carcinoid	A tumor with carcinoid morphology and less than two mitoses per 2 mm^2 (10 high power fields), lacking necrosis and 0.5 cm or larger
Atypical carcinoid	A tumor with carcinoid morphology with two to 10 mitoses per 2 mm^2 (10 high power fields) or necrosis (often punctate)
Large cell neuroendocrine carcinoma	1. A tumor with a neuroendocrine morphology (organoid nesting, palisading, rosettes, trabeculae) 2. High mitotic rate: 11 or greater per 2 mm^2 (10 high power fields), median of 70 per 2 mm^2 (10 high power fields) 3. Necrosis (often large zones) 4. Cytologic features of a non–small-cell lung cancer: large cell size, low nuclear to cytoplasmic ratio, vesicular or fine chromatin, or frequent nucleoli; some tumors have fine nuclear chromatin and lack nucleoli, but qualify as non–small-cell lung carcinoma because of large cell size and abundant cytoplasm 5. Positive immunohistochemical staining for one or more neuroendocrine markers (other than neuron-specific enolase) or neuroendocrine granules by electron microscopy
Small cell carcinoma	1. Small size (generally less than the diameter of three small resting lymphocytes) 2. Scant cytoplasm 3. Nuclei: finely granular nuclear chromatin, absent or faint nucleoli 4. High mitotic rate (11 or greater per 2 mm^2 [10 high power fields], median of 80 per 2 mm^2 [10 high power fields]) 5. Frequent necrosis often in large zones

of a 49-year-old nonsmoking man. The tumorlets were located around distorted bronchioles or embedded in fibrotic pulmonary parenchyma with a distinctive infiltrative appearance. The cells forming the tumorlets were strongly argyrophilic, and by immunohistochemistry, expressed calcitonin, serotonin, gastrin-releasing polypeptide, and vasoactive intestinal polypeptide. A case of lymph node metastasis has been reported in a person whose lung contained tumorlets.[99]

Typical Carcinoid

In 1882, Mueller[100] described a bronchial carcinoid observed at autopsy. In 1930, Kramer[101] described clinically a bronchial carcinoid under the misnomer "adenoma of the bronchus." In 1937, Hamperl[102] recognized the similarities between bronchial carcinoids and gastrointestinal carcinoids that had been described by Oberndorfer[103] in 1907, who coined the term *carcinoid* to mean a carcinoma-like neoplasm.

Most typical carcinoids present as single neoplasms in the large bronchi immediately beneath the surface of intact bronchial epithelium. Rarely, they occur in the trachea[104] and occasionally they may occur in the peripheral airways or parenchyma,[105] or as multiple discrete masss.[106,107] In a large series of pulmonary carcinoid tumors, Abdi et al.[108] reported an incidence of 21.2% (11/52) for peripheral lesions.

Macroscopically, typical carcinoids are intraluminal, yellow-tan, well demarcated, and often invade the adjacent pulmonary parenchyma (Fig. 36.10). When they occur centrally within the bronchi, they are covered by

A 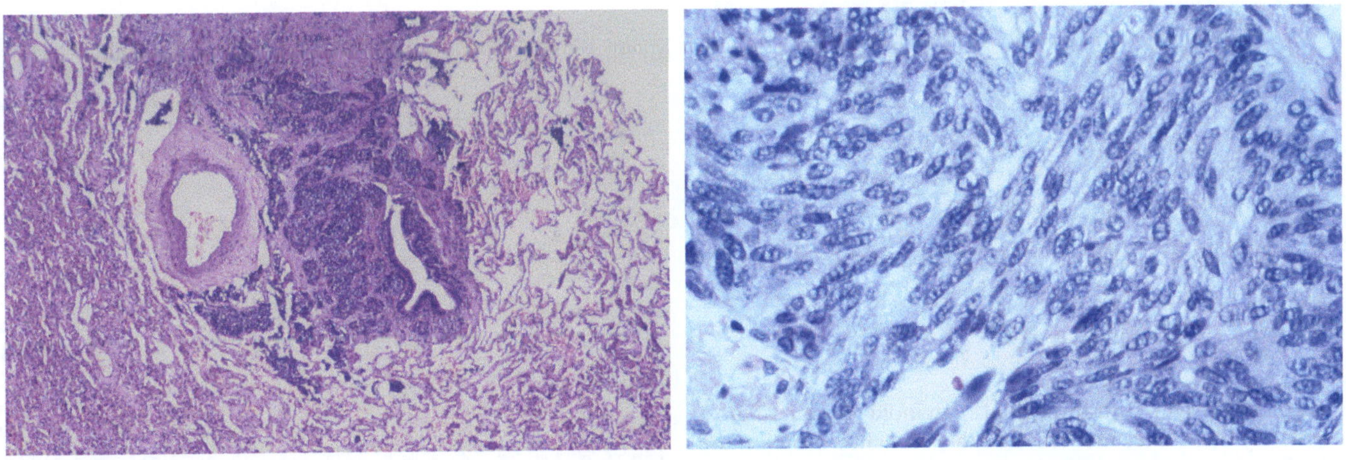 B

FIGURE 36.9. **(A)** Proliferation of neuroendocrine cells in region of distorted small airways is characteristic of this tumorlet. **(B)** Spindle pattern of neuroendocrine cells in tumorlet.

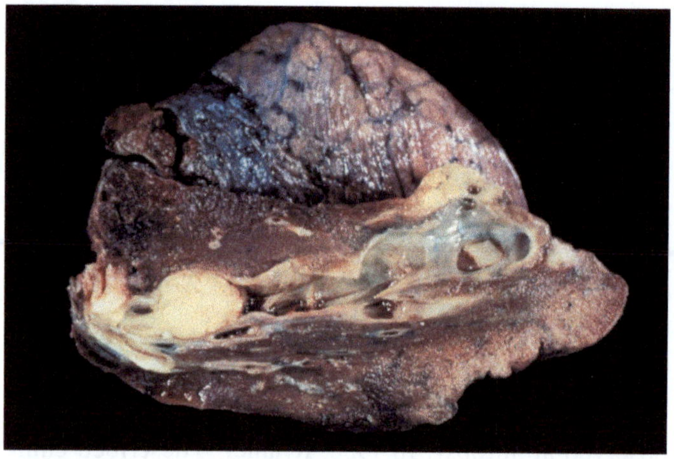

FIGURE 36.10. Obstructive intrabronchial carcinoid tumor with postobstructive bronchiectasis. (See also Chapter 5, Fig. 5.24 in Volume I).

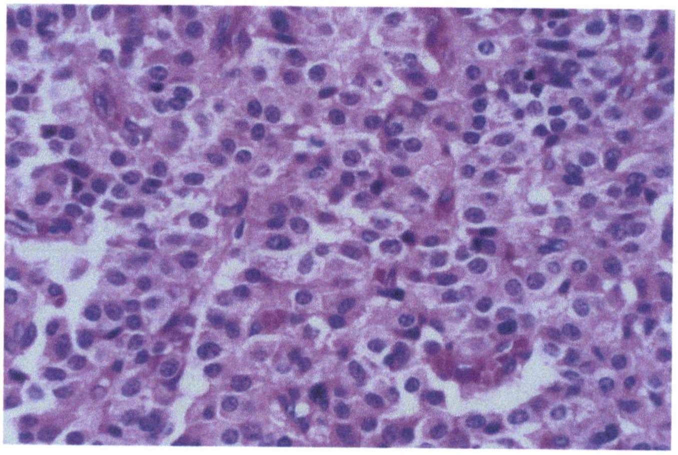

FIGURE 36.12. Uniform cellular appearance of bronchopulmonary carcinoid. Cells arranged in somewhat trabecular pattern.

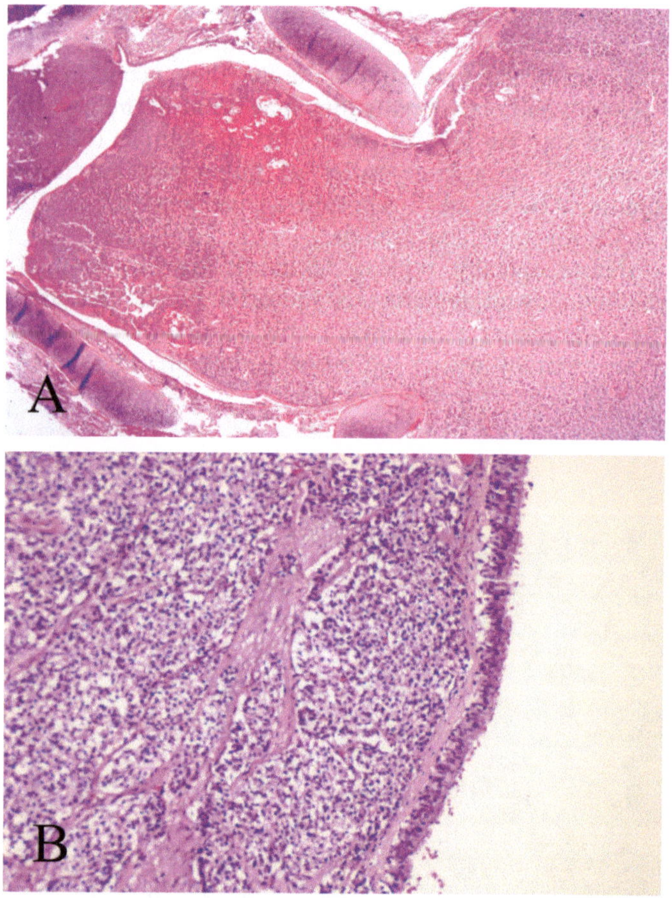

FIGURE 36.11. **(A)** Intrabronchial carcinoid tumor almost completely obliterates the lumen of this bronchus. Note on the right deep extension through the bronchial wall. **(B)** At greater magnification, intrabronchial typical carcinoid is covered by thickened basement membrane and respiratory mucosal epithelium.

respiratory epithelium or metaplastic squamous epithelium (Fig. 36.11; see also Chapter 34, Fig. 34.9). They show a wide variety of histologic growth patterns,[109,110] including trabecular, insular, papillary, interstitial, solid, and spindle (Figs. 36.12 to 36.15). Ranchod and Levine[111] reported a clinicopathologic evaluation of 35 cases of spindle cell carcinoid tumors of lung. Of interest was the finding of a disproportionate number (10/35) in the right-middle lobe. The tumors ranged from 7 mm to 4 cm in greatest dimension, and 29 of 35 (83%) were less than 2 cm in diameter. Most were in a subpleural location and the spindle cells were sometimes arranged in an organoid pattern (Fig. 36.14).

An oncocytic variety of typical carcinoid was reported by Sklar et al.[112] in 1980; since then several reports of

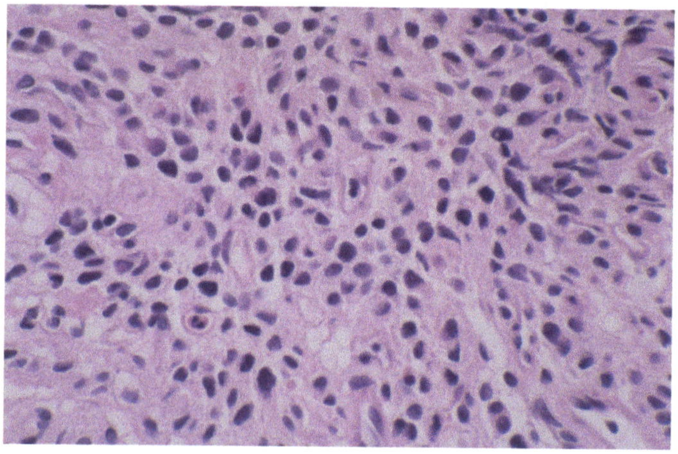

FIGURE 36.13. Carcinoid tumor of bronchus in which tumor cells are somewhat haphazardly arranged in solid growth pattern.

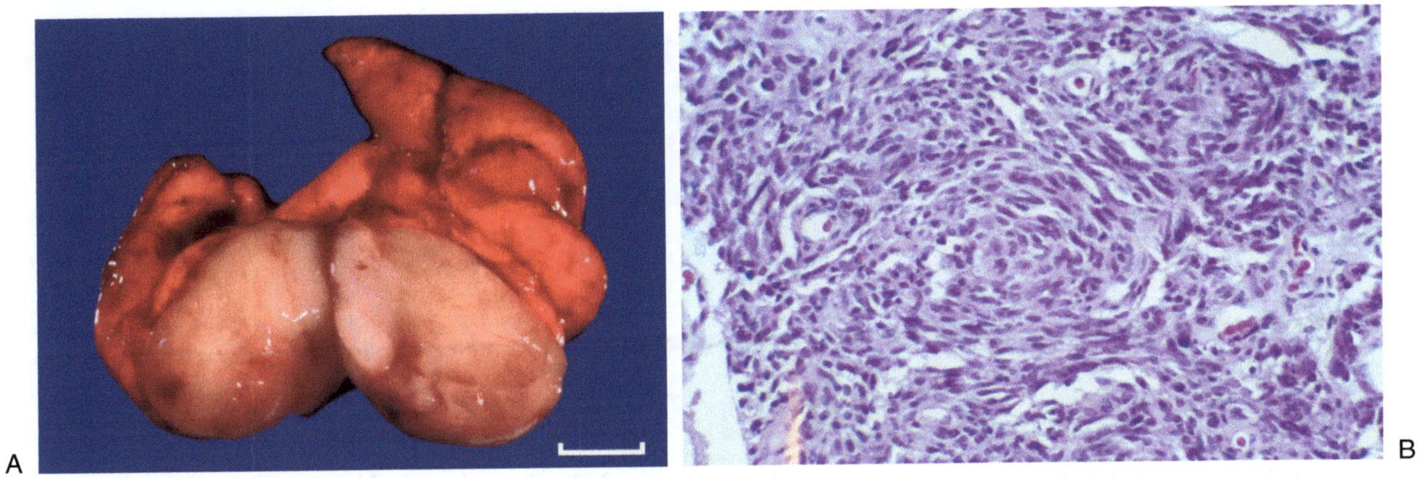

FIGURE 36.14. **(A)** Peripheral carcinoid tumor. A well-circumscribed yellow-tan mass is situated immediately subjacent to the visceral pleura (scale equals 1 cm). **(B)** Peripheral carcinoid composed of spindle-shaped cells.

oncocytic bronchial carcinoids have appeared in the literature.[113–115] These are in contrast to a bronchial oncocytoma[116] in that they are composed of neuroendocrine cells and often show a transition from a typical carcinoid into an oncocytic variety (Figs. 36.16 and 36.17) (see Chapter 38). Rare melanocytic carcinoids (Fig. 36.18) have also been described in which the tumor cells contain both melanosomes and neurosecretory granules.[117,118] Carlson and Dickersin[119] reported an intriguing case of a melanotic paraganglioid carcinoid tumor. They thoroughly reviewed the well-known fact that melanin production occurs in a wide variety of neuroendocrine neoplasms, and suggested that coexistent melanocytic and neuroendocrine differentiation was not surprising because melanocytes are functional elements of the dispersed neuroendocrine system. They cited the observation of Barbareschi et al.[120] that 36% of bronchial carcinoids contained S-100 protein–positive sustentacular cells, and suggested these sustentacular cells (Schwann cells) were neoplastic and therefore suggested such neoplasms be named paraganglioid carcinoid tumors, a name previously proposed by Capella et al.[121] In their case, Carlson and Dickersin[119] demonstrated that sustentacular cells showed melanocytic differentiation and reviewed literature reporting that such cells can show neuroendocrine differentiation. Typical carcinoid may also be associated with cartilage and bone formation[93,94] (Fig. 36.19), with amyloid deposition[93,94] (Fig. 36.20), and may show intracellular mucin or exhibit a clear cell pattern[122] (Fig. 36.21).

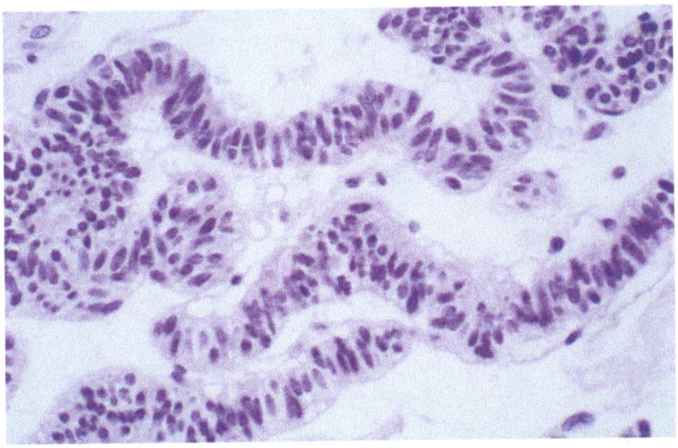

FIGURE 36.15. Carcinoid tumor composed of tall columnar cells. As in most typical carcinoids, the neoplastic cells are relatively uniform and mitoses are absent.

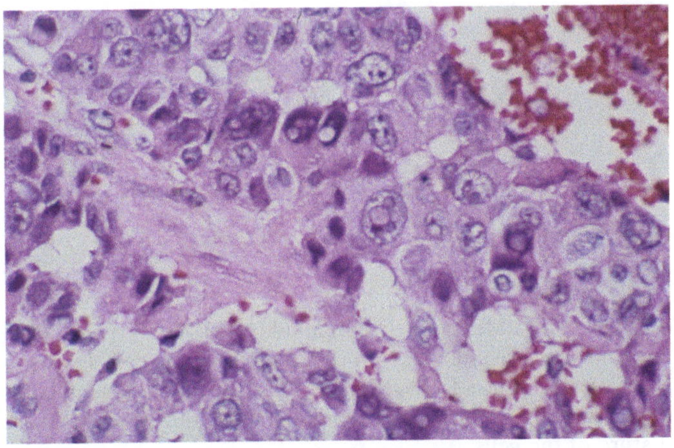

FIGURE 36.16. Region of bronchopulmonary carcinoid shows transition from typical carcinoid (left) into oncocytic variety (right).

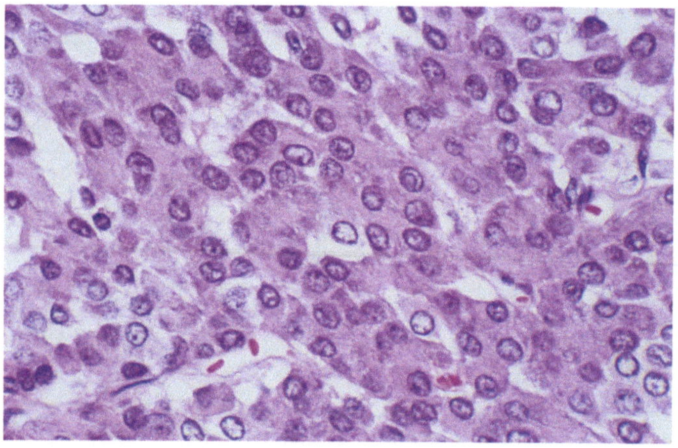

Figure 36.17. Oncocytic carcinoid composed of relatively large cells with abundant cytoplasm.

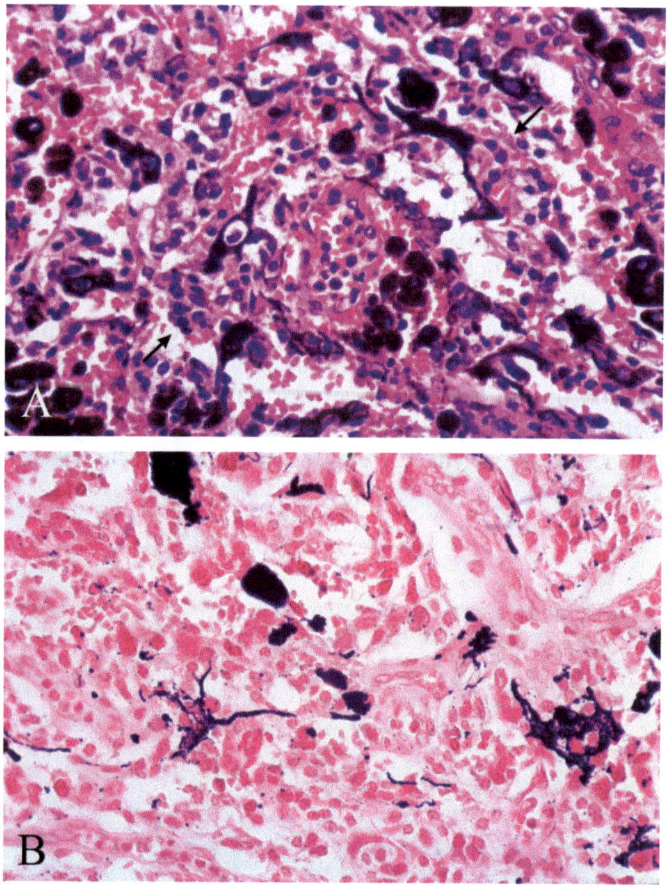

Figure 36.18. Melanocytic carcinoid. **(A)** Deeply pigmented melanocytes are intermixed with neuroendocrine cells (arrows) of typical carcinoid. **(B)** Fontana-Masson stain for melanin highlights the melanocytic component. Note the dendritic nature of the cells.

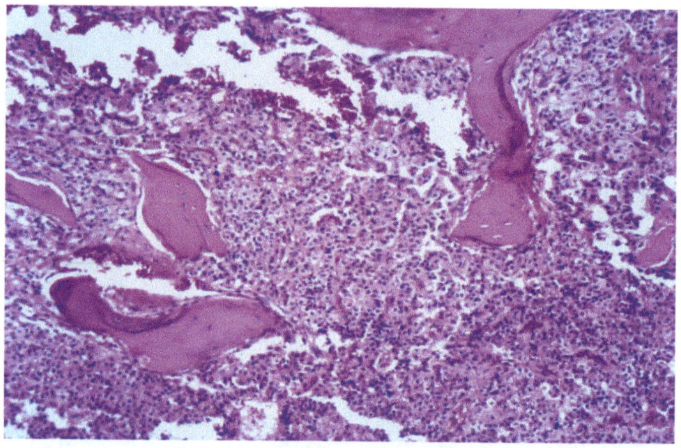

Figure 36.19. Typical carcinoid with spicules of lamellar bone.

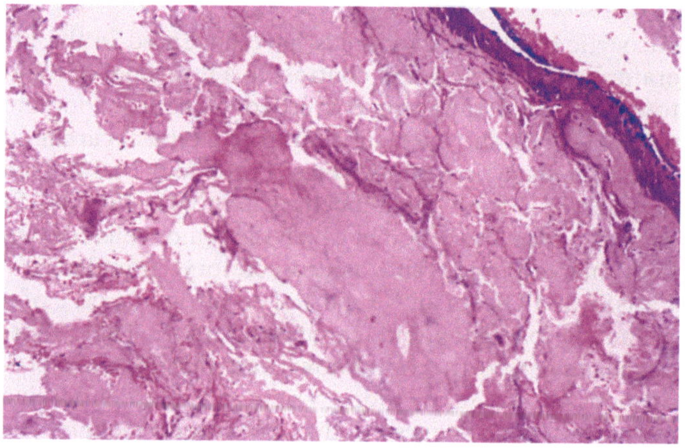

Figure 36.20. Typical carcinoid with amyloid stromal deposits.

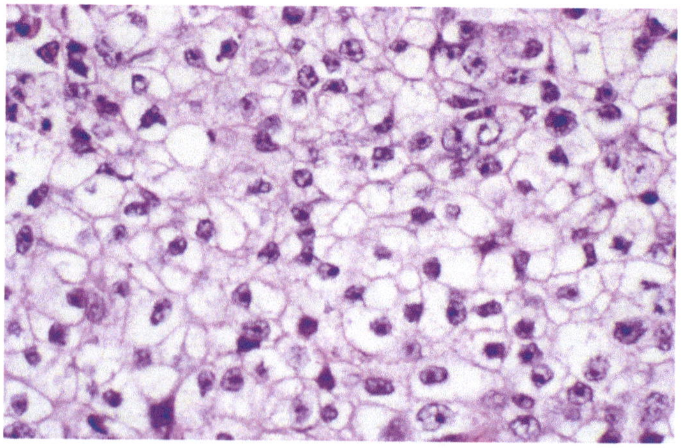

Figure 36.21. Typical carcinoid with clear cell pattern.

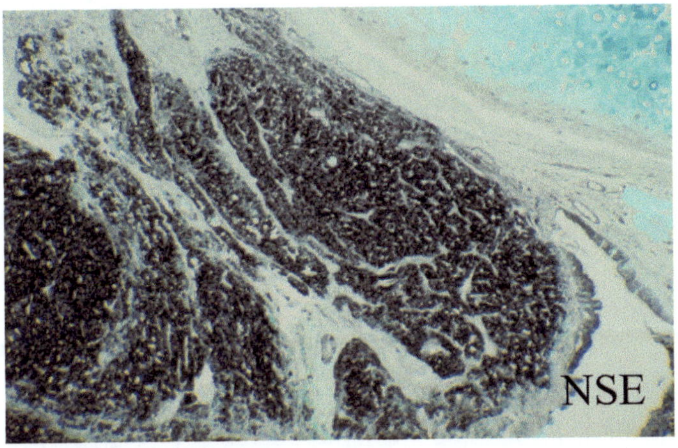

FIGURE 36.22. Intrabronchial carcinoid shown in this figure displays intense immunostaining (*black*) for neuron-specific enolase (NSE).

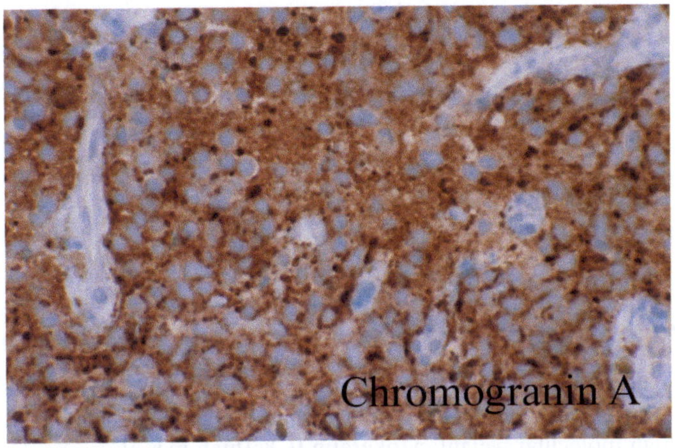

FIGURE 36.24. This typical carcinoid tumor shows intense immunostaining for chromogranin A.

Immunohistochemically, bronchial carcinoids express neuron-specific enolase (Fig. 36.22), synaptophysin (Fig. 36.23), and chromogranin A (Fig. 36.24). The intensity of the chromogranin reaction varies from one bronchial carcinoid to another and roughly correlates with the number of neuroendocrine granules demonstrated by electron microscopy in the cytoplasm of the tumor cells. In my experience, nearly all typical bronchial carcinoids express low molecular weight cytokeratin (Fig. 36.25) and may occasionally express high molecular weight keratin (Fig. 36.26). Typical bronchial carcinoids not infrequently express vimentin, as demonstrated by immunohistochemistry, which may occur as punctate staining (Fig. 36.27). In some instances, vimentin is the only intermediate filament identified in the neoplastic cells, although most coexpress vimentin and keratin. Although typical carcinoids have been reported to contain neurofilament protein, I have been unable to demonstrate this intermediate filament in formalin- or alcohol-based (methacarn-) fixed tissue. As previously discussed, this may be related to whether the neurofilament epitope is phosphorylated. Approximately 50% of typical carcinoids express carcinoembryonic antigen and epithelial membrane antigen. They may express any of the neuropeptides or other substances listed in Table 36.1. Approximately 25% to 50% of typical carcinoids show S-100 protein–positive cells admixed with the tumor cells (Fig. 36.28). These are called sustentacular cells and ultrastructurally have the appearance of Schwann cells (Fig. 36.29). In my experience, most typical pulmonary carcinoids do not express TTF-1.

Ultrastructurally, bronchial carcinoids are composed of uniform cells, the shape of which corresponds relatively well with their histologic appearance. The tumor cells resemble the cells forming neuroepithelial bodies, containing numerous, although variable numbers of, dense-core neuroendocrine granules and frequent lysosomes (Fig. 36.30). The nuclei of the tumor cells are relatively uniform, are composed of varying amounts of euchromatin and

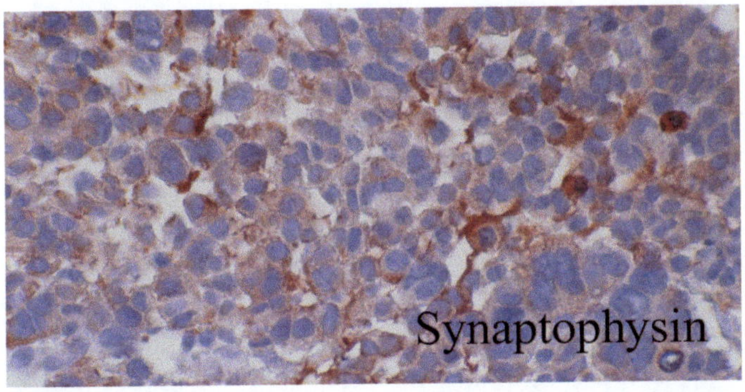

FIGURE 36.23. Centrally located typical carcinoid expressing synaptophysin.

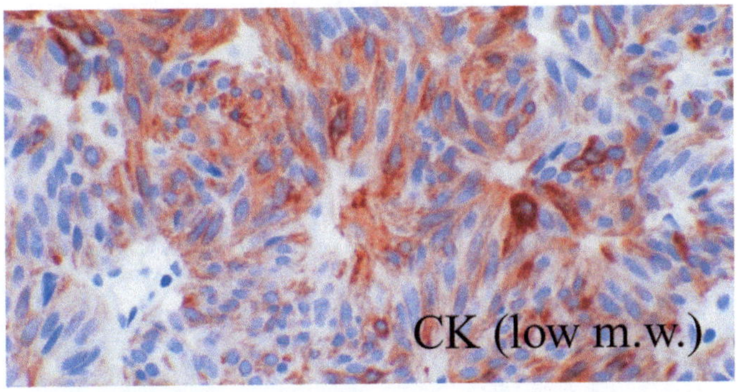

FIGURE 36.25. Nearly all typical bronchopulmonary carcinoids show immunostaining for low molecular weight, simple epithelial cytokeratin [CK (low m.w.)].

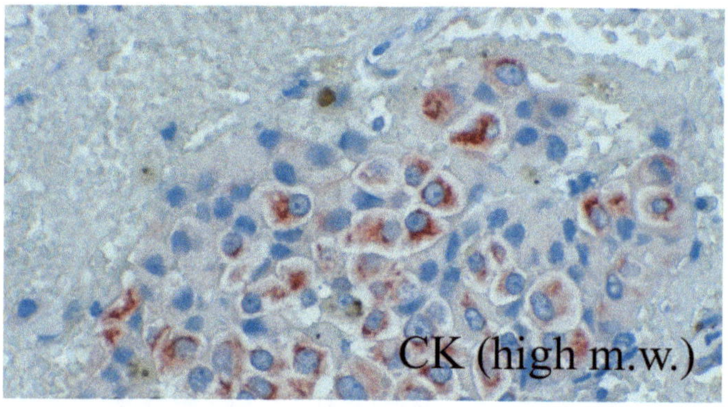

FIGURE 36.26. Typical bronchial carcinoids occasionally express high molecular weight cytokeratin [CK (high m.w.)].

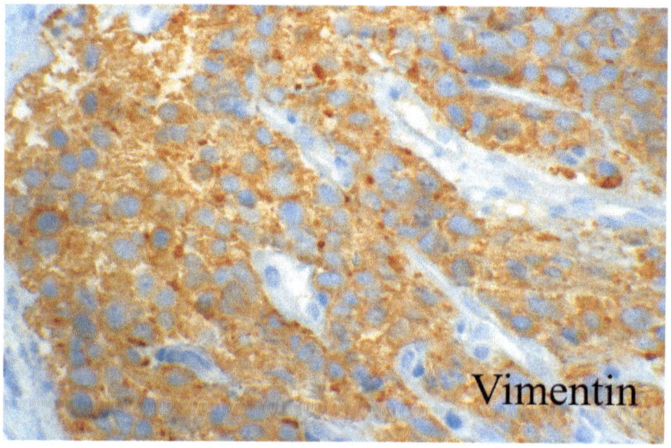

FIGURE 36.27. Typical bronchial carcinoid tumor shows focal, somewhat punctate immunostaining for vimentin.

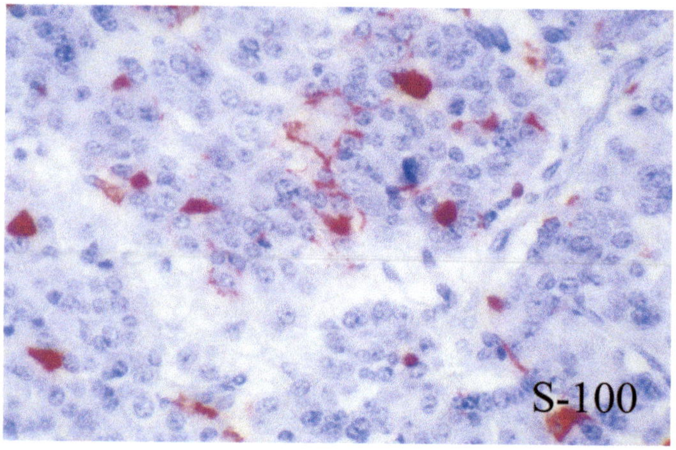

FIGURE 36.28. Many typical bronchopulmonary carcinoids contain focal S-100–positive dendritic cells resembling sustentacular cells.

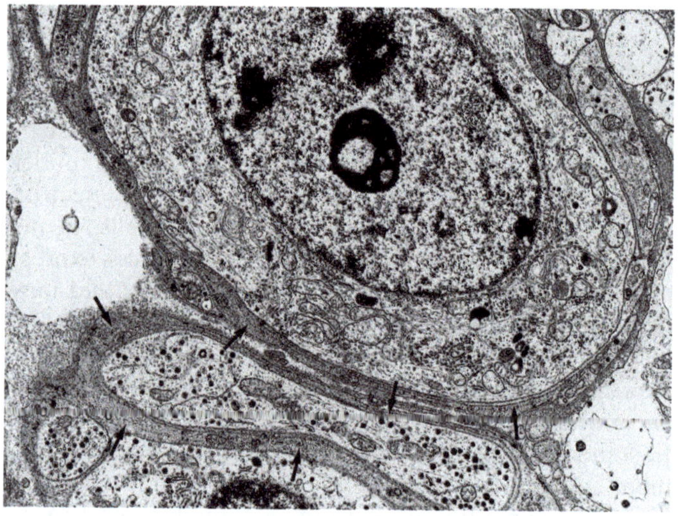

FIGURE 36.29. S-100–positive cells shown in Figure 36.28 correspond to Schwann cells that wrap around tumor cells (*arrow*). ×16,000.

A

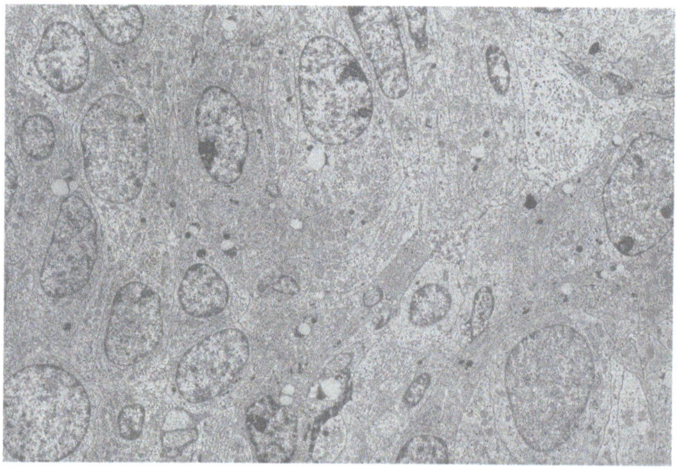

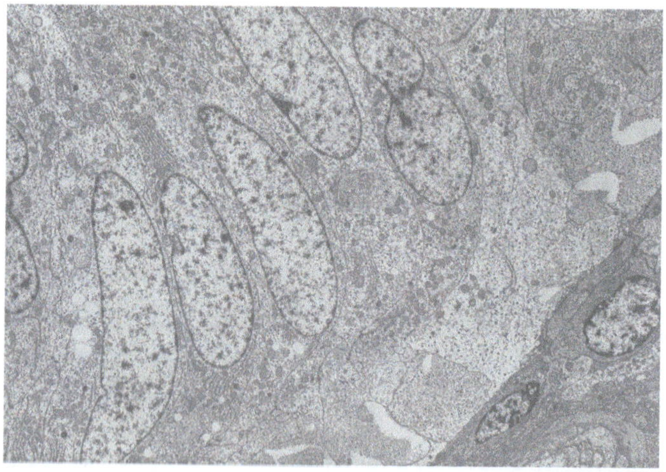

B

FIGURE 36.30. **(A)** Spindle cell carcinoid composed of uniform spindle-shaped cells contain numerous neuroendocrine granules in cytoplasm. Note also numerous lysosomes (ceroid pigment) in cytoplasm of tumor cells. ×4100. **(B)** Ultrastructural appearance of carcinoid shown in FIGURE 36.15. Note density of neuroendocrine granules in cytoplasm. ×4100.

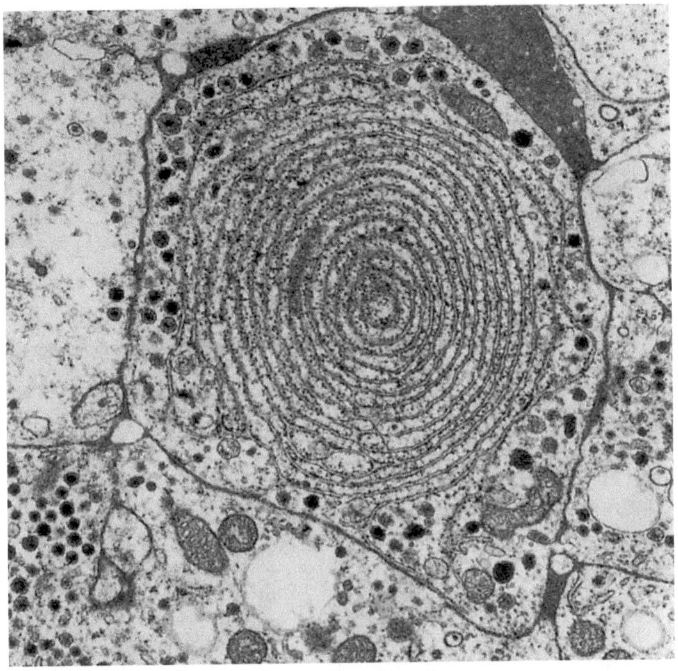

FIGURE 36.31. Many carcinoids contain parallel arrays of rough endoplasmic reticulum in their cytoplasm. ×26,500.

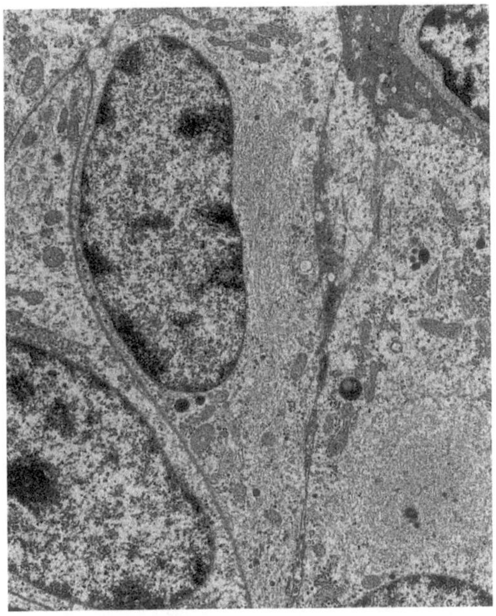

FIGURE 36.32. As in other neuroendocrine tumors, paranuclear aggregates of intermediate filaments, probably corresponding to keratin or neurofilament, may be present. ×6000.

heterochromatin, and have inconspicuous or absent nucleoli. Some typical carcinoids contain nuclei with a moderate degree of convolution. The tumor cells show processes that may be more pronounced in the spindle cell variant and that contain microtubules and intermediate filaments. The cytoplasm of typical carcinoids contains a moderate number of mitochondria, short profiles of rough endoplasmic reticulum that may be arranged in parallel stacks (Fig. 36.31), and prominent, often paranuclear, aggregates of intermediate filaments[123] (Fig. 36.32). Many carcinoids form distinct glands (Fig. 36.33) and may show multidirectional differentiation with mucous granules in their apical cytoplasm.

Atypical Carcinoid

In 1972, Arrigoni et al.[124] described 23 neoplasms they referred to as atypical carcinoids, identified in a review of lesions that had been categorized in their files as bronchial carcinoids. Subsequent reports of this type of neoplasm have appeared in the literature and they have been variously termed malignant carcinoids,[125] well-differentiated neuroendocrine carcinoma,[126] peripheral small cell carcinoma of lung resembling carcinoid tumor,[127] and Kulchitsky cell carcinoma.[128] The descriptions of this neoplasm have been remarkably similar. In contrast to typical bronchial carcinoids, atypical carcinoids occur in the periphery of the lung in more than 60% of cases. Like typical carcinoids, they are usually yellow-tan and often well demarcated. Histologically, atypical carcinoids usually have an organoid appearance, especially at their periphery (Figs. 36.34 and 36.35). The organoid nests are usually separated by fibrous bands that can be quite prominent (Fig. 36.36). The organoid nests of cells frequently show palisading of their peripheral cell layer (Fig. 36.37) and, compared to a typical carcinoid, show more

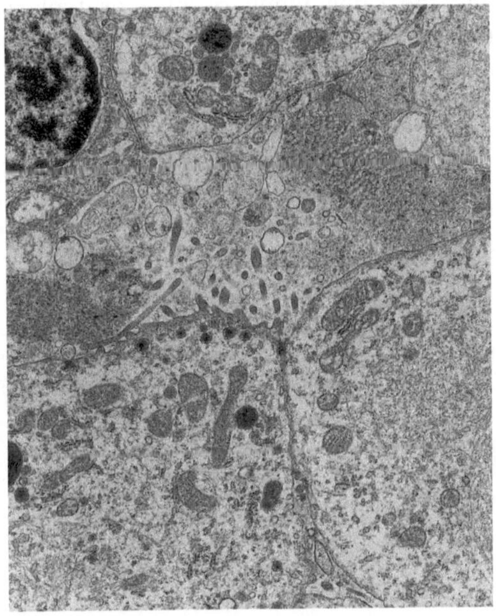

FIGURE 36.33. Some carcinoids form distinct glands with microvilli projecting into gland lumina. ×26,500.

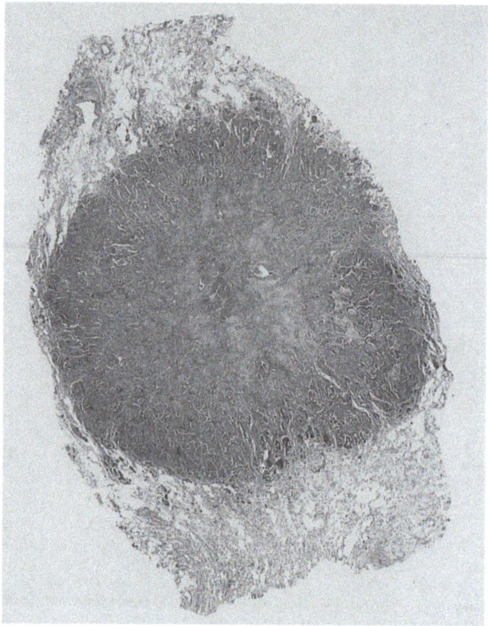

FIGURE 36.34. Well-demarcated, peripherally located, atypical carcinoid.

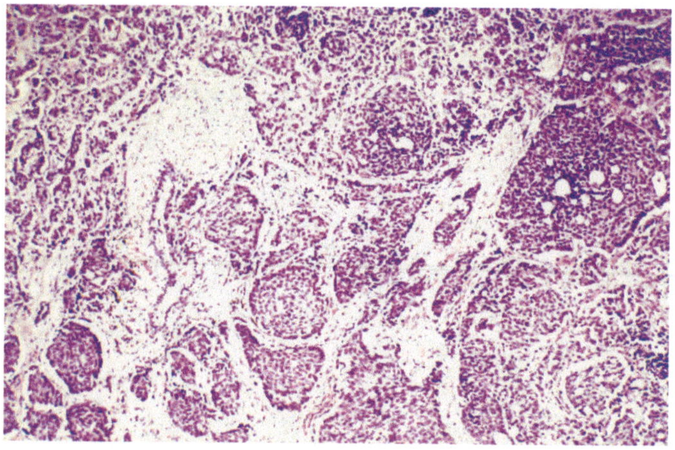

FIGURE 36.36. Organoid nests of tumor cells form this atypical carcinoid, frequently separated by fibrous tissue bands.

pleomorphism and mitoses as well as focal necrosis (Figs. 36.38 to 36.40). They may show focal gland formation (Fig. 36.41) and may be mucin positive. As described by the WHO, atypical carcinoids have 2 to 10 mitoses per mm^2 (10 high-power fields [HPFs]). A mitotic count in this range has been designated as a critical diagnostic feature.

Immunohistochemically, atypical carcinoids show essentially the same immunoprofile as typical carcinoids. Immunostaining for neuron-specific enolase frequently outlines them rather vividly (Fig. 36.42). They

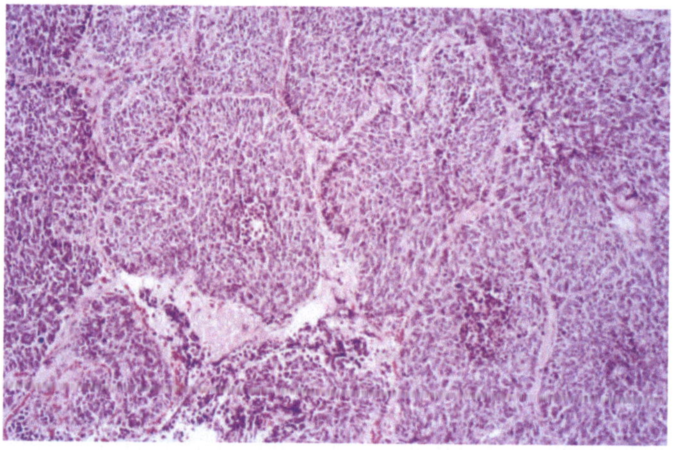

FIGURE 36.37. Palisading of peripheral cell layer is frequent feature of atypical carcinoids.

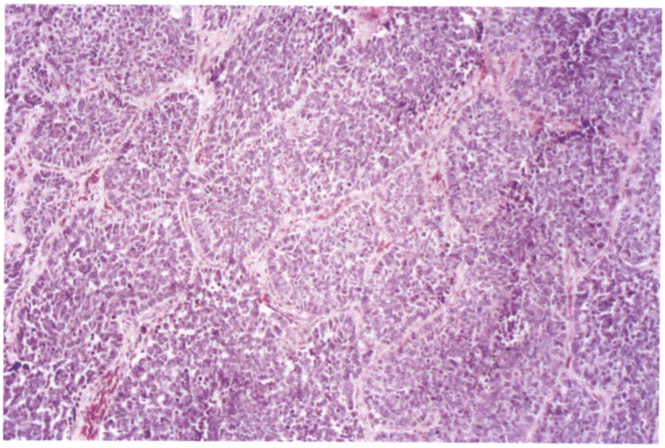

FIGURE 36.35. Atypical carcinoids usually have organoid pattern especially at periphery.

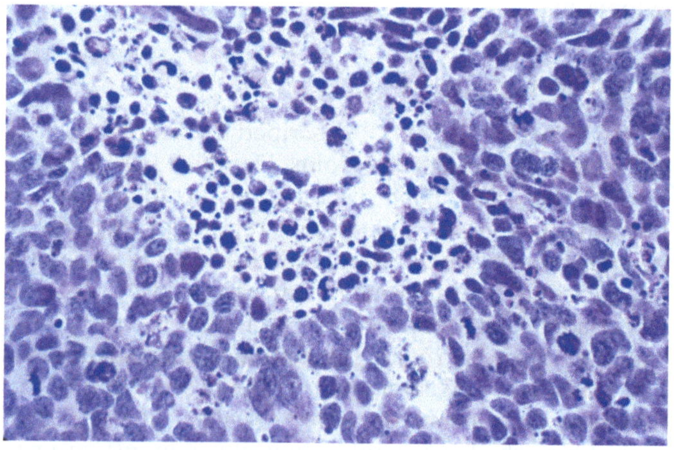

FIGURE 36.38. Atypical carcinoids frequently show focal necrosis.

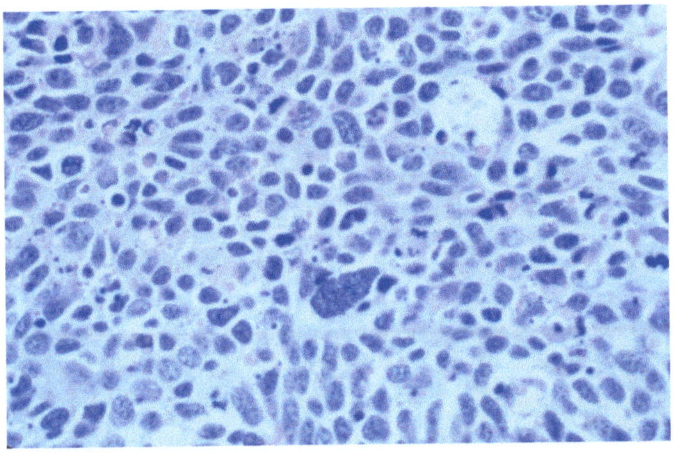

FIGURE 36.39. Cellular pleomorphism, not seen in typical carcinoids, is characteristic feature of atypical carcinoids. Note occasional tumor giant cell.

immunostain for low molecular weight cytokeratin (Fig. 36.43) and may focally express high molecular weight cytokeratin (Fig. 36.44), carcinoembryonic antigen (Fig. 36.45), and epithelial membrane antigen (Fig. 36.46). More than 50% express TTF-1 (Fig. 36.47).

Ultrastructurally, atypical carcinoids display more variability in cell size and shape than typical carcinoids, have fewer neuroendocrine granules than typical carcinoids (Fig. 36.48), occasionally have nucleoli (Fig. 36.49), and may have highly convoluted nuclei (Fig. 36.50).

Tsutsumi et al.[129] described a lung neoplasm they diagnosed as an atypical carcinoid; they described the primary neoplasm as showing carcinoid-like histology and large cell transformation in bone metastases. We observed giant neuroendocrine tumor cells in several primary lung neoplasms fulfilling the criteria of atypical carcinoids.[130]

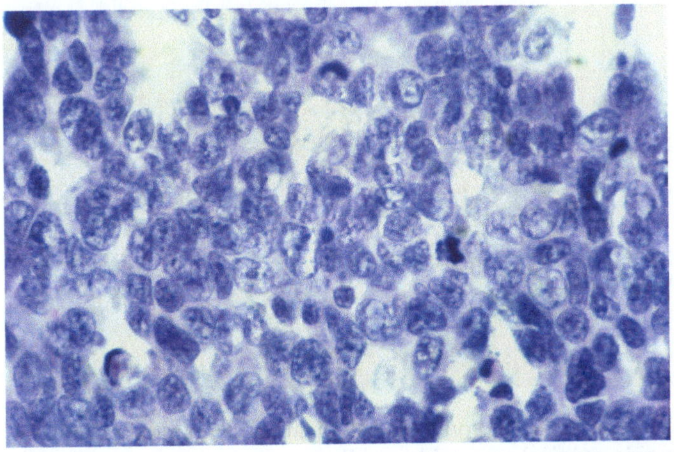

FIGURE 36.40. Most atypical carcinoids show significant mitotic activity.

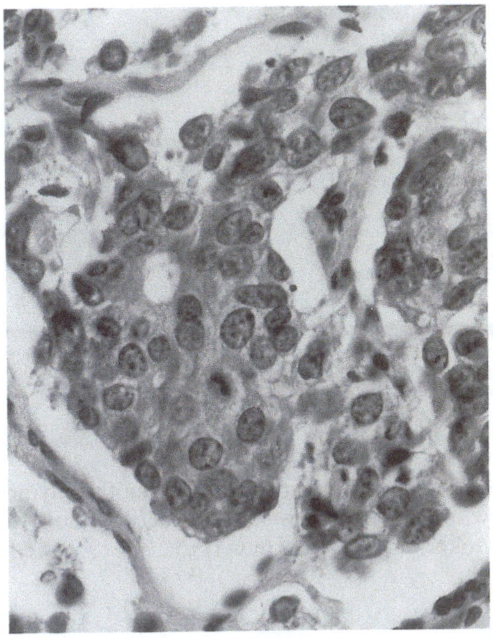

FIGURE 36.41. Focal gland formation and mucin production are features of some atypical carcinoids.

Large Cell Neuroendocrine Carcinoma

In 1978, Gould and Chejfec[131] demonstrated ultrastructurally and biochemically that some tumors diagnosed histologically as large cell undifferentiated carcinoma

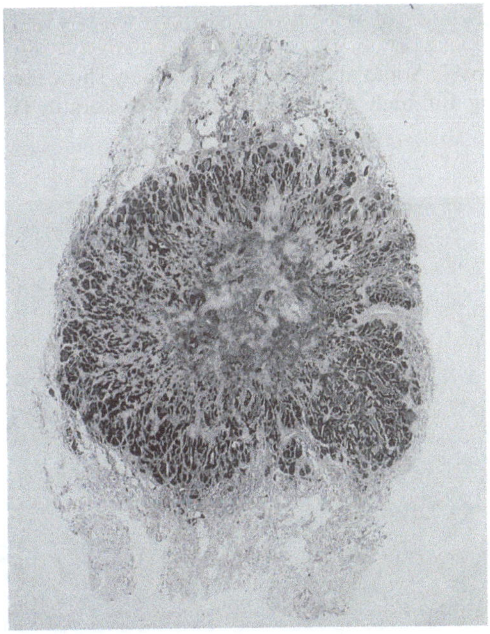

FIGURE 36.42. Similar to other bronchopulmonary neuroendocrine neoplasms, atypical carcinoids show intense immunostaining (*black*) for neuron-specific enolase (NSE).

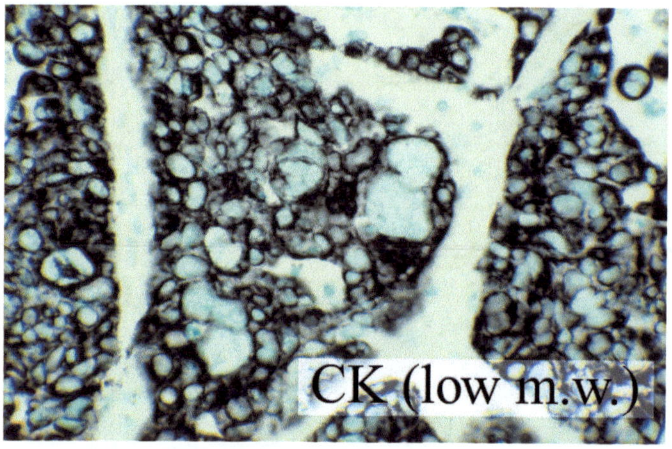

FIGURE 36.43. Nests of tumor cells forming this atypical carcinoid show intense immunostaining (*black*) for low molecular weight cytokeratin [CK (low m.w.)].

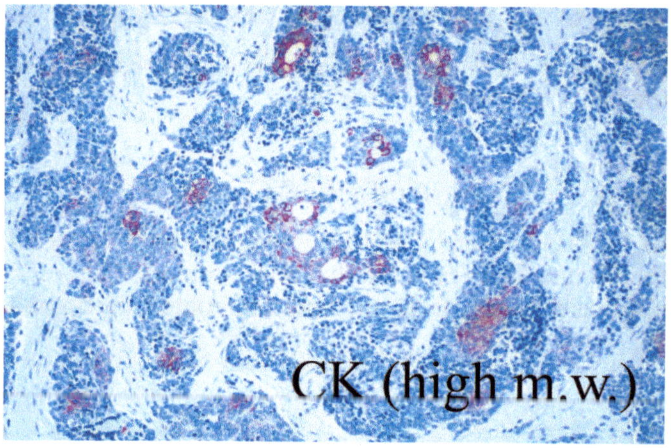

FIGURE 36.44. Some atypical carcinoids may show focal immunostaining for high molecular weight cytokeratin [CK (high m.w.)].

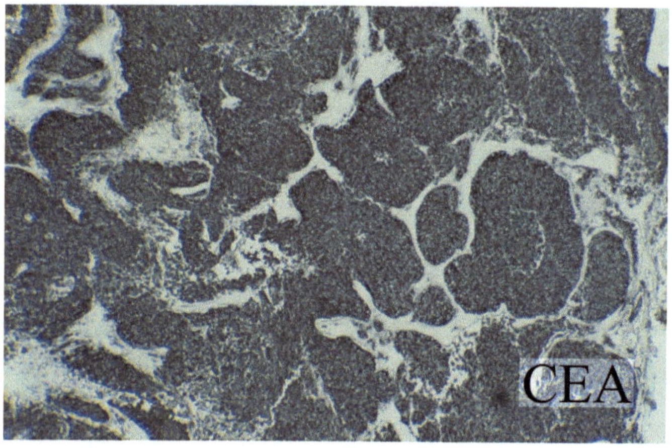

FIGURE 36.45. Approximately 50% of all neuroendocrine lung tumors, including this atypical carcinoid, show immunostaining (*black*) for carcinoembryonic antigen (CEA).

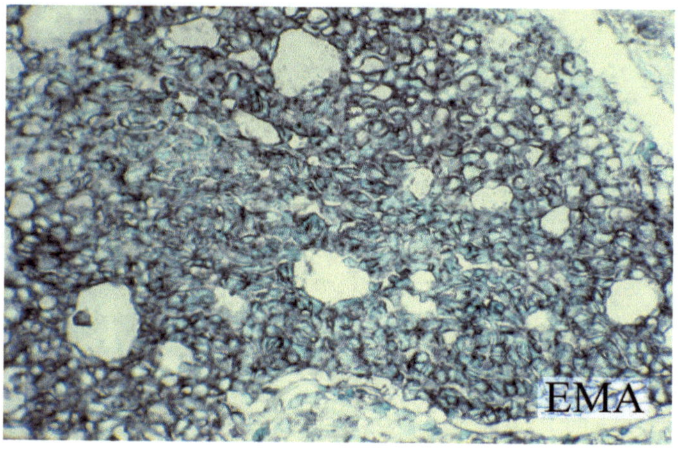

FIGURE 36.46. Many typical carcinoids and atypical carcinoids express epithelial membrane antigen (EMA) (*black*).

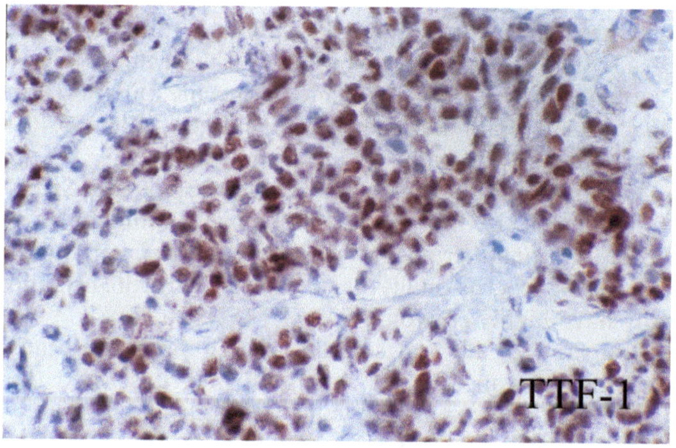

FIGURE 36.47. More than 50% of atypical carcinoids express thyroid transcription factor-1 (TTF-1).

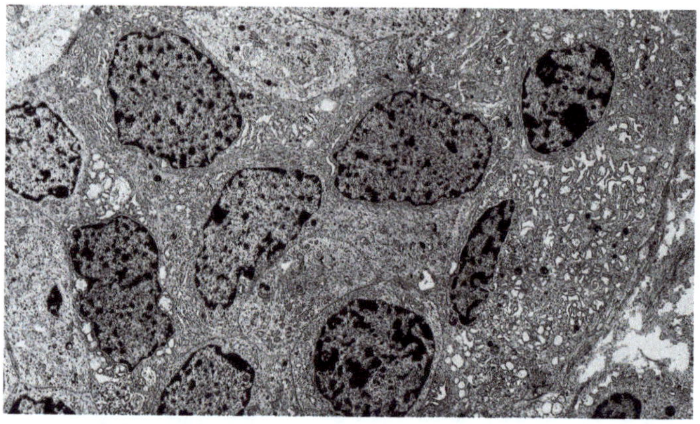

FIGURE 36.48. In contrast to typical bronchopulmonary carcinoids, atypical carcinoids usually contain fewer neuroendocrine granules in their cytoplasm when examined ultrastructurally. ×4100.

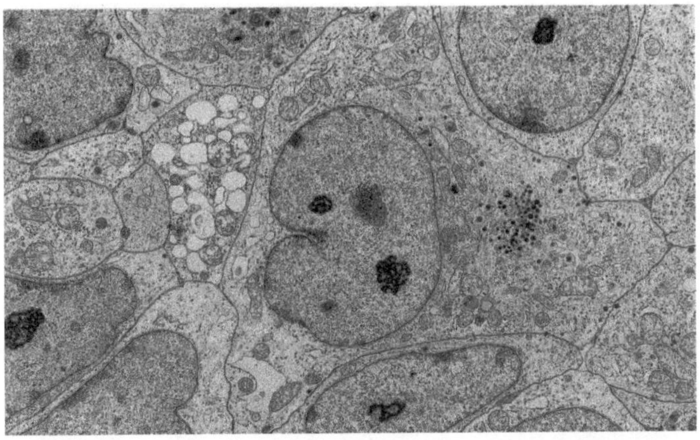

FIGURE 36.49. Some atypical carcinoids have small but distinct nucleoli, a feature usually not seen in small cell lung carcinomas. ×4100.

represented neuroendocrine carcinomas. In 1981 McDowell et al.[132] reported seven cases that had been diagnosed as squamous carcinoma, adenocarcinoma, or large cell undifferentiated carcinoma in which neoplastic cells contained neuroendocrine granules when examined by electron microscopy and contained serotonin when examined biochemically. In 1985, Hammond and Sause[133] reported eight large cell neuroendocrine carcinomas, seven of which had been diagnosed histologically as large cell undifferentiated carcinomas. Their report was followed by that of Neal et a1.,[134] who described 19 atypical endocrine tumors of the lung, which represented 9% of the 247 tumors they studied: four had been diagnosed histologically as poorly differentiated carcinoma; five as poorly differentiated adenocarcinoma; two as undifferentiated non–small-cell, non–large-cell carcinoma; six as large cell undifferentiated carcinoma; and one each as adenocarcinoma and poorly differentiated adenosquamous carcinoma.

In 1989, Barbareschi et al.[135] reported a case of large cell neuroendocrine carcinoma of the lung in a 70-year-old man who was found on a routine chest radiograph to have a "coin" lesion in the left upper lobe. The neoplasm was extensively necrotic and was initially diagnosed as a large cell undifferentiated carcinoma. The primary tumor and metastatic tumor in bone showed immunostaining for chromogranin, keratin, synaptophysin, and calcitonin. The tumor was described as being composed in part of frequent giant anaplastic cells.

Travis et al.[136] reported on 35 primary neuroendocrine neoplasms of the lung, including 20 typical carcinoids, six atypical carcinoids, five large cell neuroendocrine carcinomas, and four small cell lung carcinomas. The patients with large cell neuroendocrine carcinomas of the lung were between 35 and 75 years old, with a mean age of 59 years and a median age of 64 years; all were heavy cigarette smokers. The large cell neuroendocrine carcinomas ranged between 2.4 to 4 cm in diameter; three neoplasms were stage I and 2 were stage III-B. The criteria Travis et al. used to diagnose large cell neuroendocrine carcinoma were (1) a tumor with a neuroendocrine appearance by light microscopy that included an organoid, trabecular, palisading, or rosette pattern; (2) large cells, with most cells greater than the nuclear diameter of three small resting lymphocytes, a low nuclear-to-cytoplasmic ratio, polygonal-shaped cells, finely granular eosinophilic cytoplasm with an eosinophilic hue, coarse nuclear chromatin, and frequent nucleoli; (3) a mitotic rate greater than 10 mitoses per 10 HPFs; (4) necrosis; and (5) neuroendocrine features by immunohistochemistry or electron microscopy.

Travis et al.[136] stated that compared to small cell lung carcinoma, the tumor cells were larger and had abundant eosinophilic cytoplasm. The mitotic rate averaged 66 per 10 HPFs, which was considerably higher than that seen in atypical carcinoids. Nucleoli were stated to be prominent in two cases, and faint or focal in three cases. DNA encrustation of vascular elastic tissue was not observed. Ultrastructurally, neuroendocrine granules were observed in four cases examined and varied between 100 to 270 nm in diameter. Glandular differentiation was prominent by electron microscopy in one case, and numerous desmosomes, which the authors interpreted to represent squamous differentiation, were seen in one case. By immunohistochemistry, five of five cases immunostained for neuron-specific enolase and carcinoembryonic antigen, and four of four cases were positive for keratin. Two of five tumors expressed synaptophysin and bombesin; one of five neoplasms was positive for adrenocorticotropic hormone (ACTH); and one of four expressed calcitonin and "big" ACTH.

Wick et al.[137] compared 12 primary large cell carcinomas of the lung showing neuroendocrine differentiation with 15 large cell undifferentiated carcinomas that lacked

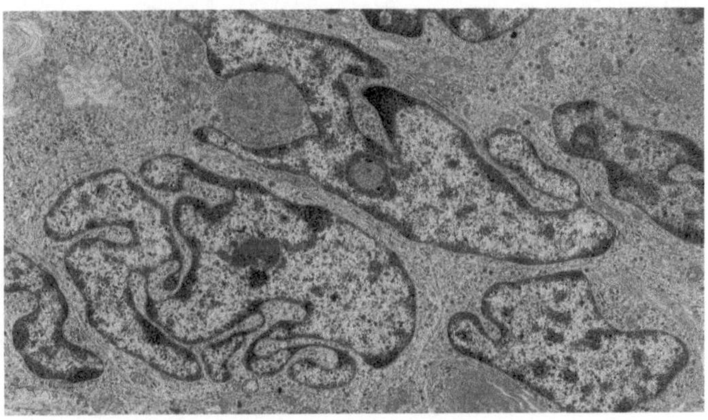

FIGURE 36.50. Some atypical carcinoids are formed by cells with highly convoluted nuclei. ×16,000.

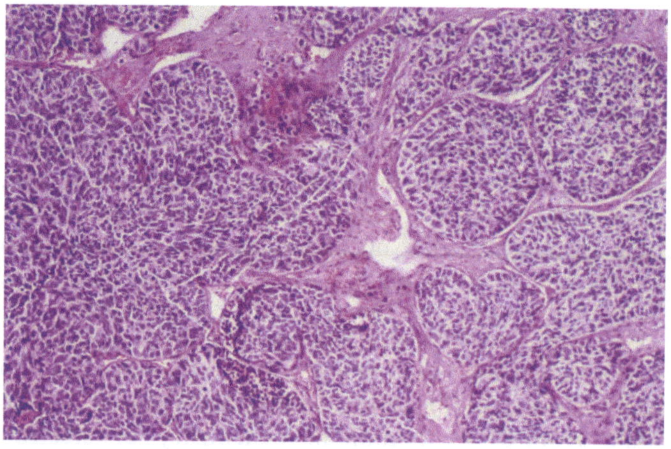

FIGURE 36.51. Large cell neuroendocrine carcinoma exhibits organoid pattern at low magnification.

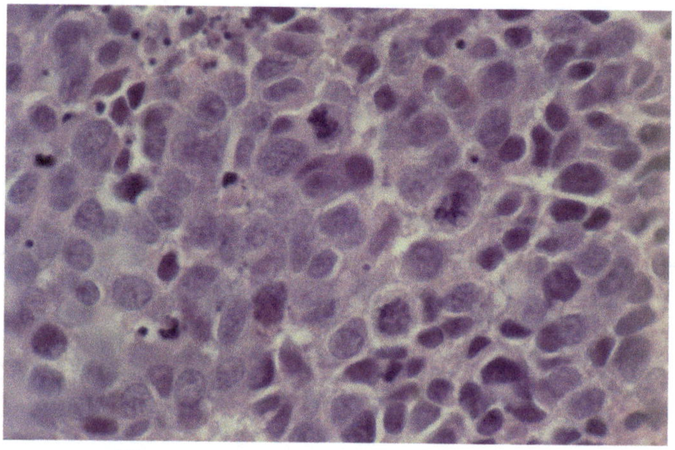

FIGURE 36.53. Histologic appearance of large cell neuroendocrine carcinoma.

neuroendocrine differentiation. Large cell neuroendocrine carcinomas were defined by immunostaining for neuron-specific enolase, Leu7, synaptophysin, or chromogranin-A, and by the presence of neurosecretory granules identified ultrastructurally. Wick et al. found large cell carcinomas with neuroendocrine features to have a significantly worse prognosis than large cell carcinomas without neuroendocrine features, and suggested large cell neuroendocrine carcinomas were probably underdiagnosed.

Mooi et al.[138] reported 11 cases of resected primary NSCLC that histologically were stated to show bronchial carcinoid or small cell lung carcinoma features. Immunohistochemically, all tumors were positive for neuron-specific enolase and protein gene product 9.5, and ultrastructurally six of seven cases examined contained dense-core neuroendocrine type granules; these findings indicated neuroendocrine differentiation. The authors suggested the histologic appearance of the tumors also indicated neuroendocrine differentiation, which could perhaps be valuable in treatment and prognosis. In this series, all neoplasms were in the upper lobes and all but one patient expired within 15 months after surgery.

Large cell neuroendocrine lung neoplasms are most commonly located peripherally or in the mid-lung field and are usually greater than 3 cm in maximum dimension. Histologically, large cell neuroendocrine carcinomas frequently exhibit a neuroendocrine pattern, and at low magnification resemble a carcinoid or an atypical carcinoid (Figs. 36.51 and 36.52). As described by Travis et al.,[136] large cell neuroendocrine carcinomas have a variable cytologic appearance. As shown in Figures 36.53, 36.54, many are composed of large cells with large vesicular nuclei and prominent nucleoli. Neoplasms with

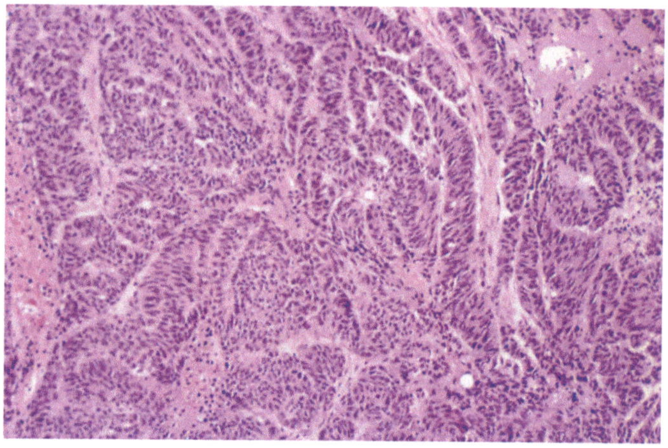

FIGURE 36.52. Large cell neuroendocrine carcinoma shows organoid and trabecular pattern.

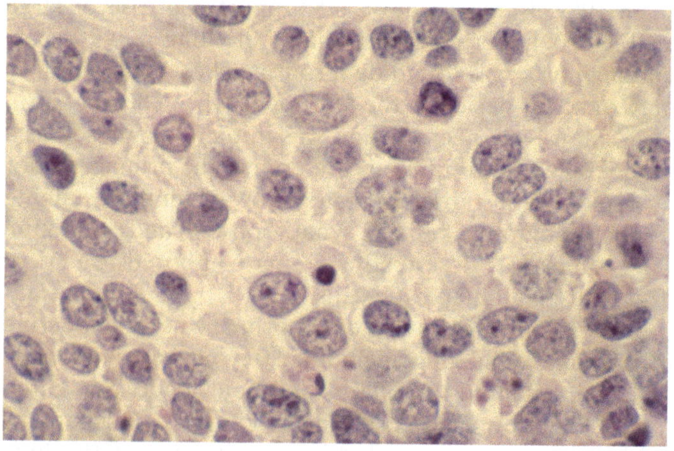

FIGURE 36.54. Large cell neuroendocrine carcinoma. Note large vesicular nuclei and prominent nucleoli.

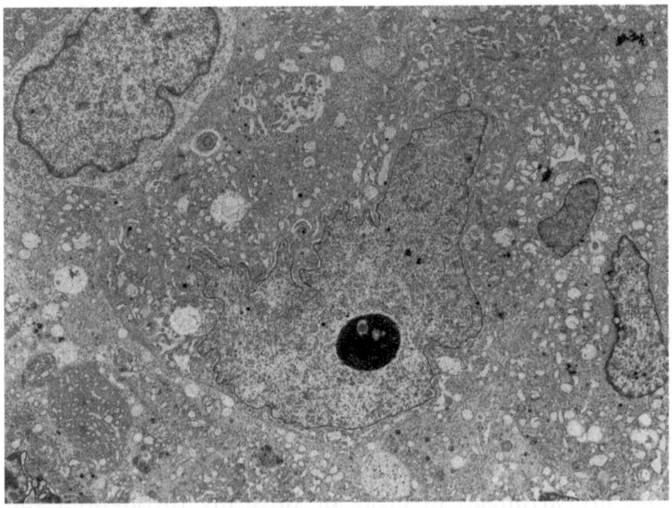

FIGURE 36.55. Ultrastructural appearance of large cell neuroendocrine carcinoma. Note large irregularly shaped nucleus and prominent nucleolus. Tumor cells contain more neuroendocrine granules than most small cell neuroendocrine carcinomas. ×16,000.

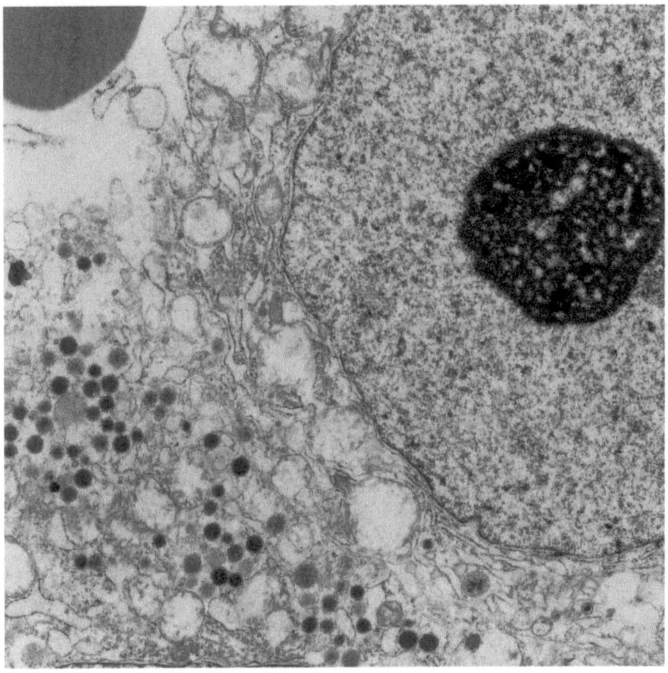

FIGURE 36.56. Portion of single large cell neuroendocrine tumor cell. Note huge nucleolus and numerous neuroendocrine granules in cytoplasm. ×43,000.

this appearance are easily confused with nonneuroendocrine large cell undifferentiated carcinomas. Other large cell neuroendocrine carcinomas are composed of cells that are large but have nuclear cytologic features resembling small cell lung carcinoma with small clumps of chromatin and absent or small nucleoli. The ultrastructural appearance of large cell neuroendocrine neoplasms usually correlates with their cytologic features. Those with large nucleoli cytologically have large nucleoli ultrastructurally (Fig. 36.55). They typically have a few cellular processes and variable numbers of dense-core neuroendocrine granules (Fig. 36.56). Those in which nuclei lack prominent nucleoli cytologically resemble "large" small cell lung carcinomas ultrastructurally, except that they have fewer processes and usually have more cytoplasmic organelles, including neuroendocrine granules (Fig. 36.57). We evaluated one large cell neuroendocrine carcinoma that contained perinuclear aggregates of intermediate filaments similar to those seen in typical carcinoids (Fig. 36.58). Large cell neuroendocrine lung carcinomas usually show processes ultrastructurally. Immunohistochemically, they usually express low and high molecular weight cytokeratin, neuron-specific enolase, carcinoembryonic antigen, synaptophysin, chromogranin A, and some substances shown in Table 36.1.

Small Cell Lung Carcinoma

Small cell carcinoma makes up approximately 20% to 25% of common lung neoplasms and in the past was frequently referred to as oat cell carcinoma or small cell neuroendocrine carcinoma. This neoplasm was initially thought to represent a sarcoma or lymphoma and it was not until 1926 that it was recognized as an epithelial neoplasm.[139] Small cell carcinoma was initially classified with large cell carcinoma of the lung as an anaplastic

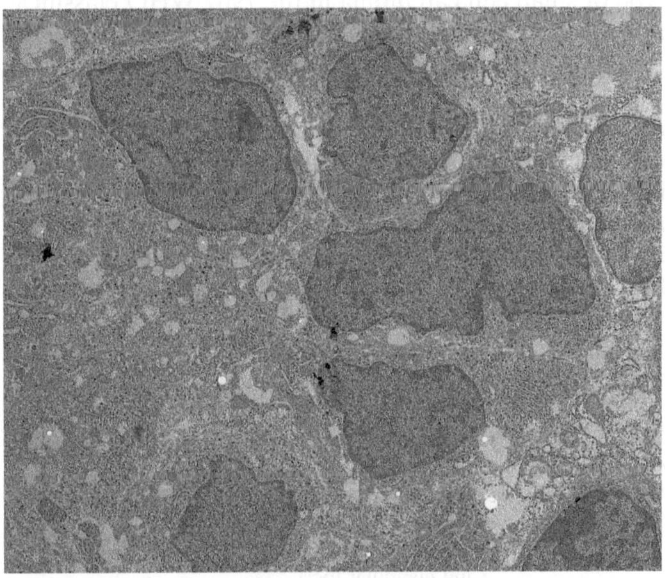

FIGURE 36.57. Large cell neuroendocrine carcinoma composed of large cells with large nuclei with absent or small nucleoli. These neoplastic cells resemble those of a "large" small cell neuroendocrine carcinoma. ×10,400.

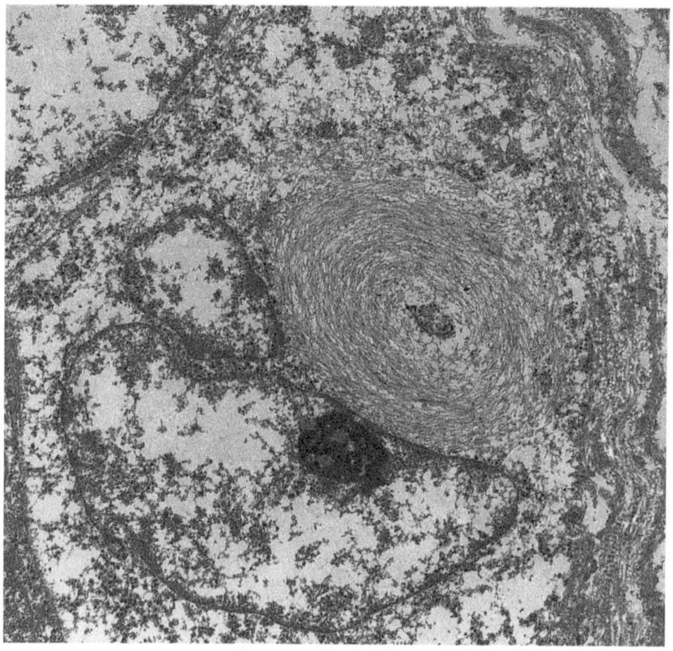

FIGURE 36.58. Ultrastructurally, large cell neuroendocrine carcinoma contains perinuclear aggregates of intermediate filaments, an occasional finding in neuroendocrine carcinomas. ×26,000.

carcinoma.[140] The evolution of small cell carcinoma is shown in Table 36.5.[141–145]

The 1967 WHO's classification of lung cancer[142] divided small cell carcinoma into three categories: (1) oat cell carcinoma, which was referred to as a lymphocyte-like type of small cell carcinoma in the 1967 WHO classification of lung tumors and was characterized as a tumor composed of small round uniform cells approximately 1.5- to threefold larger than a lymphocyte with dense round oval nuclei and sparse cytoplasm; (2) small cell carcinoma, intermediate cell type, which was characterized as being composed of polygonal or fusiform cells less regular in appearance than oat cell carcinoma and having more cytoplasm than oat cell carcinoma; and (3) combined oat cell carcinoma, characterized by a combination of a definite oat cell carcinoma and squamous cell carcinoma or adenocarcinoma.

In 1985, Yesner[145] and the other members of the pathology committee of the International Association for the Study of Lung Cancer stated there was no significant biologic difference between the oat cell subtype and intermediate subtype of small cell undifferentiated carcinoma. They suggested that the terms *oat cell, lymphocyte-like*, and *intermediate* be discarded and be replaced with the term *small cell carcinoma* to refer to such undifferentiated tumors that had no significant non–small-cell elements. They suggested that two variants of small cell lung carcinoma be recognized: (1) mixed small cell–large cell carcinoma, which is a neoplasm composed of small cells with a significant population of large cells that are arranged in nests or diffusely throughout the tumor; and (2) combined small cell carcinoma, composed of a combination of small cell carcinoma and neoplastic squamous or adenocarcinoma. The 1999 WHO[93] and 2004 WHO[94] classifications adopted these suggestions. Azzopardi's[146] 1959 light microscopic description of oat cell carcinoma remains excellent. Small cell lung carcinoma was reviewed in detail in 1983 by Yesner[147] and by Carter.[148]

Stuart-Harris et al.[149] applied this new classification scheme to 124 cases of SCLC. A specimen for histologic examination was available in 59 cases, a specimen for cytologic correlation in 91 cases, and a specimen for ultrastructural examination in 60 cases. Of the 124 cases, 120 were classified as small cell carcinoma, two as mixed small cell–large cell carcinoma, and two as combined small cell carcinoma. There was concordance by the three pathologists who reviewed the slides in all cases except one. The authors concluded their study confirmed that small cell carcinoma accounted for more than 90% of untreated cases of SCLC, and that mixed small cell–large cell carcinoma was perhaps less common than previously proposed.

Yesner[147] stated that small cell lung carcinomas may show transitions into large cell carcinomas, adenocarcinomas, squamous carcinomas, or combinations of these categories. In his study of 205 tumors diagnosed at biopsy

TABLE 36.5. Evolution of the classification of small cell lung carcinoma

Kreyberg 1962	WHO 1967	1973 WPL WHO 1981	IASLC 1998	WHO/IASLC 1999
Oat cell	Lymphocyte-like	Oat cell	Pure small cell lung cancer	Small cell lung cancer
Polygonal	Polygonal	Intermediate		
	Fusiform		Mixed (with large cells)	
	Other (containing squamous and glandular foci)	Combined	Combined	Combined small cell lung cancer (containing any other non–small-cell lung cancer component)

WHO, World Health Organization; WPL, Working Party for Therapy of Lung Cancer; IASLC, International Association for the Study of Lung Cancer.

Source: Nicholson et al.,[232] with permission from Lippincott Williams & Wilkins.

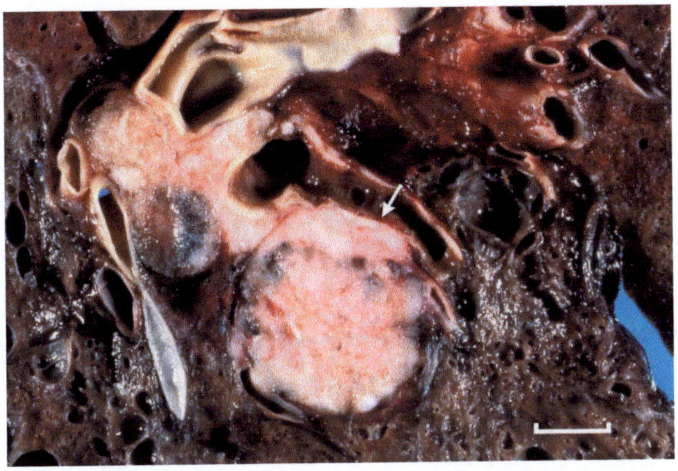

FIGURE 36.59. Central region of lung shows involvement of regional lymph nodes and hilar soft tissue by small cell lung carcinoma. Note focal invasion of the bronchus (arrow) but lack of endobronchial extension (scale equals 1 cm). (Courtesy of Carol Farver, MD, Cleveland Clinic Foundation.)

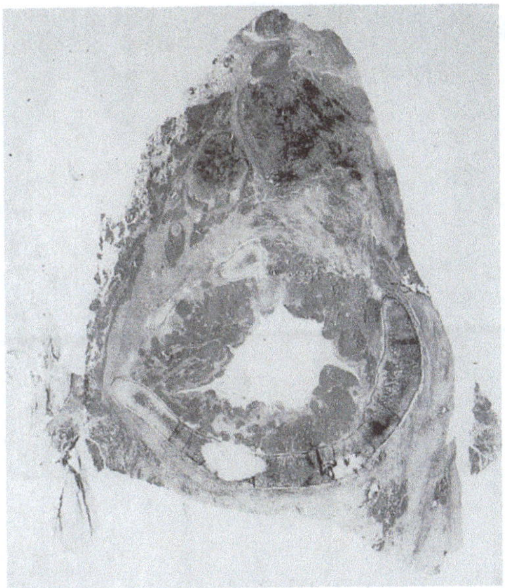

FIGURE 36.61. Small cell lung carcinoma invades directly into bronchial wall.

as small cell carcinoma, approximately 20% of treated and untreated patients' tumors showed a different histology at autopsy, representing either a combined small cell tumor or a non–small-cell tumor (see their Table 1). This is in keeping with the cell culture work of Gazdar et al.[150] who found that small cell carcinomas converted into large cell carcinomas without neuroendocrine features after 2 years in continuous culture.

Macroscopically, small cell lung carcinomas are centrally located in more than 90% of cases. The tumor tends to be soft and whitish gray with multifocal necrosis. Small cell carcinoma tends to surround and constrict the major bronchi, extensively spread within the lung in a lymphangitic pattern, and directly invade and metastasize to regional lymph nodes (Fig. 36.59). Occasionally small cell carcinoma presents as a relatively small bronchial tumor (Figs. 36.60 and 36.61). Small cell lung carcinomas frequently metastasize and may present as liver failure secondary to metastatic tumor (Fig. 36.62), or occasionally be associated with Cushing's syndrome because of ACTH production by the tumor (Fig. 36.63).

Microscopically, small cell carcinomas have round or fusiform nuclei with a ground-glass or stippled chromatin pattern and small usually indistinct nucleoli (Figs. 36.64 to 36.67). Some small cell lung carcinomas are composed of slightly larger cells with larger nuclei, occasional nucleoli, and more abundant cytoplasm; these correspond to those categorized as intermediate small cell

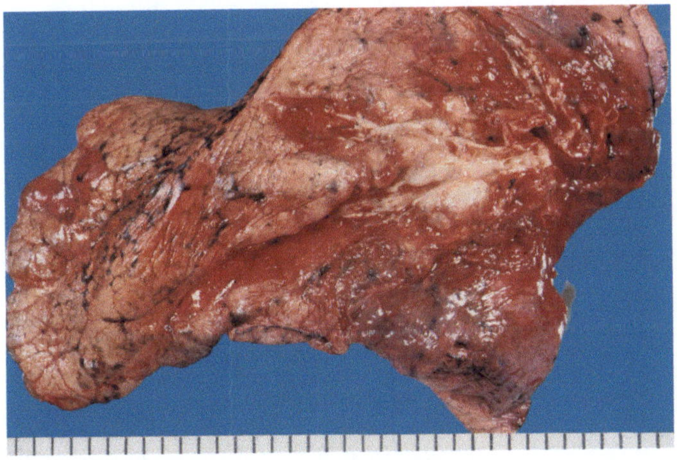

FIGURE 36.60. Left-upper lobe shows relatively small tumor in parabronchial distribution but without occlusion of lumen of bronchus.

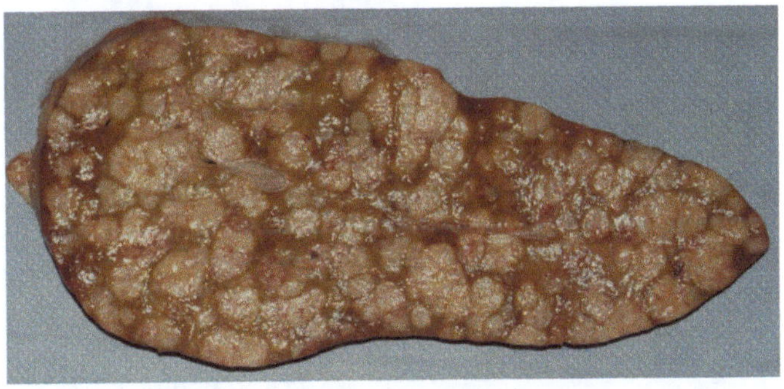

FIGURE 36.62. Some patients with small cell lung carcinoma present with liver failure caused by massive metastases to liver.

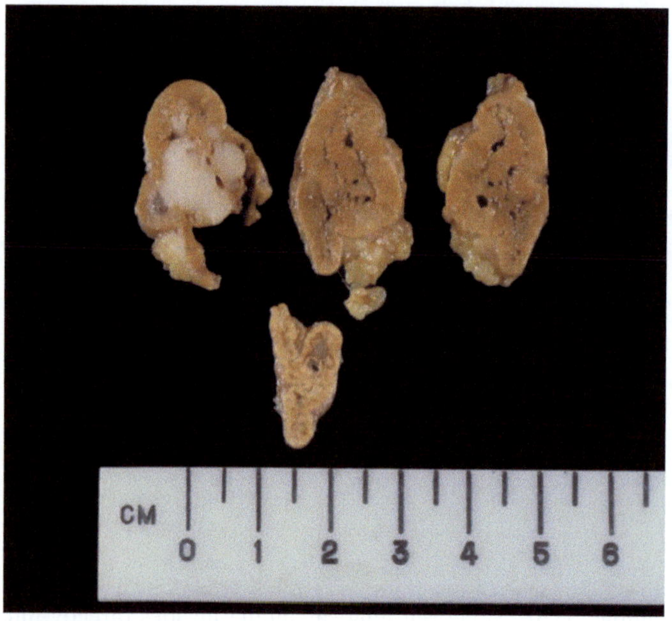

FIGURE 36.63. Some small cell lung carcinomas produce adrenocorticotropic hormone (ACTH). This ACTH-producing small cell neuroendocrine carcinoma has metastasized to the adrenal gland, resulting in adrenal cortical hyperplasia secondary to ACTH production. Normal adrenal gland at bottom. (Courtesy of Dr. John Bolen, Virginia Mason Medical Center, Seattle, WA.)

carcinomas by the 1973 World Health Organization (Figs. 36.68A–D), although some might classify these neoplasms as large cell neuroendocrine carcinomas. Small cell neuroendocrine lung carcinomas frequently show large areas of necrosis (Fig. 36.69) with nuclear chromatin impregnation of elastic tissue of vessels (so-called Azzopardi phenomenon) (Figs. 36.70 and 36.71). As shown in Figures 36.66 and 36.67, the neoplastic cells have a high mitotic

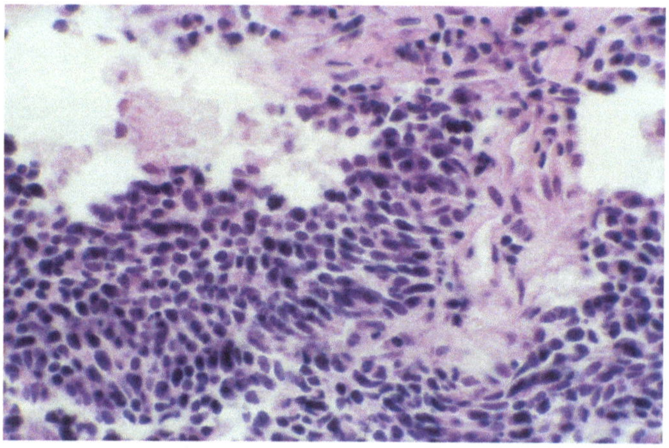

FIGURE 36.64. Small cell lung carcinoma composed predominantly of fusiform cells. Note necrosis and frequent mitoses.

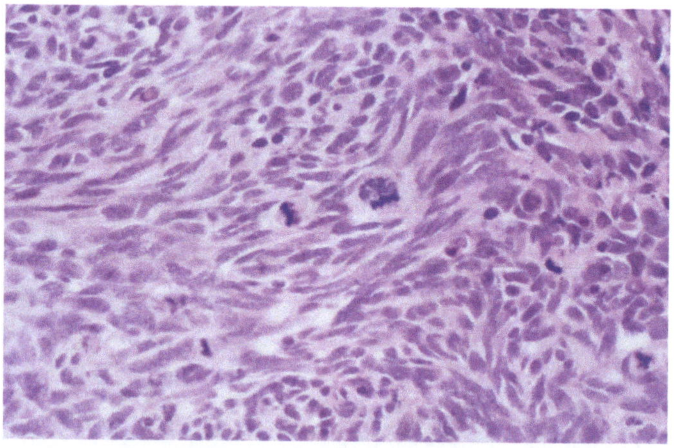

FIGURE 36.65. Another example of small cell neuroendocrine carcinoma composed mostly of spindle cells.

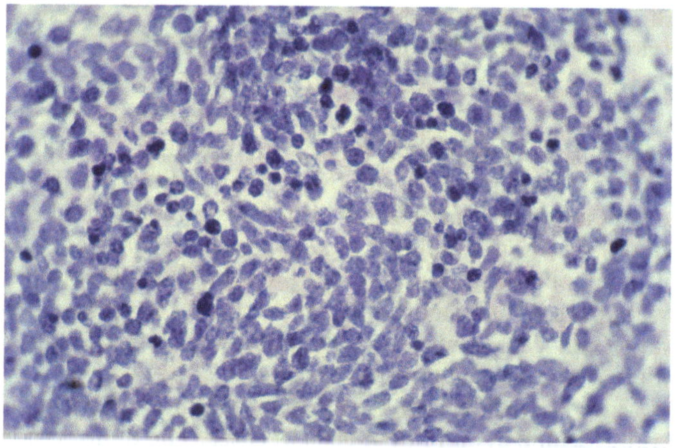

FIGURE 36.66. Small cell lung carcinoma cells show high nuclear cytoplasmic ratio, nuclear molding, and high mitotic rate. In this tumor the cells are predominantly round, superficially resembling lymphocytes.

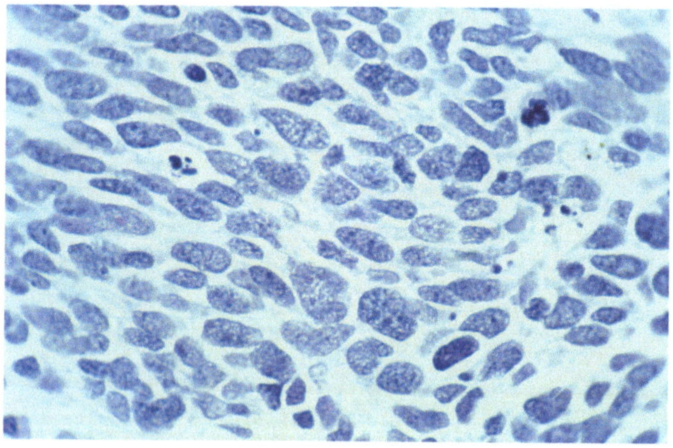

FIGURE 36.67. Greatly magnified small cell neuroendocrine carcinoma. Note large nuclei, inconspicuous cytoplasm; finely granular chromatin pattern; and absent nucleoli.

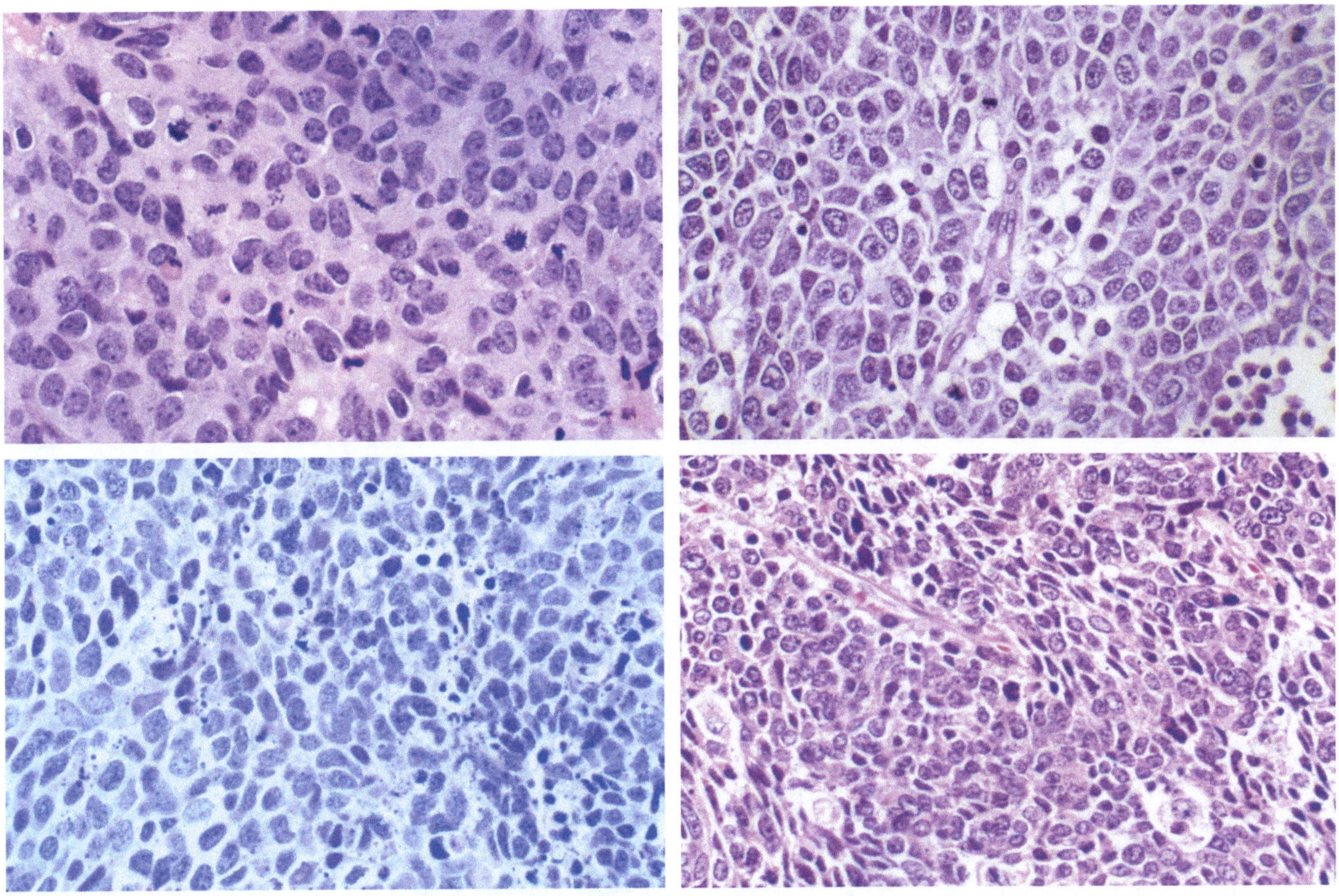

FIGURES 36.68. **(A–D)** Examples of small cell lung carcinomas that would be classified as intermediate type in the 1973 World Health Organization categorization. Note slightly larger size of cells and larger nuclei, occasionally having small nucleoli.

rate. Some small cell neuroendocrine carcinomas have a tendency to aggregate around small blood vessels (Fig. 36.72) and frequently show perineural space invasion (Fig. 36.73). An occasional small cell lung carcinoma contains tumor giant cells (Fig. 36.74).

In transbronchial biopsies, the neoplastic cells can be relatively well preserved (Figs. 36.75 and 36.76), although there is often a great deal of artifactual distortion, including crush artifact (Fig. 36.77). When the biopsy is

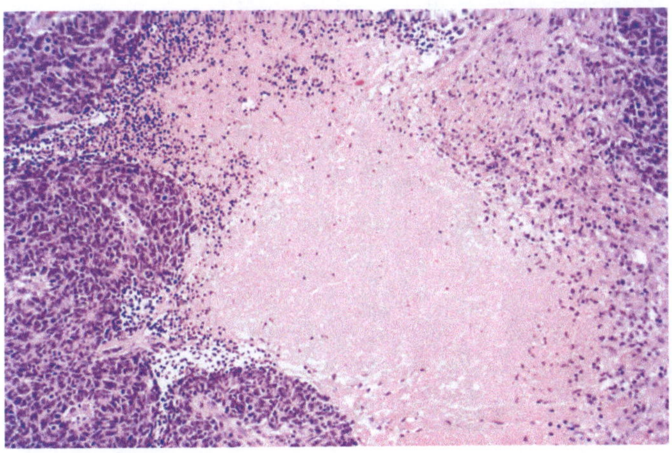

FIGURE 36.69. Many small cell neuroendocrine carcinomas are mostly necrotic.

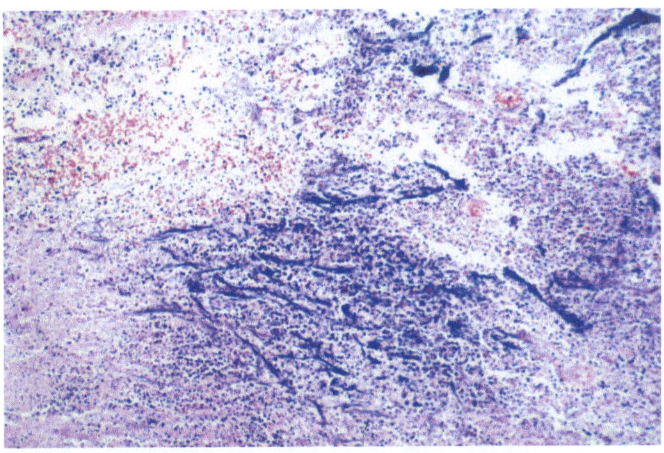

FIGURE 36.70. Mostly necrotic small cell lung carcinoma shows prominent nuclear encrustation of elastic tissue of small blood vessels (Azzopardi phenomenon).

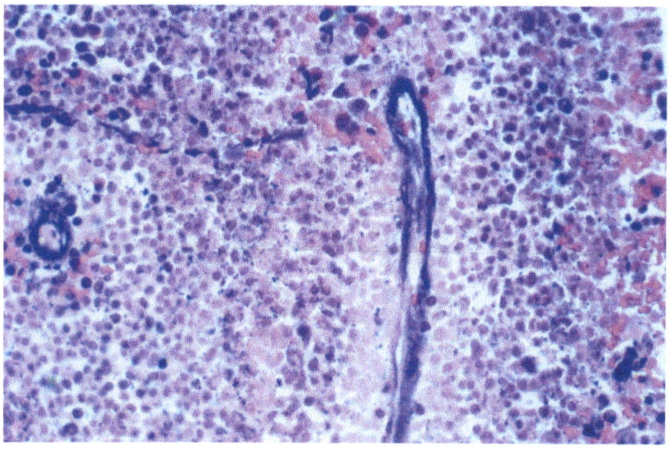

FIGURE 36.71. Greater magnification of tumor shown in Figure 36.70 shows nuclear encrustation of elastic tissue of small blood vessel.

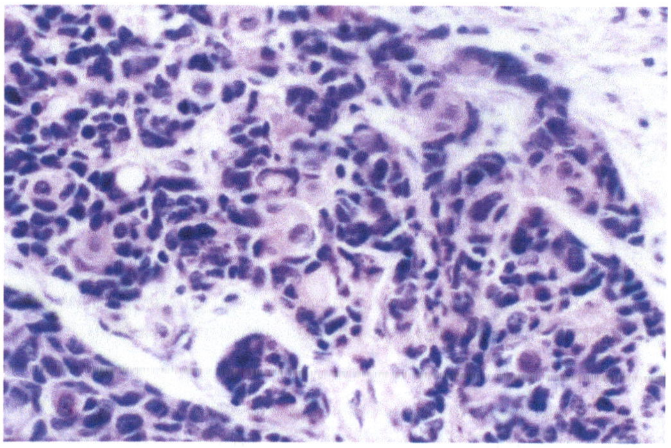

FIGURE 36.72. Some small cell lung carcinomas show aggregation of tumor cells around small blood vessels.

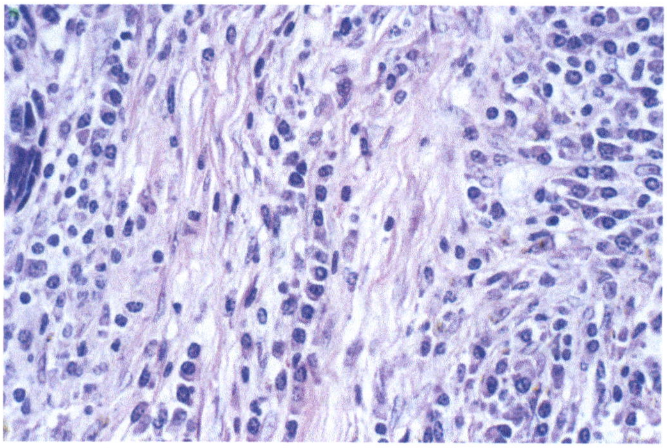

FIGURE 36.73. Perineural space invasion by small cell lung carcinoma is frequent.

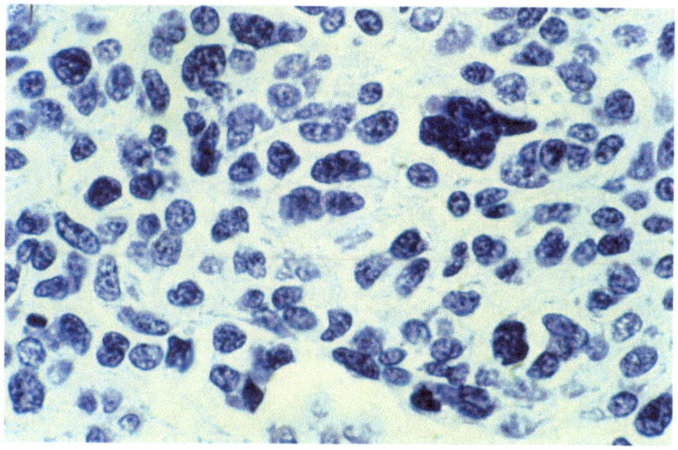

FIGURE 36.74. Some small undifferentiated neuroendocrine carcinomas contain occasional tumor giant cells.

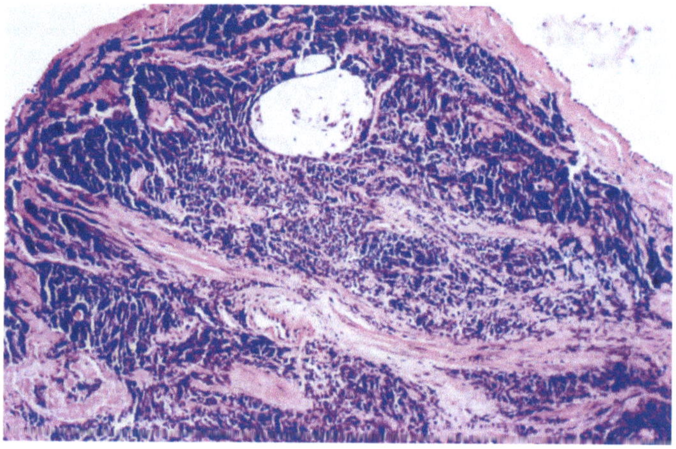

FIGURE 36.75. Transbronchial biopsy of small cell lung carcinoma. Tumor cells frequently appose respiratory mucosal epithelium and may induce squamous metaplasia, but do not usually invade through the surface epithelium.

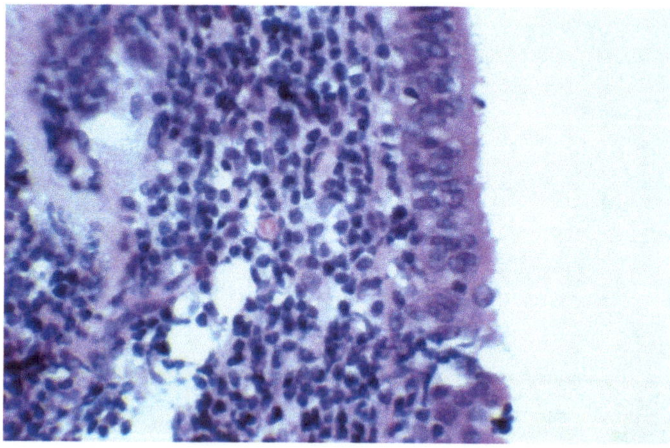

FIGURE 36.76. Transbronchial biopsy shows infiltrating small cell lung carcinoma. Tumor cells are dying and have degenerated hyperchromatic nuclei. The overlying mucosa is not invaded.

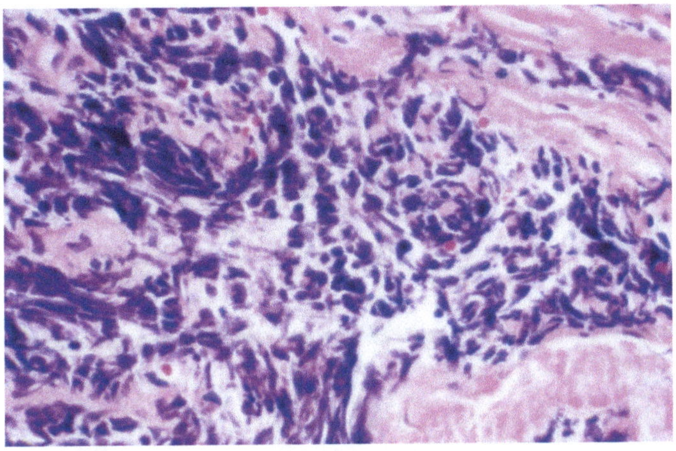

FIGURE 36.77. Crush artifact is a common finding when small cell lung carcinomas are biopsied endoscopically. A definitive diagnosis may not be possible when only crush artifact is present.

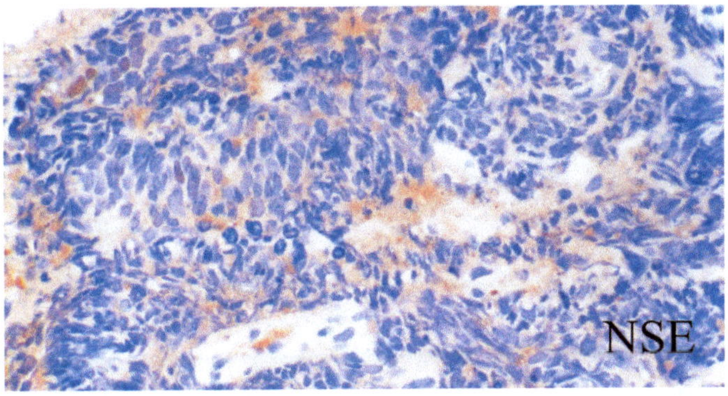

FIGURE 36.79. Small cell neuroendocrine carcinomas typically express neuron-specific enolase (NSE) immunohistochemically.

distorted by crush artifact and lacks well-preserved cells, an unequivocal diagnosis often cannot be rendered. In such specimens examined ultrastructurally, an accurate, unequivocal diagnosis is often possible by identifying membrane-bound, dense-core neuroendocrine granules. As discussed later, immunohistochemical evaluation can often support a definitive diagnosis.

Immunohistochemically, most small cell neuroendocrine carcinomas express low molecular weight cytokeratin, which is frequently distributed in a punctate streaky pattern within neoplastic cells (Fig. 36.78). In my experience, small cell lung carcinomas usually do not express high molecular weight cytokeratin. They routinely express neuron-specific enolase (Fig. 36.79) and synaptophysin (Fig. 36.80), and may show immunostaining for carcinoembryonic antigen (Fig. 36.81) and epithelial membrane

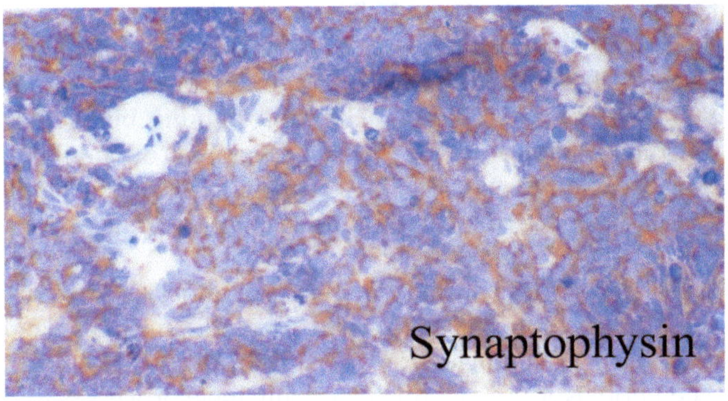

FIGURE 36.80. Most small cell neuroendocrine carcinomas express synaptophysin.

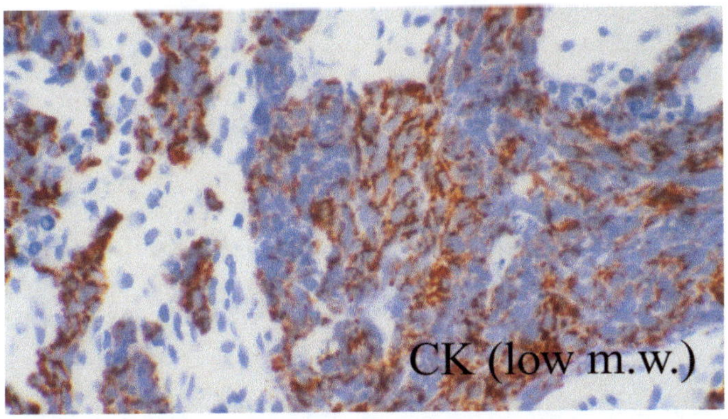

FIGURE 36.78. Low molecular weight cytokeratin [CK (low m. w.)] is present in nearly all small cell neuroendocrine carcinomas examined using avidin-biotin immunoperoxidase technique.

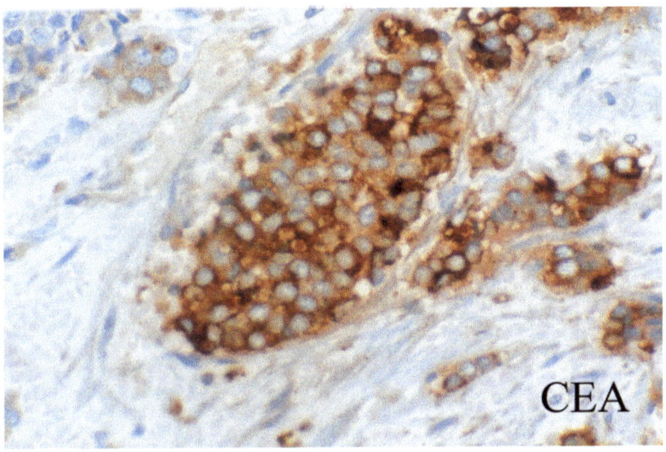

FIGURE 36.81. Approximately one half of small cell lung carcinomas immunostain for carcinoembryonic antigen (CEA).

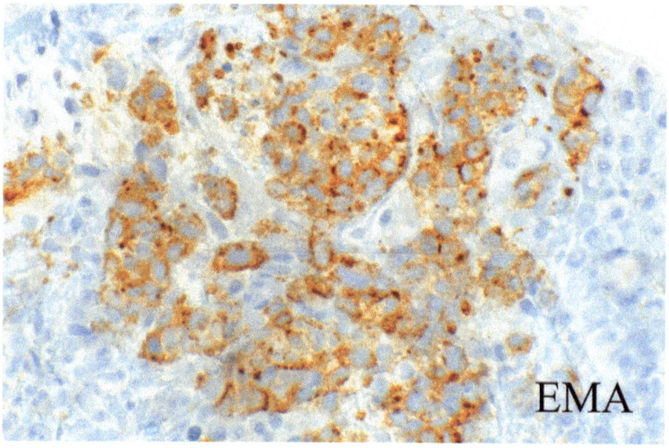

FIGURE 36.82. Immunostaining for epithelial membrane antigen (EMA) is seen in some small cell neuroendocrine lung carcinomas.

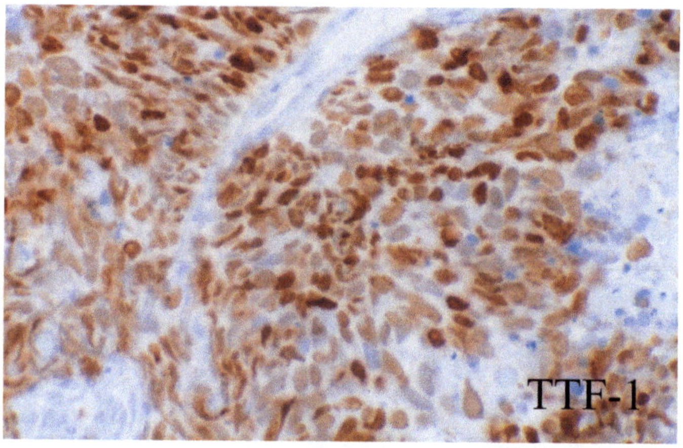

FIGURE 36.84. Over 90% of small cell lung carcinomas show nuclear immunostaining for TTF-1.

antigen (Fig. 36.82). They may also show immunostaining for chromogranin (Fig. 36.83), which is usually not as intense as seen in typical and atypical carcinoids and in large cell neuroendocrine carcinomas. Over 90% of SCLCs express TTF-1, the immunostaining being in a nuclear distribution (Fig. 36.84). Over half of small cell lung carcinomas express CD117 (c-Kit) (Fig. 36.85). Small cell neuroendocrine carcinomas may also contain any of the substances listed in Table 36.1.

Ultrastructurally, small cell neuroendocrine carcinomas are composed of small, round, unspecialized cells with high nuclear/cytoplasmic ratios (Fig. 36.86). The neoplastic cells characteristically have processes that frequently contain microtubules and neuroendocrine granules (Fig. 36.87). Some small cell neuroendocrine carcinomas are interconnected by desmosomes (Fig. 36.88) and show occasional tonofilaments (Fig. 36.89). Figure 36.90 represents a small cell neuroendocrine carcinoma with a slight degree of crush artifact. Even with this distortion, cell processes with neuroendocrine granules are obvious.

Combined Small Cell-Large Cell Neuroendocrine Carcinomas

Combined small cell-large cell neuroendocrine carcinomas exist and are composed of small undifferentiated cells like one sees in SCLC admixed with large cells scattered among the smaller cells or in distinct nests. As discussed later (see Approach to the Diagnosis of Neuroendocrine Lung Neoplasms: Variabilities and Pitfalls) the size of neoplastic cells is somewhat in the eyes of the beholder. Fushimi et al.[151] performed a retrospective evaluation of pathologic specimens from 430 patients

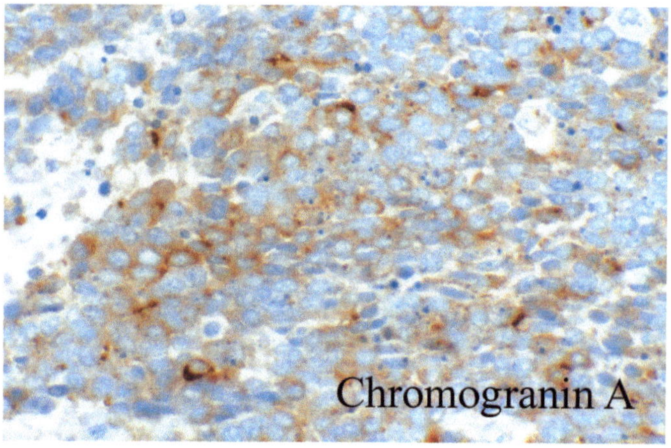

FIGURE 36.83. Approximately 20% to 50% of small cell lung carcinomas show immunostaining for chromogranin A.

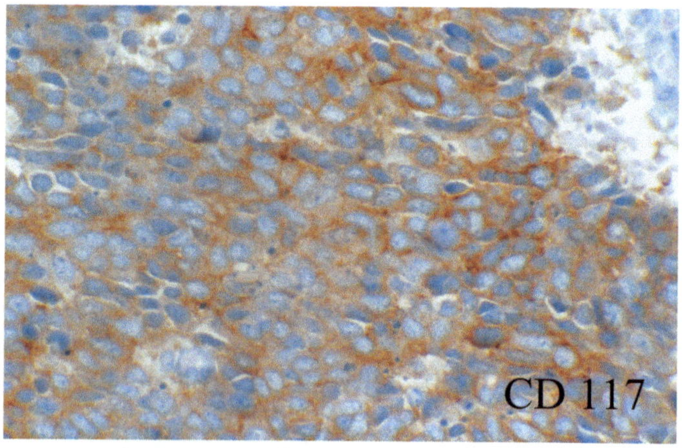

FIGURE 36.85. The majority of small cell lung carcinomas express CD117 (c-Kit).

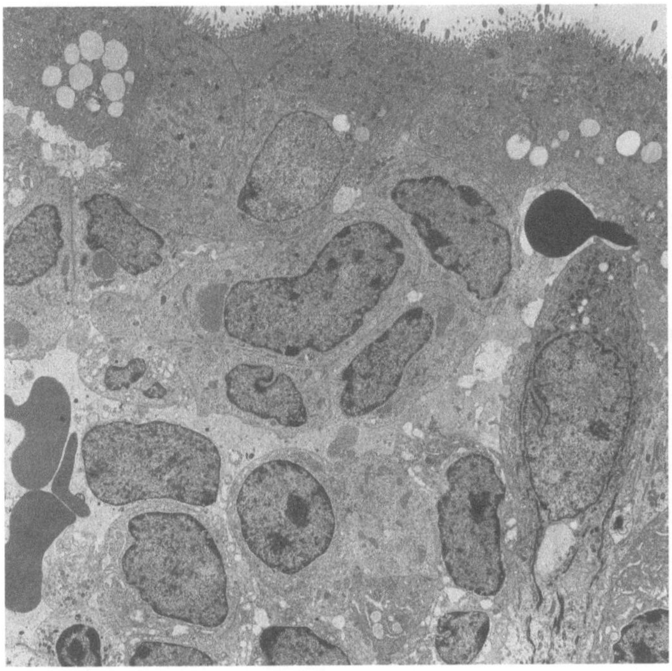

A

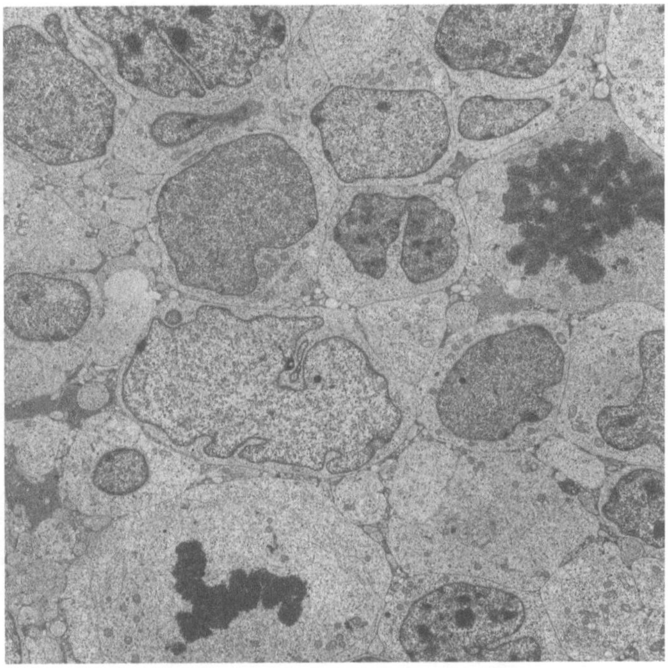

B

FIGURES 36.86. **(A,B)** Typical ultrastructural appearance of small cell neuroendocrine carcinomas. Cells have high nuclear cytoplasmic ratios with small amount of unspecialized cytoplasm. Nuclei generally lack nucleoli. Note mitoses in **(B)**. **(A)** ×4100; **(B)** ×6400.

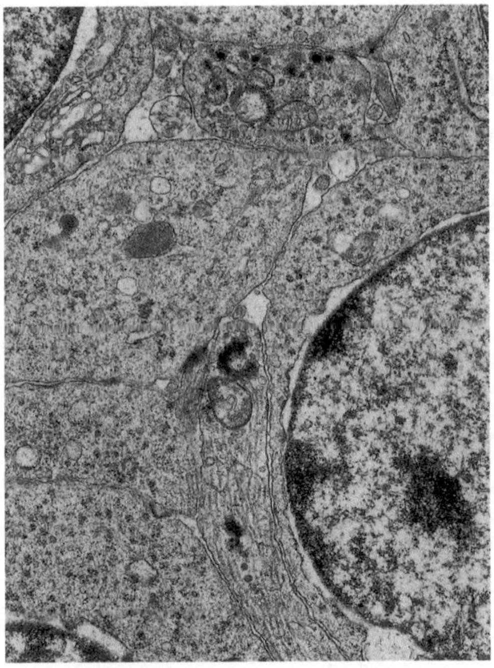

FIGURE 36.87. Neoplastic cells usually have processes containing microtubules and neuroendocrine granules. ×16,000.

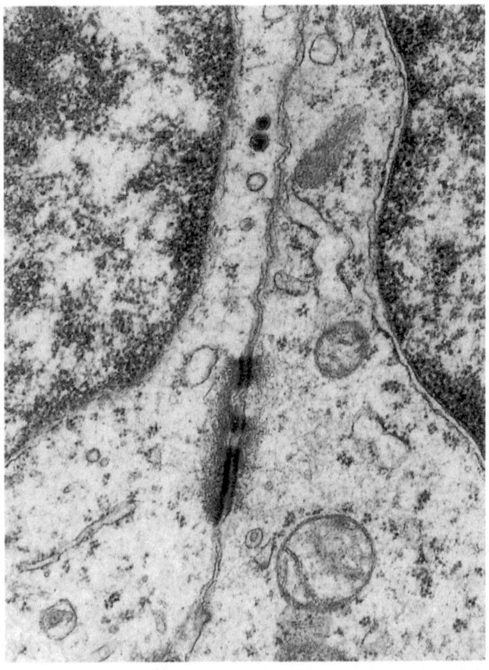

FIGURE 36.88. Small cell undifferentiated carcinoma cells are occasionally interconnected by desmosomes. Note neuroendocrine granule in cytoplasm. ×26,500.

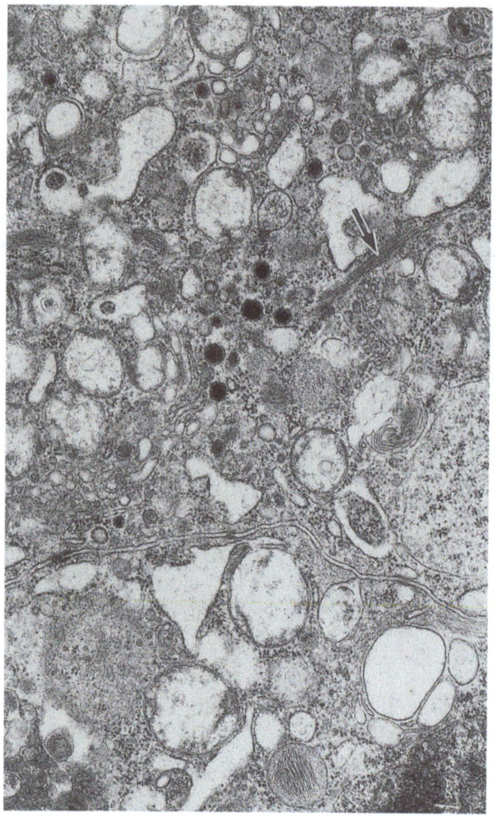

FIGURE 36.89. Some small cell neuroendocrine carcinomas contain tonofilaments in cytoplasm (*arrow*). ×26,500.

with small cell carcinoma of the lung. They defined mixed small cell–large cell carcinoma as neoplasms containing aggregates of, or individual, large cells interspersed among tumor cells with the characteristic features of a small cell lung carcinoma. The large cells were defined histologically as having varying amounts of slightly eosinophilic cytoplasm showing distinct margins, and having large vesicular nuclei with distinct nucleoli. In cytologic specimens obtained by brushings or aspiration, the large cells occurred singly or in groups, and were described as having cyanophilic or amphophilic cytoplasm, and round vesicular nuclei and prominent nucleoli. In sputum cytologic specimens, the large cells were observed singly or in loose clusters among the small cells, and were stated to show condensation of nuclear chromatin and shrinkage of cytoplasm, because of degenerative changes. In a review of the 430 cases, Fushimi et al. observed a frequency of mixed small cell–large cell carcinoma in 25 of 299 (8.4%) biopsy specimens, 75 of 400 (18.8%) cytologic specimens obtained by brushings or fine-needle aspiration biopsy, and in eight of 232 (3.4%) sputum cytology specimens. Fushimi et al. reported that whatever the diagnostic method, patients with mixed small cell–large cell carcinoma exhibited a lesser response to therapy and had a worse prognosis than those with homogeneous small cell

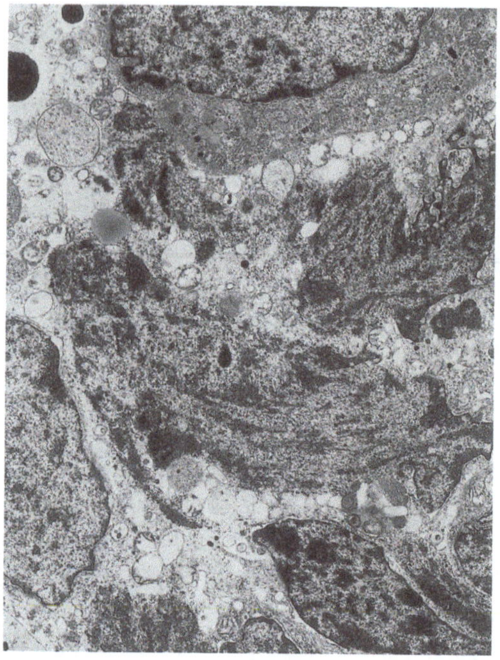

FIGURE 36.90. Ultrastructural appearance of tumor cells showing a slight degree of crush artifact. ×6400.

lung carcinoma. In the 2004 WHO classification, mixed small cell–large cell neuroendocrine carcinoma falls under the diagnostic category of combined small cell carcinoma (see below).

Combined Small Cell–Non–Small-Cell Lung Neoplasms

Occasionally, combined small cell–non–small-cell lung neoplasms are encountered composed of a small cell neuroendocrine carcinoma and a squamous carcinoma (Fig. 36.91), an adenocarcinoma (Fig. 36.92), or a large cell undifferentiated carcinoma (Fig. 36.93). The

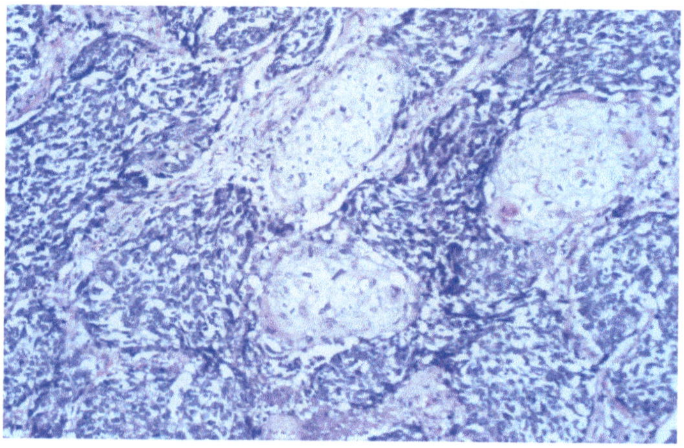

FIGURE 36.91. Combined small cell lung carcinoma with squamous cell carcinoma.

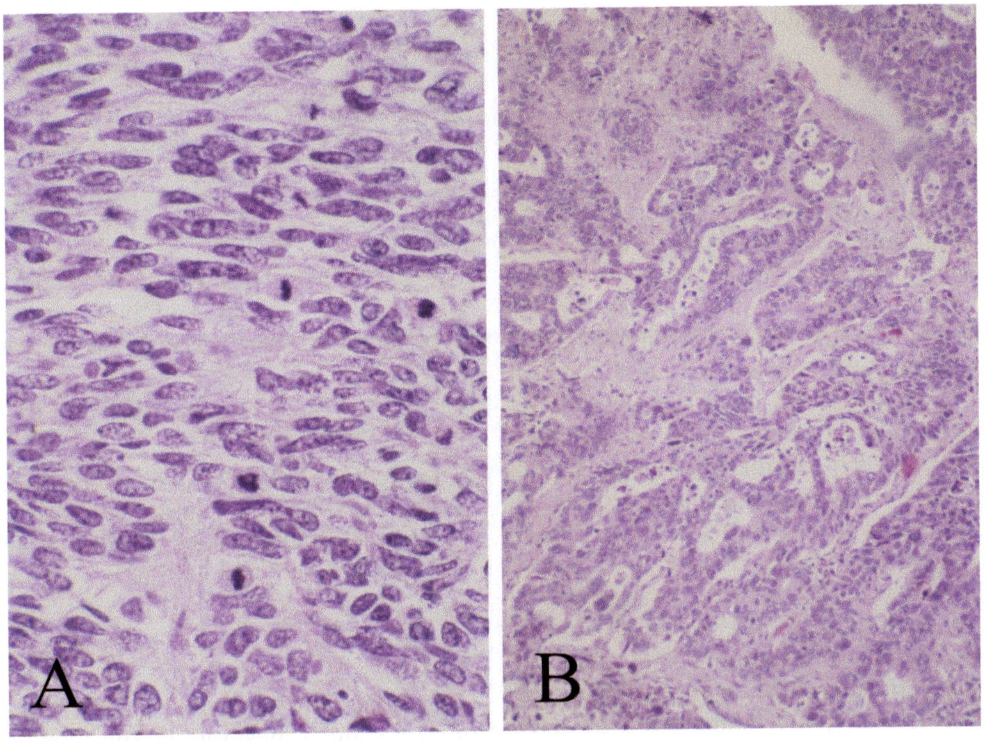

FIGURE 36.92. Combined small cell lung carcinoma **(A)** with primary pulmonary adenocarcinoma **(B)**. ×200.

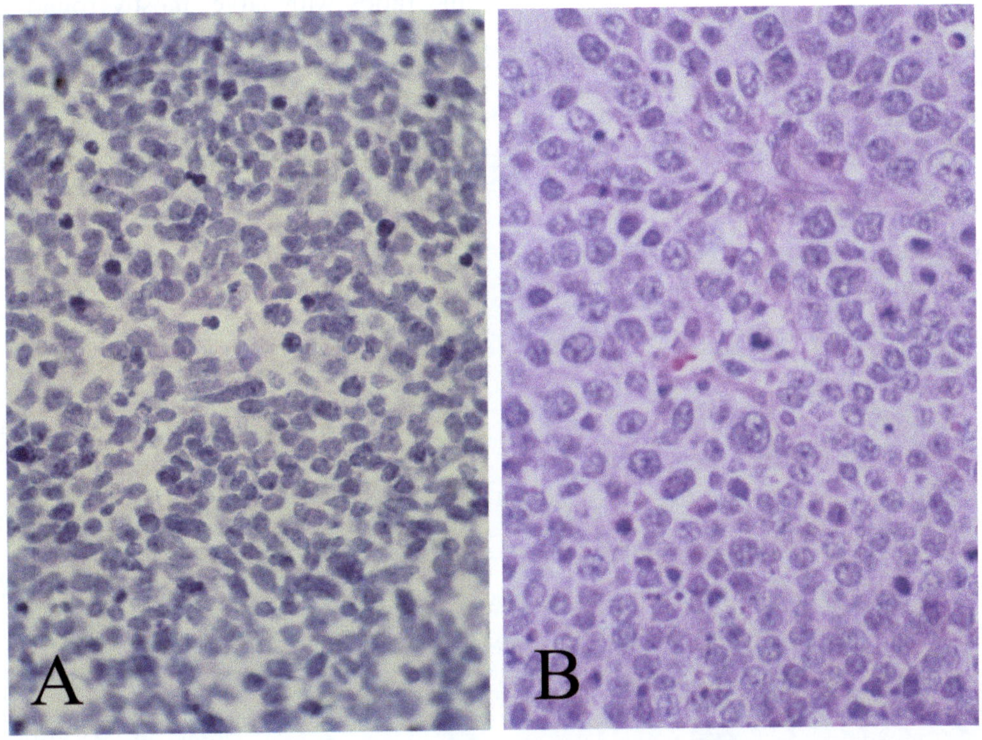

FIGURE 36.93. Combined small cell lung carcinoma **(A)** with large cell undifferentiated carcinoma **(B)**. ×200.

non–small-cell component should comprise at least 10% of the tumor.

Unusual Neuroendocrine Lung Neoplasms

Case 1 (Anemone Tumor)

A 65-year-old man with no history of cigarette smoking was scratched by a cat in January 1987. Shortly thereafter, he noticed enlarging lymph nodes in the right axilla. Computed tomography (CT) scan of the chest demonstrated right axillary and supraclavicular lymphadenopathy, and a chest radiograph showed moderate pleural thickening at the right apex and lateral aspects of the chest. A biopsy of the axillary lymph node was obtained. The lymph node was nearly completely replaced by a highly cellular malignant neoplasm composed of small, medium, and occasionally giant tumor cells (Fig. 36.94). No squamous or glandular differentiation was noted. Mitoses were relatively frequent, varying between one to three per HPF (10 to 30 per 10 HPFs). The neoplastic cells showed diffuse cytoplasmic immunostaining for low molecular weight keratin and chromogranin (Figs. 36.95 and 36.96). Ultrastructurally, the tumor was composed of round cells closely associated with one another. The cells had large nuclei with occasional indentations, and most cells had long microvilli arising from the cell surface (Fig. 36.97). The cytoplasm of most cells contained dense-core neuroendocrine granules (Fig. 36.98). Ultrastructurally, this tumor had the features of what is referred to as an *anemone tumor*.[152] Subsequent studies have shown the anemone morphology encompassing transitional cell carcinoma, squamous cell carcinoma, and lymphoma.[153–157]

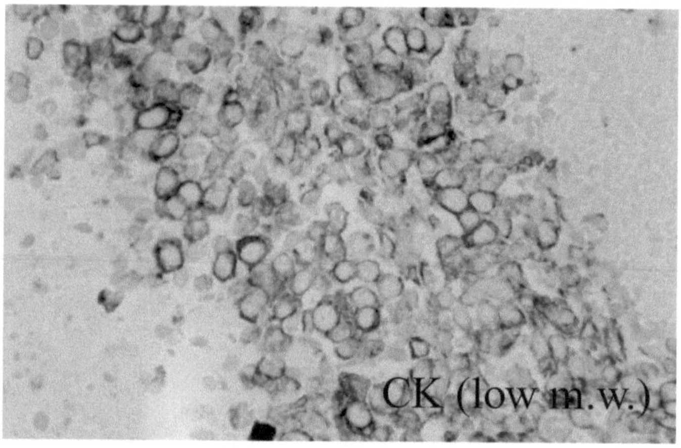

FIGURE 36.95. Metastatic neuroendocrine carcinoma from lung with anemone tumor features. Neoplastic cells showed diffuse cytoplasmic immunostaining for low molecular weight keratin [CK (low m.w.)].

Case 2 (Primitive Neuroectodermal Tumor)

A 64-year-old man with a history of cigarette smoking was evaluated for a 6-month history of sinus problems. He was found to have an elevated erythrocyte sedimentation rate, and a chest radiograph showed a right hilar and right lower lobe mass. Evaluation showed no evidence of a primary neoplasm elsewhere. A needle aspiration biopsy was performed. The fine-needle aspiration biopsy showed degenerating malignant cells with high nuclear/cytoplasmic ratios with large, mostly round nuclei and small nucleoli or prominent chromocenters (Fig. 36.99). Mitoses were frequent, varying between four and five per HPF (40 to 50 per 10 HPFs). The neoplastic cells showed no immunostaining for low molecular weight keratin, chromogranin, vimentin, or neuron-specific enolase. Ultrastructural evaluation showed round to polygonal cells with extensive cytoplasmic processes that contained numerous microtubules and microfilaments (Figs. 36.100 and 36.101). A rare structure consistent with a neuroen-

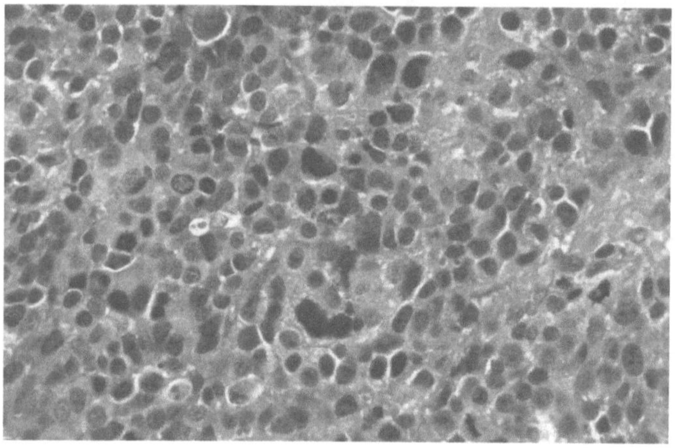

FIGURE 36.94. Metastatic neuroendocrine carcinoma from lung with anemone tumor features. Tumor is composed of variably sized and shaped cells and some tumor giant cells.

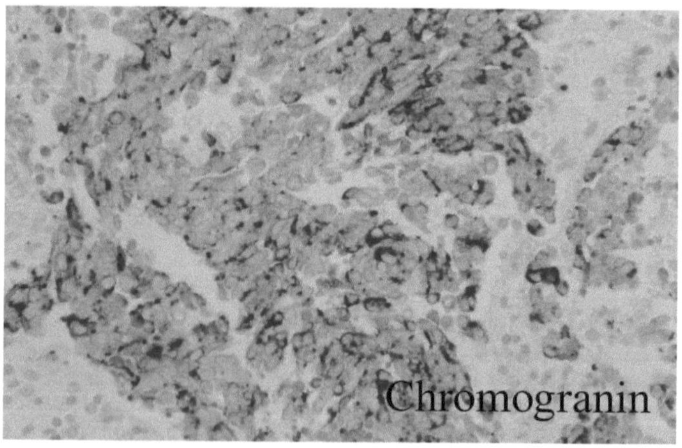

FIGURE 36.96. Metastatic neuroendocrine carcinoma from lung with anemone tumor features. Neoplastic cells showed diffuse cytoplasmic immunostaining for chromogranin.

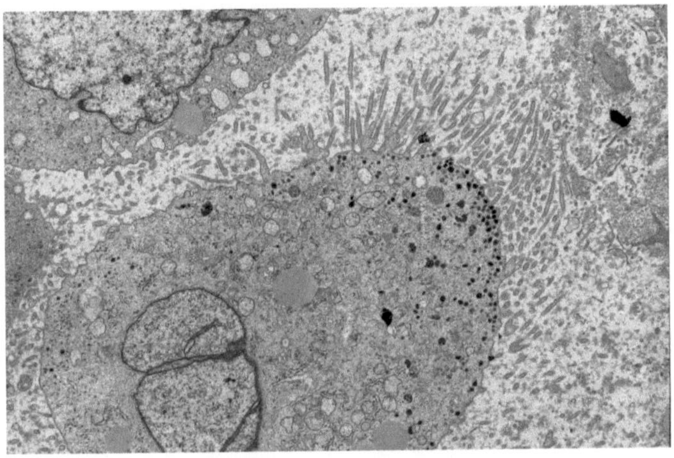

FIGURE 36.97. Metastatic neuroendocrine carcinoma of lung with anemone tumor features. Ultrastructurally, the tumor was composed of round cells closely associated with one another. The cells had large nuclei with occasional indentation and most cells had long microvilli arising from the cell surface. ×4000. (From The Unusual Spectrum of Neuroendocrine Lung Neoplams; Samuel Hammar, Dawn Bockus, Franque Remington et al. Ultrastructural Pathology, Volume 13, Issue 5, 1989. Reprinted by permission of Taylor & Francis Ltd.)

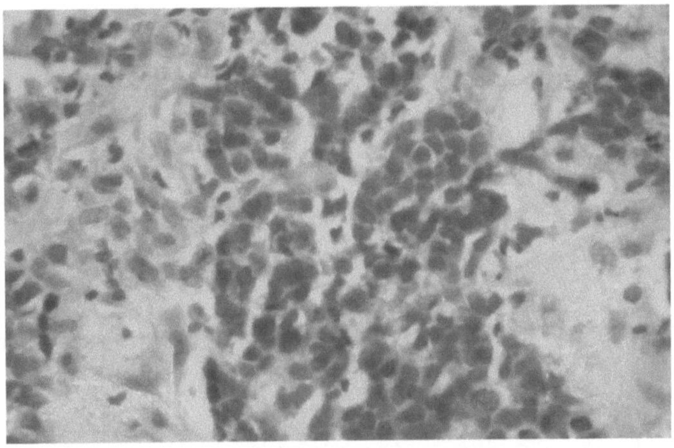

FIGURE 36.99. Primary primitive neuroectodermal tumor of lung. Aspiration biopsy specimen showed numerous degenerating, round tumor cells with high nuclear/cytoplasmic ratios.

docrine granule was identified. The neoplastic cells had the features of a rare neoplasm referred to as a *primitive neuroectodermal tumor*. This tumor primarily involves the chest wall but occasionally has been reported in the parenchyma of the lung.[158] These tumors most frequently occur in young adults or children (see Chapter 42).

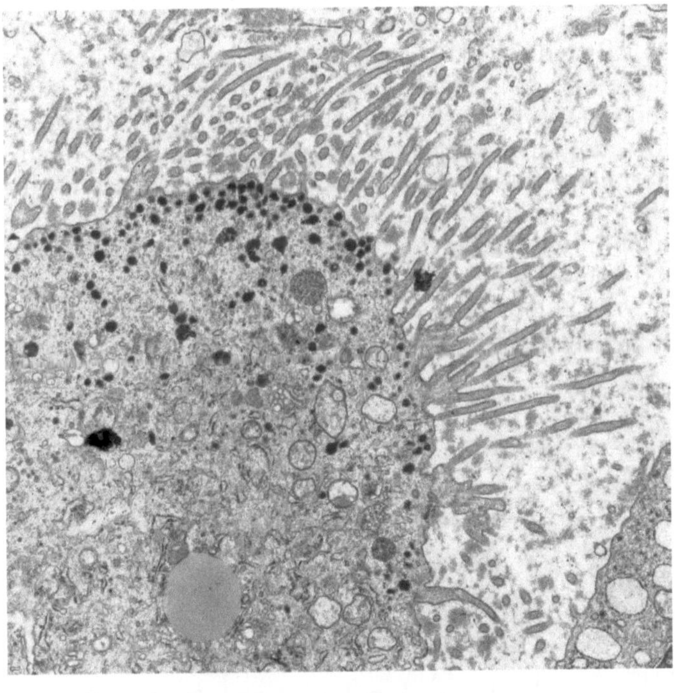

FIGURE 36.98. Metastatic neuroendocrine carcinoma of lung with anemone tumor features. The cytoplasm of most cells contained dense-core neuroendocrine granules. ×15,000. (From The Unusual Spectrum of Neuroendocrine Lung Neoplams; Samuel Hammar, Dawn Bockus, Franque Remington et al. Ultrastructural Pathology, Volume 13, Issue 5, 1989. Reprinted by permission of Taylor & Francis Ltd.)

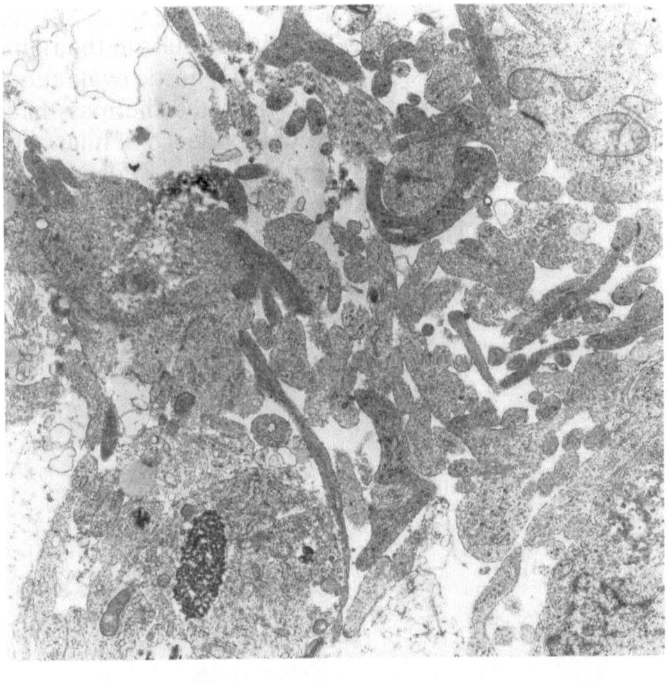

FIGURE 36.100. Primary primitive neuroectodermal tumor of lung. Ultrastructural evaluation showed round to polygonal cells with extensive cytoplasmic processes that contained numerous microtubules and microfilaments. ×6000. (From The Unusual Spectrum of Neuroendocrine Lung Neoplams; Samuel Hammar, Dawn Bockus, Franque Remington et al. Ultrastructural Pathology, Volume 13, Issue 5, 1989. Reprinted by permission of Taylor & Francis Ltd.)

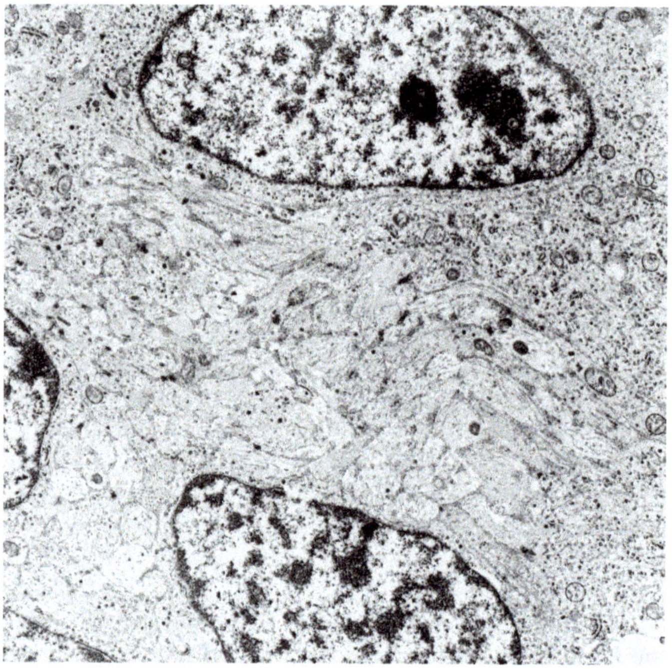

FIGURE 36.101. At greater magnification, these cytoplasmic processes contain numerous microtubules with some intermediate filaments probably representing neurofilaments. ×25,000.

Case 3 (Pulmonary Blastoma with Neuroendocrine Differentiation)

A 29-year-old woman had a history of a mass in the right lower lobe for 4 years. She refused diagnostic evaluation of the mass until 1988, when it was noted the mass had increased in size and that there was evidence of hilar and mediastinal adenopathy. A right lower lobe wedge resection with biopsy of hilar and mediastinal lymph nodes was performed. The tumor measured 5 cm in diameter and was well demarcated, being yellow-white. Histologically, it was composed of numerous glandular structures of varying sizes made up of a pseudostratified layer of cells with clear cytoplasm (Fig. 36.102). These glandular structures were admixed with stromal cells resembling cellular mesenchyme. The histologic appearance was characteristic of a pulmonary blastoma. In areas, the tumor had a different pattern, being composed of cells that showed no glandular differentiation that ranged from small and round to large and spindle shaped (Figs. 36.103 and 36.104). The tumor cells showed between three and four mitoses per HPF in these areas. They showed low-intensity cytoplasmic immunostaining for low molecular weight keratin and low-intensity immunostaining for neuron-specific enolase, being negative for chromogranin A. Ultrastructurally, the cells were relatively primitive, having few cytoplasmic organelles, but did exhibit cellular processes and many cells contained

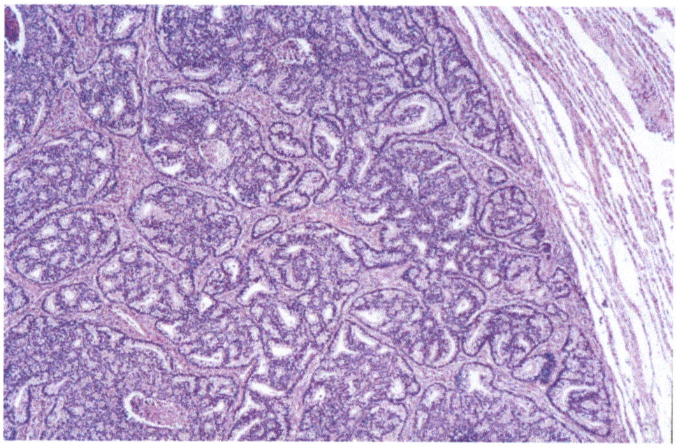

FIGURE 36.102. Pulmonary blastoma with focal neuroendocrine differentiation. Most of this tumor was composed of complex glandular structures made up of pseudostratified layer of columnar epithelial cells that frequently showed clear cytoplasm (well-differentiated fetal adenocarcinoma pattern).

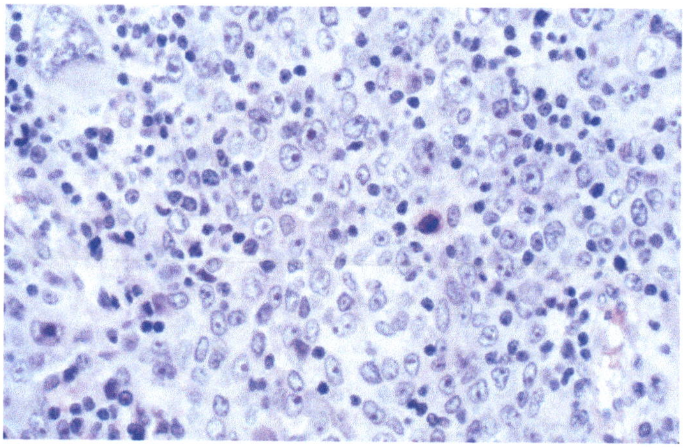

FIGURE 36.103. Pulmonary blastoma with focal neuroendocrine differentiation. Portion of tumor was composed of medium-sized round cells and elongated spindle-shaped cells that lacked differentiation.

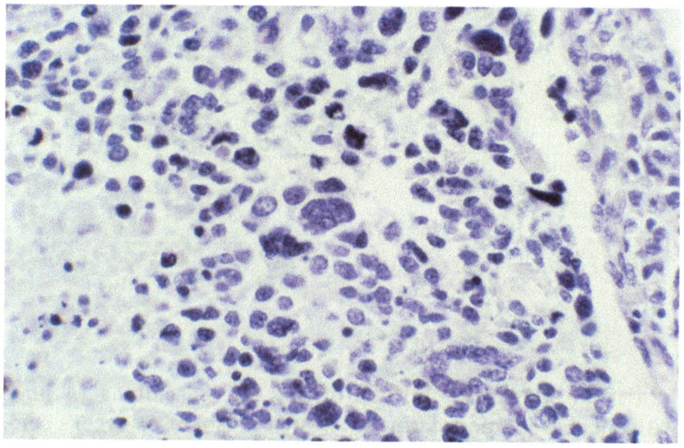

FIGURE 36.104. Pulmonary blastoma with focal neuroendocrine differentiation. Admixed with round and spindle-shaped cells were a moderate number of tumor giant cells.

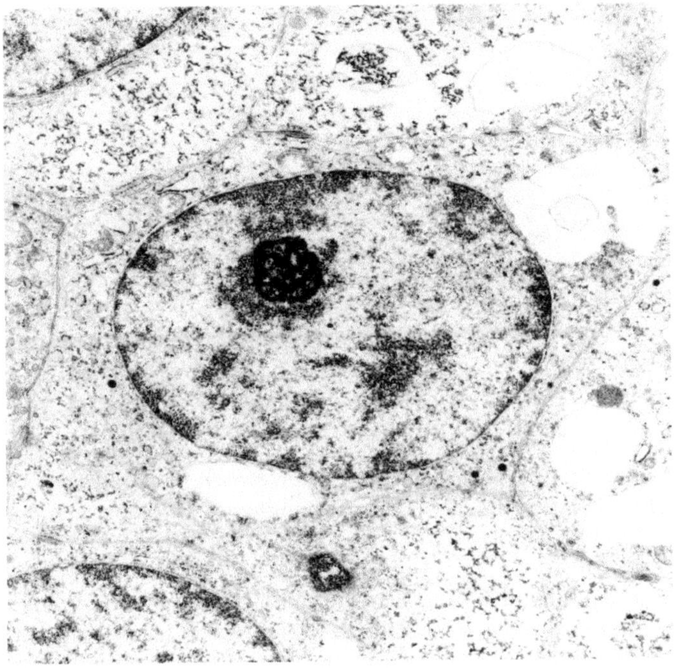

FIGURE 36.105. Pulmonary blastoma with focal neuroendocrine differentiation. Ultrastructurally, these tumor cells show distinct dense-core granules consistent with dense-core neuroendocrine granules. (From The Unusual Spectrum of Neuroendocrine Lung Neoplams; Samuel Hammar, Dawn Bockus, Franque Remington et al. Ultrastructural Pathology, Volume 13, Issue 5, 1989. Reprinted by permission of Taylor & Francis Ltd.)

dense-core neuroendocrine-type granules (Fig. 36.105). The neuroendocrine nature of these cells was confirmed by the uranaffin reaction (Fig. 36.106). Pulmonary blastomas are rare neoplasms that typically show glandular differentiation admixed with cellular mesenchyme. They occasionally show neuroendocrine differentiation, as reported in the Armed Forces Institute of Pathology (AFIP) fascicle, "Tumors of the Lower Respiratory Tract"[159] (see Chapter 37).

Case 4 (Neuroendocrine Carcinoma)

A 73-year-old woman with a 70+ pack-year history of cigarette smoking presented with acute onset of pleuritic pain in the right lateral chest. A chest radiograph showed a rib fracture of the sixth rib laterally and a solitary pulmonary nodule measuring 1.5 cm in diameter. The nodule had not been observed in a previous chest radiograph. A CT scan of the thorax showed two pulmonary nodules, one measuring 1.2 × 1.5 cm in the peripheral mid-lung field close to the major fissure, and the other measuring 7 mm in diameter in a subpleural location in the right mid-peripheral lung field a few millimeters below the larger nodule. A right upper and right middle lobectomy were performed. The tumors were relatively well demarcated and composed of cells that had an organoid appearance (Fig. 36.107). There was frequent palisading of the peripheral cell layer forming these

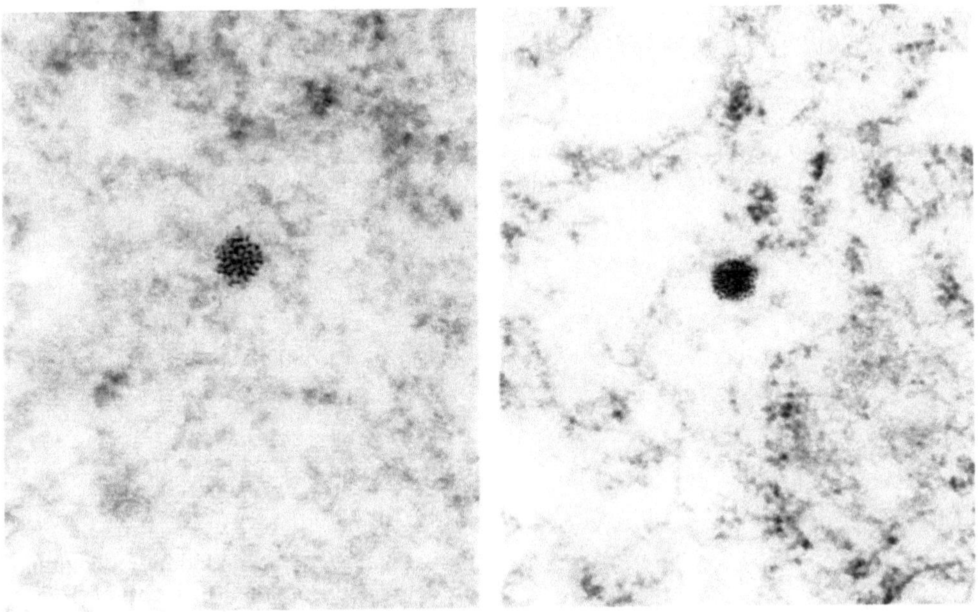

A B

FIGURE 36.106. Pulmonary blastoma with focal neuroendocrine differentiation. **(A)** A uranaffin reaction was run on dedifferentiated portion of tumor and granules showed positive reaction. **(B)** Note their distinct granularity. ×52,000. (From The Unusual Spectrum of Neuroendocrine Lung Neoplams; Samuel Hammar, Dawn Bockus, Franque Remington et al. Ultrastructural Pathology, Volume 13, Issue 5, 1989. Reprinted by permission of Taylor & Francis Ltd.)

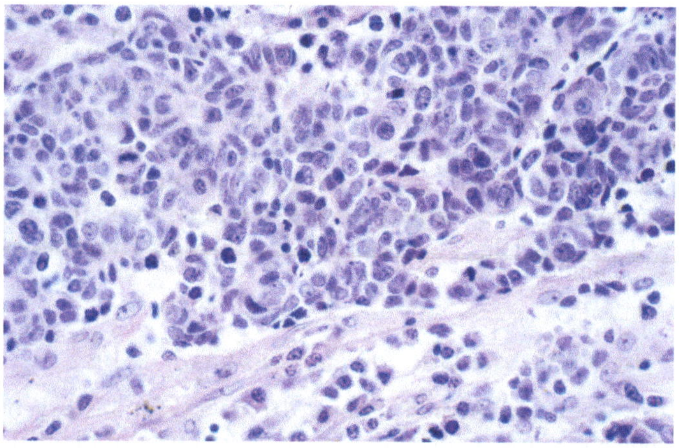

FIGURE 36.107. Neuroendocrine carcinoma. Tumor was composed predominantly of nests of small to medium-sized cells with prominent palisading of peripheral cell layer.

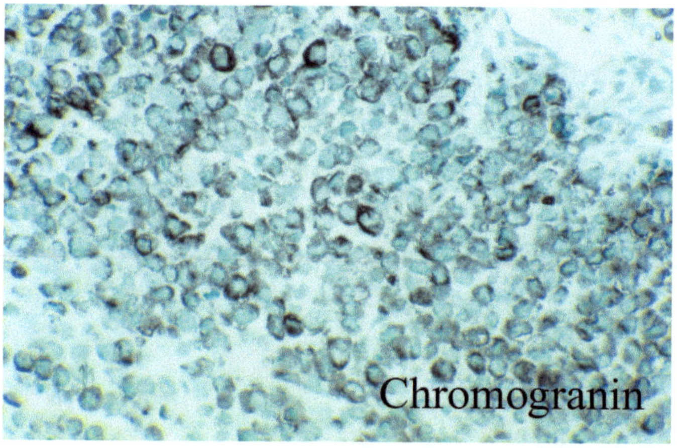

FIGURE 36.109. Neuroendocrine carcinoma. A moderate number of neoplastic cells show immunostaining for chromogranin.

nests. In many areas, distinct tumor giant cells were identified (Fig. 36.108). Immunohistochemical evaluation showed intense immunostaining for low molecular weight keratin, epithelial membrane antigen, carcinoembryonic antigen, and neuron-specific enolase. A moderate number of the neoplastic cells showed immunostaining for chromogranin A (Fig. 36.109). Ultrastructural evaluation showed considerable variation in the size and shape of the cells. Some were small and round and others were large and occasionally spindle shaped (Figs. 36.110 and 36.111). Occasional tumor giant cells were seen. Neuroendocrine granules were observed in some cells and were relatively small, measuring up to 150 nm in diameter (Fig. 36.112). This tumor was diagnosed as a neuroendocrine carcinoma, possibly representing an atypical carcinoid.

Case 5 (Amphicrine Carcinoma)

A 46-year-old woman with no history of cigarette smoking developed chest discomfort and coughing. A chest radiograph showed a nodule that had been present in this woman's lung for about 10 years. As judged from the previous chest radiograph, the nodule had increased in size and a resection was performed. Histologically, the tumor had a relatively uniform, somewhat adenoid cystic-like pattern (Fig. 36.113). A mucicarmine stain was negative. A Pasqual stain for neuroendocrine granules was

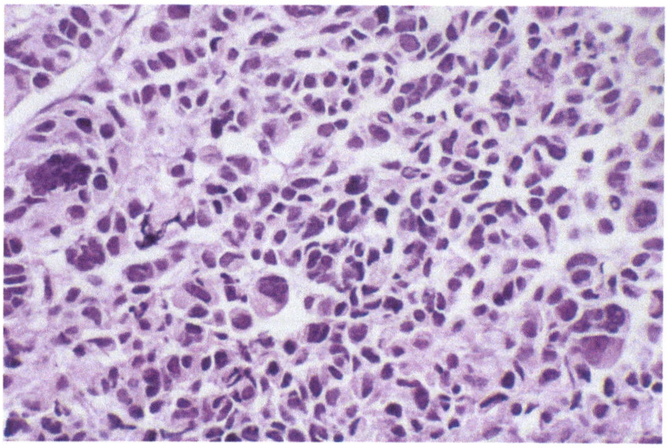

FIGURE 36.108. Neuroendocrine carcinoma. In many areas of tumor, large tumor giant cells were present.

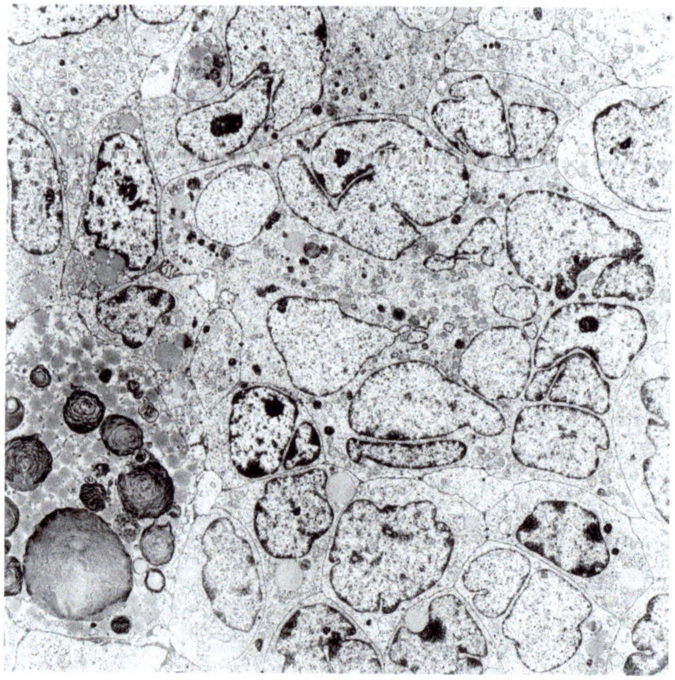

FIGURE 36.110. Neuroendocrine carcinoma. Tumor is composed predominantly of small to medium-sized cells with moderate amount of cytoplasm. Admixed with these cells are numerous tumor giant cells that have hyperlobed nuclei. ×4100. (From The Unusual Spectrum of Neuroendocrine Lung Neoplams; Samuel Hammar, Dawn Bockus, Franque Remington et al. Ultrastructural Pathology, Volume 13, Issue 5, 1989. Reprinted by permission of Taylor & Francis Ltd.)

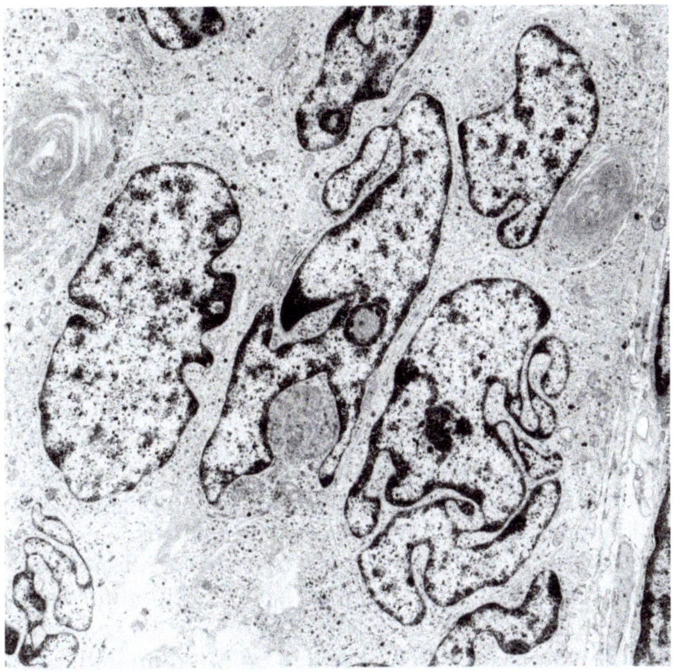

FIGURE 36.111. Neuroendocrine carcinoma. Ultrastructural evaluation shows considerable variation in the size and shape of the cells. Some are small and round and others are large and spindle-shaped with hyperconvoluted nuclei. ×4100.

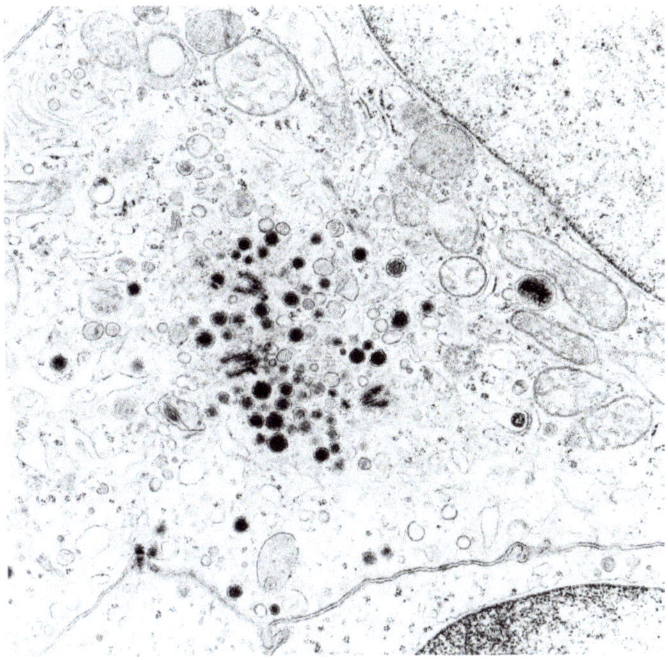

FIGURE 36.112. Neuroendocrine carcinoma. Relatively few tumor cells contain neuroendocrine granules, but those that do often contain them in significant numbers. ×25,500. (From The Unusual Spectrum of Neuroendocrine Lung Neoplams; Samuel Hammar, Dawn Bockus, Franque Remington et al. Ultrastructural Pathology, Volume 13, Issue 5, 1989. Reprinted by permission of Taylor & Francis Ltd.)

equivocal. Immunohistochemically, the tumor cells showed immunostaining for neuron-specific enolase but no immunostaining for chromogranin A. Ultrastructural examination of the tissue retrieved from paraffin block showed moderate degenerative changes. The cells forming the glandular like structures showed a pseudostratified layer of columnar cells with their apical portions showing short microvilli projecting into gland lumina with underlying prominent microfilaments (Fig. 36.114). At the basal portions of the cells were numerous dense-core membrane-bound granules that resembled neuroendocrine granules (Fig. 36.115). The neoplasm was initially thought to be a carcinoid on the basis of its appearance by light microscopy. The negative stain for chromogranin, however, ruled against that diagnosis. Based on the evidence of apical secretory-type differentiation and the basal neuroendocrine-type features, the tumor was thought to represent an amphicrine carcinoma. Amphicrine carcinomas were described by Chejfec et al[160] in 1985. These neoplasms occur in the lung, GI tract, and other parts of the body.[161]

Neuroendocrine Differentiation in Non–Small-Cell Lung Carcinomas

Visscher et al.[162] evaluated frozen unfixed tissue sections from 56 poorly differentiated non–small-cell primary lung neoplasms with monoclonal antibodies against chromogranin-A, synaptophysin, S-100 protein, keratin, vimentin, and neurofilament antigens. Histologically, neuroendocrine features were stated to be absent in these neoplasms. Immunostaining for chromogranin-A or synaptophysin was identified in five of 17 (29%) large cell

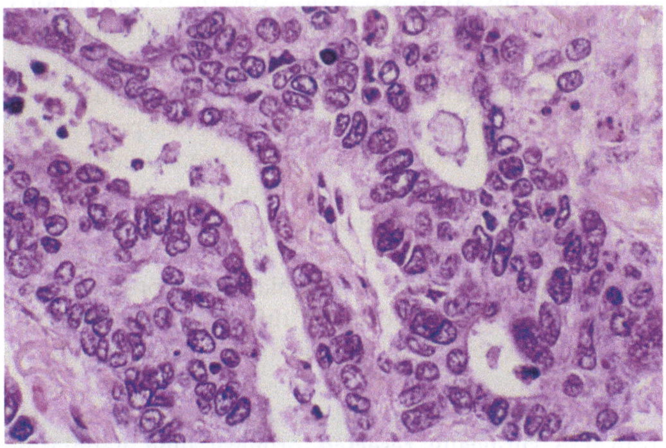

FIGURE 36.113. Primary amphicrine carcinoma of lung. Tumor had somewhat adenoid cystic-like pattern, being composed of uniform cells forming small glandular-like spaces and often containing eosinophilic material.

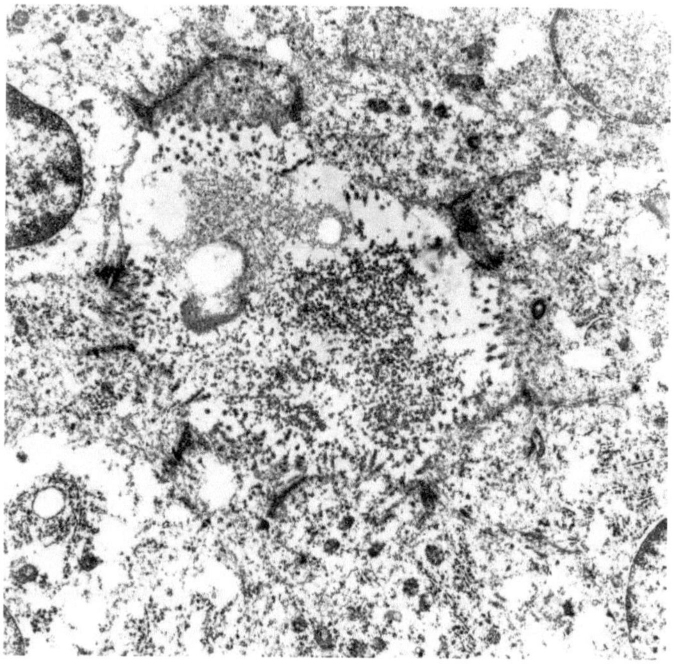

FIGURE 36.114. Primary amphicrine carcinoma of lung. Neoplastic cells show distinct gland formation with cells being connected to one another by junctional complexes. Short microvilli with underlying prominent microfilaments are inserted into gland lumina. ×10,500.

undifferentiated carcinomas and in four of 19 (21%) poorly differentiated adenocarcinomas. Diffuse intense immunostaining for synaptophysin was present in two large cell undifferentiated carcinomas and one poorly differentiated adenocarcinoma. Vimentin or neurofilament expression was observed in 10 of 17 (59%) large cell undifferentiated carcinomas, 10 of 19 (53%) poorly differentiated adenocarcinomas, and accompanied neuroendocrine markers in eight of nine (89%) cases. Synaptophysin was expressed in only one of 20 (5%) poorly differentiated squamous carcinomas and vimentin was observed in two of 20 (10%) squamous cell carcinomas. The authors concluded that (1) immunohistologic evidence of neuroendocrine differentiation was present in a significant number of large cell undifferentiated carcinomas and poorly differentiated adenocarcinomas, and was rare in poorly differentiated squamous carcinomas; (2) neuroendocrine differentiation was often accompanied by heterogeneous intermediate filament expression; and (3) divergent neuroendocrine differentiation was not necessarily reflected in the histologic features of the tumor.

Linnoila et al.[163] evaluated paraffin-embedded sections from 113 surgically resected primary lung neoplasms with antibodies against chromogranin-A, Leu7, neuron-specific enolase, serotonin, bombesin, calcitonin, ACTH, vasopressin, neurotensin, carcinoembryonic antigen, keratin, vimentin, and neurofilaments. They found that (1) the majority of carcinoids and small cell lung carcinomas expressed multiple neuroendocrine markers in a high percentage of tumor cells; (2) approximately 50% of NSCLCs contained subpopulations of tumor cells expressing neuroendocrine markers; and (3) occasional NSCLCs showed immunostaining patterns indistinguishable from small cell lung carcinomas. Neuroendocrine markers were more commonly expressed in large cell undifferentiated carcinomas and adenocarcinomas than in squamous carcinomas.

Loy et al.[164] evaluated 66 neoplasms that had been examined ultrastructurally with a battery of neuroendocrine markers, including neuron-specific enolase, chromogranin A, Leu7, and synaptophysin, and with a nonneuroendocrine marker B72.3. They studied 11 small cell carcinomas, four low-grade neuroendocrine carcinomas (atypical carcinoids?), two large cell carcinomas with neuroendocrine differentiation (large cell neuroendocrine carcinomas?), 26 adenocarcinomas, 10 squamous cell carcinomas, and 11 large cell undifferentiated carcinomas. Four of 10 squamous carcinomas, three of 26 adenocarcinomas, and one of 11 large cell undifferentiated carcinomas showed immunostaining for Leu7. Six of 10 squamous carcinomas, 15 of 26 adenocarcinomas, and

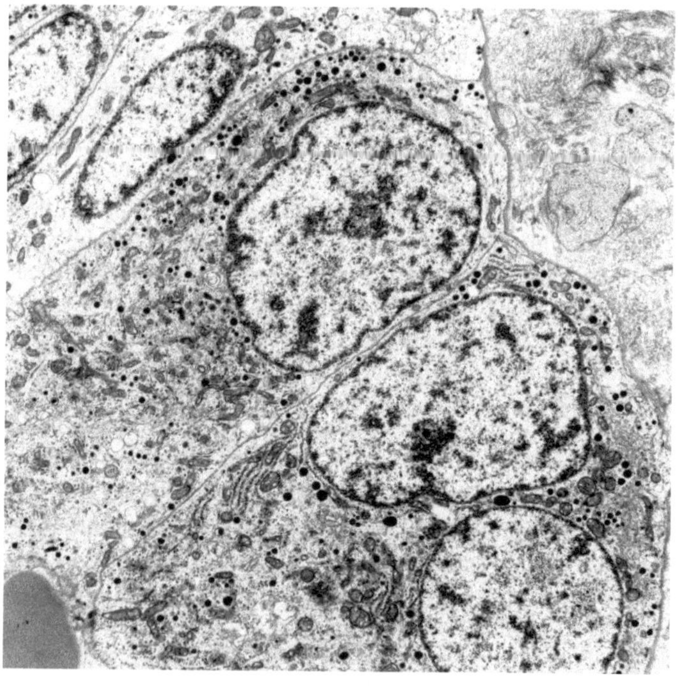

FIGURE 36.115. Primary amphicrine carcinoma of lung. At base of tumor cells are distinct dense-core granules that resemble neuroendocrine granules. Note basal lamina surrounding tumor cells. ×10,500. (From The Unusual Spectrum of Neuroendocrine Lung Neoplams; Samuel Hammar, Dawn Bockus, Franque Remington et al. Ultrastructural Pathology, Volume 13, Issue 5, 1989. Reprinted by permission of Taylor & Francis Ltd.)

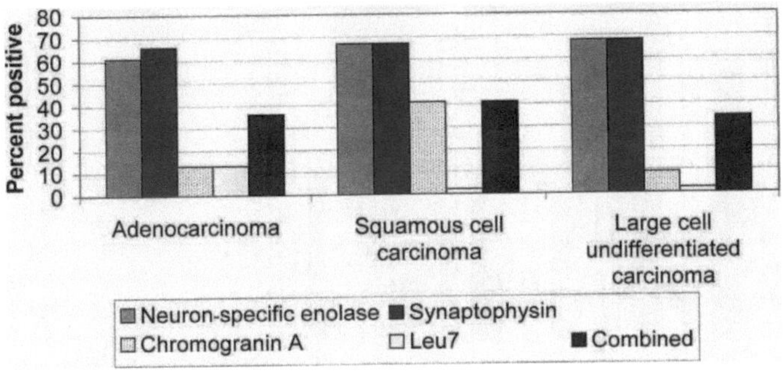

FIGURE 36.116. Immunohistogram showing summary of expression of neuroendocrine markers in histologically diagnosed nonneuroendocrine neoplasms.

seven of 11 large cell undifferentiated carcinomas showed immunostaining for neuron-specific enolase. Six of 10 squamous carcinomas, 16 of 26 adenocarcinomas, and seven of 11 large cell undifferentiated carcinomas showed immunostaining for synaptophysin. Overall, 34 of 47 (72%) carcinomas without neuroendocrine histologic features expressed at least one neuroendocrine immunohistochemical marker. Nineteen of 19 (100%) neuroendocrine carcinomas expressed at least one neuroendocrine marker.

Schleusener and Tazelaar[165] evaluated 107 patients with stage IIIA, stage IIIB, and stage IV NSCLCs (62 adenocarcinomas, 22 squamous cell carcinomas, 18 large cell carcinomas, five adenosquamous carcinomas) immunohistochemically with antibodies against keratin, synaptophysin, Leu7, and chromogranin A. Keratin was used as a control and was positive in 99.1% of cases. Thirty-five percent of adenocarcinomas, 41% of squamous cell carcinomas, and 33% of large cell carcinomas expressed at least one neuroendocrine marker. Somewhat surprising was the finding of increased survival in patients whose tumors expressed one or more neuroendocrine markers; however, there was no correlation between neuroendocrine markers and response to chemotherapy.

The bottom line for pathologists is that nonneuroendocrine lung neoplasms (adenocarcinoma, squamous cell carcinoma, and large cell undifferentiated carcinoma) may express neuroendocrine markers by immunohistochemistry. A summary of these studies showing the frequency of expression of chromogranin A, synaptophysin, neuron-specific enolase, and Leu7 is shown in Figure 36.116.

The question arises as to whether large cell undifferentiated lung carcinomas and poorly differentiated adenocarcinomas showing neuroendocrine features by immunohistochemistry should be classified as large cell neuroendocrine carcinomas. This is not an easy question to answer and perhaps some large cell undifferentiated carcinomas should be classified as large cell neuroendocrine carcinomas, especially if they showed the histologic features as outlined by Travis et al.[136] However, Travis et al. referred to such neoplasms as NSCLCs with neuroendocrine features, and indicated they represented 10% to 15% of NSCLCs but did not have the histologic/cytologic features of neuroendocrine neoplasms.

Immunohistochemical Features of Neuroendocrine Lung Cancers

The immunohistochemical features of neuroendocrine cells have been extensively illustrated in this chapter. Pulmonary neuroendocrine tumors and their immunohistochemical reactions are listed in Table 36.6 and shown in Figure 36.117. In general, neuroendocrine neoplasms that are better differentiated, such as typical carcinoids, show more intense immunostaining for the relatively specific neuroendocrine markers such as synaptophysin and chromogranin-A than the more poorly different-

TABLE 36.6. Immunohistochemical features of neuroendocrine lung neoplasms and nonneuroendocrine lung neoplasms

Type of neoplasm	AE1/AE3 keratin	CK5/6	CK7	CK8	CK20	Vimentin	p63	NSE	SYN	CGA	NCAM	TTF-1	CD117
Typical carcinoid	+	N	+/–	+	–/+	+/–	N	+	+	+	+	–/+	–/+
Atypical carcinoid	+	N	+/–	+	–/+	+/–	N	+	+	+	+	–/+	–/+
Large cell neuroendocrine carcinoma	+	–/+	+/–	+	–/+	–/+	N	+/–	+/–	+/–	+/–	+/–	–/+
Small cell lung carcinoma	+	R	+/–	+/–	–/+	–/+	N	+/–	+/–	+/–	+/–	+/–	+/–
Squamous carcinoma	+	+/–	–/+	–/+	R	–/+	+/–	R	R	R	R	R	N
Adenocarcinoma	+	–/+	+/–	+/–	–/+	–/+	N	–/+	–/+	–/+	–/+	–/+	N
Large cell undifferentiated carcinoma	+	–/+	+/–	+/–	–/+	–/+	N	–/+	–/+	–/+	–/+	–/+	N

Antigens tested: CK, cytokeratin; NSE, neuron-specific enolase; SYN, synaptophysin; CGA, chromogranin A; TTF-1, thyroid transcription factor-1.

Immunoreactivity results: +:,almost always positive; +/–, variable staining, mostly positive; –/+, variable staining, mostly negative; R, rare cells positive; N, almost always negative.

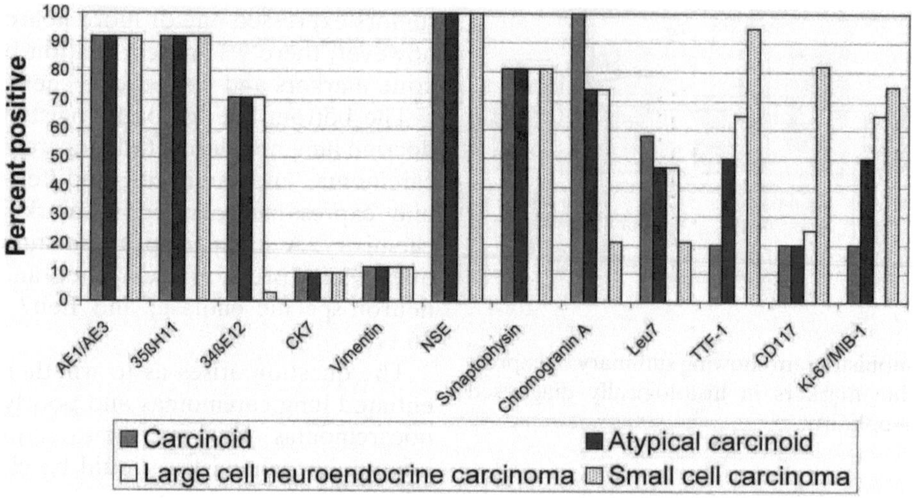

FIGURE 36.117. Immunohistogram of neuroendocrine lung carcinomas.

iated neuroendocrine carcinomas such as large cell neuroendocrine carcinoma and SCLC. More recent studies concerning the immunohistochemical features of neuroendocrine and nonneuroendocrine neoplasms are discussed below.

In 1998, Jiang et al.[166] reviewed 766 surgically resected lung cancers and were able to diagnose 22 (2.87%) neuroendocrine carcinomas subsequently confirmed by immunostaining for multiple neuroendocrine markers. Each tumor showed positive reactivity for at least three general neuroendocrine markers and 12 (54.5%) were positive for neuroendocrine hormones. Of interest, 18 had been initially classified as NSCLCs. Of the 22 cases, 21 (95.5%) expressed neuron-specific enolase, 12 (54.5%) expressed chromogranin-A, and 16 (72.7%) expressed NCAM. Of the various hormones, five (22.7%) expressed progastrin releasing peptide, 10 (45.5%) expressed calcitonin, eight (36.4%) expressed human chorionic gonadotropin, four (18.2%) expressed 5-hydroxytryptamine (5-HT; serotonin), nine (40.9%) expressed somatostatin, one (4.5%) expressed pancreatic polypeptide, five (22.7%) expressed ACTH, and four (18.2%) expressed calcitonin gene-related peptide. The authors concluded the most difficult factor in diagnosing large cell neuroendocrine carcinoma was the recognition of its light microscopic neuroendocrine features.

In 2000, Lyda and Weiss[167] immunostained 142 primary lung carcinomas for B72.3, 34ßE12 (cytokeratins 1, 5, 10, 14), cytokeratin 7, cytokeratin 17, synaptophysin, and chromogranin-A to determine the utility of the neuroendocrine markers and epithelial markers in diagnosing primary lung cancers. Among neuroendocrine carcinomas (small cell carcinoma and large cell neuroendocrine carcinoma), 84% (37 of 44) large cell and small cell neuroendocrine carcinomas expressed chromogranin-A; 58% (21 of 36) of small cell lung carcinomas and six of six large cell neuroendocrine carcinomas expressed synaptophysin; 5% (two of 43) expressed 34ßE12 keratin; 9% (four of 44) expressed CK7; and 5% (two of 37) of small cell carcinomas and 50% (three of six) of large cell neuroendocrine carcinomas were B72.3 positive. Among 98 nonneuroendocrine carcinomas, 5% (five of 98) were chromogranin-A positive; 3% (three of 98) were synaptophysin positive; 97% (95 of 98) were 34ßE12 or CK7 positive; and 99% (97 of 98) were either keratin, 34ßE12, CK7, or B72.3 positive. The authors concluded that an antibody panel consisting of CK7, 34ßE12, chromogranin-A, and synaptophysin separated 132 of the 141 (94%) of the primary lung cancers into two groups of nonneuroendocrine or neuroendocrine carcinomas, respectively (Table 36.7).

Agoff et al.[168] evaluated TTF-1 expression by immunohistochemistry in 49 gastrointestinal carcinoids, 15 pancreatic islet cell tumors, 21 paragangliomas, eight medullary thyroid carcinomas, extrapulmonary small cell carcinomas of the uterine cervix (seven cases), prostate (four cases), and bladder (four cases), six Merkel cell carcinomas, and one renal carcinoma. TTF-1 expression was not found in the gastrointestinal carcinoids, pancreatic islet cell tumors, paragangliomas, or Merkel cell carcinomas. All medullary thyroid carcinomas expressed TTF-1, and 44% of nonpulmonary small cell carcinomas, including four of four prostate, two of four bladder, and one of seven cervical small cell carcinomas expressed TTF-1. The authors concluded TTF-1 expression was not specific for small cell carcinomas of pulmonary origin and should not be used to distinguish primary from metastatic small cell carcinomas in extrapulmonary sites.

Cheuk et al.[169] evaluated TTF-1 and CK20 staining in small cell lung carcinomas and Merkel cell carcinomas. They found TTF-1 expression in 82.7% of pulmonary

TABLE 36.7. Immunoreactivity with 34BE12, keratin 7, chromogranin, and synaptophysin in lung carcinomas

Combinations*	Non–small-cell (n = 98)	Small cell (n = 37)	Large cell neuroendocrine (n = 6)
34BE12+/ANY CK7 or NE	64 (65%)	0	0
34BE12–/CK7+/NE–	27 (28%)	0	0
34BE12–/CK7–/NE+	0	30 (81%)	4
34BE12–/CK7+/NE+	3 (3%) Reactivity with chromogranin or synaptophysin ≥10% 0/3	2 (5%) Reactivity with chromogranin or synaptophysin ≥30% 2/2	2 Reactivity with chromogranin or synaptophysin ≥30% 2/2
34BE12–/CK7–/NE–	4 (4%) B72.3+ ¾	5 (14%) B72.3+ 1/5	0

*34BE12+, ≥10% cells +; CK7+, ≥30% cells + with keratin 7; NE+, ≥1% cells + with chromogranin or synaptophysin.
Source: Lyda and Weiss.[167] Copyright 2000, with permission from Elsevier.

small cell carcinomas, 42% of extrapulmonary small cell carcinomas, and 0% of Merkel cell carcinomas. Cytokeratin 20 was consistently negative in pulmonary small cell carcinomas and positive in only 4% of extrapulmonary small cell carcinomas, being expressed in 100% of Merkel cell carcinomas. The authors concluded immunostaining for TTF-1, especially when combined with immunostaining for CK20, could aid in the distinction between Merkel cell carcinoma and both pulmonary and extrapulmonary small cell carcinomas.

In 2002, Sturm et al.[50] evaluated 227 neuroendocrine proliferations and neoplasms for TTF-1 expression. Immunostaining was detected in 47 of 55 (85.5%) SCLCs, in 31 of 64 (48%) large cell neuroendocrine carcinomas, in 0 of 15 neuroendocrine hyperplasias, in 0 of 23 tumorlets, 0 of 27 typical carcinoids, and 0 of 23 atypical carcinoids. In 19 of 20 (95%) combined SCLCs and combined large cell neuroendocrine carcinomas, TTF-1 was expressed in neuroendocrine and nonneuroendocrine components of the tumor. The authors concluded that their findings challenged the concept of a spectrum of neuroendocrine neoplasms and suggested the findings lent credence to the alternative hypothesis of a common derivation for small cell lung carcinoma and NSCLC.

Chang et al.[170] evaluated TTF-1 expression in 510 primary lung cancers and 107 metastatic neoplasms. TTF-1 was detectable in four of 99 (4%) squamous cell carcinomas, 169 of 176 (96%) solitary adenocarcinomas, 34 of 34 (100%) of multifocal adenocarcinomas, one of one (100%) signet ring adenocarcinomas, 16 of 20 (80%) mucinous adenocarcinomas, 23 of 23 (100%) nonmucinous bronchioloalveolar cell carcinomas, 19 of 36 (53%) small cell carcinomas, and 39 of 44 (89%) sclerosing hemangiomas. TTF-1 was not expressed in eight typical carcinoids, three atypical carcinoids, 23 pleomorphic carcinomas, 25 lymphoepithelial-like carcinomas, the sarcomatous component of one pseudomesotheliomatous carcinoma or in one mesothelioma. In four combined small cell carcinomas and in 12 adenosquamous carcinomas, TTF-1 was expressed in the adenocarcinoma component. TTF-1 expression was absent in 125 patients with metastatic carcinomas other than lung carcinomas metastatic to cervical lymph nodes, brain, and bone.

Rossi et al.[171] evaluated TTF-1, CK7, 34ßE12 (high molecular weight keratin), and CD56/NCAM expression in 45 large cell carcinomas of the lung. The cases were stated to consist of neoplastic proliferations composed of large cells with abundant cytoplasm, vesicular nuclei, and prominent nucleoli. Twenty-seven of 45 (60%) were subclassified as adenocarcinomas, of which 24 of 27 expressed TTF-1 and CK7 while three of 27 showed expression of CK7 only. Ten of 45 (22%) that were classified as squamous cell carcinomas showed immunostaining only for 34ßE12. Four of 45 (9%) classified as large cell carcinomas with neuroendocrine differentiation showed CD56 expression, variable expression for TTF-1 and CK7, and no immunostaining for 34ßE12. Four neoplasms coexpressed CK7 and 34ßE12, and one neoplasm showed no immunostaining. The surgically resected tumors were stated to match exactly with the corresponding original biopsy specimen in 21 of 23 cases. CD56 expression was stated to be a reliable marker in confirming a diagnosis of large cell neuroendocrine carcinoma. The authors concluded that their proposed set of four commercially available markers could help subclassify large cell carcinomas, even in small biopsy material.

Somewhat along the same line, Zhang et al.[172] selected a panel of antibodies consisting of TTF-1, p63, high molecular weight keratin, and p16 (INK4A) that was highly effective in distinguishing between small cell lung carcinoma and poorly differentiated squamous cell carcinoma. The panel was also stated to facilitate the diagnosis of combined small cell and non–small-cell carcinomas (Table 36.8).

Saqi et al.[51] evaluated the usefulness of CDX2 and TTF-1 in differentiating gastrointestinal from pulmonary carcinoids. The vast majority of the gastrointestinal carcinoids expressed CDX2 and none of the 15 pulmonary carcinoids showed immunostaining for CDX2. Eight of

TABLE 36.8. Immunohistochemical reactivities of small cell carcinomas and poorly differentiated squamous cell carcinomas

	Negative	Low	Intermediate	High
Small cell carcinomas (n = 28)				
Thyroid transcription factor-1	2 (7.1%)	—	—	26 (92.9%)
p63	28 (100%)	—	—	—
High molecular weight keratin	28 (100%)	—	—	—
p16 (INK4A)	—	1 (3.6%)	—	27 (96.4%)
Poorly differentiated squamous cell carcinomas (n = 28)				
Thyroid transcription factor-1	27 (96.4%)	1 (3.6%)	—	—
p63	—	—	—	28 (100%)
High molecular weight keratin	—	—	—	28 (100%)
p16 (INK4A)	13 (46.4%)	6 (21.4%)	7 (25.0%)	2 (7.1%)

Source: Zhang et al.,[172] with permission from Modern Pathology/USCAP.

15 (53%) pulmonary carcinoids stained with TTF-1, but none of the gastrointestinal carcinoids expressed TTF-1. The authors concluded that CDX2 and TTF-1 had a high specificity for gastrointestinal and pulmonary carcinoids, respectively.

Butnor et al.[54] evaluated CD117 expression in a variety of pulmonary tumors, and found CD117 was expressed in 82% of 11 SCLCs and 25% of four large cell neuroendocrine carcinomas, but was not expressed in 22 squamous carcinomas, 23 adenocarcinomas, 11 typical pulmonary carcinoids, 19 pleural mesotheliomas, and six localized fibrous tumors of the pleura. With respect to neuroendocrine lung neoplasms, CD117 expression was seen only in high-grade neuroendocrine lung cancers, namely, SCLC and large cell neuroendocrine carcinoma.

In conclusion, most studies show that immunohistochemistry is a reliable methodology in distinguishing neuroendocrine from nonneuroendocrine neoplasms, although there is a certain degree of overlap, and one has to be careful in interpreting the staining results.

Genetic Studies (See Also Chapter 33)

Onuki et al.[173] evaluated 10 typical carcinoids, 11 atypical carcinoids, 18 large cell neuroendocrine lung carcinomas, and 20 small cell lung carcinomas for loss of heterozygosity (LOH) of 10 chromosomal regions frequently deleted in lung neoplasms and for mutations of *p53* and *ras* genes. A relatively high incidence of LOH at the *meni* gene was common in all neuroendocrine lung neoplasms. Except for *ras* gene mutations, the majority of the changes occurred in small and large cell carcinomas, and at a lower frequency in carcinoids. The incidence of LOH and *p53* gene abnormalities increased with increasing malignant features. There were different patterns of *p53* gene mutations between atypical carcinoids and high-grade neuroendocrine neoplasms.

Giard et al.[174] evaluated 36 lung cancer cell lines, 14 SCLCs and 22 NSCLCs using 399-fluorescent microsatellite markers from the ABI prism linkage mapping set on an ABI sequence genotyper. In lung cancer cell lines, at least 17 to 22 chromosomal regions with frequent allelic loss were involved, suggesting the same number of putative tumor suppressor genes were inactivated. Both SCLC and NSCLC frequently underwent different specific genetic alterations. Clusters of tumor suppressor genes were inactivated together. The authors stated that these data provided global estimates of the genetic changes leading to lung cancer and would be useful for the positional cloning of new tumor suppressor genes.

Hiroshima et al.[175] evaluated 22 patients with stage I large cell neuroendocrine carcinoma, 11 patients with SCLC and 12 patients with classic large cell carcinoma for genetic alterations with special emphasis on large cell neuroendocrine carcinoma. LOH at TP53 and 13q14 was observed in most patients, and LOH at D3S1295, D3S1234, and D5S407 was significantly higher in patients with large cell neuroendocrine carcinoma and SCLC than in patients with classic large cell carcinoma. LOH at D5S422 was more frequently found in patients with classic large cell carcinoma and SCLC than in patients with large cell neuroendocrine carcinoma. Expression of p16 protein was observed more frequently in SCLC than in classic large cell carcinoma and large cell neuroendocrine carcinoma. Hypermethylation of the *p16* gene was observed more frequently in large cell neuroendocrine carcinoma than in SCLC. Patients who had allelic losses at D3S1234 and D10S1686 had a worse prognosis compared to patients without allelic losses at these sites. The authors concluded that genetic alterations found in large cell neuroendocrine carcinoma were similar to those of SCLC, although allelic losses at 5q and abnormalities in the *p16* gene could differentiate large cell neuroendocrine carcinoma from SCLC.

Peng et al.[176] evaluated 16 cases of large cell neuroendocrine carcinomas based on expression of at least one of three neuroendocrine markers (chromogranin-A, synaptophysin, and neural cell adhesion molecules) and nine cases diagnosed as large cell carcinomas with neuroendocrine morphology. These nine cases had been previously diagnosed as large cell carcinoma (five cases), poorly differentiated squamous cell carcinoma (three cases), and adenocarcinoma (one case). These 25 cases were evaluated immunohistochemically for 34ßE12, keratin L1, vimentin, TTF-1, surfactant protein A, carcinoembryonic antigen, and FHIT, and for cell cycle regulator proteins p16, RB, p53, p21, cyclin D1, and 14-3-3 sigma. LOH was evaluated on the 3p arm of three microsatellite polymorphic markers: 3p14.2, 3p21.3, and 3p25. RB expression and simultaneous overexpression of p16 was characteristic of large cell neuroendocrine carcinoma but not large cell carcinoma with neuroendocrine morphology. In G_2/M cell cycle regulation, 14-3-3 sigma was markedly reduced in large cell neuroendocrine carcinoma. The authors concluded large cell neuroendocrine carcinoma was similar to SCLC but different from large cell carcinoma with neuroendocrine morphology. However, LOH analysis using microsatellite markers showed a high frequency of LOH at 3p in large cell neuroendocrine carcinoma, large cell carcinoma with neuroendocrine morphology, and SCLC. The authors also concluded that morphologic neuroendocrine differentiation might not be identical to biologic differentiation in large cell carcinomas of lung.

Approach to the Diagnosis of Neuroendocrine Lung Neoplasms: Variabilities and Pitfalls

With the publication of criteria for diagnosing neuroendocrine lung cancers,[93,94] there is more agreement in making a diagnosis of a specific neuroendocrine tumor. However, problems exist, especially in diagnosing atypical carcinoids, large cell neuroendocrine carcinomas, and SCLCs. Some of this disagreement has to do with perception of size and shapes of cells. As perhaps best exemplified when classifying non-Hodgkin's malignant lymphoma, there is often considerable variation in opinion among trained, experienced pathologists as to what is a large cell and what is a small cell. With respect to lung neoplasms, this is best illustrated by a case report published several years ago.[177] The case concerned a 47-year-old man with a 4-cm mass in the hilum of the left lung, a 1.5-cm nodule at the left heart border, and right inguinal and axillary masses. The right axillary mass was biopsied and was diagnosed as showing metastatic large cell undifferentiated carcinoma. The patient was treated with lomustine at 130 mg/m^2 in 6-week cycles for 2 years. His tumor completely disappeared and he was free of disease 4 years after diagnosis and treatment.

Several weeks after this article appeared in publication, a letter to the editor of the journal in which the report appeared raised concern that the neoplasm reported as a metastatic large cell undifferentiated carcinoma was a malignant lymphoma, probably a diffuse histiocytic lymphoma.[178] Dr. Gerald Vosika,[179] the author of the report, sent the slides of the biopsied tumor to three experts who offered their opinions as to the correct histologic diagnosis of the tumor. Dr. Mary Matthews opined that the neoplasm was a small cell undifferentiated carcinoma, intermediate cell type. Dr. Raymond Yesner stated: "The overall impression is that of an intermediate small cell carcinoma which is showing some large cell characteristic—i.e., 22/40"; 22 refers to intermediate small undifferentiated carcinoma, and 40 to large cell undifferentiated carcinoma. Dr. Juan Rosai stated: "It is a very undifferentiated tumor, and the differential diagnosis is between oat cell carcinoma and large cell undifferentiated carcinoma. Although I admit there is room for disagreement, I definitely favor the diagnosis of oat cell carcinoma because of the architectural pattern and nuclear shape."

In my opinion, this case report strongly suggests that even among experienced pathologists, the size of neoplastic cells is to a certain extent in the eyes of the beholder, which can cause problems in classification of lung neoplasms, especially neuroendocrine lung neoplasms. In the nine cases we published in 1989 concerning neuroendocrine lung neoplasms,[130] a considerable difference of opinion occurred in classification, even with knowledge of the ultrastructural and immunohistochemical features of the tumor cells.

Marchevsky et al.[180] evaluated 5-µm-thick H&E-stained sections from 28 surgically resected high-grade pulmonary neuroendocrine carcinomas, including 16 SCLCs and 12 large cell neuroendocrine carcinomas. Morphometry demonstrated considerable nuclear size overlap in the high-grade neoplasms. Approximately one third of SCLCs exhibited considerable numbers of neoplastic cells that were larger than three normal lymphocytes, and four of 12 large cell neuroendocrine carcinomas had a predominant number of small cells. The authors concluded that the rule that the large cell-lymphocyte size ratio greater than 3 helped distinguish large from small cell neoplastic cells was confirmed in only nine of 28 cases. Based on their studies, the authors suggested the use of more generic terminology such as "high grade neuroendocrine carcinoma" or "grade 3 neuroendocrine carcinoma" for SCLC and large cell neuroendocrine carcinoma.

Travis et al.[181] attempted to validate the current classification of neuroendocrine lung tumors (typical carci-

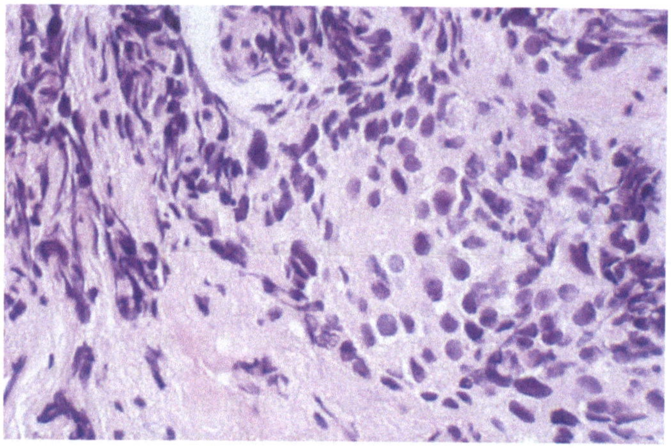

FIGURE 36.118. Carcinoid tumor simulating small cell lung carcinoma on transbronchial biopsy. This transbronchial biopsy specimen showed an infiltrate of small cells that showed mild crush artifact.

noid, atypical carcinoid, large cell neuroendocrine carcinoma, and SCLC). The authors studied 40 neuroendocrine tumors retrieved from the AFIP files, independently evaluated by five lung pathologists, and classified as one of the four entities. The participants were provided with a set of tables summarizing the criteria for differentiating the four major categories. A consensus diagnosis was achieved in 40 cases (100%), a majority agreement in 31 of 40 cases (78%), and a unanimous agreement in 22 of 40 cases (55%). Unanimous agreement occurred in seven small cell carcinomas (70%), seven typical carcinoids (58%), four atypical carcinoids (50%), and four large cell neuroendocrine carcinomas (40%). Majority diagnosis was achieved in 11 of 12 (92%) typical carcinoids, nine of 10 (90%) small cell carcinomas, six of eight (75%) atypical carcinoids, and five of 10 (50%) large cell neuroendocrine carcinomas. The authors concluded the classification of neuroendocrine lung tumors was most reproducible for typical carcinoids and SCLCs, but less reproducible for atypical carcinoids and large cell neuroendocrine carcinomas. The authors stated the results indicated a need for more careful definition and application of criteria for typical carcinoids vs. atypical carcinoids and small cell carcinoma vs. large cell neuroendocrine carcinoma.

Along the same lines as Marchevsky et al.,[180] Lin et al.[182] used the proliferation marker MIB-1 to determine low-grade versus high-grade neuroendocrine carcinomas. The authors found that all low-grade neuroendocrine lung neoplasms showed MIB-1 immunoreactivity in less than 25% of the neoplastic cells in contrast to high-grade neuroendocrine neoplasms that showed MIB-1 immunoreactivity in greater than 50% of the neoplastic cells.

Pelosi et al.[183] studied bronchial biopsies from seven patients with typical or atypical carcinoid tumors that had been overdiagnosed as small cell carcinomas by bronchial biopsy evaluation. Bronchial biopsies from nine consecutive SCLCs were used as control cases for histologic and immunohistochemical evaluation using cytokeratins, chromogranin A, synaptophysin, Ki-67, and TTF-1. Typical carcinoid tumors presented as either central or peripheral lesions composed of cells with granular, sometimes coarse chromatin pattern, high levels of chromogranin-A/synaptophysin immunoreactivity, and low (less than 20%) Ki-67 labeling index. The tumor stroma contained thin-walled blood vessels. Small cell carcinomas showed central tumor location, finely dispersed nuclear chromatin, lower levels of chromogranin-A/synaptophysin, and high (greater than 50%) Ki-67 labeling index. The stroma contained thick-walled blood vessels with glomeruloid configuration. The authors concluded, judging from their study, that there was an overdiagnosis of typical lung carcinoid neoplasms as small cell carcinomas in small crushed bronchial biopsy specimens. This was stated to be a significant worldwide problem. Pelosi et al. stated that careful evaluation of H&E-stained sections remained the most important tool for the differential diagnosis, with the evaluation of the tumor cell proliferative index as the most useful ancillary technique.

I saw three such cases in 2005. The first was of a 70-year-old man who was diagnosed as having a small cell carcinoma on bronchial biopsy (Fig. 36.118). The tumor cells were fairly uniform and showed some crush artifact and distortion, but in the best preserved areas did not show any significant mitotic activity. Immunohistochemical staining showed intense staining for chromogranin A (Fig. 36.119) and synaptophysin (Fig. 36.120), and showed no immunostaining for TTF-1. The Ki-67 analysis showed

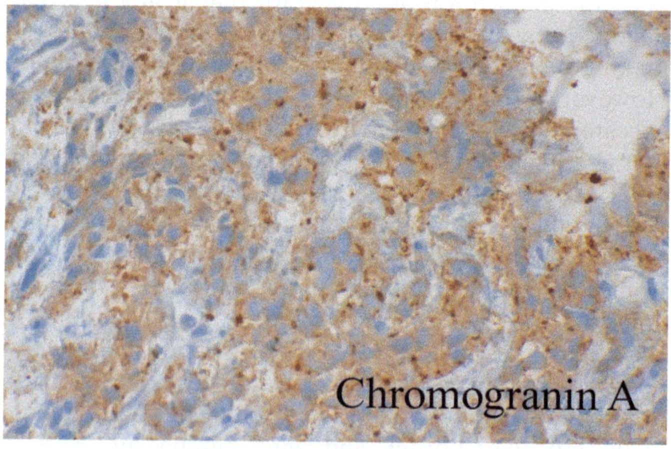

FIGURE 36.119. The neoplastic cells shown in Figure 36.118 display intense cytoplasmic immunostaining for chromogranin A.

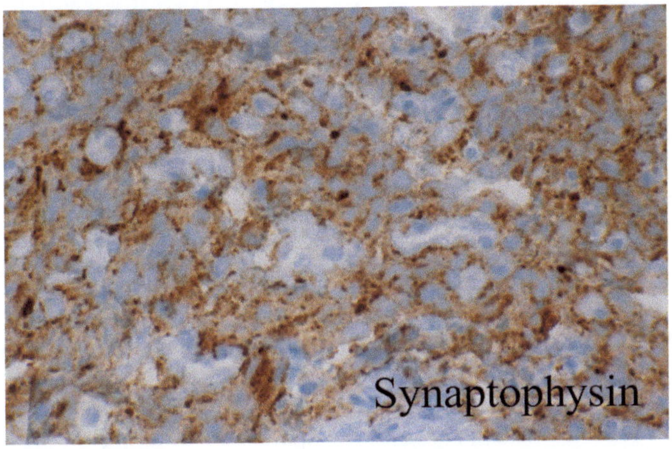

FIGURE 36.120. The neoplastic cells shown in Figure 36.118 display intense cytoplasmic immunostaining for synaptophysin.

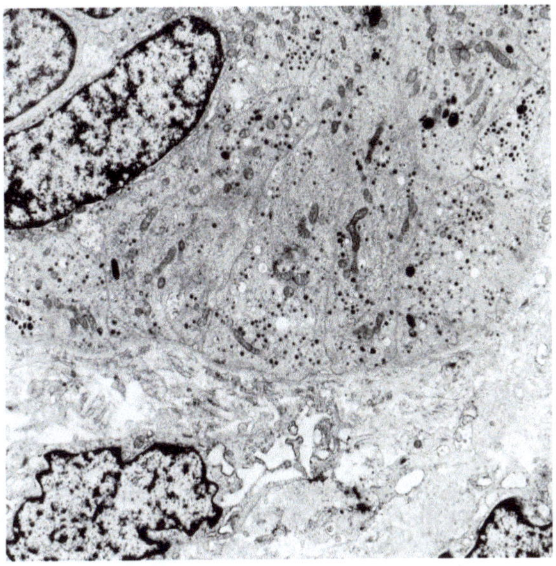

FIGURE 36.122. Ultrastructurally, the neoplastic cells contained numerous dense-core neuroendocrine granules, the expected finding in typical carcinoids. ×4500.

a proliferative index of less than approximately 15% (Fig. 36.121), which strongly indicated the diagnosis of a typical carcinoid. When examined by electron microscopy, the tumor cells contained numerous dense core granules (Fig. 36.122). In my opinion the intensity of the chromogranin A and synaptophysin reaction and lack of staining for TTF-1 are additional factors that can help prevent this misdiagnosis.

Differential Diagnosis

In today's medical environment, a greater number of less invasive procedures are being done, and the pathologist is faced with making accurate diagnoses on smaller tissue samples. As discussed, it is often helpful to have tissue available for immunohistochemical and ultrastructural examination. In my experience this has been most useful in evaluating transbronchial biopsy specimens, fine-needle aspiration biopsy specimens, and malignant cells in pleural fluid.

Lymphoma

Figure 36.123 shows a transbronchial biopsy composed of bronchial mucosa with an infiltrate of small cells in the lamina propria. When immunostained for low molecular

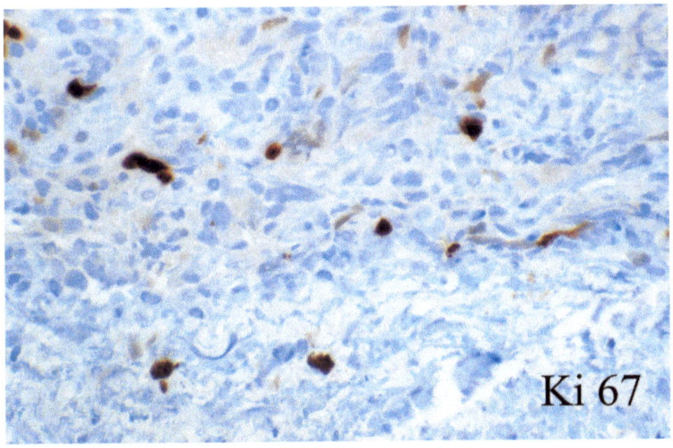

FIGURE 36.121. The neoplastic cells shown in Figure 36.118 show a low proliferative index of about 15% when stained for Ki-67.

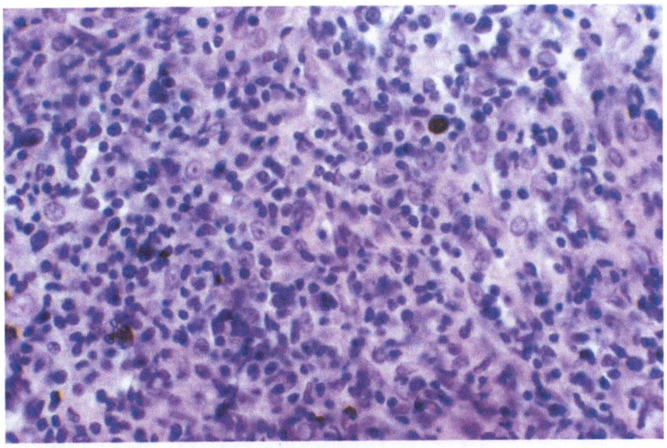

FIGURE 36.123. Small lymphocytic lymphoma simulating small cell lung carcinoma on transbronchial biopsy. This transbronchial biopsy specimen shows an infiltrate of relatively uniform small cells with a low mitotic rate.

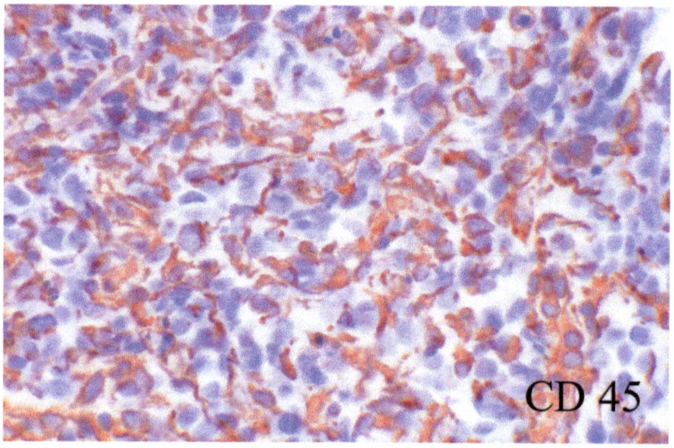

FIGURE 36.124. The small cells show moderately intense cytoplasmic immunostaining for CD45 (leukocyte common antigen), strongly suggesting the diagnosis of a B-cell small lymphocytic lymphoma/leukemia.

weight cytokeratin, the tumor cells showed no immunostaining, but were intensely positive for leukocyte common antigen (Fig. 36.124) and CD20 (Fig. 36.125), strongly suggesting the diagnosis of a B-cell lymphoma (see Chapter 32).

Small Cell Squamous Carcinoma

Another small cell lung neoplasm that can be confused with SCLC is small cell squamous carcinoma (Fig. 36.126), which characteristically immunostains for CK5/6 (Fig. 36.127), high molecular weight keratin (34ßE12) (Fig. 36.128), and p63 (Fig. 36.129). The neoplastic cells usually show no immunostaining for TTF-1 (see also Fig. 35.33 in Chapter 35).

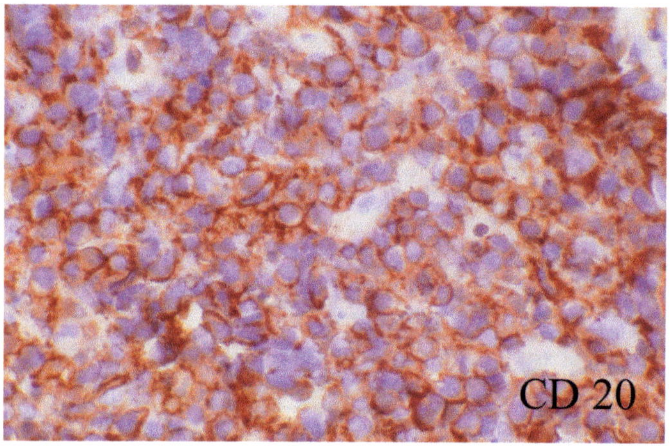

FIGURE 36.125. The small cells show moderately intense cytoplasmic immunostaining for CD20 (B-cell antigen), also strongly suggesting the diagnosis of a B-cell small lymphocytic lymphoma/leukemia.

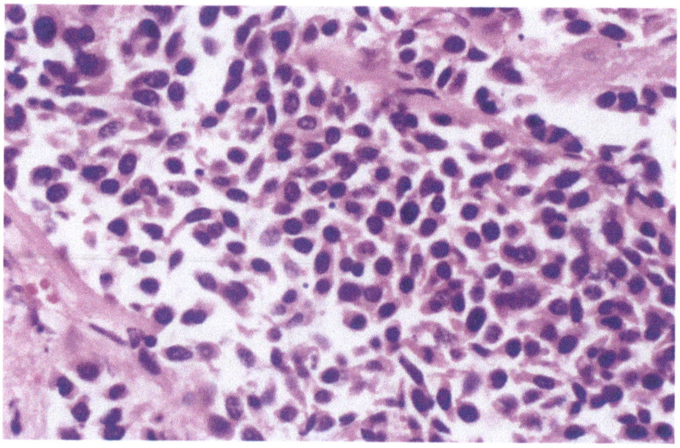

FIGURE 36.126. Small cell squamous carcinoma. This neoplasm is composed of small cells that resemble neoplastic neuroendocrine cells.

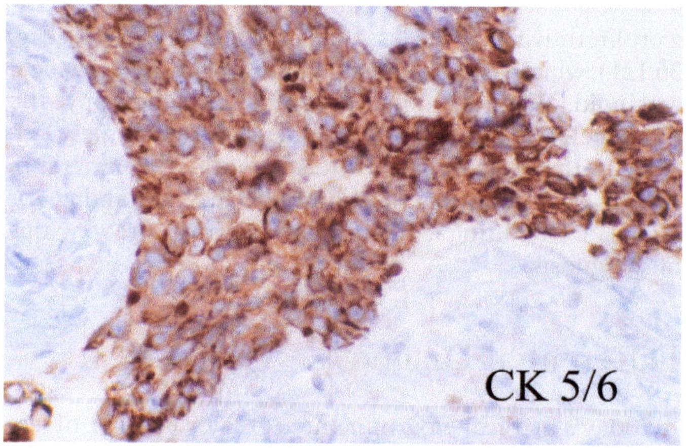

FIGURE 36.127. The neoplasm in Figure 36.126 shows immunostaining for CK5/6.

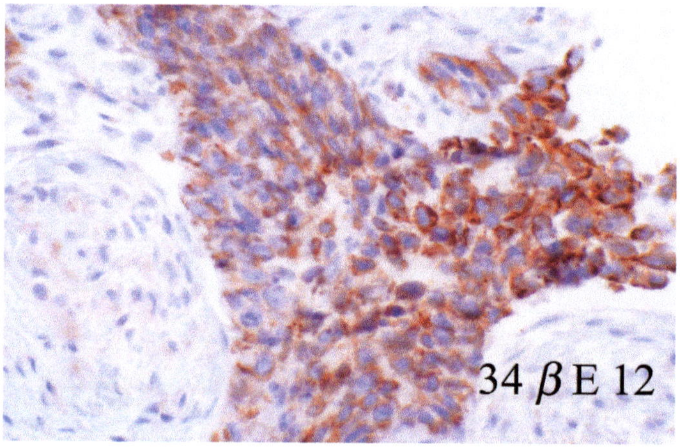

FIGURE 36.128. The neoplasm in Figure 36.126 shows cytoplasmic immunostaining for 34βE12 (high molecular weight keratin).

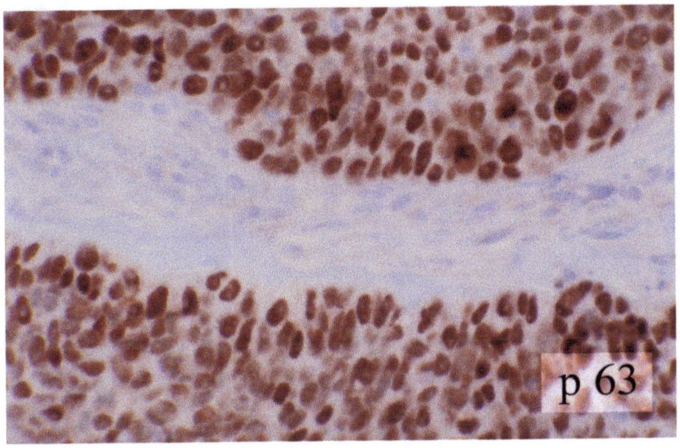

FIGURE 36.129. The neoplasm in Figure 36.126 shows immunostaining for p63.

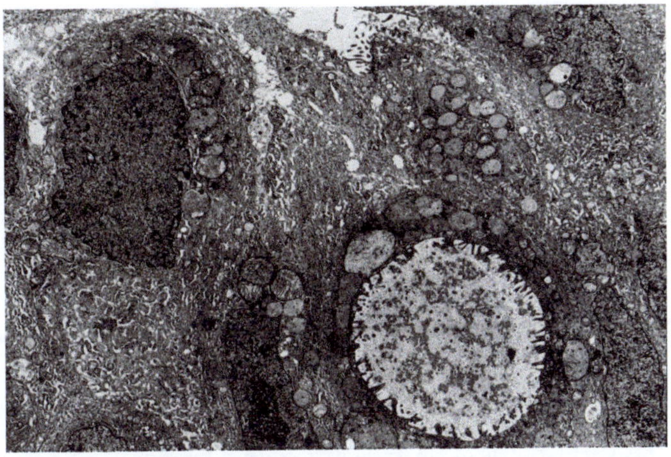

FIGURE 36.131. The neoplasm in Figure 36.130 shows glandular differentiation when examined ultrastructurally. ×4500.

Small Cell Adenocarcinoma

Small cell adenocarcinomas (Fig. 36.130) can also be confused with SCLC. Both can express TTF-1 and carcinoembryonic antigen. Ultrastructurally, the adenocarcinomas show glandular differentiation (Fig. 36.131).

Basaloid Carcinoma

Another small cell neoplasm that can be confused with SCLC is basaloid carcinoma. Basaloid carcinoma has been described in detail by Brambilla et al.[184] Basaloid carcinomas frequently show neuroendocrine features such as an organoid, trabecular, or rosette growth pattern (Fig. 36.132A) and are frequently composed of small cells (Fig. 36.132B) that can be confused with neuroendocrine cells. They usually do not express neuroendocrine markers, although rarely can express NCAM and chromogranin A. They typically show peripheral palisading (Fig. 36.132C) and a high mitotic rate (Fig. 36.132D) (see also Fig. 35.59 in Chapter 35).

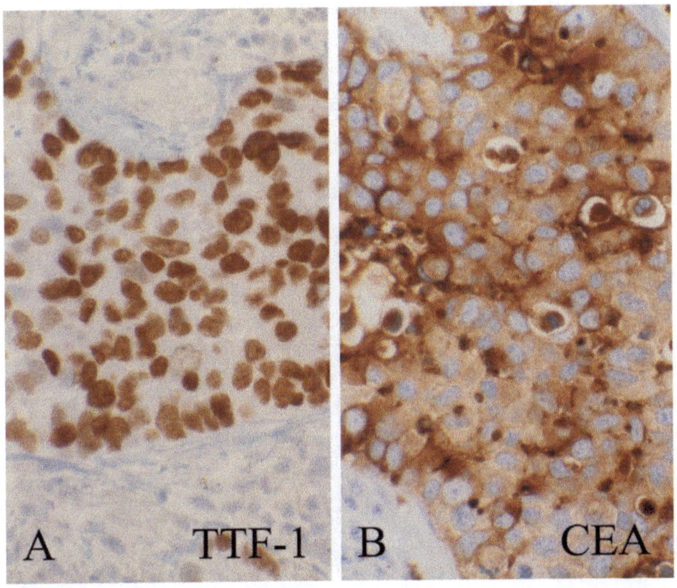

FIGURE 36.130. Small cell adenocarcinoma. This small cell neoplasm shows immunostaining for TTF-1 **(A)** and CEA **(B)**.

Pleural Neoplasms

Rarely, neuroendocrine lung neoplasms present as pleural neoplasms. VanHengel et al.[185] described a 73-year-old man who at autopsy had an atypical carcinoid that showed diffuse pleural spread suggestive of a pleural mesothelioma.

Falconieri et al.[186] described four cases of SCLC in male cigarette smokers that presented like pleural mesotheliomas. The authors stated SCLC should be added to the group of pseudomesotheliomatous lung cancer.

My group has submitted for publication a large series of pseudomesotheliomatous lung neoplasms that included three cases of SCLC[187] (see Chapter 27). One must also remember that there is a small cell mesothelioma that can be confused with SCLC (Figs. 36.133A and 36.133B), and that mesotheliomas occasionally express neuroendocrine markers by immunohistochemistry (see Chapter 43).[188]

Metastatic Carcinoma

Metastatic carcinoma should always be considered in the differential diagnosis of any lung cancer. As previously indicated, most common primary lung tumors occur as

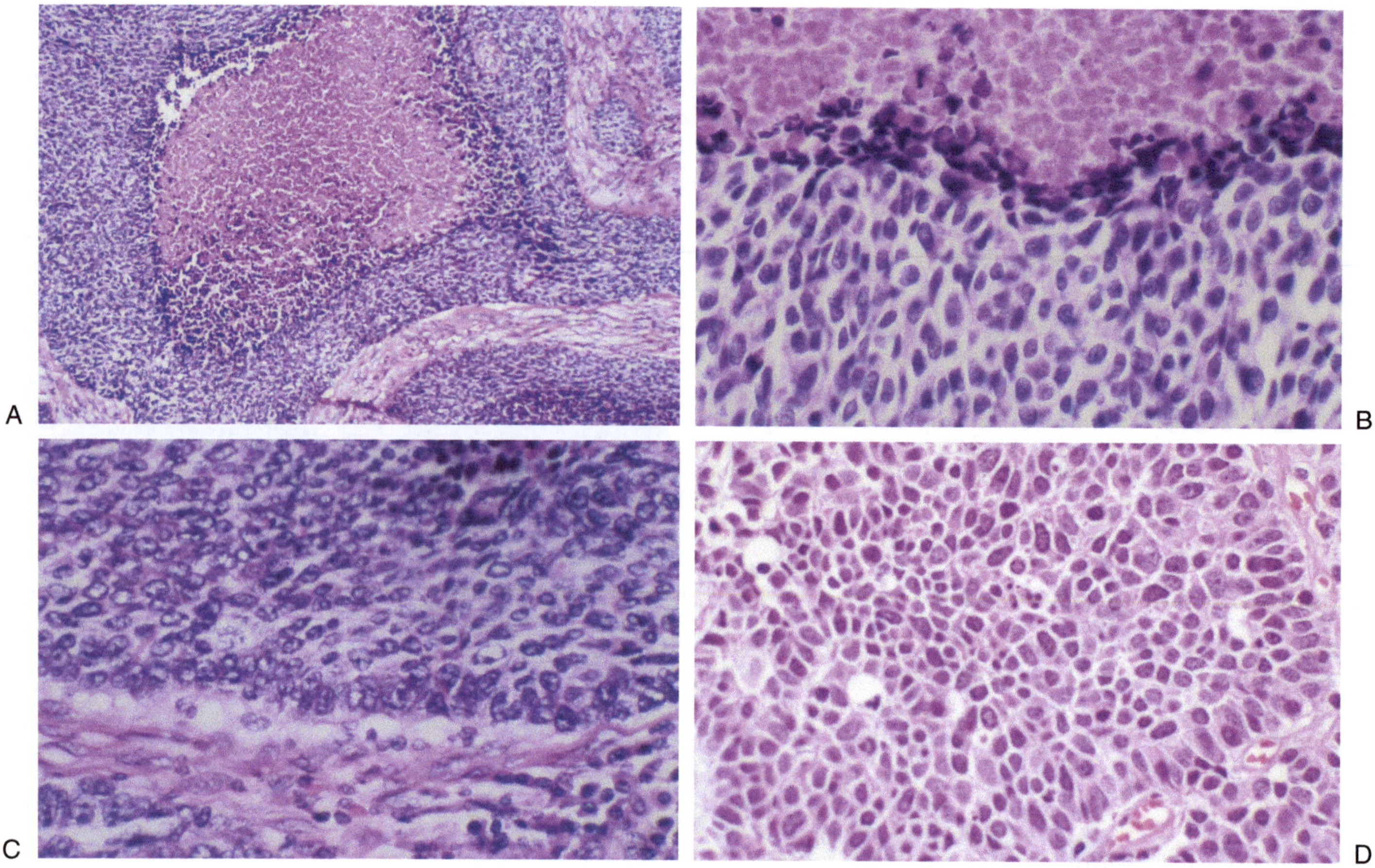

FIGURE 36.132. **(A–D)** This basaloid carcinoma has low magnification features of a neuroendocrine carcinoma. Most basaloid carcinomas are composed of small cells that can be confused with neoplastic neuroendocrine cells. Many basaloid carcinomas show palisading of the peripheral cell layer. Most basaloid carcinomas show a high mitotic rate.

single masses in the lung with the exception of some bronchioloalveolar cell carcinomas and epithelioid hemangioendotheliomas (see Chapter 44). In small specimens, it may be impossible to distinguish between primary and metastatic tumors. The role of immunohistochemistry in discriminating metastatic Merkel cell carcinoma from neuroendocrine lung tumors has been previously discussed and is also considered in Chapter 44.

In summary, neuroendocrine lung neoplasms are morphologically diverse. They can be approached in a logical

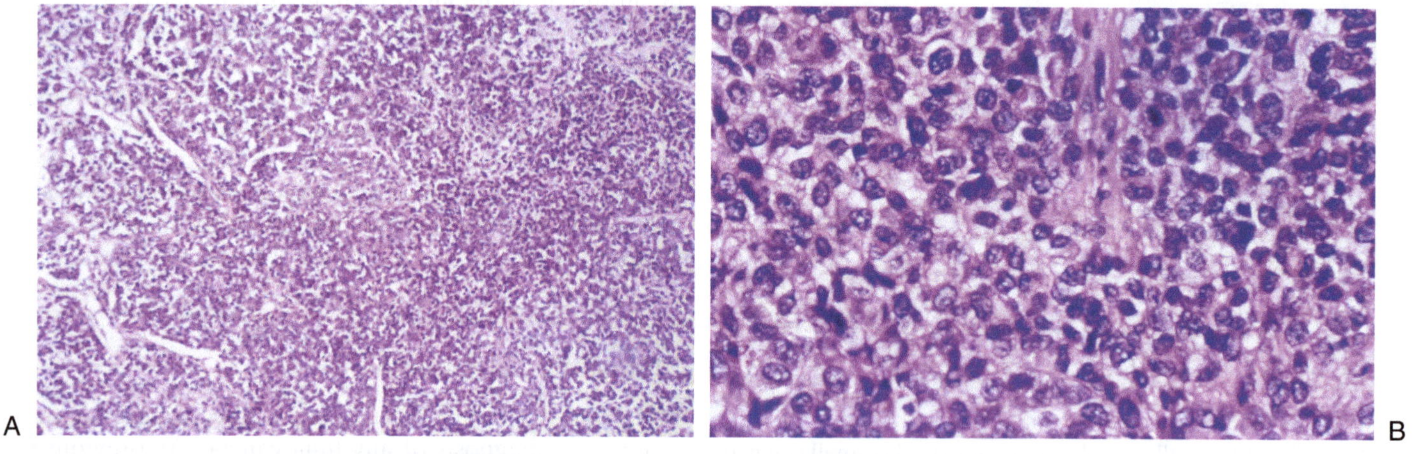

FIGURE 36.133. **(A,B)** Small cell pleural mesotheliomas can be confused with small cell lung cancer.

manner if considered in the differential diagnosis. Most typical carcinoids are diagnosed with ease. Atypical carcinoids are not infrequently misdiagnosed as small cell or large cell neuroendocrine carcinomas. Attention to the precise criteria for diagnosing neuroendocrine lung neoplasms and the use of immunohistochemistry (including Ki-67-MIB) and electron microscopy as adjuvant techniques assist in making a specific diagnosis.

Precise classification of high-grade neuroendocrine carcinomas (SCLC, large cell neuroendocrine carcinoma) is important because of the potential differences in treatment between them and NSCLCs.

Clinicopathologic Correlations

Patients with lung cancer usually present with nonspecific symptoms and signs. Chute et al.[189] studied the presenting symptoms of 1539 lung cancer patients according to their cell type and stage. They found the most common presenting symptoms were weight loss (46% of patients), cough (45%), dyspnea (37%), weakness (34%), chest pain (27%), and hemoptysis (27%). They found the presence of symptoms was directly related to the stage of the disease, with patients having a more advanced stage being more likely to have symptoms. They found no relationship between symptomatology and the histologic type of lung cancer.

Patients with primary lung cancer can present with a variety of extrathoracic signs and symptoms.[190] Many of the neurologic and metabolic manifestations of lung cancer are caused by neuroendocrine lung neoplasms. As reviewed by Yesner,[55] neuroendocrine lung tumors and occasionally nonneuroendocrine lung neoplasms produce ectopic hormones. Squamous cell carcinoma, for example, frequently produces a parathyroid hormone–like substance that may cause hypercalcemia. Some lung carcinomas, especially large cell undifferentiated carcinoma, produce human chorionic gonadotropin, which can be demonstrated biochemically in the patient's serum and immunohistochemically in the tumor cells.

Lung carcinomas may present as metastatic disease, with the brain, bone, and liver being frequent sites for metastatic lung cancers. It is not uncommon for patients with lung cancer to present with primary signs and symptoms referable to metastases in these organs, such as a patient presenting with liver failure resulting from extensive metastatic small cell undifferentiated carcinoma in the liver.

Prognosis

The biologic behavior of the neuroendocrine tumors of the lung is somewhat variable. An overview of the clinicopathologic features of neuroendocrine tumors of the lung is shown in Table 36.3. The most important factor in predicting the outcome of a patient with a malignant common lung neoplasm is the stage of the tumor.[191,192] Even in small cell neuroendocrine carcinoma of the lung, the stage of the disease is the most important factor in predicting survival.[193]

Typical and Atypical Carcinoids

Typical bronchopulmonary carcinoids generally occur in a younger age group than atypical carcinoids, small cell neuroendocrine carcinomas, or large cell neuroendocrine carcinomas. Approximately 5% to 10% of bronchial carcinoids metastasize to regional lymph nodes.[194–196] Five-year survival rates in patients with bronchial carcinoids are between 90% and 95%.[194,195] Even the presence of lymph node metastases does not necessarily imply a bad prognosis, although McCaughan et al.[196] found that disease-free survival at 5 and 10 years in 19 patients who had regional lymph node metastases was 74% and 53%, respectively, compared to 96% and 84%, respectively, in those patients with bronchopulmonary carcinoid tumors who did not have lymph node metastases. Lymphatic invasion in typical carcinoids can be dramatic (Fig. 36.134) with accompanying lymph node metastases (Fig. 36.135).

Thunnissen et al.[197] found that nodal metastases in typical bronchopulmonary carcinoids were directly related to tumor size and mean nuclear area of the neoplastic cells. The mean diameter of bronchopulmonary carcinoids that did not metastasize was 1.9 cm (standard deviation, 1.1 cm), versus 4.7 cm (standard deviation, 2.0 cm) in those that did metastasize. The mean nuclear area in the nonmetastasizing carcinoids was 34.7 μm^2 (standard deviation, 9.8 μm^2) versus 38.2 μm^2 (standard deviation, 7.7 μm^2) in the metastasizing carcinoids.

Warren and Gould[198] reported the long-term follow-up of 27 typical bronchial carcinoids for at least 10 years after curative resection. They found lymph node metastases in two patients at the time of surgery. Distant metastases were found in two patients at 5 and 10 years after surgery. Bone metastases involving the humerus were observed in both patients. Both patients were treated with radiotherapy and chemotherapy in one. One patient died of an unrelated cause 10 years after surgery and the other patient was alive 19 years after surgery. The demonstration of ACTH and related opiopeptides was not associated with a more aggressive course and was not associated with nodal metastases. Warren and Gould concluded that long-term survival was the rule even in cases of typical carcinoids with distant metastases.

In their study of 35 spindle cell carcinoid tumors of the lung, Ranchod and Levine[111] found lymph node metastases in seven patients (in two cases the metastases were observed only microscopically) and bony metastases in

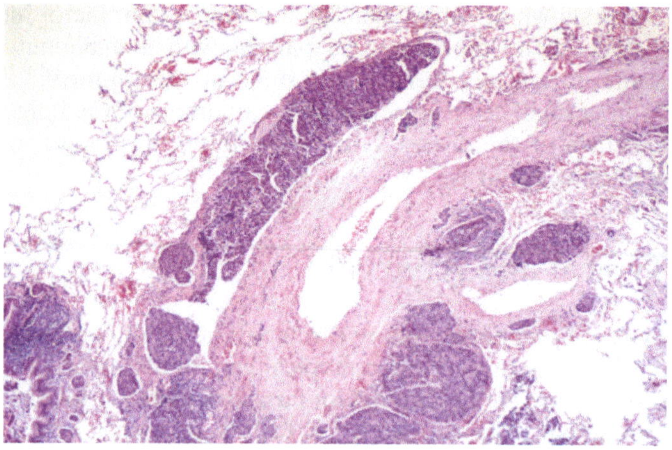

FIGURE 36.134. This typical carcinoid showed extensive lymphatic invasion.

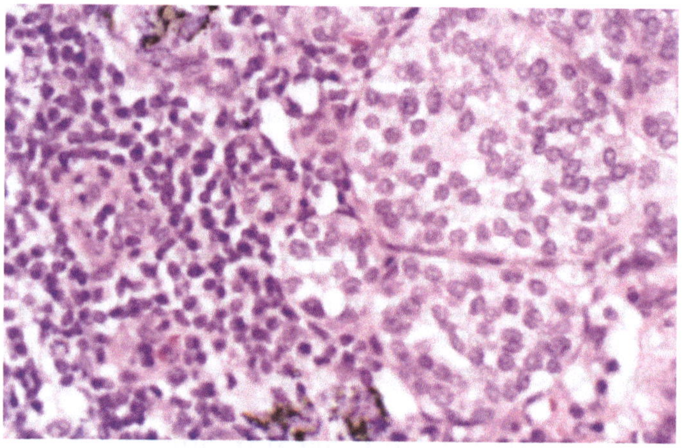

FIGURE 36.135. The typical carcinoid shown in Figure 36.134 showed extensive lymphatic invasion and lymph node metastases in the subcortical sinuses.

one patient. Follow-up information was available in 22 of 35 patients for 1 to 13 years, and no other sites of metastases were observed. None of the 22 patients followed died of their tumors.

Of the 35 neuroendocrine neoplasms reported by Travis et al.,[136] 20 were typical carcinoids. The patients with typical carcinoids had a mean age of 46.4 years and a median age of 46 years. Thirteen of the 20 typical carcinoids were associated with Cushing syndrome, and hilar lymph node metastases were identified in four cases. Of the 20 patients, death occurred in a patient with ACTH production by the tumor because of a cardiac arrhythmia in the immediate postoperative period. The remaining 19 patients were alive with a mean follow-up of 2.16 years (range, 0.33–13 years).

In their clinicopathologic analysis of 52 patients with typical carcinoid tumors of lung, Abdi et a1.[108] reported that 11 were located peripherally in the lung. The mean age of the patients with peripheral carcinoid tumors was 60.2 years, and nine of 10 patients were female. The mean tumor size of the peripheral carcinoids was 2.39 cm (range, 1.0–5.0 cm), and there were regional lymph node metastases in three of 11 cases. Except for cases of peripheral carcinoid tumors diagnosed incidentally at autopsy, all patients were alive and disease-free 1 to 6 years after surgery.

El-Naggar et al.[199] performed a clinicopathologic and flow cytometric evaluation of 33 typical carcinoids and 14 atypical carcinoids. The mean age of the patients with typical carcinoids was 52.3 years. Of the 33 typical carcinoids, 32 were centrally located and one was peripheral. Lymph node metastases occurred in three cases. Twenty-six of the typical carcinoids were less than 3 cm in diameter and seven were greater than 3 cm in diameter. Only one patient with a histologically diagnosed typical carcinoid, showing diploid DNA and a proliferative index of 5.0%, died of disease.

In the Yousem and Taylor[200] clinicopathologic and DNA analysis of 12 typical carcinoids and seven atypical carcinoids, 11 patients with typical carcinoids were alive with no evidence of disease between 1 and 46 months after diagnosis (one patient was lost to follow-up).

Bernstein et al.[201] described a case of typical bronchial carcinoid originating in the right-mainstem bronchus of a 35-year-old nonsmoking woman. The right lung was resected and the bronchial margin of resection showed no evidence of tumor and no metastases were noted in the hilar lymph nodes. The patient presented 18 years later with superior vena cava obstruction and carcinoid syndrome from a recurrence of the tumor. She was treated with radiotherapy and had a dramatic response, with resolution of her symptoms from superior vena caval obstruction and a drop in her 5-hydroxy indole acetic acid (HIAA) to normal levels.

Greengard et al.[202] evaluated 10 pulmonary carcinoid tumors for a variety of enzymes to determine the growth rate of these neoplasms. Uridine kinase to thymidine ratios were five times higher in typical carcinoids than in pulmonary carcinomas, and the concentration of α-glutamyl transpeptidase was lower in the 10 pulmonary carcinoids than in 35 pulmonary adenocarcinomas and 11 squamous carcinomas. Thymidine kinase, which bears a quantitative inverse correlation to volume doubling time, was present in lower titers in nine typical carcinoids than in six small cell carcinomas of lung. The authors concluded that because of relatively long doubling times, most typical carcinoids required a longer time (40.5 years) to reach a clinically detectable size than did carcinomas (17.8 years). The data also suggested that typical carcinoids had a prenatal or early childhood inception.

Vadasz et al.[203] evaluated 120 patients who were surgically treated for typical carcinoid tumors between 1976 and 1986. The authors found that atypia, tumor size, localization, history, and regional lymph node metastases failed to give clear information for prognosis. The authors stated that carcinoid and small cell carcinomas could be differentiated by immunostaining for chromogranin and by flow cytometry, but none of these methods was suitable for differential diagnosis within the typical carcinoid group. Resection by thoracotomy was stated to be the only treatment of choice and provided an excellent result with a 5-year survival rate of 90% and a low hospital mortality rate of 0.8%. The authors stated that parenchyma-sparing resections were to be encouraged. In their study, 67 typical carcinoids had a central location and 16 were larger than 3 cm in diameter. In 61 patients, distal parenchymal destruction was observed due to chronic obstruction. Two carcinoids were stated to have been located in the anterior mediastinum. Seven patients had hilar lymph node metastases but none of the 120 patients had distant metastases at the time of surgery. With flow cytometry, 88% (21 of 24) showed euploidy and there was no connection between ploidy and the oncopathologic criteria. Nineteen of 20 SCLCs displayed aneuploidy. The authors suggested the aneuploid, "very" atypical carcinoids with rapid fatal prognosis referred to in some articles may not represent real carcinoids but other neuroendocrine tumors such as SCLC.

Ducrocq et al.[204] evaluated 139 consecutive patients between 1976 and 1996 who underwent thoracotomy for typical bronchopulmonary carcinoid tumors. The tumors were stated to have been located centrally in 102 of 139 cases (73.4%). Staging was pT1 in 107 patients (77.0%) and pT2 in 32 (23.0%). Thirteen patients (9.4%) had nodal metastases. Seventeen patients (12.2%) were stated to have died during follow-up, but only three deaths were related to disease. The overall survival rate at 5, 10, and 15 years was stated to be 92.4%, 88.3%, and 76.4%, respectively. Estimated disease-free survival was 100% at 5 years and 91.4% at 10 and 15 years. The estimated survival of patients with lymph node metastases was stated to be 100% at 5, 10, and 15 years. Univariate analysis failed to demonstrate any prognostic significance for sex, tumor size, tumor location, and type of resection. The authors concluded the data confirmed an excellent prognosis after complete resection for typical bronchopulmonary carcinoid tumors, including those that showed lymph node metastases. The authors stated that parenchymal-saving resection was preferred.

Slodkowska et al.[205] referred to the article by Travis et al.[206] for a variety of clinical and histologic features that revised the histologic criteria for differentiating atypical carcinoid from typical carcinoid and proposed a range of mitotic counts between 2 and 20 per 10 HPFs for atypical carcinoids. The authors stated that between 1978 and 1997, 77 resected pulmonary carcinoids were reclassified as typical or atypical according to Travis et al.'s histologic criteria. The authors identified 62 typical carcinoids and 15 atypical carcinoids. Of the 77 patients who entered the study, 29 (38%) were males and 48 (62%) were females with a mean age of 43 years and an age range between 18 and 75 years. Forty-six patients underwent lobectomies, 16 bilobectomies, 12 pneumonectomies, and three wedge resections. The patients with typical carcinoid were stated to be younger than those with atypical carcinoids. Typical carcinoids were significantly smaller than atypical carcinoids. The mean diameter for typical versus atypical carcinoids was 24 mm versus 33 mm. Fifty-four (87%) typical carcinoids and all atypical carcinoids had a central location. The time of observation ranged from 2 months to 18½ years. Two patients with typical carcinoid died due to tumor progression, and three died due to other causes. Regional lymph node metastases occurred in 10% of typical carcinoids and 33% of atypical carcinoids. Heterotopic bone formation was found in 11 (18%) typical carcinoids and two (13%) atypical carcinoids. Peripheral carcinoids showed a spindle-cell morphology.

Thomas et al.[207] stated typical pulmonary carcinoids were well-differentiated neuroendocrine tumors associated with good patient survival rates, whereas atypical carcinoids were more aggressive and had worse survival rates. The authors stated that because tumors rarely involved thoracic lymph nodes at presentation, it was unknown to what extent the presence of thoracic lymph node metastases at the time of diagnosis influenced patient survival. The authors evaluated 517 patients between 1976 and 1997, of whom 36 had involvement of regional thoracic lymph nodes but without distant metastatic disease. The authors stated that after reclassification according to the current WHO criteria for neuroendocrine tumors, 23 patients had typical carcinoid tumors with thoracic lymph node involvement. At last follow-up, 19 patients had no evidence of disease, two patients had developed systemic metastases and were still alive, and two patients had died. Eleven patients had atypical carcinoid tumors with thoracic lymph node involvement. At last follow-up, four patients had no evidence of disease, seven patients had developed systemic metastases with a median interval of 17 months, and six of these seven patients died shortly thereafter. Two patients had been reclassified as having large cell neuroendocrine carcinoma at the time of review, both of whom had developed systemic metastases and had died. The authors concluded that patients with atypical pulmonary carcinoid tumors with regional lymph node metastases had a high likelihood of developing recurrent disease if treated with surgical resection alone and had a significantly worse outcome compared to those patients with typical carcinoid tumors with thoracic lymph node involvement. There was no statement in the article that the patients who had typical carcinoid and lymph node metastases received any type of adjuvant chemotherapy. It appears that thoracic lymph node involvement in patients with typical carcinoid is usually not a significant finding.

Fink et al.[208] evaluated the characteristic features and outcomes of 142 cases of pulmonary carcinoid tumors, of which 128 were classified as typical carcinoids and 14 as atypical carcinoids. The authors calculated an annual incidence of 2.3 to 2.8 cases per one million population, with a female-to-male ratio of 1.6:1. The prevalence of smoking was stated to be similar to that found in the general population in patients with typical carcinoids and twice as high in the patients with atypical carcinoids. Bronchial obstruction was stated to be the most common presenting symptom, and signs included obstructive pneumonia, pleuritic pain, atelectasis, and dyspnea. Carcinoid syndrome was stated to be extremely rare and occurred in only one patient with metastatic disease. Most neoplasms (68%) arose in major bronchi, and diagnosis was made using fiberoptic bronchoscopy in 52% of patients without evidence of endobronchial hemorrhage. Nodal involvement and distant metastases occurred in 57% and 21%, respectively, in the atypical group, and 10% and 3%, respectively, in the typical group. The respective 5-year survival rates for patients with typical and atypical tumors were 89% and 75%, and the 10-year survival rates were 82% and 56%. The authors reviewed the literature and reported data on five different studies (Table 36.9).

Schmid et al.[209] evaluated 120 neuroendocrine lung tumors, including typical carcinoids, atypical carcinoids, and high-grade neuroendocrine carcinomas consisting of SCLCs and large cell neuroendocrine carcinomas, for the presence of lymphovascular invasion by immunostaining for podoplanin and CD34. Lymphovascular invasion was correlated with clinicopathologic parameters, and its prognostic relevance was evaluated. Lymphatic vessels were stated to have been identified exclusively at the tumor invasion front, whereas blood capillaries were also seen within the tumors. Lymphatic vessels as well as lymphatic and blood vessel invasion was present in patients with high-grade neuroendocrine tumors and advanced tumor stages, closely associated with lymph node metastases (Table 36.10). The authors concluded that infiltration of peritumor lymphatic vessels played a crucial role in the progression of neuroendocrine tumors and had a greater impact than intratumoral and peritumoral blood vessel invasion. The authors concluded that immunohistologic evaluation of the vessel status of resected tumors was clinically important because of the strong correlation between lymphatic invasion and lymph node involvement. The authors suggested that this information could serve as a basis for further therapeutic approaches and decisions. The authors stated that, as suspected by Travis et al., the presence of vessel invasion alone did not allow for a distinction between different neuroendocrine tumors. As far as I can determine, there was no proof that the lymphatic invasion had an adverse effect on patients who had typical carcinoids.

From the foregoing it is readily apparent that the biologic behavior of atypical carcinoids is significantly different than that of typical carcinoids. Several papers have been published concerning the pathologic and clinical features of atypical carcinoids. Most of them discussed the clinicopathologic features of these neoplasms, specifically how they differ from typical carcinoids and SCLCs. Many studies have reported on the flow cytometric analysis of these neoplasms. An excellent editorial overview of atypical carcinoid neoplasms of the lung was published by Yousem[210] in 1991.

TABLE 36.9. Lung carcinoid neoplasms: data collected from large series in the literature

					Location, %		Histology, %		Surgery, %		Survival, %	
Source	Year	Patients, No.	Mean age (years)	Female/ male ratio	Central	Peripheral	Typical	Atypical	Lobectomy	Pneumonectomy	5-year	10-year
Hurt and Bates	1984	79	47	1.1/1	97	3	99	1	66	13	96	94
McCaughon et al	1985	124	55	1.2/1	37	63	81	19	42	11	92	77
Bertelsen et al	1985	82	45	1.1/1	79	21	79	21	54	6	88	85
Harpole et al	1992	126	53	1/1.2	55	45	66	34	50	12	78	71
Gould et al	1998	87	55	1/1.3		Not available	74	26	69	7	89*	
Fink et al	2000	142	52	1.6/1	68	32	90	10	56	16	87	79
Total		640	52	1.1/1	64	36	81	19	55	11	88	81

*Four-year survival.
Source: Fink et al.,[208] with permission.

TABLE 36.10. Lymphatic/vascular invasion of neuroendocrine lung neoplasms: cross-table of tumor type and different types of vessel invasion and tumor stage, lymph node, and distant metastases ($n = 120$)

		Tumor stage				Lymph node metastases			Distant metastases		
Tumor type	Type of vessel invasion	pT1	pT2	pT3	pT4	Absent	pN1	pN2	No	Yes	Total
Typical carcinoid	Absent	38 (31.7%)	8 (6.7%)	—	—	44 (36.7%)	2 (166%)	—	45 (37.5%)	1 (0.8%)	46 (38.3%)
	LVI	3 (2.5%)	2 (1.7%)	—	—	2 (1.7%)	2 (1.7%)	1 (0.8%)	5 (4.2%)	—	5 (4.2%)
	BVI	2 (1.7%)	1 (0.8%)	—	—	3 (2.5%)	—	—	3 (2.5%)	—	3 (2.5%)
	Both	2 (1.7%)	—	—	—	—	2 (1.7%)	—	1 (0.8%)	1 (0.8%)	2 (1.7%)
	Total	45 (37.5%)	11 (9.2%)	—	—	49 (40.8%)	6 (5.0%)	1 (0.8%)	54 (45.0%)	2 (1.7%)	56 (46.7%)
Atypical carcinoid	Absent	4 (3.3%)	3 (2.5%)	—	1 (0.8%)	8 (6.7%)	—	—	8 (6.7%)	—	8 (6.7%)
	LVI	3 (2.5%)	1 (0.8%)	—	2 (1.7%)	2 (1.7%)	3 (2.5%)	1 (0.8%)	4 (3.3%)	2 (1.7%)	6 (5.0%)
	BVI	—	1 (0.8%)	—	—	1 (0.8%)	—	—	—	1 (0.8%)	1 (0.8%)
	Both	1 (0.8%)	—	—	2 (1.7%)	—	1 (0.8%)	2 (1.7%)	1 (0.8%)	2 (1.7%)	3 (2.5%)
	Total	8 (5.7%)	5 (4.2%)	—	5 (4.2%)	11 (9.2%)	4 (3.3%)	3 (2.5%)	13 (10.8%)	5 (4.2%)	18 (15.0%)
Small cell lung cancer	Absent	8 (5.7%)	1 (0.8%)	—	1 (0.8%)	10 (8.3%)	—	—	7 (5.8%)	3 (2.5%)	10 (8.3%)
	LVI	3 (2.5%)	8 (6.7%)	1 (0.8%)	3 (2.5%)	1 (0.8%)	7 (5.8%)	7 (5.8%)	7 (5.8%)	8 (6.7%)	15 (12.5%)
	BVI	—	1 (0.8%)	—	—	1 (0.8%)	—	—	—	1 (0.8%)	1 (0.8%)
	Both	2 (1.7%)	3 (2.5%)	—	—	1 (0.9%)	1 (0.8%)	3 (2.5%)	1 (0.8%)	4 (3.3%)	5 (4.2%)
	Total	13 (10.8%)	13 (10.8%)	1 (0.8%)	4 (3.3%)	13 (10.8%)	8 (6.7%)	10 (8.3%)	15 (12.5%)	16 (13.3%)	31 (25.8%)
Large cell neuroendocrine carcinoma	Absent	3 (2.5%)	4 (3.3%)	—	—	7 (5.8%)	—	—	5 (4.2%)	2 (1.7%)	7
	LVI	—	5 (4.2%)	—	—	—	3 (2.5%)	2 (1.7%)	1 (0.8%)	4 (3.3%)	5
	BVI	1 (0.8%)	—	—	—	1 (0.8%)	—	—	1 (0.8%)	—	1
	Both Total	2 (1.7%)	—	—	—	—	2 (1.7%)	—	—	2 (1.7%)	2
		6 (5.0%)	9 (7.5%)	—	—	8 (6.7%)	5 (4.2%)	2 (1.7%)	7 (5.8%)	8 (6.7%)	15 (12.5%)
Total		72 (60.0%)	38 (31.7%)	1 (0.8%)	9 (7.5%)	81 (67.5%)	23 (19.2%)	16 (13.3%)	89 (74.2%)	31 (25.8%)	120 (100%)

LVI, lymphatic vessel invasion; BVI, blood vessel invasion.
Source: Schmid et al.,[209] with permission from Lippincott Williams & Wilkins.

Small Cell Carcinoma Versus Atypical Carcinoid

Warren et al.[211] reevaluated the clinicopathologic features of 50 cases of surgically resected small cell carcinomas. Thirty-four cases were confirmed to be correctly diagnosed as small cell carcinomas, but in 12 cases the diagnosis was changed to well-differentiated carcinoma (atypical carcinoid). They found that seven of 11 patients (64%) with T1N0, T2N0 well-differentiated neuroendocrine carcinomas (atypical carcinoid) survived more than 1 year, and six of eight patients (75%) survived more than 2 years. They concluded that well-differentiated neuroendocrine carcinoma (atypical carcinoid) was distinctly less aggressive and had a much better prognosis than SCLC.

Several investigators have evaluated the DNA index and S phase of neuroendocrine neoplasms with an emphasis on atypical carcinoids. Larsimont et al.[212] analyzed 18 typical carcinoids, six atypical carcinoids, and 11 SCLCs with a cell image processor. They found a significant increase in DNA content from typical carcinoids to SCLCs, with atypical carcinoids showing an intermediate value. They found the nuclei of atypical carcinoids to be significantly larger than those of typical carcinoids and similar to SCLCs. They found an increased chromatin condensation in atypical carcinoids versus typical carcinoids, and less condensation than in small cell carcinomas of the lung. This correlated with the observation of a progressive increase in hyperchromatism of nuclei from typical carcinoid to small cell carcinoma.

Yousem and Taylor[200] compared the DNA index and S phase of 12 typical carcinoids to eight atypical carcinoids (see their Table 1) using a cell image analyzer. They found the patients with atypical carcinoids were older (mean age, 52.2 years). Three of 12 typical carcinoids had an abnormal DNA content: one diploid/tetraploid, one tetraploid, and one aneuploid. All three neoplasms had a benign behavior and were not different in any way from the other typical carcinoids. Four of eight atypical carcinoids had aneuploid DNA indices and one had a hypodiploid DNA index. Aneuploid tumors were found to commonly show vascular invasion. Typical carcinoids had low proliferation indices, except for two cases that were slightly elevated (12.5% and 27.6%). In contrast, atypical carcinoids showed a higher proliferative index range (7.5% to 45.3%; mean 19.3%). The percentage of cells in S-G_2M phase generally correlated with mitotic rate identified in histologic sections. Yousem and Taylor concluded that although atypical carcinoids were more frequently aneuploid, DNA ploidy could not be used independently to assess malignant potential.

Lequaglie et al.[213] evaluated 19 patients diagnosed as having well-differentiated neuroendocrine carcinoma (atypical carcinoid). The patients were between 50 and 77 years old and 83% were cigarette smokers. Sixteen of 19 resected tumors were stage I, three were stage II, and one was stage IIIa. Five patients were treated with adjuvant chemotherapy and one was given regional radiotherapy. The tumor recurred in 10 patients, including four who had been given adjuvant treatment and six with stage I disease. Metastases did not correlate with pathologic stage, and the brain was the first site of metastases in seven cases. Sixty-eight percent of patients with stage I disease were alive after 100 months, and surgery was stated to be curative in more than half of patients with localized disease. Memoli[214] discussed the findings of Lequaglie et al. and reviewed the entity of well-differentiated neuroendocrine carcinoma (atypical carcinoid), indicating it had "come of age" and was a distinct clinicopathologic entity that should be recognized by pathologists.

Jackson-York et al.[215] evaluated the DNA content of nuclei from 53 primary and locally metastatic pulmonary neuroendocrine neoplasms. Nine of 22 (41%) well-differentiated neuroendocrine carcinomas (atypical carcinoids) were aneuploid. In contrast, 17 of 20 (85%) small cell neuroendocrine carcinomas and eight of 11 (73%) large cell neuroendocrine carcinomas (intermediate cell neuroendocrine carcinomas) were aneuploid. When evaluated as a single group, patients having tumors with a diploid DNA index had a longer survival than those having neoplasms with an aneuploid DNA index. However, the DNA index was not a statistically significant indicator of survival when cases with limited-stage disease were analyzed. Patients with well-differentiated neuroendocrine carcinoma (atypical carcinoid) had a significantly longer survival than those with small cell neuroendocrine carcinoma or large cell neuroendocrine carcinoma (see their Table 1).

El-Naggar et al.[199] analyzed 47 bronchopulmonary carcinoids, of which 33 (70.2%) were typical carcinoids and 14 (29.8%) were atypical carcinoids, by flow cytometry. Thirty neoplasms (63.8%) had a diploid DNA content; of these, 27 (90%) were typical carcinoids and 3 (10%) were atypical carcinoids. Of the 17 neoplasms (36.2%) that had an aneuploid DNA index, six (35.3%) were typical carcinoids and 11 (64.7%) were atypical carcinoids. The DNA indices of the aneuploid neoplasms ranged from 1.15 to 1.98 (mean, 1.35); 39 (83%) of the carcinoids had an S-phase percentage less than 7, and eight (17%) had an S-phase percentage equal to or greater than 7. The proliferative index (S phase) was higher among the aneuploid neoplasms (7.5 ± 3.6 standard deviation [SD]) than the diploid neoplasms (5.1 ± 1.3 SD). Only one patient with a typical carcinoid, a diploid DNA index, and an S-phase fraction of 5.0% died of disease. All three patients with atypical carcinoids who had a diploid DNA index were alive at last follow-up; and eight of 11 patients with an aneuploid, histologically atypical carcinoid were dead of disease. Multifactorial regression analysis revealed that histologic category (typical versus atypical) and DNA content were equally important independent prognostic factors. Additional significant prognostic factors included the size of the neoplasm and the presence of vascular invasion.

Travis et al.[136] performed flow cytometric analysis on 20 typical carcinoids, six atypical carcinoids, five large cell neuroendocrine carcinomas, and four small cell undifferentiated carcinomas. Eighteen of 20 typical carcinoids were diploid, one was aneuploid, and one was tetraploid. Of the atypical carcinoids, five were diploid and one was aneuploid. Three of five large cell neuroendocrine carcinomas were aneuploid, one was diploid, and the data in one case were not interpretable. Three of four small cell undifferentiated carcinomas were aneuploid and one was diploid. The proliferative index (S phase) for 14 diploid typical carcinoids ranged between 3.5% and 9.97% (average, 6.9%). In the other four diploid typical carcinoid tumors, the S-phase fraction was respectively 10.36%, 11.59%, 12.71%, and 18.36%. Interestingly, the proliferative index in the aneuploid and tetraploid typical carcinoids was 2.40% and 3.75%, respectively. In two diploid atypical carcinoids, the proliferative index was slightly greater than 10%, but in three diploid atypical carcinoids the proliferative index was less than or equal to 6%. In three aneuploid large cell neuroendocrine carcinomas, the proliferative index was 30.09%, 25.10%, and 5.15%, respectively. In the one diploid large cell neuroendocrine carcinoma, the S phase was 26.30%. The S phase was 9.76% and 29%, respectively, in two aneuploid small cell undifferentiated neuroendocrine carcinomas and 26.30% in one diploid small cell carcinoma. Travis et al.[136] did not find any ancillary techniques (immunohistochemistry, electron microscopy, DNA index–S- phase percentage) that provided an advantage over light microscopy for the classification or prognosis of pulmonary neuroendocrine neoplasms.

Large Cell Neuroendocrine Carcinomas

As already briefly discussed, large cell neuroendocrine neoplasms seem to pursue a more aggressive course than large cell undifferentiated carcinomas that do not have neuroendocrine features. Several other studies have performed clinicopathologic correlations on large cell neuroendocrine carcinomas. Jiang et al.[166] evaluated 22 cases of large cell neuroendocrine carcinomas that had been identified retrospectively. Eighteen had been classified as NSCLC, suggesting they were difficult to diagnose. The authors stated the most difficult diagnostic factor in diagnosing large cell neuroendocrine carcinomas was recognition of their light microscopic neuroendocrine features. The authors stated large cell neuroendocrine carcinoma needed to be distinguished not only from atypical carcinoid and SCLC, but also from common NSCLCs. The authors stated that, histologically, when an organoid architecture was subtle or absent, the rosette-like structure was the best marker for recognition of neuroendocrine differentiation. Nineteen of 22 large cell neuroendocrine carcinomas occurred in males and three in females. At the time of operation, the median age was 63.2 years with the range being 51 to 77 years. Ten cases were anatomic stage I, two were anatomic stage II, nine were anatomic stage IIIA, and one was anatomic stage IIIB. Twenty patients were treated by lobectomy, one by pneumonectomy, and one by segmentectomy. Eight patients received postoperative radiation therapy and three received chemotherapy. Follow-up information was available for 17 cases. One- and 5-year survival rates were 58.8% and 44.8%, respectively, compared to 86.2% and 54.4% for patients with NSCLCs. The difference in survivability was stated to be significant at a level of $p = .046$.

Jung et al.[216] evaluated 11 patients who were identified retrospectively as having large cell neuroendocrine carcinoma, of which eight occurred in men and three in women, with a mean age of 63 and an age range of 44 to 77 years. Chest CT scan was stated to have shown peripheral mass or nodule in eight cases and a central mass with distal atelectasis in three cases. Six tumors were accompanied by mediastinal and hilar adenopathy. All resected tumors were stated to have shown variable necrosis. Endogenous lipoid pneumonia and tumor emboli in two patients appeared by CT scan as areas of ground-glass opacity surrounding the tumor. Mediastinal lymph node metastases were identified in three (27%) patients. Pathologic staging of 11 patients was stage IB in six patients, stage IIA in one patient, stage IIB in one patient, stage IIIA in two patients, and stage IIIB in one patient. Follow-up data showed extrathoracic metastases in four patients at a mean follow-up of 15 months. One patient died from metastases 5 months after surgery. The authors concluded the CT scan findings of large cell neuroendocrine carcinoma of the lung were nonspecific and similar to those of other NSCLCs, with extrathoracic metastases being seen in approximately one third of patients in follow-up.

Mazieres et al.[217] reported on 18 consecutive resected cases of large cell neuroendocrine carcinoma, all patients being men, with a median age of 63 years. Eight cases were anatomic stage I, eight anatomic stage II, and two anatomic stage IIIA. All patients were treated as NSCLC and underwent surgery without adjuvant treatment except for postoperative radiotherapy for N2 or T3 disease. One patient was stated to have died of postoperative complications, and 13 patients relapsed with distant metastases that occurred in 10 patients within 6 months after surgery. The 1-year survival rate was 27%, and the survival rate at the end of follow-up was 22%, which was less than expected for comparable stage NSCLCs. Survival was stated to have not been influenced by lymph node status or by pathologic or molecular findings. Among the 10 evaluable patients with metastatic disease who received palliative platin-etoposide chemotherapy, only two had a partial tumor response (20%). The authors stated that standard treatment for NSCLC was ineffective when applied to patients with large cell neuroendocrine carcinoma, even in those with localized disease.

Between 1989 and 1999, Paci et al.[218] performed a retrospective assessment of cases of large cell neuroendocrine carcinoma. They identified 48 patients, 41 men and seven women, with an average age of 63.7 years. Twenty-nine patients (60.4%) had pathologic stage I disease, 11 (22.9%) had pathologic stage II disease, seven (14.6%) had pathologic stage IIIA disease, and one (2.1%) had pathologic stage IIIB disease. Two patients were stated to have undergone adjuvant chemotherapy, and two underwent mediastinal radiotherapy for N2 disease. No death was reported in the perioperative period. The median follow-up was 5 years and the actuarial survival for the entire group was 60.4% at 1 year, 27.5% at 3 years, and 21.2% at 5 years. The actuarial survival of accurately staged, stage I patients at 5 years was 27%. The authors stated that their findings suggested that treating large cell neuroendocrine carcinoma by applying treatment for NSCLC was associated with a prognosis that was worse than that for NSCLC, even in patients with low pathologic stages.

Doddoli et al.[219] evaluated 123 patients diagnosed with neuroendocrine carcinomas between 1989 and 2001 that were surgically treated with a curative intent at a single institution; 20 patients (18 men and two women, with a median age of 62 years) were diagnosed as having large cell neuroendocrine carcinoma, according to criteria derived from the 1999 WHO classification. Four patients had a preoperative diagnosis of large cell neuroendocrine carcinoma. The resections included 14 lobectomies and six pneumonectomies; there were no postoperative deaths. Four patients had stage I disease, four had stage II disease, nine had stage III disease, and three had stage IV disease. At a median follow-up at 46 months, 13 patients had died from general recurrence and seven patients were still alive. Median time to progression was 9 months, with a range of 1 to 54 months. The 5-year survival rate was 36%, with the median being 49 months. The survival rate was stated to be negatively influenced by disease stage, the presence of metastatic lymph node involvement, and vessel invasion. The authors concluded that large cell neuroendocrine carcinoma occurred predominantly in men, and that an accurate tissue diagnosis was rarely obtained preoperatively. The authors stated that although overall survival after resection was substantial, large cell neuroendocrine carcinoma frequently showed pathologic features of occult metastatic disease, such as lymph node involvement, vessel invasion, or both.

Small Cell Carcinoma

Small cell lung carcinoma is the most aggressive neuroendocrine tumor and perhaps the most aggressive common lung tumor, although approximately 20% of patients with SCLC limited to the thorax are alive at 2 years. Small cell carcinoma of the lung usually arises in the central region, although it may rarely present as a solitary pulmonary nodule. Quoix et al.[220] reviewed the cases of 408 individuals who were diagnosed as SCLC and identified 25 cases in which the neoplasm radiographically was a solitary pulmonary nodule. Pathologic review of these 25 cases confirmed 15 (60%) as small cell carcinoma (10 intermediate cell type, four oat cell, and one indeterminate). Of the 15 solitary pulmonary nodules, 10 were resected and five were treated with chemotherapy/radiotherapy; postoperative chemotherapy was given to most of the resected patients. The median survival of patients whose SCLC presented as a solitary pulmonary nodule was 24 months compared to 11 months for SCLC with limited disease and 3 months for those with extensive disease.

Kreisman et al.[221] reviewed SCLC presenting as a solitary pulmonary nodule. They defined a solitary pulmonary nodule as a single spherical or oval intrapulmonary density not exceeding 6 cm in greatest diameter. Patients with radiographic or pathologic evidence of hilar or mediastinal adenopathy were excluded. As reviewed, 4% to 12% of all solitary pulmonary nodules were SCLCs. The therapy currently recommended for a SCLC presenting as a solitary pulmonary nodule is surgery followed by adjuvant chemotherapy or radiation therapy.

Shepherd et al.[222] reported that patients with small cell carcinoma who had very limited disease, as defined by a negative mediastinoscopy or negative chest radiograph for mediastinal tumor, had a significantly better survival than those with more extensive (but still limited) SCLC.

Gephardt et al.[223] described the clinicopathologic features of 17 cases of surgically resected peripheral small cell carcinoma. The tumors were between 0.9 and 3.5 cm in diameter (mean, 2.1 cm) and histologically were predominantly mixed intermediate cell type with foci of oat cell carcinoma. Seven (41%) of the patients died of intrathoracic carcinoma or metastatic carcinoma involving the brain, with an average survival of 1.7 years. Of the patients whose tumor was stated to have an oat cell component histologically, five (71%) died of metastatic or recurrent disease. Of the 10 patients without definite foci of oat cell carcinoma, two (20%) patients died of recurrent or metastatic disease. This report is somewhat confusing in that Gephardt et al. referred to these neoplasms as atypical carcinoids.

Fraire et al.[224] reviewed 149 cases of patients with primary lung neoplasms with recorded diagnoses of SCLC (114 cases) and undifferentiated carcinoma (35 cases). Part of this study was to test the new classification scheme for SCLC as proposed by the Pathology Section of the International Association for the Study of Lung Cancer. The neoplasms were classified into the three categories (classic, pure small cell; mixed small cell, large cell; or combined small cell/adenocarcinoma or small cell/squamous carcinoma), and were clinically staged as local, regional, or distant. Consensus diagnosis was achieved in 144 (96.6%) of 149 cases. Of these 144 cases, 124 were classified as SCLC, with 115 (92.8%) as pure small cell, five (4.0%) as mixed small cell, and four (3.2%) as combined. Twenty cases were reclassified as NSCLCs. Adequate staging data were available for 123 of 124 cases, of which 27 (22.0%) were local, 22 (17.9%) were regional, and 74 (60.2%) were distant. The median length of survival based on histologic subtype was 225, 110, and 203 days for the small, mixed, and combined subtypes, respectively. For stage, the median length of survival was 428 days for local disease, 251 days for regional disease, and 111 days for distant disease. Fraire et al. concluded that stage was the major determinant in survival in SCLC. The mixed histologic type had significantly longer survival times than small or combined subtypes.

Bepler et al.[225] evaluated the relevance of histologic subtyping in SCLC. They evaluated pathologic specimens from 249 patients with SCLC that were classified into oat cell type, pure intermediate cell type, or small cell–large cell type; 170 specimens (68%) were classified as oat cell carcinoma, including 30 (18%) with mixed oat cell/intermediate cell features, 66 (39%) with intermediate cell features, and 13 (5%) with mixed small cell–large cell features. Two-year survival rates were 7%, 11%, and 15% for pure small cell, mixed small cell, and combined small cell, respectively. Bepler et al. concluded that histologic subtypes of SCLC were not distinct entities of clinical relevance, and that prognostic and therapeutic decisions could not be based on histologic subtypes.

Crown et al.[226] performed a retrospective analysis of 81 SCLC patients to determine what factors had prognostic significance for long-term survival, which was defined as disease-free survival for at least 5 years from the initiation of therapy. Six patients, five females (6.2%) and one male (1%), four with limited disease and two with extensive disease, were long-term survivors (73 to 96+ months from onset of therapy). Female gender and occurrence of herpes zoster were the only variables that were positively correlated with 5-year survival. Herpes zoster infection occurred at a median of 10 months from the inception of therapy, which supported the contention that herpes zoster acted as an immune stimulant or as a marker for intensity of treatment.

Albain et al.[227] formed a database of 2501 patients consecutively enrolled in SCLC trials since 1976 to determine the predictors of 2-year and 5-year survival in limited-stage disease and 1-year and 2-year survival in extensive-stage disease. Sixty-three patients with limited disease survived at least 5 years. Of these, there were 33 asymptomatic patients with no recurrent disease: six with recurrent SCLC, three of whom died; seven who died of non–cancer-related causes or unknown causes; three who died of second primary lung cancer; and 14 alive with persistent central nervous system symptoms and signs, possibly caused by prophylactic brain radiation. Fifty-one patients with extensive disease survived for 2 years or longer. Of these, 25 died of recurrent SCLC. The majority of the long-term survivors had either a single metastatic site or metastases limited to the opposite side of the chest or regional lymph nodes. Multivariate analysis supported the conclusion that aggressive combined modality, concurrent induction therapy, and favorable prognostic variables independently contributed to improved long-term survival in patients with limited disease.

Oud et al.[228] performed image and flow DNA cytometry on isolated nuclei from paraffin-embedded tumor tissue of patients with small cell carcinoma of the lung. Tissue was obtained from 14 patients, and in two patients tissue was obtained by both surgery and at autopsy. The authors found that image cytometry was more reliable than flow cytometry in identifying different cell populations. More important, they found that ploidy determination was not useful in predicting survival.

Funa et al.[229] performed in-situ hybridization for the expression of c-*myc* and N-*myc* oncogenes on initial biopsies from 15 untreated patients with primary lung cancer. The increased expression of N-*myc* oncogenes in SCLC was strongly associated with a poor response to chemotherapy, rapid tumor growth, and short survival.

Copple et al.[230] examined tumors ultrastructurally from 33 patients who had been diagnosed by light microscopy as small cell carcinoma of lung. They separated the tumors into four major groups based on ultrastructural criteria, such as whether or not they had neuroendocrine features, for example, neuroendocrine granules. They found that the complete and partial response rates to systemic chemotherapy, with or without radiation, was not significantly different in any of the four groups on the basis of ultrastructural findings. However, Vollmer et al.[231] studied 52 cases of oat cell carcinoma by electron microscopy and related the ultrastructural findings to tumor stage in patient survival. They found that only the type of cell junction between the tumor cells was of prognostic importance with respect to survival. Patients whose tumors showed intermediate junctions, and especially those with desmosomes, had a significantly greater chance to have more localized disease and a potentially resectable tumor, and subsequently a longer survival than those without these types of junctions. They found that the median survival periods for those with no identifiable junctions, intermediate junctions, or desmosomes was 6.4, 8.2, and 11.3 months, respectively. They indicated, however, that the ultrastructural subclassification was not as important as that obtained from careful clinical staging, a conclusion that we had previously reached.[193]

Nicholson et al.[232] reported on 100 cases of SCLC in which surgical biopsies or resections were available for evaluation. These cases came from the Armed Forces Institute of Pathology and the pathology panel of the International Association for the Study of Lung Cancer. The authors stated that SCLC currently accounted for 15% to 25% of invasive lung cancers worldwide, and approximately 45,000 new cases are diagnosed annually in the United States. The authors stated that SCLC was differentiated from all other types of lung cancer by a clinical and histopathologic profile that was distinctive from all other types, which were collectively called NSCLCs. Small cell lung cancers were stated to have been found almost exclusively in smokers, had rapid doubling time, pursued a more aggressive clinical course than NSCLC, and were often disseminated at the time of presentation.

The clinical features of these 100 patients are listed in Table 36.11. Light microscopic features of the resected tumors are listed in Table 36.12. Of interest, the nested or organoid pattern was most common (94% of cases) and peripheral palisading of tumor cells was seen in 72% of cases. A sheet-like growth pattern was a dominant pattern in only 34% of the cases. In two cases, there was marked cellular dyscohesion so that lymphoma was considered in the differential diagnosis. Other markers of neuroendocrine morphology included trabecular growth and rosette formation. Most cases were stated to have demonstrated a combination of patterns with variable distribution. Large areas of necrosis were stated to have been identified in 56% of cases. Immunohistochemical features of the neoplasms are shown in Table 36.13. Chromogranin was identified in 46 of 80 cases (58%) and

TABLE 36.11. Clinical features of small cell lung carcinoma

Feature	No.	Comment
Age	100	Range = 30–87; mean = 64
Gender	100	Male = 67; female = 33
Race	32	White = 27; black = 4; Hispanic = 1
Tobacco smoking	43	Yes = 41; no = 2; pack-year range = 25–60
Referral diagnosis	55	SCLC = 22; AC = 10; LCNEC = 6; NE carcinoma, NOS = 5; PD carcinoma, NOS = 12
Surgical procedure	82	Lobectomy = 49 Pneumonectomy = 11 Wedge excision = 13 Lymph node biopsy = 9
Chemotherapy	29	Yes = 23; no = 6
Radiation	19	Yes = 19
Length of follow-up	100	Range = 0.71–6.5 years; mean 2.5 years
Tumor size	65	Range = 0.5–0.9 cm; mean 3.0 cm
Tumor location	77	Central = 40; peripheral = 37
Tumor distribution	81	Right upper lobe = 14; right middle lobe = 9; right lower lobe = 10 Right hilum = 7 Left upper lobe = 21; left lower lobe = 13; Left, NOS = 4 Mediastinum = 3
Stage	99	I = 45; II = 20; III = 21; IV = 13
Survival	100	Dead of disease = 82; alive = 18
2-year survival by stage	99	Stage I & II = 50%; stage III & IV = 7%
5-year survival by stage	99	Stage I & II = 14%; stage II & IV – 7%
Macroscopic description	63	Well-circumscribed = 46; endobronchial = 9; subpleural = 5; apical = 1; cavitation/cystic degeneration = 2

LCNEC, large cell neuroendocrine carcinoma; N, number of patients with information available; NE, neuroendocrine; NOS, not otherwise specified; PD, poorly differentiated; SCLC, small cell lung cancer.
Source: Nicholson et al.,[232] with permission from Lippincott Williams & Wilkins.

TABLE 36.12. Light microscopic features of small cell carcinoma

	Histologic feature	Percent of cases
Number of slides examined in each case		Range = 1–17 Mean = 3
Growth pattern	Nested/organoid	94
	Peripheral palisading	72
	Sheet-like	34
	Trabecular	46
	Rosettes	36
Crush artifact	Present	14
	Minimal	7
	Absent	69
Necrosis	Extensive	78
	Punctate foci	9
	Inconspicuous	10
Azzopardi effect		8
Apoptosis		100
Tumor stroma	Fine septa	50
	Broad fibrous bands	43
	Primitive myxoid stroma	1
	Granulomas	5
	Calcification	5
	Metaplastic bone	1
Vascular invasion		42

Source: Nicholson et al.,[232] with permission from Lippincott Williams & Wilkins.

synaptophysin was identified in 41 of 72 cases (57%). Twenty-eight percent of the cases of SCLC showed combinations with NSCLC, with large cell carcinoma the most common, followed by adenocarcinoma and squamous cell carcinoma. The authors stated that because of the frequency of a few scattered large cells in small cell carcinoma, they arbitrarily recommended that at least 10% of the tumor show large cell carcinoma before the subclassification of combined small cell–large cell carcinoma was made. The authors stated combined SCLC was easily recognized if additional components consisted of adenocarcinoma or squamous carcinoma. The authors listed the histologic criteria for the distinction of SCLC from large cell neuroendocrine carcinoma and found that stage remained the only predictor of prognosis. However, I feel there is a fair amount of overlap between small cell and large cell neuroendocrine carcinoma, even though in Table 36.14, the histologic features seem fairly distinctly different.

As pointed out by Nicholson et al.,[232] most SCLCs are diagnosed on transbronchial biopsy specimens in which it is difficult to determine the growth pattern. I have recently evaluated a resected SCLC that showed an impressive neuroendocrine architecture (Fig. 36.136).

Other General Studies of Neuroendocrine Carcinomas

Additional studies have evaluated the clinicopathologic features of neuroendocrine lung neoplasms. Travis et al.[206] studied 200 neuroendocrine lung tumors to critically evaluate the Arrigoni histologic criteria for atypical carcinoids and, using statistical analysis, to delimit more rigorously an intermediate survival between atypical carcinoids and typical carcinoids and high-grade neuroendocrine tumors (i.e., large cell neuroendocrine carcinomas and SCLC). The optimal mitotic range for atypical carcinoid was stated to be two to 10 mitoses per 2 mm^2 of viable tumor (10 HPFs). Based on this finding, the authors separated mitoses into three categories (<2; 2 to 10; and ≥11 mitoses per 10 HPFs) and performed Cox multivariate analysis for all 200 neuroendocrine tumors. Mitotic counts were stated to have been the only independent predictor of prognosis. Based on this analysis, the authors proposed that atypical carcinoid be defined as a tumor with neuroendocrine morphology with mitotic counts between 2 and 10 mitoses per 2 mm^2 of viable tumor (10 HPFs), or with coagulative necrosis. Using these criteria, the 200 neuroendocrine tumors were classified as 51 typical carcinoids, 62 atypical carcinoids, 37 large cell neuroendocrine carcinomas, and 50 SCLCs. The 5- and 10-year survival rates were 87% and

TABLE 36.13. Immunohistochemistry results of small cell lung cancer

			Distribution of staining				Intensity of staining		
Stain	No. of cases stained	Total positive (%)	≤25% positive	26–50% positive	51–75% positive	76–100% positive	Weak (1+)	Moderate (2+)	Strong (3+)
Cytokeratin	70	70 (100)	7	6	13	44	2	22	46
Chromogranin	80	46 (58)	16	13	11	6	4	16	25
Synaptophysin	72	41 (57)	7	5	17	12	10	18	13
Leu 7	64	17 (27)	8	4	3	2	3	5	9

Source: Nicholson et al.,[232] with permission from Lippincott Williams & Wilkins.

TABLE 36.14. Histologic criteria for distinction of small cell lung cancer from large cell neuroendocrine carcinoma

Histologic feature	Small cell carcinoma	Large cell carcinoma
Cell size	Smaller (<3 resting small lymphocytes)	Larger
Nuclear/cytoplasmic ratio	Higher	Lower
Nuclear chromatin	Finely granular, uniform	Coarsely granular or vesicular less uniform
Nucleoli	Absent or inconspicuous	Often (not always) present, may be prominent or faint
Nuclear molding	Characteristic	Uncharacteristic
Fusiform shape	Common	Uncommon
Polygonal shape with ample pink cytoplasm	Uncharacteristic	Characteristic
Nuclear smear	Frequent	Uncommon
Basophilic staining of vessels and stroma	Occasional	Rare

Source: Nicholson et al.,[232] with permission from Lippincott Williams & Wilkins.

87% for typical carcinoids, 56% and 35% for atypical carcinoids, 27% and 9% for large cell neuroendocrine carcinomas, and 9% and 5% for SCLCs. After stratification for stage, survival for atypical carcinoid was stated to be significantly worse than survival for typical carcinoid ($p<.001$). Survival for large cell neuroendocrine carcinoma and SCLC was stated to be significantly worse than for atypical carcinoid, and the survival for large cell neuroendocrine carcinoma was no different than that for SCLC.

Garcia-Yuste et al.[233] evaluated 361 cases of neuroendocrine lung neoplasms that were treated surgically between 1980 and 1997. According to Dresler's criteria, the cases were categorized into grade 1 (typical carcinoid), grade 2 (atypical carcinoid), grade 3 large cell type, and grade 3 small cell type. Of 361 cases, 261 were grade 1, 43 were grade 2, and 22 of the large cell type and 35 of the small cell type were grade 3. Five-year survival was 96% for grade 1 typical carcinoid, 72% for grade 2 atypical carcinoid, 21% for grade 3 large cell type, and 14% for grade 3 small cell type. The authors stated there was a significant difference between typical and atypical carcinoids for mean age, tumor size, nodal metastases, and recurrence. The authors stated it could be concluded that there was a progressive deterioration of tumor organization from typical and atypical carcinoids to small cell carcinoma, and that this organization constituted a continuous spectrum. The authors stated that in their judgment, the future investigation of neuroendocrine tumors should focus on the study of the different genetic anomalies, together with evident or occult neuroendocrine differentiation, to help explain the behavior of the distinct tumor groups.

Huang et al.[234] stated pulmonary neuroendocrine carcinomas were a relatively common neoplasm and were currently divided into four major categories: typical carcinoid, atypical carcinoid, SCLC, and large cell neuroendocrine carcinoma. The authors stated that typical carcinoids and atypical carcinoids accounted for about 2% of all lung neoplasms and undifferentiated small cell carcinomas accounted for 20%. The incidence of these neoplasms was stated to be rising. The objective of the study was to provide clinicopathologic evidence to streamline and clarify the histomorphologic criteria for

A 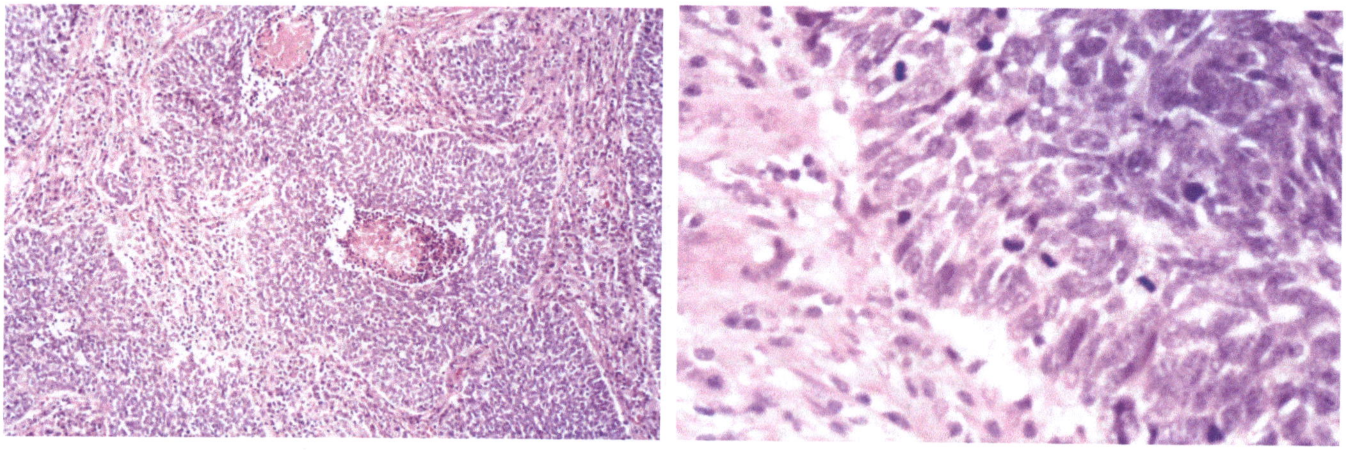 B

FIGURE 36.136. **(A,B)** Small cell lung cancer that shows an impressive neuroendocrine architecture, which might be misinterpreted as carcinoid tumor.

diagnosing neuroendocrine lung tumors, emphasizing the prognostic implications. The authors analyzed 234 cases of primary pulmonary neuroendocrine tumors and thoroughly studied 50 cases of tumors resected between 1986 and 1995. The authors stated they agreed with many of the previous investigators that these tumors were all malignant and potentially aggressive.

Based on the accumulated data, the authors modified the Gould criteria and reclassified the tumors into five types: (1) well-differentiated neuroendocrine carcinoma, otherwise called typical carcinoid (14 cases with less than 1 mitosis per 10 HPFs with or without minimal necrosis); (2) moderately differentiated neuroendocrine carcinoma, otherwise called low-grade atypical carcinoid (six cases with less than 10 mitoses per 10 HPFs and necrosis evident at high magnification); (3) poorly differentiated neuroendocrine carcinoma, otherwise called high-grade atypical carcinoid (10 cases with more than 10 mitoses per 10 HPFs and necrosis evident at low-power magnification); (4) undifferentiated large cell neuroendocrine carcinoma (five cases with more than 30 mitoses per 10 HPFs and marked necrosis); and (5) undifferentiated SCLC (15 cases with more than 30 mitoses per 10 HPFs and marked necrosis). Five-year survival rates were 93%, 83%, 70%, 60%, and 40% for well, moderately, and poorly differentiated, and undifferentiated large cell and small cell neuroendocrine carcinomas, respectively. The authors found metastases in 28% of typical carcinoids in this retrospective review, a figure higher than previously reported. The authors stated that using a grading system such as described in their article, they found their classification of pulmonary neuroendocrine carcinomas as well, moderately, poorly differentiated, or undifferentiated provided prognostic information and avoided misleading terms and concepts. This classification scheme has not caught on in the mainstream of pulmonary pathology.

Skuladottir et al.[235] studied a cancer registry-based analysis of patients in Denmark in whom bronchial neuroendocrine tumors were diagnosed between 1978 and 1997 with follow-up until December 31, 1999; 105 patients were diagnosed with typical carcinoid, 192 patients with atypical carcinoids, 50 patients with large cell neuroendocrine carcinoma, and 11,998 patients with small cell carcinoma. The recorded incidence of neuroendocrine tumors other than small cell carcinoma increased by twofold among men and by threefold in women during the study period, while the incidence of small cell carcinoma decreased among men and leveled off among women. The prognosis of patients with bronchial neuroendocrine tumors varied with the degree of malignancy. The 5-year survival rate was 87% for patients with typical carcinoids, 44% for patients with atypical carcinoids, 15% for patients with large cell neuroendocrine carcinomas, and 2% for patients with SCLC. The authors stated that in Denmark, the incidence of neuroendocrine tumors was increasing. They stated that their findings supported the pathologic classification of neuroendocrine tumors into a spectrum ranging from low-grade typical carcinoid, intermediate grade atypical carcinoid, to the two highly malignant pathologic entities: large cell neuroendocrine carcinoma and SCLC. The authors stated more research was needed to establish the etiologic factors in the development of bronchial carcinoids.

Conclusion

Neuroendocrine lung neoplasms represent a diverse group of neoplasms showing neuroendocrine differentiation, ranging from low-grade typical carcinoids to highly malignant large cell neuroendocrine carcinomas and SCLCs. The pathologic criteria for diagnosing these neoplasms is relatively straightforward, although problems occasionally arise in differentiating atypical carcinoids from large cell neuroendocrine carcinomas and SCLCs. A proposal to categorize these neoplasms into three grades—low (typical carcinoid), intermediate (atypical carcinoid), and high (large cell neuroendocrine carcinoma, SCLC)—is reasonable. A specific problem to be avoided is misdiagnosing typical carcinoids as SCLCs on transbronchial biopsy specimens. The clinicopathologic features of these neoplasms have been extensively reviewed, showing that most typical carcinoids have an excellent prognosis, even with lymphatic invasion and lymph node metastases. Atypical carcinoids are significantly more aggressive than typical carcinoids, although not as lethal as large cell neuroendocrine carcinomas and SCLCs.

References

1. Feyrter F. Ueber diffuse endokrine epitheliate organe. Zentralbl Inn Med 1938;59:545–561.
2. Pearse AGE. The cytochemistry and ultrastructure of polypeptide hormone-producing cells of the APUD series and the embryologic, physiologic and pathologic implications of this concept. J Histochem Cytochem 1969;17:303–313.
3. Pearse AGE, Takor T. Embyrology of the diffuse neuroendocrine system and its relationship to the common peptides. Fed Proc 1979;38:2288–2294.
4. Pearse AGE. The diffuse neuroendocrine system: an extension of the APUD concept. In: Taylor S, ed. Endocrinology. London: Heinemann, 1972:145.
5. Gould VE, DeLellis RA. The neuroendocrine cell system: its tumors, hyperplasias, and dysplasias. In: Silverberg SG, ed. Principles and practice of surgical pathology. New York: Wiley, 1983:1488–1501.
6. Gould VE, Moll R, Moll I, Lee I, Franke WW. Neuroendocrine (Merkel) cells of the skin: hyperplasias, dysplasias and neoplasms. Lab Invest 1985;52:334–353.

7. Gould VE, Linnoila RI, Memoli VA, Warren WH. Neuroendocrine components of the bronchopulmonary tract: hyperplasias, dysplasias, and neoplasms. Lab Invest 1983; 49:519–537.
8. Gould VE, Wiedenmann B, Lee I, et al. Synaptophysin expression in neuroendocrine neoplasms as determined by immunocytochemistry. Am J Pathol 1987;126: 243–257.
9. Hammar S, Gould VE. Neuroendocrine neoplasms. In: Azar HA, ed. Pathology of human neoplasms: an atlas of diagnostic electron microscopy and immunohistochemistry. New York: Raven Press, 1988:333–404.
10. Barnes PJ, Baranivk JN, Belvisi MG. Neuropeptides in the respiratory tract. Am Rev Respir Dis 1991;144(1):1187–1198; (2):1391–1399.
11. Haimoto H, Takahashi Y, Koshikawa T, Nagura H, Kato K. Immunohistochemical localization of γ-enolase in normal human tissues other than nervous and neuroendocrine tissues. Lab Invest 1985;52:257–263.
12. Pahlman S, Esscher T, Nilsson K. Expression of γ-subunit of enolase, neuron-specific enolase in human nonneuroendocrine tumors and derived cell lines. Lab Invest 1986;54: 554–560.
13. Vinores SA, Bonnin JM, Rubinstein LJ, Marangos PJ. Immunohistochemical demonstration of neuron-specific enolase in neoplasms of the CNS and other tissues. Arch Pathol Lab Med 1984;120:186–192.
14. Bergh J, Escher T, Steinholtz L, Nilsson K, Pahlman S. Immunocytochemical demonstration of neuron-specific enolase (NSE) in human lung cancers. Am J Clin Pathol 1985;84:1–7.
15. Said JW, Vimadalal S, Nash G, et al. Immunoreactive neuron-specific enolase, bombesin, and chromogranin as markers for neuroendocrine lung tumors. Hum Pathol 1985;16:236–240.
16. Schmechel DE. γ-subunit of the glycolytic enzyme enolase: nonspecific or neuron specific? Lab Invest 1985; 52:239–242.
17. O'Connor DT, Burton D, Deftos LJ. Immunoreactive human chromogranin A in diverse polypeptide hormone producing human tumors and normal endocrine tissues. J Clin Endocrinol Metab 1983;57:1084–1086.
18. Lloyd RV, Wilson BS, Kovacs K, Ryan N. Immunohistochemical localization of chromogranin in human hypophyses and pituitary adenomas. Arch Pathol Lab Med 1985; 109:515–517.
19. McNutt MA, Bolen JW. Adenomatous tumor of the middle ear. Am J Clin Pathol 1985;84:541–547.
20. Bussolati G, Gugliotta P, Sapino A, Eusebi V, Lloyd R. Chromogranin-reactive endocrine cells in argyrophilic carcinomas ("carcinoids") from normal tissue of the breast. Am J Pathol 1985;120:186–192.
21. O'Connor DT, Deftos LJ. Secretion of chromogranin A by peptide-producing endocrine neoplasms. N Engl J Med 1986;314:1145–1151.
22. Lloyd RV, Sisson JC, Shapiro B, Verhofstad AAJ. Immunohistochemical localization of epinephrine, norepinephrine, catecholamine-synthesizing enzymes and chromogranin in neuroendocrine cells and tumors. Am J Pathol 1986;125:45–54.
23. Banks P, Helle K. The release of protein from the stimulated adrenal medulla. Biochem J 1965;97:40C–41C.
24. Angeletti RH. Chromogranins and neuroendocrine secretion. Lab Invest 1986;55:387–390.
25. Wilson BS, Lloyd RV. Detection of chromogranin in neuroendocrine cells with a monoclonal antibody. Am J Pathol 1984;115:458–468.
26. Lauweryns JM, vanRanst K, Lloyd RV, et al. Chromogranin in bronchopulmonary neuroendocrine cells: immunohistochemical detection in human, monkey and pig respiratory mucosa. J Histochem Cytochem 1987;35:113–118.
27. Mukai M, Torikata C, Iri H, et al. Expression of neurofilament triplet proteins in human neural tumor: an immunohistochemical study of paraganglioma, ganglioneuroma, ganglioneuroblastoma and neuroblastoma. Am J Pathol 1986;122:28–36.
28. Shah IA, Schlageter M, Netto D. Immunoreactivity of neurofilament proteins in neuroendocrine neoplasms. Mod Pathol 1991;4:215–219.
29. Leoncini P, DeMarco EB, Bugnoli M, Mencarelli C, Vindigni C, Cintorino M. Expression of phosphorylated and non-phosphorylated neurofilament subunits and cytokeratins in neuroendocrine lung tumors. Pathol Res Pract 1989;185:848–855.
30. Jahn B, Schibler W, Ouimet C, et al. A 38,000 dalton membrane protein (p38) present in synaptic vesicles. Proc Natl Acad Sci USA 1985;82:4137–4141.
31. Gould VE, Lee I, Wiedenmann B, Moll R, Chejfec G, Franke WW. Synaptophysin: a novel marker for neurons, certain neuroendocrine cells and their neoplasms. Hum Pathol 1986;17:979–983.
32. Bunn P, Linnoila I, Minna J, Carney D, Gazdar AF. Small cell cancer, endocrine cells of the fetal bronchus, and other neuroendocrine cells express Leu7 antigenic determinant present on natural killer cells. Blood 1985;65:764–768.
33. Tsutsumi Y. Leu7 immunoreactivity as a histochemical marker for paraffin-embedded neuroendocrine tumors. Acta Histochem Cytochem 1984;17:15.
34. Tischler AS, Mobtaker H, Mann K, et al. Anti-lymphocyte monoclonal antibody HNK-1 (Leu7) recognizes a constituent of neuroendocrine matrix. Lab Invest I986;54:64A.
35. Komminoth P, Roth J, Lackie PM, Bitter-Suermann D, Heitz PU. Polysialic acid of the neural cell adhesion molecule distinguishes small cell lung carcinoma from carcinoids. Am J Pathol 1991;139:297–304.
36. Kibbelaar RE, Moolenaar CEC, Michalides RJAM, Bitter-Suermann D, Addis BJ, Mooi WJ. Expression of the embryonal neural cell adhesion molecular N-CAM in lung carcinoma. Diagnostic usefulness of monoclonal antibody 735 for the distinction between small cell lung cancer and non-small cell lung cancer. J Pathol 1989;159:23–28.
37. Moolenaar CE, Muller EJ, Schol DJ. Expression of neural cell adhesion molecule-related sialoglycoprotein in small cell lung cancer, and neuroblastoma cell lines H69 and CHP-212. Cancer Res 1990;50:1102–1106.
38. Stahlman M, Gray M, Whitsett J. Expression of thyroid transcription factor 1 (TTF-1) in fetal and neonatal human lung. J Histochem Cytochem 1996;44:673–678.

39. Lazzaro D, Price M, DeFelice M, et al. The transcription factor 1 is expressed at the onset of thyroid and lung morphogenesis and in restricted regions of the fetal brain. Development 1991;113:1093–1104.
40. Holzinger A, Dingle S, Bejarano P, et al. Monoclonal antibody to thyroid transcription factor-1: production, characterization, and usefulness in tumor diagnosis. Hybridoma 1996;15:49–53.
41. DiLoreto C, DiLauro V, Puglisi F, et al. Immunohistochemical expression of tissue specific transcription factor-1 in lung carcinoma. J Clin Pathol 1997;50:30–32.
42. Fabbro D, DiLoreto C, Stamerra O, et al. TTF-1 expression in human lung tumours. Eur J Cancer 1996;32A: 512–517.
43. Harlamert H, Mira J, Bejarano P, et al. Thyroid transcription factor-1 and cytokeratins 7 and 20 in pulmonary and breast carcinoma. Acta Cytol 1998;42:1382–1388.
44. Byrd-Gloster A, Khoor A, Glass L, et al. Differential expression of thyroid transcription factor 1 in small cell lung carcinoma and Merkel cell tumor. Hum Pathol 2000;31:58–62.
45. Folpe A, Gown A, Lamps L, et al. Thyroid transcription factor-1: immunohistochemical evaluation in pulmonary neuroendocrine tumors. Mod Pathol 1999;12:5–8.
46. Hanly A, Elgart G, Jorda M, et al. Analysis of thyroid transcription factor-1 and cytokeratin 20 separates Merkel cell carcinoma from small cell carcinoma of lung. J Cutan Pathol 2000;27:118–120.
47. Kaufmann O, Dietel M. Expression of thyroid transcription factor-1 in pulmonary and extrapulmonary small cell carcinomas and other neuroendocrine carcinomas of various primary sites. Histopathology 2000;36: 415–429.
48. Sturm N, Lanteujoul S, Lavierriere M, et al. Thyroid transcription factor-1 (TTF-1) and cytokeratin 1, 5, 10, 14 (34betaE12) expression in basaloid and large cell neuroendocrine carcinomas of the lung. Hum Pathol 2001;32: 918–925.
49. Oliveira A, Tazelaar H, Myers J, et al. Thyroid transcription factor-1 distinguishes metastatic pulmonary from well-differentiated neuroendocrine tumors of other sites. Am J Surg Pathol 2001;25:815–819.
50. Sturm N, Rossi G, Lanteujoul S, et al. Expression of thyroid transcription factor-1 in the spectrum of neuroendocrine cell lung proliferations with special interest in carcinoids. Hum Pathol 2002;33:175–182.
51. Saqi A, Alexis D, Remotti F, et al. Usefulness of CDX2 and TTF-1 in differentiating gastrointestinal from pulmonary carcinoids. Am J Clin Pathol 2005;123:394–404.
52. Lonardo F, Pass HI, Lucas DR. Immunohistochemistry frequently detects c-Kit expression in pulmonary small cell carcinoma and may help select clinical subsets for a novel form of chemotherapy. Appl Immunohist Mol Morphol 2003;11:51–55.
53. Casali C, Stefani A, Rossi G, et al. The prognostic role of c-Kit protein expression in resected large cell neuroendocrine carcinoma of the lung. Ann Thorac Surg 2004;77: 252–253.
54. Butnor KJ, Burchette JL, Sporn TA, Hammar SP, Roggli VL. The spectrum of c-Kit (CD117) immunoreactivity in lung and pleural tumors: a study of 96 cases using a single-source antibody with a review of the literature. Arch Pathol Lab Med 2004;128:538–543.
55. Yesner R. Spectrum of lung cancer and ectopic hormones. Pathol Annu 1978;13(pt 1):217–240.
56. Kahn HJ, Garrido A, Huang S-N, Baumal R. Intermediate filaments and tumor diagnosis. Lab Invest 1983; 49:509.
57. Lehto V-P, Stenman S, Miettinen M, Dahl D, Virtanen I. Expression of a neural type of intermediate filament as a distinguishing feature between oat cell carcinoma and other lung cancers. Am J Pathol 1983;110:113–118.
58. VanMuijen GNP, Ruiter DJ, Leeuwen CV, Prins FA, Rietsema K, Warnaar SO. Cytokeratin and neurofilament in lung carcinomas. Am J Pathol 1984;116:363–369.
59. Lehto V-P, Miettinen M, Dahl D, Virtanen I. Bronchial carcinoid cells contain neural-type intermediate filaments. Cancer (Philadelphia) 1984;54:624–628.
60. Clark RK, Miettinen M, Leij L, Damjanov I. Terminally differentiated derivatives of pulmonary small cell carcinomas may contain neurofilaments. Lab Invest 1985;53:243–244.
61. Broers J, Huysmans A, Moesker O, Vooijs P, Ramaekers F, Wagenaar S. Small cell lung cancer contains intermediate filaments of the cytokeratin type. Lab Invest 1985;52: 113–114.
62. Moll R, Franke WW, Schiller DL, et al. The catalogue of human cytokeratins. Patterns of expression in normal epithelia, tumors and cultured cells. Cell 1982;31: 11–24.
63. Cooper D, Schermer A, Sun T-T. Classification of human epithelia and their neoplasms using monoclonal antibodies to keratins: strategies, applications and limitations. Lab Invest 1985;52:243–256.
64. Gown AM, Gabbiani G. Intermediate-sized (10-nm) filaments in human tumors. In: DeLellis, RA, ed. Advances in immunohistochemistry. New York: Masson, 1984:89–109.
65. Miettinen M, Lehto V-P, Virtanen I. Antibodies to intermediate filament proteins in the diagnosis and classification of human tumors. Ultrastruct Pathol 1984;7:83–107.
66. Moll R, Cowin P, Kapprell H-P, Franke WW. Desmosomal proteins: new markers for identification and classification of tumors. Lab Invest 1986;54:4–25.
67. Funa K, Gazdar AF, Minna JD, Linnoila RI. Paucity of B2-microglobulin expression on small cell lung cancer, bronchial carcinoids, and certain other neuroendocrine tumors. Lab Invest 1986;55:186–192.
68. Payne CM, Nagle RB, Borduin V. Methods in laboratory investigation: an ultrastructural cytochemical stain specific for neuroendocrine neoplasms. Lab Invest 1984;51:350–365.
69. Nagle RB, Payne CM, Clark VA. Comparison of the usefulness of histochemistry and ultrastructural cytochemistry in the identification of neuroendocrine neoplasms. Am J Clin Pathol 1986;85:289–296.
70. Gould VE, Benditt EP. Ultrastructural and functional relationships of some human endocrine tumors. Pathol Annu 1973;8:205–230.
71. Gould VE. Neuroendocrinomas and neuroendocrine carcinomas: APUD-cell system neoplasms and their

aberrant secretory activities. Pathol Annu 1977;12(pt 2): 33–62.
72. Sunday ME, Choi N, Spindel ER, Chin WW, Mark EJ. Gastrin-releasing peptide gene expression in small cell and large cell undifferentiated carcinomas. Hum Pathol 1991; 22:1030–1039.
73. Hamid Q, Corrin B, Sheppard MN, Polak JM. Localization of chromogranin mRNA in small cell carcinoma of the lung. J Pathol 1991;163:293–297.
74. Frohlich F. Die "Helle Zelle" der Bronchialschleimhaut and ihre Beziehungen zum Problem der Chemoreceptoren. Frankfurt Ztschr Z Pathol 1949;60:517–559.
75. Feyrter F. Zur Pathologic des argyrophilen Helle-Zell-Organes im Bronchialbaum des Menschen. Virchows Arch 1954;325:723–732.
76. Bensch KG, Gordon GB, Miller LR. Studies on the bronchial counterpart of the Kultschitzky (argentaffin) cell and innervation of bronchial glands. J Ultrastruct Res 1965;12:668–686.
77. Bensch KG, Gordon GB, Miller LR. Electron microscopic and biochemical studies on the bronchial carcinoid tumor. Cancer 1965;18:592–602.
78. Gmelich JT, Bensch KG, Liebow AA. Cells of Kultschitzky type in bronchioles and their relation to the origin of peripheral carcinoid tumor. Lab Invest 1967;17: 88–98.
79. Lauweryns JM, Cokelaere M. Theunynck PK. Neuroepithelial bodies in the respiratory mucosa of various mammals: a light optical, histochemical, and ultrastructural investigation. Z Zellforsch Mikrosk Anat 1972;135:569–592.
80. Lauweryns JM, Goddeeris P. Neuroepithelial bodies in the human child and adult lung. Am Rev Respir Dis 1975; 111:469–476.
81. Johnson DE, Loch JE, Elde RP, Thompson TR. Pulmonary neuroendocrine cells in bronchopulmonary dysplasia and hyaline membrane disease. Pediatr Res 1982;16:446–454.
82. Johnson DE, Wobken JD, Landrum BG. Changes in bombesin, calcitonin and serotonin immunoreactive pulmonary neuroendocrine cells in cystic fibrosis and after prolonged mechanical ventilation. Am Rev Respir Dis 1988;137:123–131.
83. Stahlman MT, Gray ME. Ontogeny of neuroendocrine cells in human fetal lung. I. An electron microscopic study. Lab Invest 1984;51:449–463.
84. Stahlman MT, Kasselberg AG, Orth DN, Gray ME. Ontogeny of neuroendocrine cells in human fetal lung. II. An immunohistochemical study. Lab Invest 1985;52:52–60.
85. Spindel ER, Sunday ME, Hofler H, Wolfe HJ, Habener JF, Chin WW. Transient elevation of messenger RNA encoding gastrin releasing peptide, a putative pulmonary growth factor in human fetal lung. J Clin Invest 1987;80: 1172–1179.
86. Sobol RE, O'Connor DT, Addison J, Suchocki K, Royston I, Deftos LJ. Elevated serum chromogranin A levels in small cell lung carcinoma. Ann Intern Med 1986;1095: 698–700.
87. Gosney JR, Sissons MCJ, Allibone RO, Blakely AF. Pulmonary endocrine cells in chronic bronchitis and emphysema. J Pathol 1989;157:127–133.
88. Aguayo SM, King TE Jr, Waldron JA Jr, Sherritt KM, Kane MA, Miller YE. Increased pulmonary neuroendocrine cells with bombesin-like immunoreactivity in adults with eosinophilic granuloma. J Clin Invest 1989;86:838–844.
89. Aguayo SM, Kane MA, King TE Jr, Schwarz MI, Graver L, Miller YE. Increased levels of bombesin-like peptides in the lower respiratory tract of asymptomatic cigarette smokers. J Clin Invest 1989;84:1105–1113.
90. Tabassian AR, Nylen ES, Linnoila RI, Snider RH, Cassidy MM, Becker KL. Stimulation of hamster pulmonary neuroendocrine cells and associated peptides by repeated exposure to cigarette smoke. Am Rev Respir Dis 1989;140: 436–440.
91. Aguayo SM, Miller YE, Waldron JA Jr, et al. Brief report: Idiopathic diffuse hyperplasia of pulmonary neuroendocrine cells and airways disease. N Engl J Med 1992;327: 1285–1288.
92. Benfreld JR. Neuroendocrine neoplasms of the lung. J Thorac Cardiovasc Surg 1990;100:628–629.
93. Travis WD, Colby TV, Corrin B, et al. Histological typing of lung and pleural tumors. In collaboration with L.H. Sobin and pathologists from 14 countries. World Health Organization International Classification of Tumours. 3rd ed. Berlin, Heidelberg, New York: Springer-Verlag, 1999.
94. Travis WD, Brambilla E, Muller-Hermelink HG, Harris CC, eds. Pathology and genetics: tumours of the lung, pleura, thymus and heart. Lyon: IARC Press, 2004.
95. Whitwell F. Tumorlets of the lung. J Pathol Bacteriol 1955;70:529–541.
96. Churg A, Warnock ML. Pulmonary tumorlet: A form of peripheral carcinoid. Cancer (Philadelphia) 1976;37: 1469–1477.
97. Miller MA, Mark J, Kanarek D. Multiple peripheral pulmonary carcinoids and tumorlets of carcinoid type, with restrictive and obstructive lung disease. Am J Med 1978;65:373–378.
98. Pelosi G, Zancanaro C, Sbubo L, Bresaola E, Martignoni G, Bontempini L. Development of innumerable neuroendocrine tumorlets in pulmonary lobe scarred by intralobar sequestration: Immunohistochemical and ultrastructural study of an unusual case. Arch Pathol Lab Med 1992;116:1167–1174.
99. D'Aggti VD, Perzin KH. Carcinoid tumorlets of the lung with metastasis to a peribronchial lymph node: report of a case and review of the literature. Cancer (Philadelphia) 1985;55:2472–2476.
100. Mueller H. Zur Untersuchungsgeschichte der bronchialen Weiterungen. Inaug Diss Halle, 1882.
101. Kramer R. Adenoma of bronchus. Ann Otol Rhinol Laryngol 1930;39:689–695.
102. Hamperl H. Uber gutartige Bronchialtumoren. Virchows Arch [Pathol Anat] 1937;300:1937:46–88.
103. Oberndorfer S. Karzinoide Tumoren des Diinndarms. Frankfurt Zeitschr Pathol 1907;1:426–432.
104. Briselli M, Mark GJ, Grillo HC. Tracheal carcinoids. Cancer (Philadelphia) 1978;42:2870–2879.
105. Bonikos DS, Bensch KG, Jamplis RW. Peripheral pulmonary carcinoid tumors. Cancer (Philadelphia) 1976;37: 1977–1998.

106. Felton WL, Liebow AA, Lindskog GE. Peripheral and multiple bronchial adenomas. Cancer (Philadelphia) 1953; 6:555–567.
107. Skinner C, Ewen SWB. Carcinoid lung: diffuse pulmonary infiltration by a multifocal bronchial carcinoid. Thorax 1976;31:212–219.
108. Abdi EA, Goel R, Bishop S, Bain GO. Peripheral carcinoid tumours of the lung: A clinicopathological study. J Surg Oncol 1988;39:190–196.
109. Carter D, Eggleston JC, Carcinoid tumors. In: Tumors of the lower respiratory tract. Atlas of tumor pathology, 2d Ser., Fasc. 17. Washington, DC: Armed Forces Institute of Pathology, 1980:162–188.
110. Mark EJ, Quay SC, Dickensin GR. Papillary carcinoid tumor of the lung. Cancer (Philadelphia) 1981;48:316–324.
111. Ranchod M, Levine GD. Spindle cell carcinoid tumors of the lung: a clinicopathologic study of 35 cases. Am J Surg Pathol 1980;4:315–331.
112. Sklar JL, Churg A, Bensch KG. Oncocytic carcinoid tumor of the lung. Am J Surg Pathol 1980;4:287–292.
113. Sajjad SM, Mackay B, Lukeman JM. Oncocytic carcinoid tumor of the lung. Ultrastruct Pathol 1980;1:171–176.
114. Scharifker D, Marchevsky A. Oncocytic carcinoid of lung: an ultrastructural analysis. Cancer (Philadelphia) 1981;47: 530–532.
115. Ghadially FN, Block HJ. Oncocytic carcinoid of the lung. J Submicrosc Cytol 1985;17:435–442.
116. Santos-Briz, Terron J, Sastre R, Romero L, Valle A. Oncocytoma of the lung. Cancer 1977;40:1330–1336.
117. Cebelin MS. Melanocytic bronchial carcinoid tumor. Cancer (Philadelphia) 1980;46:1843–1848.
118. Grazer R, Cohen SM, Jacobs JB, Lucas P. Melanin-containing peripheral carcinoid of the lung. Am J Surg Pathol 1982;6:73–78.
119. Carlson JA, Dickersin GR. Melanocytic paraganglioid carcinoid tumor: a case report and review of the literature. Ultrastruct Pathol 1993;17:353–372.
120. Barbareschi M, Frigo B, Mosca L, et al. Bronchial carcinoids with S100 positive sustentacular cells. Pathol Res Pract 1990;186:212–217.
121. Capella C, Gabrielli M, Polak JM, Buffa R, Solcia E. Ultrastructural and histological study of 11 bronchial carcinoids. Virchows Arch Pathol Anat [A] 1979;381:313–329.
122. Gaffey MJ, Mills SE, Frierson HF Jr, et al. Pulmonary clear cell carcinoid tumor; another entity in the differential diagnosis of pulmonary clear cell neoplasia. Am J Surg Pathol 1998;22:1020–1025.
123. Barbareschi M, Frigo B, Cristina S, Valentini L, Leonardi E, Mosca L. Bronchial carcinoid with paranuclear fibrillary inclusions related to cytokeratins and vimentin. Virchows Arch [A] Pathol Anat 1989;415:31–36.
124. Arrigoni MG, Woolner LB, Bernatz PE. Atypical carcinoid tumors of the lung. J Thorac Cardiovasc Surg 1972;64: 413121.
125. Leschke H. Über nur regionär bösartige and über krebsig entartete Bronchusadenome bzw. Carcinoide. Virchows Arch [Path Anat] 1956;328:635–657.
126. Warren WH, Memoli VA, Gould VE. Immunohistochemical and ultrastructural analysis of bronchopulmonary neuroendocrine neoplasms. II. Well-differentiated neuroendocrine carcinomas. Ultrastruct Pathol 1984;7:185–199.
127. Mark EJ, Ramirez JF. Peripheral small-cell carcinoma of the lung resembling carcinoid tumor: A clinical and pathologic study of 14 cases. Arch Pathol Lab Med 1985;109: 263–269.
128. Paladugu RR, Benfield JR, Pak HY, Ross RK, Teplitz RL. Bronchopulmonary Kulchitzky cell carcinomas. Cancer (Philadelphia) 1985;55:1303–1311.
129. Tsutsumi Y, Yazaki K, Yoshioka K. Atypical carcinoid tumor of the lung, associated with giant cell transformation in bone metastases.
130. Hammar S, Bockus D, Remington F, Cooper L. The unusual spectrum of neuroendocrine lung neoplasms. Ultra Pathol 1989;13(5,6):515–560.
131. Gould VE, Chejfec G. Ultrastructural and biochemical analysis of pulmonary "undifferentiated" carcinomas. Hum Pathol 1978;9:377–384.
132. McDowell EM, Wilson TS, Trump BF. Atypical endocrine tumors of the lung. Arch Pathol Lab Med 1981;105: 20–28.
133. Hammond ME, Sause WT. Large cell neuroendocrine tumors of the lung: Clinical significance and histopathologic definition. Cancer (Philadelphia) 1985;56:1624–1629.
134. Neal MH, Kosinki R, Cohen P, Orenstein JM. Atypical endocrine tumors of the lung: a histologic, ultrastructural and clinical study of 19 cases. Hum Pathol 1986;17:1264–1277.
135. Barbareschi M, Mariscotti C, Barberis M, Frigo B, Mosca L. Large cell neuroendocrine carcinoma of the lung. Tumori 1989;75:583–588.
136. Travis WD, Linnoila I, Tsokos MG, et al. Neuroendocrine tumors of the lung with proposed criteria for large cell neuroendocrine carcinoma: an ultrastructural, immunohistochemical and flow cytometric study of 35 cases. Am J Surg Pathol 1991;15:529–533.
137. Wick MR, Berg LC, Hertz MI. Large cell carcinoma of the lung with neuroendocrine differentiation; a comparison with large cell "undifferentiated" pulmonary tumors. Am J Clin Pathol 1992;987:796–805.
138. Mooi WJ, Dewar A, Springall D, Polak JM, Addis BJ. Non-small cell lung carcinomas with neuroendocrine features: a light microscopic, immunohistochemical and ultrastructural study of 11 cases. Histopathology 1988;13: 329–337.
139. Bernard WG. The nature of the "oat-celled sarcoma" of the mediastinum. J Pathol Bacteriol 1926;29:241–244.
140. Gibbon JH Jr, Nealon TF Jr. Neoplasms of the lungs and trachea. In: Gibbon JH Jr, ed. Surgery of the chest. Philadelphia: Saunders, 1962:484.
141. Kreyberg L. Histological lung cancer types. Acta Pathol Microbiol Scand [A]1962;157(suppl):1.
142. World Health Organization. Histological typing of lung tumors. Geneva: World Health Organization, 1967.
143. The World Health Organization histological typing of lung tumors. 2d ed. Am J Clin Pathol 1982;77:123–136.
144. Hirsch FR, Matthews MJ, Aisner S, et al. Histopathologic classification of small cell lung cancer: changing concepts and terminology. Cancer 1988;62:973–977.

145. Yesner R. Classification of lung-cancer histology. N Engl J Med 1985;312:652–653.
146. Azzopardi JG. Oat-cell carcinoma of the bronchus. J Pathol Bacteriol 1959;78:513–519.
147. Yesner R. Small cell tumors of the lung. Am J Surg Pathol 1983;7:775–785.
148. Carter D. Small-cell carcinoma of the lung. Am J Surg Pathol 1983;7:787–795.
149. Stuart-Harris R, Boyer M, Greenberg M, Stevens S, Yung T. The histopathological classification of small cell lung cancer: application of the IASLC classification in 124 cases. Lung Cancer 1992;8:63–70.
150. Gazdar AF, Carney DN, Baylin SB, et al. Small cell carcinoma of the lung. Altered morphological, biological and biochemical characteristics in long term cultures and heterotransplanted tumors. Proc Am Assoc Cancer Res 1980;21:51.
151. Fushimi H, Kihui M, Morino H, et al. Detection of large cell component in small cell lung carcinoma by combined cytologic and histologic examinations and its clinical implications. Cancer (Philadelphia) 1992;70:599–605.
152. Sibley R, Rosai J, Froehlich W. A case for the panel: anemone cell tumor. Ultrastruct Pathol 1980;1:449–453.
153. Sobrinho-Simoes M, Nesland JM, Johannessen JV. The mystery of the anemone cell tumor. Ultrastruct Pathol 1985;8:3–4.
154. Taxy JB, Almanasser IT. Anemone cell (villiform) tumors: electron microscopy and immunohistochemistry of five cases. Ultrastruct Pathol 1984;7:143–150.
155. Wirt DP, Nagle RB, et al. The probable origin of an anemone cell tumor: metastatic transitional cell carcinoma producing HCG. Ultrastruct Pathol 1984;7:277–288.
156. Osborne BM, Mackay B, Butler JJ, et al. Large cell lymphoma with microvillus-like projections: an ultrastructural study. Am J Clin Pathol 1983;79:443–450.
157. Phillips JI, Murray J, Verhaart S. Squamous cell carcinoma with anemone cell features. Ultrastruct Pathol 1987;11: 47–52.
158. Colby TV, Koss MN, Travis WD. Tumors of the lower respiratory tract. Atlas of Tumor Pathology. Washington, DC: AFIP, 1995:310–311.
159. Colby TV, Koss MN, Travis WD. Tumors of the lower respiratory tract. Atlas of Tumor Pathology. Washington, DC: AFIP, 1995:313.
160. Chejfec G, Capella C, Socia E, et al. Amphicrine cells, dysplasias and neoplasias. Cancer 1985;56:2683–2690.
161. Hammar SP, Insalaco SJ, Lee RB, et al. Amphicrine carcinoma of the uterine cervix. Am J Surg Pathol 1992;97: 516–522.
162. Visscher DW, Zarbo RJ, Trojanowski JQ, Sakr W, Crissman JD. Neuroendocrine differentiation in poorly-differentiated lung carcinomas: a light microscopic and immunohistologic study. Mod Pathol 1990;3:508–512.
163. Linnoila RI, Mulshine JL, Steinberg SM, et al. Neuroendocrine differentiation in endocrine and nonendocrine lung carcinomas. Am J Clin Pathol 1988;90:641–652.
164. Loy TS, Darkow GVD, Quesenberry JT. Immunostaining in the diagnosis of pulmonary neuroendocrine carcinomas: an immunohistochemical study with ultrastructural correlations. Am J Surg Pathol 1995;19:173–182.
165. Schleusener JT, Tazelaar HD, Jung S, et al. Neuroendocrine differentiation is an independent prognostic factor in chemotherapy-treated non-small cell lung carcinoma. Cancer 1996;77:1284–1291.
166. Jiang S, Kameya T, Shoji M, et al. Large cell neuroendocrine carcinoma of the lung: a histologic and immunohistochemical study of 22 cases. Am J Surg Pathol 1998; 22:526–536.
167. Lyda MH, Weiss LM. Immunoreactivity for epithelial and neuroendocrine antibodies are useful in the differential diagnosis of lung carcinomas. Hum Pathol 2000;31: 980–987.
168. Agoff SN, Lamps LW, Philip AT, et al. Thyroid transcription factor-1 is expressed in extrapulmonary small cell carcinomas but not in other extrapulmonary neuroendocrine tumors. Mod Pathol 2000;13:238–242.
169. Cheuk W, Kwan MY, Suster S, et al. Immunostaining for thyroid transcription factor-1 and cytokeratin 20 aids in the distinction of small cell carcinoma from Merkel cell carcinoma, but not pulmonary from extrapulmonary small cell carcinomas. Arch Path Lab Med 2001;125:228–231.
170. Chang Y, Lee Y, Liao Y, et al. The utility and limitation of thyroid transcription factor-1 protein in primary and metastatic pulmonary neoplasms. Lung Cancer 2004;44: 149–157.
171. Rossi G, Marchioni A, Milani M, et al. TTF-1, cytokeratin 7, 34betaE12 and CD56/NCAM immunostaining in the subclassification of large cell carcinomas of the lung. Am J Clin Pathol 2004;122:884–893.
172. Zhang H, Cagle PT, Allen TC, et al. Distinction of pulmonary small cell carcinoma from poorly differentiated squamous cell carcinoma: an immunohistochemical approach. Mod Pathol 2005;18:111–118.
173. Onuki N, Wistuba II, Travis WD, et al. Genetic changes in the spectrum of neuroendocrine lung tumors. Cancer 1999;85:600–607.
174. Giard L, Zochbauer-Muller S, Virmani AK, et al. Genome-wide allelotyping of lung cancer identifies new regions of allelic loss, differences between small cell lung cancer and non-small cell lung cancer and loci clustering. Cancer Research 2000;60:4894–4906.
175. Hiroshima K, Iyoda A, Shibuya K, et al. Genetic alterations in early stage pulmonary large cell neuroendocrine carcinoma. Cancer 2004;100:1190–1198.
176. Peng W, Sano T, Oyama T, et al. Large cell neuroendocrine carcinoma of the lung: a comparison with large cell carcinoma with neuroendocrine morphology and small cell carcinoma. Lung Cancer 2005;47:225–233.
177. Vosika GJ. Large cell bronchogenic carcinoma: Prolonged disease-free survival following chemotherapy. JAMA 1979;241:594–595.
178. Gibbs FA. Lymphoma versus carcinoma. JAMA 1979; 242:514.
179. Vosika GJ. Large cell–small cell bronchogenic carcinoma. JAMA 1979;242:1259–1260.
180. Marchevsky AM, Gal AA, Shah S, et al. Morphometry confirms the presence of considerable nuclear size overlap between "small cells" and "large cells" in high-grade pulmonary neuroendocrine neoplasms. Am J Clin Pathol 2001;116:466–472.

181. Travis WD, Gal AA, Colby TV, et al. Reproducibility of neuroendocrine lung tumor classification. Hum Pathol 1998;29:272–279.
182. Lin O, Olgac S, Green I, et al. Immunohistochemical staining of cytologic smears with MIB-1 helps distinguish low-grade from high-grade neuroendocrine neoplasms. Am J Clin Pathol 2003;120:209–216.
183. Pelosi G, Rodriguez J, Viale G, et al. Typical and atypical carcinoid tumor overdiagnosed as small cell carcinoma on biopsy specimens: a major pitfall in the management of lung cancer patients. Am J Surg Pathol 2005;29:179–187.
184. Brambilla E. Basaloid carcinoma of the lung. In: Corrin B, ed. Pathology of lung tumors. New York: Churchill-Livingstone, 1997;71–82.
185. vanHengel P, vanGeffen F, Kazzaz BA, Heyerman HG. Atypical carcinoid presenting as mesothelioma. Neth J Med 2001;58:185–190.
186. Falconieri G, Zanconati F, Bossani R, DiBonito L. Small cell carcinoma of lung simulating pleural mesothelioma: report of 4 cases with autopsy confirmation. Path Res Pract 1995;191:1147–1152.
187. Hammar SP, Robb JA, Yokoo H, Dodson RF, Henderson D. Pseudomesotheliomatous lung cancer: a neoplasm frequently associated with asbestos exposure. (Submitted for publication).
188. Hurlimann J. Desmin and neural marker expression in mesothelial cells and mesotheliomas. Hum Pathol 1994; 25:753–757.
189. Chute CG, Greenberg ER, Baron J, Korson R, Baker J, Yates J. Presenting conditions of 1539 population-based lung cancer patients by cell type and stage in New Hampshire and Vermont. Cancer (Philadelphia) 1985;56:2107–2111.
190. Andersen HA, Bernatz PE. Extrathoracic manifestations of bronchogenic carcinoma. Med Clin North Am 1964; 48:921–931.
191. Mountain CF, Lukeman JM, Hammar S, et al. Lung cancer classification: the relationship of disease extent and cell type to survival in a trial population. J Surg Oncol 1987; 35:147–156.
192. Feld R, Rubinstein LV, Weisenberger TH, and the Lung Cancer Study Group. Sites of resected stage 1 non-small cell lung cancer: a guide for future studies. J Clin Oncol 1984;2:1352–1358.
193. Li W, Hammar SP, Jolly PC, et al. Unpredictable course of small cell undifferentiated lung carcinoma. J Thorac Cardiovasc Surg 1981;81:34–43.
194. Okike N, Bernatz PE, Woolner LB. Carcinoid tumors of the lung. Ann Thorac Surg 1976;22:270–275.
195. Brandt B, Heintz SE, Rose EF, Ehrenhaft JL. Bronchial carcinoid tumors. Ann Thorac Surg 1984;38:63–65.
196. McCaughan BC, Martini N, Bains MS. Bronchial carcinoids: review of 124 cases. J Thorac Cardiovasc Surg 1985;89:8–17.
197. Thunnissen FBJM, van Eijk J, Baak JPA, et al. Bronchopulmonary carcinoids and regional node metastases: a quantitative pathologic investigation. Am J Pathol 1988; 132:119–122.
198. Warren WH, Gould VE. Long-term follow-up of classical bronchial carcinoid tumors. Scand J Thor Cardiovase Surg 1990;24:125–130.
199. El-Naggar A, Ballance W, Abdul-Karim FW, et al. Typical and atypical bronchopulmonary carcinoids: a clinicopathologic and flow cytometric study. Am J Clin Pathol 1991; 95:828–834.
200. Yousem SA, Taylor SR. Typical and atypical carcinoid tumors of lung: a clinicopathologic and DNA analysis of 20 tumors. Mod Pathol 1990;3:502–507.
201. Bernstein C, McGoey J, Lertzman M. Recurrent bronchial carcinoid tumor. Chest 1989;95:693–694.
202. Greengard O, Head JF, Goldberg SI, Kirschner PA. Pulmonary carcinoid tumors: enzymic discriminants, growth rate and early age of inception. Cancer Res 1986; 46:2600–2605.
203. Vadasz P, Palffy G, Egervary M, Schaff Z. Diagnosis and treatment of bronchial carcinoid tumors: clinical and pathological review of 120 operated patients. Eur J Cardiothorac Surg 1993;7:8–11.
204. Ducrocq X, Thomas P, Massard G, et al. Operative risk and prognostic factors of typical bronchial carcinoid tumors. Ann Thorac Surg 1998;65:1410–1414.
205. Slodkowska J, Langfort R, Rudzinski P, Kupis W. Typical and atypical carcinoids—pathologic and clinical analysis of 77 cases. Pneumonol Alergol Pol 1998;66:297–303.
206. Travis WD, Rush W, Flieder DB, et al. Survival analysis of 200 pulmonary neuroendocrine tumors with clarification of criteria for atypical carcinoid and its separation from typical carcinoid. Am J Surg Pathol 1998;22:934–944.
207. Thomas CF Jr., Tazelaar HD, Jett JR. Typical and atypical pulmonary carcinoids: outcome in patients presenting with regional lymph node involvement. Chest 2001;119: 1143–1150.
208. Fink G, Krelbaum T, Yellin A, et al. Pulmonary carcinoid: presentation, diagnosis and outcome in 142 cases in Israel and review of 640 cases from the literature. Chest 2001; 119:1647–1651.
209. Schmid K, Birner P, Gravenhorst V, et al. Prognostic value of lymphatic and blood vessel invasion in neuroendocrine tumors of the lung. Am J Surg Pathol 2005;29: 324–328.
210. Yousem SA. Pulmonary carcinoid tumors and well differentiated neuroendocrine carcinomas: Is there room for atypical carcinoid? Am J Cln Pathol 1991;95:828–834.
211. Warren WH, Memoli VA, Jordan AG, Gould VE. Reevaluation of pulmonary neoplasms as small cell neuroendocrine carcinomas. Cancer 1990;65:1003–1010.
212. Larsimont D, Kiss R, deLaunoit Y, Melamed MR. Characterization of the morphonuclear features and DNA ploidy of typical and atypical carcinoids and small cell carcinomas of the lung. Am J Clin Pathol 1990;94:378–373.
213. Lequaglie C, Patriarca C, Cataldo I, Muscolino G, Preda F, Ravasi G. Prognosis of resected well-differentiated neuroendocrine carcinoma of the lung. Chest 1991;100: 1053–1056.
214. Memoli VA. Well-differentiated neuroendocrine carcinoma: a designation comes of age. Chest 1991;100:892.
215. Jackson-York GL, Davis GH, Warren WH, Gould VE, Memoli VA. Flow cytometric DNA content analysis in neuroendocrine carcinoma of the lung: correlation with

survival and histologic subtype. Cancer (Philadelphia) 1991;68:374–379.
216. Jung KJ, Lee KS, Han J, et al. Large cell neuroendocrine carcinoma of the lung: clinical, CT and pathologic findings in 11 patients. J Thorac Imaging 2001;16:156–162.
217. Mazieres J, Daste G, Molinier L, et al. Large cell neuroendocrine carcinoma of the lung: pathological study and clinical outcome of 18 resected cases. Lung Cancer 2002; 37:287–292.
218. Paci M, Cavazza A, Annessi V, et al. Large cell neuroendocrine carcinoma of the lung: a 10-year clinicopathologic retrospective study. Ann Thorac Surg 2004;77:1163–1167.
219. Doddoli C, Barlesi F, Chetaille B, et al. Large cell neuroendocrine carcinoma of the lung: an aggressive disease potentially treatable with surgery. Ann Thorac Surg 2004; 77:1168–1172.
220. Quoix E, Fraser R, Wolkove N, Finkelstein H, Kreisman H. Small cell lung cancer presenting as a solitary pulmonary nodule. Cancer (Philadelphia) 1990;66:577–582.
221. Kreisman H, Wolkove N, Quoix E. Small cell lung cancer presenting as a solitary pulmonary nodule. Chest 1992; 101:225–229.
222. Shepherd FA, Ginsberg R, Evans WK, Haddad R, Feld R, DeBoer G. "Very limited" small cell lung cancer: Results of nonsurgical treatment. Proc Am Soc Clin Oncol 1984; 3:223–228.
223. Gephardt GN, Grady KJ, Ahmad M, Tubbs RR, Mehta AC, Shepard KV. Peripheral small cell undifferentiated carcinoma of the lung: clinicopathologic features of 17 cases. Cancer (Philadelphia) 1988;61:1002–1008.
224. Fraire AE, Johnson EH, Yesner R, Zhang XB, Spjut HJ, Greenberg SD. Prognostic significance of histopathologic subtype and stage in small cell lung cancer. Hum Pathol 1992;23:520–528.
225. Bepler G, Neumann K, Holle R, Havemann K, Kalbfleisch H. Clinical relevance of histologic subtyping in small cell lung cancer. Cancer (Philadelphia) 1989;64:74–79.
226. Crown JPA, Chahinian AP, Jaffrey IS, Glidewell OJ, Kaneko M, Holland JR. Predictors of 5-year survival and curability in small cell lung cancer. Cancer (Philadelphia) 1990;66:382–386.
227. Albain KS, Crowley JJ, Livingston RB. Long-term survival and toxicity in small cell lung cancer: Expanded Southwest Oncology Group experience. Chest 1991;99: 1425–1432.
228. Oud PS, Pahlplatz MM, Beck LM, Wiersma-Van Tilburg A, Wagenaar SJ, Vooijs GP. Image and flow DNA cytometry of small cell carernoma of the lung. Cancer (Philadelphia) 1989;64:1304–1309.
229. Funa K, Steinholtz L, Nov E, Bergh J. Increased expression of N-*myc* in human small cell lung cancer biopsies predicts lack of response to chemotherapy. Am J Clin Pathol 1987; 88:216–220.
230. Copple B, Wright SE, Moatamed F. Electron microscopy in small cell lung carcinomas: clinical correlation. J Clin Oncol 1984;2:910–916.
231. Vollmer RT, Shelburne JD, Iglehart JD. Intercellular junctions and tumor stage in small cell carcinoma of the lung. Hum Pathol 1986;18:22–27.
232. Nicholson SA, Beasley MB, Brambilla E, et al. Small cell lung carcinoma (SCLC): a clinicopathologic study of 100 cases with surgical specimens. Am J Surg Pathol 2002;26: 1184–1197.
233. Garcia-Yuste M, Matilla JM, Alvarez-Gago T, et al. Prognostic factors in neuroendocrine lung tumors: a Spanish Multicenter Study. Ann Thorac Surg 2000;70:258–263.
234. Huang Q, Muzitansky A, Mark EJ. Pulmonary neuroendocrine carcinomas: a review of 234 cases and a statistical analysis of 50 cases treated at one institution using a simple clinicopathologic classification. Arch Pathol Lab Med 2002;126:545–553.
235. Skuladottir H, Hirsch FR, Hansen HH, Olsen JH. Pulmonary neuroendocrine tumors: incidence and prognosis of histological subtypes. A population-based study in Denmark. Lung Cancer 2002;37:127–135.

37 Sarcomatoid Carcinoma: Pleomorphic Carcinoma, Spindle Cell Carcinoma, Giant Cell Carcinoma, Carcinosarcoma, and Pulmonary Blastoma

Philip Hasleton

Definition

The 2004 World Health Organization (WHO) classification of lung tumors[1] defines sarcomatoid carcinomas as a group of poorly differentiated, non–small-cell lung carcinomas that contain a component of sarcoma or sarcoma-like (spindle or giant cell) differentiation. Five subgroups are currently recognized: pleomorphic carcinoma, spindle cell carcinoma, giant cell carcinoma, carcinosarcoma, and pulmonary blastoma. These entities have been considered separately previously. The WHO does not recommend the use of the terms *homologous* or *heterologous*, as proposed by Wick et al.[2] These tumors are rare, accounting for approximately between 0.3% and 1.3% of all lung malignancies.[1]

The unifying concept of sarcomatoid carcinoma (SC) embracing all, or most, of the above tumor types has some appeal *(vide infra)*. In such poorly differentiated tumors, there is a narrow dividing line between carcinoma and sarcoma. It will be seen later that some sarcomas may be focally cytokeratin-positive, whereas SC stains diffusely with this antibody. The 1999 WHO classification[3] proposal that cytokeratin positivity should be used for diagnosis in these undifferentiated carcinomas is no longer valid. The 2004 WHO[1] classification stated, "Expression of epithelial markers in the spindle and/or giant cell components of pleomorphic carcinoma is not required for diagnosis, so long as there is a component of squamous, adeno or large cell carcinoma." When pure spindle cell carcinomas fail to stain with an epithelial marker, such as multiple cytokeratin and epithelial membrane antigen (EMA) antibodies, differentiation from a primary or secondary sarcoma is difficult.

Nappi et al.[4] demonstrated both cytokeratin and smooth muscle actin (SMA) staining in their cases of pulmonary sarcomatoid carcinomas. There is probably a continuum, not only between some of the tumors clustered under SC, but also between carcinoma and sarcoma. The problem is the inclusion of pulmonary blastoma under the SC umbrella. There are several reasons for this. Biphasic pulmonary blastoma is seen in younger patients than the other groups of sarcomatoid carcinomas *(vide infra)*. It has a distinctive histologic pattern, with a well-differentiated fetal adenocarcinoma (WDFA) component or a glandular structure, which is very often neuroendocrine-positive and contains morules, amidst blastomatous tissue. Finally, there are β-catenin abnormalities, which appear specific for pulmonary blastoma.[5,6] Because this is the rarest entity of the group, further studies are needed to determine if pulmonary blastoma should be separated from SC.

The entities encompassed under SC are described separately in this chapter, since the data were extracted from the literature describing these rare tumors. In time, as more series of SC are described, it may be possible to "lump" all of them together.

Sarcomatoid Carcinoma (Pleomorphic Carcinoma, Spindle Cell Carcinoma)

A total of 14 studies described this entity,[4,7–19] with 314 cases. A few have included carcinosarcomas in their data and these have been separated. Just under half of the cases described were in two series.[12,13] A further 68 were described by Pelosi et al.,[9] and Nakajima et al.[15] Fishback et al.'s[12] study, based on Armed Forces Institute of Pathology (AFIP) material, set the standard for the concept of this entity.

Epidemiology

The male-to-female ratio in the published series was 4.4:1. The age range was 33 to 83 years, with a mean of 51.4 years; 91.3% of the patients smoked. In many cases the site of the tumor is not recorded, but where documented the right lung was affected in 58.9% of cases and the left in 41.1%. In the American series,[12] 65% of the tumors were located in the upper lobe, whereas in the European one[13] this figure fell to 48%. Most tumors were in the right upper lobe. The right lung predominance is most probably due to the increased area on that side.

Clinical and Radiologic Features

The clinical features are cough, dyspnea, hemoptysis, chest pain, fever, and metastatic disease; 18% of patients are asymptomatic and are detected on a routine chest radiograph.[12] Radiology shows irregularly marginated, often spiculated, masses, which in some cases show variable radiologic attenuation, thought to reflect intratumoral hemorrhage or necrosis. There is no dense calcification. In some cases the borders are relatively well circumscribed, but there is chest wall invasion (Fig. 37.1). Some tumors are hilar or midzonal but most are peripheral.[4]

Pathology

Macroscopic Appearance

In the literature, 91.5% of these tumors were peripheral and the remainder had endobronchial components or were entirely endobronchial. Sizes ranged from 1.0 to 30cm, with a mean of 7.8cm. The color was varyingly stated to be white, yellow, purple, or creamy, and the texture as gritty or mucoid (Fig. 37.2). Necrosis, which is likely to give rise to the yellow color and hemorrhage, was frequent. Some studies described circumscribed tumors and others described their cases as poorly circumscribed. Chest wall invasion was common.

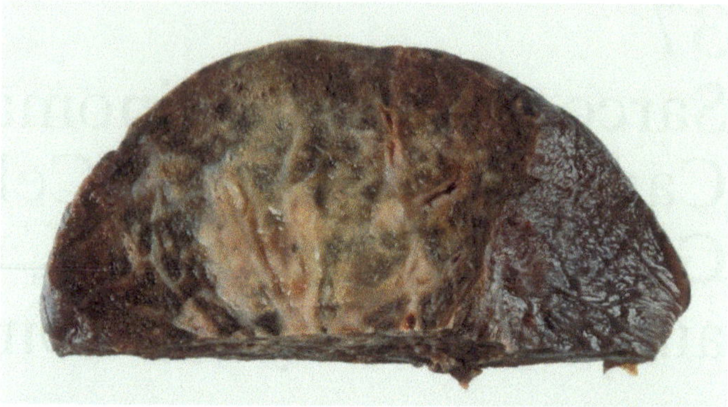

FIGURE 37.2. Cut surface of the lung showing an ill-defined tumour, with apparent spread along bronchial walls and lymphatics.

Histopathology

Fishback et al.[12] classified the histologic components as adenocarcinoma, spindle cell carcinoma, squamous cell carcinoma, large cell carcinoma, giant cell carcinoma, clear cell carcinoma, and small cell carcinoma. Essentially, pleomorphic carcinoma is a poorly differentiated, mainly, non–small-cell carcinoma, that is, squamous, adeno, or large cell carcinoma with spindle cells or giant cells, or a carcinoma consisting only of spindle or giant cells. The distribution of these cell types is given in Figure 37.3. These authors classified cases of giant cell carcinoma, when the tumor cells had abundant cytoplasm, containing multiple nuclei or a single large pleomorphic nucleus. The giant cell component had to be greater than 10% of the cell population for inclusion. Cases were classified as spindle cell carcinoma if greater than 10% of the tumor was composed of fusiform malignant cells. The spindle cells also had to react positively to one or more

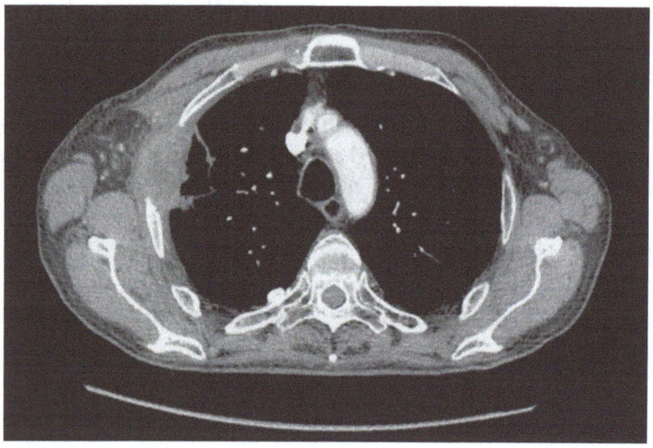

FIGURE 37.1. A pleomorphic carcinoma, with squamous differentiation and chest wall invasion, as evidenced by invasion of a rib. There is focal cystic change. (Courtesy of Dr. Paul Taylor, Consultant Radiologist, Manchester Royal Infirmary.)

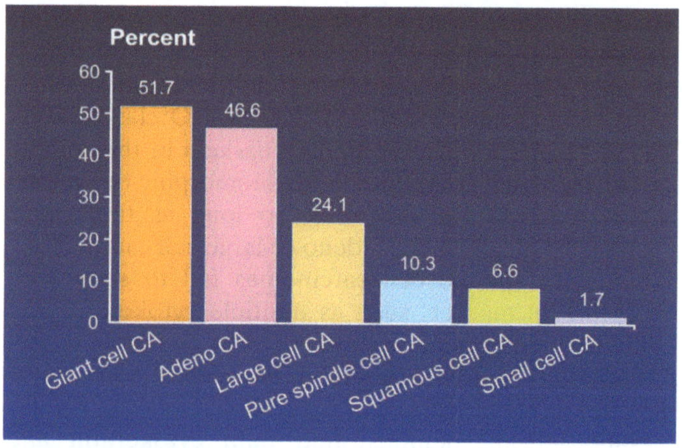

FIGURE 37.3. Other types of tumor components seen in a series of sarcomatoid carcinomas. (From Fishback et al.,[12] with permission from John Wiley & Sons.)

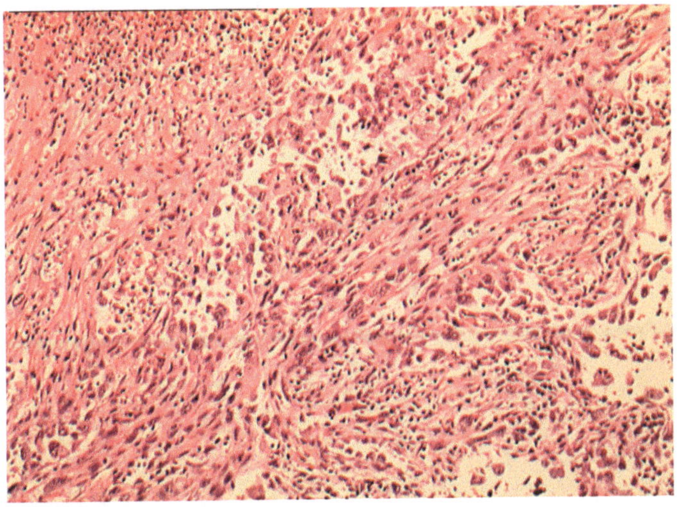

FIGURE 37.4. Sarcomatoid carcinoma with foci of poorly differentiated adenocarcinoma.

of three epithelial markers: keratin, carcinoembryonic antigen (CEA), and EMA. These authors used AE1/3, hybritech/monoclonal keratin (DAKO, Carpinteria, CA) at a dilution of 1:200. All their antibodies were produced by DAKO, a problem for comparison with other studies that did not use the same manufacturer.

Rossi et al.[13] included cases if they fulfilled one of the following histologic criteria:

1. The presence of at least 10% sarcomatoid (malignant spindle or giant cells)
2. True sarcomatous (malignant chondroid, osteoid, or muscle) components in an otherwise conventional, non–small-cell carcinoma
3. Immunoreactivity for at a least a broad-spectrum epithelial marker (MNF 116, CAM 5.2, AE1/AE3, or EMA) in the monophasic malignant, spindle, or giant cell neoplasm.

Their series included 4% carcinosarcomas and 1.3% pulmonary blastomas, which as can be seen from the above discussion confounds the classification of these tumors. Fishback et al.[12] excluded these entities.

Spindle cell carcinoma was present most often in association with giant cell and adenocarcinoma (Fig. 37.4) and less frequently with large cell and squamous cell carcinoma. Nappi et al.[4] demonstrated moderately to well-differentiated squamous cell carcinoma in 14 of 21 cases of spindle cell carcinoma. The most infrequent association was with small cell carcinoma in Fishback et al.'s[12] data. The malignant spindle cell component consisted of fusiform cells with eosinophilic cytoplasm (Fig. 37.5) The spindle cells varied from an epithelioid to cells with an innocuous and slender morphology. In some cases the ends of the spindle cells were surrounded by dense collagen, giving a fibroblastic appearance. The fusiform cells were arranged in sheets, fascicles, or occasionally a storiform pattern. In the Rossi et al.[13] study, some of the spindle cell carcinomas had moderately atypical nuclei and grew in long fascicles with a vague herringbone pattern, resembling fibrosarcoma. The authors did not identify a solely giant cell component in association with squamous cell carcinoma.

The nuclei varied with the cell type. Large epithelioid cells showed large nuclei with prominent nucleoli. Slender cells had smaller nuclei and often no nucleoli. Chromatin was usually vesicular or coarse and hyperchromatic; 53% of the tumors showed vascular invasion.

There was a mild to moderate inflammatory infiltrate of lymphocytes, amidst the spindle-shaped tumor cells. Rarely eosinophils were present. Rossi et al.[13] described cases with "appreciable" numbers of lymphocytes, plasma cells, and eosinophils, admixed with these spindle cell elements. They noted that such tumors mimicked an inflammatory pseudotumor or a follicular dendritic sarcoma. In one case atypical spindle cells dissected the alveolar septum associated with extravasated erythrocytes and superficially simulated angiosarcoma (Fig. 37.6).[20] (See also Fig. 35.29 in Chapter 35).

Wick et al.[7] described cases of inflammatory sarcomatoid carcinoma with lymphocytes and plasma cells (Fig. 37.7). The spindle cells had modest pleomorphism and a vesicular and storiform pattern, with a partially myxoid matrix. There was an irregular, spiculated interface with the surrounding lung and invasion of the bronchial submucosa. The nuclei in the tumor cells were relatively uniform and the spindle cells had up to two mitoses per 10 high power fields. There were no foci of squamous cell carcinoma. Inflammatory myofibroblastic tumor could not be differentiated from this entity on frozen section. Cytokeratin was positive in spindle cell carcinomas but negative in inflammatory myofibroblastic tumors, which are positive for smooth muscle actin (Fig. 37.8).

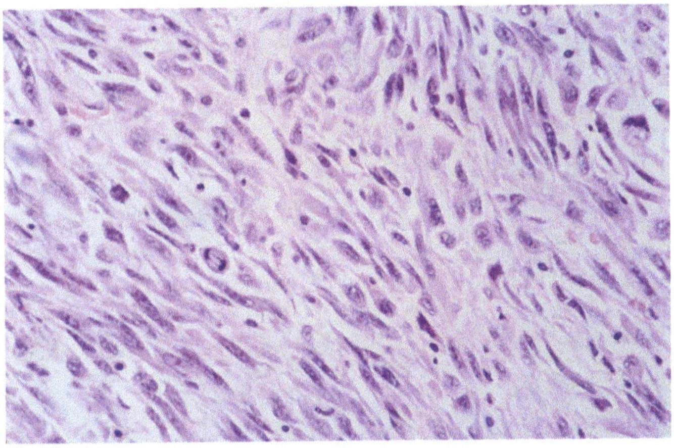

FIGURE 37.5. Sarcomatoid carcinoma with easily identified mitoses, focal nuclear pleomorphism and ample cytoplasm.

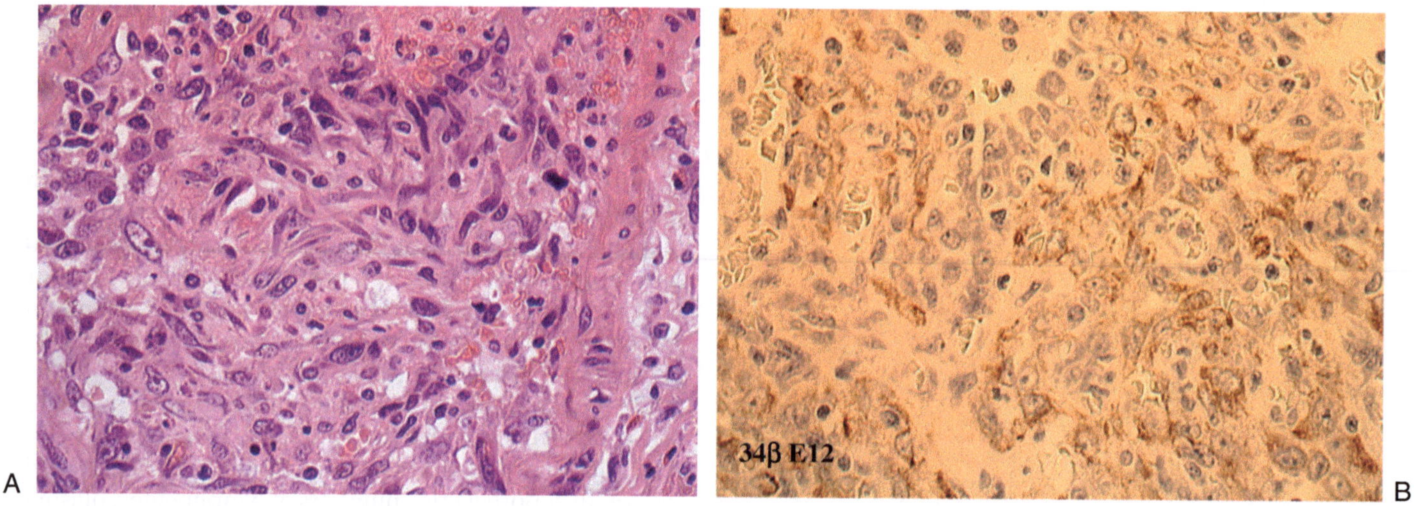

FIGURE 37.6. **(A)** Pseudoangiomatous carcinoma with intracytoplasmic vacuoles and some nuclear pleomorphism. **(B)** Pseudoangiomatous carcinoma staining positively with an anti-34βE12 antibody. Endothelial markers were negative. (Immunoperoxidase.)

The differentiation of spindle cell carcinoma from a desmoplastic stroma can be difficult. In many cases the fibrous stroma is bland (Fig. 37.9). If the cells are relatively plump and show nuclear atypia with mitoses, there is little problem. However, if there is abundant collagen associated with the spindle cells, it may be impossible to differentiate the spindle cell carcinoma from a desmoplastic stroma, based solely on light microscopy. Immunohistochemistry comes to the fore in such cases.

The giant cell component of pleomorphic carcinoma showed abundant cytoplasm in the tumor giant cells with multiple nuclei or a single large, pleomorphic nucleus (Fig. 37.10). The nucleus usually measured more than the diameter of four small resting lymphocytes. The nucleus was usually much larger, with bizarre shapes. They were hyperchromatic and had dense basophilic or vesicular chromatin. Nucleoli were frequent and prominent. There were occasional, eosinophilic, hyaline cytoplasmic globules in the tumor cells. The giant cells occasionally resembled syncytiotrophoblast or choriocarcinoma but no cases of giant cell carcinoma with osteoclast-like giant cells were seen. A solely giant cell component was never seen in association with squamous cell carcinoma in Rossi et al.'s[13] series.

Necrosis was common, including infarct-like tumor necrosis, neutrophilic microabscesses, and xanthogranulomatous changes with cholesterol clefts, associated with a dense acute inflammatory infiltrate.

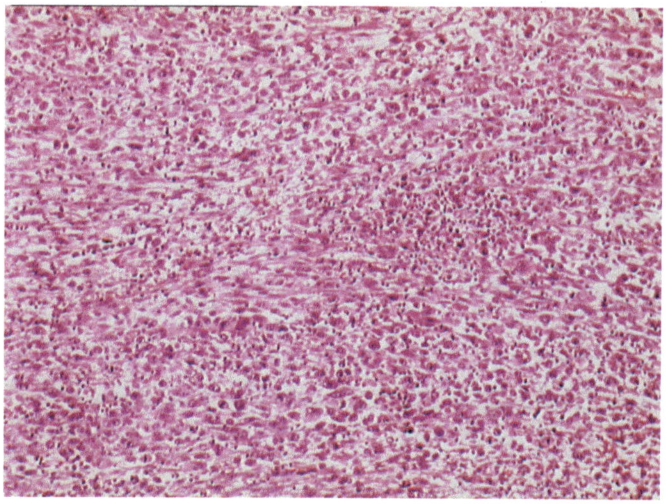

FIGURE 37.7. Sarcomatoid carcinoma with a marked inflammatory component.

Immunohistochemistry

Cytokeratins, including AE1/3, MAK–6, CAM 5.2, and MNF 116, were positive in nearly all of the cases documented. If one cytokeratin, such as AE1/3, was negative (it was positive in 36 of 37 of the Fishback series), then other markers, such as CEA or EMA, were positive. Vimentin was often positive but this varied between series. Desmin and S-100 were often negative, but in some series less than 5% of the cells were positive for SMA.[9] Neuroendocrine markers, such as chromogranin and synaptophysin, were negative.

Thyroid transcription factor-1 (TTF-1) was positive in 35% (seven of 20 cases) of pure spindle carcinoma or giant cell carcinomas. The carcinomatous component of pleomorphic carcinomas showed immunoreactivity for TTF-1 in 30 of 51 cases (58.8%) (12 of 14 adenocarcinomas, 13 of 18 large cell, four of five adenocarcinomas/large cell, and one of two adenosquamous). This antibody was negative in squamous cell carcinomas.[13] In only three

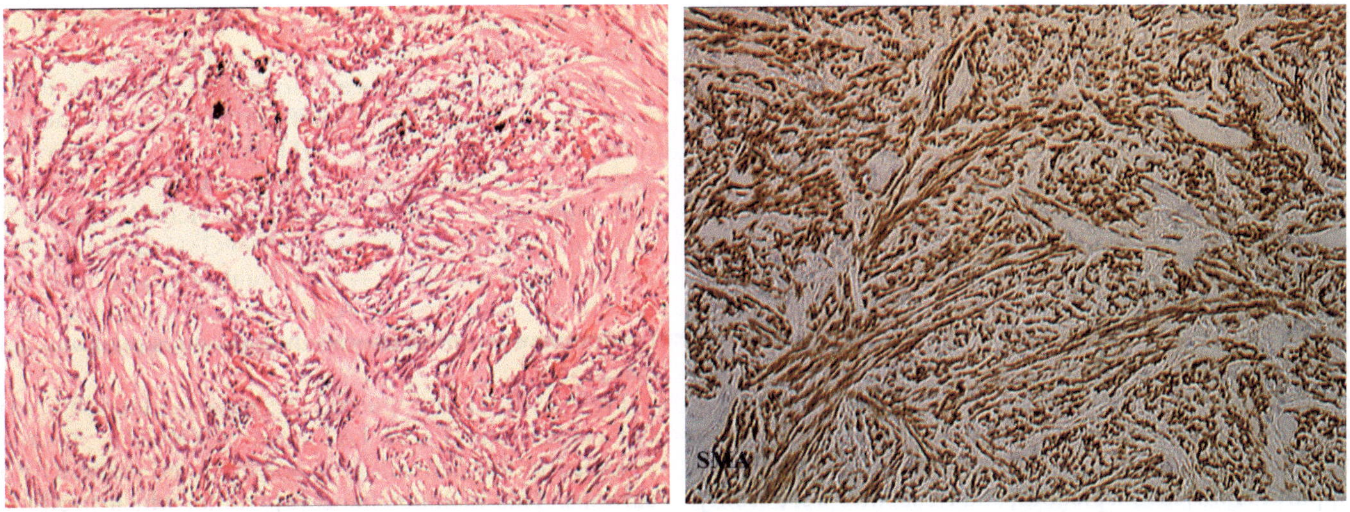

A B

FIGURE 37.8. **(A)** Inflammatory myofibroblastic tumor with bland collagen and an intraalveolar component. **(B)** Another area of the tumour in **A** stained by immunoperoxidase with an anti–smooth muscle actin antibody. Cytokeratin stains were negative.

pleomorphic carcinomas with an adenocarcinomatous component did the associated malignant spindle cells not react with TTF-1. The authors used TTF-1 made by DAKO in a 1:100 dilution.

The carcinomatous components in pleomorphic carcinomas reacted moderately with CK7 in 39 of 51 (76.5%) of cases, whereas spindle and/or giant cells showed positive staining in 32 (62.7%) cases. In tumors with a CK7-negative epithelial component, the sarcomatoid cells were also negative. Positive staining for CK7 in the epithelial component was seen in all pleomorphic carcinomas containing adenocarcinoma. The corresponding sarcomatoid component was positive in all but two cases.

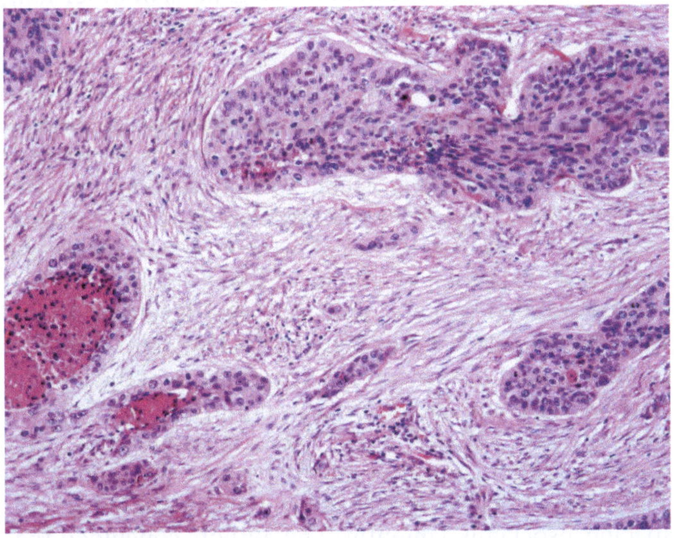

FIGURE 37.9. Non–small-cell carcinoma, which is sharply demarcated from a bland stroma, unlike a sarcomatoid carcinoma, where both elements merge.

Five out of 12 (41.7%) pleomorphic carcinomas with a squamous component were weakly positive in the latter cells. Large cell carcinomatous foci in sarcomatoid carcinoma showed positivity, as did the pleomorphic carcinomatous component. Our experience is that TTF-1 is almost invariably negative in SC.[21] This is mirrored by Lucas et al.,[22] who, using immunohistochemistry, could not distinguish sarcomatoid mesothelioma from SC with pleural invasion.

SP-A, a monoclonal antibody that recognizes 34 to 37 kDa and 62 kDa human surfactant apoproteins located on normal and hyperplastic type II pneumocytes, was negative in carcinomas composed only of spindle or giant cells[13]; 20 of 41 pleomorphic carcinomas with an epithelial component were positive for SP-A, especially in adenocarcinomas (12 of 14). Moderate positivity was found in

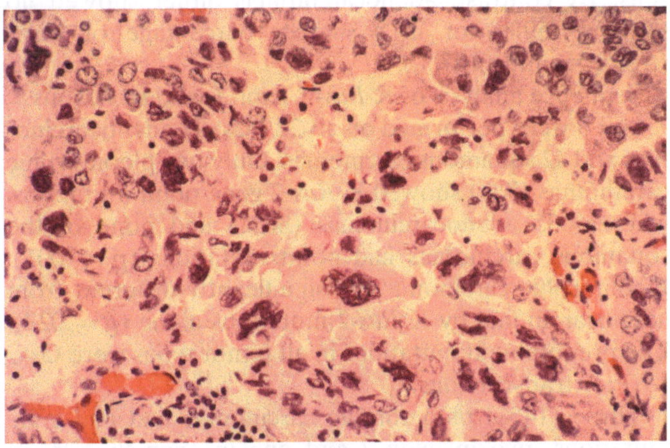

FIGURE 37.10. Giant cell carcinoma focus in a sarcomatoid carcinoma. No sarcomatoid elements are seen in this image.

the sarcomatoid components in only three pleomorphic carcinomas associated with adenocarcinoma.[13]

Electron Microscopy

Electron microscopic studies have been few.[4,8,14,16] In spindle cell carcinoma, tumor cells have a uniform morphology with fusiform, elongated shapes admixed with plump, round cells. The cells were cohesive and showed scant fibrous tissue. The nuclei were large with irregular contours and showed occasional enfolding of the nuclear membrane. There were dense aggregates of intermediate-sized filaments (8 to 12 nm), which condensed along cell borders giving rise to well-developed tonofilaments.[16] Rough endoplasmic reticulum and Golgi apparatus was inconspicuous, and lysosomes were scanty. The intercellular attachments were desmosomal in type, but primitive and immature cell junctions were also present. Ro et al.'s[8] study also found a moderate number of mitochondria. In their cases there was cytokeratin positivity in the sarcomatoid components. In one of Humphrey et al.'s[14] cases, Z bands and M lines were seen in rhabdomyoblastic cytoplasm. These findings are not representative of sarcomatoid carcinomas, since many of Fishback et al.'s [12] cases had an adenocarcinomatous component.

Genetic Studies in Pleomorphic Carcinoma

There have been few genetic studies of this tumor, probably due to its rarity.[10,23] A 1996 study evaluated the mutation rate of K-*Ras*-2 and *p53* genes.[23] *p53* staining showed only weak positivity in 86% of pleomorphic carcinomas, whereas staining was strong in 52% of squamous carcinomas and 27% of adenocarcinomas. In the pleomorphic carcinomas (PCs), nuclear staining was usually present in both spindle and giant cells, but in three cases it was limited to the giant cells. By contrast, adenocarcinomas either showed no staining (59%) or in a smaller percentage of cases strong staining (27%).

Sequence analysis of K-*Ras*-2, exon 1, and *p53* exons 5, 7, and 8 were performed on all 22 PCs; 97 adenocarcinomas and 42 squamous carcinomas. Only two pleomorphic carcinomas (9%) showed K-*Ras*-2 gene point mutations, whereas 35 adenocarcinomas (36%) and none of the squamous carcinomas had point mutations ($p < .001$). Pleomorphic carcinoma was significantly different from adenocarcinoma by K-*Ras*-2 mutations alone ($p = .027$). The predominant mutations in all tumor types were G:C → T:A transversions.

Three (14%) pleomorphic carcinomas had *p53* gene mutations, two in exon 7 and one in exon 8; 27% of adenocarcinomas were mutated, and 10 of 13 were in exon 8; 18 squamous cell carcinomas (43%) were mutated, and 11 of these mutations were also on exon 8. The spectrum of mutations between pleomorphic carcinoma on the one hand and adenocarcinoma and squamous carcinoma on the other, were significantly different, when all tumors were compared ($p < .01$). When pleomorphic and squamous carcinomas were compared, near significance was achieved ($p = .093$). Two of the pleomorphic carcinoma mutations were of the A:T → G:C transition type and the third was G:C → A:T transition type. This was in contrast to G:C → T:A transversion mutations, seen predominantly in adenocarcinoma and squamous cell carcinoma.

Przygodzki et al.[10] studied the tumor susceptibility of the cytochrome P-450 1A1 gene (*CYP1A1*), which is involved in the activation of polycyclic aromatic hydrocarbons. This includes benzo[*a*]pyrene, which produces DNA-damaging epoxides that lead to G:C → T:A point mutations. Isoleucine-valine and valine-valine genotypes of the *CYP1A1* exon 7 polymorphism are associated with the increased risk of lung cancer in certain populations. There are several polymorphisms at the *CYP1A1* gene. The polymorphism in exon 7, at codon 462 (*CYP1A1*2*), alters the protein of its heme-binding region by replacing an isoleucine with a valine.[24]

Przygodzki et al.'s [10] study utilized the Fishback[12] classification. The frequency of isoleucine/valine heterozygotes in pleomorphic carcinoma is markedly greater than seen among the baseline white population ($p < .001$), as well as compared with other studies of adenocarcinoma, large cell, or squamous cell carcinomas of the lung.[23,25] This heterozygote genotype of the *CYP1A1* gene occurred in 76% of pleomorphic carcinomas. These results suggest that epoxide-adduct–mediated carcinogenesis may be more important in the pathogenesis of pleomorphic carcinoma than in the genesis of other lung cancers. Unfortunately, we have no data on the other subsets of SC.

The epithelial malignant component of pleomorphic carcinoma consistently showed upregulation of the cell cycle inhibitors, $p21^{Waf1}$ and $p27^{Kip1}$, and of the tumor suppressor gene *FHIT*, a molecule related to apoptosis. The pleomorphic component predominantly expressed mesenchymal cytoskeletal proteins (vimentin, smooth muscle actin, and occasionally desmin) as well as fascin, a cell motility-related protein, and increased levels of microvascular density.[9] Fascin is a 55-kDa actin-bundling protein that induces membrane protrusions at the leading edge of cells and increases cell motility of normal and transformed epithelial cells.[26–30] Fascin immunoreactivity was independent of tumor growth pattern, size, and stage. The mesenchymal cytoskeletal proteins identified are not specific, especially vimentin. The authors concluded that epithelial and sarcomatoid cells in pleomorphic carcinoma are differently regulated at the cellular level. They were studying the tumor at one moment of time (i.e., resection), and it is not possible to say if cells had gained or lost phenotypes. They could not exclude that some of the molecules studied were not downstream covariants, and that other genes were involved in the genesis of these tumors. It is difficult to marry this explanation with the ultrastructural finding of coexpression of tono- and myofilaments in the same cell, as well as the monoclonal nature of some of the subgroups of SC, as detailed in the relevant sections below.

Metastatic Sites

The common metastatic sites, when documented in SC, are lymph nodes; pleura, where it may mimic mesothelioma[22]; chest wall; diaphragm; and as a perinephric mass. In Fishback et al.'s[12] series, 11.6% of cases had metastases at diagnosis and a further 30% at death.

Prognostic Factors and Survival

Stage is a critical factor in determining survival[12,13] (Fig. 37.11). For such a poorly differentiated carcinoma, most cases (59.9%) were stage I, 16.3% of cases were stage II, 19.4% were stage III, and 4.4% were stage IV. Any tumor greater than stage I or greater than 5 cm in diameter[12] had a poor prognosis (Table 37.1). Nakajima et al.[15] found the following were adverse factors: stage II or greater, lymph node metastases, tumor size greater than 5 cm in diameter, and pleural invasion. Between 65.3% and 77% of patients were dead in 7 days to 6 years.[12,13]

The mean survival in stage I was 31 months, in stage II was 10.5 months, and in stage III was 9 months.[13] In Fishback et al.'s[12] series, 12% of stage I patients survived at least 12 years. Survival was better after lobectomy and radiotherapy (13.4 months) than following extended wedge resections, after which all patients were dead in a mean of 5.3 months,[4] but the number of cases studied was small. The mean survival determined from the literature was 19.6 months but survival figures are difficult to interpret as different treatments have been given.

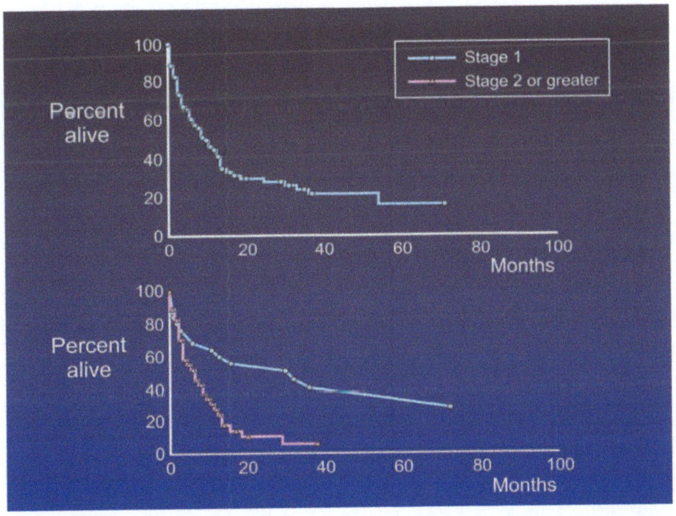

FIGURE 37.11. Survival in a series of pleomorphic carcinomas. (From Fishback et al.,[12] with permission from John Wiley & Sons.)

TABLE 37.1. Relative risk of decreased survival in pleomorphic carcinoma

Factor	*p*-value	Relative risk
Univariate Cox model results		
Size >5 cm	.0248	2.079
Stage >1	.0062	2.435
Metastases	.0039	3.263
N > 0	.0019	3.181
Multivariate Cox model results		
N > 0	.0057	3.058

Source: Fishback et al.,[12] with permission from John Wiley & Sons.

Giant Cell Carcinoma

A total of 19 studies were found in the literature describing this entity.[31–49] Some cases in the Fishback et al.[12] series are not included in this section.

Epidemiology

There were 166 cases with a male-to-female ratio of 5.9:1, which is a larger male ratio than in SC, but more cases of the latter entity have been described. The age range was 21 to 82 years, with a mean of 54.9 years, similar to SC. Where smoking is mentioned, 59.9% of patients smoked; this tumor has been related to smoking.[50]

Clinical and Radiologic Findings

The symptoms related to giant cell carcinoma are hemoptysis, cough, weakness, weight loss, anemia, hemiplegia, metastases, uremia due to ureteric involvement, fever, dyspnea, pleural effusion, and back pain. Some cases were asymptomatic but this was a smaller number than seen in SC. Rare cases were described with increased breast tenderness due to β-human chorionic gonadotropin (β HCG) production *(vide infra)*.[49] Leukocytosis was relatively common, and one case presented with a perforated jejunum.[37]

Radiologically the lesions were either oval or round, with a smooth contour and sharply defined borders. A few cases had lobar consolidation, cavitation, or an associated pleural effusion. Hilar or paratracheal metastases were apparent on x-ray in eight of 14 patients.[42]

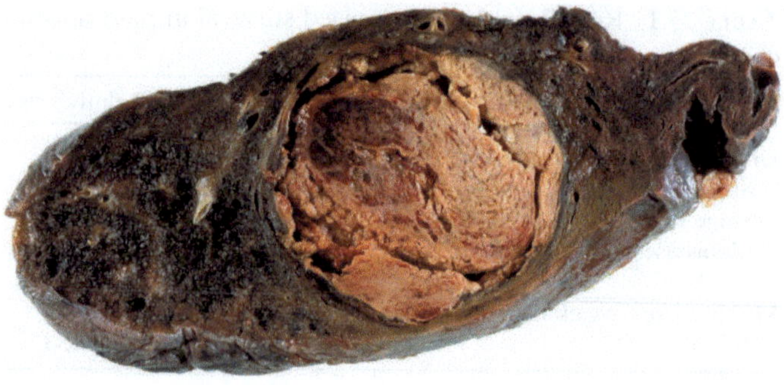

FIGURE 37.12. Macroscopic specimen of a giant cell carcinoma, as a well-defined, focally hemorrhagic and necrotic tumor.

Pathology

Macroscopic Appearance

The disease was commoner in the right lung than in the left, with a ratio of 1.3:1. It was more frequent in the upper than the lower lobes, by a ratio of 2.3:1. One case presented as multiple nodules.[39] The disease was more commonly peripheral. Tumor size ranged from 1.3 to 14cm, with a mean of 6.4cm. The colors varied, reflecting the presence of necrosis or hemorrhage. The commonest color described is gray. When necrosis or hemorrhage was present, the tumor was yellow, tan, or red (Fig. 37.12). Some cases showed cavitation.

Histopathology

There are relatively few series describing pure giant cell carcinomas, in keeping with the Fishback et al.[12] and Rossi et al.[13] papers, where in the latter only three of 75 cases were pure giant cell carcinoma. Fishback et al. described only two cases (2.1%) of pure giant cell carcinoma. Addis et al.[44] found that only one of 10 cases were pure giant cell. Another had mixtures of giant and spindle cell elements and the remaining eight had giant cell carcinoma and adenocarcinoma. These are now better classified as pleomorphic carcinomas.

The giant cells varied from 50 to 120μm in diameter with prominent nucleoli (Fig. 37.13).[34] They were multinucleated cells with five to 50 nuclei and had varying patterns, being horseshoe, central, or with no definite nuclear chromatin distribution. Some papers have described mitoses, which vary from two to 28/high power fields (HPFs), with a mean of eight.[48]

The cytoplasm is foamy or deeply eosinophilic and sometimes finely vacuolated. Necrosis can be prominent. A prominent feature is the discohesive nature of the giant cells, which often grow inside alveoli and infiltrate lymphatics, blood vessels, or nodes. Guillan et al.[34] described pseudosarcomatous cells but provided little evidence as to their percentage. This series is probably describing SC, rather than pure giant cell carcinoma. The validity of their study is further doubted by their inclusion of cases with foci of WDFA or keratinization. Some tumor cells resembled rhabdomyoblasts, lipoblasts, or osteoclasts, but histochemical stains failed to reveal the cell of origin, apart from Sudan IV.[31] However, most of Nash and Stout's cases were postmortem, and some of the cells could have been lipid-laden macrophages, related to the tumor necrosis or bronchial obstruction.[34]

A distinctive feature of this tumor is neutrophil and erythrocyte phagocytosis and emperipolesis (Fig. 37.13). The phagocytic activity of giant cell carcinoma probably represents tumor cell–tumor cell emperipolesis or leukocyte–tumor emperipolesis.[51,52] Emperipolesis means "inside round-about wandering."[52] The "inner" cell appears to be in the vacuole of the "outer" cell, and a permanent connection of the vacuole with the external membrane may or may not be present.[51]

Immunohistochemistry

Few studies describe the immunohistochemistry, since most predate the introduction of this technique and the tumor is very rare.

Prasad et al.[48] described cytokeratin-negativity in the giant cells, though vimentin was positive in all cases. CD68 was positive in the giant cells and they confirmed the lack of epithelial differentiation by electron microscopy. Addis et al.[44] described peripheral CAM 5.2 positivity in the giant and other cells in two of six cases. Epithelial membrane antigen was negative in the giant cells, and there was strong paranuclear vimentin staining in giant and other cells. Attanoos et al.[47] showed CEA was positive and membranous in giant cell carcinoma, and β-HCG was seen in 26% of cases. In a parallel series of 100 cases

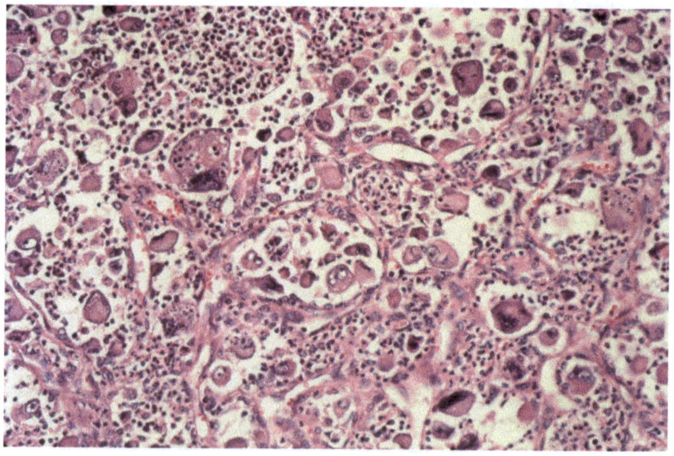

FIGURE 37.13. Giant cell carcinoma with focal cells showing emperipolesis. There is much inflammation throughout the image.

of squamous and adenocarcinomas, the authors noted that 36% of adenocarcinomas showed β-HCG positivity. None of their patients had symptoms related to the excess β-HCG production, such as gynecomastia or testicular atrophy. There was no association in their series between β-HCG–positive cells and extent of the giant cell formation, tumor stage, or survival.

Electron Microscopy

Electron microscopy findings are described in several studies.[39,40,44,45] Tumor giant cells had bizarre nuclear notching. Nucleoli were prominent and occasional nuclear inclusions were seen. Aggregations of several pairs of centrioles were frequent, occasionally associated with aggregates of irregular, dense threads or granules. Mitochondria were abundant, and in some cases there were electron-dense, membrane-bound structures, up to several hundred nanometers in size. Tonofilament bundles were present in varying numbers of cases. Addis et al.[44] demonstrated peripheral CAM 5.2 positivity, and four of their six cases had large aggregates of filaments, arranged in closely packed skeins. These were located close to the nucleus, correlating with the strong paranuclear vimentin staining. Fine background fibrils were seen in most cases. Junctional contacts between cells and basement membrane were identified. Some authors did not detect or mention microvilli,[39,45] but others did.[44] Desmosomes were seen in varying degrees of differentiation.

Genetic Studies in Giant Cell Carcinoma

There is a case report of a rearranged *c-myc* gene in a giant cell carcinoma of lung. Unfortunately, there is no description of the pathology, so it is impossible to determine if this is a "pure" giant cell carcinoma. The rearrangement was found in the region about 6 kilobase pairs upstream of the *c-myc* gene. The breakpoint was joined to a sequence carrying a Long interspersed element-1 (Line 1 [L1]) family member, located on chromosome 8. A region carrying an L1 family member located on chromosome 8 was joined to the *c-myc* gene through interstitial deletion, inversion, or translocation within the chromosome.[53]

Metastatic Sites

Metastases, in descending order of frequency, are to the contralateral lung, parietal pleura, adrenals, regional lymph nodes, diaphragm, kidneys, soft tissue, liver, bone, myocardium, pericardium, brain (including cerebellum), spinal cord, spleen, and thyroid.[34] Mesenteric, hepatic, supraclavicular and inguinal nodes may be involved, as well as ovaries, fallopian tubes, retroperitoneum, subcutis, pituitary, bowel, and testes.[31,35] This can be a rapidly growing tumor, with chest wall metastases doubling in size every 36 hours.[35]

Prognosis

The prognosis varied according to the treatment, but favorable growth patterns in a small series were absence of lymphovascular permeation, a size of 3 cm or less, a lymphoplasmacytic reaction, and stages I and II.[45,46] Not all patients behaved predictably; one of nine died 6½ years after local irradiation. A patient with adrenal metastases, detected 2 years postresection, was alive 8 years later.[48] This author documented four patients who were alive and well with no evidence of disease at periods between 0.5 and 11 years.

The survival time ranged from 1 to 116 months, with an average of 26 months in the published papers. Ginsberg et al.[46] described cases with stages I or II with no disease, 3 to 13 months postsurgery, and five of 16 (31.3%) were alive and well, with no disease, at periods ranging from 20 to 116 months. The largest series[47] documented 25 cases in stage I, 12 in stage II, 20 in stage III, and nine in stage IV.

Carcinosarcoma

There are few descriptions of this entity.[54–60] A 1985 retrospective study of 48 cases described, in most of the cases, pleomorphic carcinoma.[55] In this study the sentinel case was a needle biopsy, without immunohistochemistry. The literature review described eight true carcinosarcomas, two with cartilage, four with osteoid, and one each with osteosarcoma or rhabdomyosarcomatous foci. There was one blastoma.

The largest recent series is that of Koss et al.,[56] who describe 66 cases and compare this entity with some of the same cases of pleomorphic carcinoma studied by Fishback et al.[12]

Epidemiology

The male-to-female ratio is 4.8:1. The age range is 21 to 84 years, with a mean of 68.2 years. In the papers studied, 57 of 79 patients (72.2%) smoked, but many of the smoking histories were unavailable. One patient was a retired builder with no significant asbestos exposure.[57] Another had worked as a welder,[59] and one had associated asbestosis.[58]

Clinical and Radiologic Findings

The symptoms were cough (39% of patients), chest pain (26%), hemoptysis (18%), weight loss (5%), pneumonia

(5%), dyspnea (12%), and malaise (2%). Occasional clinical features included empyema, fever, pathologic fractures of the right hip and left ninth rib, and one patient who presented with cerebral metastases. A third of the patients in Koss et al.'s[56] series were asymptomatic. The anatomic localization was limited, but the right upper lobe was involved in five cases, the right middle lobe in three, the right lower lobe in seven, the left upper lobe in four, and the left lower lobe in three.

Koss et al. describe 60% of the tumors in the upper and 40% in the lower lobe; 34% were central tumors and 38% peripheral. In the remaining cases it was difficult to specify the site of origin. In other papers, four tumors were central, six peripheral, and two were mixed.

Chest radiographs usually showed a well-demarcated, lobulated solitary mass, as well as other nodules in a few cases. Computed tomography (CT) scan reflects these findings, as well as showing focal calcification and occasionally a pleural effusion.[56,57,61] Unlike SC, chest wall invasion is not a feature of the cases described.

Pathology

Macroscopic Appearance

These tumors vary in size from 2 to 16cm, with a mean of 5.9cm. The colors range from white to gray, or tan/red with hemorrhagic or yellow foci. The latter colors reflect hemorrhage and necrosis. They are described as firm, rubbery, or fleshy and may cavitate. The large size of some of the tumors or lack of information about location prevented accurate identification as to whether they were endobronchial or peripheral in 42% of cases. Where these data were available, 16 of 38 (42%) were endobronchial and 22 of 38 (58%) were peripheral.[56] The few endobronchial lesions were accurately described as "cast-like within airways, cauliflower or polypoid." Bronchial involvement, the authors note, could be due to secondary invasion of the major airways.

Histopathology

Koss et al.[56] excluded from their series 24 cases that had no differentiation regarding bone, cartilage, or skeletal muscle, as well as cases with no carcinoma (1) or too few slides for evaluation (2). One case was reclassified as a biphasic synovial sarcoma.

These authors also studied 33 cases of SC. For inclusion in this group, the spindle cell population had to be greater or equal to 25% to 50% of the mesenchymal cell population. Fifteen cases had a giant cell component but it was always less than 25% of the tumor population. Cases of PC with a predominance of giant cells or pure spindle cell carcinoma without a differentiated carcinomatous component were omitted. Carcinomatous components were often seen at the periphery of the tumor. The most frequent type of carcinoma in carcinosarcoma was squamous (47% of cases), whereas in their study of PC cases and also the study of Fishback et al.,[12] adenocarcinoma was commonest. Adenocarcinoma was seen in 32% of carcinosarcomas, while the next commonest epithelial components were adenosquamous (20%) and large cell carcinoma (1%), respectively. Koss et al.[56] stress the problem of sampling. Where squamous carcinoma was present, foci of clear cell and basaloid carcinoma were described. Adenocarcinoma also had clear cells (one case) and a bronchioloalveolar pattern (three cases) at the tumor periphery. No morules were seen in the 18% of cases that had fetal type epithelium. None of these cases met the authors' criteria for a blastoma, because there were no areas of WDFA or mesenchyme.

This series also described malignant bone (in 46% of cases) (Fig. 37.14), cartilage (64%) (Fig. 37.15), and skeletal muscle (53%). The commonest solitary mesenchymal components were rhabdomyoblasts. Seventeen cases (26%) had only this component as the sarcomatous focus. Many tumors (51%) had more than one differentiated stromal component. In addition, there was a background of less differentiated spindle cell, round cell, myxosarcoma, and hemangiopericytomatous sarcoma in many cases. Malignant, osteoclast-like giant cells were seen in 11 cases. Pleomorphic tumor giant cells were seen in several cases, with a storiform pattern in one. Malignant stroma formed the bulk of carcinosarcomas, and only small foci of carcinoma were seen. In other cases the epithelial cells showed nuclear pleomorphism.

An unusual case of SC in a 52-year-old woman, where the sarcomatous component was rhabdomyosarcoma and the carcinomatous component was an atypical carcinoid, has been described.[62] The sarcomatous compo-

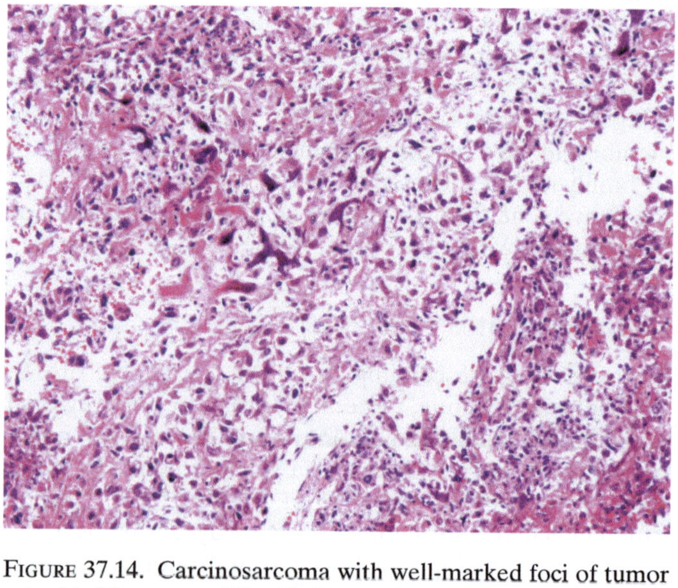

FIGURE 37.14. Carcinosarcoma with well-marked foci of tumor osteoid. (Courtesy of Dr. K. Kerr, Aberdeen, Scotland.)

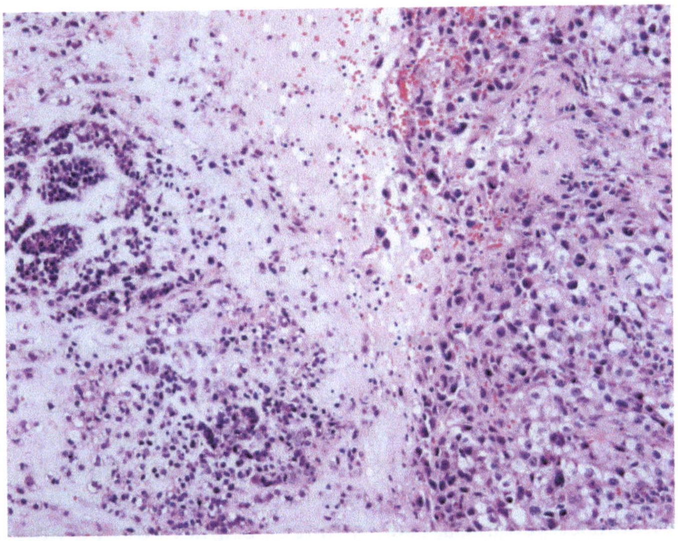

FIGURE 37.15. Carcinosarcoma with well-marked foci of tumor chondroid on the left and pleomorphic carcinoma on the right. (Courtesy of Dr. K. Kerr, Aberdeen, Scotland.)

nent was strongly positive for myoglobin. Myofibrils and Z band formation were identified in the sarcomatous component.

Immunohistochemistry

In all their cases cytokeratin was positive in the epithelial component and in 28% of the stromal component. S-100, desmin, actin, and myoglobin were negative in the epithelial component, but all these antibodies were identified in the stromal component, S-100 (67% of cases) and desmin (56%) being the commonest, while actin (54%) and myoglobin (42%) were less commonly expressed. In every case with rhabdomyoblasts, at least one muscle marker was positive. In five cases with rhabdomyoblasts on hematoxylin and eosin (H&E)-stained sections, there was insufficient material for immunohistochemistry but cross-striations were shown in each case.

Wick et al.,[2] by means of double-labeling in two of their cases, showed that mesenchymal cells simultaneously demonstrated rhabdomyoblastic and cytokeratin expression. In Koss et al.'s[56] series the spindle cell elements were cytokeratin-negative, vimentin-positive. and negative for desmin and smooth muscle actin. Ishida et al.[54] described EMA and CEA positivity in all the carcinomatous components; in the sarcomatous, two of eight were CEA-positive and three of eight vimentin-positive. The authors did not utilize rhabdomyoblastic markers.

Genetic Studies

Dacic et al.[60] noted extensive allelic loss, especially 3b, 5q, and 17p. The highest frequencies for loss of heterozygosity (LOH) were in 3p 26.1 (OGG1), 5q 21 (APCMCC), and 17p 13 (p53) in both epithelial and mesenchymal components. In one of six cases, both tumor components showed identical patterns of allelic loss or retention of all informative microsatellite markers. Four of the six cases showed one or two (two of six cases) additional allelic losses, more commonly in the mesenchymal component, that were not present in the epithelium. In contrast, allelic losses within epithelial components, not present in the mesenchymal foci, were seen in only one case. The homogeneity of allelic loss in both epithelial and mesenchymal components suggested a monoclonal origin of these two morphogenetically distinct elements. This is due to either continuous genetic progression or genetic diversion, during clonal evolution of these foci.

Metastatic Sites

The sites involved by metastases were lymph nodes; kidney; bone, including the ribs, femur, scapula, tibia, humerus, and thorax; liver; lung; spleen; gastrointestinal tract[56]; and brain.[58] In 25 of 66 of Koss et al.'s[56] cases, lymph nodes were the commonest metastatic site.

Prognosis

A tumor of 6 cm or less suggests a good prognosis. Disease stage was not related to outcome, different from pleomorphic carcinoma. However, in Koss et al.'s[56] carcinosarcoma series, 25% of cases had no staging data. Koss et al. compared carcinosarcoma with pleomorphic carcinoma. More carcinosarcomas were endobronchial, but the number of pleomorphic carcinomas for comparison was small. Carcinosarcomas were 3.1 times more likely to have a squamous component, 2.6 times less likely to have an adenocarcinomatous component, and 1.3 times less likely to have a large cell component. There was no significant difference in the 5-year survival rate between the two groups of patients, being 21.3% in carcinosarcoma and 15% in pleomorphic carcinoma.

Thirty-nine cases in the collected cases were stage I, 17 were stage II, five were stage III, and four were stage IV.

Pulmonary Blastoma

This is a misapplied term in this literature. Some cases are WDFAs, others are carcinosarcomas, and still others are pleuropulmonary blastomas. To be included in this section as a pulmonary blastoma, a tumor had to have, either described or illustrated, WDFA-type glands (described below), or a stroma, consisting of small polygonal cells, which in some areas may be spindle-like. In some cases there was striated muscle and cartilage. Rare blastomas with a prominent mesenchymal component of rhabdomyoblasts have been described.[63]

Twenty-nine papers were found, producing 88 cases.[5,6,64–90] Patients presenting before the age of 12 years were largely excluded, as most of these are probably pleuropulmonary blastomas. This entity was first recognized in 1989, and there are over 100 cases in the pleuropulmonary blastoma registry (www.pbbregistry.org). As defined by the 2004 WHO classification,[1] solid pleuropulmonary blastomas may occupy an entire lobe or lung. In a minority the mass has arisen from the visceral or parietal pleura, including the dome of the diaphragm. In the solid variant of pleuropulmonary blastoma, while respiratory epithelium may be entrapped within the tumor, neoplastic epithelial elements have not yet been identified. This is in contrast to the classic pulmonary blastoma, which has been divided by Koss et al.[75] into WDFA and pulmonary blastoma. The remainder of this section addresses the more traditional adult-type pulmonary blastoma. The reader is referred to Chapter 42 for further consideration of pleuropulmonary blastoma.

Clinical and Radiologic Features

There is a slight male predominance with a ratio of 1.33:1, which is different from SC. The age range is 16 to 77 years, with a mean of 49.5 years. Therefore, in age it differs little from giant cell carcinoma or pleomorphic carcinoma. The mean age of patients with carcinosarcoma is older, at 68.4. However, the median age of pulmonary blastoma in one large series is in the 40s.[75]

Smoking histories, where present, showed that 28 of 33 (85%) patients smoked. The tumor may involve a lobe or an entire lung. There is a predominance of upper versus the lower lobes, in a ratio of 2.2:1. Sixteen patients had the tumor in the right upper lobe, eight in the right middle lobe, seven in the right lower lobe, 14 in the left upper lobe, 10 in the left lower lobe, 34 in the right lung, and 25 in the left lung.

Most tumors were peripheral, several were central, and four mixed cases were seen. Ramos et al.[89] described a 16-year-old boy with fever, left-sided chest pain, cough, and white sputum. During bronchoscopy he coughed up some thick, violaceous tissue, histologically confirmed as pulmonary blastoma. These tumors may present at an advanced stage, having infiltrated the pleura and extended to the mediastinum. They may be asymptomatic, accounting for 17% of cases in one series.[75] Cough, hemoptysis, and chest pain were frequent findings. Some patients had dyspnea, weight loss, pneumonia, effusion, fever, and malaise. One patient had an elevated serum α- fetoprotein (AFP) (45 μg/L) but a normal serum CEA and β-HCG. A right ovarian cyst in this patient[80] had an AFP level of 4.5 μg/L. This case is possibly a carcinosarcoma. Siegel et al.[76] described two cases without an elevated serum AFP with histologic yolk sac elements. One could have been a primary thymic yolk sac tumor. The initial chest radiograph did not mention any increased thymic size, but this is an insensitive measure of an anterior mediastinal mass. There was an apparent delay between the x-ray and the surgery, but the time interval was not noted. This case was excluded because no mesenchyme was described.

One patient[91] presented with sudden onset of left-sided chest pain and an elevated temperature, was symptomless for 3 months, and then became hemiplegic. Another presented with severe dyspnea, chest pain, and a hemothorax.[79] A patient detected following soft tissue trauma and presenting with neck swelling has been documented.[73]

Most patients present radiologically with unilateral masses and, rarely, multiple nodules. The tumor is a well-circumscribed mass, usually in the periphery or mid-lung, less commonly in the hilum or central lung, or involving both the hilum and periphery. Occasionally the tumor may be lobulated or irregular in outline. Cavitation, atelectasis, regional lymphadenopathy, and pleural effusion are uncommon.

Pathology

Macroscopic Appearance

The tumors varied considerably in size, from 0.58 to 27 cm, with a mean of 6.4 cm. Macroscopically, the tumor is round, sometimes multilobulated, and well demarcated (Fig. 37.16), with a pseudocapsule of lung and bronchus, which may be invaded. On cut surface the tumor is glistening, rubbery, occasionally partly cystic, and it has a white or tan, yellow, brown, black, or hemorrhagic coloration.

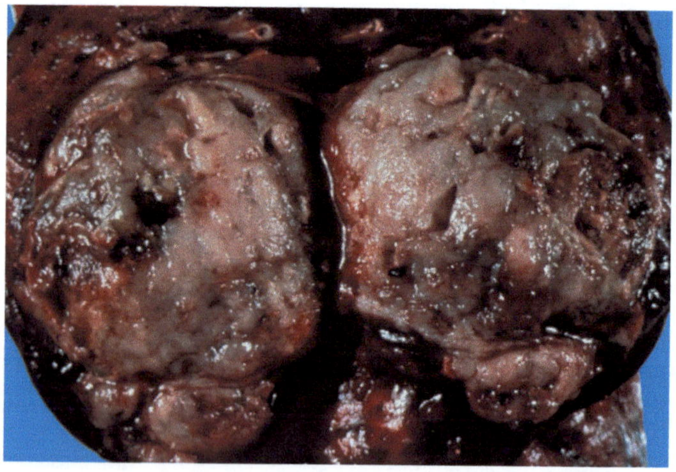

FIGURE 37.16. Macroscopic image of a pulmonary blastoma. (Courtesy of Dr. M. Koss, Los Angeles, CA, and the editor of *Cancer*.)

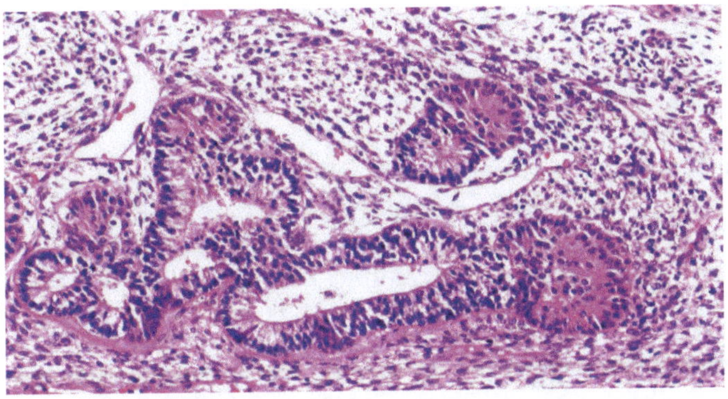

FIGURE 37.17. Pulmonary blastoma with morules in the epithelial element and an edematous mesenchymal component to the tumor.

Histopathology

Histology showed endometrioid glands. Most tumors had solid cords, ribbons, or nests, sometimes with a basaloid pattern with minute rosette-like glands. In these areas the features were those of WDFA, with varying numbers of morules (Fig. 37.17; see also Fig. 36.102 in Chapter 36) of squamoid cells with biotin-rich, optically clear nuclei. Occasionally there was squamous differentiation with abundant keratin or ghost cells resembling craniopharyngioma.[5] There are sub- or supranuclear cytoplasmic vacuoles, containing glycogen, as shown by periodic acid-Schiff (PAS) positivity. The epithelial cells have large nuclei and prominent nucleoli. There is no intracytoplasmic mucin. An abrupt transition from an epithelial to a mesenchymal component was noted (Fig. 37.18). The stroma is embryonic or primitive, with small oval or spindle cells in a myxoid matrix, which is seen usually away from the glandular component (see also Figs. 36.103 and 36.104 in Chapter 36). Immature striated muscle or cartilage was seen in 25% of Koss et al.'s[75] series, and immature bone in 13%. Mitoses were common and there was often extensive necrosis. The frequency of the histologic features in one series is summarized in Table 37.2.

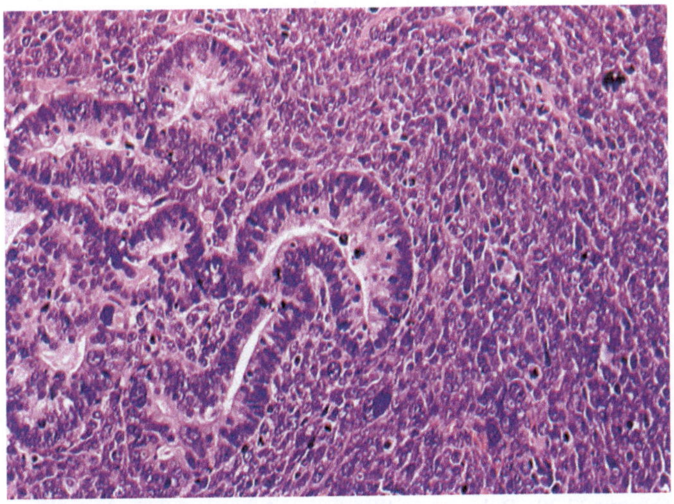

FIGURE 37.18. Pulmonary blastoma with a well-differentiated adenocarcinomatous component surrounded by and well delineated from the compact mesenchyme.

TABLE 37.2. Histologic features of pulmonary blastoma

Subtype	Biphasic blastoma No. (%)
No. of cases	24
Mean size (range) (cm)	10.2 (2–27)
Solitary/multiple	20/4
Subpleural	16 (67)
Intrabronchial	7 (29)
Well-circumscribed	14 (67)
Endometrioid (≥75% of epithelium)	5 (21)
Solid cords of cells	16 (67)
Adenocarcinoma (>0% of epithelium)	10 (36)
Undifferentiated sheets of cells	13 (54)
Morules	12 (43)
Necrosis (≥25% of tumor)	12 (50)
No. of mitoses/10 HPF	24
Tumor giant cells	6 (21)
Embryonic stroma (≥1+)	20 (83)
Adult sarcoma (≥1+)	20 (83)
Striated muscle present	6 (25)
Cartilage present	6 (25)
Bone present	3 (13)
Lymph node metastasis	3
Pathologic stage	
1	19
>1	3

HPF, high-power field.
Source: Koss et al.,[75] with permission from John Wiley & Sons.

An unusual blastoma with numerous rhabdomyoblasts, located diffusely throughout the mesenchyme, has been documented.[63]

Two cases have been described as mixed pulmonary blastoma and carcinosarcoma,[92,93] but both contained foci of well-differentiated squamous cell carcinoma, not a usual feature of pulmonary blastoma.

Necrosis is common, and some cases may show invasion of parietal pleura, bronchi, and vascular walls. There is a background myxoid stroma, which may be prominent in some cases. The epithelium is nonciliated, and may be simple, stratified, cuboidal, or columnar. Some reports describe many mitoses in the epithelium, others few. In areas the epithelial cells may form solid cores or islands. A fibrous capsule has been mentioned and may have microcalcification.[80]

Cytology

Cytology reports are few, and show highly cellular smears with two cell types on fine-needle aspirate.[73] The predominant cell had scanty cytoplasm, was round to ovoid or spindle-shaped, and one to three times the

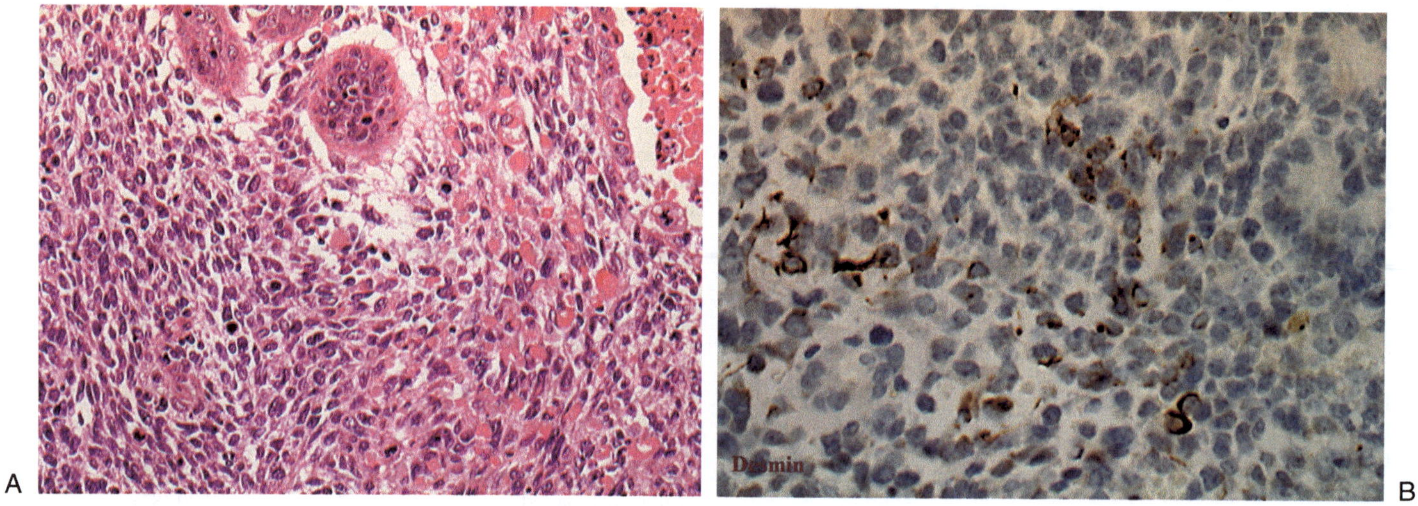

FIGURE 37.19. **(A)** Pulmonary blastoma with a mesenchymal component, which shows focal rhabdomyoblastic differentiation. **(B)** Same case, stained with an antidesmin antibody by immunoperoxidase, showing focal cytoplasmic positivity.

size of an erythrocyte. The nuclei had slightly irregular borders, stippled chromatin, and indistinct nucleoli. These poorly differentiated cells occurred both singly and in variably sized clusters, where they were haphazardly crowded within distinct boundaries. Slightly larger, round to ovoid or columnar cells were less abundant. These cells had a moderate amount of cyanophilic or amphophilic cytoplasm, and some contained cytoplasmic vacuoles. This second type of cell occurred in clusters. Such clusters had smooth borders and elongated branching or acinar configurations in some areas, consistent with a glandular origin. Cytologic diagnosis of this tumor, in view of its biphasic nature, could lead to erroneous diagnoses.

Immunohistochemistry

There have been very few studies using TTF-1. One identified TTF-1 in the epithelial component, as well as cytokeratin, CEA, and synaptophysin.[90] The stroma only was positive for vimentin. P53 was identified in isolated cells. The presence of cytokeratin in the epithelium is a fairly standard finding. Rhabdomyoblasts are shown by a positive myoglobin, present in relatively few cells, but most cells are highlighted by desmin or actin (Fig. 37.19). Epithelial cells also stain with EMA, as well as sialosylate Lewis X (SLEX).[78] These authors also demonstrated that some epithelial cells were positive for neuron-specific enolase (NSE), chromogranin A, and 6H7 (an antibody with a similar domain to neural cell adhesion molecule [NCAM]). No calcitonin, gastrin-releasing peptide (GRP), or 5-hydroxytryptamine (5-HT) was identified in any case.

Nuclear/cytoplasmic (N/C) localization of β-catenin in both epithelial and mesenchymal elements, especially in budding glands and morules, has been recently documented (Fig. 37.20).[5] There was diminished membranous expression and no significant nuclear or cytoplasmic expression in the epithelial component of four cases of "carcinosarcoma" with a high- grade, clear cell adenocarcinoma with fetal lung features as the epithelial component. There was absent or focal N/C expression in the mesenchymal component. The presence of the β-catenin related to mutational analysis of exon 3 of the β-catenin gene (*vide infra*).

Electron Microscopy

Several papers describe the electron microscopy of pulmonary blastoma.[63,67,77] The epithelial cells had intercellular junctions, separated from the stroma by a discrete

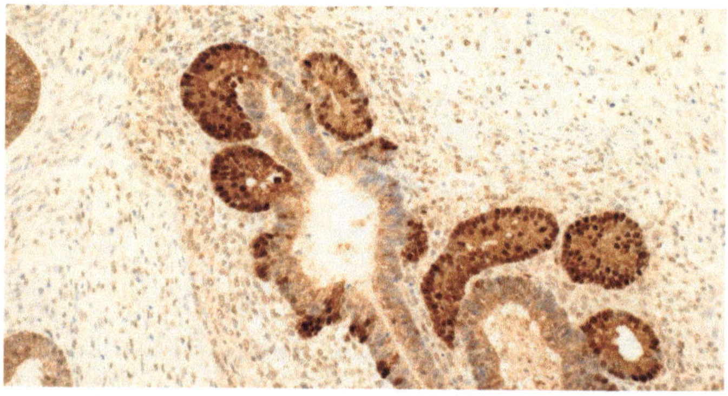

FIGURE 37.20. Pulmonary blastoma, showing β-catenin nuclear and cytoplasmic positivity. (Courtesy of Dr. Nakatani, Chiba, Japan, and the editor of the *American Journal of Surgical Pathology*.)

basal lamina. Glycogen was present in these cells and nonspecific organelles. No mucous granules were recognized, but neuroendocrine granules were identified in some epithelial cells (see Figs. 36.105 and 36.106 in Chapter 36). The apical cell membrane had occasional microvillus projections. Rarely cilia and centrioles were associated with basal bodies. In more solid areas the epithelial cells were closely opposed to each other by a simple plasma membrane, joined by desmosomes. The ovoid, irregularly shaped nuclei contained diffusely dispersed chromatin, and inside the epithelium were scanty cytoplasmic organelles, consisting mainly of free ribosomes and rare mitochondria, rough endoplasmic reticulum, lipid droplets, microfilaments, and electron-dense membrane-bound lysosomal bodies.

Mesenchymal cells had scanty cytoplasmic organelles with little rough endoplasmic reticulum, mitochondria, and lysosomal bodies. Most of the cytoplasm consisted of free ribosomes and polyribosomes. In the rhabdomyoblasts, there were interlacing bundles of thick (myosin) and thin (actin) filaments with I bands, Z lines, and light H bands with M lines. Numerous glycogen particles were observed.[63] Other organelles in the myoblasts included mitochondria, scattered lipid bodies, and short, dilated, profiles of rough-surfaced endoplasmic reticulum.

Genetic Studies

Two studies examined β-catenin and its mutations in pulmonary blastomas.[5,6] Sekine et al.[6] demonstrated β-catenin mutations in three WDFAs and two pulmonary blastomas with morules. All mutations were missense mutations producing substitution of serine/threonine residues at glycogen synthetase kinase (GSK)-3β-phosphorylation sites or of amino acids flanking one of these serine/threonine residues. No pulmonary blastomas without morules or clear cell adenocarcinoma with fetal features had mutations. Epithelial cells showed overexpression of β catenin. Mesenchymal cells, after microdissection, showed the same mutations. All neuroendocrine cells accumulated β-catenin, but there were β-catenin–positive or –negative neuroendocrine cells. On immunohistochemistry, β-catenin staining was both nuclear and cytoplasmic (Fig. 37.20). Frequent genetic alterations leading to β-catenin mutations have been reported in tumors with morules and biotin-rich nuclei, including pancreatoblastoma and endometrioid adenocarcinoma.[94–97]

β-catenin mutation is rare in lung cancers, being present in one of 90 primary lung cancers and three of 76 lung cancer cell lines.[98] In two studies, no mutations were identified among 93 and 13 lung carcinomas, respectively.[99,100] Sekine et al.[6] thought the high prevalence of β-catenin mutations in pulmonary blastomas with morules was a distinctive genetic feature in these lung tumors.

β-catenin, originally identified as one of the cell-cell adhesion molecules, including cadherins, catenins, and actin, is an important component of the Wnt signaling pathway.[101] The Wnt signaling pathways are involved in differentiation processes during embryonic development and lead to tumor formation, when aberrantly activated.[6] In classic pulmonary blastomas the epithelial cells showed predominantly nuclear/cytoplasmic expression of β-catenin. Membranous expression was typically diminished. Budding glands and morules showed intense nucleocytoplasmic expression. Nakatani et al.[5] demonstrated that the blastic cells also expressed β-catenin in their nuclei and cytoplasm, though less intensely than the cells composing the budding glands and morules. The staining intensity generally diminished as cells matured in the center to the periphery of the blastic cell island. In contrast all carcinosarcomas had a normal membranous localization of β-catenin in the epithelium. The staining intensity decreased in the epithelial components as they became less differentiated and merged with the sarcomatous component.

Mutation analysis of exon 3 of the β-catenin gene showed three of four pulmonary blastomas harbored missense point mutations.[5] Two mutations affected codon 37, and one affected codons 13 and 29, all leading to a TCT → TTT change (S37F and S29F). All mutations were heterozygous. None of their carcinosarcomas showed this mutation. These studies provide evidence that both the epithelial and mesenchymal components of pulmonary blastoma are monoclonal.

Two studies examined *p53* in pulmonary blastomas.[83,88] In the first study, five of 12 (42%) of pulmonary blastomas had *p53* gene mutations by immunohistochemistry and molecular analysis, whereas no WDFAs had such mutations. Of the five tumors with *p53* gene mutations, suggested by a single-strand confirmational polymorphism (SSCP) analysis and confirmed by sequencing, two contained transversion mutations and three transition mutations. Of the three tumors with transition mutations, two of the transitions were located at CpG dinucleotides and one tumor contained a double transition within the same codon, producing a single amino acid change.[88]

One of the transversions identified was G:C → T:A, typical of benzpyrene exposure. This patient had a heavy smoking history, though such a history was present in all patients with mutations. The predominance of a single mutant band in both SSCP and sequencing gels suggested the presence of a single clonal population in the tumor, with a slight admixture of normal (unmutated inflammatory or stromal cells). The sequencing data from Bodner and Koss's paper showed TGC → CGC transition codon 182, TGT → TTT tranversion codon 238, CGT → TGT transition codon 273, CCG → ACG tranversion condon 152, and GCC → ACT double-transition codon 161. No WDFA contained mutations. These authors thought the histologic distinction between biphasic blastoma and WDFA had prognostic significance, as shown previously by Koss et al. The 10-year survival of the latter tumor was 80%, but of biphasic blastoma was only 20%. Because the series was so small, it was impossible to draw any conclusions about the independent significance of *p53* mutations on survival, metastases, and stage of disease.

Pacinda et al.[83] stained pulmonary blastomas, WDFAs, and bronchogenic carcinomas for p53 and MDM2. MDM2 gene product interacts with *p53* and regulates its tumor suppressor function.[102] The MDM2 protein is associated with *p53* in an autoregulatory mechanism and may account for a loss of *p53* tumor-suppressor activity, even when the p53 protein is not mutated. Only one of three pulmonary blastomas stained for p53. Two of the three WDFAs stained for p53 and all stained for *MDM2*. Two of three pleuropulmonary blastomas stained only for *MDM2*. The authors concluded that the immunostaining patterns for p53 and MDM2 in adult types of pulmonary blastomas, but not pleuropulmonary blastomas, appeared similar for those of bronchogenic carcinoma. This suggested that adult-type pulmonary blastomas, but not childhood pleuropulmonary blastomas, may have a similar pathogenesis to bronchogenic carcinoma. This conclusion is not confirmed by the β-catenin data presented above or in Bodner and Koss's study.

K-*ras* mutations are absent in pulmonary blastoma and WDFA[103]; 30% to 44% of adenocarcinomas show K-*ras* mutations,[104,105] as do SC and squamous carcinomas.[106,107]

Metastases

In Koss et al.'s[75] series, three of 22 patients had metastases at diagnosis; 10 patients (43%) had recurrent tumor, and in 12 patients (52%) disseminated tumor caused death. The site of the recurrent tumor, in descending order, was the brain, mediastinum, lung/pleura, diaphragm, heart, liver, soft tissue, and extremities. Lymph node metastases were seen in 40% of a small surgical series.[65] Other sites of involvement are bone marrow and hip,[72] cerebrum,[91] spine, ribs, and intercostal muscles.[64]

Prognosis

The average survival, after initial recurrence, was 11 months (range, 2–32 months). Tumor size related to outcome, neoplasms less than 5 cm having a more favorable prognosis. Recurrence indicated a less favorable prognosis. Based on previous studies, two thirds of patients died within 2 years of diagnosis, 16% survived 5 years, and 8% survived 10 years. Stage was important in determining prognosis, since stage I blastomas reported in the literature had a 5-year survival of approximately 25%. Patients who were treated tended to survive longer. Cutler et al.[86] reviewed the literature after describing a patient who was alive and well 7 years, following subtotal resection, radiotherapy, and three cycles of chemotherapy with cisplatin and etoposide.

Where documented, most patients are stage I (24); four were stage II, four were stage III, and one was stage IV. In many cases it was impossible to determine the stage of the tumor.

Differential Diagnosis of Sarcomatoid Carcinoma

Pleomorphic Carcinoma

The differential diagnosis is wide, and consideration must be given to both benign and malignant conditions.

Inflammatory Myofibroblastic Tumor

Typically, inflammatory myofibroblastic tumors (IMTs) consist of relatively bland, sometimes modestly atypical spindle cells, arranged in fascicles with a haphazard or storiform pattern (see Chapters 39 and 42). There may be an inflammatory component, which can also be seen in pleomorphic carcinoma.[7] Inflammatory myofibroblastic tumors may show vascular and bronchial invasion, as well as infiltrating pleura,[108] soft tissues of the chest wall,[109] mediastinum,[110,111] and thoracic vertebra.[112]

Differentiation of IMT from an SC should not be made on frozen section. If there is doubt, immunohistochemistry will help. Inflammatory myofibroblastic tumor is cytokeratin and epithelial membrane antigen negative; the converse is true of SC. However, I have seen one IMT that was positive for cytokeratin. Focal cytokeratin immunoreactivity was seen in more than 33% of extrapulmonary IMTs.[113]

Inflammatory myofibroblastic tumor may undergo malignant change, and a combination of atypia, ganglion-like cells, p53 expression, and DNA ploidy analysis may be useful in identifying these.[114] Histologic features associated with poor prognosis in IMT include focal invasion, vascular invasion, increased cellularity, nuclear pleomorphism with bizarre giant cells, a mitotic rate greater than 3 per 50 high power fields, and necrosis.[1] Abnormalities of the *ALK* gene, p80, and chromosomal rearrangements of 2p23 suggest recurrence.[115]

Idiopathic Fibroinflammatory (Fibrosing/Sclerosing) Mediastinal Lesions

These lesions often present with pulmonary symptoms and may extend into the lung (see Chapter 21). They consist of acellular dense collagen with occasional lymphoid follicles. Spindle and inflammatory cells are absent whereas dystrophic calcification is common.[116]

Primary Pulmonary Malignant Fibrous Histiocytoma

Primary pulmonary malignant fibrous histiocytoma (MFH) is a rare lesion, if it exists at all (see Chapter 39). The new WHO classification does not mention this condition as a separate heading in the pulmonary section. The histologic features are indistinguishable from some pulmonary SC. There are occasional reports of keratin-positivity in this tumor,[117] and it is difficult, if not impossible, to differentiate MFH from SC. Most pulmonary sarcomas, whether primary or secondary, do not show diffuse cytokeratin-positivity *(vide infra)*.

In a review of 22 cases of primary malignant fibrohistiocytoma of lung,[118] all 18 cases studied by immunohistochemistry failed to express cytoplasmic keratin or S-100 protein. The keratin employed was not mentioned. As this study is from 1987, newer cytokeratin antibodies are available for detection of epithelial differentiation. When considering MFH, a secondary tumor should be sought.

Malignant Endobronchial Myxoid Tumor

This is a very rare salivary gland tumor, which has an origin in the tracheobronchial tree. Few cases have been described in detail.

Secondary Carcinoma

Tumors metastatic from the breast, prostate, gallbladder, pancreas, and thyroid enter the differential diagnosis of SC. Monoclonal antibodies are likely to give limited help, since in poorly differentiated tumors, antigens such as estrogen receptors and prostate-specific antigen are less likely to be expressed. In most cases, a primary site will be known.

Non–Small-Cell Carcinoma

There is a gradation between spindle cell, squamous carcinoma, adenocarcinoma with sarcomatoid foci, non–small-cell carcinoma (see Chapter 35), and SC. In SC with an epithelial component, cytokeratin 7, TTF-1, and surfactant protein-A were positive in the sarcomatoid component in 62.7%, 43.1%, and 5.9% of the cases, respectively.[13] These markers were negative in the sarcomatous foci of carcinosarcomas and pulmonary blastoma. One of the most specific markers, TTF-1, was positive in less than half the cases studied.

Thymic Tumors

It may be difficult to distinguish primary thymic from primary lung tumors (see Chapter 41). A CT scan may be of help in showing where the largest bulk of tumor resides. Morphology and TTF-1 staining may help in well-differentiated thymomas, which typically show few mitoses. Intraepithelial lymphocytes, if present, are immature T cells, which are CD1A, CD4, CD5, CD8, CD99, and TdT positive.[1]

Primary squamous cell carcinoma of the thymus is documented. A thymic origin of neoplastic squamous cells may be detected by CD5, CD70, and CD117 positivity.[119,120] Primary thymic SC is uncommon.[121] Heterologous elements may be observed, with rhabdomyosarcomatous foci. Cases studied for CD5 have been negative for this marker.[122,123] Differentiation of this primary thymic from a primary pulmonary tumor may be impossible.

Pulmonary Neuroendocrine Tumors

Pulmonary neuroendocrine tumors (see Chapter 36) may have a spindle cell pattern and should always be considered in the differential diagnosis of spindle cell carcinoma, but neuroendocrine markers will be positive. In atypical carcinoids, the number of mitoses ranges from 2 to 10 mitoses per 2 mm^2 or 10 high power fields, lower than in SC.

Mesothelioma and Other Pleural Tumors

Differentiation of a SC of the lung from a pleomorphic pleural mesothelioma may be difficult (see Chapter 43). Calretinin and CK5/6 are often negative in poorly differentiated epithelioid mesotheliomas. No cases of SC or pleomorphic malignant pleural mesothelioma were positive for TTF-1.[21] Calretinin was both sensitive in 81% and highly specific in 94% for identifying mesothelioma. CK5/6 had moderate sensitivity (75%) and specificity of 59%.

In sarcomatoid mesothelioma, when the mesothelial markers are often negative, the diagnosis is a clinical, radiologic, and pathologic synthesis. A firm diagnosis is impossible if no desmoplastic foci are seen. Synovial sarcoma *(vide infra)*, which has a different growth pattern and is often monophasic, may affect the pleura. Primary thymic epithelial tumors may also be identified in the pleura, and in this site they show variable nuclear and cytoplasmic expression.[124] Rare cases or synchronous diffuse malignant mesothelioma and carcinomas may be identified in asbestos-exposed individuals.[125] In this series none of the tumors was pleomorphic.

Solitary malignant fibrous tumors may present in the pleura, and rare cases are cytokeratin-positive.[126] The benign variant may also be primary in the lung and shows no necrosis or mitotic activity, causing little problem in differential diagnosis. CD34 is the most reliable immunohistochemical marker of solitary fibrous tumor, but it is less reliable at the malignant end of the spectrum.

Sarcomas

Primary pulmonary sarcomas (see Chapters 40 and 41) are rare, but included in this group is monophasic synovial sarcoma, which can be primary in the lung. This tumor has a distinct vesicular pattern and, characteristically, there is TX;18, p11.2:q11.2, or *SYT-SSX1* or *SYT–SSXT2* gene fusion. Most synovial sarcomas are immunoreactivefor cytokeratins and epithelial membrane antigen. In monophasic tumors the immunoreactivity may be scanty. Synovial sarcoma expresses CK7 and CK19. These markers are generally negative in other spindle cell sarcomas. Bcl2 and CD99 are frequently positive.[127–129] Leiomyosarcoma, malignant peripheral nerve sheath tumor, Ewing's sarcoma, and angiosarcoma should also be considered in the differential, as they may all be focally cytokeratin-positive. Pseudoangiosarcomatous carcinoma[20] may be confused on H&E staining with an angiosarcoma, but the former is negative for vascular markers and in my limited experience 34βE12 is a valuable discriminant. Secondary spindle cell renal carcinoma and secondary melanoma should be considered in the differential diagnosis.

Small Cell Carcinoma

Small cell carcinoma (see Chapter 36) should be considered in the differential when it has spindle or giant cells. Neuroendocrine markers will help with diagnosis.

Rhabdoid Features Associated with Large Cell Carcinoma of Lung

These cells have a vesicular nucleus with prominent nucleoli and large intracytoplasmic pale eosinophilic globules, positive for cytokeratin and vimentin[130] (see Chapter 35).

Germ Cell Tumor and Teratoma

While these entities are much commoner in the thymus, they have rarely been described in the lung (see Chapter 41). The diagnosis of a primary germ cell tumor requires the absence of a testicular or ovarian tumor. Thymic tumors spread hematogenously to the lung in nearly 40% of cases.[131] Typical mediastinal yolk sac tumors have solid and microcystic patterns, hyaline globules, and Schiller-Duval bodies. There may be an endodermal sinus pattern and foci, with marked spindling of tumor cells. Choriocarcinoma, a variant of yolk sac tumor, shows syncytio- and cytotrophoblasts. They may be difficult to distinguish from giant cell carcinomas, and are positive for cytokeratins but negative for PLAP (placental alkaline phosphatase), AFP, CEA, CD30, and vimentin. There may be β-HCG expression in the syncytiotrophoblast. β-HCG and AFP are positive in most germ cell tumors. These markers are negative in mature teratomas.

Carcinosarcoma

Secondary carcinosarcoma arising from the uterus, hypopharynx, or esophagus should be considered. Other sites include the salivary gland, thyroid, thymus, breast, skin, stomach, liver, gallbladder, small intestine, pancreas, colon, anus, kidney, renal pelvis, lower urogenital tract including ureters, and adrenal gland.[132] Osteoclastic giant cells are seen in a variety of carcinomas and sarcomas that lack bone, such as SC and leiomyosarcoma. Pure giant cell carcinomas of the lung are exceedingly rare.

Pulmonary Blastoma

Pleuropulmonary Blastoma

Pleuropulmonary blastomas may be purely cystic, characterized by a multicystic structure lined by respiratory epithelium (see Chapter 42). Beneath this there is a population of small primitive malignant cells, with or without rhabdomyofibroblastic differentiation. Others may be solid, with overgrowth of the septal stroma by sheets of primitive cells without any differentiation. Pleuropulmonary blastoma has no neoplastic epithelium, and no WDFA pattern, as seen in a typical pulmonary blastoma. Most cases are seen around 2 years of age, and the upper limit of patients described with pleuropulmonary blastoma is 12 years.

Well-Differentiated Fetal Adenocarcinoma

This is an important differential diagnosis and it contains no mesenchyme (see Chapter 35).

Teratoma

Though extremely rare in the lung, teratoma does not have mesenchymal undifferentiated foci (see Chapter 41).

Hamartoma

This has well-differentiated foci of bone, adipose tissue, and mature respiratory epithelium (see Chapter 40).

Myxoid Liposarcoma

This tumor has well-differentiated areas of fat and a myxoid background (see Chapter 40).

Myxoma of the Pleura

This is a rare pleural primary tumor.[133]

Histogenesis

Theories of the histogenesis of biphasic tumors have been well summarized by McCluggage,[134] who reviewed the uterine carcinosarcoma literature. He considered the tumor to be a metaplastic carcinoma. The same histogenetic principles underlie the current concepts of SC and pulmonary blastoma. There are four main theories regarding the histogenesis of carcinosarcomas:

1. The collision theory, suggesting the carcinoma and sarcoma are two independent neoplasms.
2. The combination theory, suggesting both components are derived from a single stem cell that undergoes divergent differentiation early in the evolution of the tumor.
3. The conversion theory, which suggests that the sarcomatous element derives from the carcinoma during the evolution of the tumor.
4. The composition theory, suggesting that the spindle cell component is a pseudosarcomatous stromal reaction to the presence of a carcinoma.

The last theory is excluded, since the sarcomatoid component is histologically malignant. In view of the data given earlier in the chapter, confirming that biphasic tumors are monoclonal, the collision theory appears to have little credibility. The evidence includes clinical, histopathologic, immunohistochemical, ultrastructural, and molecular data.

Conclusion

Tobacco smoking is the major causative factor in most of the tumors discussed in this chapter. There is a tendency for pulmonary blastoma to differentiate itself from the other tumors because of differences in age at presentation and an almost equal incidence in males and females. In addition, this tumor has a characteristic histology, immunohistochemical pattern of staining, and molecular features. Since this group of tumors is rare, these studies need to be repeated on some of the other tumors, such as carcinosarcoma. This is probably one of the rarest tumors of this group, if strict criteria for diagnosis are used.

Acknowledgments. I wish to thank the following colleagues for their kindness in being so generous with material: Drs. Koss and Travis, whose papers have greatly illuminated this difficult area, have been very forthcoming in provision of material. Drs. Koss and Nakatani have also been open-handed in giving me their rare cases so that the chapter could have these excellent illustrations. The problems with the photography are mine.

References

1. Travis WD, Brambilla E, Muller-Hermelink HK, Harris CC. World Health Organization classification of tumours. Pathology and genetics of tumours of the lung, pleura, thymus and heart. Lyon: IARC Press, 2004:51.
2. Wick MR, Ritter JH, Humphrey PA. Sarcomatoid carcinomas of the lung: a clinicopathologic review. Am J Clin Pathol 1997;108(1):40–53.
3. Travis W, et al. WHO international histological classification of tumours: histological typing of lung and pleural tumours. 3rd ed. New York: Springer Verlag, 1999.
4. Nappi O, et al. Biphasic and monophasic sarcomatoid carcinomas of the lung. A reappraisal of "carcinosarcomas" and "spindle-cell carcinomas." Am J Clin Pathol 1994; 102(3):331–340.
5. Nakatani Y, et al. Aberrant nuclear/cytoplasmic localization and gene mutation of beta-catenin in classic pulmonary blastoma: beta-catenin immunostaining is useful for distinguishing between classic pulmonary blastoma and a blastomatoid variant of carcinosarcoma. Am J Surg Pathol 2004;28(7):921–927.
6. Sekine S, et al. Beta-catenin mutations in pulmonary blastomas: association with morule formation. J Pathol 2003; 200(2):214–221.
7. Wick MR, Ritter JH, Nappi O. Inflammatory sarcomatoid carcinoma of the lung: report of three cases and clinicopathologic comparison with inflammatory pseudotumors in adult patients. Hum Pathol 1995;26(9):1014–1021.
8. Ro JY, et al. Sarcomatoid carcinoma of the lung. Immunohistochemical and ultrastructural studies of 14 cases. Cancer 1992;69(2):376–386.
9. Pelosi G, et al. Pleomorphic carcinomas of the lung show a selective distribution of gene products involved in cell differentiation, cell cycle control, tumor growth, and tumor cell motility: a clinicopathologic and immunohistochemical study of 31 cases. Am J Surg Pathol 2003;27(9): 1203–1215.
10. Przygodzki RM, Koss MN, O'Leary TJ. Pleomorphic (giant and/or spindle cell) carcinoma of lung shows a high percentage of variant CYP1A12. Mol Diagn 2001;6(2):109–115.
11. Holst VA, et al. p53 and K-ras mutational genotyping in pulmonary carcinosarcoma, spindle cell carcinoma, and pulmonary blastoma: implications for histogenesis. Am J Surg Pathol 1997;21(7):801–811.
12. Fishback NF, et al. Pleomorphic (spindle/giant cell) carcinoma of the lung. A clinicopathologic correlation of 78 cases. Cancer 1994;73(12):2936–2945.
13. Rossi G, et al. Pulmonary carcinomas with pleomorphic, sarcomatoid, or sarcomatous elements: a clinicopathologic and immunohistochemical study of 75 cases. Am J Surg Pathol 2003;27(3):311–324.
14. Humphrey PA, et al. Pulmonary carcinomas with a sarcomatoid element: an immunocytochemical and ultrastructural analysis. Hum Pathol 1988;19(2):155–165.
15. Nakajima M, et al. Sarcomatoid carcinoma of the lung: a clinicopathologic study of 37 cases. Cancer 1999;86(4): 608–616.
16. Suster S, Huszar M, Herczeg E. Spindle cell squamous carcinoma of the lung. Immunocytochemical and ultrastructural study of a case. Histopathology 1987;11(8):871–878.
17. Matsui K, Kitagawa M, Miwa A. Lung carcinoma with spindle cell components: sixteen cases examined by

immunohistochemistry. Hum Pathol 1992;23(11):1289–1297.
18. Krefting I, et al. Pleomorphic carcinoma (spindle and giant cell) of the lung. Md Med J 1994;43:787–790.
19. Lucas DR, Pass HP, Lonardo F. Peripheral sarcomatoid (spindle cell/pleomorphic) carcinoma of lung; propensity for pleural and chest wall invasion and immunoprofile indistinguishable from sarcomatoid mesothelioma. Mod Pathol 2003;16:310A.
20. Banerjee SS, et al. Pseudoangiosarcomatous carcinoma: a clinicopathological study of seven cases. Histopathology 1992;21(1):13–23.
21. King JE. Clinicopathological studies of pleural mesothelioma. Southampton: (Personal Communication), 2004.
22. Lucas DR, et al. Sarcomatoid mesothelioma and its histological mimics: a comparative immunohistochemical study. Histopathology 2003;42(3):270–279.
23. Przygodzki R, et al. Pleomorphic (giant and spindle cell) carcinoma is genetically distinct from adenocarcinoma and squamous cell carcinoma by K-ras-2 and p53 analysis. Am J Clin Pathol 1996;106(4):487–492.
24. Cascorbi I, Brockmoller J, Roots I. A C4887A polymorphism in exon 7 of human CYP1A1: population frequency, mutation linkages, and impact on lung cancer susceptibility. Cancer Res 1996;56(21):4965–4969.
25. Przygodzki RM, et al. p53 mutation spectrum in relation to GSTM1, CYP1A1 and CYP2E1 in surgically treated patients with non-small cell lung cancer. Pharmacogenetics 1998;8(6):503–511.
26. Fischer D, et al. Cell-adhesive responses to tenascin-C splice variants involve formation of fascin microspikes. Mol Biol Cell 1997;8(10):2055–2075.
27. Tao YS, et al. beta-Catenin associates with the actin-bundling protein fascin in a noncadherin complex. J Cell Biol 1996;134(5):1271–1281.
28. Tilney LG, et al. Why are two different cross-linkers necessary for actin bundle formation in vivo and what does each cross-link contribute? J Cell Biol 1998;143(1):121–133.
29. Tseng Y, et al. Micromechanics and ultrastructure of actin filament networks crosslinked by human fascin: a comparison with alpha-actinin. J Mol Biol 2001;310(2):351–366.
30. Yamashiro S, et al. Fascin, an actin-bundling protein, induces membrane protrusions and increases cell motility of epithelial cells. Mol Biol Cell 1998;9:993–1006.
31. Nash AD, Stout AP. Giant cell carcinoma of the lung; report of 5 cases. Cancer 1958;11(2):369–376.
32. Hellstrom HR, Fisher ER. Giant cell carcinoma of lung. Cancer 1963;16:1080–1088.
33. Flanagan P, Roeckel IE. Giant cell carcinoma of the lung. Anatomic and clinical correlation. Am J Med 1964;36:214–221.
34. Guillan RA, Zelman S. Giant-cell carcinoma of the lung. Am J Clin Pathol 1966;46:427–432.
35. Lerner HJ. Giant cell carcinoma of the lung. Review of literature and report of five cases. Arch Surg 1967;94(6):891–894.
36. Dailey JE, Marcuse PM. Gonadotropin secreting giant cell carcinoma of the lung. Cancer 1969;24(2):388–396.
37. Wellmann KF, Chafiian Y, Edelman E. Small bowel perforation from solitary metastasis of clinically undetected pulmonary giant cell carcinoma. Am J Gastroenterol 1969;51(2):145–150.
38. Razzuk MA, et al. Pulmonary giant cell carcinoma. Ann Thorac Surg 1976;21(6):540–545.
39. Wang NS, et al. Giant cell carcinoma of the lung. A light and electron microscopic study. Hum Pathol 1976;7(1):3–16.
40. Takenaga A, et al. Giant cell carcinoma of the lung: comparative studies of the same cancer cells by light microscopy and scanning electron microscopy. Acta Cytol 1980;24(3):190–196.
41. Kodama T, et al. Large cell carcinoma of the lung—ultrastructural and immunohistochemical studies. Jpn J Clin Oncol 1985;15(2):431–441.
42. Shin MS, et al. Giant cell carcinoma of the lung. Clinical and roentgenographic manifestations. Chest 1986;89(3):366–369.
43. Nakahashi H, et al. Undifferentiated carcinoma of the lung with osteoclast-like giant cells. Jpn J Surg 1987;17(3):199–203.
44. Addis BJ, Dewar A, Thurlow NP. Giant cell carcinoma of the lung—immunohistochemical and ultrastructural evidence of dedifferentiation. J Pathol 1988;155(3):231–240.
45. Horie A, et al. Clinicopathological study of pulmonary giant cell carcinomas with reference to prognosis of patients. J UOEH 1991;13(2):125–134.
46. Ginsberg SS, et al. Giant cell carcinoma of the lung. Cancer 1992;70(3):606–610.
47. Attanoos RL, et al. Pulmonary giant cell carcinoma: pathological entity or morphological phenotype? Histopathology 1998;32(3):225–231.
48. Prasad AR, et al. Primary giant cell tumors of the lung. Mod Pathol 2001;14:225A.
49. Yaturu S, et al. Gynecomastia attributable to human chorionic gonadotropin-secreting giant cell carcinoma of lung. Endocr Pract 2003;9(3):233–235.
50. Depue RH, Ballard BR. Pulmonary giant cell carcinoma: the relation to smoking. Br J Cancer 19891;60(4):599–600.
51. Chemnitz J, Bichel P. Tumour cell-tumour cell emperipolesis studied by transmission electron microscopy. Exp Cell Res 1973;82(2):319–324.
52. Humble JG, Jayne WH, Pulvertaft RJ. Biological interaction between lymphocytes and other cells. Br J Haematol 1956;2(3):283–294.
53. Iizuka M, et al. Joining of the c-myc gene and a line 1 family member on chromosome 8 in a human primary giant cell carcinoma of the lung. Cancer Res 1990;50(11):3345–3350.
54. Ishida T, et al. Carcinosarcoma and spindle cell carcinoma of the lung. Clinicopathologic and immunohistochemical studies. J Thorac Cardiovasc Surg 1990;100(6):844–852.
55. Cabarcos A, Gomez Dorronsoro M, Lobo Beristain JL. Pulmonary carcinosarcoma: a case study and review of the literature. Br J Dis Chest 1985;79(1):83–94.
56. Koss MN, Hochholzer L, Frommelt RA. Carcinosarcomas of the lung: a clinicopathologic study of 66 patients. Am J Surg Pathol 1999;23(12):1514–1526.
57. Reynolds S, et al. Carcinosarcoma of the lung: an unusual cause of empyema. Respir Med 1995;89(1):73–75.

58. Farrell DJ, Cooper PN, Malcolm AJ, Carcinosarcoma of lung associated with asbestosis. Histopathology 1995;27(5): 484–486.
59. Pankowski J, et al. Carcinosarcoma of the lung. Report of three cases. J Cardiovasc Surg (Torino) 1998;39(1):121–125.
60. Dacic S, et al. Molecular pathogenesis of pulmonary carcinosarcoma as determined by microdissection-based allelotyping. Am J Surg Pathol 2002;26(4):510–516.
61. Eng J, Sabanathan S. Carcinosarcoma of the lung with gastrointestinal metastasis. Case report. Scand J Thorac Cardiovasc Surg 1992;26(2):161–162.
62. Rainosek DE, et al. Sarcomatoid carcinoma of the lung. A case with atypical carcinoid and rhabdomyosarcomatous components. Am J Clin Pathol 1994;102(3):360–364.
63. Heckman CJ, et al. Pulmonary blastoma with rhabdomyosarcomatous differentiation: an electron microscopic and immunohistochemical study. Am J Surg Pathol 1988; 12(1):35–40.
64. Peacock MJ, Whitwell F. Pulmonary blastoma. Thorax 1976;31(2):197–204.
65. Jacobsen M, Francis D. Pulmonary blastoma. A clinicopathological study of eleven cases. Acta Pathol Microbiol Scand [A] 1980;88(3):151–160.
66. Medbery CA 3rd, et al. Pulmonary blastoma. Case report and literature review of chemotherapy experience. Cancer 1984;53(11):2413–2416.
67. Marcus PB, Dieb TM, Martin JH. Pulmonary blastoma: an ultrastructural study emphasizing intestinal differentiation in lung tumors. Cancer 1982;49(9):1829–1833.
68. Korbi S, et al. Pulmonary blastoma. Immunohistochemical and ultrastructural studies of a case. Histopathology 1987; 11(7):753–760.
69. Addis BJ, Corrin B. Pulmonary blastoma, carcinosarcoma and spindle-cell carcinoma: an immunohistochemical study of keratin intermediate filaments. J Pathol 1985;147(4): 291–301.
70. Berean K, et al. Immunohistochemical characterization of pulmonary blastoma. Am J Clin Pathol 1988;89(6):773–777.
71. Weisbrod GL, Chamberlain DW, Tao LC. Pulmonary blastoma, report of three cases and a review of the literature. J Can Assoc Radiol 1988;39:130–136.
72. Cohen RE, et al. Pulmonary blastoma with malignant melanoma component. Arch Pathol Lab Med 1990; 114(10):1076–1078.
73. Cosgrove MM, Chandrasoma PT, Martin SE. Diagnosis of pulmonary blastoma by fine-needle aspiration biopsy: cytologic and immunocytochemical findings. Diagn Cytopathol 1991;7(1):83–87.
74. Yousem SA, et al. Pulmonary blastoma. An immunohistochemical analysis with comparison with fetal lung in its pseudoglandular stage. Am J Clin Pathol 1990;93(2): 167–175.
75. Koss MN, Hochholzer L, O'Leary T. Pulmonary blastomas. Cancer 1991;67(9):2368–2381.
76. Siegel RJ, et al. Pulmonary blastoma with germ cell (yolk sac) differentiation: report of two cases. Mod Pathol 1991; 4(5):566–570.
77. McCann MP, Fu YS, Kay S. Pulmonary blastoma: A light and electron microscopic study. Cancer 1976;38(2): 789–797.
78. Inoue H, et al. Pulmonary blastoma. Comparison between its epithelial components and fetal bronchial epithelium. Acta Pathol Jpn 1992;42(12):884–892.
79. Vassilopoulos PP, et al. Pulmonary blastoma presenting with massive hemothorax. Chest 1992;102(2):649–650.
80. Miller RR, Champagne K, Murray RC. Primary pulmonary germ cell tumor with blastomatous differentiation. Chest 1994;106(5):1595–1596.
81. Yang P, et al. Pulmonary blastoma: an ultrastructural and immunohistochemical study with special reference to nuclear filament aggregation. Ultrastruct Pathol 1995;19(6): 501–509.
82. Novotny JE, Huiras CM. Resection and adjuvant chemotherapy of pulmonary blastoma: a case report. Cancer 1995;76(9):1537–1539.
83. Pacinda SJ, et al. p53 and MDM2 immunostaining in pulmonary blastomas and bronchogenic carcinomas. Hum Pathol 1996;27(6):542–546.
84. LeMense GP, Reed CE, Silvestri GA. Pulmonary blastoma: a rare lung malignancy. Lung Cancer 1996;15(2): 233–237.
85. Theegarten D, Zorn M, Philippou S. Proliferative activity, p53 accumulation and neoangiogenesis in pulmonary carcinosarcomas and pulmonary blastomas. Gen Diagn Pathol 1998;143(5–6):265–270.
86. Cutler CS, et al. Pulmonary blastoma: case report of a patient with a 7-year remission and review of chemotherapy experience in the world literature. Cancer 1998;82(3): 462–467.
87. Robert J, et al. Pulmonary blastoma: report of five cases and identification of clinical features suggestive of the disease. Eur J Cardiothorac Surg 2002;22(5):708–711.
88. Bodner SM, Koss MN. Mutations in the p53 gene in pulmonary blastomas: immunohistochemical and molecular studies. Hum Pathol 1996;27(11):1117–1123.
89. Ramos SG, Rezende GG, Faccio AA. A rare presentation of biphasic pulmonary blastoma. Arch Pathol Lab Med 2002;126(7):875–876.
90. Garcia-Escudero A, et al. Thyroid transcription factor-1 expression in pulmonary blastoma. Histopathology 2004; 44(5):507–508.
91. Barson AJ, Jones AW, Lodge KV. Pulmonary blastoma. J Clin Pathol 1968;21(4):480–485.
92. Olenick SJ, Fan CC, Ryoo JW. Mixed pulmonary blastoma and carcinosarcoma. Histopathology 1994;25(2):171–174.
93. Roth JA, Elguezabal A. Pulmonary blastoma evolving into carcinosarcoma. A case study. Am J Surg Pathol 1978; 2(4):407–413.
94. Tanaka Y, et al. Pancreatoblastoma: optically clear nuclei in squamoid corpuscles are rich in biotin. Mod Pathol 1998;11(10):945–949.
95. Abraham SC, et al. Distinctive molecular genetic alterations in sporadic and familial adenomatous polyposis-associated pancreatoblastomas: frequent alterations in the APC/beta-catenin pathway and chromosome 11p. Am J Pathol 2001;159(5):1619–1627.

96. Tsujimoto M, Noguchi M, Taki I. Immunohistochemical and electron microscopic study of the intranuclear inclusion bodies containing biotin in the ovarian endometrioid carcinoma. J Clin Electron Microsc 1991;24:783–784.
97. Saegusa M, Okayasu I. Frequent nuclear beta-catenin accumulation and associated mutations in endometrioid-type endometrial and ovarian carcinomas with squamous differentiation. J Pathol 2001;194(1):59–67.
98. Shigemitsu K, et al. Genetic alteration of the beta-catenin gene (CTNNB1) in human lung cancer and malignant mesothelioma and identification of a new 3p21.3 homozygous deletion. Oncogene 2001;20(31):4249–4257.
99. Ueda M, et al. Mutations of the beta- and gamma-catenin genes are uncommon in human lung, breast, kidney, cervical and ovarian carcinomas. Br J Cancer 2001;85(1): 64–68.
100. Hommura F, et al. Increased expression of beta-catenin predicts better prognosis in nonsmall cell lung carcinomas. Cancer 2002;94(3):752–758.
101. Behrens J. Control of beta-catenin signaling in tumor development. Ann N Y Acad Sci 2000;910:21–33; discussion 33–35.
102. Momand J, et al. The mdm-2 oncogene product forms a complex with the p53 protein and inhibits p53–mediated transactivation. Cell 1992;69(7):1237–1245.
103. Holst V, et al. p53 and K-ras mutational genotyping in pulmonary carcinosarcoma, spindle cell carcinoma, and pulmonary blastoma: implications for histogenesis. Am J Surg Pathol 1997;21(7):801–811.
104. Mountain CF. New prognostic factors in lung cancer. Biologic prophets of cancer cell aggression. Chest 1995; 108(1):246–254.
105. Rodenhuis S, et al. Mutational activation of the K-ras oncogene. A possible pathogenetic factor in adenocarcinoma of the lung. N Engl J Med 1987;317(15):929–935.
106. Rosell R, et al. Prognostic impact of mutated K-ras gene in surgically resected non-small cell lung cancer patients. Oncogene 1993;8(9):2407–2412.
107. vonRohr A, et al. Point mutations in codon 12 of the K-ras oncogene: incidence and clinical significance in patients with non-small cell lung cancer (meeting abstract). Ann Oncol 1992;3(suppl 5):9.
108. Makela V, Mattila S, Makinen J. Plasma cell granuloma (histiocytoma) of the lung and pleura. Report on three cases. Acta Pathol Microbiol Scand [A] 1972;80(5): 634–640.
109. Muraoka S, et al. Plasma cell granuloma of the lung with extrapulmonal extension. Immunohistochemical and electron microscopic studies. Acta Pathol Jpn 1985;35(4): 933–944.
110. Hutchins GM, Eggleston JC. Unusual presentation of pulmonary inflammatory pseudotumor (plasma cell granuloma) as esophageal obstruction. Am J Gastroenterol 1979;71(5):501–504.
111. Kim I, et al. Inflammatory pseudotumor of the lung manifesting as a posterior mediastinal mass. Pediatr Radiol 1992;22(6):467–468.
112. Hong HY, Castelli MJ, Walloch JL. Pulmonary plasma cell granuloma (inflammatory pseudotumor) with invasion of thoracic vertebra. Mt Sinai J Med 1990;57(2):117–121.
113. Coffin CM, et al. Extrapulmonary inflammatory myofibroblastic tumor (inflammatory pseudotumor). A clinicopathologic and immunohistochemical study of 84 cases. Am J Surg Pathol 1995;19(8):859–872.
114. Hussong JW, et al. Comparison of DNA ploidy, histologic, and immunohistochemical findings with clinical outcome in inflammatory myofibroblastic tumors. Mod Pathol 1999;12(3):279–286.
115. Coffin CM, et al. ALK1 and p80 expression and chromosomal rearrangements involving 2p23 in inflammatory myofibroblastic tumor. Mod Pathol 2001;14(6):569–576.
116. Flieder DB, Suster S, Moran CA. Idiopathic fibroinflammatory (fibrosing/sclerosing) lesions of the mediastinum: a study of 30 cases with emphasis on morphologic heterogeneity. Mod Pathol 1999;12(3):257–264.
117. Litzky LA, Brooks JJ. Cytokeratin immunoreactivity in malignant fibrous histiocytoma and spindle cell tumors: comparison between frozen and paraffin-embedded tissues. Mod Pathol 1992;5(1):30–34.
118. Yousem SA, Hochholzer L. Malignant fibrous histiocytoma of the lung. Cancer 1987;60(10):2532–2541.
119. Fukayama M, et al. Pulmonary and pleural thymoma. Diagnostic application of lymphocyte markers to the thymoma of unusual site. Am J Clin Pathol 1988;89(5): 617–621.
120. Hishima T, et al. CD70 expression in thymic carcinoma. Am J Surg Pathol 2000;24(5):742–746.
121. Suster S, Rosai J. Thymic carcinoma. A clinicopathologic study of 60 cases. Cancer 1991;67(4):1025–1032.
122. Kuo TT, Chan JK. Thymic carcinoma arising in thymoma is associated with alterations in immunohistochemical profile. Am J Surg Pathol 1998;22(12):1474–1481.
123. Suster S, Moran CA. Spindle cell thymic carcinoma: clinicopathologic and immunohistochemical study of a distinctive variant of primary thymic epithelial neoplasm. Am J Surg Pathol 1999;23(6):691–700.
124. Attanoos RL, et al. Primary thymic epithelial tumours of the pleura mimicking malignant mesothelioma. Histopathology 2002;41(1):42–49.
125. Attanoos RL, Thomas DH, Gibbs AR. Synchronous diffuse malignant mesothelioma and carcinomas in asbestos-exposed individuals. Histopathology 2003;43(4):387–3 92.
126. Cavazza A, et al. Cytokeratin-positive malignant solitary fibrous tumour of the pleura: an unusual pitfall in the diagnosis of pleural spindle cell neoplasms. Histopathology 2003;43(6):606–608.
127. Dei Tos A, et al. Immunohistochemical demonstration of glycoprotein p30/32 mic2 (CD99) in synovial sarcoma: a potential cause of diagnostic confusion. Appl Immunohistochem 1995;3:168–173.
128. Suster S, Fisher C, Moran C. Expression of bcl-2 oncoprotein in benign and malignant spindle cell tumors of soft tissue, skin, serosal surfaces, and gastrointestinal tract. Am J Surg Pathol 1998;22:863–872.
129. Renshaw A. O-13 (CD99) in spindle-cell tumors—reactivity with hemangiopericytoma, solitary fibrous tumor,

synovial sarcoma, and meningioma but rarely with sarcomatoid mesothelioma. Appl Immunohistochem 1995;3: 250–256.
130. Cavazza A, et al. Lung tumors with a rhabdoid phenotype. Am J Clin Pathol 1996;105(2):182–188.
131. Dueland S, et al. Treatment and outcome of patients with extragonadal germ cell tumours—the Norwegian Radium Hospital's experience 1979–1994. Br J Cancer 1998;77(2): 329–335.
132. Guarino M, et al. Sarcomatoid carcinomas: pathological and histopathogenetic considerations. Pathology 1996; 28(4):298–305.
133. Hasleton PS, et al. Pleural myxoma associated with a pulmonary squamous cell carcinoma. Respir Med 1989;83(5): 443–444.
134. McCluggage WG. Malignant biphasic uterine tumours: carcinosarcomas or metaplastic carcinomas? J Clin Pathol 2002;55(5):321–325.

38 Tracheobronchial Tumors of the Salivary Gland Type

Armando E. Fraire and David H. Dail

Tumors derived from the submucosal glands of the tracheobronchial tree are currently known as tumors of the salivary gland type. Most but not all of the tumors occurring in the major and minor salivary glands of the head and neck are known to occur in the respiratory tract. In the past, the term *bronchial adenoma* has been used to designate a group of slow-growing neoplasms, many of which arise from the bronchial glands of the respiratory tract. This is unfortunate since some of these so-called adenomas are in fact low-grade malignancies. Therefore, the term *bronchial adenoma* is to be discouraged and will not be used in this chapter.

Under the term *tumors of tracheobronchial (salivary) gland origin* we discuss the following benign and malignant tumors of the tracheobronchial glands: pleomorphic adenomas, mucoepidermoid tumors, adenoid cystic carcinomas, mucous gland adenomas, acinic cell tumors, pulmonary oncocytomas, epithelial-myoepithelial tumors, and polymorphous low-grade adenocarcinomas. In addition, in a section titled Other Tumors Believed to Be of Salivary Gland Origin, we discuss adenosquamous carcinoma with amyloid stroma, sebaceous carcinoma, sialadenoma papilliferum, and pneumocytic adenomyoepithelioma.

Pleomorphic Adenoma

Pleomorphic adenomas also known as mixed tumors are distinctly uncommon in the lung. Earlier cases were reported in the 1960s,[1] and by the early 1990s 16 cases had been described in the trachea and 12 cases in the bronchi and lungs.[2–14] These tumors occur in adults ages 47 to 74 with a mean of 68 years, and affect men and women about equally with only a slight female predominance. In an extensive review of the literature from 1922 to 1978, Ma et al.[3] documented 14 cases in the trachea and more were added by 1988.[5] In this tracheal location these tumors occur in more men than women by a factor of 2:1; they have occurred in the age range of 26 to 76, with a mean age of 50 years, and some have acted in a malignant fashion. In whatever location, they should appear similar to those occurring more frequently in the head and neck and be similar in terms of their immunohistochemical staining features. Productive cough and intermittent dyspnea are manifestations of tracheal tumors. Other symptoms are hemoptysis, wheezing, and recurrent respiratory infections. In some patients the symptomatology may resemble that of bronchial asthma. Parenchymal tumors are clinically silent, and some are discovered on chest radiographs obtained for other reason. Those in the trachea can be visualized endoscopically or by computed tomography (CT) imaging (Fig. 38.1).

Endobronchial or tracheal pleomorphic adenomas are usually soft to rubbery, polypoid nodular masses ranging from 1.5 to 16 cm in diameter, covered by intact respiratory epithelium. The cut surfaces are gray-white and shiny owing to their myxoid content. The gross appearance of parenchymal tumors, on the other hand, has not been well described but is said to mimic the appearance of these tumors in the salivary glands of the head and neck. Computed tomography imaging recapitulates the gross appearances of these tumors and can be of help to the surgeon in preoperatively planning the resection.

Microscopically these tumors appear in the assorted patterns seen in the mixed tumors of the salivary glands. They have abundant glandular epithelial and stromal components (Figs. 38.2 and 38.3), with varying degrees of differentiation of the stroma into other elements such as myxoid tissue or cartilage. Characteristically, a gradual merging pattern between the epithelial and stromal components is noted in most tumors (Figs. 38.4 to 38.6). The epithelial cells are usually arranged in tubules or cell clusters, and have an angulated form and sometimes line-flattened small ducts. Mitoses and necrosis are infrequent in pleomorphic adenomas. Adenomas made up exclusively of glandular elements and showing no evidence of

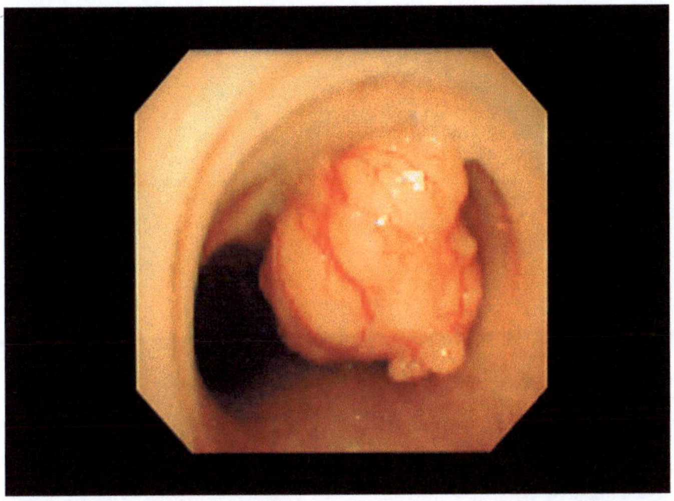

FIGURE 38.1. Pleomorphic adenoma of the trachea. Note sessile lobulated yellow tan endotracheal mass showing congested criss-crossing capillary blood vessels. (Courtesy of Dr. Jay S. Fleitman, Northhampton, MA.)

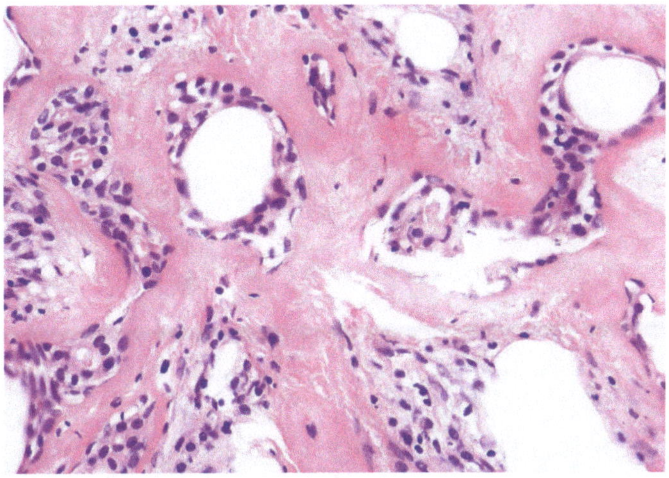

FIGURE 38.3. This area of a pleomorphic adenoma displays epithelial-lined tubules surrounded by trabecular strands of hypocellular collagenized fibrous stroma.

mesenchymal-like tissue are known as monomorphic adenomas. Well known in the salivary glands, these subtypes of pleomorphic adenomas (with the exception of oncocytoma later described in this chapter) are distinctly uncommon in the respiratory tract.[15] Pleomorphic adenomas are usually S-100 protein, cytokeratin, actin, glial fibrillary acidic protein, and vimentin positive. Ang and colleagues[16] have called attention to pulmonary pleomorphic adenomas with a high proliferative index, mainly in their epithelial component, and immunoreactivity to tumor suppressor gene product p16, and have suggested that p16 along with high proliferative indices may help to predict aggressive behavior.

In addition to metastases from primary salivary gland tumors, the differential diagnosis primarily includes mucoepidermoid tumors and adenoid cystic carcinomas as well as biphasic tumors such as carcinosarcomas and some unclassifiable bronchial gland tumors. The presence of foci of squamous cell carcinoma, tubulopapillary adenocarcinoma, or angioinvasion along with preserved features of pleomorphic adenomas helps to differentiate malignant mixed tumors (also known as carcinoma ex pleomorphic adenomas) from ordinary pleomorphic adenomas.[17] The presence of any frankly sarcomatous stroma excludes pleomorphic adenoma and should initiate a workup for either a primary or metastatic malignant tumor. Major differential features among pleomorphic

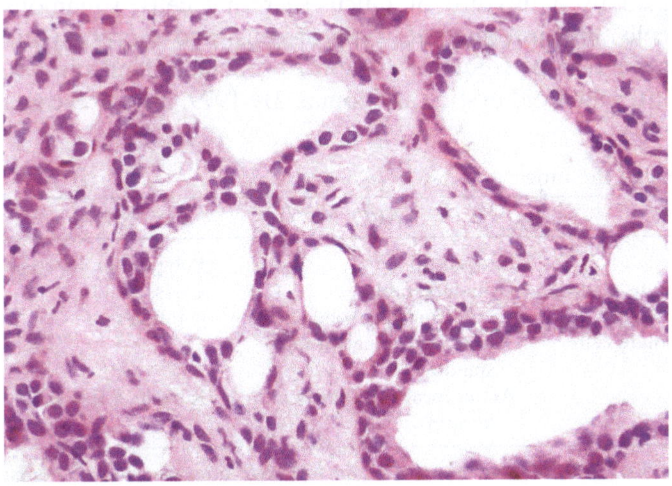

FIGURE 38.2. Pleomorphic adenoma showing well-defined tubular epithelial components.

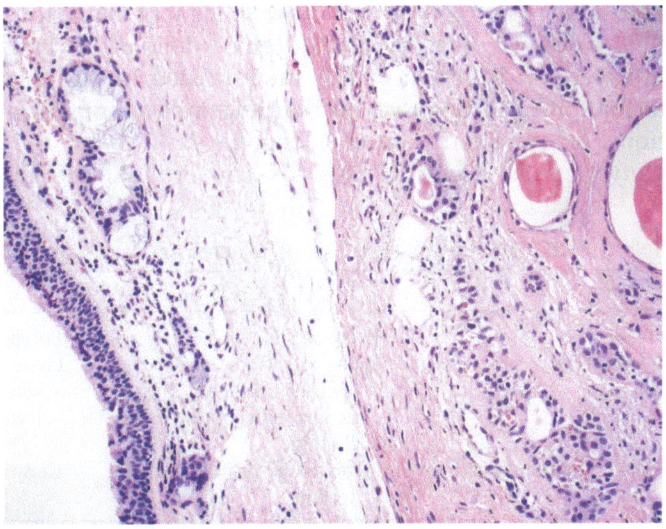

FIGURE 38.4. This subepithelial well-defined pleomorphic adenoma shows few dilated tubules containing eosinophilic coagulum.

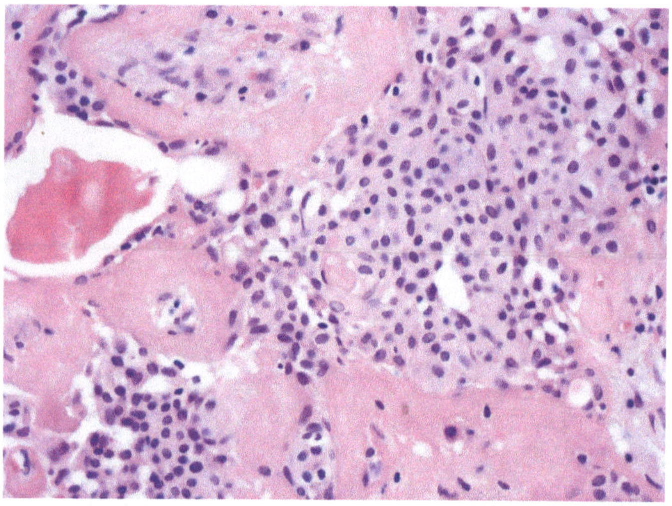

FIGURE 38.5. This area of a pleomorphic adenoma shows a group of basophilic somewhat elongated cells with a myoepithelial appearance.

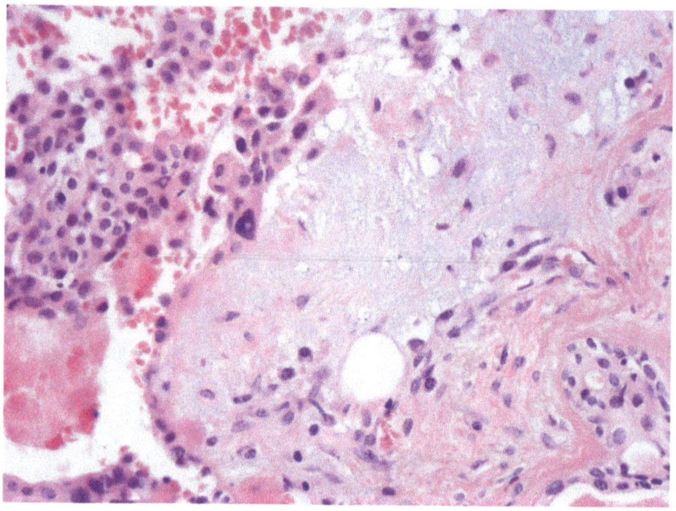

FIGURE 38.6. A centrally placed area of myxoid change is evident in this illustration of a pleomorphic adenoma. Note myoepithelial cells in the left upper corner.

adenomas, mucoepidermoid tumors, adenoid cystic carcinomas, and mucous gland adenomas are shown in Table 38.1.[18] An example of the above-cited monomorphic variant of pleomorphic adenoma showing cords and sheets of uniform epithelial cells with focal S-100 protein positivity was described 1993.[15] The main differential of this variant is with the equally rare pulmonary paraganglioma.[17] Immunostains for S-100 protein, chromogranin, and other neuroendocrine markers assist in making the distinction.

Pleomorphic adenomas may recur many years after surgical resection.[1] Recurrences have been reported at the line of resection and in the opposite lung. Other recurrences have been reported in a lumbar vertebra[6]; one other was reported to show malignant behavior.[8] One case of a primary pleomorphic adenoma of lung reported by Takeuchi et al.[19] metastasized to multiple distant sites. In this case no rearrangements, amplifications, or overexpression of oncogenes *bcl-2, c-erb B-2, c-myc,* L-*myc,* N-*myc,* H-*ras,* or K-*ras* were found. Likewise, immunohistochemistry failed to show aberrance in expression of tumor suppressor gene products Rb, p16, or p53. The authors suggested unknown mechanisms as responsible for the aggressiveness of the metastasizing pleomorphic adenoma.[19] As with other tracheobronchial gland-derived tumors, those reported outside the trachea and bronchi raise the possibility of metastases to the lung.[20,21] The lung is relatively infrequently the destination for such metastasizing mixed tumors; in the series by Wenig et al.,[20] only two of 11 tumors spreading from the main salivary glands had pulmonary metastases.

Mucoepidermoid Tumors

Mucoepidermoid tumors are microscopically characterized by a mixture of mucus-secreting cells, squamous cells, and intermediate type of cells, and represent the second most frequent group of bronchial gland tumors, after adenoid cystic carcinomas. By 1979, about 80 cases

TABLE 38.1. Comparative analysis of selected salivary gland tumors of the lung

Features	PA (MT)	MET	ACC	MGA
Gross	Polypoid	Polypoid	Heaped up	Polypoid or spherical
Microscopic	Biphasic pattern, cords, ducts, solid sheets, myxoid stroma with spindle cells, cartilage	Cysts, mucous glands, squamous cells, intermediate cells	Cylinders, tubules, cribriforming, solid sheets, myxoid stroma without spindle cells	Cysts, glands, tubules
Positive immunoreactivity	Actin, S-100 protein, GFAP, keratin	Keratin	Actin, focal S-100 protein, keratin	Keratin, CEA, EMA

PA (MT), pleomorphic adenoma/mixed tumor; MET, mucoepidermoid tumors; ACC, adenoid cystic carcinomas; MGA, mucous gland adenoma; GFAP, glial fibrillary acidic protein; CEA, carcinoembryonic antigen; EMA, epithelial membrane antigen.

Source: Colby TV, Koss MN, Travis WD. Tumors of the lower respiratory tract. AFIP atlas of tumor pathology. Third series. Washington, DC: Armed Forces Institute of Pathology/American Registry of Pathology, 1995, with permission.

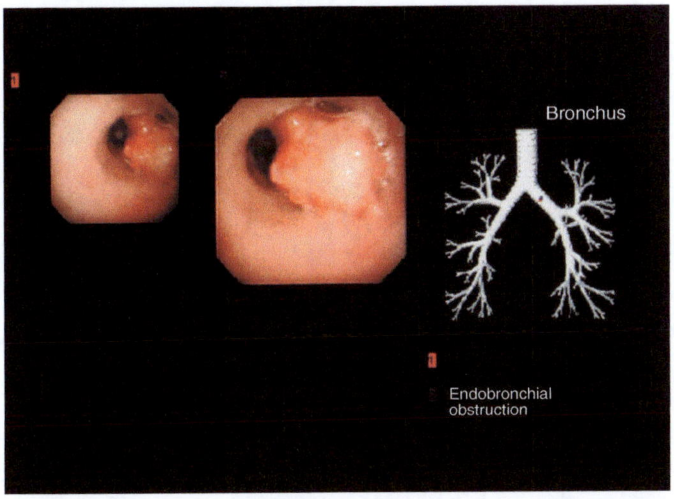

FIGURE 38.7. Endoscopic view of a mucoepidermoid tumor of the left main stem bronchus. Note broadly attached tumor mass with a knobby surface and glistening yellow pink mucosa. (Courtesy of Dr. Scott Kopec, University of Massachusetts Medical School, Worcester, MA.)

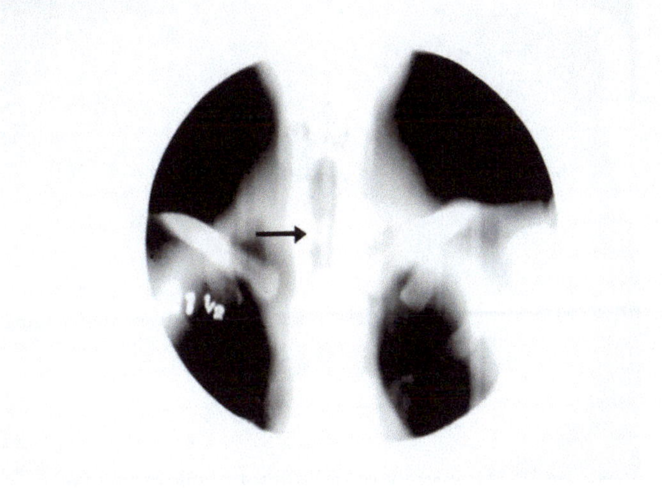

FIGURE 38.8. Radiographic image (tomogram) of a mucoepidermoid tumor of the trachea. The tumor impinges upon the contour of the trachea. (Courtesy of Dr. Jerry Balikian, University of Massachusetts Medical School, Worcester, MA.)

of mucoepidermoid tumors in the bronchi,[22] but only a few in the trachea, had been reported.[23–25] Several larger series of mucoepidermoid tumors in bronchi have been described, including 18 cases by Heitmiller et al.[26] and 58 cases by Yousem and Hochholzer.[27] The age distribution of mucoepidermoid tumors is wide, with cases occurring in individuals 4 to 78 years, with about two thirds in the age range 45 to 70. Cases in children under the age of 14 represent about 10% to 15% of all reported patients.[28,29] In Spencer's[6] series, seven of eight cases occurred under the age of 21, even though his consultation practice was not predominantly pediatric. Some childhood cases occur in association with pulmonary congenital malformations such as congenital atresia of the left upper lobe, while others have been reported in children and adolescents of Hispanic descent.[30–32] There is about an equal sex incidence, although some series show a slight male and others a slight female predominance. Endoscopic and tomographic appearances of tumors in the airways are shown in Figures 38.7 and 38.8, respectively.

On chest radiographs, mucoepidermoid tumors of the lung most often appear as centrally located masses with signs of postobstructive pneumonia or peripheral atelectasis.[33] In a study of 12 patients by Kim and collaborators,[33] four were pulmonary and eight were tracheobronchial. Six were lobulated and six were oval shaped. Punctate calcification was seen in six cases. Pathologically, two distinct groups of mucoepidermoid tumors are recognized: the low-grade tumors occur in children and younger adults and are usually benign in their behavior, and the high-grade tumors, which are less common than the low grade, are apt to occur in older adults and carry a poorer prognosis.[34] The grading is based on histology (necrosis, mitoses, and nuclear pleomorphism) as well as on the basis of gross appearance.[34]

Grossly, mucoepidermoid tumors, especially the lower-grade ones, are usually polypoid in the bronchi, and the higher-grade lesions are less polypoid than the low-grade lesions (Figs. 38.9 to 38.11). They do not extend in as linear a fashion along the wall of the airways as do adenoid cystic carcinomas, discussed later in this chapter.

Microscopically, the low-grade lesions show significant heritage to bronchial glands, with abundant mucinous

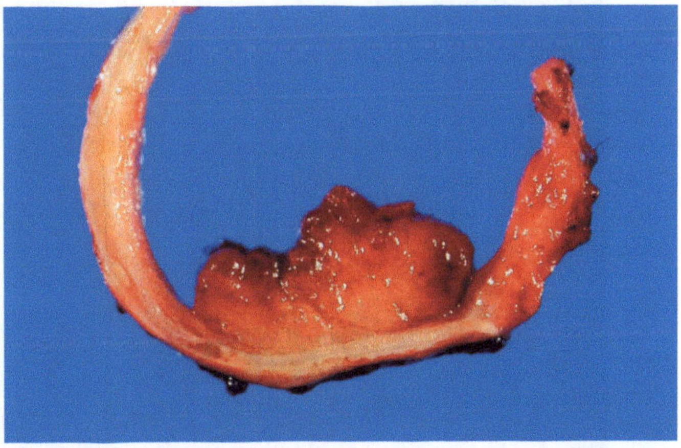

FIGURE 38.9. Mucoepidermoid tumor, endotracheal type. Note polypoid nonocclusive growth at endoluminal surface of the trachea. (Courtesy of Dr. Andrew H. Fischer, University of Massachusetts Medical School, Worcester, MA.)

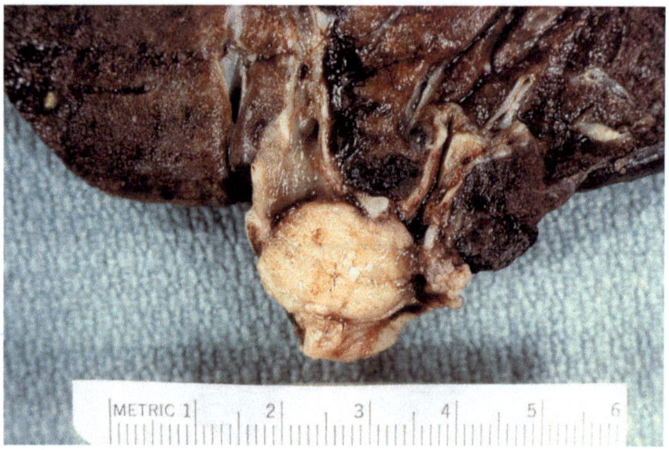

FIGURE 38.10. Mucoepidermoid tumor, endobronchial type. Note near-total obstruction of bronchial lumen by spheroidal yellow white tumor mass.

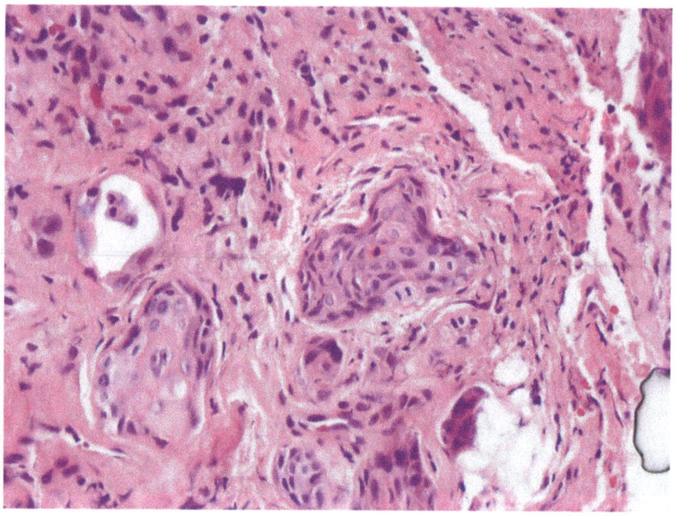

FIGURE 38.12. Mucoepidermoid tumor. Note islands of squamous epithelial cells and mucin-producing glandular epithelium.

cysts staining with acidic, weakly acidic, and neutral mucosubstance stains, as well as goblet cells. These cyst-like spaces or goblet cells may be predominant within the tumor. The mucoepidermoid nature is determined by more solid collections of nonkeratinizing squamoid or transitional cells or bland pale cells adjacent to these cysts, sometimes arranged as small nests or larger sheets. Some of these cells appear intermediate between glandular and true squamous cells (Figs. 38.12 to 38.14). Focal keratinization may or may not be present but is generally rare.[27] Rare mitoses are present in the low-grade lesions, and some of these tumors overlap with those described as mucous gland adenomas. The high-grade lesions have an abundance of solid sheets of intermediate cells. Clear or oncocytic cells are seen in low- and high-grade lesions. Rarely, giant cells are also seen in the high-grade ones.[35] Increasing pleomorphism and mitotic rate along with necrosis are seen in higher grade lesions. Ultrastructural findings generally recapitulate findings at the light microscopic level. Gross, microscopic, and ultrastructural differences between low- and high-grade mucoepidermoid tumors of the bronchus are summarized in Table 38.2.[36]

The differential diagnosis in the higher grade lesions is primarily with poorly differentiated squamous carcinoma, especially when the few mucin pools that may be present are missed and when the intermediate character of these cells is not readily apparent. Significant keratinization

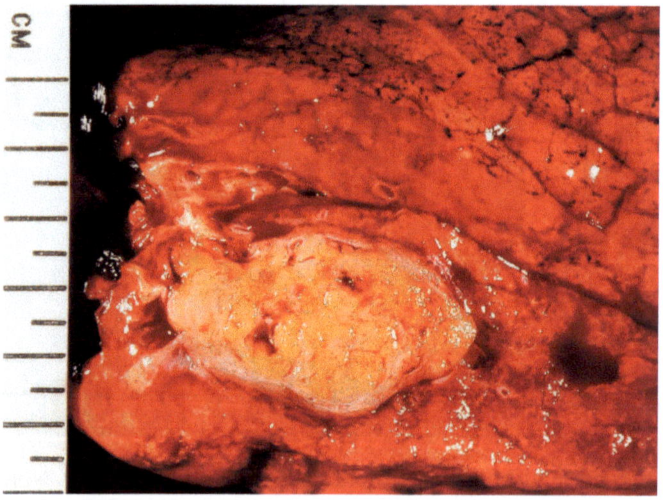

FIGURE 38.11. Mucoepidermoid tumor, parenchymal type. Note yellow-gray well-outlined tumor.

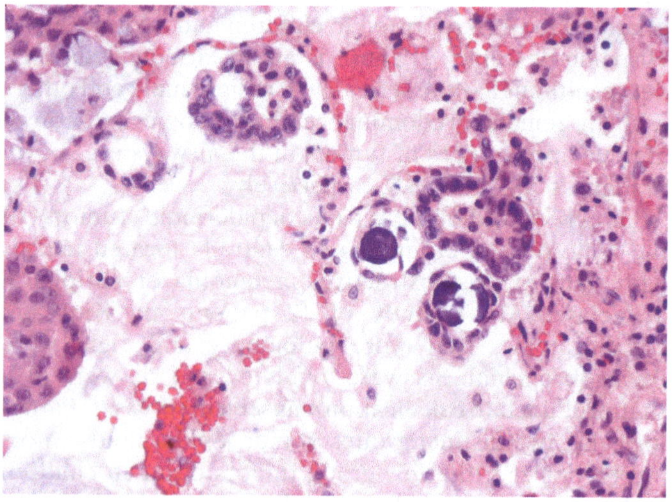

FIGURE 38.13. Mucoepidermoid tumor showing calcified spherules within glandular elements and an island of squamoid intermediate-looking cells on the left.

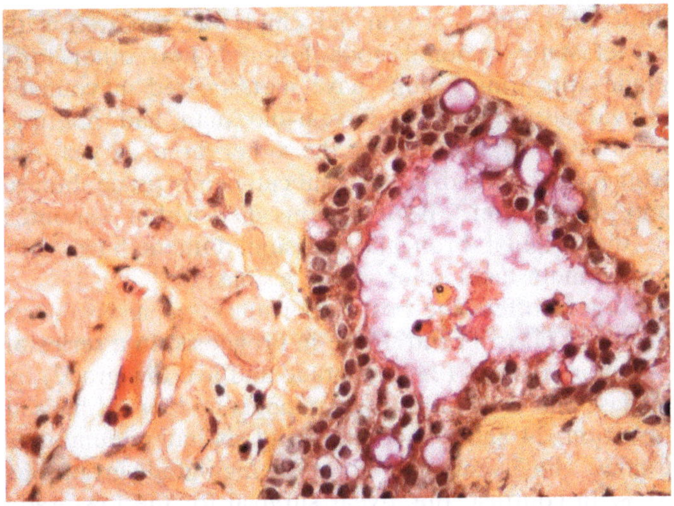

FIGURE 38.14. Mucoepidermoid tumor showing areas of mucicarmine-positive intracellular and extracellular material.

should make one consider squamous or adenosquamous carcinoma a more likely diagnosis. Ultrastructural study can assist in the identification of rare variants of mucoepidermoid tumors. In a case of papillary variant of mucoepidermoid carcinoma occurring in a 89-year-old woman, Guillou and associates[37] identified mucous cells, transitional cells, and ciliated cells by electron microscopy. The mucous cells contained mucous secretory granules, rough endoplasmic reticulum, mitochondria in moderate numbers, and scattered bundles of intermediate filaments.

Adenosquamous carcinomas are in the differential diagnosis of both low- and high grade tumors but primarily for the higher-grade lesions. Adenosquamous carcinomas are aggressive tumors that usually do not center on bronchi, tend to occur peripherally in the lung, and usually are large and without the sheet-like transitional cells of mucoepidermoid tumors. Some tumors overlap, however. Heitmiller et al.[26] have actually suggested that adenosquamous carcinomas and mucoepidermoid tumors are part of a continuum. Even the high-grade mucoepidermoid tumors tend to fare better than the more conventional types of lung cancer, so attempts at differentiation, if possible, are helpful. One peripheral mucoepidermoid tumor has been described but is perhaps better considered adenosquamous carcinoma.[38] A unique variant of mucoepidermoid tumor with a striking lymphoplasmacytic component, recently reported by Shilo et al.,[39] needs to be differentiated from low-grade pulmonary lymphomas. In this variant, the lymphoplasmacytic component is believed to be akin to lymphoid infiltrates in tumors of the major salivary glands, which are regarded as tumor-associated lymphoid proliferations.[39] In their series of six patients, Shilo et al.'s initial diagnostic consideration included a host of entities such as inflammatory pseudotumors, mucoepidermoid tumors metastatic to lymph nodes, and, in one instance, lymphoma of lung. The authors suggest that in most cases the clinical presentation is of a localized lesion, and the presence of a neoplastic epithelial component and clonality studies should help to exclude lymphoma from the differential.[39]

Cytology plays a limited role in the differential diagnosis of mucoepidermoid carcinomas but sometimes can suggest the diagnosis. Intermediate cells may be seen in low-grade tumors. Cytologically, high-grade mucoepidermoid tumors are indistinguishable from adenosquamous carcinomas. Segletes et al.[40] stress the difficulties in differentiating high-grade mucoepidermoid tumors from adenosquamous carcinomas. Presence of cells showing glandular and intermediate/squamoid differentiation are helpful cytopathologic hints.[40]

To date, Yousem and Hochholzer[27] have published the largest series of mucoepidermoid tumors of the lung. Their series, which included 45 low-grade and 13 high-grade lesions, is worth discussing in some detail. Their low-grade group consisted of 27 women and 18 men, despite the male predominance of their Armed Forces Institute of Pathology database.[27] The group age range was 9 to 78 years, averaging 34.8 years; seven (16%) were younger than 20, and 25 (56%) younger than 30 years of age, and only four were over 60 at the time of resection. Of interest, 89% were symptomatic, usually with cough, pneumonia, fever, or hemoptysis. Tobacco was smoked by 41%. Chest radiographs showed a solitary mass in 29 (64%), focal pneumonic consolidation in 15 (33%), and in one (2%) the chest radiograph was normal. Upper lobe bronchi were more often involved (59%) than lower lobe bronchi. Some 60% were predominantly glandular, 36% were of equal admixture, and 4% were predominantly solid. There was only mild nuclear pleomorphism; mitoses were rare, fewer than

TABLE 38.2. Low- vs. high-grade mucoepidermoid tumors

Features	Low grade	High grade
Gross	Polypoid, exophytic minimal or no extension into lung	Less polypoid, extending into lung tissue
Microscopic	Sheets of monomorphic cells, no or few mitoses, numerous mucous glands, no necrosis	Sheets of atypical cells, fewer glands, necrosis
Ultrastructure	Numerous goblet cells, prominent glandular lumina, rare transitional cells, rare squamous cells	Rare goblet cells, infrequent lumens, abundant transitional cells rare squamous cells

Source: Modified from Barsky et al.[36] Copyright 1983, by American Cancer Society. With permission of Wiley-Liss, Inc., a subsidiary of John Wiley & Sons, Inc.

1 per 20 high power fields (HPFs), and no necrosis was seen. Calcification of extracellular mucin was noted in 10 (22%) and ossification in four (9%); no invasion was identified in three (7%).

In this series, the high-grade group included 13 patients, with an age range of 13 to 67 years (average, 44.5), with four less than 20 years and five more than 60 years of age. Ten patients were symptomatic. Of interest, there were fewer symptoms in this group than in the low-grade mucoepidermoid group, probably related to the prominent endobronchial polypoid protrusion of the low-grade group with less wall invasion. This interpretation was supported by the presence of obstructive pneumonia in only one (8%), and lung infiltration in six (46%) of these high-grade cases. Tumor size varied from 1.5 to 4 cm, averaging 2.75 cm. Histologically, a solid appearance predominated in seven, mixed in three, and predominantly glandular in three. There was moderate to marked cytologic atypia, and mitotic activity averaged four per 10 HPFs; necrosis was present in almost half and spread to hilar nodes was seen in two. Patients in this group who had recurrences were all 58 years of age or older, and death from this tumor occurred in about one third of this age group. There were no histologic criteria within the high-grade group that distinguished those that did poorly. Attention was drawn in this series to some less common cellular patterns, as described in mucoepidermoid tumors of the salivary glands of the head and neck, including oncocytic change, clear cell change, focally dense hyaline sclerosis, and the colloid quality to some of the pools of intracystic mucin.[41–44]

Another (previously cited) series by Heitmiller and associates[26] described 18 patients—15 low grade and three high grade. This series confirmed the foregoing findings except that two of their three high-grade cases could not be resected, and one had extensive hilar and mediastinal lymph node spread; all three (17%) in this group died of their tumors.

In the past mucoepidermoid tumors have been considered by some to be so low grade as to be called benign, but as noted earlier high-grade lesions are well known to occur. Reichle and Rosemond[45] reviewed 29 cases in 1966. Metastases of this tumor from the lung were not described until 1961, by Ozlu et al.,[46] and in 1962 by Dowling et al.[47] Healey et al.[48] described criteria for low-grade and high-grade mucoepidermoid tumors in the salivary gland system, and in the next year Turnbull and associates[49] published 12 cases occurring in the lung, all high-grade mucoepidermoid tumors, five presenting with metastases by the time of diagnosis, and seven developing metastases shortly thereafter. The average duration of symptoms to death in these patients varied from 6 to 18 months, and the average survival was 9.8 months. Mucoepidermoid tumors in children are almost all benign in their behavior, and it was not until 1984 that a 4-year-old child was reported with a metastatic regional node lesion.[29] Two other low-grade–appearing lesions have metastasized in younger individuals; one in a 26-year-old man had multiple metastases to skin,[50] and the other in a 32-year-old woman had spread to skin, subcutaneous tissue, bones, and pericardium.[36] Both patients died within 3 months of the original bronchial excision. Others have confirmed metastases in low-grade lesions.[27,47,51]

Surgery offers the best opportunity for survival, but histology plays a central role in prognosis. In a series of 34 reported cases (29 high grade and five low grade) by Vadasz and Egervary,[52] four patients underwent limited resection, 24 had lobectomies, and six had pneumonectomies. The 5-year survival for the high-grade group was 31%. In contrast, the 5-year survival for the low-grade group amounted to 80%.

Adenoid Cystic Carcinomas

Within the tracheobronchial system, adenoid cystic carcinomas are the most common salivary-type gland tumors of the trachea, accounting for 20% to 35% of tracheal tumors and 75% to 80% of all tracheobronchial gland tumors.[53–58] Within the lung parenchyma adenoid cystic carcinomas are much less common. In some instances, a peripheral (apical) pulmonary location may result in the development of a Pancoast syndrome.[59] In a series of 12 cases, nine were located in the trachea and three in the mainstem bronchi.[60] When in the lung, they are usually in the central bronchi and are infrequent more distally, unless they represent metastases from another site.[61,62] They may present as nodules within, or a generalized constriction of, the major airways. They have a tendency to grow in linear fashion along the tracheobronchial walls or to form nodular growth that may ulcerate the mucosa.[63–65] This tendency is in contrast to carcinoid tumors and mucoepidermoid tumors, which have a tendency to be nodular.[63]

Patients range in age from 18 to 82 years, with an average in most series of 45 to 47 years. Men and women are about equally represented, and tobacco exposure is not a risk factor. Symptoms, usually resulting from partial airway obstruction, include wheezing, progressive shortness of breath, and hemoptysis. Hemoptysis is caused by surface ulceration, but may also be related to effects of more distal obstruction. Other obstructive symptoms may include chronic cough, which becomes more productive, fever, and general cachexia in advanced cases.

Grossly, the tumor masses are rubbery to quite firm and pink-tan to gray-white. Although the masses are always infiltrative, Nomori et al.[66] have divided these into three groups: first, those that are grossly polypoid with

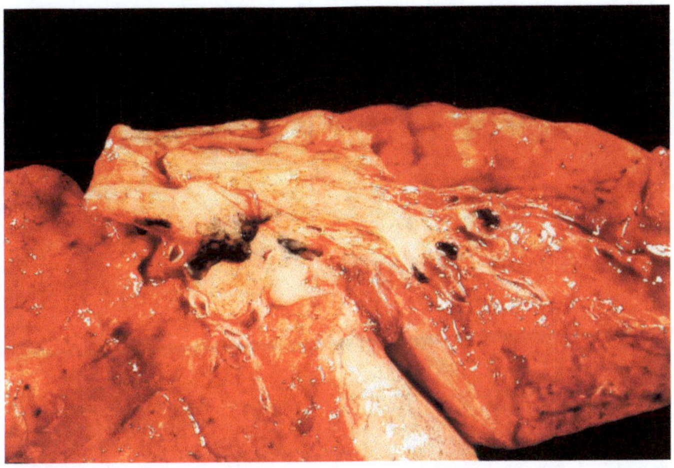

FIGURE 38.15. Adenoid cystic carcinoma. A tumor mass extends into lower lobe from mainstem bronchus. Extensions into upper lobe show dense cores of tumor with minimal evidence of patent bronchial lumina.

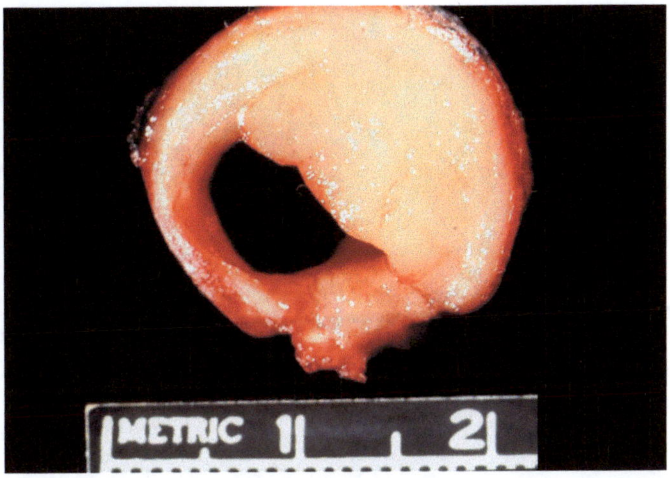

FIGURE 38.16. Adenoid cystic carcinoma of the airway. Note significant eccentric narrowing of lumen by an expanding tumor mass showing a pale yellow smooth cut surface. (Courtesy of Dr. Eugene J. Mark, Massachusetts General Hospital, Boston, MA.)

minimum infiltration of walls, which are usually less aggressive; second, those that are both polypoid and infiltrative, which are intermediate in behavior; and third, those that are predominantly infiltrative and extraluminal, which are the most aggressive. Sometimes it is difficult to identify remnant lumina in the airways (Fig. 38.15). Direct extension into adjacent structures, including nodes, may occur, usually in higher-grade solid tumors. High-grade tumors have a greater tendency toward radial spread to adjacent lung than linear spread along the bronchi and trachea.[66] Lung tumors usually infiltrate the adjacent lung in continuity with the edge of infiltration, but may have lymphatic extension away from the main tumor mass. Because of late detection of many of these tumors, spread may be more extensive than at first anticipated. Those in the airways may grow endoluminally (Fig. 38.16).

Histologically, these tumors may infiltrate bronchi in a radial fashion and encase blood vessels. They appear identical to those in the salivary gland tissue, with compact nuclei, a relatively high nuclear/cytoplasmic ratio, cysts rather evenly contoured but of varying caliber within larger tubules of tumor, and a stroma that is often hyalinized. Mitoses and necrosis are uncommon. The larger cystic spaces contain hyaluronidase-sensitive, Alcian-blue–positive mucin, while the small rather indistinct true glandular spaces contain periodic acid-Schiff (PAS) positive, diastase-resistant, neutral to weakly acidic mucin. A combined Alcian blue/PAS stain nicely highlights these characteristics. Duplicated and thickened PAS-positive basal lamina often surrounds the columns of tumor cells.

Three different microscopic patterns are recognized in the respiratory tract as in the salivary glands[66–69]: the well-differentiated tubular-trabecular pattern; the most typical intermediate cribriform-microcystic pattern, with no more than 20% solid component; and a poorly differentiated pattern with greater than a 20% solid component (Figs. 38.17 to 38.20). In general, the histologic

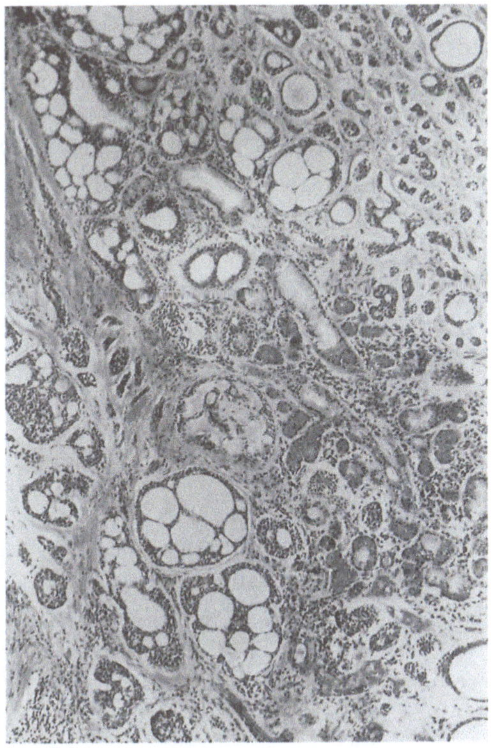

FIGURE 38.17. Adenoid cystic carcinoma. Typical-appearing tumor showing cribriform and tubular features.

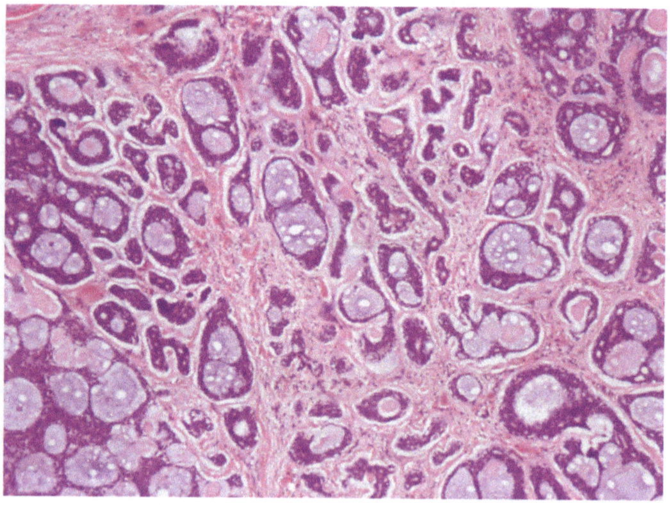

FIGURE 38.18. Adenoid cystic carcinoma. An area showing a predominant tubular pattern.

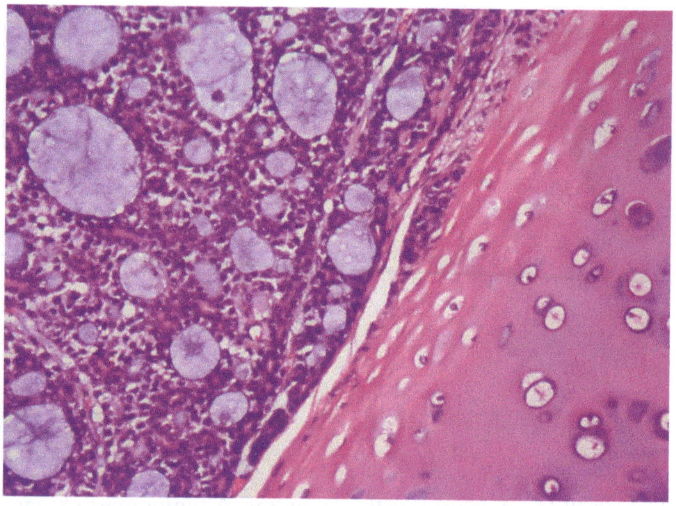

FIGURE 38.20. Adenoid cystic carcinoma. This area shows tumor adjacent to but not invading bronchial cartilage.

grades compare with the three gross appearances described. Lung tumors have an interesting tendency to form linear strands around nerves (Fig. 38.21), as is characteristic of these tumors elsewhere. The previously noted PAS-positive material seen within glands is also seen on hematoxylin and eosin (H&E) stains (Fig. 38.22). The cartilage may be easily circumvented by the tumor, but cartilaginous erosion also occurs. Lymphatic spaces may be infiltrated, and the nodes may be directly infiltrated eccentrically toward the side of the tumor mass. As noted in the Nomori et al.[66] series, normal tracheobronchial glands have serous components, but not much mucous components. Acinar cells stain for S-100 protein, lactoferrin, and cytokeratin, while myoepithelial cells of the acini and epithelial cells of the ducts stain intensely for cytokeratins and p63. Myoepithelial cells also stain positively for smooth muscle actin. The tubular and cribriform components of adenoid cystic carcinoma stain positively but variably for S-100 protein, lactoferrin, and cytokeratin. The solid components do not stain for these antigens. A similar immunoperoxidase study of five tracheobronchial adenoid cystic carcinomas by Ishida et al.[70] generally confirmed these findings. Albers and associates[71] studied 14 cases of tracheobronchial adenoid cystic carcinoma and stained them with CD117, and found that 13 of 13 cases tested

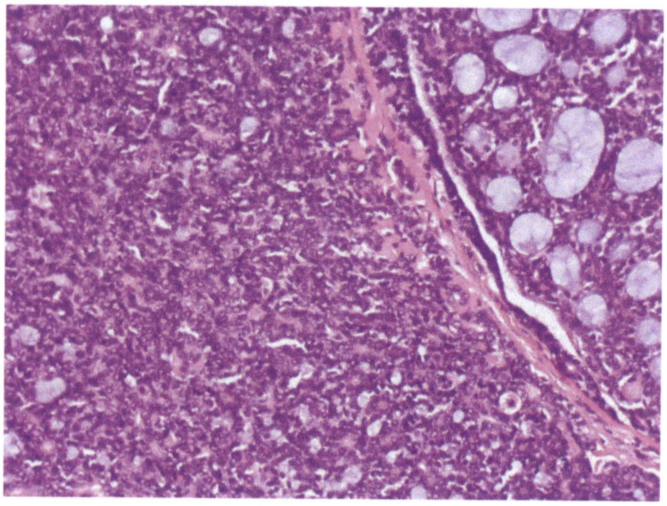

FIGURE 38.19. Adenoid cystic carcinoma. An area showing confluent nearly solidified tubular components.

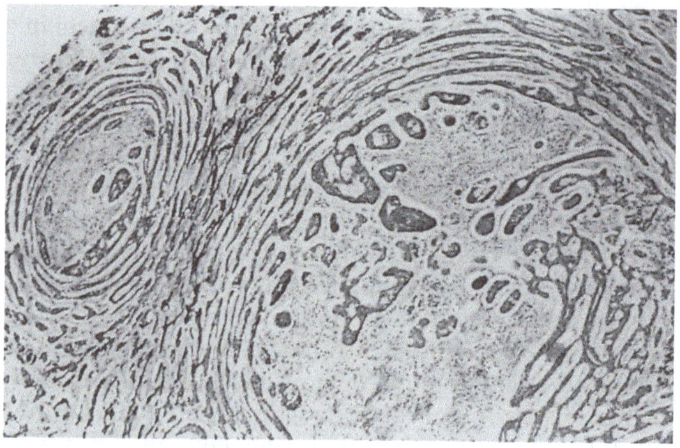

FIGURE 38.21. Adenoid cystic carcinoma. Typical peri- and intraneural tumor infiltration of this tumor occurs in the lung as elsewhere.

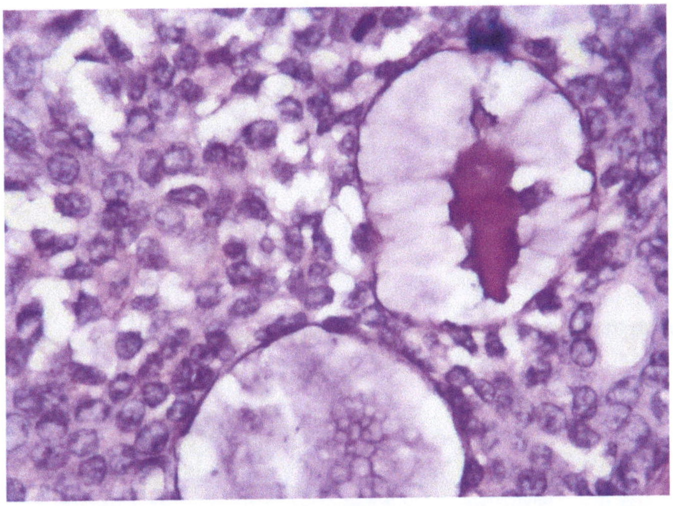

FIGURE 38.22. Adenoid cystic carcinoma. Deeply basophilic magenta-colored proteinaceous material fills a glandular space.

for CD117 were positive. The CD117 positivity was luminal and uniform in pattern. This suggests a possible use of CD117 as a potential marker for adenoid cystic carcinoma but with no correlation to histologic tumor grade.

Adenoid cystic carcinomas are occasionally diagnosed by aspiration cytology, but the material is usually submucosal, so an abrasive or extractive technique must be used to improve the diagnostic yield. Cytomorphologic features that may be helpful in the cytodiagnosis of adenoid cystic carcinomas include tridimensional clusters of basaloid cells and hyaline basement membrane material forming cylinders or spheres that are sharply demarcated from the tumor cells.[39,72]

The differential diagnosis often includes other carcinomas, mostly adenocarcinomas. The monotony of the tumor cells and their generally stiff-appearing mucinous spaces and separation by often hyalinized stroma are helpful indicators of adenoid cystic carcinoma when they are present. Some poorly differentiated carcinomas suggest they may have been adenoid cystic carcinomas, but we prefer calling them poorly differentiated adenocarcinomas with focal adenoid cystic areas. When more solid sheets of tumor cells are seen, adenoid cystic carcinoma may be mistaken for small cell carcinoma, but the chromatin pattern is not as homogeneous and there is more euchromatin evident than in small cell carcinoma. Also, they do not have as much nuclear crowding or molding, and individually infiltrating cells are not as predominant in adenoid cystic carcinomas as in small cell carcinomas. Finding focal areas of typical adenoid cystic carcinoma will help in difficult cases as they are required for an adenoid cystic carcinoma diagnosis and are not seen in small cell carcinoma. In difficult cases, assessment of the solid areas with neuroendocrine markers (such as CD56, chromogranin, and synaptophysin) will be of help to exclude small cell carcinoma occurring in combination with glandular components. Differentiation should also be made with metastatic adenoid cystic carcinomas to the lung, which in contrast to primary lesions are usually peripheral, small, and multiple. Metastatic adenoid cystic carcinomas may be some of the more slowly growing metastases to lung and rarely may show spontaneous regression.[73]

Occasional metastases have been described to regional nodes,[74] and rare extrathoracic spread may occur in liver, bone, adrenal glands, and kidney.[6] When the tumor is resectable long survival may result, but late local recurrences are a problem, and have occurred up to 17 years later in the bronchi[75] and 25 and 30 years later in the trachea.[76] Tumor stage at diagnosis plays an important role in predicting the clinical outcome.[77] In a series of 16 cases reported by Moran et al.,[77] clinical follow-up in six of the 16 patients showed that three were alive at 60, 120, and 144 months, and the other three were alive but with recurrence at 24, 60, and 180 months.

A 32-year experience with the outcome of 38 patients with adenoid cystic carcinoma presented by Maziak and collaborators[78] confirms the tendency for late local recurrence as characteristic of these tumors but suggests that excellent long-term palliation can be achieved after both complete and incomplete resections of tumors located in the airways. In the Maziak study, all patients were found to have local invasion beyond the wall of the trachea on pathologic examination. Forty-four percent of the patients had metachronous hematogenous metastases, and 33% had pulmonary metastases. Half of the resections performed were complete and potentially curative. Two patients died within 30 days of surgery. The remaining 14 had a mean survival of 9.8 years. Of the 16 patients undergoing incomplete resection, one died in the perioperative period, and 15 had a survival of 7.5 years. Mean survival in the six patients treated with primary radiation was 6.2 years. Those with pulmonary metastases had a mean survival of 37 months from the diagnosis of metastases. Radiotherapy may help to shrink the tumor mass, but nonsurgical cure is difficult, if possible at all. Obtaining clear surgical margins may be difficult at attempted resection, because the tumor tends to spread along the course of the bronchus or trachea, often well beyond that grossly visible, and even CT scans tend to underestimate the extent of intramural spread.[79] Perhaps some of the newer treatment protocols with neutron beam therapy or combined radiotherapy and chemotherapy may be helpful. Yttrium-aluminum-garnet (YAG) laser therapy may help preserve luminal patency in unresectable cases.

Mucous Gland Adenomas

Mucous gland adenomas are rare, benign epithelial and solitary tumors of the tracheobronchial tree.[80] Mucous gland adenomas have variously been referred to as adenomatous polyps, adenomas of mucous gland type, bronchial cystadenomas, and papillary cystadenomas. Only rarely have these tumors been described in the lower trachea[81] or more peripherally than the major bronchi.[82,83] Radiographic and CT findings in these rare tumors have not been well defined. The CT findings in two cases studied by Kwon et al.[84] indicated well-demarcated intraluminal masses manifesting as an air-meniscus sign or abutting the bronchus. However, in another study, radiographic findings included a greater variety of changes including infiltrating types, smooth nodular forms, and coin lesions.[80] Endoscopically, they appear as pink, mound-like structures (Fig. 38.23). Grossly, these tumors show a round, smooth, light-colored, and exophytic appearance. They range from 0.8 to 6.8cm and most are in the middle or lower lobes. They tend to have a gelatinous appearance.[80]

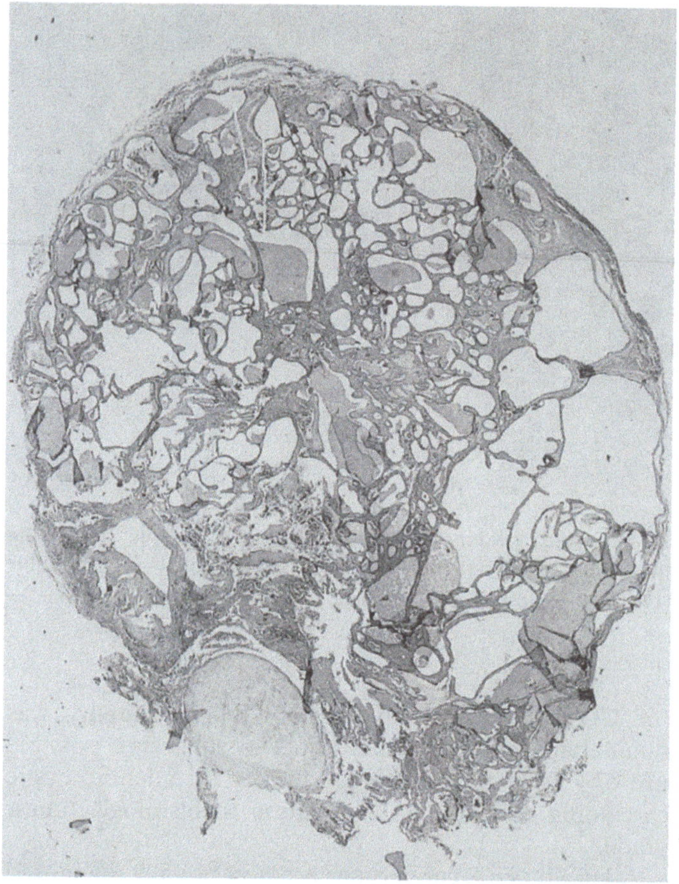

Figure 38.24. Mucous gland adenoma. Note multiple colloid-filled cystic spaces of varying diameter within a polypoid structure. An island of cartilage is present at bottom.

The histopathology suggests three different groups of mucous gland adenomas, all with varying but generally prominent cystic change. The first group consists of fairly orderly tubular glands lined by single columnar mucous cells, often surrounded by some chronic inflammatory reaction separating the tubules. They do not appear histologically complex or aggressive and may well be designated as mucinous tubular adenomas. Examples of this type are the cases reported by Ramsey and Reimann,[85] Gilman et al.,[86] and Kroe and Pitcock.[87] Whether some of the low-grade mucinous cystadenomas/cystadenocarcinomas described in Chapter 35 belong in this category is unclear. They are characterized by their distinct appearance.

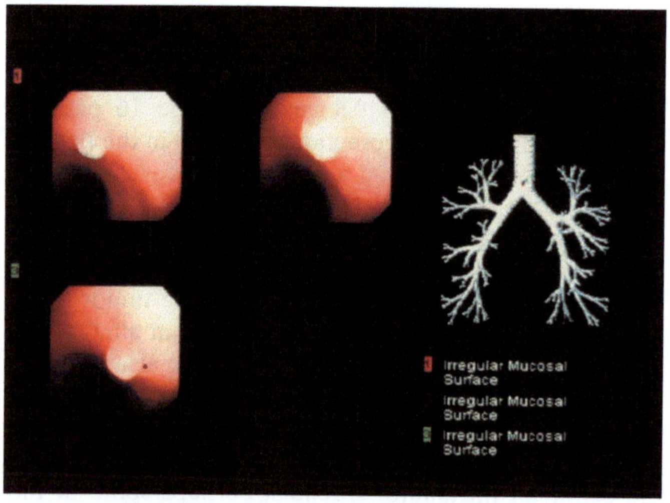

Figure 38.23. Mucous gland adenoma. Endoscopic view of mucous gland adenoma in the lower trachea, just above the bifurcation. Note small mound-like pink-white structure. (Courtesy of Dr. Richard Irwin, University of Massachusetts Medical School, Worcester, MA.)

The second group is composed of papillary and cystic adenomas, sometimes with a predominance of one pattern over another, but cystic in at least some parts. The papillary components tend to favor the luminal borders, and the cystic component is preserved toward the cartilage side of these submucosal tumor masses. The cells lining both areas are usually columnar, cuboidal, and rather monotonous, or may be more squamoid or flattened in appearance, particularly those lining enlarging cysts (Figs. 38.24 and 38.25). Fluid filling these cysts is usually homogeneous and appears dense and eosinophilic, sometimes like colloid. Examples of these in the literature are the cases of Allen et al.[83] and several reported by Spencer et al.[6]

The third group is close to the lowest grade mucoepidermoid tumors, as reported by Rosenblum and Klein[88] and Emory et al.[89] These contain small mucinous spaces with some "intermediate" cell types, possibly intercalated duct-type cells. In one case, tumor was expectorated

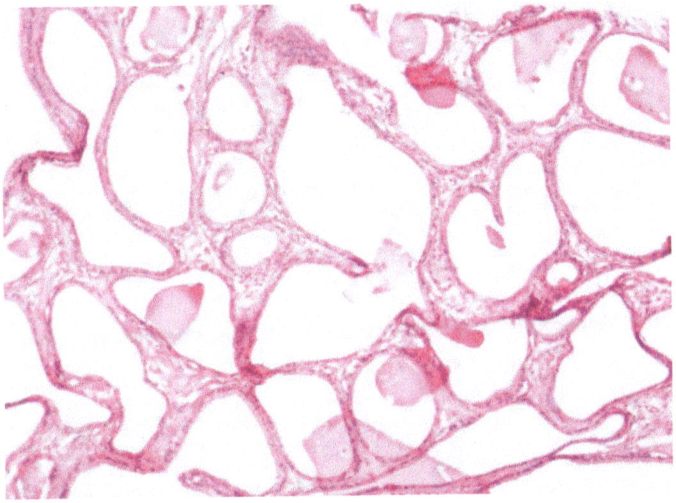

FIGURE 38.25. A closer view of the mucous gland adenoma shown in the preceding figure shows cystically dilated spaces lined by flat to low cuboidal epithelium.

during suctioning.[88] These are so low grade in histologic appearance as to suggest an adenoma designation.

Epithelial cells show immunoreactivity to epithelial membrane antigen (EMA), blood group substances, and cytokeratin. Cyst contents are positive for carcinoembryonic antigen and stromal cells for keratin. Proliferating cell nuclear antigen and Ki-67 show a low level of proliferative activity as compared to low-grade malignancies.[80] Electron microscopy shows myoepithelial cells and mucous cells with relatively uniform nuclei resembling low-grade mucoepidermoid carcinoma.[80]

Differential diagnosis includes mucoepidermoid tumors, particularly those with dominant cystic changes and low-grade mucinous adenocarcinomas. The presence of glycogen-rich intermediate cells with squamous differentiation aid in the differentiation from mucoepidermoid tumors.[80] The absence of cytologic atypia, mitoses, and focal necrosis assists in distinguishing mucous gland adenoma from low-grade mucinous adenocarcinoma and other adenocarcinomas. Clara or alveolar cell papillomas described elsewhere mostly arise in and grow on lung parenchyma and generally do not have cystic spaces, although some overlap may occur.[84] Mucous gland adenomas with greatly attenuated lining epithelium may resemble cystic lymphangiomas. In these instances appropriate use of endothelial markers will assist in making the distinction.

Histopathologic findings in mucous gland adenomas support the conclusion that they are benign tumors.[80] Complete excision of the tumor and the involved lung area usually results in cure. Nonetheless, because patients with these tumors can experience recurrent bouts of pneumonia and other bronchial problems, appropriate diagnosis and early treatment is important.[80]

Acinic Cell Tumors

Originally described in the salivary glands of the head and neck, these rare but interesting neoplasms are made up of epithelial cells resembling serous acinar cells of the major and minor salivary glands. The first case of acinic cell tumor primary in the lung was reported by Fechner et al.[90] Their patient, a 63-year-old man, had a 4.2-cm pale tan tumor in the right lower lobe. The tumor was not connected to the bronchus, and the cells were indistinguishable from those of acinic cell tumors of the salivary gland.[90] Since then, several additional cases have been described.[91–95] The age range for this tumor is 12 to 75, averaging 38 years. About 60% occur in women, and most are asymptomatic, with a rare case presenting with persistent cough. These carcinomas are usually discrete and may be found either centrally or peripherally.

Grossly, acinic cell tumors are well circumscribed but lack a capsule. They are generally 1 to 5 cm in diameter and tan-white or yellow, nonnecrotic and nonhemorraghic, and soft to rubbery in consistency. Some are endobronchial and polypoid (Fig. 38.26). Microscopically they are composed of sheets of medium to large cohesive granular cells with varying degrees of stromal fibrosis. Fibrous septa sometimes divide islands of tumor cells, and this pattern suggests an almost organoid appearance (Figs. 38.27 and 38.28). There is the same histologic variation within the lung tumors as seen in tumors of salivary glands. As is the case with acinic cell tumors primary in salivary gland of the head and neck, intrapulmonary acinic cell tumors may show acinar, cystic, and papillocystic architectural patterns.[96–99] Rare

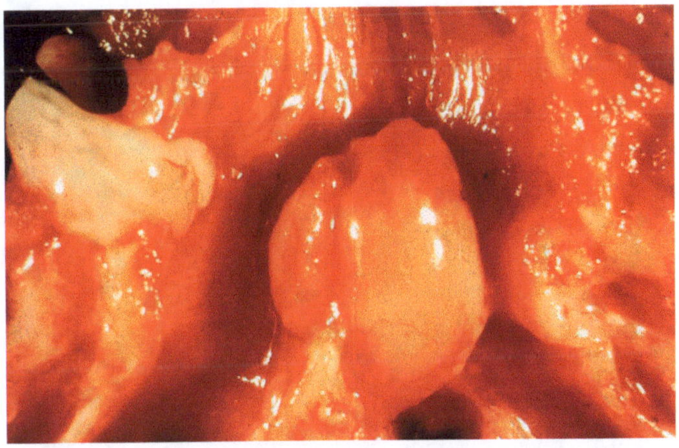

FIGURE 38.26. Acinic cell tumor. A yellow pink nodular mass with a smooth shiny surface lies at bifurcation of bronchi. (Courtesy of A.A. Liebow, Pulmonary Pathology collection, San Diego, CA; original contributor, J.R. Henneford, MD, Columbus Hospital, Great Falls, MT.)

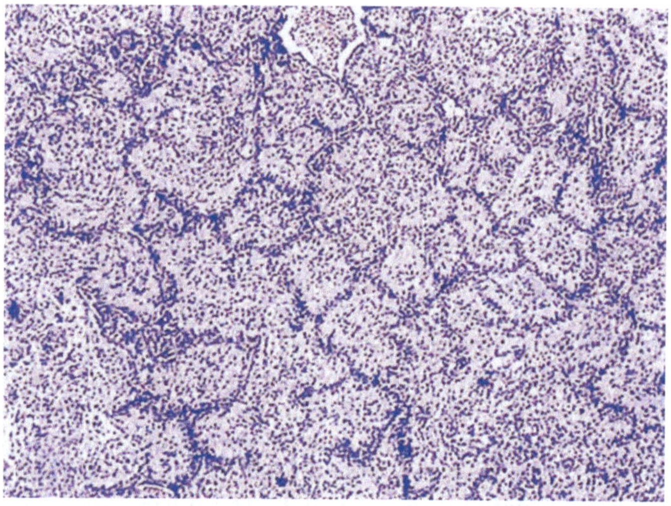

FIGURE 38.27. Acinic cell tumor. Note groups of small cells separated by fibrous septa, which confer on the tumor an organoid appearance. (Courtesy of Dr. H.-Y. Lee, Singapore General Hospital, Singapore. From Lee et al.,[104] with permission.)

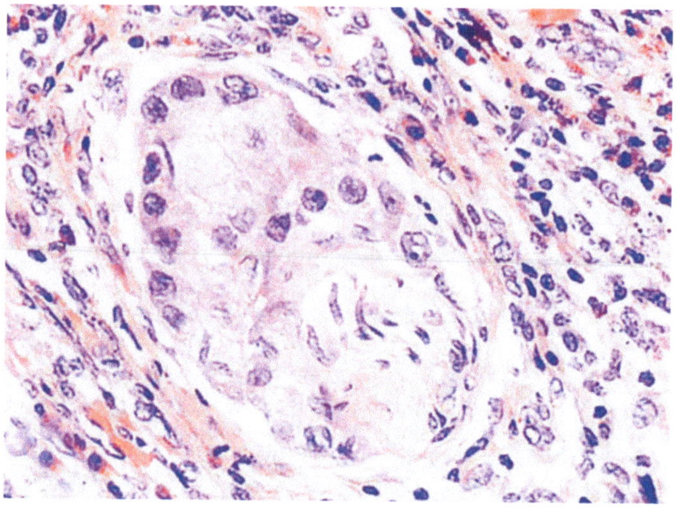

FIGURE 38.29. Acinic cell tumor. Tumor cells encase a nerve twig. (Courtesy of Dr. H.-Y. Lee, Singapore General Hospital, Singapore. From Lee et al.,[104] with permission.)

cases may show encasing of nerve twigs by tumor cells (Fig. 38.29). There may be clear cell change, variation of cell size, or tubular formations and prominent oncocytic change. The tumor cells are PAS positive (Fig. 38.30). However, only one of five cases in the series of Moran et al.[95] stained vividly with PAS or PAS diastase, and the tumors had a lower content of amylase than normal acinar cells. Electron microscopy (EM) shows typical serous-type cytoplasmic zymogen granules.[95] Other EM features include secretory granules and surface microvilli (Fig. 38.31). These tumors are strongly cytokeratin and EMA positive, and negative for vimentin, S-100 protein, and chromogranin.[95]

In the differential diagnosis of these lesions are clear to granular cell PAS-positive lesions, including benign clear cell "sugar" tumors, primary clear cell carcinoma of lung, glycogen-rich bronchioloalveolar carcinomas, metastatic acinic cell tumors, granular cell tumors from the head and neck, and metastatic renal cell carcinomas. The clinical history is helpful in excluding metastases from salivary gland lesions as pulmonary metastases usually occur after discovery of the primary malignancy. With

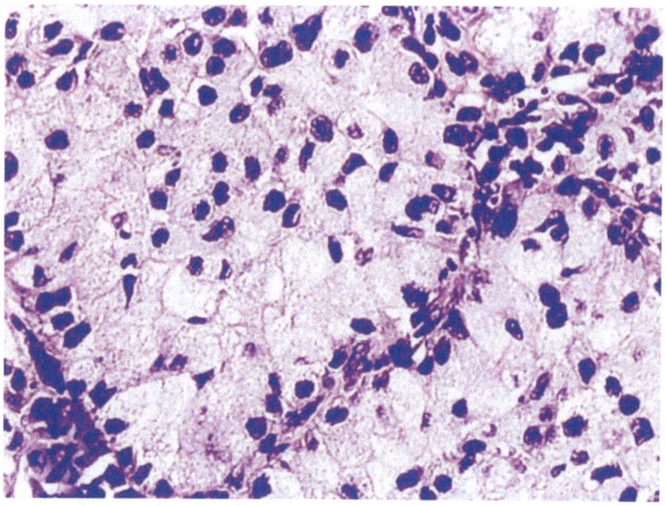

FIGURE 38.28. Acinic cell tumor. Uniform round darkly staining nuclei and abundant finely granular cytoplasm. (Courtesy of Dr. H.-Y. Lee, Singapore General Hospital, Singapore. From Lee et al.,[104] with permission.)

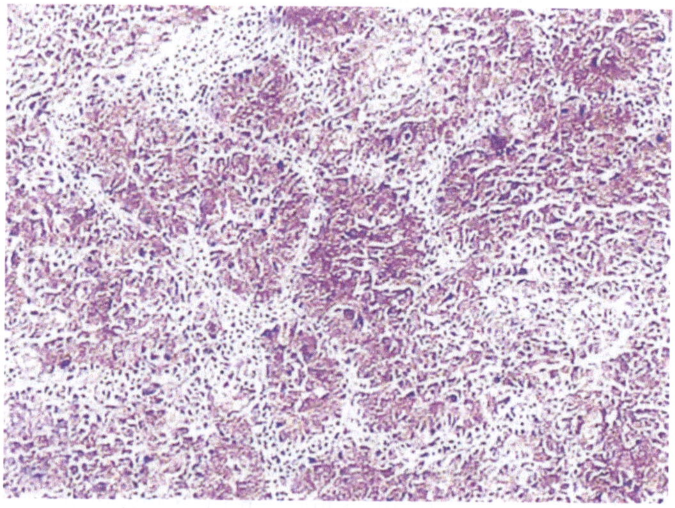

FIGURE 38.30. Acinic cell tumor. Periodic acid-Schiff stain highlighting cytoplasmic granules within tumor cells. (Courtesy of Dr. H.-Y. Lee, Singapore General Hospital, Singapore. From Lee et al.,[104] with permission.)

head and neck primaries, however, metastases can occur many years later despite a noninvasive and benign-appearing primary source.[98–100] Renal cell carcinoma has coexistent lipid and glycogen, the latter digests with diastase, and these tumors are often focally necrotic and more invasive than acinic carcinomas. Benign clear cell "sugar" tumors of lung are HMB-45 positive, do not usually stain with epithelial markers, and their PAS-positivity digests with diastase. They also have a sinusoidal vascular pattern and are more typically clear than granular. Primary clear cell carcinomas of lung have mitoses, usually more pleomorphic large cells, may have glycogen but no post-diastase PAS-positivity, and these same characteristics apply to glycogen-rich variants of bronchioloalveolar carcinomas. Electron microscopy may help in difficult cases.

Histiocytomas and granular cell tumors enter the differential. Cytokeratin positivity helps to exclude the former while ultrastructural evidence of autophagic lysomes differentiates the latter.[101] Other possibilities in the differential diagnosis discussed by Moran et al.[95] are oncocytic lesions such as carcinoid tumors and other metastatic clear and papillary carcinomas from thyroid, parathyroid, adrenal, or liver primaries. Electron microscopy is very helpful in confirming the diagnosis. The finding of large dark electron dense granules corresponding to zymogen is regarded as characteristic but not pathognomonic. Secretory granules with central electron-dense condensation are shown in Figure 38.31. A case in point is the patient described by Miura et al.,[102] whose tumor had cytoplasmic zymogenic granules larger than 600 nm in diameter, but was argyrophilic and serotonin positive, and was most likely, therefore, a carcinoid tumor.[102]

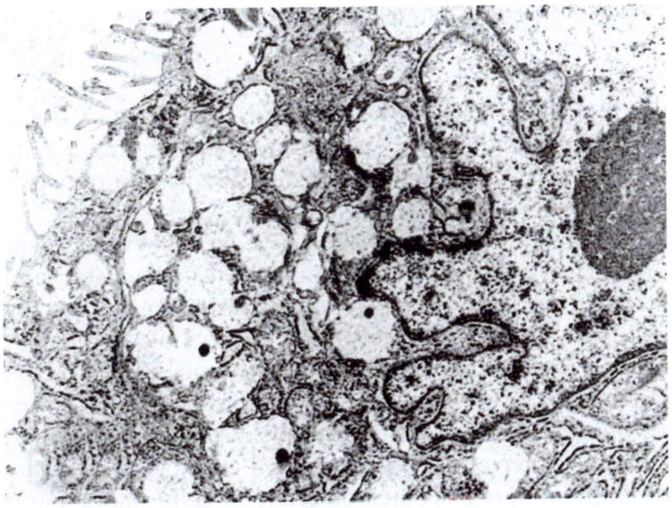

FIGURE 38.31. Acinic cell tumor. Ultrastructural appearance of tumor cells showing abundant secretory granules containing flocculent material with central or eccentric electron dense condensations. Rare homogeneous electron dense granules and surface microvilli are present (EM). (Courtesy of Dr. H.-Y. Lee, Singapore General Hospital, Singapore. From Lee et al.,[104] with permission.)

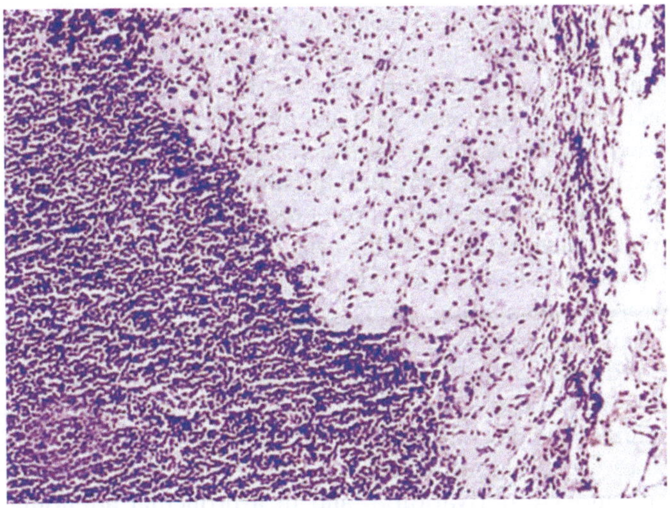

FIGURE 38.32. Acinic cell tumor. Tumor cells metastatic to the periphery of a lymph node. (Courtesy of Dr. H.-Y. Lee, Singapore General Hospital, Singapore. From Lee et al.,[104] with permission.)

Acinic cell tumors of the lung are not prone to metastasize, and their overall clinical evolution is favorable. In a review of 18 patients published by Ukoha and collaborators,[103] only one had documented metastases. The patient, a 64 year-old man, presented with an asymptomatic lung mass. At surgery, there was involvement of an interlobar (N1) lymph node, but nodes in higher stations were not involved. A further case of primary acinic cell carcinoma with metastasis to a hilar (N1) lymph node was recently reported by Lee and associates[104] (Fig. 38.32). Their patient, a 30-year-old woman, had presented with a $10 \times 6 \times 2$ cm subpleural mass in the lower lobe of the right lung, which was incidentally found on a routine chest radiograph. Of interest, this tumor also showed evidence of perineural invasion.

Pulmonary Oncocytic Change and Oncocytomas

Nonneoplastic oncocytic change of the respiratory tract is a common histopathologic finding and may be more frequent than generally appreciated. This view is supported by anecdotal observations and also by documented studies such as Matsuba et al.'s[105] finding of oncocytic change in 30 of 33 examined lungs. Oncocytic change is usually found in the respiratory mucous membrane and most particularly in the bronchial glands. This change is usually not present in patients under age 33 years, and increases in incidence with age beyond that point. As in other locations, these changes are oxyphilic in nature because of greatly increased numbers of mitochondria.[106] This change most likely represents a curious form of age-related degeneration within cells or a form of metaplasia. Oncocytic change also known as oncocytosis has also been in association with some carcinoid tumors,[106–111] glomus tumors of the trachea,[112] and some bronchial gland adenomas.[113] It is also seen in mucoepidermoid tumors, and, in one series of these tumors, oncocytic change was described as significant in nine of 53 (17%) cases.[27,114] It has also been noted in an adenoma of type II pneumocyte derivation,[115] and in a bronchial adenoma with polymorphous features.[116] In addition, oncocytic change is well known to occur in the salivary glands of the head and neck. Very thorough sampling and special procedures help distinguish these entities. The term, as used here, should be limited to those cases with only oncocytes throughout, and, on electron microscopy, abundant mitochondria and absence of neurosecretory features.

Oncocytomas, also known as oxyphilic adenomas may be viewed as localized nodular areas of oncocytic change (Fig. 38.33). It is not known whether oncocytomas arise de novo or in the setting of oncocytic hyperplasia. Although oncocytomas of salivary gland account for some 0.8% to 2% of all salivary gland tumors, they are very rare in the lung according to the ultramicroscopic features outlined above.

Fechner and Bentinck[117] in 1973 were the first to describe an acceptable case in a lung studied by electron microscopy. Black[118] had earlier described a case under this name, but he illustrated larger serous-appearing granules in the cytoplasm, and perhaps this tumor is better thought of as a variant of acinic cell carcinoma. Oncocytomas have been reported in the lung as well as in the airways and have been confirmed ultrastructurally by several authors.[119–122]

Oncocytomas are composed of large uniform polygonal cells with relatively small round nuclei containing prominent basophilic nuclei (Fig. 38.34). The cells have prominent granular eosinophilic cytoplasm and are arranged in solid sheets surrounded by thin delicate fibrous stroma containing small blood vessels. In few areas a glandular component may be seen, but solid areas may predominate and may have associated lymphoid infiltrates (Fig. 38.35). The cells are mucin negative by electron microscopy. In addition to mitochondria, organized structures with central lumina can be seen. Numerous desmosomes keep these cells together. As noted above, neurosecretory granules are lacking. Cytologic features such as clusters of monotonous syncytial-like epithelial cells with abundant amphophilic cytoplasm and

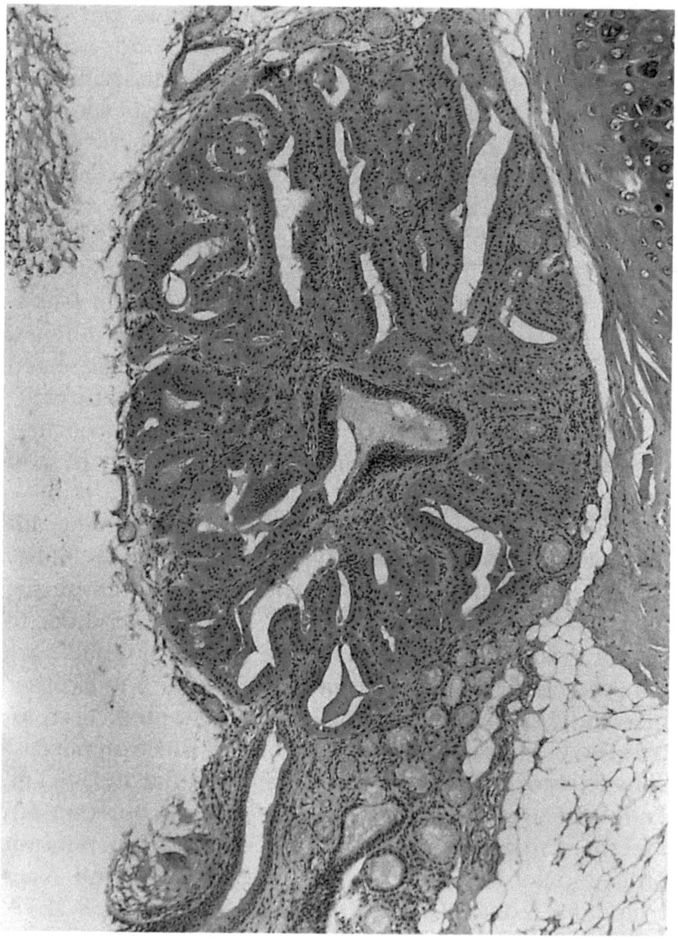

FIGURE 38.33. Oncocytoma, small 3-mm nodular tumor in bronchial wall surrounds an intercalated duct in submucosa of bronchus. Note cartilage on right upper corner.

small single round to oval uniform-looking nuclei may assist in the diagnosis. A case diagnosed by fine-needle aspiration (FNA) cytology was described by Laforga and Aranda.[123]

The main differential diagnosis is the oncocytic variant of carcinoid tumors. Both immunohistochemistry and electron microscopy are extremely useful in making the distinction. The presence of any appreciable number of electron-dense, membrane-bound granules by electron microscopy or positivity for CD56, chromogranin, or synaptophysin should cast doubt on the diagnosis of oncocytoma. Other entities that warrant consideration in the differential diagnosis include granular cell tumors, paragangliomas, and sclerosing hemangiomas, particularly in cases where these tumors may show focal oncocytic differentiation.

The biologic behavior of oncocytomas is not known, but most tumors are regarded as benign. One case reported by Tashiro et al.[124] was described as locally infiltrative.

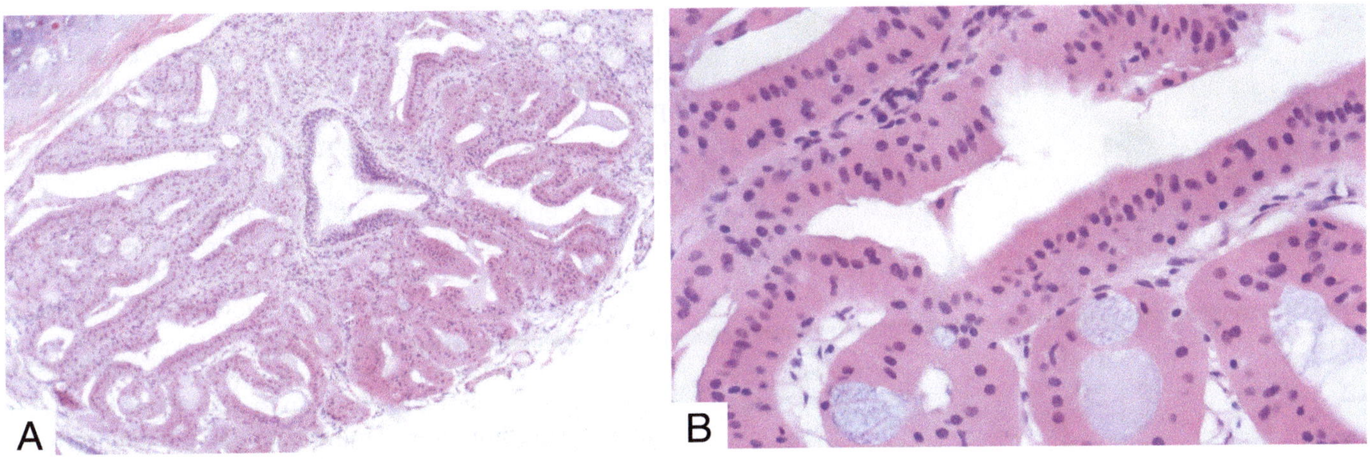

FIGURE 38.34. **(A,B)** Oncocytoma. Closer views of the preceding tumor showing intercalated duct and mucous (goblet) cells interspersed among large polygonal cells with abundant eosinophilic cytoplasm and uniform small dark nuclei.

Myoepithelioma and Epithelial-Myoepithelial Tumors

Myoepitheliomas are rare spindle cell neoplasms that may be viewed as monomorphic variants of pleomorphic adenomas lacking ductal epithelial components. Strickler et al.[125] described a myoepithelioma of the lung presenting as a circumscribed tan, parenchymal nodule occurring in a man. Microscopically, it consisted of sheets, nodules, and interdigitating fascicles of spindle and oval cells. The tumor cells contained glycogen but not mucin, and reacted with antibodies to S-100 protein and actin but not keratin. A myxoid or chondroid matrix containing stellate cells was present in some areas but no actual epithelial cells were found. The diagnosis was supported by finding numerous fine, parallel, 6-nm cytoplasmic filaments by electron microscopy consistent with myofilaments. There were also desmosomes, macula adherens, and a discontinuous basal lamina, as well as cytoplasmic glycogen. These ultrastructural features were consistent with a myoepithelial phenotype.[125]

Epithelial-myoepithelial tumors differ from myoepitheliomas. In contrast to the monomorphic appearance of myoepitheliomas, epithelial-myoepithelial tumors are composed of two types of neoplastic cells: epithelial cells in the form of tubules, and spindle-shaped myoepithelial cells forming compact masses or surrounding the epithelial tubules. Primary endobronchial neoplasms with histologic features of epithelial-myoepithelial carcinoma of the salivary gland have been reported by Nistal et al.[126] and Hayes et al.[127] These authors called attention to white, usually exophytic tumors, 2 to 3 cm in greatest dimensions, and showing proliferation of epithelial cells that formed tubules and sheets of myoepithelial cells with clear cytoplasm surrounding the tubules. Like their salivary gland counterparts, the epithelial cells marked positively for cytokeratin and were negative for S-100 protein and actin. In contrast, the myoepithelial cells were positive for S-100 protein and actin and negative for cytokeratin.[126,127] The case reported by Hayes et al. also showed a prominent spindle-cell component, which was S-100 protein positive and thought to be derived from myoepithelial cells. While the tumor depicted by Nistal et al. demonstrated scant mitoses, minimal atypia, and no evidence of metastasis, the case of Hayes et al. showed focal areas of marked cellular atypia in both the glandular and spindle cell components. Mitoses, nuclear pleomorphism, and mitotic figures were abundant in these areas.[126,127]

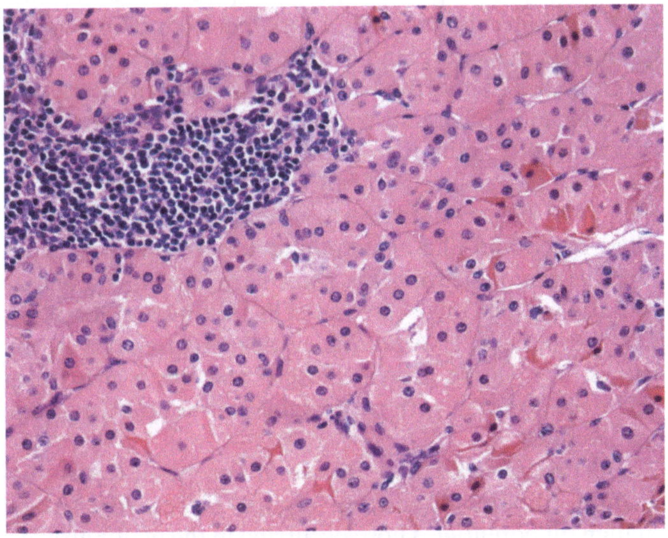

FIGURE 38.35. Oncocytoma. Detail of a solid area of an oncocytoma with a lymphoid aggregate on the upper left.

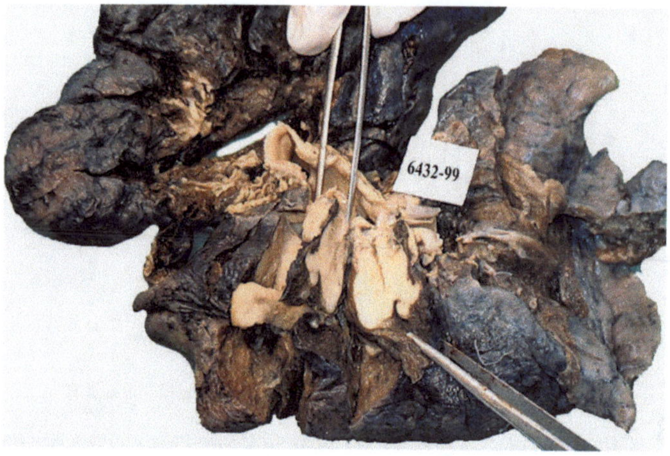

FIGURE 38.36. Epithelial-myoepithelial tumor. Note relatively well-outlined gray-white mass in the bronchus, with parenchymal extension. (Courtesy of Dr. Latifa Doganay et al., Trakya University, Edirne, Turkey. From Doganay et al.,[132] with permission.)

The differential diagnosis is wide and includes metastasis from clear cell carcinoma from the kidney, clear cell (sugar) tumor of lung, glandular forms of carcinoid tumor, bronchioloalveolar carcinoma with myoepithelial cells, and adenosquamous carcinoma.[128,129] Because of the prominent glandular appearance of some epithelial-myoepithelial carcinomas, they can also mimic conventional adenocarcinoma of lung. Demonstration of a myoepithelial immunophenotype (p63 and smooth muscle actin) is helpful in making the distinction. A case reported by Pelosi et al.[130] showed such immunoreactivity of the myoepithelial cells for p63. In addition, epithelial-myoepithelial carcinoma must be differentiated from pleomorphic adenoma, mucous gland adenoma, and adenoid cystic carcinoma. Pleomorphic adenoma is exceedingly rare in the lung and is characterized by a myxochondroid matrix or chondroid nodules in addition to mixtures of ductal and myoepithelial cells.[130] Mucous gland adenoma should be taken into account because of cystically dilated glands filled by colloid-like eosinophilic material. However, in mucous gland adenoma the glands are lined by columnar to flattened mucous-secreting cells lacking a myoepithelial component.[130] Adenoid cystic carcinoma typically shows an invasive growth pattern and has a cribriform architecture often with remarkable perineural lymphatic involvement.

The prognosis of these tumors is uncertain. Recent literature contains conflicting reports in regard to their malignant potential. Those occurring in the major airways appear to have a worse outcome than those found in the lung. Ru and associates,[131] reporting on a case of a p53 and c-kit (CD117) positive tumor, indicated that in 20 bronchial cases thus far reported 14 were malignant. Pelosi and collaborators,[130] on the other hand, believe the malignant potential of these tumors has not been defined and favor the use of a noncommittal term, such as pulmonary epithelial–myoepithelial tumor of unproven malignant potential, for tumors occurring in the lung. These authors base their assertion on the survival of one patient of their own and their review of six additional patients collected from the literature. In these six patients, there was no evidence of recurrence or metastasis but the follow-up was relatively short, up to only 49 months. This of course did not allow a more aggressive behavior to be excluded, over time.

An additional well-documented case was described by Doganay et al.[132] Their patient, a 73-year-old man, had a left hilar mass (Fig. 38.36) made up of tubules and solid epithelial nests in a hyalinized stroma. The tubular structures were double layered, having an inner layer of cuboidal cells and an outer rim of myoepithelial cells with clear cytoplasm (Figs. 38.37 to 38.39). The cells were mucicarmine positive and were immunoreactive for EMA, high molecular cytokeratin, and the S-100 protein (Fig. 38.40). Doganay et al. summarized the collective experience with these tumors up to 2004 (Table 38.3). Because of the uncertainty about the behavior of these tumors, complete surgical excision would appear to be advisable.

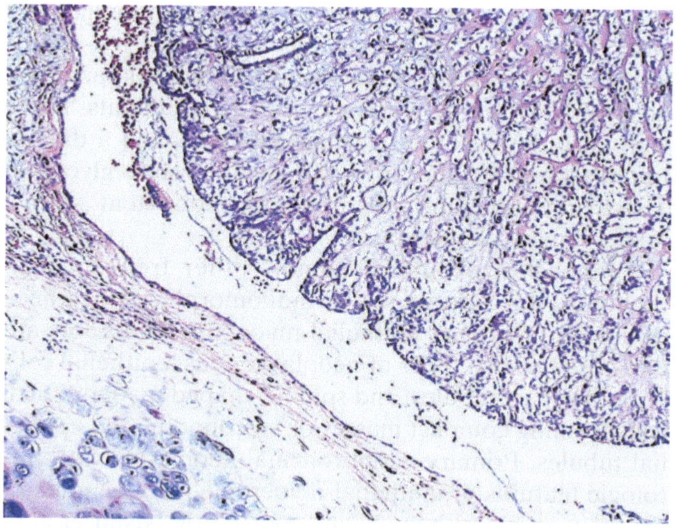

FIGURE 38.37. Epithelial-myoepithelial tumor. Intrabronchial polypoid mass covered by bronchial epithelium. (Courtesy of Dr. Latifa Doganay et al., Trakya University, Edirne, Turkey. From Doganay et al.,[132] with permission.)

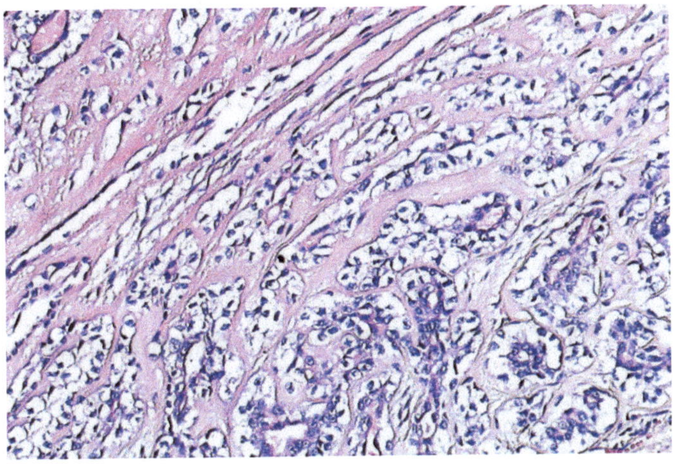

FIGURE 38.38. Epithelial-myoepithelial tumor. Note epithelial tubules in a hyalinized stroma. (Courtesy of Dr. Latifa Doganay et al., Trakya University, Edirne, Turkey. From Doganay et al.,[132] with permission.)

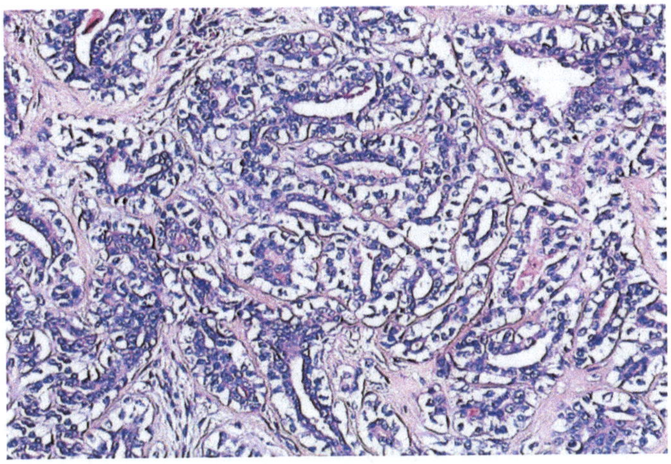

FIGURE 38.39. Epithelial-myoepithelial tumor. Note tubular structures with an inner layer of cuboidal epithelial cells and an outer rim of myoepithelial cells with clear cytoplasm. (Courtesy of Dr. Latifa Doganay et al., Trakya University, Edirne, Turkey. From Doganay et al.,[132] with permission.)

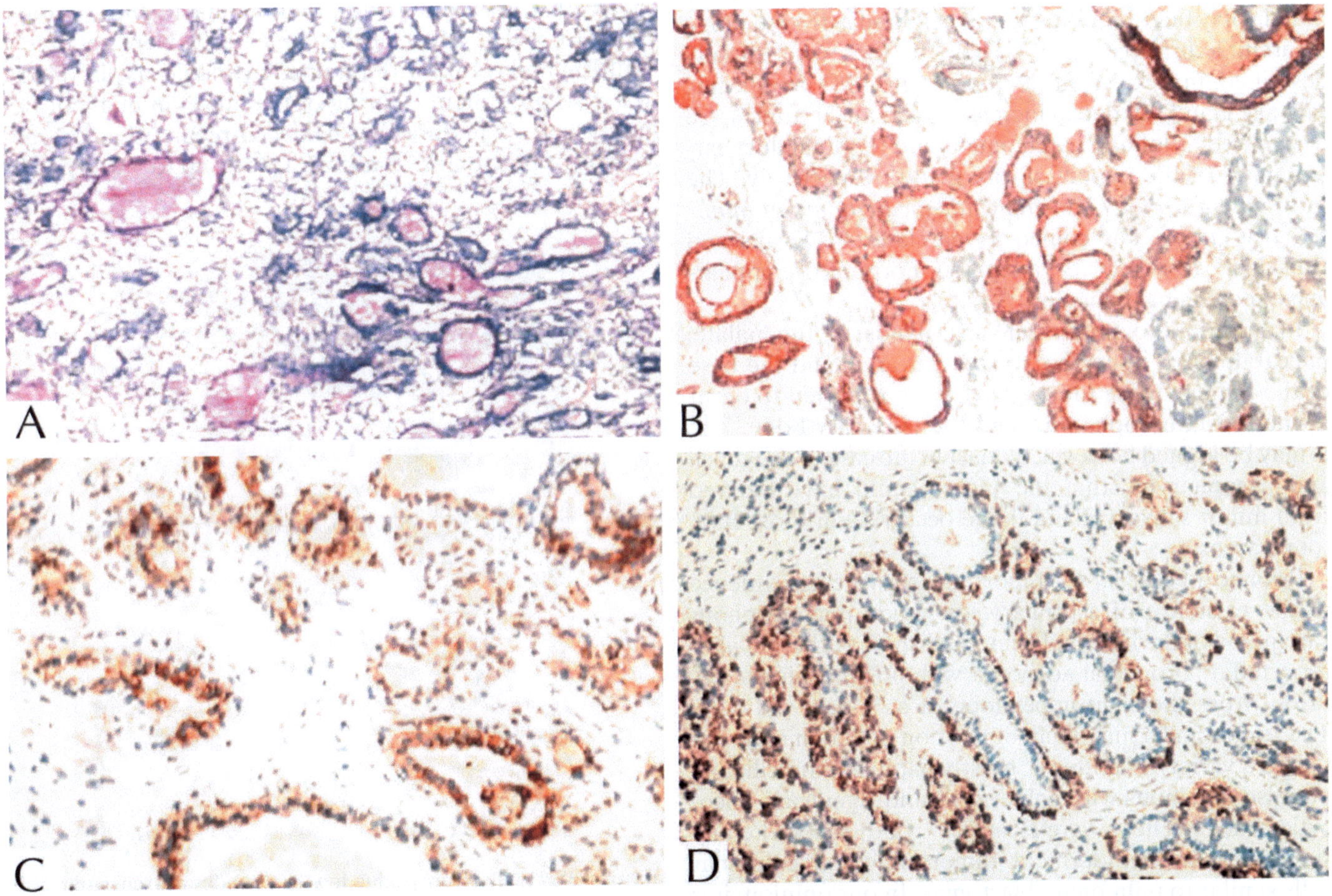

FIGURE 38.40. Epithelial-myoepithelial tumor. **(A)** Mucicarmine positivity. **(B)** Immunoreactivity to epithelial membrane antigen. **(C)** Immunoreactivity to high molecular weight cytokeratin. **(D)** Immunoreactivity to S100–protein. (Courtesy of Dr. Latifa Doganay et al., Trakya University, Edirne, Turkey. From Doganay et al.,[132] with permission.)

TABLE 38.3. Literature review: pulmonary tumors composed of epithelial and myoepithelial cells

Source	Sex/age	Location	Size (mm)	Diagnosis	Follow-up
Horinouchi	F/57	Trachea	22	EMT	NA
Nistal	F/55	Right upper lobar bronchus	20	EMT	24 months, alive and well
Tsuji	M/66	Right intermediate bronchus and parenchyma	160	Adenomyoepithelioma	36 months, dead of unrelated reason
Wilson	F/55	Lateral basal segment bronchus	39	EMC	7 months, alive and well
Shanks	M/67	Left lower lobar bronchus	13	EMC	Lost to follow-up
Ryska	F/47	Right upper lobar bronchus	NA	EMC	13 months, alive and well
Pelosi	M/47	Left upper lobar bronchus	15	EMT of unproven malignant potential	6 months, alive and well
Doganay	N/73	Left lower lobar bronchus and parenchyma	50	EMC	34 months, alive and well

EMC, epithelial-myoepithelial carcinoma; EMT, epithelial-myoepithelial tumor; NA, not available.
Source: Modified from Doganay et al.,[132] with permission.

Low-Grade Adenocarcinomas with Polymorphous Features

Polymorphous low-grade adenocarcinomas are low-grade malignant infiltrative tumors of the minor salivary glands that display bland-looking tumor cells and a diverse range of architectural patterns.[133] These tumors were initially described in two separate reports in 1983 as specific salivary gland adenocarcinomas, which at the time were designated as lobular carcinoma[134] and terminal duct carcinoma[135] of the minor salivary gland, respectively. The term *polymorphous low-grade adenocarcinoma of minor salivary glands* was coined a year later by Evans and Batsakis[136] to reflect its variegated morphologic appearance and clinical behavior.[134–136]

In addition to minor salivary glands of the palate, buccal mucosa, upper lip, retromolar area, and the base of the tongue, these tumors have been reported to occur in the tonsil, nasopharynx, and the maxillary bone.[137–139] It may be argued however, at least in the case of the tonsil and nasopharynx, that the tumor could have derived from minor salivary gland tissue occurring in those anatomic areas.

Prior to Lee et al.'s[133] report, no convincing evidence of the existence of a primary low-grade polymorphous carcinoma of the lung had been published. Akhtar et al.[116] reported a "bronchial adenoma with polymorphous features" from the right-upper lobe of a 35-year-old man. The tumor had a maximum dimension of 2.5 cm and contained a variety of patterns, mostly papillary and ciliated, but also mucinous with goblet cells and significant oncocytic change. There were clear cells, both sheet-like and similar to mucoepidermoid tumors and tall columnar cells similar to pulmonary blastomas. In our opinion, it is doubtful that this case represented a bona fide example of low-grade polymorphous adenocarcinoma. The case recently reported by Lee and associates occurred in a 56-year-old woman presenting with two peripherally located lung tumoral lesions. Histologically, the lesions showed a variety of architectural patterns including tubular, glandular, trabecular, solid, microcystic, and papillary formations. In focal areas, there was a suggestion of an adenoid cystic carcinoma-like appearance; however, this was not the predominant feature[133] (Figs. 38.41 to 38.43). Most of the tumor cells were relatively uniform and round with minimal cytologic atypia. There was also prominent clearing of the nuclei in many of the tumor cells, a feature that has been regarded as characteristic of this tumor. A mitotic rate of up to 3 to 4 per 10

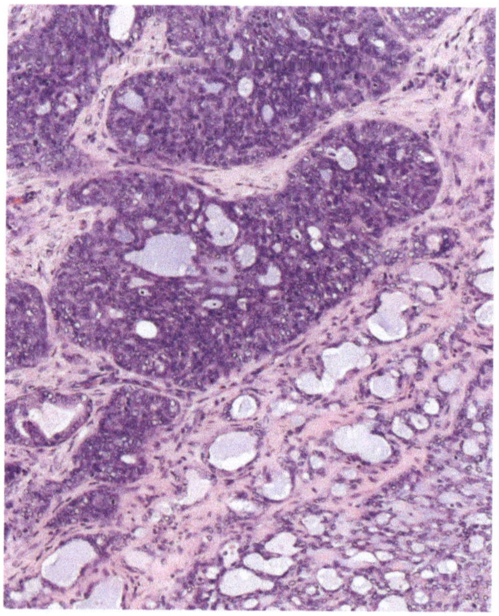

FIGURE 38.41. Polymorphous low-grade adenocarcinoma. This view shows a variety of patterns, including glandular, microcystic, and some near-solid areas reminiscent of an adenoid cystic carcinoma. (Courtesy of Dr. Victor K.M. Lee et al., Singapore General Hospital. From Lee et al.,[133] with permission from Westminster Publications, Inc.)

HPFs was found. Lymphovascular or perineural invasion was not identified. The background stroma had areas with a sclerotic and myxoid appearance. Definite cartilaginous differentiation, however, was not seen.[133] The gradual merging pattern between stroma and epithelial components characteristic of a pleomorphic adenoma was not identified. The mediastinal lymph node did not show evidence of metastatic tumor. The epithelial tumor cells were diffusely and strongly positive for cytokeratin 7. Cytokeratin 20, thyroid transcription factor-1, and smooth muscle actin were negative. This compares with immunohistochemical patterns in tumors originating in the minor salivary glands. Lee and associates[133] do not make the assertion that their case represents a lung primary. In fact, they favor a metastatic tumor from a silent or regressed primary site tumor. Nevertheless, the morphology of their tumor and the absence of an obvious primary argue for the possibility of a lung primary.

The differential diagnosis includes pleomorphic adenoma, adenoid cystic carcinoma, and mucoepidermoid tumors. Unlike these tumors, pleomorphic adenomas are noninfiltrative, well-circumscribed tumors consisting of biphasic population of epithelial and myoepithelial cells within a chondromyxoid stroma. Pleomorphic adenomas do not demonstrate perineural or stromal invasion. Polymorphous low-grade carcinomas lack tubules with two cell layers, lobules of cartilage, and glial fibrillary acidic protein immunostaining.[133] Adenoid cystic carcinoma shows more angular, pleomorphic nuclei, and increased mitotic activity compared with the nuclei in polymorphous low-grade carcinomas, which are slightly larger, rounder, and more uniform. The cytoplasm of the tumor cells is usually more eosinophilic in these tumors, whereas it is clearer in adenoid cystic carcinomas. Adenoid cystic carcinomas show EMA staining confined to the glandular lumina, and weak and patchy S-100 protein staining. In contrast, polymorphous carcinomas show more diffuse EMA staining and more intense staining for S-100 protein. Polymorphous low-grade carcinomas can also be distinguished from adenoid cystic carcinomas by their lower proliferative index.[133] Mucoepidermoid carcinoma is considered in the differential diagnosis of primary salivary gland tumor of the lung. However, polymorphous low-grade carcinomas do not show definite squamoid or intermediate cells that are distinctive for mucoepidermoid carcinoma.[133]

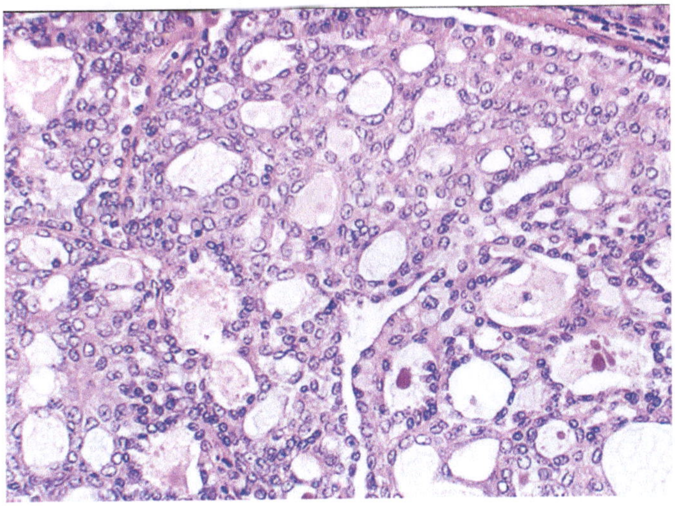

FIGURE 38.42. Polymorphous low-grade adenocarcinoma. In this area the tumor has a distinct glandular pattern with a bland cytologic appearance demonstrating characteristic clearing of nuclei. (Courtesy of Dr. Victor K.M. Lee et al., Singapore General Hospital. From Lee et al.,[133] with permission from Westminster Publications, Inc.)

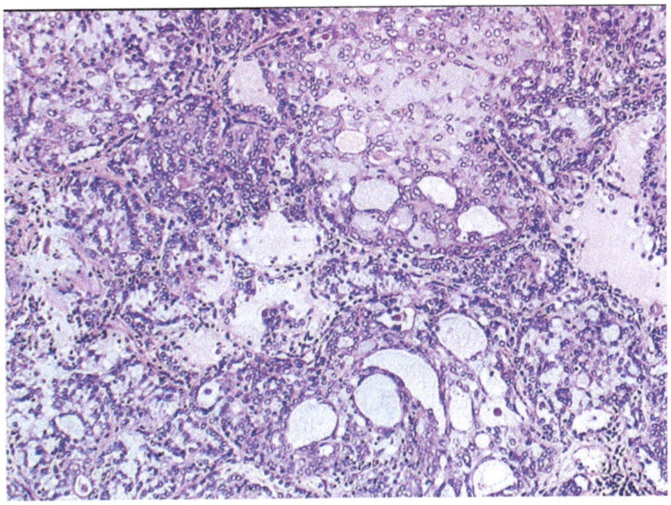

FIGURE 38.43. Polymorphous low-grade adenocarcinoma. This area shows solid and cribriform patterns reminiscent of an adenoid cystic carcinoma. (Courtesy of Dr. Victor K.M. Lee et al., Singapore General Hospital. From Lee et al.,[133] with permission from Westminster Publications, Inc.)

Primary low-grade polymorphous tumors in the salivary glands are said to be more aggressive when presenting with a prominent papillary component or when they undergo "dedifferentiation,"[140] but this occurrence has not been reported in the lung. The prognosis of low-grade polymorphous tumors when primary in the lung is not known.

Other Tumors Believed to Be of Salivary Gland Origin

Less well known tumors of the respiratory tract believed by some to be of salivary gland origin include adenosquamous carcinoma variants with amyloid stroma, sebaceous carcinomas, sialadenoma papilliferum, and pneumocytic adenomyoepithelioma.

Adenosquamous carcinomas are discussed at greater length in Chapter 35. Here we only briefly refer to two unique cases of adenosquamous carcinomas reported by Yousem,[141] which showed histologic, ultrastructural, and immunohistochemical features, including S-100 positivity, suggesting myoepithelial differentiation and an analogy to salivary gland neoplasms, particularly adenoid cystic carcinoma. However, the issue of whether or not these tumors represent separate entities from high-grade mucoepidermoid tumor remains a matter of contention. Histologic features that help to distinguish adenosquamous carcinomas from high-grade mucoepidermoid carcinoma are a peripheral location, presence of an in-situ carcinomatous component, and the absence of a low-grade mucoepidermoid pattern in adenosquamous carcinomas.

Sebaceous carcinomas of the lung are exceedingly rare. They are most often seen in the face around the eye, the eyelid, salivary glands, and the upper digestive tract.[142–144] A well-documented case of sebaceous carcinoma of the lung was described by Borczuk and associates.[145] Their patient, a 78-year-old man, presented with a mass in the left lower lung found during an evaluation for weight loss. The surgically resected tumor was characterized by a lobulated and infolded architecture with alternating undulating light and dark zones. Microscopically, two cellular components were evident in the tumor. One component was basaloid and the other was a layer of cells with cytoplasmic vacuolization (Fig. 38.44). The vacuolated cells were PAS diastase and mucicarmine negative and strongly oil red O positive. Ultrastructurally, lipid-filled vacuoles were identified (Fig. 38.45). The

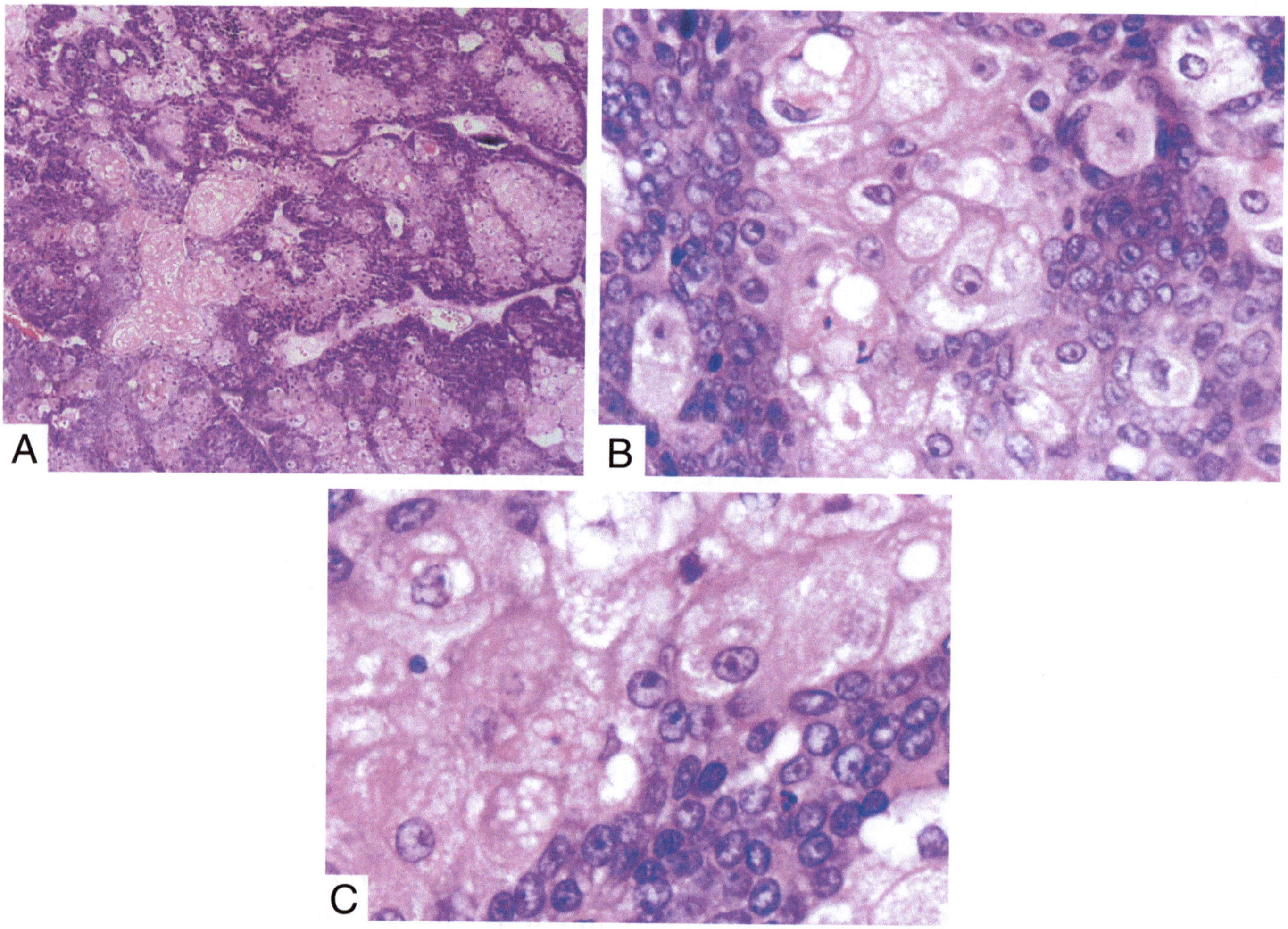

FIGURE 38.44. **(A)** Sebaceous carcinoma. Lobulated tumor with an infolded architecture with light and dark zones, indicating differences in nuclear/cytoplasmic ratios. **(B)** A higher magnification showing basaloid-type cells with uniform, vesicular nuclei, and scant cytoplasm, and differentiation toward a cell with a similar nucleus but abundant cytoplasm filled with small vesicles. **(C)** Note features of sebaceous differentiation, (sharp cytoplasmic borders and abundant small vesicles). (Courtesy of Dr. Alain C. Borczuk, Columbia Presbyterian Medical Center, New York. From Borczuk et al.,[145] with permission. Copyright 2002 by Lippincott Williams & Wilkins.)

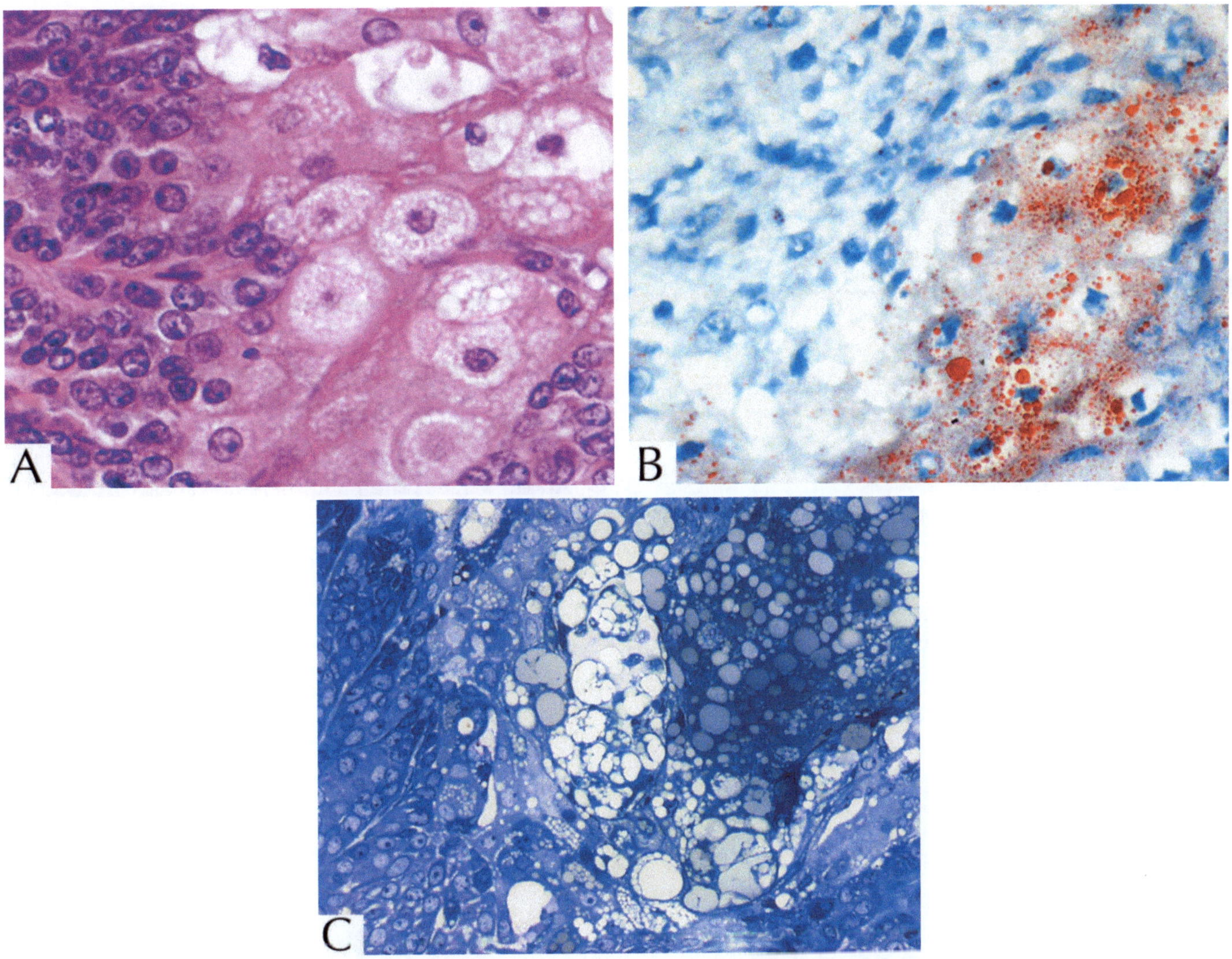

FIGURE 38.45. **(A)** Sebaceous carcinoma. Note transition from basaloid cells to cells with abundant cytoplasm. **(B)** Oil red O stain for lipid was performed on a frozen section, and a similar area to that in **A** is shown. **(C)** Electron microscopy. Note progressive increase in vacuolization. The vacuoles are filled with gray semi-opaque material consistent with lipid (osmium tetroxide post fixed, toluidine blue stain. (Courtesy of Dr. Alain C. Borczuk, Columbia Presbyterian Medical Center, New York. From Borczuk et al.,[145] with permission. Copyright 2002 by Lippincott Williams & Wilkins.)

authors considered three possible histogenetic mechanisms: (1) a salivary gland type of tumor with sebaceous differentiation, (2) a squamous cell carcinoma with sebaceous differentiation, and (3) a primary sebaceous carcinoma of the lung. The authors searched for a possible extrapulmonary sebaceous carcinoma with metastasis to the lung but none was found. At 3 years after surgical resection, the patient was alive and with no apparent disease.

Sialadenoma papilliferum, a tumor believed to be of minor salivary gland origin, occurs rarely in the oral cavity and is akin to Warthin's tumor of the parotid gland and papillary syringocystadenomas of the skin.[146,147] In the palate, its most usual location, sialadenoma papilliferum presents as an exophytic mass of well-differentiated squamous epithelium covering glandular components made up of cleft-like cystic spaces.[148] Some of the glandular components contain oncocytic cells and some show squamous metaplasia.[146–148] A case of pulmonary sialadenoma papilliferum was described by Bobos et al.[149] The patient, a 53-year-old man was incidentally found to have a mass lesion in the right lung by chest radiograph and CT scan (Fig. 38.46A,B). The surgically resected specimen showed an exophytic papillary lesion protruding from the apical bronchus of the right lower lobe (Fig. 38.46C). Microscopically the tumor was made of complex papillary structures. The papillary structures were covered by a double row of

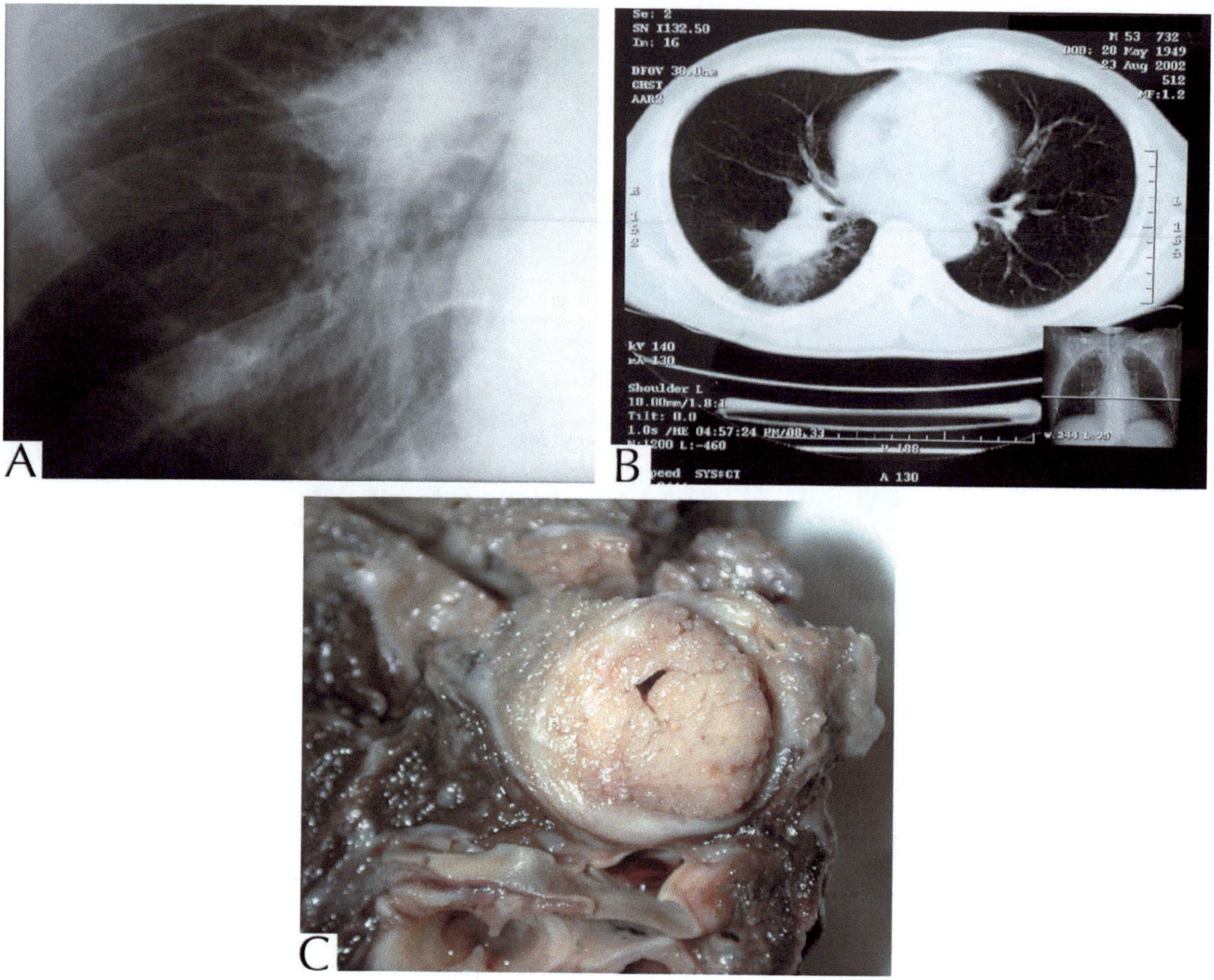

FIGURE 38.46. Sialadenoma papilliferum. Radiographic and gross pathologic findings. **(A)** Plain chest x-ray showing a plaque lesion in the lower lobe of the right lung. **(B)** Computed tomography scan of the chest confirming the presence of an area of consolidation. **(C)** Exophytic papillary lesion protruding at the cut surface of the apical bronchus of the right lower lobe. (Courtesy of Dr. Mattheos Bobos, Aristotle University Medical School, Thessaloniki, Greece. From Bobos et al.,[149] with permission from Springer.)

epithelial and myoepithelial cells. Within some of the papillary structures there were gland-like structures containing eosinophilic material (Fig. 38.47). The myoepithelial cells were S-100 protein, cytokeratin and α-smooth muscle actin positive. The epithelial cells were cytokeratin and S-100 protein positive (Table 38.4). The biologic behavior of this tumor is not known. Bobos et al.'s patient was said to be well at 8 months following surgical resection.

Pneumocytic adenomyoepithelioma was recently described and reported as a distinct type of salivary gland–type tumor with pneumocytic differentiation.[150] Pneumocytic adenomyoepithelioma shows tripartite features with elements of epithelial, myoepithelial and pneumocyte differentiation. In a series of five cases, Chang and associates[150] reported a female predominance and ages ranging from 52 to 63 years. The tumors were circumscribed, 0.8 to 2.6 cm in diameter, and showed glandular and spindle cell components. The glands were filled with colloid-like material and had an inner layer of epithelial cells with pneumocyte characteristics, being immunoreactive for pancytokeratin, surfactant apoprotein, and thyroid transcription factor-1. These epithelial cells were surrounded by an outer layer of myoepithelial cells merging with foci of spindled-shaped cells. Cells in this outer layer were immunoreactive for calponin, caldesmon, smooth

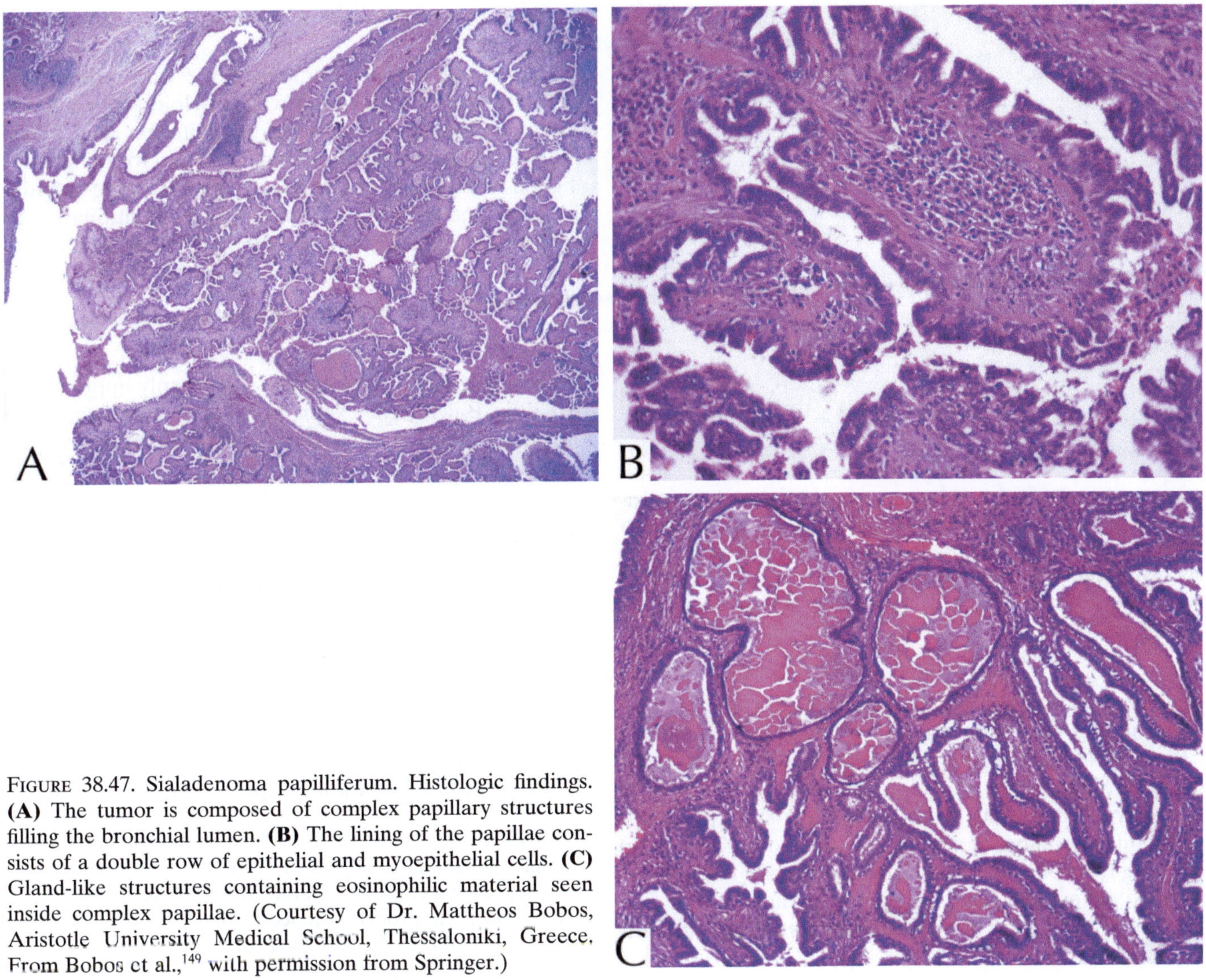

FIGURE 38.47. Sialadenoma papilliferum. Histologic findings. **(A)** The tumor is composed of complex papillary structures filling the bronchial lumen. **(B)** The lining of the papillae consists of a double row of epithelial and myoepithelial cells. **(C)** Gland-like structures containing eosinophilic material seen inside complex papillae. (Courtesy of Dr. Mattheos Bobos, Aristotle University Medical School, Thessaloniki, Greece. From Bobos et al.,[149] with permission from Springer.)

TABLE 38.4. Immunhistochemical findings in sialadenoma papilliferum of bronchus (comparison with bronchial glands and respiratory epithelium)

	Sialadenoma papilliferum		Bronchial glands		
Immunohistochemical stains	Epithelium	Myoepithelium	Epithelium	Myoepithelium	Respiratory epithelium
CAM 5.2	Positive foci	Rare positive	Positive	Focally positive	Positive
Cytokeratin 7	Positive	Focally positive	Positive	Focally positive	Positive
Cytokeratin 17	Rare positive	Focally positive	Negative	Positive	Focally positive
Cytokeratin 19	Positive	Positive	Positive	Positive	Positive
Cytokeratin 20	Negative	Negative	Negative	Negative	Negative
EMA	Positive	Negative	Focally positive	Negative	Positive
SMA	Negative	Positive	Negative	Positive	Negative
S-100 protein	Mostly positive	Mostly positive	Focally positive	Positive	Negative
GFAP	Negative	Focally positive	Negative	Negative	Negative

EMA, epithelial membrane antigen; SMA, α-smooth muscle actin; GFAP, glial fibrillary acidic protein.
Source: Courtesy of Dr. Mattheos Bobos, Aristotle University Medical School, Thessaloniki, Greece. From Bobos et al.,[149] with permission from Springer.

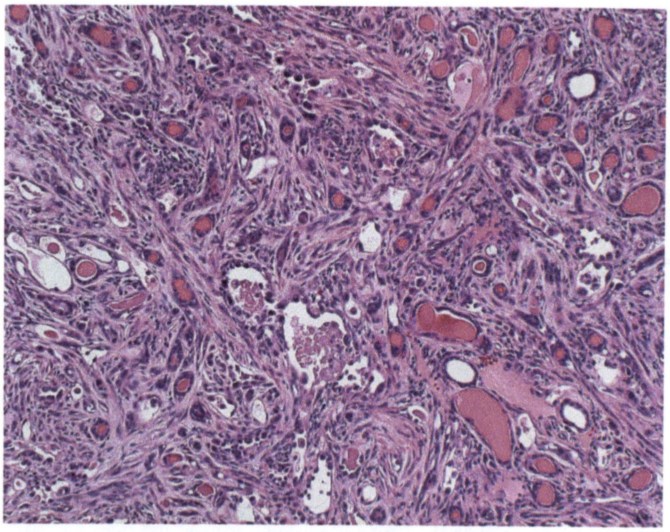

FIGURE 38.48. Pneumocytic adenomyoepithelioma. Note glandular structures, some filled with eosinophilic material (which stained immunohistochemically for surfactant protein A), lined by plump cuboidal cells, intermingling and merging with spindled cells. (Courtesy of Dr. Tiffany Chang et al., University of Chicago, Chicago, IL.)

muscle actin, S-100 protein, high molecular weight cytokeratin, and p63, supporting their myoepithelial nature (Figs. 38.48 and 38.49). The authors concluded these tumors differ from all previously recognized salivary gland-type neoplasms of lung and have aptly proposed the name pneumocytic adenomyoepithelioma. Follow-up ranging from 5 to 172 months from diagnosis has thus far shown no evidence of recurrence in any of the five patients; however, in one of the five patients, a postoperative CT scan revealed additional smaller bilateral nodules in the lung.

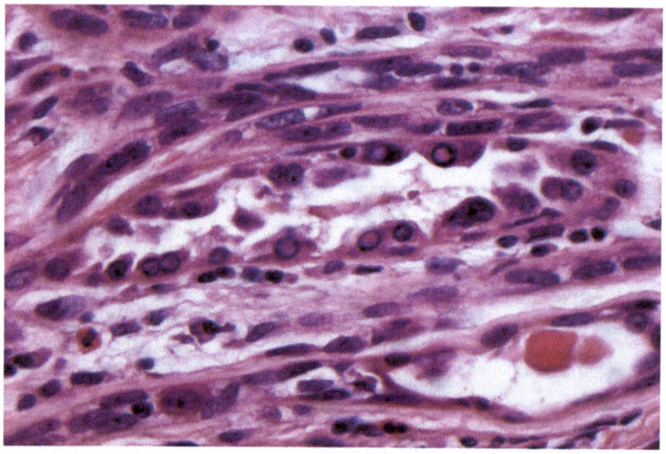

FIGURE 38.49. Pneumocytic cells with intranuclear pseudoinclusions lining a gland in pneumocytic adenomyoepithelioma. There is mild atypia of the cells, but only rare mitoses are present (not shown here). (Courtesy of Dr. Tiffany Chang et al., University of Chicago, Chicago, IL.)

While these unusual tumors of the respiratory tract (adenosquamous carcinoma with amyloid stroma, sebaceous carcinoma, sialadenoma papilliferum, and pneumocytic adenomyoepithelioma) appear to be closely aligned with tumors of the salivary glands, more cumulative data and experience derived from additional cases will be needed to determine whether or not they represent valid and separate tumoral entities in the respiratory tract.

Acknowledgments. The authors are deeply appreciative of Karen Balcius for expert secretarial assistance, Rob Carlin for photography, and Andy Dzaugis and Rosemary Leary for bibliographic support.

References

1. Payne WS, Schier J, Woolner LB. Mixed tumors of the bronchus (salivary gland type). J Thorac Cardiovasc Surg 1965;49:663–668.
2. Kay S, Brooks JW. Benign mixed tumor of the trachea with seven-year follow-up. Cancer 1970;25:1178–1182.
3. Ma CK, Fine G, Lewis J, Lee MW. Benign mixed tumor of the trachea. Cancer 1979;44:2260–2266.
4. Sano T, Hirose T, Hizawa K, et al. A case of pleomorphic adenoma of the trachea. Jpn J Clin Oncol 1984;14: 93–88.
5. Hemmi A, Hiraoka H, Mori Y, et al. Malignant pleomorphic adenoma (malignant mixed tumor) of the trachea. Report of a case. Acta Pathol Jpn 1988;38:1215–1226.
6. Spencer H. Bronchial mucous gland tumors. Virchows Arch (Pathol Anat) 1979;383:101–115.
7. Davis PW, Briggs JC, Seal RM, et al. Benign and malignant mixed tumors of the lung. Thorax 1972;27:657–673.
8. Ushizima H, Fujiwara K, Yamaguchi T, et al. A case of lung cancer of malignant mixed tumor origin. Gan No Rinsho 1975;21:1330–1336.
9. Nakamura M, Shimosato Y, Kameya T, et al. Two cases of bronchial gland "mixed tumor" of the salivary gland type. Lung Cancer 1977;17:47–57.
10. Ebihara Y, Fukushima N, Asakuma Y. Double primary lung cancers: with special reference to their exfoliative cytology and to the rare, malignant "mixed" tumor of the salivary-gland type. Acta Cytol 1980;24:212–223.
11. Wright ES, Pike E, Couves CM. Unusual tumours of the lung. J Surg Oncol 1983;24:23–29.
12. Clarke PJ, Dunnill MS, Gunning AJ. Mixed tumours of the lung: a report of three cases. Br J Dis Chest 1986; 80–87.
13. Sakamoto H, Uda H, Tanaka T, et al. Pleomorphic adenoma in the periphery of the lung. Arch Pathol Lab Med 1991;115:393–396.
14. Mori M, Furuya K, Kimura T, et al. Mixed tumor of salivary gland type arising in the bronchus. Ann Thorac Surg 1991;52:1322–1324.

15. Horinouchi H, Ishihara T, Kawamura M et al. Epithelial-myoepithelial tumor of the tracheal glands. J Clin Pathol 1993;46:185–187.
16. Ang KL, Dhanapuneni VR, Morgan WE, et al. Primary pulmonary pleomorphic adenoma. An immunohistochemical study and review of the literature. Arch Pathol Lab Med 2003:127:621–622.
17. Hasleton, PS. Benign lung tumors and their malignant counterparts. In: Hasleton PS, ed. Spencer's pathology of the lung. 5th ed. New York, St. Louis, San Francisco: McGraw Hill, 1996:892–895.
18. Colby TV, Koss MN, Travis WD. Tumors of the lower respiratory tract. AFIP atlas of tumor pathology. Washington, DC: Armed Forces Institute of Pathology, 1994:70.
19. Takeuchi E, Shimizu E, Sano N, et al. A case of pleomorphic adenoma of the lung with multiple distant metastasis—observation on its oncogenic and tumor suppressor gene expression. Anticancer Res 1998;18: 2015–2020.
20. Wenig BM, Hitchcock CL, Gnepp DR. Metastasizing mixed tumor of salivary glands: a clinicopathologic and flow cytometric analysis. Am J Surg Pathol 1992;16: 845–858.
21 Sim DW, Maran AG, Harris D. Metastatic salivary pleomorphic adenoma. J Laryngol Otol 1990;104:45–47.
22. Klacsmann PG, Olson JL, Eggleston JC. Mucoepidermoid carcinoma of the bronchus: an electron microscopic study of the low grade and high grade variants. Cancer 1979; 43:1720–1733.
23. Trentini GP, Palmieri B. Mucoepidermoid tumor of the trachea. Chest 1972;62:336–338.
24. Leonardi HK, Jung-Legg Y, Legg MA, et al. Tracheobronchial mucoepidermoid carcinoma. J Thorac Cardiovasc Surg 1978;76:431–438.
25. Fraser RS, Müller NL, Colman N, Paré PD. Diagnosis of diseases of the chest. Philadelphia: WB Saunders, 1999:1258.
26. Heitmiller RF, Mathisen DJ, Ferry JA, et al. Mucoepidermoid lung tumors. Ann Thorac Surg 1989;47:394–399.
27. Yousem SA, Hochholzer L. Mucoepidermoid tumors of the lung. Cancer 1987;60:1346–1352.
28. Torres, AM, Rickman, F.C. Childhood tracheobronchial mucoepidermoid carcinoma. A case report and review of the literature. J Pediatr Surg 1988; 23:367–370.
29. Seo IS, Warren J, Mirkin D, et al. Mucoepidermoid carcinoma of the bronchus in a 4-year-old child: a high-grade variant with lymph node metastases. Cancer 1984;53: 1600–1604.
30. Pandya A, Matthews S. Case Report. Mucoepidermoid carcinoma in a patient with congenital agenesis of the left upper lobe. Br J Radiol 2003;76:339–342.
31. Welsh JH, Maxson T, Jaksk T, et al. Tracheobronchial mucoepidermoid carcinoma in childhood and adolescence: case report and review of the literature. Int J Pediatr Pulmonol 1998;45:265–273.
32. Smiddy PF, Abdulmanaf ZM, Roberts IF, et al. Endobronchial mucoepidermoid carcinoma in childhood. Case report and literature review. Clin Radiol 2000:647–649 (on-line publication).
33. Kim TS, Lee KS, Han J, et al. Mucoepidermoid carcinoma of the tracheobronchial tree: radiographic and CT findings in 12 patients. Radiology 1999;212:643–648.
34. Hasleton PS. Benign lung tumors and their malignant counterparts. In: Hasleton PS, ed. Spencer's pathology of the lung. 5th ed. New York, St. Louis, San Francisco: McGraw-Hill, 1996:921.
35. Matsuo K, Irie J, Tsuchiyama H, et al. A high-grade malignancy bronchial mucoepidermoid carcinoma with features of giant cell carcinoma. Acta Pathol Jpn 1986; 36:293–300.
36. Barsky SH, Martinse, Matthews M, et al. "Low grade" mucoepidermoid carcinoma of the bronchus with "high grade" clinical behavior. Cancer (Philadelphia) 1983:51: 1505–1509.
37. Guillou L, DeLuze P, Zysset F, et al. Papillary variant of low grade mucoepidermoid carcinoma—an unusual bronchial neoplasm. Am J Clin Pathol 1994;101: 269–274.
38. Green LK, Gallion TL, Gyorkey F. Peripheral mucoepidermoid tumour of the lung. Thorax 1991;46:65–66.
39. Shilo K, Foss RD, Franks TJ, et al. Pulmonary mucoepidermoid carcinoma with prominent tumor-associated lymphoid proliferation. Am J Surg Pathol 2005;29: 407–411.
40. Segletes LA., Steffee CH, Geisinger KR. Cytology of primary pulmonary mucoepidermoid and adenoid cystic carcinoma. A report of 4 cases. Acta Cytol 1999;43: 1091–1097.
41. Stafford JR, Pollock J, Wenzel BC. Oncocytic mucoepidermoid tumor of the bronchus. Cancer 1984;54:94–99.
42. Seo IS, Warfel KA, Tomich CE, et al. Clear cell carcinoma of the larynx: a variant of mucoepidermoid carcinoma. Am J Otolaryngol 1980;89:168–172.
43. Stewart FW, Foote FW Jr, Becker, WF. Mucoepidermoid tumors of the salivary glands. Ann Surg 1945;122: 820–824.
44. Lack EE, Harris GBC, Erakles AJ, et al. Primary bronchial tumors in childhood. Cancer 1983;51:494–497.
45. Reichle FA, Rosemond GP. Mucoepidermoid tumors of the bronchus. J Thorac Cardiovasc Surg 1966; 51:443–448.
46. Ozlu C, Christopherson WM, Allen JD Jr. Mucoepidermoid tumors of the bronchus. J Thorac Cardiovasc Surg 1961;42:24–31.
47. Dowling EA, Miller RE, Johnson EM, et al. Mucoepidermoid tumors of the bronchi. Surgery 1962;52:600–609.
48. Healey WV, Perzin KH, Smith L. Mucoepidermoid carcinoma of salivary gland: classification, clinical-pathologic correlation, and results of treatment. Cancer (Philadelphia) 1970;26:368–388.
49. Turnbull AD, Huvos AG, Goodner JT, et al. Mucoepidermoid tumors of bronchial glands. Cancer 1971;28: 539–544.
50. Metcalf JS, Maize JC, Shaw EB. Bronchial mucoepidermoid carcinoma metastatic to skin: report of a case and review of the literature. Cancer (Philadelphia) 1986;58: 2556–2559.
51. Conlan AA, Payne WS, Woolner LB, et al. Adenoid cystic carcinoma (cylindroma) and mucoepidermoid carcinoma

of the bronchus. Factors affecting survival. J Thorac Cardiovasc Surg 1978;76:369–377.
52. Vadasz P, Egervary M. Mucoepidermoid bronchial tumors: a review of 34 operated cases. Eur J Cardiothorac Surg 2000;17:566–569.
53. Houston HE, Payne WS, Harrison EG Jr, et al. Primary cancers of the trachea. Arch Surg 1969;99:132–140.
54. Hadju SL, Huvos AG, Goodner JT, et al. Carcinoma of the trachea. Clinico Pathologic Study of 41 cases. Cancer 1970;25:1448–1456.
55. Enterline HT, Schoenberg HW. Carcinoma (cylindromatous type) of trachea and bronchi and bronchial adenoma; a comparative study. Cancer 954;7:663–670.
56. Markel SF, Abell MR, Haight C, et al. Neoplasms of bronchus commonly designated as adenomas. Cancer 1964;17: 590–608.
57. Olmedo G, Rosenberg M, Fonseca R. Primary tumors of the trachea. Clinicopathologic features and surgical results. Chest 1982;81:701–706.
58. Li W, Ellerbrock NA, Libshitz HI. Primary malignant tumors of the trachea. A radiologic and clinical study. Cancer 1990;66:894–896.
59. Hatton MQF, Allen MB, Cooke NJ. Pancoast Syndrome: an unusual presentation of adenoid cystic carcinoma. Eur Respir J 1993;6:271–272.
60. Nomori H, Kaseda S, Kobayashi K, et al. Adenoid cystic carcinoma of the trachea and main-stem bronchus. J Thorac Cardiovasc Surg 1988;96:271–277.
61. Okura T, Shiode M, Tanaka R, et al. A case of peripheral adenoid cystic carcinoma (in Japanese). Nippon Kyobu Shikkan Gakkai Zasshi 1990;28:773–776.
62. Gallagher CG, Stark R, Teskey J, et al. Atypical manifestations of pulmonary adenoid cystic carcinoma. Br J Dis Chest 1986;80:396–399.
63. Payne WS, Fontana RS, Woolner LB. Bronchial tumors originating from mucous glands: current classification and unusual manifestations. Med Clin North Am 1968;48: 945–960.
64. Corrin B. Pathology of the lungs. London, Edinburgh, New York: Churchill-Livingstone, 2000:513.
65. Reid JD. Adenoid cystic carcinoma (cylindroma) of the bronchial tree. Cancer 1952;5:685–694.
66. Nomori H, Kaseda S, Kobayashi K, et al. Adenoid cystic carcinoma of the trachea and mainstem bronchus. J Thorac Cardiovasc Surg 1988;96:271–277.
67. Nascimento AG, Amaral ALP, Prado LAF, et al. Adenoid cystic carcinoma of salivary glands. Cancer 1986;57: 312–319.
68. Matsuba HM, Spector GJ, Thawley SE, et al. Adenoid cystic salivary gland carcinoma. Cancer 1986;57:519–524.
69. Eby LS, Johnson DS, Barker HW. Adenoid cystic carcinoma of the head and neck. Cancer (Philadelphia) 1972;29:1160–1168.
70. Ishida T, Nishino T, Oka T, et al. Adenoid cystic carcinoma of the tracheobronchial tree: clinicopathology and immunohistochemistry. J Surg Oncol 1989;41: 52–59.
71. Albers E, Lawrie T, Harrell JH, et al. Tracheobronchial adenoid cystic carcinoma. A clinico pathologic study of 14 cases. Chest 2004; 125:1160–1165.
72. Qiu S, Nampoothirs MM, Zaharopoulos P, et al. Primary pulmonary adenoid cystic carcinoma: report of a case diagnosed by fine needle aspiration cytology. Diagn Cytopathol 2004;30:51–56.
73. Grillet B, Demedts MD, Roelens J, et al. Spontaneous regression of lung metastases of adenoid cystic carcinoma. Chest 1984;85:289–291.
74. Heilbrunn A, Crosby IK. Adenocystic carcinoma and mucoepidermoid carcinomas of the tracheobronchial tree. Chest 1972;61:145–149.
75. Wilkins EW, Darling RC, Soutter L, et al. A continuing clinical survey of adenomas of the trachea and bronchus in a general hospital. J Thorac Cardiovasc Surg 1963; 46:279–291.
76. Houston HE, Payne WS, Harrison EG, et al. Primary cancers of the trachea. Arch Surg 1969;99:132–140.
77. Moran CA, Suster S, Koss MN. Primary adenoid cystic carcinoma of the lung: a clinico pathologic and immunohistochemical study of 16 cases. Cancer 1994;73: 1390–1397.
78. Maziak DE, Todd TRJ, Keshavjee SH, et al. Adenoid cystic carcinoma of the airway: thirty two year experience. J Thoracic Cardiovasc Surg 1996;112:1522–1532.
79. Spizamy DL, Shepard JO, McLoud TC, et al. CT of adenoid cystic carcinoma of the trachea. AJR 1986; 146:1129–1132.
80. England EM, Hochholzer L. Truly benign "bronchial adenoma" Report of 10 cases of mucous gland adenoma with immunohistochemical and ultrastructural findings. Am J Surg Pathol 1995;19:887–899.
81. Ferguson CJ, Cleeland JA. Mucous gland adenoma of the trachea: case report and literature review. J Thorac Cardiovasc Surg 1988;95:347–350.
82. Weinberger MA, Katz S, Davis EW. Peripheral bronchial adenoma of mucous gland type. J Thorac Surg 1955; 29:626–635.
83. Allen MS, Jr, Marsh WL Jr, Greissinger WT. Mucus gland adenoma of the bronchus. J Thorac Cardiovasc Surg 1974;67:966–968.
84. Kwon JW, Goo JM, Seo JB, et al. Mucous gland adenoma of the bronchus. CT findings in two patients. J Comput Assist Tomogr 1999;23:758–760.
85. Ramsey JH, Reimann DL. Bronchial adenomas arising in mucous glands. Am J Pathol 1953;29:339–352.
86. Gilman RA, Klassen KP, Scarpelli DG. Mucous gland adenoma of the bronchus. Amer J Clin Pathol 1956; 26:151–154.
87. Kroe DJ, Pitcock JA. Benign mucous gland adenoma of the bronchus. Arch Pathol 1967;84:539–540.
88. Rosenblum P, Klein RI. Adenomatous polyp of the right main bronchus producing atelectasis. J Pediatr 1935; 7:791–796.
89. Emory WB, Mitchell WT, Jr, Hatch HG, Jr. Mucous gland adenoma of the bronchus. Am Rev Respir Dis 1973; 108:1407–1410.
90. Fechner RE, Bentinck BR, Askew JB, Jr. Acinic cell tumor of the lung: a histologic and ultrastructural study. Cancer 1972;29:501–508.
91. Katz DR, Bubis JJ. Acinic cell tumor of the bronchus. Cancer 1976;38:830–832.

92. Gharpure KJ, Deshpande RK, Vishweshvara RN, et al. Acinic cell tumor of the bronchus (a case report). Indian J Cancer 1985;22:152–156.
93. Heard BE, Dewar A, Firman RK, et al. One very rare and one new tracheal tumor found by electron microscopy: glomus tumour and acinic cell tumour resembling carcinoid tumours by light microscopy. Thorax 1982;37:97–103.
94. Yoshida K, Koyama J, Matsui T. Acinic cell tumor of the bronchial gland (in Japanese). Nippon Geka Gakkai Zasshi 1989;90:1810–1813.
95. Moran CA, Suster S, Koss MN. Acinic cell carcinoma of the lung ("Fechner tumor"): a clinicopathologic, immunohistochemical and ultrastructural study of five cases. Am J Surg Pathol 1992;16:1039–1050.
96. Ellis GL, Corio RL. Acinic cell adenocarcinoma. A clinicopathologic analysis of 294 cases. Cancer 1983;52: 542–549.
97. Grage TB, Lober PH, Arhleger SW. Acinic cell carcinoma of the parotid gland. A clinicopathologic review of eleven cases. Am J Surg 1961;102:765–768.
98. Eneroth CM, Hamberger CA, Jakobsson PA. Malignancy of acinic cell carcinoma. Ann Otol Rhinol Laryngol 1966;75:780–792.
99. Eneroth CM, Jakobsson PA, Blank C. Acinic cell carcinoma of the parotid gland. Cancer 1966;19: 1761–1772.
100. Sidhu GS, Forrester EM. Acinic cell carcinoma: long-term survival after pulmonary metastases. Light and electron microscopic study. Cancer 1977;40:756–765.
101. Colby TV, Koss MN, Travis WD. Tumors of the lower respiratory tract. AFIP atlas of tumor pathology. Washington, DC: Armed Forces Institute of Pathology, 1994:85.
102. Miura K, Moringa S, Horiuchi M, et al. Bronchial carcinoid tumor mimicking acinic cell tumor. Acta Pathol Jpn 1988;38:523–530.
103. Ukoha OO, Quartararo P, Carter D, et al. Acinic cell carcinoma of the lung with metastasis to lymph nodes. Chest 1999; 115:591–595.
104. Lee H-Y, Mancer K, Koong H-N. Primary acinic cell carcinoma of the lung with lymph node metastasis. Arch Pathol Lab Med 2003;127:e216–e219.
105. Matsuba K, Takazawa T, Thurlbeck WM. Oncocytes in human bronchial mucous glands. Thorax 1972;27: 181–184.
106. Ritter JH, Nappi O. Oxyphillic proliferations of the respiratory tract and paranasal sinuses. Semin Diagn Pathol 1999, 16:105–116.
107. Sklar JL, Churg A, Bensch KG. Oncocytic carcinoid tumor of the lung. Am J Surg Pathol 1980;4:287–292.
108. Sajjad SM, Mackay B, Lukeman JM. Oncocytic carcinoid tumor of the lung. Ultrastruct Pathol 1980;1:171–176.
109. Walter P, Waarter A, Morand G. Carcinoide oncocytaire bronchique. Virchows Arch [A] 1978;379:85–97.
110. Scharifker D, Marchevsky A. Oncocytic carcinoid of lung: an ultrastructural analysis. Cancer 1981;47:530–532.
111. Ghadially FN, Block HJ. Oncocytic carcinoid of the lung. J Submicrosc Cytol 1985;17:435–442.
112. Shin DH, Park SS, Lee JH, et al. Oncocytic glomus tumor of the trachea. Chest 1990;98:1021–1023.
113. Heard BE, Corrin B, Dewar A. Pathology of seven mucous cell adenomas of the bronchial glands with particular reference to ultrastructure. Histopathology 1985;9: 687–701.
114. Stafford JR, Pollock J, Wenzel BC. Oncocytic mucoepidermoid tumor of the bronchus. Cancer 1984;54:94–99.
115. Fine G, Chang CH. Adenoma of type 2 pneumocytes with oncocytic features. Arch Pathol Lab Med 1991;115: 797–801.
116. Akhtar M, Young I, Reyes F. Bronchial adenoma with polymorphous features. Cancer 1974; 33:1572–1576.
117. Fechner RE, Bentinck BR. Ultrastructure of bronchial oncocytoma. Cancer 1973;31:1451–1456.
118. Black WC, III. Pulmonary oncocytoma. Cancer 1969; 23:1347–1357.
119. Santos-Briz A, Terron J, Sastre R, et al. Oncocytoma of the lung. Cancer 1977;40:1330–1336.
120. Tesluk H. Pulmonary oncocytoma. J Surg Oncol 1985; 29:173–175.
121. Warter A, Walter P, Sabountchi M, et al. Oncocytic bronchial adenoma. Virchows Arch [A] 1981;392:231–239.
122. Cwierzyk TA, Glasberg SS, Virshup MA, et al. Pulmonary oncocytoma: report of a case with cytologic, histologic and electron microscopic study. Acta Cytol 1985;29:620–623.
123. LaForga JBM, Aranda FI. Multicentric oncocytoma of the lung diagnosed by fine-needle aspiration. Diagn Cytopathol 1999;21:51–54.
124. Tashiro Y, Iwata Y, Nabae T, et al. Pulmonary oncocytoma: report of a case in conjunction with an immunohistochemical and ultrastructural study. Pathol Int 1995; 45:448–451.
125. Strickler JG, Hegstrom J, Thomas MJ, et al. Myoepithelioma of the lung. Arch Pathol Lab Med 1987;111: 1082–1085.
126. Nistal M, Garcia Viera M, Martinez-Garcia C, et al. Epithelial-myoepithelial tumors of the bronchus. Am J Surg Pathol 1994;18:421–425.
127. Hayes MMM, Van der Westhuizen NG, Forgie R. Malignant mixed tumor of the bronchus: a biphasic neoplasm of epithelial and myoepithelial cells. Mod Pathol 1993; 6:85–88.
128. Ohori NP Uncommon endobronchial neoplasms. In: Cagle PT, ed. Diagnostic pulmonary pathology. New York, Basel: Marcel Dekker, 2000:685–717.
129. Ryska A, Kerekes Z, Hovorkova E, et al. Epithelial-myoepithelial carcinoma of the bronchus. Pathol Res Pract 1998;194:431–435.
130. Pelosi G, Fraggetta F, Maffini F, et al. Pulmonary epithelial-myoepithelial tumor of unproven malignant potential. Report of a case and review of the literature. Modern Pathol 2001;14:521–526.
131. Ru K, Srivastava A, Tischler AS. Bronchial epithelial-myoepithelial carcinoma. Arch Pathol Lab Med 2004;128:92–94.
132. Doganay L, Bilgi S, Ozdil A, et al. Epithelial-myoepithelial carcinoma of the lung. Arch Pathol Lab Med 2004;127: e177–e180.
133. Lee VKM, McCaughan BC, Scolyer RA. Polymorphous low grade adenocarcinoma in the lung: a case report. Int J Surg Pathol 2004;12:287–292.

134. Freedman PD, Lumerman H. Lobular carcinoma of intraoral minor salivary gland origin. Report of twelve cases. Oral Surg Oral Med Oral Pathol 1983;56: 157–165.
135. Batsakis JG, Pinkston GR, Luna MA, et al. Adenocarcinomas of the oral cavity: a clinicopathologic study of terminal duct carcinomas. J Laryngol Otol 1983;97: 825–835.
136. Evans HL, Batsakis JG. Polymorphous low-grade adenocarcinoma of minor salivary glands: a study of 14 cases of a distinctive neoplasm. Cancer 1984;53:935–942.
137. Pittman CB, Zitsch RP III. Polymorphous low-grade adenocarcinoma of the tonsil: report of a case and review of the literature. Am J Otolaryngol 2002;23: 297–299.
138. Sato T, Indo H, Takasaki T, et al. A rare case of intraosseous polymorphous low-grade adenocarcinoma (PLGA) of the maxilla. Dentomaxillofac Radiol 2001; 30:184–187.
139. Lengyel E, Somogyi A, Godeny M, et al. Polymorphous low-gra de adenocarcinoma of the nasopharynx. Case report and review of the literature. Strahlenther Onkol 2000;176:40–42.
140. Hannen EJ, Bulten J, Festen J, et al. Polymorphous low grade adenocarcinoma with distant metastases and deletions on chromosome 6q23–ater and 11q 23–ater: a case report. J Clin Pathol 2000;53:942–945.
141. Yousem SA. Pulmonary adenosquamous carcinoma with amyloid-like stroma. Mod Pathol 1989;2:240–246.
142. Batsakis JG, Littler ER, Leahy MS. Sebaceous cell lesion of the head and neck. Arch Otolaryngol 1972; 95:171–157.
143. Knepp DR. Sebaceous neoplasms of salivary gland origin. Pathol Annu 1983;18:71–102.
144. Assor D. Epidermoid carcinoma with sebaceous differentiation in the vallecula; report of a case. Am J Clin Pathol 1974;63:891–894.
145. Borczuk CA, Sha KK, Hisler ES, et al. Sebaceous carcinoma of the lung: histologic and immunohistochemical characterization of an unusual pulmonary neoplasm. Report of a case and review of the literature. Am J Surg Pathol 2002;26:795–798.
146. Fantasia JE, Nocco CE, Lally ET. Ultrastructure of sialadenoma papilliferum. Arch Pathol Lab Med 1986; 110:523–527.
147. Freedman PD, Lumerman H. Sialadenoma papilliferum. Report of two cases. Oral Surg Oral Med Oral Pathol 1978;45:88–94.
148. Rosai J. Oral cavity and oropharynx. In: Rosai and Ackerman's surgical pathology. Edinburgh, London, New York: Mosby, 2004:260.
149. Bobos M, Hytiroglou P, Karkavelas G, et al. Sialadenoma papilliferum of bronchus. Virchows Arch 2003;443: 695–699.
150. Chang T, Husain AN, Colby T, et al. Pneumocytic adenoepithelioma: a distinctive lung tumor with epithelial, myoepithelial, and pnenmocytic differentiation. Am J Surg Pathol 2007;31:562–568.

39
Mesenchymal Tumors, Part I: Tumors of Fibrous, Fibrohistiocytic, and Muscle Origin

Armando E. Fraire and David H. Dail

Tumors of Fibrous and Fibrohistiocytic Origin

Tumors generally regarded as fibrous or fibrohistiocytic in nature include inflammatory pseudotumors (inflammatory myofibroblastic tumors), intrapulmonary localized fibrous tumors, cystic fibrohistiocytic tumors, cystic mesenchymal hamartomas, malignant fibrous histiocytomas, and fibrosarcomas. In recognition of their greater frequency in the pleura, localized fibrous tumors (LFTs) are primarily discussed in Chapter 43 on pleural neoplasms; in this chapter only the intrapulmonary variants of LFTs are considered. Likewise, in view of their greater frequency in younger age groups, inflammatory myofibroblastic tumors and congenital peribronchial myofibroblastic tumors are discussed in Chapter 42 on pediatric tumors.

Inflammatory Pseudotumor (Inflammatory Myofibroblastic Tumor)

Inflammatory pseudotumors (IPT) and inflammatory myofibroblastic tumor (IMT) are but two of several other names (e.g., plasma cell granuloma, fibrous histiocytoma, fibroxanthoma, pseudosarcomatous myofibroblastic tumor) given to pulmonary lesions that are histologically similar to localized areas of organizing pneumonia. Characteristically, these lesions show filling of air spaces by plump fibroblastic cells, foamy histiocytes, and chronic inflammatory cells such as lymphocytes and plasma cells.[1–6]

In 1999, the World Health Organization (WHO) regarded these two terms (IPT and IMT) as synonyms and jointly described them as "fibroblastic or myofibroblastic proliferations with a varying infiltrate of inflammatory cells, typically plasma cells, lymphocytes and/or foamy histiocytes. The lesions may range from a primary myofibroblastic or fibroxanthomatous appearance to one that has a heavy infiltrate of plasma cells."[7] There is, however, an increasing body of evidence that supports the notion that these two processes may in fact represent separate and distinct entities, albeit with some degree of overlapping clinical and histopathologic features. For instance, the more aggressive tumors designated as IMTs are more apt to occur in children, to be clonal in nature (as evidenced by chromosome 2 alterations at the 2p23 location of the *ALK* gene and translocation of this gene to chromosome 9, creating *ALK* gene fusion products),[8–12] and to represent true neoplasms with a potential for local invasion and recurrence.[9,12] The less aggressive lesions designated as IPTs have a broader age distribution, lack clonality, and are most likely to represent postpneumonic reactive processes, as evidenced by antecedent respiratory infections in about one third of the cases and a benign follow-up in the majority of cases.[5,6] In accord with these realities, the WHO in 2004 now considers IMTs to be "subsets of the broader category of inflammatory pseudotumors" and defines them as "tumoral lesions composed of variable mixtures of collagen, inflammatory cells and usually bland spindle cells showing myofibroblastic differentiation."[8] Inflammatory myofibroblastic tumors in children are fully discussed in Chapter 42.

Although IPTs have a wider age distribution, most patients are under the age of 40 and many are children.[13] About half of the patients are asymptomatic, but some present with cough, hemoptysis, chest pain, or shortness of breath.[13] Some cases may come to attention only as a chance radiologic finding.[13] On chest x-ray, IPTs typically present as solitary, peripherally located, sharply circumscribed masses with an anatomic bias for the lower lobes.[4] In a series of 52 cases reported by Agrons et al.,[4] 11 (21.2%) cases showed atypical features including airway invasion and extension beyond the lung into hilar and mediastinal structures or even the chest wall and major vascular structures, again suggesting some degree of behavioral overlap with IMTs.[4,11]

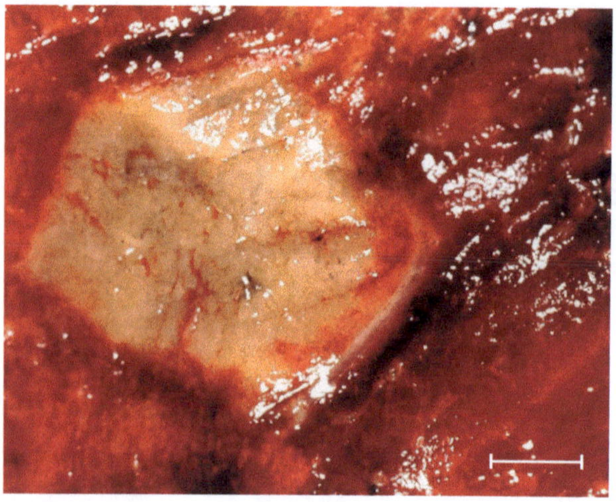

FIGURE 39.1. Inflammatory pseudotumor. Gross appearance, note yellow tan color of the lesion. Cm scale. (Courtesy of Dr. Eugene Mark, Massachusetts General Hospital, Boston, MA.)

Grossly, IPTs vary considerably in size from 0.5 to 36 cm in diameter, with 70% in the range 0.5 to 6 cm, 20% greater than 6 to 10 cm, and 10% larger than 10 cm. They usually have relatively well-defined margins without true encapsulation (Fig. 39.1). Their color and texture vary depending on the predominant cell population. Those with more fibroblasts are firmer and gray-white, those with an increased number of plasma cells are tan and rubbery, and those with abundant fat-filled macrophages assume a more brilliant yellow-orange color and are softer and more friable. Central necrosis may be found focally, and grossly identified calcification or hemorrhage has been reported but is infrequent.

In Matsubara et al.'s[5,6] series of 32 cases, three major histopathologic patterns were encountered: (1) organizing pneumonia pattern (44%), (2) fibrous histiocytoma pattern (44%), and (3) lymphoplasmacytic pattern. In practice, there is considerable overlap among the three histopathologic patterns, and most appear to represent sequelae of preexisting pneumonic processes. Microscopic features common to all IPTs include partial or complete obliteration of the fine alveolar framework of the lung, although an occasional invaded vessel or entrapped bronchus or bronchiole can be identified within an otherwise diffusely involved area of lung. The architecture of the lung as noted is usually lost, although some remnant of entrapped metaplastic cuboidal cell-lined air spaces often persists. The borders are rather sharp, with only focal interstitial spread. There may be minor reactions of inflammatory infiltrate or macrophage response and nearby giant cells of the Touton type may be present as well. As noted above, some IPTs are composed predominantly of plump spindle cells and others of plasma cells (Fig. 39.2). However, tumors with a predominance of plasma cells (and lymphocytes) may also have a background of bland spindle cell proliferation. The spindle cells have large vesicular nuclei and generally run in the same direction as their neighbors, but can form some intertwining fascicles and occasionally a storiform pattern. The storiform pattern is much more evident when the spindle cells become thinner, and the inflammatory cell reaction is less prominent. Mitoses are commonly seen but are not atypical. The stromal cells can also become increasingly hyalinized and have a cytoplasmic appearance between fibrillar and waxy. Plasma cells are seen scattered among the spindle cells, often in small aggregates, but sometimes number up to 100 per group. There is a scattering of lymphocytes with these plasma cells, but the lymphocytes may form a greater percentage of the inflammatory cell reaction. In one case described by Mark et al.[14] the fibrohistiocytic cells had positive staining for vimentin and negative staining for keratin. Scattered Langerhans cells within the lesion stained positively for S-100 protein.[14] In Ledet et al.'s[12] series, most IPTs were p53 negative.

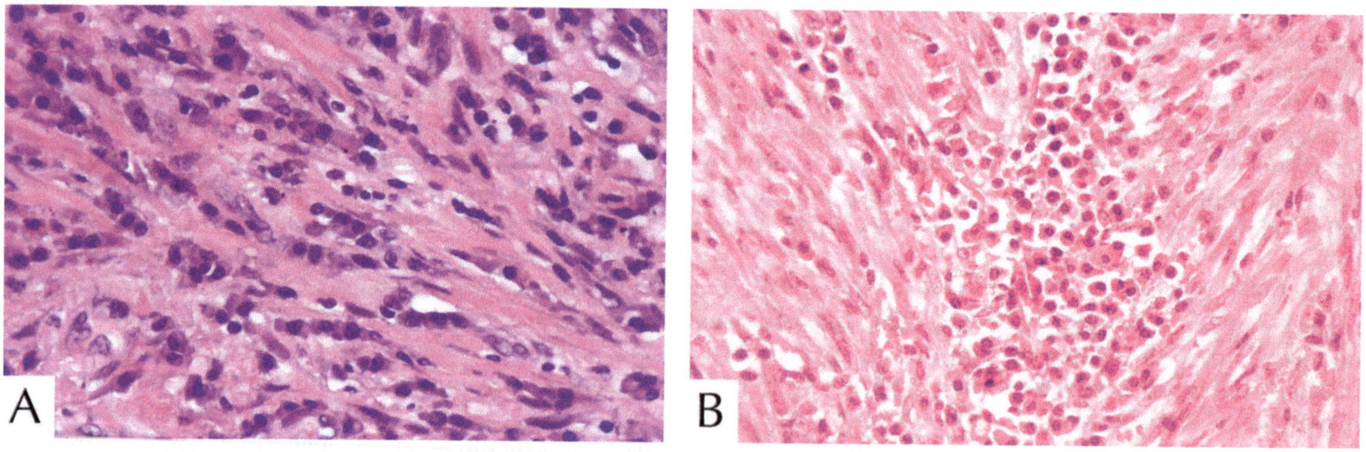

FIGURE 39.2. Inflammatory pseudotumor. **(A)** Fibroblastic pattern. **(B)** Plasma cell granuloma pattern.

Because of its variable histologic appearance, the differential diagnosis of IPT is multifaceted.[5] The plasma cell granuloma variant in particular may resemble plasmacytoma or even lymphoma. Some cases with a predominance of lymphoid cells may resemble lymphocytic interstitial pneumonia (LIP). Appropriate use of B- and T-lymphoid markers and light chain restriction studies help to distinguish IPT from lymphomas and plasmacytomas, respectively. Lymphocytic interstitial pneumonia can be distinguished by its preservation of the underlying lung architecture, its location within the interstitium, and its clinical association with Sjögren's syndrome or immune deficiency states (see Chapter 32). The fibrous histiocytoma variant may mimic malignant fibrous histiocytoma (MFH) or sarcomatoid carcinoma. Marked cellular atypia, frequent mitoses, and extreme pleomorphism should skew the diagnosis toward MFH. Immunostains positive for pancytokeratin would favor sarcomatoid carcinoma over inflammatory pseudotumor.[1–6] Ledet and associates[12] have evaluated the usefulness of p53 immunostaining in the distinction between IPT and sarcomas involving the lung. In their study, eight solitary IPTs and seven sarcomas involving the lung (two malignant fibrous histiocytomas, one fibrosarcoma, one alveolar soft part sarcoma, two high-grade sarcomas not otherwise specified, and a sarcoma developing 10 years following irradiation of an inflammatory pseudotumor) were examined for the p53 protein product by immunohistochemistry. All eight solitary IPTs were negative for the p53 protein product while four of the seven sarcomas (including the postirradiation sarcoma) were immunopositive, suggesting an important role of this tumor marker in the differentiation between IPTs and selected sarcomas involving the lung.[12]

Most cases of IPT tend to remain stable over time, and spontaneous regression has been reported in the literature.[5] Some reported cases have shown decreased tumor size following treatment with corticosteroids or irradiation therapy.[5] However, the treatment of choice appears to be complete surgical resection. Long-term follow-up after successful surgical resection (in the absence of complications such as invasion into adjacent structures) has demonstrated a benign course in 90% or more of the cases.[5,6]

Intrapulmonary Localized Fibrous Tumor

Localized fibrous tumors, also known as solitary fibrous tumors, are most common in the pleura and are discussed at greater length in Chapter 43.[15–19] In addition to the pleura, they also occur in the trachea, mediastinum, pericardium, peritoneum, liver, thyroid, nasal cavity, paranasal sinuses, and other sites, but only rarely do these tumors occur within the lung.[20–22] Here we discuss only the intrapulmonary variants.

Tumors formerly designated as hemangiopericytomas share considerable histopathologic features with LFTs, and the boundaries between these two entities have become increasingly blurred.[23–25] In the respiratory tract and particularly in the pleuropulmonary region, it is difficult to discern clinical and histopathologic characteristics that would help to differentiate pleural from pulmonary LFTs, and in fact some authors discuss them in a combined fashion as pleuropulmonary LFTs.[26] Few studies have specifically focused on intrapulmonary LFTs, some under the older rubric of pulmonary hemangiopericytoma.[20,22,27,28] Most reports are studies of single cases, and two reports include three cases each.[20,27] The three patients described by Yousem and Flynn[20] are a man aged 71 and two women aged 55 and 82 years. Two of the patients were asymptomatic and had their tumors incidentally discovered as coin lesions on chest radiographs. The other patient was symptomatic and presented with persistent cough and early morning sputum production. Paraneoplastic syndromes can occur in association with these tumors and include hypoglycemia, hypertension, and pulmonary osteoarthropathy.[28] A unique case presented by Wu and coworkers[28] was of a patient with a large pulmonary tumor mass, gingival bleeding, hematuria, hemoptysis, and coagulopathy manifested as prolonged prothrombin and partial thromboplastin times. This coagulopathy cleared following surgery with normalization of coagulation parameters.

Grossly, as in the pleura, these tumors are firm, well-circumscribed yellow-tan to gray-white, sometimes with areas of necrosis and focal hemorrhage (Fig. 39.3). About 10% are multiple, usually with smaller nodules in the same lobe. Tumors larger than 8.0 cm with necrosis and

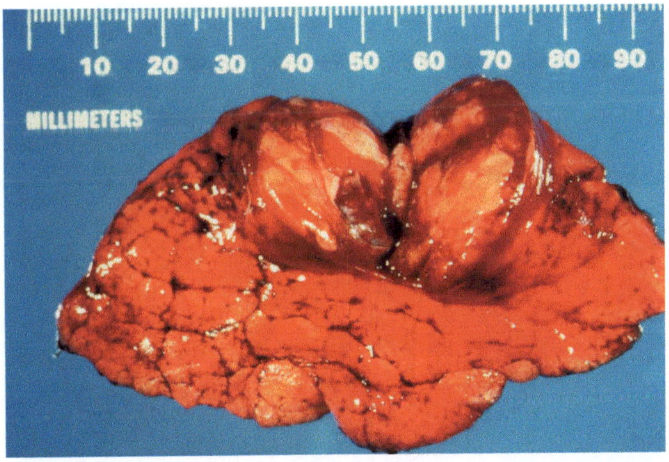

FIGURE 39.3. Intrapulmonary localized fibrous tumor. Note well-circumscribed subpleural nodular mass with a yellow reddish cut surface. (Courtesy of Dr. Sam Yousem, University of Pittsburgh Medical Center. From Yousem and Flynn.[20] Copyright © 1988, American Society of Clinical Pathologists, with permission.)

hemorrhage are likely to be malignant. Localized fibrous tumors have similar histopathologic and immunohistochemical features regardless of their site of origin. Microscopically, the most characteristic and required pattern for diagnosis is the "patternless" pattern in which the fibroblastic tumor cells are haphazardly arranged in fascicles lacking any specific architectural orientation pattern and often showing entrapped spaces lined by bronchiolar type of epithelium (Figs. 39.4 and 39.5). They may also have a vascular hemangiopericytoma-like pattern with acute angled bifurcations of sinusoidal spaces known as "antler-like" structures, and at times this pattern of growth may predominate (see discussion on vascular tumors in Chapter 40). There may be narrow collagen bands between the tumor cells and these spaces, or it may appear that the tumor cells form these spaces. The neoplastic cells are usually rather monotonous and differ from the blander appearance of low-grade neoplasms in being round to oval, often with indistinct cytoplasmic borders by light microscopy. Sometimes the intervening stroma becomes hyalinized. Like their pleural and soft tissue counterparts, intrapulmonary localized fibrous tumors are positive immunohistochemically for vimentin, Bcl-2, CD99, and CD34, and are negative for cytokeratin.[23] In the series of Yousem and Flynn,[20] the tumors were negative when immunostained for desmin, epithelial membrane antigen, and S-100 protein.

Major entities to be distinguished include localized malignant fibrous mesothelioma, MFH, and pulmonary fibrosarcoma. Localized malignant mesotheliomas as their diffuse malignant counterparts are cytokeratin positive, while LFTs are uniformly negative. The MFHs are usually large tumors with extensive necrosis and vascular

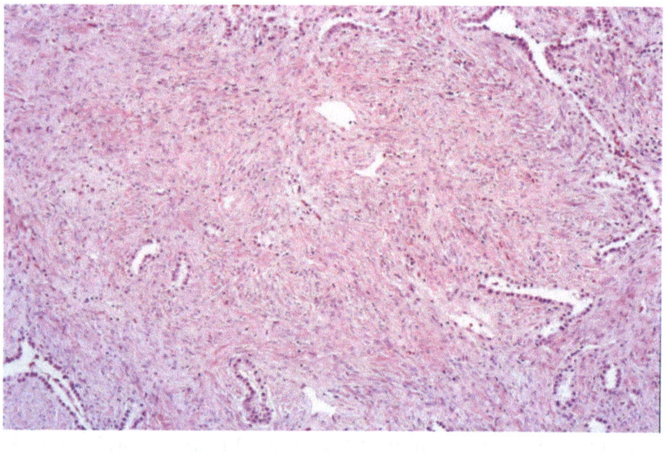

FIGURE 39.4. Localized fibrous tumor, low-power view. Note fibroblastic proliferation and multiple cleft-like spaces representing trapped bronchiolar lined structures. (From Yousem and Flynn.[20] Copyright © 1988, American Society of Clinical Pathologists, with permission.)

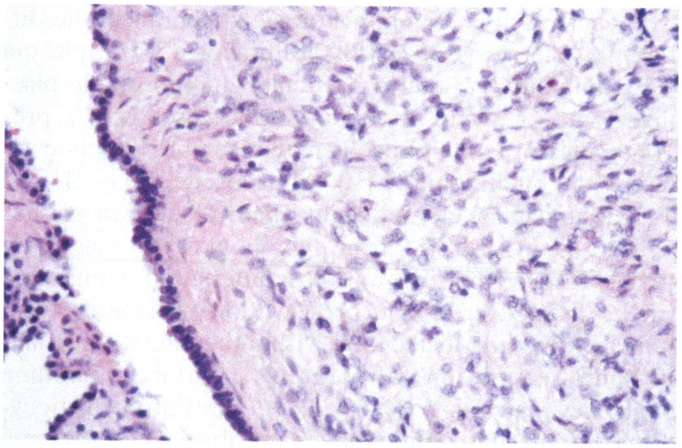

FIGURE 39.5. Localized fibrous tumor, closer view showing bronchiolar like spaces within a fibroblastic proliferation showing the typical pattern-less pattern. (Courtesy of Dr. Sam Yousem, University of Pittsburgh Medical Center. From Yousem and Flynn.[20] Copyright © 1988, American Society of Clinical Pathologists, with permission.)

invasion. Histopathologically, they lack the patternless pattern of LFTs and show areas with storiform arrangement of tumor cells.[20] Fibrosarcoma has a prominent herringbone pattern, and frequent mitoses (greater than five per 10 high-power fields [HPFs]).[20] Inflammatory pseudotumors described earlier show rich inflammatory cell infiltrates consisting of plasma cells, lymphocytes and bland-looking spindle-shaped fibrohistiocytic cells.[20] Most LFTs follow a benign course but malignant cases do occur. Predictors of malignant behavior include size greater than 8.0 cm, gross hemorrhage, necrosis, cellular pleomorphism, and a high mitotic count.[20] Immunostaining with cell proliferation markers such as Ki-67 are also useful in the differentiation of benign from malignant tumors. Surgery is the treatment of choice but is not curative in all cases. Of the three patients reported by Hansen et al.,[27] two were alive at 7 and 18 years after surgical excision without evidence of recurrence or metastatic disease, but one had recurrence of the tumor within 22 months.

Cystic Fibrohistiocytic Tumors

These exceedingly rare lung tumors are characterized by their fibrous proliferative features and uncertain histogenesis.[29] In four cases reported by Osborn and coworkers,[29] the tumors were typically composed of multiple nodules with variable degree of cystic change and an intervening stroma showing histologic features of a cellular fibrohistiocytic proliferation. While the histogenesis is poorly understood, there is some evidence to suggest that these lesions may represent metastases from indolent cutaneous neoplasms such as cellular fibrous histiocytomas or dermatofibrosarcoma protuberans.[30–33]

TABLE 39.1. Clinical data on cases of cellular fibrous histiocytic proliferations in the lungs

Case	Sex	Age*	Symptoms	Radiologic or gross description	Previous cutaneous lesions	Follow-up
1	Male	38	Hemoptysis	Bilateral opacities, many nodular and cavitating	None identified	Alive with disease at 2 years
2	Male	54	Hemoptysis	Bilateral opacities, many nodular and cavitating	Cellular fibrohistiocytic lesion removed 23 years earlier	Alive with disease at 4 years
3	Male	35	Not known	Bilateral cystic lung nodules	None identified	Alive with disease at 1 year
4	Male	29	Pneumonia Pneumothorax	Multiple bilateral cavitary lesions	History of CFH on back 10 years previously	Not known
5	Male	65	Asymptomatic, found on routine CXR	Multiple bilateral nodular opacities	None identified	Alive with disease at 2 years
6	Male	30	Dyspnea Pneumothorax	Bilateral nodular opacities	Recurrent dermatofibroma on the back 5 years previously	Alive with disease at 20 years
7	Male	25	Hemoptysis	Bilateral diffuse cysts	None identified	Alive with disease at 5 years
8	Female	30	Pneumothorax	Bilateral cystic lesions	Dermatofibrosarcoma protruberans removed 17 years previously	Not known
9	Male	19	Not known	Not known (cystic on pathology)	CFH 1.5 years previously	Alive, free of disease at 4 years
10	Male	40	Not known	Not known (cystic on pathology)	CFH 7 years previously	Alive with disease at 8 years
11	Male	35	Fatigue	Multiple masses, not cystic	CFH 2 years previously	Not known

*Age is at presentation of symptoms.
CFH, cellular fibrous histiocytoma; CXR, chest radiograph.
Source: Osborn et al.,[29] with permission from Blackwell Publishing Ltd.

Prior to the report of Osborn et al. of four cases, Joseph et al.,[34] who gave this entity its name, had described two patients with similar lesions. The two patients were men. One was a 65-year-old with bilateral multiple nodules growing slightly for 2 years that focally were found to be cystic on open lung biopsy. The other was a 30-year-old with multiple and rather dramatic partially fluid-filled bilateral cysts who developed recurrent pneumothoraces and air emboli to the brain while traveling on an extended airplane flight. He was followed for 20 years with only slow enlargement of the lung nodules. These authors referred to another possible case by Holden et al.,[35] in which the patient, a 25-year-old man who had one cyst at the beginning of observation, had developed multiple bilateral cysts over a period of 2 years. The walls of the cyst were composed of fibroblastic cells arranged in a storiform manner, similar in appearance to those of dermatofibroma of the skin but believed by the authors to be hamartomatous in nature.

The demographics of the cases reported by Osborn and colleagues[29] are similar. All four patients were men, ages 35 to 54 years. Two patients had a history of a cutaneous fibrohistiocytic lesion in the chest wall, respectively excised 10 and 23 years prior to presentation with lung disease. Demographics emphasizing a clear male gender predominance and clinical data for all cases reported in the literature are summarized in Table 39.1. Computed tomography (CT) imaging showed multiple bilateral cystic lung lesions in all four patients with nodular cavitating opacities seen on high-resolution CT scans (Fig. 39.6). Microscopically, variably dilated thin-walled cystic air spaces were lined by cuboidal epithelium with an underlying layer of mildly pleomorphic spindle cells with slightly wavy morphology and storiform architecture, admixed with inflammatory cells (Fig. 39.7). The tumor cells stained for CD68 in three of four cases and all cases were negative for CD34. Table 39.2 summarizes the immunohistochemical data reported by Osborn et al.

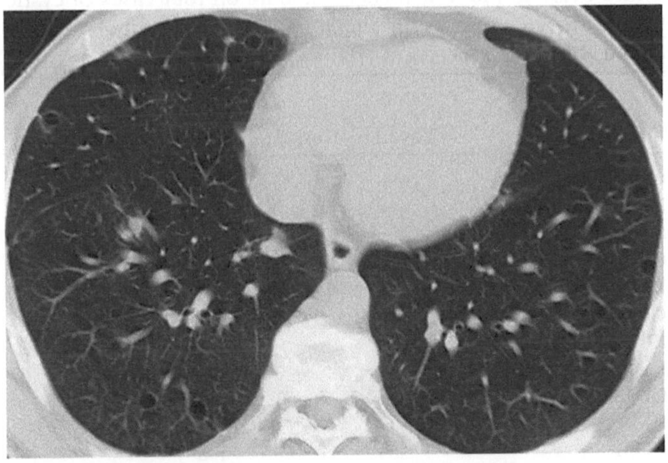

FIGURE 39.6. Cystic fibrohistiocytic tumor. High-resolution CT scan showing several poorly defined nodules with cavitation, largest 8.0mm in diameter. (From Osborn et al.,[29] with permission from Blackwell Publishing Ltd.)

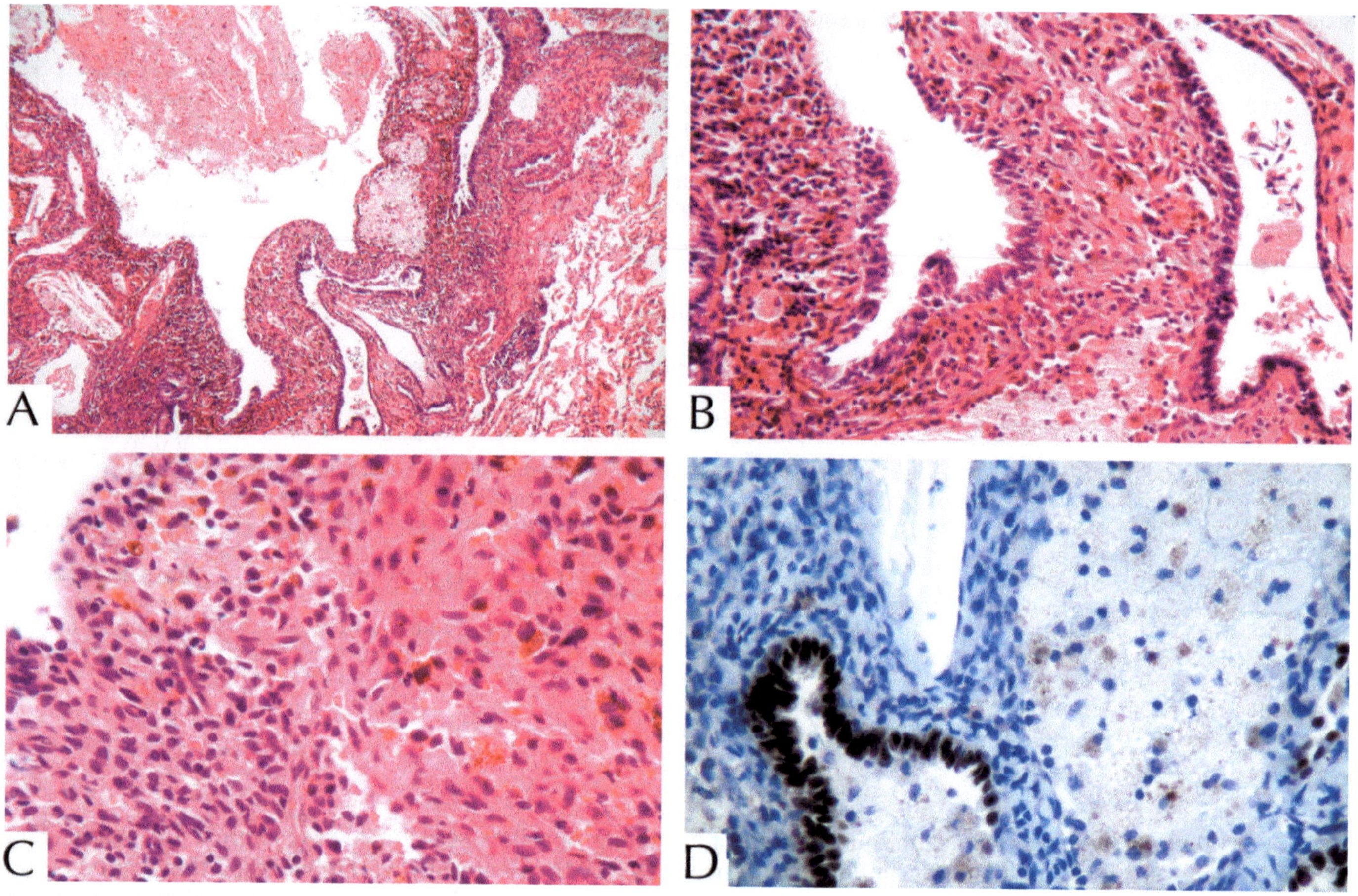

FIGURE 39.7. Cystic fibrohistiocytic tumor. **(A)** Note multicystic nodule with some cysts being empty and others containing foamy macrophages, cholesterol clefts, or proteinaceous debris. **(B)** At higher power, a fibrohistiocytic proliferation can be seen within the interstitium. **(C)** The spindle cells contain variable amounts of eosinophilic cytoplasm and are admixed with lymphocytes and some hemosiderin-laden macrophages. **(D)** Thyroid transcription factor-1 (TTF-1) stain shows that the cysts are lined by type 2 pneumocytes. (From Osborn et al.,[29] with permission from Blackwell Publishing Ltd.)

TABLE 39.2. Immunohistochemical data on four cases of cystic fibrohistiocytic tumors in the lung and one dermal cellular fibrous histiocytoma

				Case 4*	
Immunostain	Case 1	Case 2	Case 3	Lung	Skin
Cytokeratin	–	–	–	–	–
Desmin	–	–	–	n/a	–
Smooth muscle actin	–	–	–	–	–
CD34	–	–	–	–	–
TTF-1	–	–	n/a	–	–
CD68	+	+	+	–	+
S-100 protein	–	–	n/a	–	–
Factor VIII	–	–	n/a	–	–
CD1a	–	–	n/a	–	–
EMA	–	–	n/a	–	–
CD31	–		n/a	–	–

*Case 4 was resected 10 years previously.
TTF-1, thyroid transcription factor-1; EMA, epithelial membrane antigen; n /a, not available.
Source: Osborn et al.,[29] with permission from Blackwell Publishing Ltd.

The clinical differential diagnosis of pulmonary cystic fibrohistiocytic lesions as reviewed by Joseph et al.[34] includes necrotizing inflammatory reactions, lung abscesses, cavitary pneumocystis infection or other cavitary infections, bullous emphysema, cylindrical bronchiectasis, pneumatoceles, congenital lung cysts, eosinophilic granuloma, lymphangioleiomyomatosis, and other neoplastic lesions such as mesenchymal cystic hamartoma, and some cases of papillomatosis and metastases, such as those of cavitary sarcomas. The main histologic distinctions, however, are with mesenchymal cystic hamartomas and low-grade metastatic sarcomas to the lung (see Chapter 44). Thin-walled cavities have been reported in low-grade leiomyosarcomas, endometrial stromal sarcomas, and synovial sarcomas.[31,32] Immunhistochemistry for smooth muscle actin, desmin, CD10, and estrogen and progesterone receptors, along with a thorough clinical history may assist in some cases. Any positivity for desmin or smooth muscle actin would favor low-grade leiomyosarcoma, while positivity for CD10 and hormone receptors would skew the diagnosis in the direction of low-grade endometrial sarcoma. As noted in Table 39.2, CD68 positivity can be seen in about 75% of cases of fibrohistiocytic tumors examined by Osborn and associates.

Until further experience is gained, it seems prudent to regard cystic fibrohistiocytic tumors as neoplasms of indolent nature, possibly metastatic in origin. The closely allied and somewhat overlapping lesion known as mesenchymal cystic hamartoma is discussed below.

Mesenchymal Cystic Hamartoma

Mesenchymal cystic hamartomas are characterized by cystic nodules containing bands of primitive undifferentiated mesenchymal cells lined by cuboidal respiratory epithelium. Three of the five patients reported by Mark[36] were male and two were female, and their ages ranged from 18 months to 54 years. Four of the five patients had tumors that were multifocal, and all were slow growing, solid when small, and becoming cystic when they had reached 1 cm or so in diameter. One of the patients, a 34-year-old woman who had an 8-cm umbilical cyst composed of similar tissue with atypical features, had been the subject of a clinical pathologic conference.[37] These patients presented with hemoptysis, pneumothorax, hemothorax, pleuritic pain, or mild to moderate dyspnea. Initial chest radiographs showed one large cyst in three cases, multiple bilateral nodules in one, and a cyst and bilateral nodules in one. Two initially thought to have unilateral disease developed bilateral lesions after many months, and the larger cysts occasionally had fluid levels. Computed tomography scans helped highlight the cystic quality and also detected more lesions than were seen by plain films.[36] All the patients were alive at the time of the report except for the oldest, who was 53 at the time of diagnosis, and who died 28 years later at age 81 in an auto accident, with no evidence of other tumor; no autopsy was done.

Histopathologically, all five patients had cystic lung lesions ranging from 5 to 10 cm. In three cases the walls were thin and pliant, and in two they were thick and scarred. The lesions were lined by either normal ciliated respiratory epithelium or bland epithelium with squamous metaplasia. These linings in the smaller lesions could be traced in continuity with the adjacent respiratory bronchioles.[36] Tumor nodules less than 5 mm were mostly hypocellular and nodular, but even then were associated with a plexiform airway configuration. Those 5 to 10 mm in diameter were nodular and cystic, and those larger than 10 mm were mostly cystic. Only two patients had the entire spectrum of nodules, cystic nodules, and cysts. A typical cyst showing an epithelial lining, a cellular subepithelial cambium layer, and a looser, less cellular connective tissue layer beneath the cambium layer is shown in Figure 39.8.

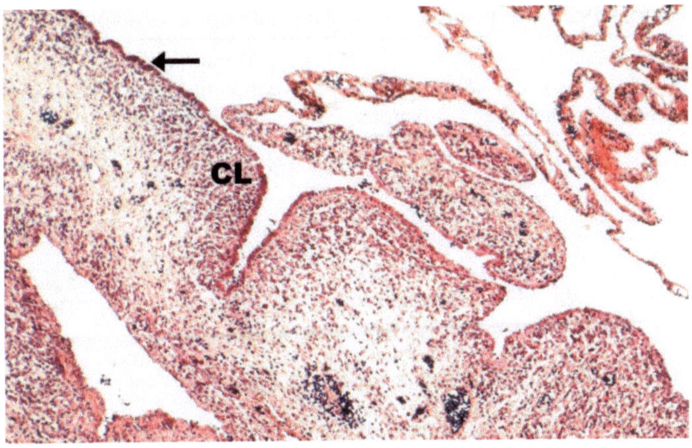

FIGURE 39.8. Mesenchymal cystic hamartoma. Cystic lesion with a cambium layer (CL), an epithelial lining (arrow), and unaffected lung tissue on the right upper corner. (Courtesy of Dr. Eugene Mark, Massachusetts General Hospital, Boston, MA. From Mark.[36] Copyright © 1986, Massachusetts Medical Society. All rights reserved.)

The diagnosis of mesenchymal cystic hamartoma is based entirely on histology, as little if any data are available in regard to immunohistochemistry or electron microscopy. The differential diagnosis is wide and includes the previously discussed cystic fibrohistiocytic tumors, diverse conditions such as regenerative changes of the lung, cystic adenomatoid malformation, cystic bronchiectasis, eosinophilic granuloma, thoracic endometriosis, cystic rhabdomyosarcoma, metastatic uterine stromal sarcoma, and lymphangioleiomyomatosis.[38–41] Follow-up has shown these lesions to be of low level of aggressivity. Four of the five patients reported by Mark[36] had progressive cysts but only two had symptoms. The oldest patient was followed 28 years; the others had been followed 2 to 4 years. One case, with an 8-cm umbilical nodule, was described in follow-up by Abrams and associates.[38] Although the initial history indicated that the patient had benign uterine pathology and a hysterectomy,[37,38] upon review of this pathology, however, it was noted that there was a low-grade endometrial stromal sarcoma extending into the round ligament, identical to both the umbilical and lung lesions. A similar companion case was presented by Abrams et al. with a 1-cm cystic nodule in the lung. Several other cases of metastatic low-grade microcystic endometrial stromal sarcomas in lung have been reported but have a somewhat different appearance, and the spectrum of uterine stromal sarcomas has been reviewed.[39] The two cases reported by Abrams et al. were both desmin positive. Of interest, the case by Holden et al.[35] has also been referred to as a possible benign fibrohistiocytic tumor and also as a cyst with hamartomatous features. Others that appear similar were described in the pediatric literature as malignant neoplasms arising in a cystic

TABLE 39.3. Clinical and radiographic features of five patients with mesenchymal cystic hamartomas*

Patient	Age	Sex	Signs or symptoms	Duration of symptoms before thoracotomy	Original pathologic diagnosis	Chest radiograph		Follow-up
						Initial	Later	
1	34	F	Hemothorax	A few days	Sequestration	Cyst in left lower lobe; vessels from mediastinum to cyst	Multiple cysts in both lungs and scarring	4 years: dyspnea on moderate exertion: metastatic nodule resected
2	28	M	Hemoptysis	3 years	Bronchogenic cyst	Cyst in right apex	Multiple cysts in both lungs	2 years: mild infrequent hemoptysis
3	42	F	Pneumothorax	A few days	Eosinophilic granuloma	Cyst in right lung and a few small nodules	Persistent nodules in both lungs	2 years: alive and well
4	$1\frac{1}{2}$	M	Dyspnea	A few days	Cystic rhabdomyosarcoma	Cyst in left lower lobe compressing left upper lobe	No disease	4 years: alive and well
5	53	F	None	No symptoms; nodules on x-ray 6 years before thoracotomy	Intrapulmonary mesothelioma	Several nodules in right and left lungs, largest 1.5 cm	Increase in size and number of nodules	28 years: died in automobile accident

Source: Mark.[36]

hamartoma, as rhabdomyosarcoma, or as blastomas of childhood.[35,40–43] One patient of Hedlund et al.[40] with abundant mitoses was alive and free of tumor 12 years after diagnosis. Overall, the prognosis appears to be good in most patients, with only rare deaths secondary to massive hemoptysis. Demographics, symptomatology, radiographic findings, pathologic features, and clinical follow-up of the five cases reported by Mark[36] are summarized in Table 39.3.

Fibrous Histiocytoma

Regarded as the benign counterpart of malignant fibrous histiocytoma, fibrous histiocytoma of the respiratory tract is a rare neoplasm that is histologically characterized by storiform arrangements of spindle-shaped fibrohistiocytic cells. Noncutaneous forms occur in muscle, mesentery, kidney, trachea, and the lung.[44,45] Fibrous histiocytomas in the lung and the tracheobronchial tree overlap with tumors described as "pulmonary fibromas" and an occasional one overlaps with the fibrous histiocytoma variant of inflammatory pseudotumors.[6,46–49] (see Inflammatory Pseudotumor above). Fibrous histiocytomas have been included in the description of several series of fibrous tumors, including 14 cases by Matsubara et al.,[6] three cases by Gal and coworkers,[50] and 2 cases by Sajjad et al.[51] The series of Gal and colleagues included 15 cases of pulmonary inflammatory pseudotumors and 13 cases of tumors previously designated as malignant fibrous histiocytoma, suggesting a spectrum of disease.

Grossly, fibrous histiocytomas are well-outlined parenchymal masses with a white yellowish color (Fig. 39.9). Some lesions may be endobronchial and may result in occlusion of the airway, particularly in children.[48] Fibrous histiocytomas may also occur in the trachea, and seven of nine reported cases in this location were benign.[47,48] Most occurred in young women and were polypoid in configuration. Most fibrous histiocytomas of the trachea occupy the upper third for reasons that are unknown. One tracheal case reported in a postradiation-treated patient was

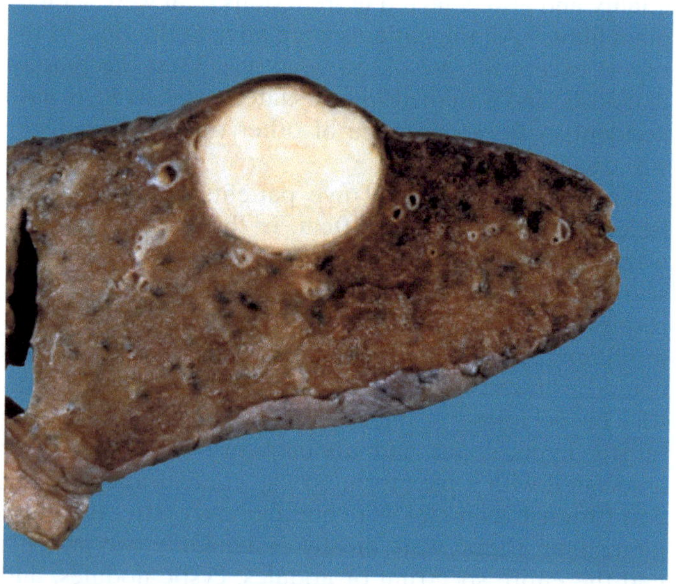

FIGURE 39.9. Fibrous histiocytoma of lung, gross appearance. Note round well-demarcated intraparenchymal mass. The mass is firm white with a faint yellow hue. (Courtesy of Dr. Eugene J. Mark.)

of higher grade.[52] Microscopically, these lesions include a histologic spectrum of tumors similar to fibrous histiocytomas in other organs or tissues, with storiform arrangement of spindle cells and showing varying degrees of cellularity or fibrosis. The spindle tumor cells are generally bland-looking with vesicular nuclei and eosinophilic cytoplasm. In other areas, histiocytic cells with small nuclei and abundant foamy cytoplasm predominate (Figs. 39.10 and 39.11). Desmin, S-100 protein, and epithelial markers such as cytokeratin are usually negative. Sometimes there is confusion between benign and malignant lesions in this category of tumors, but the greatest pitfall is with intermediate forms. Intermediate lesions with increased mitoses may overlap with the lesion described by Tan-Liu and coworkers[53] as invasive fibrous tumors of the tracheobronchial tree.

The differential diagnosis includes solitary fibrous tumors, invasive fibrous tumors of the trachea, inflammatory myofibroblastic tumors, and malignant fibrous histiocytoma, as well as localized areas of reactive fibrohistiocytic proliferations secondary to infectious processes. In contrast to localized fibrous tumors, these lesions are usually CD34 negative and are devoid of the typical patternless microscopic architecture that characterizes such tumors. Invasive fibrous tumors of the respiratory tract as described by Tan-Liu et al.[53] lack histiocytic xanthomatous cells or the intimately admixed inflammatory infiltrate of inflammatory pseudotumors or fibrous histiocytomas. The malignant variants discussed next in this chapter show considerable cellular atypia and mitotic activity and are easy to distinguish, but, as noted earlier, intermediate, diagnostically challenging forms do exist. Infectious processes can be differentiated by virtue of areas of admixed acute and chronic inflammation with or without granulomatous reaction. The clinical setting also aids in making the distinction.

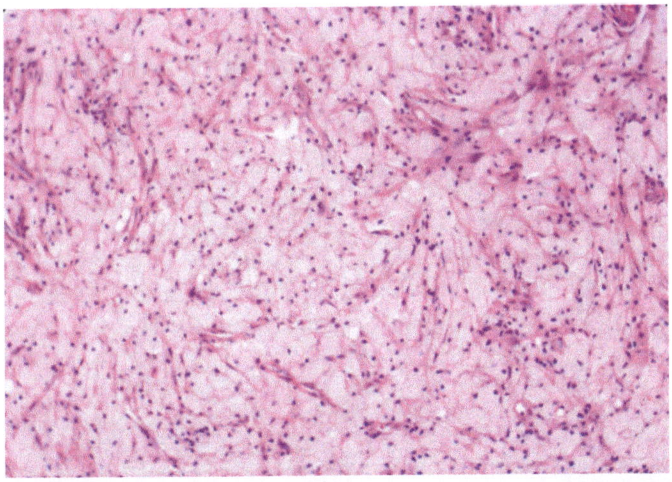

FIGURE 39.10. Fibrous histiocytoma, low-power view. Note predominance of uniform looking pale histiocytes with small nuclei and criss-crossing fibrous bands.

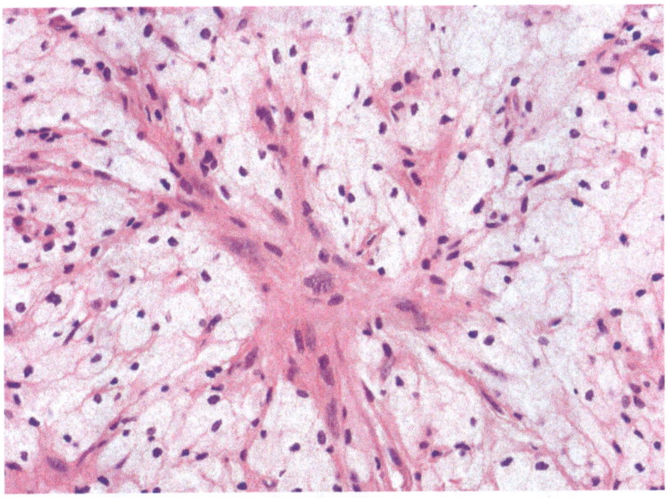

FIGURE 39.11. Fibrous histiocytoma, closer view. Note central stellate fibrous component and bland-looking histiocytes with foamy cytoplasm and small nuclei.

Malignant Fibrous Histiocytoma (Undifferentiated Sarcoma)

Currently regarded as an undifferentiated sarcoma,[54] MFH is characterized histologically by heterogeneous cell populations that include histiocytes, fibroblasts, pleomorphic giant cells, and undifferentiated mesenchymal cells.[55] Synonyms used in the past for these tumors include fibroxanthosarcoma and malignant fibrous xanthoma. More recently these tumors have been classified by the WHO as pleomorphic MFH or undifferentiated high-grade pleomorphic sarcoma.[54] While common in the soft tissues of the retroperitoneum, trunk, and extremities, these aggressive tumors are distinctly uncommon in the lung.[55] Malignant fibrous histiocytomas often present in the sixth or seventh decade of life and show no sex predilection. About one third of patients have cough, chest pain, hemoptysis, or weight loss. The other two thirds are said to be asymptomatic.[55] Chest radiographs may disclose single or multiple nodular masses. Grossly, these tumors tend to be large with reported sizes of up to 6 to 7 cm.[56] Some, however, can be considerably larger and become confluent. On cut surface, they are lobular, tan to white, and may have some cavitated areas (Fig. 39.12).

Microscopically, MFHs show varying degrees of spindled and storiform patterns, with pleomorphic sometimes bizarre multinucleate giant cells (Fig. 39.13). Necrosis is frequent, and lymphocytes may be found scattered among

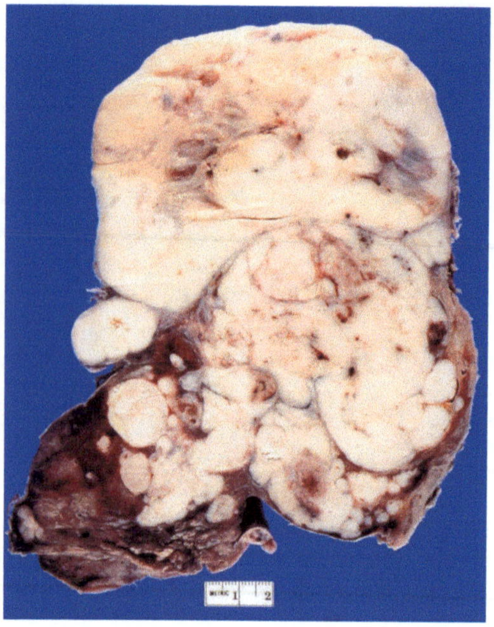

FIGURE 39.12. Malignant fibrous histiocytoma. Note multiple large parenchymal and hilar tumor nodules.

tumor cells. Some cases have myxoid areas, and in at least one case myxoid areas were dominant.[57] Mitoses are usually numerous, easily identified, and often atypical, probably relating to the highly aggressive nature of these tumors. In general, these tumors in the lung conform to their diagnostic patterns in soft tissue, and variant patterns are being described in a similar fashion as those in the soft tissues.[58–60] As always, one must exclude a source from outside the lungs, of which sarcomatoid renal cell carcinoma is particularly relevant, having an undifferentiated sarcoma pattern noted in 26 of 42 (62%) cases of primary sarcomatoid renal cell carcinoma in one series.[61] Some cases of spindle cell squamous carcinoma have been confused with these tumors in the lung. In fact, among 14 patients with sarcomatoid carcinomas of the lung, Ro et al.[61,62] reported an MFH pattern in nine (64%) of these tumors.

Immunohistochemistry may assist in differentiating MFH from other primary or secondary spindle cell tumors of the lung, including spindle cell carcinomas, carcinosarcomas, and sarcomatoid mesotheliomas as well as other types of sarcomas.[63] Often MFHs are immunopositive for vimentin, α_1-antitrypsin, α_1-antichymotrypsin, lysozyme, and CD68. Of these markers, CD68 appears to be the most valuable, but caution is needed since the expression of CD68 can be seen in a variety of nonhistiocytic tumors. Caution is further needed when considering these so-called histiocytic markers as proof of a histiocytic lineage.[64] In fact, some experts now suggest that MFH lacks a definable line of differentiation, supporting the concept that these tumors represent examples of undifferentiated sarcomas.[64] In general, MFHs can be expected to be immunonegative for cytokeratin, epithelial membrane antigen, desmin, S-100 protein, and muscle-specific actin, but occasional cases may be focally positive for these antigens, particularly actin.[63] By electron microscopy, these tumors show “histiocytic features” with cells containing lysosomes and fat droplets, and other cells with more fibroblastic and myofibroblastic differentiation. These tumors, however, should not have tonofilaments, well-formed desmosomes, intracellular lumina, secretory vacuoles, or basal lamina, as these would be indicators of poorly differentiated carcinomas or poorly differentiated tumors of other types.[65,66]

Diagnostic criteria include (1) demonstration of storiform, pleomorphic, or fascicular growth patterns; (2) predominantly spindle cell proliferation; (3) variable number of large cells resembling histiocytes, usually accompanied by pleomorphic multinucleated giant cells; (4) absence of morphologic features of other sarcomatous differentiation; (5) absence of features to suggest anaplastic carcinoma; and (6) exclusion, as best as possible, of potential sources of metastasis from other locations. In addition to metastatic sarcomas and spindle squamous cell carcinomas, these tumors need to be distinguished from inflammatory myofibroblastic tumors. Inflammatory myofibroblastic tumors usually lack frankly malignant features and abnormal mitoses. The prognosis is generally poor, although 5- to 10-year survival rates have been reported by Yousem and Hochholzer[65] and Lee and associates.[66] It is generally agreed that adjunctive chemotherapy and irradiation are ineffective in controlling growth of these tumors. Aggressive surgery remains the mainstay of treatment.[67]

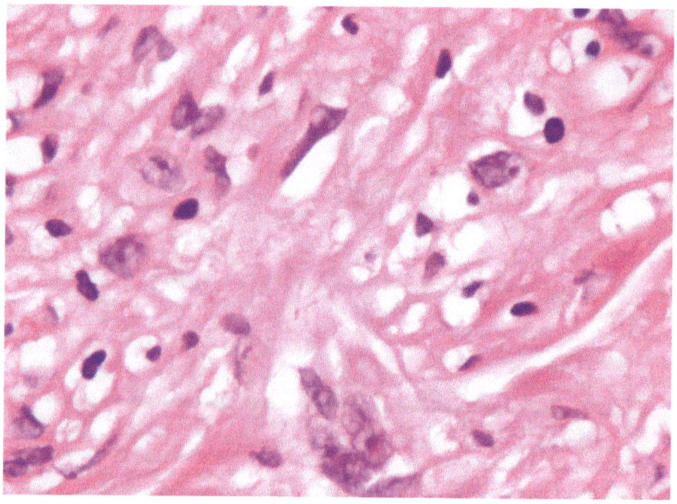

FIGURE 39.13. Malignant fibrous histiocytoma. Note atypical bizarre, and sometimes multinucleated histiocytoid cells.

Fibrosarcoma

This exceedingly rare malignant tumor of the lung occurs in the large airways of younger individuals but tends to localize in the parenchyma in older individuals. It is difficult to estimate the true frequency of fibrosarcomas since composite sarcomas and carcinosarcomas may initially present as monophasic malignancies. We have seen an 11.0-cm tumor thought to be a fibrosarcoma of lung that on further sectioning showed a transition to squamous cell carcinoma. Other tumors believed to be fibrosarcoma may actually represent sarcomatoid carcinoma. With these caveats in mind, bona fide fibrosarcomas of lung do occur and in some series are said to represent about 20% of all primary pulmonary sarcomas.[68]

Endobronchial fibrosarcomas arise from larger bronchi and may be visible on bronchoscopic examination. Parenchymal fibrosarcomas, on the other hand, do not significantly differ from other pulmonary sarcomas and present as well-defined masses made of fleshy grayish white tissue (Fig. 39.14). The microscopic hallmark of these tumors is a proliferation of fibroblastic spindle cells without any evidence of specialized cellular differentiation.[69] The spindle cells arrange themselves in broad fascicles and lie in a background of collagenized stroma (Fig. 39.15). In areas, a herringbone type of pattern can be discerned. As in other sarcomas, increased cellularity, necrosis, and unusual mitotic activity can be seen. Mitotic counts vary from three or less per 10 HPFs to 8 to 40 per 10 HPFs.[70] Reticulum stains show a fine network of fibers around individual tumor cells. The tumor cells are vimentin positive and cytokeratin negative.[70] Immunostains for desmin, actin, S-100 protein, and other myogenous and neural markers are negative.[71–73] The main differential diagnosis is with metastatic sarcomas, particularly monophasic synovial sarcomas and other spindle cell sarcomas such as leiomyosarcomas and neurofibrosarcomas. Cytokeratin positivity is useful in distinguishing synovial sarcomas. Immunostains for smooth muscle actin and S-100 protein can assist with the distinction from leiomyosarcomas and neurofibrosarcomas. Fine-needle aspiration cytology and core biopsy of discrete pulmonary masses are said to be reliable methods to establish the diagnosis.[73]

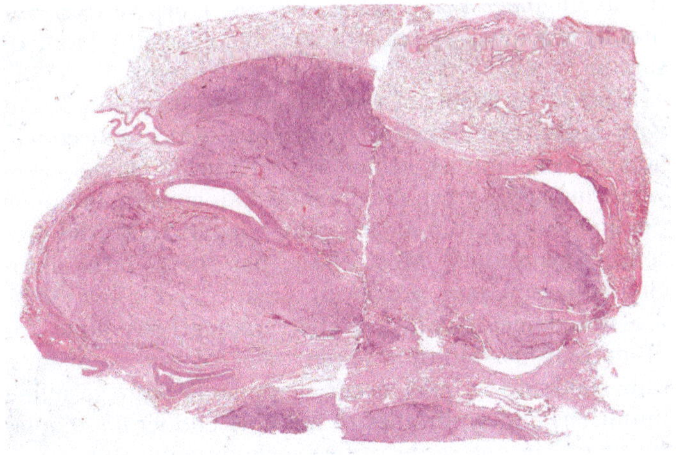

Figure 39.14. Fibrosarcoma, subgross mount. Note nodular mass encasing large vein, left midfield. (Courtesy of Dr. Eugene J. Mark.)

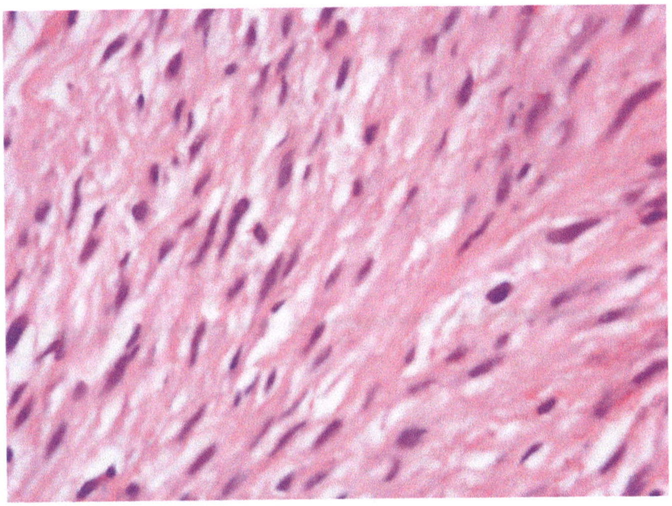

Figure 39.15. Fibrosarcoma. Cellular area showing streams of elongated hyperchromic cells. An extensive panel of immunostains showed immunoreactivity to vimentin only.

The prognosis is poor, with high-mortality rates and low long-term survivals. Surgery is said to be the treatment of choice, but chemotherapy and radiotherapy can be used for nonresectable cases.[70] Recurrences have been reported as early as 15 months following resection.[68]

Tumors of Muscle Origin

This section discusses tumors and tumor-like proliferations considered to be of smooth or striated muscle derivation. The former include microscopic nodular smooth muscle proliferations, solitary leiomyomas, benign metastasizing leiomyomas, leiomyosarcomas, lymphangioleiomyomatosis, and glomus tumors. The latter encompass rhabdomyomas, rhabdomyomatous dysplasia, and rhabdomyosarcomas. Tumors and tumor-like proliferations of striated muscle derivation are more common in children and are discussed at greater length in Chapter 42.

Nodular Smooth Muscle Proliferation and Leiomyoma

Nodular microscopic smooth muscle proliferations of benign nature that are predominantly made up of native smooth muscle fibers are occasionally found in lungs of

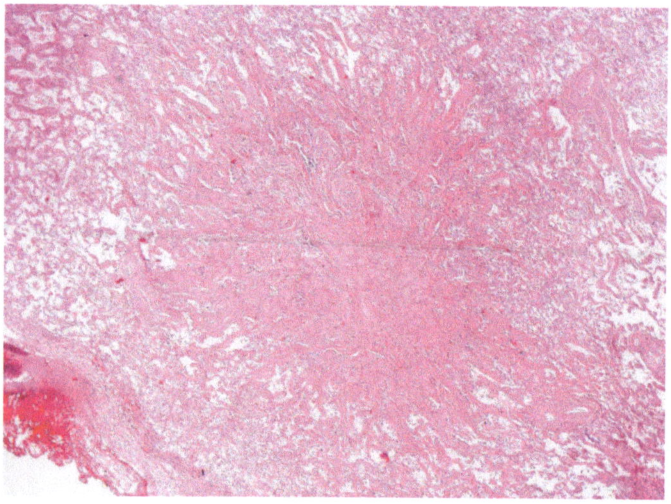

FIGURE 39.16. Smooth muscle proliferation, nodular type.

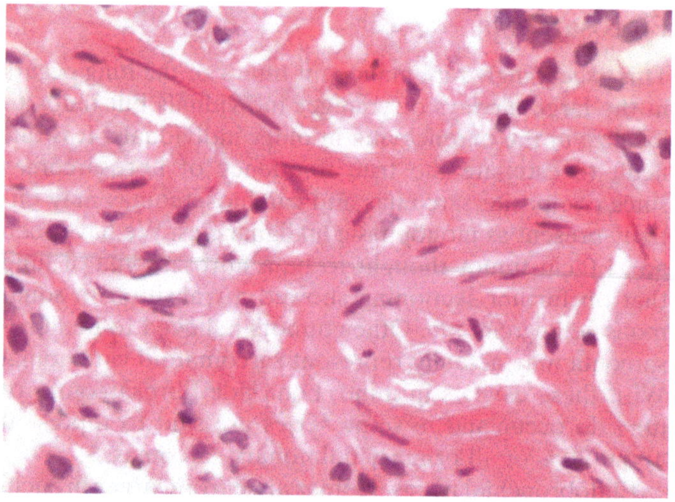

FIGURE 39.18. Smooth muscle proliferation, diffuse type, usually seen in the setting of (advanced) interstitial lung disease.

patients with congestive heart failure. These proliferations differ from hamartomas that usually do not contain significant amounts of smooth muscle and from leiomyomas primarily because of their size. These proliferations, illustrated in Figures 39.16 and 39.17, may be found around centrilobular bronchioles and may represent a localized form of reactive hyperplasia of smooth muscle.[74–76] These proliferations differ from the more diffuse smooth muscle hyperplasia that is seen in lungs affected with diffuse interstitial pulmonary fibrosis (Fig. 39.18), primarily on account of their localized nature and their lack of association with honeycombing. We have also seen localized proliferation of smooth muscle in association with lymphoid aggregates and sometimes in areas of lung that are entirely normal.[74–76] Their significance is minimal except as having a possible confounding role in the diagnosis of hamartomas, small leiomyomas, and the so-called minute meningothelial-like bodies (see Chapter 41).

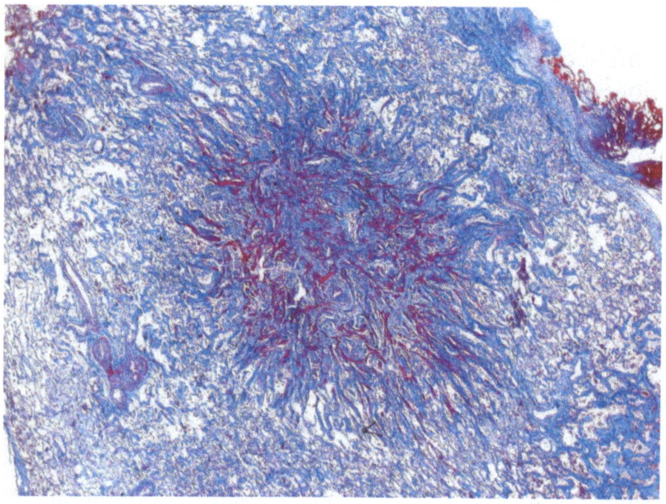

FIGURE 39.17. Same nodule of smooth muscle proliferation as in Figure 39.16. Trichrome stain.

Leiomyomas are benign tumors made up of smooth muscle cells. While common in the uterus, esophagus, and other sites, they are quite rare in the respiratory tract, accounting for less than 2% of benign pulmonary tumors.[77–80] They occur in the tracheobronchial tree and in the lung itself. Several reviews of solitary leiomyomas are available.[78,79] Most authors caution that some of the parenchymal smooth muscle nodules in women may represent benign metastasizing leiomyomas, as discussed in the following section, and some have suggested that women being considered for this diagnosis have their uteri carefully examined.[79] Solitary low-grade smooth muscle metastases are difficult to distinguish from primary leiomyomas. One third of all patients with bronchial or parenchymal leiomyomas are less than 20 years old, with the average age being in the mid-30s. Tracheal leiomyomas have a mean age of 40 years, in contrast to leiomyosarcomas, which have a mean age of 50 years.[78]

Most leiomyomas of the trachea and bronchi present with irritative and obstructive symptoms including cough, hemoptysis, and shortness of breath. In some cases wheezing is the presenting manifestation, while in others pneumothorax from air trapping appears to be the presenting symptom.[77] Most of the peripheral intraparenchymal leiomyomas are asymptomatic, and in over 90% are noted incidentally on chest radiographs done for other reasons. Multiple leiomyomas of the esophagus, lung, and uterus may occur in patients with germline mutations and syndromes of multiple endocrine neoplasia type I. In one series of five such patients, all patients were females and had varying combinations of these tumors. Germline mutations were detected in tumors from all five women.[81]

Grossly, leiomyomas of the trachea and main bronchi present as broad-based polypoid growths. They range from 1.0 to 2.5 cm while their malignant counterparts are larger, measuring from 2.0 to 8.0 cm. Larger lesions may mechanically obstruct the airways. Parenchymal lesions may have a fibrous whorled appearance resembling uterine leiomyomas, and others may be soft and fleshy. Microscopically these tumors are made up of intersecting bundles of spindle-shaped cells with eosinophilic fibrillary cytoplasm and elongated cigar-shaped nuclei with blunted ends similar to those seen in leiomyomas elsewhere (Figs. 39.19 and 39.20). Mitotic figures are rarely seen and when present are not numerous. Tumor necrosis is usually not found, and when present should raise the question of a low-grade sarcoma. Trichrome stain highlights smooth muscle cells in red brown color and renders blue the background collagenous matrix. Leiomyomas are smooth muscle actin, desmin, caldesmon, and calponin positive. Immunostains for cytokeratin and S-100 protein are negative.[80,82,83] Chromosomal analysis of leiomyomas of soft tissue in a substantial number of cases has failed to show karyotypic aberrations, but 25% of them have shown evidence of balanced translocations.[84]

Distinguishing leiomyomas from fibromas, neurofibromas, or neurilemomas by light microscopy alone is sometimes challenging. However, immunoperoxidase stains with discriminating antigens are most helpful. In particular, smooth muscle actin and desmin along with S-100 protein can assist in the differential diagnosis. Electron microscopy also is of assistance in difficult cases. As reported by Cramer et al.[85] and Silverman and Kay,[86] typical leiomyomas show basal lamina, plasmalemmal hemidesmosomes, pinocytotic vesicles, and thin cytoplasmic filaments. The prognosis of solitary leiomyomas is favorable. Sleeve resection of tumors in main stem bronchi has been reported.[87] Complete surgical excision is regarded as curative.

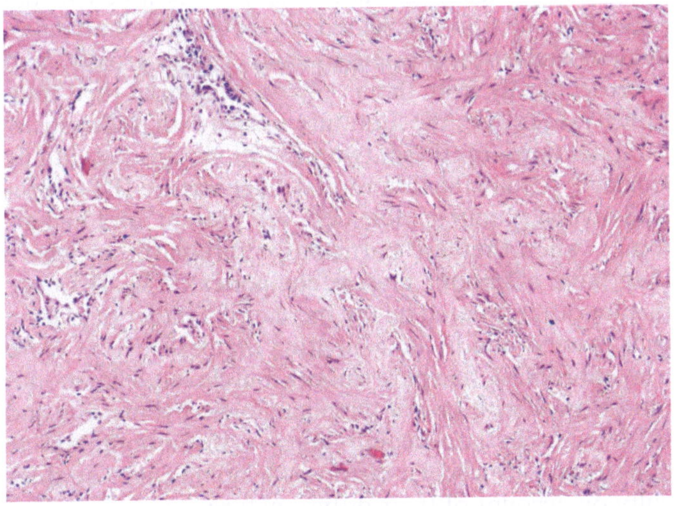

Figure 39.19. Leiomyoma, low-power view showing a spindle cell proliferation with a collagenized stroma.

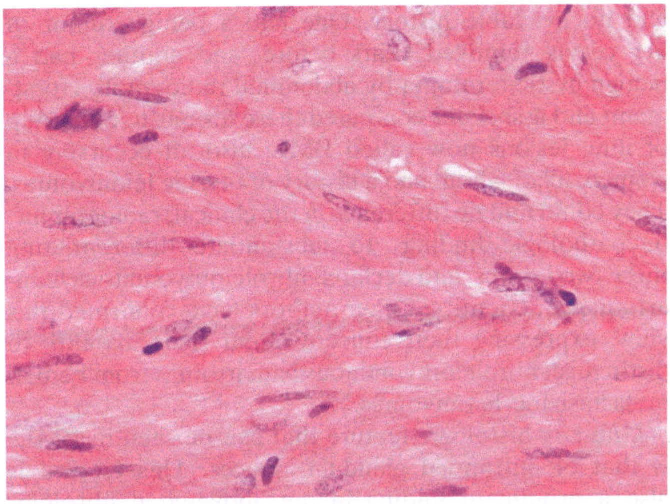

Figure 39.20. Leiomyoma, very hypocellular area with cells showing few cigar-shaped nuclei with blunted ends.

Benign Metastasizing Leiomyoma

Benign metastasizing leiomyoma (BML) is a term that has been used for distinctive multiple nodules of mature-looking, well-differentiated smooth muscle tissue occurring in the lung, usually in women, many of whom have a history of previous or concomitant leiomyomas in the uterus.[88] Benign metastasizing leiomyomas fundamentally differ from solitary leiomyomas only in regard to their multiplicity and show considerable overlap with another entity characterized by smooth muscle proliferation in the abdominal cavity, known as disseminated peritoneal leiomyomatosis (DPL).[89] DPL, also known as *leiomyomatosis peritonealis disseminata*, is a rare, benign condition in which typical uterine leiomyomas are associated with multiple small nodules of smooth muscle distributed throughout the omentum and (both visceral and parietal layers of) the peritonenum.[89] The simultaneous occurrence of BML and DPL has been recorded, and both conditions respond to hormone ablative therapy, suggesting a shared pathogenetic mechanism[84,89] (see below).

In the past, there has been much confusion between BML and another smooth muscle proliferation disorder known as fibroleiomyomatous hamartoma. Up to 1977, 14 cases of these fibroleiomyomatous hamartomas had been reported in the literature.[90] In the cases described by Horstmann et al.,[90] the patients were all women aged 30 to 74 years with a mean of 47 years. The women were usually asymptomatic and had bilateral lung nodules. Eight of these women had histories of myomectomies or hysterectomies for leiomyomata, and four had no available history. One had a benign tumor of her cervix removed years before, and another had a benign cystic teratoma by abdominal radiograph. Horstmann and associates compared these lesions to the group of lung lesions now called BML, also all occurring in women, all of whom had a history of uterine leiomyomas. They could find no difference in the clinical, radiographic, or pathologic findings to substantiate differentiating these two lesions, and declared fibroleiomyomatous hamartomas a nonentity. Other authors have confirmed this view, expressing their concern about their inability to distinguish fibroleiomyomatous hamartomas from benign metastasizing leiomyomas.[91,92]

One key histologic feature that can be seen in BMLs is that of entrapped glandular spaces. This feature is also a prominent finding in the above-cited fibroleiomyomatous hamartoma.[91] Glandular spaces, however, are not exclusively seen in these lesions. Some leiomyomas may become so hyalinized as to make their cell or origin difficult to determine, yet still show air-space entrapment. Metaplastic alveolar lining and entrapped bronchiolar space lining cells are also common in slowly growing lesions, and represent a background response and not an inherent component of the tumor. Such entrapped alveolar and bronchiolar epithelial elements can also be seen in hamartomas and sclerosing hemangiomas as well as inflammatory pseudotumors and benign clear cell (sugar) tumors of the lung. On careful serial section examinations, these entrapped glandular structures have been shown to be continuous with the lining of nearby air spaces.[93] Herrera et al.[94] studied these spaces by electron microscopy in a case of metastasizing smooth muscle tumor of lung that occurred 31 years after the patient had a hysterectomy for low-grade leiomyosarcoma. These authors found ultrastructural characteristics of entrapped alveoli and bronchiolar mucosa.

Wolff and associates[95] in 1979 further expanded the concept of metastasizing low-grade smooth muscle nodules in the lung in a report of six women and three men. They required the nodules of smooth muscle in the lung to have entrapped glandular spaces as described above. In five of the six women, uterine leiomyomas were identified, and for the other woman there was no available history. Of the three men, leiomyosarcomas were respectively documented in the saphenous vein, diaphragm, and probably the gluteal region. Wolff et al. carefully quantitated mitoses, both in the metastatic lesions and in the primary sites when tissue from primary lesions was available, using the mitotic counting methods of Kempson[96] and Norris.[97] Although mitoses were infrequent in the smooth muscle lesions of the lung, they could always identify them. The mitotic rate in the primary lesions varies, but many qualified as benign smooth muscle proliferations by standard criteria.[95]

Summarizing 21 cases from the A.A. Liebow Pulmonary Pathology Collection, Tench and coworkers[98] identified all patients as women aged 31 to 65 years, all with a history of hysterectomy 3 to 20 years (mean, 10 years) previously. In 18 of the 21 cases, benign leiomyomas were described in the uteri, but histologic slides of the uterine lesions were too infrequent for meaningful evaluation. From background material in this study, all but one had multiple bilateral nodules on chest radiographs; the other had a perihilar mass. Three of these patients had lung nodules detected 16, 19, and 20 years, respectively, after their hysterectomies.[99] These patients usually had lung nodules radiographically and pathologically that measured 0.3 to 4.0cm in greatest dimension and were enucleated easily from the lung tissue. Ninety-four percent of these cases histologically showed entrapment of metaplastic glandular lining cells.[99]

Clinically, most if not all cases are asymptomatic, but exceptions do occur. Two interesting cases exemplify the sometimes very long clinical evolution of these tumors. One case reported by Popock et al.[100] described a woman who at age 41 had her uterus removed for three large leiomyomas that had been present for nearly 15 years. She died 21 years later (36 years after the initial detection of a large uterus) of hemorrhagic pancreatitis. She had multiple lung nodules measuring up to 2.0cm at the time of hysterectomy, which had grown to 5cm at the time of autopsy and had become predominantly cystic. The other case described by Uyama and associates[91] had lung lesions noted on the chest radiograph, gradually increasing in size over a 20-year period. (See Chapter 44, Fig. 44.5).

These tumors are made up of fusiform cells with fibrillary eosinophilic cytoplasm and blunt-ended nuclei showing dispersed chromatin. Mitoses and necrosis are not seen, but areas of fibrosis with or without entrapped alveolar or bronchiolar epithelial elements are evident in some cases (Figs. 39.21 and 39.22).[101] As noted in the preceding section dedicated to solitary leiomyomas, benign metastasizing leiomyomas differ grossly and microscopically from them only on account of their multiplicity. Likewise, the literature indicates that ultrastructural features of these two conditions are essentially similar.[86] Also in the differential diagnosis are IPTs, especially when plump spindle cells are present, and hamartomas, when they are particularly fibroblastic or where they have a smooth muscle component. The IPTs are further differentiated by the increased number of plasma cells present and by documenting the basic cell as more a myofibroblast than pure smooth muscle cell. The smooth muscle proliferations of lymphangioleiomyomatosis and those seen in honeycomb lungs with smooth muscle hyperplasia ("muscular cirrhosis") should cause no difficulty on account of their diffuse nature.

Are these lesions in the lung benign or malignant? Only since the 1970s have pathologists begun to reliably

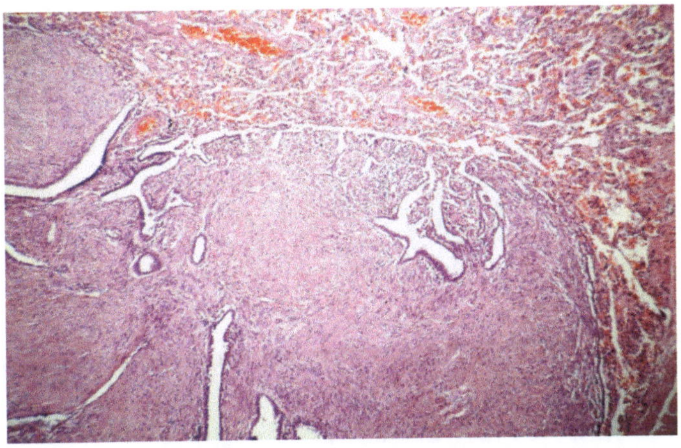

FIGURE 39.21. Benign metastasizing leiomyoma. One of multiple discrete nodules of smooth muscle in lung parenchyma. Note epithelial-lined clefts. (Courtesy of Dr. Joseph F. Tomashefski, Jr., MetroHealth Medical Center, Cleveland, OH.) (See also Chapter 44, Figs. 44.19A,B).

use mitotic counting methods to determine low-grade or high-grade activity in uterine smooth muscle tumors. Even as done by both Wolff and associates[95] and Gal and coworkers,[80] many were benign or low grade by this method. One must then question whether sampling was adequate, whether the lesions became less mitotically active after an initial growth phase with metastases, or perhaps whether fragments of smooth muscle can embolize as such and not truly represent malignancy. In the event of embolization, BML needs to be distinguished from intravenous leiomyomatosis (IL). A rare, peculiar gynecologic condition, IL is characterized by growth of mature smooth muscle in the uterus and within pelvic veins,[102] with the potential to disseminate hematogenously beyond the pelvis. As is the case with BML, IL is associated with uterine leiomyomas and may in fact arise from them. Rosai[102] believes that there may be a histogenetic relationship between IL and endometrial stromal sarcoma. It is also possible that given the shared features of BML and IL (uterine tumors of smooth muscle nature and propensity to disseminate via the bloodstream), there may be a kinship between these two conditions as well. One surgically excised IL with embolization to the right heart, documented by trichrome and smooth muscle actin stains, was presented by Soberanis-Torruco et al.[103] and is shown in Figure 39.23.

Currently, these lesions are regarded as tumoral lesions with a clonal (neoplastic) nature.[84] Using comparative genomic analysis and X-chromosome inactivation studies, Tietze and colleagues[84] determined a monoclonal origin for both uterine and pulmonary tumors occurring in the case of their patient, a 42-year-old woman who had multiple myometrial leiomyomas and who 4 years following hysterectomy had developed numerous smooth muscle nodules in her lungs. This study is significant, as it provides evidence to support the suggestion that such pulmonary nodules in patients with previous uterine leiomyomas are indeed metastatic.

Despite their neoplastic nature, the prognosis of BMLs is favorable. Cases of regression, spontaneous or in response to hormonal manipulation, have been reported. Middle-aged women may experience regression of their tumors with the onset of menopause.[101] The patient reported by Tietze et al.[84] was treated with surgical excision of her lung nodules and with agonists of gonadotropin-releasing hormone with complete tumor regression

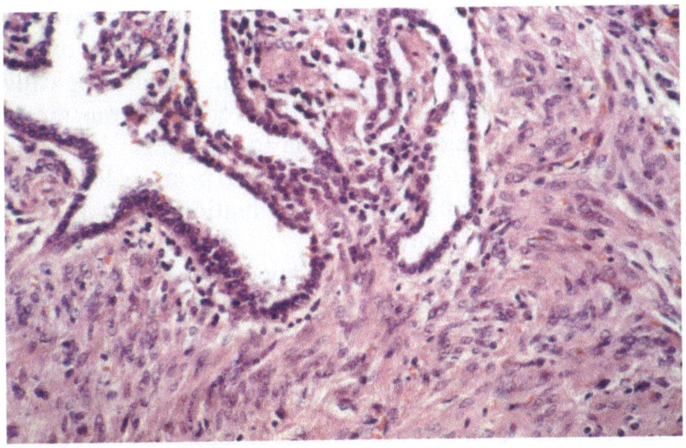

FIGURE 39.22. Benign metastasizing leiomyoma. Closer view of preceding image showing plump spindle-shaped smooth muscle cells and epithelial-lined clefts representing entrapped respiratory epithelium. (Courtesy of Dr. Joseph F. Tomashefski, Jr., MetroHealth Medical Center, Cleveland, OH.)

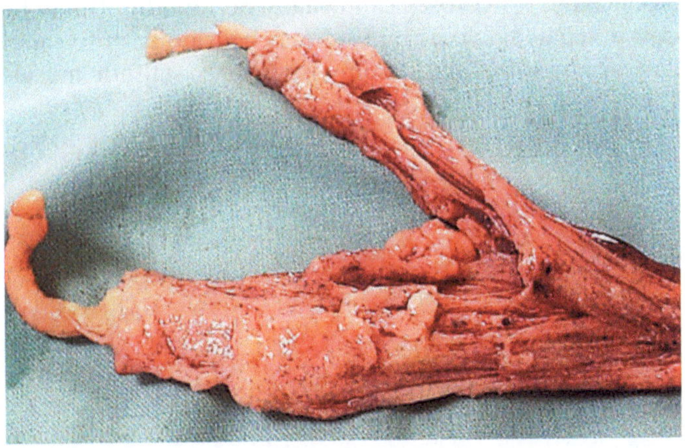

FIGURE 39.23. Benign intravenous leiomyomatosis. This surgically removed specimen shows an elongated branching structure. Microscopically, this lesion was composed of benign, smooth muscle cells positive for smooth muscle actin. (Courtesy of Drs. Carlos N. Soberanis-Torruco and Maria E. Cortes Gutierrez, Hospital Juarez de Mexico, Mexico City. From Soberanis-Torruco et al.,[103] with permission.)

by CT scan of chest and was free of pulmonary recurrences at 24 months postoperatively.

Leiomyosarcoma

Leiomyosarcoma is a malignant tumor composed of cells showing distinct smooth muscle features.[104] Leiomyosarcoma of the lung is quite rare, with fewer than 100 cases reported in the literature.[105] In a review of 80 rare pulmonary neoplasms at the Mayo Clinic by Miller and Allen,[106] only three (4%) were leiomyosarcomas. Most patients are middle-aged to elderly, but some are children.[107] Cases in children are apt to be associated with HIV infection, solid organ transplantation, and certain forms of congenital immune compromise. Almost all extrapulmonary leiomyosarcomas display complex and unbalanced karyotypic aberrations, but genetic data for primary leiomyosarcomas of the lung appear to be nonexistent.[84,108]

Most primary leiomyosarcomas of the lung are round, well-circumscribed intraparenchymal fleshy masses that can be up to 24cm in diameter and may invade the chest wall. Their color varies from gray to white to tan. Necrosis and hemorrhage may be seen grossly in larger tumors. Cystic change may be present, and about one sixth occur as polypoid endobronchial masses frequently showing superficial ulceration and hemorrhage.[104–107] Microscopically, these tumors have the histopathologic features of leiomyosarcomas occurring elsewhere (Fig. 39.24). Intersecting bundles of spindle-shaped cells occasionally arranged in storiform, palisaded, or hemangiopericytoma-like patterns can be seen. Areas of hyalinization, hypocellularity, and coagulative necrosis are frequent in larger tumors. The nuclei are characteristically elongated and blunt-ended. Nuclear hyperchromatism may be pronounced.[104–108] Mitoses can usually be found but may be few and patchy. Some mitoses may be tripolar or tetrapolar. As in soft tissue leiomyosarcomas, smooth muscle actin, smooth muscle myosin, and desmin are positive in pulmonary leiomyosarcomas (Fig. 39.25). However, these are not absolutely specific for smooth muscle, and positivity for all of these markers is more supportive of leiomyosarcoma than positivity for one marker or the other. Dedifferentiated areas may be negative for smooth muscle actin and desmin, but total negativity for both in a tumor would cast doubt on the diagnosis of leiomyosarcoma. Stains that may be positive, at least focally, include cytokeratin, epithelial membrane antigen, CD34, and S-100 protein.[108] Immunohistochemical studies in 16 of 18 cases of primary pulmonary leiomyosarcomas reported by Moran and coworkers[109] indicate that 12 were positive for smooth muscle actin and five were positive for desmin. Coexpression for actin or desmin and cytokeratin was identified in three of the 16 cases, and none was positive for S-100 protein. As in tumors of the soft tissue, diagnosis of leiomyosarcoma should not be made on the basis of immunostains in the absence of appropriate histomorphologic features.[108] Cellular examples of benign metastasizing leiomyoma are histologically (and conceptually) difficult to differentiate from metastatic low-grade leiomyosarcoma to the lungs[110] (and by extension difficult to differentiate from primary lung leiomyosarcoma) requiring careful evaluation of any uterine tumors that may be present.

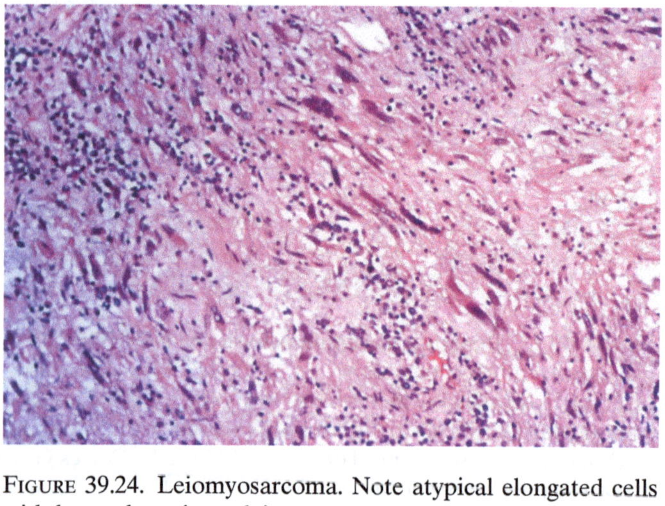

FIGURE 39.24. Leiomyosarcoma. Note atypical elongated cells with hyperchromic nuclei.

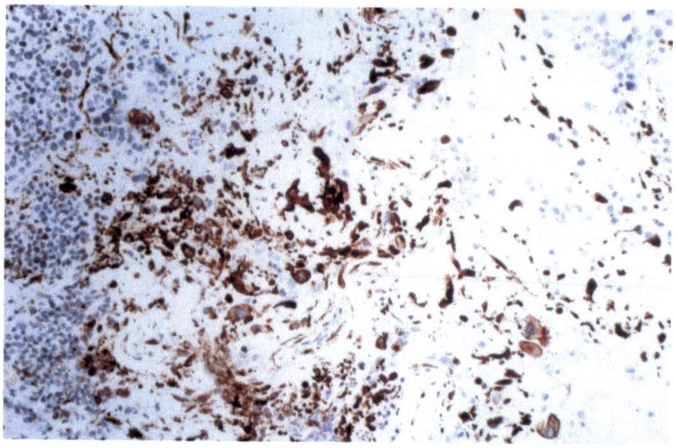

FIGURE 39.25. Leiomyosarcoma. Note strong immunoreactivity of tumor cells to smooth muscle actin.

The degree of aggressiveness appears to depend on the histologic grade of the tumor and particularly the number of mitoses. Gal et al.[80] proposed a minimum of five mitoses per 50HPFs to distinguish leiomyosarcomas from leiomyomas in the lung, but also pointed out that pleomorphism in the absence of increased mitoses was also cause for concern. In their series, leiomyosarcomas were characterized by greater than 22 mitoses per 50HPFs, moderate to high cellularity, moderate to high atypia, necrosis, and hemorrhage. Vascular invasion and epithelioid features were present in one case each.[80,107] As noted earlier, most leiomyosarcomas occur in the middle aged and the elderly, and in these groups survival rates at 5 years range from 50% to 64%. In contrast, leiomyosarcomas in children are usually of low-grade malignancy.[111–114]

Lymphangioleiomyomatosis

Lymphangioleiomyomatosis (LAM) is a rare, peculiar, rather spectacular, and often lethal disease that primarily affects the lungs and the axial thoracoabdominal lymphatic system of women of child-bearing age; its histopathologic hallmark is a widespread interstitial proliferation of immature myoid cells with a striking associated degree of cystic change. While the vast majority of patients with LAM are women, an exceptional well-documented case has been reported in a man.[115] Lymphangioleiomyomatosis is regarded as a neoplasm, although it is not a tumor mass as such. While LAM was originally described as lymphangioleiomyoma in the earlier literature, the reader of earlier articles should not think that LAM represents a tumor mass. It is distinct from pulmonary cystic lymphangiomas such as cystic hygromas that occur in neck and mediastinum, and distinct from lymphangiomatosis, a condition characterized by dilated lymphatic spaces with little or no smooth muscle proliferation of their walls. Lymphangioleiomyomatosis is also to be distinguished from primary lymphangiectasia, which is described in Chapter 40, and from benign metastasizing leiomyoma, which is described earlier in this chapter. There is debate whether LAM is hamartomatous or truly neoplastic. However, evidence pointing to recurrence of the disease in transplanted lungs would support the latter view.[116] The areas involved by LAM are central in the body, namely the mediastinal and periaortic lymph nodes, rarely clavicular and inguinal nodes, the main periaortic lymphatic duct–ductus lymphaticus–thoracic duct, and the lungs, bilaterally. When associated with tuberous sclerosis (see below), other organs such as skin, kidney, and brain may be involved by lesions of nonlymphangioleiomyomatous nature.

Lymphangioleiomyomatosis was first described within the clinical setting of tuberous sclerosis (TS) by Lautenbacher[117] in 1918, and was later reported without the syndrome of TS by two sets of authors in 1937, Burrell and Ross[118] and von Stössel,[119] and was further discussed in 1942 by Rosendal[120] and later by Laipply and Sherrick.[121] These writers better outlined the features of the disease and believed it to be a nonmalignant condition calling it "angiomyomatous hyperplasia" of the lung. In 1966, Cornog and Enterline[122] suggested LAM might be a multiple hamartomatous lesion. The earlier literature is well reviewed by these authors and by Harris et al.[123] Two other important LAM review series are available, one by Corrin et al.[124] published in 1975, noting 34 cases in the literature at that time and adding 23 previously unpublished cases, and the other by Taylor and collaborators[125] in 1990 reviewing 32 cases accumulated from the files at Mayo Clinic and Stanford; both of these series are excellent and warrant careful review by the interested reader. The interested reader may also want to review recent contributions on the pathogenesis of LAM by Kalassian et al.[126] in 1997, Matsui and coworkers[127,128] in 2000, Taveira-DaSilva[129] in 2001, Kumaki et al.[130] in 2002, and Evans et al.[131] and Kumasaka et al.[132] in 2004 (see below).

Tuberous sclerosis, an autosomal dominant disease with variable penetrance affecting 1 in 10,000 people, is associated with LAM in about 1% of patients.[133–135] It is associated with one of two tumor suppressor genes, *TSC1* (chromosome 9q 34) and *TSC2* (chromosome 15p 13.3).[136] Patients with TS may present with a variety of anatomicoclinical manifestations including renal angiomyolipomas, renal cell carcinomas, cutaneous angiofibromas, mental retardation, seizures, cerebral tubers, retinal and cardiac hamartomas, as well as pulmonary changes of LAM. Radiographically and anatomically, LAM seen within the context of TS is identical to sporadic LAM (Figs. 39.26 and 39.27). Pulmonary pathologic changes in TS in addition to LAM are basically limited to those seen in association with multifocal micronodular pneumocyte hyperplasia (MMPH).[135,137]

A peculiar epithelial cell proliferation in the lungs of patients, MMPH distinctively occurs in the lungs of patients with TS but is also known to be present in some cases of sporadic LAM.[133,135,137] The MMPH lesions are characterized by multiple nodular, generally well-demarcated aggregates of bland epithelial cells ranging in size from 1 to 3 mm. These epithelial cells have been identified

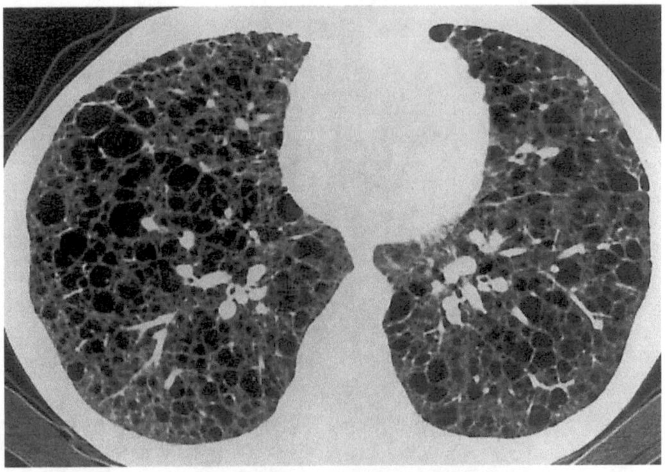

FIGURE 39.26. Lymphangioleiomyomatosis in tuberous sclerosis. High-resolution computed tomography (CT) shows many cysts throughout lungs. (Courtesy of Dr. J.D. Godwin, University of Washington Shool of Medicine, Seattle, WA. From Stern et al.,[140] with permission from the Radiological Society of North America.)

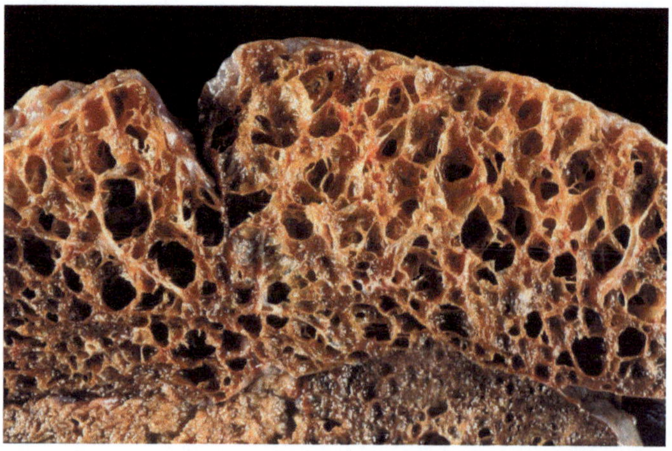

FIGURE 39.27. Lymphangioleiomyomatosis. Gross appearance, note rigid fibrous walls separating cysts of varying sizes. (Courtesy of Dr. Helmut Popper, University of Graz, Austria.)

as type II pneumocytes (Fig. 39.28) and are immunoreactive for cytokeratin, epithelial membrane antigen, and surfactant apoprotein but negative for HMB-45, hormone receptors, and smooth muscle markers.[133,135,137] This condition is regarded as an innocuous hamartomatous proliferation as documented in a series of 14 patients with MMPH in which no deaths occurred that were attributable to the condition.[135]

As noted above, lung changes in cases of TS with lung disease are identical to those seen in sporadic LAM, and LAM has been considered a *forme fruste* of TS.[138–146] In fact, there are multiple cases that show clinical and anatomicopathologic overlap between TS and LAM (Table 39.4). Cases with tuberous sclerosis with lung disease are predominantly seen in women of reproductive age. Authors arguing that this is a separate disease note that TS cases have less nodal involvement and less chylous

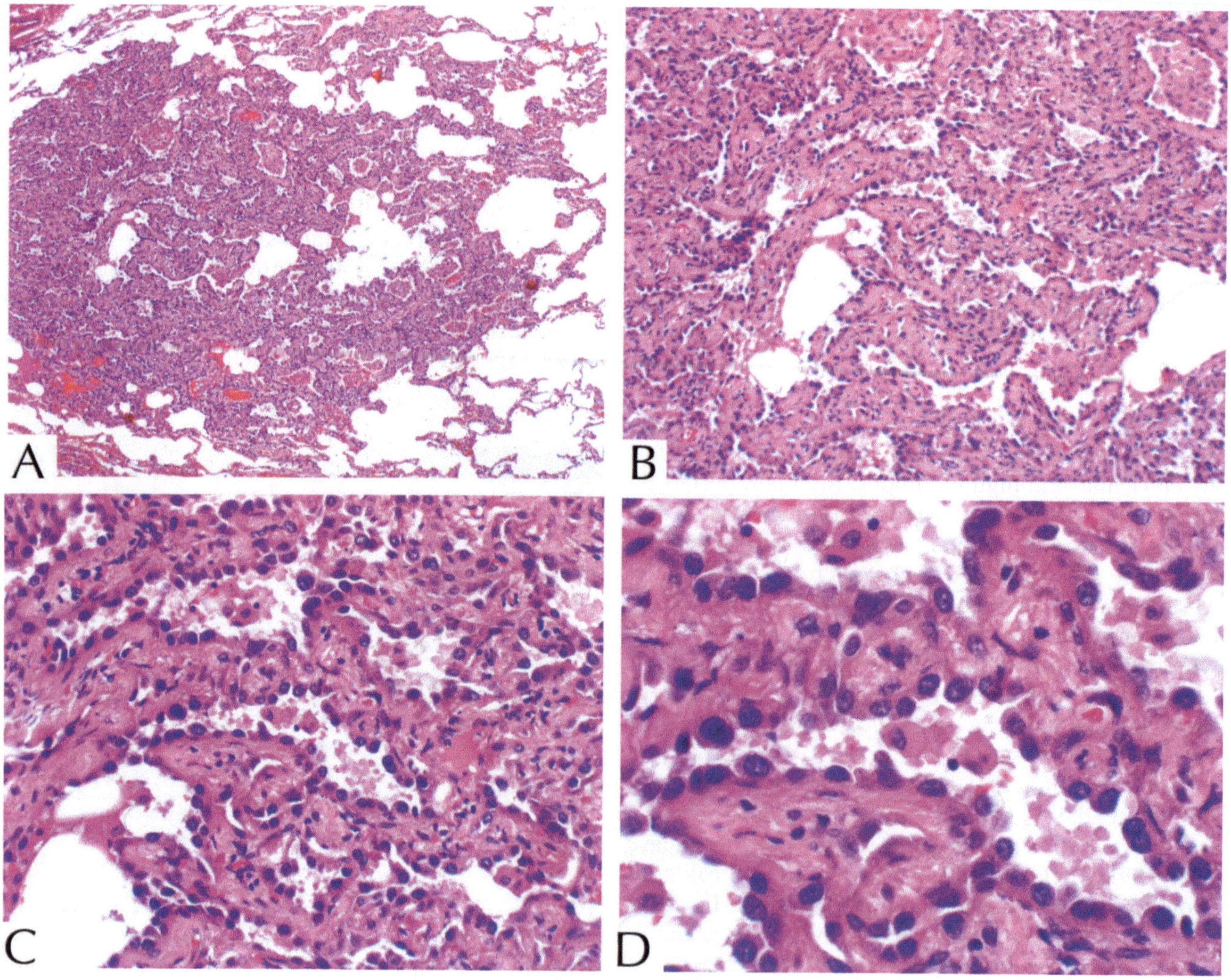

FIGURE 39.28. Multifocal micronodular pneumocyte hyperplasia. **(A)** Low-power view of well-defined nodular aggregate of epithelial cells. **(B–D)** On increasing magnification the cells, particularly those lining cleft like spaces correspond to type II pneumocytes. (Courtesy of Dr. Thomas V. Colby, Mayo Clinic, Scottsdale, AZ.)

TABLE 39.4. Comparative analysis of clinical and demographic data for tuberous sclerosis, tuberous sclerosis with lung disease, and lymphangioleiomyomatosis

Parameter	TS	TS with lung disease	LAM
Age	<20	21–50	18–61
Sex	Male and female	Female only	Female only*
Family history	50%	20–25%	–
Nodes involved	0	19%	67%
Chylothorax	0	6%	67–74%
Pneumothorax	0	3–50%	30–43%
Mental retardation	46–90%+	20–45%	0
Seizures	70–93%	20–62%	0
Brain plaques	Many	55%	0
Skin lesions	60–90%	84–90%	0
Renal angiomyolipomas	40–80%	73–77%	15%
Complete triad	28% to many	19–52%	0

*One case reported in a man since this table was put together, see text.
TS, tuberous sclerosis; LAM, lymphangioleiomyomatosis.

pleural effusion than those that occur in typical LAM. One might wonder whether the diseases are detected earlier because these patients generally are under closer medical observation, but in the review of Silverstein et al.[147] their average age at diagnosis was 33 years, identical to those in the large series of sporadic LAM by Taylor et al.[125] This remains unexplained, but the pathology is identical and, with the exception of the degree of nodal involvement and pleural effusion, they appear very much alike.

In those cases with TS and lung involvement, it is interesting that the patients are older than the others, who, when they have the full-blown spectrum of TS, often die by the age of 20 years. Also, the general group of TS has equal sex incidence and is diagnosed at an earlier age. The incidence of those with TS having lung disease is generally quoted as 0.1% to 1.0%,[148] and in a study of 355 patients at Mayo Clinic followed with TS, 49 have died, 40 from the effects of tuberous sclerosis, of whom four died of the effects of LAM out of 10 (3%) of the total group who had this disease.[149] More frequently death results from renal disease from angiomyolipomas or cysts, or brain disease from involvement with tubers or seizures. In only one instance, of four generations involved with TS, were a mother and a daughter both afflicted with lung disease—LAM.[148] Rarely, LAM is associated with multiple other non–TS-associated types of abnormalities,[149] and in two cases there have been hyperplastic parathyroid tissue,[149,150] in another there were noncaseating granulomas,[151] and a unique case had hemopericardium.[152] These are all probably within the background spectrum of disease unrelated to LAM. Of course, overlap is more frequently seen with those entities that are a part of the TS complex.

Lymphangioleiomyomatosis is currently regarded by the WHO as a member of the broad family of tumors known as PEComas, derived from perivascular epithelioid cells (PECs).[153] The PEC cells are distinctive perivascular cells with myoid features characterized immunohistochemically for positivity for HMB-45, Melan-A, and the microphthalmia transcription factor.[153] Other immunostains positive in PEC cells are tyrosinase, smooth muscle actin, muscle myosin, and calponin.[153] Members of the PEComa family other than LAM include renal angiomyolipomas, clear cell "sugar" tumors of the lung, and clear cell myomelanocytic tumors of the falciform ligament/ligamentum teres, among others.[153]

The pathogenesis and molecular biology of LAM remain poorly understood. However, recent studies looking at the role of matrix metalloproteinases (MMPs), telomerase, vascular growth factors, and transforming growth factor-β1 (TGF-β1) have shed some light on some pathogenetic mechanisms leading to the formation of the complex mix of proliferative and destructive lung lesions that are so characteristic of LAM.[127,130–132] The nodular lesions of LAM made up of small spindly cells with properties of smooth muscle cells are regarded as proliferative lesions, while the cystic lesions that predominate in later stages of the disease are regarded as destructive lesions.[127,130–132] Matrix metalloproteinases have been shown to play a role in the development of destructive pulmonary lesions in LAM.[128] One study aiming to evaluate the role of activated MMPs in LAM used enzyme activation techniques, immunohistochemistry, and confocal microscopy to localize α-smooth muscle actin, proliferating cell nuclear antigen, HMB-45 antigen, and membrane type 1 MMP (MT1-MMP), MT2-MMP, and MT3-MMP in lung tissues from 10 women with LAM.[128] The study demonstrated an association between cellular proliferation and the presence of MMP-1 in LAM cells while suggesting a possible role of MMP-2 and MMP-1 in the destruction of lung tissue in this disorder.[128]

Telomerase synthesizes nucleotide hexameric repeats (telomeres) at the ends of chromosomes, replacing base sequences that are lost from these sites during each mitotic cycle and protecting these cells against the action of exonucleases and ligases. Therefore, telomerase is essential for maintaining cellular replication.[130] To evaluate the role of telomerase in the proliferation of smooth muscle cells in LAM, Kumaki et al.[130] performed immunostaining and in-situ hybridization studies to identify telomerase protein and messenger RNA (mRNA) in pulmonary and extrapulmonary lesions of 22 women with LAM. Immunoreactivity and hybridization signals for telomerase were found in 5% to 20% of LAM cells, suggesting that telomerase-positive cells may constitute the source of renewal of smooth muscle cells in LAM.[130] In

TABLE 39.5. Clinical and radiographic findings in 32 women with lymphangioleiomyomatosis

	Number of women (%)	
	At onset	During course
Symptoms		
Dyspnea		
Resting	0	13 (41)
Exertional	15 (47)	30 (94)
Cough	4 (12)	13 (41)
Chest pain	4 (12)	11 (34)
Chyloptysis	0	1 (3)
Hemoptysis	3 (9)	14 (44)
Findings		
Pneumothorax	17 (53)	26 (81)
Chylothorax	0	9 (28)
Wheezing	0	3 (10)
Chylous ascites	1 (3)	2 (6)
Chest radiography		
Normal	1 (3)	0
Reticulonodular change	15 (47)	30 (94)
Cysts or bullae	4 (12)	13 (41)
Effusion	0	9 (29)
Pneumothorax	17 (53)	26 (81)
Hyperinflation	0	8 (25)

Source: Taylor et al.,[125] with permission. Copyright © 1990, Massachusetts Medical Society. All rights reserved.

addition to abnormal smooth muscle cell proliferation, there is evidence of proliferation of lymphatic endothelial cells as well as an increased level of angiogenesis in LAM.[132] Kumasaka et al.[132] examined lymphangiogenesis in LAM using immunohistochemistry for vascular endothelial growth factors (VEGFs) Flt-4 (VEGF receptor 3 [VEGFR-3]) and VEGF-C. In their study, LAM cells demonstrated reactivity against anti–VEGF-C antibody at varying intensities. A significant correlation was further noted between the degree of lymphangiogenesis in LAM or VEGF-C expression in LAM cells.[132]

Transforming growth factor-β1 is a potent cytokine known to promote mesenchymal cell proliferation, contributing to the regulation of synthesis of fibronectin, a major component of extracellular matrix.[131] Using lung biopsy specimens from 13 women known to contain pathologic LAM cells, Evans and coworkers[131] studied the immunohistochemical expression of TGF-β1 and fibronectin. In this study, strong expression of both TGF-β1 and fibronectin was found in highly cellular regions, suggesting that the proliferation of aberrant myoid cells in LAM may be associated with altered regional expression of both TGF-β1 and fibronectin.

In most published series patients with LAM are all women and generally of reproductive age. While most of them are diagnosed between 30 and 35 years of age, exceptions do occur at both ends of life. For instance, in the series of Taylor and associates,[125] two patients were postmenopausal, and of note both were receiving exogenous estrogens. The clinical presentation is varied but is typified by dyspnea, hemoptysis, and chylous pleural effusions as well as pneumothoraces. These signs and symptoms are readily explained by overproliferation of smooth muscle cells around lymphatic channels, respiratory bronchioles, veins, and venules, resulting in impaired drainage of lymph, airway constriction, and hemorrhage, respectively. Pneumothorax was the major presenting finding in about 50% of patients and eventually occurred in about 80% over the course of the disease in the series by Taylor et al.,[125] and was present in 43% of the cases personally reviewed by them and 35% of those in the literature (Table 39.5). Chylous pleural effusion may result when only regional lymph nodes are involved without lung involvement, but pneumothorax by definition requires lung involvement. Nodes were involved with smooth muscle proliferation replacement of the lymphoid tissue in the mediastinum in 69% of the cases and in retroperitoneum in 50% of the cases with lung involvement in a series by Silverstein and coworkers,[147] and most, but not all, of those with node involvement do have lung changes. Rarely, chyloptysis (the expectoration of chyle fluid) has been also noted.[124,125] Hemoptysis is quite frequent in LAM and has been reported in up to 79% of patients.[124,125] An excellent comparative analysis of the prevalence of pneumothorax, pleural effusions, and hemoptysis as they occur in LAM and other pulmonary disorders such as emphysema and sarcoidosis is graphically shown in Figure 39.29.[154] This analysis con-

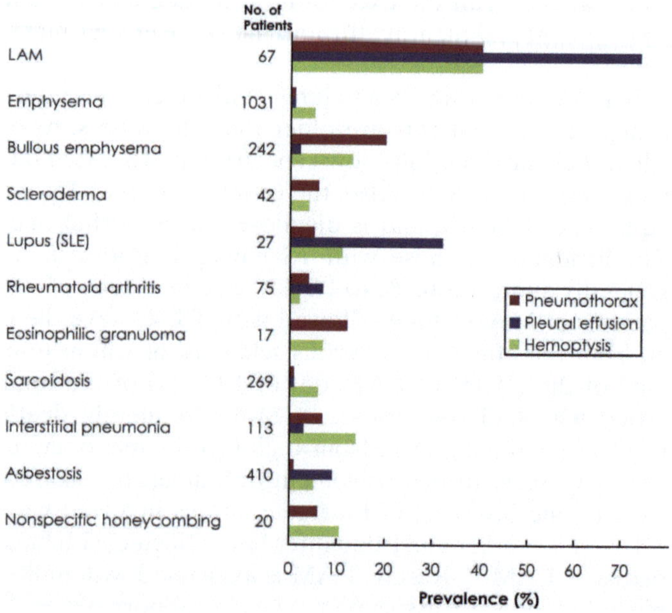

FIGURE 39.29. Lymphangioleiomyomatosis. Incidence of pneumothorax, hemoptysis and chylous pleural effusion graphed in relation to several other respiratory diseases. LAM, lymphangioleiomyomatosis; SLE, systemic lupus erythematosus. (From Carrington et al.,[154] with permission.)

ducted by Carrington et al.[154] showed that the 39.3% prevalence of hemoptysis in LAM was exceeded only by that among patients not shown in Figure 39.29 who had pulmonary vascular disease, pulmonary idiopathic hemosiderosis, or Goodpasture's syndrome.[154]

As indicated earlier, and as shown in Table 39.6, some of the presenting symptoms and signs in LAM (particularly chylous effusions) can be explained by the involvement with overgrowth of smooth muscle around lymphatic walls. This overgrowth can also be seen in (mediastinal) lymph nodes, a location where lymphatic spaces and their walls are usually unrecognizable or difficult to detail, but with proliferating smooth muscle the lymphoid tissue becomes quite atrophic and the nodes no longer function well as lymphatic drainage pathways, causing some obstruction and leading to the development of chylous effusions. The thoracic duct is similarly involved. Within the lung, the smooth muscle proliferates around lymphatic walls and causes further obstruction to flow of chyle, especially around respiratory bronchioles, and can lead to air-filled cyst formation. As the cysts form next to respiratory bronchioles, the respiratory bronchioles often lose the tethering effect of the adjacent lung tissue, and airflow entrapment occurs with enlarging cysts. Cyst formation is accompanied by degeneration of parenchymal connective tissue, both collagen and elastic tissue, in a fashion similar to cyst formation in emphysema and histiocytosis. Some of the cysts in the subpleural area may rupture and cause pneumothoraces. Lymphatic wall smooth muscle proliferation about venules and veins leads to their obstruction, causing bleeding and hemoptysis and hemosiderin deposits.[155]

Radiographic examination of the chest most frequently shows pneumothorax, as this is the most common presenting finding, but rarely the lungs may be normal (Fig. 39.30). Cysts may be outlined by slight thickening around their edges. Of interest, Kerley B lines on chest radiographs, indicating thickening of the interlobular septa, are not as frequently reported as would be expected by the incidence of chylous pleural effusion. The cysts are dramatically shown by CT scan, vary from small to large, involve all areas of lung fields, from superior to inferior and central to peripheral, and correlate with the gross findings rather nicely. The walls of the cysts vary from being imperceptible to 2 mm in thickness and correlate with the findings by histology. Of interest, bronchography contrast material does not fill the cysts. At times enlarged lymph nodes are seen with CT scans, having been described in four of seven patients in one series, while only one was suggested on plain film in this series. Also confirmed on CT scan are pneumothoraces, pleural fluid, and sometimes pericardial fluid. Pulmonary function tests show obstructive changes earlier and a mixture of obstructive and restrictive changes in later stages, with some diffusion defects that have been described as rather significant. Of interest, in the large series by Taylor and colleagues[125] the only patients presenting with restrictive defects were those having had tube thoracostomies or pleurodesis, but restriction developed later in others.

The gross appearance of the lungs in LAM is characteristic. At surgery, particularly in well-developed cases, the lungs are found to contain multiple air-filled cysts forming protruding dome-shaped pleural areas in all lobes, and the surgeon might describe a weeping of chylous fluid from cobblestone-like pleural surfaces (Fig. 39.31). The lungs are brownish in color, on account of their often significant amount of hemosiderin pigment, and are essentially replaced by cysts of varying sizes, although in earlier stages of involvement, normal lung parenchyma between the cysts may be seen. These cysts vary usually from quite small to about 3 cm, although rarely, isolated cysts up to 6 cm have been described (Fig. 39.32). In end-stage disease, the lungs are volumi-

TABLE 39.6. Clinical, physiologic, and radiographic consequences of pathologic changes seen in lymphangioleiomyomatosis

Pathologic features	Consequences: Clinical	Consequences: Physiologic	Consequences: Radiographic
Hyperplasia of smooth muscle along lymphatic routes with lymphatic obstruction	Rupture of lymphatics with chylous effusion, ascites, chyloptysis, abdominal masses	Decreased lung volume from effusion	Reticulonodular pattern, abnormal lymphangiogram, pleural effusions, coarse reticulation
Venous obstruction with focal hemorrhage and hemosiderosis	Hemoptysis, dyspnea	Uneven perfusion, ventilation/perfusion mismatch Hypoxemia and decreased diffusing capacity of the lung	Reversible coarse infiltration
Bronchiolar obstruction, distal alveolar lesions, emphysema	Emphysema, recurrent pneumothorax, dyspnea	Increased TLC and RV, airflow obstruction, uneven ventilation, and ventilation/perfusion mismatch	Enlarged lung volumes, "microcysts", pneumothorax

RV, residual volume; TLC, total lung capacity.
Source: Carrington et al.,[154] with permission.

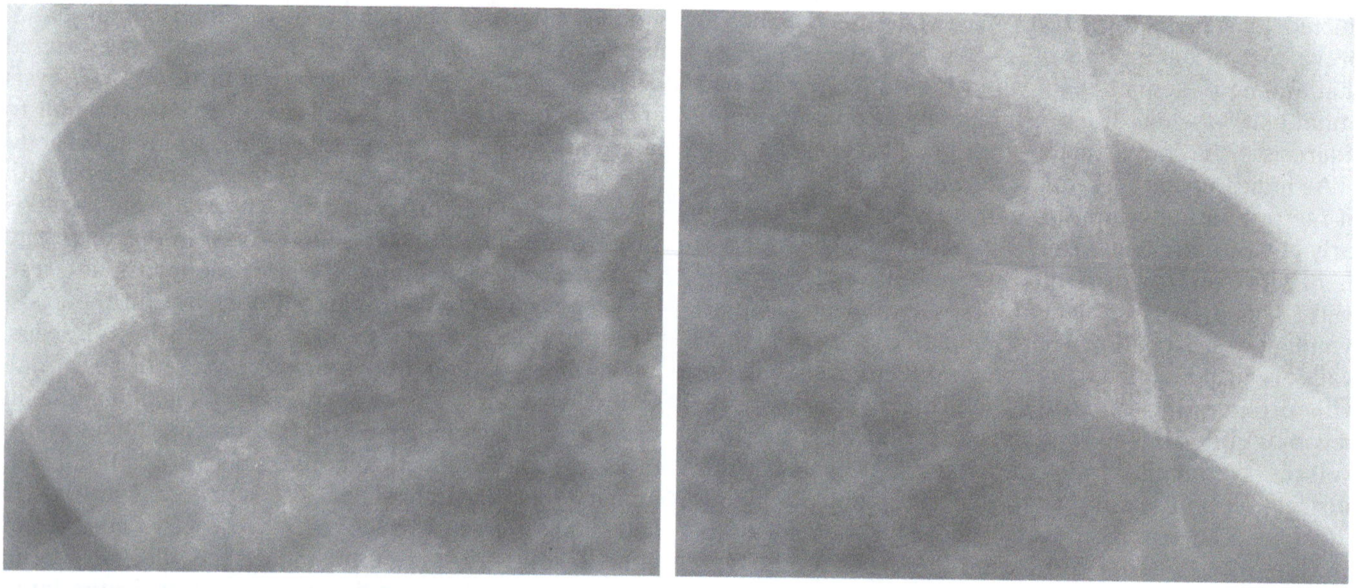

FIGURE 39.30. Lymphangioleiomyomatosis. Radiographs of chest in a 25-year-old woman with biopsy-proven disease. Early cystic change is seen bilaterally. **(A)** Expanded right lung. **(B)** Pneumothorax seen in left side of chest.

nous. The regional lymph nodes are rubbery, and the thoracic duct may also be rubbery, quite thickened, and cigar shaped due to the formation of lymphangioleiomyomatous nodules (see below).

Microscopically, cystic change is a striking feature. The cystic spaces of LAM are lined by variable numbers of small spindly myoid cells that are seen in and around small airways, lymphatic channels, pleura, and interlobular septa. The small spindly myoid cells, also known as LAM cells, represent phenotypically immature smooth muscle cells (Fig. 39.33). In some cases there is focally smooth muscle accentuation in the subpleural zone in the region of lymphatics, similar to the smooth muscle that can be seen in lymph nodes. Lymphatic spaces are dilated, and there can be variable degrees of hemosiderin and fresh blood, sometimes to rather extraordinary degrees

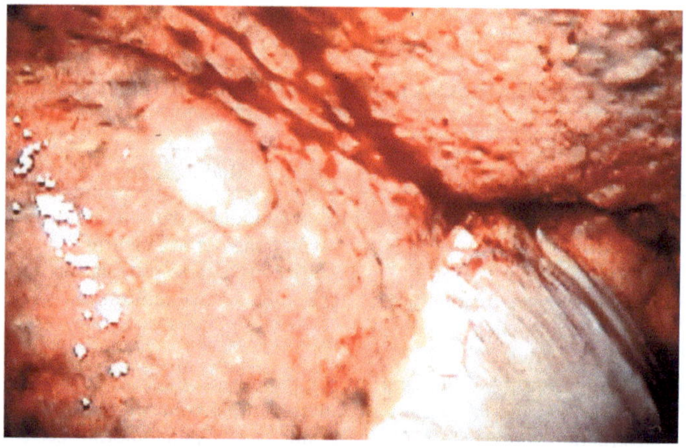

FIGURE 39.31. Videothoracoscopic view of visceral pleura in LAM. Note cobblestone appearance due to subpleural air cysts and dilated lymphatics. (Courtesy of Dr. Angelina Bautista Parma Hospital, Parma, OH.)

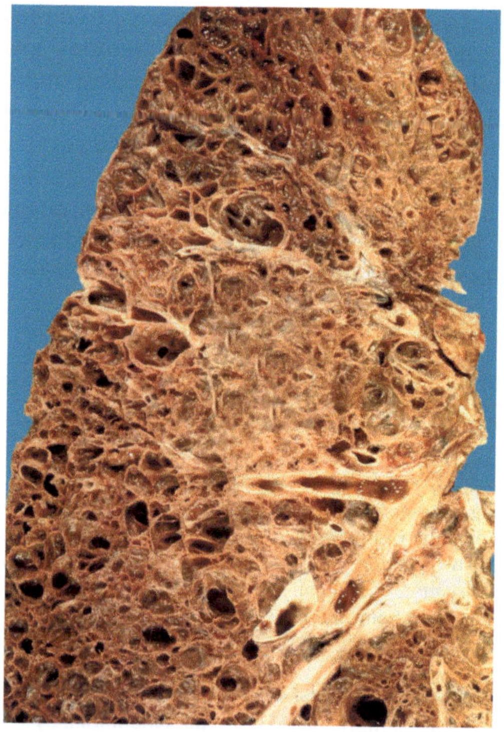

FIGURE 39.32. Lymphangioleiomyomatosis. Gross appearance, note innumerable cysts throughout. (Courtesy of Dr. J.E. Yi, Curator, the A.A. Leibow Pulmonary Pathology Collection, San Diego, CA.)

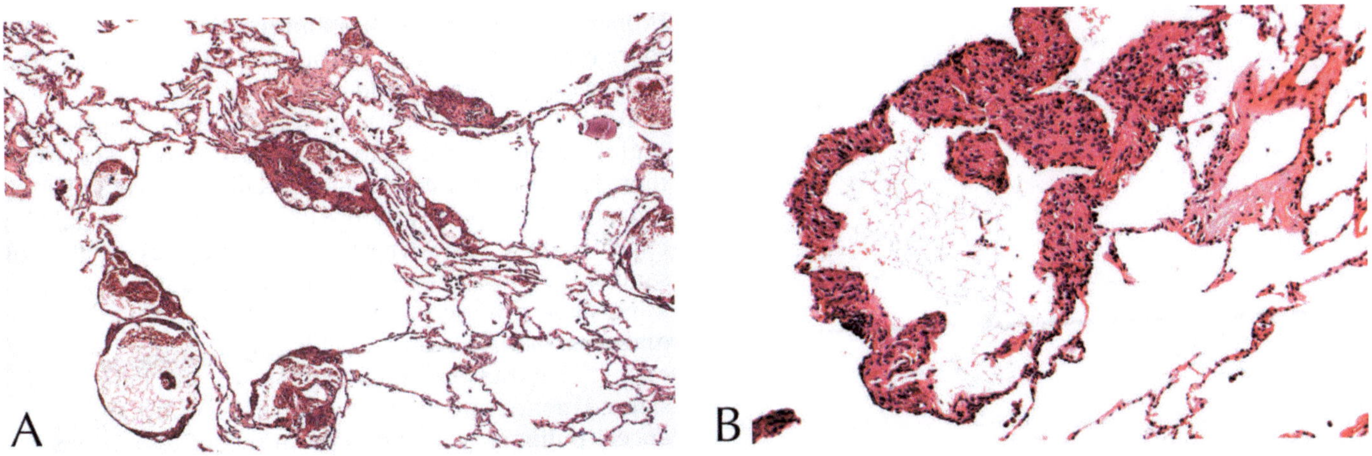

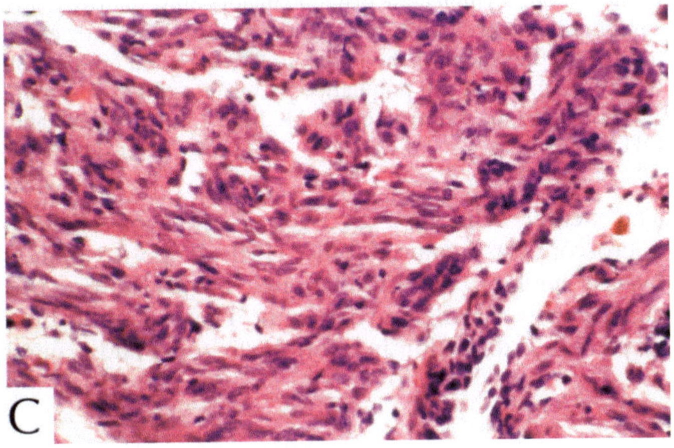

FIGURE 39.33. Lymphangioleiomyomatosis. **(A,B)** Note varying densities of smooth muscle cell proliferation with formation of cystic spaces. **(C)** Closer view of spindle shaped smooth muscle cells with dark nuclei. (**A,B** courtesy of Dr. Helmut Popper, University of Graz, Graz, Austria.)

(Fig. 39.34). Occasionally there is iron encrustation of elastic tissue from this iron accumulation (see Chapter 21). Venous elastica is disrupted in areas of myomatous infiltration (Fig. 39.35). Nodal involvement by LAM cells is rare but does occur. When significant, the proliferation of LAM cells results in effacement of the nodal architecture and depletion of native lymphoid cells (Fig. 39.36). The smooth muscle proliferations of LAM stain vividly with smooth muscle actin, HMB-45, and are generally estrogen or progesterone receptor positive (Fig. 39.37).

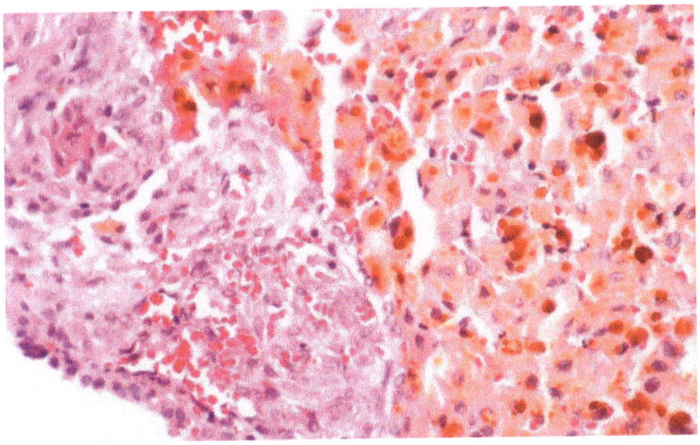

FIGURE 39.34. Lymphangioleiomyomatosis. Note intraalveolar hemosiderin-laden macrophages adjacent to a focus of perivenous infiltration by myoid LAM cells. (Courtesy of Dr. Joseph F. Tomashefski, Jr., MetroHealth Medical Center, Cleveland, OH.)

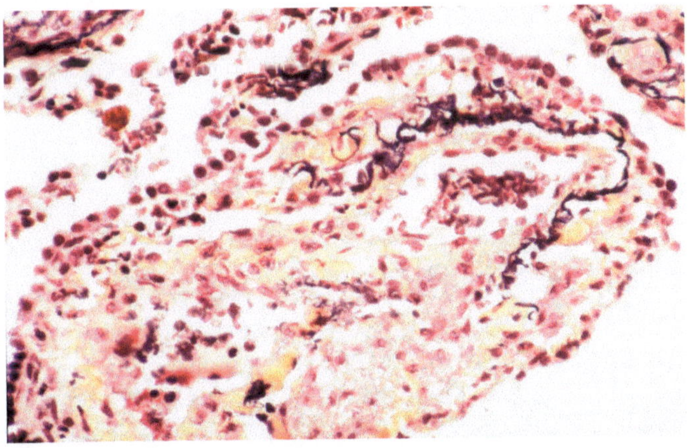

FIGURE 39.35. Lymphangioleiomyomatosis. Note small vein infiltrated by smooth muscle cells with disruption and partial loss of the elastic lamina (Movat pentachrome stain). (Courtesy of Dr. Joseph F. Tomashefski, Jr., MetroHealth Medical Center, Cleveland, OH.)

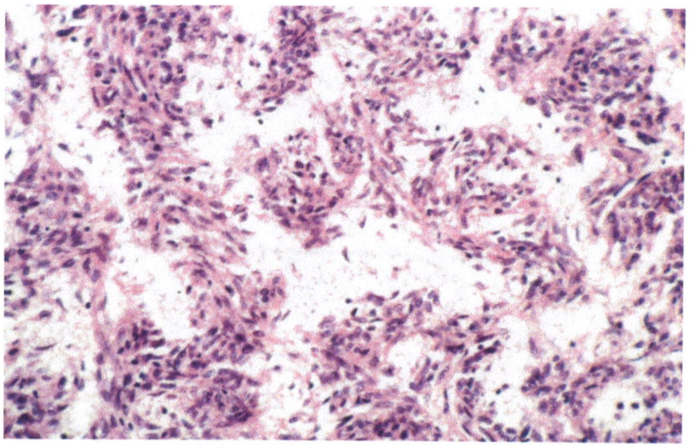

FIGURE 39.36. Lymph node in lymphangioleiomyomatosis. Note smooth muscle proliferation along the walls of lymphatic channels with effacement of the nodal architecture and eradication of native lymphoid cell population. (Courtesy of Dr. Joseph F. Tomashefski, Jr., MetroHealth Medical Center, Cleveland, OH.)

The clearer cells have glycogen in them on electron microscopy, and stain focally HMB-45 positive, in a fashion similar to the smooth muscle focally showing this change in renal angiomyolipomas. There may be lymphatic space dilatation in interlobular septa and around bronchopulmonary bundles and in pleura. Occasionally there is intraalveolar edema, but this is less striking in the usual case than one would expect.

Open video-assisted thoracoscopic lung biopsies are preferred and often used to make the diagnosis. However, there is a limited role for transbronchial biopsies in LAM. Because of the patchy nature of this disease, it would be expected that some transbronchial biopsies would not sample the characteristic lesions. Nonetheless, if proliferating smooth muscle is present in a typical pattern, the diagnosis of LAM can be made. In the series by Taylor et al.,[125] five transbronchial biopsies were all initially considered nondiagnostic, but upon review by an experienced pulmonary pathologist, three of the five were considered diagnostic. HMB-45 immunopositivity may also be helpful in this regard.

In the differential diagnosis, radiographically at least, are emphysema and pulmonary Langerhans cell histiocytosis; both can form cysts, usually thin-walled in emphysema, and usually representing cavities admixed with nodules in Langerhans cell histiocytosis, the latter characteristic helping to distinguish this disease from LAM.[156,157] Both of these occur in smokers and have more of a mid- and upper-lung-field predominance. Langerhans cell histiocytosis can occur in the same age group as LAM, but Langerhans cell histiocytosis is usually of equal

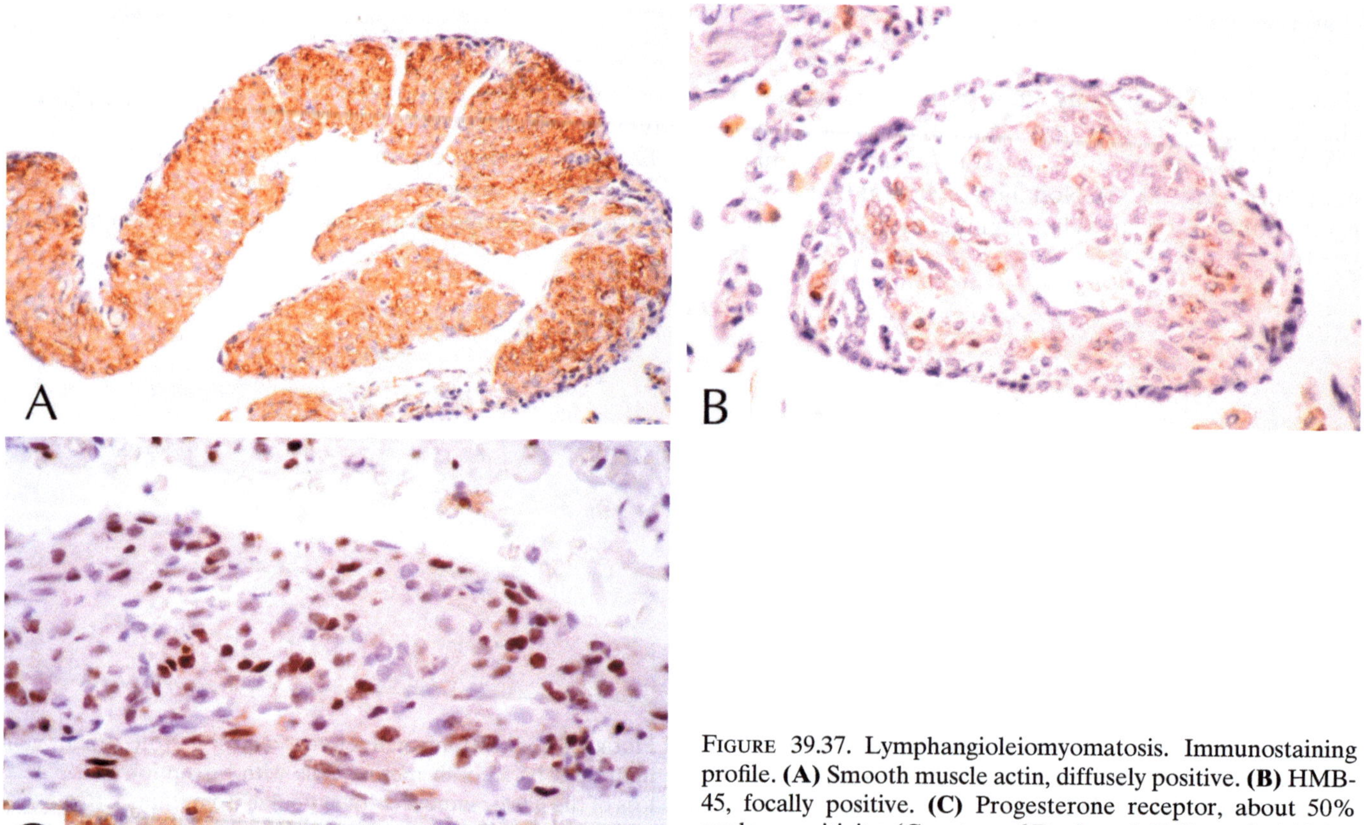

FIGURE 39.37. Lymphangioleiomyomatosis. Immunostaining profile. **(A)** Smooth muscle actin, diffusely positive. **(B)** HMB-45, focally positive. **(C)** Progesterone receptor, about 50% nuclear positivity. (Courtesy of Dr. Joseph F. Tomashefski, Jr., MetroHealth Medical Center, Cleveland, OH.)

sex distribution while LAM is decidedly more common in women, there being only one bona fide case of LAM reported in a man.[115] Moreover, a significant smoking history may be elicited in most patients with Langerhans cell histiocytosis (see Chapter 16).

Also in the differential diagnosis of cysts is interstitial pulmonary fibrosis with honeycombing. In this instance, the fibrosis favors mid- and lower lung fields, and is worse in the subpleural zones; histologically, the cysts are filled with mucus, often representing dilated bronchioles with destruction of surrounding alveoli giving the appearance of "simplification of peripheral lung." There are more chronic inflammatory cells in the interstitium, polymorphonuclear neutrophilic (PMN) leukocytes are seen within the mucus of the dilated cystic spaces, and the interstitial tissue is composed of usually dense fibrous tissue, sometimes with younger, more myxomatous, components. There may be smooth muscle proliferation, but this is in discrete bundles in the interstitium itself; this has been termed "muscularization of lung" and appears to be a reaction of smooth muscle to contraction. Interstitial fibrosis can be patchy, but usually is more confluent, the cysts are not as delicate as those with LAM, and the stroma is spindle cell in LAM in contrast to mature fibrosis and inflammatory reactions. Also, toward the end stage, fibrotic lungs are often contracted, whereas those of LAM are expanded. In LAM, the cysts are seen everywhere, are thin-walled, and vary in caliber. The cysts in LAM are air filled and there is not the usual inflammatory reaction seen with fibrosis. The intervening lung parenchyma is relatively normal between the LAM cysts instead of being densely fibrotic.

If veins are heavily involved, there may be some confusion with primary (idiopathic) hemosiderosis or pulmonary veno-occlusive disease, or other causes of chronic hemorrhage such as Goodpasture's disease. Lymphatic space dilatation may suggest congestive heart failure or other forms of passive failure, or possibly lymphangiectasia in younger patients. The atypia in some of the proliferating myocytes has caused some to consider LAM to be sarcoma, but the distinctive cyst formation should allow this distinction. The spindle cells are somewhat leiomyoblastic and may approach the variations seen in some angioleiomyomas. A few metastatic spindle cell sarcomas do cavitate and may appear cystic, but their walls are generally thicker and they are not limited to lymphatic walls. Benign metastasizing leiomyomas, also discussed in this chapter, should be kept in mind since some cases can become very cystic, mimicking not only LAM but also the more recently recognized lung lesion known as cystic fibrohistiocytic tumor, which has a storiform pattern and is also described earlier in this chapter.

Diffuse pulmonary lymphangiomatosis (DPL) differs from LAM both clinically and histopathologically.[158] It is characterized by diffuse proliferation of well-formed lymphatic vascular channels, with or without a minor smooth muscle component, affecting lymphatic routes of the lung (pleural, septal, bronchovascular). In contrast to LAM the smooth muscle component (when present) is HMB-45 negative, both sexes are affected, and the patients do not have emphysema-like cysts of the lung on chest radiographs.[158]

Kaposi's sarcoma (KS) can affect younger people, and this can follow lymphangitic pathways but is associated with cleftlike vascular spaces with variable amounts of blood cells in them, and in some adjacent or nearby areas it can show hemangiomatous-type lesions. Kaposi's sarcoma does not form pulmonary cysts as seen in LAM, and KS of the lung has a greater incidence in men, although this may change in the future due to changing risk factors. The individual spindle cells in LAM are larger with more abundant cytoplasm, staining vividly with actin, in contrast to the endothelial markers such as CD34 that stain KS. In addition, the proliferations in LAM consist of smooth muscle without small vascular spaces as noted in classic cases of KS.

Earlier reports emphasized a dismal prognosis for patients with LAM. Hughes and Hodder[159] in 1987 stated the problem well: "the usual course (in LAM) is one of relentless deterioration, with death from respiratory failure occurring within only a few years of presentation." Reaffirming this view, Silverstein and coworkers[160] in 1974 reported that death from respiratory insufficiency usually ensued within 4 years of the onset of the disease. Later, Corrin et al.[161] reported that most patients with LAM died within 10 years of the onset of the disease and this was the figure most quoted during the following two decades.[125] Exceptions occurred, however, and were so reported. For instance, two patients in the Taylor et al.[125] series of 32 patients had slow but marked deterioration but remained alive at 13 and 20 years after initial presentation. More recent case series' survival statistics in LAM are not as dismal, reporting significant outcome improvements as compared to the above-cited figures; perhaps reflecting an increased ability to recognize early lesions or improved therapies, chiefly through hormonal modulation and allograft transplantation.

A semiquantitative histologic score looking at the extent and degree of two microscopic features of LAM, the cystic lesions, and the degrees of infiltration of lung tissue by abnormal smooth muscle cells appears helpful in determining both the severity and the outcome of LAM.[162] This score, termed the lymphangioleiomyomatosis histologic score (LHS) by Matsui and colleagues,[162] can be of predictive value in assessing the prognosis of patients with this disease. In this scoring scheme, the histologic severity of LAM was determined on the basis of a semiquantitative estimate of the percentage of lung tissue involvement by (1) the cystic lesions and (2) the

TABLE 39.7. Survival of patients with pulmonary lymphangioleiomyomatosis in major reports

Author	Year	No. of patients	5-year survival (%)	10-year survival (%)
Silverstein et al.	1974	31	61	24
Corrin et al.	1975	23	65	30
Taylor et al.	1990	32	81	78
Kitaichi et al.	1995	46	78	40
Urban et al.	1999	64	91	79
Matsui et al	2000	105	85	71

Source: Matsui et al.,[162] with permission from Blackwell Publishing Ltd.

infiltration of lung tissue by abnormal smooth muscle cells. Scores were noted as LHS-1, LHS-2, and LHS-3 for cases with <25%, 25% to 50%, and >50% involvement by each of the two histologic features, respectively.[162] In their evaluation of the LHS score in 105 patients Matsui et al. documented 5- and 10-year survivals of 85% and 71%, respectively (Table 39.7 and Fig. 39.38). Hormonal modulation can be achieved with regimes using progesterone, tamoxifen, or luteinizing hormone–releasing hormone or by surgical ablation of the ovaries, and these therapeutic modalities further the hope of even longer survival rates.[163] Lung transplantation offers the only hope for cure, with survivals of up to 58% at 2 years. Lung transplantation, however, is not without complications. Complications include rejection, bronchiolitis obliterans, infection, and recurrence in the transplanted allografts (see Chapter 23).[116] Recurrence in one case was reported in 1997. The patient, a 31-year-old woman experienced recurrence of LAM in an allograft from a male donor.[116] In this case, non-isotopic in-situ hybridization showed that the smooth muscle proliferation seen in the allograft was of donor origin.[116]

Multicenter LAM registries that seek to enroll patients with LAM, follow their clinical course, and monitor their therapy offer additional expectations of improved management and survival through research and gathering of collective experience. One such center in the United States is sponsored by the National Heart, Lung, and Blood Institute.[126] Equally important are patient advocacy and support groups that promote patient education as well as research efforts to gain additional insight into fundamental mechanisms of the disease and to generate therapeutic strategies for this chronically progressive disease with high morbidity and still high mortality.[126] One such patient advocacy group is the Ohio-based LAM Foundation (4105 Executive Park Drive, Suite 320, Cincinnati, OH, 45241-4015; phone/fax: (513) 777 6889, (513) 777 4109; email: info@thelamfoundation.org).

Glomus Tumor

Glomus tumor is a mesenchymal neoplasm composed of cells that closely resemble the modified smooth muscle cell of the normal glomus body. Depending on the cellularity and degree of vascularity, different authors use different terms (such as glomangioma) somewhat synonymously for this low-grade lesion that is thought to be derived from neuromuscular cells of a special arteriovenous shunt in the glomus body, the Sucquet–Hoyer canal.[164] The glomus apparatus is thought to affect blood flow and to be sensitive to temperature, at least in the extremities. These lesions are not well defined in the lung and are only occasionally seen elsewhere. Outside the lung they are most often found in the extremities, particularly around the fingernails, including nail beds. They may occur in internal organs, including stomach and jejunum, colon, rectum, vagina, and cervix.[164] Most cases occur in young adults and no sex predilection has been reported, except for digital lesions, which for unknown reasons tend to predominate in women.[164]

Glomus tumors are rare in the lung, and only a few have been described in the trachea.[165–169] One case had oncocytic change, which has also been reported in cases of glomus tumors in soft tissue.[166] Among five cases

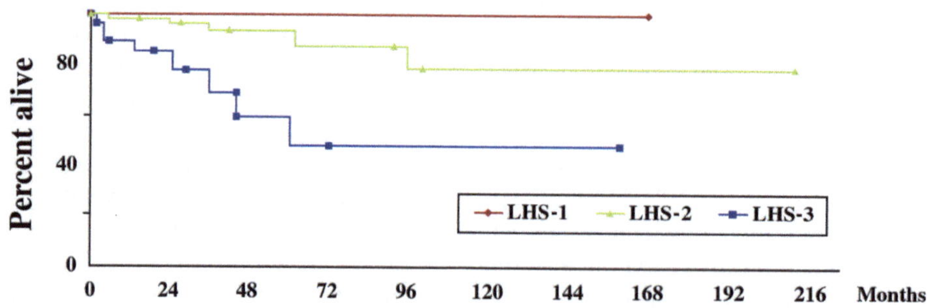

FIGURE 39.38. Kaplan-Meier survival curves of patients with pulmonary lymphangioleiomyomatosis according to the lymphangioleiomyomatosis histologic score (LHS). Patients with LHS-1 have an excellent survival. Patients with LHS-3 have the worst survival, and those with LHS-2 have an intermediate survival ($p < .002$). (From Matsui et al.,[162] with permission of Lippincott Williams & Wilkins.)

Table 39.8. Clinical, pathologic, and therapeutic characteristics of 16 patients with glomus tumors of the trachea

Age range	34–74
Male : female	14:2
Symptoms	
Hemoptysis	9
Dyspnea	8
Cough	7
Stridor or hoarseness	2
Wheeze	2
Chest pain	1
None	2
Tumor size (range) (cm)	1.2–4.5
Tumor location	
Posterior wall	16
Upper trachea	3
Middle trachea	7
Lower trachea	6
Tumor type	
Classic glomus tumor	12
Glomangioma	3
Oncocytic glomus tumor	1
Treatment	
Surgical resection	13
Bronchoscopic resection	1
Laser resection with or without radiotherapy	2

Source: Nadrous et al.,[173] with permission of Dowden Health Media.

reported by Gaertner et al.,[170] four were primary in lung and one was mediastinal. One of the four pulmonary cases was clearly malignant and was classified as a glomangiosarcoma. In some cases primary glomus tumors may coexist with esophageal tumors,[171] and a few may be clearly malignant.[170,172] Glomus tumors primary in the lung are usually asymptomatic, being discovered as coin lesions on chest radiographs, but cases presenting with hemoptysis, epigastric pain, and pneumothorax have been reported.[170] Demographics and symptomatology of glomus tumors in the trachea are shown in Table 39.8.[173] Computed tomographic virtual bronchoscopy can be of much value in assisting with the preoperative assessment of tracheal tumors (Figs. 39.39 and 39.40).[173]

Grossly, glomus tumors of the lung are well-circumscribed, multilobulated, gray to tan to red-brown tumors with a slippery glistening surface, without necrosis and sometimes having vascular spaces visible to the naked eye. Those in the trachea may present as fleshy endoluminal polypoid red masses (Fig. 39.41). Most are only a few centimeters in maximum dimensions. In the series of five cases reported by Gaertner et al.,[170] the four tumors in the lungs averaged 3.3 cm in greatest dimension. Microscopically, cells are polygonal or round, small to medium in size and rather monotonous, often having round-to-oval nuclei, with variable cytoplasmic borders (Fig. 39.42). There is no nuclear molding, nucleoli are inconspicuous, and mitoses are quite infrequent. The cytoplasm is usually granular and eosinophilic but also may be clear. There may be some variations in cellularity, with well-preserved cells near vascular spaces. The vascular spaces are ectatic and slightly irregular in shape, larger than those in hemangiopericytoma, without the acute angle divisions of "antler-like" spaces. Those with prominent vasculature may be termed glomangiomas (Fig. 39.43). Microscopic necrosis or spindle cell change is not seen. Conventional neuroendocrine markers such as chromogranin, neuron-specific enolase, and synaptophysin are negative. Vimentin and smooth muscle actin are positive (Fig. 39.44).

Glomus tumors of soft tissue typically express smooth muscle actin and have abundant pericellular type IV collagen production.[174] Caldesmon is also positive, and markers such as cytokeratin, desmin, CD34, and S-100 protein are usually negative.[174] However, in two cases described by Koss et al.,[175] there was intense diffuse (>75%) decoration of tumor cells for actin, desmin, and vimentin. In those two cases, antibodies to cytokeratin, CD34, neurofilament, chromogranin, S-100 protein, HMB-45, and myoglobin were negative. Electron microscopy of glomus tumors in the lung and bronchus show findings similar to those seen in glomus tumors elsewhere. The cells have smooth muscle features, including envelopment of individual cells by basal lamina, abundant pinocytotic vesicles, abundant intermediate filaments, and dense bodies and plaques. Nerve filaments are often seen in or near these tumor cells. In the series of Gaertner et al.,[170] the tumors did not have neurosecretory granules.

The differential diagnosis includes localized fibrous tumors, which are usually slightly more pleomorphic in cellular characteristics, CD34 positive, and show a typical patternless pattern of spindle-shaped fibroblastic cells, along with entrapped respiratory lined cleft-like intratumoral spaces. Carcinoid tumors and paragangliomas show identifiable neurosecretory features, the latter with S-100 protein–positive sustentacular cells. Leiomyosarcomas have more mitoses and more pleomorphism in spindle cell areas, and usually lack the typical ectatic vascular spaces found in glomus tumors.

Glomus tumors are said to be chiefly benign lesions. One of the four patients reported by Gaertner and associates[170] was alive and well 5 years after diagnosis. As noted, malignant tumors do occur but are exceedingly rare.[170,172] The patient with glomangiosarcoma reported by Gaertner et al. died 68 weeks after initial therapy. This malignant variant differed from the other four tumors; it was larger, measuring 9.5 cm, and showed increased mitotic activity (nine mitoses per 10 HPFs), focal necrosis, and cytologic atypia, and was associated with disseminated disease.[170] Surgical sleeve resection is particularly applicable to tumors of the main stem bronchi and trachea. Reporting on a patient with a successful surgical resection for a tracheal glomus tumor, Nadrous et al.[173] advocated the use of preoperative computed bronchoscopic mapping as an intraoperative aid to surgical resection.

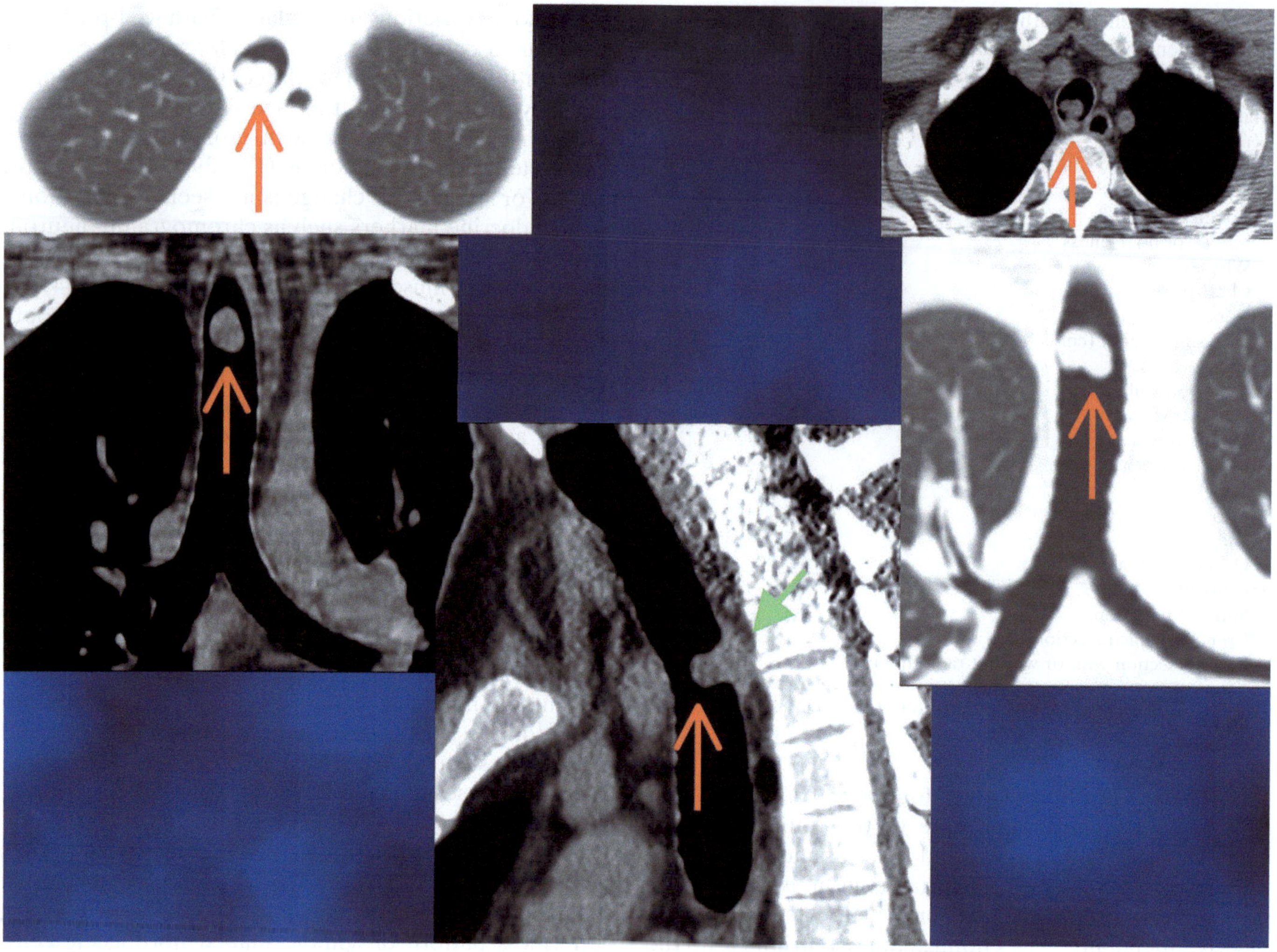

FIGURE 39.39. Glomus tumor of the trachea. Computed tomographic images showing endoluminal and extraluminal extent of the tumor. (Courtesy of Drs. H.F. Nadrous and J.R. Jett, Mayo Clinic, Rochester, MN. From Nadrous et al.,[173] with permission of Dowden Health Media.)

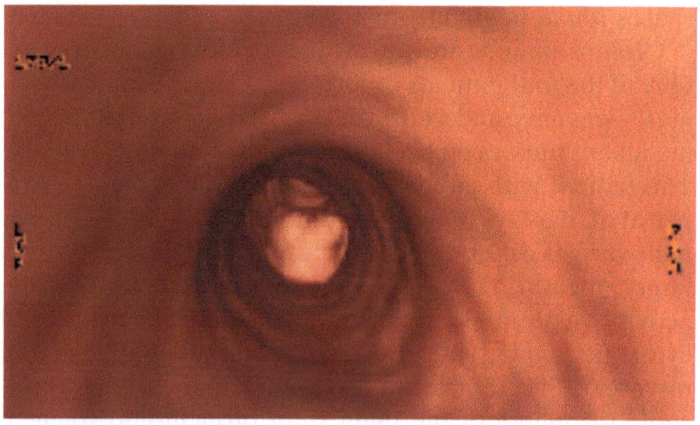

FIGURE 39.40. Glomus tumor of the trachea. Highly detailed and interactive virtual bronchoscopy showing posterior lobulated tumor. (From Nadrous et al.,[173] with permission of Dowden Health Media.)

Available follow-up in one of the two patients reported by Koss and coworkers[175] revealed that the patient, a 41-year-old man, was alive and well nearly 4 years after surgical resection. Therapeutic modalities particularly applicable to tracheal tumors are shown in Table 39.8.

Rhabdomyoma, Rhabdomyomatous Dysplasia, and Rhabdomyosarcoma

Rhabdomyomas are benign mesenchymal tumors with skeletal (striated) muscle differentiation that are classified into cardiac and extracardiac types depending on location.[176] Extracardiac rhabdomyomas occur in the head and neck area and in the larynx,[176,177] but their occurrence in the lower respiratory tract and lung has not been documented.

On the other hand, *rhabdomyomatous dysplasia* (discussed at greater length in Chapter 42) refers to the occurrence of striated muscle fibers around bronchioles,

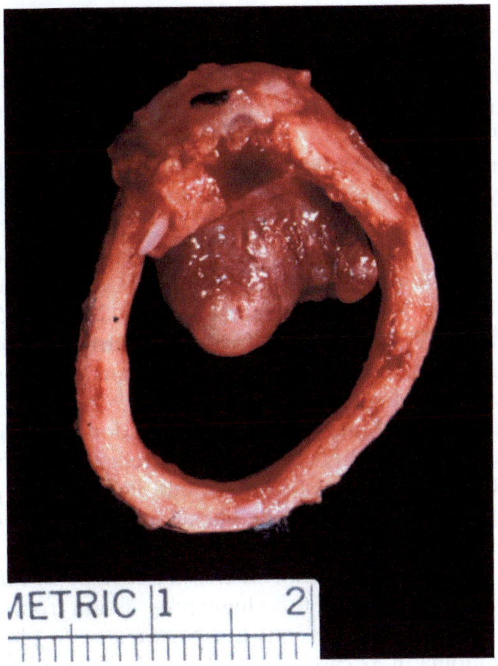

FIGURE 39.41. Glomus tumor of the trachea. Gross appearance of surgically resected specimen. Note polypoid mass arising from the posterior membranous wall. (From Nadrous et al.,[173] with permission of Dowden Health Media.)

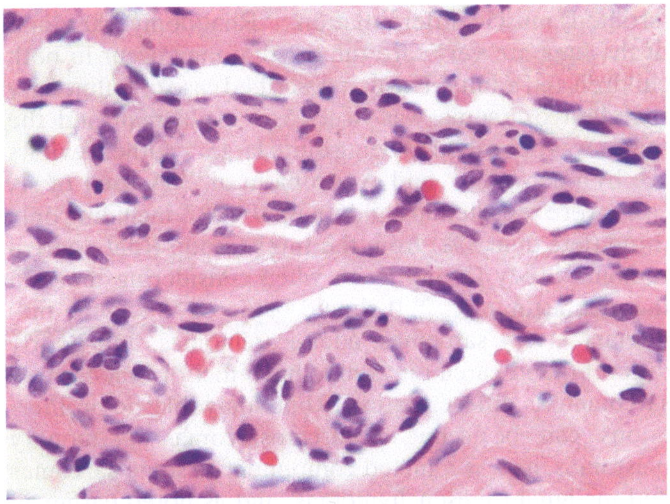

FIGURE 39.43. Glomangioma. Note vascular spaces lined by endothelial cells. Some of the spaces contain tufts of oval to round cells or scattered red blood cells.

and interlobular septa, which is well-documented, usually presenting as an incidental finding in association with other abnormalities such as congenital heart disease or cystic adenomatoid malformation of the lung. A tumorous type of rhabdomyomatous dysplasia reported by Ramaswamy et al.[178] described distinctive striated muscle tissue in the upper and lower lobes of the right lung. A critical review of the paper does not disclose the presence of discrete tumor masses despite the term *tumorous* being used in the title. A report at the turn of the 20th century by von Helsing and Zipkin, cited by Ramaswamy et al., integrated cases with striated muscle fibers in the lung in the group of "teratoids" and called them rhabdomyomas and adenorhabdomyomas. At present, with the exception of the above-cited case of a laryngeal rhabdomyoma, it would appear appropriate and prudent to say that bona fide rhabdomyoma of the lung has yet to be documented and that the anomalous occurrence of striated muscle tissue in the lung is probably best regarded as a form of tissue heterotopia.

Rhabdomyosarcomas are malignant tumors showing light microscopic and ultrastructural features of skeletal

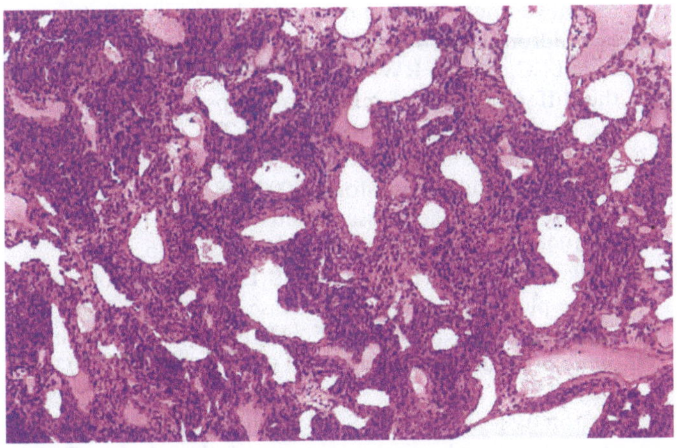

FIGURE 39.42. Glomus tumor of the trachea. Note sheets and trabeculae of uniform looking cells surrounding dilated vascular channels. (From Nadrous et al.,[173] with permission of Dowden Health Media.)

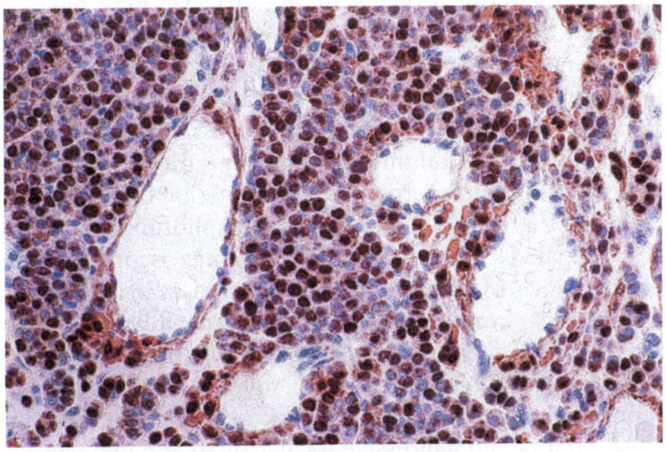

FIGURE 39.44. Glomus tumor of the trachea. Smooth muscle actin immunostain. Note staining positivity. (From Nadrouset al.,[173] with permission of Dowden Health Media.)

(striated) muscle differentiation.[179] Rhabdomyosarcomas of the lung are very rare tumors that may occur in both children and adults. The first described case of pulmonary rhabdomyosarcoma was in a 25-year-old man and the tumor was described as being quite large.[180] Other reviews are by Lee et al.[179] and Avignina et al.[181] A total of six cases were reported in children up to 1987, including only three (less than 3%) from the Inter Group Rhabdomyosarcoma Study Group, even when considering those in the mediastinum.[182,183] It should be noted that some pulmonary artery sarcomas, adenocarcinomas, and poorly differentiated carcinomas may have foci of rhabdomyosarcomatous differentiation. Rhabdomyoblastic proliferations can be seen in carcinosarcomas, pulmonary blastomas, and as a mixed component in some sarcomas and malignant mesenchymomas, and as noted earlier in the setting of cystic adenomatoid malformations. Rhabdomyoblastic differentiation can also be seen in neurogenic tumors known as triton tumors.[184]

In the respiratory tract, rhabdomyosarcomas may present in four distinct ways: (1) in the bronchus; (2) in the pulmonary trunk (i.e., pulmonary artery sarcoma); (3) associated with a congenital cystic adenomatoid malformation; and (4) as an intraparenchymal tumor.[185] It appears that rhabdomyosarcomas associated with congenital cystic malformations are more often seen in children and are better termed cystic blastomas.[185] Tumors presenting as endobronchial lesions or affecting the bronchial tree tend to show symptoms related to obstruction, whereas tumors located in periphery of the lung may present with chest pain.[185]

Grossly, intrapulmonary rhabdomyosarcomas present as solid masses with areas of hemorrhage or necrosis. The size of the tumor varies depending largely on its location. Endobronchial lesions tend to be smaller than intraparenchymal neoplasms.[185] Microscopically, embryonal and alveolar variants have been described. Some, particularly those growing in the airways, may have a botryoid appearance, with the presence of zonal layering of neoplastic cells, the so-called cambium layer. Individually, some cells may be strapped or globoid in configuration, and some may show cross-striations characteristic of skeletal muscle differentiation. Although difficult to identify, cross-striations in rhabdomyoblasts may be better visualized with phosphotungstic acid-hematoxylin (PTAH) stains. Electron microscopy reveals the presence of Z disks, linear ribosomes, or primitive junctions.[181] Immunohistochemically, negative staining for epithelial membrane antigen and cytokeratin along with positive staining for desmin, myosin, and myoglobin support the diagnosis. Prognostic data are limited in these tumors, but aggressive local growth and metastases have been documented.[179] Surgical excision is the treatment of choice with or without postoperative irradiation or chemotherapy.[179,182,183]

References

1. Anthony PP. Inflammatory pseudotumor (plasma cell granuloma) of lung, liver and other organs. Histopathology 1993;23:501–503.
2. Cerfolio RJ, Allen MS, Nascimento AG, et al. Inflammatory pseudotumors of the lung. Ann Thorac Surg 1999;67:933–936.
3. Fraire AE. Non malignant versus malignant proliferations on lung biopsy. In: Cagle PT, ed. Diagnostic pulmonary pathology. New York: Marcel-Dekker, 2000:525–545.
4. Agrons GA, Rosado-de-Christensen, Kirejczyk WM, et al. Pulmonary inflammatory pseudotumor: radiologic features. Radiology 1998;206:511–518.
5. Matsubara O, Mark EJ, Ritter JH. Pseudoneoplastic lesions of the lungs, pleural surfaces and mediastinum. In: Wick MR, Humphrey PA, Ritter JH, eds. Pathology of pseudoneoplastic lesions. Philadelphia: Lippincott-Raven, 1999:97–129.
6. Matsubara O, Tan-Liu NS, Kenney RM, et al. Inflammatory pseudotumors of the lung: progression from organizing pneumonia to fibrous histiocytoma or to plasma cell granuloma in 32 cases. Hum Pathol 1988;19:807–814.
7. Travis WD, Colby TV, Corrin B, et al. World Health Organization. International histological classification of tumours. Histological typing of lung and pleural tumours. Berlin, Heidelberg, New York: Springer, 1999:63.
8. Yousem SA, Tazelaar HD, Manabe T, Dehner LP. Inflammatory myofibroblastic tumour. In: Travis WD, Brambilla E, Müller-Hermelink HK, Harris CC, eds. World Health Organization classification of tumours. Pathology and genetics of tumours of the lung, pleura, thymus and heart. Lyon: IARC Press, 2004:105–106.
9. Snyder CS, Dell'Aguilla M, Haghighi P, et al. Clonal changes in inflammatory pseudotumor of the lung: a case report. Cancer 1995;76:1545–1549.
10. Su LD, Atayde-Perez A, Sheldon S, et al. Inflammatory myofibroblastic tumor: cytogenetic evidence supporting clonal origin. Mod Pathol 1998;11:364–368.
11. Hedlund GL, Navoy JE, Gallianai CA, et al. Aggressive manifestations of inflammatory pulmonary pseudotumor in children. Pediatr Radiology 1999;29:112–116.
12. Ledet SC, Brown RW, Cagle PT. P53 immunostaining in the differentiation of inflammatory pseudotumor involving the lung. Modern Pathol 1995;8:282–286.
13. Corrin B. Pathology of the lungs. London, Edinburgh, New York: Churchill Livingstone, 2000:588.
14. Case records of the Massachusetts General Hospital (Case 20–1994). N Engl J Med 1994;330:1439–1446.
15. Okike N, Bernatz PE, Woolner LB. Localized mesothelioma of the pleura. J Thorac Cardiovasc Surg 1978;75:363–372.
16. Scharifker D, Kaneko M. Localized fibrous "mesothelioma" of pleura (submesothelial fibroma). Cancer 1979;43:627–635.
17. Dalton WT, Zolliker AS, McCaughey WTE, Jacques J, et al. Localized primary tumors of the pleura. Cancer 1979;44:1465–1475.
18. Briselli M, Mark EJ, Dickersin GR. Solitary fibrous tumors of pleura: eight new cases and review of 360 cases in the literature. Cancer 1981;47:2678–2689.

19. Janssen JP, Wagenaar SS, Van Den Bosch JMM, et al. Benign localized mesothelioma of the pleura. Histopathology 1985;9:309–313.
20. Yousem SA, Flynn SD. Intrapulmonary localized fibrous tumor (so-called localized fibrous tumor). Am J Clin Pathol 1988;89:365–369.
21. Van de Rijn M, Lombard CM, Rouse RV, et al. Expression of CD34 by solitary fibrous tumors of the pleura, mediastinum and lung. Am J Surg Pathol 1994;18:814–820.
22. Caruso RA, La Spada F, Gaeta M. Report of an intrapulmonary fibrous tumor: fine needle aspiration cytologic findings, clinicopathological and immunohistochemical features. Diagn Cytopathol 1996;14:64–67.
23. Guillou L, Fletcher JA, Fletcher CDM, et al. Extrapleural solitary fibrous tumour and hemangiopericytoma. In: World Health Organization classification of tumours. Pathology and genetics. Tumors of soft tissue and bone. Lyon: IARC Press, 2002:86–90.
24. Brunneman RB, Ro JY, Ordonez NG, et al. Extrapleural solitary fibrous tumor: a clinicopathologic study of 24 cases. Mod Pathol 1999;12:1034–1042.
25. Hasegawa T, Matsuno Y, Shimoda T, et al. Extrathoracic solitary fibrous tumors: their histological variability and potentially aggressive behavior. Hum Pathol 1999;30: 1464–1473.
26. Wick MR, Mills SE. Benign and borderline tumors of the lungs and pleura. In: Leslie KO, Wick MR, eds. Practical pulmonary pathology. Philadelphia, Edinburgh, London: Churchill Livingstone, 2005:706–713.
27. Hansen CP, Francis D, Bertelson S. Primary hemangiopericytoma of the lung. Case report. Scand J Thorac Cardiovasc Surg 1990;24:89–92.
28. Wu Y-C, Wang L-S, Chen W, et al. Primary pulmonary malignant hemangiopericytoma associated with coagulopathy. Ann Thorac Surg 1997;64:841–843.
29. Osborn M, Mandys V, Beddow E, et al. Cystic fibrohistiocytic tumours presenting in the lung: primary or metastatic disease? Histopathology 2003;43:556–562.
30. Colby TV. Metastasizing dermatofibroma. Am J Surg Pathol 1997;21:976.
31. Colome-Grimmer MI, Evans HL. Metastasizing cellular dermatofibroma. A report of two cases. Am J Surg Pathol 1996;20:1361–1367.
32. Colby TV, Koss MN, Travis WD. Atlas of tumor pathology. Tumors of the lower respiratory tract. Washington, DC: Armed Forces Institute of Pathology, 1994:348.
33. De Hertogh G, Bergmans G, Molderex C, et al. Cutaneous cellular fibrous histiocytoma metastasizing to the lungs. Histopathology 2002;41:85–86.
34. Joseph MG, Colby TV, Swensen SJ, et al. Multiple cystic fibrohistiocytic tumors of the lung: report of two cases. Mayo Clin Proc 1990;65:192–197.
35. Holden WE, Mulkey DD, Kessler S. Multiple peripheral lung cysts and hemoptysis in an otherwise asymptomatic adult. Am Rev Respir Dis 1982;126:930–932.
36. Mark EJ. Mesenchymal cystic hamartoma of the lung. N Engl J Med 1986;315:1255–1259.
37. Case Records of the Massachusetts General Hospital (Case 32–1985). N Engl J Med 1985;313:374–382.
38. Abrams J, Talcott J, Corson JM. Pulmonary metastases in patients with low-grade endometrial stromal sarcoma: clinicopathologic findings with immunohistochemical characterization. Am J Surg Pathol 1989;13:133–140.
39. Chan KL, Crabtree GS, Lim-Tan SK, et al. Primary uterine endometrial stromal neoplasms. A clinicopathologic study of 117 cases. Am J Surg Pathol 1990;14:415–438.
40. Hedlund GL, Bisset GS, III, Bove KE. Malignant neoplasms arising in cystic hamartomas of the lung in childhood. Radiology 1989;173:77–79.
41. Weinberg AG, Currarino G, Moore GC, et al. Mesenchymal neoplasia and congenital pulmonary cysts. Pediatr Radiol 1980;9:179–182.
42. Ueda K, Gruppo R, Unger F, et al. Rhabdomyosarcoma of lung arising in congenital cystic adenomatoid malformation. Cancer 1977;40:383–388.
43. Valderrama E, Saluja G, Shende A, et al. Pulmonary blastoma: report of two cases in children. Am J Surg Pathol 1978;2:415–422.
44. Fletcher CD. Benign fibrous histiocytomas of subcutaneous and deep soft tissue: a clinicopathologic analysis of 21 cases. Am J Surg Pathol 1990;14:801–809.
45. Hakimi M, Pai RP, Fine G, et al. Fibrous histiocytoma of the trachea. Chest 1975;68:367–368.
46. Viguera JL, Pujol JL, Reboiras SD, et al. Fibrous histiocytoma of the lung. Thorax 1976;31:475–479.
47. Gonzalez-Campora R, Matilla A, Sanchez-Carrillo JJ, et al. "Benign" fibrous histiocytoma of the trachea. J Laryngol Otol 1981;93:1287–1292.
48. Tagge E, Yunis E, Chopyk J, et al. Obstructing endobronchial fibrous histiocytoma: potential for lung salvage. J Pediatr Surg 1991;26:1067–1069.
49. Spencer H. The pulmonary plasma cell/histiocytoma complex. Histopathology 1984;8:903–916.
50. Gal AA, Koss MN, Hocholzer L, et al. Prognostic factors in pulmonary inflammatory pseudotumor and malignant fibrous histiocytoma. Mod Pathol 1992;5:113A.
51. Sajjad SM, Begin LR, Dail DH, et al. Fibrous histiocytoma of lung: a clinicopathologic study of two cases. Histopathology 1981;5:325–334.
52. Louie S, Cross CE, Amott T, et al. Postirradiation malignant fibrous histiocytoma of the trachea. Am Rev Respir Dis 1987;135:761–762.
53. Tan-Liu NS, Matsubara O, Grillo HC, et al. Invasive fibrous tumor of the tracheobronchial tree: clinical and pathologic study of seven cases. Hum Pathol 1989;20:180–184.
54. Burke AP, Tazelaar H, Butany JW. Cardiac sarcomas. In: Travis WD, Brambilla E, Müller-Hermelink HK, Harris CC, eds. World Health Organization classification of tumors. Pathology and genetics of tumours of the lung, pleura, thymus and heart. Lyon: IARC Press, 2004:276–278.
55. Colby TV, Koss MN, Travis WD. Atlas of tumor pathology. Tumors of the lower respiratory tract. Washington, DC: Armed Forces Institute of Pathology, 1994:342–345.
56. Juettner FM, Popper H, Sommersguter K, et al. Malignant fibrous histiocytoma of the lung: prognosis and therapy of a rare disease; report of two cases and review of the literature. Thorac Cardiovasc Surg 1987;35:226–231.

57. Silverman JF, Coalson JJ. Primary malignant myxoid fibrous histiocytoma of the lung: light and ultrastructural examination with review of the literature. Arch Pathol Lab Med 1984;108:49–54.
58. Shah IA, Kurtz SM, Simonsen RL. Radiation-induced malignant fibrous histiocytoma of the pulmonary artery. Arch Pathol Lab Med 1991;115:921–925.
59. Kearney MM, Soule EH, Ivins JC. Malignant fibrous histiocytoma: a retrospective study of 167 cases. Cancer 1980;45:167–178.
60. Enjojii M, Hashimoto H, Tsuneyoshi M, et al. Malignant fibrous histiocytoma: a clinicopathologic study of 130 cases. Arch Pathol Jpn 1980;30:727–741.
61. Ro Jy, Ayala AG, Sella A, et al. Sarcomatoid renal cell carcinoma. Clinicopathologic study of 42 cases. Cancer 1987;59:476–526.
62. Ro Jy, Chen JL, Lee JS, et al. Sarcomatoid carcinoma of the lung. Immunohistochemical and ultrastructural studies of 14 cases. Cancer 1992;69:376–386.
63. Thurlbeck WM, Churg AM, eds. Pathology of the lung. 2nd ed. New York: Thieme, 1995:510.
64. Fletcher CDM, van der Berg E, Molenaar WM. Pleomorphic malignant fibrous histiocytoma/undifferentiated high grade pleomorphic sarcoma. In: Fletcher CDM, Unni KK, Mertens F, eds. World Health Organization classification of tumours. Pathology and genetics. Tumours of soft tissue and bone. Lyon: IARC Press, 2002:120–122.
65. Yousem SA, Hochholzer L. Malignant fibrous histiocytoma of the lung. Cancer 1987;60:2532–2541.
66. Lee JT, Shelburne JD, Linder J. Primary malignant fibrous histiocytoma of the lung: a clinicopathologic and ultrastructural study of five cases. Cancer 1984;53:1124–1130.
67. Halyard MY, Camoriano JK, Culligan JA. Malignant fibrous histiocytoma of the lung. Report of four cases and review of the literature. Cancer 1996;78:2492–2497.
68. Miller DL, Allen MS. Rare pulmonary neoplasms. Mayo Clin Proc 1993;68:492–498.
69. Leslie KO, Wick MR. Practical pulmonary pathology. A diagnostic approach. Philadelphia, Edinburgh, London: Churchill Livingstone, 2005:478.
70. Colby TV, Koss MN, Travis WD. Atlas of tumor pathology. Tumors of the lower respiratory tract. Washington, DC: Armed Forces Institute of Pathology, 1994:346–347.
71. Pettinato G, Manivel JC, Saldana MJ, et al. Primary bronchopulmonary fibrosarcoma of childhood and adolescence: recurrent of a low grade malignancy. Clinicopathologic study of five cases and review of the literature. Hum Pathol 1989;20:463–471.
72. Wick MR, Manivel JC. Primary sarcoma of the lung. In: Williams CJ, Krikorian JG, Green MR, Raghavarn D, eds. Textbook of uncommon cancer. New York: John Wiley and Sons, 1988:335–381.
73. Logrono R, Filipowicz EA, Eyzaguirre EJ, et al. Diagnosis of primary fibrosarcoma of the lung by fine needle aspiration and core biopsy. Arch Pathol Lab Med 1999;123:731–735.
74. Liebow AA, Loring WE, Felton WL, II. The musculature of the lung in chronic pulmonary disease. Am J Pathol 1953;29:885–911.
75. Heppleston AG. The pathology of honeycomb lung. Thorax 1956;11:47–53.
76. Spencer H. Pathology of the lung. 4th ed. Oxford: Pergamon, 1985:680.
77. Shahian DM, McEnany MT. Complete endobronchial excision of leiomyoma of the bronchus. J Thorac Cardiovasc Surg 1979;77:87–91.
78. Yellin A, Rosenman Y, Lieberman Y. Review of smooth muscle tumours of the lower respiratory tract. Br J Dis Chest 1984;78:337–351.
79. White SH, Ibrahim NBN, Forrester-Wood CP, et al. Leiomyomas of the lower respiratory tract. Thorax 1985;40:306–311.
80. Gal AA, Brooks JSJ, Pietra GG. Leiomyomatous neoplasms of the lung: a clinical, histologic, and immunohistochemical study. Mod Pathol 1989;2:209–215.
81. McKechy JL, Li X, Zhuang Z, et al. Multiple leiomyomas of the esophagus, lung and uterus in multiple endocrine neoplasia, type 1. Am J Pathol 2001;159:1121–1127.
82. Kayser K, Zink S, Schneider T, et al. Benign metastasizing leiomyoma of the uterus: documentation of clinical, histochemical and lectin-histochemical data of 10 cases. Virchows Arch 2000;437:289–292.
83. Esteban JM, Allen WM, Schaerf RH. Benign metastasizing leiomyoma of the uterus: histologic and immunohistochemical characterization of primary and metastatic lesions. Arch Pathol Lab Med 1999;123:960–962.
84. Tietze L, Günther K, Hörbe A, et al. Benign metastasizing leiomyoma: a cytogenetically balanced but clonal disease. Hum Pathol 2000;31:126–128.
85. Cramer SF, Meyer JC, Kraner JF, et al. Metastasizing leiomyoma of the uterus: S-phase fraction, estrogen receptor and ultrastructural. Cancer 1980;45:932–937.
86. Silverman JF, Kay S. Multiple pulmonary leiomyomatous hamartomas: report of case with ultrastructural examination. Cancer 1976;38:1199–1204.
87. Sung DF. Complete endobronchial obstruction and left non-aerated hemithorax caused by a leiomyoma: report of a case. Surg Today 1995;25:161–163.
88. Colby TV, Koss MN, Travis WD. Atlas of tumor pathology. Tumors of the lower respiratory tract. Washington, DC: Armed Forces Institute of Pathology, 1994:355–356.
89. Rosai J. Peritoneum, retroperitoneum and related structures. In: Rosai J, ed. Rosai and Ackerman's surgical pathology. 9th ed. Edinburgh, London, New York: Mosby, 2004:2386.
90. Horstmann JP, Pietra GG, Harman JA, et al. Spontaneous regression of pulmonary leiomyomas during pregnancy. Cancer 1977;39:314–321.
91. Uyama T, Monden Y, Harada K, Sumitomo M, Kimura S. Pulmonary leiomyomatosis showing endobronchial extension and giant cyst formation. Chest 1988;94:644–646.
92. Kaplan C, Katoh A, Shamato M, et al. Multiple leiomyomas of the lung: benign or malignant. Am Rev Respir Dis 1973;108:656–659.
93. Piccaluga A, Capelli A. Fibroleiomiomatosi metastatizzante dell'utero. Arch Ital Anat Istolog Patol 1967;41:99–164.
94. Herrera GA, Miles PA, Greenberg H, et al. The origin of pseudoglandular spaces in metastatic smooth muscle neo-

plasms of uterine origin: report of a case with ultrastructure and review of previous cases studied by electron microscopy. Chest 1983;83:270–274.
95. Wolff M, Silva K, Kaye G. Pulmonary metastases (with admixed epithelial elements) from smooth muscle neoplasms: report of nine cases, including three males. Am J Surg Pathol 1979;3:325–342.
96. Kempson RL. Mitosis counting II (editorial). Hum Pathol 1976;7:482–483.
97. Norris HJ. Mitosis counting III (editorial). Hum Pathol 1976;7:483–484.
98. Tench WD, Dail D, Gmelich JT, et al. Benign metastasizing leiomyomas: a review of 21 cases. Lab Invest 1978;38: 367–368(abstr).
99. Matani N. San Diego, California. Personal communication.
100. Popock E, Craig JR, Bullock WK. Metastatic uterine leiomyomata: a case report. Cancer 1976;38:2096–2100.
101. Wick MR, Mills SE. Benign and borderline tumors of the lungs and pleura. In: Leslie KO, Wick MR, eds. Practical pulmonary pathology. Philadelphia, Edinburgh, London: Churchill Livingstone, 2005:685–687.
102. Rosai J. Tumors of the uterine corpus. In: Rosai J, ed. Rosai and Ackerman's surgical pathology. 9th ed. Edinburgh, London, New York: Mosby, 2004:1607–1608.
103. Soberanis-Torruco CN, Cortes-Gutierrez ME, Parra-Soto I, et al. Leiomyomatosis intravenosa con extension a la auricula derecha. Informe de un caso. Patologia 2003;41: 225–230.
104. Yellin A, Rosenman Y, Lieberman Y. Review of smooth muscle tumours of the lower respiratory tract. Br J Dis Chest 1984;78:337–351.
105. Hasleton PS. Benign lung tumors and their malignant counterparts. In: Hasleton PS, ed. Spencer's pathology of the lung. 5th ed. New York, St. Louis, San Francisco: McGraw-Hill, 1996:954.
106. Miller DL, Allen MS. Rare pulmonary neoplasms. Mayo Clin Proc 1993;68:492–498.
107. Thurlbeck WM, Churg AM, eds. Pathology of the lung. 2nd ed. New York: Thieme, 1995:510.
108. Fletcher CDM, Uni K, Merteur F. World Health Organization classification of tumors. Pathology and genetics. Tumors of soft tissue and bone. Lyon: IARC Press, 2002: 131–134.
109. Moran CA, Suster S, Abbondanzo SL, et al. Primary leiomyosarcomas of the lung: a clinico-pathologic study of 18 cases. Mod Pathol 1997;10:122–128.
110. Travis WD, Colby TV, Corrin B, et al. World Health Organization. International classification of tumours. Histological typing of lung and pleural tumours. 3rd ed. Berlin, Heidelberg, New York: Springer, 1999:60–61.
111. Cameron WEJ. Primary sarcoma of the lung. Thorax 1975; 30:516–520.
112. Dowell AR. Primary pulmonary leiomyosarcoma: report of 2 cases and review of the literature. Ann Thorac Surg 1974;17:384–394.
113. Nascimento AG, Unni KK, Bernatz PE. Sarcomas of the lung. Mayo Clin Proc 1982;57:355–359.
114. Beluffi G, Bertolotti P, Mietta A, et al. Primary leiomyosarcoma of the lung in a girl. Pediatr Radiol 1986;16: 240–244.
115. Aubry M-C, Myers JL, Ryu JH, et al. Pulmonary lymphangioleiomyomatosis in a man. Am J Respir Crit Care Med 2000;162:749–752.
116. Bittman I, Dose TB, Müller C, et al. Lymphangioleiomyomatosis: recurrence after single lung transplantation. Hum Pathol 1997;26:1420–1423.
117. Lautenbacher R. Dysembryomes métotypiques des reins, carcinose submiliere aiguë poumon avec emphysème généralisé et doulde pneumothorax. Ann Med Intern (Paris) 1918;5:435–450.
118. Burrell LS, Ross HM. A case of chylous effusion due to leiomyosarcoma. Br J Tuberc 1937;31:38–39.
119. von Stössel E. Uber muskuläre Cirrhose der Lunge. Beitr Klin Tuberk 1937;90:432–442.
120. Rosendal T. A case of diffuse myomatosis and cyst formation in the lung. Acta Radiol 1942;23:138–146.
121. Laipply TC, Sherrick JC. Intrathoracic angiomyomatous hyperplasia associated with chronic chylothorax. Lab Invest 1958;7:387–400.
122. Cornog JL Jr, Enterline HT. Lymphangiomyoma, a benign lesion of chylous lymphatics synonymous with lymphangiopericytoma. Cancer 1966;19:1909–1930.
123. Harris JO, Waltuck BL, Swenson EW. The pathophysiology of the lungs in tuberous sclerosis. A case report and literature review. Am Rev Respir Dis 1969;100:379–387.
124. Corrin B, Liebow A, Friedman PJ. Pulmonary lymphangiomyomatosis: a review. Am J Pathol 1975;79:347–382.
125. Taylor JR, Ryv J, Colby TV, et al. Lymphangioleiomyomatosis: clinical course in 32 patients. N Engl J Med 1990; 323:1254–1260.
126. Kalassian KG, Doyle R, Kao P, et al. Pulmonary perspective: lymphangio-leiomyomatosis. New insights. Am J Respir Crit Care Med 1997;155:1187–1186.
127. Matsui K, Takeda K, Yu Z-X, et al. Down regulation of estrogen and progesterone receptors in the abnormal smooth muscle cells in pulmonary lymphangioleiomyomatosis following therapy. Am J Respir Crit Care Med 2000; 161:1002–1009.
128. Matsui K, Takeda K, Yu Z-X, et al. Role of activation of matrix metalloproteinases in the pathogenesis of pulmonary lymphangioleiomyomatosis. Arch Pathol Lab Med 2000;124:267–275.
129. Taveira-DaSilva AM, Hedin C, Stylianou M, et al. Reversible airflow obstruction, proliferation of abnormal smooth muscle cells, and impairment of gas exchange as predictors of outcome in lymphangioleiomyomatosis. Am J Respir Crit Care Med 2001; 164:1072–1076.
130. Kumaki F, Takeda K, Yu Z-X, et al. Expression of human telomerase reverse transcriptase in lymphangioleiomyomatosis. Am J Respir Crit Care Med 2002;166:187–191.
131. Evans SE, Colby TV, Ryu JH, et al. Transforming growth factor-β1 and extracellular matrix-associated fibronectin expression in Pulmonary lymphangioleiomyomatosis. Chest 2004;125:1063–1070.
132. Kumasaka T, Seyama K, Mitani K, et al. Lymphangiogenesis in lymphangio-leiomyomatosis: its implication in the progression of lymphangioleiomyomatosis. Am J Surg Pathol 2004;28:1007–1016.

133. Atkins KA, Ferguson K. Pathologic quiz case. A 23 year old woman with recurrent pneumothorax. Arch Pathol Lab Med 2000; 124:1841–1842.
134. Castro M, Shepherd C, Gomez M, et al. Pulmonary tuberous sclerosis. Chest 1995;107:189–195.
135. Muir TE, Leslie KO, Popper H, et al. Micronodular pneumocyte hyperplasia. Am J Surg Pathol 1998;22:465–472.
136. van Slegtenhorst M, de Hoogt R, Hermans C, et al. Identification of the tuberous sclerosis gene TSC1 on chromosome 9q34. Science 1997;277:805–808.
137. Popper HH, Juettner-Smolle FM, Pontgratz MG. Micronodular hyperplasia of type II pneumocytes—a new lung lesion associated with tuberous sclerosis. Histopathology 1991;16:347–54.
138. Harris JO, Waltuck BL, Swenson EW. The pathophysiology of the lungs in tuberous sclerosis. A case report and literature review. Am Rev Respir Dis 1969;100:379–387.
139. Lenoir S, Bravner M, et al. Pulmonary lymphangiomyomatosis and tuberous sclerosis: comparison and radiographic and thin-section CT findings. Radiology 1990;175:329–334.
140. Stern EJ, Webb WR, Golden JA, et al. Cystic lung disease associated with eosinophilic granuloma and tuberous sclerosis. Air trapping at dynamic ultrafast high-resolution CT. Radiology 1992;182:325–329.
141. Milledge RD, Gerald BE, Carter WJ. Pulmonary manifestations of tuberous sclerosis. Am J Roentgenol 1966;98:734–738.
142. Jao J, Gilbert S, Messer R. Lymphangiomyoma and tuberous sclerosis. Cancer 1972;29:1188–1192.
143. Monteforte WJ Jr, Kohnen PW. Angiomyolipomas in a case of lymphangiomatous syndrome: relationship to tuberous sclerosis. Cancer 1974;34:317–321.
144. Stovin PGI, Lum LC, Flower CDR, et al. The lungs in lymphangiomyomatosis and in tuberous sclerosis. Thorax 1975;30:497–509.
145. Valensi QJ. Pulmonary lymphangiomyoma, a probable forme frust of tuberous sclerosis, report of a case and survey of the literature. Am Rev Respir Dis 1973;108:1411–1415.
146. Capron F, Ameille J, Leclerq P, et al. Pulmonary lymphangioleiomyomatosis and Bourneville's tuberous sclerosis with pulmonary involvement: the same disease? Cancer 1983;52:851–855.
147. Silverstein EF, Ellis K, Wolff M, et al. Pulmonary lymphangiomyomatosis. AJR 1974;120:832–850.
148. Slingerland JM, Grossman RF, Chamberlain D, et al. Pulmonary manifestations of tuberous sclerosis in first degree relatives. Thorax 1989;44:212–214.
149. Cagnano M, Benharroch D, Geffen DB. Pulmonary lymphangioleiomyomatosis: report of a case with associated multiple soft-tissue tumors. Arch Pathol Lab Med 1991;115:1257–1259.
150. Kreisman H, Robitaille Y, Dionne GP, et al. Lymphangiomyomatosis syndrome with hyperparathyroidism: a case report. Cancer 1978;42:364–372.
151. Huml JP, Borkgren MW, Henley LB, et al. Pulmonary lymphangioleiomyomatosis associated with pulmonary parenchymal, hilar and mediastinal noncaseating granulomas. Chest 1991;100:1726–1728.
152. Fahy J, Toner M, O'Sullivan J, et al. Haemopericardium and cardiac tamponade complicating pulmonary lymphangioleiomyomatosis. Thorax 1991;46:222.
153. Folpe AL. Neoplasms with perivascular epithelioid cell differentiation (PEComas). In: Travis WD, Brambilla E, Müller-Hermelink HK, Harris CC, eds. World Health Organization classification of tumours. Pathology and genetics. Tumours of the lung, pleura, thymus and heart. Lyon: IARC Press, 2004:221–222.
154. Carrington CB, Cugell DW, Gaensler EA. Lymphangioleiomyomatosis. Physiologic–pathologic–radiologic correlations. Am Rev Respir Dis 1977;116:977–995.
155. Fukuda Y, Kawamoto M, Yamamoto A et al. Role of elastic fiber degradation in emphysema-like lesions of pulmonary lymphoangiomyomatosis. Hum Pathol 1990;21:1252–1261.
156. Brauner MW, Grenier P, Mouelhi MM, et al. Pulmonary histiocytosis X: evaluation with high-resolution CT. Radiology 1989;172:255–258.
157. Moore ADA, Godwin JD, Müller NL, et al. Pulmonary histiocytosis X: comparison of radiographic and CT findings. Radiology 1989;172:249–254.
158. Travis WD, Colby TV, Corrin B, et al. World Health Organization. International histological classification of tumours. Histological typing of lung and pleural tumors. Berlin, Heidelberg, New York: Springer, 1999:50.
159. Hughes E, Hodder RV. Pulmonary lymphangiomyomatosis complicating pregnancy: a case report. J Reprod Med 1987;32:553–557.
160. Silverstein EF, Ellis K, Wolff M, et al. Pulmonary lymphangiomyomatosis. AJR Am J Roentgenol 1974;120:832–850.
161. Corrin B, Liebow AA, Friedman PJ. Pulmonary lymphangiomyomatosis: a review. Am J Pathol 1975;79:348–382.
162. Matsui K, Beasley MB, Nelson WK, et al. Prognostic significance of pulmonary lymphangioleiomyomatosis histologic score. Am J Surg Pathol 2001;25:479–484.
163. Travis WD, Colby TV, Koss MN, et al. Atlas of non tumor pathology, first series, fascicle 2, non neoplastic disorders of the lower respiratory tract. Washington, DC: American Registry of Pathology and the Armed Forces Institute of Pathology, 2002:147–160.
164. Fletcher CDM. Diagnostic histopathology of tumors. 2nd ed. London, Edinburgh, New York: Churchill Livingstone, 2000:75–77.
165. Alt B, Huffer WE, Belchis DA. A vascular lesion with smooth muscle differentiation presenting as a coin lesion in the lung: glomus tumor versus hemangiopericytoma. Am J Clin Pathol 1983;80:765–770.
166. Slater DN, Cotton DWK, Azzopardi JG. Oncocytic glomus tumour: a new variant. Histopathology 1987;11:523–531.
167. Fabich DR, Hafez G-R. Glomangioma of the trachea. Cancer 1980;45:2337–2341.
168. Ito H, Motohiro K, Nomura S, et al. Glomus tumor of the trachea: immunohistochemical and electron microscopic studies. Pathol Res Pract 1988;183:778–784.
169. Kim YI, Kim JH, Suh J-S, et al. Glomus tumor of the trachea: report of a case with ultrastructural observation. Cancer 1989;64:881–886.
170. Gaertner EM, Steinberg DM, Huber M, et al. Pulmonary and mediastinal glomus tumors. Report of 5 cases includ-

ing a pulmonary glomangiosarcoma: a clinicopathologic study with literature review. Am J Surg Pathol 2000;24: 1105–1114.
171. Altorjay A, Arató G, Adame M, et al. Synchronous multiple glomus tumors of the esophagus and lung. Hepatogastroenterology 2003;50:687–690.
172. Hishida T, Hasegawa T, Asamura H, et al. Malignant glomus tumor of the lung. Pathol Int 2003;52:632–636.
173. Nadrous HF, Allen MS, Bartholomai BJ, et al. Glomus tumor of the trachea: value of multidetector computed tomographic virtual bronchoscopy. Mayo Clin Proc 2004;79:237–240.
174. Folpe AL. In: Fletcher CDM, Unni K, Mertens F, eds. World Health Organization classification of tumors. Pathology and genetics. Tumors of soft tissue and bone. Lyon: IARC Press, 2002:136–137.
175. Koss MN, Hochholzer L, Moran CA. Primary pulmonary glomus tumor: a clinicopathologic and immunohistochemical study of two cases. Mod Pathol 1998;11:253–258.
176. Kapadia SB, Barr FG. Rhabdomyoma. In: Fletcher DM, Unni KK, Mertens F, eds. World Health Organization classification of tumours. Pathology and genetics. Tumors of soft tissue and bone. Lyon: IARC Press, 2002:142–145.
177. Kapadia SB, Meiss JM, Frisman DM, et al. Adult rhabomyoma of the head and neck: a clinico-pathologic and immunophenotypic study. Hum Pathol 1993;24:608–617.
178. Ramaswamy A, Weyers I, Duda V, et al. A tumorous type of pulmonary rhabdomyomatous dysplasia. Pathol Res Pract 1998;194:639–642.
179. Lee SH, Rengachary SS, Paramesh J. Primary pulmonary rhabdomyosarcoma: a case report and review of the literature. Hum Pathol 1981;12:92–95.
180. Helbing C, 1898, as quoted by Drennan JM, McCormack RJM. Primary rhabdomyosarcoma of the lung. J Pathol Bacteriol 1960;79:147–149.
181. Avignina A, Elsner B, DeMarco L, et al. Pulmonary rhabdomyosarcoma with isolated small bowel metastases: a report of a case with immunohistological and ultrastructural studies. Cancer 1984;53:1948–1951.
182. Allan BT, Day DL, Dehner LP. Primary pulmonary rhabdomyosarcoma of the lung in children: report of two cases presenting with spontaneous pneumothorax. Cancer 1987;59:1005–1011.
183. Christ WM, Raney RB, Jr, Newton W, et al.; for the Intergroup Rhabdomyosarcoma Study Committee. Intrathoracic soft tissue sarcomas in children. Cancer 1982;50: 598–604.
184. Moran CA, Suster S, Koss MN. Primary malignant "triton" tumour of the lung. Histopathology 1997;30:140–144.
185. Koss M, Travis W, Moran C. Pulmonary sarcomas, blastomas, carcinosarcomas and teratomas. In: Hasleton PS, ed. Spencer's pathology of the lung. 5th ed. New York, St. Louis, San Francisco: McGraw-Hill, 1996:1070–1071.

40
Mesenchymal Tumors, Part II: Tumors of Hamartomatous, Osteochondromatous, Lipomatous, Neural, and Vascular Origin

Armando E. Fraire and David H. Dail

Pulmonary Hamartomas

Pulmonary hamartomas, also known as benign mesenchymomas (and a variety of other names such as fibrochondrolipomas and adenochondromas) represent the most common benign neoplasms of the lung. However, the true frequency of lung hamartomas is difficult to measure since some predominantly chondroid tumors may variously be reported as either chondroid hamartomas or chondromas.[1] In one series, 100 (77%) of 130 benign tumor masses of the lung were hamartomas.[2] In a study of 7972 autopsies by McDonald et al.,[1] there were 20 hamartomas, a prevalence of about one case per 400 autopsies. Hamartomas are up to four times as common in men as in women in parenchymal locations, but of more equal sex distribution in the central regions (near the hilar areas) and occur mostly in the age group from the late 30s to the early 70s, with a peak in the late 50s and early 60s.[1,3–5] However, rare cases have been described in teenagers and children. Hamartomas have not been described at earlier ages; they are not seen in infants, and do not appear to be of congenital origin. Detailed vital statistics along with histopathologic data in a large series of cases reported by Tomashefski[6] are presented in Table 40.1. Rarely hamartomas will occur in association with other lesions such as sclerosing hemangiomas.[7] Equally rare is the occurrence of an isolated (tumor to tumor) carcinomatous metastasis from an extrapulmonary tumor into a pulmonary hamartoma.[8]

The histogenesis of pulmonary hamartomas has been discussed by several authors, but most now agree they are not congenital lesions.[9] The term *hamartoma* is still used, however, to describe these lesions and is retained because of its familiarity and common usage. It is nevertheless recognized that the term *hamartoma* carries with it the implication of a congenital malformation. Whether hamartomas are reactive growths in response to some type of inflammation is unclear, but considering the number of episodes of pulmonary inflammation and the low incidence of hamartomas, and considering their solitary state compared to multifocal areas usually involved with inflammation, this is most unlikely. The surrounding lung and bronchi are usually normal when these lesions are first detected. More than likely they are benign neoplastic proliferations whose growth is controlled by unknown factors. Tomashefski[6] refers to them as benign mesenchymomas of lung, which seems a fairly good term given the peculiar combination of tissues seen microscopically.

Glandular inclusions within hamartomas are fairly common. In the past, these inclusions have caused considerable debate as to their genesis. Bateson,[10–12] in several sequential studies, has shown that the glandular component of hamartomas is caused by metaplasia of alveolar lining cells and entrapped bronchiolar cells. Several electron microscopic studies are compatible with this view.[13,14] Intranuclear inclusions have been found in the lining cells, and probably represent surfactant as in alveolar and metaplastic lining cells.[13,14] Such entrapments occur in other low-grade primary pulmonary neoplasms and even in very low grade metastases. Most hamartomas are solitary. There are, however, occasional cases of multiple cartilaginous hamartomas, and these seem to be more frequent in association with the Carney's syndrome.[15] This syndrome consists of epithelioid gastric smooth muscle tumors, either leiomyomas or leiomyosarcomas, functioning extraadrenal paragangliomas, and pulmonary chondromas (see Pulmonary Chondroma, below). The association between these diverse proliferating tissues is unclear, but the syndrome appears now to be accepted as such, and it occurs predominantly in girls and young

TABLE 40.1. Comparative features of endobronchial and parenchymal hamartomas

Features	Endobronchial (n = 17)	Parenchymal (n = 147)
Age		
Range	43–73 years	17–77 years
Mean	52.9 years	56.2 years
Sex (M/F)	9/8	92/55
Involved lung (L/R)	13/4	43/45*
Size (maximum dimension)		
Range	0.3–3.4 cm	0.3–6 cm
Mean	1.4 cm	1.7 cm
Shape	Polypoid	Spherical
Epithelial clefts		
Internal	3 (18%)	127 (86%)
Peripheral	2 (12%)	135 (92%)
Mesenchymal derivatives		
Cartilage	14 (82%)	141 (96%)
Percent cartilage		
≥90%	3 (18%)	57 (39%)
75–<90%	1 (6%)	44 (30%)
50–<75%	3 (18%)	27 (18%)
10–<50%	7 (41%)	9 (6%)
<10%	0	4 (3%)
None	3 (18%)	6 (4%)
Bone	2 (12%)	3 (2%)
Adipose tissue	14 (82%)	110 (75%)
Fibrous tissue	13 (76%)	108 (74%)
Fibroadenoma-like areas	1 (6%)	12 (8%)

Source: Tomashefski,[6] with permission of Lippincott Williams & Wilkins.
*88 cases with data available.

women under the age of 20 who may have only two of the three lesions mentioned. Gabrail and Zara[16] found a high percentage of other abnormalities in 24 cases they reviewed. They particularly noted an increased incidence of other benign tumors, mostly outside the chest, and other developmental abnormalities. In the latter group lesions such as inguinal hernias are included, and it is open to debate whether this is a developmental abnormality. We agree with these authors that more correlation is needed in a larger number of cases to determine the statistical significance of these assorted associated disorders. These authors note that many of the associated findings may overlap with Cowden's syndrome, but also that pulmonary hamartomas are not part of Cowden's multihamartoma syndrome.

There is a question as to whether hamartomas ever become malignant.[17–19] If malignant transformation occurs, it is exceedingly rare. There is an increased incidence of lung cancers in these patients, but whether this is related to a greater use of chest radiographs and follow-up is unclear. One case was stable for 37 years and then underwent "explosive sarcomatous evolution," almost totally occupying a lower lobe.[18] Another case documented a benign-appearing recurrence 5 years after a tracheal chondroma was excised. Six years after that, chondrosarcoma developed at this site and the patient died of metastases 1 year later.[19] Given the challenge of diagnosing low-grade cartilaginous lesions in other sites, this may be a better example of such a problem. In one study, clonality was evaluated in two cases of pulmonary hamartomas, and, of interest, both showed stromal cell chromosomal aberrations.[20] Further evidence of neoplastic transformation was provided by Fletcher et al.[21] In a study of 17 cases of pulmonary chondroid hamartomas, these authors identified clonal chromosomal aberrations in mesenchymal cells in 10 of the 17 reported cases. Chromosome band 12q-15 was rearranged in four cases, and one other case had a t(12:14) (q15;q24) translocation, which is identical to the translocation that is regarded as characteristic of uterine leiomyomas (see Chapter 33).

Within the past 20 years there have been two major series of hamartomas, one by van den Bosch et al.[22] and the other by Gjevre and associates.[23] The van den Bosch series provides data to support the current concept of this tumor being a benign neoplasm rather than a malformation, based on age, incidence, and progressive growth. The Gjevre study of 215 patients found a substantial number (29.3%) of patients with a concurrent neoplasm, most commonly lung carcinoma. This study, however, found no evidence of malignant transformation.

Submucosal hamartomas in the airways may erode the overlying mucosa and present with hemoptysis. Their endoscopic appearance is not distinctive (Fig. 40.1). In contrast, most parenchymal hamartomas are clinically silent and are discovered incidentally.

Radiographically, an occasional endobronchial hamartoma may present as an air-displacing mass within the air shadow of the bronchi, but most often such lesions are detected because of symptoms leading to direct

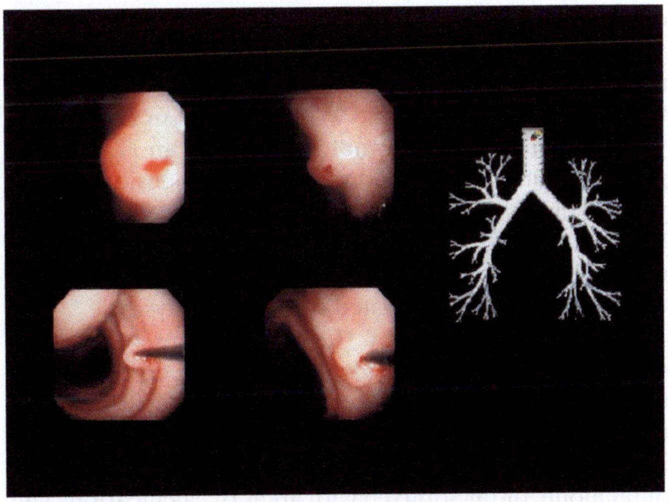

FIGURE 40.1. Hamartoma. Endoscopic view. Small spheroidal lesion covered by intact respiratory mucosa. (Courtesy of Dr. Richard Irwin, University of Massachusetts Medical School, Worcester, MA.)

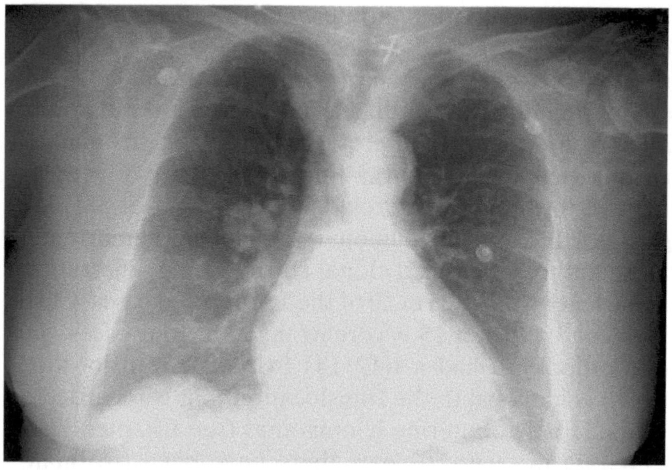

FIGURE 40.2. Hamartoma. Radiograph of chest. Note opaque round lesion in right mid-lung field.

examination of these areas. Peripheral hamartomas are often subpleural and incidental on chest radiographs. Their radiographic characteristics have been well described by Bateson and Abbott[24] as sharply defined masses, often with lobulated borders, most often subpleural, and most often less than 3 cm in diameter (Fig. 40.2). Speckled calcification can be seen on radiographs, and in one series this was seen in four (16%) of 25 cases.[9] As smaller nodular growths within the lesions are often found protruding in different directions, calcification (Fig. 40.3) in each of these protrusions may be seen as a "popcorn"-type calcification, but this occurs less frequently than originally believed.[25–27] Occasionally, areas of lesser density, especially seen at the periphery of the nodules, may be seen radiographically and are compatible with fat tissue. Some hamartomas have been noted to enlarge while under radiographic surveillance. Jensen and Schiodt[28] and Weisel et al.[29] estimated growth at about 0.5 cm in diameter per year. Sagel and Ablow[30] reported one case that grew from 1 to 2.6 cm over 1.5 years. Weinberger et al.[31] noted growth in an 11-year-old patient from 2 to 7 cm in maximum dimension over 3 years. This lesion was unusual in that it also encircled the hilar structures and required pneumonectomy for removal. In one case followed over 20 years, the tumor doubling time was estimated to be 4968 days.[32]

Computed tomography (CT) has further refined the distinction of fat and cartilage, and has been effectively used by Siegelman and associates[33] in suggesting a diagnosis of hamartoma. Their criteria include lesions 2.5 cm in diameter or less, with a smooth edge, with focal areas of fat alone, or fat admixed with areas of calcification. The presence of fat was most helpful, either alone (18 cases) or intermixed with calcification (10 cases). Seventeen cases did not have fat and could not be further classified by CT scans. Using these criteria, none of the 283 cases of primary carcinomas or any of the 72 cases of metastatic carcinomas was confused with hamartomas.

Grossly, hamartomas vary from a few millimeters to 20 cm, but most are in the range of 1 to 3 cm. They usually "pop out" from the peripheral lung tissue, are rounded, and may have small smoothly contoured irregularities on their surface. Endobronchial hamartomas are often polypoid, either sessile or with a thin pedicle. Whether peripheral or central, they are usually well circumscribed from surrounding tissue and their texture is firm, usually cartilaginous and shiny owing to myxoid changes, although there may be areas that correlate with fat. The central lesions tend to develop predominantly cartilage, and the peripheral lesions are more an admixture of fibrous tissue, cartilage, and fat (Figs. 40.4 and 40.5).

As in other anatomic sites, hamartomas of the lung consist essentially of focal excessive disorderly growth of cells and tissues that are native to a given organ. Microscopically, mature cartilage is present in most pulmonary lesions, including 82% of endobronchial and 96% of parenchymal ones.[2,6] As shown in Table 40.1, the relative proportion of cartilage also varies depending on the location of the lesion. The cartilage appears more hyaline in central lesions and more fibrohyaline in the peripheral ones. In those lesions that are predominantly made of cartilage, cartilaginous nests seem always to be surrounded by some cellular fibrous tissue, and often there are collections of mature fat cells. Sometimes other tissue components are monotonous and compose the predominant mass without cartilage, such as occurs with lipomas, and possibly fibromas and myxomas of both lung and bronchi (Figs. 40.6 and 40.7). Some consider the latter lesions discrete and others part of hamartomatous development. Rarely the fat cells have appeared atypical. Rarely there

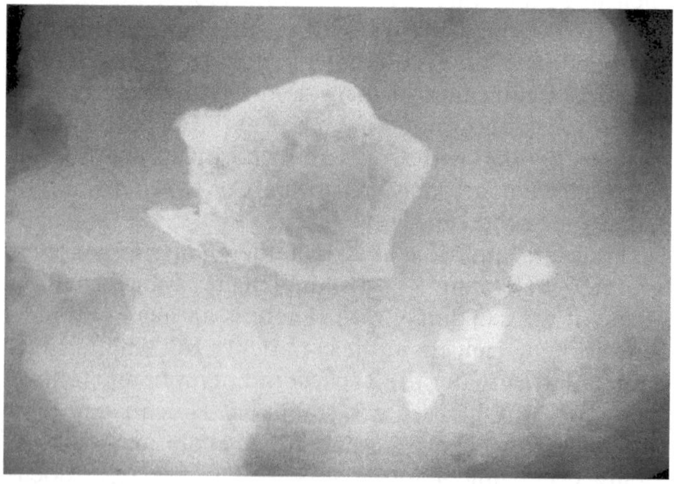

FIGURE 40.3. Hamartoma. Specimen radiograph with "popcorn" calcifications. (Courtesy of Dr. Terrence Gleason, Providence Medical Center, Seattle, WA.)

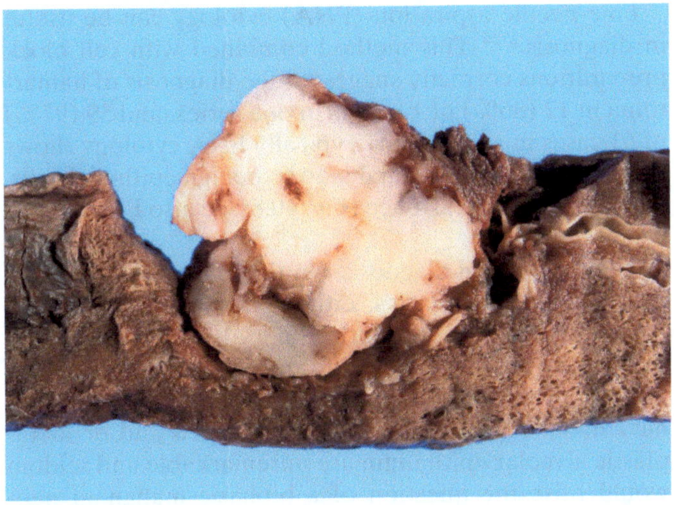

FIGURE 40.4. Parenchymal hamartoma. Surgically resected specimen corresponding to lesion illustrated in the preceding radiograph of chest (Fig. 40.2). Note tan gray, well-circumscribed lobulated growth.

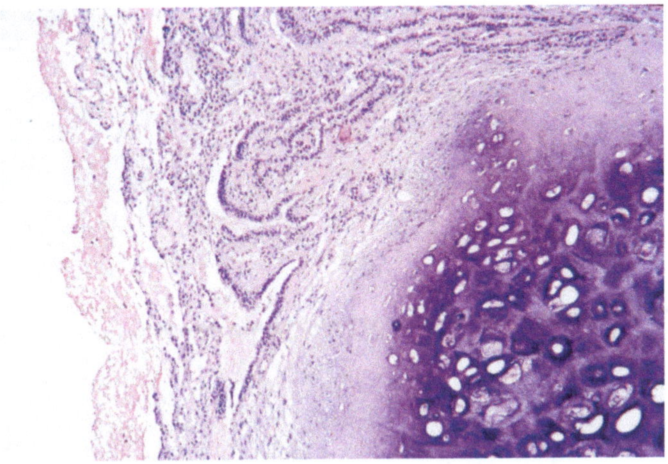

FIGURE 40.6. Hamartoma. Note prominent chondroid component on the right and epithelial lined clefts on the left.

may be bone, and occasionally entrapped vessels, bronchioles, or a variable but generally small amount of smooth muscle. The smooth muscle component, however, may be prominent in some cases, giving some lesions a fibroleiomyomatous appearance. The so-called fibroleiomyomatous hamartoma, however, is a nonentity and is now considered to represent primary or metastatic smooth muscle proliferations (see Chapter 39).

Depending on the plane of section, one can find these lesions developing in the wall of bronchioles and occasionally of small bronchi. At times native cartilage is seen in the peripheral lesions, being enveloped by the new growth. In

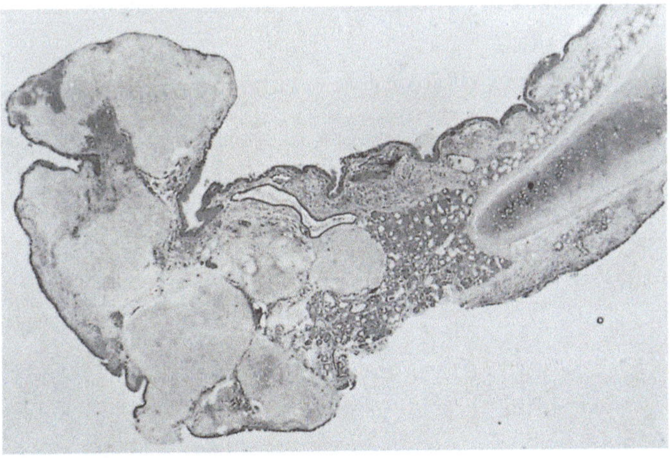

FIGURE 40.5. Polypoid endobronchial hamartoma. Grossly this nodular mass extends into major bronchus, from a site of slight thickening of adjacent bronchial wall. Multinodular areas of cartilage are unattached to the native bronchial cartilage.

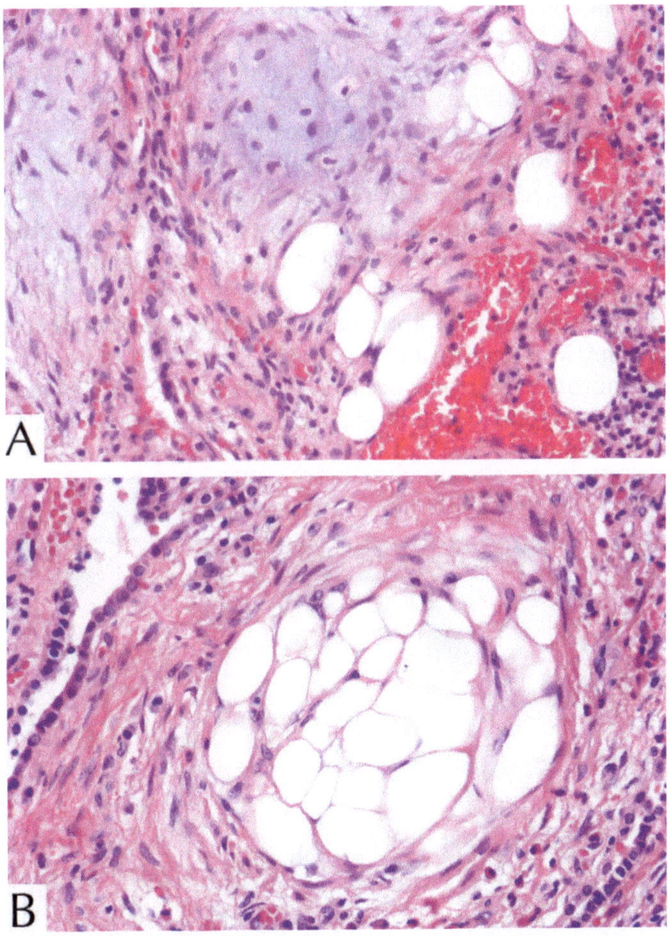

FIGURE 40.7. Hamartoma. **(A)** Note myxoid tissue component and scattered adipocytes. **(B)** Note a conglomeration of fat in a fibrous stroma and a cleft lined by cuboidal epithelium.

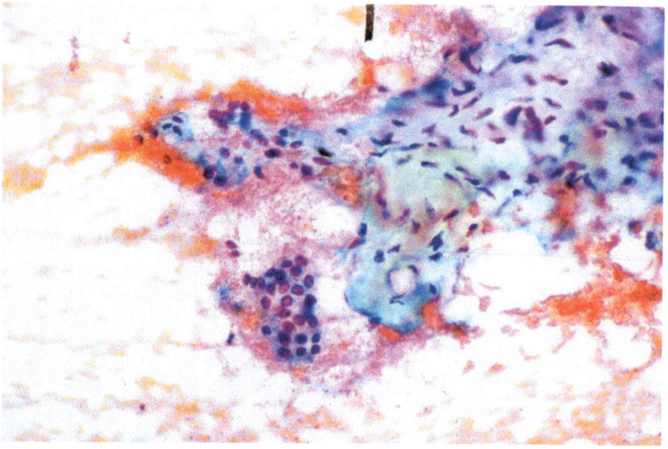

FIGURE 40.8. Hamartoma. Cytologic preparation showing myxoid mesenchymal matrix and a group of small round epithelial cells. (Courtesy of Dr. Andrew Fischer, University of Massachusetts Medical School, Worcester, MA.)

the central lesions, cartilaginous proliferations of any size may or may not show fusion with the cartilaginous rings. The previously mentioned glandular component, if present, can easily be traced from adjacent alveoli or adjacent bronchioles, and the lining cells are cuboidal to low columnar and are sometimes distorted in their course within the lesions themselves, presumably caused by irregularly proliferating mesenchyme. At times terminal bronchioles can be identified because of the cilia in their lining cells and some wisps of smooth muscle. Most of the time the lining cells appear more like metaplastic cells. As expected, the cartilaginous components are S-100 protein positive. Other components express fibronectin and types I, II, and III collagen.[34] Mukensnabl and Hadravska[35] described an unusual chondroid hamartoma occurring in association with islands of small, round to spindle-shaped cells showing neuroendocrine features.

Fine-needle aspiration (FNA) cytology can be useful in diagnosis.[25,26] This method combined with cell block preparations correctly suggested the diagnosis of hamartoma in 12 (86%) of 14 cases in one series, and 59 (97%) of 61 cases in another.[25,26] Typically FNA cytology shows a fibrillary myxoid stromal matrix, benign epithelial cells, and fragments of cartilage (Fig. 40.8; see also Fig. 45.26 in Chapter 45).

The differential diagnosis is quite limited and includes mesenchymal neoplasms, either primary or metastatic. Any evidence of significant cellular atypia, mitotic activity, or necrosis must raise the question of a primary or metastatic sarcoma. The epithelial elements of pulmonary hamartomas representing entrapped and or metaplastic alveolar epithelium are unremarkable and seldom would raise the question of a biphasic malignant neoplasm such as carcinosarcoma. Pulmonary hamartoma is a benign lesion. Simple surgical excision, sometimes enucleation of the lesion suffices, and most if not all excisions result in a cure. Laser therapy has been used for centrally located lesions.[36]

Pulmonary Chondroma

Tumors described in the past as chondromas, myxomas and fibromyomas are difficult to differentiate from pulmonary hamartomas. This difficulty arises primarily from the often prominent chondromatous component in tumors diagnosed as chondromatoid hamartoma or chondrohamartomas[1,11,24,34,35] and to a lesser degree from terminology.[1]

In our opinion, the term *chondroma* should be reserved for those rare tumors entirely or nearly entirely made up of cartilage and some bone but with no fat or muscle or any other mesenchymal component (Fig. 40.9). Chondromas are recognized as integral components of

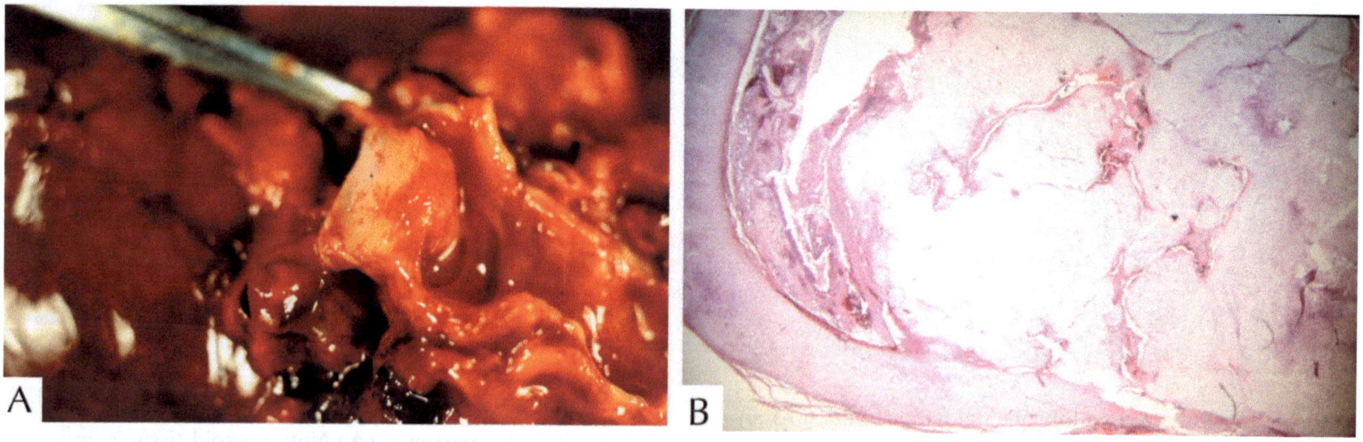

FIGURE 40.9. **(A)** Endobronchial chondroma in a bronchiectatic airway. **(B)** Microscopic view of the lesion shown in **A** with focal attachment of tumor to bronchial wall. (Courtesy of Dr. J.F. Tomashefski, Jr., MetroHealth Medical Center, Cleveland, OH.)

the Carney triad (epithelioid gastric stromal tumors, pulmonary chondroma, and extraadrenal paragangliomas),[15] and are known to occur in the larynx and major airways as well as in the lung itself. A recent paper reaffirms the separate existence of pulmonary chondromas, at least in the setting of the Carney's triad, calling attention to their sharp circumscription, their capsule, the predominance of hyaline cartilage and bone, with foci of calcification, and their lack of internal epithelium and other mesenchymal tissue elements.[37]

Chondrosarcoma

Malignant mesenchymal tumors made up of neoplastic cartilage are well documented in bone and somatic soft tissues. However, their occurrence in the larynx, conducting airways, and pulmonary parenchyma is distinctly uncommon and much less well documented. Bone and soft tissue chondrosarcomas are characterized by plump atypical chondrocytes arranged in lobular structures separated from one another by thin septa of connective tissue. In the respiratory tract their morphology is quite similar (Fig. 40.10).

Pulmonary chondrosarcomas were first described as enchondromas of lung, with the first description attributed to Wilks[38] in 1862. It is difficult if not impossible, however, to evaluate this report and many of the early cases, as criteria for the diagnosis of better-differentiated chondrosarcomas were established only by the 1940s. Some of the older cases may no longer qualify as chondrosarcomas. One must be sure that the case in question is not a case of a large hamartoma with a prominent chondromatous component or a chondroma. In a 1972 review of the subject, Morgan and Salama,[39] using very restrictive criteria (to eliminate chondrosarcomas from other sites possibly spreading to the lung), reported eight cases of chondrosarcoma, including two previously described cases with vascular invasion, one such case predominantly located in the pulmonary artery and the other involving the pulmonary vein. A few of these cases may be in the category of large vessel chondrosarcomas, but some are most likely truly parenchymal. Other cases have been described in the tracheobronchial tree, particularly in the trachea and lobar bronchi.[40,41] One must always suspect metastases if the lesions are multiple. An early case described as chondrosarcomatosis of the lung was wisely eliminated from consideration by Morgan and Salama, and is now known to be a case of epithelioid hemangioendothelioma of lung with dystrophic chondrification.[39,42] Primary chondrosarcomas occur in the pleura.[43] Hayashi and associates[44] in 1993 summarized the world literature and added a case of their own, which occurred in the major bronchus of 73-year-old man.

The clinical presentation is not unique, with most patients having nonspecific symptoms and signs such as cough, dyspnea, or chest pain.[45] As would be expected on account of their strategic anatomic location, chondrosarcomas of the conducting airways tend to manifest themselves earlier and more severely than their parenchymal counterparts.[45] Radiographically, five of the seven cases reviewed by Morgan and Salama[39] contained foci of calcification or ossification. This finding warrants caution, as there is a radiographic dictum that calcified pulmonary coin lesions are mostly benign granulomatous lesions.[46] In most cases this is true, but chondrosarcomas (and osteosarcomas) are notable exceptions.

Grossly, these tumors are variegated and nodular, with some cartilaginous, translucent gray-white areas admixed

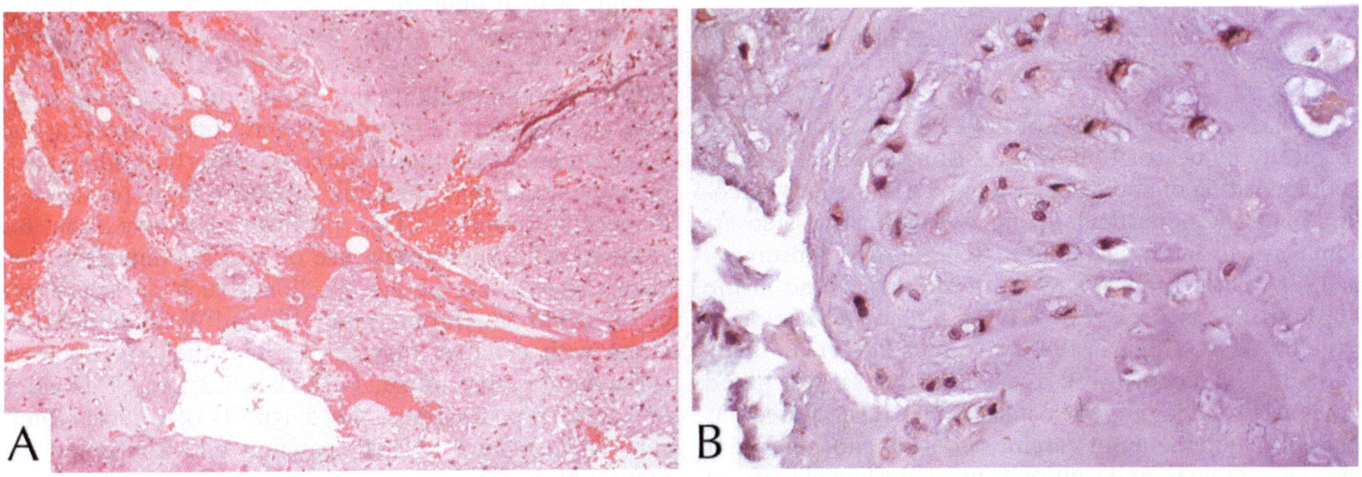

FIGURE 40.10. Chondrosarcoma. **(A)** Note distinct lobulations in this chondrosarcoma of trachea. **(B)** Chondrocytes in this field are plump and atypical.

with cystic areas, some with more densely calcified areas, and some with focal necrosis and hemorrhage. Microscopically, most are reported as rather well-differentiated chondrosarcomas made of plump atypical chondrocytes arranged in relatively well-defined lobules (Fig. 40.10). However, less well differentiated tumors do occur.[47] One such case, a mesenchymal variant of chondrosarcoma, was reported by Huang and coworkers[47] in a 40-year-old woman who had a tumor characterized by islands of atypical chondroid cells enmeshed within dense sheets of primitive small blue cells with hemangiopericytoma-like vascular components.

In addition to metastatic chondrosarcoma from distant sites and local spread from a rib primary, the differential diagnosis includes pulmonary chondromas and other tumors with chondrosarcomatous foci, such as malignant mesenchymomas, carcinosarcomas, mesotheliomas, and epithelioid hemangioendotheliomas.

Treatment consists primarily of surgical resection.[44] The prognosis is generally poor, but some chondrosarcomas may follow a protracted course over many years after surgical resection. The patient reported by Daniels et al.[41] underwent a palliative endobronchial resection of a chondrosarcoma that was followed for 3 years without further complications. Bailey and Head[43] described a patient with a presumed primary pleural chondrosarcoma with bony changes, who had a very long survival without evidence of recurrence 13 years after resection. On the other hand, Morgenroth et al.[40] reported another patient with a 6.0-cm chondrosarcoma of the left-lower-lobe bronchus, and this patient died only 8 months later with massive mediastinal nodal spread. Another patient experienced a recurrence first at the bronchial line of excision several times before spreading to the mediastinum.[48] At times a period of slow growth is noted following a very rapid increase in tumor size.[42] In one series, most patients were dead within 6 months.[41]

Osteosarcoma

Osteosarcomas are tumors of bone characterized microscopically by destruction of preexisting bone trabeculae and deposition of malignant osteoid. Extraosseous osteosarcomas and in particular primary pulmonary osteosarcomas are distinctly uncommon. Reingold and Amromin[49] in 1971 added two cases to the three they found in the literature. Later, in a review of 18 pulmonary sarcomas from the Mayo Clinic in 1982 by Nascimento et al.,[50] only two additional cases were so classified, and it was noted that each was a high-grade osteosarcoma. Osteosarcomas may be components of carcinosarcomas and malignant mesenchymomas, and caution is needed when classifying sarcomatous tumors. Occasionally, on further sampling of tumors that were originally thought to be primary osteosarcomas, epithelial areas became apparent; this was the case in two of five patients reported by Colby et al.[51] and one of two cases reported by Loose et al.,[52] the latter being a case where the epithelial nature was detected only in a mediastinal recurrence. By 1990 there was a total of only about 10 reported pulmonary cases without any malignant epithelial components.[53] These figures compare with a total of about 200 cases of extraskeletal osteosarcoma in all sites by 1987.[52] More recently Tsunezuka et al.[54] in 2004 reported a case of an osteosarcoma arising from the pulmonary artery. This case showed a prominent chondroid component and was classified as a chondromatous osteosarcoma. A further well-documented primary lung case by Sievert et al.[55] was found in the left upper lobe of a 56-year-old man. This osteoid-forming tumor with surrounding osteoblasts is illustrated in Figure 40.11.

Pulmonary osteosarcomas occur equally in men and women and are likely to be more frequent in older individuals.[56] These tumors vary from about 4 cm to massive in size. As one would expect, grossly these tumors are hard, pearly gray, and often have chalky-white opaque areas. Lobulations may be present and small cystic areas may occur. Microscopically, besides malignant osteoid (similar if not identical to that seen in primary bone tumors) and benign and malignant chondroid areas, areas of more monotonous spindle cells may intermix with some pleomorphic and more anaplastic areas. How many of these tumors should be classified as true malignant mesenchymomas is not clear.

As is the case with other pulmonary sarcomas, osteosarcomas may extend into pulmonary vessels producing tumoral emboli. In these instances, distinction from a primary osteosarcoma of the pulmonary artery as reported by Tsunezuka et al.[54] may be difficult. Other differential diagnoses include carcinosarcomas with prominent osteosarcomatous and malignant mesenchymomas with prominent osteosarcomatous components. Carcinosarcomas are more likely, however, to have distinct and prominent areas of epithelial differentiation, and this should facilitate the distinction. Malignant mesenchymomas, on the other hand, have other sarcomatous components besides osteosarcoma. Rarely, a malignant mesothelioma with osseous differentiation presents a diagnostic problem. This problem, however, can be resolved with appropriate use of positive immunohistochemical markers of mesothelioma such as calretinin, cytokeratins 5/6, thrombomodulin, and WT-1 antibodies, along with negative markers of mesothelioma such as carcinoembryonic antigen (CEA), B72.3, and CD15 (Leu M-1). In rare situations, the diagnosis of osteosarcoma can be suspected by CT scanning and confirmed by pleural biopsy.[57]

The treatment of choice is surgical resection. The prognosis, as would be expected, is poor, with most tumors

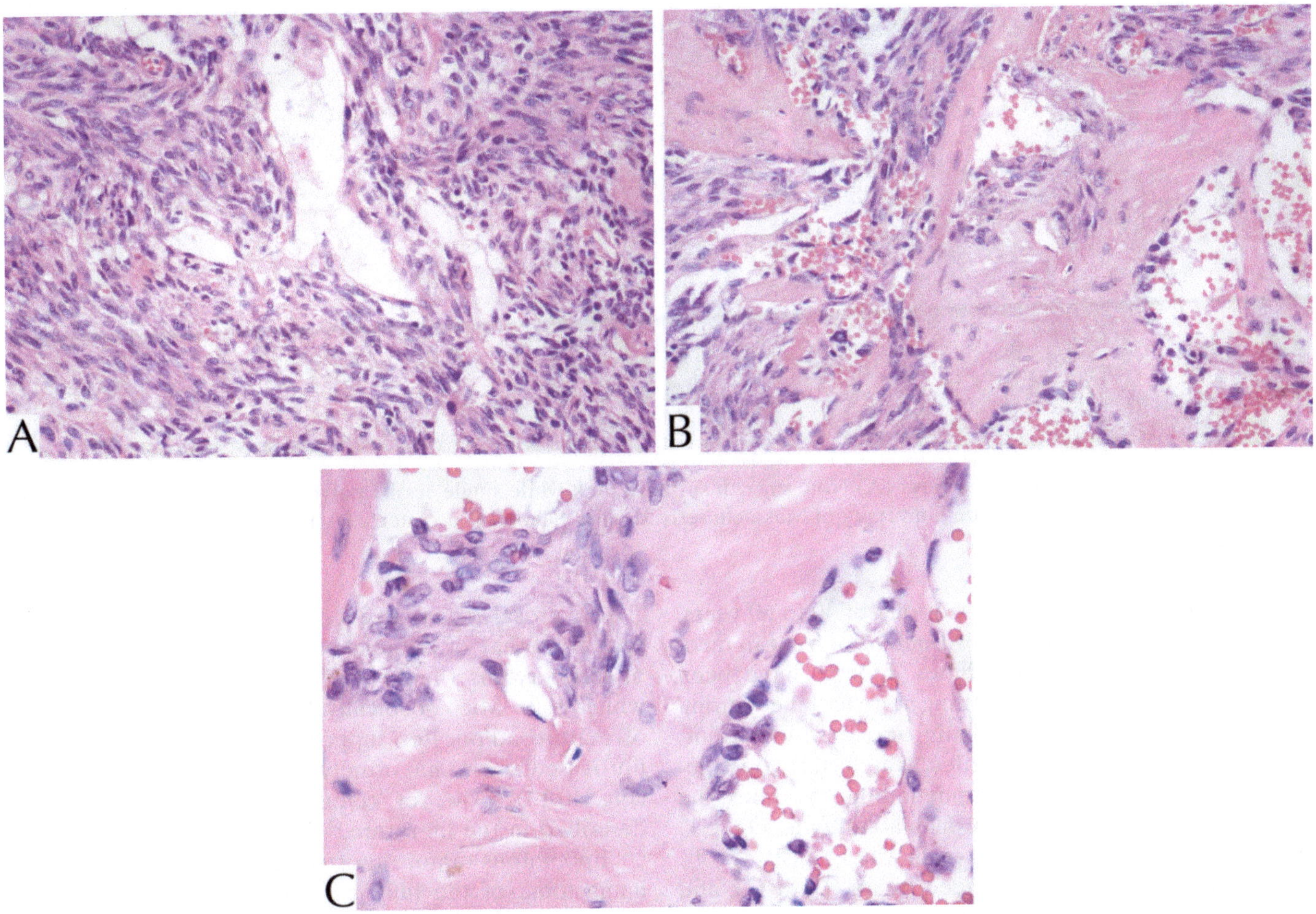

FIGURE 40.11. Primary osteosarcoma of lung. **(A)** Note cellular area resembling undifferentiated sarcoma. **(B)** In areas, eosinophilic osteoid material is evident. **(C)** Note plump highly atypical osteoblasts rimming an osteoid trabecula. (Courtesy of Drs. Maria L Evans, Laura J. Sievert and Timothy S. Loy, University of Missouri at Columbia, Columbia, MO.)

following a malignant course, with documented metastasis to the heart and regional lymph nodes.[56] Osteosarcomas arising in the pulmonary artery also carry a poor prognosis. However, intermediate levels of disease-free survival can be seen in some cases. Such was the case in Tzunezuka et al.'s[54] patient, a 58-year-old woman who was alive and free of recurrence 24 months following pneumonectomy.

Lipoma and Liposarcoma

In the lung, as in soft tissues, lipomas can be defined as benign tumors made up of mature adipocytes. Their histogenesis is not well understood, but they are believed to originate from fat cells in peribronchial tissue or from fat cells beneath the respiratory mucosa.[58] Unlike lipomas of soft tissue, lipomas of the respiratory tract are distinctly uncommon. Lipomas may occur in the bronchi, less frequently in the trachea, and occasionally in the lung parenchyma or peripherally in the subpleural zone. In the bronchi, they are submucosal and may be only submucosal or may be dumbbell shaped, extending between portions of bronchial cartilage. The true frequency of bona fide pulmonary lipomas is difficult to estimate. Lipomatous components can be seen in other pulmonary tumors such as hamartomas or angiolipomas and some of these with predominance of fat might have been reported as lipomas. Twenty-five cases were reported as lipomas by Plachta and Hershey[59] in 1962; 32 cases were further described by Crutcher and associates[60] in 1968. Additional series were published by MacArthur et al.[61] in 1977, Schraufnagel et al.,[62] and Politis et al.,[63] both in 1979. Moran et al.[64] added four cases from the Armed Forces Institute of Pathology in 1994. Altogether about 100 cases had been reported by 1994, and the actual number now may well be higher.[59–64]

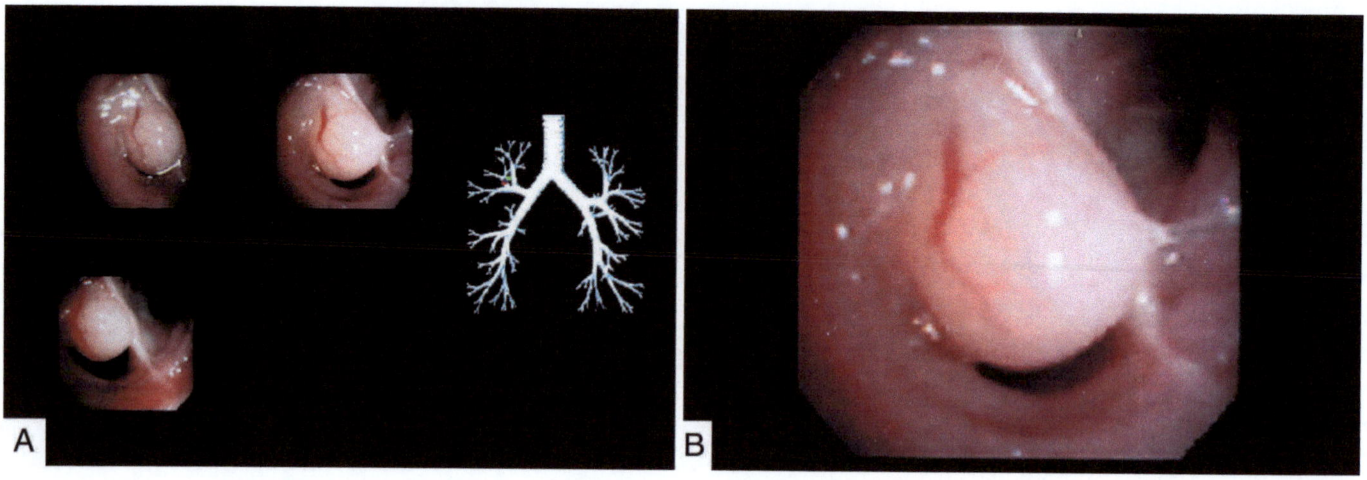

FIGURE 40.12. Lipoma, endoscopic view. **(A)** Note smooth surfaced pink white single sessile polypoid lesion. **(B)** Closer view of **A.** (Courtesy of Dr. Richard Irwin, University of Massachusetts Medical School, Worcester, MA.)

Most lipomas occur in the age group of 40 to 60 years, with a range of 29 to 64 years. About 90% occur in men, for unknown reasons. Sometimes lipomas have been noted to change in shape, becoming more flattened during deep inspiration and round again on expiration. Clinically, lipomas may become manifest as atelectasis, obstructive pneumonitis, or recurrent pneumonia. At times, the clinical picture may mimic bronchial asthma. On CT, lipomas rarely appear different from water density, probably because they are surrounded by air. Both CT and magnetic resonance imaging (MRI) can help to distinguish the fatty quality of these lesions, if they are large enough for detection and show attenuation values consistent with adipose tissue. Some lipomas have a tendency to sequester xenon.[65] Endoscopically, lipomas of the airways appear as soft mound-like submucosal prominences with smooth uniform surfaces (Fig. 40.12).

The gross appearance of lipomas in the airways is similar to that of lipomas elsewhere, often in the form of soft, circumscribed rounded protuberances of yellow white tissue. Microscopically, lipomas are made of groups of mature adipocytes supported by delicate strands of fibrovascular stroma, usually with no evidence of atypia (Fig. 40.13). However, cellular atypia may occur and is described in the literature.[66] One particularly large, 6.5-cm lipomatous tumor reported as an atypical lipomatous hamartoma of the lung by Palvio et al.[66] in 1985 had minute islands of cartilage and bone and small epithelial clefts, and was considered atypical because of atypical nuclei. Portions of cartilage have been described in other lipomas, and there is evidence that some, if not all, may be best designated as members of the family of hamartomas. In the surgically resected cases described by Moran et al.,[64] the lesions were nodular, soft, yellow, and well

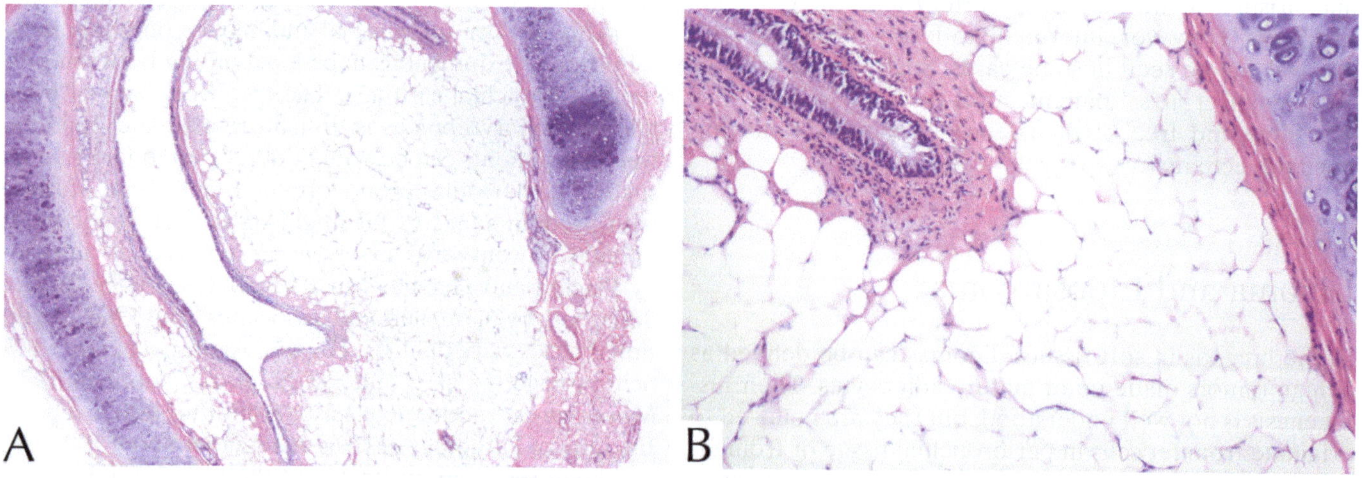

FIGURE 40.13. Lipoma. **(A)** Note endobronchial polypoid lesion. **(B)** Note mature adipocytes surrounding a glandular duct.

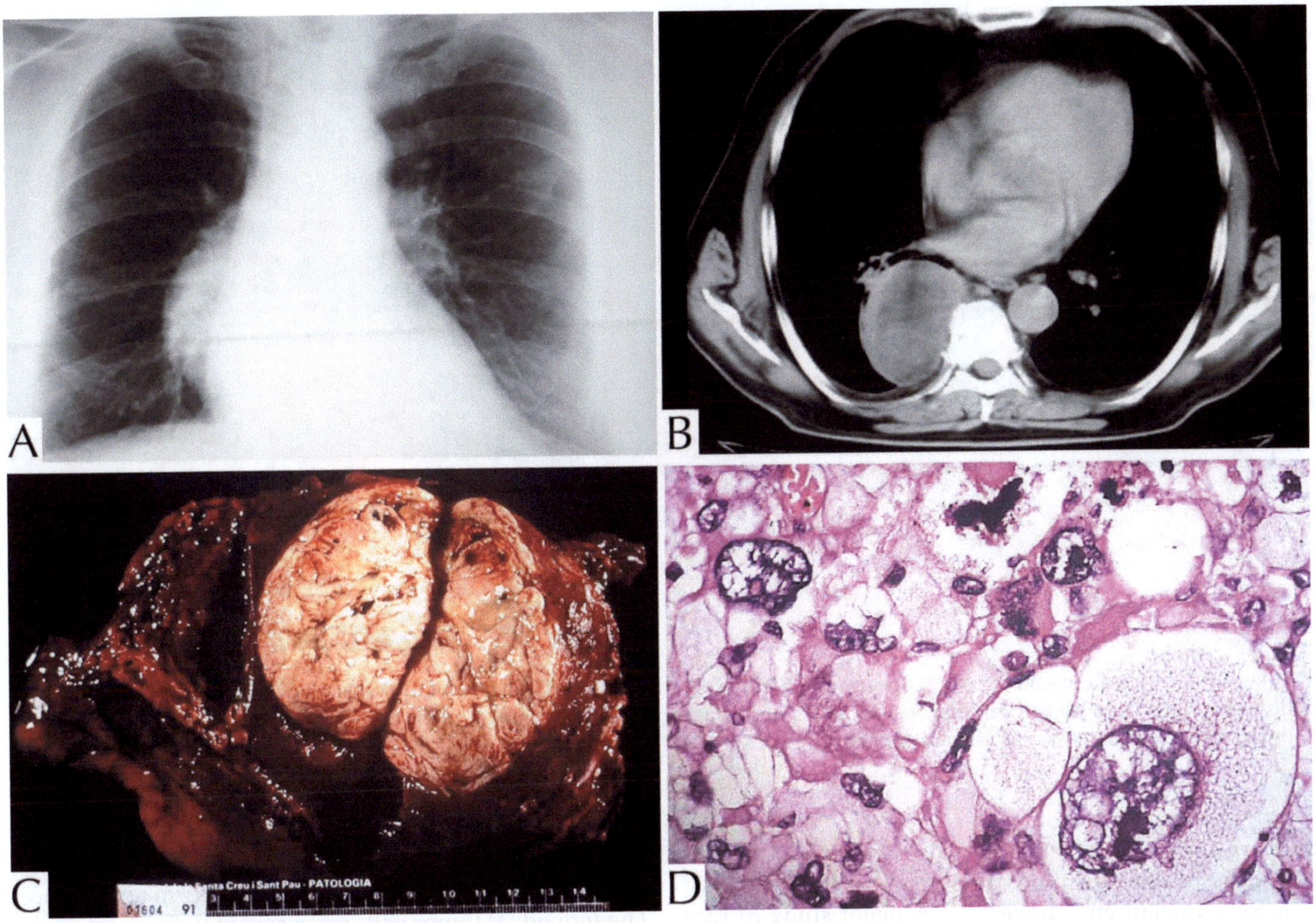

FIGURE 40.14. Liposarcoma. **(A)** Posteroanterior (PA) view of chest showing a mass in the right lower lobe. **(B)** Computed tomography (CT) image showing heterogeneous right lower mass with areas of low attenuation. **(C)** Surgically resected mass showing a lobulated yellowish cut surface reflecting high fat content. **(D)** Bizarre lipoblasts with cytoplasmic and nuclear vacuolization. (Courtesy of Dr. Ana Gimenez, Universitat Autonoma de Barcelona, Barcelona, Spain.)

circumscribed, ranging from 1.2 to 3.0cm in diameter. Microscopically, the lesions did not differ from lipomas elsewhere and were devoid of atypia. Two of the four cases showed areas of spindle cell morphology. The presence of blood vessels or bone marrow tissue elements within an otherwise typical lipoma should raise the question of angiolipoma in the former or a myelolipoma in the latter.[67]

Moran et al.[64] stressed the importance of radiographic and endoscopic evaluation with preoperative biopsy in order to guide the extent of surgery and to prevent unnecessary major surgical resections. The prognostic outlook of lipomas is good. Full recovery follows most instances of complete surgical excision. Some cases are amenable to bronchoscopic resection. Thus far malignant transformation is not known to occur. Liposarcomas do occur but are believed to arise de novo. Three cases of primary liposarcomas cited by Fraser and Paré[65] included a 9-year-old girl with adrenogenital syndrome, a 76-year-old man with a tracheal polyp, and another patient with multiple liposarcomas involving lungs, pleura, and mediastinum. A nicely illustrated case of primary pulmonary liposarcoma reported by Gimenez et al.[68] presented as a huge intrapulmonary mass with a yellow-tan color and bizarre gigantic lipoblasts (Fig. 40.14).

Neurogenic Tumors

Pulmonary neurogenic tumors such as neurofibromas, neurilemomas (schwannomas), and ganglioneuroblastomas have a light microscopic appearance similar to that of neurogenic tumors occurring elsewhere in the body. Moreover, they stain similarly with standard histochemical and immunohistochemical stains. As a group, this family of tumors is exceedingly rare in the lung, and most

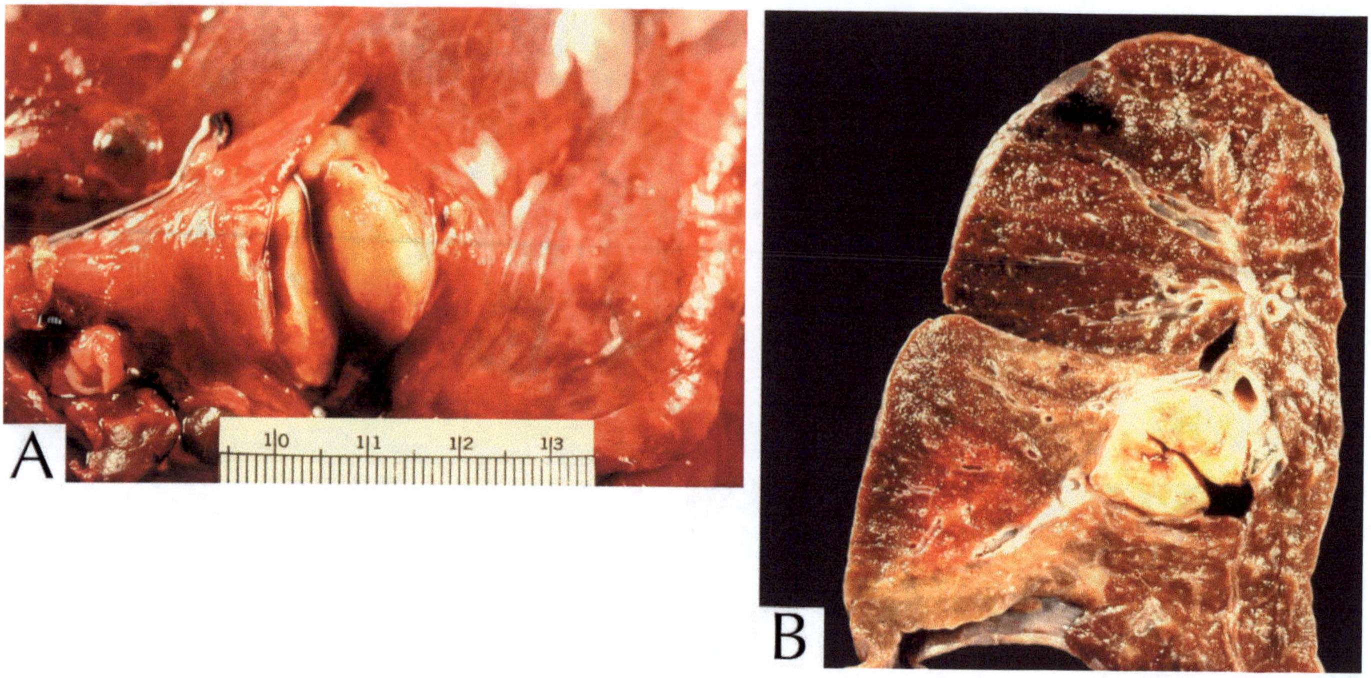

FIGURE 40.15. Neurilemoma, gross appearance. **(A)** Note yellow-gray, centrally placed nodular lesion. **(B)** Cut surface showing solid yellow mass and obstructive pneumonia at base of lung. (Courtesy of Dr. Joseph F. Tomashefski, Jr., MetroHealth Medical Center, Cleveland, OH.)

data are derived from individual case reports and reviews of the literature.[69,70] Some cases occur in the setting of von Recklinghausen's disease.[71,72] A major study of rare pulmonary neoplasms at Mayo Clinic from 1980 through 1990 identified 10,134 patients with lung cancers. Among these there were 80 (0.8%) cases that were classified as rare pulmonary neoplasms. In this group of 80 patients none had tumors of neurogenic origin.[73] In one study of 1664 patients with pulmonary tumors, neurogenic neoplasms comprised 0.2% of the cases.[69] Neurofibromas are more common than neurilemomas when presenting in the lung. In one study of 32 cases, 24 were neurofibromas and eight neurilemomas.[74]

The age at presentation ranges from 6 to 63 years old, with younger patients likely having stigmata of neurofibromatosis.[72] Radiographically, these neoplasms are usually manifested as solitary nodules and less commonly as atelectasis or obstructive pneumonitis.[74] The clinical symptomatology is driven by the size and location of the tumor. Endobronchial tumors may present with signs of airway obstruction.[75] Most pulmonary cases are asymptomatic, however, and may come to attention only as incidental findings on chest radiographs. At gross inspection, most neurofibromas and neurilemomas present as solitary nodules, but rare cases are multiple.[72] As noted, these tumors can occur in the airways or within the lung parenchyma. Those in the parenchyma are well-defined yellow masses (Fig. 40.15). Gross foci of necrosis, calcification, or cystic change may be present. Microscopically, neurofibromas of lung may have a plexiform appearance. The individual tumor cells are wavy, with fusiform nuclei much like those seen in neurofibromas of soft tissues. Likewise, neurilemomas of lung, especially those with histopathologic Antoni and Antoni B patterns, closely mimic neurilemomas elsewhere (Figs. 40.16 and 40.17). A case described by Bosch et al.[70] arose from a segmental

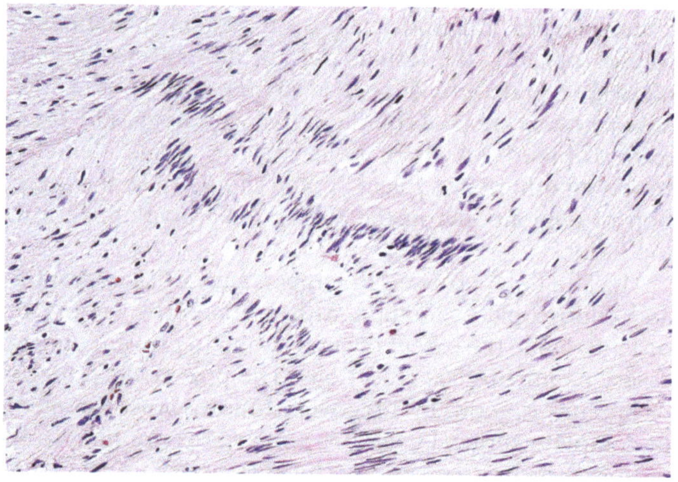

FIGURE 40.16. Neurilemoma, microscopic view of Antoni A pattern with palisading of nuclei and formation of Verocay bodies.

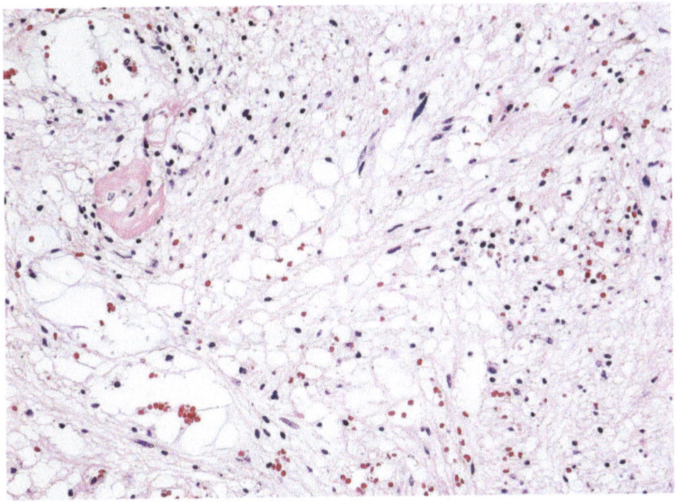

FIGURE 40.17. Neurilemoma, microscopic view of Antoni B pattern. Note hypocellularity and clear microcystic spaces.

bronchus, had a typical microscopic appearance, and was positive for S-100 protein. Ultrastructurally, the tumor cells showed elongated cells surrounded by well-preserved basal lamina and numerous cytoplasmic processes. Immunostains for thyroid transcription factor-1 (TTF-1), smooth muscle actin, and S-100 protein can assist in differentiating neurilemomas from sclerosing hemangiomas, and some leiomyomas may have a palisading effect similar to that seen in Verocay bodies of neurilemomas. Primitive neurogenic tumors such as primitive neuroectodermal tumors and malignant nerve sheath tumors are known to occur in the lung, but can be regarded as oddities due to their very infrequent occurrence. Primitive neuroectodermal tumors of the respiratory tract are described in Chapter 42 on pediatric neoplasms.

Two patients with primary pulmonary ganglioneuroblastoma with areas of neuropil and scattered ganglion cells were presented by Hochholzer and associates.[76] In these two cases, the tumor cells showed immunoreactivity for neurofilament, neuron-specific enolase, and S-100 protein. Noteworthy and stressing the extremely rare occurrence of ganglioneuroblastoma in the lung, the two cases described by these authors were identified in the files of the Armed Forces Institute of Pathology over a period of time spanning nearly five decades. Adverse reactions secondary to right to left shunting and resultant hypoxemia have been described in patients with multiple neurofibromas but not with neurilemomas or ganglioneuroblastomas.[77]

Primary pulmonary meningiomas and ependymomas are equally rare lung tumors, which are believed to be derived from ectopic neural rests in the lung. These tumors are discussed in Chapter 41. Granular cell tumors, currently believed to be of neurogenic origin, are likewise described and discussed in Chapter 41.

Malignant Mesenchymoma

The term *malignant mesenchymoma* refers to mesenchymal tumors showing two or more distinct areas of malignant mesenchymal tumor, in addition to a fibrosarcomatous component.[78] Malignant mesenchymomas may thus be viewed as the malignant counterparts to hamartomas. However, in contrast to hamartomas, malignant mesenchymomas are vanishingly rare in the lung and as noted earlier in this chapter (see Pulmonary Hamartomas), there is no conclusive evidence that hamartomas undergo malignant transformation. A subset of pediatric malignancies have in the past been referred to as malignant mesenchymomas. This designation has fallen from favor in current nosology, and such pediatric malignancies are currently known as pleuropulmonary blastomas.[79] These are discussed in Chapter 42.

True malignant mesenchymomas occur in the heart, retroperitoneum, larynx, and other sites but only rare genuine cases appear to have been published under this name in the lung.[80,81] Certainly one case published as malignant fibrous histiocytoma of the trachea qualifies,[82] as do several in the pulmonary arteries.[83–86] Of the lung cases thus far reported, one published by Kalus et al.[80] was perihilar, 4 cm in diameter, and entrapped the right-main bronchus. Microscopically, the tumor contained elements of osteosarcoma, chondrosarcoma, and rhabdomyosarcoma in addition to undifferentiated malignant areas. The adjacent hilar nodes were not involved. This tumor was incompletely excised, and the patient died 1 month later. At autopsy, tumor extended around the lower trachea and crossed the midline to involve the opposite mainstem bronchus; there was no tumor elsewhere. The prognosis, as exemplified by Kalus et al.'s case, is poor.

Hemangioma

Hemangiomas are frequently found in the liver, skin, and subcutaneous tissue. However, primary hemangiomas of the respiratory tract are exceedingly rare, arising from the bronchial wall or the lung parenchyma of newborns, children, and adults. They are by far most common and most convincingly neoplastic in newborns and children, where they represent a spectrum of capillary hemangiomas, often associated with similar lesions elsewhere.[87–90] In the lung, hemangiomas may occur in the setting of hereditary telangiectasis or Rendu-Osler-Weber syndrome. In adults, they are prone to irritation in the bronchial wall, sometimes resulting in hemoptysis.[91–93] In adults, hemangiomas

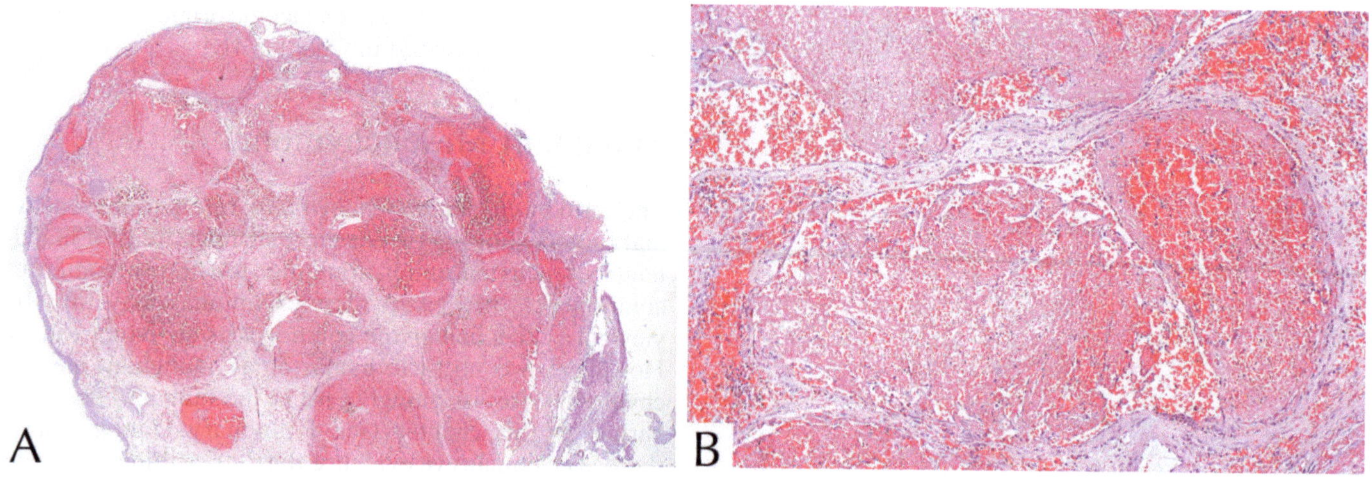

Figure 40.18. **(A,B)** Hemangioma. Polypoid endobronchial tumor showing large but thin-walled vessels and blood-filled, partially thrombosed vascular spaces.

are usually cavernous and sometimes undergo thrombosis or organizational changes.

Microscopically, pulmonary hemangiomas resemble their counterparts in the soft tissues forming poorly defined aggregates of continuous dilated vascular structures lined by CD31, CD34, and factor VIII positive endothelial cells. The vessels may be poorly formed and may lack medial components in their walls. As in other anatomic sites, lobular, racemose, and cavernous variants have been described (Figs. 40.18 to 40.20).[92–98] The diagnosis is not difficult when one sees an abnormally high concentration of blood vessels within the lung. At times, however, cystic lesions such as cystic fibrohistiocytic tumors and mesenchymal cystic hamartomas may have linings that are rich in capillary vessels, raising the question of an hemangioma. As noted below, arteriovenous malformations are tangles of enlarged thick-walled vessels that may mimic hemangioma. However, hemangiomas are generally made of vessels with thinner walls. In addition, arteriovenous malformations are more commonly found in the mid- and lower lung fields. In contrast to hemangiomas, hemangiomatosis is characterized by a proliferation of capillary-size blood vessels along preexisting pulmonary interstitium as well as in the interlobular septa and sometimes within the pleura (see Chapter 28). Rarely, an alveolar adenoma with greatly attenuated lining epithelial cells may mimic an hemangioma. However, immunostains in alveolar adenomas are positive for cytokeratin but negative for endothelial markers.

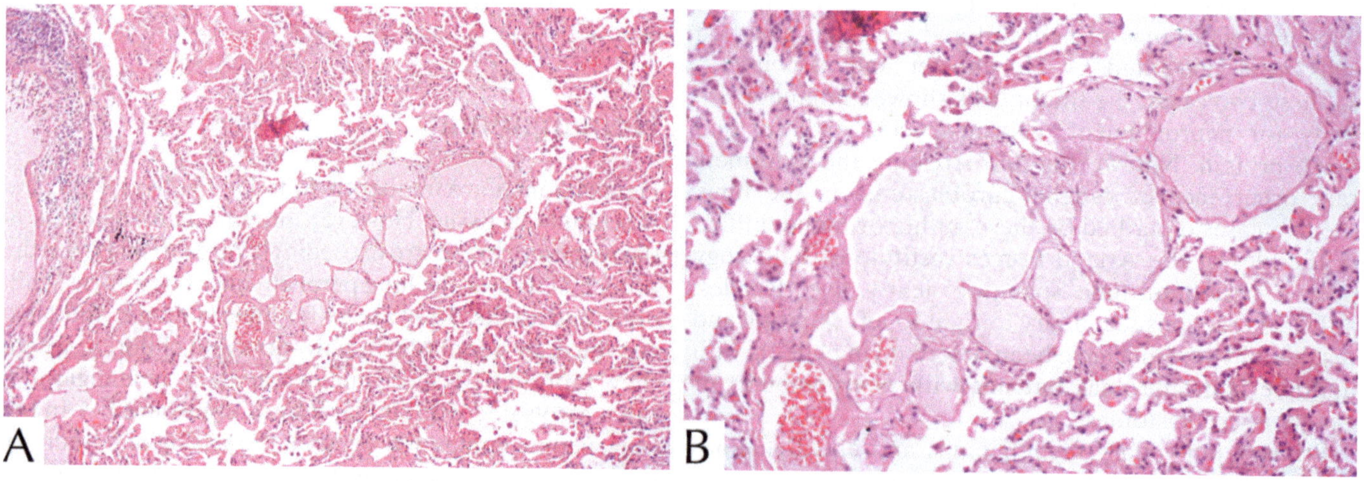

Figure 40.19. **(A,B)** Hemangioma. Intraparenchymal hemangioma showing thin-walled vascular spaces containing amorphous eosinophilic material.

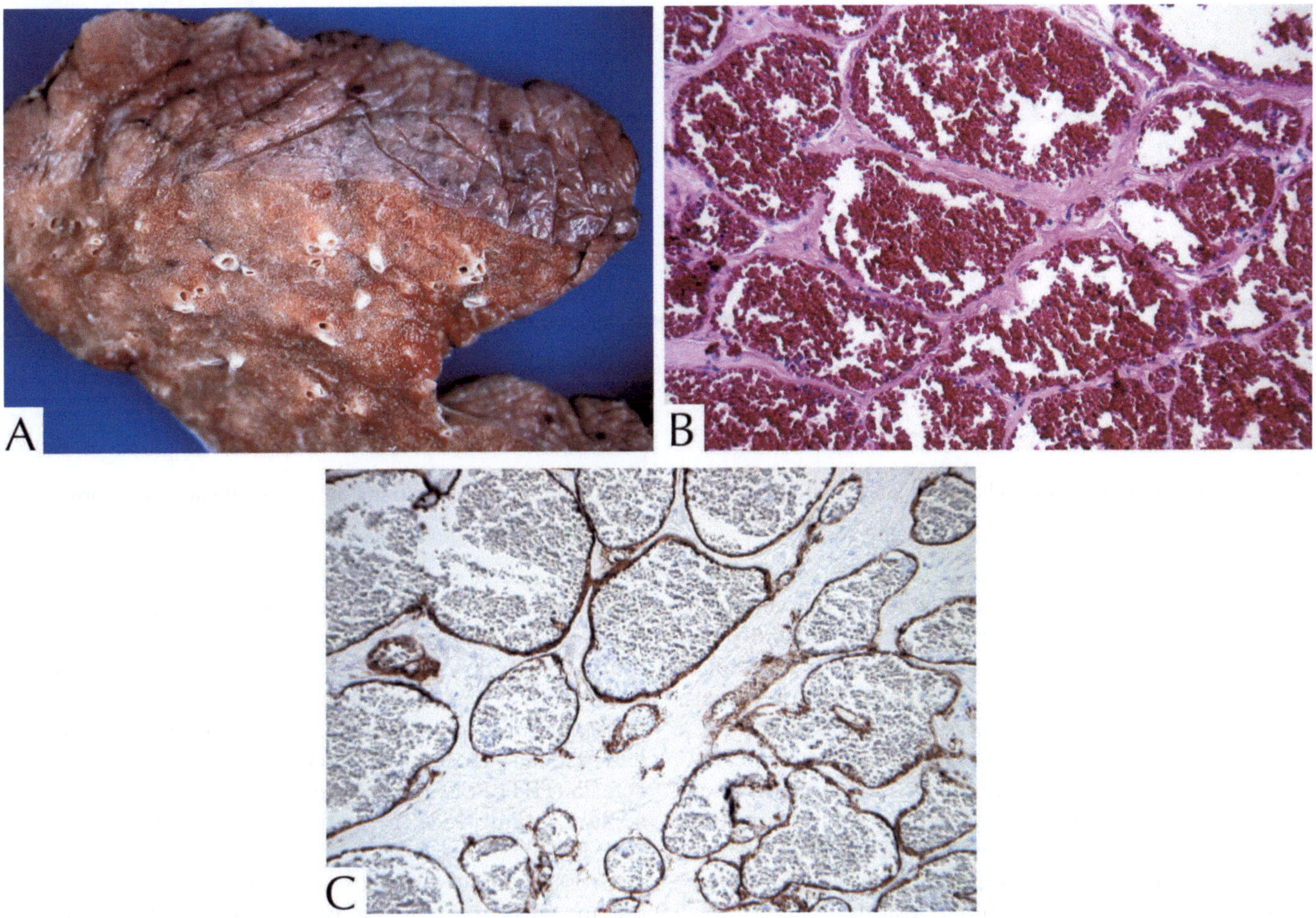

FIGURE 40.20. Cavernous hemangioma. **(A)** Note multiple small purplish hemorrhagic areas more evident on the pleural surface. **(B)** Note blood-filled dilated vascular spaces separate from one another by fibrous septa. **(C)** CD34 immunostain highlighting a single layer of flat endothelial cells lining the vascular spaces. (Courtesy of Dr. Samson W. Fine, Johns Hopkins University Hospital, Baltimore, MD.)

The prognosis is generally good but serious complications may occur. For example, hemangiomas may bleed considerably when biopsied, leading to grave complications.[99] Some cavernous variants of hemangiomas can be either asymptomatic or present with life-threatening spontaneous hemoptysis.[100] They can bleed spontaneously, as in the case reported by Rios-Zambudio et al.,[91] in which therapeutic embolization proved successful in controlling massive hemoptysis following rupture of a tracheal capillary hemangioma in a 66-year-old woman. A racemose variant of hemangioma of the bronchial artery also associated with hemoptysis was reported by Iwasaki and coworkers.[94] Their patient, a 44-year-old woman, had repeated episodes of hemoptysis. At surgery, dilated bronchial arteries with thickened walls were observed. Most authors state that surgical resection is the treatment of choice. Other important therapeutic options gaining favor are interventional radiologic techniques using endovascular embolization. This approach is particularly useful in patients who are clinically unfit to undergo surgery and those with life-threatening hemoptysis.[91]

Hemangiomatosis

This equally rare vascular proliferation is discussed at greater length in Chapter 28 on vascular diseases. Here we only call attention to some salient histopathologic features. Microscopically, hemangiomatosis is characterized by proliferation and engorgement of capillary vessels forming plexuses of small, thin-walled, dilated capillaries extending around and into the walls of larger vessels, both veins and arteries, along the preexisting pulmonary interstitium, interlobular septa, and pleura (Fig. 40.21). A characteristic feature of the disease is capillaries that

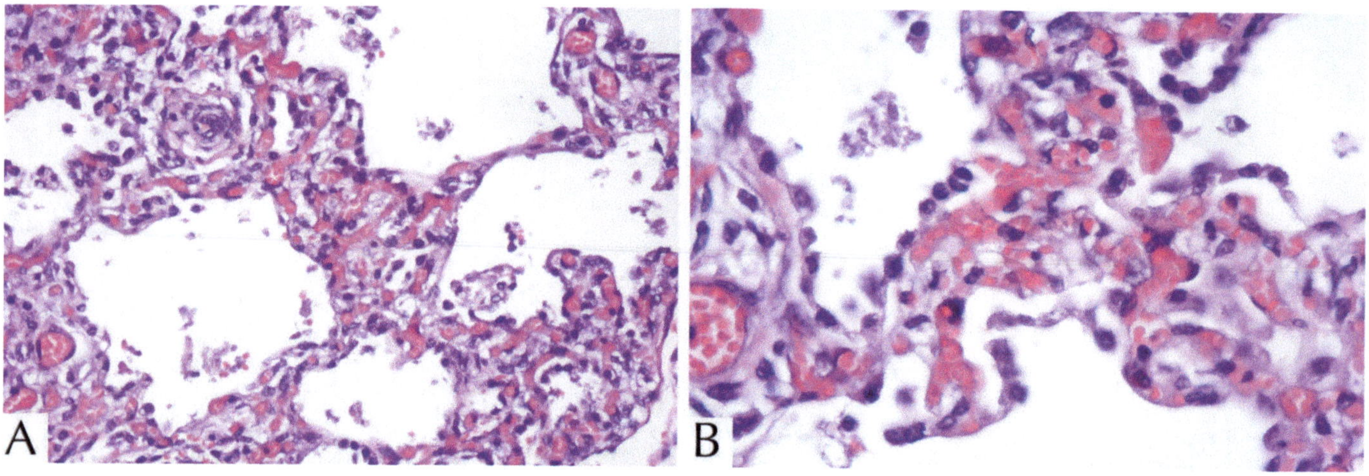

FIGURE 40.21. **(A,B)** Capillary hemangiomatosis. Note expanded interstitium containing an excess of capillary loops.

appear to fill veins and cause secondary venous occlusion.[101–103] Most reported cases describe findings of focal areas of capillary engorgement of the lung, sometimes associated with thick-walled, central or eccentric vessels, and some identify an overgrowth of vessels that is also thought characteristic. A secondary pulmonary hypertensive change is reported that involves thickening of vascular walls, including medial hypertrophy and fibrointimal proliferation, but usually not including more severe degrees of pulmonary hypertensive changes such as necrotizing, plexiform, or dilatational lesions.[101–106]

Arteriovenous Malformations

Arteriovenous malformations (AVMs) of the lung are rare vascular malformations originating from persistent anastomotic fetal capillaries. Most AVMs first manifest themselves during the second decade of life.[107,108] They are twice as common in females as they are in males, and nearly half of patients show evidence of AVMs in other organs.[109] In a review from the Mayo Clinic, most patients with AVM were asymptomatic, but some presented with (sometimes massive) hemoptysis or dyspnea, the latter resulting from right to left shunting.[110,111] Central nervous system (CNS) complications such as stroke and brain abscess may develop in the setting of paradoxical emboli. Connections with systemic vessels have been described in about 4% of the cases.[111]

The spectrum of pathologic manifestations ranges from tiny multiple telangiectatic lesions to large single or paucivascular structures, sometimes dilated and sometimes reaching aneurysmal proportions.[111] A network of vessels may be seen in some lesions showing vessels with thickened walls made up of variable amounts of smooth muscle, elastic fibers, and collagen (Fig. 40.22). The dilated appearance of some of the vessels has fostered the incorrect term *cavernous angiomas*, while aneurysmal proportions in some lesions have led to the term *arteriovenous aneurysms*.[111] Lesions with thin-walled vessels may mimic hemangiomas. In one study, 39 of 45 patients with AVMs had associated lesions of hereditary hemorrhagic telangiectasia (HHT) or Osler-Rendu-Weber disease.[110,111] Conversely, about 15% of patients with HHT may have AVMs.[110–112]

Grossly, the lower lobes are most commonly affected, but any parts of the lung may be involved. The lesions are multiple in about one third of the cases, and in one sixth the condition is bilateral.[113] Arteriovenous malformations are usually peripheral and located immediately beneath the pleura, where they may appear as areas of bluish

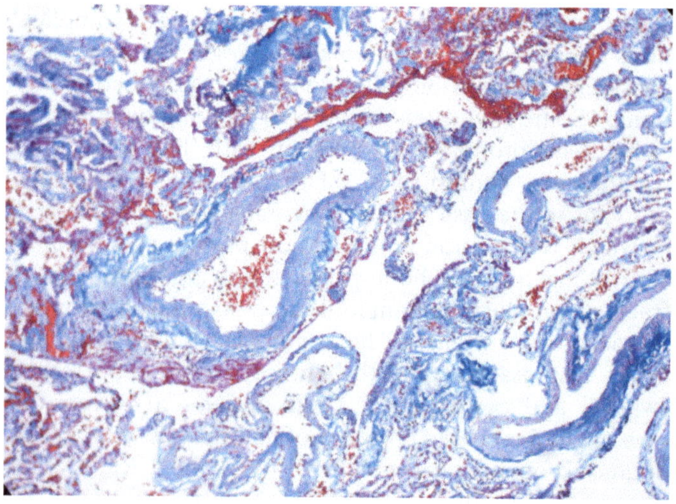

FIGURE 40.22. Arteriovenous malformation. Note conglomerate of thick-walled vessels. Trichrome stain.

swelling. When embolized they may acquire a pneumonic appearance (Fig. 40.23). Subpleural AVMs may rupture and cause hemothorax.[107] Injecting lesions with a mixture of barium and gelatin enhances the visualization and topography of the AVMs (see Chapter 1). Arteriovenous malformations may protrude endobronchially. In a case reported by Soda et al.,[114] a large tortuous artery with accompanying proliferation of tiny vessels was seen histologically beneath an intact bronchial mucosa. Arteriovenous malformation of the lung may produce single or multiple discrete nodules radiographically, but the nodules generally are inapparent after excision because the blood flows out of the vessels and the vessels themselves collapse, becoming much less visible.

Hemosiderin deposition and abnormal elastic structure of the vascular walls are clues to the correct diagnosis.[107] Pseudoarteriovenous malformations are potential diagnostic confounders. Recent in vivo or postoperative atelectasis may result in artifactual (closer) approximation of arteries and veins that simulate a vascular malformation or hemangiomatosis.[107] Other differential diagnoses include true aneurysms of the pulmonary arteries, telangiectatic lesions of the lung, and, less likely, capillary hemangiomatosis. True aneurysms show a vessel with aneurysmal dilatation of its wall, while telangiectatic lesions are not difficult to distinguish due to their thin walls (see Chapter 28). The capillary proliferation of hemangiomatosis in the walls of veins and arteries, interlobular septa, and pleura described in the previous section are not usually present in AVMs (see also Chapter 28).

Surgical excision particularly in cases associated with significant or repeated bleeding episodes is the treatment of choice. However, in recent years transcatheter embolization has become a safe, effective means of vascular occlusion and is now widely considered to be the procedure of choice for the treatment of AVMs.[115] Various types of embolic materials have been employed to achieve vascular occlusion, including polyvinyl alcohol (Ivalon), wool coils, stainless steel coils, and detachable silicone balloons.[115] Over time, steel coils may passively migrate, finding their way into the bronchi and sometimes becoming visible at endoscopy (Fig. 40.24).[116,117]

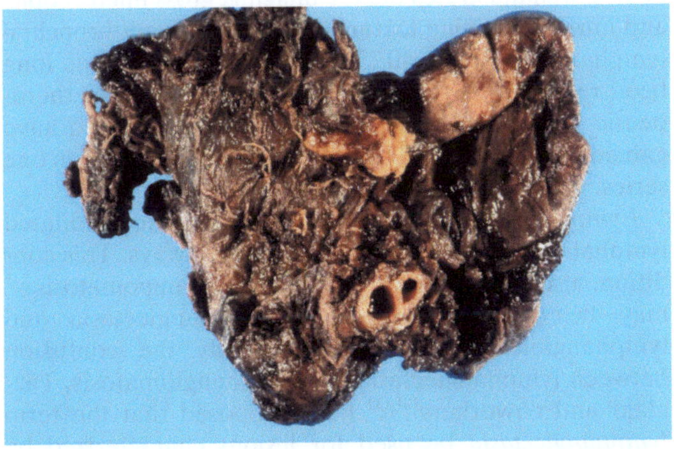

FIGURE 40.23. Arteriovenous malformation. Note solidified tan-brown area (top right) signifying an inflammatory reaction secondary to embolization.

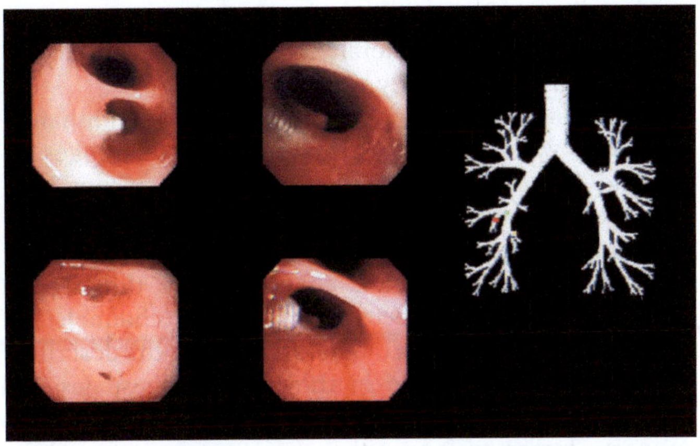

FIGURE 40.24. Migration of embolization coil. Note white cylindrical coil pushing from beneath the airway mucosa. (Courtesy of Dr. Richard Irwin, University of Massachusetts Medical School, Worcester, MA.)

Lymphangiectasia, Lymphangiomas, and Lymphangiomatosis

The term *lymphangiomatosis* has been loosely applied to a spectrum of proliferative/tumoral or localized/systemic lesions involving generally dilated lymphatic channels. As used here, the term *lymphangiomatosis* encompasses lymphangiectasia, lymphangiomas, and diffuse lymphangiomatosis.

Lymphangiectasia is most often a congenital pulmonary abnormality diagnosed in a stillborn or newborn and thought to be a persistence of dilated lymphatics in the 14th to 20th week of intrauterine development.[118] About a third of the cases are associated with cardiac anomalies, especially those retarding venous return, and this may be secondary to persistently increased lymphatic pressure[119] (see Chapter 6). Other cases are associated with a wide variety of congenital defects, and in total, about 80% are associated with congenital defects including absence of lymphatic valves.[119] Lymphangiectasia may be more generalized or occur in adults, and in both circumstances may overlap with the hemangiomatosis syndromes. Wagenaar et al.[120] and Noonan et al.[121] have suggested a classification of lymphangiectasia encompassing three variants:

limited to lung, with both pulmonary and mediastinal involvement, and a generalized variant (secondary to obstruction of pulmonary venous outflow).

Wagenaar et al.[120] reported three cases of lymphangiectasia in two adolescent boys and a young man (ages 13, 16, and 19 years), with intrapulmonary tumorous lymphangiectasia, limited to one or two lobes and the mediastinum. All three patients were asymptomatic. Their cystically dilated lymphatic channels were thin walled and followed naturally occurring lymphatic channels; the cysts were up to 1.5 cm in diameter. The authors described sporadic smooth muscle in the walls of these lesions. There were no dilated or sclerotic veins, evidence of pulmonary hypertension, either primary or secondary, intraalveolar edema, or hemosiderosis, which would indicate that these lesions were secondary.[120] In most cases, the lungs are bulky and firm and show numerous small cystic spaces, which can measure up to 5 mm in diameter (Fig. 40.25). Microscopically, elongated "cysts" are lined by a flattened endothelium and are located within interstitial connective tissue of the bronchovascular bundles, interlobular septa, and pleura (Fig. 40.26). Infrequent smooth muscle cells may be seen in their walls, and their lumina contain hypocellular eosinophilic fluid characteristic of lymph.[115] These lesions usually become evident at birth and are almost always fatal.

Lymphangiomas, also known as cystic hygromas, are congenital or developmental abnormalities, and only rarely affect the lung. As noted by Enzinger and Weiss,[118] lymphangiomas most often occur in the areas of primitive lymph sacs such as the neck and the axilla, and half or a little more of the cases are seen in newborns and infants. About 75% of cystic hygromas occur in the neck and some 20% in the axilla.[122] Only rarely has a generalized case been described with involvement of the scalp and associated chylothorax.[123] Those diagnosed in utero before 30 weeks' gestation have a high rate of morbidity and fetal death, and are usually detected during evaluation of polyhydramnios.[124] These lesions have been subclassified depending on the size of the spaces they produce. Those with grossly visible spaces of several millimeters to several centimeters have been called cystic lymphangiomas or cystic hygromas. Those with small but still dilated spaces are called cavernous lymphangiomas, and those composed of small-caliber vessels are called capillary lymphangioma, lymphangioma complex, or lymphangioma circumscripta; the latter is usually seen in the skin of adults.[125] Rare cases of lymphangiomas develop within the lung,[126–128] and even rarer cases occur in the bronchi.[129] A recent case published by Chikkamuniyappa et al.[129] well illustrates the CT imaging, gross microscopic, and immunostaining features of a solitary endobronchial lymphangioma (Fig. 40.27). Surgical resection has long been regarded as the treatment of choice. Other therapeutic modalities such as sclerotherapy appear to have gained popularity, with better than a 50% response in one series.[130]

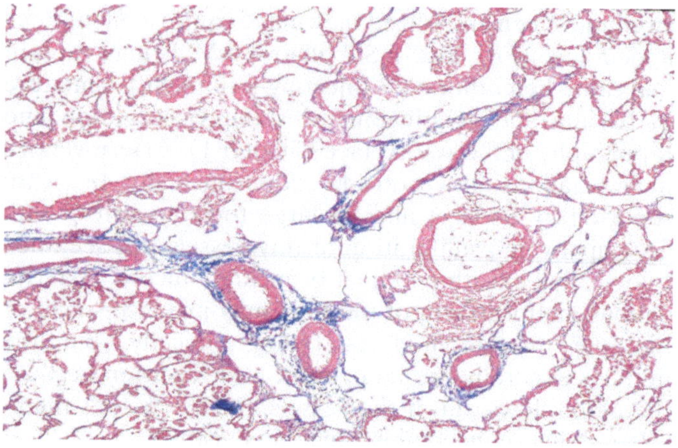

FIGURE 40.26. Lymphangiectasia. Microscopic view of lesion shown in Figure 40.25. Note dilated lymphatic channel (trichrome stain). (Courtesy of Dr. Joseph F. Tomashefski, Jr., MetroHealth Medical Center, Cleveland, OH.)

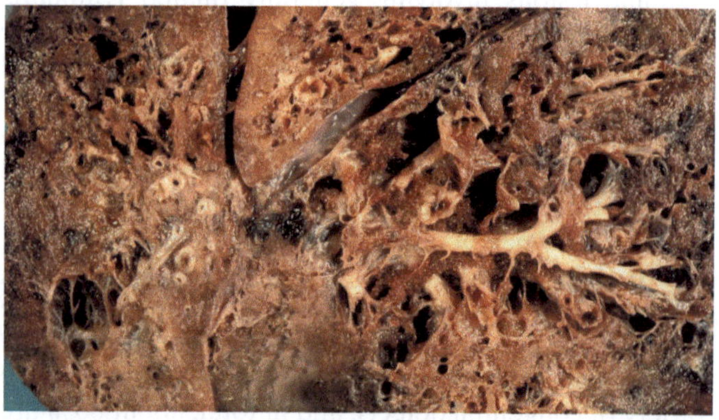

FIGURE 40.25. Congenital lymphangiectasia, gross appearance of the lesion in a patient with anomalous pulmonary venous return. Note cystically dilated lymphatic channels accompanying bronchovascular bundles. (Courtesy of Dr. Joseph F. Tomashefski, Jr., MetroHealth Medical Center, Cleveland, OH.)

Lymphangiomatosis refers to the occurrence of dilated lymphatic channels along lymphatic pathways. This condition, also known as diffuse pulmonary angiomatosis,[115] may be confused with both lymphangiectasia and lymphangioleiomyomatosis. To clarify the confusion between lymphangiectasia and lymphangiomatosis, Tazelaar and coworkers[131,132] have proposed that the term *lymphangiectasia* be used for lesions characterized by dilation of existing lymphatic channels without an increase in their number or complexity. Conversely, the term *lymphangiomatosis* could be reserved for proliferative

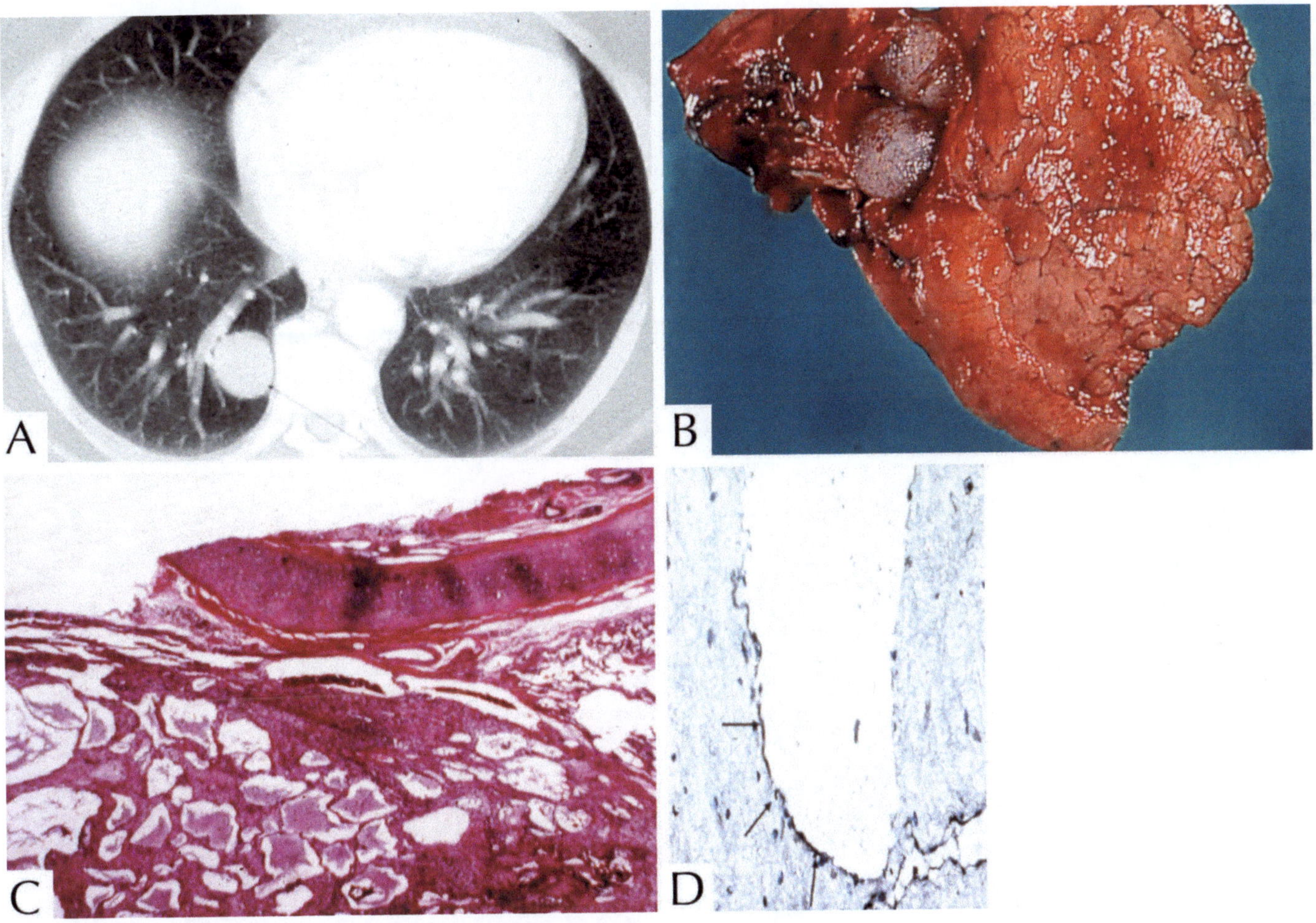

FIGURE 40.27. Lymphangioma. **(A)** A CT scan showing well-defined nodular density. **(B)** Bisected bluish glistening 2.5-cm nodule in lung. **(C)** Juxtabronchial vascular spaces of varying sizes separated by paucicellular septa. **(D)** Flat endothelial cells stained positively for CD31. (Courtesy of Dr. S. Chikkamuniyappa, University of Texas Health Science Center, San Antonio, TX.)

vascular lesions in which there is an actual increase in the number or size of lymphatic vessels. Swank and colleagues[133] in 1989 reported a case of diffuse pulmonary lymphangiomatosis mimicking lymphangioleiomyomatosis in a 20-year-old woman. This was slowly progressive over 8 years. She was noted to have absence of involvement of lymph nodes or other organs; histology showed thick-fibrous-walled, dilated subpleural lymphatics, and it was specifically noted that there was no muscle in their walls. Of interest, despite this absence of muscle, she was treated as lymphangioleiomyomatosis with medroxyprogesterone and responded well.

Tazelaar et al.[132] in 1993 described nine cases of diffuse pulmonary lymphangiomatosis, ages 1 month to 35 years. Seven of the nine patients were males and two were females; in none was there extrathoracic involvement. They described asymmetrically spaced bundles of smooth cells that stained for vimentin in nine cases, factor VIII in eight cases, actin in seven cases, and desmin in six cases. These cases were all progressive and especially aggressive in children. The authors favored a lymphatic origin for these lesions and suggested the lesions are distinct from lymphangiectasia, lymphangioleiomyomatosis, capillary hemangiomatosis, Kaposi's sarcoma, and Kaposiform hemangioendothelioma.

Microscopically, lymphangiomatosis consists of dilated lymphatic spaces along the usual lymphatic pathways. Long-standing cases may have vessels with very thickened walls that may appear empty or be filled with lymph or red blood cells (Fig. 40.28). There is some confusion and overlap between lymphangiomatosis and some cases of cavernous hemangiomatosis in the lung. Both entities are described as dilated, cavernous thick-walled spaces that follow lymphatic pathways around bronchopulmonary rays, and interlobular septa and pleura. Some are clearly empty or filled with chyle, and these should be

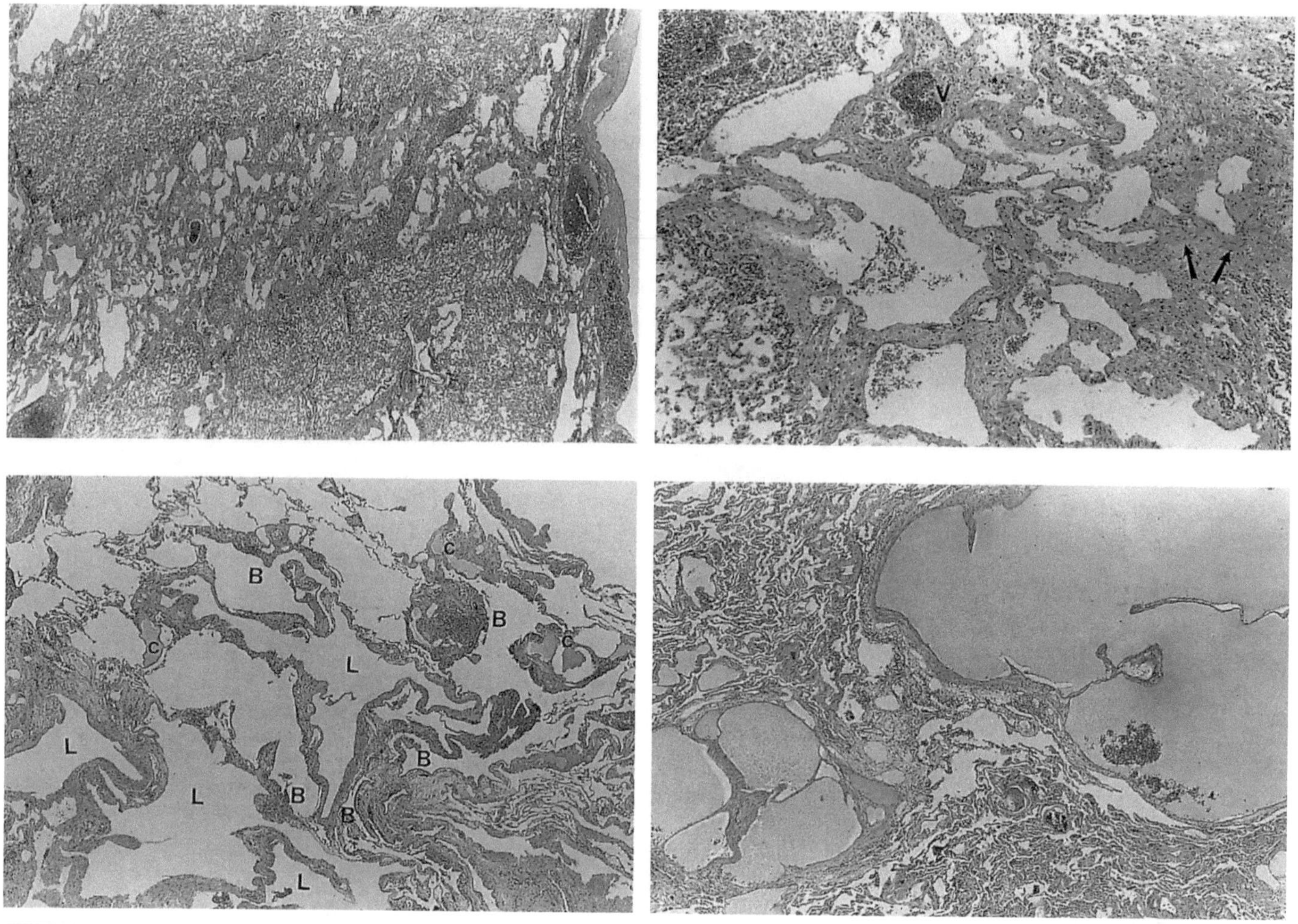

FIGURE 40.28. Lymphangiomatosis. **(A)** Dilated thick-walled lymphatic vessels in interlobular septum and pleura. **(B)** Bundles of proliferating smooth muscle (arrows); V, vein at top. **(C)** Cystically dilated lymphatic channels (L); terminal bronchioles (B); dilated, more opaque lymphatics (c). **(D)** Some spaces are filled with lymph.

identified as lymphangiomatosis. Others in the same route appear to have blood in them, and it is unclear whether this represents blood in transit or spillage into lymphatics. Koblenzer and Bukowski[134] have therefore proposed the encompassing term *angiomatosis* for these lesions.

Hemangiopericytomas (Localized Fibrous Tumors)

Hemangiopericytomas are currently designated as solitary or localized fibrous tumors. They can sometimes be massive in proportion and be readily visualized on chest x-ray (Fig. 40.29). Hemorrhage and necrosis can be seen grossly (Fig. 40.30). Microscopically these tumors are typified by the presence of thin-walled branching vascular spaces set in a fibrous stroma and involve the pleura

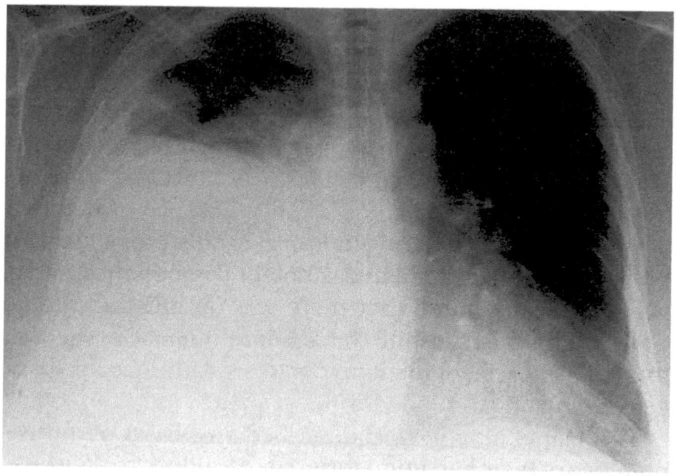

FIGURE 40.29. Hemangiopericytoma/localized fibrous tumor. Massive pulmonary tumor in the right lung of a 38-year-old woman as seen in the PA view of the chest. (Courtesy of Dr. R. Schmidt, University of Washington School of Medicine, Seattle, WA.)

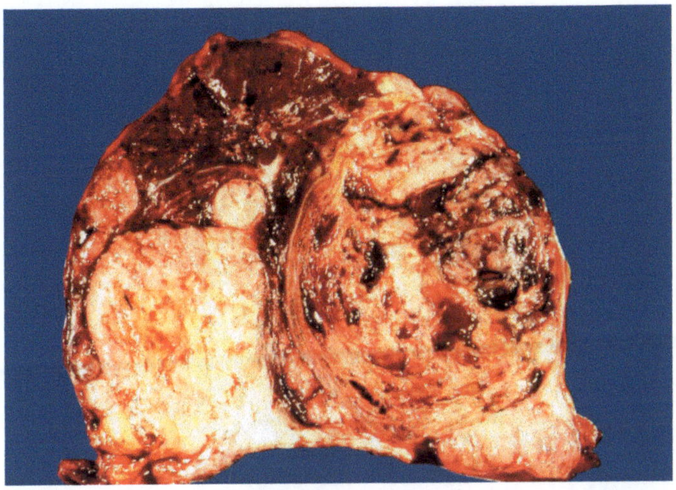

FIGURE 40.30. Hemangiopericytoma/localized fibrous tumor (same patient as in Fig. 40.29). Note large nodular tumor masses involving nearly the entire lung. Large size, hemorrhage, and necrosis usually signify malignancy (same case as Fig. 40.29).

or less commonly the lung (Fig. 40.31). They closely resemble the cellular areas of localized fibrous tumors and as noted above are currently regarded as variants of localized fibrous tumors.[135] Therefore, at least in the field of soft tissue tumors, the delineation of hemangiopericytomas as a separate and distinct entity may become obsolete since their histopathologic features as generally understood at the present time are shared by a variety of soft tissue tumors.[135] These tumors are discussed at length in Chapter 43 on pleural neoplasia and briefly in Chapter 39.

Epithelioid Hemangioendotheliomas

These low-grade angiosarcomas, also known as sclerosing interstitial vascular sarcomas, sclerosing endothelial tumors, sclerosing epithelioid angiosarcomas, and initially as intravascular bronchioloalveolar tumors, typically present in the lung as multiple nodules having a superficially chondroid appearance.[42] In addition to the lung, this morphologically unique neoplasm occurs primarily in other sites such as liver, bone, and soft tissues.[42] Further cases have been reported in brain, lymph nodes, meninges, breast, and scalp.[136–138]

The story of epithelioid hemangioendothelioma in the lung as a separate entity begins in 1975, with a report of 20 cases by Dail and Liebow.[139] These 20 cases were felt to represent an unusual variant of bronchioloalveolar tumor (BAT) with a high rate of intravascular spread, or intravascular BAT (IV-BAT). This belief was based on its multifocal bilateral nodular appearance and on a case with concurrent adenocarcinoma in the lung, with a typical bronchioloalveolar carcinoma pattern. On reflection, this latter occurrence was just a misleading independent primary (or metastatic) adenocarcinoma unrelated to this lesion. Ironically, there have been no other concurrent malignancies in the lung described with these tumors.

As with many other rare or previously undescribed entities, comparisons with known disease processes occur first, followed by application of special techniques in trying to resolve the cell of origin. The tumor was first thought to have a chondroid appearance, and an early case published by Smith et al.[42] was titled "Primary Chondrosarcomatosis of the Lung." This same case was later rejected by Morgan and Salama[39] as any type of typical chondrosarcoma, in their critical review article of primary chondrosarcomas of the lung. Its multifocal character was unlike any other chondrosarcoma. Another early case published by Farinacci et al.[140] as deciduosis of the lung occurred in a woman undergoing evaluation for an ectopic pregnancy, and in this case the tumor's appearance was somewhat like decidual tissue.

Corrin and associates[141] studied three cases of this unusual lesion by electron microscopy, and were the first to suggest that this was an endothelial-derived tumor. Weldon-Linne et al.[142] and Azumi and Churg[143] obtained similar ultrastructural results and reached similar conclusions. A case published by Ferrer-Roca[144] illustrated similar findings, but this author drew different conclusions. Weldon-Linne et al.[145] and soon thereafter Bhagavan and associates[146] stained this tumor with factor VIII–related antigen by immunoperoxidase technique, lending further support to the endothelial nature of this lesion. Both the electron micrographic and factor VIII analysis have been supported by others. Later, Dail and coworkers[147] published details on additional cases, further contributing to the fund of data on this tumor. To emphasize some of its spectrum, Yousem and Hochholzer[148] reported four cases with unusual clinical appearances, including cases presenting as an intramediastinal mass, as lymphangitic metastases simulating carcinomatosis, as diffuse pleural thickening simulating mesothelioma, and as a solitary peripheral calcified nodule in lung. Experience with nine cases reported in Japan was summarized in 1989.[149]

Pulmonary epithelioid hemangioendothelioma has a distinct predilection for women. Eighty percent of the cases occur in women and about 50% are diagnosed before the age of 40. However, cases have been documented in older and younger individuals. Considering all sites, the youngest affected patient was aged 4 years.[150] One 15-year-old girl had fairly extensive disease for her early age, with multiple lesions in the liver and lung and a bone lesion. Pulmonary epithelioid hemangioendotheliomas usually present with radiographic evidence of

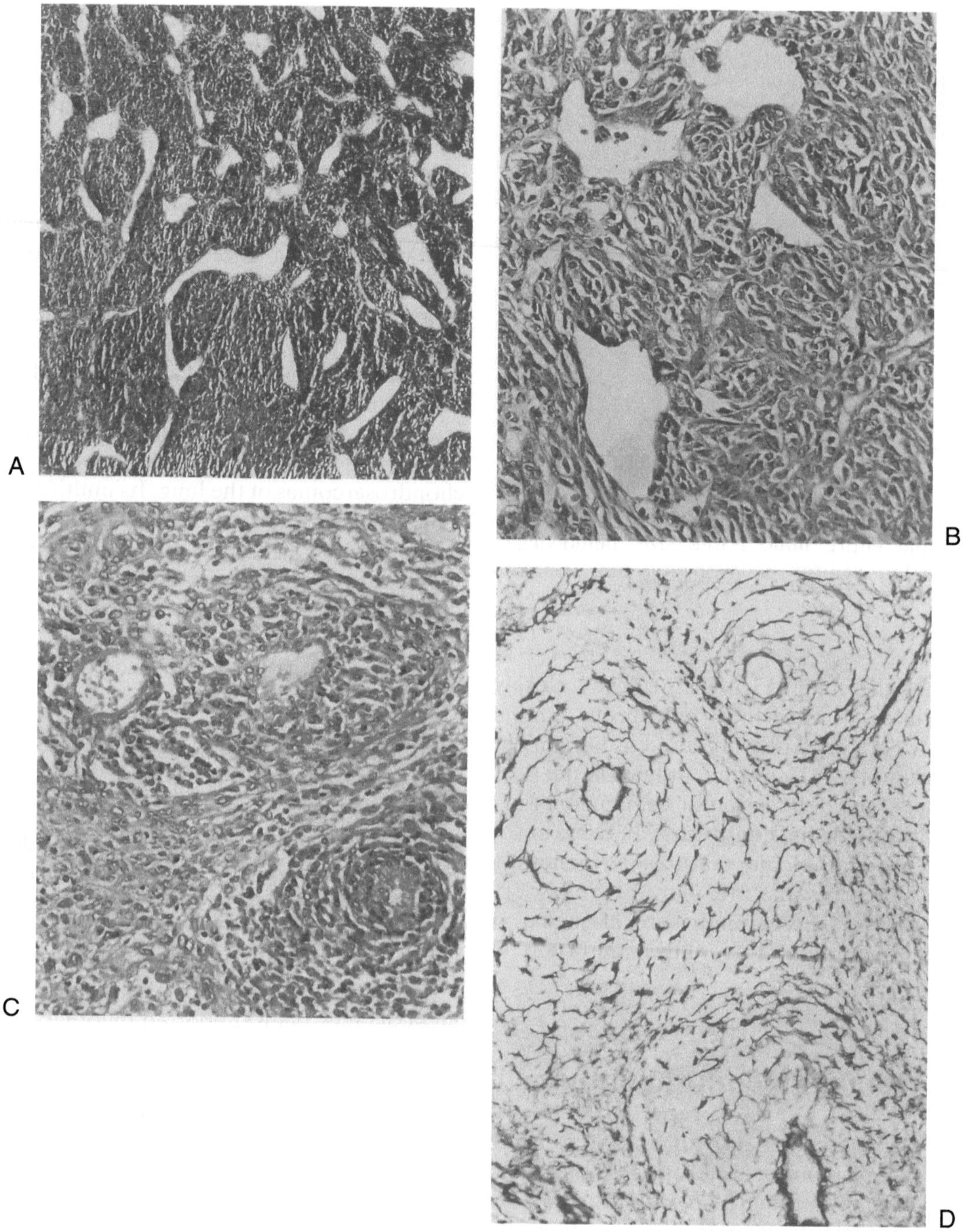

FIGURE 40.31. Hemangiopericytoma/localized fibrous tumor. **(A)** Antler-like spaces. **(B)** Cells are monotonous, round or oval. **(C)** Tumor cells surrounding vessels give original expression of cell of origin. **(D)** Typical reticulin network.

nodules, usually less than 2 cm in diameter. On chest roentgenograms, the nodules can be well or poorly defined. The nodules may enlarge slowly and in time lead to respiratory insufficiency. On CT scanning, the nodules appear to have a perivascular distribution and some may calcify.[151] Most patients are initially asymptomatic and are discovered incidentally on screening radiographs or radiographs obtained for other reasons (Fig. 40.32). A rare patient may present with dyspnea, malaise, and weight loss.[151]

The gross appearance of epithelioid hemangioendothelioma is distinctive only in its multiplicity. There are usually more nodules in the lung than are appreciated radiographically. The lesions in the lung are usually multiple, bilateral, and small, often in the range of about 1 cm and usually less than 2 cm.[147] However, some tumors may

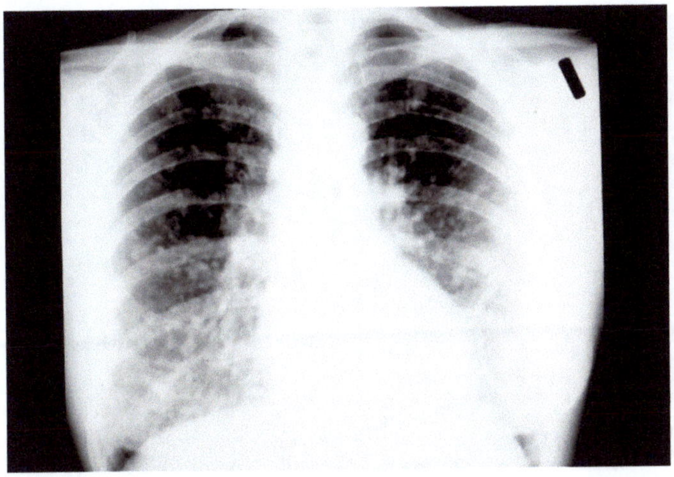

FIGURE 40.32. Epithelioid hemangioendothelioma. Chest radiograph showing multiple bilateral nodules of varying sizes.

become focally confluent (Fig. 40.33), while others may be much smaller and dot-like in appearance (Fig. 40.34). The surgeon often reports some increased number in the subpleural zone, but this may be an artifact of finding more than expected in the region of the biopsy. Pleural and pericardial spread may occur, somewhat like a mesothelioma, with encasement, thickening, and transdiaphragmatic penetration. Metastasis to regional nodes has been seen, and these show rather nodular infiltrates in the nodes.[147] The individual lesions in the lung are usually spherical, almost cartilaginous in consistency, and when sectioned usually they have a gray-white translucent viable rim with a more opaque gray-white center representing either calcification or coagulative necrosis. Calcification may be present in these necrotic zones, and may be seen radiographically.[147]

Microscopically, viable tumor is best seen at the periphery of the lung nodules. In the center of the nodules there is often coagulative necrosis (Fig. 40.35), and in the transition there are lacunar-like cell ghosts left in a dense matrix, presumably where nuclei or the last cells existed. The transition between the totally necrotic and the totally viable zone demonstrates this best, where there are a few nuclei or cells dying and dropping out. For a vascular-derived and specifically an endothelial-derived tumor, this tumor is remarkably avascular. Such tumor nodules must derive their metabolic support from diffusion rather than a capillary network of their own. The tumor cells grow in a very peculiar micropolypoid fashion, extending from alveolus to alveolus through one or several small sites, usually pores of Kohn (Fig. 40.36A). In areas tumor cells may show cytoplasmic vacuoles representing primitive vascular lumina (Fig. 40.36B). As the small micropolyps grow, they fill each alveolus to about its expected dimension, and then stop growing. They encase the adjacent and intervening alveolar septa, with the resulting effect of encased ghosts of background lung tissue, both in the viable tumor zones and in the necrotic centers. Tumor spread through pores of Kohn is not exclusively seen in these tumors. We have recently seen a cytokeratin-positive, CD31- and CD34-negative, large cell carcinoma of lung showing a micropolypoid configuration with spread through the pores of Kohn (Fig. 40.37).

There are low- and high-grade variants of epithelioid hemangioendotheliomas. The low-grade variants are easiest to diagnose because of their described conformation and their cytology showing the above-cited primitive vascular lumina illustrated in Figure 40.36B. The high-grade variants are more difficult to diagnose with certainty, and must retain many of the described characteristics to be so classified, especially to avoid overlap with other sarcomas. In low-grade variants there are exceptionally

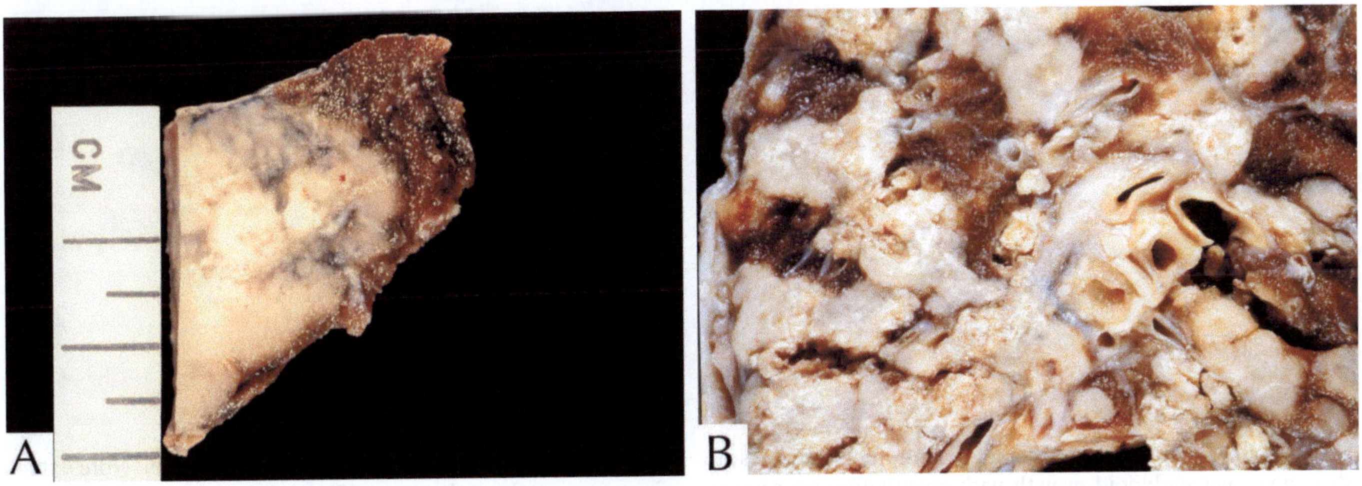

FIGURE 40.33. **(A,B)** Epithelioid hemangioendothelioma. Gross appearances. This tumor is made of focally confluent nodules.

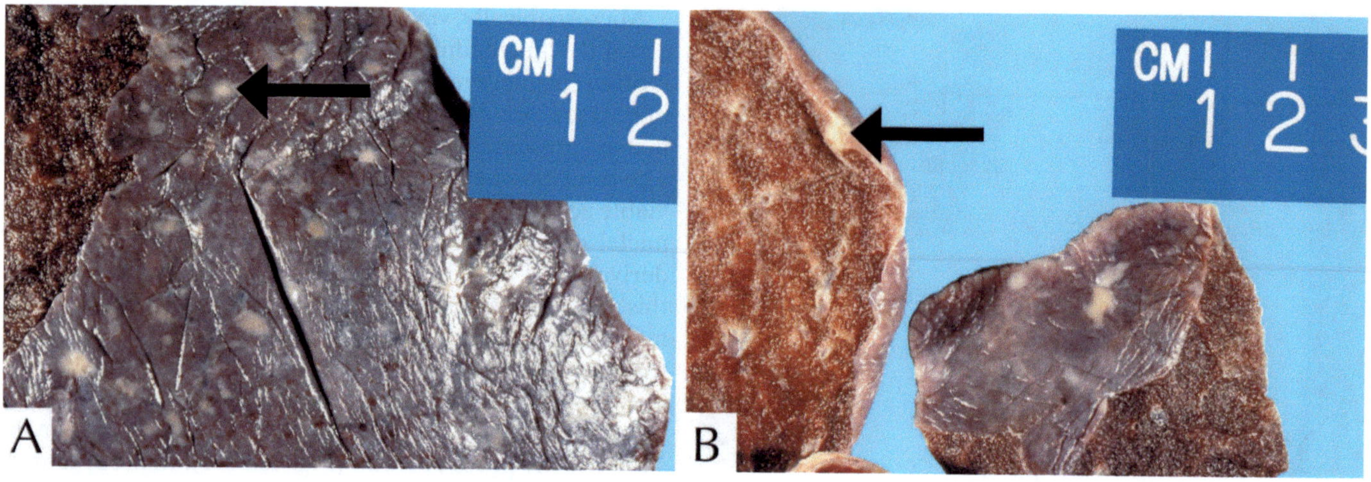

FIGURE 40.34. **(A,B)** Epithelioid hemangioendothelioma. Small subpleural whitish nodules with irregular borders (arrow). (Courtesy of Dr. Carol Farver, Cleveland Clinic, Cleveland, OH.)

rare or no mitoses. Nuclei are oval to slightly irregular, slightly convoluted, and bland appearing, and nucleoli are inconspicuous or small. Some nuclei have large eosinophilic cytoplasmic inclusions that are rather hyalinized, with only a rim of nucleus surrounding most of the inclusion.

The cytoplasm of tumor cells varies, being densely hyalinized, finely granular, fibrillar, or myxoid in nature. Cytoplasmic borders may also vary, being quite distinct, outlining polygonal cells or irregularly contoured cells, or being indistinct. The more myxoid the background, the more distinct are the individual tumor cells and the more irregular are their cytoplasmic contours. Intracytoplasmic

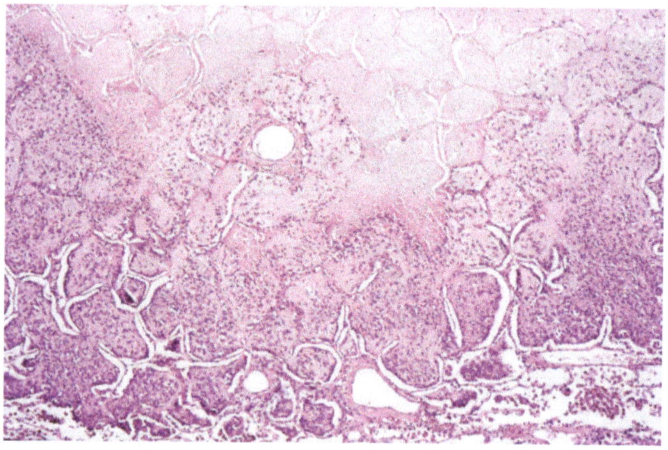

FIGURE 40.35. Epithelioid hemangioendothelioma. Note advancing micropolypoid growth with coagulative necrosis of central area.

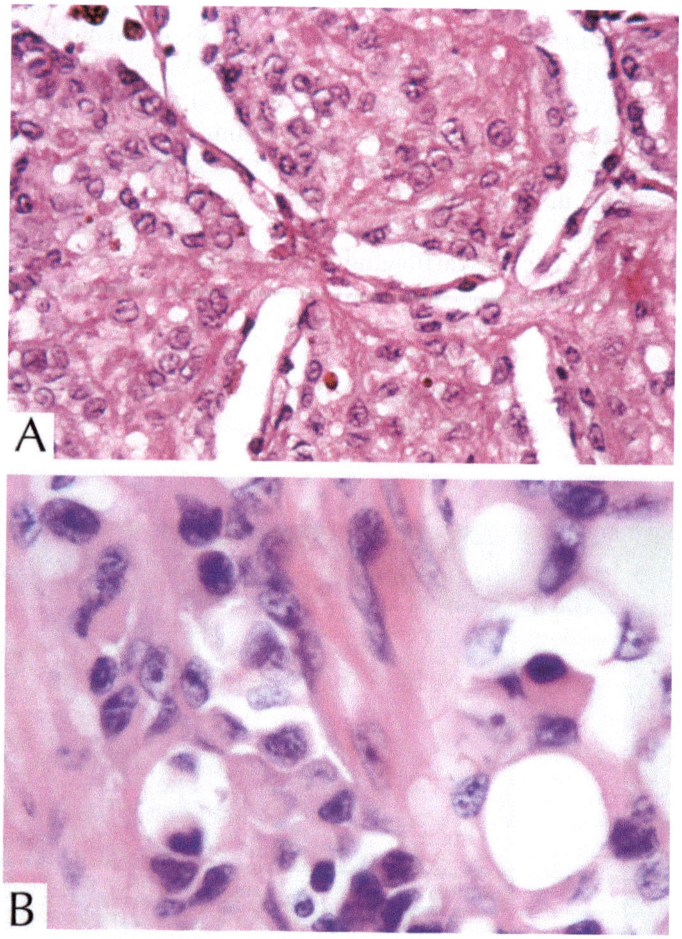

FIGURE 40.36. Epithelioid hemangioendothelioma. Note extension of tumor through pores of Kohn **(A)** and cytoplasmic vacuoles **(B)** representing primitive vascular lumina.

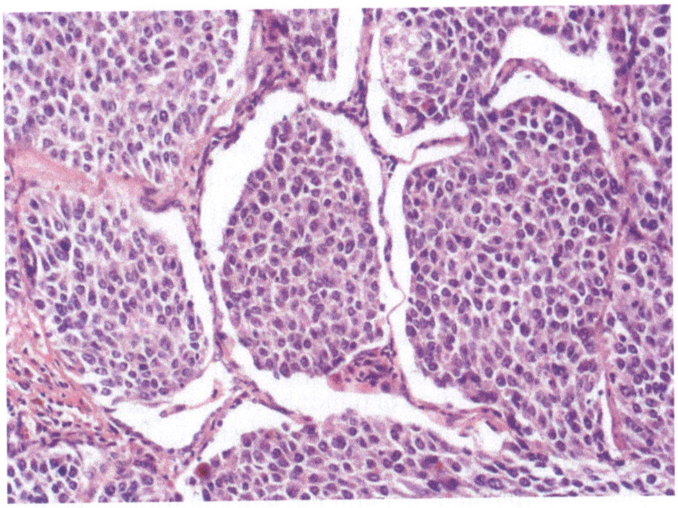

FIGURE 40.37. Large cell carcinoma. Micropolypoid intraalveolar growth of tumor cells is not exclusively seen in epithelioid hemangioendothelioma. This growth pattern was seen in a CD31- and CD34-negative large cell carcinoma showing extension through pores of Kohn.

lumina, sometimes of fair size, are seen, and are an inherent and key part of the tumor when identified. In some cases these are not obvious by light microscopy. Occasionally cytology specimens contain cells with similar features. Immunostains for factor VIII, CD31, and CD34 highlight both the cytoplasm of the tumor cells and these lumina. However, there is quite a degree of variability of staining in these lesions. The tumor cells can be estrogen and progesterone receptor positive.

In some tumors, there is retrograde extension into terminal bronchioles by plugs of tumor. Sometimes pleural spread results in characteristic nodules and positive pleural cytology. Vascular spread is also present in most lesions, often in the tumor nodules themselves, but at other times in vessels up to approximately 2 mm in diameter located away from identifiable nodules. Elastic stains may help define involved vessels in the midst of the tumor nodules. Rarely acute pulmonary hemorrhage has been described, and, at least in the mediastinum, osteoclast-like giant cells have been reported. Lymphangitic spread has also been identified. It may be in the form of elongated cells with eosinophilic cytoplasm, almost appearing as smooth muscle, or smaller groups of loosely cohesive cells that have an increased nuclear/cytoplasmic ratio and sometimes accentuate lymphatic spaces around the pulmonary artery, particularly thickening the wall. Sometimes this is seen as one-sided thickening of the vessel wall. The lymphatic spaces may be involved around the bronchopulmonary rays, interlobular septa, and pleura. The more lymphangitic spread there is, the worse the prognosis.

Electron microscopy as described by Corrin et al.[141] and others[152] shows abundant cytoplasmic intermediate filaments and a corresponding reduction in other expected organelles. The cytoplasmic membranes may have focal attachments with adjacent cells, described either as small desmosomes or as zonula adherens type. There are some pinocytotic vesicles along the cytoplasmic membranes. Although exceptions occur, usually there are no dense bodies or dense plaques as would be seen in smooth muscle. Cytoplasmic invaginations of intermediate filaments correspond with the nuclear inclusions seen at light microscopy. The cytoplasmic lumina have delicate projections of tumor cell cytoplasm extending into them. Weibel–Palade bodies have been described in a fair number of these tumors, but also have been absent in otherwise acceptable lesions when studied by electron microscopy (Fig. 40.38).[141,152,153]

The differential diagnosis of pulmonary epithelioid hemangioendothelioma includes many lesions. Practically speaking, the most common problems are with metastatic sarcomas of other types. Sarcomas, particularly leiomyosarcoma, chondrosarcoma, or osteosarcoma, and some nonsarcomatous poorly differentiated malignant tumors metastatic to the lung can have an initial micropolypoid filling of alveoli, but these tumor nodules usually rather rapidly eradicate the background lung architecture, become more spindle like, and somewhere in their mass give rise to their distinctive characteristics. In most of these sarcomas mitoses are plentiful and easily found. It is also unusual to have lung spread without being able to detect a primary source for most sarcomas. Very slowly growing metastases, such as in the case of benign metastasizing leiomyomas, usually form more solid balls with entrapment of metaplastic spaces but without preservation of the background architecture.

Another tumor to be distinguished is sclerosing hemangioma. This is usually a solitary lesion, although in a few cases multiple lesions have been described. Sclerosing hemangiomas occur in women in 82% of the cases, a percentage very close to the 80% incidence in women of pulmonary epithelioid hemangioendotheliomas. Immunostains for TTF-1 are positive, but factor VIII and other vascular markers have been negative in the tumor cells of sclerosing hemangioma, and electron microscopy appears different in that there is no evidence of endothelial differentiation. In addition, cells of sclerosing hemangiomas possess distinct cytoplasmic extensions and interdigitations with neighboring tumor cells. Lastly, by light microscopy sclerosing hemangiomas typically form larger papillae and denser areas of sclerosis, usually obliterating the lung background. These cellular proliferations carry with them a highly metaplastic alveolar type II cell covering, which causes confusion on electron micrographic and other studies. The micropolyps of epithelioid hemangioendothelioma lesions in the lung do not have a

A

B

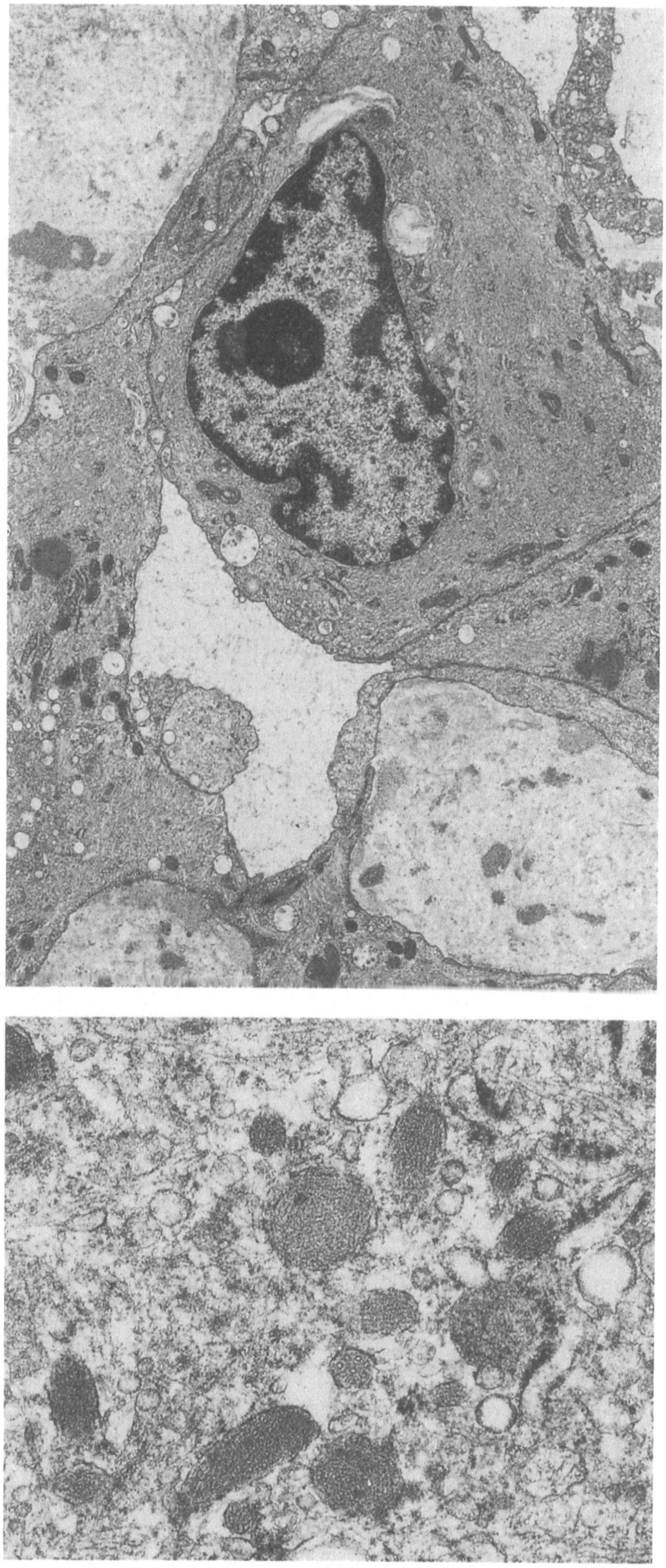

FIGURE 40.38. Epithelioid hemangioendothelioma. Ultrastructure. **(A)** Cells with abundant intermediate filaments and primitive vascular lumina. (Transmission electron microscopy [TEM].) **(B)** Weibel-Palade bodies. (TEM.)

covering of reactive alveolar type II cells, and any lesions stimulating hyperplastic alveolar type II cells must be suspicious as not being this tumor.

No effective therapy is yet known for pulmonary epithelioid hemangioendothelioma. Various attempts have been made to treat symptomatic patients, but by this time they are usually preterminal. Radiotherapy effected temporary remission in one liver tumor associated with lung nodules, but the patient died soon thereafter. The dense accumulation of stroma from the dying tumor cells may also mean that the mass effect of these lesions is not reversible to any degree, despite cell death, and only rarely has reabsorption of tumor been seen focally. Unlike most of these lesions in bone, soft tissue, or liver, lesions in the lungs cannot easily be resected because of the typical multiple and bilateral nodular infiltrates. Surgical excision was most effective in soft tissues of the extremities or for solitary internal tumors. Early experience with transplantation for these tumors in liver is now seen to be unfavorable as recurrences are frequent. In the lung, the surgeon often finds many more nodules than were radiographically appreciated.

Patients with epithelioid hemangioendotheliomas tend to be seen in one of two phases of their relationship to their tumors. One group dies within a year of diagnosis, these being the more symptomatic patients, with either more aggressive disease, or those toward the end of their natural course. However, exceptions do occur and longer survivals have been documented.[136,147] A boy 13 years old and a woman of 23 years at the time of diagnosis were alive and functioning well 20 years later despite very involved-looking chest radiographs.[136,147] Another patient died 20 years after diagnosis of slow progression of her disease. At autopsy her right ventricle was 1.4 cm thick. Death usually results from slow respiratory compromise, although one patient died with an acute pneumonia.[147] Overall, the prognosis of these tumors is very unpredictable, with life expectancies ranging from 1 to 15 years. However, spontaneous regression and some responses to chemotherapy and interferon have been reported.[154,155]

Angiosarcoma

As with other sarcomas, metastatic angiosarcoma is the most common form of this tumor seen in the lung. It may come from any site where angiosarcomas arise, including postmastectomy sites and other areas of chronic vascular stasis, and postirradiation fields, as well as in thorotrast-exposed patients, and it may arise spontaneously in such areas as head, scalp, breast, and heart.[156,157] Spencer[158] questioned whether there is any truly primary angiosarcoma in lung. Even in a group of large pulmonary vessel sarcomas, only rarely are they classified as angiosarcoma.

It is interesting that the lung is not more subject to the development of angiosarcomas, or, for that matter, other truly vascular neoplasms, considering how much of a vascular organ it is.

Due to their exceedingly low frequency, most knowledge of pulmonary angiosarcomas is derived from case reports or a handful of small series of cases. The three patients reported by Yousem[159] as presenting with angiosarcoma in the lung were all women between the ages of 22 and 30 at the time of diagnosis who had bilateral infiltrates without cardiac tumors identified. One patient later died, and no autopsy was done. The second had bilateral nodular parenchymal infiltrates and a right-atrial and right-ventricular tumor, including a possible tumor nodule in the liver, and was alive at 5 months. The third had bilateral reticulonodular infiltrates, but on clinical evaluation had no malignancy anywhere else at the time of diagnosis. Three months later she had CNS and hepatic involvement, and died 1 month later. Again, no autopsy was performed. At least the second case must be considered definitely metastatic, and the other two are suspicious as being so. Because autopsies were not available in the other two cases, a full description of the extent of these lesions will remain unknown, and Yousem acknowledged this with the words "presenting in" instead of "arising in" the lung in the article title.

A more convincing but still unusual case was described by Spragg and associates.[156] These authors reviewed the literature and noted 10 possibly primary cases, but on close review many of these cases could not be confirmed as primary pulmonary angiosarcomas. Only two cases are reported as most likely to represent primary angiosarcomas in their review.[156–159] Their added case was that of a 75-year-old man with bilateral diffuse pulmonary infiltrates, who at autopsy had diffusely hemorrhagic and heavy lungs, with the right lung weighing 2700 g and the left 1700 g. This was a diffuse process with highly pleomorphic, malignant endothelial-appearing cells forming some thin-walled vascular-like spaces, but factor VIII–related antigen by immunoperoxidase was negative. An embolus of malignant cells, appearing to have come from vascular invasion in the lung, ended up in the femoral blood supply. The only other site of malignancy was a 0.3 × 0.1 cm presumed metastatic lesion in the submucosa of the colon. These authors argued reasonably that, due to the bulk of the disease in the lung, the lung was most likely the primary site. Their patient had a prior history of industrial exposure in South African copper mines.

Overall angiosarcoma in the lungs must be regarded as a very unusual tumor. In the Mayo Clinic series these tumors represented only 10% of all primary pulmonary sarcomas.[160] In the series from the Massachusetts General Hospital, only two of 26 primary pulmonary sarcomas were angiosarcomas.[161] The median age is 45 years but with a wide range, and no sex predilection has been reported. Clinically, some patients may present with hemoptysis or syndromes akin to diffuse pulmonary hemorrhage. Others may have nonspecific symptomatology such as dyspnea and weight loss, and others yet may be entirely asymptomatic.[162] Those in the pulmonary artery tract may mimic pulmonary thromboembolic disease.[163] By gross examination, most angiosarcomas in the lung show multiple, bilateral lesions; rarely, they present as solitary masses.[164,165] More frequently, they occur as multiple nodules, and sometimes they appear as red to purple streaks along bronchovascular bundles. The lesions are often hemorrhagic.[164,165] Microscopically, the tumor may form discrete nodules or subtle interstitial infiltrates. Characteristically the tumor cells form anastomosing vascular spaces lined by cytologically atypical endothelial cells, which often have a hobnailed appearance and prominent nucleoli (Fig. 40.39).[164,165] The cells may have varying amounts of eosinophilic cytoplasm; when the cytoplasm is abundant, the tumor may be readily confused with a carcinoma.[164,165]

Angiosarcomas typically stain for one or more of the following vascular markers: factor VIII–related antigen, *Ulex europaeus*, CD31, and CD34.[164] In poorly differentiated tumors, however, it may be difficult to demonstrate staining for these vascular antigens.[164] Epithelial markers such as keratin or epithelial membrane antigen should be absent. Still, some epithelioid angiosarcomas may stain with epithelial markers such as keratin and B72.3.[164,166–169] In such cases, the diagnosis must be carefully considered using other parameters such as the vascular immunohistochemical markers, histologic features, and electron microscopy.[164] Characteristic ultrastructural features of angiosarcomas include the finding of endothelial cells with pinocytotic vesicles, lateral desmosome-like attachments, and paranuclear filaments. A basal lamina can be present around the endothelial cells, and Weibel-Palade bodies are a distinctive feature of endothelial differentiation.[164,170] Important differential diagnoses include metastatic angiosarcomas to the lung and carcinomas with pseudoangiomatous features. In these instances a thorough clinical history and appropriate use of immunohistochemistry along with vascular markers assist in making this distinction.

Extracutaneous angiosarcomas metastatic to the lungs have a differential of their own, and as reported by Bocklage and associates[171] they must be distinguished from a variety of benign and malignant tumors and other nontumoral conditions such as thromboembolic disease, alveolar hemorrhage syndrome, and benign vasoformative lesions such as capillary hemangiomatosis. These authors considered benign entities in the differential diagnosis because some lesions presented wedge-shaped morphology, presented as a subpleural mass, or showed intraalveolar proliferation of spindle cells with fibrosis and inflammation. Among malignant tumors mimicking

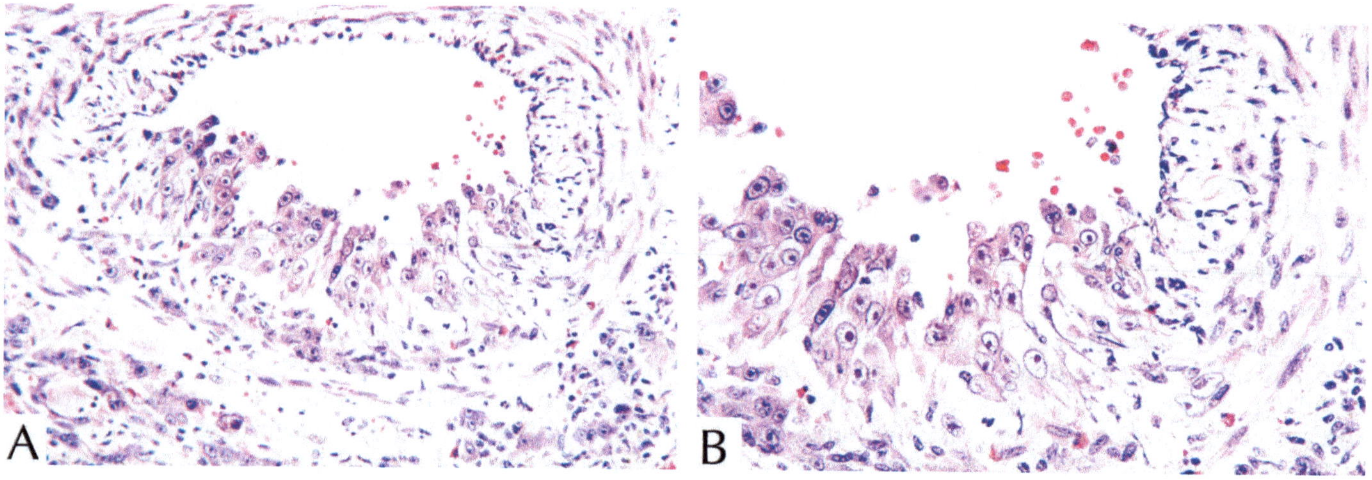

FIGURE 40.39. Angiosarcoma. **(A)** Note atypical epithelioid cell proliferation growing along the endothelial surface of a vessel. **(B)** On closer view, the cells display hobnailing, atypia, and prominent nucleoli.

extracutaneous angiosarcoma metastatic to the lung, the authors cite the following potential confounders: high-grade adenocarcinoma, malignant fibrous histiocytoma, epithelioid hemangioendothelioma, Kaposi's sarcoma, intravascular lymphoma, and melanoma.

The prognosis for angiosarcomas presenting in the lung is very poor, with an average survival of 9 months. There is no known effective therapy for angiosarcomas involving the lung. Radiation therapy, chemotherapy, and surgical resection have been attempted with little success.[162] Rare exceptions do occur however. One patient reported by Kojima et al.[172] responded to combined modality treatment consisting of radiotherapy and immunomodulation with recombinant interleukin-2. Angiosarcomas are more common as primary tumors in the pleura, and are further discussed in Chapter 43.

Pulmonary Artery Sarcomas

These rare neoplasms most often arise in or adjacent to the pulmonary artery trunk. They frequently extend more distally along the main pulmonary arteries and may embolize to the lung parenchyma.[173–177] Occasionally just one pulmonary artery is involved without spread to the pulmonary trunk. In some cases, tumor extends into, or arises from, the right ventricle, and hence the broader term *right outflow tract sarcomas* is preferred by some. One case may have arisen in an arteriovenous fistula near the right hilum, and rare ones are thought secondary to past radiotherapy.[178–180] Clinically, pulmonary artery sarcomas may present either as a single large pulmonary embolus or multiple smaller emboli, or with obvious right-heart failure, or they may present with ongoing progressive and mysterious respiratory symptoms. Many of the symptoms are related to right-heart obstruction and compromised perfusion of one or both lungs, or embolization mimicking thromboembolic disease.[181] Computed tomography, MRI, and angiography are the best ways to detect these tumors, but even with these technologies premortem diagnosis is made in about only half of the cases.[182,183]

Mandelstamm[184] is credited with the first description of outflow tract–pulmonary artery sarcoma. Twenty-one cases were summarized by Wackers et al.[173] in 1969; 37 by Shmookler et al.[174] in 1977; 60 by Bleisch and Kraus[175] in 1980; and 78 by Baker and Goodwin[176] in 1985, who then summarized the cases in the English-language literature; the review of Bleisch and Kraus covers those in the non–English-language literature. McGlennen et al.[177] in 1989 estimated about 100 cases had been reported, but it is still so rare that their experience with four cases over 15 years at a major medical center is considered a large series. Among 26 cases of primary pulmonary sarcoma reported by Keel et al.[161] in 1999, two were identified as intimal sarcoma. The later reviews are the source for most of the findings given here.

The youngest reported patient was 15 years old and the oldest 81. Sixty percent occur in the 45- to 64-year age group, and twice as many women as men are affected. Dyspnea, chest pain, and cough are the main clinical manifestations. Approximately 76% of the patients present with dyspnea, 60% with chest pain, 53% with cough, and others with assorted pulmonary obstructive and hypoxic symptoms. A rare patient may have symptoms for prolonged periods of time, and in one particular case this was 21 years.[175]

Grossly, the tumor masses most often involve the pulmonary trunk and may extend along the walls to involve either or both pulmonary arteries. They may extend in retrograde fashion and involve the pulmonic valve. Most are described as multinodular, firm, yellow-tan, and smoothly contoured (Fig. 40.40A,B). Some have grossly evident endovascular tumor polyps. Occasionally there is evidence of recent embolization from such a site, as both an acute fracture line on the proximal tumor and a distally identified companion fragment. Some endovascular tumors resemble thrombus material throughout. Some are localized to a main pulmonary artery, while direct extension grossly is noted to the lungs in 56% of the cases, and sometimes this can be traced almost to the periphery. Although usually small, nodules of metastatic tumor as large as 3 cm may be present in the lung parenchyma, and these are often bilateral. The nodules may show associated bronchial and parenchymal invasion after spread through the vascular wall, but often they are contained within the vessels. There may be other densities that represent infarcts from either growing tumor or tumor emboli or thromboemboli plugging vessels.

Microscopically, these sarcomas present with a wide spectrum of morphologic patterns, which are well summarized by McGlennen et al.[177] Some are quite cellular, others are hypocellular and more myxoid, while still others have a variegated pattern (Figs. 40,40C,D and 40.41). Most commonly the sarcomatous elements are described as undifferentiated (34%), leiomyosarcomatous (20%), rhabdomyosarcomatous (6%), fibrosarcomatous (17%), chondrosarcomatous (4%), osteosarcomatous (4%), and 6% with mixed differentiation, classifiable as malignant mesenchymomas. A lesser degree of angiosarcomatous differentiation is present than would be expected for origin in this organ, but this is also true for sarcomas arising in other large vessels, whether they be arteries or veins.[181] Some of the primary chondrosarcomas in lung may belong to this vascular group.[185,186] A few of these sarcomas of major vessel origin have large to giant pleomorphic undifferentiated cells, sometimes being multinucleate. Three to five percent have definite mixed

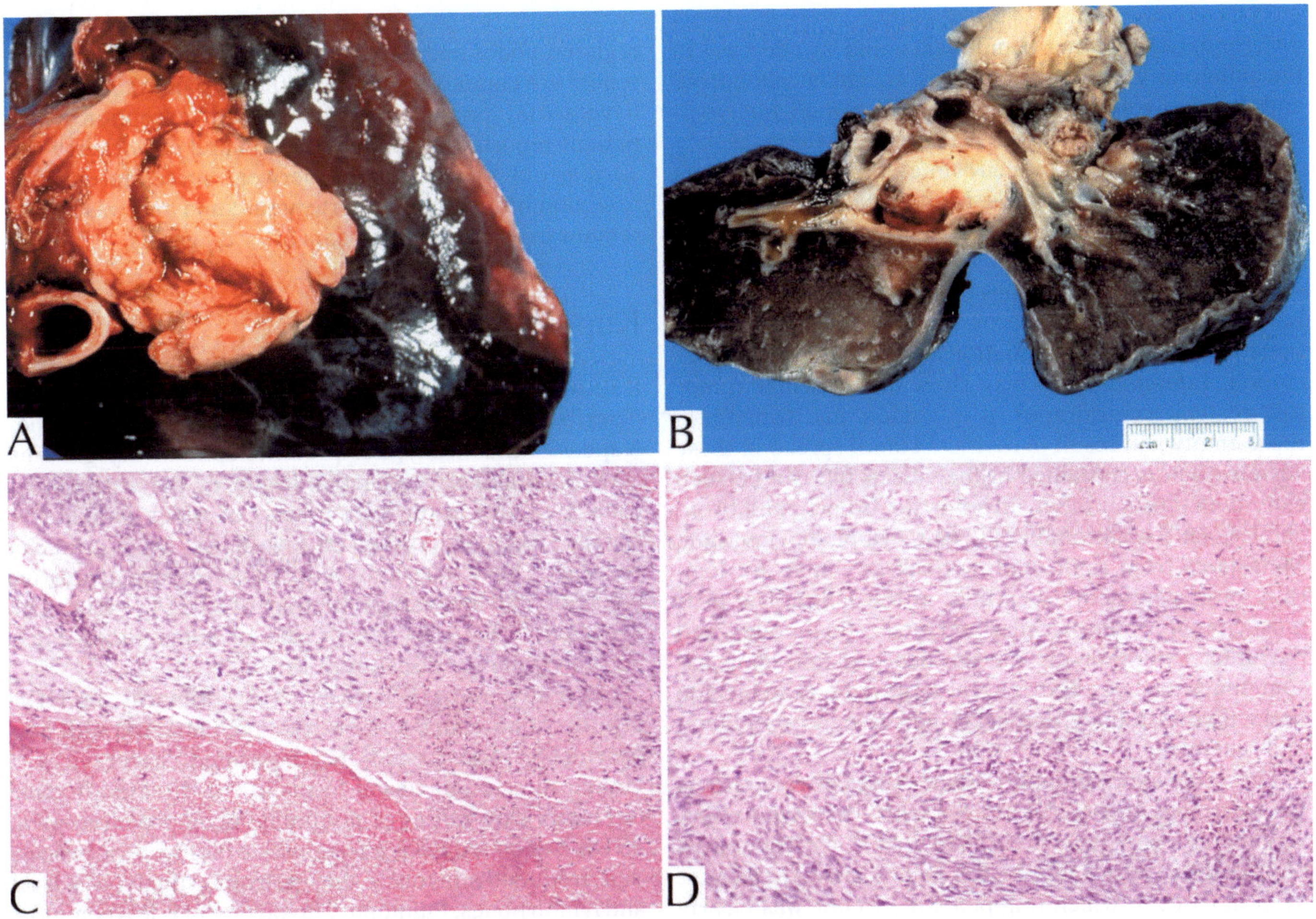

FIGURE 40.40. Pulmonary artery sarcoma. **(A,B)** Note fleshy gray-yellow intravascular mass, which greatly distends the proximal pulmonary artery. **(C,D)** Note fibrin-filled vascular lumen and wall of artery permeated by a hypercellular atypical spindle cell proliferation. (Courtesy of Dr. Arthur Tischler and Dr. Maria Moliner, Tufts University School of Medicine, Boston, MA.)

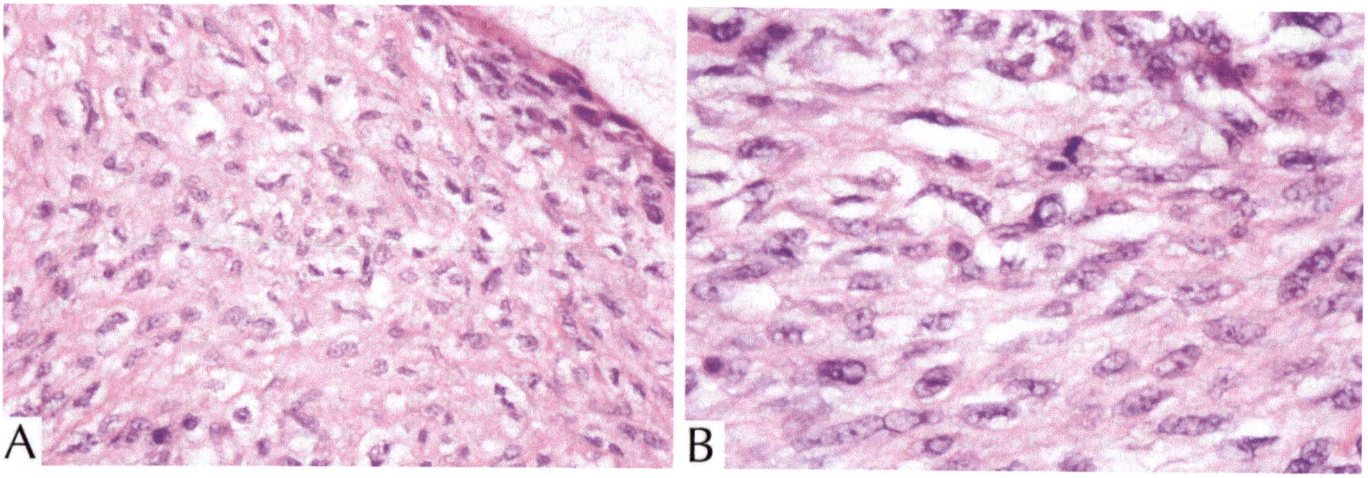

FIGURE 40.41. **(A,B)** Pulmonary artery sarcoma. Closer microscopic view of tumor shown in the preceding figure. Note hypercellularity, pleomorphism, and mitotic figures. (Courtesy of Dr. Arthur Tischer and Dr. Maria Moliner, Tufts University School of Medicine, Boston, MA.)

differentiated sarcoma components, and in one case in the pulmonary outflow there was malignant chondroid and rhabdomyoblastic change[187]; the term *malignant mesenchymoma* may be preferred for some of these.

Tumor may spread in a circumferential manner along the inner walls of the vessels. More distally there may be eccentric or concentric thickening by an admixture of tumor, fibrin, and collagen in varying proportions. In some places such thickenings appear to be collagen only, but on serial sections, nearby tumor is identified in the same vessels. A similar situation exists for carcinomatous emboli. Infarcted areas may show endovascular tumor toward their central apex of infarction, and sometimes these empty and result in cavities. Tumor spread in these vessels often is contained in the vessels but can be seen extending through them, invading the bronchi and bronchioles, and occasionally showing lymphatic invasion. Metastases from right outflow track sarcomas are logically most commonly identified in the lungs. The next most common sites are hilar and mediastinal nodes, and by direct extension the pleura, heart, diaphragm, and sometimes the liver. Extrathoracic sites of spread include brain, thyroid, kidney, adrenal gland, mesentery, jejunum, and omentum.

The prognostic outlook is poor. Surgical resection is the treatment of choice, but even when detected earlier, surgery is only rarely curative.[177,182,188] Postoperative recurrence is most often in the field nearest the tumor, even in cases in which it appears the tumor was clearly excised at first operation. The mean survival after diagnosis is about 12 months, and at that time nearly four fifths of patients have already developed metastases. Some metastases are intrapulmonary and others occur in regional nodes and outside the chest. Postsurgical recurrences are common, and chemotherapy and radiotherapy have so far proven ineffective.[175] An exception is the patient reported in 2002 by Mattoo and coworkers[181]—a 32-year-old woman who underwent successful surgical resection of a pulmonary artery sarcoma and was said to remain free of disease 5 years after diagnosis.

Kaposi's Sarcoma

Kaposi's sarcoma (KS) is a vascular sarcoma that was first described in 1872 by the Hungarian physician Moricz Kaposi.[189] Classically, KS presents as a slowly growing cutaneous and subcutaneous lesion of the extremities, usually in the lower extremities, of older individuals, usually men of Ashkenazi-Jewish or Mediterranean descent. The KS lesions tend to have low aggressive behavior, and an average life span of 8 to 14 years can be expected.[190] Patients usually die of some other cause before significant disease develops.[191]

Currently, most KS cases occur primarily in HIV-positive homosexual and bisexual men infected with herpesvirus-8, also called KS-associated herpesvirus.[192] Unlike the classic clinical forms of the disease affecting the lower extremities of nonimmunocompromised men, AIDS-associated KS is an aggressive multicentric process that frequently involves the gastrointestinal (GI) tract and lymph nodes. Pulmonary involvement is less common, affecting only about 10% of AIDS patients.[192] In women, the disease risk factors include intravenous drug use, heterosexual contact, or both, and the clinical manifestations are usually mistaken for pulmonary infection.[193] The clinical symptomatology is not specific. Fever, cough, dyspnea, and wheezing with or without hemoptysis are the usual presenting symptoms. Chest radiographs may show nodularities or diffuse infiltrates.[194] Computed tomography and MRI do not provide much additional information. Endoscopically, KS appears as bright red or bluish, slightly raised mucosal areas on the bronchial mucosa, an appearance that is regarded as diagnostic.[194]

Grossly, the surface of the lungs may show, in the visceral pleura, flat to slightly raised disk-shaped red to violaceous plaques (Fig. 40.42A,B). However, these lesions have not been described on the parietal pleura. A few changes have been noted in the lung parenchyma itself. Most striking is lymphangitic thickening by tumor with a perivascular or periseptal distribution, giving a red to red-blue discoloration to the affected tissues (Fig. 40.42C). There are sometimes nodules of red to purple to gray tumor that vary in size up to 0.5 cm. These nodules may coalesce to form larger tumor densities. The lymph nodes may be involved by spongy red-to-gray material replacing the usual translucent tan architecture. Central carbon deposition, so common in these nodes, may also be disrupted. In addition to Kaposi's sarcoma, there is also an admixture of other disease events, such as opportunistic infection and respiratory distress syndrome, and nonspecific changes that add other densities to the gross findings.

Microscopically, lesions of KS may be subtle, especially when focal. Attention should be paid to the areas of expected lymphatic routes. In the more solid regions, spindle cells are in loose fascicles with some tendency to form interdigitating fascicles (Fig. 40.43). There are slit-like spaces, often without identifiable endothelial cells or lining tumor, with abundant scattered red cells and some hemosiderin, both in these spaces and in the more solid part of the tumor. The smooth muscle of the bronchioles and pulmonary arteries may be infiltrated by tumor, giving it a thickened appearance, almost like granulation tissue. The larger bronchi show focal spindle cell and hemorrhagic proliferations in the involved submucosa. Fairly extensive acute intraalveolar hemorrhage may be present, especially at the time of death. This background of acute hemorrhage can be confusing and may possibly obscure some of the lesions that would be more obvious

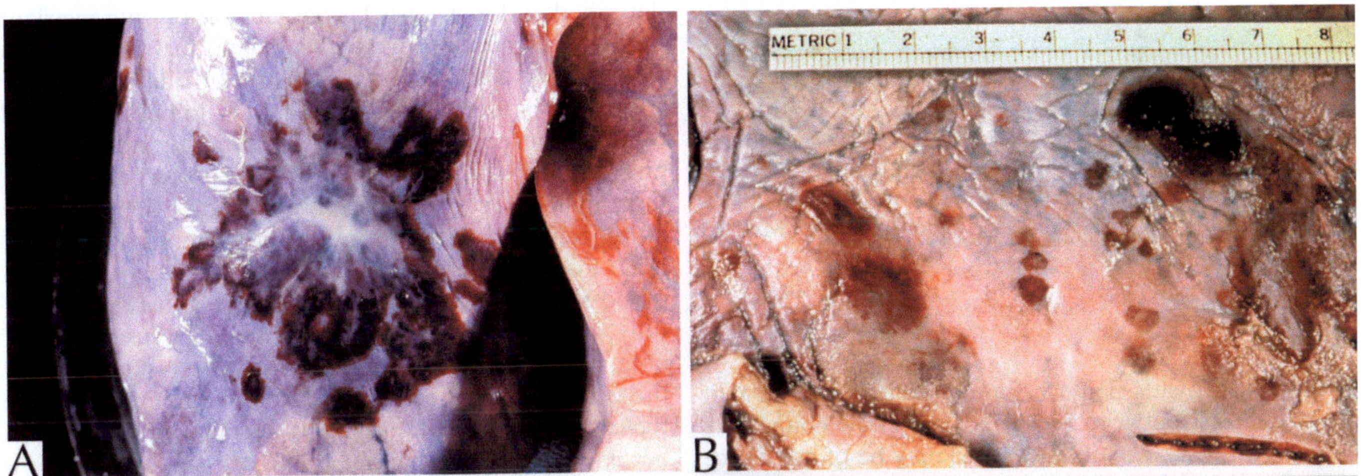

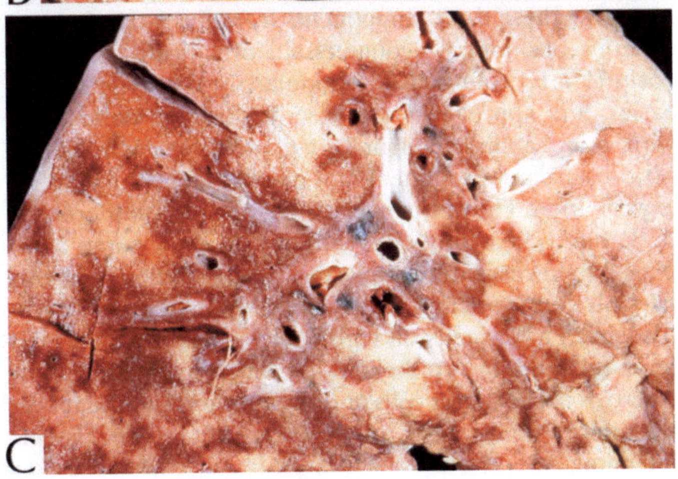

FIGURE 40.42. Kaposi's sarcoma. Gross appearance. **(A)** Note violaceous plaques on visceral pleural surface. **(B)** Reddish nodular lesion on pleural surface. **(C)** Same lesions on cut surface of lung. Note perivascular and periseptal distribution.

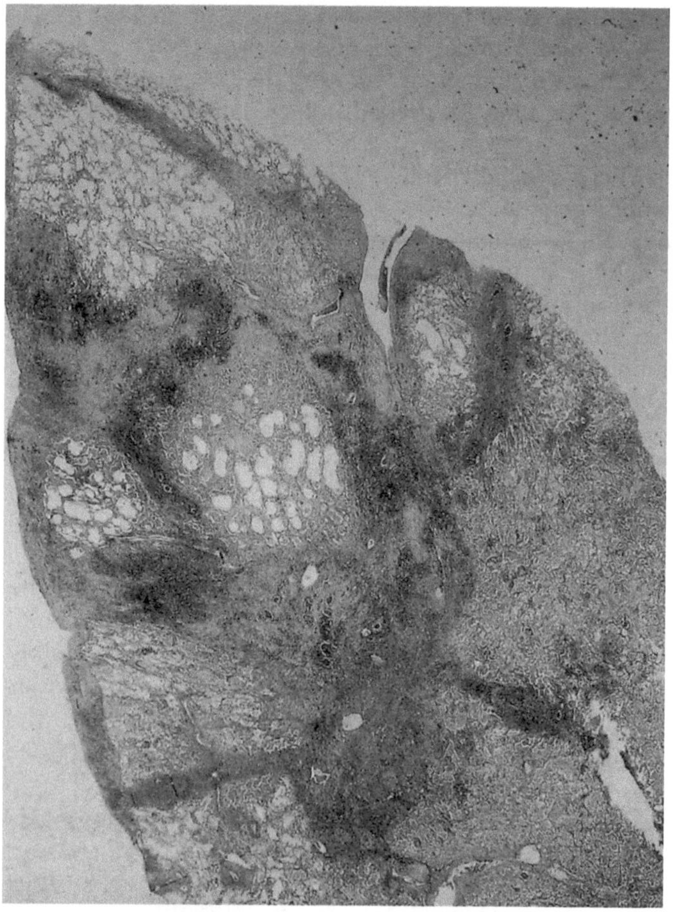

FIGURE 40.43. Kaposi's sarcoma. Lymphangitic spread, appreciated at this low power, involves bronchopulmonary rays and interlobular septa along with focal pleural involvement. (Courtesy of R. Askins and W.B. Kinglsley, Baylor University Medical Center, Dallas, TX.)

without it. Movat's pentachrome stain is one stain that offers contrast between red cells and yellow connective tissue, with black elastic tissue, and may be of assistance in sorting these three components from the rather homogeneous eosinophilic counterstain of hematoxylin and eosin (H&E) stains. In the nodular form recognition is easier, and approaches are described in the classic KS, with more abundant spindle cells and vascular clefts. Mitoses are not prominent, but may be seen with careful examination. The tumor nuclei are elongated, moderately dark, and not greatly enlarged, but do show some anaplastic features. Intracytoplasmic hyalin bodies, thought possibly to represent a stage of erythrophagocytosis, are present in a few cells on high-power examination. They tend to be in more epithelioid-appearing malignant cells. Necrosis in the tumor cells or distant lung is rarely caused by tumor, being more often the result of coexistent infection.

Several microscopic patterns of KS have been observed (Fig. 40.44). One pattern is the cavernous-angiomatous pattern, seen in the pleura and interlobular septa, or around blood vessels of the lung. Blood-filled thin-walled dilated channels are sometimes seen on only one side of a blood vessel, or focally in other lymphatic drainage areas, and should be a clue to this diagnosis. Blood should not be in the lymphatic pathways. In reactive states, the whole system should be involved equally. Dilated vessels filled with blood may account for some of the pleural plaques seen from the surface. Similar changes may occur in lymph nodes and elsewhere, both of the variant patterns and in more typical Kaposi's lesions. Early nodal spread is first seen in the subscapular sinuses, in keeping with this lymphangitic spread of this peculiar sarcoma. Thickening of a node capsule in an eccentric manner may suggest serial sections are warranted to detect KS nearby. Nodes may be so involved as to have obliteration of germinal centers, subcapsular and interfollicular sinuses, and eventually of the medullary regions, leading to enlarged but lymphoid-depleted nodes. Focally, KS may extend into adjacent fat near the nodes, or into fat adjacent to some of the more proximal main bronchi.

Another pattern of KS has been called inflammatory, early, or polymorphous Kaposi's sarcoma. This has been described in skin in early lesions, and represents a variant pattern, not necessarily a precursor to the more typical lesions. This variant lesion consists of dilated vascular spaces with more pleomorphic cells lining them, and often obscured by plasma cells, lymphocytes, macrophages, and some eosinophilic leukocytes. The same inflammatory reaction is seen in focal, and sometimes in more generalized, infiltrates in the interstitium of the lung. Focal collections of these inflammatory cells with blood should lead one to search these areas more carefully, and perhaps do serial sections if KS is suspected. Of note, plasma cells in particular have been associated with these infiltrates. These lesions blend with areas of more typical KS, and were originally recognized in the skin because of this association. Limited tissue samples provided by transbronchial biopsies may show cellular spindle cell populations that may at least allow a suspicion of KS. In these instances immunostaining and other techniques as noted below are helpful (Fig. 40.45).

The spindle cells of KS stain positively for vascular markers such as factor VIII–related antigen and CD34. Stains for vimentin may also be positive.[195] By electron microscopy, KS shows variable mixtures of endothelial cells, pericytes, fibroblasts, and myofibroblasts. Weibel-Palade bodies may be absent.[195] Identification of human herpesvirus-8 DNA (HHV-8) in bronchoalveolar lavage fluid is useful in confirming the diagnosis of tracheobronchial KS.[196] Similar assays using polymerase chain reaction technology have been found valuable in KS patients suffering from recurrent pleural effusions.[197]

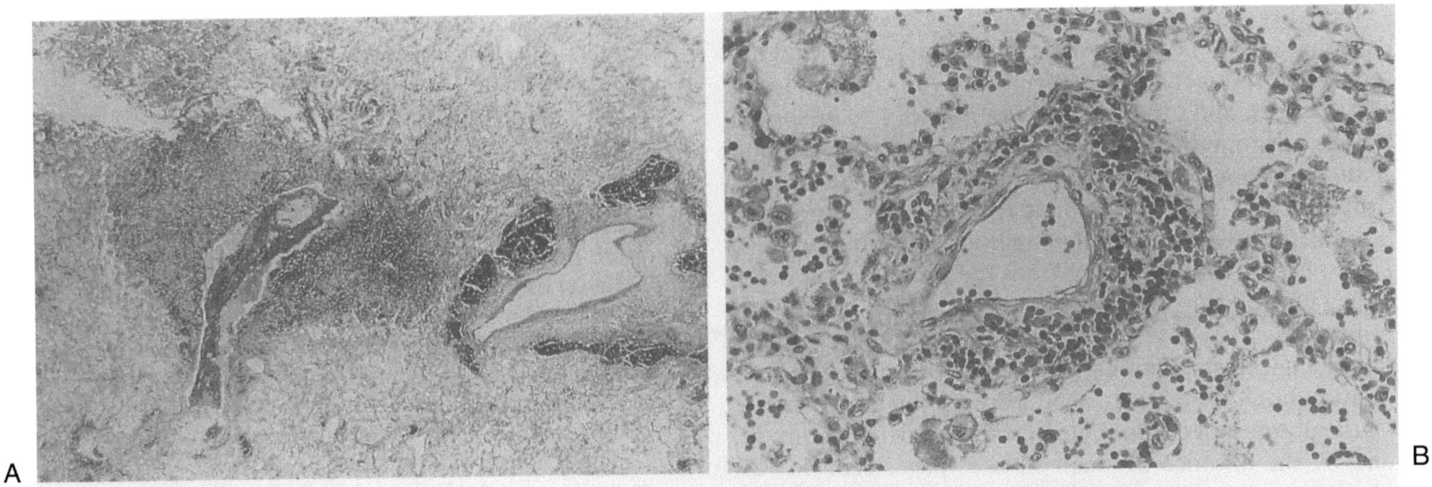

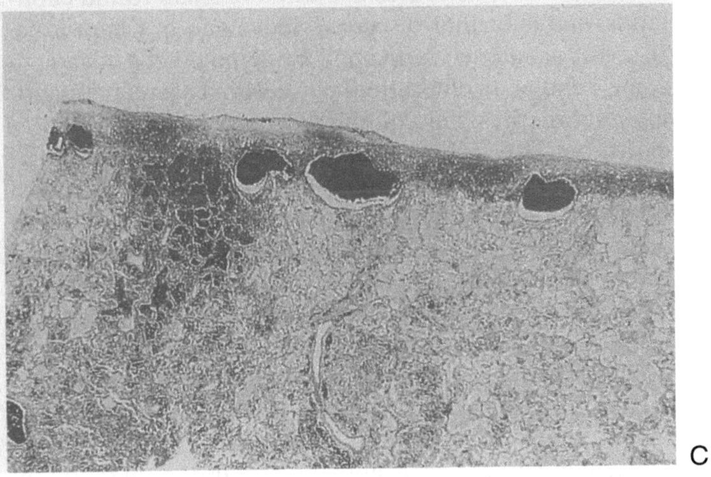

FIGURE 40.44. Kaposi's sarcoma (KS). **(A)** Combination of smaller slitlike vessels of KS presenting as a nodule on the left and as a cavernous hemangiomatous pattern on the right. **(B)** Perivascular lymphangitic spaces filled with blood. Note spared zone on the left-lower edge. **(C)** Cavernous hemangioma pattern extends to pleura and accounts for some blood-filled bleb formation grossly seen in pleura in Figure 40.43.

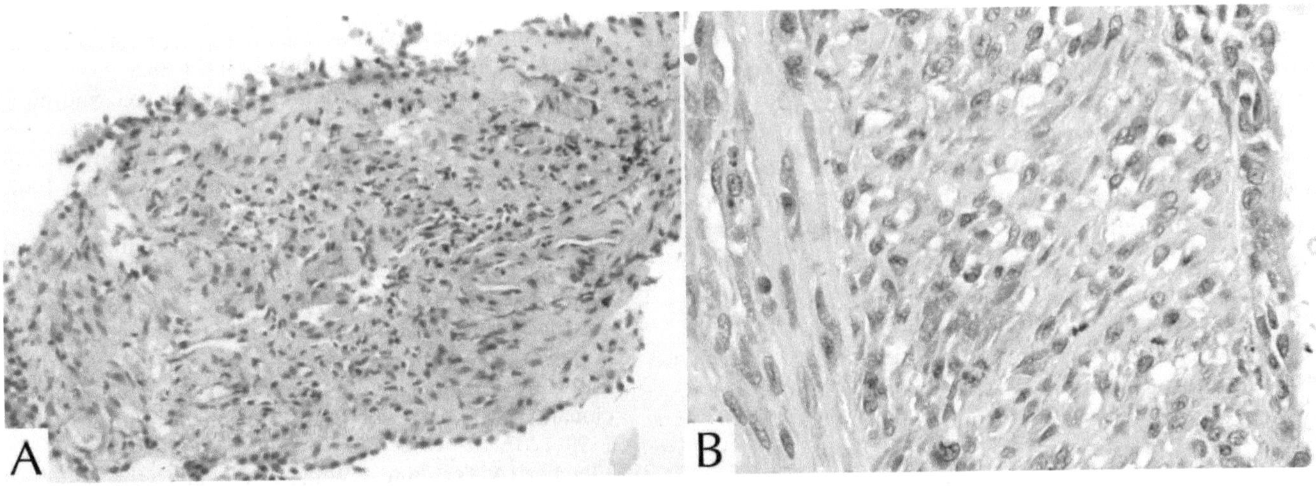

FIGURE 40.45. Kaposi's sarcoma. **(A)** Transbronchial biopsy showing denuded respiratory epithelium on top and a cellular spindle cell population on bottom. **(B)** Detail of above; note smooth muscle fibers of bronchial wall on left.

In terms of differential diagnosis, the atypical spindle cells that focally line cleft-shaped vascular spaces, and the increased red cells, in association with hemosiderin, plasma cells, and other mixed inflammatory cells, should help to distinguish KS from fibrosarcoma, granulation tissue, and other fibroblastic proliferations. The hyaline droplets that are fairly characteristic of KS are also helpful if identified. The lymphangitic distribution pattern is also useful, and is distinct from the intraalveolar organizing fibroblastic polyps, or Masson bodies, bronchiolitis obliterans, or other forms of fibrosis. Lymphangiomatosis, lymphangiectasia, lymphangioma, and other dilated lymphatics should be distinguished from dilated blood vessels by the absence of erythrocytes, clear to pink fluid content, and by the absence of small slitlike spaces seen in KS. Hemangiomatosis causes dilatation of small round capillaries, and is further discussed above and in Chapter 28. It is not usually accompanied by spindle cells, although some cellular proliferation can occur. Lymphangioleiomyomatosis has rims of spindle cells, without vascular clefts, but also follows lymphatic pathways. Lymphangioleiomyomatosis forms air cysts in the lung, whereas KS does not. Lymphangioleiomyomatosis only rarely shows acute bleeding or congestion. These two should only rarely be confused. A history of documented KS elsewhere is very helpful in establishing a firm diagnosis. Bacillary angiomatosis (BA) can cause endobronchial polyps, which basically have an angiomatous appearance mixed with inflammatory cells resembling granulation tissue.[195] However, BA fundamentally represents an unusual inflammatory histologic response to infection by a bacillary organism, *Rochalimaea henselae*.[195] This microorganism can be demonstrated by Warthin-Starry stains, electron microscopy, or immunohistochemistry (see Chapter 8).[195]

The prognosis of KS is poor. Virtually all patients with visceral involvement die within 2 years from diagnosis. However, chemotherapy and radiation therapy may provide significant palliation, particularly if used in conjunction with highly active antiretroviral therapy (HARRT).[192] Surgical excision is not a realistic option due to the multiplicity of the lesions.

Acknowledgments. The authors are deeply appreciative to Karen Balcius for expert secretarial assistance, Rob Carlin for photography, and Andy Dzaugis and Rosemary Leary for bibliographic support.

References

1. McDonald JR, Harrington SW, Clagett OT. Hamartoma (often called chondroma) of the lung. J Thorac Cardiovasc Surg 1945;14:128–143.
2. Arrigoni MG, Woodner LB, Bernat PE, et al. Benign tumors of the lung. A ten year surgical experience. J Thorac Cardiovasc Surg 1970;60:589–599.
3. Mitsudomi T, Kaneko S, Tateishi M, et al. Benign tumors and tumor-like lesions of the lung. Int Surg 1990;75:155–158.
4. Jones RC, Cleve EA. Solitary circumscribed lesions of lung: selection of cases for diagnostic thoracotomy. AMA Arch Intern Med 1954;93:842.
5. Bateson EM. So-called hamartoma of the lung: a true neoplasm of fibrous connective tissue of the bronchi. Cancer 1973;31:1458–1467.
6. Tomashefski JF Jr. Benign endobronchial mesenchymal tumors: their relationship to parenchymal pulmonary hamartomas. Am J Surg Pathol 1982;6:531–540.
7. Tanno S, Ohsaki Y, Nakao S, et al. A case of pulmonary hamartoma and sclerosing hemangioma in the same lung. Nihon Kokyuki Gakkai Zasshi 2003;41:112–116.
8. King JC, Myers J. Isolated metastasis to a pulmonary hamartoma. Am J Surg Pathol 1995;19:472–475.
9. Blair TC, McElvein RM. Hamartoma of the lung: a clinical study of 25 cases. Dis Chest 1963;44:296–302.
10. Bateson EM. Relationship between intrapulmonary and endobronchial cartilage-containing tumours (so-called hamartoma). Thorax 1965;20:447–461.
11. Bateson EM. Cartilage-containing tumours of the lung: relationship between the purely cartilaginous type (chondroma) and the mixed type (so-called hamartoma). An unusual case of multiple tumours. Thorax 1967;22:256–259.
12. Bateson EM. Histogenesis of intrapulmonary and endobronchial hamartomas and chondromas (cartilage containing tumours). A hypothesis. J Pathol 1970;101:77–83.
13. Stone FJ, Churg AM. The ultrastructure of pulmonary hamartoma. Cancer 1977;39:1064–1977.
14. Perez-Atayde AR, Seiler MW. Pulmonary hamartoma: an ultrastructural study. Cancer 1984;53:485–492.
15. Carney JA. The triad of gastric epithelioid leiomyosarcoma, functioning extra-adrenal paraganglioma, and pulmonary chondroma. Cancer 1979;43:374–382.
16. Gabrail NY, Zara BY. Pulmonary hamartoma syndrome. Chest 1990;97:962–965.
17. Hayward RH, Carabasi RJ. Malignant hamartoma of the lung: fact or fiction? J Thorac Cardiovasc Surg 1967;53:457–466.
18. Basile A, Gregoris A, Antoci B, et al. Malignant change in a benign pulmonary hamartoma. Thorax 1989;44:232–233.
19. Salminen U-S, Halttunen P, Taskinen E, et al. Recurrence and malignant transformation of endotracheal chondroma. Ann Thorac Surg 1990;49:830–832.
20. Fletcher JA, Pinkus GS, Weidner N, et al. Lineage-restricted clonality in biphasic solid tumors. Am J Pathol 1991;138:1199–1207.
21. Fletcher JA, Longtine J, Wallace K, et al. Cytogenetic and histologic findings in 17 pulmonary chondroid hamartomas. Evidence for a pathogenetic relationship with lipomas and leiomyomas. Genes Chromosomes Cancer 1995;12:220–223.
22. van den Bosch JMM, Wagenanar Sj Sc, Corrin B, et al. Mesenchymoma of the lung (so called hamartoma): a

review of 154 parenchymal and endobronchial cases. Thorax 1987;42:790–793.
23. Gjevre JA, Myers JL, Prakash UBS. Pulmonary hamartomas. Mayo Clin Proc 1996;71:14–20.
24. Bateson EM, Abbott EK. Mixed tumors of the lung or hamartochondromas: a review of cases published in the literature and a report of fifteen new cases. Clin Radiol 1960;11:232–247.
25. Hamper UM, Khouri NF, Stitik FP, et al. Pulmonary hamartoma: diagnosis by transthoracic needle aspiration biopsy. Radiology 1985;155:15–18.
26. Sinner WN. Fine-needle biopsy of hamartomas of the lung. AJR 1982;138:65–69.
27. Crouch JD, Keagy BA, Starek PJK, et al. A clinical review of patients undergoing resection for pulmonary hamartoma. Ann Surg 1988;54:297–299.
28. Jensen KG, Schiodt T. Growth conditions of hamartoma of the lung: a study based on 22 cases operated on after radiographic observation from one to 18 years. Thorax 1958;13:233–237.
29. Weisel W, Glicklich M, Landis FB. Pulmonary hamartoma, an enlarging neoplasm. Arch Surg 1955;71:128–135.
30. Sagel SS, Ablow, RC. Hamartoma: on occasion a rapidly growing tumour of the lung. Radiology 1968;91:971–979.
31. Weinberger M, Kakos GS, Kilman JW. The adult form of pulmonary hamartoma. Ann Thorac Surg 1973;15: 67–72.
32. Shinkai M, Kobayashi H, Kanoh S, et al. Pulmonary hamartoma: an unusual radiologic appearance. J Thorac Imaging 2004;19:38–40.
33. Siegelman SS, Khouri NF, Scott WW Jr, et al. Pulmonary hamartoma: CT findings. Radiology 1986;160:313–317.
34. Takemura T, Kusafuka K, Fujiwara M, et al. An immunohistochemical study of the mesenchymal and epithelial components of chondromatous hamartomas. Pathol Int 1999;49:938–946.
35. Mukensnabl P, Hadravska S. Unusual chondroid hamartoma. Histopathology 2002;41(S1):110.
36. Nakano M, Fukuda M, Sasayama K, et al. Nd-YAG laser treatment for central airway lesions. Nippon Kyobu Shikkan Gakkai Zasshi 1992;30:1007–1015.
37. Rodriguez FJ, Aubry MC, Tazelaar HD, et al. Pulmonary chondroma: a tumor associated with Carney triad and different from pulmonary hamartoma. Am J Surg Pathol 2007;31:1844–1853.
38. Wilks S. Enchondroma of the lung. Transpathol Soc (Lond) 1862;12:27–28.
39. Morgan AD, Salama FD. Primary chondrosarcoma of the lung. Case report and a review of the literature. J Thorac Cardiovasc Surg 1972;64:460–466.
40. Morgenroth A, Pfeuffer HP, Viereck HJ, et al. Primary chondrosarcoma of the left inferior lobar bronchus. Respiration 1989;56:241–244.
41. Daniels AC, George H, Strans FH. Primary chondrosarcoma of tracheobronchial tree. Arch Pathol 1967;84: 615–624.
42. Smith EAC, Cohen RV, Peale AR. Primary chondrosarcomatosis of the lung. Ann Intern Med 1960;53:838–846.
43. Bailey SC, Head HD. Pleural chondrosarcoma. Ann Thorac Surg 1990;49:996–997.
44. Hayashi T, Tsuda N, Iseki M, et al. Primary chondrosarcoma of the lung. Cancer 1993;72:69–74.
45. Colby TV, Koss MN, Travis WD. Atlas of tumor pathology. Tumors of the lower respiratory tract. Washington, DC: Armed Forces Institute of Pathology, 1994:384.
46. Abeles H, Chaves AD. The significance of calcification in pulmonary coin lesions. Radiology 1952;58:199–202.
47. Huang H-Y, Hsieh M-J, Chen W-J, et al. Primary mesenchymal chondrosarcoma of the lung. Am Thorac Surg 2002;73:1962–1964.
48. Sun C-CJ, Kroll M, Miller JE. Primary chondrosarcoma of the lung. Cancer 1982;50:1864–1866.
49. Reingold IM, Amromin GD. Extraosseous osteosarcoma of the lung. Cancer 1971:41–498.
50. Nascimento AG, Unni KK, Bernatz PE. Sarcomas of the lung. Mayo Clin Proc 1982;57:355–359.
51. Colby TV, Bilbao JE, Batifora H, et al. Primary osteosarcoma of the lung. Arch Pathol Lab Med 1989;1147–1150.
52. Loose JH, El-Naggar AK, Ro JY, et al. Primary osteosarcoma of the lung: report of two cases and review of the literature. J Thorac Cardiovasc Surg 1990;100:867–873.
53. Manivel JC, Priest JR, Watterson J, et al. Pleuropulmonary blastoma of childhood. Cancer 1988;62:1516–1526.
54. Tsunezuka Y, Oda M, Takahashi M, et al. Primary chondromatous osteosarcoma of the pulmonary artery. Ann Thorac Surg 2004;77:331–334.
55. Sievert LJ, Elwing TJ, Evans ML. Primary pulmonary osteogenic sarcoma. Skeletal Radiol 2000;29:283–285.
56. Moran CA. Mesenchymal tumors. In: Saldana MJ, ed. Pathology of pulmonary disease. Philadelphia: JB Lippincott, 1994:645–656.
57. Connolloy JP, McGuyer CA, Sageman WS, Bailey H. Intrathoracic osteosarcoma diagnosed by CT scan and pleural biopsy. Chest 1991;100:265–267.
58. Bango A, Colubs L, Molinos L, et al. Endobronchial lipomas. Respiration 1993;60:297–301.
59. Plachta A, Hershey H. Lipoma of the lung: review of literature and report of a case. Am Rev Respir Dis 1962; 86:912–916.
60. Crutcher RR, Waltuck TL, Ghosh AK. Bronchial lipoma. J Thorac Cardiovasc Surg 1968;55:422–425.
61. MacArthur CG, Cheung DL, Spiro SG. Endobronchial lipoma: a review of four cases. Br J Dis Chest 1977;71: 93–100.
62. Schraufnagel DE, Morin JE, Wang NS. Endobronchial lipoma. Chest 1979;75:97–99.
63. Politis J, Funahashi A, Gehisen J, et al. Intrathoracic lipomas: report of three cases and review of the literature with emphasis on endobronchial lipomas. J Thorac Cardiovasc Surg 1979;77:550–556.
64. Moran CA, Suster S, Koss MN. Endobronchial lipomas: a clinicopathologic study of four cases. Mod Pathol 1994; 7:212–214.
65. Fraser RS, Müller NL, Colman N, Paré PD, eds. Fraser and Paré's diagnosis of diseases of the chest. 4th ed. Philadelphia, London, Toronto: WB Saunders, 1999:386.
66. Palvio D, Egeblad K, Paulsen SM. Atypical lipomatous hamartoma of the lung. Virchows Arch [Pathol Anat] 1985;405:253–261.

67. Guinee DG, Thornberry DS, Azumi N, et al. Unique pulmonary presentation of an angiolipoma. Analysis of clinical, radiographic and histopathologic features. Am J Surg Pathol 1995;19:476–480.
68. Gimenez A, Franquet T, Prats R, et al. Unusual primary lung tumors: a radiologic-pathologic overview. Radiographics 2002;22:601–619.
69. Roviaro g, Montorsi M, Varoli F, et al. Primary pulmonary tumours of neurogenic origin. Thorax 1983;38:942–945.
70. Bosch X, Ramirez J, Font J, et al. Primary intrapulmonary benign schwannoma: a case with ultrastructural and immunohistochemical confirmation. Eur Respir J 1990;3: 234–237.
71. Bernabeu L, Gillon JC, Loison F, et al. Une cause rare de fibrose interstitielle diffuse: la maladie de Von Recklinghausen. Lille Med 1980;25:283–285.
72. Unger PD, Geller SA, Anderson PJ. Pulmonary lesions in a patient with neurofibromatosis. Arch Pathol Lab Med 1984;108:654–657.
73. Miller DL, Allen MS. Rare pulmonary neoplasms. Mayo Clin Proc 1993;68:492–498.
74. Bartley TD, Arean VM. Intrapulmonary neurogenic tumors. J Thorac Cardiovasc Surg 1965;50:114–123.
75. Miura H, Kato H, Hayata Y, et al. Solitary bronchial mucosal neuroma. Chest 1989;95:245–247.
76. Hochholzer L, Moran CA, Koss MN. Primary pulmonary ganglioneuroblastoma: a clinico-pathologic and immunohistochemical study of two cases. Ann Diagn Pathol 1998; 2:154–158.
77. O'Donohue WJ, Edland J, Mohiuddin SM, et al. Multiple pulmonary neurofibromas with hypoxemia. Occurrence due to pulmonary arteriovenous shunts within the tumors. Arch Intern Med 1986;146:1618–1619.
78. Stout AP. Mesenchymoma, the mixed tumor of mesenchymal derivatives. Ann Surg 1948;27:278–290.
79. Leslie KO, Wick MR, eds. Practical pulmonary pathology. Philadelphia: Churchill Livingstone, 2005:507–508.
80. Kalus M, Rahman F, Jenkins DE, et al. Malignant mesenchymoma of the lung. Arch Pathol 1973;95:199–202.
81. Listrom MB, Johnson FP, Black WC. Malignant mesenchymoma of the lung. Am Soc Clin Pathol AP Check Sample 1990;AP-I(4):1–4.
82. Randleman CD, Unger ER, Mansour KA. Malignant fibrous histiocytoma of the trachea. Ann Thorac Surg 1990; 50:458–459.
83. Shah IA, Kurtz SM, Simonsen RL. Radiation-induced malignant fibrous histiocytoma of the pulmonary artery. Arch Pathol Lab Med 1991;115:921–925.
84. Munk J, Griffel B, Kogan J. Primary mesenchymoma of the pulmonary artery: radiologic features. Br J Radiol 1965;38:104–111.
85. Hagstrom L. Malignant mesenchymoma in pulmonary artery and right ventricle. Acta Pathol Microbiol Scand [A] 1961;51:87–94.
86. Hohbach CHG, Mall W. Chondrosarcoma of the pulmonary artery. Beitr Pathol 1977;60:298–307.
87. Harding JR, Williams J, Seal RM. Pedunculated capillary hemangioma of the bronchus. Br J Dis Chest 1978;72: 336–342.
88. Shikhani AH, Jones mm, Marsh BR, et al. Infantile subglottic hemangiomas: an update. Ann Otol Rhinol Laryngol 1986;95:336–347.
89. Paul KP, Borner C, Muller KM, et al. Capillary hemangioma of the right main bronchus treated by sleeve resection in infancy. Am Rev Respir Dis 1991;143:876–879.
90. Burman D, Mansell PWA, Warin RP. Miliary haemangiomata in the newborn. Arch Dis Child 1967;42:193–197.
91. Rios-Zambudio A, Roca Calvo MJ, Torres Lanzas J, et al. Massive hemoptysis caused by tracheal hemangiomas treated with interventional radiology. Ann Thorac Surg 2003;75:1302–1304.
92. Sirmah M, Demirag F, Aydin E, et al. A pulmonary cavernous hemangioma causing massive hemoptysis. Ann Thorac Surg 2003;76:1275–1276.
93. Irani S, Brack T, Pfaltz M, et al. Tracheal lobular capillary hemangioma. A rare cause of recurrent hemoptysis. Chest 2003;123:2148–2149.
94. Iwasaki M, Kobayashi H, Nomoto T, et al. Primary racemose hemangioma of the bronchial artery. Intern Med 2001;40:650–653.
95. Sie KC, Tampakopoulou DA. Hemangiomas and vascular malformations of the airway. Otolaryngol Clin North Am 2000;33:209–220.
96. Fine SW, Whitney KD. Multiple cavernous hemangiomas of the lung. A case report and review of the literature. Arch Pathol Lab Med 2004;128;1439–1441.
97. Kase M, Sakamoto K, Yamagata T, et al. A case of pulmonary cavernous hemangioma: immunohistological examination revealed its endothelial cell origin. Kyobu Geka 2000;53:1055–1057.
98. Stausz J, Soltesz I. Bronchial capillary hemangioma in adults. Pathol Oncol Res 1999;5:233–234.
99. Fligner C, King County Medical Examiner's Office, Seattle, WA. Personal communication, 1992.
100. Galliani CA, Beatty JF, Grossfeld JL. Cavernous hemangioma of the lung in an infant. Pediatr Pathol 1992;12: 105–111.
101. Wagenvoort CA, Beetstra A. Spijker J. Capillary haemangiomatosis of the lung. Histopathology 1978;2:401–406.
102. Tron V, Magee F, Wright JL, et al. Pulmonary capillary hemangiomatosis. Hum Pathol 1986;17:1144–1149.
103. Faber CN, Yousem SA, Dauber JH, et al. Pulmonary capillary hemangiomatosis: a report of three cases and a review of the literature. Am Rev Respir Dis 1989;140: 808–813.
104. Oviedo A, Abramson LP, Worthington R. Congenital pulmonary capillary hemangiomatosis: report of two cases and review of the literature. Pediatr Pulmonol 2003;36: 253–256.
105. Varnholt H, Kradin R. Pulmonary capillary hemangiomatosis arising in hereditary hemorrhagic telangiectasia. Hum Pathol 2004;35:266–268.
106. Almagro P, Joaquim J, Sansume M, et al. Pulmonary capillary hemangiomatosis associated with primary pulmonary hypertension. Medicine 2002;81:417–424.
107. Anabtawi IN, Ellison RG, Ellison LT. Pulmonary arteriovenous aneurysms and fistulas. Anatomic variations, embryology, and classification. Ann Thorac Surg 1965;1: 277–285.

108. Cheung Y, Ahrens WR, Singh J. Massive hemoptysis in a child due to pulmonary arteriovenous malformation. J Emerg Med 1997;15:317–319.
109. Mark EJ, et al. Case records of the Massachusetts General Hospital. Pulmonary arteriovenous malformations. Thalamic abscess. N Engl J Med 1990;322:1139–1148.
110. Lee DW, White RI, Egglin K, et al. Embolotherapy of large pulmonary arteriovenous malformations: long term results. Ann Thorac Surg 1997;64:930–940.
111. English JC. Pulmonary vascular lesions. In: Cagle PT, ed. Diagnostic pulmonary pathology. New York and Basel: Marcel Dekker, 2000:368–369.
112. Burke cm, et al. Pulmonary arteriovenous malformations. A critical update. Am Rev Respir Dis 1986;134:334–339.
113. Corrin B. Pathology of the lungs. London, Edinburgh, New York: Churchill-Livingstone, 2000:529–530.
114. Soda H, Oka M, Kohno S, et al. Arteriovenous malformation of the bronchial artery showing endobronchial protrusion. Int Med 1995;34:797–800.
115. Fraser RS, Müller NL, Colman N, Paré PD, eds. Fraser and Paré's diagnosis of diseases of the chest. 4th ed. Philadelphia, London, Toronto: WB Saunders, 1999:662–664.
116. Abad J, Villar R, Parga g, et al. Bronchial migration of pulmonary arterial coil. Cardiovasc Intervent Radiol 1990;13:345–346.
117. Irwin R, University of Massachusetts Medical School. Personal communication, 2004.
118. Enzinger FM, Weiss SW. Soft tissue tumors. 2nd ed. St. Louis: CV Mosby, 1988:614–637.
119. Spencer H. Pathology of the lung. 4th ed. Oxford: Pergamon Press, 1985:125–129.
120. Wagenaar SJSC, Swierenga J, Wagenvoort CA. Late presentation of primary pulmonary lymphangiectasis. Thorax 1978;33:791–795.
121. Noonan JA, Walters LR, Reeves JT. Congenital pulmonary lymphangiectasis. Am J Dis Child 1970; 120:314–319.
122. Nanson EM. Lymphangioma (cystic hygroma) of the mediastinum. J Cardiovasc Surg (Torino) 1968;9:447–452.
123. Thomas HM, Shaw NJ, Weindling AM. Generalized lymphangiomatosis with chylothorax. Arch Dis Child 1990;65: 334.
124. Langer JC, Fitzgerald PG, Desa D, et al. Cervical cystic hygroma in the fetus: clinical spectrum and outcome. J Pediatr Surg 1990;25:58–61; discussion, 61–62.
125. Bill AH, Jr, Sumner DS. A unified concept of lymphangioma and cystic hygroma. Surg Gynecol Obstet 1965;120: 79–86.
126. Kim WS, Lee KS, Kim I, et al. Cystic intrapulmonary lymphangioma: HRCT findings. Pediatr Radiol 1995;25: 206–207.
127. Takahara T, Morisaki Y, Torigoe T, et al. Intrapulmonary cystic lymphangioma: report of a case. Surg Today 1998; 28:1310–1312.
128. Brown M, Pysher T, Coffin cm. Lymphangioma and congenital pulmonary lymphangiectasis: a histologic, immunohistochemical and clinicopathologic comparison. Mod Pathol 1999;12:569–575.
129. Chikkamuniyappa S, Heim-Hall S, Jajirdar J. Solitary endobronchial lymphangioma: a case report and review of the literature. Sci World J 2005;5:103–108.
130. Sanlialp I, Karnak I, Tanyel FC, et al. Sclerotherapy for lymphangioma in children. Int J Pediatr Otorhinolaryngol 2003;67:795–800.
131. Tazelaar KH, Yousem S, Saldana M, et al. Diffuse pulmonary lymphangiomatosis. Mod Pathol 1992;5: 114A(abstr).
132. Tazelaar HD, Kerr D, Yousem SA. Diffuse pulmonary lymphangiomatosis. Hum Pathol 1993;24:1313–1322.
133. Swank DW, Hepper NGG, Folkert KE, et al. Intrathoracic lymphangiomatosis mimicking lymphangioleiomyomatosis in a young woman. Mayo Clin Proc 1989;64:1264–1268.
134. Koblenzer PJ, Bukowski MJ. Angiomatosis (hamartomatous hemolymphangiomatosis): report of a case with diffuse involvement. Pediatrics 1961:28:61–76.
135. Fletcher CDM, Unni KK, Mertens F. WHO classification of tumours. Pathology and genetics. Tumours of soft tissue and bone. Lyon: IARC Press, 2004:86–90.
136. Weiss SW, Ishak KG, Dail DH, et al. Epithelioid hemangioendothelioma and related lesions. Semin Diagn Pathol 1986;3:259–287.
137. Meister P, Hoede N, Rumpelt H-J. Epithelioid hemangioendothelioma of the scalp. Pathol Res Pract 1985;180: 220–226.
138. Silva EG, Phillips J, Langer B, et al. Spindle and histiocytoid (epithelioid) hemangioendotheliomas: primary in lymph nodes. Am J Clin Pathol 1986;85:731–735.
139. Dail D, Liebow A. Intravascular bronchioloalveolar tumor. Am J Pathol 1975;78:6a–7b(abstr).
140. Farinacci CJ, Blauw AS, Jennings EM. Multifocal pulmonary lesions of possible decidual origin (so-called pulmonary deciduosis): report of a case. Am J Clin Pathol 1973; 59:508–574.
141. Corrin B, Manners B, Millard M, et al. Histogenesis of the so-called "intravascular bronchioloalveolar tumor." J Pathol 1979;128:163–167.
142. Weldon-Linne cm, Victor TA, Christ ML, et al. Angiocentric nature of the "intravascular bronchioloalveolar tumor" of the lung. An electron microscopic study. Arch Pathol Lab Med 1981;105:174–179.
143. Azumi N, Churg A. Intravascular and sclerosing bronchioloalveolar tumor. A pulmonary sarcoma of probable vascular origin. Am J Surg Pathol 1981;5:587–596.
144. Ferrer-Roca O. Intravascular and sclerosing bronchioalveolar tumor. Am J Surg Pathol 1981;5:587–596.
145. Weldon-Linne cm, Victor TA, Christ ML. Immunohistochemical identification of factor VIII-related antigen in the intravascular bronchioloalveolar tumor of the lung. Arch Pathol Lab Med 1981;105:628–629.
146. Bhagavan BS, Murthy MSN, Borfman HD, et al. Intravascular bronchioloalveolar tumor (IVBAT). A low-grade sclerosing epithelioid angiosarcoma of lung. Am J Surg Pathol 1982;6:41–52.
147. Dail DH, Liebow AA, Gmelich JT, et al. Intravascular, bronchiolar, and alveolar tumor of the lung (IVBAT): an analysis of twenty cases of a peculiar sclerosing endothelial tumor. Cancer 1983;51:452–464.
148. Yousem SA, Hochholzer L. Unusual thoracic manifestations of epithelioid hemandioendothelioma. Arch Pathol Lab Med 1987;111:459–463.

149. Shirakusa T, Yoshida M, Tsutsui M, et al. Advanced intravascular bronchioloalveolar tumor and review of reports in Japan. Respir Med 1989;85:127–132.
150. Ellis GL, Kratochvil FJ III. Epithelioid hemangioendothelioma of the head and neck: a clinicopathologic and followup study of twelve cases. Oral Surg Oral Med Oral Pathol 1986;61:61–68.
151. Fraser RS, Muller NL, Colman N, Paré PD, eds. Fraser and Paré's diagnosis of disease of the chest. 4th ed. Philadelphia, London, Toronto: WB Saunders, 1999:1339.
152. Pilotti S, Rilke F, Lombardi L, et al. Immunohistochemistry and electron microscopy of intravascular bronchioloalveolar tumor of the lung. Tumori 1983;69:283–292.
153. Nakatani Y, Aoki I, Misugi K. Immunohistochemical and ultrastructural study of early lesions of intravascular bronchioloalveolar tumor with liver involvement. Acta Pathol Jpn 1985;35:1453–1465.
154. Kitaichi M, Nagai S, Nishimura K, et al. Pulmonary epithelioid hemangioendothelioma in 21 patients, including 3 with spontaneous regression. Eur Respir J 1998;12: 89–96.
155. Cronin P, Arenberg D. Pulmonary epithelioid hemangioendothelioma: an unusual case and review of the literature. Chest 2004;125:789–793.
156. Spragg RG, Wolf PL, Haghighi P, et al. Angiosarcoma of the lung with fatal pulmonary hemorrhage. Am J Med 1983;74:1072–1076.
157. Maddox JC, Evans HL. Angiosarcoma of skin and soft tissues: a study of forty-four cases. Cancer 1981;48:1907–1921.
158. Spencer H. Pathology of the lung. 4th ed. Oxford: Pergamon Press, 1985:1000.
159. Yousem S. Angiosarcoma presenting in the lung. Arch Pathol Lab Med 1986;110:112–115.
160. Miller DL, Allen MS. Rare pulmonary neoplasms. Mayo Clin Proc 1993;68:492–498.
161. Keel SB, Bacha E, Mark EJ. Primary pulmonary sarcoma: a clinicopathologic study of 26 cases. Mod Pathol 1999; 12:1124–1131.
162. Junge K, Toens C, Peiper C, et al. Primary angiosarcoma of the lung. Chirurg 2001;72:969–972.
163. Tschirch FTC, DelGrande F, Marincek B. Angiosarcoma of the pulmonary trunk mimicking pulmonary thromboembolic disease. Acta Radiol 2003;44:504–507.
164. Hasleton PS, ed. Spencer's pathology of the lung. 5th ed. New York, St. Louis, San Francisco: McGraw-Hill, 1996: 1071–1074.
165. Nappi O, Swanson PE, Wick MR. Pseudovascular adenoid squamous cell carcinoma of the lung: clinicopathologic study of three cases and comparison with true pleuropulmonary angiosarcoma. Hum Pathol 1994;25:373–378.
166. Wenig BM, Abbondanzo SL, Heffess CS. Epithelioid angiosarcoma of the adrenal glands. A clinicopathologic study of nine cases with a discussion of the implications of finding epithelial-specific markers. Am J Surg Pathol 1994;18:62–73.
167. Alles JU, Bosslet K. Immunocytochemistry of angiosarcomas. A study of 19 cases with special emphasis on the applicability of endothelial cell specific markers to routinely prepared tissues. Am J Clin Pathol 1988;89:463–471.
168. Gray MH, Rosenberg AE, Dickersin GR, et al. Cytokeratin expression in epithelioid vascular neoplasms. Hum Pathol 1990;21:212–217.
169. Sirgi KE, Wick MR, Swanson PE. B72.3 and CD34 immunoreactivity in malignant epithelioid soft tissue tumors. Adjuncts in the recognition of endothelial neoplasms. Am J Surg Pathol 1993;17:179–185.
170. Enzinger FM, Weiss SW, eds. Soft tissue tumors. St. Louis: CV Mosby, 1995:641–677.
171. Bocklage T, Leslie K, Yousem S, et al. Extracutaneous angiosarcomas metastatic to the lungs: clinical and pathologic features of twenty-one cases. Mod Pathol 2001;14: 1216–1255.
172. Kojima K, Okamoto I, Ushijima S, et al. Successful treatment of primary pulmonary angiosarcoma. Chest 2003;124: 2397–2400.
173. Wackers FJ, van der Schoot JB, Hampe JR. Sarcoma of the pulmonary trunk associated with hemorrhagic tendency: a case report and review of the literature. Cancer 1969; 23:339–351.
174. Shmookler BM, Marsh HB, Roberts WC. Primary sarcoma of the pulmonary trunk and/or right or left main pulmonary artery: a rare cause of obstruction of right ventricular overflow. Am J Med 1977;63:263–272.
175. Bleisch VR, Kraus FT. Polypoid sarcoma of the pulmonary trunk: analysis of the literature and report of a case with leptomeric organelles and ultrastructural features of a rhabdomyosarcoma. Cancer 1980;46:314–324.
176. Baker PB, Goodwin RA. Pulmonary artery sarcomas: a review and report of a case. Arch Pathol Lab Med 1985; 109:35–39.
177. McGlennen RC, Manivel JC, Stanley SJ, et al. Pulmonary artery trunk sarcoma: a clinicopathologic, ultrastructural, and immunohistochemical study of four cases. Mod Pathol 1989;2:486–494.
178. Wang N-S, Seemayer TA, Ahmed MN, et al. Pulmonary leiomyosarcoma associated with an arteriovenous fistula. Arch Pathol 1974;98:100–105.
179. Shah IA, Kurtz SM, Simonsen RL. Radiation-induced malignant fibrous histiocytoma of the pulmonary artery. Arch Pathol Lab Med 1991;115:921–925.
180. Chowdbury L, Swerdlow MA, Jao W, et al. Post-irradiation malignant fibrous histiocytoma of the lung. Am J Clin Pathol 1980;74:820–826.
181. Mattoo A, Fedullo PF, Kapelanski D, et al. Pulmonary artery sarcoma. A case report of surgical cure and 5 year follow up. Chest 2002;122:745–747.
182. Killebrew E, Gerbode F. Leiomyosarcoma of the pulmonary artery diagnosed preoperatively by angiocardiography. J Thorac Cardiovasc Surg 1976;71:469.
183. Lyerly HK, Reves JG, Sabiston DC, Jr. Management of primary sarcomas of the pulmonary artery and reperfusion intrabronchial hemorrhage. Surg Gynecol Obstet 1986;163: 291–301.
184. Mandelstamm U. Über primare Neubildungen des Herzens. Virchows Arch Pathol Anat 1923;245:43–54.
185. Greenspan EB. Primary osteoid chondrosarcoma of the lung: report of a case. Am J Cancer 1933;18:603–609.
186. Lowell IM, Tuhy JE. Primary chondrosarcoma of the lung. J Thorac Surg 1949;18:476–483.

187. Hagström L. Malignant mesenchymoma in pulmonary artery and right ventricle. Report of a case with unusual location and histologic picture. Acta Pathol Microbiol Scand 1961;51·87–94.
188. Head HD, Flam MS, John MJ, et al. Long-term palliation of pulmonary artery sarcoma by radical excision and adjuvant therapy. Ann Thorac Surg 1992;53:332–334.
189. Kaposi M. Idiopathisches multiples Pigmentsarkom der Haut. Arch Dermatol Syphilol 1872;4:265–273.
190. Volberding D. Therapy of Kaposi's sarcoma in AIDS. Semin Oncol 1984;11:60–66.
191. Cox FH, Helwig EB. Kaposi's sarcoma. Cancer 1959;12: 289–298.
192. Aboulafia DM. The epidemiologic, pathologic and clinical features of AIDS–associated pulmonary Kaposi's sarcoma. Chest 2000;117:1128–1145.
193. Haramanti LB, Wong J. Intrathoracic Kaposi's sarcoma in women with AIDS. Chest 2000;117:410–414.
194. Corrin B, ed. Pathology of the lungs. London, Edinburgh, New York: Churchill Livingstone, 2000:534–535.
195. Hasleton PS, ed. Spencer's pathology of the lung. 5th ed. New York, St. Louis, San Francisco: McGraw-Hill, 1996: 1077–1081.
196. Tamm M, Recihen Berger F, McGandy CE, et al. Diagnosis of pulmonary Kaposi's sarcoma by detection of human herpes virus 8 in bronchioalveolar lavage. Am J Respir Crit Care Med 1998;157:458–463.
197. Bryant-Greenwood P, Sorbara L, Fillie AC, et al. Infection of mesothelial cells with herpes virus 8 in human immunodeficiency virus-infected patients with Kaposi's sarcoma, Castlemann's disease and recurrent pleural effusion. Mod Pathol 2003;16:145–153.

41
Miscellaneous Tumors and Tumor-Like Proliferations of the Lung

Armando E. Fraire and David H. Dail

This chapter discusses endometriosis, tumors, and tumor-like conditions putatively derived from ectopic tissues in the lung. These include thymomas, melanomas, bronchial nevi, meningothelial-like bodies, meningiomas, ependymomas, germ cell tumors (teratomas and choriocarcinomas), and synovial sarcomas. In addition, this chapter discusses other miscellaneous tumors and tumor-like proliferations of the lung such as sclerosing hemangiomas, alveolar and papillary adenomas, inflammatory bronchial polyps, clear cell (sugar) tumors/PEComas, granular cell tumors, paragangliomas and uncommon surface neoplasms of the airways.

Tissue Ectopias and Primary Pulmonary Tumors Derived from Ectopic Tissues

Lung tissue can rarely be found heterotopically within adjacent anatomic structures such as the diaphragm (Fig. 41.1) and occasionally within some teratomas. Conversely, heterotopic tissues can be found in the lung itself (Fig. 41.2). Ectopic tissues in the lung are most unusual, and primary pulmonary tumors derived from such ectopic tissues are even more uncommon.[1] Ectopic tissues in lung (and pleura) include liver, spleen, pancreas, thyroid, adrenal, and brain as well as endometrium.[1–5] These ectopic tissues in the lung can theoretically be derived from several sources, including embryonic remnants from nearby organ systems displaced during embryonal development, traumatic implantation from nearby anatomic sites, or embolization from distant organ systems. Almost any tissue fragment can gain access to venous systemic blood and end up in the lungs. However, most of these tissue fragments die, and apparently only a few appear to thrive or persist, under special conditions. Endometriosis, discussed next in this chapter, is particularly prone to thrive in the lung and to present in a symptomatic fashion since it affects both the lung and the pleura, and the ectopic tissue may be physiologically active causing catamenial hemoptysis or pneumothorax.[6,7]

Pulmonary Endometriosis

Known to frequently occur in the female pelvic organs and tissues from the lower abdomen, endometriosis is distinctly less common in the lung and pleura. Key early reports of pleuropulmonary endometriosis are those by Hart[8] in 1912, and Büngeler et al.[9] in 1939. Park[10] in 1954 detected microscopic fragments of both endometrial and decidual tissue in the lungs of a woman who died postpartum. Subsequently, other reports have confirmed small residual fragments in and about pulmonary vessels.[11–13] Cameron and Park[12] believed that some of the fragments seen in one of their patients were growing out from a vessel onto the alveolar septa and therefore were extravascular. Decidualization can be seen in some cases of metastasizing leiomyomas and in cycling endometriosis of the lung or pleura. Decidualization was also a term used to describe a pulmonary lesion in one reported case, before the true epithelioid hemangioendotheliomatous nature of that lesion became evident.[14]

Endometriosis has been described in lung, bronchi, pleura, and diaphragm and has been reviewed by Spencer,[15] Hibbard et al.,[16] Karpel et al.,[17] Austin et al.,[18] and Di Palo et al.[19] Reports of endometriosis affecting the respiratory tract are generally rare, and according to Di Palo and collaborators the first mention of pleuropulmonary endometriosis is found in Hart's[8] 1912 report. Subsequently, Schwartz[20] in 1938 described recurrent hemoptysis with menses (catamenial hemoptysis) in a woman with inguinal node endometriosis. Pleural endometriosis was first described in 1939 by Büngeler et al.[9] By 1981 Foster et al.[21] had summarized 65 cases of pleuropulmonary endometriosis, 11 in the lung parenchyma and 54 in pleura. In 1985 a careful review of 87 thoracic cases was conducted by Karpel et al.[17] In 1998, Flieder et al.[22] reviewed the literature and added 10 cases of their own.

The clinical presentation of endometriosis is variable but is highlighted by bleeding, which may be cyclic. In one series, however, pneumothorax was the predominant symptom occurring in 76% of the patients; hemothorax

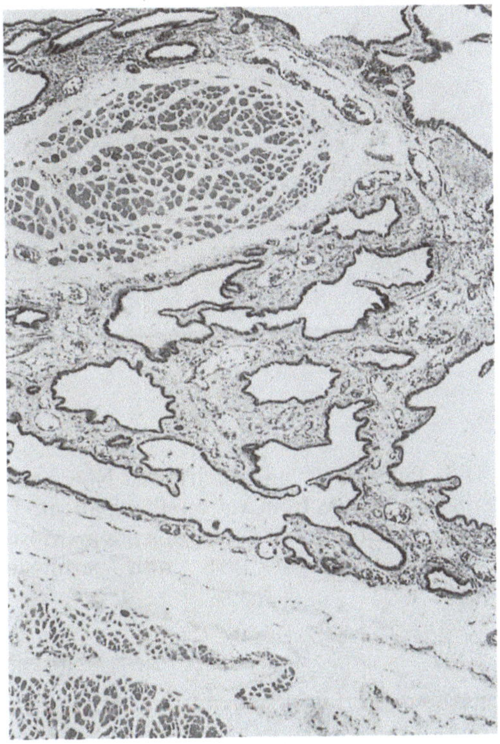

FIGURE 41.1. Ectopic lung in diaphragm. Primitive lung-like spaces with cilia are admixed with muscle fibers.

developed in 10%, hemoptysis in 8%, and asymptomatic mass lesions in the remaining 6% of patients.[17] The number of recurrent pneumothoraces can be extraordinary, and as reviewed by Karpel et al.,[17] episodes of probable pneumothorax occurred anywhere from two to 42 times per patient (averaging 14), while clinically documented pneumothorax was noted about one to 25 times per patient.[17] Of these episodes, 95% were right-sided, and a few were bilateral, while only one case occurred on the left side.[17] Of interest, pneumothorax is usually not associated with pleural effusions. Catamenial hemothorax, although it occurs less often than pneumothorax, is always right-sided in the setting of extensive pelvic endometriosis, often with ascites.[17] Right-sided pleural involvement is most often thought to result from intraabdominal fluid spreading through diaphragmatic fenestrations that are situated above the liver and its attachment to the diaphragm.[23]

Parenchymal lung involvement is probably hematogenous and, along with bronchial involvement, is most often right-sided, with some cases forming nodular hemorrhagic masses measuring up to 6 cm.[18] One exceptional case presented with bronchial occlusion.[19] Foster et al.[21] noted that pleural involvement tends to occur in younger patients (mean age, 33.6 years) who have more pelvic endometriosis than the patients with parenchymal endometriosis, whose mean age is 39 years. In patients with pleural endometriosis there is only a 10% incidence of pelvic endometriosis, whereas catamenial hemoptysis, or catamenial pain and dyspnea, respectively, occur in 82% and 18% of patients. In the lung, endometriosis may variably present as nodular masses, cystic lesions, or as involuting or "burnt out" lesions[22] (Figs. 41.3 to 41.5). In some instances, the distribution of lesions may be lymphangitic or involve the bronchovascular bundle. Of interest, the "chronological" endometrial pattern in Flieder et al.'s [22] series was proliferative in nine of the 10 cases. One of the 10 cases showed mixed proliferative and secretory features, one had an indeterminate pattern, and none was purely secretory. The clinical/demographic data of the 10 patients presented by Flieder et al. are listed in Table 41.1.[22]

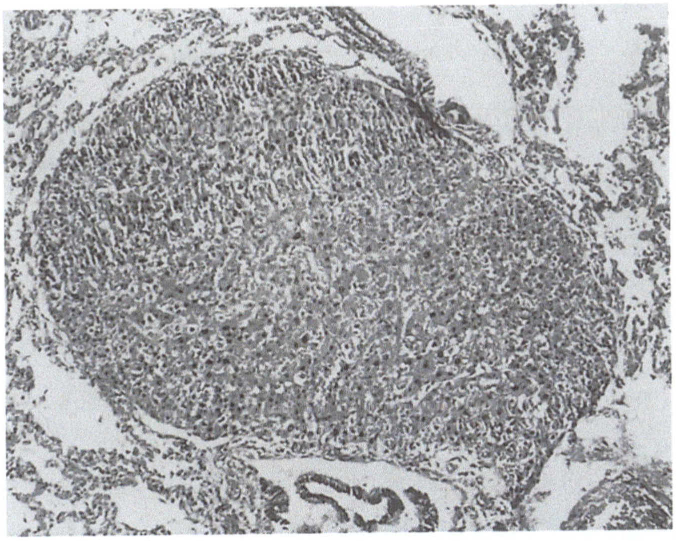

FIGURE 41.2. Ectopic adrenal in lung. The nodule appears viable. (Courtesy of Dr. H. Spencer, Pulmonary Pathology Collection, London.)

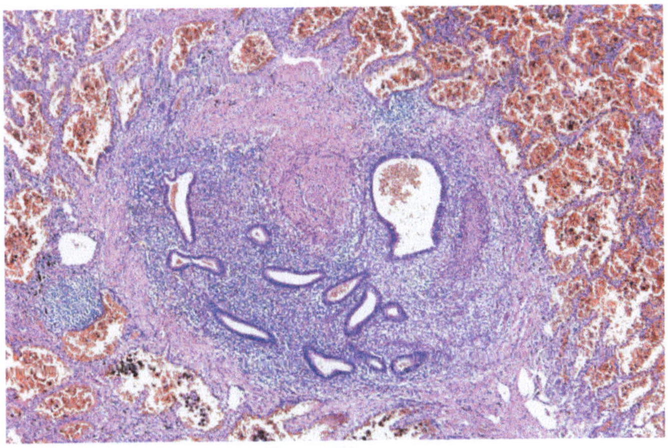

FIGURE 41.3. Pulmonary endometriosis. Note expansion of the bronchovascular bundle by a single focus of irregularly shaped endometrial glands and cellular stroma. Note also significant intraalveolar hemorrhage. (From Flieder et al.[22] Copyright 1998, with permission from Elsevier.)

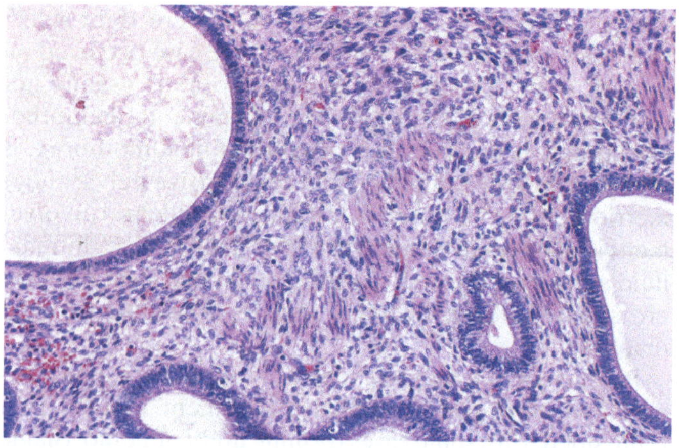

FIGURE 41.4. Pulmonary endometriosis. Closer view of another focus of endometriosis in a different patient. Note proliferative pattern and cellular stroma with bundles of smooth muscle. (Hematoxylin and eosin [H&E].) (From Flieder et al.[22] Copyright 1998, with permission from Elsevier.)

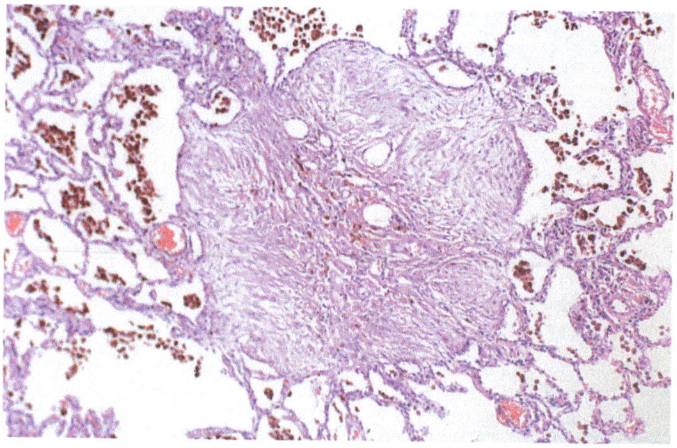

FIGURE 41.5. Pulmonary endometriosis. Note fibroblastic, hemosiderin-rich nodule from yet another patient. This most likely represents a burnt-out focus of endometriosis. (From Flieder et al.[22] Copyright 1998, with permission from Elsevier.)

TABLE 41.1. Pleuropulmonary endometriosis/deciduosis clinical data

Case No.	Age (years)	Type of lesion	Symptoms	Pelvic endometriosis	Parity*	H/O pelvic surgery	OC use	CXR	Rx	F/U
1	38	Pleural	SOB, pleuritic chest pain, hemoptysis	Yes	G2P2	C/S × 1	No	Right PTx; RLL infiltrate	Pleural decortication, Enovid	NED @ 20 years
2	38	Pleural	SOB	No	G0	No	No	Right PTx	Pleural decortication	NED @ 7 years
3	34	Pleural	SOB	No	G0	No	Yes	Right PTx	Pleural abrasion	NED @ 10 months
4	36	Pleural	None	N/A	N/A	N/A	N/A	1.0 cm subpleural nodule	Segmen-tectomy	N/A
5	74	Pulmonary	Occasional blood-tinged cough (for weeks)	No	G3P2	TAH/BSO @ 50 y.o.	Yes	3.0 cm RLL nodule	Lobectomy; Premarin	NED @ 1 year
6	36	Pulmonary	None	No	G2P2	No	N/A	1.0 cm RLL subpleural nodule	Segmentectomy	NED @ 5 years
7	35	Pulmonary	Catamenial hemoptysis for 4 months	No	G2P2	PID @ 30 y.o. D&C @ 33 y.o.	No	3.0 cm LLL opacity	Segmentectomy	NED @ 2 years
8	35	Pulmonary	Cough, dyspnea, hemoptysis for 15 months	No	G4P2	No	No	RUL consolidation during menses	Segmentectomy	N/A
9	33	Pulmonary	Catamenial hemoptysis	No	G5P3	D&C × 2 @ 32 y.o.	No	LUL density	Lobectomy	N/A
10	27	Pulmonary	Pleuritic chest pain, SOB @ week 28 of pregnancy	No	G1	No	No	Slowly evolving bilateral infiltrates × 2 years; right PTx	Open lung biopsy	Unchanged @ 5.5 years

*Number of gravida (G)/para (P).
H/O, history of; CXR, chest x-ray; OC, oral contraceptive; SOB, shortness of breath; D&C, dilation and curettage; C/S, caesarian section; TAH/BSO, total abdominal hysterectomy/bilateral salpingo-oophorectomy; PID, pelvic inflammatory disease; PTx, pneumothorax; RLL, right lower lobe; LLL, left lower lobe; LUL, left upper lobe; NED, no evidence of disease; y.o., years old; F/U, follow-up; N/A, not available.
Source: Flieder et al.[22] Copyright 1998, with permission from Elsevier.

Cytology has been helpful in making the diagnosis.[24,25] Benign columnar cells, and a few benign glands in a bloody and often hemosiderin-stained background, are very suggestive of endometriosis. Stromal cells look quite similar to alveolar macrophages or reactive mesothelial cells, and may not be of much help in diagnosis. Decidual change may occasionally be identified in cytologic and histologic specimens.

According to Flieder and associates,[22] the differential diagnosis for intrathoracic endometriosis depends mainly on the anatomic location of the lesion. In cases of pleural endometriosis, the main considerations are metastatic adenocarcinoma and mesothelial proliferations, whereas in cases of pulmonary endometriosis, the differential diagnosis includes primary and metastatic adenocarcinoma, biphasic neoplasms, and metastatic sarcomas. Recognition of a stromal component in surrounding glands should help to exclude adenocarcinoma or mesothelioma. However, epithelium in endometriosis can exhibit both architectural and cytologic atypia, and carcinoma arises in endometriosis, albeit rarely.[22] In both needle and open lung biopsies, glandular and stromal elements may be interpreted as representing biphasic lung tumors, especially well-differentiated fetal adenocarcinoma or biphasic pulmonary blastoma. Proliferative pattern epithelium with cilia, the absence of squamous morules, and negative staining for chromogranin would favor endometriosis.[22]

Metastatic uterine biphasic tumors, including adenosarcoma and malignant mixed müllerian tumor, can be excluded on the basis of clinical history and the lack of frankly malignant epithelial and stromal components. When biopsy specimens contain mostly stromal cells, morphologic differentiation from metastatic low-grade endometrial stromal sarcoma is virtually impossible. Identifying invasive tongues of tumor or vascular permeation along with a detailed clinical history should facilitate the distinction. When endometriosis is accompanied by cystic changes, it may be confused with metastatic low-grade endometrial stromal sarcoma, metastatic smooth muscle tumors, and mesenchymal cystic hamartoma.[22] Endometrial epithelium should not be confused with entrapped bronchioloalveolar epithelium in these metastatic stromal lesions, and endometrial stroma should be distinguished from primitive mesenchymal cells forming a cambium layer in mesenchymal cystic hamartoma. Mucin stains may be helpful in differentiating adenocarcinoma from endometriosis, but minute malignant lesions may not show unequivocal mucin positivity.[22]

Flieder et al.[22] report that immunostaining does not provide a clear distinction between endometriosis and malignant tumors metastatic to the lungs since identical results may be found in malignant lesions studied immunohistochemically for cytokeratin 7, cytokeratin 20, actin, estrogen receptor, progesterone receptor, and neuroendocrine markers. Flieder et al. further state that within the proper clinical context, endometriosis also should be included in the differential diagnosis of pulmonary hemorrhage. Although lobules filled with erythrocytes and hemosiderin-laden macrophages raise the possibility of pulmonary infarct or other hemorrhagic lesions like arteriovenous malformation, poorly sampled neoplasms, and systemic diseases such as Wegener's granulomatosis, Goodpasture's syndrome, and idiopathic pulmonary hemosiderosis, lung tissue should also be scrutinized for inconspicuous or minute foci of endometriosis. Unlike pulmonary endometriosis, pulmonary ectopic deciduosis may be easily confused both clinically and histologically with epithelioid hemangioendothelioma. Despite multifocality and similar morphologic features, immunohistochemistry may prove helpful because epithelioid hemangioendothelioma but not decidual tissue marks positively for vascular markers such as CD31, CD34, and factor VIII–related antigen.

Whether or not endometriosis is histologically proven, hormonal suppression of ovulation has dramatically reduced the symptoms in many of these cases, and in some cases symptoms have returned after cessation of drugs. Gonadotropin-releasing hormone agonists have shown some promise.[26,27] Surgery plays a minor role in therapy since many cases may be multifocal. However, surgical excision of limited, well-demarcated pulmonary endometriosis can offer symptomatic relief in some cases of intractable endometriosis. Terada et al.[28] reported the case of a woman with histologically proven endometriosis, successfully treated with a partial lung segmentectomy.

Pulmonary Thymomas

Extramediastinal (ectopic) thymomas may occur in the neck, trachea, thyroid, pericardium, pleura, and lung.[29–34] In the lung, these neoplasms are quite rare, with only 14 cases reported by 1989,[29–34] eight more added by Moran et al.[35] in 1995, and one additional case reported by Veynovich and associates[36] in 1997. The histogenesis of these uncommon tumors is poorly understood. Ectopic fragments of thymic tissue within the lung or transformation from a preexisting teratoma have been considered as possible mechanisms for the development of intrapulmonary thymomas. Patients with primary pulmonary thymomas are reported as having about an equal sex incidence, with ages ranging from 14 to 74 years. A fundamental requirement to validate the diagnosis of a primary pulmonary thymoma is a pulmonary mass without a mediastinal component. This requirement was fulfilled in Moran et al.'s series, in which all eight patients had clinical and radiographic evidence of an intrapulmonary mass without mediastinal involvement.

Clinical manifestations of intrapulmonary thymoma include chest pain, dyspnea, and weight loss. As is the case with some mediastinal thymomas, myasthenia gravis, pure red cell aplasia, and hypogammaglobulinemia can occur in association with some pulmonary thymomas.[29,34,36] Thy-

TABLE 41.2. World Health Organization (WHO) histologic classification of thymomas

Epithelial tumors
Thymoma
Type A (spindle cell: medullary)
Type AB (mixed)
Type B1 (lymphocyte-rich; lymphocytic; predominantly cortical; organoid)
Type B2 (cortical)
Type B3 (epithelial; atypical; squamoid; well-differentiated thymic carcinoma)
Micronodular thymoma
Metaplastic thymoma
Microscopic thymoma
Sclerosing thymoma
Lipofibroadenoma

Source: Modified from Travis et al.,[34] with permission.

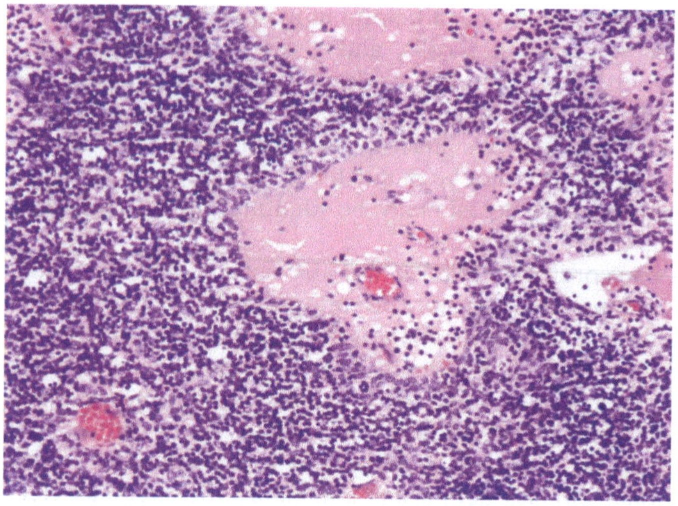

FIGURE 41.7. Mediastinal thymoma, World Health Organization (WHO) B1 type. Note vesicular space with a centrally located blood vessel. Small spindle-shaped cells are overwhelmed by a population of small lymphocytes. (Courtesy of Dr. Peter Wu, University of Massachusetts Medical School, Worcester, MA.)

momas vary from very small to 6cm in diameter, and have been subdivided into peripheral and central. Most peripheral thymomas inexplicably occur on the right side, while the central ones localize on the left side, with one exception reported by Kung et al.[31] Typically intrapulmonary thymomas are well-circumscribed solitary masses, but they may also present as multiple nodules with borders imperceptively blending into the surrounding lung parenchyma. The tumor substance is usually tan, soft, and fleshy, but it can be hemorrhagic or white and firm.[37]

Primary intrapulmonary thymomas like those originating in the mediastinum are classified histopathologically according to World Health Organization (WHO) guidelines[34] (Table 41.2). In Moran et al.'s[35] series of eight cases, the histopathology was characterized by the classic biphasic cellular composition of thymomas, that is, an admixture in varying proportions of epithelial cells and lymphocytes (Figs. 41.6 and 41.7). Four of the eight thymomas were composed of sheets of lymphocytes admixed with scattered epithelial cells that were separated by fibrous bands into lobules. Three were composed predominantly of sheets of epithelial cells admixed with scattered small lymphocytes and containing prominent perivascular spaces. In two of these thymomas, focal areas of spindling of the cells were noted. One tumor was composed predominantly of a spindle cell proliferation with perivascular spaces and numerous small lymphocytes. A unique variant reported by Srivastava et al.[38] showed a marked granulomatous reaction within an otherwise typical spindle cell thymoma (Fig. 41.8). Microscopic examination of the capsule (if a capsule is present) in thymomas is of utmost importance. In mediastinal thymomas, extension beyond the capsule or adherence to adjacent structures suggests invasiveness. In cases of intrathymic thymomas, this assessment of invasiveness

A

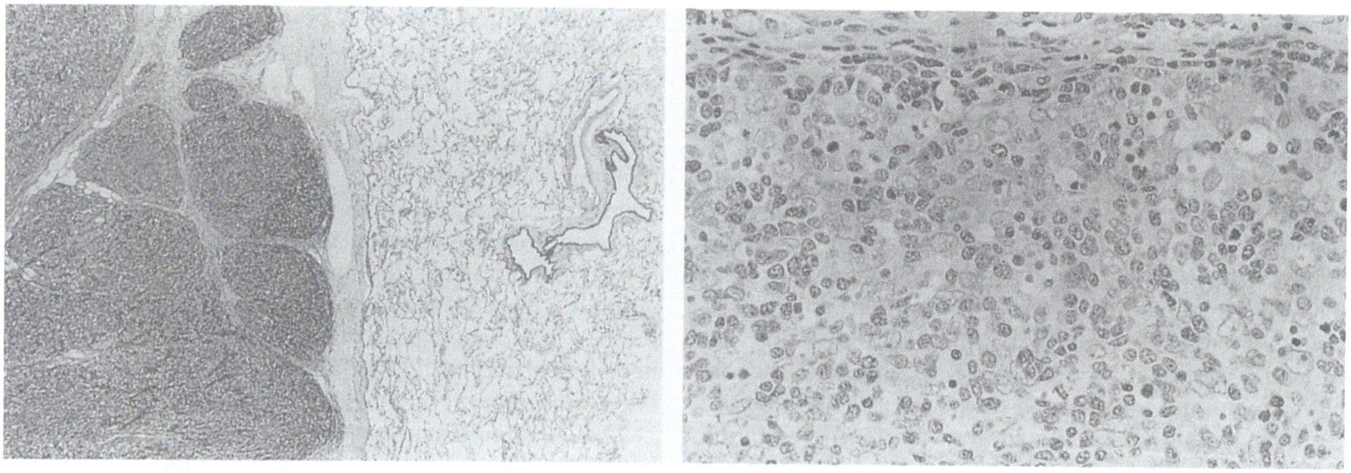

B

FIGURE 41.6. Thymoma extending into lung. **(A)** This thymoma was a primary in the mediastinum but is similar to those described in the lung. **(B)** Microscopic patterns are also similar to those in the mediastinum, but recognition by first thinking of the possibility and then conducting appropriate immunohistochemical evaluations is needed for diagnosis.

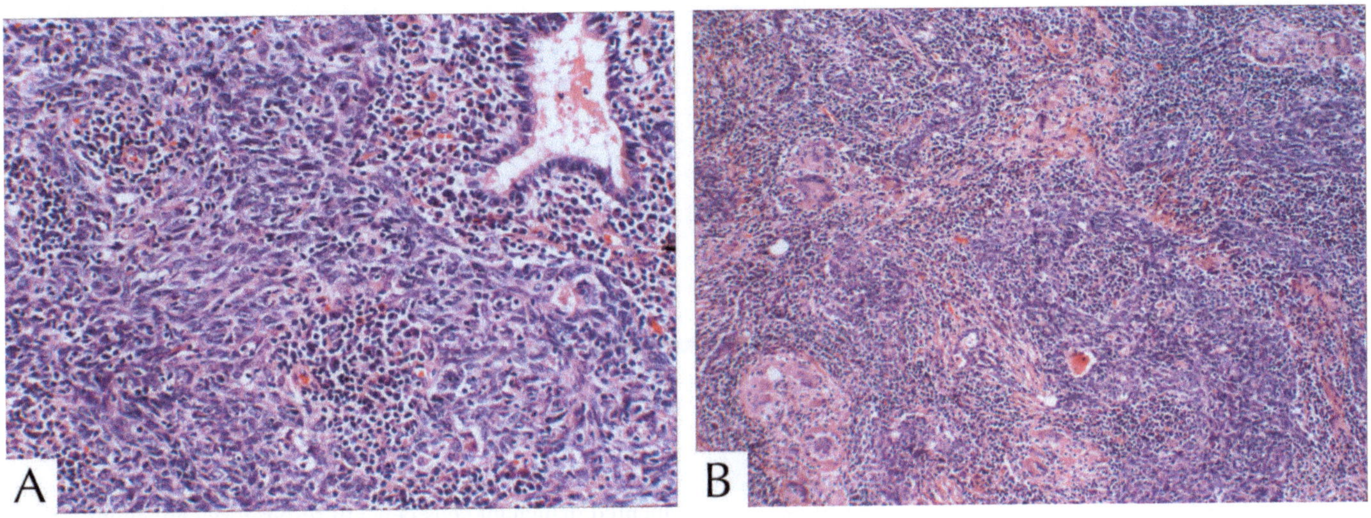

FIGURE 41.8. **(A)** This thymoma was a primary intrapulmonary spindle cell thymoma. **(B)** Note prominent granulomatous reaction and multinucleated giant cells in the left lower field. (Courtesy of Dr. A. Srivastava, New England Medical Center, Boston, MA.)

is best made by the surgeon, who is in a position to adequately evaluate adherence to adjacent structures. However, the responsibility to determine invasiveness in intrapulmonary thymomas would appear to be entirely that of the examining pathologist.

In Moran et al.'s[35] cases, stains for cytokeratin and epithelial membrane antigen (EMA) highlighted scattered epithelial cells against a rich lymphoid background. In paraffin-embedded tissues, the thymic epithelial cells of thymomas stain with epithelial markers such as keratin and the lymphocytes stain with CD45RO and UCHL-1 but not CD20.[38] Lymphocytes from intrapulmonary thymomas stain for CD4, CD8, and CD5, but not for CD20 or CD21.[37] The lymphocytes also stain for CD1a and show nuclear immunoreactivity for terminal deoxynucleotidyl transferase.[37] Thymomas are negative for actin, desmin, vimentin, and the S-100 protein. Cytokeratin subtype 5/6 is expressed by thymic epithelial cells and along with the p63 protein (a member of the p53 protein family) can be valuable in establishing a diagnosis.[39,40] The differential diagnosis, in addition to thymoma metastatic from the pleura or the mediastinum, includes malignant lymphomas, lymphocyte-rich carcinomas, spindle cell carcinomas, and pulmonary teratomas with thymic components. In practice, differentiation from these entities is not difficult. Lymphoid markers as described above and cytokeratin assist in the differential diagnosis.

The clinical course of intrapulmonary thymomas is an indolent one. These slow-growing lesions may remain asymptomatic until they reach a critical mass and cause clinical problems due to local growth or tumefaction, that is, chest pain or airway obstruction.[36] Local recurrence and distant metastasis are rare but may occur.[31,32,35,36] Surgical excision with or without postoperative radiation is regarded as the treatment of choice. In Moran et al.'s[35] series, surgically resected patients lived up to 8 years after resection, without evidence of recurrence. Ishibashi and coworkers[41] reported a case of primary intrapulmonary thymoma with invasion of the brachiocephalic vein. Complete resection of the tumor with vascular reconstruction was successfully performed with no evidence of recurrent disease 6 years later.

Primary Malignant Melanomas

Primary pulmonary melanomas are extremely rare and require rigorous exclusion of metastatic disease by means of a thorough history and an extensive dermatologic examination. Metastatic melanomas to the lung are often multiple and bilateral, and involve the parenchyma.[42] At times, however, metastatic melanomas to the lung can be solitary (Fig. 41.9). On the other hand, primary

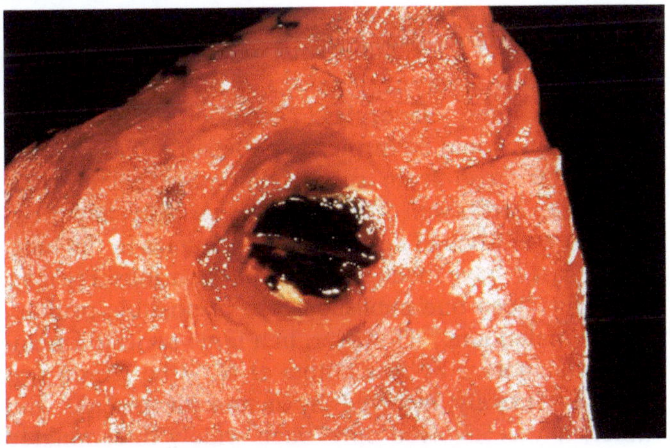

FIGURE 41.9. Metastatic melanoma to lung. Note sharply demarcated jet black nodular lesion at center. (Courtesy of Dr. Rhonda Yantiss, University of Massachusetts Medical School, Worcester, MA, and Dr. Eugene J. Mark, Massachusetts General Hospital, Boston, MA.)

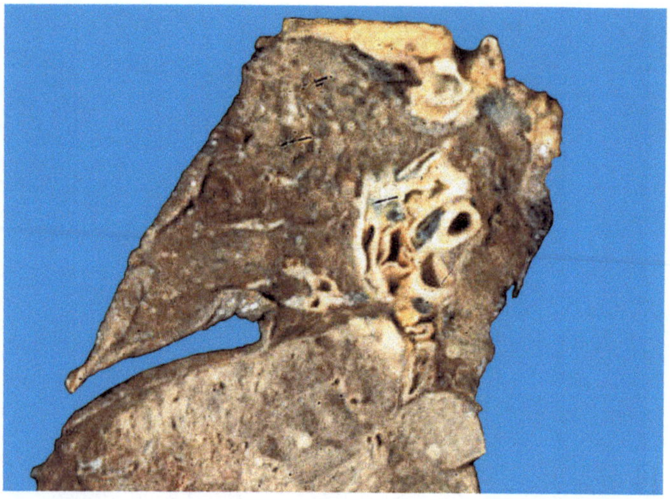

FIGURE 41.10. Primary malignant melanoma. Note small poorly defined gray black nodular area at apex with fatty adhesions. This is an atypical example. As noted in the text most primary pulmonary melanomas are endobronchial. (Courtesy of Dr. Philip T. Cagle, Methodist Hospital, Houston, TX.)

pulmonary melanomas typically arise in the bronchus and are likely to be single. Most primary bronchial melanomas are pigmented and are therefore detectable or at least suspected by bronchoscopic examination. Knowledge of radiologic imaging studies is important, since peripheral nodular melanomas are virtually always metastatic.[42] Cases of bronchial melanoma reported in the literature emphasize the relationship of the melanocytic cells to the bronchial mucosa and the demonstration of junctional activity as a sign of the neoplasm arising at that site.[42]

The histogenesis of primary pulmonary melanomas is not well understood. Cagle et al.[43] and others[44,45] have reviewed the subject. Melanin-containing cells have not been identified in normal bronchial mucosa. However, some authors hypothesize that because the lungs are an outpouching of the endodermal tube and melanomas arise in the oropharynx, larynx, and esophagus, there is the potential for melanocytes to occur in the lungs. If this is the case, it could be further hypothesized that primary melanomas arise from such pulmonary melanocytes. Some cases are as well documented as possible, and probably represent bona fide primary melanomas in the lung. Other cases have been excluded for various reasons. There has been one published case of possible primary pleural melanoma.[46] However, in a large series of metastatic melanomas by Das Gupta et al.,[47] the pleura was never exclusively involved by metastatic disease, but rather, it was involved only when widely disseminated melanoma was present in the adjacent lung.

Grossly, primary pulmonary melanomas may present as polypoid intraluminal masses of fleshy brown to black tissue. Much less commonly, primary pulmonary melanomas will be peripherally located (Fig. 41.10). The histologic features of primary pulmonary melanomas are similar to those of melanomas from other sites chiefly showing large polygonal discohesive cells with prominent nucleoli (Fig. 41.11).[42] The differential diagnosis includes poorly differentiated malignant neoplasms such as large cell lymphomas and poorly differentiated carcinomas. Immunostains for cytokeratin and lymphoid markers such as CD45 greatly facilitate the distinction from carcinomas and lymphomas, respectively. Immunostains that assist in the diagnosis of primary or metastatic melanomas include S-100 protein, HMB-45, and MART-1 immunostains (Fig. 41.12). However, caution is needed, as some other tumors such as pigmented carcinoid tumors may also contain melanin, and clear cell "sugar" tumors are positive for S-100 protein and HMB-45. The peripheral location of clear cell sugar tumors is also a useful discriminating feature.[42] Electron microscopy is useful in difficult cases, helping to identify pre-melanosomes and melanosomes in the cytoplasm of tumor cells. If present, these cytoplasmic structures are regarded as diagnostic of melanoma.

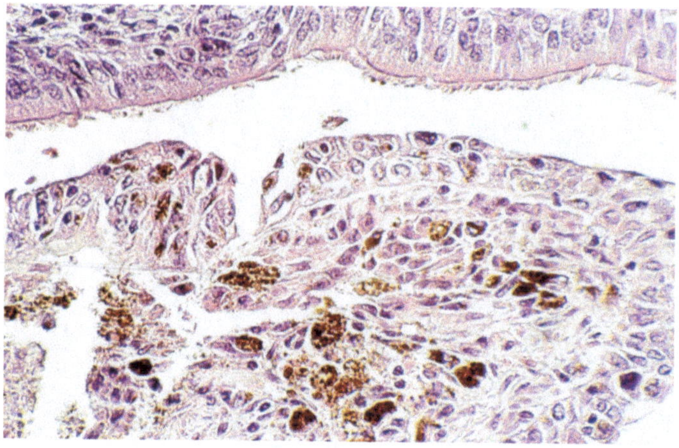

FIGURE 41.11. Primary bronchial melanoma. Note deeply pigmented malignant cells beneath respiratory epithelium.

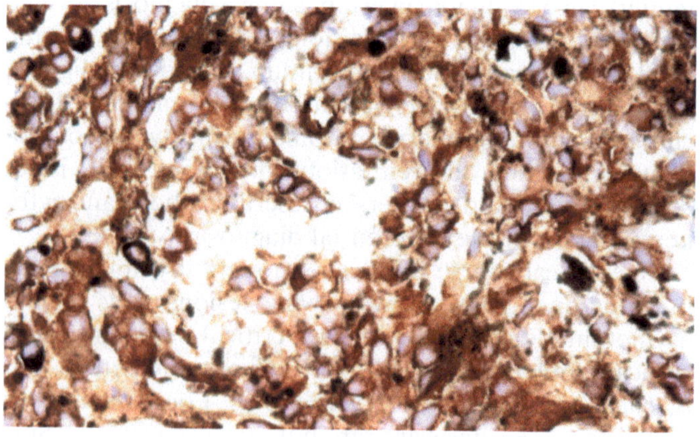

FIGURE 41.12. Primary pulmonary melanoma. Intense positive immunostaining of tumor cells with HMB-45. (Courtesy of Dr. Philip T. Cagle, Methodist Hospital, Houston, TX.)

One of the better histologic criteria used to diagnose primary melanoma on mucous membranes, analogous to cutaneous melanomas, is the presence of atypical melanocytic hyperplasia in overlying or nearby bronchial mucosa.[48] Some authors have called this junctional or lentiginous change,[49,50] and some require this change to be associated with the "dropping off" of nests of atypical melanocytes between the surface and the tumor mass.[51] This change is usually associated with squamous metaplasia, but also may be seen in ciliated respiratory epithelium, with atypical cells present in the base of the mucosa.[52] This change in adjacent mucosa has been referred to by some authors as the "melanoma flare."[53] Other cases that appear to be primary have not always had this association, so its absence does not exclude a case from being considered a true primary melanoma.

Although exceptions occur, nodular melanomas in peripheral lung tissue rarely represent primary melanomas (Fig. 41.10). Various sets of criteria have been offered by different authors at various times in attempting to refine parameters most useful in making a diagnosis of primary melanoma of lung.[48,49,54] The most reasonable of these criteria for suggesting a diagnosis of primary pulmonary melanoma appear to be the following: (1) absence of other past or present atypical-to-malignant pigmented lesions from any site; (2) a solitary lung lesion centered on a bronchus, with no evidence of any other organ involvement; and (3) in situ atypical melanocytic change of bronchial mucosa adjacent to or overlying the major tumor mass. However, establishing a diagnosis of melanoma as a primary lesion in the lung is a very challenging and often impossible task. Regressing melanomas of the skin are a well-known source of regional lymph node and widespread metastases. In the study by Das Gupta et al.,[47] 100 (10%) of 992 metastatic melanomas were initially identified to be without known primary. However, after thorough evaluation, only 37 (3.7%) remained in this category. Of these, 24 involved only one node group and 13 were widespread. None apparently was solitary in a visceral organ.

As a continuation of this study, Das Gupta and Brasfield,[55] in an autopsy series of widespread metastasis from melanoma, later noted that the lungs are subject to metastatic melanoma more often than any other organ.[56] Metastatic melanoma to lung usually consists of multiple bilateral nodules varying between several millimeters and 2.5 cm and favoring the periphery of the lungs. These metastatic nodules are most common in areas of high blood flow, specifically in the lower lobes. Metastatic melanoma less commonly affects the airways. In the series of Das Gupta et al.,[56] only one of 652 cases spread to the trachea and another to the bronchus. Forty-five spread to the lungs alone. None spread to the pleura alone. These are important statistics, as the bronchus is the source of origin of those cases that are most likely primary in the lung. Several reported cases have tumor limited only to lung or with only regional node spread. Autopsy follow-up with thorough evaluation of all possible sites is helpful when attempting to determine the primary site.[53–57] One additional histopathologic feature that can be seen in metastatic melanomas to the lung is a lepidic type of spread of tumor cells along preexisting alveolar walls in a manner that resembles that of bronchioloalveolar carcinoma (Fig. 41.13).

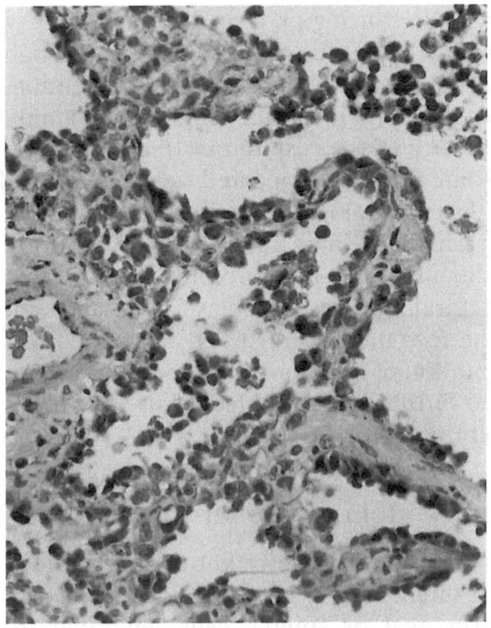

FIGURE 41.13. Metastatic melanoma. Some malignant cells lie in the interstitium, while others line air spaces in a manner reminiscent of a bronchioloalveolar carcinoma.

The prognosis of primary melanoma of lung is extremely poor. Although exceptions occur, most patients are dead within 1.5 years from diagnosis. Similar dismal results are reported by Wilson and Moran.[58] In their study of eight patients, five died of metastatic disease from 4 to 34 months after resection. However, some patients are reported as having survived up to 11 years after pneumonectomy without evidence of tumor.[59–61] In one reported case, a pulmonary lesion was diagnosed 31 years after a choroidal melanoma was excised. In another case, 3 years after a melanoma from the left cheek was excised, a patient with a right-bronchial melanoma presented with hemoptysis.[60] Recurrent hemoptyses required repeated cauterizations, and progressive involvement of the tracheobronchial system was identified during the next 10 years.[60] At autopsy there were submucosal lesions in an area just below the larynx, in the midtrachea, and in both mainstem bronchi, each with overlying atypical melanocytic hyperplasia in the tracheobronchial mucosa.[60] Perhaps this was a case of multiple primary melanomas, even though two of the three criteria noted above could not be identified.

Benign, extracutaneous, nonmucosal, nonmalignant melanocytic proliferations are known to occur in sites such as lymph nodes but are exceedingly rare in the respiratory tract. Reporting on a single patient, a 68-year-old man with a 0.4-cm blue-black nodule in the right bronchus, Ferrara and associates[62] called attention to the occurrence of a previously unrecognized and unpublished possible entity of the respiratory tract, a bronchial blue nevus. While the nevus appeared well documented on the basis of histopathology, histochemical stains (Fontana-Masson stain for melanin and Perl's stain for iron), immunohistochemistry (S-100 protein immunostain), and ultrastructural features (cytoplasmic melanosomes identified), the case must be regarded as a curiosity. Clearly, documentation of additional cases and experience will be needed to further establish blue nevus as a valid entity in the respiratory tract.

Pulmonary Meningothelial-Like Bodies

Pulmonary lesions formerly known as chemodectomas consist of small, usually microscopic nest-like aggregates of uniform oval or spindle cells separated from one another by thin strands of fibrous tissue. First described in detail by Korn and associates,[63] these small or minute bodies were detected in the lung tissue of 18 patients—four men and 14 women. In only one patient were they observed grossly; in the others they were incidental findings on microscopic examination. The authors attempted injection techniques to further study the character of these cell collections, but the techniques did not penetrate the small-caliber vessels in the center of the lesions, probably because of a technical problem, and did not show arteriovenous anastomoses. Their serial sections, however, confirmed that these bodies were centered on veins, without a significant arterial supply, and without significant capillary plexus arrangement. The authors pointed out that no systematic search or study of these bodies had been done, and it was probable that if such was carried out, the incidence would be higher. Korn et al. titled their article "Multiple Minute Pulmonary Tumors Resembling Chemodectomas," and for many years thereafter these structures were known to many as small chemodectomas. Because of the morphologic similarity of these chemodectoma-like structures to paraganglionic tissue, the authors wondered about their possible chemoreceptor function. The nesting of some of the cells initially suggested some type of oxygenated blood monitoring function.

Spencer[64] later suggested that these minute bodies might be reactive or possibly hamartomatous. Zak and Chabes[65] studied six patients, all women, and collectively called these bodies "chemodectomatosis" because of their multiplicity. Using silver staining techniques, Barroso-Moguel and Costero[66,67] identified nerve-like filaments that extended into the center of some cell balls. They stained some structures that were quite distinct, while some of the silver-staining filaments appear to be entrapped elastic fibers. Some appeared almost neuroid in arrangement, and it was unclear on the basis of follow-up studies what the fine filaments and cell ball arrangement really were. They also found some nonspecific argentaffin-positive reaction in these cells, endothelial cells, and pleural cells, but this finding remains unconfirmed by others. Follow-up by Costero et al.[68] with electron microscopy data seemed to reverse this earlier suggestion, because no nerves, nervelike features, or secretory granules could be identified. The authors wondered if they could be pleural-derived rests or hamartomas in the lung. Spain[69] published 15 cases, and was the first to draw attention to the high rate of associated acute and organizing pulmonary emboli with these bodies. Ichinose et al.[70] added 10 cases, and carefully itemized the associated conditions in these 10 and in the 46 cases reported in the literature by 1971. Of these, 29 were associated with pulmonary emboli, 30 had cardiovascular disease, and 17 had malignancy. Some patients had more than one of these associated findings. Some 91% of these patients had conditions predisposing them to thromboemboli. On histologic review, six of the 10 new cases had changes compatible with old pulmonary emboli.[70] Currently, these minute lesions are known to be more closely related to meningothelial cells and to share histologic, ultrastructural, and immunohistochemical properties with meningiomas.[71] Therefore, the previous term (chemodectoma) is no longer used or recommended.

Small meningothelial-like bodies in the lung have been found in patients of ages 12 to 91 years, but mostly in the seventh decade. This may well reflect the age range in autopsy series used to collect most of the data on these cases; they are also found in surgical excisions of middle-aged to older individuals. They are multiple in some 30% to 50% and grossly have been seen in only a few cases (Fig. 41.14). In one case, hundreds of these bodies were seen on the pleural surface.[63] Ichinose and coworkers[70]

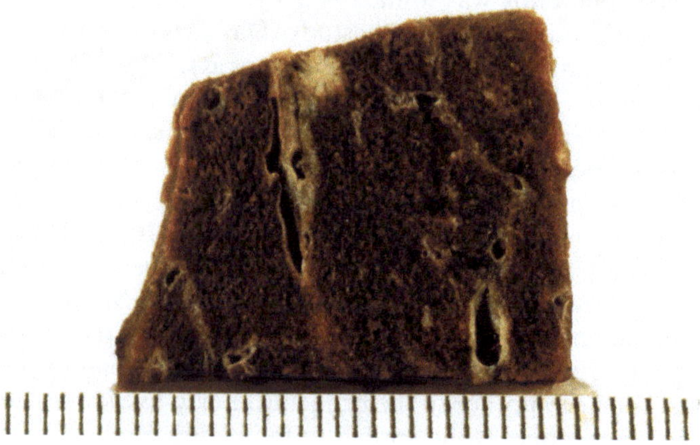

FIGURE 41.14. Meningothelial-like body at top center. Note small, flat, somewhat stellate nodule. Millimeter scale. (Courtesy of Dr. Andrew Fischer, University of Massachusetts Medical School, Worcester, MA.)

went back to the paraffin-embedded blocks and found gray specks in two of the 10 cases detected, and when they cut more tissue in five of these cases, no more bodies were found nearby. One of us (D.H.D.) found one meningothelial-like nodule grossly in the adjacent cut of a sample from a lobectomy specimen, but this was only detected after it was seen microscopically. Eighty-four percent of all cases to date have occurred in women. These bodies were thought to be more frequent toward the pleural surface, but were also found in the deep parenchyma.[63,72] In the series by Churg and Warnock,[73] in which location was identified, the bodies seemed to follow lung volume, being most frequent in the lower lobes (six of 13, 46%) and next most common in the upper lobes (five of 13, 38%), and least common in the middle lobe and lingula (two of 13, 15%). Although the sample number was small, it is interesting that in the cases of Churg and Warnock, these lesions were found to be three times more common on the right side than on the left. Those with multiple lesions were most often in adjacent lung, as a single location was given. The one case described as multiple in the series by Korn et al.[63] had grossly identifiable multiple lesions in all lobes.

The frequency of these bodies varies in different series. As noted by Korn et al.,[63] they were found in 12 of 3635 (0.3%), or at a frequency of about 1 in 300 routine autopsies. Ichinose et al.[70] found them in nine of 1828 autopsies, or about one in 200. The rate was one in 360 (0.3%) in selected autopsies in the retrospective review by Churg and Warnock,[73] but when prosectors were made aware of these lesions and asked to be alert for them, the rate rose to six in 200 (3%), or about one in 33. Considering these bodies' higher incidence in women, Churg and Warnock estimated they occurred in about one in every 20 women in their autopsy series. Spain[69] found a rate of 15 in 303 autopsies, or about one in 20. Half of his cases were selected for ischemic conditions, and the other half were a series of all autopsies followed in his hospital for 1 year. The incidence in each of these groups was not specified.

For obvious reasons, the gross morphology is not well defined. However, several authors have called attention to these bodies' multiplicity and small size, up to 1 to 2 mm and their location on the pleural surface, being gray-pink in color and having the appearance of flat or slightly raised, round to slightly irregular but sometimes stellate nodules, often occurring near interlobular septa (Fig. 41.14).[68–70] They have also been described as resembling miliary disease, ranging in size from 1 to 4 mm in maximum diameter.[68–70] Small lymphoid nodules may also be in the gross differential diagnosis, but these are usually more translucent and associated directly with lymphatic pathways. Cases of infectious miliary disease, focal micronodules of smooth muscle hyperplasia, and small metastatic tumor nodules might also be considered. Lastly, carcinoid tumorlets can be suggested by their juxtabronchiolar location.

Microscopically, these lesions vary and may be delicate or thick. As they surround veins, they are usually in the middle or peripheral portions of the lobules of the lung, but occasionally are seen to outline alveolar ducts. At low power these bodies often have a somewhat stellate shape, usually with central thickening and with retraction of nearby air spaces, giving a focal emphysema effect. These bodies may also be contained in a more linear fashion within the interstitium. Occasionally they abut the pleura or interlobular septa, but they do not extend into either of these structures. They are not seen in bronchi or in branches of pulmonary or bronchial arteries. The cells making up these proliferations have bland-looking, oval to slightly indented nuclei with finely granular chromatin and inconspicuous nucleoli. These cells have no mitoses. Their cytoplasm is usually abundant, granular, light pink, and homogeneous throughout. They have poorly defined cytoplasmic borders, and measure about 30 μm in diameter. At times they are more elongated, and appear either to form nodules or to be cut in different directions of orientation, giving some variation to the pattern. In about 20% of cases, some hemosiderin is associated with the cells in the interstitium. Tumor cells are always separated from the alveolus by a delicate crown of capillaries, and the alveolar type II cells are only minimally reactive. Perhaps the juxtaposition of capillaries prevents the usual alveolar type II cell hyperplasia seen in most interstitial thickenings. The tendency toward formation of cell nests has suggested to one group of authors that these appear like nevus cells.[70] There is, however, no suggestion of this ultrastructurally or by S-100 protein immunostaining.

Three electron microscopic studies are available, and we have studied one case. In the first, Costero et al.[68] commented on the lack of nerve or neurosecretory granule features and noted the presence of well-developed desmosomes. Two other studies, Kuhn and Askin[72] and Churg and Warnock,[73] were done almost concurrently and have shown similar architecture, and both studies reached almost identical conclusions. Both studies showed broad irregular cytoplasmic membrane processes that were closely apposed (in a "jigsaw" fashion) and generally separated by 200 Å or so, occasionally opening to some 800 Å for short distances. There were numerous well-formed desmosomes. Most of the cytoplasm was filled with 60- to 100-Å filaments oriented toward the longer axis of the cells. Our case concurred and also showed some remarkably generous cystic spaces. The Golgi apparatus was usually prominent, but other organelles, including mitochondria, were scant. A few lipid or lipofuscin granules and occasional glycogen granules were seen. Some pinocytotic vesicles were seen along the cell membranes, but there was no basement membrane material around the cells and none encapsulating the group of cells. Collagen and elastic tissue were confirmed as radiating between the tumor cells, were extracellular, and did not appear to be produced by the tumor cells themselves.

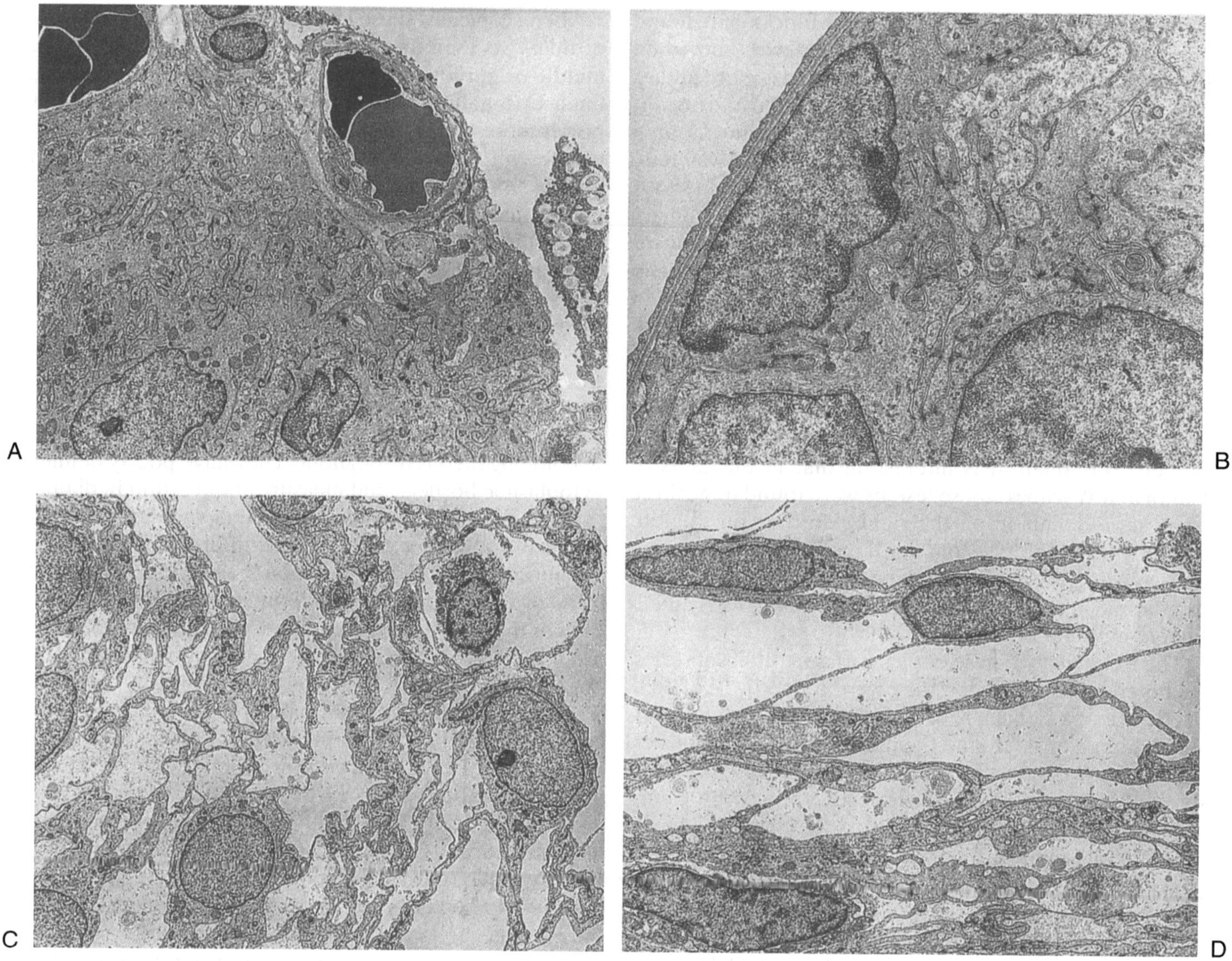

Figure 41.15. Meningothelial-like body. Ultrastructure. **(A)** Clusters of cells with highly convoluted cell mechanisms and well-developed desmosomes. **(B)** Note complex interdigitation of cell membranes and well-developed desmosomes. **(C)** Well-developed cystic spaces are evident in this view. **(D)** Sometimes these cystic spaces, similar to those seen in meningiomas are dominant in some areas. (Transmission electron microscopy [TEM].)

The more peripheral cells in the nodules were more elongated and spread around the more central tumor cells in a circumferential manner. No tumor cells infiltrated capillaries or alveolar lining cells. No nerves were seen in or near these nodules. Confirming the earlier study, no neurosecretory granules were identified. Also, there was no intracytoplasmic lumen formation to suggest angioblasts, and no Weibel–Palade bodies, but cystic spaces were present as shown in Figure 41.15. These cells look most like pia arachnoid cells of meningiomas.[72,73] They appear distinct from the ultramicroscopic appearance of both mesothelial cells and submesothelial fibroblasts.

We have used immunoperoxidase on several of these cases, and the tumor cells stain vividly with vimentin and are negative for cytokeratins, S-100 protein, and chromogranin. Recent studies have confirmed lack of reactivity for cytokeratin, S-100 protein, and neuron-specific enolase. These studies have also shown immunoreactivity for vimentin and EMA in accordance with the resemblance of these cells to meningothelial cells. The authors have also seen progesterone receptor positivity again in accord with a putative relationship of these cells to meningothelial cells and the cells of some meningiomas (Fig. 41.16).

The differential diagnosis is varied. Small neuroendocrine cell proliferations or "tumorlets," are collections of neurosecretory cells, usually in and about smaller bronchioles and terminal bronchioles, that are associated with distortion of the architecture with some scarring in these areas. These clusters of cells are neuroendocrine with appropriate stains and electron microscopy, may be mul-

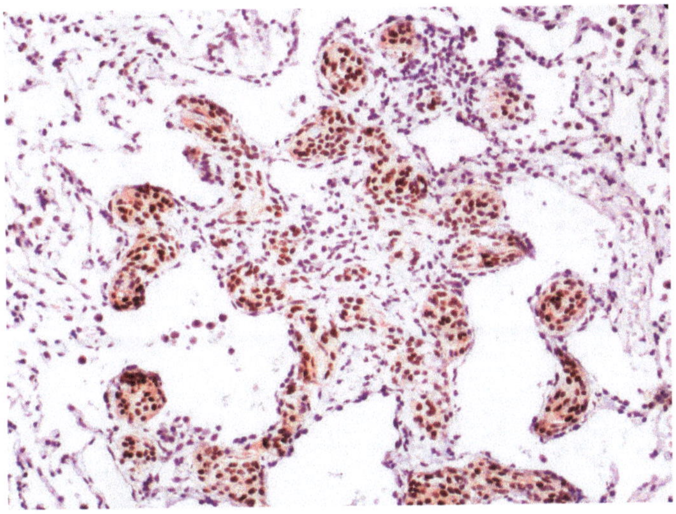

FIGURE 41.16. Meningothelial-like body showing strong nuclear positivity for progesterone receptor.

tiple, and invade the adjacent air spaces. There is a higher nuclear-to-cytoplasmic ratio, and a moderate degree of hyperchromasia with thicker chromatin and more elongated cell arrangement than in small meningothelial-like bodies. Other tumors in the differential diagnosis include benign clear cell (sugar) tumors, epithelioid hemangioendotheliomas, small sclerosing hemangiomas, metastatic paragangliomas, and small primary or metastatic meningiomas. Benign clear cell sugar tumors have larger cells that are more polygonal, glycogen rich, and are permeated by ectatic sinusoids with some collagen in their vascular walls. Clear cell (sugar) tumors form consolidated nodules, destroying the underlying lung architecture. Epithelioid hemangioendotheliomas are composed of epithelioid-appearing bland cells with granular cytoplasm filled with filaments, but these tumors proliferate predominantly in alveolar spaces, with some protrusion in a retrograde fashion in terminal bronchioles. They are also seen in vessels and have a tendency to become more spindle-like. Only rarely can interstitial tumor spread be identified, quite unlike the findings of minute meningothelial-like bodies. Small sclerosing hemangiomas can cause interstitial thickening, and even when these tumors are small they begin to have central sclerosis. Their tumor cells are apt to be more cuboidal, their cytoplasm more granular, and they stimulate overlying alveolar epithelial type II cells more than do the cells of small meningothelial-like bodies.

Are pulmonary meningothelial-like nodules tumoral processes? Are meningothelial-like bodies precursor lesions of meningiomas? Ionescu et al.[71] elegantly explored the answer to these intriguing questions (Fig. 41.17). In their study, a genotypic comparison of these bodies with meningiomas suggests that isolated lesions are most likely reactive. However, symptomatic cases with multiple lesions showed more than one loss of heterozygosity (LOH) event, suggesting a transitional stage between reactive and neoplastic proliferation (Table 41.3).[71] Whether reactive or neoplastic, these small but enigmatic pulmonary bodies thus far appear to be of no intrinsic clinical significance. However, as the resolution of modern imaging techniques continues to rise, it is possible that these bodies may act as important confounding factors in the diagnosis of radiographically visible lesions, by virtue of their resemblance to infectious miliary lesions or micronodular spread of known malignancies.

Meningiomas

Primary meningiomas in the lung are histologically similar if not identical to those arising in the intracranial cavity or the spinal canal. They are very uncommon, with only nine cases of presumed primary meningioma reported up to 1993,[74–80] and 10 more cases reported by Moran et al.[81] in 1996. Rare pulmonary meningiomas may arise in the setting of neurofibromatosis.[82] Most extracranial meningiomas involve the head and neck, and rare occurrences in the chest have been reported in the posterior mediastinum and pleura, in addition to the lung.[83–85] Metastases from intracranial meningiomas to the lung do occur, usually following surgery or postoperative recurrences. In two separate series of 56 and 113 cases of metastasizing meningiomas, the lung was identified as a site of metastasis in 60% and 61%, respectively.[86,87]

Grossly, meningiomas present as soft, well-circumscribed masses with granular white or yellow-gray cut surfaces. They are typically located in the pulmonary parenchyma and may be subpleural.[81,88] Microscopically, cases reported as primary in the lung have typical meningothelial-like patterns with whorls of spindle-shaped cells with or without psammomatous calcifications, and no mitoses or cellular pleomorphism (Fig. 41.18). However, primary pulmonary meningiomas may show atypical histopathologic features and malignant behavior.[89] One such case was reported by Prayson and Farver,[89] in which increased mitotic figures (up to 15 per 10 high power fields) and cells with nucleoli were observed. Immunostaining shows that tumor cells are negative for high and low molecular weight cytokeratins, chromogranin, neuron-specific enolase, bombesin, and desmin, but positive at least focally for S-100 protein, vimentin, and EMA.[88–90] One of several cases studied by Moran et al.,[81] a fibrous meningioma, showed focal positivity for CD34, while none showed positivity for factor VIII. One case studied by us was focally positive for progesterone receptor. The malignant case cited above was also focally positive for progesterone receptor and had an MIB-1 labeling index of 9.2%.[89] By electron microscopy, meningiomas have typical, highly interdigitated cell membranes and desmosomes.[81,89]

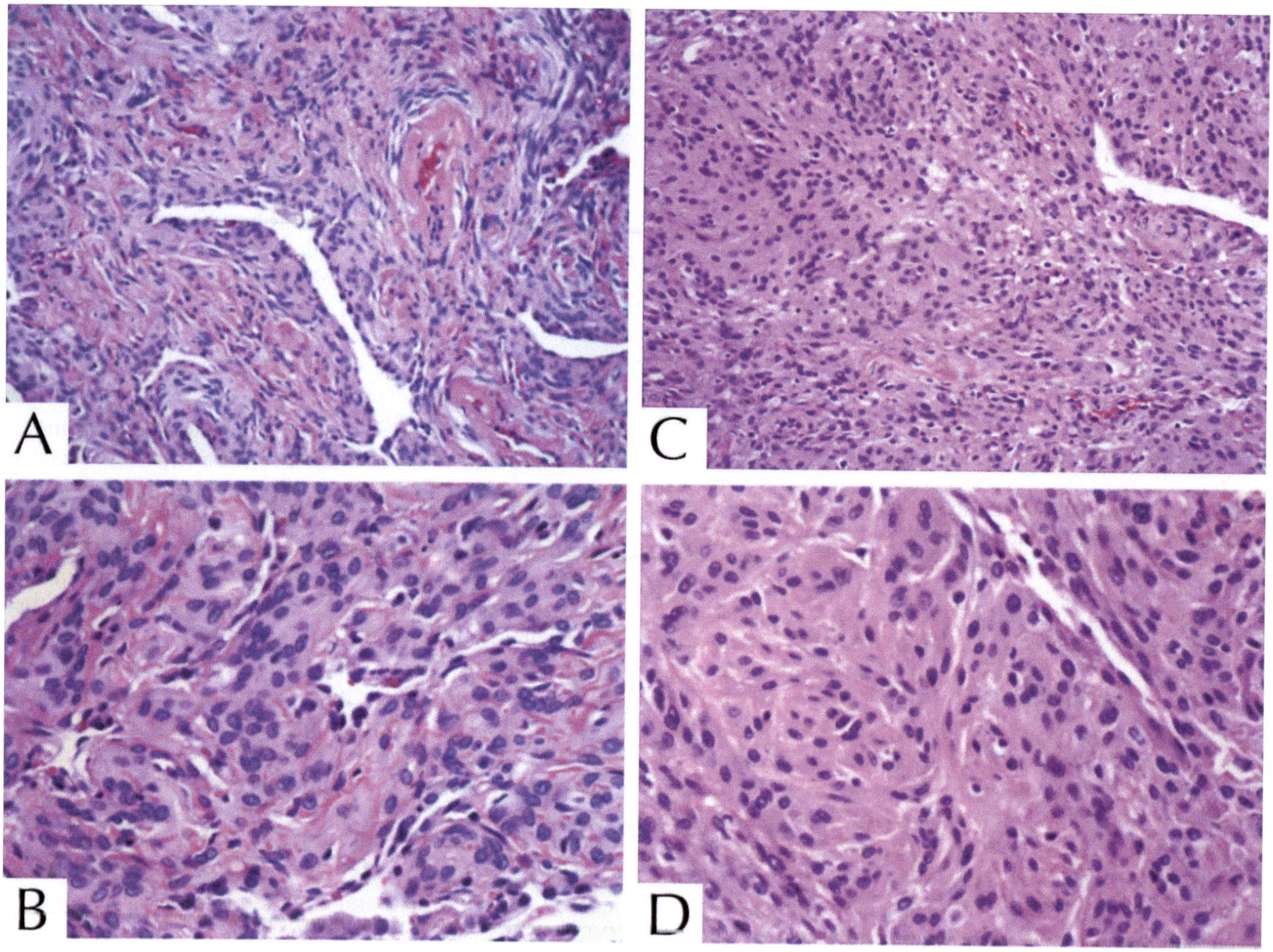

FIGURE 41.17. Meningothelial-like bodies in comparison with meningioma. Panels **A** and **B**, corresponding to a meningothelial-like body, have a histologic appearance similar to a benign meningioma shown in **C** and **D**. The nuclei in both entities are bland, oval, with inconspicuous nucleoli, and the cytoplasm is abundant eosinophilic and granular. (Courtesy of Dr. D.N. Ionescu, University of Pittsburgh Medical Center, Pittsburgh, PA.)

TABLE 41.3. Frequency of loss of heterozygosity in minute pulmonary meningothelial-like (MPMN) nodules, MPMN-omatosis syndrome, and benign meningioma

Chromosomal locus	Single MPMN		MPMN-omatosis*		Meningioma	
	Nodules	Cases	Nodules	Cases	Nodules	Cases
1p	0% 0/11	0% 0/11	4.8% 1/21	25% 1/4	44.4% 4/9	44.4% 4/9
3p	16.7% 2/12	16.7% 2/12	9.5% 2/21	50% 1/2	33.3% 3/9	33.3% 3/9
5q	0% 0/8	0% 0/8	0% 0/21	0% 0/4	0% 0/9	0% 0/9
9q	0% 0/8	0% 0/8	6.3% 1/16	33.3% 1/3	25% 1/4	25% 1/4
9p	0% 0/7	0% 0/7	7.1% 1/14	33.3% 1/3	16.7% 1/6	16.7% 1/6

(*Continued*)

Table 41.3. *Continued*

Chromosomal locus	Single MPMN		MPMN-omatosis*		Meningioma	
	Nodules	Cases	Nodules	Cases	Nodules	Cases
10q	0%	0%	4.8%	25%	11.1%	11.1%
	0/12	0/12	1/21	1/4	1/9	1/9
14q	0%	0%	0%	0%	42.9%	42.9%
	0/8	0/8	0/18	0/4	3/7	3/7
17p	10%	10%	19%	50%	0%	0%
	1/10	1/10	4/21	2/4	0/7	0/7
18q	0%	0%	0%	0%	0%	0%
	0/9	0/9	0/13	0/3	0/6	0/6
19q	0%	0%	5.6%	25%	12.5%	12.5%
	0/10	0/10	1/18	1/4	1/8	1/8
22q	10%	10%	4.8%	25%	60%	60%
	1/10	1/10	1/21	1/4	6/10	6/10

*MPMN-omatosis syndrome refers to multiple MPMNs, and is equivalent to the term *chemodectomatosis*. The term is used to distinguish it from single MPMNs.

Source: Ionescu et al.,[71] with permission from Lippincott Williams & Wilkins.

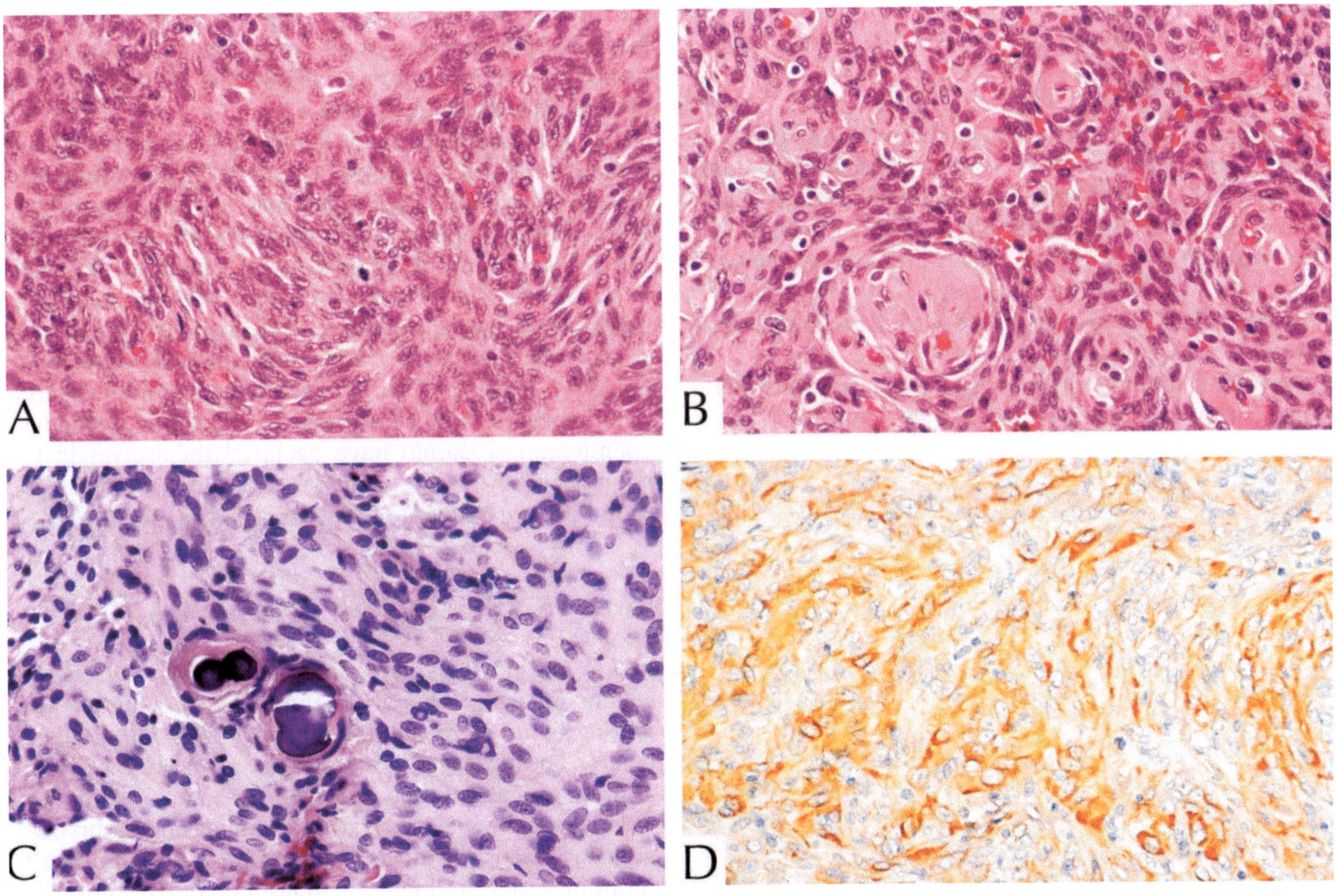

Figure 41.18. Meningioma. **(A)** Note cells with oval to round nuclei arranged in a somewhat syncytial pattern. **(B)** Same cells in a more typical whorled manner. **(C)** Areas containing calcified psammoma bodies. **(D)** Positive diffuse immunostaining with vimentin. (**A,B,D**: Courtesy of Drs. R A. Prayson and C.A. Farver, Cleveland Clinic Foundation, Cleveland, OH; **C**: Courtesy of Dr. Thomas Smith, University of Massachusetts Medical School, Worcester, MA.)

A classification scheme proposed by Hoye et al.[91] for extracranial meningiomas includes (1) meningiomas secondary to extracranial extension from intracranial primary meningiomas; (2) meningiomas originating from arachnoid cells at the borders of the nervous system, such as the cranial foramina with exodus of cranial vertebral nerves; (3) totally detached extracranial ectopic meningiomas; and (4) metastases from benign-appearing intracranial meningiomas. One might wonder whether ectopic cells (as proposed in the second category above) might be related to small meningothelial-like bodies. However, in no case of proposed primary pulmonary meningioma was there a reported increase of these types of bodies around the tumor, which may be suggestive of a field effect. Furthermore, meningiomas tend to be large and solitary as opposed to the smallness and multiplicity of meningothelial-like bodies. In addition, as reported by Ionescu et al.,[71] a high frequency of LOH in meningiomas, not shared by minute meningothelial-like bodies, seems to distinguish these two processes. Clinical follow-up in seven of the 10 cases reported by Moran et al.[81] suggested that meningiomas are amenable to surgical resection, which can be curative.

Ependymomas

Ependymomas are rare tumors derived from primitive glia.[92] Most ependymomas are intracranial in children and in the spinal cord and filum terminale in adults. Ependymomas of the central nervous system are typified by the presence of ependymal canals and a dense network of fibrillary cytoplasmic processes that condense in a collar-like fashion around blood vessels, forming structures known as perivascular pseudorosettes (Fig. 41.19).[92] Intracranial ependymomas rarely metastasize outside the central nervous system, but when they do they most commonly involve the lung. Extracranial ependymomas are exceedingly uncommon wherever they occur, including the lung, and tend to show morphologic features similar to those in the cranial cavity.[92] The most common sites of primary extracranial ependymoma are in or around the pelvis, including the sacrococcygeal region, broad ligament, mesoovarium, and the uterosacral ligament. However, cases have been reported in other anatomic sites well beyond the pelvis such as the posterior mediastinum.[93–95]

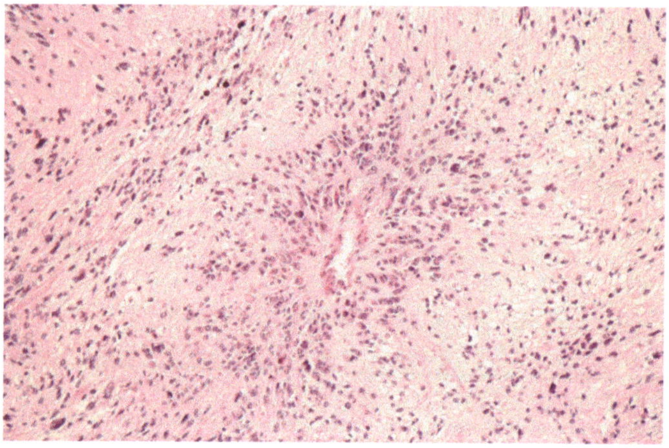

FIGURE 41.19. Ependymoma. Note pseudovascular pseudorosette with a dense collar-like network of fibrillary cytoplasmic processes. (From Crotty et al.,[93] with permission.)

Crotty et al.[93] in 1992 reported the most frequently cited case of a primary pulmonary ependymoma. Their patient had a 2-cm, right upper lobe nodule typical of ependymoma, occurring only in the lung, with clinical evaluation of the central nervous system being normal. Of interest, 30 months prior the patient had a separate nodule in the right upper lobe, somewhat more lateral, with enlarged hilar and supraclavicular lymph nodes, the latter of which was involved by biopsy-proven small cell carcinoma. Radiation and chemotherapy yielded complete resolution of all tumor. The patient subsequently died of a cerebral vascular accident in the distribution of the middle cerebral artery. Since no autopsy was performed, the possibility of an occult intracranial or other primary extrapulmonary ependymoma cannot be completely excluded in this case.

The immunohistochemical profile in Crotty and colleagues'[93] case of pulmonary ependymoma was similar to that of endocranial ependymomas showing strong positivity for glial fibrillary acidic protein and some positivity for EMA, S-100 protein, Leu-7, and vimentin, and negative reactivity for cytokeratin, synaptophysin, and chromogranin. The differential diagnosis is limited to neuroendocrine tumors that may show rosetting. As noted by Hasleton,[88] use of the above-cited neuroendocrine markers should facilitate the diagnosis. Secondary ependymomas should have declared themselves in the clinical history. Little is known about the prognosis due to the rarity of cases.

Germ Cell Tumors

The WHO classifies pulmonary germ cell tumors as miscellaneous neoplasms and defines them as tumors containing tissue elements derived from all three germ cell layers. The term *germ cell tumor*, in the lung as in the gonads, essentially encompasses teratomas and choriocarcinomas. However, teratocarcinomas and embryonal/yolk sac tumors also occur in the lung.[96,97] In contrast to teratomas, dermoid cysts of the lung consist entirely of derivatives of the ectodermal layer. This section discusses teratoma and choriocarcinoma only.

Teratomas occurring in the mediastinum outnumber those that originate in the lung, with a reported ratio of lung to mediastinal teratomas of about 1 to 30. Teratomas of the lung occur in the age group of 19 to 68 years and may contain thymic tissue; most are benign.[98] One notable exception is the case reported by Pound and Willis,[99] in which a large 9-cm lung tumor that presumably represented a congenital tumor was diagnosed in a 10-month-old infant. This tumor had spread to regional nodes and represented one of the very rare cases of truly malignant pulmonary teratomas. As noted by Jamieson and McGowan,[100] this is the only definite case of such a malignant teratomatous lesion proven by metastases. In another interesting case, an infiltrate in the upper lobe, thought to be tuberculosis, was diagnosed at age 5 years and treated, and after slow resolution of the pulmonary infiltrate, a perihilar mass persisted.[100] At age 22 years, following 6 weeks of chest pain, cough, and hemoptysis, the perihilar mass was excised and found to be a teratoma that had changed little in size in 17 years. The presenting signs and symptoms are usually those of an intrapulmonary mass. Rarely, trichoptysis (literally, the expectoration of hair) has been described with these lesions.[101,102]

Radiographically and by computed tomography several clues may suggest this tumor, but may be most helpful only in hindsight. These include calcifications or lucencies within more solid densities. Some of the lucencies detected radiographically are caused by cavitation and some by fat within the lesion. These findings are characteristic but not pathognomonic of teratoma of lung, as other lesions may also have lucent or cystic areas mixed with calcification, but confirming the densities as fat is very suggestive of teratoma or other fat-containing tumor. Teratomas are slow-growing tumors, and slow growth, if documented radiographically, is suggestive of the diagnosis. However, a definite diagnosis requires histologic confirmation.

Grossly, these tumors vary in texture and appearance, as does the spectrum of teratomas arising elsewhere, such as dermoid cysts of the ovary. Often cystic cavities are filled with either granular brown watery or flaky yellow debris. Most often identified grossly are sebum, fat, and sometimes bone (Fig. 41.20). In contrast to gonadal teratomas, teeth have not so far been reported in pulmonary lesions. Microscopically, all three germ cell layers are present. The most common component is ectodermal including skin and its appendages with pseudocystic areas containing accumulated keratin and sebum. Fat is frequent, as are fragments of tissue with gastrointestinal or respiratory tract differentiation immediately adjacent to mucosa of other types in a mature but disorderly arrangement (Fig. 41.21). Thymus and pancreas are identified with some regularity in lung teratomas.[103–105] Skeletal and smooth muscle, bone, cartilage, and brain are also identified in some. About a third of these have been called malignant, but this is based on the histologic appearance of immature cells, particularly stromal cells, and not on aggressive behavior. Only one case, as noted, has been documented to actually have metastasized, and as already noted this case was exceptional.[103–105]

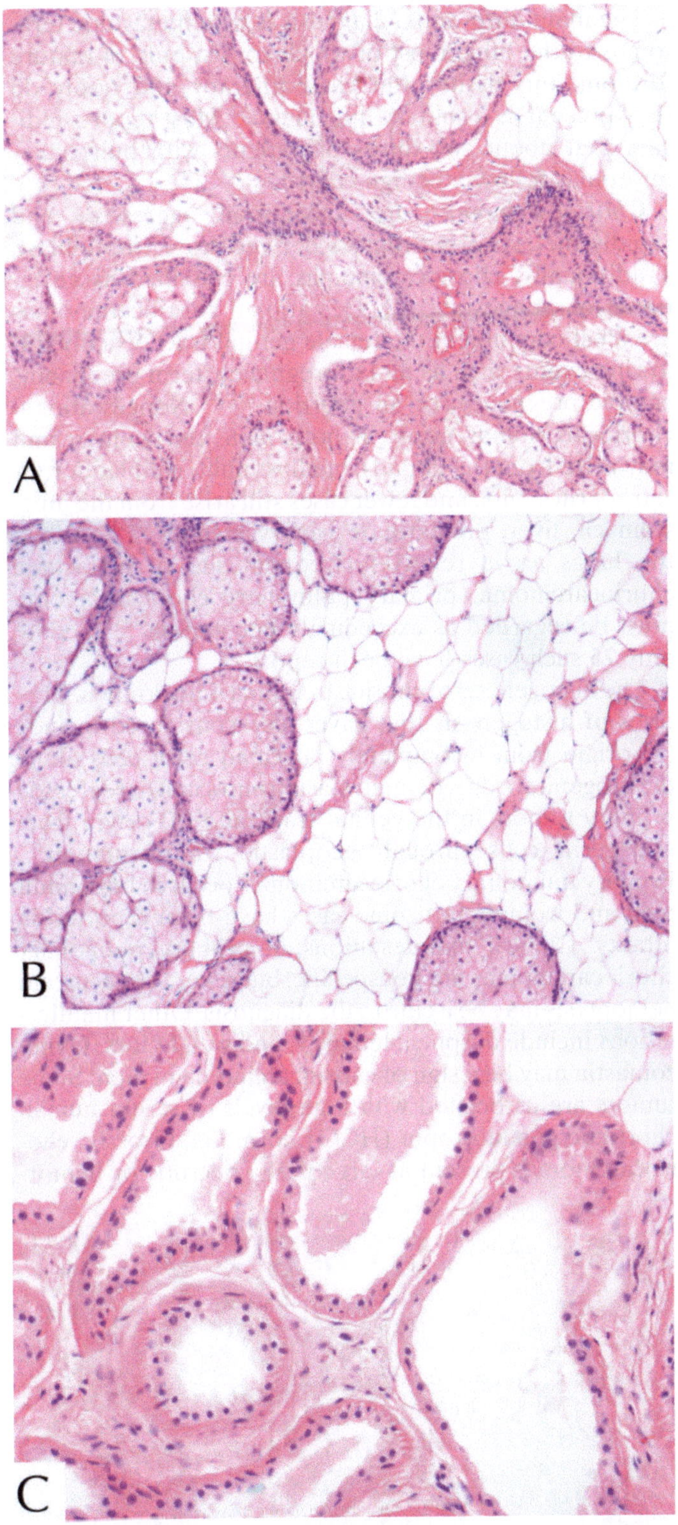

FIGURE 41.20. Teratoma. **(A)** Pilosebaceous unit. **(B)** Sebaceous glands and fat. **(C)** Apocrine glands.

The main differential diagnosis is with metastatic teratomas to the lung, most of which consist only of mature teratomatous tissue after chemotherapy and rarely do they present as a solitary lung mass.[105] Most reports indicate that about two-thirds of patients with pulmonary teratomas follow a benign course.

Choriocarcinomas are uncommon aggressive and rapidly metastasizing tumors derived from trophoblast. Traditionally, choriocarcinomas are classified as gestational or nongestational. Gestational choriocarcinomas are most common in the female genital tract, usually following events such as molar pregnancy, term pregnancy, ectopic pregnancy, or an abortion.[105–109] Nongestational choriocarcinomas occur in both men and women and may arise from the gonads, mediastinum, gallbladder, or retroperitoneum, and fewer cases still arise from the lung, stomach, liver, prostate, or urinary bladder.[106–109] While the lungs are a relatively frequent site of metastatic choriocarcinoma, primary pulmonary choriocarcinoma must be regarded as exceedingly uncommon.[106] To date only 25 such cases have been reported.

The histogenesis of choriocarcinoma is not known. Theories of histogenesis that have been considered include (1) origin from incompletely migrated germ cells along the urogenital ridge, (2) metastasis from occult or regressed primary tumors in the genital tract, and (3) origin from non–germ cells through neoplastic transformation.[106] Primary pulmonary choriocarcinomas occur in both adult men and women, but some cases have been reported in infants. Clinical manifestations of primary pulmonary choriocarcinomas are nonspecific, but severe or recurrent hemoptysis may be a clue to the diagnosis. Other manifestations include dyspnea, lethargy, and weight loss. Gynecomastia may be a sign of choriocarcinoma in men. Some tumors are associated with high levels of serum human chorionic gonadotropin (HCG) hormone. Grossly, choriocarcinomas present as large fleshy necrotic or hemorrhagic masses. Microscopically, mixtures of cytotrophoblast and syncytiotrophoblast can be seen (Fig. 41.22).[105,110] Immunohistochemical demonstration of HCG hormone is of limited value since it may be present in carcinoma of lung, particularly in giant cell carcinoma, now considered a variant of pleomorphic carcinoma.[110]

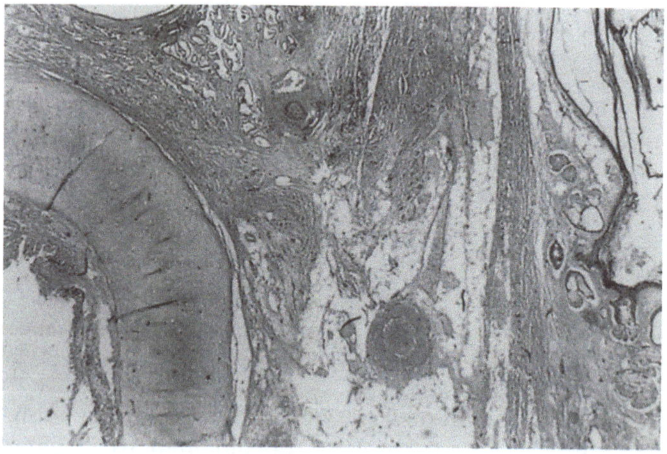

FIGURE 41.21. Teratoma. At left is bronchial structure; at right is keratinized epidermis with appendages. Fat is in the middle lower part.

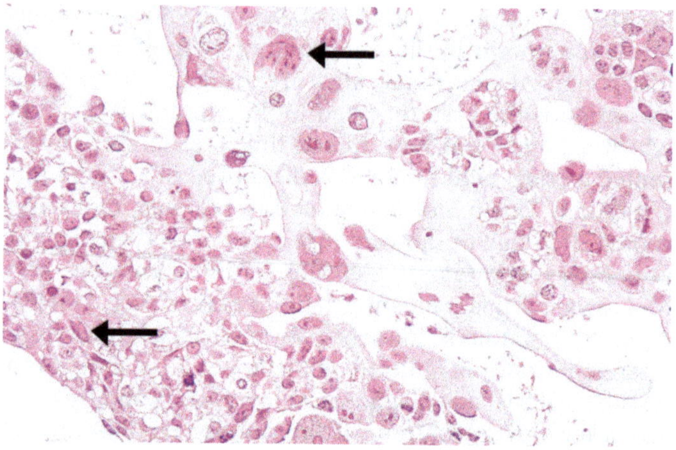

FIGURE 41.22. Choriocarcinoma primary in lung. Note syncytiotrophoblast (upper arrow) and cytotrophoblast (lower arrow).

Epidermal growth factor (EGF) and its receptor (EGFR) may play an autocrine role in the proliferation and differentiation of tumor cells of primary pulmonary choriocarcinoma as reported by Toda and coworkers.[106] In their report of a 69-year-old man with primary choriocarcinoma of the lung presenting with weight loss and hemoptysis, the tumor cells stained positively with immunostains for HCG and EGF and its receptor. Both of these growth factors are expressed in cytotrophoblast and syncytiotrophoblast of uterine choriocarcinoma, and their identification in the above-cited nongonadal (pulmonary) choriocarcinoma suggested a possible autocrine role in cell proliferation and differentiation.

The differential diagnosis includes choriocarcinoma metastatic to the lung and large cell carcinomas with ectopic production of HCG hormone. Exclusion of adenocarcinoma occurring in association with choriocarcinoma as noted by Chen et al.[111] is also a consideration in the differential diagnosis. The prognosis of primary pulmonary choriocarcinomas is poor.[112] Reported survival rates have ranged from 0 to 12 months. Some reports indicate response to multimodal therapy consisting of chemotherapy, surgery, and radiation, but reported responses to treatment have been short lived.[112–114]

Synovial Sarcomas

Synovial sarcomas rank as the fourth most common sarcomas of soft tissues.[115] They are so named because they were once believed to recapitulate synovium. However, only a small minority of them involve articular or synovial-lined spaces. Their histogenesis remains unclear, and a synovial origin has not been documented.[115,116] About four fifths of synovial sarcomas arising from soft tissues are located about the knee and ankle of children and young adults.[95] Synovial sarcomas infrequently occur in the oral cavity, larynx, lung, pleura, peritoneum, heart, and mediastinum.[117–120] An intravascular form has been recognized. Synovial sarcomas primarily in the pleura are discussed in Chapter 43 on pleural neoplasms. Here we discuss only the primary intrapulmonary variants.

Zeren and associates[121] first called attention to these peculiar tumors in an intrapulmonary location. In their 1995 report of 25 cases of monophasic synovial sarcoma derived from the files of the Armed Forces Institute of Pathology, 11 patients were men and 14 were women, with ages ranging from 16 to 77 years. The most common symptoms were chest pain, dyspnea, and hemoptysis. A year later, Roberts et al.[122] observed the X;18 translocation, which is characteristic of this neoplasm, in a surgically removed tumor from a 62-year-old woman. Three years after Roberts et al.'s report, Hisaoka and coworkers[123] detected the *SYT-SSX* fusion gene transcripts in pulmonary tumors from two women, ages 44 and 50 years. This molecular assay thus became useful for the diagnosis of tumors histologically resembling synovial sarcomas of soft tissue but occurring in unusual anatomic sites.

Most current knowledge pertaining to gross, microscopic, ultrastructural, and histochemical features of monophasic synovial sarcomas in the lung is derived from the work of Zeren and associates.[121] Briefly, in these authors' report, the tumors varied in size from 0.6 to 20 cm, and all were soft to rubbery with areas of necrosis (Fig. 41.23). Atypical spindle cell proliferation with solid growth patterns characterized the tumors microscopically (Fig. 41.24). Among 25 cases examined immunohistochemically, strong focal immunoreactivity for vimentin, EMA, and cytokeratin was observed in 25, 25, and 23 lesions, respectively. Immunostains for desmin, smooth muscle actin, and S-100 protein were all negative. In contrast to intrapulmonary synovial sarcomas, synovial sarcomas of the pleura are almost always biphasic, express carcinoembryonic antigen (CEA) and Ber EP4, and are positive for neutral mucin.[124] Ultrastructural analysis in three of the 25 cases showed spindle cells with abundant rough endoplasmic reticulum and well-developed desmosomes. The case described by Roberts et al.[122] showed similar microscopic features but with a herringbone histologic pattern, while the two cases described by Hisaoka and coworkers[123] showed distinct hemangiopericytomatous morphology. Biphasic synovial sarcomas present lesser diagnostic difficulties than do their monophasic variants.

Most intrapulmonary synovial sarcomas are monophasic and can be confused with a variety of sarcomas such as fibrosarcomas, leiomyosarcomas, and malignant schwannomas.[117] As noted earlier, cytokeratin immunostaining can be helpful in making the diagnosis and can assist with the differential diagnosis. Among 15 primary monophasic synovial sarcomas of various sites (including 12 from lung) 63% stained for cytokeratin and one stained for CEA.[117] The usefulness of cytokeratin is diminished, however, because it is not consistently found in synovial sarcomas, and other sarcomas such as epithelioid sarcomas, leiomyosarcomas, and some vascular tumors, though rarely, can also react with this immunostain.[117] Monophasic synovial sarcomas are occasionally reactive for smooth muscle actin. In difficult cases ultrastructural and cytogenetic studies can be extremely valuable. In all cases metastatic synovial sarcoma to the lung should be considered in the differential diagnosis and ruled out clinically.

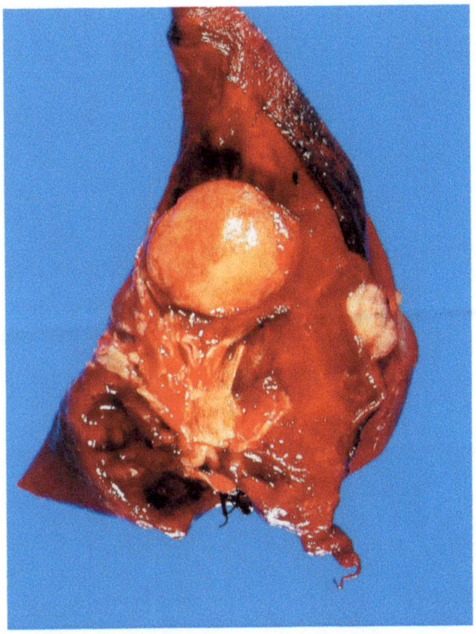

FIGURE 41.23. Synovial sarcoma. Gross appearance. Note large spheroidal tumor mass with a smooth yellow-pink surface and a smaller mass on the right. (Courtesy of Dr. Andrew Fischer, University of Massachusetts Medical School, Worcester, MA.)

Surgical resection is the treatment of choice. The prognosis is generally poor, with nearly 50% of patients dying within 2 years of diagnosis. In the series of Zeren et al.,[121] significant mortality was reported with six of 18 patients dying of their disease and some patients showing recurrence or metastases up to 7 years from diagnosis.

Sclerosing Hemangiomas

Also known as sclerosing pneumocytomas, these intriguing neoplasms have received considerable attention due to their variegated microscopic morphology, controversial histogenesis, and diagnostic difficulty. At various times, these tumors have been considered to be of vascu-

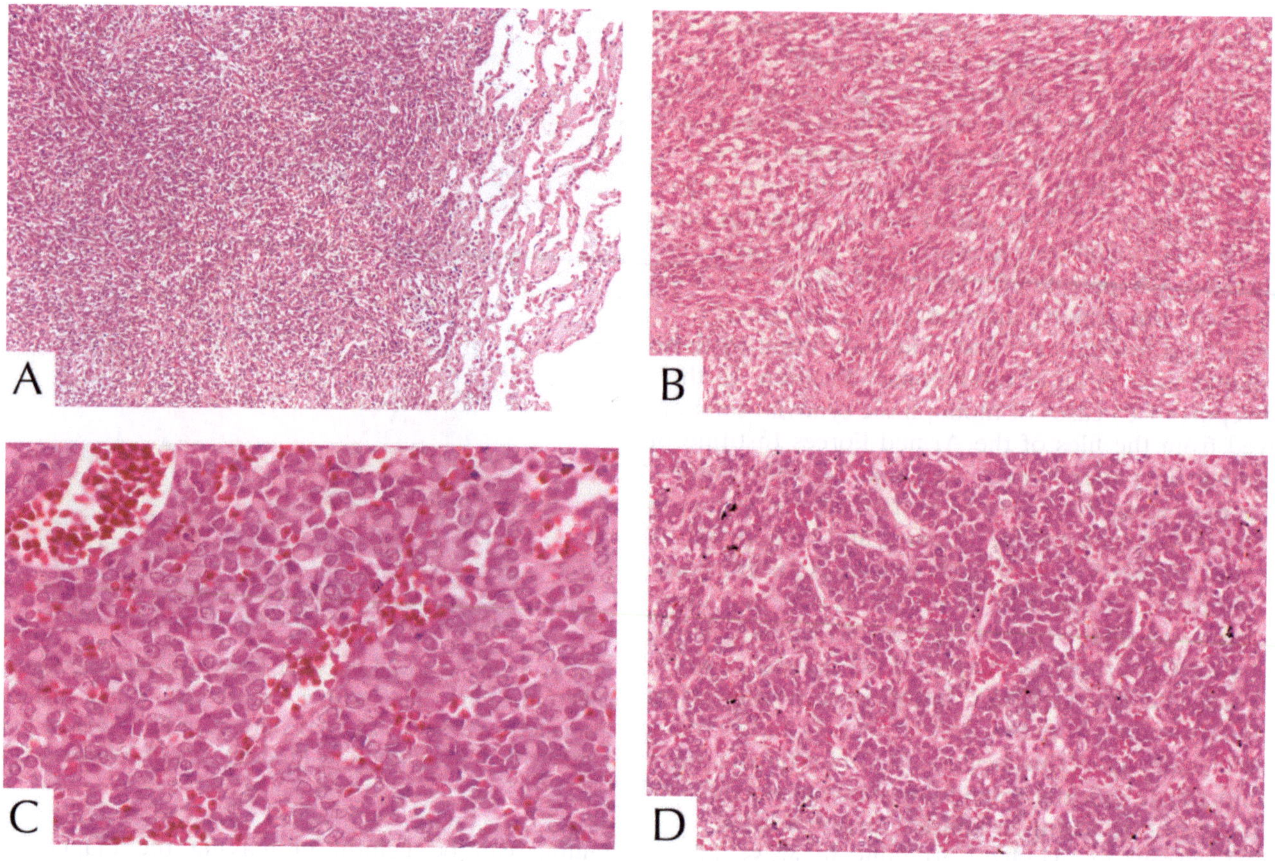

FIGURE 41.24. Synovial sarcoma. Microscopic appearance panels. **(A)** Monophasic fibrous synovial sarcoma. Note solid proliferation of spindle cells and uninvolved lung tissue on the right. **(B)** Closer view of **A**. **(C)** In this area, rhabdoid features are present. **(D)** Less well differentiated tumor showing rounded cells and a hemangiopericytomatous vascular pattern. (Courtesy of Dr. S. Okamoto and Dr. H. Hashimoto, University of Occupational and Environmental Health, Kitaki-Ushu, Japan.)

lar, mesothelial, or epithelial origin, with most recent immunohistochemical and ultrastructural evidence arguing for an epithelial origin. The story of sclerosing hemangiomas begins in the 1950s when these tumors were differentiated from the general group of histiocytomas by Liebow and Hubbell.[125] These authors described seven cases, one of which had been previously published as a capillary hemangioma of lung.[126] A large series by Katzenstein et al.[127] in 1980 described 51 cases seen in consultation by Liebow during the 17 years following his 1956 review. In 1982, Chan et al.[128] described 14 additional cases from Hong Kong collected from 1974 to 1980, 10 of them coming from one hospital. These authors wondered whether there was some environmental factor(s), such as herbs, involved in the etiology. In 1986, Spencer and Nambu[129] also noted an increase in Asian patients, and in that same year, Thomas and Lee[130] described 11 cases in Singapore. Indeed this appears to be a valid observation. Much of the earlier work on sclerosing hemangiomas came from the Orient, especially Japan.

Significantly, most patients with sclerosing hemangiomas are women, with some series being exclusively female.[128] The mean age at presentation is about 45 years, but patients have been reported from ages 15 to 83, with most cases occurring during the fifth decade of life.[131–133] Most patients with sclerosing hemangiomas are asymptomatic and come to medical attention on an incidental basis. The proportion of patients without symptoms has ranged from 50% to 90% in some series. When symptomatic, patients usually present with vague chest pain and in some instances with hemoptysis.

Chest radiographs are apt to show nodular lung lesions that enlarge, grow gradually or not at all. In the series by Katzenstein et al.,[127] 14 patients had prior radiographs demonstrating the lesion from 1 to 14 years previously, with an average of 5 years. In one of the cases in the Liebow and Hubbell[125] series, one lesion was followed radiographically for 12 years with little change. In another reported case, a lesion had been present for nearly 15 years, but no comment as to whether it had changed or not was noted in the report.[134]

Grossly, these tumoral lesions are well circumscribed and easily free up (shell out) from the adjacent lung parenchyma. They vary in color depending on the amount

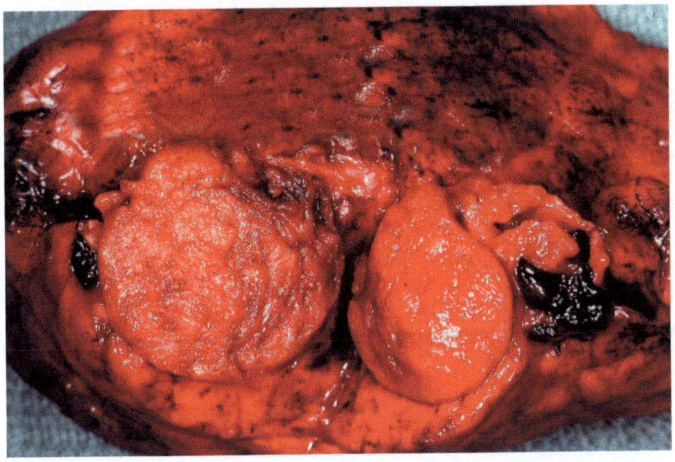

FIGURE 41.25. Sclerosing hemangioma. Gross appearance in the fresh state. Note bisected hemorrhagic nodular mass.

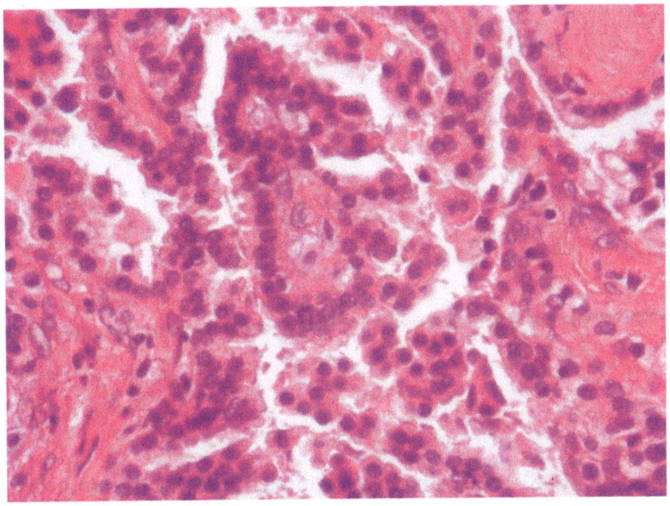

FIGURE 41.27. Sclerosing hemangioma. Note papillary fronds with distinctly separate darker cells lining the surface.

of fresh and old blood within them (Fig. 41.25). They may be gray-white or tan-yellow when relatively bloodless, with some being more intensely yellow, with increased foamy histiocytes and iron, or even dark red in those with abundant blood. Focal variegation of lighter colored tumor with zones of blood and possibly focal yellow flecks is frequently observed (Fig. 41.26). The cut surfaces show some clefts, often defined as fine or slight clefts. Sometimes these lesions have a spongy appearance, which usually coincides with blood-filled lesions that are dark red. In other cases the cut surface is granular or rubbery. The nearby lung parenchyma is compressed but does not have a true capsule, and sometimes there is a rim of red or brown discoloration near the tumor. In these cases the tumor is often also a darker color. Further away from the tumor the surrounding lung parenchyma is usually normal. In a case with multiple lesions (two nodules larger than 2 cm, and innumerable smaller ones), the histologic angiomatous pattern was seen only in the two reddish nodules measuring more than 2 cm, while all those that were less than 1 cm were described as gray-white and lacked histologic evidence of angiomatous change.

Microscopically, these tumors are quite variegated, but basically consist of two types of cells: dark surface cuboidal cells and deeper round to polygonal paler cells. Architecturally, there are some more cellular solid zones, others that are more papillary, and others that are both solid cellular and sclerotic, while others yet have more confluent sclerotic zones or angiomatous or hemorrhagic patterns (Figs. 41.27 and 41.28). Often these patterns are mixed, usually consisting of at least three types. Focal sclerosis of some parts is common but is not dominant. Any of the other described patterns may be dominant. We have seen one case with a dominant angiomatous component misinterpreted as an angiosarcoma. Occasionally, in a more solid cellular area, entrapped bronchioles are present. These tumors usually also have a slight admixture of lymphocytes, plasma cells, and mast cells. These are often scattered among the tumor cells and are confirmed by electron microscopy and special stains. Sometimes some lymphocytes, plasma cells, and histiocytes are common in the rim of interface with more normal lung tissue. Iron-stained and foamy macrophages are also seen with some regularity, and are increased in the lesions that contain bloody cysts. Foam cell change is shown in Figure 41.29.

The deeper polygonal tumor cells in the interstitium are sometimes covered by a single surface layer of slightly darker squamoid-to-cuboidal cells. At times smaller collections of cuboidal cells appear in cystic spaces and probably represent hyperplastic lining cells. Hyalinized areas may evolve from the solid, papillary, or

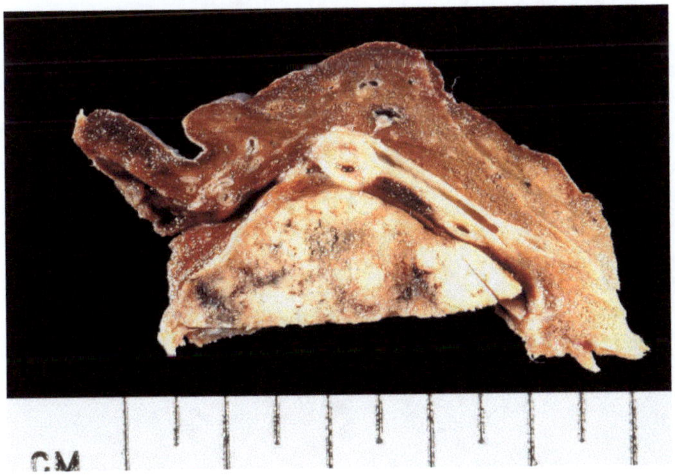

FIGURE 41.26. Sclerosing hemangioma. Gross appearance after fixation. Note variegation of texture and color in this specimen, reflecting varieties of histologic components.

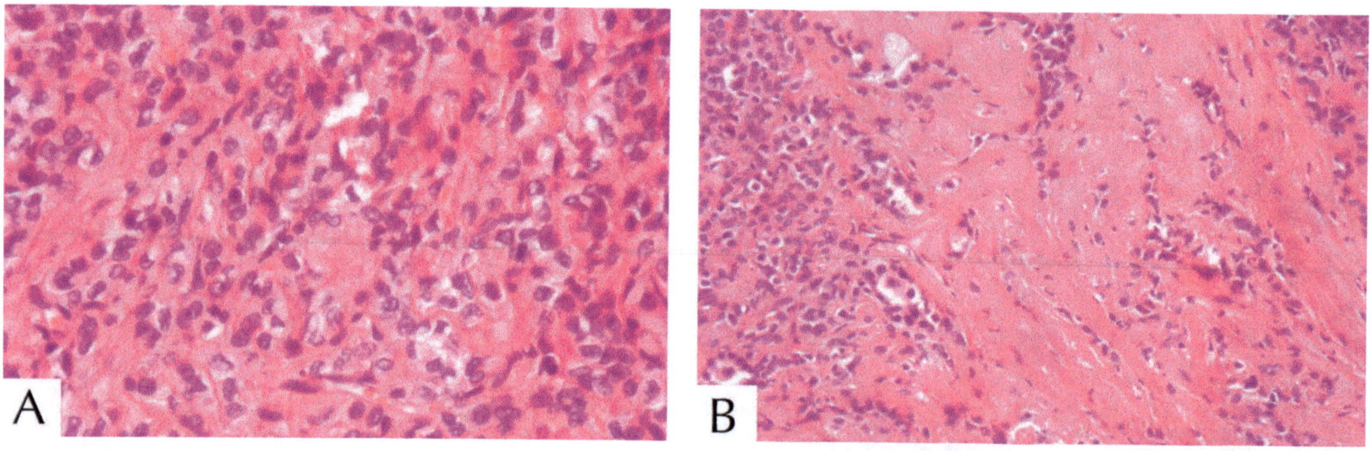

FIGURE 41.28. Sclerosing hemangioma. **(A)** Area of tumor displaying a more solid appearance. **(B)** Area of tumor with sclerosis.

hemangiomatous zones. These hyalinized areas may be more confluent and spherical with short radiating arms corresponding to adjacent papillae or connections to other tumor or adjacent lung. Longer arms of sclerosis may cause a medusa-head appearance. Occasional discoid plaques of lamellar fibrosis are seen adjacent to foci of cholesterol clefts. Central dystrophic calcification may be present in areas of hyalinization. There may be cholesterol clefts with focal giant cells around them in some areas, and often these are associated with discoid areas of lamellar fibrosis as mentioned previously. Many of the red cells appear viable, but focally they are undergoing necrosis with adjacent foamy, fat-filled, or iron-stained histiocytes and the cholesterol clefts just mentioned.

Several recent reports have documented the positivity of thyroid transcription factor-1 (TTF-1) in sclerosing hemangiomas.[135–138] Chan and Chan[135] reported TTF-1 expression in both the nuclei of surface lining cells and the pale polygonal cells of sclerosing hemangioma. In their study of nine cases, the surface lining cells were EMA, cytokeratin, and surfactant apoprotein A positive. One of the cases had mediastinal node metastasis and in this case consisting of polygonal cells only, the cells were EMA, cytokeratin, and TTF-1 positive. In difficult cases lacking one of the classic architectural patterns or one of the usual cell types, TTF-1 immunostaining can be of value. Four such cases were reported by Nicholson et al.[136] In these four unusual and difficult cases, two were

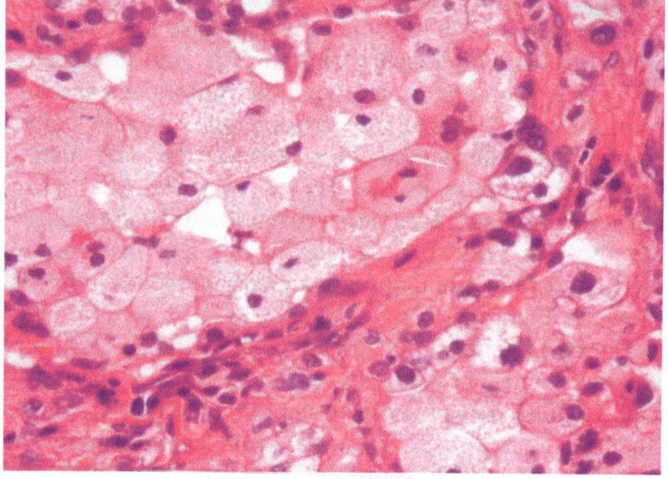

FIGURE 41.29. Sclerosing hemangioma. Area of tumor with focal foam cell change.

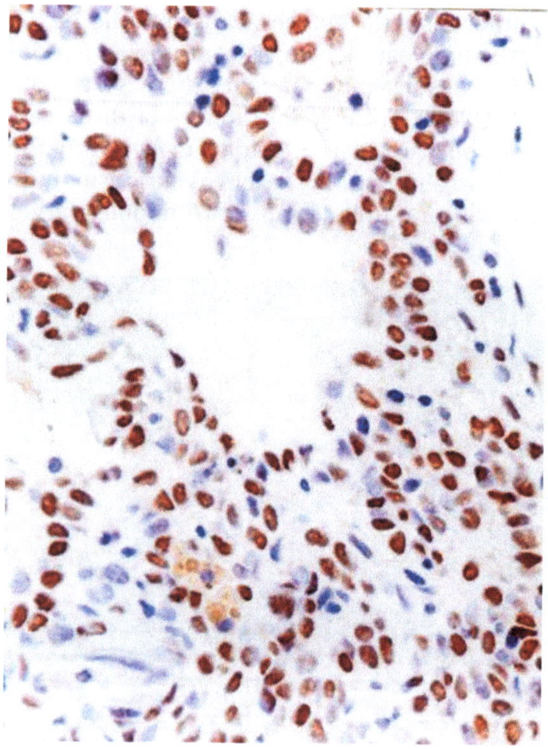

FIGURE 41.30. Sclerosing hemangioma. Note pronounced nuclear expression of thyroid transcription factor-1 (TTF-1) in both cuboidal and polygonal cells. (Courtesy of Dr. E. Wang, China Medical University, Shenyang, China.)

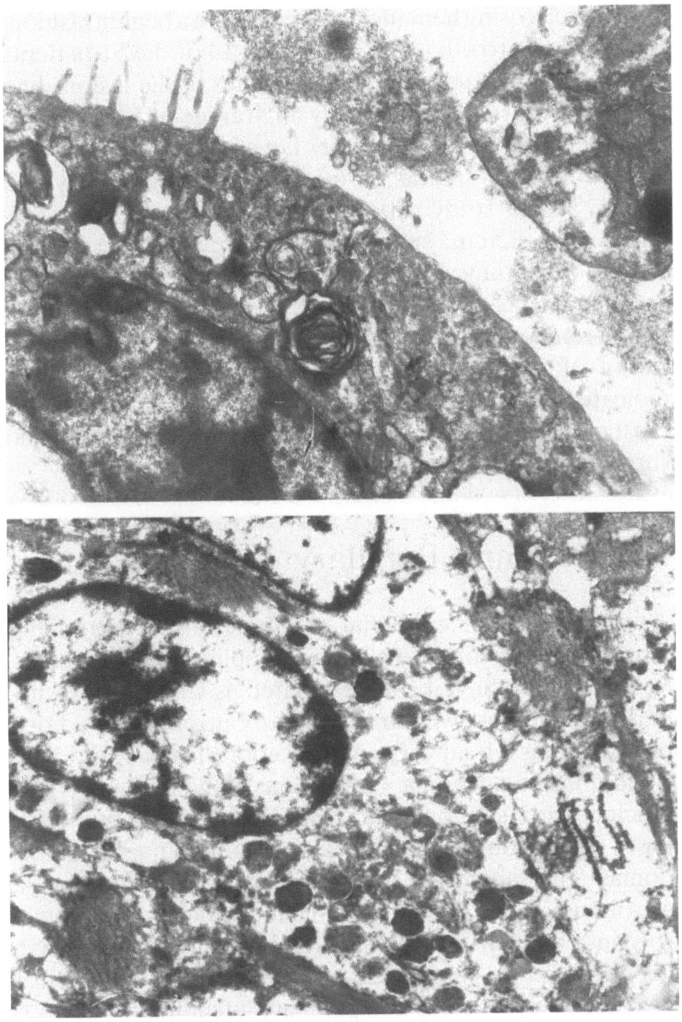

A

B

FIGURE 41.31. Sclerosing hemangioma. Ultrastructure showing differences between cuboidal and polygonal cells. **(A)** Lamellar bodies and microvilli of cuboidal cells. **(B)** Neuroendocrine granules, rough endoplasmic reticulum, and microtubules in polygonal cells. TEM. (Courtesy of Dr. E. Wang, China Medical University, Shenyang, China.)

confounded by cystic masses, one resembled an alveolar adenoma, and another had only solid components, in a metastasis to a mediastinal lymph node. A detailed analysis by Wang et al.[137] based on immunostaining for vimentin TTF-1, Surfactant Protein B (SP-B), Low Molecular Weight Cytokeratin (CK-L), EMA, CEA, neuron specific enolase, chromogranin A, synaptophysin, calcitonin, adrenocorticotropic hormone, and human growth hormone (and ultrastructural features) suggested different origins for the surface cuboidal and polygonal cells. The study showed that cuboidal cells having short microvilli and cytoplasmic lamellar bodies are strongly positive for TTF-1, SP-B, CK-L, EMA, and CEA (Fig. 41.30). In contrast, the polygonal cells (also known as round or pale cells by other authors) were strongly positive for TTF-1, vimentin, and two to three of the neuroendocrine markers cited above. Some sclerosing hemangiomas are ER and PR positive. Electron microscopy reveals key differences between cuboidal and polygonal cells including lamellar bodies and microvilli in the former and neuroendocrine granules and microtubules in the latter (Fig. 41.31). Other ultrastructural features such as finger-like cellular processes are shown in Figure 41.32.

The differential diagnosis includes benign and malignant tumors. Because of the papillary nature of these lesions, adenocarcinomas, especially the rare papillary noninvasive ones, are often considered. The papillary fronds in sclerosing hemangiomas usually vary in diameter and composition from each other more than those seen with adenocarcinomas. In the less differentiated adenocarcinomas with more solid areas, the cell pleomorphism, mitotic rate, and invasive capacities, without the multiple histologic patterns of sclerosing hemangioma, should help to make the distinction. Focal mucin production in adenocarcinoma cells is also helpful, and this can be confirmed with mucicarmine stains. The bland-appearing cell monotony in some areas of sclerosing hemangiomas and blood-filled spaces raises the possibility of highly vascularized carcinoid tumors. Usually carcinoid tumors are less papillary, although a rare exception occurs, and neuroendocrine stains are useful and easy to do. Another monotonous tumor is lobular carcinoma of breast, but this is rarely metastatic to lung as a nodule, and much more frequently metastasizes as lymphangitic spread or serosal surface spread. Pulmonary blastomas, benign clear (sugar) tumors, plasma cell granulomas, and metastases from other sites such as thyroid or kidney are not usually a problem to distinguish. Of interest, three benign epithelial localized mesotheliomas were reported in a series of 18 localized mesotheliomas; all three were found on review to be sclerosing hemangiomas.[139]

Epithelioid hemangioendotheliomas have sometimes been confused with sclerosing hemangiomas. The cells of epithelioid hemangioendothelioma usually appear bland, can be rather monotonous, and have abundant cytoplasm. Epithelioid hemangioendotheliomas tend to infiltrate the lung in a different pattern, being respective of the background alveolar architecture, while extending from one alveolus to another in a micropolypoid fashion through the pores of Kohn. They are not as papillomatous as sclerosing hemangiomas. In some cells of epithelioid hemangioendothelioma there are primitive vascular lumina. These tumor cells stain positively for vascular markers including CD34 and factor VIII antigen, and by electron microscopy the cells have endothelial characteristics, including Weibel–Palade bodies. We have seen one case of this tumor misidentified as multiple sclerosing hemangiomas. Histiocytomas may sometimes be papillary and have the admixture of inflammatory cells as seen in sclerosing hemangiomas, including the foam cells and cholesterol clefts. One must be sure to identify the tumor cell type of proliferation before making a diagnosis of sclerosing hemangioma.

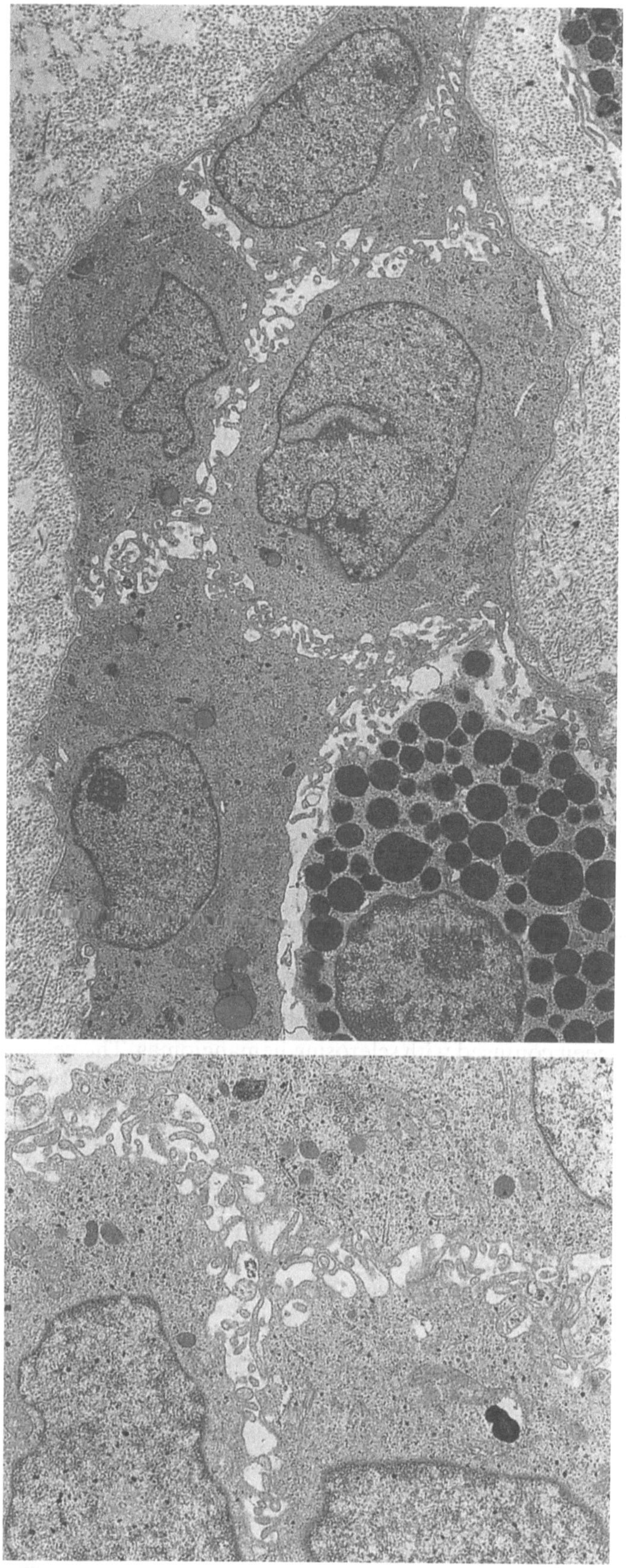

A

B

FIGURE 41.32. Sclerosing hemangioma. Ultrastructure. **(A)** Cluster of tumor cells with finger-like cell processes extending into shared common space between cells. Mast cell at bottom right. **(B)** Cell processes are better shown at higher magnification. TEM.

Most sclerosing hemangiomas behave in a benign fashion. In fact, slow growth is the norm.[140] In 14 of the 51 patients reviewed by Katzenstein and associates,[127] the lesions had been apparent radiographically an average of 5 years prior to surgery. However, rare cases have been associated with intrapulmonary spread or metastasis to regional lymph nodes.[141] One study reports nodal metastasis in tumors larger than 3.5 cm, suggesting the need to resect these tumors while they are smaller in size.[141] The significance of nodal metastasis particularly in cases of sclerosing hemangioma remains to be determined. Nonetheless, the identification of metastasis in rare cases does not necessarily indicate aggressive behavior.[141] Overall, the prognosis for most patients with sclerosing hemangioma is excellent, and surgical resection can result in a cure.

Alveolar and Papillary Adenomas

Assorted discrete epithelial prolifcrations in peripheral lung tissue have long been known as pulmonary adenomas. Some of these have been designated as Clara cell adenomas and others as alveolar adenomas. Currently, in addition to adenomas of salivary or tracheobronchial gland type (pleomorphic adenoma and mucous gland adenoma) and mucinous cystadenomas, the WHO recognizes two other types of pulmonary adenomas, alveolar and papillary adenomas. The salivary or tracheobronchial gland adenomas are discussed in Chapter 38, while mucinous cystadenomas (because of their difficult separation from mucinous cystadenocarcinoma) are discussed in Chapter 35. This section discusses only alveolar and papillary adenomas.

Alveolar adenomas are currently defined by the WHO as solitary nodules in the periphery of the lung consisting of a network of spaces lined by simple low cuboidal epithelium.[142] The intervening stroma can range from thin, inconspicuous bands of connective tissue to broad accumulations of spindle cells, sometimes with a myxoid matrix.[142] In 1986, Yousem and Hochholzer[143] published six cases of these lesions and chose to call them alveolar adenomas. The majority of their patients were asymptomatic older patients, with a mean age of 59 years. All lesions were solitary and appeared as noncalcified coin lesions on chest radiographs. Five were peripheral (three right upper lobe, two left lower lobe), subpleurally located, well circumscribed but nonencapsulated, gray-white-tan, and finely cystic, sometimes with hemorrhage in some of the cysts. They averaged 1.8 cm and easily shelled out from the surrounding lung parenchyma. In the series of 17 patients by Burke et al.,[144] the age and gender of one patient was not reported, but of the remaining 16, seven patients were men and nine were women, and their mean age was 53. Most patients were asymptomatic and had solitary lesions seen radiographically as coin lesions. Those patients who were symptomatic had nonspecific symptoms. The mean size of the lesions was 2.2 cm.

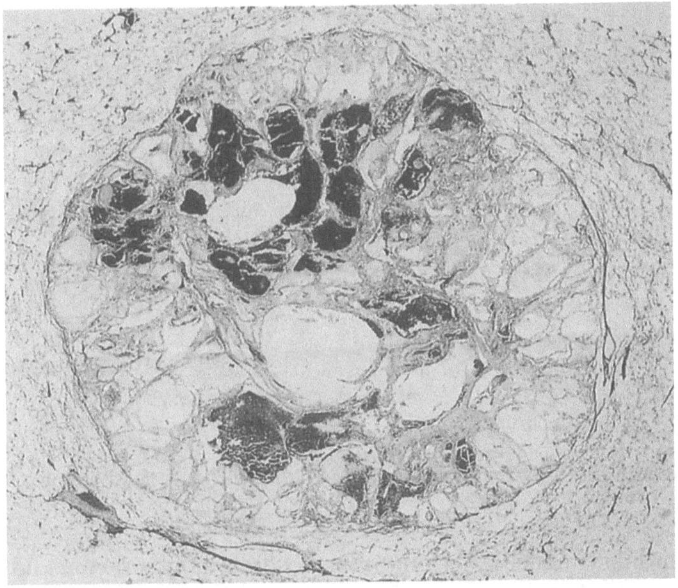
A

FIGURE 41.33 **A–C**. "Alveolar adenoma." Spherical cystic lesion. Some spaces are filled with clear fluid, others with blood (*darker areas*). **B**. Cysts are filled with flocculent material, and intervening stroma is delicate. **C**. Densest area of interstitial thickening in this example shows stellate interstitial cells mixed with some inflammatory cells, Focal cubidal lining, perhaps metaplastic alveolar lining cells (see text) at upper left; squamoid lining to right. Note dilated capillaries in loose substance of tumor.

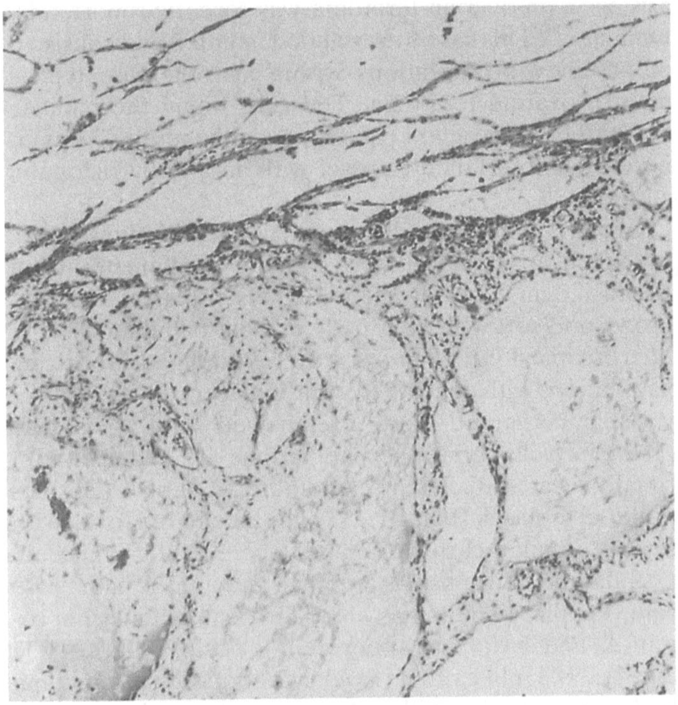
B

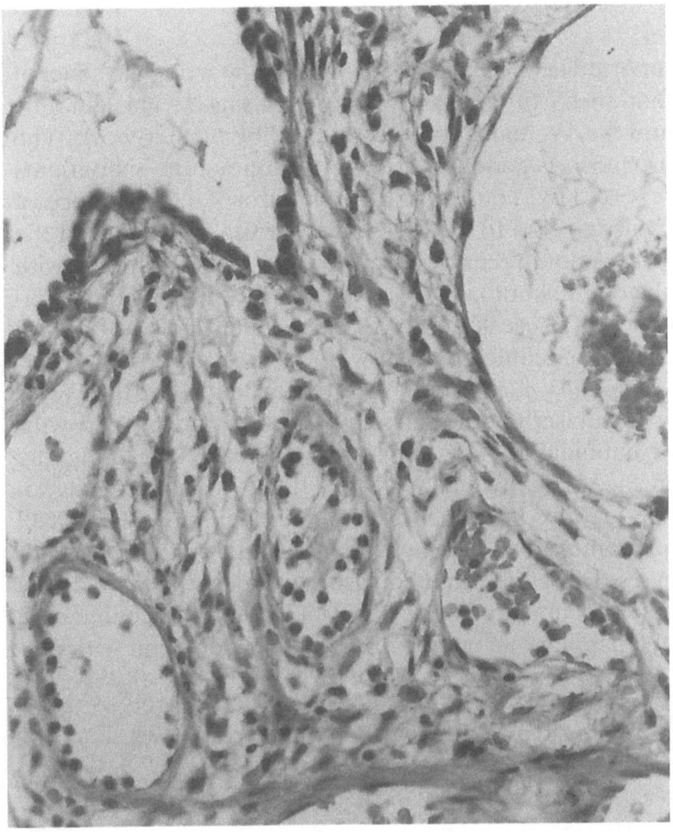
C

Microscopically, alveolar adenomas contain variously sized and contoured cystic spaces (Fig. 41.33). The interstitium shows some delicate to plump spindle cells, with some variation in cellularity between mild and moderate in degree, in a loose background, containing a few mixed macrophages, plasma cells, and lymphocytes. The epithelium lining the cystic spaces is usually inapparent or squamoid, but may be clear cell or cuboidal in type (Fig. 41.34). Centrally there may be some focal scars. No mucin is identified in the lining cells. There is no necrosis, and only a quite rare mitosis will be found. Immunohistochemical data in nine of the 17 patients reported by Burke et al.[144] indicated that all nine cases were cytokeratin positive. The CEA was evaluated in four of the nine cases and all four were positive for this marker. The main cellular constituents were type 2 pneumocytes, as evidenced by immunoreactivity for TTF-1, pro-SP-B, and pro-SP-C, and by ultrastructural analysis.

The differential diagnosis is limited, and metastatic microcystic low-grade stromal sarcomas of uterus lead the list. Some alveolar adenomas have been published in the past as lymphangiomas. Metastatic microcystic low-grade stromal sarcomas and lymphangiomas, however, can be distinguished with appropriate use of cytokeratin and endothelial markers such as CD31, CD34, and factor VIII. Abnormal pseudodiploid karyotypes have been

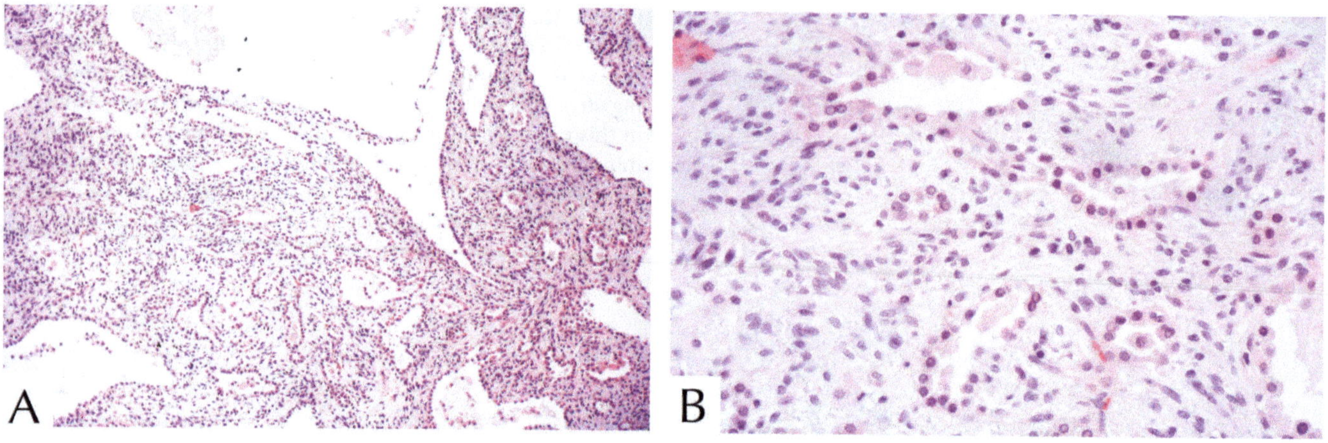

FIGURE 41.34. **(A,B)** Alveolar adenoma showing alveolar-like spaces lined by hyperplastic type 2 cells with cuboidal shape.

reported in one alveolar adenoma, supporting the concept that these tumors are true neoplasms.[142] This finding, however, remains to be confirmed by further work. The prognosis is good. On follow-up, none of the six patients reported by Yousem and Hochholzer[143] had evidence of recurrence up to 3.5 years after surgical resection. In the larger, more recently described series of 17 patients with alveolar adenomas reported by Burke et al.,[144] the benignancy of these lesions was also evident on the basis of clinical outcome and follow-up.

Papillary adenomas are currently defined by the WHO as circumscribed nodules consisting of papillary growths of cuboidal to low cuboidal epithelial cells lining the surface of fibrovascular stromal tissue.[142] Papillary adenomas are also known as bronchiolar papillomas, Clara cell adenomas, and papillary adenomas of type 2 pneumocytes. These are rare neoplasms, with less than two dozen cases documented up to 2002, including one peculiar case of a papillary adenoma occurring in association with pulmonary metastasis from an osteosarcoma in a 9-year-old boy.[145] A unique case of a papillary adenoma-like tumor arising in an ovarian teratoma was recently reported by Damiani.[146] This case was well documented and consisted of papillary proliferations within an otherwise typical mature ovarian teratoma. The cells lining the papillae were TTF-1, surfactant protein, and cytokeratin 7 immunoreactive, but failed to react with an antithyroglobulin antibody.[146]

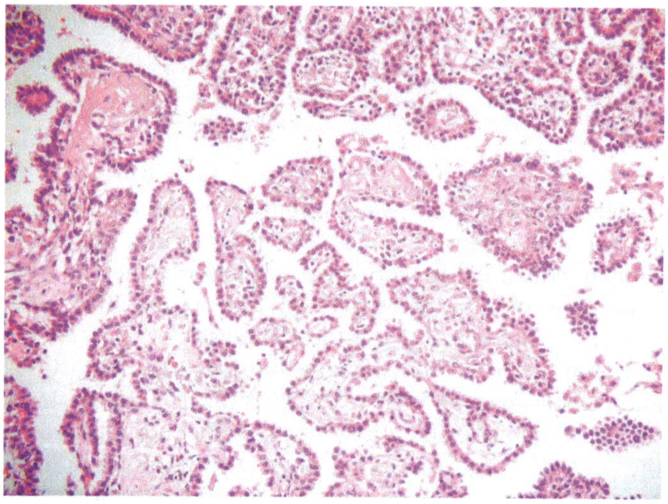

FIGURE 41.35. Papillary adenoma with surface epithelial cells and focally sclerosed hypocellular stroma. (From Sheppard et al.,[149] with permission.)

Grossly, papillary adenomas are well circumscribed, but unencapsulated tumors ranging in diameter from 1.2 to 4.0 cm. On cut section, the neoplasms are tan-brown and soft with no grossly evident papillations.[147–150] Microscopically, the tumors show well-defined, arborizing papillations with delicate to occasionally prominent fibrovascular cores and some interspersed solid areas. The epithelial cells lining the papillations are cuboidal with basally located nuclei and moderate amounts of eosinophilic cytoplasm (Fig. 41.35). The nuclei are oval with finely granular chromatin and inconspicuous nucleoli. Cellular pleomorphism is minimal, and mitotic figures are rare. Papillary adenomas are TTF-1, surfactant apoprotein A, and surfactant apoprotein B positive (Figs. 41.36 and 41.37). Unlike other papillary neoplasms, psammoma bodies have not been identified in papillary adenomas.[147–150] The cytologic features of papillary adenoma are not well characterized. One recent report suggests that the diagnosis can be suspected on cellular material obtained by transbronchial needle aspiration biopsy.[150] In this case, however, the cytologic features were rather nondescript, with the authors calling attention to tumor cells arranged in sheets of cells that contained scant or vesicular cytoplasm. Multidirectional differentiation of these tumors is evident by electron microscopy, with epithelial cells showing ultrastructural features of type 2 pneumocytes (Fig. 41.38) or bronchial ciliated cells and Clara cells.[151]

The main differential diagnosis is with nodules of benign proliferating type 2 pneumocytes as seen in patients with tuberous sclerosis, low-grade (primary or

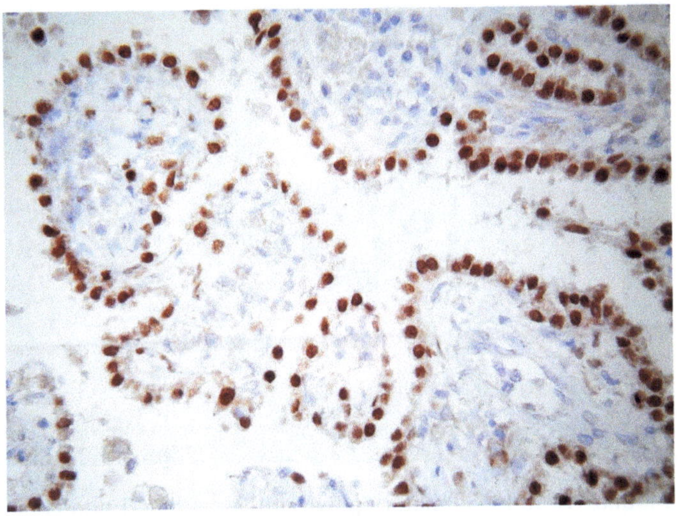

FIGURE 41.36. Papillary adenoma showing positive immunostaining of surface cells for TTF-1. (From Sheppard et al.,[149] with permission.)

metastatic) papillary carcinomas, papillary carcinoid tumors, and sclerosing hemangiomas. Nodules of type 2 pneumocytes occur in a distinct clinical setting and lack the frank papillary architecture of papillary adenomas.[152] Low-grade papillary carcinomas, either primary or metastatic, can be distinguished by the bland cytomorphology of papillary adenomas and the absence of pleomorphism, necrosis, or metastatic activity.[149] Similar to sclerosing hemangiomas, papillary adenomas can be TTF-1 positive and show papillary morphology. However, other patterns of sclerosing hemangiomas such as the vascular hemangioma-like pattern are lacking, and, more importantly, pale round cells can be seen in the papillae of sclerosing hemangioma but not in papillary adenomas. Furthermore, TTF-1 in papillary adenoma is found only in the nuclei of the surface cells, with stromal cells being negative. This is in contrast to sclerosing hemangioma, where the surface cells as well as the stromal cells stain positively with this marker.[149] Neuroendocrine markers are helpful in differentiating the rare papillary variants of carcinoid tumors from papillary adenomas.

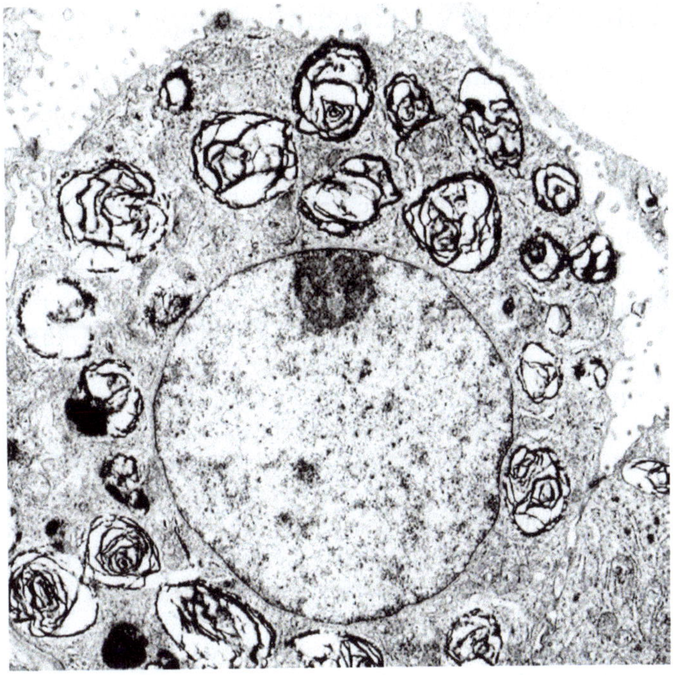

FIGURE 41.38. Papillary adenoma. Ultrastructure of tumor cells showing osmiophilic lamellar bodies similar to those found in normal type II pneumocytes. (Courtesy of Dr. Masuko Mori, Tohoku University, Sendai, Japan.)

The biologic behavior of papillary adenomas is not well characterized, but most authors emphasize their benignancy.[147] This benign behavior was documented in three patients described by Hegg et al.[147] These three patients were free of disease up to 108 months after diagnosis. However, Mori and coworkers,[153] using morphometric analysis, found features of papillary adenomas resembling those of adenocarcinomas derived from type 2 pneumocytes, suggesting a possible malignant potential for these tumors.

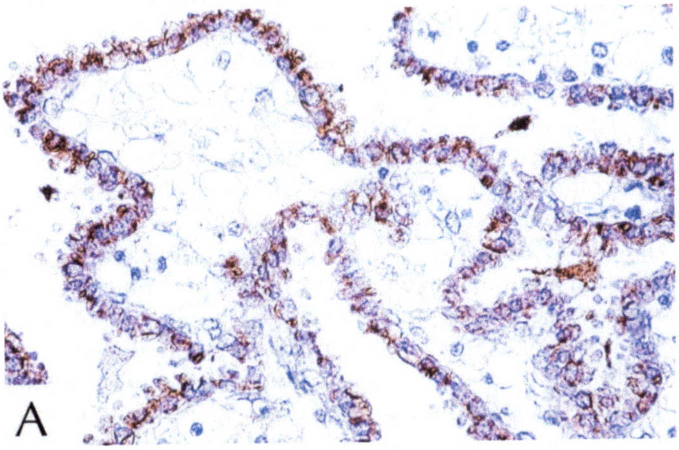

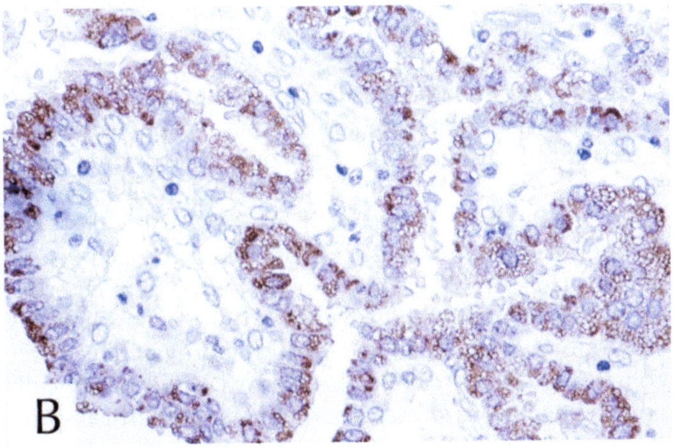

FIGURE 41.37. Papillary adenoma. Surface papillary cells showing immunoreactivity for surfactant apoprotein A **(A)** and B **(B)**, respectively. (Courtesy of Dr. Masuko Mori, Tohoku University, Sendai, Japan.)

Inflammatory Bronchial Polyps

These rare but distinct nonneoplastic inflammatory polypoid lesions of the airways may be idiopathic or associated with a variety of injurious agents to the respiratory epithelium. Chronic bronchial infection, aspiration of foreign bodies, chronic sinusitis, mycobacterial infection, inhalation injury, thermal injury, bronchial asthma, cystic fibrosis, mechanical intubation, and chronic smoke injury are some of the risk factors or clinical settings that appear to predispose to the development of these lesions.[154–158] These lesions occur in adults and less commonly in children. A review of the literature does not find a sex predilection. The lesions are usually solitary but may occasionally present as multiple lesions. The case reported by Roberts et al.[155] was grossly characterized by multiple endobronchial lesions measuring up to 4 mm throughout bronchi and bronchioles. This case occurred in association with cylindrical bronchiectasis in the setting of cystic fibrosis.

The gross appearance of these lesions after resection is not well characterized, as some of the lesions are very small and removed in even smaller pieces. Endoscopically, however, some lesions such as the one described by Niimi and coworkers[158] are said to be small, polypoid, white-colored, and smooth surfaced lesions. A solitary endotracheal inflammatory polyp visualized at endoscopy is shown in Figure 41.39. Typically, these lesions have edematous stroma that may show squamous metaplasia. Acute or chronic inflammation is a prominent histopathologic feature, and granulation tissue may be seen. The cases reported in the literature appear to fulfill these definitional criteria. Some authors, however, point to the presence of capillary blood vessels in addition to the above-described findings (Fig. 41.40A,B). Niimi et al., for example, described a lesion lined by columnar epithelium consisting of a fibrous stroma with many capillary vessels and marked infiltration by inflammatory cells, mainly lymphocytes and eosinophils. The basement membrane in this case was focally thickened and no microorganisms were identified. One of the four cases reported by McShane and coworkers[156] consisted of a single polyp covered by granulation tissue, which contained a striking array of arborizing capillaries. These capillaries were interspersed within loose fibroconnective stroma containing acute and chronic inflammatory cells. On the other hand, the case reported by Roberts et al.[155] was composed of numerous polyps filling bronchiectatic airways (Fig. 41.40C). These polyps had a complex bronchial architecture, with the surface of the polyps lined by respiratory epithelium and central fibrovascular cores containing dilated capillaries filled with red blood cells and an edematous stroma showing mild but diffuse sprinkling of chronic (mononuclear) inflammatory cells. The inflammatory cells included lymphocytes, plasma cells, and eosinophils (Fig. 41.40D,E).

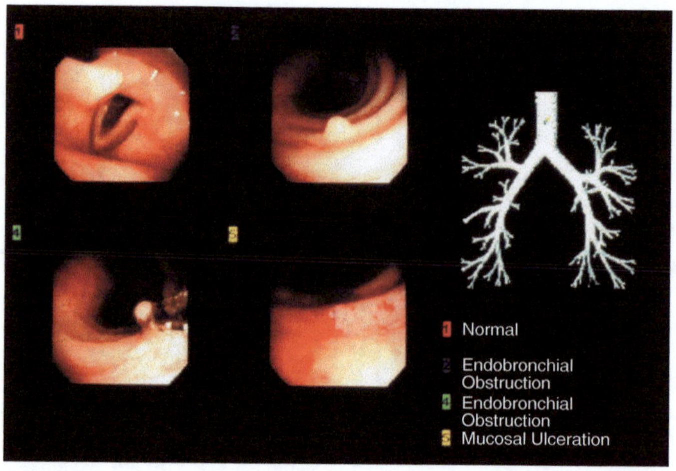

FIGURE 41.39. Inflammatory polyp of the trachea. Endoscopic view. Note small mound-like lesion on the mucosal surface of the trachea. (Courtesy of Dr. Richard Irwin, University of Massachusetts Medical School, Worcester, MA.)

The histopathologic changes, the morphologic resemblance to pyogenic granulomas occurring elsewhere, and the clinical backgrounds in which these lesions arise point to a reactive inflammatory nonneoplastic nature of these lesions, and the generally benign outcome of these lesions supports this view. However, serious complications such as airway obstruction and massive hemoptysis may occur.[157] These lesions appear curable, and several cases with successful responses to antibiotics, inhalational corticosteroids, and laser photoablation (in urgent cases of polyps obstructing the airways) have been documented.[158–160]

Benign Clear Cell (Sugar) Tumor

So named because of their rich glycogen content, pulmonary clear cell or sugar tumors were first reported in abstract form by Liebow and Castleman.[161] These tumors have attracted considerable attention and interest because of their uncertain histogenesis, unique morphology, and histochemical and immunohistochemical properties. Some cases occur in association with tuberous sclerosis and lymphangioleiomyomatosis, but most occur de novo. Since the first report, a well-detailed series of 12 cases was later published by the same authors.[162] The cases were further reviewed by Andrion et al.[163] and by Gaffey et al.[164] By 1991, about 50 cases had been published, and by now that number is likely greater.[165,166] There may be some overlap in the total number of cases published. Overall, this must still be considered a very rare lung tumor.

The cell of origin of clear cell tumor of lung has long been the source of much discussion. Liebow and Castleman[161,162] entertained the possibilities of this tumor being myoid or neuroid. They noted that the clear cell leiomyomas that might be in the differential diagnosis did not

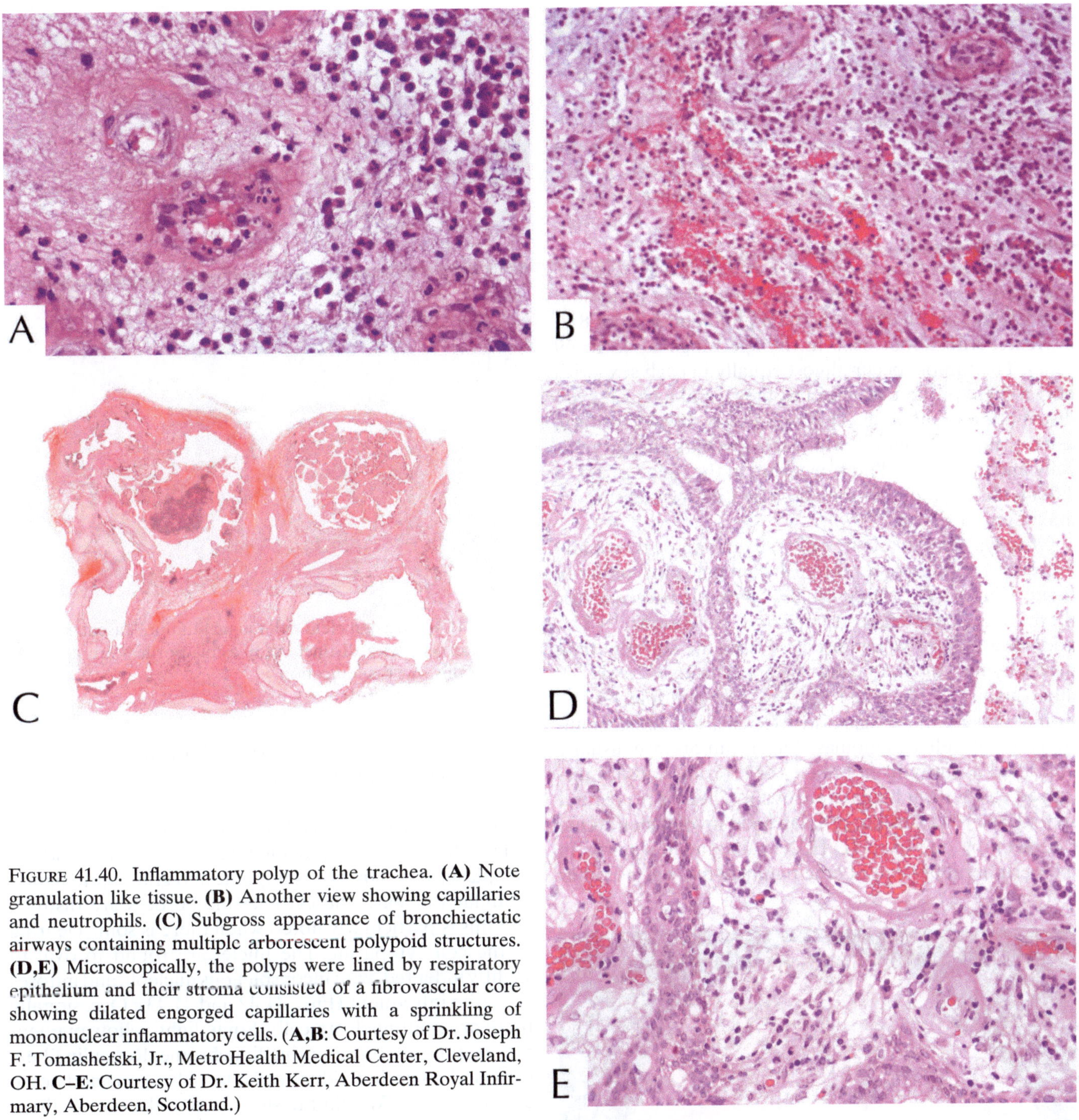

FIGURE 41.40. Inflammatory polyp of the trachea. **(A)** Note granulation like tissue. **(B)** Another view showing capillaries and neutrophils. **(C)** Subgross appearance of bronchiectatic airways containing multiple arborescent polypoid structures. **(D,E)** Microscopically, the polyps were lined by respiratory epithelium and their stroma consisted of a fibrovascular core showing dilated engorged capillaries with a sprinkling of mononuclear inflammatory cells. (**A,B**: Courtesy of Dr. Joseph F. Tomashefski, Jr., MetroHealth Medical Center, Cleveland, OH. **C–E**: Courtesy of Dr. Keith Kerr, Aberdeen Royal Infirmary, Aberdeen, Scotland.)

contain glycogen. Smooth muscle tumors would be expected to arise in association with bronchioles or pulmonary vessels, neither of which seemed to be true in this case. Liebow and Castleman continued to wonder about some smooth muscle–derived origin, as the muscle of some shellfish is rich in glycogen. Becker and Soifer[167] saw electron-dense small granules in 2% to 5% of cells, and proposed that perhaps these are variants of Kulchitsky cells. Hoch et al.[168] and others were more struck with the possibility of a smooth muscle or pericyte derivation.

Currently, clear cell "sugar" tumors of lung are recognized as neoplasms with perivascular epithelioid cell (PEC) differentiation. Mesenchymal tumors with this type of differentiation are known as PEComas and are composed of histologically and immunohistochemically distinctive perivascular epithelioid cells.[169] The PEComa family of tumors includes angiomyolipoma, lymphangioleiomyomatosis, clear cell myomelanocytic lesion of the falciform ligament/ligamentum teres, and unusual clear cell tumors of the pancreas, rectum, abdominal serosa, uterus, vulva, thigh, and heart.[169] Perivascular epithelioid cells are characterized by positivity with melanocytic markers such as HMB-45, Melan-A, tyrosinase, microphthalmia transcription factor, and muscle markers such as pan-actin, smooth muscle actin, muscle myosin, and calponin.[169] Desmin is less often positive, and cytokeratin and S-100 protein are usually negative. Likewise, immunostains for CEA are negative. The most sensitive melanocytic markers for PEComas are HMB-45, Melan-A, and microphthalmia transcription factor.[169]

Patients with these tumors are usually asymptomatic, and their tumors are likely to be found on an incidental basis. They vary in age at the time of diagnosis from 8 to 70 years, with about 66% in the age range of 45 to 69 years. The tumors occur almost equally in each sex (with only a slight predominance in women), and have an even distribution in the lung. They are almost always solitary, usually more peripheral, with even contours radiographically and grossly, and most measure in the range of 1.5 to 3.0cm, although one in the series by Liebow measured a maximum of 6.5cm.[161,162]

Grossly, benign clear cell "sugar" tumors usually present as nodules of semi-translucent pale pink-tan-gray tissue (Fig. 41.41). They usually show no necrosis, but there have been several reported exceptions.[170] The nodules are sharply circumscribed from the adjacent lung parenchyma, with no true encapsulation. Grossly or microscopically identified necrosis and multiple lesions would suggest more aggressive lesions, including metastatic renal cell carcinomas. Sugar tumors are usually described as away from bronchi or arteries, and are dislodged easily from lung parenchyma. There is no pleural spread, pleural effusion, or hilar node involvement. One case seen by one of us (D.H.D.) surrounded a nerve in the peripheral portion of lung parenchyma, but no other associations with nerve, artery, or bronchiole have been noted. They usually occur within 2cm of the pleura but do not involve the pleura.

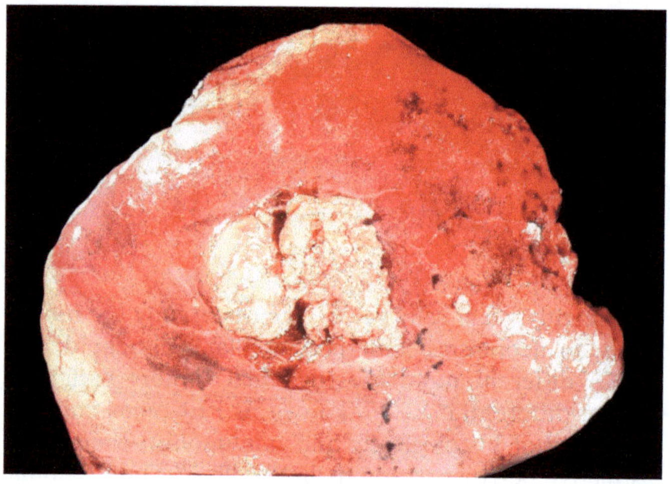

FIGURE 41.41. Benign clear cell (sugar) tumors. Gross appearance. Note well-defined gray white tumor mass at center of field. (Courtesy of Dr. Eugene J. Mark, Massachusetts General Hospital, Boston, MA.)

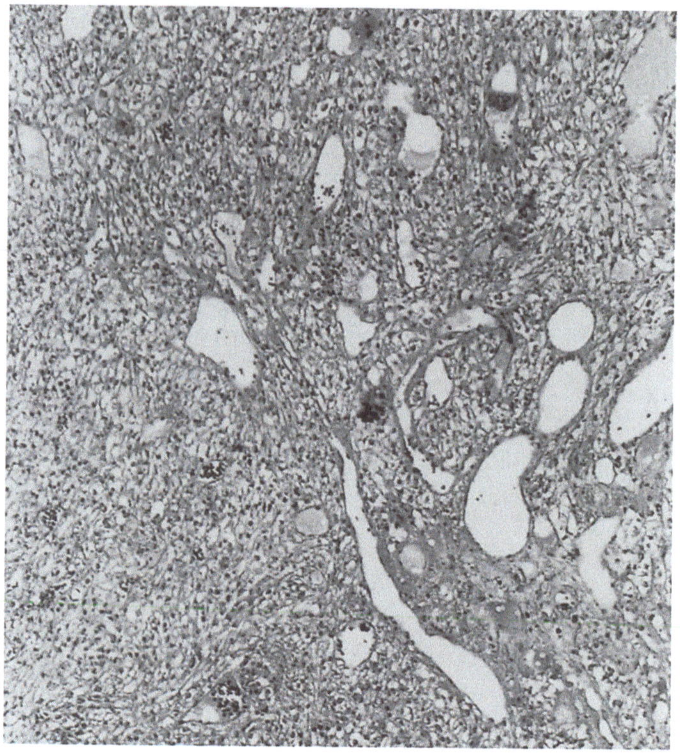

FIGURE 41.42. Benign clear cell (sugar) tumor. Vascular spaces and clear cells with distinct cytoplasmic borders are apparent at even this low magnification.

Microscopically, the cells can be moderately pleomorphic, in the fashion of a benign endocrine tumor, and the cytoplasm varies from eosinophilic and granular to lightly granular to clear. The cytoplasmic borders are distinct, and this is particularly noted when there is some clearing of the cell cytoplasm. The nuclei are round to oval to slightly indented, with inconspicuous nucleoli, and mitoses are quite infrequent (Figs. 41.42 and 41.43). Occasionally there are multinucleate cells. Some light-yellow pigment may be present, representing lipochrome. Reticulin fibers surround some individual cells, but also surround some clumps of cells. Within the substance of the tumor, there may be a few entrapped bronchioles evident at the edge, but these are usually not present throughout the tumor or in the middle of its substance. Toward the periphery there may be some small spaces with cuboidal cells that presumably are metaplastic alveolar lining cells. True acini and papillary configurations are not present in most of the tumors. Characteristically, there are dilated sinusoidal-like vascular spaces within the tumor. These sinusoidal spaces have no muscle coats. Rarely, these vessel-like walls may serve as sites of small calcification. A distinctive feature of these tumors is their high glycogen content. The periodic acid-Schiff (PAS) stain

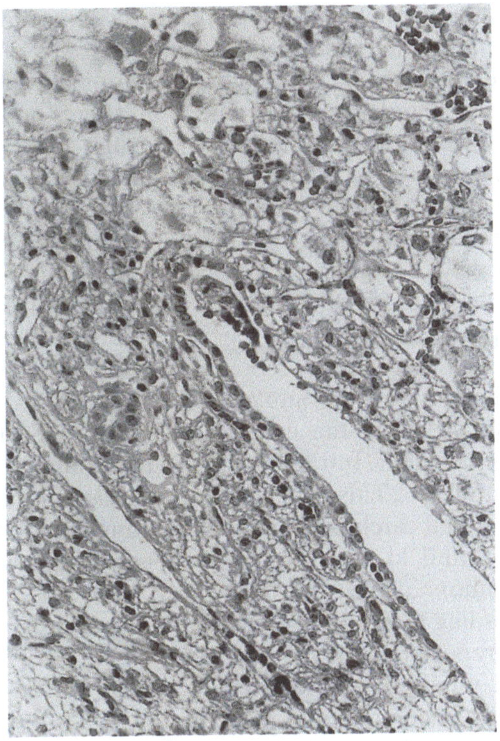

FIGURE 41.43. Benign clear cell (sugar) tumor. Note pleomorphism of cells at top of field. Dropout of glycogen leaves multiple cleared areas in the tumor cells.

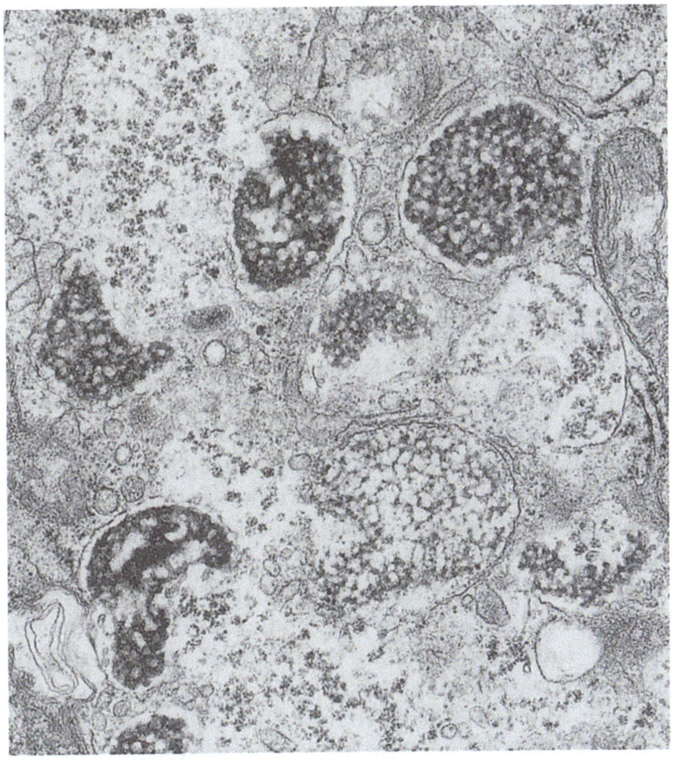

FIGURE 41.45. Benign clear cell (sugar) tumors. Ultrastructure. Note typical membrane bound glycogen globules. TEM.

before diastase is usually quite intensely positive, but this completely digests away with diastase pretreatment. There is a trace Alcian blue reaction and a moderate colloidal iron reaction. Pulmonary clear cell tumors stain consistently for HMB-45 (Fig. 41.44). Most are S-100 protein positive and cytokeratin negative. Some have been reported to be actin and CD117 positive. One case studied cytologically showed large irregular clusters of polygonal and spindle cells with vacuolated granular PAS-positive cytoplasm.[171,172]

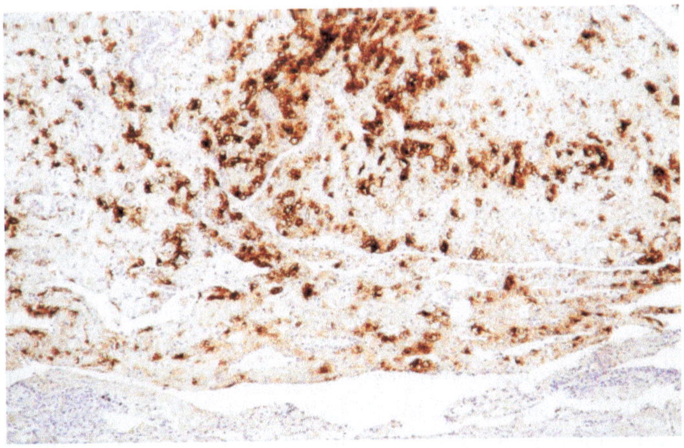

FIGURE 41.44. Benign clear cell (sugar) tumor. Intense positive reaction of tumor cells for HMB-45. (Courtesy of Dr. Bruno Murer, Venice, Italy.)

Ultrastructurally, the cells of clear cell sugar tumors are known to contain abundant free and membrane-bound glycogen (Fig. 41.45).[171] The membrane-bound glycogen appears unique to this lung tumor, although it is typically described in Pompe's disease (type II glycogenosis). In Pompe's disease, glycogen usually accumulates mainly in lysosomes, principally in the liver, because of a deficiency of acid glucosidase (acid maltase) necessary to further break down glycogen in these lysosomes. There is no evidence that sugar tumor of lung has ever occurred in a background of Pompe's disease. The only independent tumor in this disease was in a case described in the trachea with a 1-cm mixed follicular and papillary thyroid carcinoma without vascular invasion. These electron micrographic findings have been confirmed in several additional studies. Necrosis has been seen in three lesions, including one seen in consultation by A.A. Liebow, but apparently unreported, as noted by Sale and Kulander.[170,172] There was apparently a thrombus in one of the vessels near the necrotic lesion in the case not reported, but in the 4.5-cm case of Sale and Kulander that eventually metastasized, there was no evidence of thrombi near the tumor. Finding adjacent thrombi may depend on the plane of section. Rarely, cavitation may occur.

The differential diagnosis principally involves metastatic clear cell carcinomas from kidney and primary clear cell carcinomas of lung. Also to be considered are acinic cell tumors, and at times oncocytomas and other granular cell tumors. All of these lack the typical sinusoidal vascularity and glycogen positivity of benign clear cell tumors, and each has its own distinctive characteristics. Metastatic renal clear cell carcinomas can be solitary and can present before, during, or after diagnosis of renal adenocarcinomas, and may even be present many years after primary excision. Renal clear cell adenocarcinoma is one of the typical tumors that may metastasize endobronchially. Many cases of clear sugar tumor have had renal evaluations, and this may still be warranted, because of the rarity of sugar tumors and the possibility of confusion with metastatic lesions. However, there are histologic differences, including rare or no necrosis, no mitoses, no fat, little iron, and a differential reticulin pattern, that differentiate sugar tumors from metastatic renal cell carcinomas. The sinusoidal thin-walled nonmuscular vessels in clear cell tumors are also distinct from the muscular arteries supplying metastatic renal clear cell adenocarcinoma. Immunoperoxidase stains help with metastatic renal cell carcinomas, these being more vimentin, cytokeratin, and EMA positive than clear cell tumors, and in reverse, if S-100 and HMB-45 are positive, this is more typical of benign clear cell tumor.

Primary clear cell carcinomas of lung enter the differential in a major way. First recognized by Liebow and also by Walter and Pryce,[173] these tumors may mimic clear cell sugar tumors microscopically. In a study of 348 consecutive cases of lung carcinoma, Katzenstein et al.[174] aimed to determine the incidence of clear cell carcinomas, and found that clear cells were common in all major types of lung carcinomas except small cell carcinoma. Among the 348 tumors, 14 (4%) contained more than 50% clear cells, and of these 10 showed foci of epidermoid differentiation and four showed gland formation by light microscopy. The tumors with more than 50% clear cell change behaved no differently from their nonclear cell variants.[174] These authors suggested this characteristic should be considered a variation only within lung cancer proper.[174] Edwards and Carlile[175] studied six tumors considered primary clear cell carcinomas of lung by electron microscopy, and found adenocarcinoma differentiation in three and squamous differentiation in two. The other was considered a large cell anaplastic carcinoma. Edwards and Carlile found no membrane-bound glycogen in their six cancer cases. Other differential considerations include balloon clear cell melanomas and clear cell sarcomas. The former can be distinguished by the presence of significant atypia and clinical history, while actin and CD117 might be useful in differentiating clear cell tumors from clear cell sarcoma.

Of particular interest, a well-documented case by Gaffey and associates[176] of a lung tumor closely mimicking pulmonary clear cell sugar tumor was reported in a 53-year-old woman. The patient was found to have a pulmonary nodule in the left upper lobe during routine chest roentgenography. Histologically, the tumor was composed of predominantly clear to lightly eosinophilic, polygonal cells with bland nuclei arranged in sheets and nests. Nuclear pleomorphism, necrosis, vascular invasion, and mitotic figures were not seen. The tumor cells were negative for oil-red-O and PAS stains with and without diastase pretreatment on frozen and formalin-fixed sections, respectively. On immunohistochemical evaluation, the tumor cells were focally positive for cytokeratin and diffusely positive for neuron-specific enolase and chromogranin. Electron microscopy showed electron-dense, neurosecretory-type granules and variably sized vacuolated areas within the cytoplasm, the nature of which remained unclear. Intracytoplasmic glycogen or lipid was not identified.[176] This appears to be the first bona fide case of a clear cell carcinoid tumor of the lung, and it must be kept in mind in the differential diagnosis of clear cell sugar tumors of the lung.

According to Fraser et al.,[177] almost all clear cell (sugar) tumors reported in the literature have behaved in a benign fashion, unassociated with recurrence or distant spread. Surgical resection is said to be curative. However, late recurrences, after surgical removal, although extremely infrequent, may occur. A case in point is the patient reported by Sale and Kulander.[178] In this case the patient developed liver metastasis 10 years after the initial diagnosis.

Granular Cell Tumor

Initially regarded as tumors of striated muscle origin,[179–183] granular cell tumors are currently believed to be of neural origin, of either nerve sheath or Schwann cell derivation. Several reports documenting immunoreactivity to the S-100 protein and neuron-specific enolase are consistent with the purported nerve sheath derivation of these tumors.[184–186] Therefore, the older term, *granular cell myoblastoma*, is no longer used or recommended for these tumors. Granular cell tumors occur in the tongue, heart, skin, subcutaneous tissue, breast, hypopharynx, esophagus, and other sites, as well as the larynx and the lower respiratory tract.[187] Several reviews of granular cell tumors in the tracheobronchial system have been published, some under the rubric of granular cell myoblastoma. Ostermiller et al.[179] added three cases to the literature, which contained 31 such cases by 1970. Oparah and Subramanian[180] added two cases to 42 in the literature by 1976. This series was expanded and additionally reviewed in 1983 by DeClercq et al.,[181] and by 1995 the literature contained reports about 100 cases. By now that number is said to be much greater. Of interest, granular cell tumors in horses are relatively frequent and are often cited in the veterinary pathology literature.[188]

Patients with granular cell tumors are generally in their 30s and 40s, although cases in children ages 10 or younger have been documented.[185] Granular cell tumors of the tracheobronchial tree usually present with symptoms of airway irritation or obstruction, including dyspnea and hemoptysis. Obstructive symptoms were present in 94% of cases in one series.[179] One reported case was associated with hypercalcemia, which was cured following excision of the tumor.[189] Another case coexisted with a bronchogenic squamous cell carcinoma.[190] Pulmonary cases can be asymptomatic and found incidentally as coin lesions on chest radiographs.[191]

Granular cell tumors occur in the right-mainstem bronchus in 59% of the cases, left-mainstem bronchus in 36% of cases, and bilaterally in 5% of cases. They usually present as small crests or ridges, plaques, or polyps, and are generally in the range of 2 cm, but larger tumors occur. One reported case described a tumor measuring 6.5 cm.[179] Despite the large size of this tumor, there was no evidence of untoward clinical behavior. Of all cases inside and outside the chest, about 20% have multiple lesions. Of these, about 22% are multiple within the tracheobronchial system, and there were even four multicentric endobronchial cases reported from one institution.[182] The others occur with involvement of other organs, especially skin where the lesions may be multiple, but multiple cases also occur in tongue, vulva, and the esophagus. Of those that involve the carina, about 40% occur with multiple pulmonary lesions, and in another 40% the carina is involved contiguous with a lesion in the main bronchus. Despite their multicentricity, these tumors act in a benign fashion. One peculiar well-documented case was reported with multiorgan involvement in a 29-week stillborn boy.[192] The infiltrate of abnormal cells was not as nodular as expected. This case was S-100 protein negative, and compared to congenital epulis lesions, only occurring systemically. Electron microscopy was done and showed abundant lysosomes.[192] At bronchoscopy, granular cell tumors appear as endobronchial nodules at points of bifurcation, but others are flat and plaque-like. Grossly these tumors are generally soft to friable to rubbery, yellow-tan to gray, and most often limited to the tracheobronchial wall. The overlying mucosa may be intact or may be focally ulcerated with associated bleeding. Ulceration occurs most often with pedunculated tumor polyps (Fig. 41.46A,B).

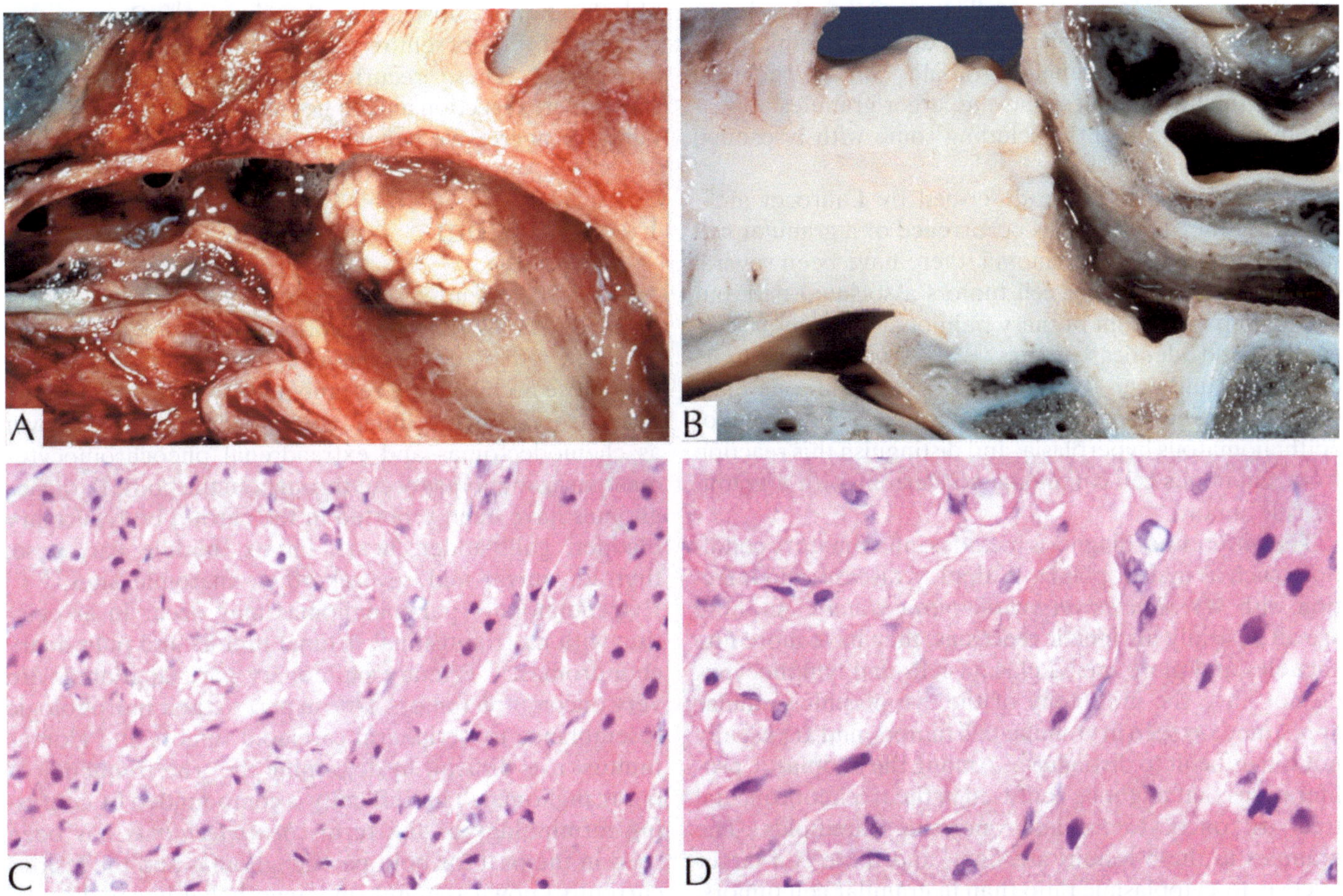

Figure 41.46. **(A)** Gross image of a granular cell tumor extending into bronchial lumen as a multilobular sessile mass. **(B)** Cross section of tumor shown in **A**, note deep extension with effacement of bronchial wall and narrowing of lumen. **(C,D)** Microscopic views of granular cell tumor, note large cells with small dark nuclei and abundant granular cytoplasm. (**A,B**: Courtesy of Dr. Joseph F. Tomashefski, Jr., MetroHealth Medical Center, Cleveland, OH.)

Microscopically, granular cell tumors are composed of monotonous large polygonal-to-elongated cells with pale eosinophilic granular cytoplasm that is also monotonous, without vacuoles or other variations, with eccentrically placed small nuclei, and very rare or no mitotic figures (Fig. 41.46C,D). The tumor cells infiltrate among submucosal glands, and some may extend between fragments of bronchial cartilage; in one reported case there was extension to the adjacent lung.[187] Squamous metaplasia of the overlying respiratory epithelium occurs in some two-thirds of the cases and sometimes is atypical, but is not as often pseudoepitheliomatous in appearance as it is in mucous membranes, tongue, or skin. The cytoplasmic granules are distinct, vary somewhat in size, and the larger ones stain with PAS and Alcian blue. By immunohistochemistry, positivity for the S-100 protein and neuron-specific enolase can be observed. A recent review of 29 cases of granular cell tumors from various sites included four laryngeal cases but no actual lung cases. In these laryngeal tumors, immunostains for the S-100 protein were positive in all four instances.[193] Interestingly, immunostains for inhibin and CD68 were also positive, suggesting that these markers also may be useful in the diagnosis in granular cell tumors of the lower airways.[193] By electron microscopy, the cytoplasmic granules vary in size. The smaller granules contain packages of even smaller granules, and the larger granules appear to have mixed contents, including some with lysosomal characteristics.[192,194]

In addition to the case described by Lauro et al.,[195] reporting the simultaneous occurrence of a granular cell tumor and small cell carcinoma, there have been several case reports of granular cell tumors associated with but usually separate from primary pulmonary squamous carcinomas and adenocarcinomas.[183,190] As with these tumors elsewhere, and even though it is less frequent, one must be aware of the potential for exuberant reactive pseudoepitheliomatous hyperplasia, and distinguish this reaction from squamous cell carcinoma concurrent with a granular cell tumor.

The differential diagnosis includes inflammatory conditions such as malakoplakia, Whipple's disease, and infection with *Mycobacterium avium–intracellulare*. As these are all basically histiocytic reactions, they have more fine vacuoles and more mixed plasma cells and lymphocytes, do not have the monotony of the cytoplasmic granular appearance as seen in granular cell tumors, and are usually not too difficult to distinguish. Among the neoplastic proliferations that might be confused in the tracheobronchial tree are oncocytomas and oncocytic carcinoids. The granules in these lesions are finer, and there is a larger nuclear-to-cytoplasmic ratio than in granular cell tumors. Neuroendocrine markers and S-100 protein immunostains as well as electron microscopic procedures help in cases where there is difficulty. Most of these oncocytic tumors infiltrate in a more obliterative manner than the delicate approach of the granular cell tumors. Adenocarcinoma variants from various sites can also have granular cytoplasm but they can be differentiated on account of their significant atypia, necrosis, or mitotic activity. Granular cell tumors in the lung and elsewhere are S-100 protein and neuron-specific enolase positive, and these stains can be used to differentiate problem cases. Transbronchial biopsies may also be very suggestive of this tumor, and cytology specimens, including sputa, washings, and brushings, may contain granular cells and be at least suspicious of granular cell tumors. Cytologically, oncocytic carcinoid may closely mimic granular cell tumors.[196]

True malignant granular cell tumors with poor outcome do occur but are exceedingly rare, with only 40 cases reported as of 2003. One such case presenting in the lung was described by Jiang et al.[197] However, for most cases the prognosis is usually excellent and complete surgical excision is regarded as curative. Some larger benign lesions located in strategically difficult areas may be difficult to extirpate. Deavers et al.[184] cite bronchoscopic removal, laser therapy, and sleeve resections as optional therapeutic modalities. Neodymium:yttrium-aluminum-garnet (Nd:YAG) laser therapy appears particularly suitable for tumors obstructing the airways.[198] Recurrences in cases of tumors removed bronchoscopically have been reported.[198] These recurrences may be secondary to incomplete resection and do not necessarily signify malignancy or aggressive behavior.

Paraganglioma

Along with ependymomas, paragangliomas are recognized by the WHO classification of pulmonary tumors under an "other" miscellaneous category. Paragangliomas bear close architectural resemblance to carcinoid tumors but have distinct cellular components.[199] Also known as chemodectomas and extraadrenal pheochromocytomas, paragangliomas occur throughout the body. Paragangliomas have been reported in the carotid body, urinary bladder, gallbladder, heart, larynx, middle ear, nose, thyroid, vulva, and several other anatomic sites.[200–204] Extrapulmonary paragangliomas may occur in association with gastrointestinal stromal tumors and pulmonary chondromas.[205] Primary pulmonary paragangliomas are very uncommon tumors. Due in part to their morphologic resemblance to peripheral carcinoid tumors and glomus tumors, it is difficult to determine the true frequency of paragangliomas. This difficulty is compounded by confusing terminology as the term *chemodectomas* has been used in the past for both paragangliomas and the lesions currently known as minute meningothelial-like bodies. To date, perhaps no more than 25 cases of paraganglioma have been reported in the literature.[200–207]

Paragangliomas of the respiratory tract may occur in the trachea or the lung parenchyma. A female predomi-

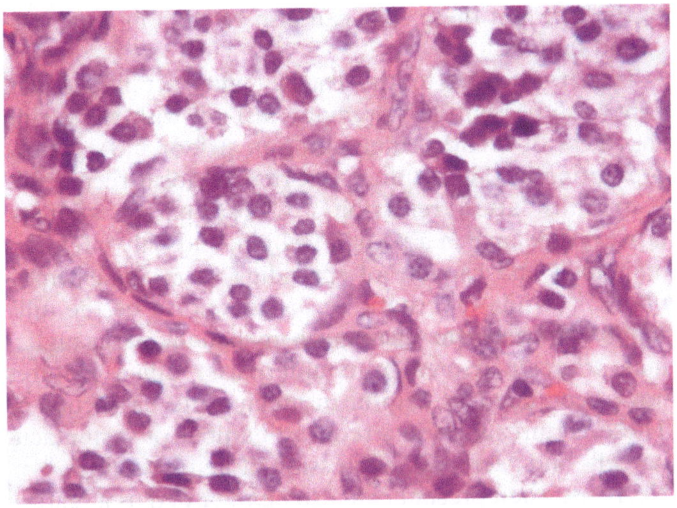

FIGURE 41.47. Paraganglioma. Note cells arranged in ball-like clusters (zellballen) and surrounding sustentacular cells.

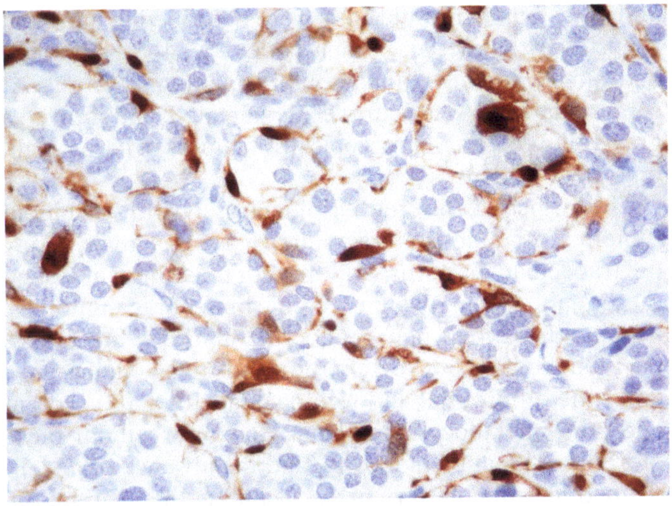

FIGURE 41.49. Paraganglioma. S-100 protein immunostain. Note positive immunostaining of sustentacular cells and negative immunostaining of tumor cells.

nance is reported for both tracheal and pulmonary tumors. Presenting symptoms are dyspnea, hemoptysis, hoarseness, dysphagia, or stridor in tracheal tumors, and cough, dyspnea, or chest pain in pulmonary tumors. Pulmonary paragangliomas are peripherally located lesions, often well outlined but without a capsule and have pink or tan cut surfaces with no connection to the airways.[200–208]

In Hangartner et al.'s[209] review, the tumors ranged from 1 to 7 cm in diameter. The tumors were well outlined with a smooth gray-pink bulging cut surface. The formation of zellballen typifies these tumors microscopically (Fig. 41.47). The chief cells within the zellballen have clear amphophilic or eosinophilic cytoplasm. Their nuclei are centrally placed with finely stippled chromatin. Surrounding these chief cells there are CD34-positive fibrovascular septa and elongated S-100–positive sustentacular cells (Figs. 41.48 and 41.49). The chief cells making the zellballen are cytokeratin negative and express a variety of neuroendocrine markers. These include chromogranin, neuron-specific enolase, and synaptophysin (Fig. 41.50). In addition to being S-100 positive, the sustentacular cells may express glial fibrillary acidic protein. Ultrastructurally, these tumors show electron-dense cytoplasmic granules, 100 to 140 μm in diameter, similar to those seen in extrapulmonary paragangliomas and carcinoid tumors of the lung.[207] The case reported by Shibahara et al.[210] was immunoreactive for CD56, chromogranin A, neuron-specific enolase, and the S-100 protein but negative for cytokeratins, calcitonin, somatostatin, and TTF-1. Cytologic features of paraganglioma have not been well characterized. Tridimensional papillary-like clusters of epithelioid cells with round to oval nuclei, evenly dispersed chromatin, micronucleoli,

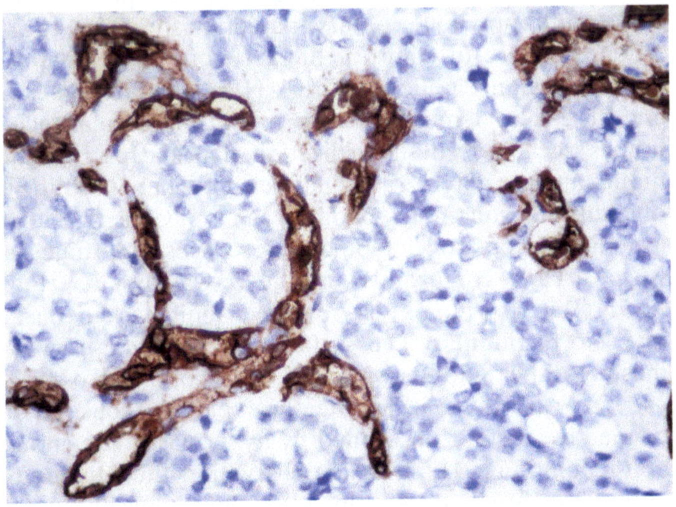

FIGURE 41.48. Paraganglioma. Note CD34 immunostain decorating fibrovascular cores partly surrounding the zellballen.

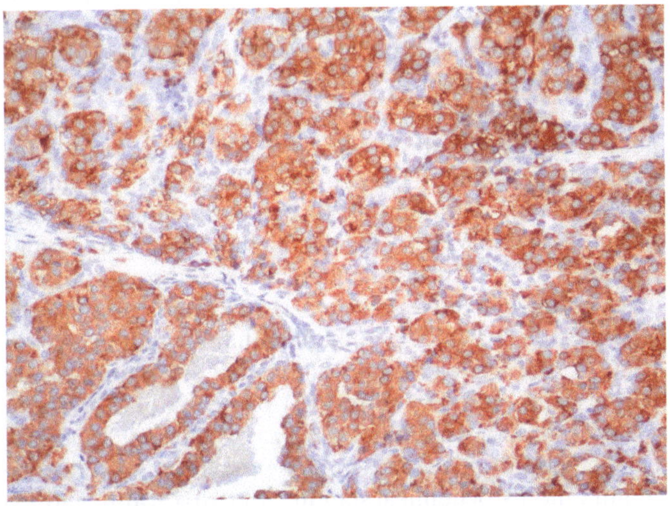

FIGURE 41.50. Paraganglioma. Chromogranin immunostain. Note positive immunostaining of tumor cells with negative immunostaining of blood vessels and sustentacular cells.

and occasional anisonucleosis were described in a patient reported by Kim et al.[211] Their patient, a 34-year-old man had an incidentally found solitary pulmonary mass. At surgery the mass was 3 cm, well demarcated, and showed a gray-yellow color. Microscopically, features of paraganglioma were evident.

The principal differential diagnosis is with carcinoid tumors. Carcinoid tumors are more apt to show ribbony or trabecular patterns and pseudorosetting, although these features can also be seen in some paragangliomas. Carcinoids express neuroendocrine markers, but unlike paragangliomas are cytokeratin positive. Melanomas enter the differential and would stain with S-100 protein and other melanocytic markers. However, cellular pleomorphism, junctional activity, and the absence of a well-defined nesting pattern may facilitate the distinction. Renal cell carcinoma may be considered when cytoplasmic clearing is prominent. However, these tumors most often lack zellballen formations and are cytokeratin and EMA positive. Acinic cell tumors, benign clear cell tumors, and glomus tumors can be differentiated with appropriate use of neuroendocrine and smooth muscle markers. An effort should always be made to exclude the possibility of paraganglioma metastatic to the lung, particularly in patients with a known paraganglioma elsewhere.

A unique case of a pulmonary paraganglioma with gangliocytic differentiation was presented by Hironaka et al.[212] The patient, a 75-year-old man, underwent surgical resection of a pulmonary mass located at the bifurcation of the lower and middle lobe bronchus. Microscopically, the resected tumor showed three different cellular elements: uniform endocrine cells in a zellballen arrangement, large ganglion-like cells within the nests of endocrine cells, and spindle-shaped cells arranged in streams surrounding the nests.[212] Each component exhibited characteristic immunohistochemical properties, which were similar to those of the corresponding neuroendocrine neoplasms: the endocrine cells were positive for CAM 5.2 cytokeratin, chromogranin A, and synaptophysin, much like a carcinoid tumor; the ganglion-like cells were positive only for neurofilament, like ganglioneuroma; and the spindle-shaped cells were positive for neurofilament and S-100 protein, like paraganglioma.[212]

Microscopic, immunohistologic, and clinical criteria outlined by the WHO[199] for the diagnosis paragangliomas include (1) a diffuse zellballen pattern throughout; (2) absence of distinctive features of carcinoid tumors such as trabecular pattern, pseudoglandular acini, foci of ossification, oncocytic change, spindle cell morphology, and perivascular pseudorosettes; (3) presence of distinctive features of paragangliomas, such as cytoplasmic vacuoles, and the cell-in-cell embracing phenomenon; (4) absence of immunohistochemical staining for cytokeratin; and (5) absence of a primary paraganglioma elsewhere.[199] The presence of S-100–positive sustentacular cells surrounding the zellballen is not a diagnostic criteria. This is due to the fact that these cells can also be seen in some carcinoid tumors.

Tumors located in the trachea may act like a ball valve and present in a dramatic fashion with worsening shortness of breath, culminating in stridor.[208] A patient presenting in this manner experienced local recurrence 9 months after resection.[208] Most paragangliomas, however, behave in a benign fashion, and only a few are malignant and capable of spreading to regional lymph nodes.[213] While metastatic spread is said to be the only reliable criterion to distinguish malignant paragangliomas from their benign counterparts, other features have been cited as helpful in making the distinction.[213] These features include a reduced number of sustentacular cells and decreased expression of neuropeptides.[214,215] Necrosis, when present can also be regarded as a feature of malignancy. Tracheotomy under local anesthesia to secure the airway followed by general anesthesia in order to surgically remove paragangliomas of the trachea has been successfully performed in patients with stridor.[208]

Uncommon Endobronchial Surface Tumors

Epithelial papillary proliferations arising from the mucosa of the tracheobronchial tree are uncommon, generally benign proliferations, currently classified by the World Health Organization as Papillomas of Squamous, Glandular or Mixed Phenotype.

Squamous Papillomas

Squamous papillary lesions of the upper respiratory tract occur in children and adults and may be either solitary or multiple.[216] A disseminated form, laryngo—tracheobronchial papillomatosis, is more likely seen in children or adolescents but may also occur in adults, particularly those with previous solitary papillomas.[216] The viral-induced nature of some of these lesions is well established. Human Papilloma Virus (HPV), usually types 6 and 11, can be demonstrated by modern molecular techniques, such as in situ hybridization, hybrid capture techniques and the polymerase chain reaction, in both solitary or multiple squamous papillomas.[217,218] Grossly, most lesions are exophytic polypoid excrescences of the mucosa with variable compromise of the airway lumina (Fig. 41.51). Rare papillomas are inverted, similar to sinonasal inverted papillomas. The surfaces of exophytic papillomas are either smooth or slightly verrucoid. Microscopically, an arborescent architectural pattern consists of connective tissue fronds lined by hyperplastic squamous epithelium (Fig. 41.52). The cells within the squamous epithelium are cytologically bland but typically show nuclear hyperchromatism, koilocytotic change or binucleation (Fig. 41.52). Variants with extensive koilocytotic

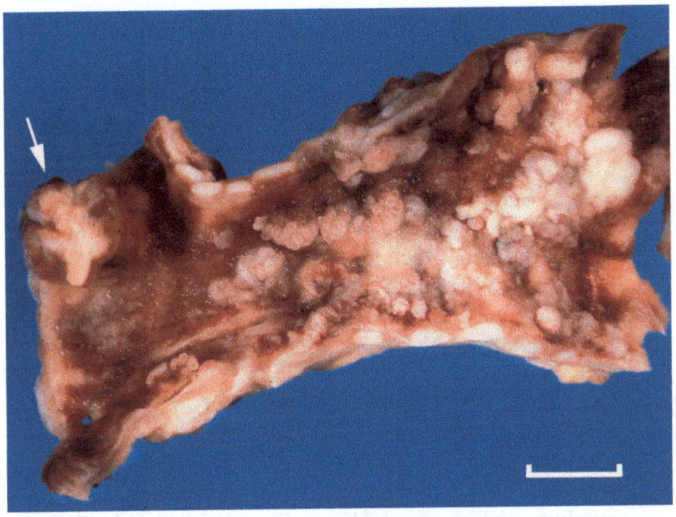

FIGURE 41.51. Juvenile tracheobronchial squamous papillomatosis. Numerous papillomatous excrescences distort the tracheal mucosal surface in this 13 year old male adolescent. Papillomas extend into the lobar bronchus (arrow). Scale equals 1 cm.

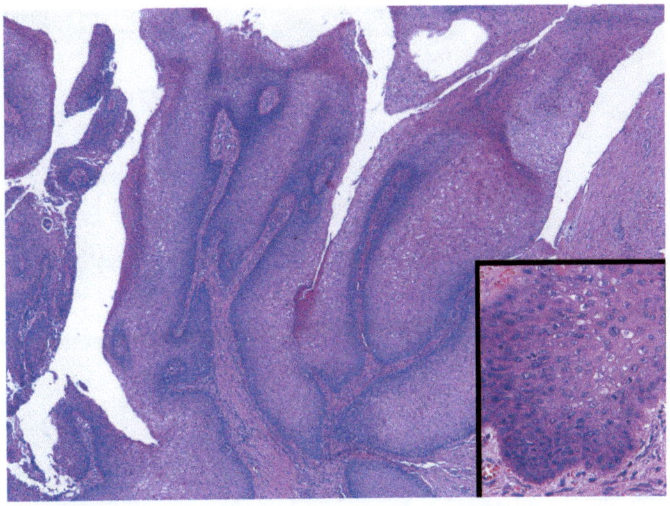

FIGURE 41.52. Squamous papilloma showing exophytic verrucous extensions of acanthotic squamous epithelium with a hyperplastic basal layer and fibrovascular stalk. Insert. Koilocytotic and dysplastic nuclear features are frequently seen in the squamous epithelium.

changes have been termed condylomatous papillomas.[219] Evaluating endobronchial biopsy specimens of squamous papillomas, especially the solitary lesions, can be hazardous. One must be cautious not to under or overextrapolate findings based on the limited tissue provided by these biopsy procedures. Both poorly differentiated and well-differentiated squamous carcinomas can appear bland in selected areas; conversely, squamous papillomas can appear atypical. It is best to diagnose ambiguous biopsies as "atypical", while discussing alternative possibilities, followed by a recommendation that a limited excision should be undertaken for endotracheal and endobronchial lesions, and that all the tissue should be submitted for histological examination, in a manner similar to villous adenoma of colon. In some lesions hyperplastic squamous epithelium extends into the neck of the subepithelial glands. This pattern of contiguous surface spread should not be interpreted as evidence of invasion (Fig. 41.53). The prognosis of squamous papillomas can be ascertained by immunohistochemical or molecular techniques. Increased expression of alpha II topoisomerase and the p53 protein product may serve as markers of malignant transformation.[220,221]

Solitary squamous papillomas behave in a clinically indolent manner and require only conservative surgical excision. Juvenile tracheobronchial papillomatosis, however, is a more serious disorder capable of extensive airway destruction, bronchiectatic cyst formation, and malignant transformation with lymphangitic spread. In cases with deep lung extension, chest radiographs show multiple cavitary lesions. Tracheostomy and repeated removal of papillomas is often required throughout the individual's lifetime. As in the larynx, radiation or chemotherapy is said to be contraindicated in patients with tracheobronchial papillomatosis.[222]

Glandular Papillomas

Also known as columnar cell papillomas, glandular papillomas are papillary tumors of the airways lined by ciliated or non -ciliated columnar epithelium[216]. In contrast to their squamous counterparts, no etiologic agents have been identified in these lesions. Glandular papillomas develop in larger conductive airways and are less common

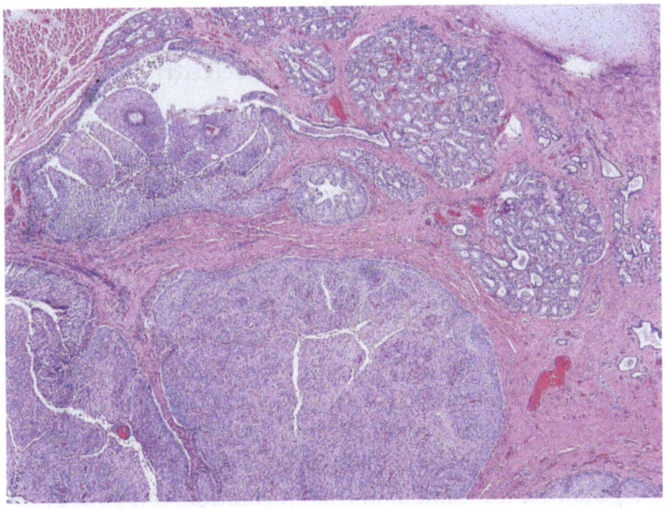

FIGURE 41.53. Papillomatous growth extends into the underlying submucosal glandular ducts in this laryngeal papilloma, a process not to be mistaken for submucosal invasion by well differentiated squamous carcinoma. Note thickened mucosal surface growth in lower portion of the field.

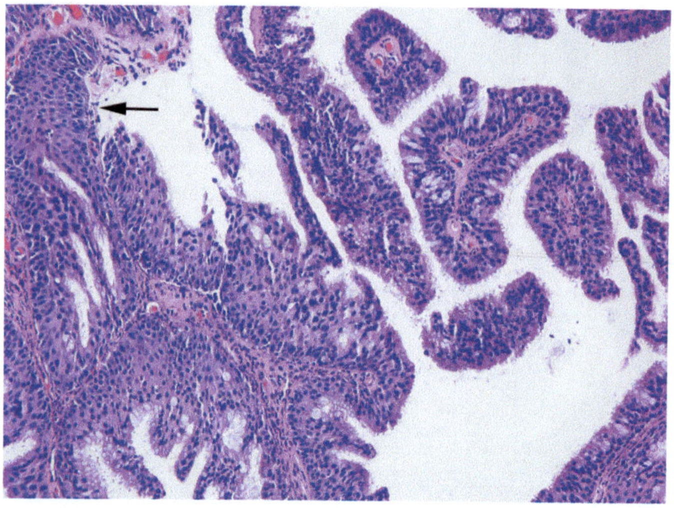

FIGURE 41.54. Mixed glandular and squamous papilloma. Non—keratinized squamous epithelium (arrow) is intermixed with ciliated and mucous epithelial cells lining papillary fronds.

than squamous papillomas. They have a wide age distribution but most occur in adults. Presenting symptoms include dyspnea, cough and hemoptysis. Most if not all glandular papillomas are solitary and disseminated forms are not known to occur. Central and peripherally located lesions are recognized, the latter are exceedingly rare and occur within the lung parenchyma.[216] Microscopically, the connective tissue fronds are lined entirely by ciliated or non -ciliated columnar epithelial cells alternating with low columnar to cuboidal cells and some goblet cells.[223,224] The columnar cells are aligned in a single orderly layer with well oriented basal nuclei. Glandular papillomas are benign, but recurrences have been reported following incomplete removal. However, in Basheda's series of eight cases, there were no reported recurrences.[224]

Mixed squamous and glandular papillomas

Previously known as transitional cell papillomas, these papillary lesions feature connective tissue fronds lined by a mixture of squamous and glandular epithelium[216] (Fig. 41.54). Only a small number of cases have been reported and no specific etiologic agent has been identified. As was the case with other papillomas, presenting respiratory symptoms are related to airway obstruction. Grossly these papillomas are sessile, granular, yellow—tan elevations of the mucosal surface. The squamous components can undergo dysplastic change, and thus the lesion has the potential for malignant transformation, but viral cytopathic effect has not been reported. Complete resection is said to be curative.

Acknowledgments. The authors are deeply appreciative to Karen Balcius for expert secretarial assistance, Rob Carlin for photography, and Andy Dzaugis and Rosemary Leary for bibliographic support.

References

1. Marchevsky AM. Lung tumors derived from ectopic tissues. Semin Diagn Pathol 1995;12:172–184.
2. Mendoza A, Voland J, Wolf P, et al. Supradiaphragmatic liver in the lung. Arch Pathol Lab Med 1986;44:1085–1086.
3. Lasser A, Wilson GL. Ectopic liver tissue mass in the thoracic cavity. Cancer 1975;36:1823–1826.
4. Jaiwalla AG, Al-Nasir NK. Splenosis pleurae. Thorax 1979; 34:123–124.
5. Kershisnik MM, Kaplan C, Craven CM, et al. Intrapulmonary neuroglial heterotopia. Arch Pathol Lab Med 1992; 116:1043–1046.
6. Ripstein CB, Rohman M, Wallach JB. Endometriosis involving the pleura. J Thorac Surg 1959;37:464–471.
7. Chung SY, Kim SJ, Kim TH, et al. Computed tomographic findings of pathologically confirmed pulmonary parenchymal endometriosis. J Comput Assist Tomogr 2005;29: 815–818.
8. Hart C. Histologisch benigne Metastasen vom bau eines Adenymioms 22 jahre nach Extirpation eines tumors der Genitalien. Frankf Z Pathol 1912;10:78.
9. Büngeler W, Fleury-Silveira D. Arg Cirug Clin Exp 1939; 3:169–187.
10. Park WW. The occurrence of decidual tissue within the lung: report of a case. J Pathol Bacteriol 1954;47:563–570.
11. Hartz PH. Occurrence of decidual-like tissue in the lung. Am J Clin Pathol 1956;26:48–51.
12. Cameron HM, Park WW. Decidual tissue within the lung. J Obstet Gynaecol Br Commonw 1965;72:748–752.
13. Lattes R, Shepard F, Tovell H, et al. Clinical and pathologic study of endometriosis. Surg Gynecol Obstet 1956;103: 552–558.
14. Farinacci CJ, Blauw AS, Jennings EM. Multifocal pulmonary lesions of possible decidual origin (so-called pulmonary deciduosis): report of a case. Am J Clin Pathol 1973; 59:508–574.
15. Spencer H. Pathology of the lung. 4th ed. London: Pergamon Press, 1985:1011–1012.
16. Hibbard LT, Schumann WR, Goldstein GE. Thoracic endometriosis: a review and report of two cases. Am J Obstet Gynecol 1981;140:227–232.
17. Karpel JP, Appel D, Merav A. Pulmonary endometriosis. Lung 1985;163:151–159.
18. Austin MB, Frierson HF Jr, Fechner RE, et al. Endometrioma of the lung presenting as hemoptysis and a large pulmonary mass. Surg Pathol 1988;1:165–169.
19. Di Palo S, Mari G, Castoldi R, Standacher C, Taccagni G, Di Carlo V. Endometriosis of the lung. Respir Med 1989; 83:255–258.
20. Schwartz OH. In: Discussion of paper by Counseller on endometriosis, a clinical and surgical review. Am J Obstet Gynecol 1938;36:887–888.
21. Foster DC, Stern JL, Buscema J, et al. Pleural and parenchymal pulmonary endometriosis. Obstet Gynecol 1981; 58:552–556.
22. Flieder DB, Moran CA, Travis WD, et al. Pleuro-pulmonary endometriosis and pulmonary ectopic decidu-

osis: a clinicopathologic and immunohistochemical study of 10 cases with emphasis on diagnostic pitfalls. Hum Pathol 1998;29:1495–1503.
23. Slasky BW, Siewers RD, Lecky JW, Zajko A, Buckholder JA. Catamenial pneumothorax: the roles of diaphragmatic defects and endometriosis. AJR 1982;138:639–643.
24. Granberg I, Willems JS. Endometriosis of lung and pleura diagnosed by aspiration biopsy. Acta Cytol 1982;26:295–297.
25. Zaatara GS, Gupta PK, Bhagavan BS, et al. Cytopathology of pleural endometriosis. Acta Cytol 1982;26:227–232.
26. Espaulella J, Armengol J, Bella F, Lain JM, Calaf J. Pulmonary endometriosis: conservative treatment with GnRH agonists. Obstet Gynecol 1991;78:535–537.
27. Koizumi T, Inagaki,Takabayashi Y, et al. Successful use of gonadotropin-releasing hormone agonist in a patient with pulmonary endometriosis. Respiration 1999;40:544–546.
28. Terada Y, Chen F, Shoji T, et al. A case of endobronchial endometriosis treated by subsegmentectomy. Chest 1999; 115:1475–1478.
29. Crane AR, Carrigan PT. Primary subpleural intrapulmonary thymoma. J Thorac Surg 1953;25:600–605.
30. Yeoh CB, Ford JH, Lattes R, et al. Intrapulmonary thymoma. J Thorac Cardiovasc Surg 1966;51:131–136.
31. Kung I, Loke SL, So SY, et al. Intrapulmonary thymoma: report of two cases. Thorax 1985;40:471–474.
32. Fukayama M, Maeda Y, Funata N, et al. Pulmonary and pleural thymoma: diagnostic application of lymphocyte markers to the thymoma of unusual site. Am J Clin Pathol 1988;89:617–621.
33. Begin LR, Eskandari J, Joncas J, et al. Epstein–Barr virus-related lymphoepithelioma-like carcinoma of the lung. J Surg Oncol 1987;36:280–283.
34. Travis WD, Brambilla E, Muller-Hermelink HK, Harris CC, eds. World Health Organization classification of tumours. Pathology and genetics. Lyon: IARC Press, 2004:146.
35. Moran CA, Suster S, Fishback NF, et al. Primary intrapulmonary thymoma. A clinicopathologic and immunohistochemical study of eight cases. Am J Surg Pathol 1995;19: 304–312.
36. Veynovich B, Masetti P, Kaplan PD, et al. Primary pulmonary thymoma. Ann Thorac Surg 1997;64:1471–1473.
37. Colby TV, Koss MN, Travis WD. Atlas of tumor pathology. Tumors of the lower respiratory tract. Washington, DC: Armed Forces Institute of Pathology, 1994:482.
38. Srivastava A, Padilla O, Alroy J, et al. Primary intrapulmonary cell thymoma with marked granulomatous reaction: report of a case with review of the literature. Int J Surg Pathol 2003;11:353–356.
39. Chu PG, Weiss LM. Expression of cytokeratin 5/6 in epithelial neoplasms. An immunohistochemical study of 509 cases. Mod Pathol 2002;15:6–10.
40. DiComo CJ, Urist MJ, Babayan I, et al. p63 expression profiles in human normal and tumor tissues. Clin Cancer Res 2002;8:494–501.
41. Ishibashi H, Takahashi S, Tomoko H, et al. Primary intrapulmonary thymoma successfully resected with vascular reconstruction. Ann Thorac Surg 2003;76:1735–1737.
42. Ohori NP. Uncommon endobronchial neoplasms. In Cagle PT, ed. Diagnostic pulmonary pathology. New York and Basel: Marcel Dekker, 2000:685–717.
43. Cagle P, Mace ML, Judge DM, et al. Pulmonary melanoma; primary versus metastatic. Chest 1984;85:125–126.
44. Taboada CF, McMurray JD, Jordan RA, et al. Primary melanoma of the lung. Chest 1972;62:629–631.
45. Carstens PHB, Kuhns JG, Ghazi C. Primary malignant melanomas of the lung and adrenal. Hum Pathol 1984; 15:910–914.
46. Smith S, Opipari MI. Primary pleural melanoma: a first reported case and literature review. J Thorac Cardiovasc Surg 1978;75:827–831.
47. Das Gupta T, Bowden L, Berg JW. Malignant melanoma of unknown primary origin. Surg Gynecol Obstet 1963;117: 341–345.
48. Allen MS Jr, Drash EC. Primary melanoma of the lung. Cancer 1968;21:154–159.
49. Allen AC, Spitz S. Malignant melanoma: a clinicopathologic analysis of the criteria for diagnosis and prognosis. Cancer 1953;6:1–45.
50. Angel R, Prades M. Primary bronchial melanomas. J Louisiana State Med Soc 1984;136:13–15.
51. Gephardt BN. Malignant melanomas of the bronchus. Hum Pathol 1981;12:671–673.
52. Robertson AJ, Sinclair DJM, Sutton PP, et al. Primary melanocarcinoma of the lower respiratory tract. Thorax 1980;35:158–159.
53. Slam R. A primary malignant melanoma of the bronchus. J Pathol Bacteriol 1963;85:121–126.
54. Jensen OA, Egedorf J. Primary malignant melanoma of the lung. Scand J Respir Dis 1967;48:127–135.
55. Das Gupta T, Brasfield R. Metastatic melanoma. A clinicopathologic study. Cancer 1964; 17:1323–1339.
56. Das Gupta TK, Brasfield RD, Paglia MA. Primary melanomas in unusual sites. Surg Gynecol Obstet 1969;128: 841–848.
57. Walter P, Fernandes C, Florange W. Melanome malin primitif pulmonaire. Ann Anat Pathol (Paris) 1972;17: 91–99.
58. Wilson RW, Moran CA. Primary melanoma of the lung: a clinicopathologic and immunohistochemical study of eight cases. Am J Surg Pathol 1995;21:1196–1202.
59. Reed RJ, Kent EM. Solitary pulmonary melanomas: two case reports. J Thorac Cardiovasc Surg 1964;48:226–231.
60. Rosenberg LM, Polanco GB, Blank S. Multiple tracheobronchial melanomas with ten-year survival. JAMA 1965; 192:717–719.
61. Reid JD, Mehta VT. Melanoma of the lower respiratory tract. Cancer 1965;19:627–631.
62. Ferrara G, Boscaino A, DeRosa G. Bronchial blue naevus. A previously unreported entity. Histopathology 1995;26: 581–583.
63. Korn D, Bensch K, Liebow AA, et al. Multiple minute pulmonary tumors resembling chemodectomas. Am J Pathol 1960;37:641–472.
64. Spencer H. Pathology of the lung. Oxford: Pergamon Press, 1962:690–692.
65. Zak FG, Chabes A. Pulmonary chemodectomatosis. JAMA 1963;183:887–889.
66. Barroso-Moguel R, Costero I. Some histochemical tests in Zak's chemodectomatosis. Am J Pathol 1964;44:17a–18a.
67. Barroso-Moguel R, Costero I. Quimiorreceptores y otras estructuras intrapulmonares argentafines relacionadas con

la regulacion de la circulacion pulmonar. Arch Inst Cardiol Mex 1968;38:337–344.
68. Costero I, Barroso-Moguel R, Martinez-Palomo A. Pleural origin of some of the supposed chemodectomoid structures of the lung. Beitr Pathol 1972; 146:351–365.
69. Spain DM. Intrapulmonary chemodectomas in subjects with organizing pulmonary thromboemboli. Am Rev Respir Dis 1967;96:1158–1164.
70. Ichinose H, Hewitt RL, Drapanas T. Minute pulmonary chemodectomas. Cancer 1971;28:692–700.
71. Ionescu DN, Sajatomi E, Aldeeb D, et al. Pulmonary meningothelial-like nodules. A genotypic comparison with meningiomas. Am J Surg Pathol 2004;28:207–214.
72. Kuhn C III, Askin FB. The fine structure of so-called minute pulmonary chemodectomas. Hum Pathol 1975;6: 681–691.
73. Churg AM, Warnock ML. So-called "minute pulmonary chemodectoma": a tumor not related to paragangliomas. Cancer 1976;37:1759–1769.
74. Kemnitz P, Spormann H, Heinrich P. Meningioma of lung: first report with light and electron microscopic findings. Ultrastruct Pathol 1982;3:359–365.
75. Chumas JC, Lorelle CA. Pulmonary meningioma. A light- and electron-microscopic study. Am J Surg Pathol 1982;6: 795–801.
76. Zhang FL, Cheng XR, Zhang XS, et al. Lung ectopic meningioma: a case report. Chin Med J 1983;96:309–311.
77. Strimlan CV, Golembiewski RS, Celko DA, et al. Primary pulmonary meningioma. Surg Neurol 1988;29:410–413.
78. Kodama K, Doi O, Higashiyama M, Horai T, et al. Primary and metastatic pulmonary meningioma. Cancer 1991;67:1412–1417.
79. Flynn DS, Yousem SA. Pulmonary meningioma: a report of two cases. Hum Pathol 1991;22:469–474.
80. Drlicek M, Grisold W, Lorber J, et al. Pulmonary meningioma: immunohistochemical and ultrastructural features. Am J Surg Pathol 1991;15:455–459.
81. Moran CA, Hochholzer L, Rush W, et al. Primary intrapulmonary meningiomas. A clinicopathologic and immunohistochemical study of 10 cases. Cancer 1996;78: 2328–2333.
82. Unger PD, Geller SA, Anderson PJ. Pulmonary lesions in a patient with neurofibromatosis. Arch Pathol Lab Med 1984;108:654–657.
83. Kepes JJ. Meningiomas in unusual sites. In: Kepes JJ, ed. Meningiomas: biology, pathology, and differential diagnosis. New York: Masson, 1982:44–47.
84. Wilson AJ, Ratliff JL, Lagios MD, et al. Mediastinal meningioma. Am J Surg Pathol 1979;3:557–562.
85. Erlandson RA. Diagnostic transmission electron microscopy of human tumors. In: Erlandson RA, ed. Monographs in diagnostic pathology. Vol. 3. New York: Masson, 1982: 125–128.
86. Karasick JL, Mullan SF. A survey of metastatic meningiomas. J Neurosurg 1974;39:206–212.
87. Stoller JK, Kavuru M, Mehta AC, et al. Intracranial meningioma metastatic to the lung. Cleve Clin J Med 1987;54: 521–527.
88. Hasleton PS. Benign lung tumors and their malignant counterparts. In Hasleton PS, ed. Spencer's pathology of the lung. 5th ed. New York, St. Louis, San Francisco: McGraw-Hill, 1996:875–989.
89. Prayson R, Farver CF. Primary pulmonary malignant meningioma. Am J Surg Pathol 1999;23:722–726.
90. Comin CE, Caldarella A, Novelli L, et al. Primary pulmonary meningioma. Report of a case and review of the literature. Tumori 2003;89:102–105.
91. Hoye SJ, Hoar CS, Murray JE. Extracranial meningioma presenting as a tumor of the neck. Am J Surg 1960;100: 486–489.
92. Rosenblum MC, Bilbao JM, Ang L-C. Neuromuscular system. In: Rosai and Ackerman's surgical pathology. 9th ed. Edinburgh, London, New York: Mosby, 2004:2461–2622.
93. Crotty TB, Hooker RP, Swenson SJ, et al. Primary malignant ependymoma of the lung. Mayo Clin Proc 1992;67: 373–378.
94. Doglioni C, Bontempini L, Luzzolino P, et al. Ependymoma of the mediastinum. Arch Pathol Lab Med 1988; 112:194–196.
95. Nobles E, Lee R, Kircher T. Mediastinal ependymoma. Hum Pathol 1991;22:94–96.
96. Hasleton P. Biphasic pulmonary neoplasms. In: Cagle PT, ed. Diagnostic pulmonary pathology. New York and Basel: Marcel-Dekker, 2000:665–683.
97. Kakkar N, Vasishta RK, Benergee AK, et al. Primary pulmonary malignant teratoma with yolk sac element associated with hematological neoplasia. Respiration 1996; 63:52–54.
98. Holt S, Deverall PB, Boddy JE. A teratoma of the lung containing thymic tissue. J Pathol 1978;126:85–89.
99. Pound AW, Willis RA. A malignant teratoma of the lung in an infant. J Pathol 1969;98:111–114.
100. Jamieson MPG, McGowan AR. Endobronchial teratoma. Thorax 1982;37:157–159.
101. Cloetta. Ober das Vorkommen einer Dermoidcyste in der Lunge. Virchow Arch Pathol Anat 1861;20:42–44 (as cited by von Mohr. Medizinsche Zietung. Berlin, 1839:S130.)
102. Laffitte H. Embryome teratoide intra-pulmonaire. Exerese en un temps. Mem Acad de Chir (Paris) 1937;63:1076–1085.
103. Day DW, Taylor SA. An intrapulmonary teratoma associated with thymic tissue. Thorax 1975;30:582–587.
104. Gonzalez-Cruzzi F. Extragonadal teratomas. Washington, DC: Armed Forces Institute of Pathology, 1982:184–186.
105. Travis WD, Colby TV, Corrin B, et al. World Health Organization. International classification of lung and pleural tumours. 3rd ed. Berlin, Heidelberg, New York: Springer, 1999.
106. Toda S, Inoue Y, Ishino T, et al. A rare case of primary pulmonary choriocarcinoma in a male: immunohistochemical detection for human chorionic gonadotrophin hormone, epidermal growth factor (EGF) and EGF-receptor. Endocr J 1995;42:655–659.
107. Abu-Farsakh H, Fraire AE. Adenocarcinoma and (extra gonadal) choriocarcinoma of the gallbladder in a young woman. Hum Pathol 1991;22:614–615.
108. Liu Z, Mira JL, Cruz-Caudillo JC. Primary gastric choriocarcinoma. Arch Pathol Lab Med 2001;125:1601–1604.
109. Arslanian A, Pischedda F, Filosso PL. Primary choriocarcinoma of the lung. J Thorac Cardiovasc Surg 2003;125: 193–196.

110. Corrin B, ed. Pathology of the lungs. London, Edinburgh, New York: Churchill Livingstone,2000:523.
111. Chen F, Tatsumi A, Numoto S. Combined choriocarcinoma and adenocarcinoma of the lung occurring in a man. Cancer 2001;91:123–129.
112. Van Nostrand KM, Lucci JA, Liao S-Y, et al. Primary lung choriocarcinoma masquerading as a metastatic gestational neoplasm. Gynecol Oncol 1994;53:361–365.
113. Sridhar KS, Saldana MJ, Thurer RJ, et al. Primary choriocarcinoma of the lung: report of a case treated with multimodality therapy and review of the literature. J Surg Oncol 1989;41:93–97.
114. Canver CC, Voytovich MC. Resection of an unsuspected primary pulmonary choriocarcinoma. Ann Thorac Surg 1996;61:1249–1251.
115. Rosenberg AE. Bone, joints and soft tissue tumors. In: Kumar V, Abbas AK, Fausto N, eds. Robbins and Cotran's pathologic basis of disease. 7th ed. Philadelphia: Elsevier-Saunders, 2005:1273–1324.
116. Rosai J. Rosai and Ackerman's surgical pathology. 9th ed. Edinburgh, London, New York: Mosby, 2004:3409–2313.
117. Ordoñez NG, Mahfouz SM, Mackay B. Synovial sarcoma: an immunohistochemical and ultrastructural study. Hum Pathol 1990;21:733–749.
118. Karn CM, Socinski MA, Fletcher JA, et al. Cardiac synovial sarcoma with translocation (X;18) associated with asbestos exposure. Cancer 1994;73:74–78.
119. Gaertuer E, Zeren EH, Fleming MV, et al. Biphasic synovial sarcoma arising in the pleural cavity. A clinicopathologic study of five cases. Am J Surg Pathol 1996;20:36–45.
120. Kashima T, Matsushita H, Kuroda M, et al. Case report: biphasic synovial sarcoma of the peritoneal cavity with t(X;18) demonstrated by reverse transcriptase polymerase chain reaction. Pathol Int 1997;47:637–641.
121. Zeren H, Moran CA, Suster S. Primary pulmonary sarcomas with features of monophasic synovial sarcoma. A clinico-pathologic study of 25 cases. Hum Pathol 1995;26:474–480.
122. Roberts CA, Seemayer TA, Neff JR. Translocation (X;18) in primary synovial sarcoma of the lung. Cancer Genet Cytogenet 1996;88:49–52.
123. Hisaoka M, Hashimoto H, Iwamasa T, et al. Primary synovial sarcoma of the lung: report of two cases confirmed by molecular detection of SYT-SSX fusion gene transcripts. Histopathology 1999;34:205–210.
124. Hammar SP. Lung and pleural neoplasms. In: Dabbs DJ, ed. Diagnostic immunohistochemistry. Philadelphia: Churchill Livingstone, 2002:267–312.
125. Liebow AA, Hubbell DS. Sclerosing hemangioma (histiocytoma, xanthoma) of the lung. Cancer 1956;9:53–75.
126. Goorwitch J, Madoff I. Capillary hemangioma of the lung. Dis Chest 1955;28:98–103.
127. Katzenstein A-LA, Gmelich JT, Carrington CB. Sclerosing hemangioma of the lung: a clinicopathologic study of 51 cases. Am J Surg Pathol 1980;4:343–356.
128. Chan KW, Gibbs AR, Lio WS, et al. Benign sclerosing pneumocytoma of the lung (sclerosing hemangioma). Thorax 1982;37:404–412.
129. Spencer H, Nambu S. Sclerosing hemangioma of the lung. Histopathology 1986;10:477–487.
130. Thomas A, Lee CN. Sclerosing haemangioma in Singapore. Ann Acad Med Singapore 1986;15:71–76.
131. Haimoto H, Tsutsumi Y, Nagura H, et al. Immunohistochemical study of so-called sclerosing haemangioma of the lung. Virchow Arch [A] 1985;407:419–430.
132. Nagata N, Dairaku M, Sueishi K, et al. Sclerosing hemangioma of the lung: an epithelial tumor composed of immunohistochemically heterogeneous cells. Am J Clin Pathol 1987;88:552–559.
133. Yousem SA, Wick MR, Singh G, et al. So-called sclerosing hemangiomas of lung: an immunohistochemical study supporting a respiratory epithelial origin. Am J Surg Pathol 1988;12:582–590.
134. Aiba M, Hirayama A, Sakurada M, et al. So-called sclerosing hemangioma of the lung with nuclear inclusion bodies: immunohistochemical study of a case. Acta Pathol Jpn 1988;38:873–881.
135. Chan ACL, Chan JKC. Pulmonary sclerosing hemangioma consistently expresses thyroid transcription factor-1 (TTF-1). A new clue to histogenesis. Am J Surg Pathol 2000;24:1531–1536.
136. Nicholson AG, Magkou C, Snead D, et al. Unusual sclerosing hemangiomas and sclerosing hemangiomas-like lesions, and the value of TTF-1 in making the diagnosis. Histopathology 2002;41:404–413.
137. Wang E, Lin D, Wang Y, et al. Immunohistochemical and ultrastructural markers suggest different origins for cuboidal and polygonal cells in pulmonary sclerosing hemangioma. Hum Pathol 2004;35:503–508.
138. Devoussoux-Shisheboran M, Hayashi T, Linnoila RI, et al. A clinicopathologic study of 100 cases of pulmonary sclerosing hemangioma with immunohistochemical studies. Am J Surg Pathol 2000;24:906–916.
139. Katzenstein A-LA, Weise DL, Fulling K, et al. So-called sclerosing hemangioma of the lung: evidence for mesothelial origin. Am J Surg Pathol 1983;7:3–16.
140. Fraser RS, Muller NL, Colman N, Paré PD, eds. Fraser and Paré's diagnosis of diseases of the chest. 4th ed. Philadelphia, London, Toronto: WB Saunders, 1999:1365.
141. Yano M, Yamakawa Y, Kiriyama M, et al. Sclerosing hemangioma with metastasis to multiple nodal stations. Ann Thorac Surg 2002;73:981–983.
142. Travis WD, Colby TV, Corrin B, et al. World Health Organization. International Histological Classification of Tumours. Histological typing of lung and pleural tumours. Berlin, Heidelberg, New York: Springer, 1999:26.
143. Yousem SA, Hochholzer L. Alveolar adenoma. Hum Pathol 1986;17:1066–1071.
144. Burke LM, Rush WI, Khoor A, et al. Alveolar adenoma: a histochemical, immunohistochemical and ultrastructural analysis of 17 cases. Hum Pathol 1999;30:158–167.
145. Neusuess A, Claviez A, Schroeter T, et al. Brief report: synchronous detection of a pulmonary papillary adenoma and lung metastasis in a patient with osteosarcoma in relapse. Med Pediatr Oncol 2002;38:125–127.
146. Damiani S. Pulmonary papillary adenoma-like tumour arising in ovarian teratoma [letter to the editor]. Virchows Arch 2004;445:96–97.
147. Hegg CA, Flint A, Singh G. Papillary adenomas of the lung. Am J Clin Pathol 1992;97:393–397.

148. Hruby NJ, Gaffey MJ, Mills SE. Miscellaneous tumors. In: Saldana M, ed. Pathology of pulmonary disease. Philadelphia: JB Lippincott, 1994:673–689.
149. Sheppard MN, Burke L, Kennedy M. TTF-1 is useful in the diagnosis of pulmonary papillary adenoma [letter to the editor]. Histopathology 2003;43:397–405.
150. Minami Y, Morishita Y, Yamamoto T, et al. Cytologic characteristics of pulmonary papillary adenoma. Acta Cytol 2004;48:342–248.
151. Colby TV, Koss MN, Travis WD. Miscellaneous benign epithelial tumors. In: Atlas of tumor pathology. Washington, DC: Armed Forces Institute of Pathology, 1994:57–63.
152. Popper HH, Jeutner-Smolle FM, Pongratz MG. Micronodular hyperplasia of type II pneumocytes—a new lung lesion associated with tuberous sclerosis. Histopathology 1991;18:347–354.
153. Mori M, Chiba R, Tezuka F, et al. Papillary adenoma of type II pneumocytes may have malignant potential. Virchows Arch 1996;428:195–200.
154. Argüelles M, Blanco I. Inflammatory bronchial polyps associated with asthma. Arch Intern Med 1983;143:570–571.
155. Roberts C, Devenny AM, Brooker R, et al. Inflammatory endobronchial polyposis with bronchiectasis in cystic fibrosis. Eur Respir J 2001;18:612–615.
156. McShane D, Nicholson AG, Goldstraw P, et al. Inflammatory endobronchial polyps in childhood. Pediatr Pulmonol 2002;34:79–84.
157. Mittelman M, Fink G, Mor R, et al. Inflammatory bronchial polyps complicated by massive hemoptysis. Eur J Respir Dis 1986;69:63–66.
158. Niimi A, Amitami R, Ikeda T, et al. Inflammatory bronchial polyps associated with asthma: resolution with inhaled corticosteroids. Eur Respir J 1995;8:1237–1239.
159. Snow N, Fratianne RB. Obstructing endobronchial inflammatory polyps: treatment and urgent laser photo ablation. Trauma 2001;150:753–754.
160. Yamagishi M, Harada H, Kurihara M, et al. Inflammatory endotracheal polyp resolved after antibiotic treatment. Respiration 1993;60:193–196.
161. Liebow AA, Castleman B. Benign "clear cell tumors" of the lung. Am J Pathol 1963;43:13a–14a(abstr).
162. Liebow AA, Castleman B. Benign clear cell ("sugar") tumors of the lung. Yale J Biol Med 1971;43:213–222.
163. Andrion A, Mazzucco G, Gugliotta P, et al. Benign clear cell ("sugar") tumor of the lung. A light microscopic, histochemical, and ultrastructural study with a review of the literature. Cancer 1985;56:2657–2663.
164. Gaffey MJ, Mills SE, Askin FB, et al. Clear cell tumor of the lung. A clinicopathologic, immunohistochemical, and ultrastructural study of eight cases. Am J Surg Pathol 1990;14:248–259.
165. Gaffey MJ, Mills SE, Zabo JR, et al. Clear cell tumor of the lung: immunohistochemical and ultrastructural evidence of melanogenesis. Am J Surg Pathol 1991;15:644–653.
166. Gal AA, Koss MN, Hochholzer L, et al. An immunohistochemical study of benign clear cell ("sugar") tumor of the lung. Arch Pathol Lab Med 1991;115:1034–1038.
167. Becker NH, Soifer I. Benign clear cell tumor ("sugar tumor") of the lung. Cancer 1971;27:712–719.
168. Hoch WS, Patchefsky AS, Takeda M, et al. Benign clear cell tumor of lung: an ultrastructural study. Cancer 1974:33:1328–1336.
169. Fletcher CDM, Unni KK, Mertens F. WHO classification of tumours. Pathology and genetics. Tumours of soft tissue and bone. Lyon: IARC Press, 2002:221.
170. Sale GE, Kulander BG. Benign clear cell tumor of lung with necrosis. Cancer 1976;37:2355–2358.
171. Lantuejoul S, Isaac S, Pinel N, et al. Clear cell tumor of the lung: an immunohistochemical and ultrastructural study supporting a pericytic differentiation. Mod Pathol 1997; 10:1001–1008.
172. Sale GE, Kulander BG. Benign clear cell ("sugar") tumor of lung. Arch Pathol Lab Med 1988;113:574.
173. Walter JB, Pryce DM. The histology of lung cancer. Thorax 1955;10:107–116.
174. Katzenstein A-LA, Prioleau PG, Askin FB. The histologic spectrum and significance of clear-cell change in lung carcinoma. Cancer 1980;45:943–947.
175. Edwards C, Carlile A. Clear cell carcinoma of the lung. J Clin Pathol 1985;38:880–885.
176. Gaffey MJ, Mills SE, Frierson HF. Pulmonary clear cell carcinoid tumor. Another entity in the differential diagnosis of pulmonary clear cell neoplasia. Am J Surg Pathol 1998;22:1020–1025.
177. Fraser RS, Muller NL, Colman N, Paré PD. Diagnosis of diseases of the chest. 4th ed. Philadelphia, London, Toronto: WB Saunders, 1999:1363–1380.
178. Sale GE, Kulander BG. "Benign" clear-cell tumor (sugar tumor) of the lung with hepatic metastases ten years after resection of pulmonary primary tumor. Arch Pathol Lab Med 1988;112:1177–1178.
179. Ostermiller WE, Comer TP, Barker WL. Endobronchial granular cell myoblastoma. Ann Thorac Surg 1970;9: 143–148.
180. Oparah SS, Subramanian VA. Granular cell myoblastoma of the bronchus: report of two cases and review of the literature. Ann Thorac Surg 1976;22:199–202.
181. DeClercq D, Van der Straeten M, Roels H. Granular cell myoblastoma of the bronchus. Eur J Respir Dis 1983; 64:72–76.
182. Redjaee B, Kumar-Rohatgi PK, Herman MA. Multicentric endobronchial granular cell myoblastoma. Chest 1990;98: 945–948.
183. Gabriel JB Jr, Thomas L, Mendoza CB, et al. Granular cell tumor of the bronchus coexisting with bronchogenic adenocarcinoma: a case report. Chest 1975;68:256–258.
184. Deavers M, Guinee D, Koss MN, et al. Granular cell tumors of the lung. Clinicopathologic study of 20 cases. Am J Surg Pathol 1995;19:627–635.
185. Abdulhamid I, Rabah R. Granular cell tumor of the bronchus. Pediatr Pulmonol 2000;30:425–428.
186. Villena V, Asencio Sanchez S, de Miguel Poch E, et al. Tracheobronchial granular cell tumors. A report of 8 cases. Arch Bronconeumol 1997;33:434–437.
187. Sobel HJ, Marquet E. Granular cells and granular cell lesions. Pathol Annu 1974;9:43–79.
188. Ohnesorge B, Gehlen H, Wohlsein P. Transendoscopic electrosurgery of an equine pulmonary granular cell tumor. Vet Surg 2002;31:375–378.

189. Gabriel JR, Jr, Thomas L, Kondlapoodi P, et al. Granular cell tumor of the bronchus: a previously unreported cause of hypercalcemia. J Surg Oncol 1983;24:338–340.
190. Hurwitx SS, Conlan AA, Gritzman MCD, et al. Coexisting granular cell myoblastoma and squamous carcinoma of the bronchus. Thorax 1982;37:292–393.
191. Hosaka T, Susuki S, Niikawa H, et al. A rare case of pulmonary granular cell tumor presenting as a coin lesion. Jpn J Thorac Cardiovasc Surg 2003;51:107–109.
192. Park SH, Kim TJ, Chi JG. Congenital granular cell tumor with systemic involvement: immunohistochemical and ultrastructural study. Arch Pathol Lab Med 1991;115: 934–938.
193. Le BH, Boyer PJ, Lewis JE, et al. Granular cell tumor. Immunohistochemical assessment of inhibin x protein gene product 9.8, S-100 protein, CD68 and Ki-67 proliferative index with clinical correlation. Arch Pathol Lab Med 2004;128:771–775.
194. Alvarez-Fernandez E, Carretero-Albinana L. Bronchial granular cell tumor: presentation of three cases with tissue culture and ultrastructural study. Arch Pathol Lab Med 1987;111:1065–1069.
195. Lauro S, Trasatti L, Bria E, et al. Malignant bronchial Abrikossoff's tumor and small cell lung cancer: a case report and review. Anticancer Res 2001;21:563–566.
196. Ogino S, Al-Kaisi N, Abdul-Karim FW. Cytopathology of oncocytic carcinoid tumor of the lung mimicking granular cell tumor. A case report. Acta Cytol 2000;44:247–250.
197. Jiang M, Anderson T, Nwogu C, et al. Pulmonary malignant granular cell tumor. World J Surg Oncol 2003; 1:22.
198. Epstein LJ, Mohsenifar Z. Use of Nd:YAG laser in endobronchial granular cell myoblastoma. Chest 1993;104: 958–960.
199. Travis WD, Colby TV, Corrin B, et al., eds. WHO international histological classification of tumours. Histological typing of lung and pleural tumours. 3rd ed. Berlin, Heidelberg, New York: Springer, 1999:57–58.
200. Singh G, Lee RE, Brooks DH. Primary pulmonary paraganglioma: report of a case and review of the literature. Cancer 1977;40:2286–2289.
201. Mostecky H, Lichtenberg J, Kalus M. A non-chromaffin paraganglioma of the lung. Thorax 1966;21:205–208.
202. Laustela E, Mattila S, Franssila K. Chemodectoma of the lung. Scand J Cardiovasc Surg 1969;3:59–62.
203. Lee YN, Hori JM. Chemodectoma of the lung. J Surg Oncol 1972;4:33–36.
204. Blessing MH, Borchard F, Lenz W. Glomustumor (sog chemodektom) der Lunge. Virchows Arch [A] 1973; 359: 315–329.
205. Scopsi L, Collins P and Muscolino G. A new observation on the Carney's triad with long follow-up period and additional tumors. Cancer Detect Prev 1999;23:435–443.
206. Lack EE. Pathology of adrenal and extraadrenal paraganglia. Philadelphia: WB Saunders, 1994:1–350.
207. Corrin B. Pathology of the lungs. London, Edinburgh, New York: Churchill Livingstone, 2000:538.
208. Jones TM, Alderson D, Sheard JDH, et al. Tracheal paraganglioma: a diagnostic dilemma culminating in a complex management problem. J Laryngol Otol 2001;115:747–749.
209. Hangartner JR, Loosemore TM, Burke M, et al. Malignant primary pulmonary paraganglioma. Thorax 1989;44:154–156.
210. Shibahara J, Goto A, Niki T, et al. Primary pulmonary paraganglioma. Report of a functioning case with immunohistochemical and ultrastructural study. Am J Surg Pathol 2004;28:825–829.
211. Kim MK, Park SH, Cho HD, et al. Fine needle aspiration cytology of primary pulmonary paraganglioma. A case report. Acta Cytol 2001;45:459–464.
212. Hironaka M, Fukayama M, Takayashiki N, et al. Pulmonary gangliocytic paraganglioma. Case report and comparative immunohistochemical study of related neuroendocrine neoplasms. Am J Surg Pathol 2001;25: 688–693.
213. Lemonick DM, Pai PB, Hines GL. Malignant primary pulmonary paraganglioma with hilar metastases [letter]. J Thorac Cardiovasc Surg 1990;99:563–564.
214. Linnoila RI, Becker RL, Steinberg SM, et al. The role of S-100 protein containing cells in the prognosis of sympathoadrenal paragangliomas. Mod Pathol 1993;6:39A.
215. Linnoila RI, Lack EE, Steinberg SM, et al. Decreased expression of neuropeptides in malignant paragangliomas: an immunohistochemical study. Hum Pathol 1988;19: 41–50.
216. Flieder D, Koss MN, Nicholson A, et al. Solitary pulmonary papillomas in adults: a clinicopathologic and in situ hybridization study of 14 cases combined with 27 cases in the literature. Am J Surg Pathol 1998;22:1328–1342.
217. Popper HH, El-Shabrawi Y, Wockel W, et al. Prognostic importance of human papillomavirus typing in squamous cell papilloma of the bronchus: comparison of in-situ hybridization and the polymerase chain reaction. Hum Pathol 1994;25:1191–1197.
218. Clavel CE, Nawrocki B, Boxxeaux B, et al. Detection of human papillomavirus DNA in bronchopulmonary carcinomas by hybrid capture II. A study of 185 tumors. Cancer 2000;88:1347–1352.
219. Trillo A, Guha A. Solitary conlylomatous papilloma of the bronchus. Arch Pathol Lab Med 1988;112:731–733.
220. Rady PL, Schnadig VJ, Weiss RL, Hughes TK, Tyring SK. Malignant transformation of recurrent respiratory papillomatosis associated with integrated human papillomavirus type II DNA and mutation of p53. Laryngoscope 1998;108:735–740.
221. Gupta D, Holla J, Layfield L. Topoisomerase alpha II, retinoblastoma gene product and p53: potential relationships with aggressive behavior and malignant transformation in recurrent respiratory papillomatosis. Appl Immunohistochm Mol Morphol 2001;9:86–91.
222. Dail DH. Uncommon Tumors. In, Pulmonary Pathology (2nd ed.), DH Dail and SP Hammar, eds. Springer–Verlag, New York, 1993, pp.1295–1303. .
223. Fraire AE, Ch 25 Non Malignant Versus Malignant Prolfieration on Lung Biopsy. In: Diagnostic Pulmonary Pathology, Cagle PT, Ed. Marcel-Dekker, Inc New York-Basel 2000, pp 525–545.
224. Basheda S, Gephardt GN, Stoller JK. Columnar papilloma of the bronchus. Case report and literature review. Am Rev Respir Dis 1991;144:1400–1402.

42
Pediatric Tumors

J. Thomas Stocker, Aliya N. Husain, and Louis P. Dehner

Some pulmonary lesions of an overtly neoplastic or quasi-neoplastic nature present in the first two decades of life proportionately less frequently than in adults. However, the major category of malignant tumors involving the lung in both children and adults is similar; that category is metastatic disease, which in adults is usually a carcinoma or melanoma and in children is rhabdomyosarcoma, osteosarcoma, Ewing sarcoma–primitive neuroectodermal tumor, germ cell neoplasms, and Wilms' tumor. Unusual sources of metastatic disease to the lungs in children include chordoma, epithelioid hemangioendothelioma, malignant fibrous histiocytoma, and neuroblastoma. The lungs are also important sites for the quasi-neoplastic processes, Langerhans cell histiocytosis (histiocytosis X), and juvenile xanthogranuloma as infiltrates or reticulonodular densities.

Only a few collected reviews or experiences exist in the literature on the topic of primary lung tumors in children. Hartman and Shochat[1] reviewed the English-language literature through 1982 on the subject; they identified 230 cases of primary tumors of the lungs in children, 79 benign and 151 malignant. Stocker[2] compiled the experience of the Armed Forces Institute of Pathology, which constitutes 166 primary pulmonary tumors in individuals 21 years of age or younger at diagnosis (Table 42.1). Malignant neoplasms were more common than benign ones in both series. Inflammatory myofibroblastic tumor (also called inflammatory pseudotumor), was the most common benign tumor, whereas carcinoid was the most common malignant neoplasm in these two series.

Inflammatory Myofibroblastic Tumor

Inflammatory myofibroblastic tumor (IMT)(also called inflammatory pseudotumor and plasma cell granuloma) is the most common primary neoplasm of the lung in children, and children account for 25% to 40% of IMTs in all age groups.[3] It presents as a mass with or without accompanying localized or generalized clinical manifestations.[4–6] Evidence to date would appear to support the conclusion that IMT is a true neoplasm as evidenced by translocations in the ALK receptor tyrosine-kinase receptor region at chromosome 2p23. In the lung approximately 50% to 80% IMTs have the translocation.[7–10]

The lung is the most frequent site of IMT, and similar tumors have been documented in the trachea or bronchus and various extrapulmonary locations including the mesentery, liver, spleen, mediastinum, central nervous system, and soft tissues.[6,11–25] More than one site may be involved in a minority of cases. When the lung is involved, there is a slight predilection for the right side[4] (Fig. 42.1). Some of the more important manifestations of pulmonary and extrapulmonary IMTs are summarized and compared in Table 42.2. When symptomatic, chief complaints include cough (44.4%), chest pain (29.6%), fever (22.2%), hemoptysis (15%), sputum (15%), and dyspnea (11.1%).[4] Interleukin-1, interleukin-6, and tumor necrosis factor, which are secreted by macrophages, fibroblasts, and other constituent cells of an IMT, may be important mediators of the accompanying systemic manifestations. IMT may be one of several types of inflammatory pseudotumors whose etiologies may include one or another infectious cause such as Epstein-Barr virus and human herpesvirus-8.

Agrons et al.[26] noted the radiographic features in 61 cases of IMT, with 52 patients (85%) having a solitary peripheral nodule or mass and 11 (18%) having extraparenchymal involvement. By computed tomography (CT), 12 lesions were of heterogeneous attenuation and five homogeneous.

Grossly, the usual appearance is of a firm, sharply circumscribed, but nonencapsulated intrapulmonary mass measuring 4 to 6cm in diameter and showing a whorled to homogeneous, grayish-white to focal yellowish-white cut surface (Fig. 42.2). An intrapulmonary mass with contiguous extension to local structures such as the pericardium, esophagus, parietal pleura, mediastinum,[27] left atrium,[28] diaphragm,[29] and regional blood vessels is

TABLE 42.1. Primary pulmonary tumors in children

Benign	
Inflammatory myofibroblastic tumor	52
Chondromatous hamartoma	3
Granular cell tumor	3
Leiomyoma	2
Bronchial chondroma	1
Teratoma	1
Total:	62
Malignant	
Bronchial	
Carcinoid	35
Mucoepidermoid carcinoma	9
Adenoid cystic carcinoma	2
Subtotal:	46
Bronchogenic carcinoma	
Adenocarcinoma	14
Squamous cell carcinoma	7
Small cell carcinoma	3
Large cell carcinoma	3
Subtotal:	27
Sarcoma	
Fibrosarcoma	8
Rhabdomyosarcoma	7
Leiomyosarcoma	6
Undifferentiated sarcoma	4
Subtotal:	25
Pulmonary blastoma	6
Total:	104

Compiled from cases seen at the Armed Forces Institute of Pathology, 1950–1989 (166 cases).
Source: Modified from Stocker,[2] with permission.

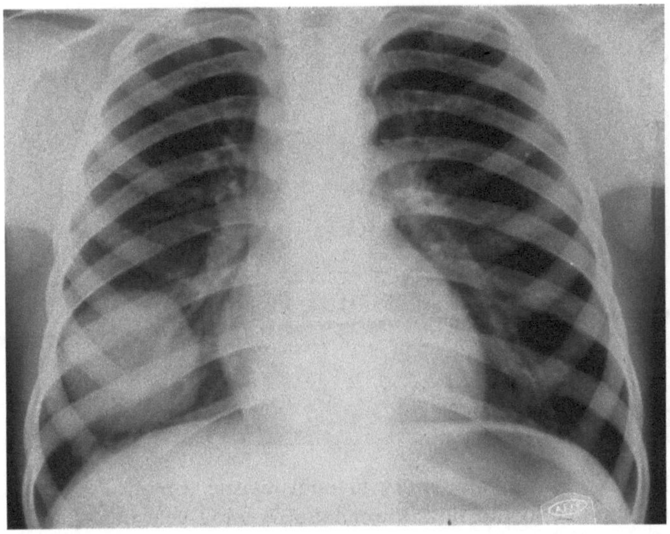

FIGURE 42.1. Inflammatory myofibroblastic tumor. The right lower lobe of a 2-year-old boy contains a mass that appears well circumscribed.

present in a minority of cases.[26,30] Calcifications are present grossly or microscopically in 25% to 30% of IMTs. Several microscopic patterns may be recognized in a single mass, although one is usually predominant (Fig. 42.3; also see also Fig. 37.8 in Chapter 37 and Fig. 39.2 in Chapter 39). Matsubara et al.[31] identified three histologic patterns: organizing pneumonia, fibrous histiocytoma, and lymphoplasmacytic type. We have seen a few cases whose predominant feature was a myxomatous stroma with a component of plasma cells rather than bundles of spindle cells with a storiform configuration. In all cases the number and distribution of lymphocytes, plasma cells, and foamy histiocytes vary from one microscopic field to another and from one tumor to another. Foamy histiocytes and a spindle cell stroma with a storiform arrangement are responsible for the fibrous histiocytoma-like pattern. The presence of neoplastic round cells is cause for concern about overt malignant transformation.

The differential diagnosis of the IMT is organizing pneumonitis, fibrous histiocytoma, sclerosing hemangioma, and smooth muscle neoplasm. If the tissue is limited in amount, it may be difficult to differentiate among these spindle cell proliferations. There is sufficient histologic overlap that some diagnostic uncertainty may still exist even after a thorough pathologic examination of the

TABLE 42.2. Comparison of pulmonary and extrapulmonary inflammatory (myofibroblastic) pseudotumors

	Pulmonary	Extrapulmonary
Age	40% in first two decades	90% in first two decades
Sex	Males = females	Slight female predominance
Presentation	30–40% asymptomatic	67% with generalized manifestations
Laboratory	Infrequently documented, but a few cases with anemia, thrombocytosis, elevated ESR, hyperglobulinemia	Anemia, thrombocytosis, elevated ESR, hyperglobulinemia in patients with abdominal tumors
Pathology	Circumscribed mass (1–12 cm) Spindle cells, plasma cells, lymphocytes Fibroblasts and myofibroblasts by EM	Circumscribed mass or polyp (2 mm–36 cm) Spindle cells, plasma cells, lymphocytes Fibroblasts and myofibroblasts by EM
Outcome	Resolution of symptoms and laboratory abnormalities, if present, in majority of cases; rarely recurs	Resolution of symptoms and laboratory abnormalities, if present, in majority of cases; rarely recurs, may persist as incompletely resected mass; one death attributed to persistence

EM, electron microscopy; ESR, erythrocyte sedimentation rate.

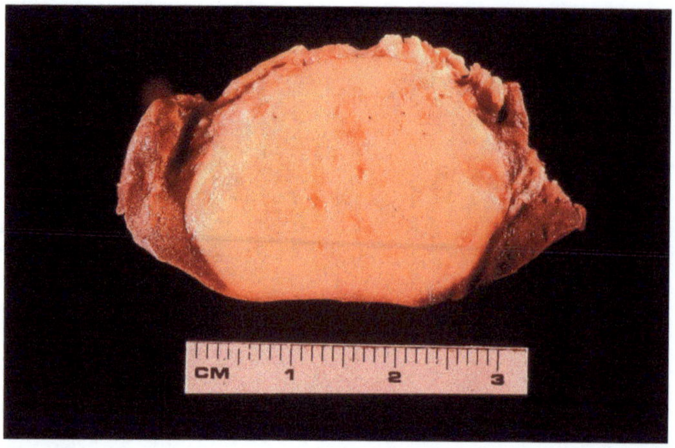

FIGURE 42.2. Inflammatory myofibroblastic tumor. The mass resected from the right-lower lobe of the 2-year-old child in Figure 42.1 was nonencapsulated and blended into adjacent lung parenchyma. Dystrophic calcification is seen in otherwise homogeneous yellow-tan surface.

resected specimen. The spindle cells in each of these lesions are predominantly myofibroblasts by electron microscopy and immunohistochemical analysis (see Fig. 37.8 in Chapter 37).[32]

Peribronchial Myofibroblastic and Smooth Muscle Tumors

Smooth muscle and peribronchial myofibroblastic tumors can have very similar histologic and immunophenotypic features with the expression of vimentin and smooth muscle actin. However, the clinical settings are often quite separate. The latter tumor is observed in neonates and may be associated with nonimmune hydrops or early-onset respiratory distress with bronchial constriction.[33,34] The peribronchial myofibroblastic tumor is a relatively firm tumor that measures between 1.5 and 14.5 cm in greatest dimension and has a gray-white to

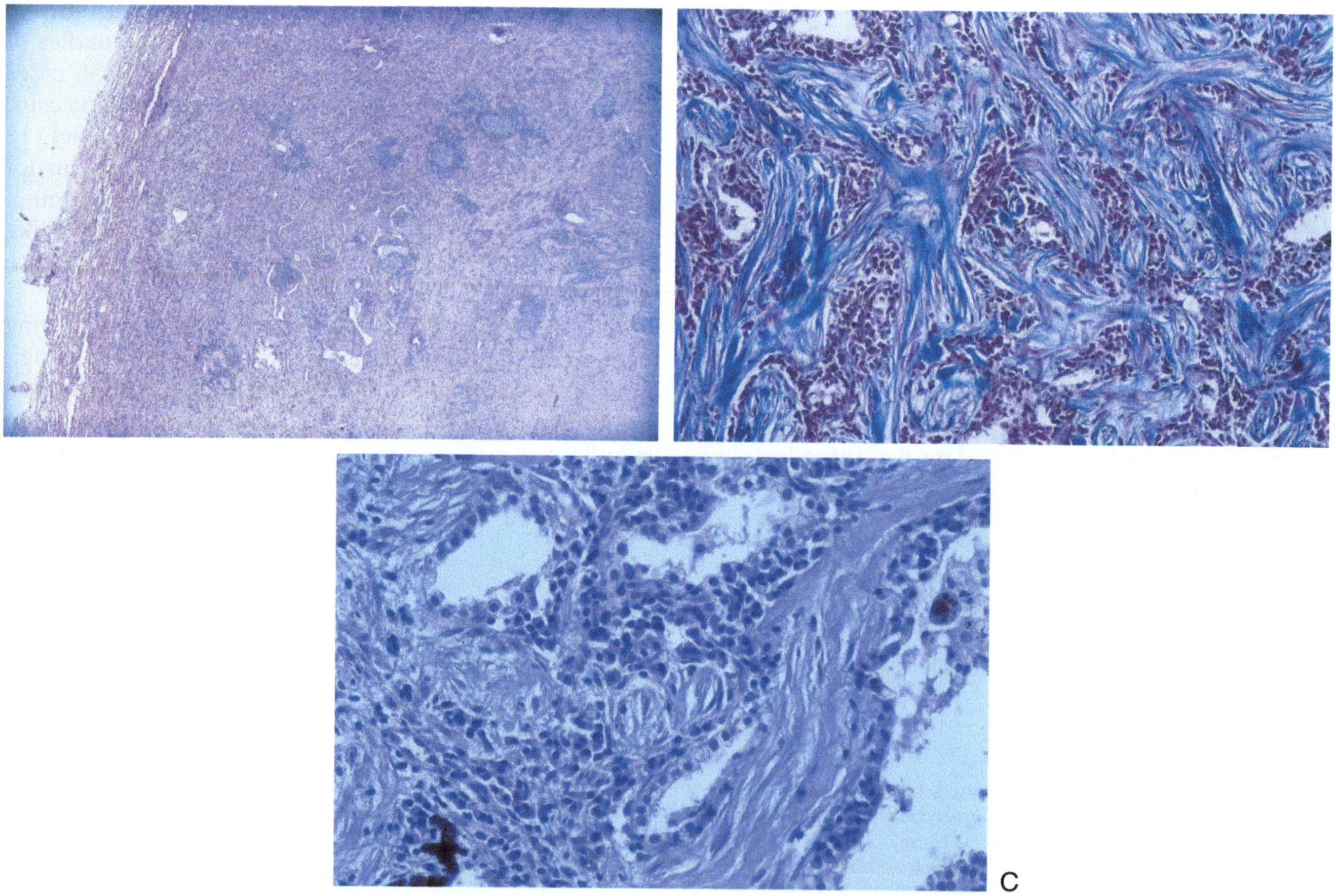

FIGURE 42.3. Inflammatory myofibroblastic tumor. **(A)** The mass is composed of loose to dense fibroblastic tissue suffused with lymphocytes and plasma cells including lymphoid follicles with germinal centers. **(B)** Broad bands of interlacing collagen separate clusters of lymphocytes and plasma cells. Masson trichrome. **(C)** An entrapped bronchiole (right) and an alveolus (upper left) lined by plump cells are separated by bands of collagen and prominent plasma cells.

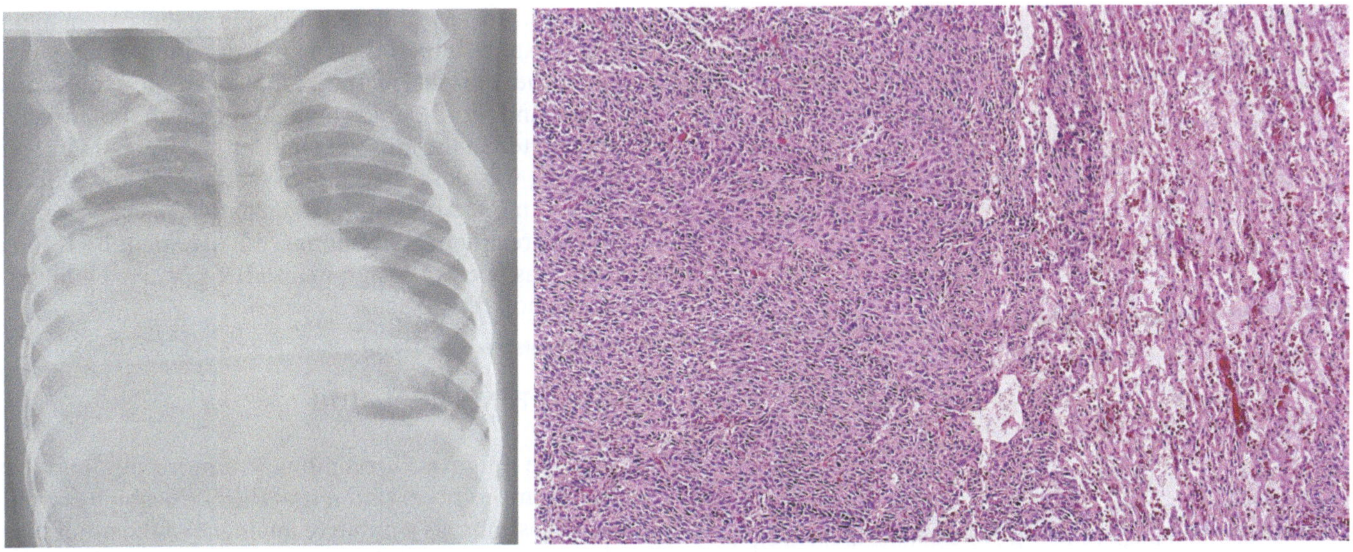

FIGURE 42.4. Congenital–infantile fibrosarcoma. **(A)** At birth this infant was noted to have respiratory distress and a large right pulmonary mass. **(B)** The mass is composed of spindle cells in a vague herringbone pattern that compresses the adjacent lung.

yellow appearance on cut surface. These neoplasms are usually well circumscribed and have rounded to lobulated contours. Focal hemorrhage and cysts are present in some tumors. A dense proliferation of uniform spindle cells with vesicular nuclei and finely granular chromatin is a consistent microscopic feature. Mitotic activity is variable and may be abundant in some cases; the mitotic figures lack atypical or bizarre characteristics. A herringbone pattern of growth is readily apparent in some but not all tumors. Staghorn vascular spaces in a background of compact spindle cells may suggest the diagnosis of hemangiopericytoma. Extramedullary hematopoiesis and cartilaginous foci may be encountered in those tumors that present in the neonatal period. With these histologic features, the tumor resembles congenital–infantile fibrosarcoma (CIF) (Fig. 42.4) and may also have the t(12;15)(p13;q25) translocation. The prognosis for these infants is excellent after successful resection.

More conventional smooth muscle tumors are rare in the lung, regardless of the age at presentation. A smooth muscle neoplasm in a child should be the cause for concern about human immunodeficiency virus (HIV)–acquired immunodeficiency syndrome (AIDS). These tumors are associated with integrated Epstein-Barr virus in the neoplastic cells.[35] The challenge with these tumors is the assignment to a benign or malignant category based on the microscopic features, which can range from quite bland with negligible mitotic activity to a more cellular spindle cell neoplasm with numerous mitotic figures. These tumors qualify as atypical smooth muscle neoplasms, if not leiomyosarcoma. The other myofibroblastic or fibromatous neoplasm of the lung is infantile myofibromatosis as the rare isolated lesion in the lung or as multiple nodules in congenital generalized myofibromatosis. Wiswell et al. (36) reviewed the literature on this topic. Isolated lung involvement appears to have a more favorable outcome, but the infants with generalized myofibroblastic tumors have a poor prognosis, usually ascribable to the pulmonary lesions (37). The histologic features of the nodules are similar to those in the skin and soft tissues with plump spindle cells in a "myxochondroid" background. At autopsy, the pulmonary veins are often partially or totally occluded by the spindle cells, which appear to arise from the subintima of the vessels. The similarities to pulmonary veno-occlusive disease are not surprising in these cases. The so-called fibroleiomyomatous hamartoma, despite its presumed pathogenesis as some type of maldevelopment, does not occur in children to the best of our knowledge.

Cartilaginous Lesions

Cartilaginous lesions are represented by the chondromatous hamartoma and chondroma (Fig. 42.5). The former is encountered principally in adults as a solitary peripheral lobulated mass. A pulmonary chondroma in a young female may be a manifestation of Carney's triad, which also includes extraadrenal paraganglioma and gastrointestinal stromal tumors.[38–40] Metastasis of a gonadal or extragonadal malignant germ cell tumor may consist almost entirely of lobules of cartilage with varying degrees of cellularity and atypia. Cartilage is a component of the so-called pleuropulmonary blastoma, bronchopulmonary fibrosarcoma, and congenital pulmonary airway malformation, type 1. Microscopically, in pleuropulmonary blastoma the cartilage has malignant features in most cases,

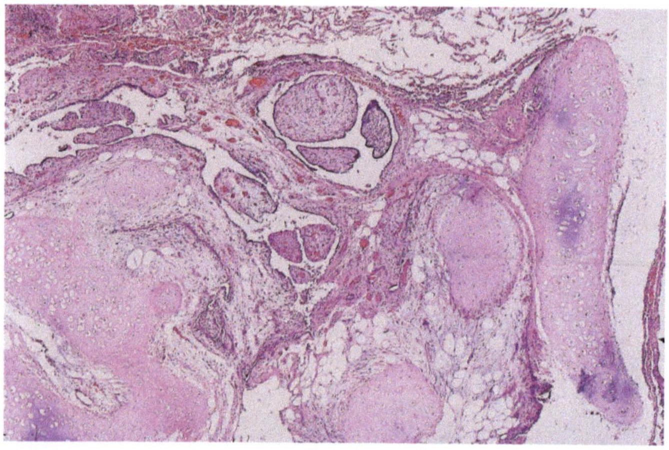

FIGURE 42.5. Chondromatous hamartoma. This peribronchial lesion is composed of islands of cartilage interspersed with fibrovascular and adipose tissue. Note epithelial-lined clefts.

whereas it is more immature or fetal appearing in the other two processes. (See also Chapter 40).

Vascular Neoplasms and Malformations

Vascular neoplasms and malformations or fistulas are in aggregate uncommon in the lung. Arteriovenous malformations are discussed elsewhere (see Chapter 40). Hemangioma or hemangioendothelioma, a relatively common type of mesenchymal neoplasm in children, is rarely encountered in the lung. When the lung is involved, the clinical features and even the gross presentation may suggest an entirely different pathologic process. Capillary-sized vascular spaces replace the parenchyma and may extend into and along existing pulmonary structures at the periphery. Individual examples of Kaposi sarcoma and epithelioid hemangioendothelioma have been reported in the lungs of children.[41,42] Kaposi sarcoma of the lung was described in a 5-year-old child with multicentric tumors; although HIV negative, she was a renal transplant recipient.[43] Pulmonary involvement by Kaposi sarcoma has been reported in an HIV-positive child with lymphadenopathic disease.[44]

Pulmonary Blastoma

One of the enigmas in pulmonary tumor pathology has been the curious observation that the classic, biphasic pulmonary blastoma, as a putative analogue of the other blastematous neoplasms of childhood, occurs predominantly in adults between the ages of 30 and 50 years with only isolated cases in childhood. Approximately 4% of classic pulmonary blastomas are diagnosed in children younger than 10 years of age. These tumors are typical pathologically in all other respects to the pulmonary blastoma in adults (see Chapter 37). The biphasic histologic pattern of fetal-appearing tubules resembling those of the pseudoglandular stage of lung development and a fibrosarcoma-like stroma is the characteristic microscopic finding. It has been suggested that the neoplasm with a pure epithelial pattern be designated as a pulmonary endodermal tumor resembling fetal lung or well-differentiated fetal adenocarcinoma, and it is part of the morphologic spectrum of the pulmonary blastoma (Fig. 42.6). Most examples of well-differentiated fetal adenocarcinoma have been reported in adults[45–47] (see Chapter 35).

A

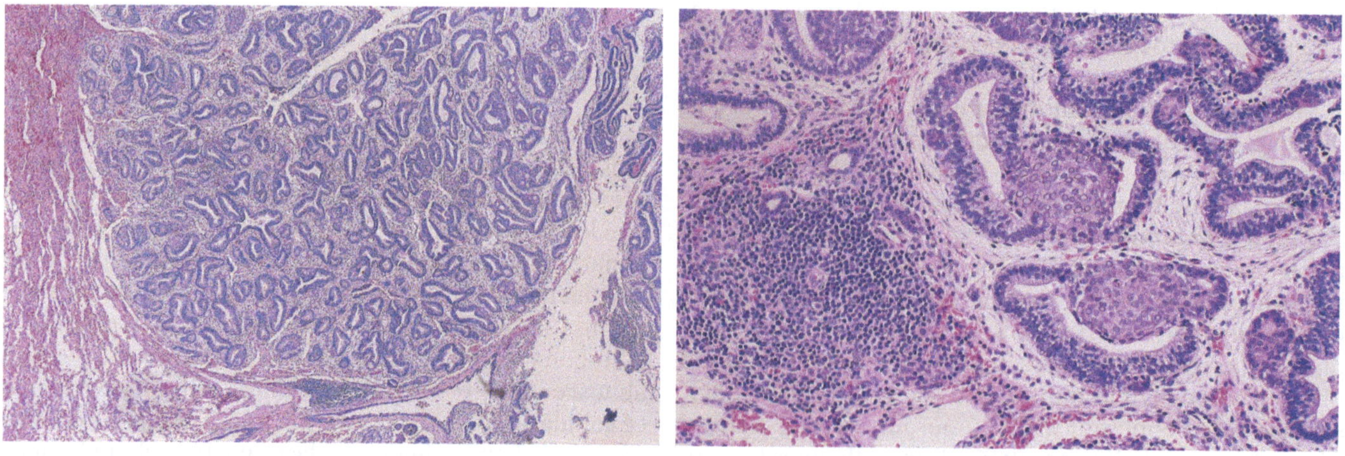

B

FIGURE 42.6. Well-differentiated fetal adenocarcinoma. **(A)** This neoplasm is composed of immature-appearing tubules and glands resembling the pseudoglandular stage of development (see Fig. 6.2 in Chapter 6). **(B)** Some of the "pseudoglands" contain morules of squamous-like epithelial cells.

Pleuropulmonary Blastoma

Pleuropulmonary blastoma (PPB) is a pure mesenchymal neoplasm of pulmonary or extrapulmonary intrathoracic origin that, unlike the classic biphasic pulmonary blastoma, occurs almost exclusively in children and should be regarded as the equivalent neoplasm to the other dysembryonic neoplasms of childhood.[10,45] Pleuropulmonary blastoma is the pulmonary blastoma of childhood.[48] Prior to 1988, examples of PPB had been reported in the literature as simply pulmonary blastoma, rhabdomyosarcoma arising in congenital pulmonary airway malformation or bronchogenic cyst, pulmonary blastoma associated with cystic lung disease, and malignant mesenchymoma in a congenital cyst.[49–51] Since the original report of PPB, we have had the opportunity to review well over 100 cases. One critical point is for the clinician and pathologist to consider the diagnosis of PPB in any infant with a presumed congenital cyst or cysts of the lung in a neonate or young infant.[52–54]

One of us (L.P.D.) has found that PPB has accounted for almost 40% of pulmonary neoplasms in children who have been seen in consultation. We have estimated that as many as 15% of all primary lung neoplasms in childhood are PPBs. Approximately 25% of cases occur in a constitutional or familial setting in which the affected children themselves or other young family members have dysembryonic or neoplastic conditions. These other neoplasms have been embryonal rhabdomyosarcoma, synovial sarcoma, and PPB in first- and second-degree relatives. Colonic polyps, cystic nephroma of the kidney, and neurofibromatosis are some of the additional associations.

The PPB typically presents in the first 4 years of life with symptoms that correlate with the age at presentation and pathologic subtype, of which there are three (types I, II, and III) (Figs. 42.7 to 42.9). Very few cases are diagnosed after 10 years of age, with a few exceptions in adolescents and young adults. In the youngest group, an asymptomatic cyst in the lung may be the only finding, or the lesion is detected after a spontaneous pneumothorax. The median age at diagnosis for the purely cystic PPB type is approximately 9 months. The cystic and solid (II) and solid (III) types are discovered in children whose median ages are 31 and 42 months, respectively. It is thought that the pathologic subtypes from type I to type III reflect tumor progression over time from the prognostically favorable type I to the unfavorable type III. Morphologic complexity and anaplasia are the pathologic correlates of tumor progression from type I and type III.

Imaging studies may reveal only the presence of a cyst or a multicystic structure that is more often in the periphery of the lung. Less often, multiple cysts or the development of new cysts after an initial resection of a solitary cyst may occur.[55] A cyst with a solid component or a mass partially filling the thorax are indicative of the type II or type III PPB, respectively. In the presence of fever and a consolidated lobe, the initial clinical presentation may be pneumonia.

The operative findings reflect the pathologic subtype, from a rather innocuous multicystic, delicately septated structure on the visceral pleura (Fig. 42.7) to a large, poorly delimited mass filling the hemithorax (Fig. 42.9). When the latter is the case, the friable mass is often hemorrhagic and necrotic. An en bloc resection is possible if the tumor is confined to the lung, but extension into the thoracic space is a common finding especially with the solid type III PPB. Infrequently, a PPB may arise on the parietal pleura or diaphragm.

Type I and type II PPBs have similar microscopic features in terms of their cystic component.[56] The epithelium lining of the cysts is usually a single layer of low cuboidal to columnar cells. The stroma contains a population of small primitive dark cells residing beneath the epithelium as a continuous mantle of cells resembling the cambium layer of a botryoid embryonal rhabdomyosarcoma (Fig. 42.7E). Alternatively, the malignant cells are small isolated collections separated by an edematous or fibrous stroma, without obvious atypical cells. Small nodules of primitive or more mature appearing cartilage are useful in alerting the examiner that the cystic structure is more than just another benign cyst. Because the tumor cells can be relatively inconspicuous in terms of density and distribution, it is necessary in some cases to examine an entire cyst microscopically. When rhabdomyoblasts with abundant eosinophilic cytoplasm are differentiated, the diagnosis of a PPB can be made with a greater sense of confidence. Immunopositivity more often than not confirms the histologic impressions of myogenic differentiation, but the absence of staining should not convey a sense that the lesion is benign, since the primitive tumor cells may only express vimentin.

The solid areas of type II and the solid type III PPB have a more complex and diverse histologic appearance, which is almost always the case in the type III PPB. Islands of blastema resembling the blastema (Fig. 42.8C) of a Wilms' tumor may merge into embryonal rhabdomyosarcomatous foci with interspersed areas of high-grade spindle cell sarcoma. Small to large nodules of cartilage are found in a substantial proportion of type III PPBs. Large anaplastic cells with bizarre mitotic figures are mainly restricted to the type III PPB (Fig. 42.9E). The latter cells display nuclear staining for p53. No type II or type III PPB has an identical microscopic appearance in terms of the distribution or dominance of one pattern over another. The solid areas of a type II PPB may only be represented by blastemal and rhabdomyosarcomatous patterns. The type III PPB is more likely to have foci of hemorrhage and necrosis.

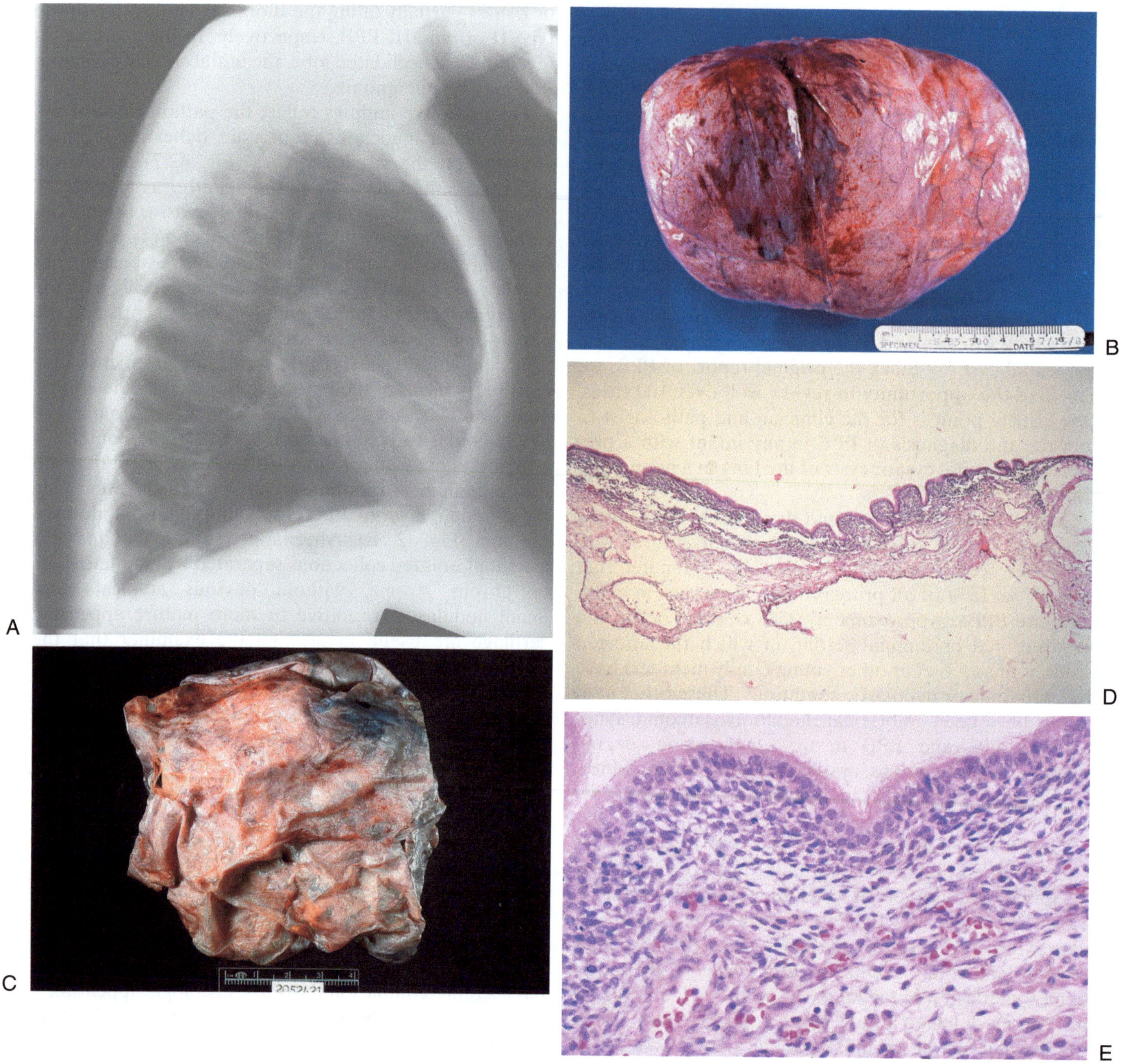

FIGURE 42.7. Pleuropulmonary blastoma, type I. **(A)** A 14-month-old boy with mild respiratory distress has a cystic lesion in the right lower lobe. **(B,C)** The resected lesion is composed of a large cyst with a thin smooth surface. No solid component was present. **(D)** The cyst wall consists of fibrovascular connective tissue covered by an epithelium that consists of ciliated columnar cells overlying a submucosal collection of "small, round blue cells." **(E)** The submucosal cells form a "cambium layer" similar to that of embryonal rhabdomyosarcoma with greater density of cells immediately beneath the mucosa and more widely separated cells further away from the mucosa.

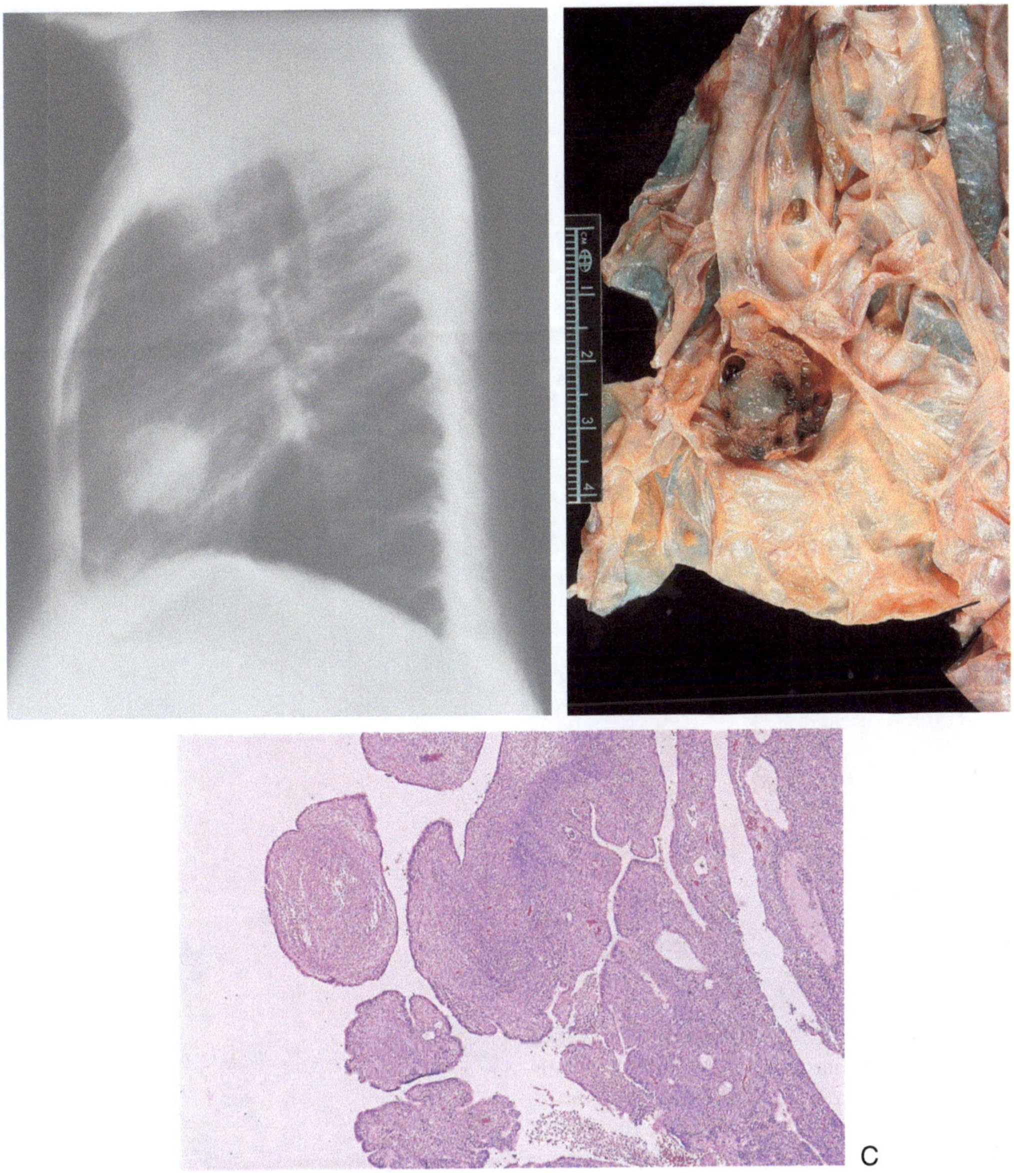

FIGURE 42.8. Pleuropulmonary blastoma, type II. **(A)** A 2-year-old boy has a cystic lesion in the left lower lobe in which a 2- to 3-cm diameter nodule is present. **(B)** The opened specimen displays a thin-walled multicystic lesion and a discrete red-tan nodule. **(C)** The nodule is composed of ciliated columnar epithelium overlying clusters of cells resembling the "blastema" of Wilms' tumor.

At diagnosis approximately 15% to 20% of PPBs are type I and the remaining 80% to 85% of cases are equally distributed between the types II and III. Based on age at presentation and observations on various cases, there is a compelling argument that a progression from type I to type III is the natural history of the PPB. Prognosis is correlated with the pathologic type, with long-term survival of greater than 80% for the type I and 50% or less for types II and III (see PPB website at www.ppbregistry.org). In addition to failure of local control of disease in the chest, hematogenous metastases to the brain and bone have been seen in 25% and 10% of cases, respectively. The brain is an important metastatic site that requires careful follow-up with appropriate imaging studies.[57] Tumor emboli to the brain are known to be the source of metastatic PPB in some cases. The metastatic lesions generally do not have the histopathologic diversity of the primary tumor.

The only consistent cytogenetic abnormality in the PPB is trisomy 8, although it is not unique to this neoplasm. Given the constitutional-familial nature of this tumor, an as yet unidentified signature mutation, likely a tumor suppressor gene, is thought to exist.

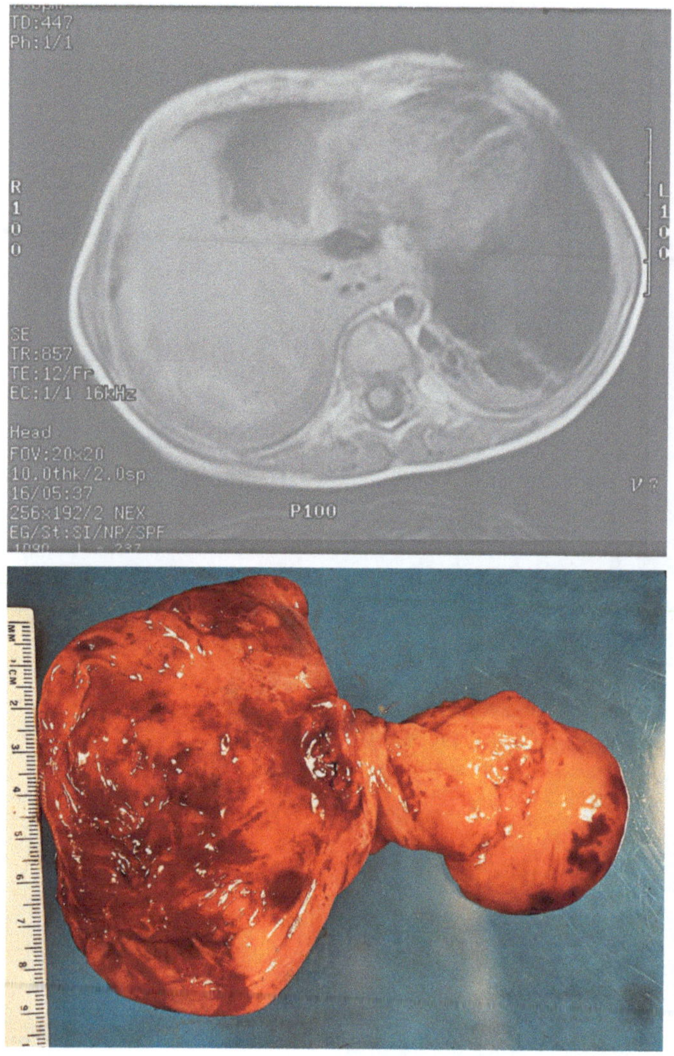

A

C

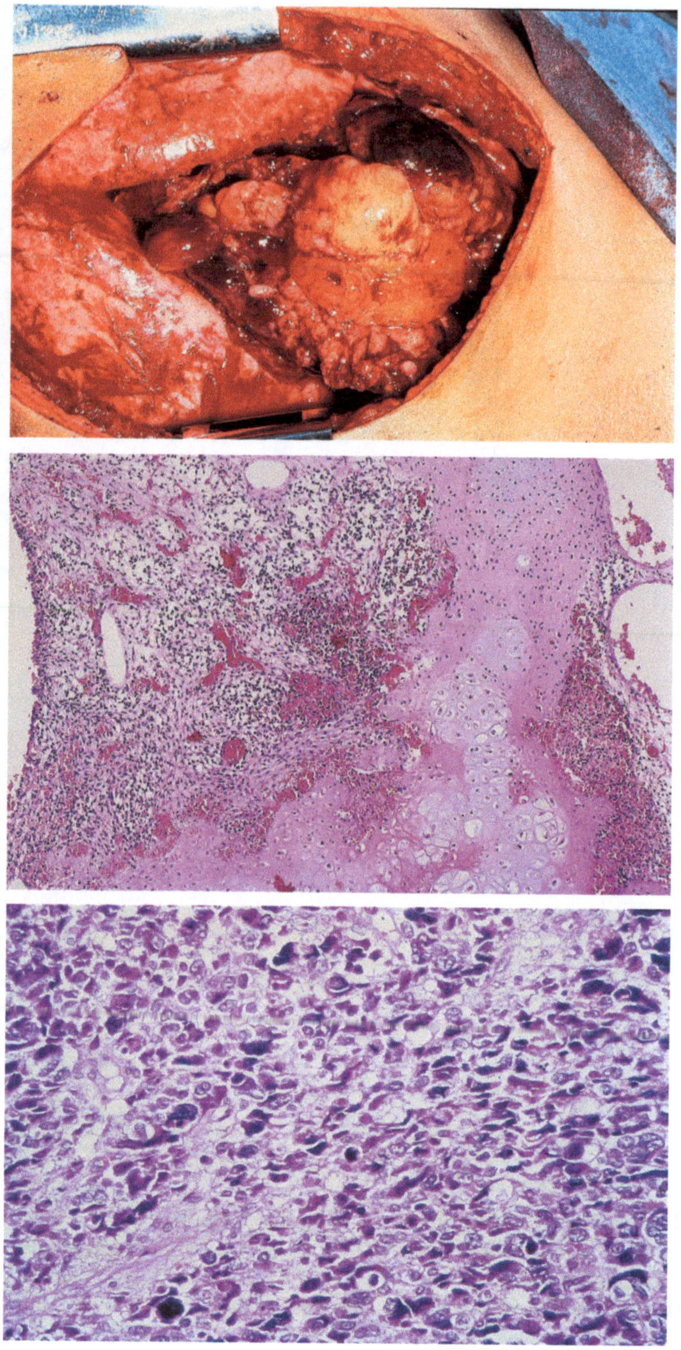

B

D

E

FIGURE 42.9. Pleuropulmonary blastoma, type III. **(A)** Computed tomography (CT) scan in a 4-year-old boy demonstrates a large right-sided pleuropulmonary mass eroding the ribs of the chest wall. **(B)** At surgery a focally hemorrhagic mass is resected. **(C)** The mass has a dumbbell shape and is composed of soft to firm red-tan tissue. **(D)** The mass consists of poorly to undifferentiated mesenchymal tissue, some of which can be identified as chondrosarcoma and fibrosarcoma. **(E)** Some areas consist of only anaplastic cells with large, irregular hyperchromatic nuclei with bizarre mitotic figures.

Other Sarcomas

Primitive neuroectodermal tumor–Ewing sarcoma (PNET-EWS) is the second most common soft tissue sarcoma in childhood and has a known predilection for the chest wall with or without direct extension into the lung. There are uncommon examples of primary pulmonary PNET-EWSs. On the chest wall or in the lung, most cases are diagnosed between 10 and 19 years of age, although we have seen cases presenting in the first 2 years of life. The PNET-EWS is characterized by its signature translocation, t(11;22)(q24;q12), in 90% or more of cases.[58] Less common is the t(21;22)(q22;q12) translocation. A malignant small cell population arranged in nests, lobules, and diffuse sheets is the prototypic microscopic appearance. Rosette formation is not present in all cases. The tumor cells are uniformly immunoreactive for vimentin and CD99 and for cytokeratin in 20% to 25% of cases.

Desmoplastic small round cell tumor (DSRCT) was first reported in the abdomen as multiple masses involving the parietal and visceral surfaces of the peritoneum. This tumor is recognized in other less common primary sites including the chest wall and lung.[59–61] There is an age predominance in older children and young adults. A characteristic nonrandom translocation, t(11;22)(p13;q12), is found in 90% to 95% of cases.[62] Nests of primitive small cells separated by a desmoplastic stroma give this neoplasm its name. However, a similar desmoplastic stroma can be seen in metastatic Wilms' tumor, rhabdomyosarcoma, and PNET-EWS. As seen from the immunophenotypic profile with reactivity for vimentin, cytokeratin, desmin, WT1, and CD99, there is some overlap with the other neoplasms in the differential diagnosis. Fluorescence in-situ hybridization or reverse-transcriptase polymerase chain reaction (RT-PCR) may be required before a final diagnosis can be made.

Rhabdomyosarcoma as a primary neoplasm of the lung, exclusive of the setting of cystic pleuropulmonary blastoma, would appear to be quite rare; however, the lungs are one of the preferred sites for metastatic involvement by embryonal and alveolar rhabdomyosarcomas[63] (Fig. 42.10). The metastases are usually multiple and have a bronchovascular distribution reflecting the hematogenous mode of spread to the lungs. Nonneoplastic skeletal muscle has been reported in the interstitium of fetal and neonatal lungs as rhabdomyomatous dysplasia, in extralobar sequestration, and type 2 congenital pulmonary airway malformation.[64–66] The presence of skeletal muscle in these instances is an example of heterotopia, because striated muscle is not normally found in the lung.

Synovial sarcoma, like PNET-EWS and DSRCT, has become the ubiquitous sarcoma with its recognition in diverse sites other than the peripheral soft tissues. The chest wall and lung are uncommon yet well-documented primary locations for this neoplasm.[67] When the synovial sarcoma is poorly differentiated, its histiologic features are similar to PNET-EWS and the other malignant small cell tumors of childhood. If the pattern is a predominantly spindle cell sarcoma or epithelial profiles, the differential diagnosis can become quite broad. The immunophenotypic profile of synovial sarcoma includes reactivity for vimentin, cytokeratin, epithelial membrane antigen, and CD99. If the tumor is poorly differentiated, cytogenetics may be necessary since the immunotype is not necessarily diagnostic in all cases. Most synovial sarcomas have the t(x;18)(p11;q11) translocation.

Whether in the lung or chest wall, we recognize that some primitive small cell neoplasms in children are not classifiable into any one of the well-established pathologic categories. These tumors are diagnosed as undifferentiated round cell sarcomas.

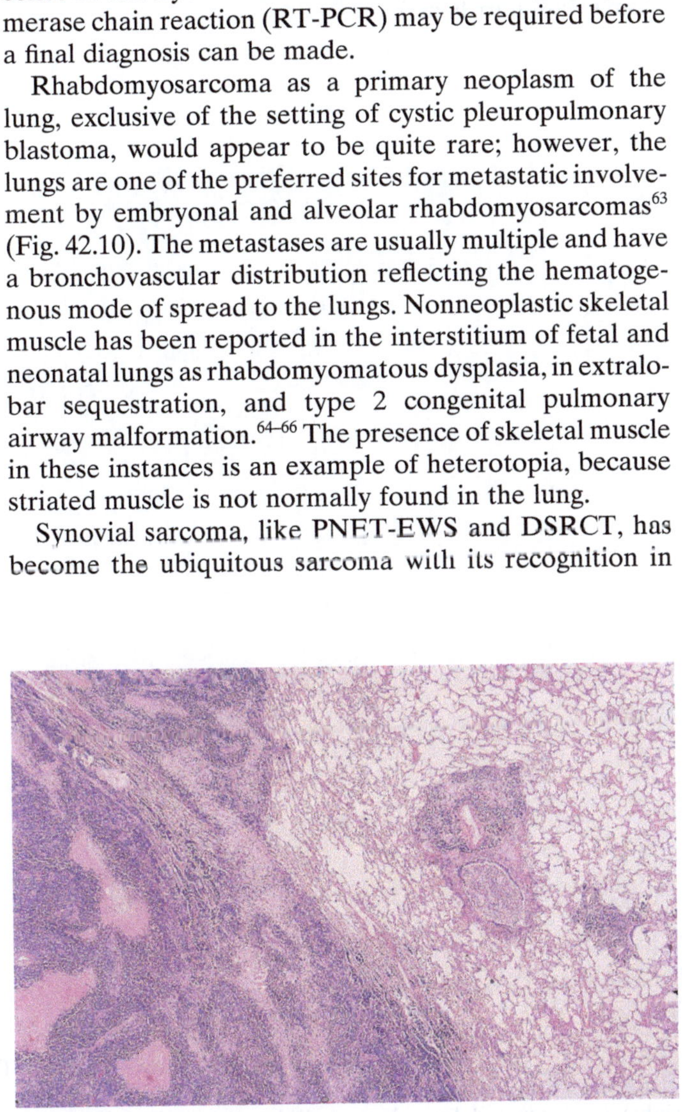

FIGURE 42.10. Rhabdomyosarcoma metastatic to lung. Multiple foci of embryonal rhabdomyosarcoma, some with areas of necrosis are present in a 5-year-old girl with her primary rhabdomyosarcoma in the neck.

Epithelial Tumors

There are few benign epithelial neoplasms of the lung other than the rare true adenomas (see Chapter 41). Among the primary nonmesenchymal malignant tumors of the lung, the bronchial gland-derived neoplasms are the most common in children (Table 42.1). Carcinoid (Fig. 42.11), mucoepidermoid carcinoma (Fig. 42.12), and adenoid cystic carcinoma, in descending order of frequency, are the three major tumor types of bronchial gland–derived tumors in children.[68] There is a report of acinic cell carcinoma in a child.[69] Bronchial carcinoid in the pediatric age group typically presents between the ages of 12 and 19 years with symptoms and signs referable to the obstruction of a major bronchus.[70,71] A yellowish submucosal mass measuring 2 to 4 cm protrudes into the lumen of a bronchus. Microscopically, cords and nests of small uniform tumor cells with minor cytologic abnormalities infiltrate around and through the bronchial cartilage. Foci of necrosis, nuclear aberrations, and pleomorphism should be viewed as evidence of a higher grade neoplasm than the typical carcinoid, which has an excellent prognosis in 80% to 90% of cases.[72] Mucoepidermoid carcinoma, although less common than carcinoid, has been well documented in the lungs of children.[70,73] Like carcinoid, the tumor presents as a central obstructive lesion of the bronchus. A broad-based, endobronchial polypoid mass measuring 2 to 3 cm is the gross appearance. Microscopically, the tumor is composed of intermediate- to high-grade squamous cells forming nests and mucin-containing glands or luminal structures filled with mucin. Adenoid cystic carcinoma of the bronchus is a

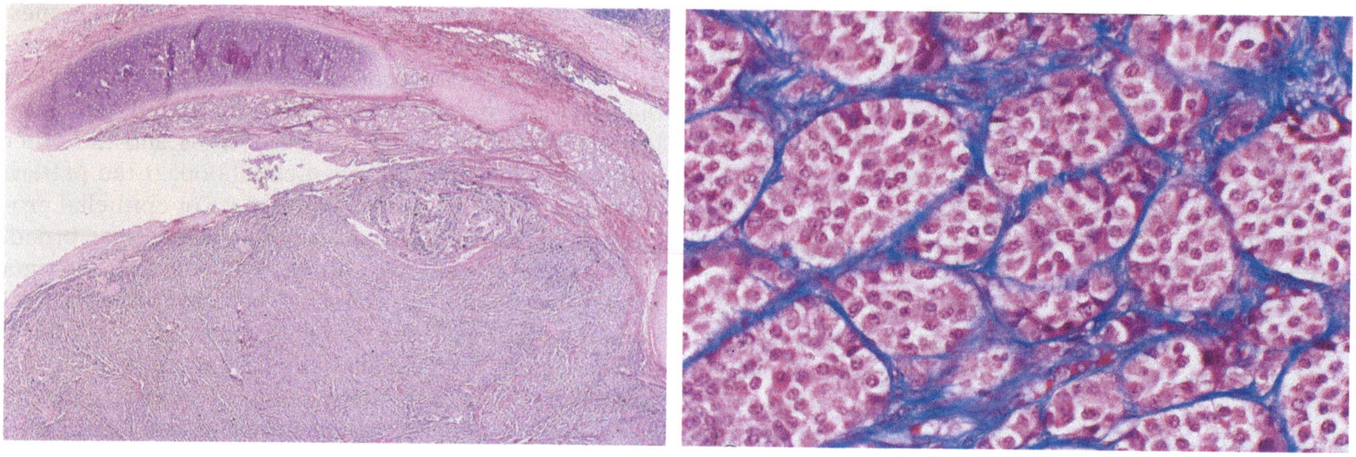

A B

FIGURE 42.11. Carcinoid tumor. **(A)** This 15-year-old boy has a bronchus largely obstructed by a homogeneous cell mass. **(B)** Thin stands of connective tissue surround small nests of neuroendocrine cells with uniform nuclei and abundant cytoplasm (Masson trichome).

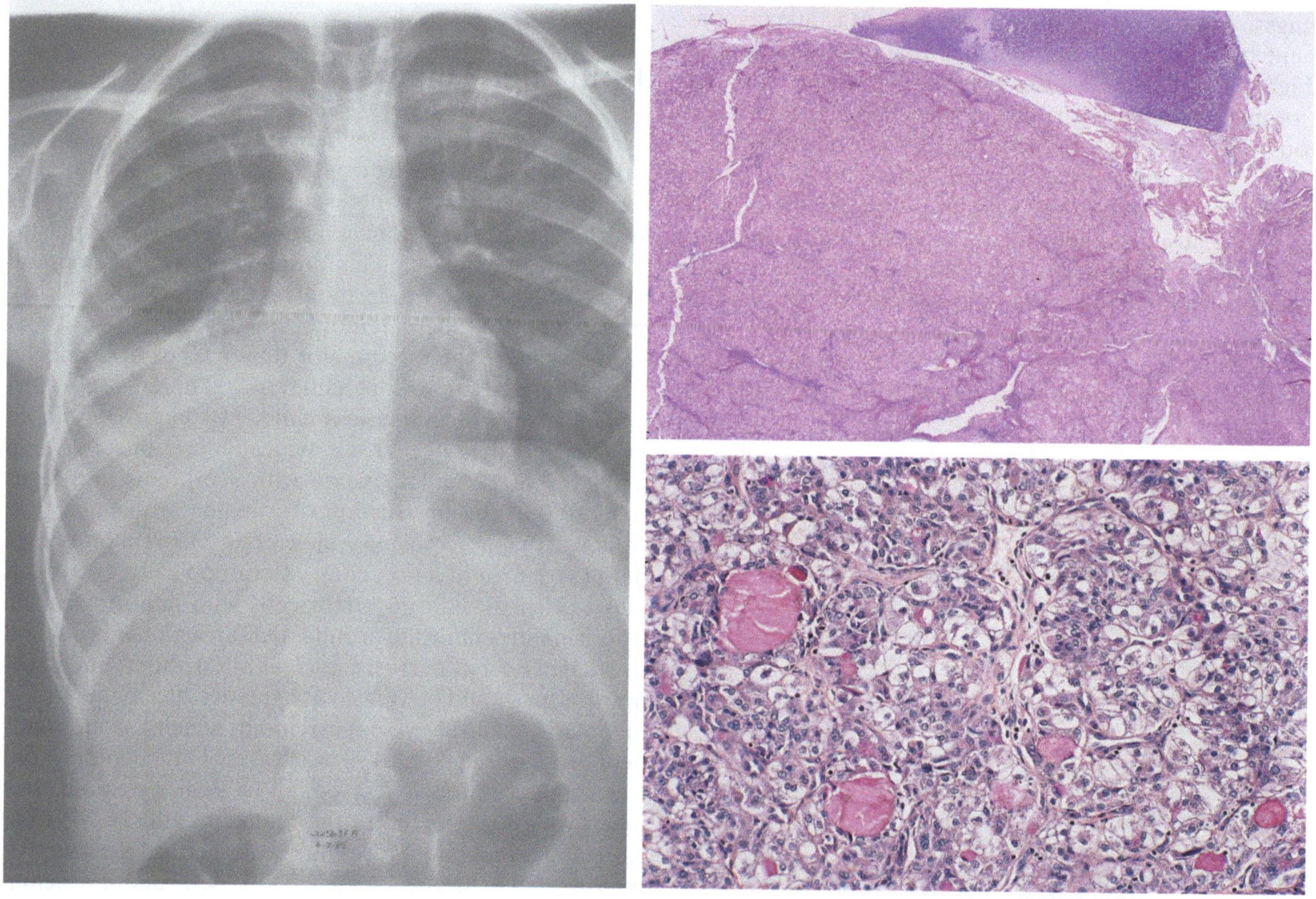

A B C

FIGURE 42.12. Mucoepidermoid carcinoma. **(A)** This 7-year-old girl presented with postobstructive pneumonia of the right lower lobe. **(B)** The bronchus (note bronchial cartilage at upper right) is obstructed by a large cellular mass. **(C)** Infiltrating neoplastic nests are composed of mucinous and intermediate squamous cells in a desmoplastic stroma. (Mucicarmine stain)

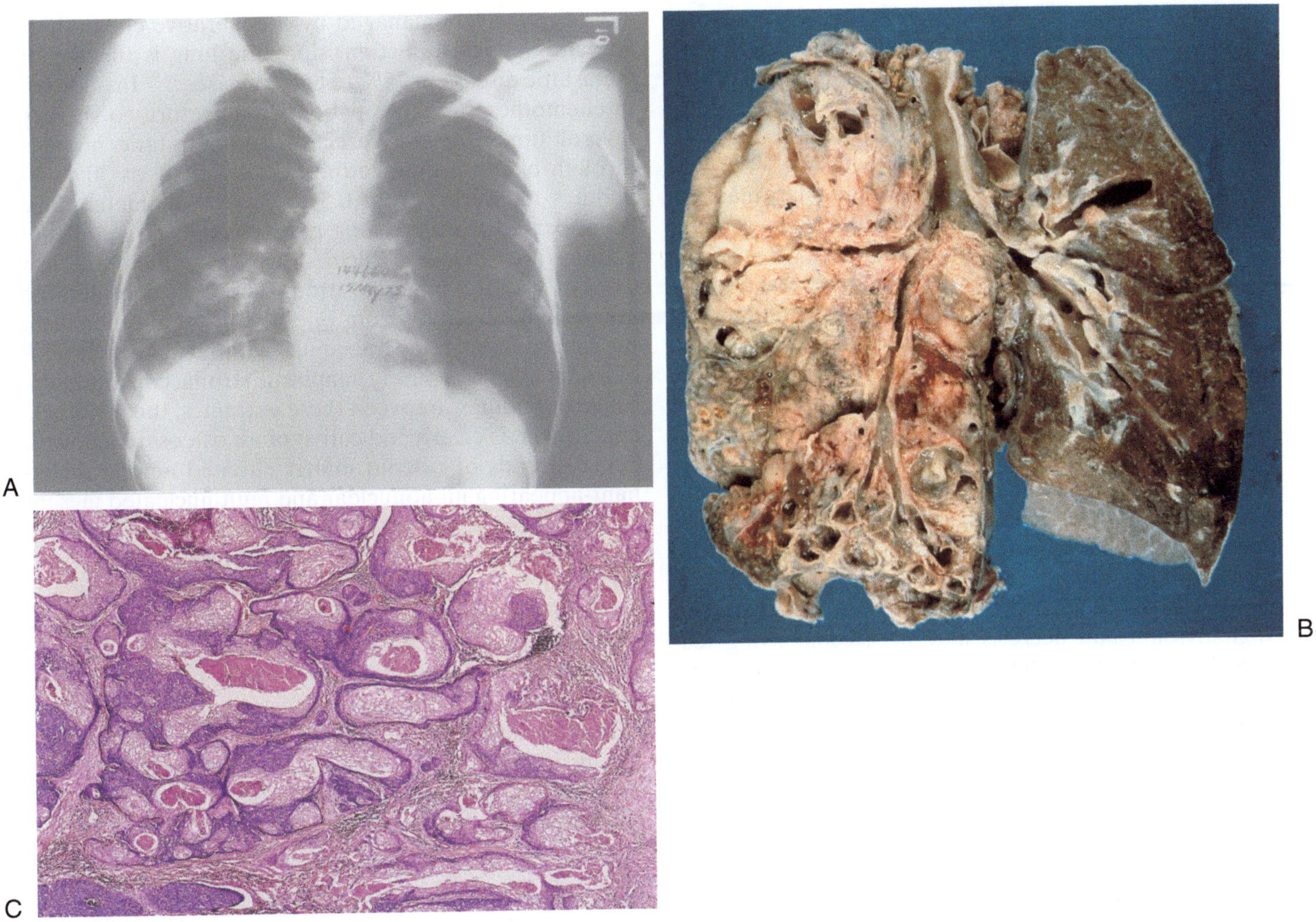

Figure 42.13. Squamous cell carcinoma. **(A)** This 10-year-old, profoundly retarded girl experienced recurrent episodes of "pneumonia" and eventually died. **(B)** Her right lung was largely replaced by firm tan tissue. **(C)** The tumor consists of well-differentiated squamous cells with clusters of keratinized material.

very uncommon neoplasm, but we have seen one example in the trachea in an 11-year-old girl.

More conventional forms of bronchogenic carcinoma (Fig. 42.13) are infrequently reported in children and young adults.[74] Examples of invasive squamous cell carcinoma have been described as a de novo neoplasm in an adolescent with a history of smoking dating to early childhood or as malignant transformation in bronchopulmonary papillomatosis.[75] Travis and associates[76] reported the occurrence of single pulmonary nodules in the lung resembling bronchioloalveolar carcinoma (BAC) in adolescent patients who had received chemotherapy. Likewise, Benjamin and Cahill[77] described a BAC in a 19-year-old man with a history of a resected congenital cystic adenomatoid malformation as an infant. Additional examples of BAC or atypical mucinous hyperplasia have been identified in the setting of adenomatoid malformations.[78–80] (See Chapter 34).

Langerhans Cell Histiocytosis and Lymphoid Neoplasms

Histiocytic and lymphoid infiltrates in the lung are not unique to children, but at least one entity, Langerhans cell histiocytosis (LCH), has a predilection for the pediatric age group. In the younger child, diffuse pulmonary involvement generally accompanies multisystem or generalized LCH.[81] The adolescent or young adult is more likely to have involvement restricted to the lung, but there are isolated cases of primary pulmonary LCH in very young children.[82] Aggregates of Langerhans cells or a more subtle infiltration of the interstitium with or without a fibrous reaction are the variable histologic findings. A stellate scar may be the only remnant of an earlier active lesion. One of several problems in histologic interpretation is the distinction of pulmonary macrophages from Langerhans cells. Also, the presence of some Langerhans cells does not guarantee a diagnosis of LCH since dendritic cells occur in any number of inflammatory reactions in the lungs. Immunohistochemistry with the demonstration of aggregates of CD1a positive cells is required for a definitive diagnosis of LCH.[83]

Lymphoproliferative disorders with pulmonary manifestations occur almost exclusively in children with a primary or secondary immunodeficiency condition.[84–87] Regardless of the specific underlying disorder, one or several nodular densities with or without cavitation are noted on imaging studies, with a differential diagnosis that includes some opportunistic pathogens.[88] When it is a lymphoproliferative process, it is usually a B-cell infiltrate, and very often Epstein-Barr virus (EBV) is detected as a primary or reactivation infection.[89,90] A lung biopsy may demonstrate one of several pathologic appearances from a polymorphous B-cell infiltrate with lymphoid cells ranging from immunoblasts to mature plasma cells. The other end of the spectrum is a monotypic infiltrate consisting of large, atypical lymphoid cells with centroblastic to immunoblastic features. Angioinvasion and necrosis may be accompanying features. It is more often the case that the latter microscopic features are correlated with monoclonality, whereas the polymorphous infiltrate is polyclonal.

Children with cystic fibrosis who are lung-allograft recipients appear to be especially vulnerable for posttransplant lymphoproliferative disorder (PTLD).[91] The latency period for the development of PTLD may be quite short in these patients. Epstein-Barr virus–associated B-cell lymphoma with angioinvasion and clinical features of lymphomatoid granulomatosis has been reported as a posttransplant complication. Only rarely does lymphomatoid granulomatosis occur in an immunologically intact child.[92,93] Anaplastic large cell lymphoma has been documented in children with diffuse infiltrates in the lung.[94] So-called lymphoid interstitial pneumonitis has been reported in children with HIV-AIDS. This proliferation involves the bronchial and mucosa associated lymphoid tissue as a hyperplasia of a polyclonal population of B lymphocytes or as a monoclonal marginal zone lymphoma. Hodgkin's lymphoma, usually in association with mediastinal disease or recurrent disease, presents as one or more nodules with or without cavitation.[95,96] A polymorphous infiltrate with few or many Reed-Sternberg cells can be diagnostically challenging on biopsy. (See also Chapter 32).

Metastatic Tumor

Metastatic tumor, as noted previously, is the type of pulmonary neoplasm from a child that is most frequently seen in our surgical pathology laboratory. Osteosarcoma to the lung is without question the malignancy that is most aggressively managed by preoperative chemotherapy and surgical resection, since the lung is the site of metastatic disease in 75% to 80% of cases.[96,97] In addition to chemotherapy, these patients may return to surgery several times for the resection of metastatic nodules through bilateral thoracotomies.[98] As many as 30 to 40 nodules measuring from 0.5 to 3 cm in diameter have been excised from the lung parenchyma.[99] Some of the nodules are obviously calcified, whereas others are firm to soft without mineralization. There is considerable microscopic diversity from one nodule to another from the same patient; bony trabeculae without an overtly neoplastic stroma to a purely anaplastic stroma constitute the range of findings. Between these extremes, the histologic appearance is clearly indicative of an osteosarcoma with dense strands of osteoid matrix situated among malignant-appearing mononuclear and multinucleated mesenchymal cells.

The malignant germ cell tumors, endodermal sinus tumor, and mixed pattern germinal neoplasms frequently produce pulmonary metastases in children with advanced clinical stage disease. Shortness of breath, chest pain, and multiple metastatic nodules in the lung of an adolescent boy or girl are the initial manifestations of a malignant germ cell tumor in a minority of patients. Other neoplasms in children that we have encountered as pulmonary metastases include nonkeratinizing squamous cell carcinoma and chordoma.

References

1. Hartman GE, Shochat SJ. Primary pulmonary neoplasms of childhood: a review. Ann Thorac Surg 1983;36:108–119.
2. Stocker JT. The respiratory tract. In: Stocker JT, Dehner LP, eds. Pediatric pathology. Philadelphia: Lippincott Williams & Wilkins, 2001:445–518.
3. Cerfolio RJ, et al. Inflammatory pseudotumors of the lung. Ann Thorac Surg 1999;67(4):933–936.
4. Kim JH, et al. Pulmonary inflammatory pseudotumor—a report of 28 cases. Korean J Intern Med 2002;17(4):252–258.
5. Sakurai H, et al. Inflammatory myofibroblastic tumor of the lung. Eur J Cardiothorac Surg 2004;25(2):155–159.
6. Narla LD, et al. Inflammatory pseudotumor. Radiographics 2003;23(3):719–729.
7. Yousem S, et al. Inflammatory myofibroblastic tumour. In: Travis W, et al., eds. Classification of tumours. Lyon: IARC Press, 2004:105–106.
8. Chun YS, et al. Pediatric inflammatory myofibroblastic tumor: anaplastic lymphoma kinase (ALK) expression and prognosis. Pediatr Blood Cancer 2005;45(6):796–801.
9. Debelenko LV, et al. Identification of CARS-ALK fusion in primary and metastatic lesions of an inflammatory myofibroblastic tumor. Lab Invest 2003;83(9):1255–1265.
10. Dehner L. Inflammatory myofibroblastic tumor: the continued definition of one type of so-called inflammatory pseudotumor. Am J Surg Pathol 2004;28:1652–1654.

11. Rodrigues M, et al. Inflammatory myofibroblastic tumor of the larynx in a 2-year-old male. ORL J Otorhinolaryngol Relat Spec 2005;67(2):101–105.
12. Seki S, et al. A clinicopathological study of inflammatory pseudotumors of the liver with special reference to vessels. Hepatogastroenterology 2004;51(58):1140–1143.
13. Pungpapong S, Geiger XJ, Raimondo M. Inflammatory myofibroblastic tumor presenting as a pancreatic mass: a case report and review of the literature. JOP 2004;5(5): 360–367.
14. Oz Puyan F, et al. Inflammatory pseudotumor of the spleen with EBV positivity: report of a case. Eur J Haematol 2004;72(4):285–291.
15. Lo OS, et al. Inflammatory pseudotumor of the liver in association with a gastrointestinal stromal tumor: a case report. World J Gastroenterol 2004;10(12):1841–1843.
16. Fang JC, Dym H. Myofibroblastic tumor of the oral cavity. A rare clinical entity. N Y State Dent J 2004;70(3):28–30.
17. Dehner LP. Inflammatory myofibroblastic tumor: the continued definition of one type of so-called inflammatory pseudotumor. Am J Surg Pathol 2004;28(12):1652–1654.
18. Dasgupta D, et al. Liver transplantation for a hilar inflammatory myofibroblastic tumor. Pediatr Transplant 2004;8(5): 517–521.
19. Browne M, et al. Inflammatory myofibroblastic tumor (inflammatory pseudotumor) of the neck infiltrating the trachea. J Pediatr Surg 2004;39(10):e1–e4.
20. Yoshida T, et al. Inflammatory pseudotumor of the liver: report of a case diagnosed by needle biopsy. Hepatol Res 2003;27(1):83–86.
21. Ueda M, et al. A case of inflammatory pseudotumor of the liver hilum successfully treated with aggressive hepatectomy. J Pediatr Surg 2003;38(11):E9–E11.
22. Thompson RJ, Barrett AM, Dildey P. Congenital multifocal inflammatory pseudotumor: a case report. J Pediatr Surg 2003;38(10):E17–E19.
23. Sobesky R, et al. Inflammatory pseudotumor of the common bile duct. Endoscopy 2003;35(8):698–700.
24. Koea JB, et al. Inflammatory pseudotumor of the liver: demographics, diagnosis, and the case for nonoperative management. J Am Coll Surg 2003;196(2):226–235.
25. Kapusta LR, et al. Inflammatory myofibroblastic tumors of the kidney: a clinicopathologic and immunohistochemical study of 12 cases. Am J Surg Pathol 2003;27(5):658–666.
26. Agrons GA, et al. Pulmonary inflammatory pseudotumor: radiologic features. Radiology 1998;206(2):511–518.
27. Hedlund GL, et al. Aggressive manifestations of inflammatory pulmonary pseudotumor in children. Pediatr Radiol 1999;29(2):112–116.
28. Berman M, et al. Pulmonary inflammatory myofibroblastic tumor invading the left atrium. Ann Thorac Surg 2003; 76(2):601–603.
29. Kato S, et al. A case report of inflammatory pseudotumor of the lung: rapid recurrence appearing as multiple lung nodules. Ann Thorac Cardiovasc Surg 2002;8(4):224–227.
30. Hajjar WA, Ashour MH, Al-Rikabi AC. Endobronchial inflammatory pseudotumor of the lung. Saudi Med J 2001; 22(4):366–368.
31. Matsubara O, et al. Inflammatory pseudotumors of the lung: progression from organizing pneumonia to fibrous histiocytoma or to plasma cell granuloma in 32 cases. Hum Pathol 1988;19(7):807–814.
32. Pettinato G, et al. Inflammatory myofibroblastic tumor (plasma cell granuloma). Clinicopathologic study of 20 cases with immunohistochemical and ultrastructural observations. Am J Clin Pathol 1990;94(5):538–546.
33. Travis W, et al. Congenital peribronchial myofibroblastic tumour. In: Travis W, et al., eds. Pathology and genetics of the lung, pleura, thymus and heart. World Health Organization classification of tumours. Lyon: IARC Press, 2004:102–103.
34. Balarezo F, Joshi V. Proliferative and neoplastic disorders in children with acquired immunodeficiency syndrome. Adv Anat Pathol 2002;9:360–370.
35. Monforte-Munoz H, Kapoor N, Saavedra J. Epstein-Barr virus associated leiomyomatosis and posttransplant lymphoproliferative disorder in a child with severe combined immunodeficiency: case report and review of the literature. Pediatr Dev Pathol 2003;6:449–457.
36 Wiswell TE, et al. Infantile myofibromatosis: the most common fibrous tumor of infancy. J Pediatr Surg 1988;23(4): 315–318.
37. Roggli VL, Kim HS, Hawkins E. Congential generalized fibromatosis with visceral involvement. A case report. Cancer 1980;45(5):954–960.
38. Valverde K, et al. Typical and atypical Carney's triad presenting with malignant hypertension and papilledema. J Pediatr Hematol Oncol 2001;23:519–524.
39. Wales P, Drab S, Kim P. An unusual case of complete Carney's triad in a 14-year-old boy. J Pediatr Surg 2002; 37:1228–1232.
40. Carney JA. Gastric stromal sarcoma, pulmonary chondroma, and extra-adrenal paraganglioma (Carney triad): natural history, adrenocortical component, and possible familial occurrence [see comments]. Mayo Clin Proc 1999; 74(6):543–552.
41. Rock MJ, et al. Epithelioid hemangioendothelioma of the lung (intravascular bronchioloalveolar tumor) in a young girl. Pediatr Pulmonol 1991;11(2):181–186.
42. Marais B, Pienaar P, Gie R. Kaposi sarcoma with upper airway obstruction and bilateral chylothoraces. Pediatri Infect Dis J 2003;22:926–928.
43. Fournet JC, et al. Multicentric Kaposi's sarcoma in a 5 year-old human immunodeficiency virus-negative renal allograft recipient. Hum Pathol 1992;23(8):956–9560.
44. Baum LG, Vinters HV. Lymphadenopathic Kaposi's sarcoma in a pediatric patient with acquired immune deficiency syndrome. Pediatr Pathol 1989;9(4):459–465.
45. Manivel JC, et al. Pleuropulmonary blastoma. The so-called pulmonary blastoma of childhood. Cancer 1988;62(8):1516–1526.
46. Nakatani Y, Dickersin GR, Mark EJ. Pulmonary endodermal tumor resembling fetal lung: a clinicopathologic study of five cases with immunohistochemical and ultrastructural characterization. Hum Pathol 1990;21(11):1097–1107.
47. DiFurio M, Auerbach A, Kaplan K. Well-differentiated fetal adenocarcinoma: rare tumor in the pediatric population. Pediatr Dev Pathol 2003;6:564–567.
48. Dehner LP. Pleuropulmonary blastoma is THE pulmonary blastoma of childhood. Semin Diagn Pathol 1994;11(2): 144–151.

49. Domizio P, et al. Malignant mesenchymoma associated with a congenital lung cyst in a child: case report and review of the literature. Pediatr Pathol 1990;10(5):785–797.
50. Weinberg AG, et al. Mesenchymal neoplasia and congenital pulmonary cysts. Pediatr Radiol 1980;9(3):179–182.
51. Holland-Moritz RM, Heyn RM. Pulmonary blastoma associated with cystic lesions in children. Med Pediatr Oncol 1984;12(2):85–88.
52. Dehner L. Beware of "'degenerating"' congenital pulmonary cysts. Pediatr Surg Int 2005;21:123–124.
53. Hill DA, Dehner LP, Ackerman LV. A cautionary note about congenital cystic adenomatoid malformation (CCAM) type 4. Am J Surg Pathol 2004;28(4):554–555; author reply 555.
54. Hasiotou M, et al. Pleuropulmonary blastoma in the area of a previously diagnosed congenital lung cyst: report of two cases. Acta Radiol 2004;45(3):289–292.
55. Picaud JC, et al. Bilateral cystic pleuropulmonary blastoma in early infancy. J Pediatr 2000;136(6):834–836.
56. Hill DA. USCAP Specialty Conference: Case 1–Type I Pleuropulmonary Blastoma. Pediatr Dev Pathol 2005;8: 77–84.
57. Serrano M, et al. Histologic predictors of central nervous system metastasis in pleuropulmonary blastoma: a pilot study (abstract 10). Mod Pathol 2005;18:303.
58. Qualman S, Morotti R. Risk assignment in pediatric soft-tissue sarcomas: an evolving molecular classification. Curr Oncol Rep 2002;4:123–130.
59. Ostoros G, et al. Desmoplastic small round cell tumour of the pleura: a case report with unusual follow-up. Lung Cancer 2002;36:333–336.
60. Parkash V, et al. Desmoplastic small round cell tumor of the pleura. Am J Surg Pathol 1995;19:659–665.
61. Syed S, et al. Desmoplastic small round cell tumor of the lung. Arch Pathol Lab Med 2002;126:1226–1228.
62. Gerald W, Haber D. The EWS-WT1 gene fusion in desmoplastic small round cell tumor. Semin Cancer Biol 2005;15: 197–205.
63. Ozcan C, et al. Primary pulmonary rhabdomyosarcoma arising within cystic adenomatoid malformation: a case report and review of the literature. J Pediatr Surg 2001; 36(7):1062–1065.
64. Hardisson D, et al. Rhabdomyomatosis of the newborn lung unassociated with other malformations. Histopathology 1997;31(5):474–479.
65. Orpen N, et al. Intralobar pulmonary sequestration with congenital cystic adematous malformation and rhabdomyomatous dysplasia. Pediatr Surg Int 2003;19(8):610–611.
66. Lienicke U, et al. Rhabdomyomatous dysplasia of the newborn lung associated with multiple congenital malformations of the heart and great vessels. Pediatr Pulmonol 2002;34(3):222–225.
67. Begueret H, et al. Primary intrathoracic synovial sarcoma: a clinicopathologic study of 40 t(x;18)-positive cases from the French Sarcoma Group and the Mesopath Group. Am J Surg Pathol 2005;29:339–346.
68. Al-Qahtani A, et al. Endobronchial tumors in children: institutional experience and literature review. J Pediatr Surg 2003;38:733–736.
69. Sabaratnam R, Anunathan R, Govender D. Acinic cell carcinoma: an unusual case of bronchial obstruction in an child. Pediatr Dev Pathol 2004;7:521–526.
70. Dehner LP. Tumors and tumor-like lesion of the lung and chest wall in childhood: clinical and pathologic review. In: Stocker JT, ed. Pediatric pulmonary disease. Washington, DC: Hemisphere, 1989:207–267.
71. Moraes T, et al. Pediatric pulmonary carcinoid: a case report and review of the literature. Pediatr Pulmonol 2003;35:318–322.
72. McKay B, Lokeman J, Ordonez N. Tumors of the lung. Philadelphia: WB Saunders, 1991:246–284.
73. Giusti R, Flores R. Mucoepidermoid carcinoma of the bronchus presenting with a negative chest x-ray and normal pulmonary function in two teenagers: two case reports and review of the literature. Pediatr Pulmonol 2004;37:81–84.
74. Icard P, et al. Primary lung cancer in young patients: a study of 82 surgically treated patients. Ann Thorac Surg 1992; 54(1):99–103.
75. Kramer SS, et al. Pulmonary manifestations of juvenile laryngotracheal papillomatosis. AJR Am J Roentgenol 1985;144(4):687–694.
76. Travis WD, et al. Pulmonary nodules resembling bronchioloalveolar carcinoma in adolescent cancer patients. Mod Pathol 1988;1(5):372–377.
77. Benjamin DR, Cahill JL. Bronchioloalveolar carcinoma of the lung and congenital cystic adenomatoid malformation. Am J Clin Pathol 1991;95(6):889–892.
78. MacSweeney F, et al. An assessment of the expanded classification of congenital cystic adenomatoid malformations and their relationship to malignant transformation. Am J Surg Pathol 2003;27(8):1139–1146.
79. Stacher E, et al. Atypical goblet cell hyperplasia in congenital cystic adenomatoid malformation as a possible preneoplasia for pulmonary adenocarcinoma in childhood: a genetic analysis. Hum Pathol 2004;35(5):565–570.
80. Granata C, et al. Bronchioloalveolar carcinoma arising in congenital cystic adenomatoid malformation in a child: a case report and review on malignancies originating in congenital cystic adenomatoid malformation. Pediatr Pulmonol 1998;25(1):62–66.
81. Colby TV, Lombard C. Histiocytosis X in the lung. Hum Pathol 1983;14(10):847–856.
82. Nondahl SR, et al. A case report and literature review of "primary" pulmonary histiocytosis X of childhood. Med Pediatr Oncol 1986;14(1):57–62.
83. Gold J, L'Heureux P, Dehner LP. Ultrastructure in the differential diagnosis of pulmonary histiocytosis and pneumocystosis. Arch Pathol Lab Med 1977;101(5):243–247.
84. Buckley R. Pulmonary complications of primary immunodeficiencies. Paediatr Respir Rev 2004;5(suppl A):S225–S233.
85. Pinkerton C, et al. Immunodeficiency-related lymphoproliferative disorders: prospective data from the United Kingdom Children's Cancer Study Group Registry. Br J Haematol 2002;118:456–461.
86. Gao S, et al. Post-transplantation lymphoproliferative disease in heart and heart-lung transplant recipients: 30-year experience at Stanford University. J Heart Lung Transplant 2003;22:505–514.

87. Swigris J, et al. Lymphoid interstitial pneumonia. A narrative review. Chest 2002;122:2150–2164.
88. Siegel M, et al. CT of posttransplantation lymphoproliferative disorder in pediatric recipients of lung allograft. AJR Am J Roentgenol 2003;181:1125–1131.
89. Tao J, Kahn L. Epstein-Barr virus-associated high-grade B-cell lymphoma of mucosal-associated lymphoid tissue in a 9-year-old boy. Arch Pathol Lab Med 2000;124:1520–1524.
90. Tao J, Valderrama E. Epstein-Barr virus-associated polymorphic B-cell lymphoproliferative disorders in the lungs of children with AIDS: a report of two cases. Am J Surg Pathol 1999;23:560–566.
91. Cohen A, et al. High incidence of posttransplant lymphoproliferative disease in pediatric patients with cystic fibrosis. Am J Respir Crit Care Med 2000;161:1252–1255.
92. Fassas A, et al. Lymphomatoid granulomatosis following autologous stem cell transplantation. Bone Marrow Transplant 1999;23:79–81.
93. Moertel C, et al. Lymphomatoid Granulomatosis after childhood acute lymphoblastic leukemia: report of effective therapy. Pediatrics 2001;107:e82.
94. Onciu M, et al. ALK-positive anaplastic large cell lymphoma with leukemic peripheral blood involvement is a clinicopathologic entity with an unfavorable prognosis. Report of three cases and review of the literature. Am J Clin Pathol 2003;120:617–625.
95. Horak E, et al. Multiple cavitating pulmonary nodules and clubbing in a 12-year-old girl. Pediatr Pulmonol 2002;34: 147–149.
96. Karnak I, et al. Pulmonary metastases in children: an analysis of surgical spectrum. Eur J Pediatr Surg 2002;12:151–158.
97. Szafranski A, Wozniak W, Rychlowska-Pruszynska M. [Pulmonary metastases in osteosarcoma patients—treatment results]. Przegl Lek 2004;61(suppl 2):24–28.
98. del Prever AB, et al. Long-term survival in high-grade axial osteosarcoma with bone and lung metastases treated with chemotherapy only. J Pediatr Hematol Oncol 2005;27(1): 42–45.
99. Torre W, Rodriguez-Spiteri N, Sierrasesumaga L. Current role for resection of thoracic metastases in children and young adults—do we need different strategies for this population? Thorac Cardiovasc Surg 2004;52(2):90–95.

43 Neoplasms of the Pleura

Samuel P. Hammar, Douglas W. Henderson, Sonja Klebe, and Ronald F. Dodson

Pleural Neoplasms

In contrast to primary lung neoplasms, primary pleural neoplasms are uncommon. Pleural neoplasms may be difficult to diagnose and must be distinguished from metastatic carcinomas and sarcomas involving the pleura, and from benign reactive processes causing pleural thickening. A correct diagnosis is important so that appropriate therapy, although it may be only palliative, can be instituted.

The most common and most frequently referenced primary pleural neoplasm is mesothelioma, which is considered a signal tumor because of its etiologic relationship to asbestos exposure. Neoplasms such as metastatic carcinomas, sarcomas, leukemia, and lymphoma may occur primarily in the pleura and must be differentiated from mesothelioma.

Mesothelioma

Definitions, History, Incidence, and Epidemiology

Definition

Mesotheliomas are tumors derived from cells forming the serosal lining of the thoracic, abdominal, and pericardial cavities (see Chapter 30).[1,2] They exhibit a wide variety of histologic patterns and may be confused with many other types of neoplasms. Former pathologic "dogma" viewed mesothelioma as a diagnosis of exclusion that could be diagnosed only by postmortem examination. It is our opinion that immunohistochemical and ultrastructural analysis of pleural neoplasms can lead to an accurate diagnosis of mesothelioma and nonmesotheliomatous neoplasms in most cases, even with small biopsy specimens.

History

Mesotheliomas are rare tumors, accounting for less than 1% of all cancer deaths in the world.[3] Two pleural tumors possibly representing mesotheliomas, as noted by Chahinian,[4] were described by Joseph Lieutaud in 1767 in a study of 3000 autopsies. E. Wagner[5] recognized mesotheliomas as a pathologic entity in 1870, and concluded that only sarcomas could be classified as primary malignant pleural tumors and that all epithelial-appearing neoplasms were metastases from an unrecognized or latent primary site. In 1924 Robertson,[6] in an article titled "'Endothelioma' of the Pleura," provided a thorough account of early reports on the clinical and pathologic features of pleural neoplasms. Of interest, one case included in the evaluation of lung cancer related to asbestos by Doll[7] was referred to as an *endothelioma*, most likely indicating this case was a mesothelioma and not a lung cancer. In 1931 Klemperer and Rabin[8] described five primary pleural neoplasms—four were localized and had mesenchymal features and one was diffuse, encasing the lung with a mixed epithelial and mesenchymal histologic appearance. Klemperer and Rabin divided primary tumors of the pleura into localized and diffuse forms, stating localized tumors originated from subpleural "areolar" tissue and were low-grade malignancies usually causing death by interference with the pulmonary circulation, and were potentially curable by surgical removal. They concluded that diffuse neoplasms of the pleura arose from the mesothelial cells lining the serosal surface and could exhibit an epithelial or mesenchymal histologic pattern.

Most cases of mesothelioma reported between 1940 and 1960 were localized.[9,10] In 1943 Wedler[11] reported a case of a diffuse mesothelioma in a person with asbestos exposure. Wedler[12] and Merewether[13] referred to tumors of the pleura in discussing cases of lung carcinoma in patients with asbestosis. It is likely that these neoplasms referred to as "tumors of the pleura" represented mesotheliomas. In the United States the first report of a diffuse mesothelioma with asbestos exposure was in 1947.[14] Even as late as the mid-20th century, some pathologists, notably Willis,[15] denied the existence of mesotheliomas. A pleural and a peritoneal mesothelioma associated with asbestosis were respectively reported in the German literature in 1953 and 1954,[16,17] and in 1960 Keal[18] reported the association of peritoneal mesotheliomas and asbestos exposure. Also in 1960 Wagner et al.[19] reported 33 cases of diffuse pleural mesothelioma in the North Western Cape Province of South Africa. Of these 33 patients, 32 had exposure to asbestos. Wagner[20,21] recounted his experience with the discovery of mesotheliomas in South Africa, and further suggested that all pleural mesotheliomas in the United States were caused by crocidolite asbestos, a suggestion with which we strongly disagree and which is not supported in the medical literature.[22,23] Smither et al.[24] and McCaughey et al.[25] recorded additional cases of asbestos-related mesothelioma in 1962, and for some of those cases the exposure appeared to have been minimal. In the same year, Wagner et al.[26,27] published studies on the mucin histochemistry of mesothelioma and on the induction of malignant mesothelioma (MM) in experimental animals by asbestos.

In 1964 and 1965 Selikoff and colleagues[28,29] linked mesotheliomas to asbestos exposure by finding that 10 of 307 consecutive deaths in asbestos insulation workers were caused by diffuse mesothelioma. Also in 1965 Newhouse and Thompson[30,31] recorded the occurrence of mesotheliomas as a consequence of domestic (household contact) asbestos exposure among those who shook out and laundered the asbestos-contaminated work clothes of their partners, and from neighborhood exposure acquired by residence in the vicinity of an asbestos factory. Most MMs reported since 1970 have been diffuse; the localized form is rare.[18,32]

By the late 1990s, the incidence of MM in some industrialized nations was comparable to that of cancer of the larynx,[33] with a death rate similar to that of renal cell carcinoma in males and uterine cancer in females.[33–37] Apart from lung cancer,[38] MM is now the most important occupational cancer among industrial workers, because of its prevalence, resistance to conventional cancer treatments, and its lethality.

The history of the medical-legal aspects of asbestos-related lung disease was discussed in detail by Motley[39] and Brodeur.[40,41] Information presented by these authors suggested that serious deleterious health effects of asbestos were known long before they were reported in the medical literature.

Incidence and Epidemiology

Mesotheliomas encountered in the early 21st century are most often a consequence of prior occupational exposure to asbestos from the 1940s through the 1970s, including end-uses of asbestos-containing materials and "bystander" (indirect) exposures.[36,42–44] The relationship between inhalation of asbestos fibers—especially one or more of the amphibole varieties—and MM is accepted by virtually all authorities as causal.[42] Because of the constancy and specificity of the asbestos–MM relationship, the incidence of mesothelioma is usually considered to reflect a society's past per capita usage of asbestos,[45–48] after allowance for a suitable latency interval between first exposure to asbestos and the subsequent rise in incidence of MM (Fig. 43.1 and Table 43.1).[47,49]

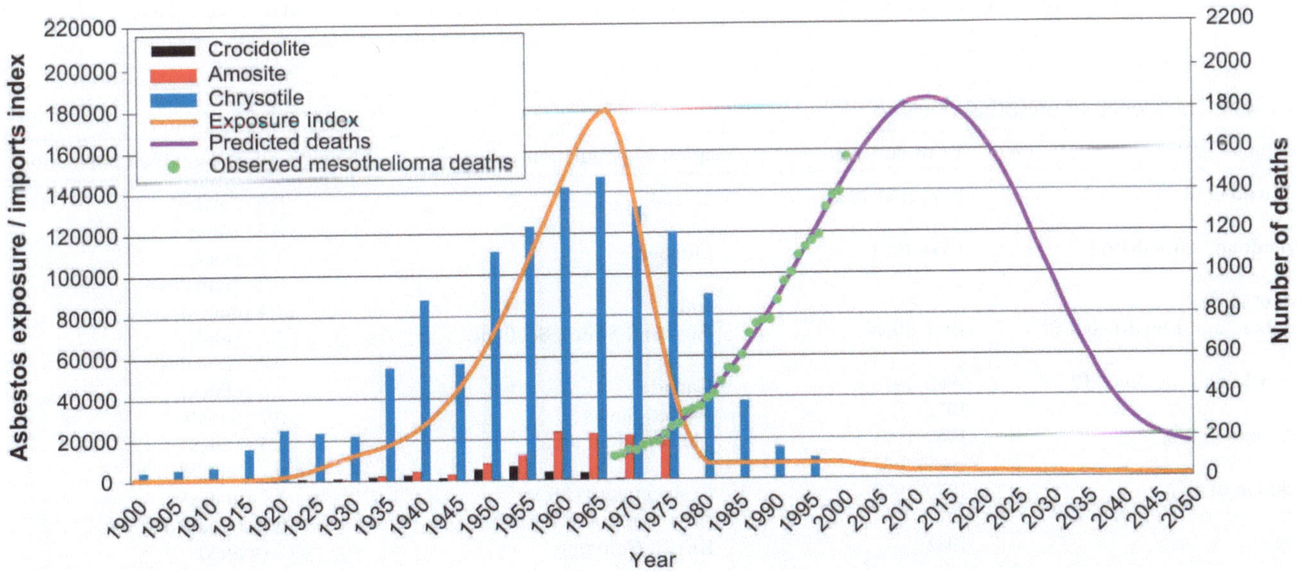

FIGURE 43.1. Observed and predicted deaths from mesothelioma in the United Kingdom, versus asbestos imports and estimated exposure indices, for men aged 20 to 89, for the years 1900 to 2050. (Modified from Health and Safety Executive [HSE]. Mesothelioma mortality in Great Britain: estimating the future burden, December 2003, with permission of the HSE.)

TABLE 43.1. Mesothelioma incidence for some countries relative to their historical per capita use of asbestos

Country	Mesothelioma incidence cases/10^6/yr	Use of asbestos in kg/capita (year)
Australia (1995)	33	4.4 (1968)
Netherlands (1995)	27	3.4 (1976)
United Kingdom (1991)	23	2.7 (1970)
Italy (1993)	22	2.5 (1975)
France (1996)	17	2.6 (1970)
Finland (1995)	15	2.2 (1970)
Germany (1997)	15	3.0 (1975)
Sweden (1995)	15	2.4 (1970)
United States (2000)	15	2.3 (1975)
Norway (1995)	14	1.9 (1970)

Source: Modified from Tossavainen.[47]

Because mesotheliomas are rare neoplasms, their exact incidence is unknown and varies among populations surveyed (Table 43.2).[50–59] The highest incidence in the world is currently in Australia.[58]

The incidence of mesothelioma in autopsy series is considerably lower. McDonald and McDonald[59] summarized the incidence in six series from eight cities between 1950 and 1970. They tabulated 165 cases in 69,302 autopsies (0.24%).

Several studies[54,56,57] documented an apparent increased incidence of MM, especially in men, during the last several decades. Hughes and Weill[60] estimated that 1500 new cases of mesothelioma were diagnosed in the United States in 1986. The increased incidence of MM is probably related to the delayed effects of an increase in occupational exposure to asbestos. Selikoff et al.[28] reported that 8% of 17,800 workers in the heat and frost insulation industry who were followed prospectively between January 1, 1967, and December 31, 1976, died of diffuse MM.[61] According to Huncharek,[62] the incidence of mesothelioma is increasing at a rate of about 10% per year for U.S. males.

The authors' experience has also suggested an increased incidence of MM that, in part, may reflect an increased awareness by pathologists of mesothelioma and of more accurate diagnostic methods such as electron microscopy and immunohistochemistry. In addition, many cases of mesothelioma in the United States come to litigation, which has made the general public more aware of mesothelioma and, in turn, has caused heightened physician awareness.

According to the Environmental Working Group,[63] there is an asbestos epidemic in America. This group reports that asbestos-related disease is responsible for the death of one in 125 American men over the age of 50, and that 10,000 Americans die each year—30 per day—from asbestos-caused diseases. At this time, the death toll is rising in nine of the 10 states with the highest number of mesotheliomas and asbestosis deaths. Between 1979 and 2001, more than 43,000 Americans died from MM. According to Price,[64] there are approximately 2500 new cases of MM annually in the U.S., 80% of which occur in men.[65] According to Price, the incidence of mesothelioma appears to be rising in men aged 45 years or older, with a maximum lifetime risk in the 1925 to 1929 cohort. The incidence of MM in women and in men less than 75 years of age is claimed to have been stable since 1983[64] (but see later discussion).

Peto et al.[66] predicted MM deaths would continue to increase for at least 15, and more likely 25, years. In the most affected cohort, men born in the 1940s, MM would

TABLE 43.2. Incidence of mesotheliomas[a]

Reference	Years surveyed	Location of population surveyed	Number of cases/million population/year
McDonald et al.[50]	1959–mid-1968	Canada	0.65 (males) 0.35 (females)
Theriault and Grand-Bois[51]	1969–1972	Quebec	1.56 (males) 0.74 (females)
Biava et al.[52]		Italy	21.4 (males)
Greenberg and Lloyd-Davies[53]	1967–1968	England, Wales, Scotland	1.88 (males) 0.42 (females)
McDonald and McDonald[54]	1960–1975 1972	Canada United States	2.8 (males) 0.7 (females)
Cutler and Young[55]	1969–1971	Metropolitan area[b]	1.5 (males) 0.7 (females)
Bruckman et al.[56]	1970–1972	Connecticut (U.S.)	1.7 (males) 0.9 (females)
Churg[57]	1982	British Columbia	17 (males) 1.9 (females)
McDonald and McDonald[59]	1950–1970	Eight cities	0.24% of 69,302 autopsies

[a]Incidence includes both pleural and peritoneal mesotheliomas, and in some instances mesotheliomas arising in ovary and male genital system.
[b]Atlanta, Birmingham, Dallas–Ft. Worth, Detroit, Pittsburgh, San Francisco–Oakland, Denver (U.S.).

account for around 1% of all deaths. In 2005 Hodgson et al.[67] stated there were 1848 mesothelioma deaths in Great Britain in 2001 and mesothelioma deaths were predicted to peak at around 1950 to 2450 per year between the years 2011 and 2015 (Fig. 43.1). The Health and Safety Executive Data[68] suggested the peak would occur earlier than originally predicted and the maximum would be approximately 2000 deaths in or around the year 2010. According to Treasure et al.,[69]

> one in every 100 men born in the 1940s will die of malignant pleural mesothelioma. . . . For a man first exposed as a teenager, who remained in a high-risk occupation such as insulation throughout his working life, the lifetime risk of mesothelioma can be as high as 1 in 5. . . . The disease is increasing in frequency. . . . We will see many more mesotheliomas in the next 25 years. In the developed world alone, 100,000 people alive will now die from it.

In Australia, mortality from MM was stated to have been increasing since 1975. Mesothelioma incidence rates are among the highest in the world, and the Australian Mesothelioma Registry received 6129 mesothelioma notifications between 1986 and 2000. Of the mesothelioma cases with past asbestos exposure, close to 89% were work-related, about 3% were not work-related, and about 8% could not be classified. Of the persons who developed work-related MM, one in three worked in the construction industry and one in five worked in the manufacturing industry.

In contrast, Roggli,[70] based on his experience, suggests that a mesothelioma epidemic was beginning to wane in the U.S. Lemen,[71] using Surveillance Epidemiology and End Results (SEER) data and International Classification of Diseases (ICD-10-TEM) coding that went into effect in 1999, stated the accuracy for reporting mesothelioma was about 80% effective, which would mean that in the U.S. there were over 6000 cases of mesothelioma per year.

Etiology

Asbestos

The association of asbestos exposure and the development of mesothelioma has been reviewed in detail.[72–74] The chronology of asbestos is shown in Box 43.1 (Figs. 43.2 and 43.3). Asbestos is the single most important causative agent of mesothelioma. Numerous

Box 43.1. The History of Asbestos

4000 BCE	Asbestos was used for wicks in lamps and candles. "Asbestos" means inextinguishable or unquenchable.
2000–3000 BCE	Embalmed bodies of Egyptian pharaohs were wrapped in asbestos cloths to offset the ravages of time.
2500 BCE	Used in Finland to strengthen clay pots.
800–900 AD	Anecdotal evidence of Charlemagne's tablecloth made from woven asbestos.
1000	Mediterranean people used chrysotile from Cyprus and tremolite from upper Italy for the fabrication of cremation clothes, mats, and wicks for temple lamps.
1300–1400	Marco Polo visited an asbestos mine in China in the latter half of the 13th century. He concluded that asbestos was a stone and lay to rest the myth that asbestos was the hair of a woolly lizard.
Early 1700s	Asbestos papers and boards were made in Italy.
1724	Benjamin Franklin brought a purse made of asbestos to England. The purse is now in the Natural History Museum.
1828	United States patent issued for asbestos insulating material used in steam engines.
1853	Asbestos helmet and jackets worn by Parisian Fire Brigade.
1866	Molded lagging material made from water, glass, and asbestos.
1896	First asbestos brake linings were made by Ferodo Ltd., in England.
1900	High pressure asbestos gaskets made by Klinger in Austria.
1913	First asbestos pipes developed in Italy.
1919	Standard corrugated sheet asbestos introduced in Australia by Hardies.
1939–1945	Wartime use included fireproof suits and parachute flares. In the film *The Wizard of Oz* in 1939, the Wicked Witch of the West appeared on a broom made of asbestos.
1945–1975	Postwar construction projects relied heavily on the use of asbestos, reaching an all-time high in 1973.
1990s	The solid fuel boosters of the space shuttle are insulated with asbestos, one of the few remaining current uses.

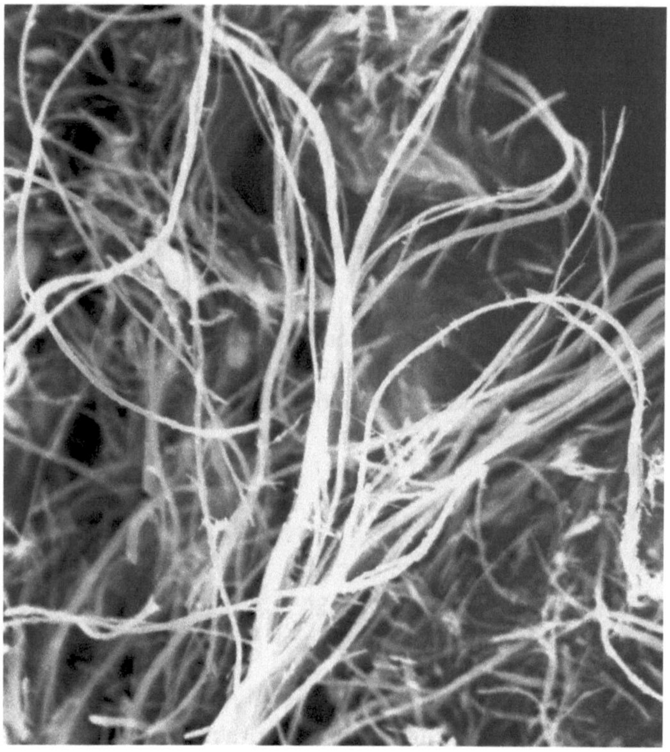

FIGURE 43.2. Canadian chrysotile fibers as visualized by scanning electron microscopy (SEM). The individual fibers are long and wavy (serpentine).

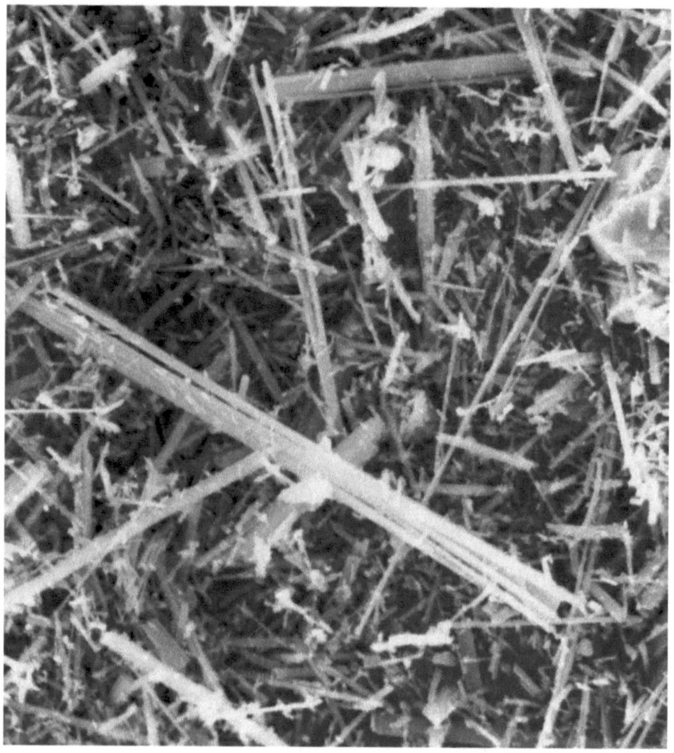

FIGURE 43.3. Scanning electron microscopy appearance of South African crocidolite fibers. In comparison to chrysotile fibers (Figure 43.2), these amphibole fibers are straight and show evidence of longitudinal splitting.

reports[31,59,75–86] have tabulated the percentage of mesothelioma cases associated with asbestos exposure (Table 43.3). The association between asbestos exposure and mesothelioma is stronger in men than in women and, in many series, very few women with mesothelioma have had a history of exposure to asbestos. The threshold amount of asbestos necessary to induce mesothelioma is unknown, although in most reports a dose–response relationship has been suggested[87,88]; that is, persons with a greater intensity and duration of exposure to asbestos have a higher incidence of mesothelioma. Small concentrations of asbestos may induce mesothelioma[89–97] (see

TABLE 43.3. Association of exposure to asbestos and incidence of mesothelioma

		Sex distribution			Cases associated with asbestos exposure		
Reference	Number of cases	Male	Unspecified	Female	Male	Unspecified	Female
Borow et al.[75]	72	64		8	55/55 (100%)		5/5 (100%)
Cochrane and Webster[76]	70		70[a]			60/70[a] (86%)	
Tagnon et al.[77]	61	61		0	45/56 (80%)		
Whitwell and Rawcliffe[78]	52	40		12	35/40 (87.5%)		8/12 (67%)
Hammar[79]	151	119		32	66/82 (80%)		10/22 (45%)
Taylor and Johnson[80]	30	23		7	17/23 (74%)		0/7 (0%)
Vogelzang et al.[81]	31	22		9	13/22 (59%)		2/9 (22%)
Newhouse and Thompson[31]	83	41		42	24/41 (59%)		17/42 (40%)
Peto et al.[82]	116	116		0	69/116 (59%)		
McDonald and McDonald[59]	557	395		162	188/344 (55%)		8/162 (5%)
Roggli et al.[83]	25	21		4	11/21 (52%)		0/4 (0%)
Oels et al.[84]	37	32		5	10/32 (31%)		0/5 (0%)
Brenner et al.[85]	123	84		39	16/84 (19%)		0/39 (0%)
Ratzer et al.[86]	31	21		10	4/31[a] (13%)		

[a]Gender not specified.

below). Malignant mesothelioma can occur via household exposure to asbestos.[98] Vianna and Polan[99] reported a relative risk of 10 for such situations compared to matched controls unexposed to asbestos. Kane et al.[100] reported 10 cases of MM in patients 40 years old or younger. In seven of the 10 cases, there was asbestos exposure—two occupational exposures and five household exposures. Cazzadori et al.[101] reported a case of pleural MM in a 37-year-old woman exposed to asbestos during childhood. From birth to age 10 she lived in a house next to an asbestos-processing factory. Asbestos exposure was confirmed by finding 0.3 asbestos bodies per milliliter in her bronchoalveolar lavage fluid. Huncharek[62] pointed out that exposure to asbestos was no longer confined to asbestos industry workers, and there were nonoccupational hazards such as household and building occupant exposures. Dodoli et al.[102] reviewed death certificates of 39,650 persons between 1975 and 1988 in Livorno, Italy and in 45,900 persons in La Spezia, Italy, between 1958 and 1988. A total of 262 cases of pleural mesothelioma were recorded, most of which occurred in persons occupationally exposed to asbestos in the shipbuilding industry. Thirteen cases of mesothelioma occurred in women who washed the asbestos-contaminated work clothes of their relatives, and six cases occurred in persons domestically exposed to asbestos, possibly from installing fireproof or nonconductive materials.

In 1997 Hammar et al.[103] reported on 103 women with mesothelioma of whom about 70 were exposed to asbestos, the most common source of asbestos exposure being domestic bystander exposure.

Proposed Nonasbestos Causes of Mesothelioma

Erionite

Theoretically, MM might develop at the site of pleural injury caused by almost any agent. Of particular interest has been a group of naturally occurring fibrous silicate minerals called zeolites. In 1975 and subsequent years, Baris and colleagues[104–108] reported that people living in Tuskoy and Karain (two small villages in central Turkey) had the highest incidence of mesothelioma in the world. In Karain, 21 of 50 deaths recorded in people over 20 years old during a 5-year period were caused by mesothelioma. People living in this region of Turkey were found to have very fine fibers of a zeolite called *erionite* in their sputum and lung tissue. These fibers were not found in similar specimens of people living in other areas of Turkey. A search for asbestos in soil, rock, and water samples was negative and it was hypothesized that airborne erionite fibers from building materials caused the mesotheliomas. Lillis[109] substantiated the findings of Baris et al. Sebastien and coworkers[110] demonstrated that 93% of ferruginous bodies from lung samples of two patients with MM from Tuskoy were formed on erionite cores. Wagner et al.[111] induced mesotheliomas in 38 of 40 rats inoculated with erionite. Rohl et al.,[112] however, were able to identify small amounts of tremolite and chrysotile in addition to erionite in environmental samples taken from Tuskoy and Karain (see Nonasbestos and Nonoccupational Mineral Fibers and Mesothelioma, below). They also reported that erionite was found in environmental samples taken from villages with no reported cases of mesothelioma. Recent studies have suggested a genetic susceptibility to mesothelioma in Turkey based on identification of mesothelioma in one village and not in another.[113,114]

Chronic Pleural Inflammation and Scarring

In 1985 Hillerdal and Berg[115] reported two patients who developed mesothelioma in regions of pleural scarring caused by tuberculosis that had been treated with pneumothorax. They reviewed the literature and found 20 additional cases of malignant tumors in pleural scars, 12 of which were found in areas of squamous carcinoma. They reported that squamous carcinoma was the most common tumor associated with scarring from chronic empyema and extrapleural pneumothorax. Malignant mesotheliomas have occurred years after chronic inflammatory lesions of the pleura; for example, chronic empyema or packing of the pleural cavity with leucite spheres as treatment for tuberculosis (so-called plombage therapy). Also, there are a few reports (about eight cases) of an association of peritoneal mesothelioma with familial Mediterranean fever (FMF), possibly related to recurrent FMF serositis.[116] Cases of this type are exceptional, and confounding factors for mesothelioma need to be addressed; for example, in relation to FMF, cases of mesothelioma have been reported in the Mediterranean littoral from white-washing of homes with tremolite-containing material, so that domestic and environmental tremolite exposure might represent a potential confounding factor for the association of FMF and mesothelioma.[117,118] In addition, most cases of postinflammatory mesothelioma with a short interval between inflammation and tumor are probably mesotheliomas that presented with a burst of inflammatory activity, perhaps related to production of cytokines or mediators of inflammation such as interleukin-8, before their final diagnosis as mesothelioma.[119,120]

Irradiation

The literature contains multiple reports of mesothelioma following exposure to ionizing radiation,[121–150] and excess rates of MM have also been reported among both Danish and German patients exposed to radio-active thorium dioxide (Thorotrast®) for radiologic procedures.[121,124,134,135]

Austin et al.[131] reported an ipsilateral malignant pleural mesothelioma in a 28-year-old woman who had a Wilms' tumor at age 4 that had been treated with nephrectomy followed by irradiation. This case is of further interest because asbestos analysis on the autopsy lung tissue found the asbestos content to be within the "normal" range (0–20 asbestos bodies/gram of wet lung tissue). Anderson et al.[132] reported a diffuse epithelial mesothelioma in a 16-year-old boy who at age 2 had received pulmonary irradiation for metastatic Wilms' tumor.

A case of mesothelioma was reported by Mizuki et al.[133] in a 75-year-old Japanese man who developed a left pleural mesothelioma 50 years after the atomic bomb was dropped on Nagasaki in 1945. However, this patient had a history of asbestos exposure at the munitions factory where he was employed as a shipbuilder for 2 years. This case emphasizes the dilemma that background asbestos exposure represents as a confounding factor for some cases associated with radiation (or other associations such as immunodeficiency); for example, in one report on mortality among 260 plutonium workers, all six mesotheliomas occurred in individuals who had also sustained asbestos exposure.[123] In the authors' files are three cases of MM following mantle irradiation for Hodgkin's disease, renal transplant, and radiotherapy for carcinoma of the vulva. Each patient, however, had background exposure to asbestos, including one patient with domestic exposure who laundered her husband's asbestos-laden work clothes.

Neugut et al.[130] carried out a retrospective study of 251,750 women with breast cancer (~25% of whom had been treated with radiation therapy [RT]) and 13,743 patients with Hodgkin's disease (~50% treated with RT), and found no evidence of an association with MM. Nonetheless, this study had two major weaknesses: (1) there appears to have been little or no pathologic verification or classification of recurrent tumors, so that given the past medical history for those patients (breast cancer, Hodgkin lymphoma), any mesotheliomas might have been misclassified as recurrent breast cancer or lymphoma; and (2) the follow-up for the patients in this study did not extend beyond 20 years, so that any mesothelioma cases developing thereafter would have been missed.

Teta et al.[151] found 26 patients with mesothelioma as second primaries based on an evaluation of 21,881 diagnoses of Hodgkin's lymphoma and 101,001 diagnoses of non-Hodgkin's lymphoma. There was stated to be a statistically increased incidence of mesothelioma, with a standardized incidence ratio (SIR) of 6.9 and a confidence interval (CI) of 1.79 to 16.87 among men with Hodgkin's lymphoma who received radiation, and a nonsignificant excess of mesothelioma among men with non-Hodgkin's lymphoma with an SIR of 1.91 and a CI of 0.77 to 3.93. Teta et al. concluded that mesothelioma rates for patients who received radiotherapy were increased for survivors of Hodgkin's lymphoma and non-Hodgkin's lymphoma. No increased incidence of mesothelioma was observed among the nonirradiated.

Travis et al.[129] carried out a study on second cancers among 40,576 testicular cancer patients with a focus on long-term survivors, and found a significantly elevated relative risk (RR) for pleural MM of 3.4 (95% CI, 1.7–5.9). The authors concluded that survivors of testicular cancer were at a statistically significantly increased risk of solid tumors for at least 35 years following treatment by either radiotherapy or chemotherapy. This study did not find any *peritoneal* mesotheliomas following radiation therapy; all of the MMs were *pleural* in location. The authors mentioned that the thorax can receive radiation as a consequence of radiotherapy for testicular cancer, but it is also worth emphasizing that the radiation field for testicular tumors is directed mainly to abdominal and paraaortic lymph nodes. Therefore, it is of interest that all the MMs in this study occurred *outside* the main radiation field, although there are at least two reports of peritoneal MM following radiotherapy for testicular cancer.[137,149]

It is well known that patients with one cancer have an increased risk of other cancers; for example, one strong risk factor for breast cancer is an antecedent cancer in the contralateral breast. The notion of innate (gene-mediated) predisposition to cancer/mesothelioma induction has also been debated by some of the authors addressing radiation and mesothelioma. For example, Shannon et al.[145] noted that the experimental data support a role for radiation in the development of pleural MM. Mesotheliomas were found in 65% of rats 1 year after intraperitoneal injection of plutonium 239 ($^{239}PuO_2$). Whether radiation acts as an independent carcinogen or whether it potentiates the effects of other carcinogenic factors such as asbestos is unclear. An overall increased incidence of pleural MM in rats exposed to irradiation and asbestos (11.8%) over those exposed to asbestos alone (3.8%) has been observed, suggesting that radiation may act as a cocarcinogen to induce MM.[139]

Shannon et al.[145] also reported the following:

> Other variables must be considered in cases negative for asbestos exposure. An obvious common denominator in each of the cases reported is a history of a previous malignancy. The incidence of metachronous multiple primary neoplasms varies from 0.2 to 12%, depending on the selection criteria for the study group. The excess rates of second neoplasms have been ascribed to a genetic predisposition for multiple cancers in several types of tumors. In particular, studies have found a two to three-fold increased incidence of second neoplasms in patients with colon, lung, breast and head and neck carcinomas as well as certain leukemias and Hodgkin's and non-Hodgkin's lymphoma. However, pleural MM as a second malignancy in cancer-prone patients does not appear to be increased in the absence of other predisposing factors. Hence, genetic predisposition is unlikely to be the sole factor in the development of MM as a second primary malignancy.

Travis et al.[129] also conclude that treatment (as opposed to genetic susceptibility to tumors) probably explains much of the observed excess tumors in testicular cancer patients, an interpretation supported by the lower risks in the first 10 years of follow-up.

Accordingly, it is our view that ionizing radiation may play a causal-contributory role in the genesis of some mesotheliomas, probably as a cofactor along with innate susceptibility to cancer development (as demonstrated by one or more antecedent cancers), with or without past asbestos exposure, but the number of such radiation-related cases is small in comparison to the burden of asbestos-related MMs, for which radiation is not a co-factor.

Malignant Mesotheliomas in Children (and the Concept of Spontaneous Mesotheliomas)

In 1985 Talerman et al.[152] reported a case of a diffuse malignant deciduoid peritoneal mesothelioma in a 13-year-old girl and reviewed the literature identifying 41 previously reported cases of mesothelioma in children. Thirty-three of the 41 previously reported cases began in the pleura, and 40 of the 41 children died 2 weeks to 21 months after diagnosis, a clinical course similar to that in adults. In many reported cases of mesothelioma in children, a history of exposure to asbestos was not documented, and in Talerman et al.'s case and in two other cases reviewed, there was no history of exposure to asbestos.

Fraire et al.[153] independently reviewed slides available of 17 children previously diagnosed as having mesothelioma. Upon review, only three cases were confirmed as mesothelioma. Therefore, they concluded mesothelioma in children might be rarer than suspected. Fraire et al.[154] conducted an extended evaluation of 80 reported cases of mesothelioma in childhood. Of the 80 cases, tissue slides were available for review in 22 cases, of which 10 were considered MM, nine nonmesothelial malignant tumors, and three malignant neoplasms of uncertain type. The authors found no relationship between childhood MM and asbestos, radiation, or isoniazid therapy. Lin-Chu et al.[155] reported a confirmed case of MM in a 19-month-old girl. In their review of the literature, they found three other cases of MM in infants. In their case, there was no information concerning exposure to asbestos.

The occurrence of mesothelioma during infancy, childhood, and adolescence supports the notion of true spontaneous mesotheliomas. Diagnosis of mesothelioma during infancy and childhood poses greater difficulties than for adults, especially the distinction from pleuropulmonary blastomas of childhood[156] and perhaps desmoplastic small round cell tumors of the pleura,[37] but there is little doubt that childhood mesotheliomas do occur. From a review of three studies, McDonald and McDonald[157] suggest that the incidence of childhood mesothelioma may be within the range of 0.5 to 1.0 case/10^7/yr.

Background Exposure to Asbestos and Background or Spontaneous Mesotheliomas: Do They Exist? It is our perception that background asbestos exposure from the environment at large represents general environmental exposure unrelated to the use of asbestos-containing materials in the workplace or at home, or from significant point sources of asbestos such as factories. We consider background exposure to include exposures related to the passive weathering of in-place asbestos-containing materials, including asbestos-cement roofing materials with very low or unmeasurably low airborne fiber concentrations, and environmental exposure derived from the brakes of passing automobiles; we exclude from "background" any exposure arising from active disturbance of any asbestos-containing materials such as asbestos-cement building products or insulation materials.

It is also important to recognize that absence of a history of asbestos exposure does not equate to absence of exposure. Many cases of seemingly background MM can be attributed to long-past forgotten or unrecognized asbestos exposures. For example, many of the cases that are encountered in our everyday or referral practice are accompanied by a clinical statement that no asbestos exposure has been identified, but subsequent and more detailed history-taking usually does yield a history of brief exposure to asbestos, and in some of those cases the mesothelioma patient was unaware that the material used (e.g., fibrous cement building materials) did in fact contain asbestos. The problem of detailed and systematic history-taking is also exemplified by some of the data in the Australian Mesothelioma Surveillance Program, in which a substantial number of the cases initially classified as having no known exposure history in fact had asbestos exposure documented upon more detailed review.[43]

The often-cited background MM rate of 1 to 2 per million person-years, was derived partly from backward extrapolation of the incidence rates in men, to the point where the rates for men and women diverged from each other, based on a presupposition that the female incidence rate for mesothelioma has been stable, and that most MMs in women represent background cases.[158] In reality, there is persuasive evidence that both of these assumptions are false: (1) in the United Kingdom the death rate for MM in females increased from 4.67/10^6/yr in 1989–1991 to 5.77 in 1995–1997,[159] and to 9.75 in 2002–2004; (2) the female incidence rate in Australia rose about threefold over a period of ~20 years; (3) Strickler et al.[160]

also recorded a rising incidence of MM in the U.S. for women aged 45 to 54 years and above, for the period 1975–1997, based on SEER data, which cover about 14% of the U.S. population; and (4) among female MM patients, up to ~75% in some series[36,161] had a history of asbestos exposure, but the exposures were occupational in only a minority (~20%),[161] so that nonoccupational exposures such as domestic (household contact) exposure constitute a much higher proportion of MM cases among women than in men.[161] As foreshadowed in the preceding discussion, Roggli et al.[161] found that the lung tissue asbestos burden was elevated in 70% of a series of female MM patients in the U.S., and the main fiber type detected was amosite, followed by tremolite and chrysotile, and the lung tissue asbestos body and fiber concentrations as a consequence of such domestic exposure approached those found with some patterns of occupational exposure.[162]

The background environmental mesothelioma incidence rate and especially the true spontaneous rate is probably substantially less than one case/10^6/yr, but the true rate can only be guessed, because no significant control adult population without asbestos fibers in lung tissue can be assembled.[163]

Hereditary Factors and the Role of Genetic Susceptibility

Mesothelioma occurs in only a minority of asbestos-exposed individuals, even in those exposed heavily to amphibole asbestos.[36] This observation might be explicable by mesothelioma induction as a chance event; that is, mesothelioma is the outcome of a multistage process involving multiple mutational and epigenetic events, so that most of those exposed to asbestos simply do not strike the correct combination of a complex set of events necessary for development of mesothelioma. Alternatively, one of the mutations induced by asbestos may be lethal to the initiated cell, so that subsequent steps cannot occur (see Molecular Pathogenesis and Pathology of Malignant Mesothelioma, below). However, alternative explanations include (1) modulation of the asbestos-imposed risk by genetic or acquired susceptibility/resistance factors,[164] or (2) a combination of randomness and predisposition.

In 1985 Lynch et al.[165] described the occurrence of epithelial mesotheliomas in two brothers who had been exposed to asbestos, and reviewed the literature citing three other reports of familial mesothelioma. Ten of 11 family members in the four families reported had a definite history of exposure to asbestos. In 1984 Martensson et al.[166] reported two pairs of siblings, a brother and sister and identical twin brothers, who developed pleural MMs. Both pairs of siblings had exposure to asbestos. We reported three brothers who had an asbestos insulation business; two developed mesotheliomas that arose in the pleura and the other brother had peritoneal mesothelioma.[167] Subsequently, one male child and one female child in this family died from pleural MM.

Other studies have evaluated hereditary factors in mesothelioma. Huncharek et al.[168] studied 39 cases of pleural mesothelioma and 259 age-matched controls to assess the possibility of influence of family history on pleural MM risk. Twenty-eight (71%) cases reported a parental history of cancer versus 114 (44%) in the control group ($p < .01$), suggesting a possible role for a family history of cancer in the development of pleural mesothelioma.

Heineman et al.[169] evaluated mesothelioma, asbestos, and reported history of cancer in first-degree relatives. Specifically, they compared reported histories of cancer in first-degree relatives of 196 patients who had a pathologic diagnosis of mesothelioma, with those from 511 deceased controls. The authors found only limited suggestive evidence that a family history of cancer may be a risk factor for mesothelioma, possibly in conjunction with asbestos exposure. Studies of small family clusters, including that of Ascoli et al.[170] in relatives working in a confectionary shop highlighted the possibility that inherited factors might be involved in the development of MM. We have seen a number of other familial cases of mesothelioma where two or more family members developed mesothelioma, usually in a setting of occupational or domestic bystander asbestos exposure (Fig. 43.4).

A larger survey conducted by Bianchi et al.[171] included 610 pleural mesotheliomas of which 40 were found to be familial. Familial mesotheliomas included 31 men and nine women with an age range of 44 to 93 with a mean of 70.7 and a median of 71.0 years. In 15 families, there were blood relations between or among the members involved. However, all patients had reported exposures to asbestos, mostly in the shipyard.

Ohar et al.[172] tried to identify a more extensive set of traits that would define a mesothelioma phenotype for the purpose of genetic analysis. They found that compared to other asbestos-exposed groups, subjects with mesothelioma were younger at first asbestos exposure, had a greater risk of second cancer diagnosis, had a longer disease latency, and had a greater risk of cancer among first-degree relatives. The authors concluded that thoracic tumor location, work exposure, male gender, long latency, early age at first exposure, presence of a second cancer, and first-degree relative with cancer defined a phenotype that distinguishes mesothelioma patients with a short survival from other asbestos-exposed individuals. They proposed this phenotype could be applied to candidate gene analysis.

Several studies have attempted to determine a cytogenetic profile for MM. Ascoli et al.[173] performed genomic

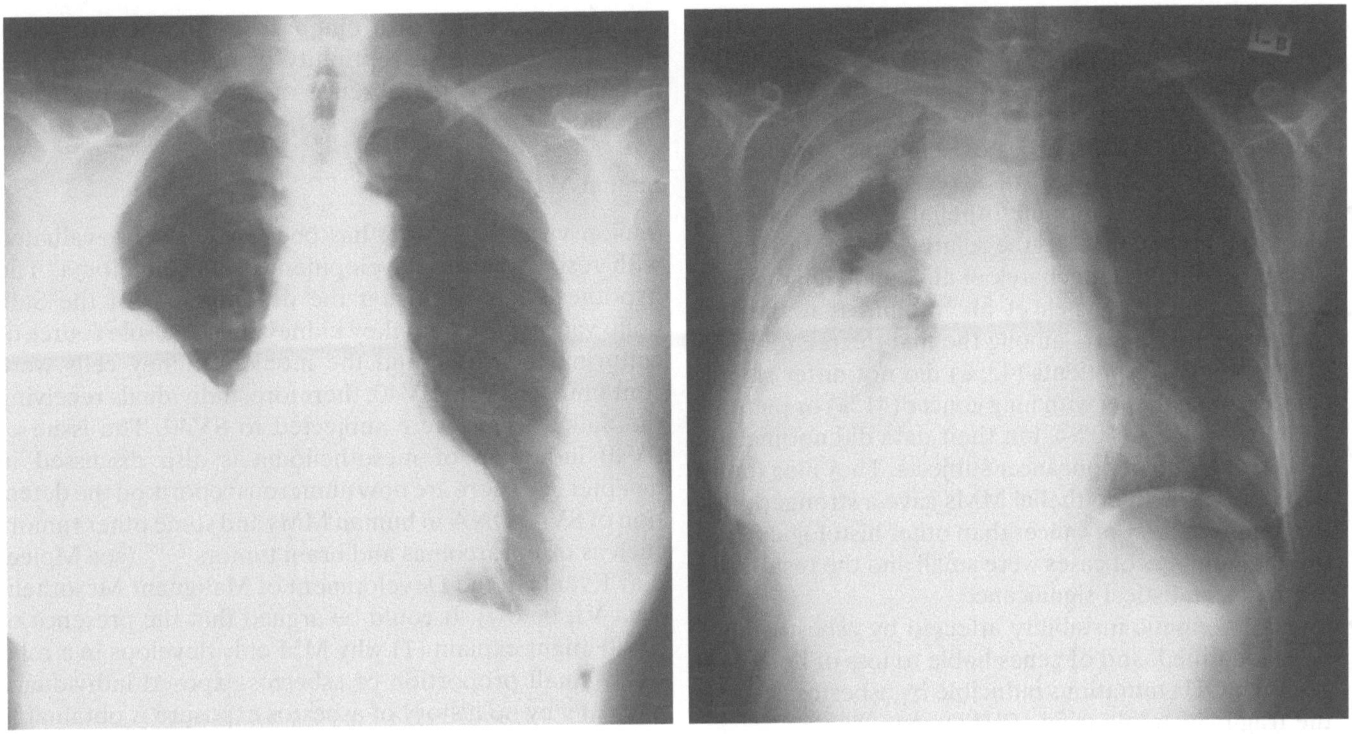

FIGURE 43.4. Familial pleural malignant mesothelioma (MMs) in a mother **(A)** and her daughter **(B)**, proven by surgical biopsy in each case. The mother often shook out and washed the asbestos-contaminated work clothes of the husband/father, and the daughter was often present in the laundry when her mother did so. The mother and daughter developed their mesotheliomas within 3 years of each other.

hybridization analysis on tumor samples from members of a family with MM of the pleura and a history of parental cancer. Their aim was to find a recurrent copy number loss indicating the chromosomal area to which a gene underlying the development of mesothelioma could be assigned according to the Knudson two-hit hypothesis. They found losses at 1p, 6q, 9p, 13q, and 14q. The copy number changes were stated to have been very similar to those reported in sporadic cases. Their findings and results from sporadic cases highlighted the importance of cloning of the genes in the loss sites at 1p, 6q, 14q, and 22q.

Musti et al.[174] described a family of three sisters affected by MM, two of which were pleural and one of which was peritoneal, and one brother who had pleural plaques. All family members were stated to have been subjected to previous asbestos exposure of environmental-residential type. DNA extracted from paraffin-embedded MM samples was used to search for chromosomal alterations by a comparative genomic hybridization (CGH) method. In two cases, a loss at 9p was found to be the only change. The loss at 9p was stated to be a frequent event in MM. The fact this anomaly was diagnosed in two sisters as the only alteration suggested this region could be the site of one or more oncosuppressor genes that could play an important role in the development of MM in inducing greater genetic susceptibility to the carcinogenic effect of asbestos.

Bianchi et al.[175] indicate that the most frequent cytogenetic abnormality in MM is loss of chromosome 22. Neurofibromatosis type 2 gene *(NF2)* is a tumor suppressor gene assigned to chromosome 22q that plays an important role in the development of familial and spontaneous tumors of neuroectodermal origin. Molecular studies have implicated *NF2* in the oncogenesis of MMs and possibly other nonneural tumors (see below).

Is There a Genetic Susceptibility to Mesothelioma Induction by Asbestos? Evidence for a component of genetic susceptibility to mesothelioma includes the following:

- There is an analogy with other cancers. From data in the Swedish Family-Cancer Database, Hemminki et al.[176] found evidence for a genetic component for a variety of cancers, among which mesothelioma is unlikely to be an exception.
- Familial clusters of MM[177,178] (Fig. 43.4) may be explicable mainly by the sharing of occupational, domestic,

environmental, and even recreational asbestos exposures among members of the same family,[179] but the development of MM among multiple different members of one family is unlikely, even when all the affected members did sustain asbestos exposure (see above discussion).

- The frequency of nonmesothelial cancers may be increased among first-degree relatives of MM patients; see above data of Huncharek et al.[168] and Heineman et al.[169] In contrast, Lynch et al.[180] found that the frequency of any cancers among the first-degree relatives of mesothelioma patients (43%) did not differ significantly from patients with lung cancer (41%) or patients with any cancers (40%), but their data did not include a control group of noncancer subjects. They also found that patients with epithelial MMs gave a stronger positive family history of cancer than other histologic types, but the numbers of cases were small and the results did not reach statistical significance.
- Sites of genomic instability affected by asbestos have been identified, and of genes liable to loss of heterozygosity (LOH) mutations inducible by asbestos, such as the fragile histidine triad *(FHIT)* gene.[181,182]
- Hirvonen et al.[183] carried out a molecular case-referent study on the glutathione-S-transferase M1 *(GSTM1)* gene and the *N*-acetyltransferase-2 *(NAT)* genotype (slow versus fast acetylators) among 145 Finnish asbestos insulators exposed to high levels of asbestos; 69 had no pulmonary disorders (controls), and 76 had either MM (n = 24), or benign pleuropulmonary disorders such as asbestosis or pleural plaques (n = 52). Hirvonen et al. found that the odds ratio (OR) for the development of either malignant or benign pulmonary disorders for individuals with a *NAT2* slow-acetylator genotype was more than double the OR for those with a *NAT2* fast-acetylator genotype (OR, 2.3; 95% CI, 1.1–4.7): for *NAT2* slow-acetylators, the OR_{MM} was 3.8 (95% CI, 1.2–14.3). Those who lacked the *GSTM1* gene and who had a *NAT2* slow-acetylator genotype had about a fivefold risk for both malignant and benign pulmonary disorders in comparison to those who had the *GSTM1* gene and a *NAT2* fast-acetylator genotype (OR, 5.1; 95% CI, 1.6–17.6). Subjects with a *GSTM1*-absent/*NAT2* slow-acetylator profile had an almost eightfold increased risk of MM (OR, 7.8; 95% CI, 1.4–78.7), although it is notable that the CI for this last result is very wide. Such findings are reviewed and discussed in greater detail by Puntoni et al.[184]
- There is evidence of species and strain susceptibility to mesothelioma among experimental animals used as models of mesotheliomagenesis. As examples, hamsters appear to be particularly susceptible to mesothelioma induction by a variety of factors, whereas rats are more resistant (and reportedly about 100-fold less susceptible to MM than humans[185]).

Nonetheless, it is worth emphasizing that it is unlikely that such genetic susceptibility would be expressed as mesothelioma in the absence of asbestos (in particular amphibole) exposure.

Simian Virus 40

Simian virus 40 (SV40) has been extensively evaluated with respect to the development of mesothelioma. The hypothesis has been that the development of the Salk polio vaccine used monkey kidney cells as a sole source of culturing the virus, and the monkey kidney cells were contaminated with SV40; therefore, individuals receiving the Salk vaccine were subjected to SV40. The issue of SV40 induction of mesothelioma is also discussed in Chapter 33. There are now numerous reports on the detection of SV40 DNA in human MMs and some other tumors such as osteosarcomas and brain tumors[186,187] (see Molecular Events in the Development of Malignant Mesothelioma VI, below). It could be argued that the presence of SV40 might explain (1) why MM only develops in a relatively small proportion of asbestos-exposed individuals, and (2) why no history of asbestos exposure is obtainable on a sizable minority of MMs. However, almost all the MMs in which SV40 DNA has been found were asbestos-associated. Existing data do not adequately address either of the two foregoing issues, for which there are alternative explanations. In other studies, SV40 or SV40 large T-antigen (Tag) could not be detected within MMs.[188] A statement on MM from the British Thoracic Society ranked the evidence for SV40 as a cofactor for mesothelioma induction as only "weak,"[189] and Lee et al.[190] argued that the relationship is unproven. In addition, an expert committee in the U.S. concluded that the evidence was insufficient either to assign or to exclude a contributory role for SV40 in the genesis of MM.[187] Two of the most recent studies suggest that there is no evidence that SV40 causes mesothelioma in humans.[191,192] Accordingly, SV40 might be regarded as a possible but unproven genetic susceptibility factor in the induction of MM by asbestos or a permissive factor for MM growth after its induction.

Immunodeficiency

Rare individual cases of MM have been recorded in association with immunodeficiency states, including HIV/AIDS, and in a renal transplant recipient.

Occupations at Risk

In national cancer registries, up to about 90% of male MM patients have a history of past asbestos exposure, especially for pleural MM, with a somewhat smaller percentage (about 60%) for patients with peritoneal MM.[193,194] Among female mesothelioma patients, about 40% to 75% have a history of asbestos exposure,[161] but

TABLE 43.4. Mesothelioma proportional mortality ratios (PMRs) in the United Kingdom, 1980–2000, by 5-year intervals, for men aged 16 to 74, according to last occupation, for the top 10 PMRs and the lowest five PMRs

Occupation	1980–1986 (excluding 1981)	1986–1990	1991–1995	1995–2000	Increased (↑) or decreased (↓) trend
Top 10 in 1995–2000					
Vehicle body builder	504	614	606	462	
Carpenter	361.5	373	361	395	
Electrical plant operator	405	163	255	295	
Metal plate worker	723	608.5	556	292	↓
Boiler operator	270	255.5	241	250	
Construction manager	180	226	185.5	195	
Metal, jewelry, electrical prod'n	105	84	167	165	↑
Construction worker	268	228	204	174	↓
Painter, decorator	137	146	168	173	
Technicians	182	124	170	158	
Lowest five in 1995–2000					
Lawyer	0.0	0.0	40	10	
Leather/shoe worker	34	39	34	11	
Clergy	46	48	60	20	
Doctor	0.0	25	37	32	
Farmer	15	28	25	32	

PMRs corrected to the nearest 0.5.
Source: HSE Statistics. Mesothelioma Occupation Statistics: Male and Female Deaths Aged 16–74 in Great Britain 1980–2000 (Excluding 1981): Table 3 in original.

the exposures are occupational in only about 20% of cases,[161] so that a higher proportion of MM cases among women is a consequence of nonoccupational exposure[161,193] (see previous discussion).

The occupations that account for the greatest absolute numbers of MMs have changed over the years from miners/millers, products manufacturers, and insulation workers, to other end-users of asbestos-containing products, including the building construction and demolition industries (Tables 43.4 and 43.5),[49] while ship construction and repair still account for substantial numbers of cases, especially in the U.S. (Table 43.5).[162]

The building construction workforce is large and comprises a heterogeneous collection of occupations and workers who vary from the self-employed, to employees of small or large corporations, and working conditions in

TABLE 43.5. Mesothelioma cases in the United States according to industry, among 1445 cases of malignant mesothelioma (MM)

Industry	Single pattern of exposure (No.)	Multiple patterns of exposure (No.)	Total (%)
Shipbuilding[a]	203	86	27.6
U.S. Navy/merchant marine	91	84	16.7
Building construction[b]	99	35	12.8
Insulation[c]	92	11	9.8
Oil/chemical	78	10	8.4
Power plant	50	10	5.7
Railways	37	16	5.1
Automotive/brake mechanic	24	27	4.9
Steel/metal/foundry/furnace	33	10	4.1
Asbestos products manufacture[d]	34	5	3.7
Paper mill	7	0	0.7
Ceramics/glass	6	0	0.6
Totals	754	294	1048

[a]Includes joiner, shipwright, rigger, sandblaster, shipfitter, electrician, painter, welder.
[b]Includes construction worker, laborer, carpenter, painter, plasterer.
[c]Includes pipe coverer (lagger), insulator, asbestos sawyer, asbestos sprayer.
[d]Includes textile and other products manufacture.
Source: Modified from Roggli et al.[162]

TABLE 43.6. Individual lifetime risk of mesothelioma (MM) in Australia by occupational groupings

Occupational group	Lifetime risk of MM (%)*
Wittenoom miner/miller	16.5
Power station worker	12
Railways laborer	6.5
Navy/merchant navy	5
Carpenter/joiner	2
Waterside worker/docker	2
Plasterer	2
Boilermaker/welder	2
Bricklayer	2
Plumber	1.5
Painter/decorator	1
Electrical fitter/mechanic/electrician	0.5
Vehicle/automobile mechanic	0.5
All Australian men	0.4
All Australian women	0.05

*To the nearest 0.5%, except for *all Australian men and women.*
Source: Modified from Leigh et al.[43]

the building industry have been poorly regulated.[42,159,195,196] In Australia, crocidolite miners/millers, power station workers, railway laborers, and naval, merchant naval, and shipyard personnel (in descending order of risk) have the highest estimated individual lifetime risks of MM (Table 43.6).[36] Even so, the number of personnel employed in each of those occupations is smaller than in the building and construction industry, so that carpenters/joiners, for example, contribute greater absolute numbers to the national MM toll, although their individual risk is less.[193]*

Statistical data for the U.K. published by the Health and Safety Executive (HSE)[44] also recorded significant numbers of mesotheliomas as a consequence of insulation materials in buildings (and elsewhere), the highest risks being the consequence of exposures related to shipbuilding, railway carriage and locomotive building, and the installation or maintenance of insulation materials in buildings or factories.

Substantial numbers of MMs—about 10% of the total, according to data from the HSE in the U.K.[49]—are now seen as a consequence of nonoccupational exposures, including occasional and transient "handyman"-type exposures related to home renovation, repairs and maintenance, and domestic exposure[197] (e.g., from shaking and laundering asbestos-contaminated work clothes[198]) and other types of occasional or nonoccupational exposures.[42,117,163,193] It is worth emphasizing, however, that not all such nonoccupational exposures necessarily represent low-dose exposures; for example, the shaking of asbestos-contaminated work clothes before laundering them can generate high peak concentrations of airborne asbestos fibers,[199,200] resulting in cumulative exposures that can approach or amount to some occupational exposures[162,201,202] (such as those recorded for electricians[162]), and some such cases have shown clinical or histologic evidence of asbestosis.[203,204] Roggli et al.[161] recorded asbestosis in three of 38 cases of mesothelioma that followed household contact exposure to asbestos (8%), and more than half had pleural plaques (Table 43.7).

Apart from some specific industries, such as former crocidolite miners/millers at the Wittenoom blue asbestos industry in Western Australia[205–207] (Figs. 43.5 to 43.8), those who assembled gas masks that contained crocidolite fibers during World War II,[208] and amosite factory workers, most asbestos exposures in the past (until about the early 1980s) involved mixtures of commercial amphibole and chrysotile fibers (e.g., in asbestos insulation and high-density asbestos-cement products), so that most mesotheliomas following end-use asbestos exposures are a consequence of mixed-fiber exposures.[42] There is also evidence that manipulations carried out on such materials resulted in preferential release of amphibole fibers as opposed to chrysotile, presumably because of differences in their physical properties. Accordingly, the proportional concentrations of the airborne fibers in the breathing zones of those exposed were not the same as the proportions in the products as manufactured; for example, in one report in Australia, the ratio of crocidolite/chrysotile fibers in the airborne dust produced by machining of asbestos-cement products was about 28:100 in comparison to 11:100 for the asbestos-cement as manufactured (about 2.5 times greater).[209]

Pleural/Peritoneal Mesothelioma Ratios

On theoretical grounds, one would expect the pleural/peritoneal ratio for true spontaneous MMs uninfluenced by any exogenous causal factor(s) to be about 1:1 or <1:1, taking into account the mesothelial surface areas for the pleural cavities combined versus the peritoneum. Although peritoneal mesotheliomas outnumber pleural MMs in some series—for example, in 86 deaths among Swedish insulation workers during the period 1970–1994, there were seven peritoneal mesotheliomas but no pleural MMs[210]—in most series and in national data, about 90% of MMs or more affect the pleura, about 9% the peritoneum, and about 1% or less the pericardium or tunica

*Data for Australia are discussed at various points in this chapter because the Australian Mesothelioma Register collated all cases of pathologically verified mesothelioma across the entire Australian population (~20 million), but following the introduction of privacy legislation, follow-up of the reported cases became more difficult and notifications to the register were suspended in 2006. However, it seems that mortality statistics and some other data will continue to be reported, from anonymous data sent from State Cancer Registries. The peak incidence of mesothelioma in Australia seems likely to occur in about 2020.

TABLE 43.7. Malignant mesothelioma (MM) pleura-to-peritoneum ratio, parietal pleural plaques and asbestosis, according to industry and occupational versus non-occupational exposures for 1445 cases of MM, in the United States

Industry/occupation	Pleura-to-peritoneum ratio	Parietal pleural plaques (%)	Asbestosis (%)
Industry			
Shipbuilding	52:1	81	26
U.S. Navy	54:1	21	11
Construction	8.6:1	34	17
Insulation	2.1:1	85	58
Oil/chemical	82:1	78	17
Power plant	17:1	85	19
Automotive	8:1	67	0
Railways	38:1	83	12
Steel/metal	9.3:1	93	27
Asbestos products mfg.	2.2:1	87	65
Paper mill	6.1	83	20
Ceramics/glass	6:0	50	0
Occupation			
Pipefitter	50:1	87	24
Boilermaker	30:1	81	24
Maintenance	26:1	80	20
Machinist	22:1	78	14
Electrician	74:1	83	27
Sheet metal	20:1	82	14
Other asbestos	5:1	33	0
Nonoccupational			
Domestic	4.3:1	57	7.9
Building occupants	1.8:1	43	0
Environmental	4:10	0	0
Other	8.5:1	46	9.5

Source: Modified from Roggli et al.[162]

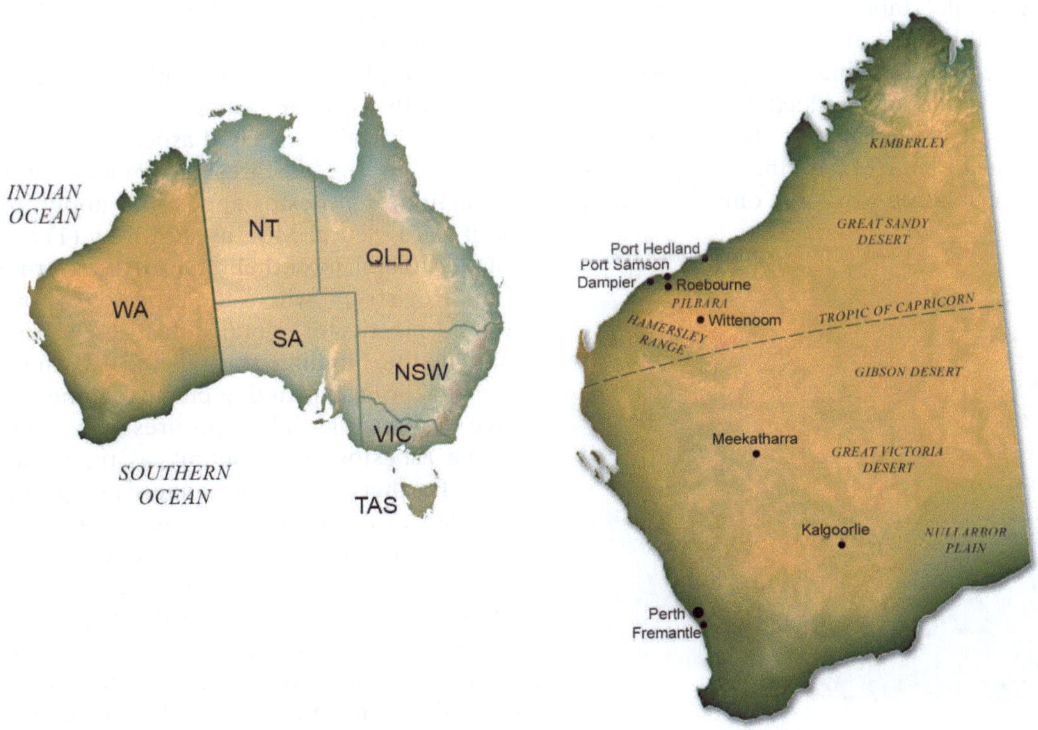

FIGURE 43.5. Schematic map of Western Australia showing Wittenoom in relation to the Tropic of Capricorn, in the Pilbara-Hamersley region, together with other regional centers and Perth. WA, Western Australia; NT, Northern Territory; SA, South Australia; NSW, New South Wales; QLD, Queensland; VIC, Victoria; TAS, Tasmania.

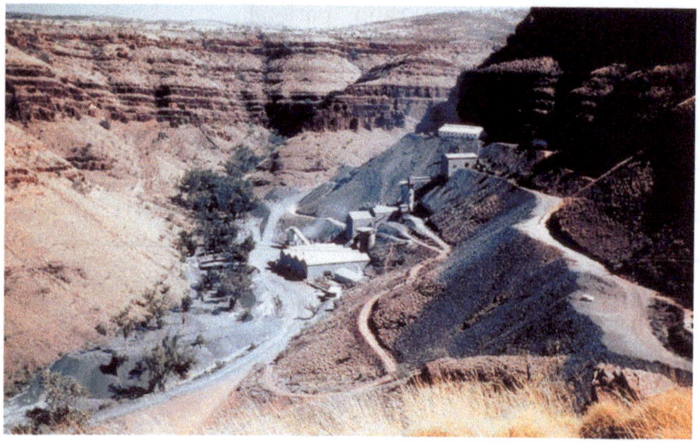

FIGURE 43.6. The Wittenoom asbestos mine and mill. The mine was located slightly to the right of the uppermost white building, in the face of the gorge. The mill has a white roof and is located near the center of the photograph. The gray-blue material represents crocidolite tailings from the mine. For scale, note the parked white automobile on an access road, near the lower right portion of this view. (Courtesy of the Asbestos Diseases Society of Australia.)

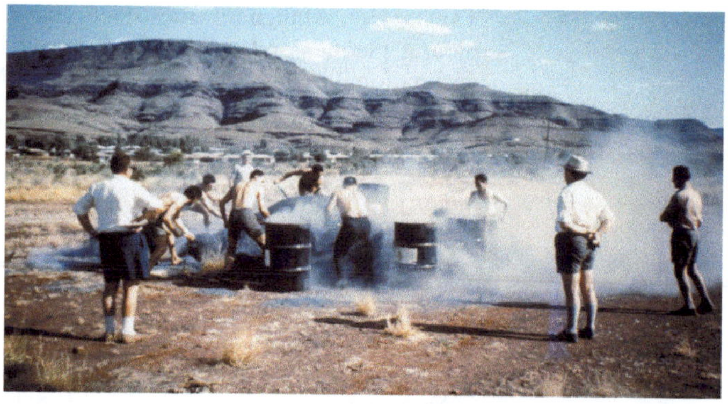

FIGURE 43.8. A race at Wittenoom to determine who could fill a 44-gallon drum with crocidolite in the shortest time. All but two of the men in this field are thought to have died from asbestos-induced cancer. The man just to the left of the 44-gallon drum closest to the observers, from which blue-gray dust is streaming, was awarded compensation in 2004 for the emotional distress induced by his work at Wittenoom, in that he had seen his brother and many of his coworkers die from mesothelioma and other asbestos-related disorders. (Courtesy of the Asbestos Diseases Society of Australia.)

vaginalis testis.[162,193,211] Accordingly, it is thought that inhalation and deposition of asbestos fibers in the lung, with subsequent translocation of fibers (especially amphibole fibers) to the pleura, followed by lesser translocation to sites beyond the pleura, skews the anatomic distribution of MM toward the pleura. In a large series of 1445 mesotheliomas, Roggli et al.[162] tabulated the pleural/peritoneal ratios for MMs (Table 43.7) and found that the smallest ratio of 1.8:1 was for building occupants, which the authors suggested would have reflected, or nearly so, the "background rate of occurrence for these tumors" (but see Hemminki and Li[212]). Even so, the MM pleura/peritoneum ratio for insulation work was only 2.1:1, despite

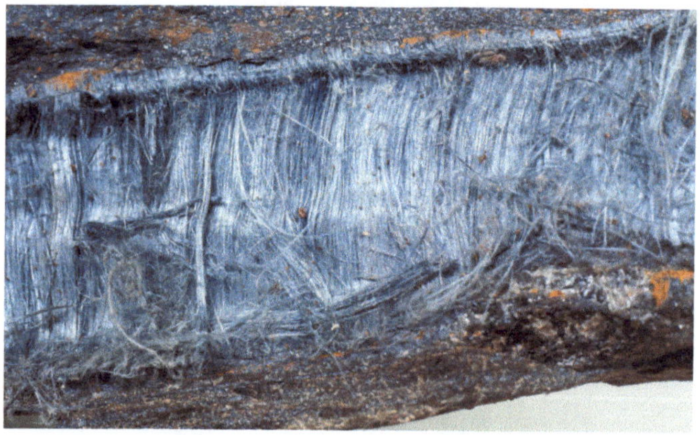

FIGURE 43.7. Wittenoom crocidolite ore. The crocidolite was disposed as thin seams, enclosed by ironstone, as shown here.

the finding of asbestosis as marker for substantial to heavy asbestos exposure in 58% of those MM cases (and pleural plaques in 85%),[162] so that insulation work appears to differ in some unknown ways from other occupational exposures. One might speculate that this reflects transport of a greater fraction of inhaled and deposited fibers from the lungs to the peritoneum than for other patterns of exposure.[213]

In general, peritoneal mesotheliomas tend to be associated with heavier asbestos exposures than pleural MMs,[214,215] with associated asbestosis in a higher proportion,[214] but the no-threshold model for mesothelioma induction by asbestos appears to apply to peritoneal as well as to pleural MM, as shown by (1) analysis of cases of peritoneal mesothelioma in the German Mesothelioma Registry,[214] where the asbestos exposures were sustained mostly in "metal industries, asbestos industries, and in the building trade"; and (2) the occurrence of mesothelioma (including peritoneal mesothelioma) relative to chrysotile-only exposures with analysis of the lung tissue asbestos fiber content, as reported by Rogers et al.[216] Furthermore, in an analysis of peritoneal MMs in Sweden using the Family-Cancer Database, Hemminki and Li[217] recorded an increasing incidence of peritoneal mesothelioma in women in Sweden (but not for men after 1985). They suggested this trend might be related "to nonoccupational exposure [to asbestos] or reasons other than asbestos." For men (among whom pleural mesotheliomas predominated), the occupational groups at greatest risk for peritoneal mesothelioma were bricklayers (SIR = 7.22) and plumbers (SIR = 5.12).

In the German Mesothelioma Registry,[214] the mean age at the time of diagnosis of peritoneal MM was about 59 years for men, whereas women were on average 4 years younger. The mean survival time was about 1 year, but in six of 38 patients longer survival times of up to 7 years were recorded. The epithelial MMs predominated, but no effect on survival time was noticed. The average latency interval was 36 years.

Latency Intervals Between the Commencement of Asbestos Exposure and the Subsequent Diagnosis of Mesothelioma

In the Australian Mesothelioma Surveillance Program, the mean latency interval was 37 years and ranged up to 75 years,[218] and the corresponding latency interval for cases of mesothelioma certified by the Dust Disease Board (DDB) in New South Wales in 2001/2002 was approximately 42 years. In a study of 557 mesothelioma cases reported in 2001 by Bianchi et al.,[219] the latency intervals ranged from 14 to 75 years, with a mean of ~49 years and a median of 51 years. Some authorities and The Helsinki Criteria[220] specify a minimum latency interval of 10 years, whereas others require a minimum interval of 15 years.

Mineral Fibers and Mesothelioma

This section focuses on the relationship between exposures to mineral fibers and the resultant observations of the development of mesothelioma.[1,2] Pleural MMs are most common,[2] although a study of lung cancer and mesothelioma in the pleura and peritoneum among Swedish insulation workers[210] found that "mesothelioma in insulation workers seems to be situated in the peritoneum more often than in the pleura."

Mesothelioma is widely considered an asbestos "marker disease." The report of the Pneumoconiosis Committee of the College of American Pathologists and the National Institute for Occupational Safety and Health (NIOSH)[221] concluded, "malignant mesothelioma of the pleura and peritoneum either are exceptionally rare or never occur in persons not exposed to asbestos."

In fact, Henderson et al.[222] concluded in an overview of attribution of asbestos-related cohorts in Australia that "no threshold of exposure (in other words a level below which there is no effect) has been delineated for asbestos-related malignancies (mesothelioma and lung cancer), but there is some evidence for a threshold for asbestosis and perhaps diffuse pleural fibrosis."

Fiber Length and Mesothelioma

Mineral fibers other than asbestos have been of concern with regard to possible induction of MM in humans.[223] An appreciable concern for exposure to nonasbestos fibers and the risk of producing disease has been based on exposures using animal models where the exposure to the dust was via intraperitoneal route[224–227] or intrapleural implants.[228,229] The common conclusion in these models is that a comparison of risk for the induction of mesothelioma indicates that on a one-to-one basis, a short fiber is less carcinogenically active than a longer, thinner fiber of the same type. Stanton et al.[228,229] acknowledged that some tested fibers that were shorter or thicker also induced mesothelioma. Pott et al.[224–227] concluded the dimensions of fibers are only one factor that enables a fiber to have the ability of inducing mesothelioma.

The Stanton hypothesis[229,230] argues that carcinogenicity is expressed mainly by long thin asbestos fibers, with lengths >5 μm and especially >8 μm, and in the range of 10 to 20 μm, and diameters <0.25 μm. Shorter fibers appear to be less carcinogenic, although it is doubtful that carcinogenicity is restricted to a critical and precise fiber length or diameter.[38] The Stanton model is supported by evidence derived from animal experiments,[231–234] but it seems likely that biopersistence of amphibole fibers may be more important for MM induction than precise fiber dimensions, and data in humans concerning fiber length and mesotheliomagenicity are equivocal.[230,235] Even so, very short-length fibers (<1 μm) appear to have comparatively little carcinogenic activity.

The majority of the existing data from human studies indicates the fibers that are likely to be relocated from the lungs to extrapulmonary sites where mesothelioma develops are short or thin fibers.[236] In studies by Dodson et al.,[236] some longer fibers (>5 μm) were shown to reach the lymph nodes and pleural areas, but the shorter fibers of chrysotile were the predominant fiber type in pleural plaques. This same observation has been made by Sebastien et al.,[237] and by Suzuki and Yuen.[235,238] Suzuki and Yuen also reported short chrysotile fibers in mesothelial tissue. Dodson et al.[239] reviewed the content of omentum and mesentery tissue from occupationally exposed individuals. While there were some longer fibers in these sites where peritoneal mesothelioma develops, the majority of asbestos burden was found to be in the form of short fibers. Boutin et al.[240] did a comparative study of asbestos burden in lung tissue and "black spots" in the parietal pleura. Their finding in the study group was that there was a prevalence of amphiboles in all sites with 22.5% of the fibers ≥5 μm in the "black spots" of pleural tissue. The authors questioned whether this accumulation of fibers indicated a preferred site for mesothelioma and pleural plaques. In a companion paper, Mitchev et al.[241] evaluated the parietal pleura of 150 consecutive necropsies of urban dwellers. The size and intensity of spots were scored and recorded, as were pleural plaques. The report stated that 92.7% of cases had detectable black spots. The study concluded that "there was no relationship between the predominant locations of black spots and hyaline pleural plaques" or the development of mesothelioma.

Nonasbestos and Nonoccupational Mineral Fibers and Mesothelioma

The risk of mesothelioma is not exclusively associated with occupational exposure to asbestos since there are reports of occurrence of mesothelioma in settings where there is no relationship to commercial asbestos exposure. These include reports from Southern Anatolia (Turkey) where causal exposures were suggested as being from environmental "asbestos most consistent with tremolite and actinolite."[242] One other famous internationally recognized area where there are appreciable environmentally induced MMs is in the Cappadocian region of Turkey.[243,244] The explanation for the causal agent in this region is environmental dust deposits of fibrous zeolite-erionite. Rohl et al.[112] found that environmental samples from the villages of Karain, Tuzkoy, and Sarihidir where mesotheliomas had been reported contained not only fibrous zeolite (erionite), but also trace (<3% by weight) to major (≥3% or more by weight) component of asbestos (chrysotile/tremolite). Fibrous outcrops of zeolite are also situated in the Western U.S. Johnson et al.[245] reported in a rat inhalation model that erionite (fibrous zeolite from the Rome, Oregon, area) could induce mesothelioma more rapidly and more frequently than asbestos.

Another example of exposure to a mineral that contains a component now recognized as a causal agent for MM is vermiculite that was mined in Libby, Montana.[246] This material was widely distributed across the U.S. to sites where it was processed into commercial products. This site and the surrounding areas are of concern, as is the "exposure pathway" from mined minerals, shipped minerals, processed minerals, and consumer exposures to asbestos- contaminated vermiculite.[247] Fibrous amphiboles, including tremolite asbestos, which contaminate vermiculite, have resulted in an appreciable loss of life due to asbestos-related diseases in Libby, not only among the miners and others working with processing and delivery of the mineral, but also within the town populace whose only contact was environmental. The previously described exposures reflect only a selected series of exposure to fibrous materials that may stimulate the development of mesothelioma once inhaled.

Identification of Tissue Markers of Past Exposure (Ferruginous Bodies and Uncoated Fibers)

Fibrous minerals in environmental or tissue samples can be assessed and quantitated by light or electron microscopy. To best interpret tissue burden of fibrous dust in individuals diagnosed with mesothelioma, it is imperative that one understands the limitations of detection with various instruments, magnifications, and preparative techniques used in such evaluation. The largest structures seen in tissue that reflect past exposure to fibrous dust (the causal agent for mesothelioma) are ferruginous bodies. These structures are representative of inhaled fibers (>10 μm) that accumulate surface deposits (to varying degrees) of iron coating along the fibrous core. A ferruginous body having a beaded structure with a clear, elongated, transparent, usually straight core is with a high degree of certainty an asbestos body (see Chapter 27).[248] Tissue sections are very insensitive indicators for determining asbestos content since random sampling and random orientation of ferruginous bodies in the plane of the sections require that many sections be reviewed before their presence can be detected, even when the tissue burden is at occupational levels.[249] Roggli and Pratt[249] stated that the sensitivity for quantitating ferruginous bodies increases greatly when the equivalent of many tissue blocks are digested. Several laboratories have defined a burden of asbestos bodies in tissue from the general population that falls in the range of 0 to 20 ferruginous bodies per gram of wet tissue.[250–253]

The use of light microscopy for the detection of uncoated asbestos fibers in tissue is of essentially no value since they are invisible with rare exception. Even when asbestos fibers are numerous only the larger fibers are seen. Langer et al.[254] stated, "The optical microscope delivers a select, biased population" (i.e., larger fibers thicker than 0.5 μm in diameter). The detection and identification of asbestos fibers isolated from tissue can be more readily done with the scanning electron microscope, but with inherent limitations when compared to the capability of the analytical transmission electron microscope (ATEM) as a counting tool,[255] which enables viewing the thinnest/shortest fiber and can confirm a fiber as asbestos based on morphology, elemental composition (chemistry), and crystalline structure (selected area diffraction). The following concepts may be helpful in interpreting data on tissue fiber content in individuals with mesothelioma:

1. The dust burden within a tissue sample represents that portion of the dust that has not been cleared by the time of evaluation. This skews the analysis toward larger inhaled structures, since the smaller ones are more easily cleared over time. This concept is highly relevant for chrysotile, since chrysotile is predominantly inhaled as a short fiber due to its innate physical curvature (Fig. 43.2).
2. The number of isolated ferruginous bodies (morphologically compatible with asbestos bodies) per gram of tissue, determined by tissue digestion, can be reasonably compared between different studies.

3. Low magnification counts of fibers by scanning electron microscopy (SEM) or transmission electron microscopy (TEM) potentially excludes long/thin asbestos fibers, particularly those of chrysotile.[255]

4. An exclusion of fibers <5 µm in a counting strategy, even when the resolution capability of the ATEM is used can result in exclusion of the vast majority of asbestos within tissue samples from lung and, even more dramatically, from extrapulmonary sites.

Much of the chrysotile burden in tissue can be missed due to items 3 and 4.

Studies Defining Mineral Fiber Content in Mesothelioma Patients

In a series of studies using tissue digestion, Roggli et al.[83] quantified ferruginous bodies using light microscopy and detected fibers (>5 µm in length) with SEM. In 25 cases of mesothelioma, Roggli et al. analyzed core material of ferruginous bodies and quantified their numbers per gram of tissue. They found the number of ferruginous bodies fell between the number in tissue from patients with asbestosis and controls. Those cases where ferruginous body counts overlapped with counts found in tissue from the general population often lacked an identifiable occupational exposure to asbestos. The cores of 88 of the 90 ferruginous bodies were found to be amphibole asbestos, with only two asbestos bodies having chrysotile cores.[256] A review of fiber exposures and disease by Roggli[257] concluded, "Mesothelioma may occur with fiber burdens considerably less than those necessary to produce asbestosis." Srebro and Roggli[258] reviewed the tissue burden of five cases with pleural mesothelioma and two with asbestosis. The study found that tremolite asbestos, although not commercially of interest, is a component of some commercially exploited chrysotile veins and vermiculite and talc veins. Their conclusion from the tissue evaluation was that "modest elevations of tremolite content in some of their mesothelioma cases suggest that at least for some susceptible individuals, moderate exposures to tremolite-contaminated dust can produce malignant pleural mesothelioma."

Srebro et al.[259] quantified ferruginous bodies and uncoated fibers in 18 mesothelioma cases in which the tissue burden of ferruginous bodies fell within a "control" population (0–20 asbestos bodies (AB)/g wet tissue). The findings indicated that "electron microscopic analysis of pulmonary mineral fibers may be required to differentiate asbestos-related mesotheliomas from non-asbestos-related cases when AB counts are within the range of background values."

In a synopsis of observations regarding tissue burden from 396 cases of MM, 28 of which were peritoneal, Roggli[260] concluded that the highest levels of fiber burden "occurred in patients who also had asbestosis, which was found in 12% of pleural and 43% of peritoneal cases." He concluded that the average lung fiber burden was higher in peritoneal cases than in pleural cases, a point that is not in agreement with data from our laboratories.[23,261] The observation was also made that approximately 70% of female mesothelioma cases had elevated fiber burden and many had exposure via household contact to an individual with occupational exposure to asbestos. The analysis strategy incorporating SEM included fibers that were detected and were >5 µm in length.

Paoletti et al.[262] reported a high number of pleural mesotheliomas in eastern Sicily. The study included residents who purportedly "never had any relevant exposure to asbestos during their professional lives." However, samples from quarries and building materials commonly used in the area yielded amphibole fibers, as well as the same type of tremolite-actinolite fibers as in lung tissue of a mesothelioma patient. In a similar environmental exposure, Langer et al.[263] reported that four small villages in northwestern Greece had levels of malignant pleural mesothelioma which accounted for "1% of the total mortality from 1981–1985." They reported fibers found in the lungs in individuals with so-called "Metsovo (Greece) lung" consisted of asbestiform tremolite that was identical to the fibers found in the whitewash once used in the area.

Howel et al.[264] reviewed the mineral fiber content and routes of exposure to asbestos associated with mesothelioma in a region of England. They concluded, "The study has confirmed previous results of higher concentrations of asbestos fibers in cases than controls, and has shown that this is still found in subjects with little evidence of occupational and para-occupational exposure. The overlap in concentrations of retained asbestos for different groups of subjects did not suggest a clear cut-off value."

One of the few places where anthophyllite has been mined for commercial utilization is in Finland. Karjalainen et al.[265] reviewed the clinical status of 999 Finnish anthophyllite miners. Three of the individuals died from pleural MM and one from peritoneal mesothelioma. The latency period from onset of employment until diagnosis was from 39 to 58 years. Such a long latency period is not unusual in asbestos-exposed individuals.[23,261] Tissue analysis was conducted on tissue from three individuals with the findings by ATEM being from 270 to 1100 million fibers per gram of dry tissue. This information is important in light of the discussions regarding the carcinogenicity of fibers based on a concept of long/thin fibers being the most dangerous, since individual anthophyllite fibers are among the thickest in diameter of all the amphiboles. Tuomi et al.[266] reported on tissue burden in 19 mesothelioma cases and 15 randomly selected autopsy cases from Finland. The technique used SEM analysis of lung tissue. The "fiber concentration ranged from 0.5 to 370 million fibers per gram of dry tissue in the mesothelioma group and from <0.1 to 3.2 million fibers per gram of dry tissue in the autopsy group. . . . In the lungs of the six mesothelioma patients, anthophyllite was the main fiber type."

While most reports of individuals with MM involve a long period from first exposure, there are reports of mesothelioma developing in young people. Andrion et al.[267] reported a case of peritoneal mesothelioma in a 17-year-old boy. They analyzed lung tissue and found 510,000 asbestos fiber per gram of dry lung tissue, of which 62% were chrysotile and 38% were tremolite. It was suggested that "the tremolite fibres were probably due to environmental exposure to contaminated cosmetic talc."

Glickman et al.[268] reported a study of 18 histologically confirmed cases of canine mesothelioma. The "lung tissue from three dogs with mesothelioma and one dog with squamous cell carcinoma of the lung had higher levels of chrysotile asbestos fibers than lung tissue from control dogs." Such findings raise the question as to whether environmental/secondary exposures to mineral fibers in family members were similar to that of their pets.

It is appropriate to focus on publications that have reviewed mineral fiber content in mesothelioma cases from Canada since 90+% of asbestos used in commercial products in the U.S. came from mines in Canada. Canadian chrysotile has been reported to have a small component of fibrous tremolite asbestos. An evaluation for tremolite was conducted on a *Union Internationale Contre le Cancer* (UICC-B) sample of chrysotile. This sample was composed of chrysotile obtained from several mines in Canada with the percentage based on percent of total mined commercial product. Over 20,000 fibers were analyzed by ATEM and all asbestos fibers observed were chrysotile.[269] This finding is of considerable importance since chrysotile has been shown to induce mesotheliomas in animal models.[227,270] There is confusion as to the ore of which mines contain tremolite and what percent is tremolite.[271] Adding to the confusion is the doctoral dissertation by De[272] stating that crocidolite existed in the adjacent mineral formations to the mined veins of chrysotile.

There are several publications with the same theme regarding chrysotile and risk of MM. Churg[273] evaluated what he considered to be 53 "acceptable" cases of chrysotile-induced mesothelioma, 41 of which were in individuals exposed to chrysotile mine dust that was considered by Churg to be naturally contaminated with tremolite. Ten cases were in individuals who worked in industries where "suspicion of amosite or crocidolite contamination [was] high." His conclusion at that time was that "although chrysotile asbestos can produce mesothelioma in man, the total number of such cases is small and the required doses extremely large." He further concluded,

> The data [were] consistent with the idea that mesotheliomas seen in chrysotile miners and some secondary industry workers [was] produced by the tremolite contained in the chrysotile ore, but that the short length and low aspect ratio of the tremolite [made] its carcinogenicity quite low. However, these data are very indirect, and a role for the chrysotile fiber itself is still possible.

In another study from Churg et al.'s[274] laboratory, an evaluation of lung tissue from 94 long-term chrysotile miners and millers from the region of Thetford Mines, Quebec, was conducted. The conclusion was that "mesothelioma, airway fibrosis, and asbestosis were strongly associated with a high tremolite fiber concentration, whereas pleural plaques and carcinoma of the lung showed no relationship to tremolite burden." They stated,

> Total fiber size measures (total fiber length/g and others) showed differences similar to fiber concentration for mesothelioma, airways fibrosis, and asbestosis, but no one measure was clearly better than another or better than fiber concentration. We conclude that, in this population of heavily exposed chrysotile miners and millers, the presence of airways fibrosis and asbestosis and, probably, mesothelioma reflects high tremolite burden. Whether chrysotile fibers themselves play a role in disease induction remains uncertain.

Another report from Canada evaluated the fiber content in 50 workers seeking compensation from the Workers' Compensation Board of Quebec for pleural or peritoneal mesothelioma.[275] Twelve in the study group were from Asbestos Township (chrysotile mining region) and 11 were from the chrysotile mining region of Thetford Mines. The remaining 27 worked in various nonmining industries. The fiber types found in the three groups were different: "The lungs of workers from Thetford Mines [contained] only chrysotile and tremolite; those from Asbestos Township [contained] chrysotile, tremolite, amosite, and crocidolite; and those in other industries [contained] largely amosite and crocidolite."

Begin et al.[276] reviewed 120 cases referred to the Quebec Workman's Commission Board for work-related compensation of industrial disease. The individuals were divided into three groups. The first consisted of 50 cases from the manufacturing and industrial application sector (primary industry, group 1); 50 cases from the manufacturing industrial application sector (secondary industry, group 2); and 21 from industries where asbestos was not a major work material, often an "incidental" material (tertiary industry, group 3). They reported

> [the] incidence of new cases in each group documenting the general incremental trend in all groups, with the sharpest rises in group 3. In the mining towns of Thetford and Asbestos, the incidence of mesothelioma was proportional to the workforce, thus suggesting that the tremolite air contamination, which [was] 7× higher in Thetford, may not be a significant determinant of the disease in these workers. The incidence of the disease in these chrysotile miners and millers was 62.5 cases per million

per year for the 1980–1990 period in Quebec. The incidence of pleural mesothelioma in chrysotile miners and millers, although not as high as in crocidolite workers, [was] well above the North American male rate. Comparative analyses of incidence of the disease in the two mining towns suggest that tremolite contamination may not be a determining factor in these chrysotile workers.

Langer and McCaughey[277] analyzed lung tissue from an individual whose "sole exposure to asbestos was to chrysotile form during brake maintenance and repairs." Contrary to the concept that chrysotile clears from the lung, these investigators found unaltered chrysotile in the analysis in the form of chrysotile fibrils <1 μm and some >5 μm in length. There were no amphiboles found in the tissue; thus the data were consistent with the occupational history of exposure.

Nolan et al.[278] evaluated the fiber burden by ATEM in five lung cancer cases from Quebec, Canada, and one case of an American worker who developed pleural mesothelioma. Interestingly, the predominant fiber type in the tissue from the American worker was chrysotile, and it was present at a "concentration of 300 times that of the average total fiber content of the Canadian case." Furthermore, "the fiber length distribution of the chrysotile recovered from the U.S. mesothelioma case was indistinguishable from that of chrysotile specimens known to produce mesotheliomas in rats. It was also found that the characteristics of the calcium-magnesium-iron silicate fibers present in all six cases were not readily comparable to tremolite asbestos specimens known to induce mesotheliomas in animals." The longest chrysotile fiber found was 33 μm, with 99% of the fibers identified being chrysotile. No commercial amphiboles were found in the analysis and only 1.5% of the 883 fibers sized were reported as being ≥5 μm in length. An important observation was made that when studies report findings based on fibers ≥5 μm in length, a bias toward tremolite may be introduced since the fiber length distributions in this study indicate a difference between chrysotile and the CaMgFe fibers found in the samples. Eleven percent of the latter were ≥5 μm in length, and the mean of the three reference chrysotile specimens was 1.3%.[278]

Churg and Vedal[279] evaluated tissue samples from 144 shipyard workers and insulators in the Pacific Northwest. Amosite (the majority fiber type) was reported to be found in all lungs, while tremolite and chrysotile were found in most lungs. "No relationship was found between the concentration of chrysotile or tremolite and any disease. Analysis of fiber size measures (length, width, aspect ratio, surface, mass) showed that pleural plaques were strongly associated with high aspect ratio amosite fibers and suggested mesotheliomas were associated with low aspect ratio amosite fibers." They concluded that differences in fiber burden and disease exist when comparing mesothelioma in chrysotile miners and millers and shipyard workers, in that mesothelioma appears to occur at much lower amosite burdens than does asbestosis, "in contrast with the situation previously reported for chrysotile-induced mesothelioma."

McDonald et al.[280] reported on the fiber content of lung tissue from individuals with mesothelioma who were 50 years of age or younger at time of diagnosis. There were 69 males and four females. "Incremental risk examined in a linear model was as highly significant for all amphiboles together as individually. Short, medium and long amphibole fibers were all associated with increased risk in relation to length. In this young age group, amosite and crocidolite fibers could account for about 80% of cases of mesothelioma, and tremolite for some 7%." There was some increased risk with chrysotile, but that was determined to fall short of statistical significance.

Leigh and Driscoll[193] reviewed cases of MM in Australia. They reported that Australia had a history of asbestos mining extending over 100 years, and Australia was the world's highest user per capita of asbestos in the 1950s, with the highest reported national rates of mesothelioma in the world. A review of tissue burden in cases of mesothelioma without documented exposure to asbestos found asbestos in 80% of lung fiber burdens as determined by ATEM of >200,000 fibers >2 μm length per gram of dry lung. They noted the high rate of MM in Australia was related to high past use of asbestos, which was reflected in the findings of elevated tissue levels from previously unrecognized exposures.

Workplace exposures to asbestos often involve exposure to several types of asbestos. There are several reported settings where exposures are overwhelmingly limited to one type of asbestos. Such occurred in facilities where manufacturers were creating filters for cigarettes from crocidolite asbestos. In 1987 Talcot et al.[281] reported that mesotheliomas had been observed in three employees in such a facility. In 1989 Talcot et al.[282] reported that 15 of 33 deaths associated within the cohort were from cancer and five were due to MM. Tissue was referred to our laboratory from two individuals who worked in the facility and died from pleural mesotheliomas.[283] The lung tissue from each individual was found to contain large numbers of ferruginous bodies as well as asbestos fibers, the vast majority of which were crocidolite. Nearly all of the ferruginous bodies analyzed also had crocidolite cores. Dodson and Hammar[284] reported a case in which a housewife developed pleural mesothelioma and the only known contact with asbestos was a history of smoking crocidolite-filtered cigarettes. Crocidolite fibers were identified by ATEM in digested samples from this individual's lung and lymph node tissue, in which anthophyllite and tremolite fibers were also found.

Another rather isolated exposure to a type of mineral fiber (amosite asbestos) occurred in an asbestos pipe insulation plant. The uniqueness of the exposure was that no other type of asbestos was ever documented as having been used in this isolated facility. Levin et al.[285] reviewed the status of former workers in the facility and determined that as of 1998, there were four deaths from pleural mesothelioma and two from peritoneal mesothelioma among a cohort of 1130 individuals. An interesting aspect of employment at the facility was that, historically, individuals often worked for only short periods of time before leaving the facility.

We have published findings in over 200 cases of mesothelioma referred to our labs for evaluation. Ferruginous body concentrations and uncoated asbestos fiber burden as defined on a count scheme by ATEM included fibers >0.5 µm in length. Dodson et al.[23] evaluated the asbestos content in 55 mesothelioma cases from the Northwestern U.S. The area has appreciable heritage in shipbuilding and repair, and thus it was not a surprise that the most common finding was amosite fibers in all but two lung samples (96.4%); 18 individuals had over one million amosite fibers per gram of dry tissue, and 46 of the 55 individuals had an average asbestos body burden of over 1000 asbestos bodies per gram of dry tissue. Analysis of the cores of ferruginous bodies indicated that most were formed on amphiboles: 92.9% were found to have amosite cores, 2.9% crocidolite cores, 1% tremolite cores, 0.4% anthophyllite cores, 0.4% actinolite cores, and 0.1% chrysotile cores. The common observation was that the positive lung samples often reflected a mixed asbestos exposure. The other commercial asbestos fibers were crocidolite in 40% of cases and chrysotile in 56.4% of cases. Five cases were diagnosed as having a primary mesothelioma of the peritoneum. Peritoneal mesotheliomas have traditionally been associated with a higher asbestos burden than pleural MMs. However, the five cases in this study did not follow this pattern, showing a range from high fiber burden to very low fiber burden. In another study by Dodson et al.,[261] cases of peritoneal mesothelioma did not follow the general rule of association with the highest fiber burdens.

A possible explanation for the relatively low fiber counts by Dodson et al.[261] may lie in the manner in which the counts were performed. Most asbestos fibers in human lung are less than 5 µm in length and are therefore not reported in many studies that include only the longer or thicker population of fibers in lung tissue. Both studies concluded that most fibers found in the lung tissue would not have been seen if screened by light microscopy or SEM.[23,261] The study from the Northwest cohort also found that 26 of the cases had appreciable ferruginous body and uncoated fiber burdens but did not have pathologically definable asbestosis.[23] All but three cases from the Northwestern cohort had levels of ferruginous bodies higher than that considered in our laboratory as representing general population levels (20 ferruginous bodies per gram of wet tissue). However, in the second study, 13 cases had ferruginous body levels within those considered as reflective of tissue from the general population.[261] This implies the importance of combining the data regarding uncoated fiber burden and ferruginous body burden when attempting to define past exposure and a causal relationship of that exposure to asbestos and mesothelioma.

A similar trend was seen in a study of tissue burden of ferruginous bodies and uncoated asbestos fibers in 15 cases of mesothelioma in women[286]; 13 of 15 samples contained ferruginous bodies and, as with the two previous studies, amosite was the most commonly found form (80% of cases). However, unlike the other studies, the second most commonly found form of asbestos was tremolite (60% of cases). There was a considerable drop in overall tissue burden of uncoated asbestos fibers in the lower half of the study group when compared with the levels found in the lower half of the other two mesothelioma study groups. Seven individuals had bystander exposure from contact with contaminated clothing of a spouse or family member.

The common findings in all three study groups were the presence of mixed types of asbestos. The lung tissue in some cases of mesothelioma in each group had low overall tissue burden of asbestos.

The transport and deposition of asbestos fibers in extrapulmonary sites was evaluated in another study from our laboratory.[239] These individuals resided in the shipyard building/repair areas of the Northwest. Ferruginous bodies were found in 18 lung samples, five mesentery samples, and two omentum samples. The common fiber type in the lung (95% of cases positive), mesentery (65%), and omentum (70%) was amosite. Chrysotile was found in 50% of lung samples. Chrysotile was the second most common form of asbestos found in the extrapulmonary sites; 25% of the mesentery and three omentum samples were positive for chrysotile. Crocidolite was found in 25% of lung samples, 15% of mesentery samples, and 5% of the omentum samples. In the amosite-exposed individuals, the predictors of the likelihood of finding an asbestos fiber in the extrapulmonary sites included the presence and numbers of ferruginous bodies and total asbestos fibers in the lung. The relevance of the findings was couched in the fact that the individual studies had appreciable amphiboles in the lung tissue and the parameters may well change in a heavily exposed chrysotile cohort.

Mesothelioma is a rare tumor that, based on the previous data, clearly is related to the exposure to fibrous minerals, and in most instances, Peto et al.[287] correctly observed, "the great majority of mesotheliomas are caused by asbestos" and a "country's mesothelioma rate is therefore a quantitative indicator of its population's past exposure—mainly occupationally—to asbestos."

Asbestos Fiber Types and Dose, and Mesothelioma Risk and Induction

It is well known that there exists a dose-response causal relationship between asbestos exposure and MM, for any fiber type or mixture[39] (Table 43.8).[288] In addition, the amphibole varieties of asbestos are substantially more potent for MM induction than chrysotile[42,288] (Table 43.9),[289] and an extensive review by Hodgson and Darnton[93] on the dose-response relationships between asbestos and mesothelioma risk estimated that the relative potencies for crocidolite, amosite, and chrysotile for mesothelioma induction are roughly 500:100:1, respectively. However, in a subsequent analysis from Australia, based on lung tissue amphibole fiber concentrations allowing for clearance half-lives, Leigh and Robinson[43] calculated the potency ratios to be 26:14:1, respectively, and another set of potency ratios cited in the literature is 30:15:1, respectively.[42]

The factors that determine these differential potencies are sometimes summarized as the three D's: dose, dimensions, and durability (i.e., biopersistence in tissue).[42] Because of their wavy characteristics, chrysotile fibers appear to be trapped more readily within the upper airways and central bronchi than amphibole fibers (Figs. 43.2 and 43.3).[290] In the circumstances of air flow through tubular airways, fibers tend to be concentrated in the central regions of the airway lumen where flow is laminar, with the long axes of fibers parallel to the direction of flow, and fractional deposition of fibers is determined by straight versus curly fiber characteristics and by the diameter of the fibers, rather than their length.[290] Accordingly, Middleton et al.[291] found that the fraction of chrysotile deposited in rats was in the range of 17% to 36% of crocidolite at varying inhaled concentrations, and the deposited fraction of amosite was 65% of crocidolite. Other studies did not detect such differences, but there appears to be general agreement that for exposures in experimental animals lasting for 6 weeks or longer, the relative retention of amphibole fibers is greater than for chrysotile.[290] Fibers and particles most likely to be deposited are those with an aerodynamic equivalent diameter in the range of about 1 to 5 μm, and the sites of greatest deposition are the bifurcations of terminal bronchioles.[290]

TABLE 43.8. Mesothelioma rates in groups exposed occupationally to asbestos, according to fiber types and duration

Fiber type	Industry	Duration (years since first employed)	Rate per 10^6 person-years
Mixed fiber exposure: crocidolite, amosite, and chrysotile	Textile manufacture and insulation	20–24	1520
		25–30	1710
		31+	3180
Mixed fiber exposure: mainly amosite	Insulation workers	20–24	290
		25–29	1550
		30–34	2760
		35–39	6300
		40–44	6330
		45+	8110
Mixed fiber exposure: crocidolite and chrysotile	Fibrous cement manufacture	20–24	2700
		25–29	6300
		30–34	9600
Chrysotile, some crocidolite	Textile manufacture	20–24	108
		25–29	143
		30–34	1156
		35–39	493
		40+	1774
Amosite	Insulation manufacture	20–24	744
		25–29	2623
		30–34	5078
		35+	1842
Mixed fiber exposure	Dockyards	20–24	120
		25–29	410
		30–34	220
		35–40	370
		40–44	1240
		45–49	1510
Crocidolite	Mining and milling	20–24	900
		25–29	2200
		30–34	3000
		35–39	7000

Source: Modified from de Klerk NH, Armstrong BK. The epidemiology of asbestos and mesothelioma. In: Henderson DW, Shilkin KB, Langlois SL, Whitaker D, eds. Malignant mesothelioma, pp. 223–250. Copyright 1992 by Hemisphere. Reproduced with permission of Informa Healthcare Books via Copyright Clearance Center. (See same reference for detailed reference listing.)

TABLE 43.9. Different mineral fibers, their properties, and MM risks

Fiber	MM risk	Aspect ratio[a]	Biopersistence	Human exposure
Erionite (E)	High	High	Persistent	Environmental and residential (Turkey)
Amphibole asbestos				
Crocidolite (C)	High	High	Persistent	Occupational, nonoccupational
Amosite (A)	High but less than C, E	High but less than C	Persistent	Occupational, nonoccupational
Tremolite (T)	Probably high, ?≤C	As for A	Persistent	Environmental, some occupational
Anthophyllite	Low	Fairly low	Persistent	Environmental, formerly restricted occupational (Finland)
Chrysotile	Low, not zero (disputed)	Low	Poor; less than all above	Occupational, nonoccupational
Fiberglass	Zero	Low	Probably poor	Occupational
Ceramic/MMMF	Not documented in humans	High to low	Probably as for amphiboles	Experimental

[a]Length : diameter ratio.
MMMF, man-made mineral fibers.
Source: Modified from Hammar.[289]

Once deposited, amphibole fibers are more persistent in tissues than chrysotile. The clearance half-life in lung tissue has been estimated at 5 to 10 years for crocidolite[292,293] (clearance rate is about 10% to 15% per year) and up to 20 years for amosite fibers,[279] in comparison to 90 to 110 days for chrysotile (although one study[294] recorded a longer clearance half-life of about 8 years for long chrysotile fibers among chrysotile miners/millers in Quebec). Clearance appears to be more effective for short than long fibers—although de Klerk et al.[293] could find no difference between the clearance rates for long and short crocidolite fibers—so that the length of retained fibers increases with time after exposure.[290] Clearance for chrysotile appears to involve both longitudinal and transverse splitting and solubilization of fibers, so that such cleavage can increase the number of fibers per unit weight of lung even after cessation of exposure, before further clearance of fibers accompanied by a diminution in their numbers.[38,295]

To induce MM, deposited asbestos fibers presumably must first translocate to the pleura from the lung where they are deposited initially, but we know of no data on the precise mechanisms and rates at which translocation occurs in humans. However, Boutin et al.[240] demonstrated that asbestos fibers are concentrated in parietal pleural "black spots" located near stomata on the parietal pleura. Amphiboles outnumbered chrysotile in all samples, and 22.5% of fibers in black spots were ≥5 µm in length, which might explain in part why the parietal pleura seems to be the target site for both MM and plaques, and why chrysotile is less potent than the amphiboles (whereas chrysotile appears to be no less potent than the amphiboles when fibers are implanted directly into the pleural cavity of experimental animals). Other studies have demonstrated the presence or even a predominance of chrysotile fibers in human pleural tissue (e.g., see the World Health Organization monograph Environmental Health Criteria 203: Chrysotile Asbestos,[92] pp. 64–65).

Translocation may take place by either migration of naked amphibole fibers, or by ingestion of the fibers by macrophages followed by subsequent transport along lymphatic vessels to the subpleural lymphatic channels.[290] Nonetheless, it seems worth emphasizing that studies on the persistence and clearance of fibers discussed above have focused on lung tissue, obviously not the site where MMs develop, and there appear to be no systematic data for humans on the clearance rates for fibers translocated to the pleura.

The relationship between asbestos inhalation and the subsequent risk of mesothelioma can be expressed by the Peto model and its various modifications[288,296]:

$$I = k \cdot f \cdot (t^{p} - [t - d]^{p})$$

where I is the incidence; k depends on fiber type, mix, size, and other site-specific variables; f is the intensity of exposure in fibers/mL; t is the time in years following exposure; and d is the exposure in years. For the purposes of modeling, variations of the basic equation have been proposed to account for latency period, multiple periods of exposure, weightings for different fiber types in the exposure history, and clearance rates.[297] From the Peto model and its modifications, the following deductions can be inferred:

- Early exposures to asbestos are more significant for MM induction than later exposures, other factors being equal.
- When there are multiple episodes of exposure, each increment of exposure within an acceptable latency interval produces a corresponding increment in the risk/incidence of MM, dependent on the time of the exposure, its magnitude, and the types of asbestos fiber involved. This issue was discussed at some length in the World Trade Organization (WTO) report on asbestos (specifically chrysotile),[42] and the dose-response relationship between asbestos and mesothelioma was illus-

trated in tabular form by de Klerk and Armstrong in 1992[288] (Table 43.8).

Is a Threshold or Minimal Level of Asbestos Exposure/Inhalation Required for Mesothelioma Induction?

No minimum threshold dose of inhaled asbestos has been delineated below which there is no increase in the risk of mesothelioma.[92,93,176,189,212,217] In a study on time trends and occupational risk factors for pleural mesothelioma in Sweden, based on the Swedish Family-Cancer Database, Hemminki and Li[212] found an increasing age-adjusted incidence of pleural mesothelioma over the period 1961–1998, not only for occupations expected to be associated with asbestos exposure (manual and blue-collar workers), but also in professional groups and even farmers.

In relation to the no-threshold model for mesothelioma induction by asbestos, reviews and several case-control studies from Europe are of particular relevance and include the following:

- A review by Hillerdal[163] on mesothelioma related to nonoccupational asbestos exposure was published in 1999. It is of particular interest in relation to mesotheliomas as a consequence of low-level exposures to asbestos.
- A review and meta-analysis by Bourdès et al.[298] of the risk of pleural mesothelioma from environmental exposure to asbestos was published in 2000. These authors identified eight relevant studies on the risk of pleural mesothelioma from household or neighborhood exposures to asbestos. These studies did not include the case-control studies outlined below. These authors found that the RRs of pleural mesothelioma for household exposure ranged between 4.0 and 23.7, with a summary risk estimate of 8.1 (95% CI, 5.3–12). For neighborhood exposures, the RRs ranged between 5.1 and 9.3 with a summary estimate of 7.0 (95% CI, 4.7–11). This analysis appears to be in reasonable agreement with the studies by Magnani et al.[299,300] and Rödelsperger et al.[301] (see below). Bourdès et al.[298] commented that their data were insufficient to estimate the magnitude of excess risk at the levels of environmental exposure commonly experienced by the general population in industrial countries (in other words, from the general environment).
- In a case-referent study reported from France by Iwatsubo et al.,[91] it was found that the odds ratio for mesothelioma (OR_{MM}) was 4.2 with low-dose exposures in the range of 0.5 to 0.99 fibers/mL-years (fiber-years). In this study, there was a clear dose-response trend from no exposure, through levels of 0.001 to 0.49 fiber-years, 0.5 to 0.99 fiber-years, 1.0 to 9.9 fiber-years, and >10 fiber-years with age and socioeconomic, class-adjusted ORs (RRs) of 1.0 (for no exposure), 1.2, 4.2, 5.2, and 6.7, respectively. Although the OR_{MM} of 1.2 at 0.001 to 0.49 fiber-years did not achieve statistical significance, further calculations show a highly significant trend. Furthermore, it has been suggested that this study lacked statistical power because the number of subjects was too small to detect an $OR_{MM} = 1.2$ at the usual scientific level of significance. Accordingly, this study[91] is not inconsistent with a no-threshold model.
- In a case-referent study reported from Germany by Rödelsperger et al.,[301] the OR_{MM} was >4.5 with lung tissue asbestos fiber concentrations in the range of 100,000 to 200,000 fibers longer than 5 µm per gram of dry lung tissue, and an OR_{MM} of about 2 or more was recorded for lower lung tissue asbestos fiber concentrations, in the range of 50,000 to 100,000 fibers longer than 5 µm per gram dry lung.
- In a meticulous case-referent analysis published in 2001 using individualized estimates of exposures, Rödelsperger et al.[94] found that the OR_{MM} was 7.9 with low exposures in the range of anything more than 0 to 0.15 fibers/mL-years (>0–0.15 fiber-years). Similar findings were reported by Magnani et al.[299]
- In a population-based study on the distribution of mesothelioma in California, after attempted allowance for occupational exposures, Pan et al.[302] reported an apparent direct correlation between the odds of mesothelioma and proximity of residence according to the distribution of ultramafic rocks in the general environment (serpentinite/ultramafic rocks in California contain mainly chrysotile, with some other forms of asbestos in some areas, such as tremolite). These authors found about a 6% reduction in the odds of mesothelioma for residence for every 10 km further away from the ultramafic rocks.
- As set forth in their review on dose-response relationships between asbestos and mesothelioma, Hodgson and Darnton[93] estimated that a cumulative exposure of 1.0 fiber/mL-year for crocidolite yields a lifetime risk "best" estimate of about 650 mesothelioma deaths/100,000 (range = 250–1500), 90/100,000 for amosite (range = 15–300), and 5/100,000 for chrysotile (range = 1–20). For a cumulative exposure of 0.1 fibers/mL-years, these authors set forth a best estimate of about 100 deaths per 100,000 exposed for crocidolite, with a highest arguable estimate of 350 and a lowest of 25; for amosite, the corresponding figures were 15 deaths per 100,000, with a highest arguable estimate of 80 and lowest of 2; at this level of exposure, the risk for chrysotile was "probably insignificant," with a highest arguable estimate of four deaths per 100,000. For a cumulative exposure of 0.01 fibers/mL-years, the best estimate was about 20 deaths per 100,000 exposed for crocidolite, with a highest arguable estimate of 100 and a lowest of two; for amosite, the corresponding figures

were three deaths per 100,000, with a highest arguable estimate of 20 and lowest that was "insignificant"; at this level of exposure, the risk for chrysotile was "probably insignificant," with a highest arguable estimate of 1 death per 100,000.

One point also worth emphasizing is that the estimated RRs, ORs, SIRs, or proportional mortality ratios (PMRs) for cohort and case-control studies on mesothelioma represent cases in excess of any background risk from background exposures; in all cohort and case-control studies, the control group represents a comparable group of individuals with background (or greater[303]) levels of asbestos in their lungs, so that the risks delineated by such studies represent risks in excess of no exposure and background exposure.[44]

In line with these considerations, the Industrial Injuries Advisory Council (IIAC) in the U.K. set forth in 2005 a comment concerning causation of mesothelioma,[304] similar to and reaffirming the criteria for causation originally set out in 1996:

> Mesothelioma is a rare disease in the general population almost always caused by asbestos, so that attribution to occupation is far more straightforward [than lung cancer] and does not require epidemiological evidence. . . . The last IIAC review of asbestos-related diseases in 1996 . . . recommended that benefit for mesothelioma be awarded for claimants in any occupation involving asbestos exposure at a level above that commonly found in the environment at large. . . . The Council recommends that the prescription for [mesothelioma] should remain unchanged.

Commercial Chrysotile and Mesothelioma: Can Chrysotile-Only Exposure Induce Mesothelioma?

Chrysotile represented about 95% of past production and usage of asbestos, and it is still mined in particular in Russia (the world's largest producer), Canada (the world's largest exporter), Brazil, China, and Zimbabwe; small chrysotile mines also operated at some times in other nations, such as the U.S. and Australia.

There appears to be general but not universal agreement that commercial chrysotile as exemplified by the chrysotile mined and milled in Quebec has the capacity to induce mesothelioma, not only in experimental animals but also in humans. Nonetheless, Canadian chrysotile contains trace amounts of tremolite, including fibrous tremolite (a noncommercial amphibole), as a contaminant. The amount of tremolite appears to vary from one sample to another, but is generally <1%. Some authorities claim that the occurrence of mesotheliomas among the Quebec chrysotile miners and millers is a consequence not of the chrysotile per se but rather of the coexistent trace quantities of tremolite. The amphibole hypothesis,[305,306] which argues that chrysotile itself has little or no mesotheliomagenicity and that mesotheliomas following chrysotile exposure are a consequence of the admixed commercial or trace contaminant noncommercial amphibole fibers, remains the subject of dispute.[306–312]

Analysis of the asbestos fiber content of lung tissue from the cohort of Quebec chrysotile miners/millers has consistently demonstrated disproportionately high concentrations of tremolite in comparison to chrysotile (Table 43.10).[313] This appears to represent a bioaccumulation phenomenon whereby chrysotile is cleared from lung tissue more rapidly than the tremolite, so that the tremolite not only persists but increases in proportional concentration. In this respect, the tremolite content of the lung tissue can be used as an index of past chrysotile-only exposures, and some claim that the incidence of mesotheliomas in the same cohort can be related directly to the tremolite content.[313,314]

Mesotheliomas related to the use of tremolite in whitewash or stucco have been reported in Turkey,[315,316] Greece,[118] Cyprus, Corsica,[317] and New Caledonia[318,319] (see also Schneider and Woitowitz[117]). Tremolite has also been implicated in lung cancer and mesothelioma induction among vermiculite miners in Montana,[320,321] who were exposed only to tremolite-actinolite fibers.

Table 43.10. Asbestos fiber concentrations in lungs at autopsy from 21 mesothelioma cases among Quebec chrysotile miners and millers (fibers per microgram [μg]; geometric means)

Place of employment	No. of cases	Chrysotile	Tremolite	Crocidolite	Amosite
Mines and mills					
Thetford Mines	14	12.8	104.1	0	0
Asbestos	5	4.3	7.5	1.7	0.3
Factory					
Asbestos	2	2.1	0.5	6.4	0.3

Source: Modified from McDonald et al.,[313] Table 2 in the original reference; see also Table 1 in the original. In calculating geometric means, a zero count has been replaced by half the detectable limit. For crocidolite and amosite, all counts were zero; i.e., below the detection limit. For fiber counts/g lung tissue, multiply the raw figures by 10^6.

Case[322] has extensively reviewed the biohazards of tremolite, including epidemiologic investigations in humans and experimental data on animal models. He also favored the expression chrysotile/tremolite for Quebec chrysotile, but is of the opinion that it is the tremolite component that causes mesothelioma.

The Quebec Chrysotile Cohort

In an analysis of mesotheliomas among the Quebec chrysotile miners and millers, up to 1997, McDonald et al.[313,314] reported 38 mesotheliomas, most of which occurred after prolonged and heavy exposure, especially at the mine where the greatest concentrations of trace tremolite occurred (Thetford). In comparison to the Thetford main complex, relatively few mesotheliomas occurred among workers at the Asbestos mine and mill (23 versus eight), despite nearly equivalent person-years of observation. In addition, asbestos fiber analysis on lung tissue demonstrated crocidolite and amosite in five of the eight cases from the mine and mill at Asbestos and in two out of the five mesotheliomas from the Asbestos factory (Table 43.11).[313]

The clear implication of this study is that the risk of MM was related strongly to years of service in the central area at Thetford where geologic factors "would probably result in tremolite, some in fibrous form, being mined with the ore."[313] In addition, the MM rate for miners and millers was >2.5 times higher at Thetford mines (excluding the smallest mines) than at Asbestos, and this difference was also attributed to differences in the amount of fibrous tremolite in the ores. Despite these differences within the cohort for the distribution of MM related to chrysotile and tremolite (and also to crocidolite and amosite at the Asbestos factory and the Asbestos mine and mill), the results clearly indicate that Quebec chrysotile has the capacity for mesothelioma induction. The abstract describes 25 MMs from the Thetford mines,[313] representing a mesothelioma rate of 337 per million person-years, substantially (almost 20-fold) higher than the incidence rate of about 17 cases/10^6/yr for men in British Colombia and the U.S. in 1982 and 1973–1984, respectively, and well above the often-cited MM "background" rate of 1 to 2 cases/10^6/yr.

In the final two paragraphs of the paper, McDonald et al.[313] commented, "The tremolite hypothesis, if correct, has several important implications. First, it supports the widely but not universally held view that most, if not all, asbestos-related mesotheliomas are caused by amphibole fibers. This in turn points to fiber durability and biopersistence as critical factors in aetiology."

A report from the *Institut National de Santé du Québec* pointed out that the average annual rate of increase in the incidence of MM in Quebec during the period 1982–1996 was 5% for men, and that work in the (chrysotile) mines was associated with 35% of a total of 691 cases of asbestos-related diseases (MM, asbestosis, and lung cancer).[323] An earlier report from the same institute found that average adjusted incidence rates for pleural MM were 32% and 92% higher for men and women, respectively, in Quebec "than those of Canadian men and women in all other provinces combined."[324] The second (2005) institute report also commented that multiple criteria for causation "show that chrysotile is carcinogenic" and that "safe use of asbestos is difficult, perhaps impossible, in industries such as construction, renovation, and asbestos processing."[323]

Mesotheliomas have also been produced in experimental animals by implantation and inhalation of chrysotile (presumably also containing trace amounts of tremolite). Mesotheliomas can also be induced in rats by intraperitoneal injection of chrysotile, with evidence of a dose-response effect.[227]

Other Chrysotile-Exposed Cohorts and Studies

In addition to the Quebec chrysotile miners and millers, mesotheliomas have also been reported among other workforces apparently exposed to chrysotile only, with much smaller amounts of contaminant tremolite.

Even so, it is doubtful whether chrysotile exists in the complete absence of contaminant amphiboles. For example, Yano et al.[325] reported a 25-year longitudinal cohort study on male asbestos workers exposed to

TABLE 43.11. Mesotheliomas among Quebec chrysotile miners and millers, 1997

	Number of mesothelioma deaths	Person-years (thousands)	Mesothelioma rate (per million person years)
Thetford Mines:			
Main complex and the oldest of the smaller mines	23	65.14	353
The five smallest mines	1	6.01	266
Asbestos:			
Mine and mill	8	60.64	132
Factory	5	10.84	462

Source: Modified from McDonald et al.[313]

Table 43.12. Mesotheliomas according to types of exposures to asbestos in Saxony-Anhalt

	Amphiboles	Amphiboles and chrysotile	Chrysotile; possible amphiboles	Chrysotile	Mean values
Age at beginning of exposure	25	28	28	34	28
Duration of exposure	16	21	19	14	19
Latent period (years)	40	40	41	31	38
Age of person dying of mesothelioma	65	68	69	65	66
Number of mesotheliomas	135	279	331	67	Total = 812

Note: All types of application of asbestos with common addition of chrysotile fall under the heading *Chrysotile*; *possible amphiboles* when previous admixture of amphiboles could not be definitely excluded.
Source: Modified from Sturm et al.[336,337]

chrysotile in Chongqin, China. The factory used only Sichuanese chrysotile that was claimed to be virtually amphibole-free (<0.001% tremolite, below the detection limit of the assays). Nonetheless, subsequent investigations reported by Tossavainen et al.[326,327] using acid-alkali digestion of the bulk samples of chrysotile[328] or from analysis of the lung tissue asbestos fiber types have demonstrated that tremolite or anthophyllite is in fact present in both Russian and Chinese chrysotile (including chrysotile from the two Sichuanese mines that apparently supplied the factory studied by Yano et al.[325]).

Russia

Although precise figures for the mesothelioma incidence in the Urals region (Uralasbest) in Russia, where chrysotile is mined,[329–331] are difficult to procure, Kogan[332] commented in a textbook on occupational lung diseases published in 1998, that in the Middle Ural mountains, the main asbestos mining region in Russia, the mortality from mesothelioma over a 10-year period was sixfold higher than the average rate in the Sverdlovsk region, an area where there was negligible asbestos mining. Most of those with mesothelioma had worked at the asbestos mining and milling plants, or had lived in an adjacent town near old and very "dusty" mills.

Other Central and Eastern European Nations

One might expect data on mesothelioma incidence in Central and Eastern European countries to be of interest, from an assumption that some of them would have imported mainly chrysotile from Russia until the breakup of the Soviet Union. Unfortunately, it is difficult to evaluate national mesothelioma statistics because a number of these countries also imported amphibole asbestos.[333–335]

The Former German Democratic Republic (GDR)

Sturm et al.[336,337] have published data on asbestos-related diseases and asbestos types in the German State of Saxony-Anhalt. They report that the asbestos used in the GDR was essentially "pure" chrysotile from the Soviet Union, with a small amount (approximately 7%) of long-fiber chrysotile from Canada. In addition to these imports of chrysotile asbestos, smaller quantities of amphibole asbestos were imported.

Between 1960 and 1990, a total of 1082 mesotheliomas was recorded in Saxony-Anhalt, and these included 843 "proven asbestos-accepted mesotheliomas." Table 43.12, as modified from Sturm et al.[336,337] gives a breakdown of 812 cases for which adequate data were available: 67 were said to follow exposure to chrysotile only, and 331 were associated with "chrysotile; possible amphiboles."

China

Yano et al.[338] reported on lung cancer incidence in a Chongqin cohort of 515 male asbestos workers heavily exposed to chrysotile claimed to contain <0.001% tremolite (see preceding discussion in this chapter); two mesotheliomas over 11,850 person-years of observation occurred in this cohort. Assuming this rate to be representative, it would amount to 170 mesotheliomas/10^6/yr (about half the rate for the Quebec chrysotile miners/millers at the Thetford mines main complex[313]).

In a retrospective cohort mortality study of 1227 men employed at a chrysotile mine in Hebei Province of China before 1972, there were three deaths from mesothelioma.[92]

Other Countries

A few isolated cases of mesothelioma in chrysotile textile workers or in asbestos miners and millers have been reported from the U.S.[339,340] and Zimbabwe,[92] respectively.

Chrysotile Content of Human Lung Tissue from Mesothelioma Patients

Morinaga et al.[341] detected asbestos fibers in 19 of 23 cases of mesothelioma studied. Amphibole fibers were found in 13 cases, but six were found to have only chrysotile fibers (five pleural mesotheliomas and one peritoneal mesothelioma). Nonetheless, the methodology for this study was unimpressive, with relatively small numbers of fibers analyzed.

TABLE 43.13. Distribution of fiber concentrations: transmission electron microscopic analysis, chrysotile only (all lengths)

Fibers/gram (F/g) dry lung		Mesothelioma cases No.	Mesothelioma cases %	Controls No.	Controls %	Odds ratio (95% confidence interval)
F/g	0–200,000	12	48.0	26	83.9	
Log_{10} (F/g)	5.3–5.5	1	4.0	2	6.5	1.08 (0–17.95)
	5.5–6	7	28.0	3	9.7	8.67 (1.77–48.14)
	6–6.5	3	12.0			
	6.5–7	1	4.0			
	7–8	1	4.0			$\chi^2_1 = 9.80$ ($p < .0005$)

Source: Modified from Rogers et al.[216]

A 1991 paper by Rogers et al.[216] recorded a substantial number of mesothelioma patients in whom the only detectable type of asbestos was chrysotile (Table 43.13), with evidence of a dose-response effect as reflected in a trend to an increasing OR_{MM} at a relatively low fiber concentration of $\leq 10^6$ fibers per gram dry lung tissue ($\log_{10} = 5.5$–6; OR = 8.67).

More recently, Yarborough[342] has argued that chrysotile fibers found in the lung tissue of MM patients are unrelated to causation of the MM; the implication is that because of rapid clearance of chrysotile fibers, with a correspondingly short half-life, and the known long latency between first exposure to asbestos and the subsequent clinical development of the mesothelioma, any parenchymal fibers must have been deposited more proximately in time, after mesotheliomagenesis began; that is, neither the presence nor the absence of chrysotile fibers would be considered as evidence of causation. This argument overlooks the fact that chrysotile fibers *are* found in the parenchymal tissue of asbestos-exposed individuals, years and even decades after cessation of asbestos exposure. In this regard, it must be remembered that the clearance times represent *half-lives*, not absolute clearance times (see also the preceding discussion on mesotheliomas in Quebec).

Chrysotile-Only Exposure: Asbestos and Mesothelioma Among Automotive and Brake Mechanics

Before bans in many countries in the 1990s and early 2000s on the use of any type of asbestos, but on a continuing basis in some nations, vehicular brake blocks and linings contained substantial amounts of commercial chrysotile (within the range of about 30% to 70% by weight[343]), mostly from Canada, bound in a resinous matrix.[343] Since the 1970s there have been concerns over the potential for dust derived from the brake materials[344,345] to be inhaled by automotive mechanics, with the potential for mesothelioma induction, and individual case reports of MM among automotive/garage mechanics have been published,[277,346] yet workers in the friction products manufacturing industry appeared to have a low risk of MM.[42,347–350]

Braking of automobiles generates high temperatures in the brake drums/linings, up to about 700°C or more, and at this temperature a high proportion (up to about 98%) of the chrysotile undergoes degradation and recrystallization to form the mineral forsterite,[344,345] which is not implicated in mesothelioma induction. Nonetheless, asbestos fibers, mainly short fibers[351] but including a small proportion of long fibers,[92] remain within the dust created within worn brake linings. In addition, it is a truism that heat-related changes do not apply to work on or with new brake linings/pads.

In August 1975, NIOSH in the U.S. Department of Health, Education and Welfare issued a communication to alert the country to "recently gathered information indicating a potential health hazard for persons exposed to asbestos during the servicing of motor vehicle brake and clutch assemblies." This communiqué indicated that average peak airborne fiber concentrations for "blow-out of automobile drum brake assemblies, grinding of used truck brake linings and bevelling of new truck brake linings" were 10.5, 3.75, and 37.3 fibers/mL, respectively (for fibers longer than 5 μm). Analysis of brake drum dust (worn linings) demonstrated that almost all of the fibers were shorter than 0.4 μm in length. The same communiqué stated that the "present findings indicate that enough asbestos is preserved to produce significant exposures during certain brake servicing procedures."

A 1998 monograph from the World Health Organization/International Programme on Chemical Safety (WHO/IPCS), entitled "Environmental Health Criteria 203: Chrysotile Asbestos,"[92] reviewed studies on airborne dust concentrations produced by blowing out worn brake linings with a compressed air hose or from grinding new brake blocks/linings, and commented that recent findings are probably not applicable to the airborne fiber concentrations from these types of work in the past. For example, the WHO/IPCS monograph stated that during "early" years when poor or no control measures were used, there was "high total dust exposure," especially during grinding of brakes and the use of compressed air to blow off dust, but lower levels "were measured when engineering controls were introduced."

The same WHO/IPCS monograph set forth the mean airborne asbestos fiber concentrations measured during maintenance and replacement of brakes. Studies carried out in 1976 revealed mean concentrations of 3.8 fibers/mL for grinding truck brakes and 15.9 fibers/mL for blowing out brakes. Different studies carried out in the same year also found a mean airborne fiber concentration of 3.8 fibers/mL for grinding brake blocks, 16 fibers/mL for blowing out the brakes, and 2.5 fibers/mL for "dry brushing." Subsequent studies have generally found lower airborne fiber concentrations, but one investigation carried out in 1985 found that blowing off and grinding brakes produced a mean airborne fiber concentration of 6.25 fibers/mL. Other investigations also recorded elevated airborne fiber concentrations from such maintenance and replacement work on brakes,[344,345,352] whereas later studies recorded lower[353,354] or no significant[351] elevations of airborne fiber concentrations.[343] Furthermore, in Germany, Rödelsperger et al.[355] recorded the presence of long fibers 5 μm or more in length in the airborne dust.

A study by Butnor et al.[356] on lung tissue fiber analysis for 10 cases of MM among brake mechanics found that the individuals with elevated fiber counts had "excess" commercial amphibole fibers in their lung parenchyma and that elevated levels of noncommercial amphibole fibers—such as tremolite as a marker for chrysotile, or anthophyllite or actinolite—were found only in those who also had elevated levels of commercial amphibole fibers, leading to the conclusion that those subjects had "unrecognized" exposures other than the brake dust exposure. However, this study concerned only a small number of MM cases associated with exposure to brake dust, with no analysis of MM risk relative to parenchymal asbestos fiber concentrations.

In addition, one of these cases was evaluated by Dodson et al.[357] by ATEM, which found high concentrations of chrysotile in parenchymal lung tissue and two chrysotile asbestos-cored asbestos bodies.

Several reviews have argued that there is no increased risk among automotive mechanics,[343,358–360] These publications have been funded by the automotive industry, related to litigation in the U.S.[343,361] Those same reviews have also been criticized by Egilman and Billings[361] on a number of grounds and, in generic sense, by Egilman and Bohme[362] and Gennaro and Tomatis.[363] These latter three reviews can be regarded as adversarial or polemical, but they do raise substantive issues of risk assessment such as stratifying cumulative exposures within the group being studied in order to avoid underestimating the risk for those exposed or, conversely, overestimating the risk for those not, or only minimally, exposed.[364]

In addition, to evaluate any risk cogently, a distinction should be made between work on worn (heat-altered) versus work with new brake linings and, perhaps, between those who worked with brake materials for passenger cars as opposed to those who worked with brake materials for heavy vehicles (trucks).

It is well known that death certificates are a poor measure of disease outcome because of their inherent limitations, and studies that rely on death certificate diagnoses are subject to error as was pointed out by Paustenbach et al.[343] relative to the Connecticut friction products study. Death certificates simply may not list the disease under investigation (e.g., mesothelioma). It is also essential that all cases of the disease in question are captured by the study: this is a major problem when the duration of the study is short and cannot allow for the long latencies that underpin MM induction by asbestos. Another issue that must be taken into account is ensuring that the control reference population is truly unexposed in order not to underestimate the risk of disease in the exposed group.[303] A further question is whether the individual studies reviewed had the statistical power to detect small increments in risk if they did exist.[38,365]

Data in Australia point to an increased risk of mesothelioma among brake mechanics. The Australian Mesothelioma Register (AMR) Report for 2002 lists 59 cases of mesothelioma for the exposure category *brake linings–made/repaired* (single exposure only) and a further 19 cases for the same class of exposure but with multiple patterns of exposure, giving a total of 78 cases.[36,43,193,366] Taking into account census data for automotive mechanics in Australia, it has been estimated that brake mechanics have a MM rate of at least 20 cases per million person-years, as discussed in the Dispute Settlement Report for the WTO[42] (i.e., a risk that is up to about 20-fold greater than the background risk of mesothelioma). In addition, it has been noted that the increase in the number of cases of mesothelioma apparently related to work on brake linings roughly parallels the increase in the number of cases of mesothelioma related to other occupations that involved asbestos exposure.[367]

As of 2007, the AMR data constitute the strongest evidence for an increased risk of mesothelioma among brake mechanics who ground and chamfered new brake pads/linings/blocks, but those figures have been criticized as inferior in probative value to formal epidemiologic studies (an issue debated at some length in the WTO report on chrysotile[42]). In terms of science, the question of whether automotive mechanics—and especially dedicated brake mechanics with protracted exposures to dust derived from the grinding/chamfering of new brake blocks/linings—have an increased risk of MM remains unresolved and contentious.

Summary

- The association between asbestos inhalation and the development of MM fulfills all of the Bradford Hill criteria[368] for the establishment of causality, in terms of the strength, consistency and specificity of the association, biologic gradient (dose-response), relationship in time, experimental evidence, reasoning by analogy, bioplausibility, and coherence of the evidence (and its apparent resistance to falsification[369,370]).
- All forms of asbestos have the capacity to induce MM, but the commercial amphiboles crocidolite and amosite are substantially more potent on a fiber-for-fiber basis than chrysotile (white asbestos). The exact ratio of potencies for crocidolite, amosite, and chrysotile remain somewhat uncertain, with different ratios being cited in the literature.
- No lower (minimum) threshold level of exposure to asbestos has been delineated below which there is no increase in the risk of MM, and most authorities approach causation of mesothelioma by asbestos from the perspective of a no-threshold model.
- From the Peto model and its modifications, the risk of MM can be related to cumulative asbestos exposure (assessed from the intensity, frequency, and duration of exposure) multiplied by time in years raised to about the cubic or 4th power), so that other factors being equal, the time elapsed following commencement of exposure is a major probability factor for risk; that is, early exposures are more significant for MM risk than later exposures, other factors remaining constant.
- Epidemiologic studies indicate that there is no increase in the risk of MM for at least 10 years following the commencement of exposure, and the Helsinki criteria,[220] for example, adopt a minimal 10-year latency interval in order to assign causation of MM to asbestos; other authorities require a minimum latency interval of 15 years.
- One factor that emerges from the Peto model and its modifications is that when there are multiple asbestos exposures, each contributes to cumulative exposure and hence to the risk and causation of MM, within an appropriate latency interval.
- Asbestos alone appears capable of acting as a *complete* carcinogen for the mesothelium. As such, asbestos and the secondary reactions associated with its inhalation are apparently sufficient over time to elicit malignant transformation of the mesothelium.
- Only a minority of those exposed even heavily to asbestos develops MM, even after heavy exposures to amphibole asbestos. This has given rise to the notion that there may be a possible genetic predisposition to MM.

The Molecular Pathogenesis and Pathology of Malignant Mesothelioma

The mechanisms whereby asbestos fibers induce malignant transformation of mesothelial cells have long remained elusive, despite extensive investigation.[371–374] Nonetheless, there have been substantial advances in uncovering some of the mechanisms for the induction of MM, and these appear comparable to the multiple steps implicated in the development of other cancers. It is now recognized that asbestos fibers themselves are carcinogenic,[37] mainly by indirect mechanisms, and that malignant transformation is a multistage process, correlating with the known long latency interval between the first exposure to airborne asbestos fibers and the subsequent diagnosis of the MM (see later discussion). However, no single molecular event or series of events can explain all MMs, and most studies have investigated only single steps in what appears to be a highly complex sequence of cellular and molecular events (Fig. 43.9).

Malignant mesotheliomas do not commonly show mutations in oncogenes, but rather multiple alterations in

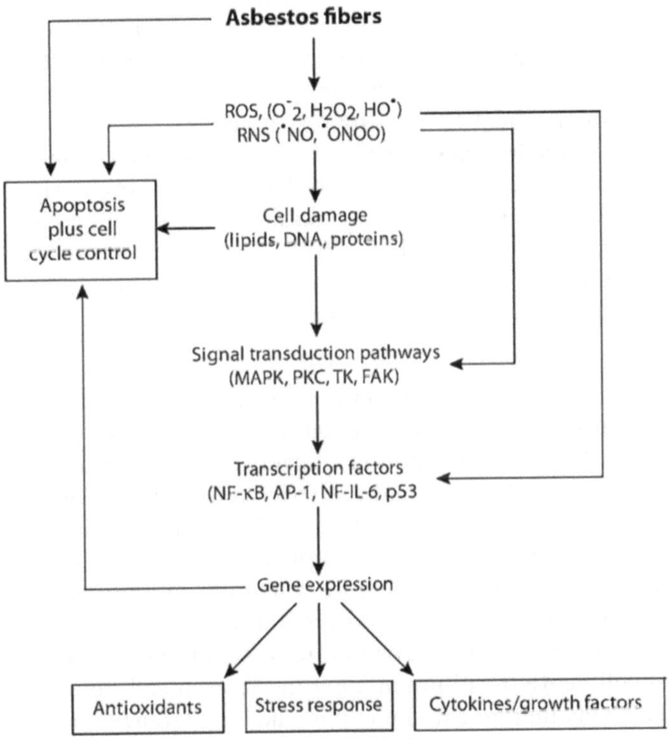

FIGURE 43.9. Mechanisms of asbestos-induced pleuropulmonary toxicity. Schematic illustration of the likely pathways involved in asbestos-induced damage. ROS, reactive oxygen species; RNS, reactive nitrogen species; MAPK, mitogen-activated protein kinase; PKC, protein kinase C; TK, tyrosine kinase; FAK, focal adhesion kinase; NF, nuclear factor; IL, interleukin. See text. (Modified from Kamp and Weitzman.[371])

Box 43.2. Important Definitions (see also Chapter 33)

Oncogenes: Genes that stimulate cell growth under normal conditions, to allow for continuous turnover of tissues such as skin and gastrointestinal epithelia. They are analogous to the accelerator in a car. A mutation of these genes is comparable to a "stuck accelerator" that is independent of the driver's action: forward motion continues, even if the driver removes his foot from the accelerator. Cells with defective oncogenes continue to grow, even in the absence of valid growth stimuli. Examples of classical oncogenes are *bcl-2* and *ras*. In malignant mesotheliomas, mutations of oncogenes are rare.

Tumor suppressor genes: A car with a "stuck accelerator" may still be stopped using the brakes; because the ability to brake is vitally important, there are several to choose from (brake pedal, hand brakes, gears). Similarly, cells possess multiple mechanisms that regulate cell proliferation and restrict cell numbers, either by promoting programmed cell death (apoptosis) or by inhibiting progression through the cell cycle, and slowing mitotic activity. Examples of classical tumor suppressor genes are *p53*, *pRb* (the gene inactivated in retinoblastoma), and *p16*^{INK4a}, which inhibits cyclin-dependent kinases, therefore preventing completion of the cell cycle. Many of the mutations found in malignant mesotheliomas affect tumor suppressor genes.

DNA repair genes: Even a car with functional brakes and accelerator needs to be serviced regularly. Repair genes themselves do not control cell proliferation directly; they simply fix mutations in all genes. If repair genes are defective, there is an increased rate of mutations in all genes.

tumor suppressor genes, most of which are regulated by a complex network of regulators with several backup loops. This type of mutation interferes with the regulatory mechanisms that normally restrict cell numbers and is therefore akin to "defective brakes" (Box 43.2; see Chapter 33).[375] There are multiple regulatory backups, so that there is a requirement for a number of mutations in several genes, and this type of mutation initially produces little increase in cell growth rate. Instead, there is a lack of cell death, resulting in a net increase in cell numbers. This may help to explain in part the long latency interval between exposure and clinically evident disease.

Molecular Events in the Development of Mesothelioma I: Physical Interaction Between Fibers and Cells

Asbestos fibers may exert their carcinogenic effects on mesothelial cells by direct and indirect mechanisms. Direct effects are related to the physical interaction of fibers with target cells or by the generation of free radicals and reactive oxygen species (ROS) at the surface of fibers. Indirect effects are related to an inflammatory response to fibers, including the generation of factors, such as ROS and cytokines as a consequence of attempted but incomplete phagocytosis of fibers by macrophages ("frustrated phagocytosis").[376] There is now substantial scientific evidence for the indirect model, as discussed in several reviews.[371,372,376–378]

Direct genotoxic effects following exposure to asbestos fibers include chromosome mis-segregation, disruption of the mitotic spindle, the formation of aneuploid and polyploid cells, and disruption of nuclei. The formation of micronuclei as a result of DNA disruption is also common. There is experimental evidence, based on in vitro cell culture experiments, that asbestos fibers can interact directly with the mitotic spindle, resulting in aneuploidy.[379,380] Asbestos also has been shown to induce structural and numerical chromosomal alterations in cultured human mesothelial cells[381] (see Molecular Events in the Development of Mesothelioma III). In some of these processes, the particle state and fiber dimensions are considered important parameters in the generation of the genotoxic effects.[382] According to the Stanton hypothesis,[229,383] long, thin fibers appear to be more carcinogenic than short fibers (see above).

Molecular Events in the Development of Mesothelioma II: Free Radicals

Indirect Toxic Effects

Some of the very early steps in the malignant transformation of mesothelial cells are related to oxido-reduction processes generated by fibers.[382] It is now widely accepted that a key process in the development of MM is the production of free radicals, including ROS[371,372,376–378,382] (Fig. 43.9; Box 43.3). This process is neither unique nor specific to MM, and free radicals are implicated in carcinogenesis of many tumors; for example, some carcinogenic polycyclic aromatic hydrocarbons (PAHs) in cigarette smoke are known to generate showers of free radicals,[384] and the mutagenicity of ionizing radiation is related predominantly to the generation of free radicals in tissues (see Chapter 33).

As reviewed by Kamp and Weitzman[371] (Fig. 43.9; Box 43.3), there is abundant evidence that free radicals such as ROS, including hydrogen peroxide (H_2O_2), the superoxide anion (O_2^-), the hydroxyl radical ($HO^\bullet$), and singlet oxygen (O), as well as reactive nitrogen species (RNS), are important mediators of asbestos-induced tissue injury, including MM induction. The RNS include nitric oxide ($^\bullet NO$) and peroxynitrite ($^\bullet ONOO$). The ROS (notably $HO^\bullet$) and RNS (notably $^\bullet ONOO$) can affect a variety of macromolecules, with multiple genotoxic effects and

Box 43.3. Reactive Oxygen Species (ROS)

ROS, including free radicals, are thought to play an important role in the molecular pathogenesis of a number of tumors, including MM. ROS include hydrogen peroxide (H_2O_2), the hydroxyl radical (HO^-), and superoxide anion (O_{2-}). Reactive nitrogen species (RNS) are also thought to play a role.

All types of asbestos contain iron cations, either as part of their crystalline lattice structure (crocidolite and amosite), or as a surface impurity (chrysotile). ROS may be generated at the surface of asbestos fibers by chemical reactions catalyzed by the iron component of the fibers or they may be released by macrophages that have partially engulfed the fibers. Cell damage may be related to the peroxidation of phospholipids, such as those present in cell membranes, or by direct damage to DNA and other macromolecules.

The Fenton reaction is the primary reaction involved in OH^- formation, but free radicals may be produced by the Haber-Weiss reaction in the presence of iron (as present on chrysotile), resulting in generation of hydrogen peroxide (H_2O_2).

1. $Fe^{2+} + H_2O_2 \rightarrow Fe^{3+} + OH^- + OH^\bullet$ (Fenton reaction)
2. $Fe^{3+} + O_{2-} \leftrightarrow Fe^{2+} + O_2$
3. $2O_{2-} + 2H^+ \rightarrow H_2O_2 + O_{2-}$
4. $H_2O_2 + Fe^{2+} \rightarrow OH^- + OH^\bullet + Fe^{3+}$ (iron-catalyzed Haber-Weiss reaction)

activation of signaling cascades. The free radicals may originate either at the surface of the asbestos fibers or they may be released by macrophages that have partially phagocytosed long fibers.[378]

All varieties of asbestos have iron either as a component of the crystalline lattice (crocidolite and amosite) or as a surface impurity (chrysotile has a low but significant surface iron component as a contaminant). The iron associated with asbestos is thought to generate ROS partly by the Fenton reaction ($Fe^{2+} + H_2O_2 \rightarrow Fe^{3+} + HO^- + HO^\bullet$). In addition, H_2O_2 can be converted to $HO^\bullet$ by the iron-catalyzed Haber-Weiss reaction (Box 43.3), and iron is also thought to catalyze alkoxyl radical production from inorganic hydroperoxides. The process of free radical production can also involve other highly reactive molecules such as ferryl or perferryl species. In relation to mutations inducible by iron ions, it has been found that Fe^{2+}-treated DNA shows a 20- to 80-fold greater frequency of mutations, and these mutations appear to include G→C transversions, C→T transitions, and G→T transversions.[385] Such observations may also account in part for the greater carcinogenicity of crocidolite and amosite than chrysotile for the mesothelium. The importance of iron contaminants for cytotoxicity and mutagenic potential has also been demonstrated for erionite in an in vitro system.[386] Even so, the total amount of breakage of plasmid DNA in a cell-free system was not directly associated with the amount of iron released by the fibers, and iron reactivity alone cannot explain all the DNA damage observed.[382] Instead, fiber characteristics such as size, availability of calcium, and the state of cells nearby appear to be important for malignant transformation.

Most studies on free radicals and ROS have been carried out on in vitro systems, such as cell cultures or cell-free systems, and this approach cannot examine the role of secondary ROS released by macrophages during phagocytosis. Reactive oxygen species have an extremely short half-life. and therefore physical proximity of DNA and cell membranes susceptible to the damage by ROS is a prerequisite for damage to occur. As instructive as those studies are, it is likely that a significant proportion of the cell damage in vivo is actually induced by oxido-reduction secondary to inflammatory cellular processes, and phagocytosis in particular. The damage is likely to be transmitted via secondary molecules that are more stable than ROS. This is supported by the fact that asbestos fibers can induce the release of ROS from neutrophils and macrophages.[387] When incubated with neutrophils in vitro, crocidolite, amosite, and chrysotile fibers induce greater release of lactate dehydrogenase than rockwool, glasswool, or ceramic fibers.[387] Experimental studies have also shown that crocidolite, amosite, and chrysotile fibers appear to produce significantly greater amounts of HO^- from mixtures of neutrophils and asbestos fibers than from mixtures of such cells and man-made fibers such as rockwool, glasswool, and ceramic fibers. It appears that asbestos fibers are more efficient for stimulation of ROS from phagocytic cells than are nonfibrous mineral dusts.[387]

In this context it seems worth reiterating that small fibers can be successfully phagocytosed, whereas large fibers are resistant to complete phagocytosis because of their dimensions, and such "frustrated phagocytosis" yields abundant ROS. This partly supports the Stanton hypothesis, but it seems to be the biopersistence of fibers resistant to clearance by inflammatory or other processes that is important for MM induction, rather than a precise and critical fiber dimension per se.

Interference with Apoptosis

Asbestos fibers and ROS induce apoptosis in cultured normal mesothelial cells (Fig. 43.9).[388–391] One function of apoptosis is the elimination of severely damaged cells, including cells that may have undergone some of the steps potentially leading to malignant transformation. Apoptosis is therefore one of the protective mechanisms against

Box 43.4. Control Mechanisms of the Normal Cell Cycle and Loss of Control in MM

The cell cycle is a tightly controlled process, with the greatest level of control being exerted at the transition from the G_1 to the S phase. The S, G_2, and M phases are largely autonomous ,and the only opportunity for DNA repair or induction of apoptosis in the case of irretrievable damage is during the transition from G_1 to S. Two of the major pathways altered by mutations in MM are involved in the regulation of transition from G_1 to S phase: these are the retinoblastoma gene product (pRb) pathway and the p53 pathway. (See diagram below and The Cell Cycle in Chapter 33).

The regulatory proteins p14^{ARF} and p16^{INK4} are each encoded by CDKN2A/ARF at 9p.21, a locus commonly mutated in MM, resulting in loss of control of cell cycle progression and loss of an initiating stimulus of apoptosis. However, in a normal cell, there are numerous regulatory interactions and backups between these two major pathways of growth control. For example, the transcription factor E2F-1 also induces transcription of p16^{INK4}, resulting in stabilization of pRb and inhibition of E2F-1 itself in a classical negative feedback loop. Therefore, deletion or mutation of both p14^{ARF} and p16^{INK4} in the same cell is likely to have a synergistic disruptive effect, rather than simply an additive effect, on cell cycle and growth control.

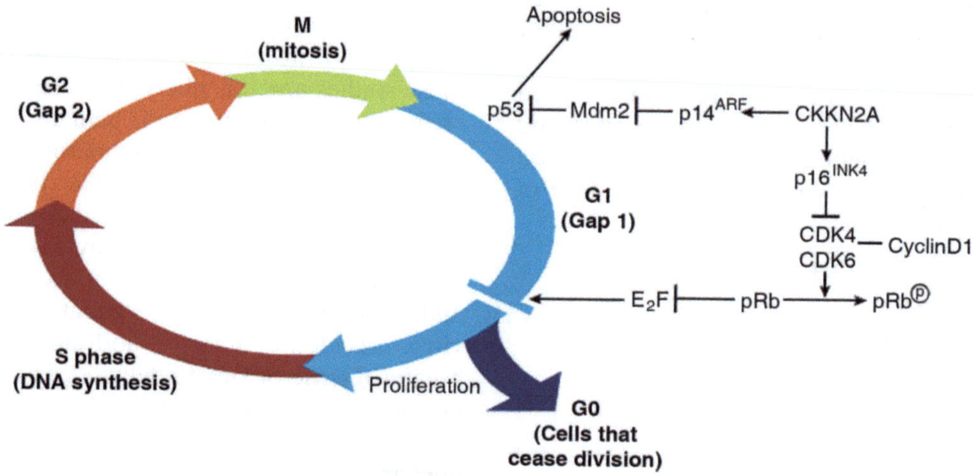

the development of tumors (Boxes 43.4 and 43.5). In contrast, MM cell lines are highly resistant to asbestos-induced and ROS-induced apoptosis.[391] This effect is not related to expression of Bcl-2, an important regulator of apoptosis that is mutated in many tumors, but the mechanism underlying this resistance is not understood at present.

Direct Activation of Transcription Pathways

Induction of the mitogen-activated protein kinase (MAPK) signaling pathways occurs in response to exposure to asbestos and appears to be related to ROS. This cascade includes signal transcription factors such as nuclear factor κB (NF-κB),[371] which triggers activation of a number of genes involved in cell proliferation and apoptosis, including cytokines, growth factors, and adhesion molecules as well as proto-oncogenes such as c-*myc*. Reactive oxygen species also induce expression of the AP1 transcription factors c-*fos* and c-*jun*, both of which are also proto-oncogenes[392] implicated in malignant transformation. However, recent experiments investigating protein expression and phosphorylation status (activity) of the extracellular-regulated kinase (ERK), the c-*jun* amino-terminal kinase (JNK), and the high-osmolarity glycerol response kinase (p38) in fresh frozen reactive mesothelium and MM specimens did not detect significant differences between reactive mesothelium and MM.[393] Although there is undoubtedly upregulation of these genes, there is insufficient experimental evidence at present to conclude that MAPK activation contributes significantly to malignant transformation.

Molecular Events in the Development of Mesothelioma III: Chromosome and Gene Alterations, and Disruption of Cell Pathways

The capacity of asbestos to induce mesothelioma in experimental animals was established as early as the 1960s by inhalation/installation and direct implantation experiments, where chrysotile was found to be about equipotent with the amphiboles when implanted directly

Box 43.5. Apoptosis

The term *apoptosis* is of Greek origin, meaning "falling off" and is used to describe the process that leads to controlled self-induced cell death. Apoptosis plays an important role in the morphogenesis of developing organisms, as well as maintaining homeostasis in adult organisms. In addition, apoptosis allows deletion of damaged and potentially dangerous cells, such as cells that contain irreparable DNA damage, infected cells or autoreactive immune cells. (See sections Cell Death and Survival, and Apoptosis in Chapter 33.)

There are many potential pathways that may lead to apoptosis, and some of those that have been investigated in MM are illustrated below.

The role of p53 is central. Activated p53 may arrest the cell cycle, via upregulation of p21, a cyclin-dependent kinase, which has been found to be altered in some MMs. Depending on the cell type, p21 may not only induce cell cycle arrest, but also initiate apoptosis directly. In addition, p21 phosphorylates merlin, the gene product of the *NF2* gene at chromosome 22, which has been found mutated in a significant number of MM. Phosphorylation decreases function of merlin, which is thought to act as a tumor suppressor gene, although the exact mechanism is not well understood as yet.

In addition, there are alternative pathways to apoptosis via the mitochondrial-bound proteins Bax and Bak, which are opposed by the antiapoptotic protein Bcl-2. This pathway is commonly affected in malignant tumors, but there is currently insufficient evidence to suggest that it plays a major role in the development of MM.

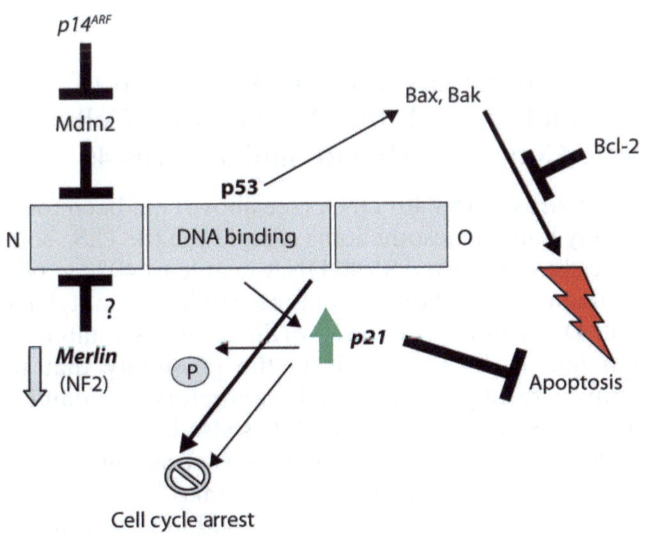

into the pleural cavities. More recently, in vitro studies have yielded significant information, and it has been established that asbestos has clastogenic and genotoxic effects in cells.[37] Asbestos fibers have been shown to induce chromosomal aberrations, anaphase-telophase abnormalities, and sister chromatid exchanges in cultured rodent and human cells. Both crocidolite and chrysotile have been shown to disturb cell division, resulting in aneuploidy or polyploidy. However, although asbestos was found to induce clonally aneuploid cells with abnormal banding patterns in vitro, these alterations were insufficient to render the cells tumorigenic.[394]

Studies on the chromosomal profile of MMs have demonstrated multiple abnormalities, usually more than 10 clonal abnormalities in any one case, although no consistent or specific chromosomal abnormality has been identified. Nonetheless, recurrent chromosomal abnormalities are common in MM, deletions being the most common chromosomal alterations,[395–402] including deletions in chromosome arms 1p, 3p, 4q, 6q, 9p, 13q, 14q, 15q, and 22q where the neurofibromatosis 2 *(NF2)* gene is located.[403–407] The most frequent numerical change is monosomy of chromosome 22[395]; gains are less common, but gains of chromosomes 5, 7, and 20 have been described.[37] Comparative genomic hybridization (CGH) studies have shown multiple chromosome abnormalities in most of the tumors analyzed, with no consistent or specific abnormality.[397,402]

Combinations of such cytogenetic abnormalities can be found in most MMs, and all are present in about 25%.[37] Loss of heterozygosity has also been demonstrated on chromosome 1, as have allelic deletions on chromosomes 3, 4, and 6 as well as 15 (where *RAD51*, a tumor suppressor gene that participates in the repair of breaks in double-stranded DNA, is located at 15.q.15.1[37]). Deletion of p16^{INK4A} has also been demonstrated at 9p.21, in about 85% of MM cell lines and about 22% of primary MMs.[37] In a study on transgenic mice carrying the *lacI* reporter gene, Rihn et al.[408] also found evidence suggestive of a decrease in DNA repair in crocidolite-treated animals.

It is worth noting that most of the studies investigating the molecular basis for MM were carried out using epithelial mesotheliomas, although some studies did not distinguish between the different types of mesotheliomas. This may affect some of the results and may explain some contradictory results in different studies.

Most of the recurring mutations seem to affect tumor suppressor genes and growth factors, rather than oncogenes. Although no specific chromosomal or genomic abnormality has been demonstrated in MM, it has been recognized that the disruption of certain cellular *pathways* is a recurring event. Therefore, it is useful to think of MMs as being characterized and unified by disruption of those pathways, rather than by mutations of specific genes.

Molecular Events in the Development of Mesothelioma IV: Interference with Cell Cycle Control and Apoptosis: *p53*

Because the induction of MM represents a multistep process that requires progressive accumulation of mutations, the pathways that prevent this occurrence in healthy cells play a pivotal role. The tumor suppressor gene *p53*, sometimes termed "the guardian of the genome," initiates cell cycle arrest or programmed cell death in response to cellular damage and stress (Boxes 43.4 and 43.5; also see The Cell Cycle in Chapter 33).

Mutations of the gene encoding *p53* (usually point mutations leading to an inactive form of p53) are well characterized and are known to play a role in the carcinogenesis of many tumors, but are rarely identifiable in mesotheliomas. For example, mutations in *p53* itself or the tumor gene *RAS*, which is known to interfere with p53 concentrations and which is commonly mutated in lung cancer,[179] are not common in mesotheliomas.[409,410] Even so, whereas mutations in *p53* itself are rarely described in mesotheliomas, the p53 pathway is commonly affected. The high frequency of deletions at the 9p.21 locus corresponds to loss of functional activity of a number of critical proteins involved in the p53 and pRB pathways, namely $p14^{ARF}$, as well as the CDK inhibitors $p16^{INK4a}$ (and, to a lesser extent, $p15^{INK4b}$).

The protein $p14^{ARF}$ induces p53. The level of p53 in unstressed cells is low, maintained by degradation of p53 and suppression of its transcriptional activity by binding of Mdm2. Mdm2 effectively counteracts p53 tumor suppressor activity. Mdm2 activity is blocked by $p14^{ARF}$, and $p14^{ARF}$ acts as a positive regulator for *p53*. Therefore, functional loss of $p14^{ARF}$, as seen in many MMs, results in lack of functional p53 because of unopposed Mdm2. This results in a loss of the ability of the cell to arrest the cell cycle and or undergo apoptosis in response to cell damage sustained, for example, by ROS. Unless the cell damage is lethal, the mutated cell undergoes uninhibited growth.

This has been exploited in several experimental models, where transfection of cultured human mesothelioma cell lines with an adenovirus vector expressing $p14^{ARF}$ resulted in increase of functional p53, and therefore cell cycle arrest and slowing of tumor growth.[411–414]

Molecular Events in the Development of Mesothelioma V: Cell Cycle Control: *pRb*

The gene product of the retinoblastoma gene, *pRb*, is the prototypical tumor suppressor gene. It is part of the cyclin-dependent kinase-cyclinD1/INK4/pRb/E2F cascade, and mutations in this cascade have been identified in more than 80% of human neoplasms.[415] Active pRb is hypophosphorylated and binds to transcription factors, E2F-1 in particular, and inactivates them. Phosphorylation renders pRb inactive, so that the transcription factors become active and DNA synthesis is initiated. Members of the INK4 family (CDK inhibitors $p16^{INK4a}$ and $p15^{INK4b}$) inhibit phosphorylation of *pRb*, by interaction with cyclin-dependent kinases, maintaining the binding of transcription factors to *pRb* and preventing transcription. The cells remain in G_1 phase and do not progress through the cell cycle (Box 43.4). Cyclin-dependent kinases act as checkpoints that prevent transition into the next cell cycle phase, and loss of CDK inhibitors results in uncontrolled cell proliferation (see The Cell Cycle in Chapter 33).

Mutations in this cascade can occur within the effector proteins, such as pRb itself, as in the case of retinoblastoma. In MM and MM cell lines, expression of the wild-type pRb is mostly maintained. In contrast, there is deletion or mutation of the upstream regulators, $p16^{INK4a}$ and $p15^{INK4b}$. When $p16^{INK4a}$ is replaced in human mesothelioma cells by adenovirus gene transfer, and functional protein expressed, arrest of the cell cycle occurs via inhibition of pRb phosphorylation. The end result is diminished cell growth, and, eventually, death of the transfected cells.[411,414] This approach may have some therapeutic potential.

It becomes clear at this stage that there are many interconnections of the pathways that are commonly altered in MM. The intimate association of p53 and pRb pathways does not end with the shared site that expresses $p16^{INK4a}$, $p15^{INK4b}$, and $p14^{ARF}$. In addition, transcription of p21WAF/CIP1 is induced by p53, and p21 then may act as an inhibitor of cyclin-dependent kinases involved in the pRb pathway, causing cell cycle arrest (rather than apoptosis). The expression of p21 appears to have prognostic significance in MM, and increased expression of p21 is associated with improved survival.[416]

Molecular Events in the Development of Mesothelioma VI: Interference with Cell Cycle Control: pRb and Simian Virus 40

Simian virus 40 (SV40) DNA (see above) has been found in many human mesothelioma samples: in the U.S., some studies have reported SV40 DNA in at least 40% to 60% of human mesotheliomas, but other studies did not detect SV40 DNA in any tumors[417] or in cell lines established from human MM,[192,418] raising the possibility that the positive results represented laboratory contamination.[418,419] Simian virus 40 DNA has also been found in a number of other tumors, including osteosarcomas, brain tumors, and papillary thyroid carcinomas.[420,421]

Two epidemiologic studies published in 1998 found no evidence of an increased rate of bone or brain tumors, or mesothelioma, 30 years after the use of polio vaccines contaminated with SV40.[422,423] In a later study stratified for age, Strickler et al.[160] found that the incidence of pleural mesothelioma remained stable or declined in younger age groups with a high probability of having received the SV40-contaminated vaccine, whereas the incidence rose in the oldest age groups with a low probability of inoculation with the contaminated vaccine. The evidence on SV40 and human cancer, including four epidemiologic studies, has been reviewed systematically by Shah.[424]

Simian virus 40 encodes two tumor antigens, large T and small t; SV40 causes interference with cell cycle regulation, in part by the blocking of p53 via its SV40 large T antigen (SV40 LT), but SV40 LT also interacts with pRb. These interactions result in inactivation of proteins with tumor suppressor activity, via two pathways that are commonly disrupted "upstream" by other mechanisms in MM. Interference with either pathway is sufficient to induce tumors, because a mutant SV40 LT which cannot bind p53 is still capable of transforming cells lacking p53.[192] The t antigen has also been implicated in the oncogenic activity of SV40 via binding to phosphatase 2A, but its role is less well established.[192]

There is no doubt that SV40 can be oncogenic under certain conditions. In particular, this DNA virus has been shown to induce mesotheliomas when injected into the heart or pleura of hamsters.[425] In addition, SV40 also transforms human cells in tissue culture, and these cells show extensive DNA damage. Although it appears certain that SV40 can induce tumors in animal models and in vitro, this does not seem to contribute to an understanding of MM carcinogenesis in humans.

The ATCC cell line Met-5A (www.atcc.org) comprises nonneoplastic human mesothelial cells that have been immortalized by transfection with a plasmid containing the SV40 early region DNA. Met-5A cells, one of the standard human mesothelial cell lines used in many experiments investigating MM, have a single copy of SV40 early region DNA integrated in their genome. They express SV40 large T antigen, and they maintain mesothelial cell characteristics, such as sensitivity to the cytotoxic effects of asbestos fibers. However, when injected into nude mice, these cells are nontumorigenic, providing evidence that SV40 alone is insufficient to induce MM.[426]

Asbestos alone fails to induce the transformation of these human mesothelial cells in vitro, but if interleukin-1β (IL-1β) and tumor necrosis factor-α (TNF-α) are added (simulating the release of these major cytokines by macrophages after inhalation of asbestos), they contribute to erionite-induced transformation of the MeT-5A cells in vitro. These cells could only be transformed when exposed to a combination of cytokines and erionite, or at least two cytokines together without erionite, for at least 4 months in vitro. The findings presented here suggest that IL-1β and TNF-α play a significant role in the pathogenesis of mesothelioma, and that it might be desirable to block or inhibit cytokine secretion in high-risk populations to prevent mesothelioma.[427]

As discussed above, both of the pathways that are subject to inactivation by SV40 are usually already mutated further upstream in MM. For example, loss of effective pRb control in human MM already results from the near-universal deletion of $p16^{INK4a}$; therefore, an argument can be adduced that SV40 LT is not necessary for inactivation of pRb in MM, and that it may not contribute to tumor development.[428] Also, since SV40 LT acts downstream from both $p16^{INK4a}$ and $p14^{ARF}$, the effect would be expected to be more akin to a point mutation in these major tumor suppressor proteins. Therefore, one would expect much faster tumor growth, and the long latency of MM argues against a significant role for SV40 in human MMs.

Finally, other polyomaviruses, such as JC virus, which have been shown to be oncogenic in animal models could not be detected in significant numbers of MMs.[429]

Molecular Events in the Development of Mesothelioma VII: SV40: Other Effects

There is evidence that SV40 may induce some growth factors, including vascular endothelial growth factor (VEGF),[430,431] which has been found to play an important role in the growth of MM.[432] It is therefore possible that SV40 creates a favorable environment for the accelerated growth of MM. Some authors believe that VEGF shows potential as a prognostic indicator,[433] whereas others deny that VEGF predicts prognosis.[434]

At present, a significant role for SV40 in the induction of MM is far from accepted and appears unlikely, despite the undisputed fact that this virus has oncogenic capacity in some models. In particular, epidemiologic data make it unlikely that SV40 can act as the single causative agent inducing MM. Rather, it appears likely that SV40 may contribute to a permissive environment that may favor tumor growth. Finally, crocidolite asbestos has been shown to mediate transfection of human mesothelial cells by plasmid DNA containing SV40 sequences, and it is possible that exposure to asbestos simply facilitates entry of SV40 into affected cells, and that in fact the frequent finding of SV40 sequences in MM is a consequence of exposure to asbestos.[394]

Molecular Events in the Development of Mesothelioma VIII: Interference with the p53 Pathway: The Role of Wilms' Tumor 1 (*WT1*)

WT1 is a tumor-suppressor gene expressed in the developing kidney, whose inactivation leads to the development of Wilms' tumor, a pediatric kidney cancer. *WT1* is expressed in normal mesothelium and in most epithelial mesotheliomas. *WT1* mutations have been found to be expressed in mesothelioma,[428,435] although this is disputed by others who believe mutations to be exceptional.[37] In contrast, lung carcinomas rarely express WT1, and this has led to the use of WT1 antibodies for diagnosis of epithelial MM, although there is some debate in the literature about their usefulness.[436,437]

WT1 encodes a transcription factor that binds to the early growth response gene 1 *(EGR1)* consensus sequence and suppresses transcription of early growth response genes including insulin-like growth factor-I (IGF-I) receptor and epidermal growth factor receptor (EGFR).[438] It is therefore conceivable that mutation of *WT1* could lead to increased growth factor release, creating a favorable environment for tumor growth. WT1 also interferes with the p53 pathway, because the tumor-suppressor gene *p53* physically associates with WT1. The interaction between WT1 and p53 modulates their respective capacity to transactivate their respective targets. Unexpectedly, in the absence of p53 (as would be the case in MM cells), WT1 acts as a potent transcriptional *activator* of the EGFR-1 site,[439] so that even normal WT1 could potentially lose its tumor-suppressant attributes in this environment. Nonetheless, no correlation between WT1 expression and expression of growth factors has been demonstrated so far in MM.[440] Even so, the interaction among p53, WT1, and growth factors appears to play a role in the growth of MM, and we have found antibodies against WT1 to be useful for diagnosis in many cases.

Molecular Events in the Development of Mesothelioma IX: NF2 Inactivation and Mesothelioma

The neurofibromatosis 2 (NFS)-encoded protein belongs to the ERM (ezrin-radixin-moesin) family of cytoskeleton-membrane linkers.[438] The protein encoded by NF2 is a tumor suppressor protein called merlin (for mesosin-ezrin-radixin-like protein) or schwannomin, which functions as a negative growth regulator, and it is known that inactivating mutations in *NF2* predispose humans to tumors. Some of its tumor suppressor properties are probably associated with contact-mediated growth inhibition. Mutations of the *NF2* gene or reduced expression of the gene product are an extremely common finding in MM,[405,407,441] but not in lung cancers.[37] There are several connections of merlin with the p53 pathway (Box 43.5). First, merlin increases p53 stability by inducing degradation of the p53 inhibitor Mdm2. In addition, merlin appears to mediate an increase of p53-mediated transcriptional activity. As mentioned in Box 43.5 and above, there is already a connection of *NF2* with the p53 pathway, as p53 induces p21, a cyclin-dependent kinase, which phosphorylates merlin.[442] This diminishes the function of merlin and acts as a negative feedback loop. However, there is nearly ubiquitous loss of $p14^{ARF}$ in MM, resulting in lack of p53 and lack of induction of p21, so that this pathway is unlikely to play a major role.

Furthermore, patients with NF2 appear to have no increase in the risk of MM. This implies that the tumor suppressor gene *NF2*, despite the common presence of mutations or deletions in MM, is likely to play a permissive or supportive role in the development of MM, rather than being an initiator of tumorigenesis (similar to *WT1* and SV40). Similar observations have been made in other hereditary cancers where tumor suppressor genes are affected; for example, *Rb-1* is commonly mutated in nonhereditary small cell carcinomas of lung, but patients with hereditary retinoblastoma do not have an increased risk for developing small cell carcinoma of lung. It has been proposed that, depending of the tissue type, further pathogenetic stimuli are required.[443]

Molecular Events in the Development of Mesothelioma X: *FHIT*

The fragile histidine triad *(FHIT)* tumor suppressor gene located at 3p14.2 appears to represent a site of genomic fragility relevant to carcinogenesis,[181,444–446] including the pathogenesis of MM.[182] FHIT protein is expressed in most nonneoplastic tissues, and the highest levels of expression occur in epithelial cells. FHIT appears to be subject to deletion or LOH by cigarette smoke and asbestos.[101,103,111,115] Diminished expression of FHIT has been recorded in up to 80% of cigarette smoke–associated lung cancers,[444] and in both asbestos-associated lung cancers (69%) and nonexposed cases (59%) in one study,[181] and in 54% of mesotheliomas.[182] The limited data available suggest a frequent decrease of FHIT protein expression, thus supporting the significance of FHIT inactivation in development of MM.

Molecular Events in the Development of Mesothelioma XI: Growth Factors/Cytokines

There is now a large body of evidence that growth factor signaling, and in particular EGFR signaling, plays a key role in tumor growth. Consisting of complex cascades of interactions, the EGFR signaling system is one of the most extensively studied signaling pathways (Fig. 43.10). As discussed above, disruption of regulation of apoptosis plays a major role in MM development, and there are complex interactions between growth factor signaling and apoptosis control. The intracellular mechanisms of interactions between EGF and apoptosis pathways are incompletely understood, but many of them involve the

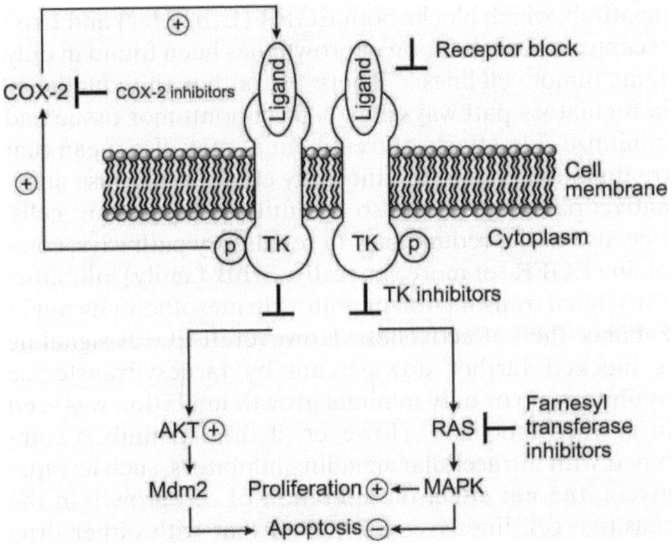

FIGURE 43.10. The epidermal growth factor receptor domain and its interaction with signaling pathways and cyclooxygenase-2 (COX-2), and potential targets for therapeutic intervention.

kinase Akt (see PI3K/Akt/mTOR Pathway in Chapter 33), which is activated downstream of many growth factors not limited to EGF. Another pathway involves RAS signaling (Box 43.6). These signaling pathways have been the focus of targeted treatment attempts (see also Chapter 33, section on Ras/Raf-1/Mitogen activated protein kinase pathway).

Epidermal growth factor receptor signaling has been recognized as a key step in MM growth and it has been suggested that control of cell survival through EGFR activation is conditional, in the sense that it is crucial for tumor cell survival but not for survival of normal mesothelial cells. Specifically, normal epithelial cells are provided with a full complement of physiologic cell-cell contacts and cell-matrix interactions that lessen their dependence on survival signals provided by the EGFR. In contrast, malignant tumor cells faced with inadequate cell-matrix contacts are thought to depend critically on EGFR activation for survival, making them more susceptible to apoptosis induction by EGFR blockade. This was the basis for focusing research efforts on developing potential clinical treatments for MM, based on blocking EGFR signaling, but it now appears that redundant control of cell survival by the EGFR and extracellular matrix/cell adhesion receptors remains, to a degree, enabled in tumor cells. This is at least in part the result of shared signal transduction pathways controlling apoptosis (Fig. 43.9), and these complex interactions are discussed below.

In addition, growth factors are also involved in the regulation of matrix metalloproteinases (MMPs), a group of enzymes involved in dissolution of extracellular matrix that enable cell growth and vascularization under normal circumstances, and in tumors play a key role in cell invasion and metastasis.

The Epidermal Growth Factor Receptor Transforming Growth Factor-α Loop

Epidermal growth factor receptor belongs to the ErbB family of receptor tyrosine kinases, which has recently gained prominence because of the mutations found in a group of breast carcinomas, which then may be selectively treated with specific tyrosine kinase inhibitors, such as Herceptin. This family of receptors includes EGFR (ErbBHer1), ErbB2-Her2/neu, Her3, and Her4. Epidermal growth factor receptor is a transmembrane glycoprotein that consists of the extracellular ligand-binding domain, a transmembrane component, the intracellular tyrosine kinase functional domain, and a COOH-terminal region containing autophosphorylation sites (Fig. 43.10). Phosphorylation at the COOH-terminal tail initiates a cellular signaling pathway that regulates fundamental cellular processes such as proliferation, migration, differentiation, and survival.

Epidermal growth factor receptor on the cell surface presents as an inactive monomer that is activated by binding of specific ligands, including EGF and transforming growth factor-α (Fig. 43.10). The activated EGFR monomer can pair with another EGFR to form an active homodimer, or an EGFR receptor monomer may pair with another member of the ErbB receptor family, such as Her2/neu, to create a heterodimer.

Ligand binding induces the intrinsic protein-tyrosine kinase activity of EGFR, initiating a signal transduction

Box 43.6. Cell Signaling Pathways and RAS

RAS pathways are involved in cell signaling pathways that control cytoskeletal integrity, cell proliferation, cell–matrix interactions, apoptosis, and cell migration. RAS is a G protein (a small guanosine triphosphatase [GTPase]) that alternates between two conformations: activated or inactivated. Mutations in the *ras* family of proto-oncogenes (e.g., H-*ras*, N-*ras*, and K-*ras*) are present in 20% to 30% of all human tumors, but are not common in MM.[47] Despite this, the RAS pathway may still be affected indirectly (e.g., by increased EGFR expression), and downstream modulation and inhibiting of RAS signaling may inhibit growth and promote apoptosis. Farnesylation is necessary to attach RAS to the cell membrane. Without this attachment to the cell membrane, RAS cannot transfer signals from membrane receptors, and this is the rationale for treatment attempts with farnesyltransferase inhibitors.

cascade. This involves the MAPK, Akt, and JNK pathways, among others (see relevant sections in Chapter 33). Increased proliferation is achieved by promoting cell cycle progression at the level of the G_1-phase, and inhibiting apoptosis, and the net effect is tissue growth. The kinase activity can also result in autophosphorylation of the COOH terminal region, as mentioned above, resulting in activation of proteins distinct from those activated by the kinase signaling cascade directly. These proteins include regulatory proteins involved in cell matrix continuity and play a role in maintaining cell-cell and cell-matrix interaction, disturbance of which may lead to loss of contact inhibition and increased invasiveness.

There has been convincing evidence that expression of EGFR at the protein and transcriptional level is increased in MM in comparison to reactive mesothelial proliferations or normal mesothelial cells.[447–449] The EGFR ligands that have been shown to play a role in the pathogenesis of MM include EGF and TGF-α. Binding of TGF-α induces an autocrine feedback loop resulting in increased EGFR expression and increased proliferation. Phosphorylation of EGFR[450] and an increase in expression of TGF-α is observed early after exposure to asbestos,[451] and cell growth can be inhibited under those circumstances by antibodies to TGF-α. In addition, there appears to be a correlation between the expression of EGFR and the carcinogenicity of the fibers used.[452] Furthermore, autophosphorylation of EGFR can be induced by asbestos fibers directly in vitro, with long fibers being more effective than short fibers.[453] It can be argued that the ongoing inflammatory response directed at the asbestos fibers in vivo provides an ongoing source for TGF-α, and in effect delivers a continuous growth stimulus.

Selective inhibition of EGFR signaling by the small molecule inhibitor gefitinib (ZD1839) in models using mesothelioma cell lines in vitro results in reduced growth of tumor cells of some cell lines. In most cell lines this effect appears to be cytostatic, rather than cytotoxic, as evidenced by a lack of increase in the apoptotic fraction,[454] although there was an increase in apoptosis in another cell line.[455] However, the main effect of EGFR blockade appears to be arrest of the cells in the G_1/S phase.[456] A similar effect resulting in reduction of tumor volume has also been reported in an in vivo murine model of mesothelioma. Inhibition of EGFR signaling was effective in reducing tumor size if used alone, with an increased effect if used in conjunction with radiation.[457] It appears that selective blockade of the EGFR pathway at the ligand level in solid tumors limits tumor cell survival rather than survival of normal tissues, as alternative pathways of apoptosis control and cell proliferation are intact in the normal tissues, making EGFR pathway blockade an attractive potential treatment modality for MM.[458] More recently, use has been made of lapatinib, which blocks both EGFR (Erb1-Her) and Erb2 receptors, but inhibition of growth has been found in only some tumor cell lines.[456] Therefore, although redundancy in regulatory pathways may protect nontumor tissue and minimize side effects of treatment, it may also mean that treatment may not be sufficiently effective because alternative pathways can also be utilized by tumor cells. Because of the redundancy in regulatory pathways, combining EGFR (or more generally, ErbB-family) inhibitors with signal transduction inhibitors in mesothelioma might enhance their effectiveness. However, if EGFR signaling is blocked further downstream by farnesyltransferase inhibitors, no or only minimal growth inhibition was seen in in vitro models.[449] However, if the lapatinib is combined with intracellular signaling inhibitors, such as rapamycin, the net effect on inhibition of cell growth in the sensitive cell lines is greater than that with either drug alone.[456]

Only some of the mesothelioma cell lines tested in vitro were sensitive to treatment targeting the EGFR pathways, and this is reflected in the results of recent clinical trials. Use of alternative pathways appears to occur in vivo, and to date, clinical trials with oral gefitinib have been disappointing.[459,460] This may have been expected, because EGFR status has not been identified as an independent prognostic factor, presumably due to this redundancy in regulatory pathways. In addition, EGFR expression in MM seems to correlate with epithelioid histology, and it would be desirable to differentiate clinical treatment groups according to the histologic subtype of MM. Combination of EGFR inhibitors and intracellular signaling inhibitors has been proposed for future clinical trials.[456]

The Epidermal Growth Factor Receptor–Cyclooxygenase-2 Loop

Apart from these fairly direct effects on growth, EGFR is also involved in a second autocrine feedback loop via cyclooxygenase-2 (COX-2), with EGFR increasing COX-2 transcription, and COX-2 increasing EGFR transcription, in turn (Fig. 43.10). Cyclooxygenase-2 expression has been proposed as an independent negative prognostic factor,[461–463] although other investigators claim that COX-2 expression indicated improved survival.[464] Inhibition of COX-2 may be achieved by nonspecific nonsteroidal antiinflammatory drugs (NSAIDs) such as acetylsalicylic acid or indomethacin, or more selectively by the COX-2 inhibitor NS-398 or celecoxib (Fig. 43.10).

Cyclooxygenase-2 has been implicated in carcinogenesis by way of downregulation of cell-mediated immunity and promotion of angiogenesis, and COX-2–expressing cancer cell lines are associated with increased proliferation and invasive potential. Cyclooxygenase-2 overexpression has been noted in many solid tumors, and expression has recently also been shown in MM,[462,465,466] as well as reactive mesothelial proliferations.[466] Selective inhibition of COX-2 with the COX-2 inhibitor NS-398 in vitro revealed dose- and time-dependent antiproliferative activity,[466] and similarly, the selective COX-2 inhibitor celecoxib reduced in vitro proliferation of several MM cell lines obtained from previously untreated patients. In addition, there was increased MM cell apoptosis that involved decreased Akt phosphorylation, loss of bcl-2, survivin protein expression, and caspase-3 activation.[467] Simultaneous application of VEGF rescued apoptosis and Akt phosphorylation, but if anti-VEGF antibodies were also given, this effect was abrogated. This finding highlights the complex interaction and cross-regulation between the different growth factors, all leading to tight control of apoptosis.

Vascular Endothelial Growth Factor

Vascular endothelial growth factor is a potent angiogenic factor, involved in the growth and metastasis of neoplasms by stimulating stromal vascular growth. There is overexpression of VEGF and VEGF-C in MM,[430,434,468–470] but this also occurs in some reactive conditions. Although some studies claim negative prognostic significance associated with VEGF expression, this has not been confirmed by all investigators.[471] In MM, VEGF is expressed along with the VEGF receptor flt-1.[472] The production of the growth factors by tumors is a widespread phenomenon, but the coexpression of receptors and formation of an autocrine loop, as seen in MM, is less common. This pathway appears to be effective in promoting tumor growth, as VEGF also has been shown to increase proliferation of MM by directly stimulating tumor growth in a dose-dependent manner.[432] Blocking of the autocrine loop by antibodies against VEGF receptor or antisense oligonucleotides that act as inhibitors of VEGF and VEGF-C has been shown to inhibit MM cell growth in vitro.[473] Also, if there is a role for SV40 as a driving agent for MM development, it may be through VEGF activation.[430,474]

Tumor Necrosis Factor-α

Tumor necrosis factor-α is a potent initiator of apoptosis, but paradoxically, in some cases, it can inhibit apoptosis by upregulation of survival-inducing proteins, including members of the so-called inhibitors of apoptosis (IAP) family. Interestingly, raised serum levels of TNF-α have been found in those individuals exposed to asbestos who would eventually develop a thoracic malignancy.[475] The secretion of TNF-α may also aid in explaining a paradox: crocidolite asbestos is cytotoxic, and in isolation fails to transform primary human mesothelial cells, causing extensive cell death instead. In in vitro experiments, treatment with TNF-α significantly reduced crocidolite cytotoxicity and promoted cell survival, thus increasing the pool of asbestos-damaged cells susceptible to malignant transformation.[476] In vivo, macrophages are a potential source of TNF-α, and secretion of TNF-α has been linked with fiber length, with longer more carcinogenic fibers inducing higher levels of secretion.[476,477]

Inhibitors of Apoptosis Proteins and Tumor Necrosis Factor-α

The family of IAPs includes the proteins IAP-1, IAP-2, livin, and survivin. These are proteins that can block apoptosis. There is increased expression of survivin in MM (but also in some inflammatory conditions),[478,479] and this appears to have some prognostic significance in predicting poorer outcome.[479] Anti-survivin oligonucleotides could inhibit survivin activity in vitro in cell lines expressing survivin, resulting in apoptosis, whereas apoptosis could not be induced in the survivin-negative cell line LRK1A by antisense oligonucleotides. Therefore, downregulation of survivin by a targeted antisense oligonucleotide could represent an effective gene therapy approach to the treatment of mesothelioma. Tumor necrosis factor-α has been shown to increase expression of IAP-1, IAP-2, and XIAP in MM in vitro.[480] Inhibitors of apoptosis may therefore represent an additional target for treatment attempts in clinical trials.

Growth Factors and Extracellular Matrix Interaction

Malignant mesotheliomas express a wide range of MMPs in comparison to normal pleura[481–484] (Box 43.7). Matrix

> **Box 43.7. Extracellular Matrix and Matrix Metalloproteinases**
>
> Extracellular matrix proteins and interaction play an important role in maintaining tissue integrity. Mutations and activations of some of these enzymes that can dissolve extracellular matrix are essential steps for a tumor to promote angiogenesis, and acquire invasiveness and metastatic potential. Numerous mutations of matrix proteins have been described in MM. Matrix metalloproteases (MMPs) are a family of zinc-dependent enzymes that dissolve extracellular matrix and seem to play a particularly important role in tumor cell invasion and metastasis. Most of the enzymes are secreted as inactive proenzymes and activated by cleavage of the N-terminal sequence. They are directly negatively regulated by tissue inhibitors of metalloproteinases (TIMPs), and growth factors and angiogenic factors such as TGF-α, EGF, and COX-2 activate MMPs.

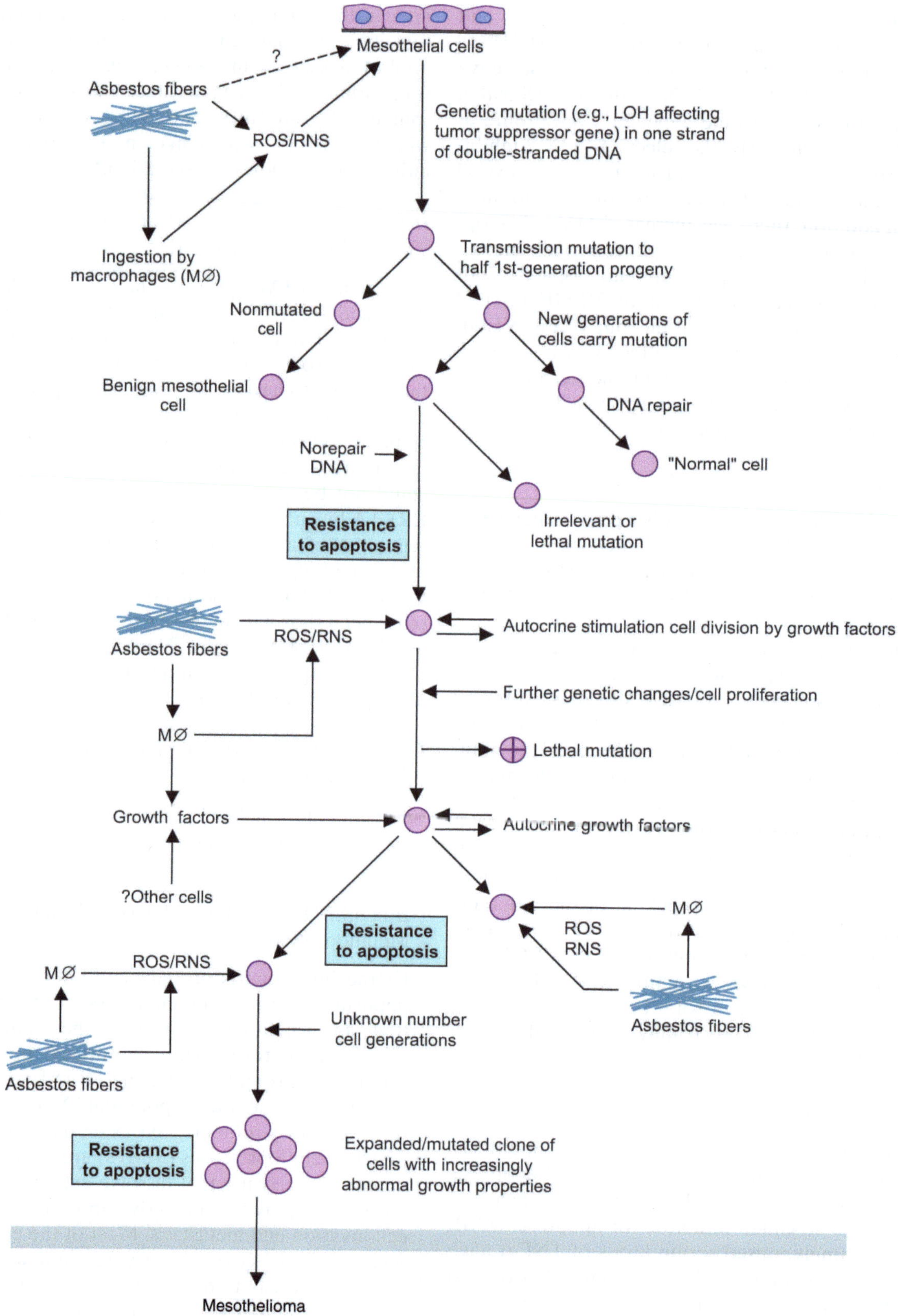

FIGURE 43.11. Schematic overview of possible or likely events leading to the development of MM, extending over multiple generations of mesothelial cells.

metalloproteinase-2 was found to be the predominant gelatinase in a study of 16 tumors,[483] but MMP-2 expression was not induced by the growth factors EGF or TGF-α,[485] and there was no correlation with expression of COX-2. Instead, ligation of EGFR increases MMP-3 and MMP-9 production,[482,485] and the increase in MMP could be blocked in vitro by the tyrosine kinase inhibitor genistein.[485] This increase in MMP expression was associated with enhanced cell motility, and this may play a role in acquiring invasive potential. In addition, MMP-1, which may be induced by platelet-derived growth factor (PDGF) and TGF-α, has been shown to increase mesothelial cell motility and possibly play a role in invasiveness.[482]

Hoang et al.[486] found an 826-fold increased expression of matriptase, a trypsin-like protease, in epithelioid MM cells. Matriptase messenger RNA (mRNA) has been "characterized as an extracellular matrix-degrading protease system that may function as an epithelial membrane activator for other proteases and latent growth factors involved in cancer cell growth, invasion, and metastasis."[164] Hoang et al. also found upregulation of insulin-like growth factor exon I (IGF-I), which has also been found to act as an autocrine growth factor for normal and neoplastic mesothelial cells, and IGF-I also drives mesothelial cell differentiation toward a fibroblast-like morphology.[164] Strong expression of the c-*sis* gene (PDGF B-chain) has also been recorded in comparison to normal mesothelial cells.[487,488]

Molecular Events in the Development of Mesothelioma XII: Mesothelial Cell Kinetics and Proliferation

Although some authorities have invoked a multipotential subserosal cell as the stem cell for repair of mesothelial injury and for the histogenesis of MM, studies on the repair of mesothelial cell damage that does not include disruption of the basal lamina or other submesothelial tissues indicate that repair is effected by mesothelial cells themselves by a process of proliferation, migration, and probably detachment and reimplantation. The concept of mesothelioma in situ[489,490] has also redirected attention to the mesothelium itself as the target site for mesothelioma induction.

It is known that in the resting mesothelium in the rat, about 1% of the mesothelial cells are in the S-phase of the mitotic cycle (0.5–3.0%, and about 0.16–0.25% in the mouse); however, about 60% to 80% of the cells go into the S-phase within 1 to 2 days of a superficial injury that denudes the mesothelium, with proliferation of mesothelial cells that then move across the denuded surface to reestablish continuity of the mesothelial layer in about 8 to 10 days.[491–494] (A single mesothelial cell has been observed by time-lapse cinephotography to travel a distance of up to 75 μm within the space of 3 hours).[492,493,495] It appears that about 30% of resting mesothelial cells turnover about every 10 days, and "inflammatory" stimuli and asbestos fibers have the effect of increasing the rate of turnover. Suppose, however, that the resting rate remains unchanged after asbestos fibers reach the pleural membrane, and that the turnover rate is 10 to 20 days for 30% of the mesothelial cell population, so that the time for the entire population to be renewed is about 35 to 65 days; this means that the pleural mesothelium renews itself about six to 10 times each year.

The mean lag time between first exposure to asbestos and the diagnosis of MM is about 35 to 45 years (rounding off to the nearest 5 years). Suppose also that a mesothelioma comes into existence as such about 5 years before diagnosis. During the preceding 30 years there would be some 180 to 300 generations of mesothelial cells for an average MM case. Even if the first mesothelioma cell came into existence only 5 years after exposure, one can calculate that some 30 to 50 generations of mesothelial cells would have passed before the MM would have come into existence. Figure 43.11 presents a schematic overview of the types of events that are considered likely in the development of MM, over multiple generations of mesothelial cells.

Pathologic Features of Malignant Pleural Mesothelioma

Macroscopic Features of Pleural Mesothelioma

Most patients with pleural mesotheliomas present with shortness of breath due to a pleural effusion on the side of the tumor. When these patients are evaluated by video-assisted thoracoscopic surgery or by an open thoracotomy, the visceral and parietal pleura are often found to be studded by multiple nodules ranging in size from less than 1 mm to about 1 cm. (Fig. 43.12). As time progresses, the small nodules coalesce to form a solid tumor that encases the lung and obliterates the pleural cavity (Fig. 43.13). In most instances, the tumor is thicker at the base of the thoracic cavity than at the apex. The tumor not infrequently invades the lung parenchyma and chest wall (Fig. 43.14). Mesotheliomas frequently become nodular and sometimes can present as large nodules within the lung parenchyma (Fig. 43.14). Mesotheliomas frequently metastasize to lymph nodes, causing their enlargement. Occasionally, metastatic mesothelioma to bronchopulmonary, hilar, and mediastinal lymph nodes produces a hilar mass that can be mistaken for a primary lung cancer (Fig. 43.15).

Approximately 25% to 30% of pleural mesotheliomas invade the parietal and, occasionally, visceral pericardium, and sometimes there is massive involvement of the heart

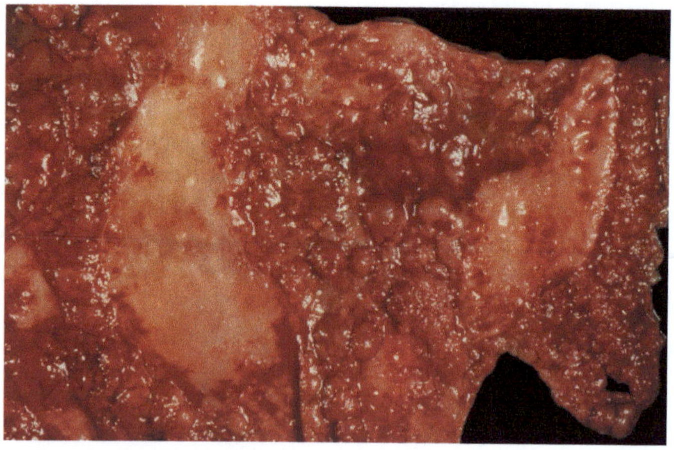

FIGURE 43.12. The parietal pleura is studded by <1- to 5-mm tumor nodules of mesothelioma. The pleura is also involved by larger hyaline pleural plaque characteristic of plaque caused by asbestos.

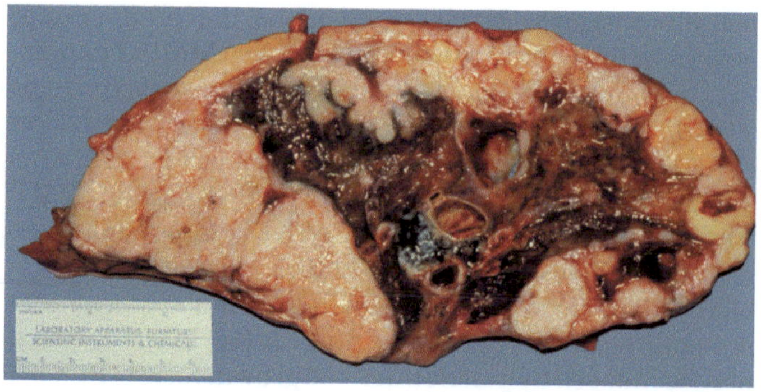

FIGURE 43.14. Pleural mesotheliomas frequently invade lung parenchyma and chest wall. Note also the nodular growth pattern, which is typical of most mesotheliomas.

with replacement of a sizable portion of the myocardium by tumor (Fig. 43.16). Rarely secondary tumor encasement of the heart is so thick as to simulate a primary pericardial mesothelioma. In this situation it may be difficult to determine whether a tumor showing both pleural and pericardial involvement is a primary pericardial mesothelioma or a primary pleural mesothelioma (Fig. 43.16).

Some epithelial mesotheliomas produce excess amounts of hyaluronic acid that can result in cyst formation within the tumor (Fig. 43.17). Occasionally, such tumors will invade the lung to the point that one cannot recognize normal pulmonary parenchyma. Outward growth into the mediastinal fat with metastasis to mediastinal lymph nodes is characteristic (Fig. 43.15).

The most common site of intrathoracic metastasis of pleural mesothelioma is to bronchopulmonary, hilar, and mediastinal lymph nodes. The next most common metastatic site is the contralateral pleural surface. Sometimes, mesotheliomas metastasize outside the chest cavity, such as to the adrenal gland. On the other hand, peritoneal mesotheliomas may metastasize to the pleural surfaces, producing a relatively thin, whitish film that encases the lung (Fig. 43.18).

Because most mesotheliomas are caused by asbestos, it is common to see mesotheliomas in association with hyaline pleural plaques that involve the lateral and diaphragmatic parietal pleura (Fig. 43.12). Mesotheliomas can directly invade or encase the plaque.

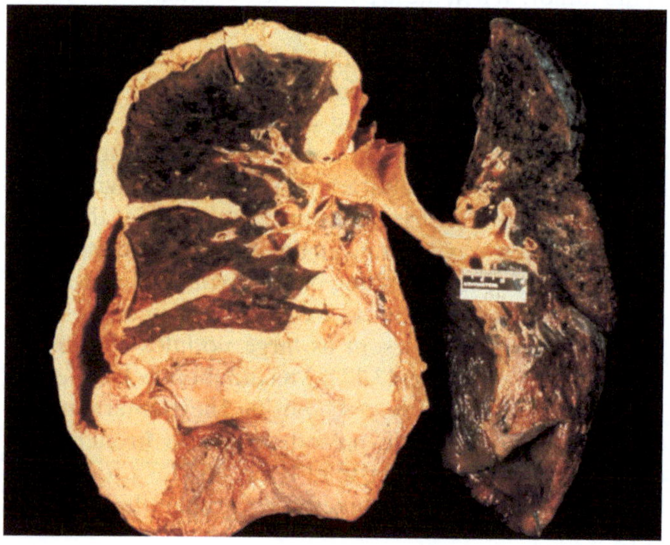

FIGURE 43.13. Right pleural mesothelioma showing encasement of lung by rind of tumor, which, like most mesotheliomas, is thicker at the base (diaphragmatic surface) than at the apex.

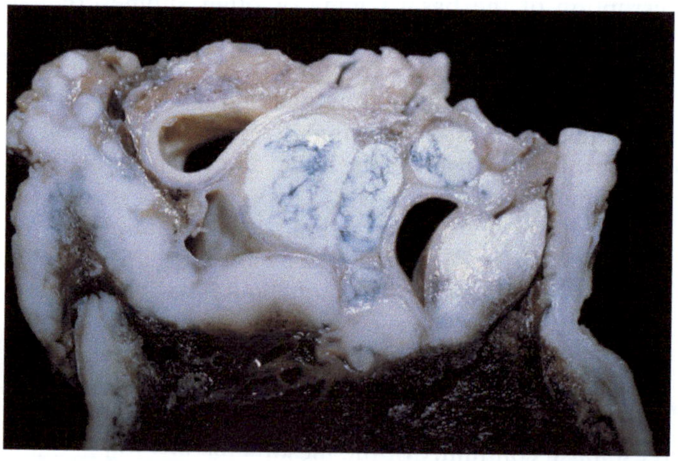

FIGURE 43.15. Pleural mesotheliomas not infrequently metastasize to hilar, bronchopulmonary, and mediastinal lymph nodes producing what is seen radiographically as a hilar mass.

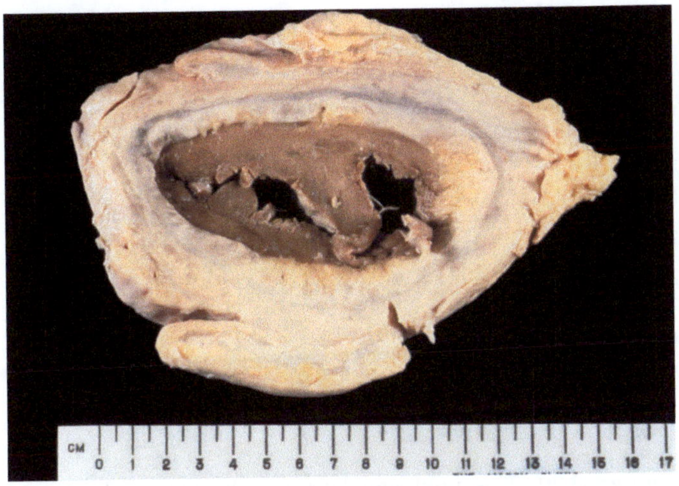

FIGURE 43.16. Pleural mesotheliomas may directly invade the pericardium and myocardium and may replace a significant portion of the myocardium. In some instances, it is difficult to tell if the pericardial involvement is an invasion or metastasis of a pleural mesothelioma or a primary pericardial mesothelioma.

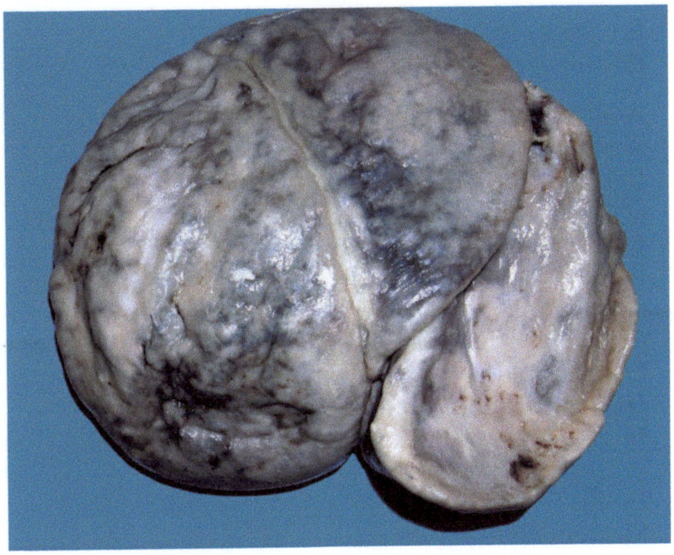

FIGURE 43.18. The lungs are coated by a thin rind of grayish-white tissue that represents a metastasis from a peritoneal mesothelioma.

Histologic Features and Classification of Pleural Mesothelioma

Mesotheliomas show a wide variety of histologic patterns and can resemble many other types of malignant neoplasms.[38,495–503] The application of immunohistochemistry and electron microscopy to percutaneous and open pleural biopsy-obtained tumor specimens or neoplastic cells in pleural fluid is often necessary to render a diagnosis of mesothelioma versus some other type of neoplasm.

The simplest histologic classification of mesothelioma encompasses three general categories: epithelial (epithelioid) mesothelioma, sarcomatoid (fibrous, sarcomatous) mesothelioma, and biphasic (mixed epithelial-sarcomatoid) mesothelioma. Desmoplastic mesothelioma, a form of sarcomatoid mesothelioma, is sometimes put into a separate subtype because it has such a unique morphology. A more detailed, expanded classification includes epithelial mesothelioma, sarcomatoid mesothelioma, biphasic mesothelioma, transitional mesothelioma, and pleomorphic mesothelioma. Within each of these categories, especially that of epithelial mesothelioma, there are additional histologic variants. Some of the more recognizable variants are listed in Box 43.8 and are discussed separately below.

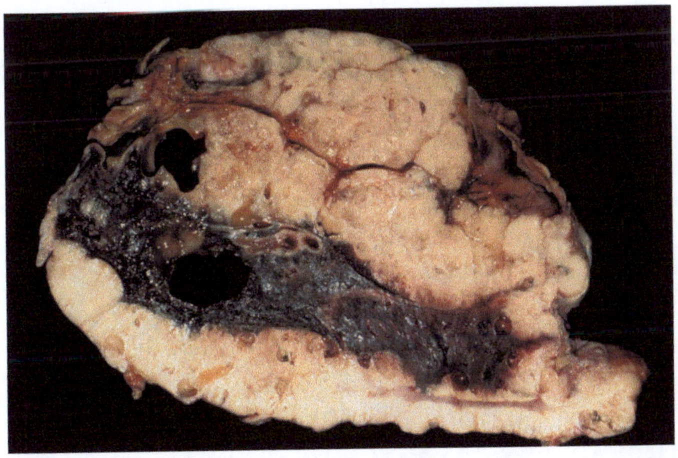

FIGURE 43.17. Some epithelial mesotheliomas produce excess amounts of hyaluronic acid/proteoglycan, producing cysts filled with this material.

Epithelial Mesothelioma

Epithelial mesotheliomas are the most frequently diagnosed histologic type of mesothelioma and show a wide variation in histologic patterns (Box 43.8). It is not uncommon to see more than one histologic pattern (subtype) of epithelial mesothelioma in any given mesothelioma. The more tissue one has to evaluate, the more likely one will see additional subtypes or a biphasic pattern.

The tubulopapillary pattern is the most common epithelial subtype, being composed of relatively uniform cuboidal to rectangular cells with centrally located round nuclei that form distinct papillary structures containing a fibrovascular core or small tubular structures when cut in cross section (Figs. 43.19 and 43.20). They may be associated with psammomatous calcification (Fig. 43.20), which is a nonspecific histologic feature and can be seen in any papillary neoplasm. Occasionally, individual tubulopapillary epithelial mesotheliomas are composed of large,

Box 43.8. Epithelial Mesothelioma (Histologic Subtypes)

- Adenoid cystic
- Adenomatoid
- Bakery roll
- Clear cell
- Deciduoid
- Diffuse—not otherwise specified
- Gaucher-like
- Glandular/acinar
- Glomeruloid
- Histiocytoid/epithelioid
- In association with excess amounts of hyaluronic acid or proteoglycan
- In situ
- Macrocystic
- Microcystic
- Mucin positive
- Placentoid
- Pleomorphic
- Poorly differentiated
- Rhabdoid
- Signet ring
- Single file
- Small cell
- Tubulopapillary
- Well-differentiated papillary

more pleomorphic, cells with large nuclei and prominent nucleoli (Fig. 43.21).

Epithelial mesotheliomas may form predominantly glandular/acinar structures that vary in size and shape and be histologically identical to adenocarcinomas

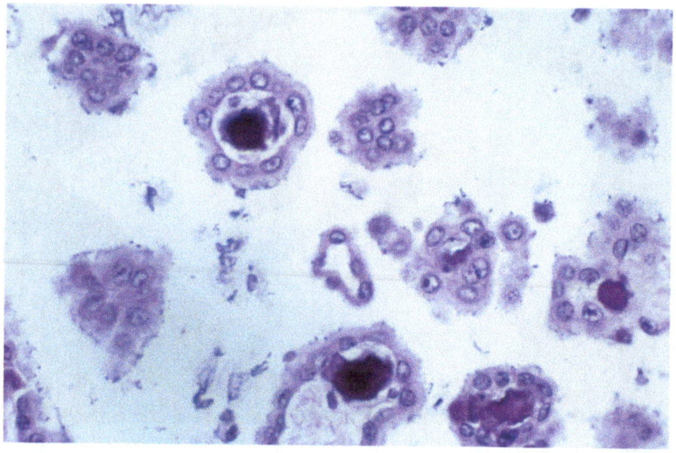

FIGURE 43.20. This tubulopapillary epithelial mesothelioma was associated with numerous psammoma bodies.

(Fig. 43.22). Sometimes the glandular/acinar epithelial mesotheliomas are composed of large columnar cells and resemble mucus-producing adenocarcinomas (Fig. 43.23).

Mesotheliomas are not infrequently composed of round histiocytoid cells that vary in size. The smaller-sized cells have an epithelioid/histiocytoid morphology resembling alveolar macrophages (Fig. 43.24). These cells have round nuclei and often large nucleoli and have abundant glassy eosinophilic cytoplasm on hematoxylin and eosin (H&E)–stained sections (Fig. 43.25). They not infrequently show periodic acid-Schiff (PAS)-positive staining that is sensitive to diastase, indicating glycogen in the cytoplasm of these cells. As we have reported,[304] round cell mesothelioma encompasses a spectrum based on cell size, the large-cell end of which is referred to as a *deciduoid mesothelioma*. Deciduoid mesotheliomas are com-

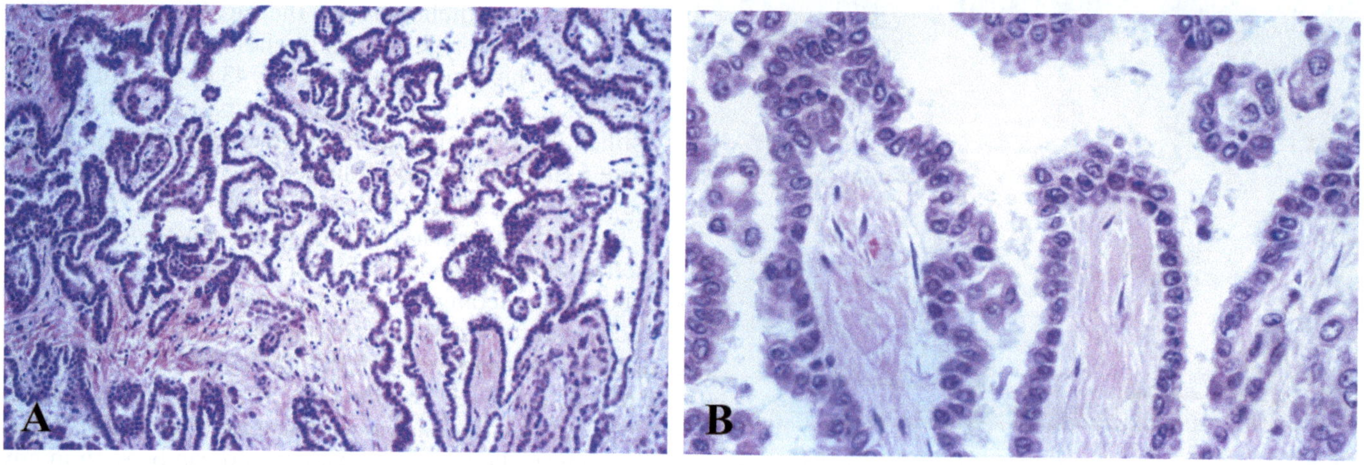

FIGURE 43.19. **(A)** This epithelial mesothelioma shows a tubulopapillary pattern. **(B)** Greater magnification showing fibrovascular cores that are covered by fairly uniform cuboidal epithelial cells.

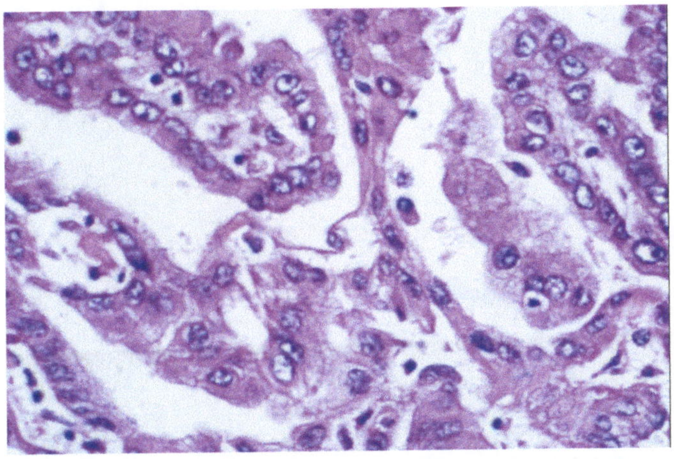

FIGURE 43.21. Some tubulopapillary epithelial mesotheliomas are composed of large cells with large nuclei and prominent nucleoli.

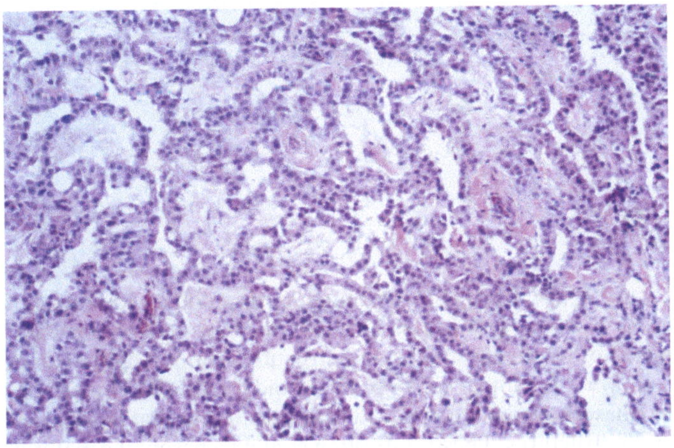

FIGURE 43.22. This epithelial mesothelioma shows a complex glandular (acinar) structure, resembling an adenocarcinoma.

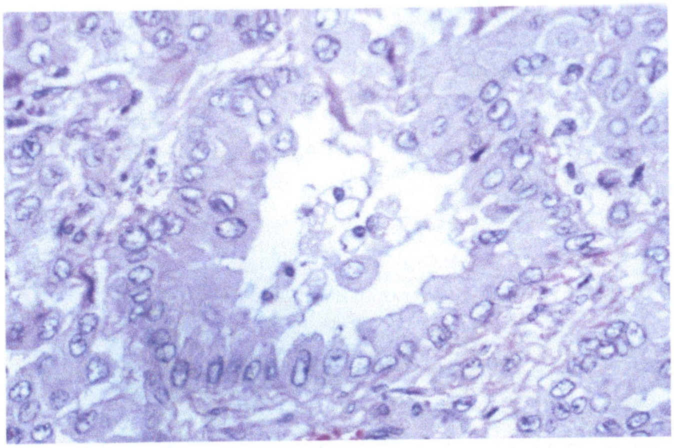

FIGURE 43.23. This epithelial mesothelioma is composed of tall cells suggestive of mucus production.

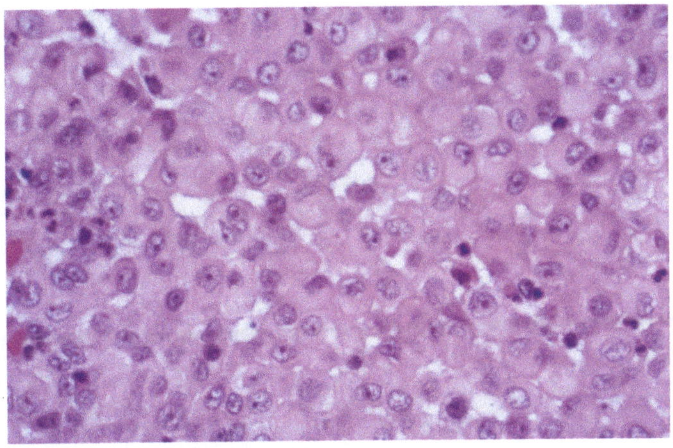

FIGURE 43.24. Diffuse sheets of uniform round tumor cells resemble histiocytes.

posed of cells that resemble progestationally stimulated endometrial stromal cells or cells seen in placental tissue (i.e., deciduoid cells). Occasionally, round cell mesotheliomas exhibit a rhabdoid morphology with the nucleus of the cell toward the cell membrane with intracytoplasmic eosinophilic inclusions that represent intermediate filaments (Fig. 43.26).

Not infrequently, epithelial mesotheliomas are composed of cystic structures ranging from an adenoid cystic morphology (Fig. 43.27) to cells organized as microcystic or macrocystic structures. The microcystic morphology appears as small cysts usually formed by somewhat attenuated squamoid-appearing cells (Fig. 43.28A). The same type of cell also forms the larger macrocystic structures (Fig. 43.28B). Some mesotheliomas are formed by cells that contain intracytoplasmic vacuoles that may impart a signet ring morphology (Fig. 43.29).

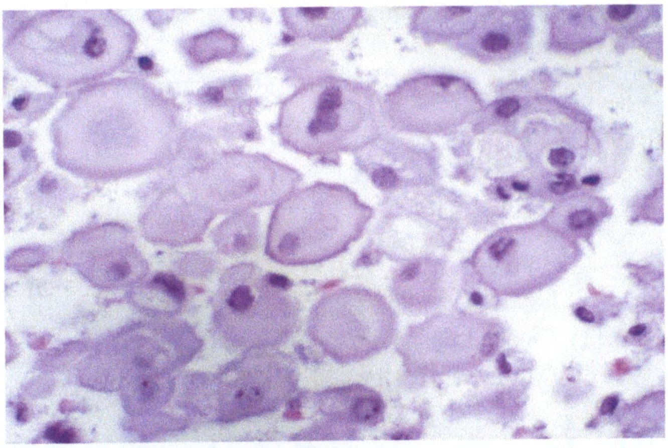

FIGURE 43.25. This mesothelioma is composed of large round cells with mostly centrally located nuclei and abundant, glossy eosinophilic cytoplasm. This is referred to as a *deciduoid mesothelioma* because of its resemblance to decidualized endometrial stromal cells.

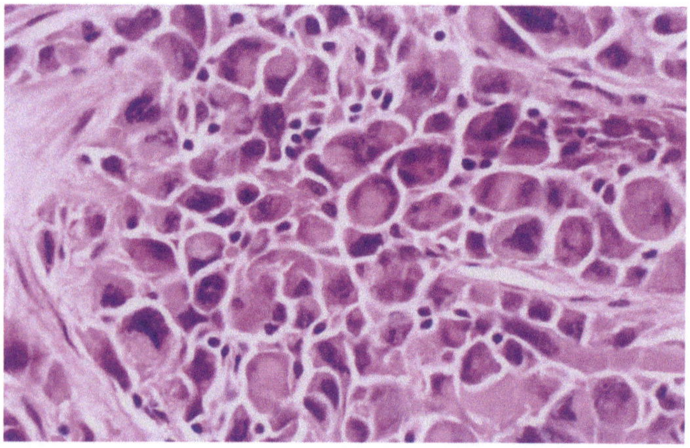

Figure 43.26. Some round cell mesotheliomas are composed of cells exhibiting a rhabdoid morphology with nuclei at the edge of the cell in association with nodular-appearing eosinophilic cytoplasm.

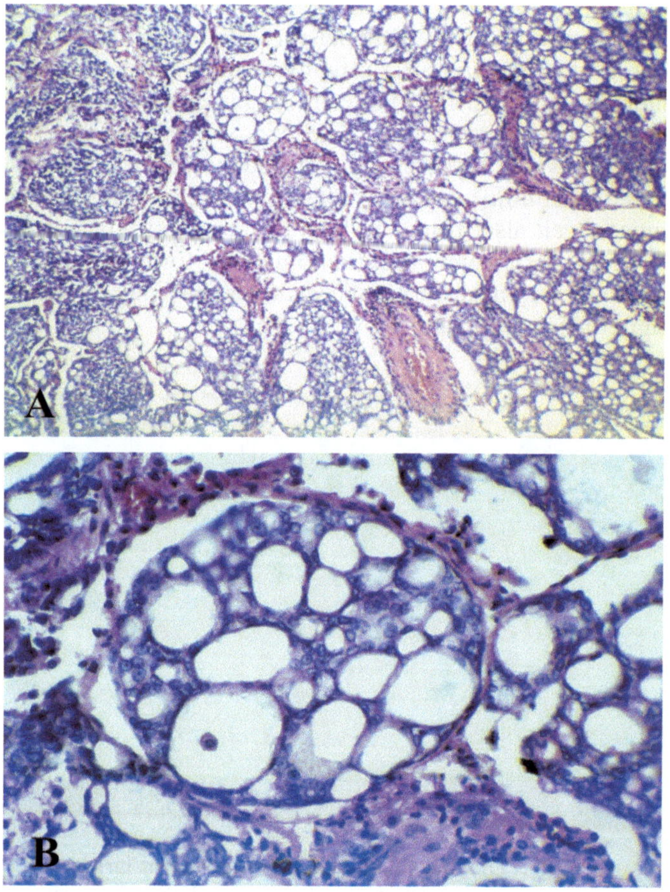

Figure 43.27. **(A,B)** Some epithelial mesotheliomas produce an adenoid-cystic pattern resembling adenoid-cystic carcinoma.

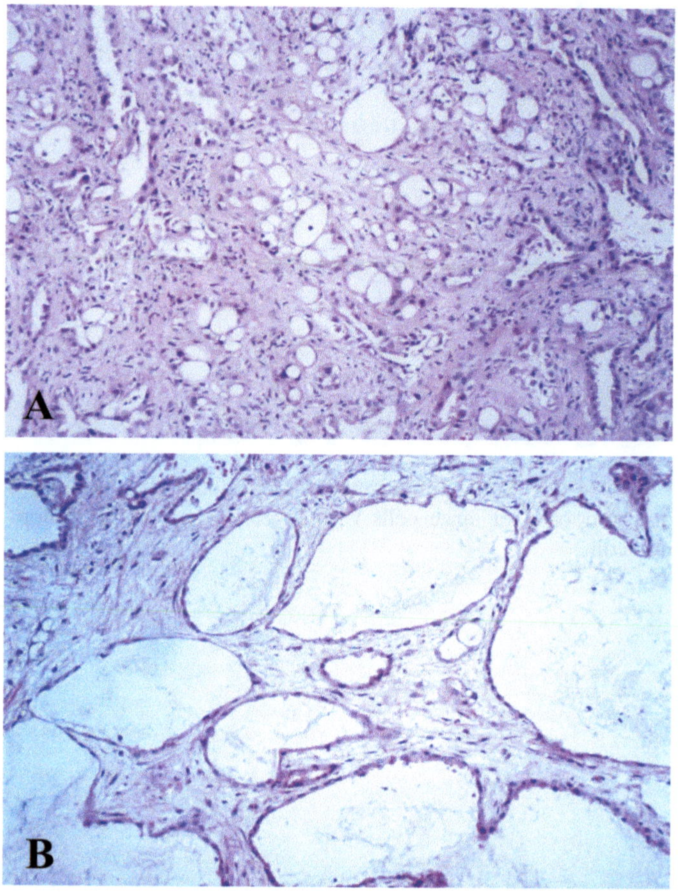

Figure 43.28. Epithelial mesotheliomas exhibit a wide-range of cystic patterns. **(A)** In this example, the mesothelioma is composed of relatively small cystic structures formed by flattened, somewhat squamoid cells and by cuboidal cells. **(B)** This epithelial mesothelioma is composed of flattened cells that form larger cystic structures. These cysts often contain a basophilic material in them that represents hyaluronic acid or proteoglycans.

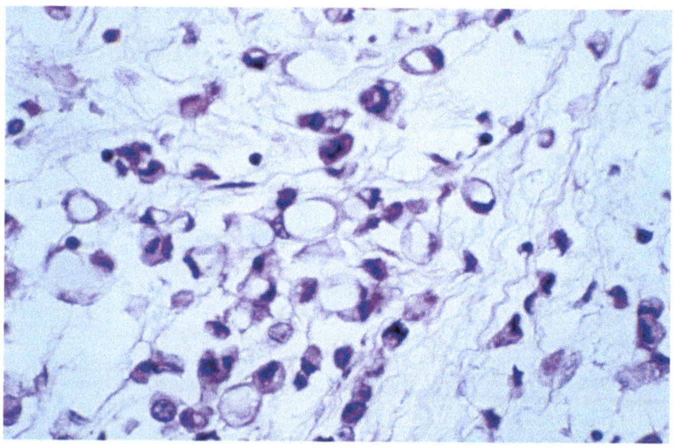

Figure 43.29. Occasional mesotheliomas are formed by cells that contain intracytoplasmic vacuoles. Some cells have a signet-ring morphology.

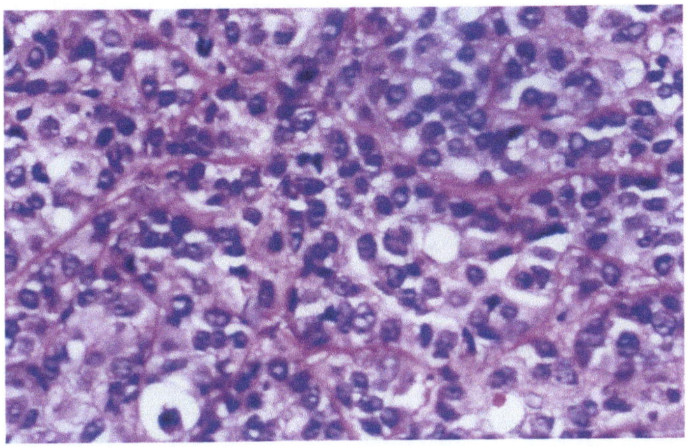

FIGURE 43.30. An uncommon epithelial mesothelioma is composed of small cells that resemble cells of neuroendocrine carcinomas.

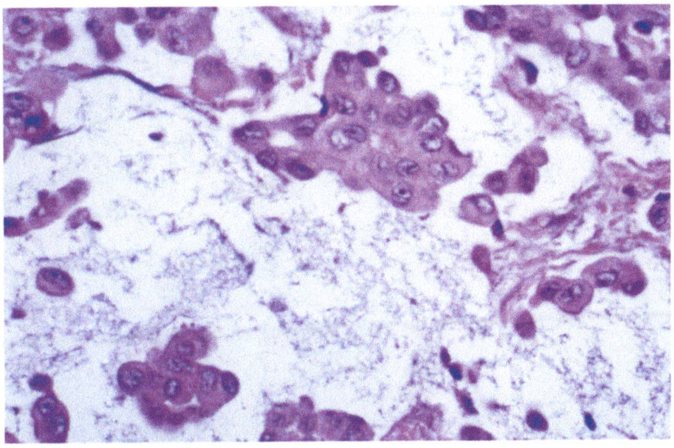

FIGURE 43.32. This epithelial mesothelioma produced large excess amounts of hyaluronic acid/proteoglycan that separates the neoplastic cells. Granular gray material surrounds the tumor cells.

An uncommon type of epithelial mesothelioma referred to as a small cell mesothelioma closely resembles small cell neuroendocrine lung cancers. These mesotheliomas are usually arranged in diffuse solid sheets of small cells (Fig. 43.30) and are discussed in detail below (see Rare/Unusual Mesotheliomas or Mesothelial Proliferations). A probable subtype of small cell mesothelioma is what we describe as glomeruloid mesothelioma, in which the small cells are arranged into structures that resemble renal glomeruli (Fig. 43.31).

Approximately 10% to 20% of epithelial mesotheliomas produce excess amounts of hyaluronic acid or proteoglycan (Figs. 43.32 and 43.33) that can be identified with an Alcian blue or colloidal iron stain. Pretreatment of the tissue sections with hyaluronidase usually decreases the intensity of, but often does not completely eliminate, the colloidal iron and Alcian blue staining (Fig. 43.33). Hyaluronic acid frequently crystallizes, which is best seen ultrastructurally (see Ultrastructural Features of Mesotheliomas, below). Histologically, this material is grayish-blue and sometimes forms distinct crystalloid structures (Fig. 43.34).

In contrast to epithelial mesotheliomas that produce hyaluronic acid and proteoglycan, pulmonary adenocarcinomas contain intracellular mucosubstances that usually stain with a neutral mucosubstance stain such as PAS-diastase stain or with a slightly acidic mucosubstance stain such as Mayer's mucicarmine. We found that pulmonary adenocarcinomas that stain positive with PAS-diastase and mucicarmine also stain intensely positive with an Alcian blue or colloidal iron stain.[505]

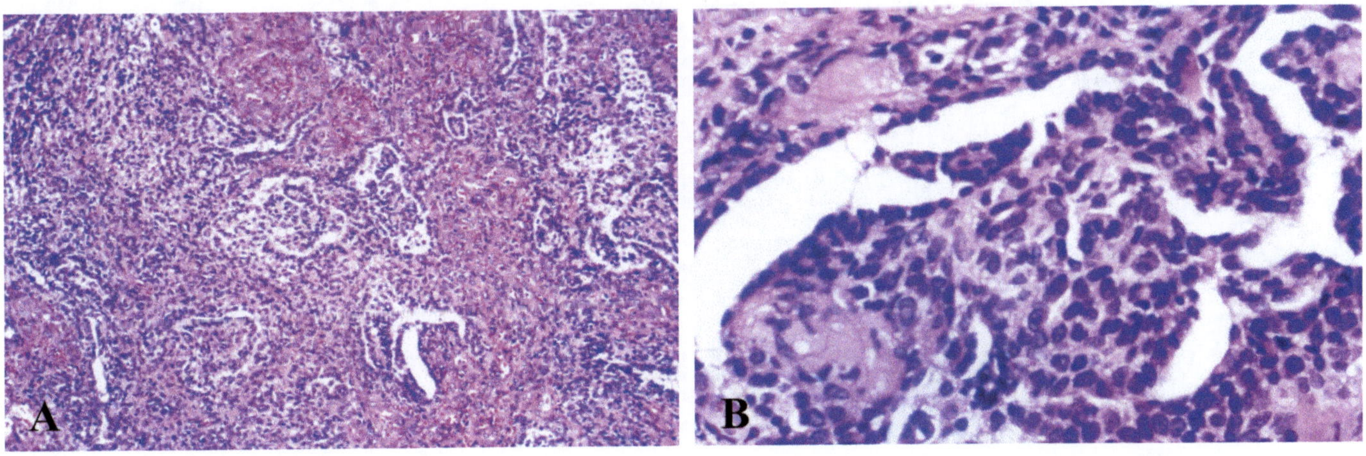

FIGURE 43.31. **(A,B)** A variant of small cell mesothelioma is composed of small cells that produce structures that resemble glomeruli.

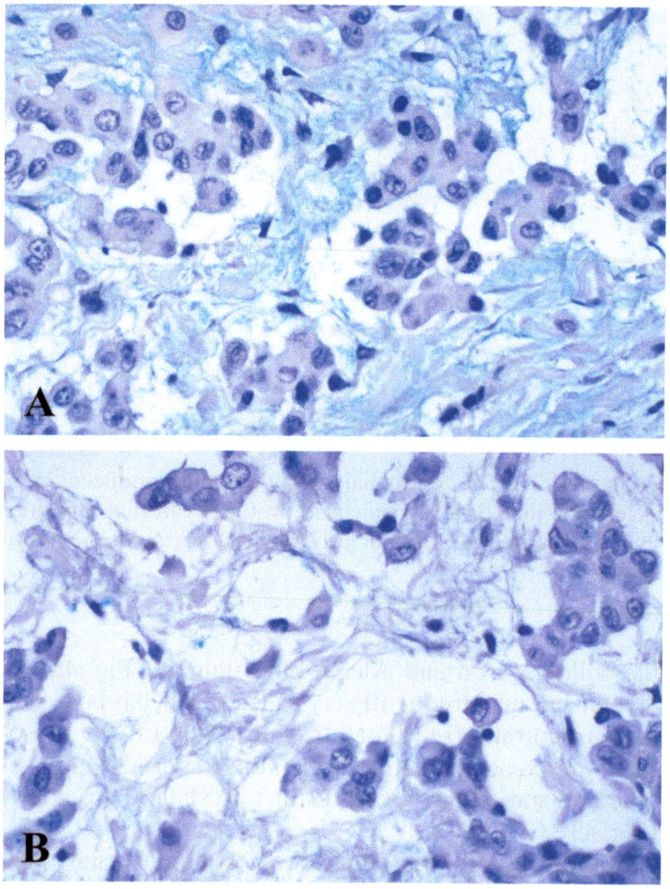

FIGURE 43.33. **(A)** Alcian blue–stained section shows intense bluish staining of the hyaluronic acid/proteoglycan. **(B)** When pretreated with hyaluronidase, the Alcian blue staining material is decreased in intensity or totally abolished.

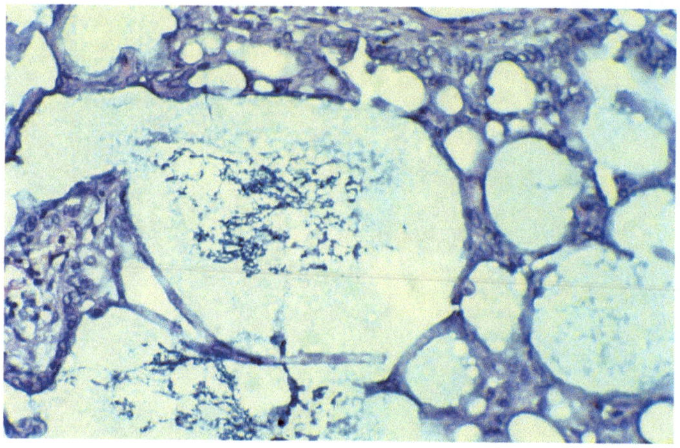

FIGURE 43.34. Crystallized proteoglycan in the cystic structures of an epithelial mesothelioma.

Some mesotheliomas are composed of relatively small, uniform cells that infiltrate in a single file arrangement and resemble lobular breast carcinomas. This type of pattern can be extensive (Fig. 43.35). Rare epithelial mesotheliomas are composed of relatively uniform cells that form concentric rolls (bakery roll pattern) (Fig. 43.36) or resemble chorionic villi (placentoid mesotheliomas) (Fig. 43.37). Rarely focal areas of squamous differentiation (Fig. 43.38) occur, which perhaps is not surprising given that reactive nonneoplastic mesothelial cells show squamous metaplasia. Some epithelial mesotheliomas are composed of cells that have clear cytoplasm (clear cell mesotheliomas) (Fig. 43.39). This clearing is usually caused by glycogen, but has been reported by Ordóñez

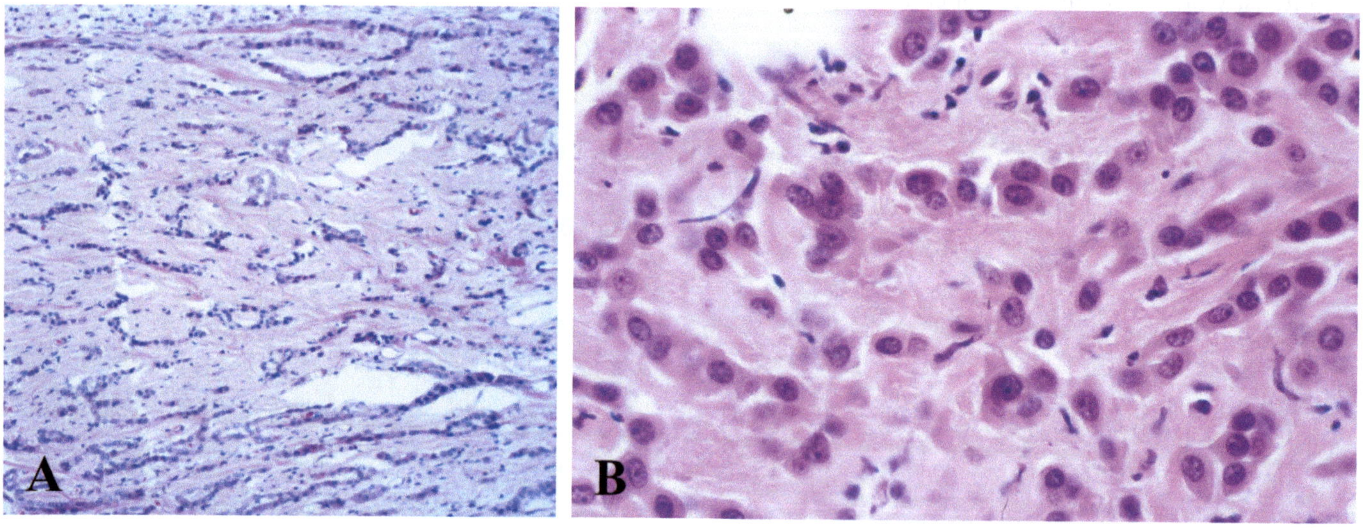

FIGURE 43.35. **(A,B)** Some epithelial mesotheliomas are composed of cells that infiltrate stroma in a single file arrangement reminiscent of infiltrating lobular carcinoma of breast.

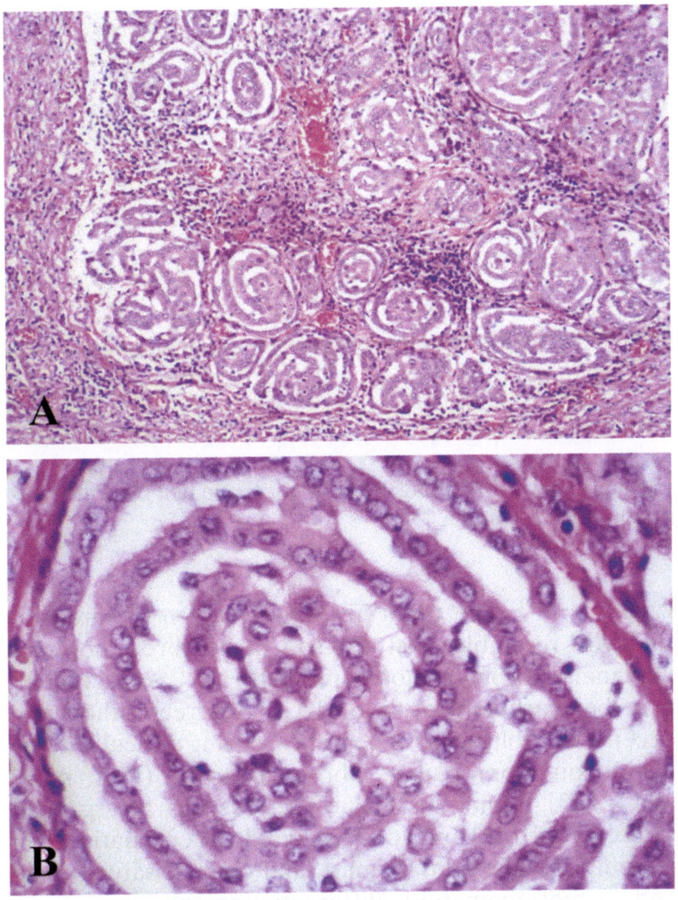

FIGURE 43.36. **(A,B)** Epithelial mesothelioma composed of uniform cells may arrange themselves in a circular pattern resembling a bakery roll.

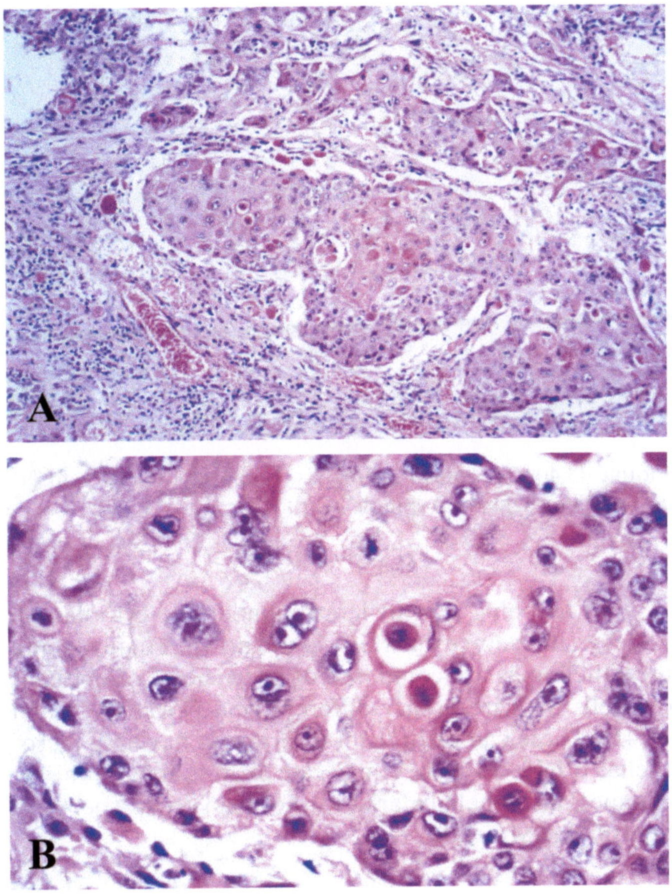

FIGURE 43.38. **(A,B)** This epithelial mesothelioma shows focal squamous differentiation. Finding squamous epithelium does not necessarily indicate metastatic squamous carcinoma.

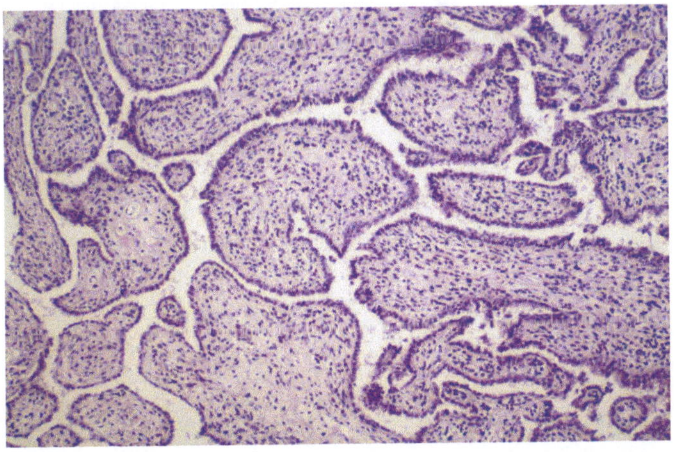

FIGURE 43.37. Occasional epithelial mesotheliomas are composed of cells that form structures that resemble chorionic villi.

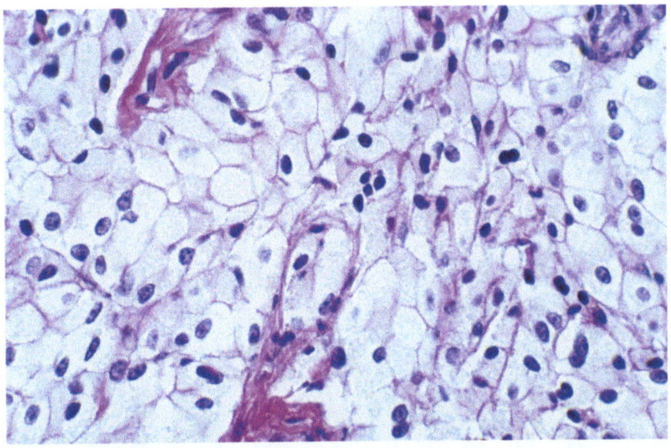

FIGURE 43.39. Some epithelial mesotheliomas are composed of cells that have clear cytoplasm usually due to glycogen accumulation. These may resemble metastatic clear cell carcinoma of the kidney.

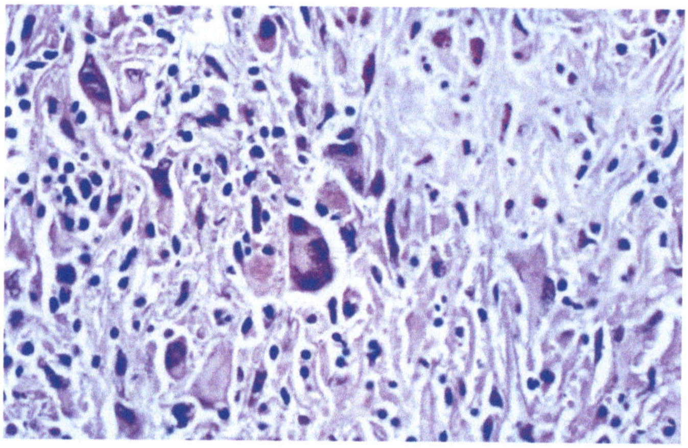

FIGURE 43.40. This mesothelioma is composed of poorly differentiated epithelial and spindle cells.

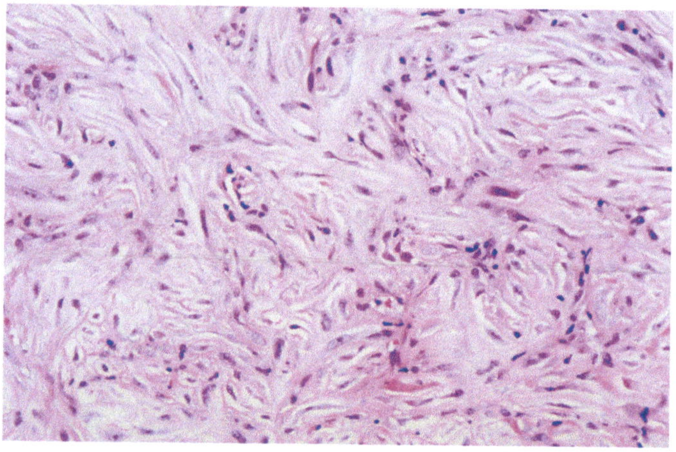

FIGURE 43.42. Fibrocollagenous tumor tissue in a pleural sarcomatoid mesothelioma.

et al.[506] as being due to large numbers of cytoplasmic vesicles, the source of which is unknown. Finally, some mesotheliomas are composed of solid sheets of epithelioid cells that are poorly differentiated (Figs. 43.40 and 43.41). These can be difficult to prove as having a mesothelial origin since they may not express immunohistochemical mesothelial markers other than broad-spectrum keratin and vimentin.

Sarcomatoid Mesothelioma of the Pleura

Pleural sarcomatoid MMs, as defined by either complete absence of epithelial tissue in an adequate biopsy or less than 10% of epithelial tissue,[37] represent about 10% of pleural MMs, within a reported range of about 7% to 22%.[37,211,503,507] The usual histologic pattern of sarcomatoid MM resembles that of a soft tissue fibrosarcoma or malignant fibrous histiocytoma (MFH).[211] Some tumors may be extremely pleomorphic,[503] whereas others are deceptively "bland" in appearance, posing difficulty in the distinction from benign fibrous pleuritis (Figs. 43.42 and 43.43). Other histologic patterns characteristic of sarcomatoid MM include leiomyoid differentiation[508,509] (resembling leiomyosarcoma), and chondrosarcomatoid and osteosarcomatoid differentiation on rare occasions.[38,211,503] Patterns resembling neurogenic sarcoma and rhabdomyosarcoma have also been described,[211] as has a focal hemangiopericytic architecture (which requires distinction from a localized fibrous tumor of the pleura and from a pleural synovial sarcoma; see later discussion). In

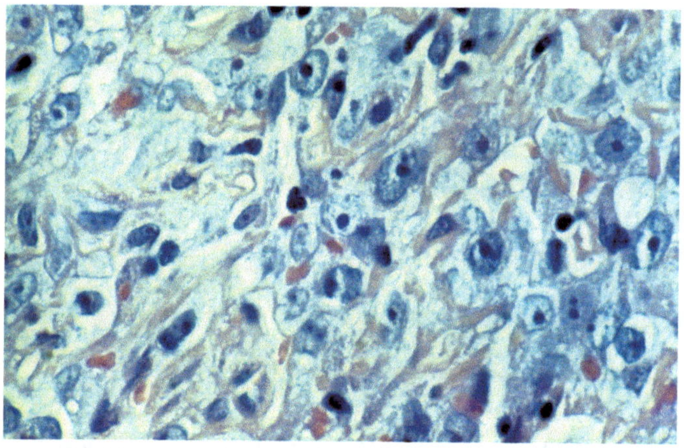

FIGURE 43.41. This mesothelioma is composed of plump, somewhat spindle-shaped cells with large nuclei and prominent nucleoli. (Alcian blue stain.)

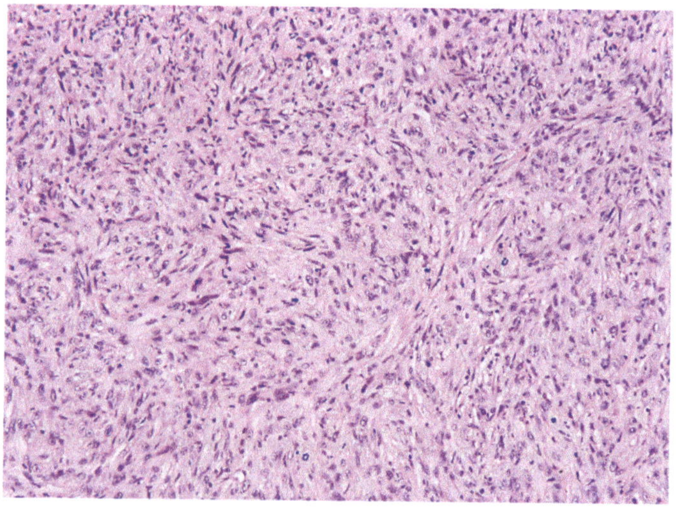

FIGURE 43.43. Pleural sarcomatoid mesothelioma. The neoplastic tissue has a focal storiform architecture and the overall appearances resemble those of malignant fibrous histiocytoma.

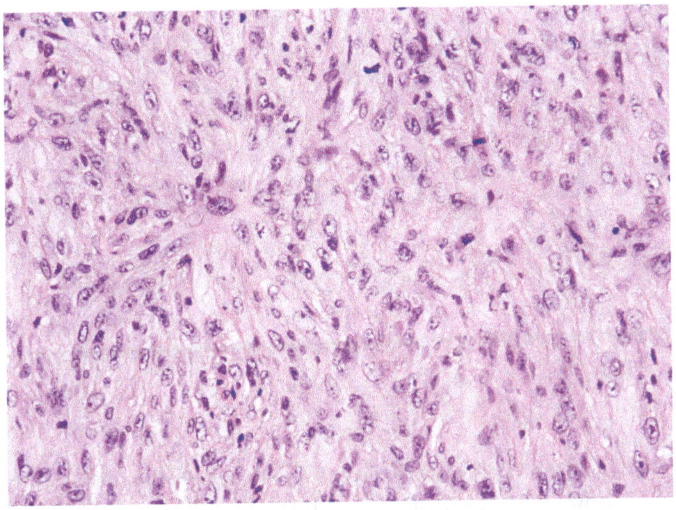

FIGURE 43.44. Pleural sarcomatoid mesothelioma. (Same case as in Fig. 43.43.) The storiform architecture of the tumor is shown at higher magnification. Mitotic figures are also evident.

the Australian Mesothelioma Surveillance Program, an MFH-like appearance was the most common histologic pattern, and cytokeratin expression by the tumor cells was usually detectable (Figs. 43.44 and 43.45).

The immunohistochemical repertoire of sarcomatoid MMs is usually more restricted than epithelial MMs, and immunohistochemistry is less decisive in diagnosis.[507] It is unusual for the positive markers of mesothelial differentiation—useful for the diagnosis of epithelial and biphasic MMs—to be expressed. In this regard, the most valuable and common pattern of antigen expression is that of strong cytokeratin expression (which also aids in the important assessment of invasion),[119,507] but cytokeratin-negative sarcomatoid MMs are well described.[37,211,503,510] Attanoos et al.[511] identified calretinin expression in only 39% of a series of 31 sarcomatoid MMs (usually focal and patchy in distribution in our experience), cytokeratin (CK) 5/6 expression in only 29%, and pan-CK expression in about 75%. Nonetheless, the combination of calretinin and CK expression was highly specific for mesothelioma in their series of 31 cases, and was not found in nonmesothelial sarcomas.

Hinterberger et al.[512] performed a tissue microarray-based analysis for calretinin and podoplanin (D2-40 antigen) expression in 341 MMs (112 epithelioid MMs, 46 sarcomatoid MMs, and 183 biphasic tumors): 91% of the epithelial MMs showed calretinin expression, as opposed to 57% of sarcomatoid tumor areas; for D2-40, the figures were 66% and 30%, respectively. The combination of calretinin and D2-40 increased the sensitivity in epithelioid areas to 0.96, and to 0.66 in sarcomatoid areas.[512]

We encounter numerous referred cases of sarcomatoid mesotheliomas where the diagnosis has been considered doubtful because of failure to demonstrate expression of calretinin, CK5/6 or with Hector Battifora Mesothelial Epitope (HBME-1), whereas this is far from unusual with sarcomatoid MMs. It is also worth emphasizing that CK expression in some sarcomatoid mesotheliomas is patchy in distribution, with areas of intense CK expression interrupted by extensive regions where CK expression is undetectable. The confidence index for a diagnosis of sarcomatoid MM is roughly proportional to the size of the biopsy and is least when the biopsy is small (for example, a core biopsy).

It is also worth emphasizing that considerable and sometimes high-grade cytologic atypia can be found superficially in some cases of benign fibrous pleuritis, presumably representing reactive atypical myofibroblasts. In some cases this pattern of atypia poses considerable diagnostic difficulties, but in our experience such cytologic atypia restricted to the superficial (subsurface) zone of pleural fibrous lesions is of little or no significance for a diagnosis of MM.[503,513] On the other hand, in our experience the most cellular and atypical areas of sarcomatoid MMs are usually found at the deep advancing margin of the tumor, as opposed to the superficial zone (in other words, a reversal of the zonal pattern found in benign fibroinflammatory disorders of the pleura).[503]

In our experience, the following criteria, not all of which need be encountered in any one case, are useful for the diagnosis of sarcomatoid mesothelioma:

- A confluent growth pattern of the tumor along the pleura, whether the lesion shows CK expression or not, although localized sarcomatoid MMs do occur. In limited biopsy specimens the anatomic distribution and

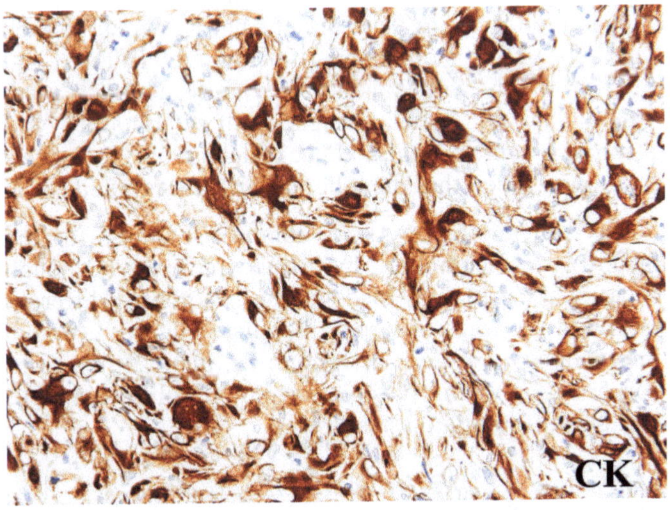

FIGURE 43.45. Pleural sarcomatoid mesothelioma. (Same case as in Figs. 43.43 and 43.44. Strong expression of low molecular weight cytokeratins (CK) by the fibroblastoid tumor cells.

localization of the lesion may not be readily apparent. In this circumstance, the findings on radiologic investigation, including computed tomography (CT) scans, can substitute as a useful surrogate for gross assessment.

- Sarcomas of extraserosal soft tissue or bone, sarcomatoid renal cell carcinoma, and amelanotic spindle cell melanoma should be excluded on clinical grounds, including organ imaging studies such as ultrasound or CT scans, or (importantly) from consideration of the past medical history of the patient in question.
- Cellularity, cytologic atypia and pleomorphism, and a mitotic index that are excessive for a benign fibrous lesion of the pleura; in other words, tissue that is overtly sarcomatoid in the context of lesions of the pleura, with exclusion of reactive serosal fibrosis (benign fibrous pleuritis), from the histologic appearances of the lesion in question, including the zonal pattern.
- Focal tumor necrosis.
- The presence of invasion[119,503,513]: it is our experience that most sarcomatoid mesotheliomas show an insinuative pattern of invasion into subpleural adipose tissue (and occasionally deeper structures), whereby the spindle-shaped cells insinuate between individual adipocytes, splaying them apart and incorporating them into the advancing margin of the tumor (see discussion of desmoplastic sarcomatoid mesothelioma of the pleura).
- In the case of localized tumors in particular, a malignant solitary fibrous tumor (SFT) requires exclusion, from the gross morphology of the lesion, or by immunohistochemical studies for CKs, CD34, bcl-2, and CD99, but on rare occasions it may be impossible to distinguish between a localized sarcomatoid MM and SFT because of discordant immunohistochemical staining (see later discussion).
- Usually, intense CK expression by the tumor, as revealed by immunostaining using either a pan-CK cocktail such as AE1/AE3 or on staining for low molecular weight CKs, which also aids in the assessment of invasion,[38,119,507,514–516], but a diagnosis of sarcomatoid MM remains tenable in the absence of detectable CK expression, provided that the other criteria are fulfilled.

Electron microscopy is of limited usefulness for the diagnosis of sarcomatoid MM in our experience. Although occasional cases show evidence of mesothelial differentiation in the form of serpentine microvilli, desmosomal intercellular junctions, or tonofibrils, many other cases comprise only fibroblastoid or myofibroblastoid cells without differentiating features.[211]

Heterologous Differentiation in Sarcomatoid Malignant Mesotheliomas

The distinction between pleural sarcomatoid MM with osseous differentiation and osteogenic sarcoma arising in relation to the rib or chest wall soft tissues (extraosseous osteosarcoma) can pose difficulties (Fig. 43.46). Analogous considerations apply to chondroid tumors.

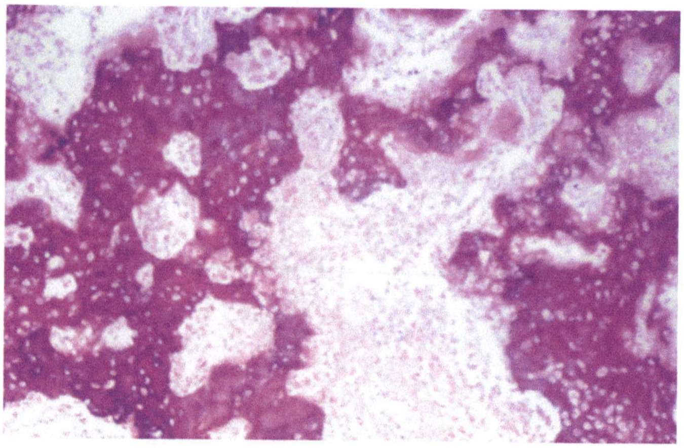

FIGURE 43.46. This mesothelioma showing variable differentiation shows fairly extensive bone formation in the sarcomatoid portion of the mesothelioma.

As mentioned previously, strong expression of CKs by a pleura-based sarcomatoid tumor is a strong indicator of MM. However, CK expression may be depleted in areas of heterologous differentiation, and in this regard the growth pattern of the tumor within the pleura is (again) of considerable value in the differential diagnosis. Confluent pleura-based heterologous sarcomatoid tumors in adults, whether liposarcomatous, chondrosarcomatoid, or osteosarcoma-like,[503] which is radiologically indistinguishable from MM, in our opinion should be designated as pleural MMs, whereas heterologous sarcomatoid tumors arising in relation to chest wall tissue are characteristically localized, without confluence along the pleura itself.

On the other hand, given the distinctive status of epithelioid hemangioendothelioma of the pleura (see later discussion) and pleural angiosarcoma of conventional type,[517] we would not designate those latter two tumors as MMs, because (1) unlike mesotheliomas, angiosarcomas affect the pericardium predominantly, although an origin from other serosal membranes is recorded; (2) serosal involvement as part of an angiosarcoma may constitute part of angiosarcoma of the heart with intramyocardial or intracavitary components, or a multifocal angiosarcoma affecting multiple sites such as the skin, deep soft tissues, liver, and spleen; and (3) so far as we are aware, conventional (nonepithelioid and vasoformative) endothelial differentiation is not part of the documented histologic repertoire of a biphasic or sarcomatoid mesothelioma. (In this context, it is worth recalling that some authors[518,519] use the term *angiosarcoma* interchangeably with *epithelioid hemangioendothelioma* for epithelioid endothelial sarcomas of the pleura.)

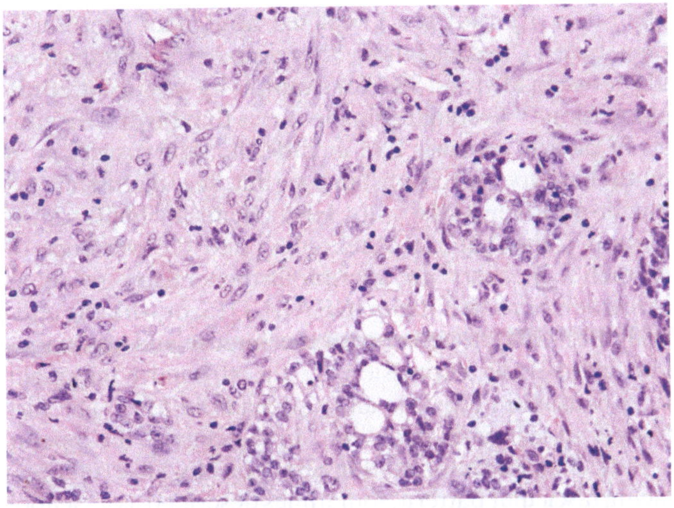

FIGURE 43.47. Biphasic pleural malignant mesothelioma. The epithelial component is represented by circumscribed aggregates of epithelioid cells with rudimentary tubuloacinar structures, seen in the right half of the field illustrated. The spindle-cell stromal tissue shows about the minimal cellularity and atypia required for designation of the stromal component as sarcomatoid (as opposed to a cellular reactive stroma in an epithelial mesothelioma). Note the pleomorphism of some of the stromal cells in the upper left and lower left areas of this field. Compare with Figs. 43.42 to 43.44 in the sarcomatoid section.

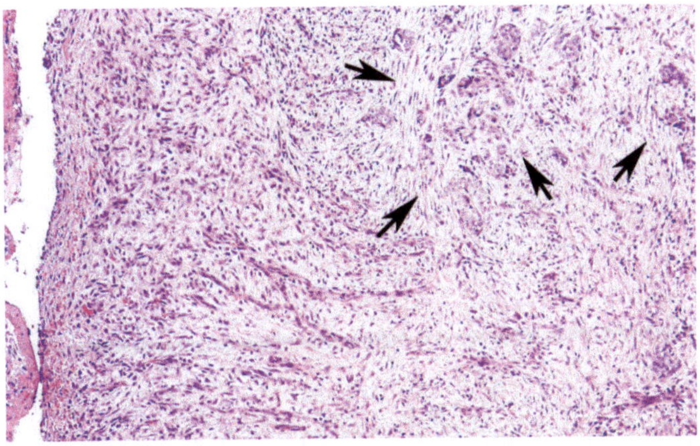

FIGURE 43.48. As opposed to a stromal sarcomatoid component required for diagnosis of a biphasic mesothelioma, this figure depicts an invasive epithelial mesothelioma, with small rounded aggregates of epithelial cells (arrows), surrounded by a prominent reactive stroma. The reactive character of the stroma is indicated by the small parallel blood vessels, orientated almost perpendicular to the free surface of the pleura, and the greater cellularity in the subsurface zone as opposed to the deeper tissues comprising the reactive stroma (a "top heavy" zonal architecture characteristic of a pleural inflammatory process).

Biphasic Malignant Mesothelioma

A mixed (biphasic) epithelial and mesenchymal architecture is perhaps the most distinctive histologic picture encountered with MMs[516]: about 30% of MMs[37,211] within a reported range of 24% to 35%,[37,211,503] But it is worth emphasizing that a mixed histologic pattern can also be encountered, with nonmesothelial tumors affecting the pleural cavities, most notably primary synovial sarcoma of the pleura and secondary spread from a spindle cell carcinoma (carcinosarcoma) of lung, as well as biphasic pulmonary blastoma. Subclassification of MM as biphasic requires that unequivocal epithelial and mesenchymal elements are identifiable, and that each shows malignant features in conventional H&E-stained sections (Fig. 43.47), thereby excluding (1) cellular but not obviously malignant stromal tissue in an epithelial MM (Fig. 43.48); and (2) incorporation of benign alveolar epithelium into a sarcomatoid mesothelioma as it invades into lung parenchyma (staining for thyroid transcription factor-1 [TTF-1] is invaluable in this situation but requires critical evaluation of the histologic distribution of TTF-1–positive epithelial cells, to ensure that a biphasic or sarcomatoid MM is not misdiagnosed as a spindle cell carcinoma of lung).

The appearances of the epithelial component by light microscopy, immunohistochemistry, and electron microscopy are essentially indistinguishable from those of entirely epithelial MMs, and the same considerations apply to the appearances of the sarcomatoid component,[516] which usually resembles either fibrosarcoma or MFH, with heterologous patterns of differentiation on rare occasions (Figs. 43.49 and 43.50). Nonetheless,

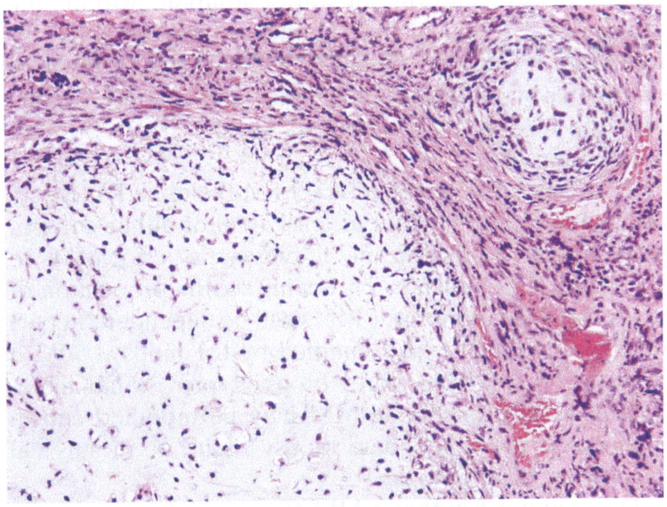

FIGURE 43.49. Heterologous chondroid differentiation in the stromal tissue of a biphasic mesothelioma.

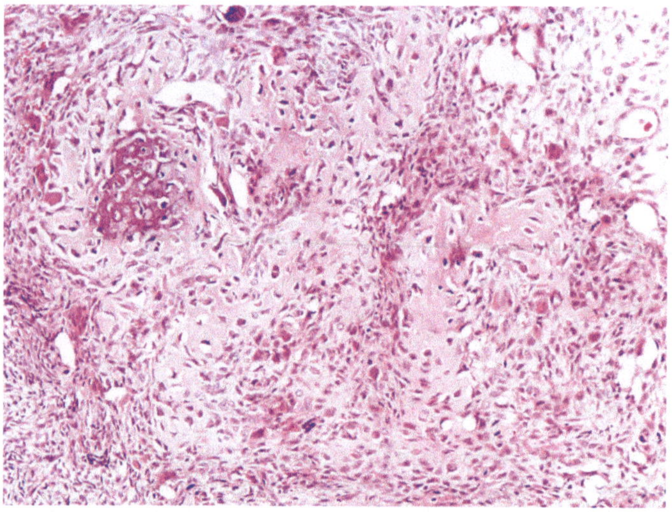

FIGURE 43.50. Heterologous osteoid and bone in the stromal tissue of a biphasic malignant mesothelioma.

the relative proportions of each component in a biphasic MM are highly variable, as are the distribution and the appearances of each component, from one case to another. The tumor may show an intermingling of each of the epithelial and sarcomatoid components, but in other cases and even in different areas of the same tissue sample, the two components may be reasonably discrete (Fig. 43.47), with an abrupt transition from one component to the other.[211,516] As for epithelial and sarcomatoid mesotheliomas, respectively, there may also be considerable histologic variation within each component in a single case, so that tubulopapillary areas and sheets of pleomorphic cells may be encountered within the epithelial component, whereas the sarcomatoid component may vary from cellular and pleomorphic—resembling either fibrosarcoma or MFH—to hypocellular desmoplastic tissue. Heterologous patterns of differentiation within the sarcomatoid tissue include chondroid and osseous differentiation (Figs. 43.49 and 43.50),[211,520] and focal rhabdomyoblastic differentiation was encountered in one biphasic MM in the Australian Mesothelioma Surveillance Program.[211]

At present, the International Mesothelioma Panel recommends arbitrarily that at least 10% of either component should be recognizable in biopsy tissue for MMs to be classified as biphasic. This being so, the proportion of cases classified as biphasic MMs will be dependent in part on the amount of tissue sampled by the biopsy.[516] With limited (for example, core) biopsies, provisional histologic classification of the MM may be modified subsequently by more adequate biopsy tissue or in surgical specimens, or at autopsy.

Distinction of biphasic MM from a biphasic synovial sarcoma (SSa)[521–526] can pose considerable difficulties, especially when the tumor is widely distributed within the pleural cavity (but see Localized Malignant Mesothelioma, below), because there is overlap in the immunoprofile between MM and SSa, for example by way of calretinin expression.[527] Distinguishing features that favor a diagnosis of pleural biphasic SSa include the demonstration of epithelial-type mucosubstances (but see discussion on mucin-positive MMs[505] in Histochemical Features of Pleural Epithelial Mesotheliomas) and the presence of epithelial markers on immunohistochemistry (such as carcinoembryonic antigen [CEA], CD15, or with the antibody Ber-EP4), together with less intense and less extensive cytokeratin expression by the stromal component than is usual in biphasic and sarcomatoid MM. The histologic appearances also differ. In this regard, the bipolar spindle-shaped cells found in SSa typically have an interlacing fascicular pattern, sometimes described as a "school of fish" appearance, in contrast to the fibrosarcomatoid or MFH-like pattern of the stromal component in most biphasic MMs. Synovial sarcoma is also characterized by the t(X;18) translocation,[526,528–531] whereas biphasic mesothelioma is not.

When they spread into the pleura, spindle cell (sarcomatoid) carcinomas of lung (carcinosarcomas)[532] can also pose considerable problems in differential diagnosis, but the radiologic demonstration of an intrapulmonary mass lesion with appearances characteristic of a primary lung cancer can aid considerably in this distinction, together with expression of epithelial-type markers such as CEA, CD15, or Ber-EP4 antigen in the epithelial component of such carcinosarcomas,[532] in the absence of calretinin or CK5/6 expression. Biphasic pulmonary blastomas[533,534] are distinguishable from biphasic MM by their predominantly intrapulmonary localization (although they can spread to the pleura), by their histologic resemblance to fetal lung parenchyma (with an embryonal appearance for the stromal component, which often shows focal chondroid differentiation), and by the resemblance of the epithelial component to endometrial glands (see Figs. 37.18 and 37.19 in Chapter 37). In addition, some pulmonary blastomas show focal expression of CD117.[535]

Transitional Mesothelioma

Transitional mesothelioma refers to a histologic type of mesothelioma that has features transitional between epithelial and sarcomatoid. These were described in 1986.[536] Some mesotheliomas described by Dardick et al.[537] as poorly differentiated mesotheliomas would fit into this category. These mesotheliomas are composed of large, polygonal to plump, occasionally spindle-shaped cells arranged in nests or showing no distinct pattern (Fig. 43.51A,B). These mesotheliomas typically express broad-spectrum keratin (Fig. 43.51C) and vimentin (Fig. 43.51D). These neoplasms usually do not show

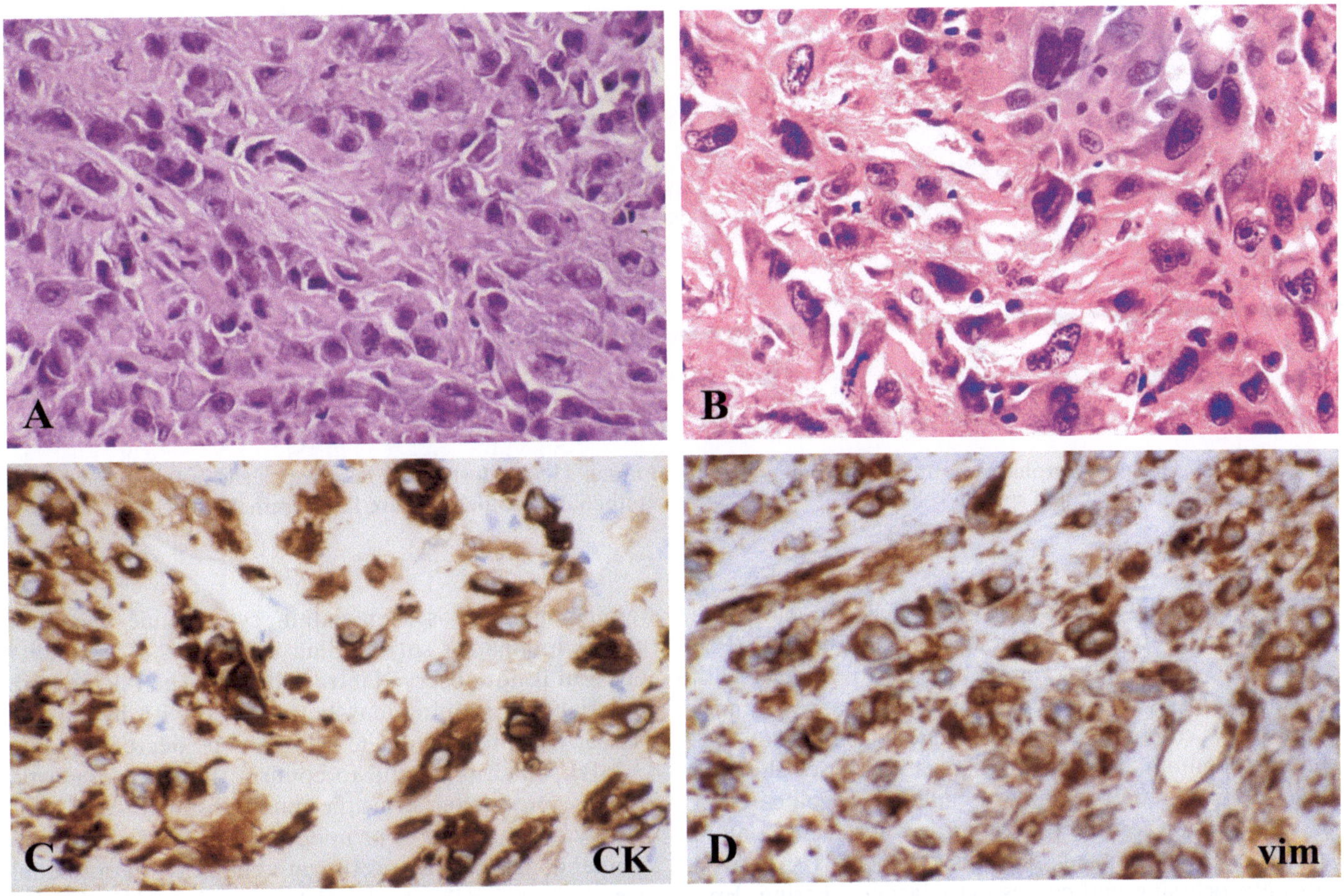

FIGURE 43.51. **(A,B)** Transitional mesotheliomas are composed of epithelioid and spindle cells as seen in these images. **(C)** Transitional mesotheliomas show intense cytoplasmic immunostaining for broad-spectrum (AE1/AE3) keratin. **(D)** As shown in this image, vimentin (vim) is typically expressed in all transitional mesotheliomas.

mesothelial-specific markers and the ultrastructural features are nonspecific.

Pleomorphic Mesothelioma

Pleomorphic mesotheliomas are composed of large, undifferentiated, irregularly shaped cells often having an epithelioid or sarcomatoid morphology. These pleomorphic mesotheliomas (Figs. 43.52 to 43.54) characteristically express broad-spectrum keratin and vimentin, and occasionally other markers of mesothelial differentiation such as CK5/6, calretinin, mesothelin, and epithelial membrane antigen (EMA).

Mesotheliomas Showing Variable Differentiation

In cases where the specimen is large, such as pleural pneumonectomy specimens or autopsy specimens, it is not uncommon to see several different histologic patterns of mesothelial differentiation (Fig. 43.55). This variation can span the entire histologic, immunohistochemical, and ultrastructural expression seen in MM.

Histochemical Features of Pleural Epithelial Mesothelioma

Several standard histochemical tests for the demonstration of carbohydrate/mucopolysaccharide substances are occasionally useful in differentiating epithelial mesotheliomas from other malignant tumors, primarily pulmonary adenocarcinomas and other mucin-producing adenocarcinomas. The two main substances to be considered are mucin and glycogen. *Mucin* is a somewhat vague term and is frequently used synonymously with mucopolysaccharide, glycoprotein, proteoglycan, glycosaminoglycan, mucosubstance, and glycoconjugate. *Glycoconjugate* is the term preferred by some[538]; we prefer *mucosubstance*. The protein portion of a glycoprotein mucosubstance is synthesized in the rough endoplasmic reticulum, and the carbohydrate portion is added in the Golgi apparatus. Mucosubstances can be divided into highly acidic, weakly acidic, or neutral mucosubstances.

Glycogen is observed in the cytoplasm of epithelial mesotheliomas in up to 50% of cases and readily stains

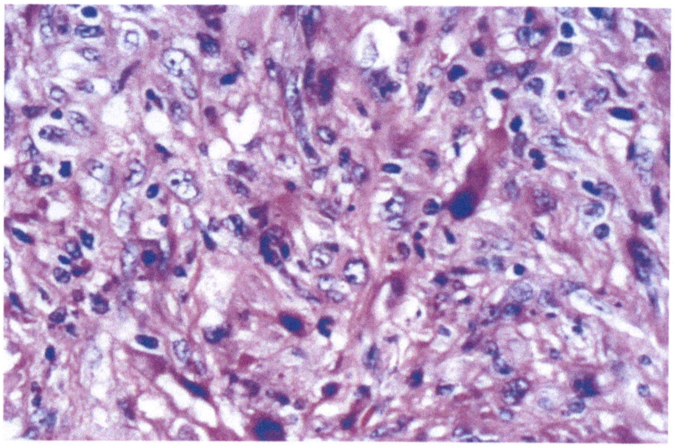

FIGURE 43.52. This pleomorphic mesothelioma is composed of large atypical epithelioid and spindle cells.

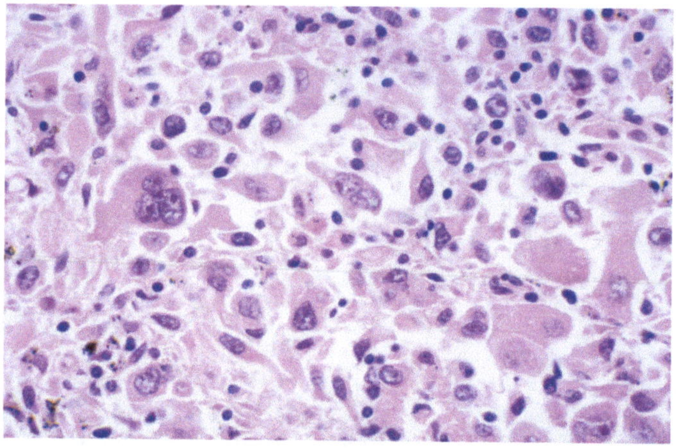

FIGURE 43.54. Most of the neoplastic cells in this pleomorphic epithelial mesothelioma are large epithelioid cells.

with PAS reagent (Fig. 43.56). The glycogen can cause mesotheliomas to have a clear cell morphology (Fig. 43.39) and is usually removed by pretreatment with diastase. This is a nonspecific finding because primary pulmonary carcinomas such as adenocarcinomas frequently contain glycogen, especially those showing degenerative changes. Many so-called clear cell carcinomas of the lung represent neoplasms whose cells contain significant amounts of glycogen, which is removed during processing and causes cytoplasmic clearing. Epithelial mesotheliomas containing significant quantities of glycogen may or may not exhibit a clear cell histologic pattern.

Approximately 20% of epithelial mesotheliomas produce highly acidic mucosubstances, namely, hyaluronic acid and proteoglycan, which can be identified with Alcian blue or colloidal iron stain (Fig. 43.33A). The bluish-staining material is seen within cytoplasmic vacuoles, tubular lumina, or surrounding aggregates of epithelial cells, but is not observed intracellularly. The Alcian blue colloidal iron staining may be removed with hyaluronidase or the intensity of the stain may be decreased (Fig. 43.33B), which is helpful to confirm that the neoplastic cells are producing an acidic mucosubstance consistent with hyaluronic acid or proteoglycan. A note of caution: stromal connective tissue surrounding nests of epithelial mesothelioma cells can be rich in hyaluronic acid and thus misinterpreted as a positive reaction.

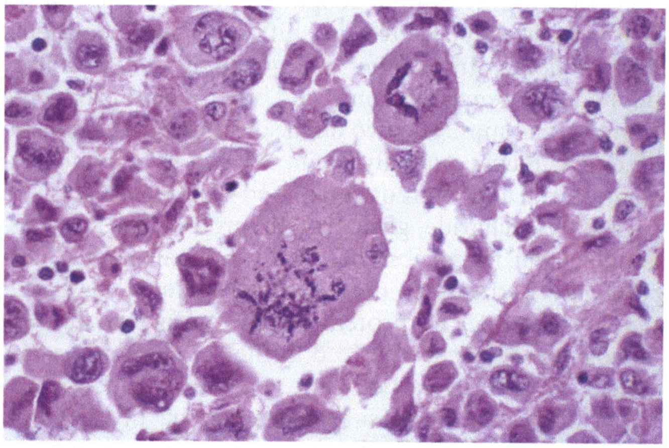

FIGURE 43.53. This epithelioid pleomorphic mesothelioma contains occasional tumor giant cells with abnormal mitoses.

Approximately 65% to 70% of pulmonary adenocarcinomas show intracytoplasmic staining for neutral or weakly acidic mucosubstance that can be identified by PAS-diastase (PAS-D; pretreatment with diastase removes glycogen) or Mayer's mucicarmine. As we reported, most pulmonary adenocarcinomas that show intracytoplasmic staining with PAS-D (Fig. 43.57) or Mayer's mucicarmine (Fig. 43.58) also show Alcian blue/colloidal iron-positive staining at pH 2.5 (Fig. 43.59).[505] The positive-staining glycoprotein material is resistant to pretreatment with hyaluronidase.

Hammar et al.[505] compared the histochemical and immunohistochemical staining reactions of 10 epithelial mesotheliomas (diagnosis documented by ultrastructural examination) that were mucicarmine-positive and compared them with 10 pulmonary adenocarcinomas. The adenocarcinomas were all primary "nodular" lung adenocarcinomas that were mucicarmine-positive. The mucicarmine and PAS-D staining reaction in epithelial mesotheliomas resulted from hyaluronic acid production by these neoplasms. When the tissue sections were pretreated with hyaluronidase, the intensity of staining reactions with mucicarmine and PAS-D usually decreased or disappeared. In some cases, specifically those that showed intracellular droplet-like staining, the staining reaction

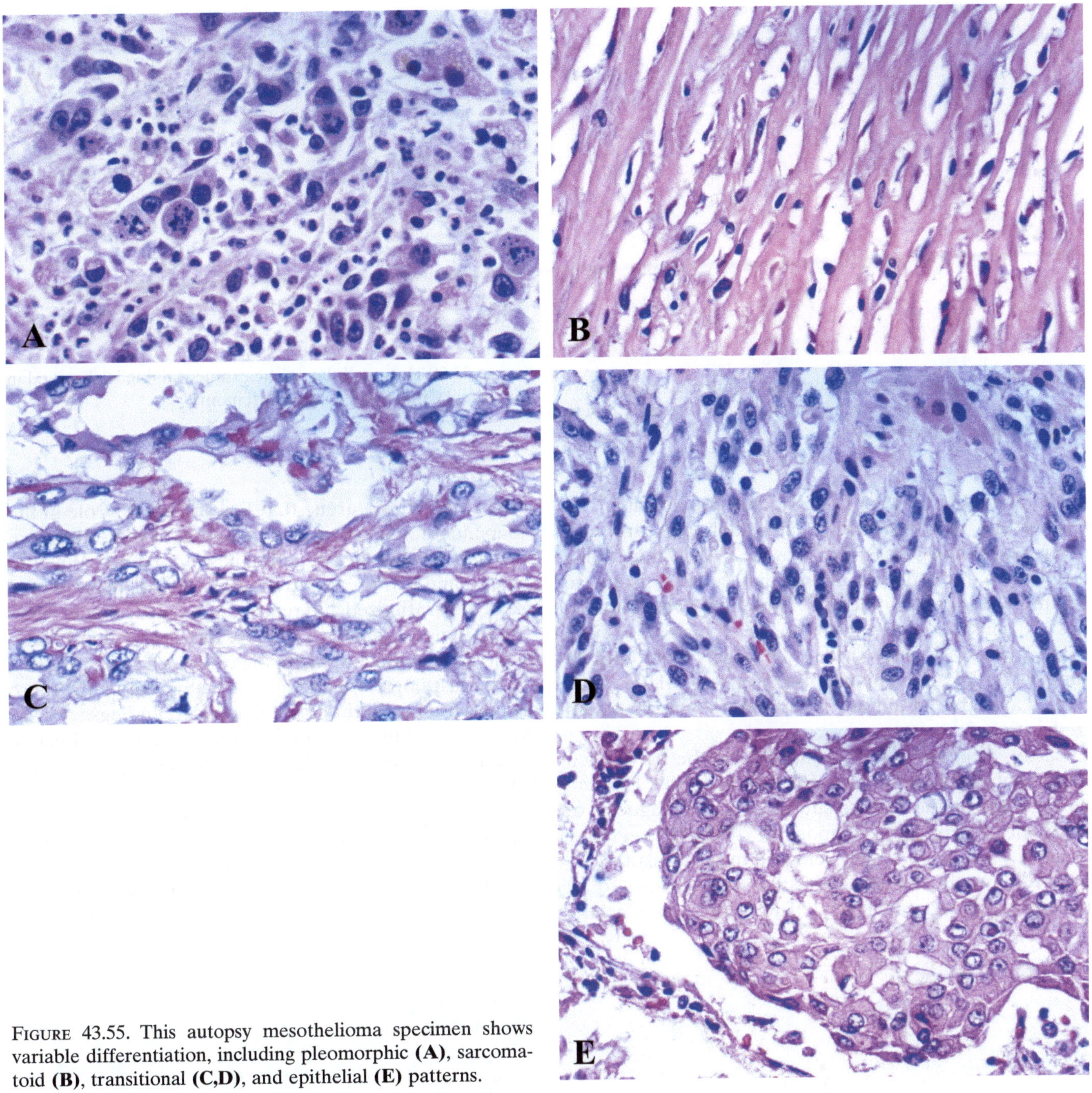

FIGURE 43.55. This autopsy mesothelioma specimen shows variable differentiation, including pleomorphic **(A)**, sarcomatoid **(B)**, transitional **(C,D)**, and epithelial **(E)** patterns.

was not eradicated. All mucin-positive epithelial mesotheliomas we have examined contained crystalloid structures that are described in the section on mucin-positive epithelial mesotheliomas.

Immunohistochemical Features of Pleural Mesothelioma

The cytologic or biopsy diagnosis of MM can be problematic and requires the use of ancillary techniques more frequently than for most other epithelioid tumors and as a routine procedure. As a historical development, supplemental special stains for mucins, including stains for neutral and acidic mucosubstances, notably hyaluronic acid before and after hyaluronidase digestion, have been supplemented in turn, and largely supplanted by, immunohistochemistry.[37] Many adenocarcinomas that commonly spread to the pleura, such as those originating in the breast, may not produce significant amounts of mucin (about 60% to 75% of adenocarcinomas of lung produce

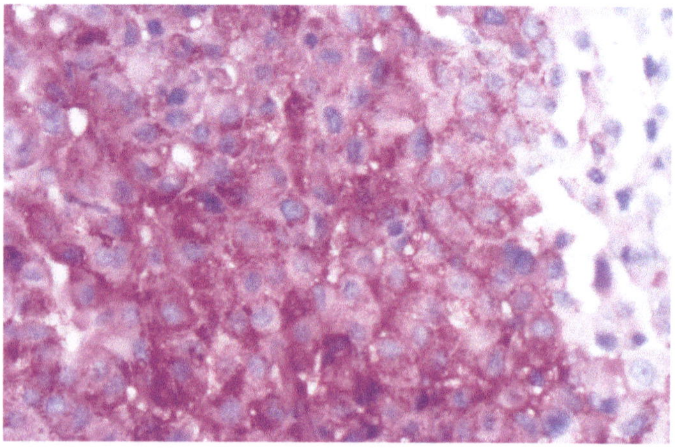

FIGURE 43.56. A significant percentage of epithelial mesotheliomas contain cytoplasmic glycogen that can be shown by a periodic acid-Schiff (PAS) stain.

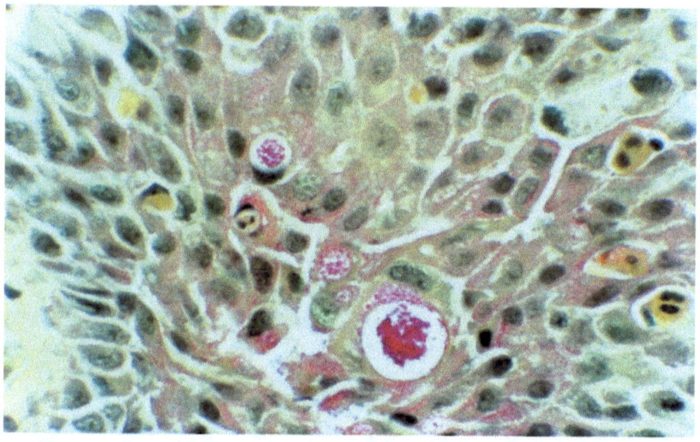

FIGURE 43.58. Intracellular mucicarmine staining is observed in this primary pulmonary adenocarcinoma.

mucin stainable by PAS-D or mucicarmine stains[227,505]). Conversely, mucin-producing mesotheliomas are well described, although rare,[505,539,540] as are PAS-D mucin-like droplets in hyperplastic mesothelial cells, resistant to hyaluronidase pretreatment.[119] Therefore, some authorities[37,541] consider mucin stains to be of limited or little value in diagnosis and to have been largely if not entirely superseded by the immunohistochemical (IHC) techniques available in almost all laboratories in industrialized nations.[542]

Lastly, electron microscopy (EM) can be used when uncertainties remain concerning the diagnosis; EM can be regarded as the "gold standard" for the diagnosis of MMs with an epithelial component,[211,543] but in everyday practice it has been largely replaced in most institutions by IHC investigation (a diminished role aggravated by the closure of many diagnostic EM units). Nonetheless, some authorities[544] argue that EM still plays a role in the independent validation of a diagnosis of mesothelioma, particularly when investigating new antibodies. We continue to find EM useful, often decisively so, including the use of deparaffinized and reprocessed biopsy tissue, when (1) the sample is small (e.g., those that are predominantly cytologic in character, including cell-block preparations); (2) the histologic appearances are atypical; or (3) there are discordant immunohistochemical findings.[213,543] In these circumstances, EM remains an extremely effective ancillary methodology for the diagnosis of epithelial MMs.[213,543,545]

Obviously, the character of the diagnostic problem is dependent on the morphology of the neoplasm. For an epithelioid tumor, the main distinction is between epithelial MM and secondary adenocarcinoma: spread to the pleura is common, with adenocarcinomas arising in

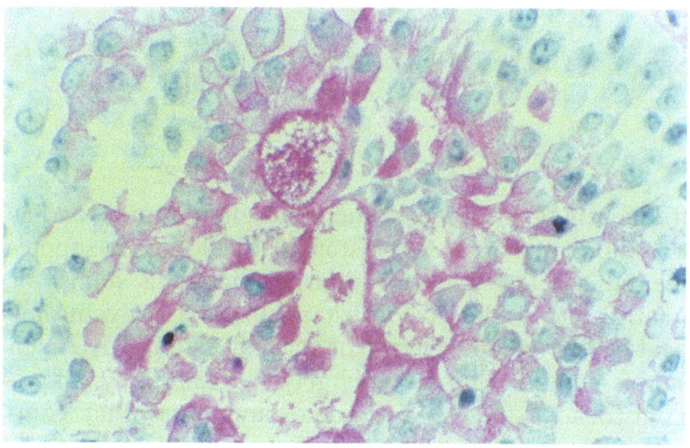

FIGURE 43.57. This pulmonary adenocarcinoma shows intracellular PAS-diastase histochemical staining.

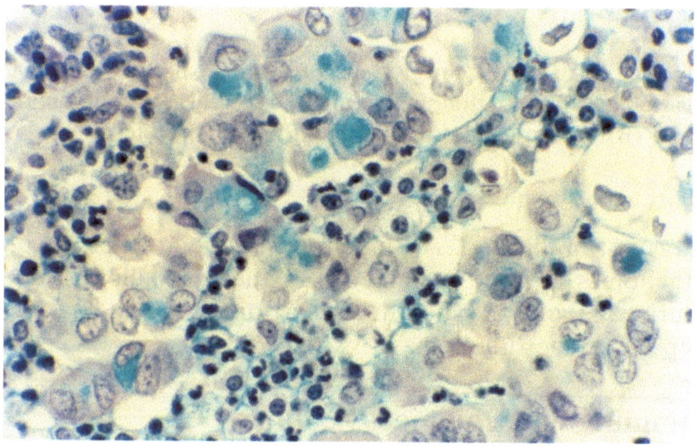

FIGURE 43.59. Alcian blue and colloidal iron are seen in this primary pulmonary adenocarcinoma and are resistant to hyaluronidase predigestion.

various anatomic sites, especially lung and breast, as discussed in a later section of this chapter. For sarcomatoid tumors, the situation is somewhat different, and the differential diagnosis includes solitary fibrous tumor, sarcomas (primary or secondary and including biphasic and monophasic synovial sarcoma), as well as spindle cell carcinoma and other neoplasms where the neoplastic cells can assume a spindle cell morphology (such as renal cell carcinoma and melanoma). Most of the published IHC studies on MM focus on epithelial or biphasic MMs. Immunohistochemistry has a far more restricted role in the diagnosis of sarcomatoid and desmoplastic MMs, but most coexpress broad-spectrum cytokeratins and vimentin.[511,546,547] A further diagnostic difficulty includes the differential diagnosis of (atypical) mesothelial hyperplasia and MM, and ancillary studies may also be of some value for that distinction, although this issue remains the subject of controversy. Finally, some antibodies may also prove useful once a diagnosis of MM has been established, as predictors of prognosis, and this seems to be represent an area of increasing interest.[544–554] In summary, there are three broad indications for immunohistochemistry:

1. The differential diagnosis between MM and other tumors
2. The discrimination between MM and reactive mesothelial hyperplasia
3. The prediction of prognosis

Despite extensive investigations, no definitive mesothelioma-specific antibody has been generated to date (as is the case for most other cancers). Given the protean phenotypic repertoire of MMs, this seems unsurprising. The antibodies currently available can be subdivided into the following broad categories:

1. *Antibodies useful for the positive identification of (epithelioid) mesothelial cells,* and of variable specificity and sensitivity: Although calretinin appears to have high specificity for mesothelial cells, other markers of lesser specificity such as cytokeratin 5/6 are still useful in the differential diagnosis, because some cancers are distinguishable from MM by their histologic appearances or by the expression of some markers and nonexpression of other mesothelial cell markers.

2. *Exclusionary antibodies that are characteristically negative in MMs and that are more frequently and consistently expressed by carcinomas:* Examples include CEA, CD15 (Leu-M1 antigen), and TTF-1 whenever adenocarcinoma of the lung is part of the differential diagnosis. The choice of antibodies in this class can be tailored to the specific circumstances of the case at issue: for example, in a patient with a history of prostatic adenocarcinoma, antibodies against prostate-specific antigen and prostatic acid phosphatase can be added, and in a patient with a background of colorectal cancer, antibodies against CK7 and CK20 can be used in addition to immunostaining for CEA.

3. *Antibodies that can decorate both mesothelial cells and carcinoma cells with reasonable frequency and that have restricted, little, or no discriminatory value in terms of a binary positive or negative result:* An example is immunostaining for EMA. Although positive in MMs and various carcinomas, some such antibodies show differences in the staining pattern between MM and carcinoma (for example, EMA and HBME-1).

4. *Antibodies directed against intermediate filament proteins, most notably cytokeratins (CKs), usually demonstrable in MMs of all histologic types and carcinomas:* Although pan-CK antibodies such as AE1/AE3 have little discriminatory value in general, they assume significance in certain circumstances, such as (a) exclusion of a lymphoma when it is in the differential diagnosis; (b) CK expression by a pleura-based sarcomatoid tumor resembling malignant fibrous histiocytoma or a collagen-rich pleural tumor can provide supportive or confirmatory evidence for a diagnosis of sarcomatoid or desmoplastic mesothelioma; (c) CK5/6 expression by a pleural epithelioid tumor can support a diagnosis of MM with an epithelial component and, substantially less often, a sarcomatoid MM; and (d) as a means to highlight the presence or absence of invasion.

5. *Antibodies that may be of probabilistic value in the discrimination between reactive mesothelial hyperplasia and epithelioid MM.*

6. *Antibodies that may be useful as predictors of prognosis.*

Because no single 100% sensitive and 100% specific antibody has been found, panels of antibodies that include both positive and negative markers are employed. Importantly, those antibodies do not by themselves consistently distinguish between benign and malignant lesions, and application of basic principles of tumor diagnosis is still required. The possible contribution of immunohistochemistry differs according on the diagnostic dilemma at hand.

The reproducibility of immunohistologic diagnosis of MM was examined in the late 1990s by a group of Italian pathologists with an interest in asbestos-related diseases, and they concluded that "the information additionally contributed by IHC did not seem to change the pathologists' diagnoses very much compared with those made by routine H&E [staining]. . . . Careful scrutiny of routinely stained preparations still remains the most rewarding component of the diagnostic pathway."[555] However, all the pathologists involved in that study were experienced in the assessment of asbestos-related disorders, whereas many pathologists do not encounter significant numbers of MM, and it is conceivable that in this particular study

Table 43.14. Markers usually positive in epithelial or biphasic mesothelioma

Positive mesothelial markers	Comment
Calretinin	Currently regarded as the most sensitive and specific marker for mesothelial differentiation
CK5/6	Sensitive and specific for differential diagnosis of epithelial MM versus adenocarcinoma, but not suitable to distinguish ovarian serous and squamous cell carcinoma
WT-1	Good sensitivity and specificity for epithelial mesotheliomas, but possible difficulties with autopsy material; cross-reactivity with renal cell carcinoma is not a problem
D2-40 (Podoplanin)	Similar sensitivities and specificities to calretinin, but less extensively studied
Thrombomodulin	Very variable in literature, but we consider it useful in the distinction of MM from metastatic adenocarcinoma; also avoids misdiagnosis of epithelioid hemangioendothelioma
HBME-1	Variably regarded, but we have found useful if only membrane labeling is considered positive and if dilution is sufficient (1:5000 to 1:15,000)
CD44S	High sensitivity but low specificity
Mesothelin	Some consider it useful (if negative, epithelial MM less likely), but we have found no advantage over calretinin and other positive markers

Table 43.15. Markers usually negative in (epithelial or biphasic) mesothelioma

Markers positive in carcinoma (negative in mesothelioma)	Comments
CEA	Very useful for differential diagnosis of MM and adenocarcinoma but usually negative in renal cell carcinoma and ovarian/peritoneal serous carcinoma
CD15 (Leu-M1)	Well characterized and we consider it a good discriminator; useful in the distinction from renal cell carcinoma (most are positive), but it does not reliably identify squamous cell carcinomas
B72.3	Variable reports, but we (and others) continue its use; sensitivity and specificity of 93% and 80%, respectively (meta-analysis)
Ber-EP4 and MOC31	Both antibodies recognize the same antigen; less reliable than CEA or BG-8, and we have found some labeling of mesotheliomas, but may be useful in certain situations, for example with metastatic breast carcinoma and pleural synovial sarcoma
BG-8	Reliable in distinction of MM and adenocarcinoma, labels 80% of squamous cell carcinomas, but does not label renal cell carcinomas
TTF-1	Useful for differential diagnosis of MM and lung adenocarcinoma; highly specific, but lack of labeling does not exclude lung adenocarcinoma, and squamous cell carcinomas of lung usually do not stain

the experience of the investigators resulted in an underestimation of the role of IHC in the diagnosis of MM Also, it is unclear how the diagnosis of MM was confirmed, other than by consensus among observers.

We believe that IHC plays an important and often crucial role in the diagnosis of MM and that it routinely contributes to the diagnosis. We have encountered mesotheliomas misdiagnosed as adenocarcinoma histologically and vice versa (pseudomesotheliomatous adenocarcinoma [PMAC]; see later discussion), where the correct final diagnosis was achieved mainly by immunohistochemistry. Although MM and PMAC represent lethal diseases refractory to treatment and with similar mean/median survival times measured in a few months only following diagnosis, we routinely employ carefully considered panels of antibodies, believing the distinction to be important, not least because of the medicolegal implications, but also for strictly scientific reasons.

The considerations presented here are limited to commercially available antibodies that can be used on paraffin-embedded tissues. Apart from the antibodies listed in Tables 43.14 to 43.16, there are many more that have been described in the literature,[556–558] but if they are not commercially available or their use is limited to frozen section material, they are not considered here in detail.

Table 43.16. Other useful markers in the diagnosis of pleural malignant mesothelioma

Antibody	Utility/comment
CK7/CK20	Limited value to ascertain origin of secondary adenocarcinoma; not useful for discrimination between mesothelioma and adenocarcinoma; MM may be CK7+/CK20– or CK7+/CK20+
p63	Useful marker to distinguish MM from squamous cell carcinoma
Gross cystic disease fluid protein (GCDFP)	Limited usefulness to distinguish MM from metastatic breast carcinoma; low sensitivity but high specificity
CD10	Not specific enough to distinguish MM and renal cell carcinoma, because up to 54% of MM are positive
Estrogen receptor (ER)	Useful to distinguish MM from serous carcinoma of ovary or peritoneum and breast carcinoma
Progesterone receptor (PR)	In conjunction with ER, useful to distinguish MM from serous carcinoma of ovary or peritoneum and breast carcinoma
p53	Possibly some limited use in distinguishing reactive mesothelial hyperplasia and MM

There have been numerous studies comparing the usefulness of various panels of antibodies, and different laboratories have recorded different results. For example, some studies have found calretinin to be of little use or "worthless,"[436,559,560] but others have found it to be at least useful[561,562] or even highly sensitive and specific.[511,563,564] Much of the discordance between studies can be explained by the following factors:

1. The use of different materials for assessment (histologic sections of surgical specimens versus autopsy material,[565] versus cell blocks prepared from effusion fluids).
2. The clones of antibodies used: for example, one group that had found immunostaining for calretinin to be "useless" when a Chemicon guinea pig antibody was used, rather than the Zymed or Dako antibodies, remarked that when the Zymed antibody was used, it was the "preferred marker in identifying mesothelial cells in cytological samples, showing the highest sensitivity for mesothelial cells."[566]
3. Methodologic differences, including different dilutions (ranging between 1:50[563] and 1:8000[567] or even more), the use or nonuse of antigen retrieval methods, and, if used, different retrieval methods, incubation temperatures, and times.
4. Variation in what type and intensity of labeling is considered positive in the histologic assessment. For example, in some of the earlier studies on calretinin, cytoplasmic staining was considered positive, leading to the assessment that a high proportion of carcinomas showed positive staining, but when more restrictive criteria were used and nuclear staining was required for a positive result irrespective of cytoplasmic staining, high specificity ensued.[563] In an editorial comment on two successive papers on the IHC assessment of MM versus adenocarcinoma, Ordóñez[568] and Riera et al.,[569] published in the same issue of the same journal in 1997, Wick[570] pointed out that the two papers reached "somewhat divergent conclusions," although both affirmed the value of CEA, TAG-72 (recognized by the B72.3 antibody), and CD15 for the diagnosis of adenocarcinoma, but they differed over the usefulness of Ber-EP4. Ordóñez did not evaluate calretinin, whereas Riera et al. did. They also reached somewhat different conclusions concerning the value of HBME-1 and thrombomodulin. These differences were explicable at least in part by methodology. Among other factors mentioned by Wick, Ordóñez preselected the cases for study on the basis of "strong cytoplasmic staining for keratin"; Riera et al. used epitope retrieval for some probes, whereas Ordóñez did not, except for thrombomodulin; Ordóñez did not set forth specific criteria for a positive result, except that the staining was graded semiquantitatively (1+, corresponding to 1% to 25% of the cells, to 4+ amounting to >76%, and staining of <1% was considered equivocal), whereas Riera et al. considered weak staining of <10% of cells to be a negative result, although intense staining of any number of cells was designated as positive, and their semiquantitative grading system also differed, so that staining of 10% to 25% of cells was assigned to grade 1.

Some such difficulties were highlighted in a published exchange of letters and views on the subject,[571–573] highlighting the differences in approach even among those publishing actively in the field. Finally, despite the large number of studies on this subject, there are only few that attempted to weigh the usefulness of the antibodies in a statistically meaningful manner, for example by using logistic regression or decision tree analysis,[574–577] as opposed to a simple listing of the specificity and sensitivity for each individual antibody.

There are numerous current reviews suggesting various panels of antibodies[547,563,578–581] and meta-analysis has been carried out in an attempt to provide guidance,[547] but the validity of meta-analysis is limited, taking into account the heterogeneity in the methodologic variables in those analyses. The same principle applies to the Web site for Immunoquery,[582] which provides suggested IHC panels for differential diagnosis based on the published literature. Although an immensely useful database, its optimal use requires a critical and discriminatory approach. Finally, studies evaluating the potential use of new antibodies are difficult to interpret. Few provide independent validation of the diagnosis of MM, for example by EM, but if only morphologically unequivocal cases are included, this selective approach may not coincide with the true relative proportion of positive tumors, and thus skew the results. Some recent studies have attempted to overcome this particular problem by using tissue microarrays of both epithelial and sarcomatoid areas of tumors separately, to gain a better understanding of IHC staining profiles of the tumors as a whole.[512] Similarly, some of the studies comparing the immunoprofiles of epithelial MMs versus adenocarcinomas with spread into the pleura either (1) pooled carcinomas arising at different primary sites within the class of *adenocarcinoma*, or (2) used sections of the primary carcinoma rather than the actual pleural deposits.

It is worth mentioning at the outset that no literature review can replace one's own experience and knowledge of the techniques applied in one's own laboratory. In view of the versatility in appearance displayed by MM, it is not surprising that no unique and reproducible immunoprofile has been established that encompasses all types of MM, and that knowledge of immunophenotype of the morphologic subtype of lesion in question, and its differential diagnosis, is necessary to choose the most appropriate studies and for interpretation of the results. One of the most common scenarios that we

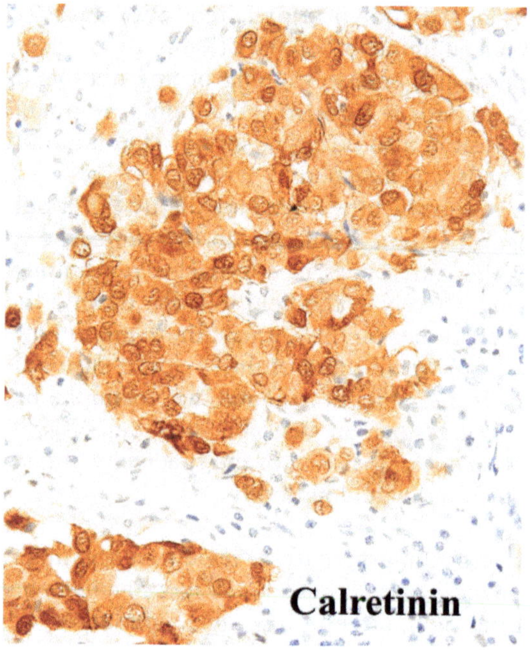

FIGURE 43.60. Pleural epithelial mesothelioma, labeled for calretinin. In addition to the labeling of the cytoplasm, there is convincing decoration of the nuclei of the neoplastic cells. Nuclear labeling of this type or more intense is required for designation of calretinin labeling as positive. If the nuclei are unlabeled, we classify the result as negative.

experience in consultation is a pleural spindle cell lesion with a clinical appearance of mesothelioma but that lacks labeling for the mesothelioma markers—not a surprising finding given the small proportion of sarcomatoid MMs that shows detectable expression of markers such as calretinin, CK5/6, and other mesothelial cell markers. This necessity for familiarity with the strengths of one's own laboratory as well as the specific diagnostic problems with an individual lesion are reflected in the reluctance of both the International Mesothelioma Panel and the Association of Directors of Anatomic and Surgical Pathology (ADASP) to suggest definitive panels of antibodies. Instead, they recommend a panel that includes at least two mesothelial-related antibodies and two antibodies that are commonly negative in mesothelioma, supplemented by immunostaining for cytokeratins in the case of the International Mesothelioma Panel.[37,583] Consequently, the opinions expressed here are largely based on our diagnostic experience with the antibodies suggested, as well as consideration of the current literature.

The discussion in this section focuses on epithelial MMs and the epithelial component of biphasic MMs. The role of immunohistochemistry in the diagnosis of sarcomatoid and desmoplastic MMs is discussed elsewhere in this chapter.

Positive Immunohistochemical Markers for Mesothelial Cells

Calretinin

Calretinin is a 29-kDa calcium-binding protein that belongs to the same family of EF-hand proteins as S-100, and that is thought to play a role in calcium-dependent cell signaling.[584] Typically expressed in the nervous system, it is also found in normal and neoplastic mesothelium.[585–587] There are a number of clones of antibodies available, and we have found the Zymed and the Dako antibodies to be particularly useful. As mentioned above, calretinin has had very variable reports, but we have found this antibody to be highly sensitive, on the order of 98% with a diagnostic accuracy of 95% (unpublished observations). Patchy cytoplasmic staining with this antibody may be observed in some metastatic adenocarcinomas, but if only nuclear staining in tumor cells is considered positive, the diagnostic accuracy of this antibody is high (Fig. 43.60). Calretinin is currently regarded as the most sensitive and specific marker for mesothelioma, and this is reflected by publications that advocate the use of this antibody as a primary antibody in suggested panels.[577,581,588,589] There is some evidence to suggest a complementary role for this antibody if used together with D2-40, particularly in spindle cell lesions.[512]

Cytokeratin 5/6

The use of differential cytokeratin (CK) subtypes, such as CK5/6[590], is of diagnostic value (Fig. 43.61). Initial

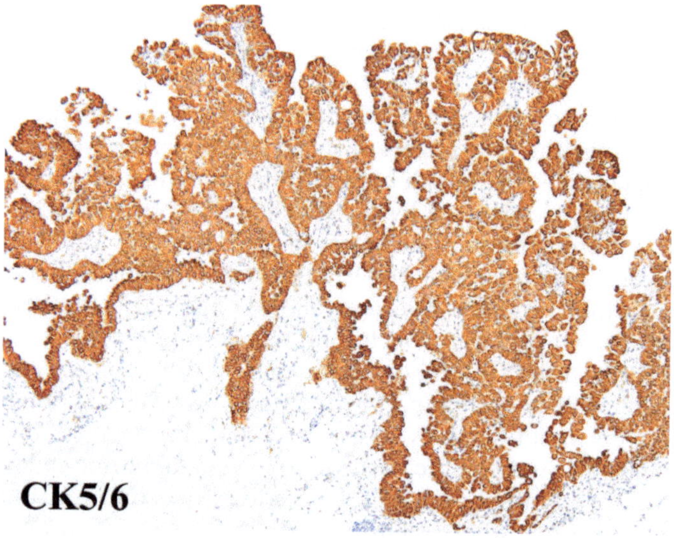

FIGURE 43.61. Exophytic mesothelioma, epithelial in type and in situ in distribution in this micrograph (superficial but undoubted invasion was found in other areas of the same biopsy). Positive labeling of the lesional cells for CK5/6.

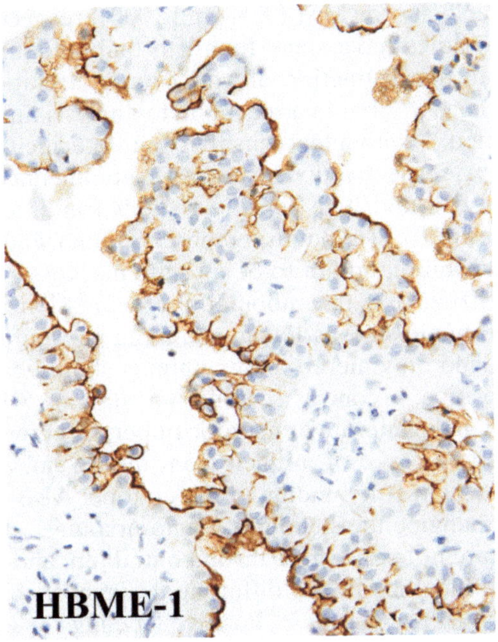

FIGURE 43.62. This tumor shows the positive linear membrane-related labeling characteristic of mesothelial cells and mesotheliomas. Although the diagnostic value of HBME-1 labeling has been questioned, we still find HBME-1 to be one of the most useful markers for epithelial mesothelial cells, provided that the antibody is used at high dilution (1:5000 to 1:15,000 in our laboratories). At higher concentrations, HBME-1 labels a variety of other tumors, although the reaction pattern in such circumstances is often cytoplasmic, rather than the linear pattern shown here.

reports of close to 100% sensitivity and specificity[564] of labeling for CK5/6 for the diagnosis of MM require reevaluation in the light of subsequent data,[547] but nonetheless, we have found this antibody useful for the diagnosis of MM and distinction from adenocarcinoma of lung in particular, although it is not reliable for distinction from ovarian serous or metastatic squamous carcinoma,[564,547,590,591] endometrial adenocarcinomas, and urothelial neoplasms.[592]

HBME-1

HBME-1 is a monoclonal antibody raised from the human mesothelial cell line SPC111. The exact antigen is not known but appears to be associated with microvilli. Reported sensitivities (66% to 100%[436,593]) and specificities (15% to 91%[594,595]) vary widely, but so does the concentration at which this antibody is used: 1:100 and 1:250 and 1:1500 are described,[563,588] and the commercial manufacturer (Dako, Denmark) recommends a dilution of 1:50 to 1:100. However, we have found that high dilutions of this antibody, in the range of 1:5000 to 1:15,000, are required for optimal results.[37,119,507] If used at sufficient dilution, and if only membranous labeling in a distribution similar to that seen with thrombomodulin or EMA is considered positive (Fig. 43.62), we have found a sensitivity of 91% and accuracy of 79% for the positive recognition of epithelial MMs with this antibody (unpublished observations). In a review of published papers, the overall sensitivity and specificity were 85% and 43%, respectively.[547] Unlike Ordóñez,[581] who regards this antibody as "not useful," we continue to find it helpful.

WT1 Protein

This protein is normally expressed by some fetal tissues as well as adult mesothelium and can be detected in up to 93% of epithelial mesotheliomas,[436,527,563,596–598] with overall sensitivity and specificity estimated as 77% and 96%, respectively, in a review of published studies.[547] However, many ovarian tumors also show labeling.[599] Another potential problem with this antibody appears to be that reactivity is significantly reduced or even completely absent in postmortem material compared to surgical specimens, and it is unclear whether this is related to fixation technique or tissue degradation.[436,565] Furthermore, some authors have expressed concern regarding labeling of renal cell carcinoma (RCC) and suggest that RCC should be specifically excluded by radiologic means,[542] but in a comparative study WT1 expression was seen in only 4% of RCCs of clear cell type.[600] We have found nuclear labeling for WT1 to be a very useful marker (Fig. 43.63), particularly in male patients, for the

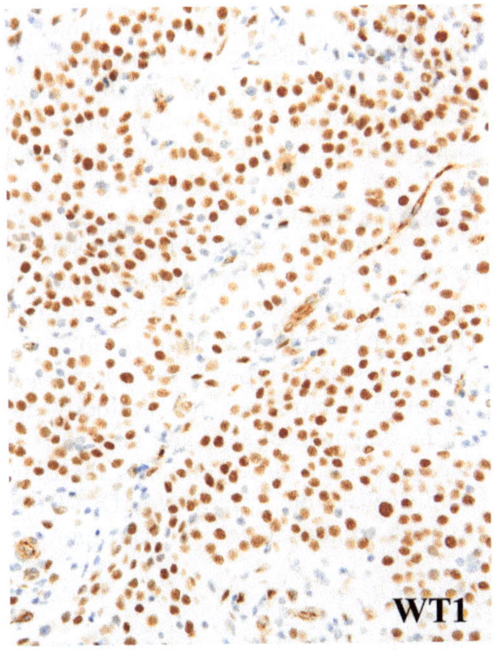

FIGURE 43.63. Epithelial mesothelioma of the pleura, immunolabeled for WT1; the labeling is almost exclusively nuclear in distribution.

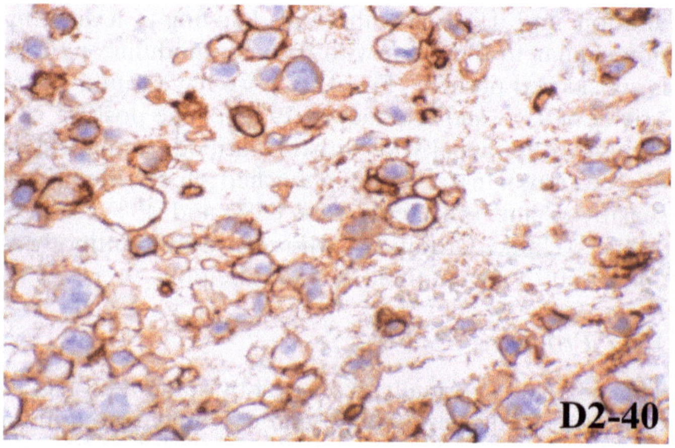

FIGURE 43.64. This epithelial mesothelioma shows cell membrane expression for D2–40.

distinction of MM from lung adenocarcinoma, where there is no possibility of metastatic ovarian carcinoma.

Podoplanin/D2-40

D2-40 is a monoclonal antibody that is directed against an M2 protein derived from germ cell tumors and that was found to specifically bind to human podoplanin, making it a useful marker for lymphatic endothelium.[601] It was noted that normal, reactive, and neoplastic mesothelial cells show labeling, and the usefulness of this antibody for the diagnosis of MM has been investigated.[580,602–604] Up to 100% of epithelial MMs investigated showed membrane staining,[604] but there was labeling of other cell types, including metastatic adenocarcinoma. Some authors suggest that membrane staining is specific for D2-40,[604] whereas others found both membrane and cytoplasmic labeling in metastatic carcinoma cells, with membranous labeling being particularly prominent in metastatic ovarian carcinoma.[605] Labeling in sarcomatoid mesotheliomas appears less reliable, with sensitivities of 27%[604] to 58%.[512] Most authors emphasize that only linear membrane staining should be regarded as positive in this context (Fig. 43.64), but since podoplanin expression is found in numerous tissue types,[601] further cross-reactions may be discovered. However, this antibody does show promise in the diagnosis of MM and may be particularly useful in conjunction with calretinin in the diagnosis of pleural spindle cell lesions.[512] However, D2-40 in isolation appears to have no advantage over calretinin.

Thrombomodulin

Thrombomodulin (CD141) is a 75-kDa glycoprotein that is expressed by mesothelium, vascular endothelium, synovium, and placental syncytiotrophoblast.[606–608] In early studies it was found to have very high sensitivity and specificity for MM (92% and 100%, respectively).[606] Many studies have since found thrombomodulin to be useful in the distinction of MM from metastatic adenocarcinoma,[588,609] but in a recent meta-analysis this was not confirmed,[547] with a low sensitivity and specificity of 61% and 80%, respectively. However, we among many others have also found high sensitivity (91%) and acceptable accuracy (79%) (unpublished observations), and we consider thrombomodulin to be a useful marker. It is worth emphasizing that thrombomodulin expression in viable cells is manifested as linear membranous staining (Fig. 43.65), and only membranous staining should be considered positive. In contrast, cytoplasmic staining, which may be seen in degenerate or necrotic tumor, is thought to due to passive uptake of antigen from the serum, and does not represent true binding to the epitope. Also, epithelioid hemangioendotheliomas, angiosarcomas, and squamous carcinomas express thrombomodulin, and this may cause difficulties in the differential diagnosis of pleural spindle cell neoplasms.[511] Positive labeling for thrombomodulin in the absence of detectable labeling for other mesothelial or carcinoma-related markers raises the distinct possibility of an epithelioid hemangioendothelioma,

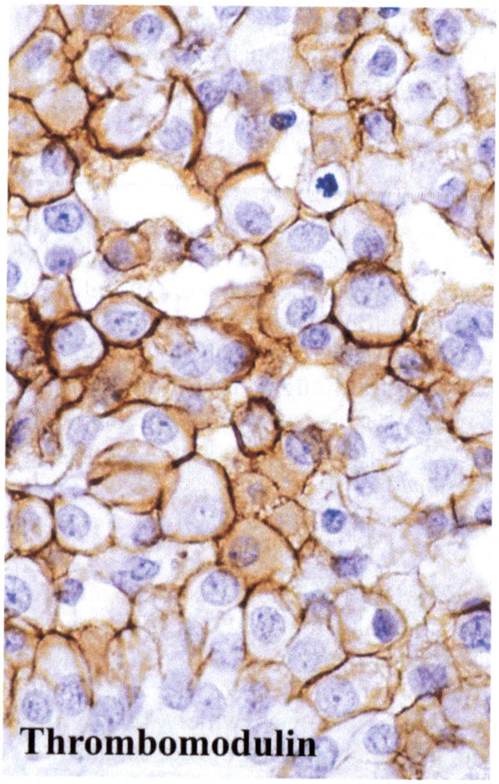

FIGURE 43.65. Pleural epithelial mesothelioma, immunolabeled for thrombomodulin. Characteristically, the labeling is linear and membrane-related, with a "chicken wire" pattern in this area.

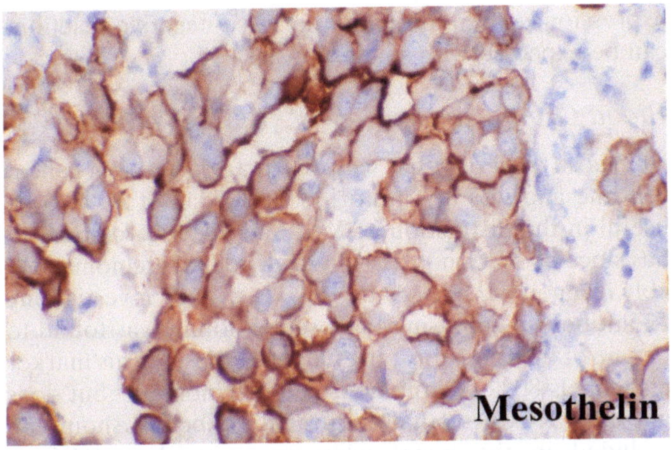

FIGURE 43.66. Fairly intense cell membrane staining for mesothelin is seen in this epithelial mesothelioma.

which can be confirmed by labeling for endothelial markers such as CD31 and von Willebrand factor.

Mesothelin

Mesothelin is a 40-kDa surface glycoprotein that was generated using an ovarian cell line, and it has been reported to be expressed on the surface of normal, reactive, and malignant mesothelial cells (Fig. 43.66).[610] There have been several studies investigating the usefulness of this marker for the diagnosis of mesothelioma.[563,579,580,600,611–614] Some authors describe high sensitivity and specificity for epithelial MMs with no labeling of the metastatic adenocarcinomas investigated,[610] but other investigators found positive labeling in up to 39% of lung adenocarcinomas.[611–613] However, it is worth mentioning that the latter studies utilized a different commercially available clone of antibody. This antibody also shows positive labeling of squamous cell carcinomas of lung, pancreatic carcinomas, and ovarian tumors,[611,615] but no labeling of RCCs where it may play a limited role in the distinction of MM from RCC.[600] In view of the overall low specificity but apparently high sensitivity of this antibody for epithelial mesothelioma in all of the studies published, it has been suggested that a *lack* of labeling could be considered an indication *against* a diagnosis of mesothelioma. In view of the fact that there are now several mesothelioma-related antibodies available that show higher sensitivity and specificity, we consider this antibody to be rather limited in its usefulness.

CD44S

This 85- to 90-kDa transmembrane glycoprotein is expressed by many hematopoietic and lymphoid cells. This protein acts as a receptor for hyaluronic acid as well as facilitating lymphocyte interaction with endothelial cells. After initial encouraging reports describing labeling of up to 92% of mesothelioma cell lines,[616] later studies showed overall disappointing results with fairly high sensitivity (90–100%) but low specificity.[588,609,617]

There are now numerous mesothelial-related markers available, so much so that one might question the need for further markers in this area.[618]

Exclusionary Markers: Characteristically Positive in Adenocarcinomas and Negative in Mesotheliomas

Carcinoembryonic Antigen

Carcinoembryonic antigen is an oncofetal glycoprotein not normally expressed by mesothelial cells but commonly expressed by lung and other adenocarcinomas, most notably colorectal carcinomas. It was the first widely accepted marker to aid in the distinction of MM and adenocarcinoma[619] and remains one of the best of the exclusionary markers.[577,581,589]

In a survey of 598 diffuse MMs comprising 21 separate reports, Henderson et al.[211] found that only 58 (10%) were reactive with antibodies to CEA, whereas 359 of 404 pulmonary adenocarcinomas were CEA positive (89%), and that in those mesotheliomas that are reactive with antibodies to CEA, the staining is usually focal and weak. Polyclonal CEA antibodies (PoAbs) were used in some of the early studies and resulted in some nonspecific staining due to cross-reactions,[211] but an analysis of recent data found a sensitivity of 81% and specificity of 97%.[547]

The significance of immunolabeling for CEA for the diagnosis or exclusion of mesothelioma can be summarized as follows:[119]

1. Intense or extensive cytoplasmic or membrane-accentuated immunoreactivity for CEA is highly characteristic of adenocarcinoma or other carcinomas, and is strong evidence against a diagnosis of mesothelioma.[211]
2. Because CEA is undetectable in 10% to 15% of pulmonary adenocarcinomas and in most serous papillary carcinomas, both ovarian and extraovarian, a negative result on immunolabeling for CEA is not decisive by itself.
3. Numerous CEA polyclonal and monoclonal antibodies are in existence, with different sensitivities and specificities for CEA, so that the results can vary from one study to another. Dejmek and Hjerpe[620] compared patterns of reactivity for CEA in a series of 61 mesotheliomas of different histologic subtypes, using a single PoAb (Dako) and five monoclonal antibodies (MoAbs). Thirteen of the mesotheliomas (21%) were labeled with the CEA PoAb. The staining was focal in 11 cases, and diffuse in two. Four of the five CEA MoAbs were reactive

with variable but smaller proportions of the mesotheliomas (one to seven out of 61 cases). Only the Dako MoAb was unreactive with all mesotheliomas, whereas it decorated 15 of 20 adenocarcinomas.

4. Nonspecific staining with CEA antibodies can be encountered in mesotheliomas and other tumors, including uptake of the antibody in areas of tumor necrosis or in benign alveolar remnants incorporated into mesotheliomas invading lung. False-positive labeling has also been recorded in mesotheliomas with a high content of hyaluronic acid, and this was abolished by pretreatment of sections with hyaluronidase[621]; protracted trypsinization of sections may also lead to nonspecific labeling.[622] Accordingly, interpretation of a positive result for a tumor that resembles MM in all other respects requires some caution. We routinely monitor each immunoreaction with both positive and negative controls and consider only unequivocal labeling of viable tumor remote from any areas of necrosis to be significant.[119]

Cluster of Differentiation 15 (CD15; Clone Leu-M1)

CD15 is a complex cluster of cell surface glycoproteins and glycolipids that share the terminal Lewis^x antigen, a human myelomonocytic antigen. The CD15 antigen is present on more than 95% of mature peripheral blood eosinophils and neutrophils and is present at low density on circulating monocytes. There are over 90 clones of antibodies assigned to CD15 and eight alternate names for CD15. The discussion here is limited to the clone Leu-M1.

CD15 is one of the oldest and best characterized markers for adenocarcinoma and has been used for the distinction from mesothelioma for over 20 years.[623,624] It has established itself in the panels used in most laboratories, although some authors report positivity in up to 32% of MMs.[527,625] In addition, one study using "logic" regression concluded that despite high sensitivity and specificity, some of the newer antibodies such as BG8 and MOC31 are more suitable for the positive identification of adenocarcinoma.[563] We and others have found that MM is only rarely positive for CD15[559,581,626,627] and consider it to represent a useful discriminator. It is also useful in the distinction of MM from RCC, most of which are positive,[600,628] but it does not reliably identify squamous cell carcinomas.[629] Sheibani et al.[623,624] and Battifora[515] found that CD15 was undetectable in all 127 mesotheliomas investigated, whereas it was expressed by 199 out of 268 adenocarcinomas (74%). Wick et al.[627] reported quite decisive results: CD15 was found in all 52 pulmonary adenocarcinomas studied, but none of 51 epithelial mesotheliomas. Battifora has pointed out that pulmonary adenocarcinomas express CD15 more often than adenocarcinomas originating in other sites. He also cautioned that CD15 expression is often focal and that false-negative reactions can be expected with small biopsies.

Blood Group Antigen Lewis^y (BG8 Clone)

BG8 is an antibody that was raised against a lung cancer cell line and was first reported by Jordan et al.[630] to be useful in the distinction of MM and adenocarcinoma. It has since been found to distinguish adenocarcinoma reliably from epithelioid MM.[547,569,631] In a study investigating 12 antibodies and using logic regression, it was found to be one of the three most useful antibodies.[563] This marker also labels 80% of squamous cell carcinomas[632] but does not label RCCs, so that additional antibodies should be included in the panel whenever secondary RCC is suspected.[600]

Antibodies Directed Against Epithelial Cell Adhesion Molecule, Including Ber-EP4 and MOC31

The epithelial cell adhesion molecule (Ep-CAM), which was discovered in the early 1980s, is a type I transmembrane glycoprotein. Expression has been detected at the basolateral membrane of the majority of epithelial tissues, including transitional cell epithelium, but Ep-CAM expression appears to be absent in mature squamous stratified epithelium and in hepatocytes[633–635]; Ep-CAM has also been identified in carcinomas of ovary, colon, breast, kidney, and lung.[634,636] In squamous cell carcinomas, Ep-CAM expression is absent, as detected by the Ber-EP4 antibody.[637]

There are now numerous clones of antibodies commercially available: among those extensively investigated for the distinction between MM and metastatic carcinoma are Ber-EP4 and MOC31, both of which identify the EGF-1–like domain of Ep-CAM.[634] Among the lesser known clones not as extensively studied are HEA125 (also identifying the EGF-1 like domain of Ep-CAM)[638] and AUA1.[634,639,640] Some reports identified high specificity for adenocarcinomas, with no labeling of any of the eight mesotheliomas included in a pilot study using AUA1,[641] but later reports revealed labeling of up to 21% of mesotheliomas,[641] and currently this antibody is not widely recommended for this role.

A meta-analysis of published reports found 80% specificity and 90% sensitivity for Ber-EP4 in the distinction between MM and adenocarcinoma, and 93% sensitivity and specificity for MOC31.[547] An evaluation of 12 antibodies using logic regression included MOC31 in the final three-antibody panel, which reportedly provided 96% sensitivity and specificity for the distinction of MM from adenocarcinoma.[563] Despite these encouraging reports in the literature, in our practice we have removed both Ber-EP4 and MOC31 from our routine mesothelioma proto-

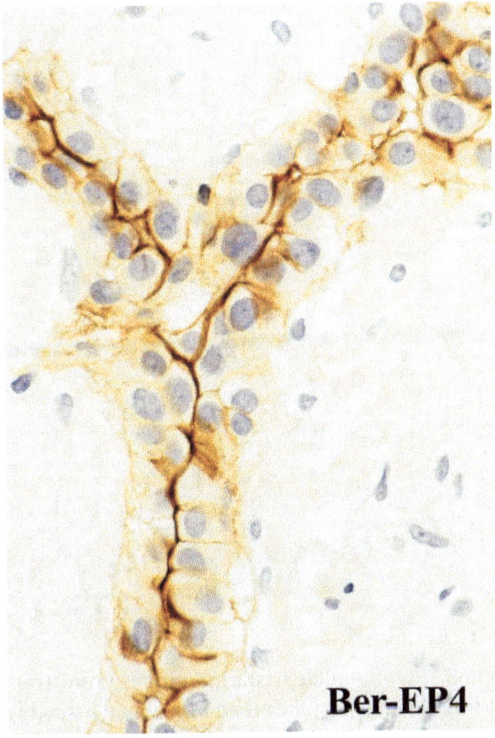

FIGURE 43.67. Pleural malignant mesothelioma. Positive linear immunolabeling with Ber-EP4. No immunohistochemical marker is entirely specific or sensitive for mesothelial cells versus carcinoma cells.

col because in our laboratory each labeled a significant proportion of mesotheliomas (up to about 20–30% with Ber-EP4; Fig. 43.67).

B72.3

The antibody B72.3 identifies the tumor-associated protein TAG-72, a complex glycoprotein expressed in breast carcinoma lines, and has long been used as a positive adenocarcinoma marker, with numerous studies investigating this antibody for the distinction of adenocarcinoma from MM.[627] The published reports have been very variable, with some reporting labeling of more than 40% of MM,[642] and only 50% of adenocarcinomas,[643] in contrast to others that described virtually no labeling of mesotheliomas with this antibody.[579,580] We, like many others, have found acceptable sensitivity and specificity with this antibody, which has been found to be positive in about 85% of lung adenocarcinomas,[625,632,644,645] with overall sensitivity and specificity of 93% and 80%, respectively, as assessed by meta-analysis. In our experience, labeling of epithelial MMs by B72.3 is distinctly uncommon, about three MMs among a few hundred cases tested. In one of the positive cases, the labeling appeared to correlate spatially with prominent lakes of glycogen in the mesothelioma cell cytoplasm as visualized by EM.[119]

E-Cadherin

Cadherins are part of a family of cell adhesion molecules that present as membrane-bound heterodimers. E-cadherins are though to be preferentially expressed by epithelial tissues, in contrast to N-cadherins, which are considered to be preferentially expressed by neural crest tissue. E-cadherin is normally present as a complex with β-catenin, which plays an important role in the *WNT* pathway (the pathway mutated in familial adenomatous polyposis (FAP) and many other malignancies). Some reports see value in using either expression of E-cadherin alone as an adenocarcinoma marker,[646] or assessing differential patterns of expression of E-cadherin (in lung adenocarcinomas) versus expression of N-cadherins (in MM),[560,647] but we, like some others,[579] have found labeling of a significant proportion of mesotheliomas, and a meta-analysis found an overall sensitivity and specificity of 86% and 83%, respectively. With other more reliable markers being available, we have discontinued the routine use of this antibody for this application.

Thyroid Transcription Factor-1

Thyroid transcription factor-1 is a member of the family of homeodomain (HD) transcription factors and is involved in the regulation of genes expressed within the thyroid, lung, and brain, including those that encode thyroglobulin, Clara cell secretory protein, and surfactant proteins.[648] Gene targeting experiments among others have demonstrated that expression of TTF-1 is essential for morphogenesis of the thyroid, lung, and ventral forebrain; TTF-1 knockout mice lack these organs,[648] and suppression of TTF-1 translation inhibits "lung branching morphogenesis."[649] Thyroid transcription factor-1 is expressed at the onset of thyroid differentiation; TTF-1 mRNA is detectable in the endodermal cells of the thyroid rudiment in the rat embryo and precedes the expression of two other known target genes by 5 days.[650] Thyroid transcription factor-1 mRNA and protein are also present at the earliest stages of lung differentiation and are later confined to the bronchial epithelium. In the brain, TTF-1 appears to be restricted to structures of diencephalic origin, including the developing neurohypophysis.[650]

Stahlman et al.[651] studied the IHC localization of TTF-1 in the lungs of 24 human fetuses at 11 to 23 weeks' gestation, three infants without pulmonary pathology at 36 to 42 weeks, and 24 infants aged 2 days to 6.5 months with hyaline membrane disease or bronchopulmonary dysplasia. Thyroid transcription factor-1 was detected in fetal lung epithelial cell nuclei by 11 weeks' gestation. By 17 weeks, labeling was present in scattered nonciliated columnar and cuboidal cells. Throughout gestation, nuclear staining for TTF-1 was prominent in airways that abutted pleural, peribronchial, and perivascular connective tissue, and was less prominent in centers of lobules. At term, TTF-1 was detected primarily in type II pneumocytes.

In adult normal human lung, TTF-1 expression is restricted to bronchial and alveolar epithelium.[652] Fabbro et al.[652] found TTF-1 expression in seven of 29 cases of non–small-cell lung carcinoma, representing a subset. Curiously, TTF-1 was not expressed in carcinoid tumors, but was "always" expressed in small cell lung carcinomas.[652]

Subsequent studies have shown that TTF-1 is expressed in the nuclei of primary lung (and thyroid follicular) adenocarcinomas and small cell carcinomas, but not in colorectal or breast carcinomas.[653] The specificity and sensitivity of TTF-1 for the diagnosis of adenocarcinomas (and other carcinomas) of lung versus carcinomas of extrapulmonary origin, versus MM, and for the subclassification of lung carcinomas have subsequently been reported in numerous studies.[547,559,579,580,631,654–660] Most such investigations have demonstrated labeling of about 70% to 90% of lung adenocarcinomas for TTF-1,[559,579,655,657–659,661] with a specificity of up to 100%,[547] in comparison to a smaller proportion of large cell carcinomas (~25%[661]) or nonneuroendocrine large cell carcinomas (~50%[659]). Ordóñez[579] found that none of 50 MMs labeled for TTF-1. Our experience is comparable: 4/45 epithelial MMs labeled for TTF-1 (9%) and equivocal labeling at most was found in a further 9%. We consider that definite or strong nuclear labeling in a pleural epithelial tumor represents strong evidence against a diagnosis of epithelial MM (Fig. 43.68) and in favor of an adenocarcinoma of bronchopulmonary origin.

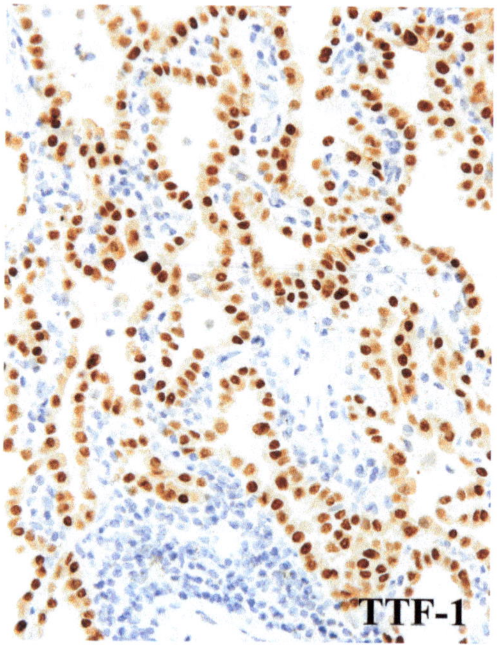

Figure 43.68. Strong nuclear staining for thyroid transcription factor-1 (TTF-1), in a peripheral and localized bronchioloalveolar adenocarcinoma (BAC), nonmucinous type, in an 88-year-old man, treated by wedge resection. Nuclear staining for TTF-1 in a pleural tumor is strong evidence against a diagnosis of mesothelioma.

Antibodies that Decorate both Mesothelial Cells and Carcinoma Cells with Reasonable Frequency: Cytokeratins, Epithelial Membrane Antigen, and CA125

Cytokeratins are discussed in a later section.

Epithelial Membrane Antigen

Epithelial membrane antigen (EMA) is a membrane-bound glycosylated phosphoprotein anchored to the apical surface of many epithelia by a transmembrane domain, with the degree of glycosylation varying according to the cell type. It is thought to play a role in the adhesive function of cell-to-cell interaction, including metastasis. Increased expression, aberrant (intracellular) localization, and changes in glycosylation patterns have been associated with carcinomas.

Epithelial membrane antigen is frequently expressed by adenocarcinomas and epithelial MMs alike, but differences in the distribution of staining make this a useful marker. Adenocarcinomas are usually characterized by cytoplasmic staining, whereas epithelial MMs generally show strong, thick, and circumferential membrane-related staining in up to 97% of cases (Fig. 43.69).[588,662–664] Labeling of the atypical cells in this characteristic linear distribution with antibodies based on clone E29 (for example, the Dako antibody) has also been found useful for the distinction between MM and nonmalignant mesothelial proliferations, both in surgical specimens and in cell-block material prepared from effusion fluids.[665–670] This antibody has been extensively studied in effusion fluid cytology[671] and aids in the differentiation of mesothelioma from reactive mesothelial hyperplasia, where labeling is usually undetectable or weak.[402,664,672–678] Although none of the reactive effusions showed staining in this pattern, about 75% of MMs or more in some studies[489,674,678,679] showed this pattern of EMA labeling, resulting in high specificity but low sensitivity. We have found labeling of tumor cells for EMA (E29 clone) to be a useful probabilistic indicator of malignancy, most notably in cells recovered from effusion fluids, but we have encountered numerous tissue biopsies of proven invasive epithelial MMs where there was either no labeling for EMA or where EMA staining was confined to the superficial zone of the tumor tissue, with undetectable staining in the deeper zones.

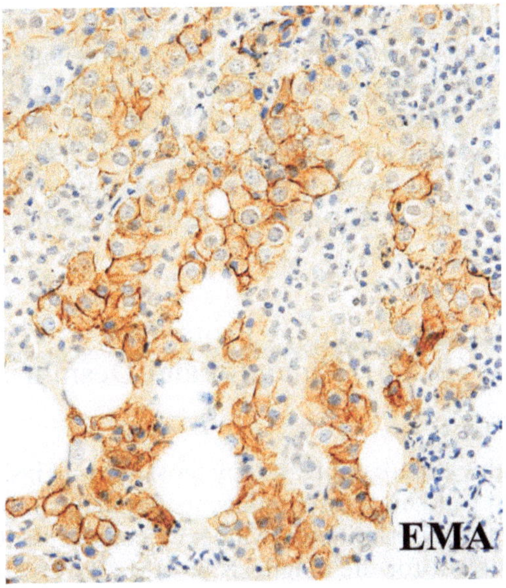

FIGURE 43.69. Pleural malignant mesothelioma, epithelial type. The neoplastic cells, including those invading into subpleural fat, show predominant linear membrane-related labeling for epithelial membrane antigen (EMA), with lesser staining of the tumor cell cytoplasm. Although we have encountered many invasive mesotheliomas that were EMA-negative, as seen in tissue biopsies, it is our experience that the presence of strong thick linear membrane-related labeling for EMA is a probability marker for mesothelioma as opposed to a benign reactive mesothelial hyperplasia, provided that the antibody used is based on the E29 clone (see text). Although not sufficient by itself for diagnosis of mesothelioma as distinct from a reactive mesothelial proliferation, EMA expression in this pattern is an indicator for close follow-up and further investigation of the patient.

CA125

It is well established that immunolabeling of tissue sections for CA125 has no value in the discrimination between MM and adenocarcinomas developing at different anatomic sites, such as those arising in the ovary, lung, and breast.[567,593,680,681] As examples, Bateman et al.[593] found that 15/17 cases of MM labeled for CA125 (88%) in comparison to 7/14 cases of secondary adenocarcinoma in lung and pleura (50%). Attanoos et al.[567] observed positive immunostaining for CA125 in 19/20 ovarian papillary serous adenocarcinomas (95%) and 2/3 primary peritoneal serous adenocarcinomas, in comparison to 8/32 peritoneal MMs (all in females). In a further study from Japan on 90 epithelial MMs and 51 adenocarcinomas of lung, Kushitani et al.[680] found that 85% of the MMs and 80% of the adenocarcinomas were positive for CA125. Finally, in another study based on effusion fluids, Zhu and Michael[681] reported positive staining of all 20 metastatic ovarian carcinomas for CA125, in comparison to 8/13 adenocarcinomas of lung (62%) and 6/13 cases of metastatic breast carcinoma (46%). In all such cases, staining for CA125 is membrane-related.

Therefore, immunostaining of cytology or biopsy samples has essentially no value as a diagnostic discriminator between MM and adenocarcinomas of lung, breast, or ovary. But there is evidence that measurement of serum CA125 levels is a useful and sensitive marker for assessment of the progression of MM and its prognosis, or for the response of MM to treatment. Hedman et al.[682] found that serum CA125 concentrations increased as the disease progressed, whereas stable disease was accompanied by a decrease in CA125 levels. In a study from Turkey on 11 peritoneal MMs, Kebapci et al.[683] found that the mean serum CA125 level was 230 U/mL, within a range of 19 to 1000 U/mL (the normal reference range for this study was 1.2–32 U/mL). In a later study from Italy on 60 cases of peritoneal MM, Baratti et al.[684] recorded a baseline diagnostic sensitivity of 53% for serum CA125 in the MM patients. Forty-six of the patients underwent cytoreductive surgery (CRS) with intraperitoneal hyperthermic perfusion (IPHP): following "adequate" CRS and IPHP, the serum CA125 became negative in 21/22 patients who had elevated baseline levels, but it remained elevated in all nine patients with grossly persistent MM. Elevated CA125 levels developed in all 12 patients who developed progressive disease after CRS and IPHP.

Therefore, there is reasonable evidence that serum CA125 levels represent a sensitive but nonspecific marker for MM, and that serial measurements of the serum levels are a useful means to monitor the progression and prognosis of MM or its response to therapeutic measures, especially when the results are correlated with other serum markers such as soluble mesothelin-related protein (SMRP) and osteopontin (see Serum Osteopontin Levels, below).

Markers of Possible Use for the Distinction of Benign Mesothelial Proliferations Versus MM: EMA, bcl-2, p53, and CD56 (NCAM)

Epithelial Membrane Antigen

The value of IHC staining for EMA in the discrimination between benign versus malignant mesothelial proliferations is discussed above.

Bcl-2

Bcl-2 is a proto-oncogene with a 26-kDa gene product that inhibits apoptosis and therefore promotes survival of individual cells. As discussed earlier, detectable overexpression[478] and direct mutations of *bcl-2* in MM are rare,[391] unlike many other tumors, including follicular lymphoma and even lung carcinoma,[685–687] where overexpression is commonly observed and may be linked to poorer prognosis. Only a small proportion of MMs has been shown to label with antibodies against *bcl-2*, and none of the "reactive" cases labeled.[665,688] Nonetheless, because only a small percentage of MMs immunolabeled, the IHC detection of *bcl-2* seems to be insufficiently sensitive in isolation to be useful for routine diagnostic work to distinguish MM and reactive pleural lesions,[689,690] although it might find some role as part of a panel, for specific problematic cases.

p53

The tumor suppressor gene *p53* induces cell cycle arrest and is maintained at low levels in normal unstressed cells. Stress may induce increased levels of p53 and result in cell cycle arrest and apoptosis. Because of its short half-life, p53 is rarely detectable in normal cells, but paradoxically, increased levels of p53 are commonly expressed in malignant tumors. This is not due to an increase in functional p53 but rather to mutations that render p53 nonfunctional and resistant to degradation. Such mutations of *p53* are only rarely seen in MM,[410] but the *p53* pathway is affected by numerous mutations.

Studies report the presence of p53 in between 25% and 97% of MMs, whereas p53 was found in between 0% and 82% of reactive mesothelial lesions examined.[689–700] In view of the variability in results, use of this antibody for the distinction of benign from malignant mesothelial lesions seems questionable, but warrants further investigation. A relationship between *p53* expression and prognosis has not been identified.

Neural Cell Adhesion Molecules: CD56

The neural cell adhesion molecules (NCAMs) corresponding to CD56 antigen represent a family of closely related cell surface glycoproteins that are thought to play a role in the development of neural cells and the interactions between them. In a study of 16 MMs that included "all three subtypes" in comparison to normal mesothelial cells and a single specimen of pleural mesothelium, Kettunen et al.[699] found that gene expression for NCAM L1 *(L1CAM)* was upregulated mainly in biphasic MMs in comparison to the reference samples. On IHC analysis of tissue microarrays from 47 MMs (26 epithelial, six biphasic, and 15 sarcomatoid), they also recorded significant *p*-values for *L1CAM* when antigen expression levels for epithelial MM were compared with sarcomatoid MMs.

Lantuéjoul et al.[700] studied 26 cases of epithelial, biphasic, and sarcomatoid MM for NCAM reactivity using the 123C3 antibody in comparison to normal mesothelium and 50 non–small-cell lung carcinomas divided equally between adenocarcinomas and squamous cell carcinomas. Although normal mesothelium was negative, NCAM expression was recorded in 19 of the 26 MMs (73%), including all histologic types. Although this finding raises the possibility that CD56 immunoreactivity might prove useful for the discrimination between benign mesothelial proliferations versus MM, there is too little information on NCAM/CD56 expression in MM and mesothelial hyperplasia to justify inclusion of NCAM/CD56 antibodies (such as that based on clone 1B6) in routine diagnostic protocols until further and more extensive studies become available.

Intermediate Filament Proteins: Cytokeratins (Except CK5/6), Vimentin and Desmin

Cytokeratins

Although CKs are expressed by most MMs (Figs. 43.51C and 43.61) and most carcinomas, so that their simple presence is of no discriminatory value, we consider IHC staining important for the diagnosis of MM and we routinely include a CK antibody in our IHC protocol, for two reasons: to highlight invasion, and for the diagnosis of sarcomatoid mesothelioma.[119] Provided that tissue fixation is prompt and adequate and IHC procedures are carried out correctly, CKs are detectable in most MMs, especially with the use of monoclonal antibodies to a CK cocktail or low molecular weight CKs,[37,119,211,626] and trypsinized sections or other techniques are used for epitope enhancement or retrieval.[119] CK7 is expressed by almost all MMs, and CK20 by about 10%.[37] Within this context, immunostaining for pan-CKs, CK8/18 (Fig. 43.70), or CK7 demonstrates CKs in (1) the overwhelming majority of neoplastic cells in virtually all epithelial mesotheliomas, (2) the epithelial component and usually but not always the sarcomatoid component of biphasic mesothe-

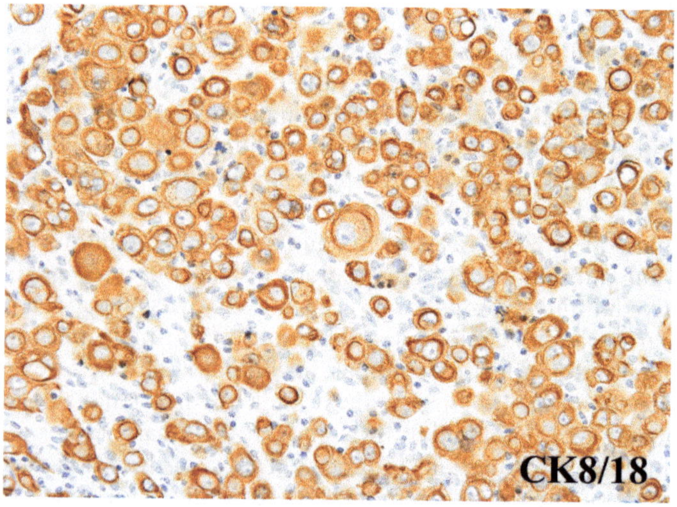

FIGURE 43.70. Pleural malignant mesothelioma, epithelial type, immunolabeled for cytokeratins 8/18 (CAM5.2). There is moderately strong labeling of almost all tumor cells, and some show a perinuclear wreath of intensified labeling.

lioma, and (3) most spindle cells in most but not all sarcomatoid mesotheliomas (see later discussion of sarcomatoid MM in the section Ultrastructural Features of Mesotheliomas). As reviewed by Henderson et al.,[119] CKs were reported in all 137 mesotheliomas comprising nine separate series, in all 94 mesotheliomas in three separate studies that used an antibody against low molecular weight CKs, and in 81 of 94 MMs (86%) with an antibody against high molecular weight CKs. With the use of a broad-spectrum antibody, Mayall et al.[508] identified CKs in 92% and 100% of their epithelial and mixed mesotheliomas, respectively. Lower rates of CK expression in some series seem to be explicable in part by the use of antibodies that recognize stratum corneum keratins, prolonged formalin fixation with loss of immunogenicity, or the use of nontrypsinized sections.[119]

Coexpression of CKs and Vimentin

Vimentin-cytokeratin co-synthesis is characteristic of sarcomatoid, desmoplastic, and transitional MMs and the spindle-cell component of biphasic MM.[119] Mayall et al.[508] identified vimentin in 54% and 74% of epithelial and mixed MMs, respectively, and in 87% of sarcomatoid MMs.

Most sarcomas and other sarcomatoid tumors, and many carcinomas, including metastatic carcinomas and carcinoma cells in effusion fluids,[701] express vimentin so that vimentin by itself is of little or no value in the diagnosis of mesothelioma.[119] Nonetheless, immunolabeling for vimentin in pleura-based tumors is sometimes worthwhile as a check on the immunogenicity of the tissue, and failure to demonstrate vimentin may point to degradation of epitopes, perhaps as a consequence of prolonged fixation.[119]

In addition, disproportionately strong vimentin staining in an epithelioid pleural tumor that shows no or only weak to moderate expression of CKs is an indicator to proceed to immunostaining for CD31 or other markers of endothelial differentiation (epithelioid hemangioendothelioma), especially if the mesothelial cell markers other than thrombomodulin are negative. When investigating a sarcomatoid tumor, it is also worth recalling that sporadic examples of other mesenchymal tumors that express CKs have been also been documented and include malignant fibrous histiocytoma, and smooth muscle cell tumors,[119] but in such instances CK expression is usually weak to moderate at most and is usually confined to a small proportion of the tumor cell population.[119]

Desmin

Desmin is a type III intermediate filament found near the Z-line in sarcomeres. It is only expressed in vertebrates. Scoones and Richman[702] studied desmin and α-smooth muscle actin (α-SMA) in paraffin-embedded biopsy tissue from 10 cases of reactive mesothelial hyperplasia (recurrent pneumothoraces) versus 38 mesotheliomas (27 predominantly epithelioid, four predominantly sarcomatoid, and seven mixed). The reactive hyperplasias expressed desmin and α-SMA more often than mesotheliomas. Similar findings were reported by Attanoos et al.,[689] who found that 85% of reactive mesothelial hyperplasia expressed desmin, but only 10% of mesotheliomas. Mayall et al.[508] detected desmin in 10% of biphasic mesotheliomas, but all of their epithelial or sarcomatoid tumors were negative.

Other Markers

Increased nuclear labeling for the transcription factor *β-catenin*, which is normally found in complex with the cell surface glycoprotein E-cadherin, may be useful in the distinction of reactive and malignant mesothelial proliferations and shows some promise in effusion fluids,[703] but further studies are necessary to further assess its utility in this context.

Labeling for the *X-linked inhibitor of apoptosis proteins* (XIAPs) also shows some promise in distinguishing benign from reactive pleural effusions, although this can be positive in mesotheliomas as well as some (but not all) metastatic adenocarcinomas, colonic adenocarcinomas being a notable exception.[704]

P glycoprotein (also known as p170) plays a role in cell membrane transport, and expression has been associated with resistance to chemotherapy.[689,705,706] Normal mesothelium has not been found to express this protein, but expression has been found in a high proportion of MMs, with no demonstrated effect on patient survival.[705] The overall sensitivity of this antibody for malignancy is relatively low at 52%; however, if labeling is present specificity is high, at about 92%.

GLUT-1[689] is part of a family of transmembranous glucose transporters, which facilitate the entry of glucose into cells. It is largely undetectable by immunohistochemistry in normal epithelial tissues and benign tumors, but is expressed in a variety of malignancies. In a study on pleural effusion fluids, GLUT-1 was expressed in 72% (28 of 39) of cases of malignant effusions: 100% from the ovary, 91% from the lung, 67% from the gastrointestinal tract, and 12% from the breast, but none (0/25) of the benign effusions expressed GLUT-1.[707] Thus, the expression of GLUT-1 appears to be a potentially useful marker of malignant transformation, but additional investigations are required to assess this marker further.

In rare instances, unusual substances have been demonstrated immunohistochemically in mesotheliomas. Okamoto et al.[708] reported two neoplasms consistent with primary pleural mesotheliomas that contained anaplastic tumor giant cells that demonstrated human chorionic gonadotropin on immunohistochemistry.

TABLE 43.17. Markers potentially useful in the distinction of reactive and malignant mesothelial proliferations

Antibody	Utility/comment
EMA (clone E29)	Strong, diffuse, linear labeling supports diagnosis of malignancy
p53	Sensitive but not very specific; labeling may support diagnosis of malignancy
Bcl-2	Specific but not very sensitive; labeling may support diagnosis of malignancy
Desmin	Positive in reactive lesions (and in some MMs with sarcomatoid features)

McAuley et al.[709] evaluated a patient with MM who had hypercalcemia and an elevated serum concentration of parathyroid-like hormone. They also evaluated nine epithelial mesotheliomas for parathyroid-like peptide and found abundant immunopositive cells in eight of nine cases. They also observed parathyroid-like peptide immunoreactivity in normal and reactive epithelial mesothelial cells.

Markers Related to Prognosis

A high proliferative index as assessed by *Mib-1* labeling has been found to be associated with a poorer prognosis in MM.[550] However, because there appears to be correlation between Mib-1 labeling index and the subtype of MM, the possibility that this represents poor survival associated with tumor type cannot be excluded.[549,550] Also, a mitotic activity index, assessed by direct count of mitotic figures, was not found to be an independent prognostic factor.[470]

Expression of the proliferation-associated antigen *p27*, which blocks progression of the cell cycle to mitosis, was also found to be related to prognosis, with lower expression being predictive of poorer survival,[554] but interestingly, and somewhat surprisingly, this was not linked to mitotic indices, so that the mechanism of action for p27 in this context appears uncertain.

Apart from being used as indicator of malignancy, labeling for XIAPs has also been suggested to predict poorer response to apoptosis-inducing chemotherapy regimens. Development and testing of XIAP-blocking drugs is underway, but further studies are needed before the value of this investigation can be assessed.[704]

Unsurprisingly, increased expression of *vascular endothelial growth factor* (VEGF), which may be triggered by tumor necrosis and which is an established growth factor for MM, has also been identified to predict a poorer outcome.[470]

The value of serial serum estimations of CA125 as a marker for progression of MM and hence prognosis, or its response to treatment, was discussed earlier in this section on immunohistochemistry.

Currently, it appears that although a number of markers are under investigation, no clinically or therapeutically useful marker has emerged.

Recommended Panel

The various antibodies/markers for MM diagnosis discussed in the preceding text (and some others) are summarized in Tables 43.14 to 43.18.[436,527,547,552,559,563,564,569,577,579–581,588–591,593–598,600,602–604,606,609–613,617,623–632,642–645,655,658,689–692,710–719] As also indicated in that discussion, we consider that an optimal approach to the IHC evaluation of possible or suspected mesothelioma entails each laboratory establishing its own protocol from proven cases of MM and non-MM lesions, and validating its methodology for each immunoreaction. Like the International Mesothelioma Panel,[37] we believe a reasonable and systematic first-line protocol would include the following:

- Immunostaining for CKs, for example, pan-CKs, CK8/18, or CK7
- Epithelial membrane antigen (EMA)
- *At least two mesothelial cell markers,* from a panel that would include calretinin as the most useful and specific marker at present, and one of the following: CK5/6, HBME-1, WT-1, podoplanin/D2-40, or perhaps thrombomodulin (the last also useful as an endothelial marker) (Table 43.18)
- *At least two carcinoma-related markers:* CEA, CD15 (Leu-M1 antigen), B72.3, BG-8, and TTF-1[648–656,661] (now standard in many protocols)

TABLE 43.18. Summary of immunoreactivity of malignant mesotheliomas with an epithelial component versus adenocarcinoma of lung

Tumor	CKs	CK5/6	CALR	HBME-1	WT1	TM	D2-40	MT	EMA	CEA	CD15	B72.3	BerEP4 MOC31	TTF-1
Malignant mesothelioma	+	+	+	+*	+	+	+	+	+*	0	0	0	0/+	0
Lung adenocarcinoma	+	0	0	0/+**	0	±	0	±	+**	+	+	+/0	+	+

CK, cytokeratins (AE1/AE3, CK8/18, CK7); CALR, calretinin; WT1, Wilms' tumor-1 antigen; TM, thrombomodulin; D2-40, podoplanin antibody; MT, mesothelin; EMA, epithelial membrane antigen; CEA, carcinoembryonic antigen; CD15, Leu-M1 antigen; TTF-1, thyroid transcription factor-1; +, usually positive; 0, usually negative; ±, may be positive or negative; *, linear, membrane-related; **, cytoplasmic.

In the event of discordant or equivocal findings, other members of each group can be added, or one can proceed to EM (for example, when there is one major discordant immunoreaction such as positive labeling for CEA, or two discordant reactions with antibodies of lesser specificity, such as Ber-EP4 or MOC31).

If the IHC protocol shows that the lesion is a carcinoma, the following labels can then be used according to the specific circumstances of the case:

- The CK7/CK20 profile[655,710]
- Others depending on the clinical background (e.g., prostate-specific antigen and prostatic acid phosphatase, especially if there is a suspicion or a past history of prostate cancer; CD99 and bcl-2 for biphasic tumors where synovial sarcoma enters the differential diagnosis; CD10, erythropoietin and RCC antigen if there is a suspicion of secondary RCC[711]; CD31, CD34, factor VIII–related antigen whenever epithelioid hemangioendothelioma enters into the differential diagnosis; and S-100 protein, HMB-45, and melan A if there is a suspicion of secondary melanoma (CK-negative tumor)

For pleura-based sarcomatoid tumors, the following simplified protocol can be used:

- Pan-CKs or low molecular weight CKs, ± vimentin
- ±CK5/6, calretinin (negative in about 50% of sarcomatoid mesotheliomas or more)
- CD34, bcl-2, CD99 (if the differential diagnosis includes solitary fibrous tumor)
- Ber-EP4, other carcinoma-related markers, bcl-2, CD99 (if the differential diagnosis includes synovial sarcoma)
- Others depending on the clinical background

Ultrastructural Features of Mesotheliomas

Several reports in the literature have illustrated the ultrastructural features of mesotheliomas.[79,720,721] Similarly, the ultrastructural features of primary lung neoplasms have been described extensively. In our experience, epithelial mesotheliomas have ultrastructural features that can be used to differentiate them from pulmonary adenocarcinomas and other primary lung carcinomas. The converse is also true: pulmonary adenocarcinomas and other primary lung carcinomas have electron microscopic features that can be used to differentiate them from epithelial mesotheliomas. This does not mean that every epithelial mesothelioma or every primary pulmonary carcinoma looks identical by electron microscopy, but there are enough ultrastructural differences to allow their separation.

Ultrastructurally, well and moderately well differentiated epithelial mesotheliomas are formed by cuboidal, polygonal, columnar, and round cells that are often connected to each other by well-formed desmosomes and junctional complexes (Fig. 43.71). Tumor cell nuclei are round, occasionally indented, and have medium-sized nucleoli. Their cytoplasm contains numerous mitochondria, short profiles of rough endoplasmic reticulum, and numerous intermediate filaments that are often aggregated into tonofilaments, which insert into large desmosomes connecting the cells together (Fig. 43.72). The most conspicuous ultrastructural feature of neoplastic epithelial mesothelial cells is the presence of numerous long, slender, sinuous microvilli that arise from the cell membrane (Fig. 43.73). These are often referred to as bushy microvilli. The neoplastic mesothelial cells are characteristically separated from the fibrovascular tissue by a well-defined basal lamina that is often infolded and is associated with micropinocytotic vesicles in the cell membrane of the adjacent mesothelial cells (Fig. 43.74). Epithelioid mesotheliomas composed of round cells have ultrastructural features similar to those of tubulopapillary mesotheliomas. They have long cell-surface microvilli, numerous cytoplasmic intermediate filaments, including tonofilaments, and aggregates of cytoplasmic glycogen (Fig. 43.75). Some mesotheliomas show microvillus-matrix interaction in which the microvilli of an

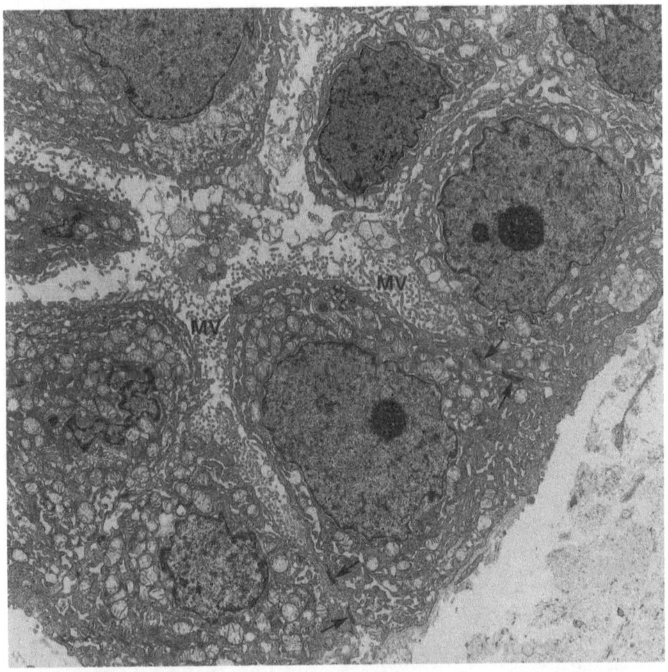

FIGURE 43.71. Electron micrograph shows representative region of tubulopapillary mesothelioma. Tumor cells are similar in size and shape and are connected to each other by well-formed desmosomes (arrows). Round nuclei located near center of cell have medium-sized nucleoli. Cytoplasm contains numerous mitochondria and other organelles. Note microvilli (MV) arising from cell surface.

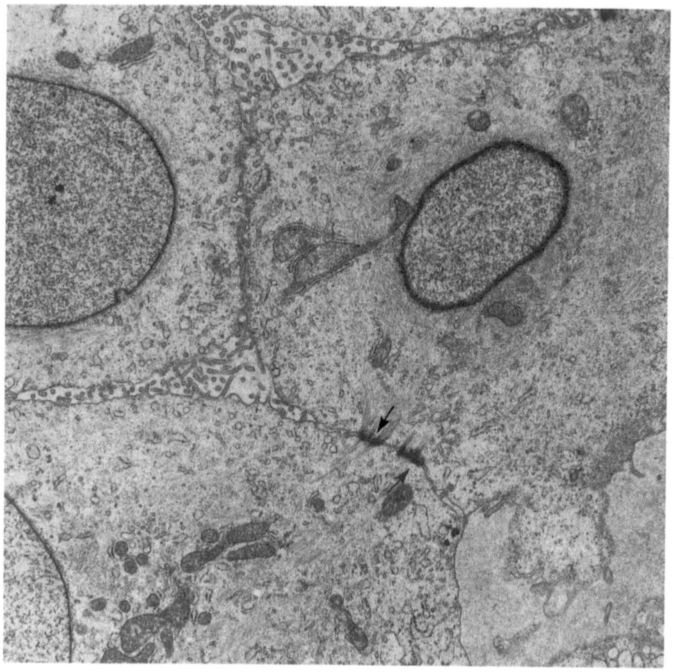

FIGURE 43.72. Mesothelial cells are usually connected by large desmosomes into which intermediate filaments insert (arrows).

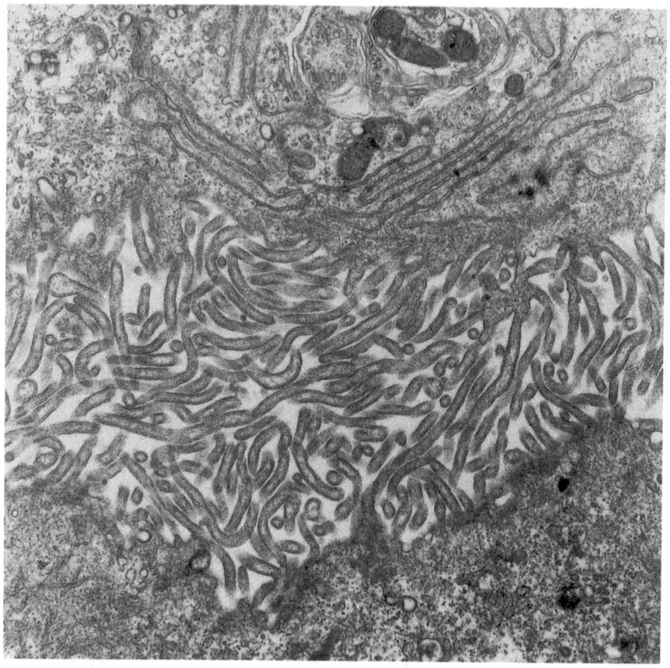

FIGURE 43.73. Most characteristic feature of epithelial mesothelioma cells is long sinuous microvilli. These have length-to-width ratios averaging 10 to 15, significantly greater than the length-to-width ratio of microvilli of pulmonary adenocarcinomas, and are not covered by a fuzzy glycocalyx.

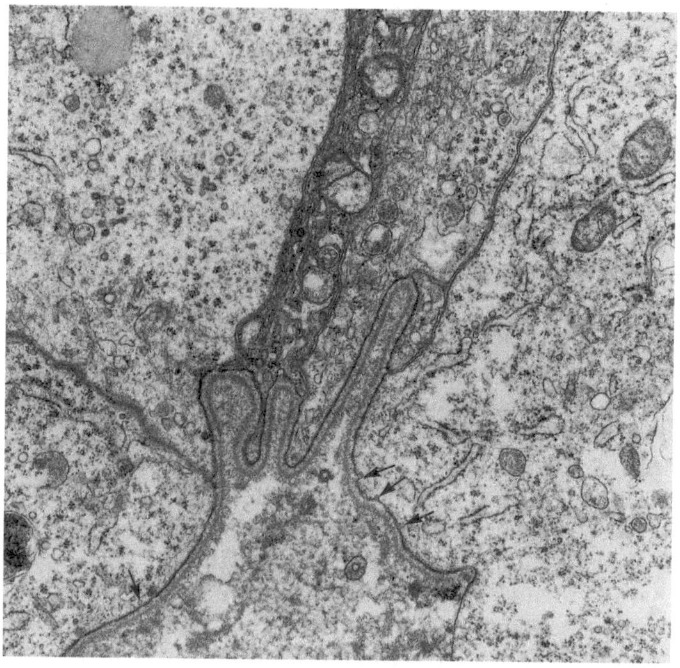

FIGURE 43.74. Portions of several mesothelioma cells show invagination of their cytoplasm and investment by basal lamina. Note micropinocytotic vesicles in cell membrane of tumor cells (arrows).

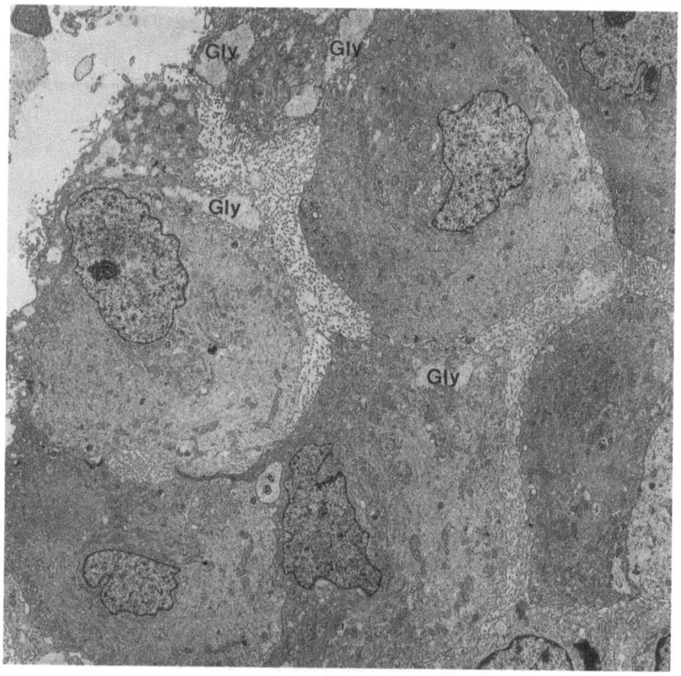

FIGURE 43.75. Ultrastructural appearance of epithelioid mesothelioma. Cells are round with abundant intracellular intermediate filaments and aggregates of glycogen (Gly).

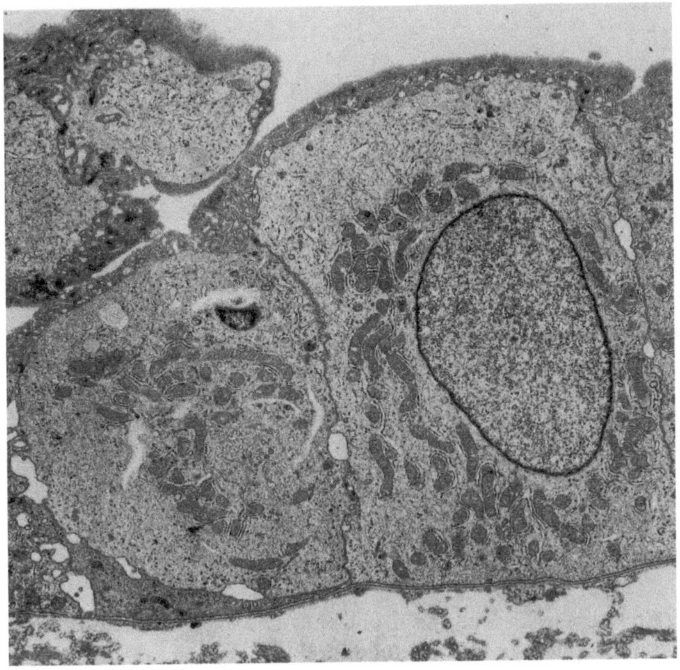

FIGURE 43.76. Some epithelial mesotheliomas produce hyaluronic acid. This is not seen within cytoplasm of tumor cells but appears as medium electron-dense material on cell surface in which microvilli are "embedded."

epithelial mesothelioma directly penetrate into adjacent collagen fibrils.

Approximately 20% of epithelial mesotheliomas produce a mucosubstance, hyaluronic acid and proteoglycan, that can be identified ultrastructurally as a medium electron-dense material associated with the cell microvilli (Fig. 43.76). This material is often seen in intracellular neolumina and often crystallizes (Fig. 43.77). Hyaluronic acid may form scroll-like crystalline structures (Fig. 43.78). Mesotheliomas that show the crystalloid material typically are "mucin-positive," showing intracellular PAS-D, mucicarmine, hyaluronidase-resistant and Alcian blue/colloidal iron-hyaluronidase–resistant material.

Sarcomatoid MMs have variable ultrastructural features. The tumor cells may resemble fibroblasts (Fig. 43.79), containing short profiles of distended rough endoplasmic reticulum, a prominent Golgi apparatus, and occasionally inspissated electron-dense material in the cisterna of the rough endoplasmic reticulum. Other sarcomatoid MMs show more variability in size and shape (Fig. 43.80) and occasionally show epithelial differentiation in the form of well-formed intercellular junctions (Fig. 43.81), basal lamina formation (Fig. 43.82), and tonofilaments (Fig. 43.83). They may even show a few microvilli arising from the cell surface (Fig. 43.80). Some sarcomatoid mesotheliomas have an ultrastructural appearance resembling myofibroblasts, containing peripherally located actin filaments and centrally located short profiles of rough endoplasmic reticulum[722] (Fig. 43.84). Desmoplastic MMs have variable ultrastructural features, being composed of cells that resemble fibroblasts or myofibroblasts.

Transitional mesotheliomas are composed of cells with electron microscopic features of both epithelial and mesenchymal cells. The tumor cells are frequently connected to each other by relatively well-formed intercellular junctions, have aggregated mitochondria, and have cytoplasmic intermediate filaments that may represent vimentin (Fig. 43.85). In some tumor cells, thin actin filaments are observed in association with the cell membrane. The tumor cells typically do not show the long, sinuous microvilli observed in better differentiated epithelial mesotheliomas.

The epithelial component of biphasic mesotheliomas shows the ultrastructural features of epithelial mesotheliomas with long bushy cell-surface microvilli and abundant intracellular tonofilaments and other organelles. The sarcomatoid portion is composed of cells with electron microscopic characteristics of sarcomatoid MMs. In transition zones, the tumor cells may have an ultrastructural appearance transitional between cells expressing epithelial features and other cells expressing sarcomatoid features.

Most of the controversy concerning the ultrastructural features of mesotheliomas has centered around epithelial

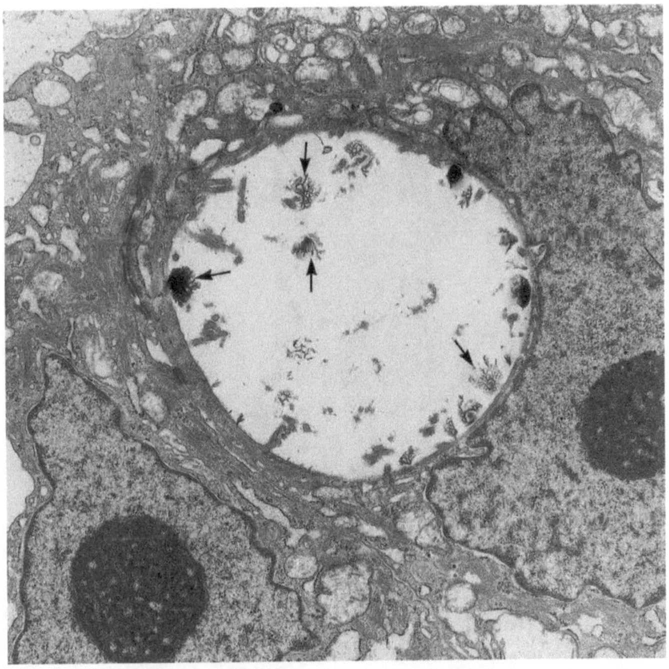

FIGURE 43.77. Intracellular lumen in mesothelioma cell shows crystallized mucosubstance (arrows) that has a fern-like appearance.

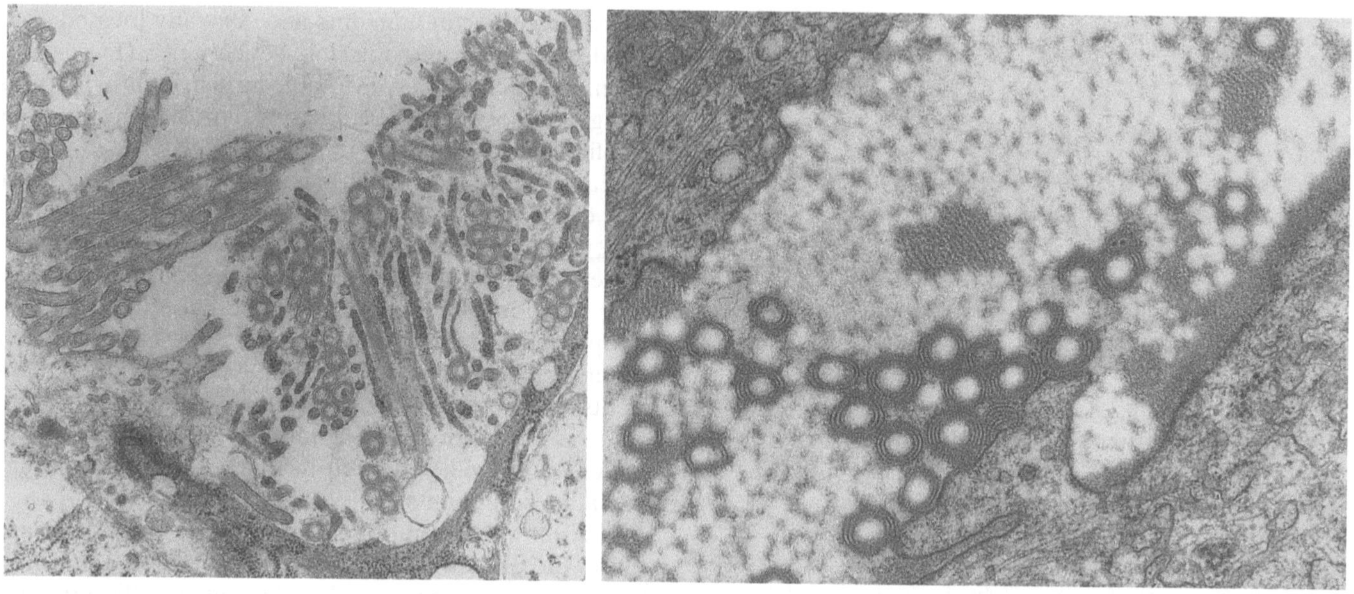

A B

FIGURE 43.78. **(A)** In this hyaluronic acid–producing epithelial mesothelioma, hyaluronic acid crystallized to form hollow tubular structures with a scroll-like appearance on cross section. **(B)** In cross section, the hyaluronic acid crystals have a scroll-like morphology and resemble hollow chrysotile fibrils.

mesotheliomas, specifically with respect to whether they can be differentiated ultrastructurally from pulmonary adenocarcinomas or other types of adenocarcinomas. Warhol et al.[723] and Warhol and Corson[724] studied quantitatively the difference between the microvilli of epithelial mesotheliomas and pulmonary and breast adenocarcinomas. They found the mean length-to-diameter ratio of epithelial mesothelioma microvilli was 15.7, whereas pulmonary adenocarcinoma microvilli had a length-to-diameter ratio of 8.7. Burns et al.[725] found

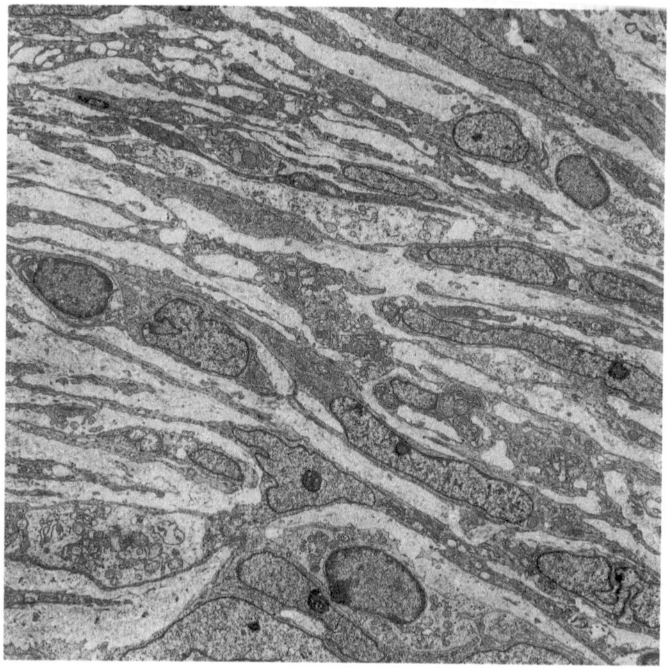

FIGURE 43.79. Sarcomatoid mesothelioma composed of spindle cells that resemble fibroblasts.

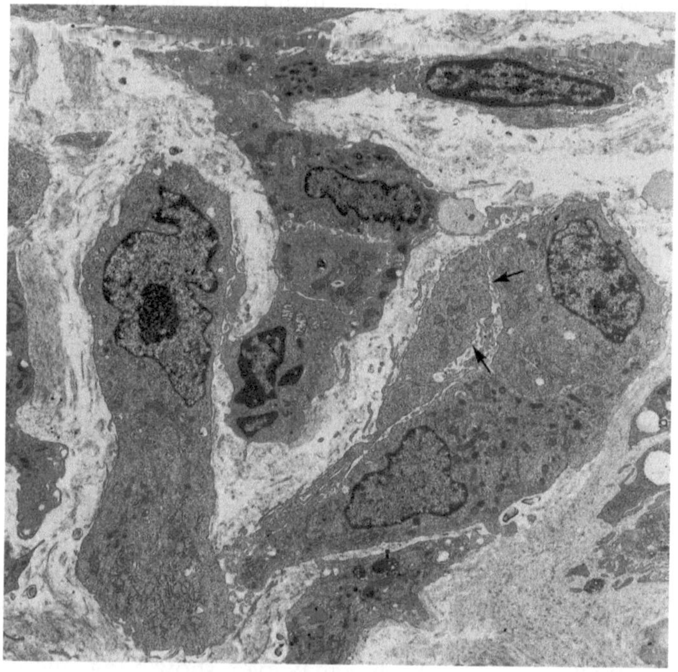

FIGURE 43.80. Sarcomatoid mesothelioma composed mostly of spindle-shaped cells with large nuclei. An occasional cell shows a few cell-surface microvilli (arrows).

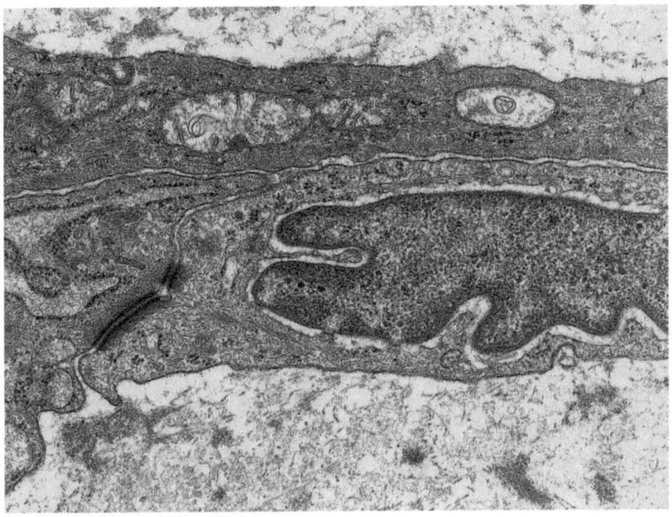

FIGURE 43.81. Some neoplastic cells in this sarcomatoid mesothelioma are connected to each other by well-formed desmosomes.

similar results with a mean length-to-diameter ratio of 11.44 for seven epithelial mesotheliomas and 5.39 for three pulmonary adenocarcinomas. Warhol and colleagues also found epithelial mesotheliomas had more cytoplasmic tonofilaments than pulmonary adenocarcinomas. Hammar et al.[79,669] have emphasized the overall difference in the pattern of the microvilli of epithelial mesotheliomas and pulmonary adenocarcinomas. As

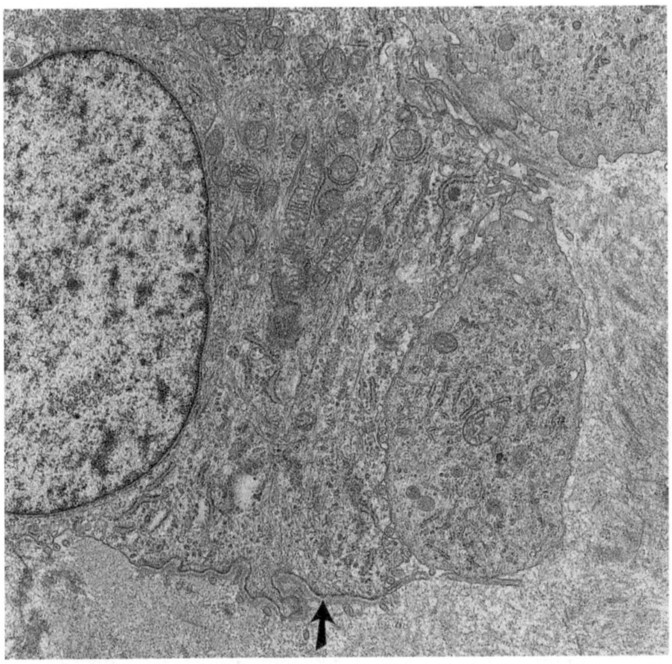

FIGURE 43.82. Some neoplastic cells forming this sarcomatoid mesothelioma are surrounded by basal lamina (arrow).

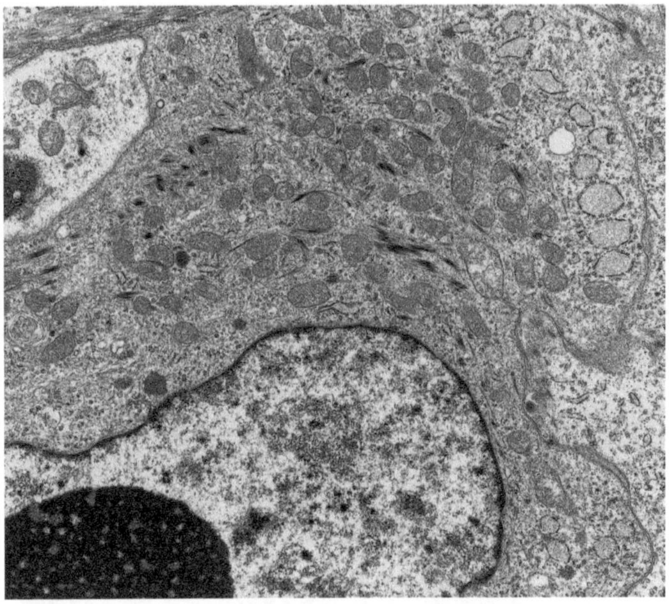

FIGURE 43.83. In this sarcomatoid mesothelioma, many neoplastic cells contain aggregates of intermediate filaments in their cytoplasm consistent with tonofilaments.

shown, the microvilli of epithelial mesotheliomas are numerous, long, and sinuous, whereas the microvilli of pulmonary adenocarcinomas are frequently short, straight, and covered by a fuzzy glycocalyx. We do not

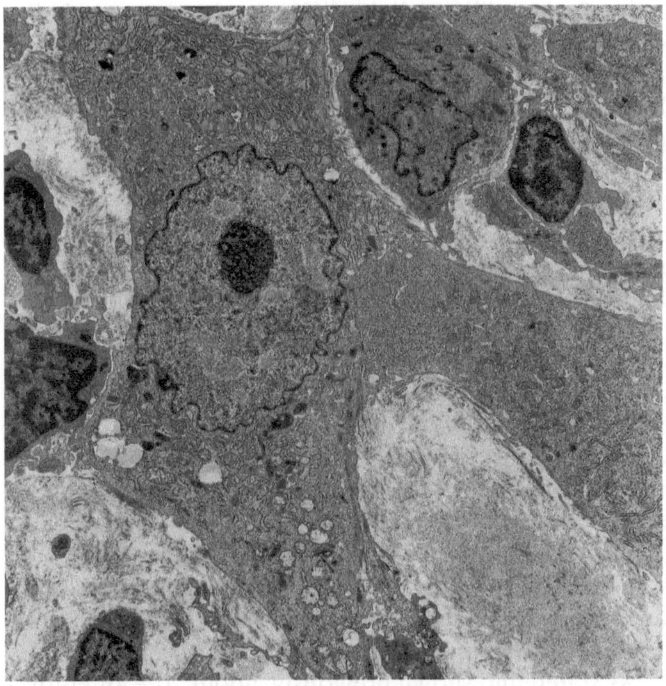

FIGURE 43.84. Some cells of this sarcomatoid mesothelioma have ultrastructural features of myofibroblasts, with peripherally located thin filaments consistent with actin filaments and abundant short profiles of rough endoplasmic reticulum.

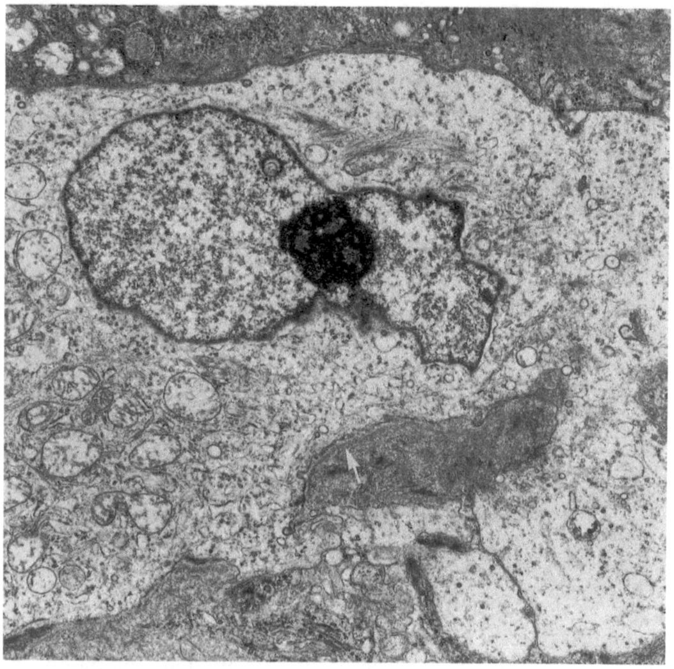

FIGURE 43.85. Transitional mesothelioma composed of large polygonal cells with large nuclei and relatively nonspecialized cytoplasm. A few intermediate filaments in cell cytoplasm resemble tonofilaments. Note focal basal lamina (arrow).

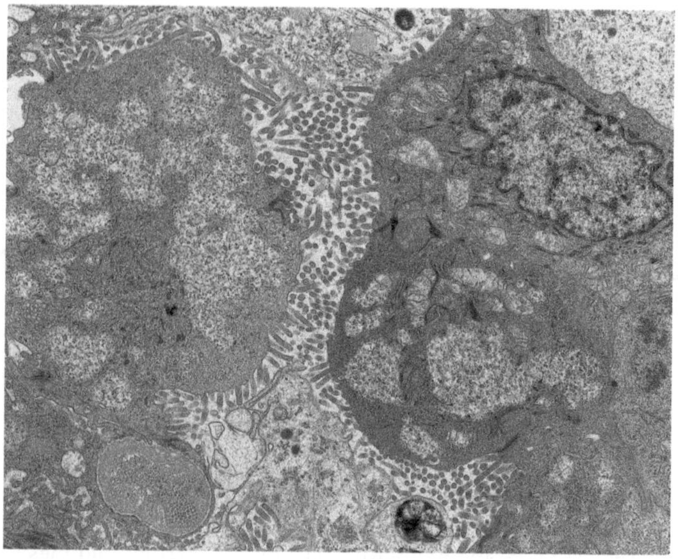

FIGURE 43.86. Peripheral pulmonary adenocarcinoma had long slender microvilli resembling those seen in epithelial mesothelioma.

believe it is necessary to determine the length-to-width ratio of microvilli to tell the difference between epithelial mesothelioma and pulmonary adenocarcinoma. Determining the length-width ratio is difficult because the long, thin, sinuous microvilli are usually not in the same plane of section, and the entire length cannot be measured. Rare pulmonary adenocarcinomas exist that have relatively long microvilli and at first glance may resemble an epithelial mesothelioma (Fig. 43.86), but on closer inspection are covered by fuzzy microvilli (Fig. 43.87), a finding incompatible with an epithelial mesothelioma.

There are other ultrastructural differences between epithelial MMs and pulmonary adenocarcinomas. The cells forming epithelial mesotheliomas and pulmonary adenocarcinomas are connected to each other by intercellular junctions. Where the tumor cells form glands, they are attached by junctional complexes and elsewhere are connected predominantly by desmosomes. As a general rule, the desmosomes connecting mesothelioma tumor cells are larger than those connecting pulmonary adenocarcinoma cells. This observation has been confirmed by a semiquantitative study.[726]

As stated and shown previously, about 20% of epithelial mesotheliomas produce hyaluronic acid, which can be identified ultrastructurally as a medium-electron-dense material in which the cell microvilli appear embedded. Hyaluronic acid–producing mesotheliomas do not contain mucosubstance granules in their cytoplasm, which is in contrast to the 60% to 75% of pulmonary adenocarcinomas that are mucus-producing and contain cytoplasmic mucous granules of variable size and density that are often associated with a prominent terminal web. Pulmonary adenocarcinomas of Clara cell or type II pneumocyte origin frequently contain cytoplasmic multivesicular bodies and lamellar bodies. These structures are infre-

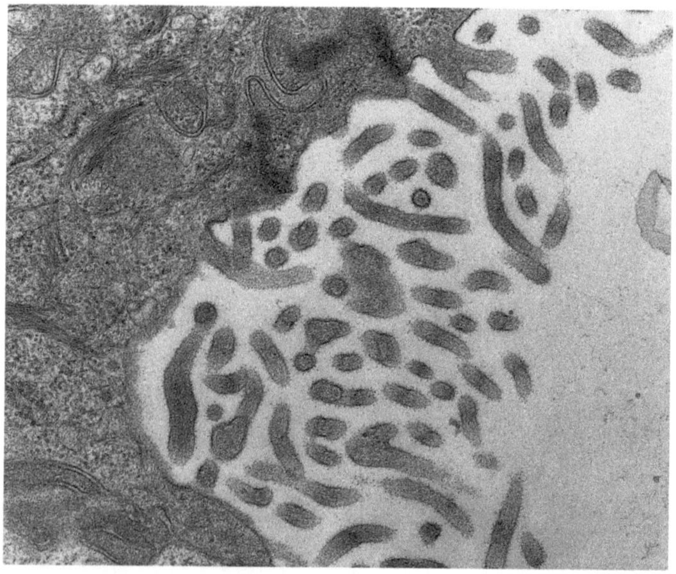

FIGURE 43.87. At greater magnification, long microvilli of neoplastic cells were covered by fuzzy glycocalyx, a finding not seen in epithelial mesothelioma.

TABLE 43.19. Comparison of the ultrastructural features of epithelial mesothelioma and pulmonary adenocarcinoma

Ultrastructural features	Epithelial mesothelioma	Pulmonary adenocarcinoma
Microvilli	Long, sinuous, smooth	Short, usually straight; covered by fuzzy glycocalyx
Intercellular junctions	Junctional complexes; large desmosomes	Junctional complexes; small desmosomes
Mucosubstance production	No mucosubstance granules in cytoplasm; mucosubstance on cell surface; crystallization	Mucous granules in cytoplasm; glycocalyceal bodies; mucus in gland lumen
Cytoplasmic intermediate filaments	Abundant; often in a perinuclear distribution; tonofilaments frequent	Common; often distributed throughout cytoplasm; tonofilaments variable
Cytoplasmic inclusions	Infrequent; some lysosomes	Frequent; multivesicular bodies and lamellar bodies frequent in bronchioloalveolar cell carcinoma

quently seen in epithelial mesotheliomas. A comparison of some of the ultrastructural features of epithelial mesotheliomas and pulmonary adenocarcinomas is shown in Table 43.19.

Cytogenetic and Molecular Features in Mesothelial Cell Proliferations

Cytogenetic abnormalities are commonly found in MMs. Tiainen et al.[727] performed successful cytogenetic analyses on cells obtained from solid tumors and from pleural effusions in 34 of 38 patients with MM. Clonal chromosomal abnormalities were detected in 25 patients, the majority being complex and heterogeneous with no chromosome abnormality specific to mesothelioma. Nine patients had normal karyotypes or nonclonal chromosomal abnormalities. Translocations and deletions involving a breakpoint at 1p11-p22 were the most common structural abnormality. The number of copies of chromosome 7 short arms was inversely correlated with survival, and a high concentration of asbestos fibers in the lung tissue was associated with partial or total loss of chromosomes 1 and 4, and a breakpoint at 1p11-p22.

Hagemeijer et al.[728] evaluated 40 confirmed cases of MM, in 90% of cases using malignant cells in pleural fluid. A normal karyotype was found in nine cases, and complex karyotypic abnormalities were identified in 30 cases. The chromosomal changes were all complex and heterogeneous, with no consistent specific abnormality found. Two main patterns of nonrandom abnormalities were found: (1) loss of chromosomes 4 and 22, 9p and 30p in the most abnormal cases, corresponding to a hypodiploid and for hypotetraploid modal chromosome number; and (2) gain of chromosomes 7, 5, and 20 with deletion or rearrangement of 3p.

Hicks[729] recently reviewed the biologic, cytogenetic, and molecular factors in mesotheliomas and mesothelial cell proliferations. As Hicks pointed out, these types of studies have been performed in an attempt to identify specific, nonrandom alterations that may be useful in diagnosing mesotheliomas and mesothelial cell proliferations. Hicks and others have reported that karyotyping mesotheliomas has not provided any specific diagnostic abnormalities. The changes one sees are listed in Tables 1 and 2 of Hicks's review article (see also the discussion of chromosomal abnormalities in Molecular Events in the Development of Mesothelioma III, above.)

Davidson et al.[730] reported on chemokine receptors expressed on malignant or benign mesothelial cells. They concluded that chemokine receptors were widely expressed on leukocytes in MM and reactive mesothelial effusions, but were rarely found on normal cells of mesothelial origin. The findings were stated to argue against an autocrine chemokine pathway in MM. An increased monocyte infiltration and higher expression of chemokine receptors in these cells in MM effusions could possibly have tumor-promoting rather than inhibiting effects.

Jaurand[731] reported on asbestos, chromosomal deletions, and tumor suppressor gene alterations in human MM, and found the most frequent alterations were on chromosome losses involving chromosomes 1, 3, and 9 (most often p arm), and chromosomes 6, 13, 14, 15, and 22 (most often q arm). Chromosomal gains were reported on chromosome 5 and 7 (most often on the p arm).

Janne[732] developed two proteomic methods to identify potential therapeutic targets. The first had to do with a pan-receptor tyrosine kinase and the second had to do with activators of the PI3K/Akt pathway.

Christensen et al.[733] reported on asbestos burden and epigenetic silencing in pleural MM and found that asbestos induced a pronounced epigenetic silencing of tumor suppressor genes in a fashion directly related to measurable lung function burden. They stated that this novel tumorigenic mechanism of action for asbestos had not been previously described and could help understand the role of asbestos in the development of MM, as well as the clinical course (see Molecular Pathogenesis and Pathology of Malignant Mesothelioma).

Rihn[734] evaluated oxidative stress gene modulation in pleural mesotheliomas as assessed by microarray and found dozens of overexpressed genes in mesothelioma that promoted local invasion; protected cells against oxidative stress; and counteracted the anticancer therapies. Rihn concluded the portrait of normal and cancerous

TABLE 43.20. DNA indices and proliferative rates of malignant mesotheliomas versus reactive mesothelial cells and other nonmesothelial malignant neoplasms

Study	Malignant mesothelioma					Reactive mesothelial cells					Non-mesothelioma malignant neoplasms				
	No. of cases/ specimens	DNA index		S phase		No. of cases/ specimens	DNA index		S phase		No. of cases/ specimens	DNA index		S phase	
		Diploid	Aneuploid	≤6%	>6%		Diploid	Aneuploid	≤6%	>6%		Diploid	Aneuploid	≤6%	>6%
Croonen et al.[736]	13[a]	10	3[b]	ND	ND	45[a]	40	5[c]	ND	ND	29[a]	7[d]	22	ND	ND
Hafiz et al.[737]	18[e]	30.5±[f]	7.2[f]	ND	ND	14[e]	15.2[f]	±2.9[f]	ND	ND	—				
Frierson et al.[738]	19[g]	9	10[i]	ND	ND	28[h]	28	0	ND	ND					
Burmer et al.[739]	46[j]	30[k]	15[l]	23[m]	22[m]	—	—	—	—	—	31[n]	4[o]	27[o]	15[p]	15[p]
Dazzi et al.[740]	70[q]	3[r]	34[r]	19[s]	36[s]	—	—	—	—						
Tierney et al.[741]	25[t]	u	U	ND	ND	11[t]	u	u	ND	ND	20[t]	—	20	ND	ND
El-Naggar et al.[742]	23[v]	18	6[w]	x	x				—	—	41[y]	5[z]	36[z]	aa	aa
Esteban and Sheibani[743]	45[bb]	30	5	cc	5[cc]	—	—	—	—	—	41[dd]	10	31	ee	ee

[a]Malignant cells in pleural/peritoneal fluids.
[b]Autopsy diagnosis was lung adenocarcinoma in two cases.
[c]In two of 54 cases there was an associated malignancy, but no evidence of malignancy on follow-up.
[d]In one case a primary tumor was not identified, and there was no evidence of recurrence or metastases.
[e]Cells in pleural or peritoneal fluid.
[f]Mean DNA content of 50 mesothelial cells in arbitrary absorbance units as determined by analysis of Feulgen-stained cells. The DNA content of mesothelial cells was compared to the DNA content of lymphocytes.
[g]Deparaffinized malignant epithelial mesothelioma.
[h]Reactive cells in pleural or peritoneal effusions.
[i]None of the malignant epithelial mesotheliomas had multiple aneuploid peaks.
[j]Of the 46 mesotheliomas, 30 were epithelial, five were sarcomatous, and 11 were biphasic
[k]Diploid or near-diploid.
[l]All but two of the aneuploid mesotheliomas exhibited a single aneuploid peak. No significant difference between percentage of aneuploid mesotheliomas according to histologic type.
[m]Only "fresh" tissue specimens were analyzed and one case could not be evaluated. Average S phase for diploid mesotheliomas was 5.0% (17 cases) and 8.7% for aneuploid mesotheliomas (10 cases). No significant correlation between S phase and histologic subtype.
[n]Seven primary pulmonary adenocarcinomas; six primary poorly differentiated squamous carcinomas; three primary poorly differentiated carcinomas, not otherwise specified; four primary lung sarcomas; three metastatic sarcomas; four metastatic breast carcinomas; and four metastatic renal cell carcinomas.
[o]Nonmesothelioma malignant tumors that were diploid included one primary pulmonary adenocarcinoma, one metastatic renal cell carcinoma, one primary pulmonary sarcoma, and one metastatic sarcoma.
[p]One case could not be analyzed.
[q]168 paraffin-embedded tissue specimens from 70 patients with malignant pleural mesothelioma, 31 epithelial mesotheliomas, 21 sarcomatoid mesotheliomas, and 18 biphasic mesotheliomas.
[r]37 cases diploid or near-diploid, 34 cases aneuploid or multi-aneuploid.
[s]Phase % could be calculated in 55 cases. Range was 0.8–16.1%, median S phase was 6%.
[t]Feulgen stained nuclei of 100 tumor cells/reactive cells were measured using a DNA image analyzer. Lymphocyte nuclei were used as controls. Aneuploidy determined by measuring 5*c* exceeding rate (5*c*ER), which was defined as the percentage of aneuploid cells having a DNA content >5*c* where diploid = 2*c*. Previous studies suggested a 5*c*ER or greater than 0.1 was malignant. In this study, a 5*c*ER of 1 was used as a cutoff for malignancy.
[u]Information not given. Using the cutoff of 1 for 5*c*ER (see footnote t), 14 "mesothelial" cases were classified as benign, and 22 as malignant, which equated to a false-negative rate of 57% and a false-positive rate of 23%. All of the nonmesothelial tumors had a 5*c*ER >1, which indicated they were aneuploid.
[v]All cases were of pleural origin and had epithelial histology. Tumor tissue from multiple blocks were analyzed.
[w]The mesotheliomas that were aneuploid exhibited a "solid" growth pattern.
[x]S + G_2M of 18 diploid mesotheliomas was 5.83 ± 2.62 SD. S + G_2M of five aneuploid mesotheliomas was 5.0 ± 1.23 SD.
[z]Of the 36 aneuploid pulmonary adenocarcinomas, 31 were well to moderately differentiated, and five were poorly differentiated. Of the five diploid pulmonary adenocarcinomas, four were well to moderately differentiated, and one was poorly differentiated.
[aa]SG_2M of 5 diploid pulmonary adenocarcinomas was 12 ± 7.48 SD. SG_2M for 36 aneuploid pulmonary adenocarcinomas was 16.42 ± 10.21 SD.
[bb]Thirty-one epithelial mesotheliomas, six sarcomatoid mesotheliomas, eight biphasic mesotheliomas. Five of the 45 mesotheliomas could not be analyzed because the histograms obtained were uninterpretable; five other cases of mesothelioma were excluded because the coefficients of variation were >9.
[cc]Not all cases could be analyzed; in most aneuploid mesotheliomas the S phase could not be determined. Five (17) of the diploid mesotheliomas had an S phase >10%.
[dd]All cases were pulmonary adenocarcinomas.
[ee]Nine of the diploid adenocarcinomas had an S phase >10%.
ND, not done.

pleura achieved at the mRNA level seemed meaningful for the understanding of asbestos-mediated carcinogenesis, and for mesothelioma stratification and management. Rihn stated mesothelioma markers described in the study should improve the accuracy of mesothelioma diagnosis and therapy.

Bahnassy et al.[735] evaluated the role of $p14^{ARF}$, $p16^{INK4A}$, and their related genes in MM and concluded that pleural MM is a complex disease characterized by multiple genetic aberrations in the cell cycle regulatory genes. The authors identified regulatory genes that seemed to play a role in the pathogenesis of mesothelioma and also other pathways that were involved in the progression and survival of mesothelioma.

DNA Analysis and Proliferative Index in Malignant Mesothelioma

DNA concentrations or proliferative rates have been evaluated in reactive mesothelial cell proliferations and in MMs[736–743] (Table 43.20). Croonen et al.[736] concluded that mesotheliomas were usually DNA-euploid, whereas most adenocarcinomas were aneuploid. Hafiz et al.,[737] using cytophotometry to evaluate the DNA content of cells in Feulgen-stained sections of effusion specimens, found the mean DNA content of malignant mesothelial cells (30.5 ± 7.2) was significantly higher than the mean DNA content of reactive mesothelial cells (15.2 ± 2.9). Frierson et al.[738] determined that 53% of epithelial mesotheliomas were aneuploid, but considered that the finding of DNA aneuploid cells in an effusion specimen supported the diagnosis of MM. Burmer et al.[739] found most MMs to be DNA diploid with low to intermediate proliferative rates, whereas 85% of primary lung carcinomas were DNA aneuploid and had high proliferative rates.

In the study of Dazzi et al.,[740] 38.6% of mesotheliomas were diploid and 61.4% were aneuploid, and a higher percentage of epithelial mesotheliomas were diploid. The authors found no significant difference in survival in the patients whose mesotheliomas were aneuploid versus diploid. Patients whose tumor showed an S-phase percentage greater than the median of 6% had a significantly shorter survival than those whose tumors had a lower S-phase percentage. Tierney et al.[741] determined DNA cellular concentrations using DNA image analysis of Feulgen-stained tissue sections. These authors concluded that mesothelial lesions appeared to have a wide range of ploidy values regardless of their biologic behavior, and that ploidy could not be used as a reliable diagnostic index in diagnosing primary mesothelial tumors.

El-Naggar et al.[742] analyzed epithelial mesotheliomas by flow cytometry and compared them with pulmonary adenocarcinomas, and found that 80% of pulmonary adenocarcinomas and 100% of pleural mesotheliomas showed a homogeneous DNA ploidy; 78% of epithelial mesotheliomas were diploid, whereas 88% of pulmonary adenocarcinomas were aneuploid. The proliferative fraction (S-phase percentage) of aneuploid adenocarcinomas was significantly greater than aneuploid epithelial MMs, leading the authors to conclude that the DNA indices of epithelial mesotheliomas were significantly different from pulmonary adenocarcinomas. Esteban and Sheibani,[743] in their flow cytometric analysis, found that 14% of mesotheliomas were aneuploid; in contrast, 75% of pulmonary adenocarcinomas were aneuploid. These authors recommended that ploidy analysis should be used in diagnostically difficult cases of possible mesothelioma.

More recently, Cakir et al.[744] evaluated cell proliferation rate and telomerase activity in the differential diagnosis between benign and malignant mesothelial cell proliferations. By means of immunohistochemical analysis for Ki-67 and human telomerase reverse transcriptase (hTERT), the mean value of Ki-67 proliferation index in MMs was found to be significantly higher than that of benign mesothelial lesions. Ki-67 immunohistochemistry was reported to have a sensitivity of 74%, a specificity of 86%, and a positive predictive value of 94% in detecting MM. The hTERT immunohistochemistry detected MM with a sensitivity and specificity of 68%. The authors suggested that immunohistochemistry profiling for Ki-67 and hTERT was useful in differentiating malignant and benign mesothelial lesions in routine formalin-fixed, paraffin-embedded material.

Rare/Unusual Mesotheliomas or Mesothelial Proliferations

Benign Mesothelial Inclusions in Lymph Nodes

Although regional lymph node metastases can occur with pleural MMs—to axillary, cervical, bronchial, mediastinal, and retroperitoneal lymph nodes—as part of late-stage disease (for example, as an autopsy finding[211]) or even as a presenting manifestation.[745–748] Such metastatic deposits require distinction from benign mesothelial inclusions within subpleural, bronchial, or mediastinal lymph nodes,[119,749,750] related to chronic inflammatory processes affecting the pleura (and occasionally other serosal membranes). In some cases, the reactive mesothelial cell inclusions are confined to or concentrated within the subcapsular sinuses (Fig. 43.88), but deeper extension into lymph node tissue is also recorded and no clear criteria for histologic discrimination between benign inclusions of this type and metastatic MMs have been delineated. Accordingly, the International Mesothelioma

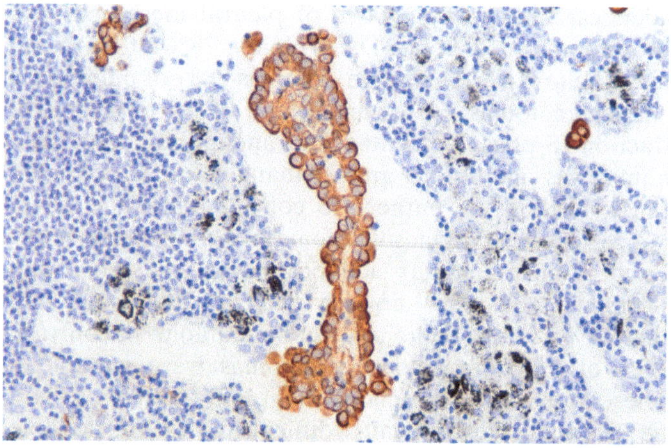

FIGURE 43.88. One of multiple benign mesothelial inclusions with a papillary architecture found in bronchial lymph nodes in an elderly woman who had undergone pneumonectomy for treatment of a non–small-cell carcinoma of lung. The mesothelial cells are concentrated within sinusoids. Their identity as mesothelial inclusions was established in this case by immunohistochemistry and by electron microscopic examination of deparaffinized tissue.

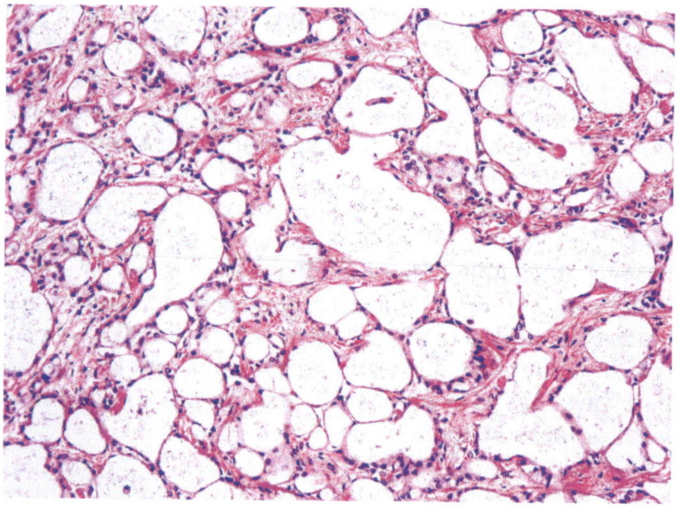

FIGURE 43.89. Pleural adenomatoid tumor discovered as an incidental autopsy finding in an elderly man. The tumor consists entirely of microcystic spaces lined by attenuated cells, with a sparse intervening fibrocollagenous stroma.

Panel[37] recommends that a diagnosis of metastatic mesothelioma within lymph nodes should be supported by one or both of the following criteria: (1) a diagnostic biopsy of the corresponding serosal membrane, or (2) radiologic evidence supportive of an underlying pleural mesothelioma (such as diffuse pleural thickening with encasement of the lung, accompanied by evidence of nodularity).

Adenomatoid Tumor of the Pleura

Characteristically, adenomatoid tumors represent benign mesothelial tumors that develop in relation to the reproductive tract of either males (testis/epididymis[751]) or females (uterus[752]). In these locations they are often clinically silent lesions, although they can produce clinically detectable localized mass lesions (especially in relation to the testis/epididymis).

On gross examination, adenomatoid tumor is a nonencapsulated and usually poorly delineated firm, pale yellow mass. Histologic examination reveals unencapsulated lesions that comprise multiple microcystic spaces and complex tubules, embedded within a fibrous stroma and lined by flattened epithelial-type cells that express immunohistochemical markers of mesothelial differentiation. The differential diagnosis includes lymphangioma, and it is important to emphasize that the antibody D2-40 labels both lymphatic endothelium and mesothelial cells.[632,753]

Pleural adenomatoid tumors[37,754,755] (Fig. 43.89) are exceedingly rare and typically represent small and clinically silent lesions.[37] The major differential diagnosis for pleural adenomatoid tumor is that of a conventional MM with focal or extensive microcystic change producing an adenomatoid appearance (Fig. 43.90; also see Figs. 43.27 and 43.28). Accordingly, the following criteria for the diagnosis of pleural adenomatoid tumor are suggested[37]:

- The tumor typically is a lesion found incidentally either in surgery (thoracoscopy or thoracotomy) carried out for other reasons[755] or at autopsy (Fig. 43.89); that is, there should be no clinical manifestations such as a

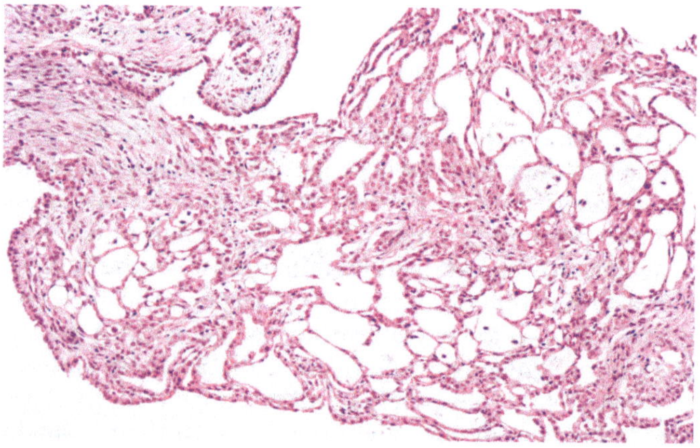

FIGURE 43.90. Pleural malignant mesothelioma with focal microcystic (adenomatoid) features, in a woman in her 30s, who had sustained childhood environmental exposure to crocidolite at Wittenoom in Western Australia. In its advanced clinical stage, this mesothelioma showed prominent transdiaphragmatic spread into the peritoneum, with intractable ascites.

pleural effusion directly attributable to the adenomatoid tumor.

- The tumor is a small localized lesion; the International Mesothelioma Panel has suggested that it should be less than 5 mm in greatest dimension,[37] but occasionally it may be larger (Fig. 43.89).
- The histologic appearance is of a benign adenomatoid tumor throughout. It is recommended that the entire lesion be embedded and sectioned, with no areas characteristic of conventional MM of epithelial type.[37] Tumors that show areas of conventional MM with either focal or extensive adenomatoid features should be designated as a conventional MM showing microcystic change (Fig. 43.90).
- The phenotype should conform to a mesothelial lesion on either immunohistochemistry or electron microscopy, or both.
- The differential diagnosis in the pleura also includes an epithelioid hemangioendothelioma, from which adenomatoid tumors are distinguishable by absence of labeling for markers of endothelial differentiation (CD31, CD34, and factor VIII–related antigen[37]). In addition, although some epithelioid hemangioendotheliomas show weak to moderate expression of cytokeratins, most do not, whereas adenomatoid tumors characteristically show moderate to strong cytokeratin expression, like other mesothelial lesions.

Well-Differentiated Papillary Mesothelioma

Well-differentiated papillary mesothelioma (WDPM) is well recognized in the peritoneum, usually in middle-aged women.[756–767] The median age in the series of 22 cases reported by Daya and McCaughey[759] was 40 years (range, 25–69 years), and 18 of the 22 patients were women. A WDPM may represent either solitary and localized lesions or multifocal tumors, and it generally measures about 5 to 20 mm in diameter. Some authors consider the localized lesions to be benign and amenable to cure by local resection,[757,764,768] whereas others designate WDPMs as tumors of borderline or attenuated malignant potential,[758,763] with an indolent natural history[765] even when they are multifocal.[762] Even so, one of 14 cases so diagnosed by Butnor et al.[767] pursued an aggressive clinical course. Rare examples of WDPM have also been encountered in the pericardium,[769] the tunica vaginalis testis,[767,768] and the pleura.[766,767,770]

Butnor et al.[767] reported 14 cases of WDPM, seven of which affected the pleura, six in the peritoneum, and one in the tunica vaginalis. Eleven of the patients were men and three were women (presumably reflecting a selected group of patients, as expected for a tertiary referral center), with an average age of 58 years (range, 32–82 years). Six of the patients had a history of asbestos exposure. Of nine cases with complete follow-up, six had clinically indolent disease, but one case pursued an aggressive course. The authors concluded that WDPM represents "a rare variant of mesothelioma with a variable clinical prognosis . . . etiologically related to asbestos exposure in some cases" (whereas peritoneal WDPMs affecting young to middle-aged women are typically not associated with a background of asbestos exposure).

Subsequently, Galateau-Sallé et al.[770] reported a series of 24 cases that were classified as WDPM affecting the pleura, in 11 men and 13 women, with a mean age of 60 years (range, 31–79 years). The cases were selected on the basis of a "relatively uniform spreading of papillary formations with very limited or no invasion." In 10 cases, invasion was present at the time of diagnosis "but was strictly limited to the submesothelial layers," with no extension into lung parenchyma or subpleural adipose tissue. However, the histologic appearances of the tumors "in 2 cases at the time of progression of the disease was like . . . [that] of conventional epithelioid mesothelioma." Twenty-two of the cases presented with pleural effusion, hemorrhagic in some, and accompanied by pneumothoraces in two patients, and only one was an incidental finding. Nine cases had radiologic evidence of "thin focal pleural thickening" and the oldest patient showed contraction of the affected hemithorax. The findings at thoracoscopy for six patients were those of multiple small (millimeter-sized) nodules over the parietal or visceral pleura, producing a "velvety" appearance. With progression of disease, pleural nodularity developed, sometimes with encasement of the lung, and in one case there was dissemination into the peritoneum. Eleven of the patients had a history of asbestos exposure, occupational in character except for two patients with household contact (domestic exposure). Among 11 patients with follow-up data for a minimum of 24 months, the average survival was 74 months (range, 36–180 months) with a 10-year survival rate of almost 31%, in comparison to an average survival of about 10 months for 1248 paired patients with conventional MM.

We have encountered occasional cases of pleural mesothelioma where areas histologically indistinguishable from WDPM coexisted with other areas characteristic of conventional MM of epithelial type.

Here is our approach to these lesions:

- The diagnosis of *apparently benign, well-differentiated papillary mesothelioma* should be restricted to such solitary and localized terms when they are discovered as an incidental finding at thoracoscopy, thoracotomy, at autopsy, with no clinical symptoms or an effusion directly attributable to the lesion itself, and when the lesions comprise papillary to club-shaped processes with a core of fibrovascular tissue covered by a layer of bland mesothelial cells, with no evidence of invasion (Fig. 43.91). Benign WDPMs so diagnosed do

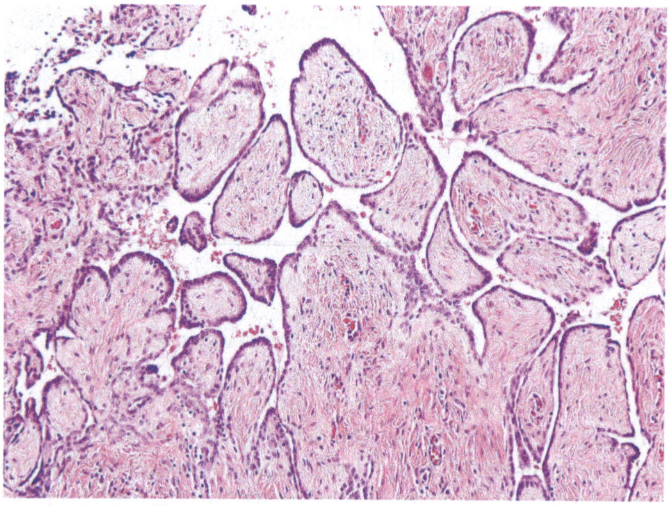

FIGURE 43.91. Well-differentiated papillary mesothelioma (WDPM) of the peritoneum, discovered incidentally at laparotomy carried out for other reasons; this lesion comprised this pattern of tissue entirely and was noninvasive in character.

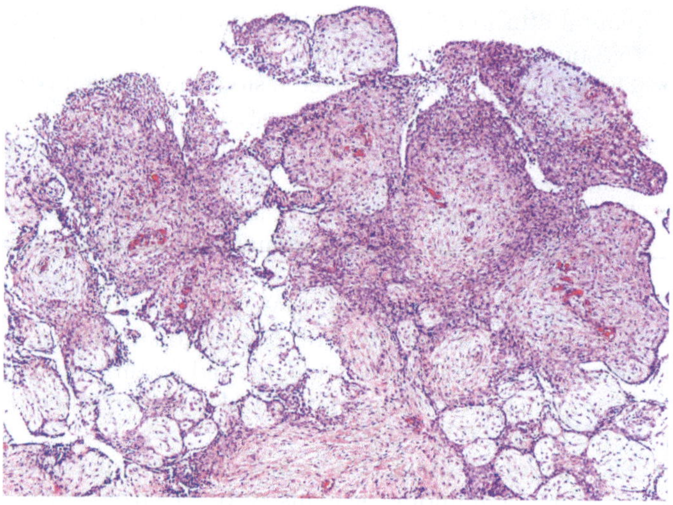

FIGURE 43.92. Pleural mesothelioma with areas of WDPM. Multilayering of the mesothelium covering some of the WDPM formations.

not require radical surgery or chemotherapy,[762] but instead should simply be observed by way of clinical follow-up.

- Multifocal pleural tumors with features of WDPM (Figs. 43.92 and 43.93), when associated with pleural effusion or pleural thickening, frequently pursue a progressive clinical course even when they are only minimally and superficially invasive, with significant morbidity and mortality[770]; however, evidence indicates that the WDPM appearances are associated with a more indolent course than pleural MM, with longer survivals in most cases.
- When areas of WDPM are admixed with other areas of invasive mesothelioma, where the appearances would allow a diagnosis of conventional MM in the absence of the WDPM-like foci, we diagnose such lesions as a pleural MM with WDPM-like areas. The WDPM-like tissue may point to a more indolent clinical course than ordinary pleural MMs. In this regard, the natural history of WDPM in terms of survival times seems to be related directly to the proportion of the WDPM-like tissue, and inversely to the extent of the lesion(s) and their invasiveness.

Noninvasive Atypical Mesothelial Proliferations: The Concept of Mesothelioma In Situ and Discrimination Between Early-Stage Mesothelioma and Reactive Mesothelial Hyperplasia

In the 1980s Bolen et al.[536,771] proposed a multipotential subserosal fibroblastoid cell as the stem cell for mesothelial healing and regeneration, and as the progenitor cell for mesothelioma development, and proposed that an origin of mesothelioma from such subserosal cells could account for the bidirectional differentiation characteristic of biphasic mesotheliomas. As an alternative model,

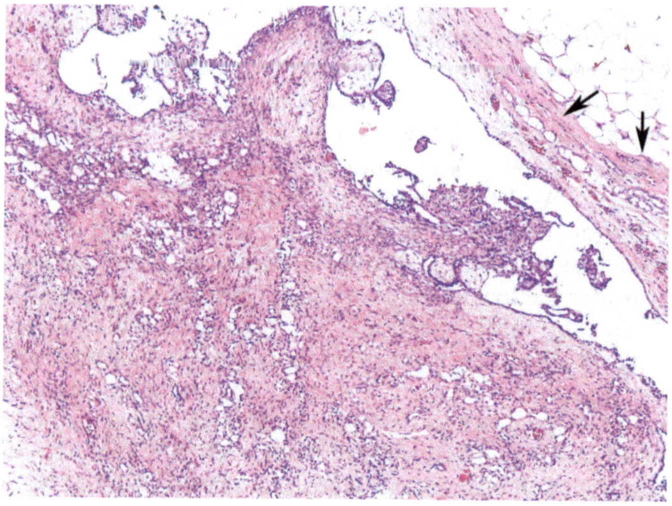

FIGURE 43.93. Pleural mesothelioma with WDPM-like areas. (Same case as in Fig. 43.92.) The apparent invasion in the lower part of this field is explicable in part by an en face appearance resulting from a tangential plane of section, but not entirely so, taking into account the extent of the epithelial-type tumor within the submesothelial fibrous tissue. En profile infiltration into the pleural fibrous tissue is also evident, where there is no suggestion of an oblique plane of section (arrows), and there were multiple other areas of undoubted invasion into the pleural fibrous layer.

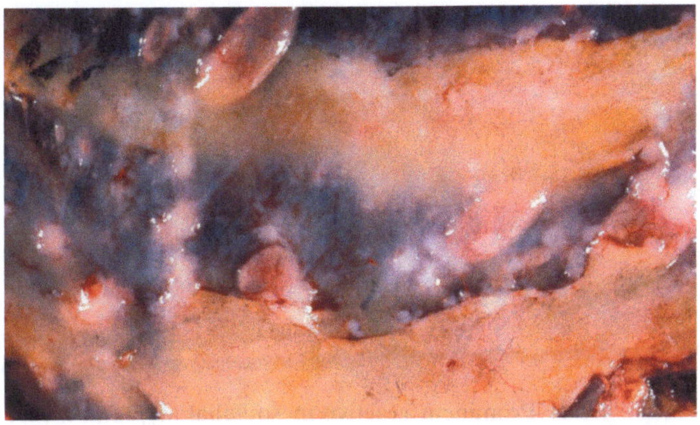

FIGURE 43.94. Pleurectomy specimen from a patient who presented with a massive pleural effusion. No distinctive abnormality was seen at thoracoscopy, but multiple random biopsies revealed an extensive atypical mesothelial proliferation, in situ in most areas of the biopsies, but with small foci of invasion. A pleurectomy was subsequently carried out, and in the surgical specimen, small foci of white invasive tumor were found, some of which extended into subpleural adipose tissue. The entire pleurectomy specimen was examined as a series of Swiss roll sections, and the areas devoid of invasive mesothelioma were seen to show extensive in situ mesothelial atypia.

Whitaker et al.[489] advanced the concept of mesothelioma in situ, based in part on experimental models of mesothelial healing following injury that did not disrupt the submesothelial basal lamina,[492,493,495,] and on their observation of a number of cases of apparently early-stage MM of epithelial type, where mesothelial atypia appeared to be predominantly in situ, in the absence of any radiologic or gross anatomic evidence of pleural thickening or nodularity. This being so, Whitaker's group[489,679] suggested that mesothelioma in situ could be defined as the replacement of benign surface mesothelium by mesothelial cells with markers of malignancy. The problem was to define an acceptable and consistently reproducible marker of neoplastic change. Accordingly, they described 22 cases of pleural disease characterized by atypical and predominantly in situ mesothelial proliferation.[489] The cases had presented in conventional fashion with a pleural effusion with either no identifiable pleural tumor or only tiny nodules at thoracoscopy (Fig. 43.94), and the diagnosis in a number of cases was established by existing cytologic criteria. Whitaker et al.[489] suggested that the markers for MM in situ in pleural biopsies included the following[119,490]:

- *Absence of background inflammation* as a potential drive for reactive mesothelial hyperplasia (to which one could add the clinical absence of any underlying cause or association for pleural inflammation and reactive mesothelial proliferation).
- *An abnormal architecture of the mesothelium at the surface of the affected pleural tissue.* The architectural abnormalities included noninvasive, linear, papillary and tubulopapillary patterns, sometimes with a complex exophytic architecture (Fig. 43.95). Whitaker's group[679] emphasized that a prominent papillary pattern of mesothelial proliferation in pleural biopsies is a disturbing feature, not usually seen with reactive mesothelial hyperplasias (although this observation does not apply to mesothelial proliferations affecting the peritoneum and in relation to the omentum in particular).
- Substantial cytologic atypia (Fig. 43.95B), but Whitaker's group also considered that other cases might occur where there is substantially less cytologic atypia, so that such cases would be diagnosable (if at all) only by ancillary techniques. Among these techniques they included strong linear labeling for EMA or areas occupied by silver labeling of nucleolar organizing regions (AgNORs), in excess of the areas found in proven benign reactive mesothelial proliferations.
- In relation to labeling for EMA, Whitaker et al.[489] found that 17 of 22 cases showed thick linear labeling

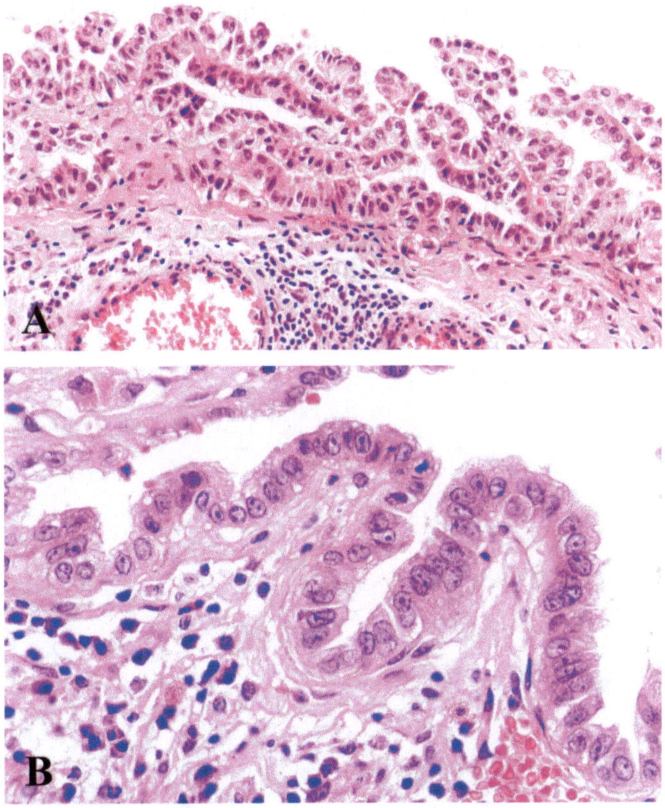

FIGURE 43.95. **(A)** Atypical mesothelial proliferation seen in a pleural biopsy, with an exophytic papillary architecture at the surface. **(B)** Same pleural biopsy illustrating the mesothelial atypia at higher magnification.

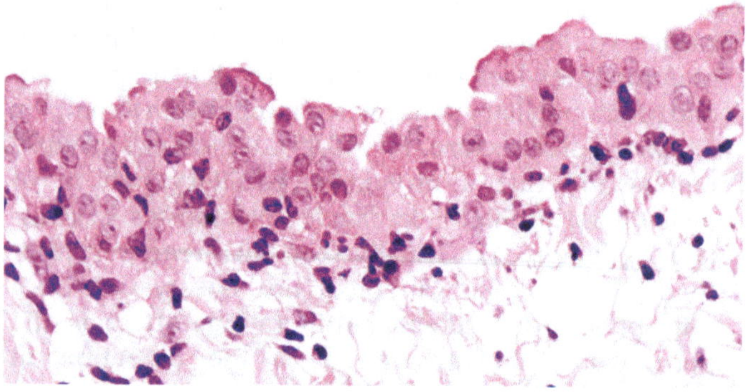

Figure 43.96. Example of benign reactive mesothelial proliferation in a pleural biopsy taken from a patient with proven lung cancer. Compare with Figure 43.95B.

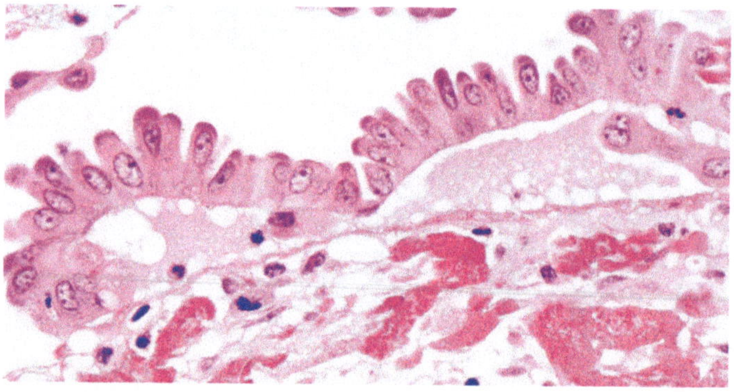

Figure 43.98. Prominent reactive mesothelial atypia in a case of organizing fibrinous pericarditis. Fibrinous exudate is evident in the lower half of this field.

of the mesothelial cells for EMA, whereas proven benign reactive mesothelial proliferations usually showed no significant labeling or only patchy weak labeling, as studied in the same laboratory.[119] (On the other hand, we emphasize that in tissue biopsies, a substantial proportion of cases of invasive mesothelioma may show no detectable immunohistochemical labeling for EMA.) Saad et al.[671] investigated EMA expression in 20 cases of reactive mesothelial proliferation (RMP) versus 20 cases of MM, using antibodies based on the Mc5 and E29 clones. For the Mc5 clone, there was positive staining in 14/20 cases of MM (70%) and 12/20 cases of RMP (60%); for the E29 clone, the corresponding results were 15/20 for MM (75%) and 0/20 for RMP. For the E29 clone, the sensitivity and specificity for MM were 75% and 100%, respectively. The authors concluded that EMA antibodies based on the E29 clone are a reliable discriminator between RMP and MM. Simon et al.[402] also commented on this pattern of EMA labeling as a discriminator between benign RMPs and areas of seemingly in situ MM.

Nonetheless, because it is known that there is overlap in the degree of cytologic atypia between benign reactive mesothelial proliferations (Figs. 43.96 to 43.98) versus mesothelioma[37,490,503,513] (Fig. 43.95), Whitaker et al.[489] and Henderson et al.[119] emphasized that the only consistently reliable marker for mesothelioma as opposed to RMP is the presence of acceptable neoplastic invasion in the same biopsy, or a different biopsy taken at a different time, or at autopsy (Figs. 43.99 to 43.103). Accordingly, Henderson et al. commented in 1997:

We caution against rash or premature diagnosis of mesothelioma in situ from conventional light microscopy examination of

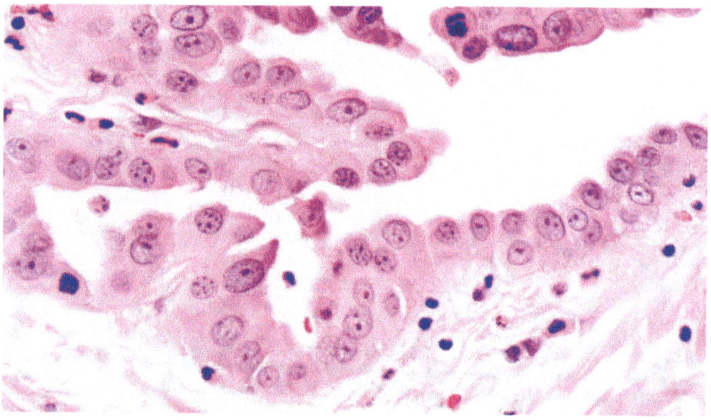

Figure 43.97. Extreme reactive mesothelial atypia as seen in the visceral and parietal layers of the pleura, in an apical wedge resection specimen of lung and in the pleura, from a man in his 20s, with a history or recurrent pneumothoraces on the same side.

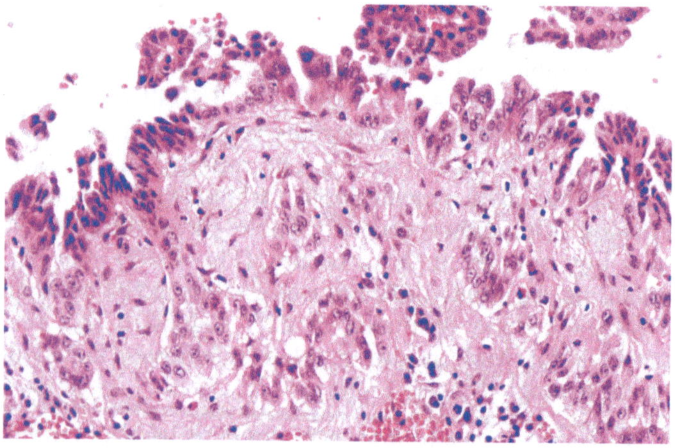

Figure 43.99. Different area of the same biopsy shown in Figure 43.95. Foci of infiltration into the submesothelial fibrous tissue are evident, so that the findings overall were interpreted as those of an exophytic-papillary mesothelioma in situ with multiple foci of superficially invasive mesothelioma.

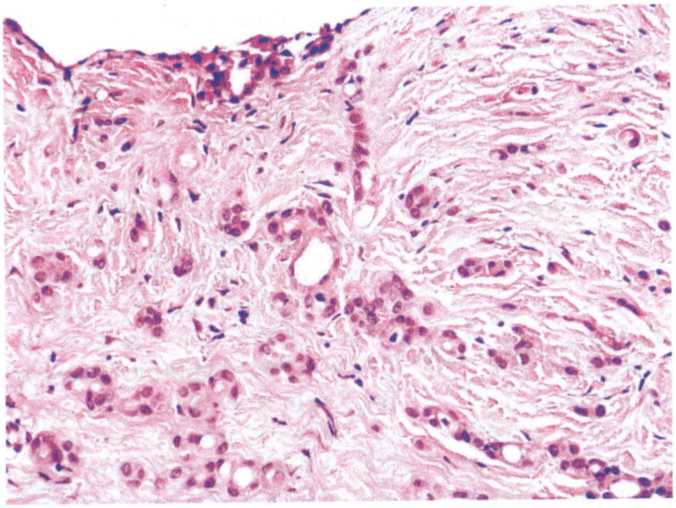

FIGURE 43.100. Early-stage invasive mesothelioma of epithelial type, with infiltration of the submesothelial fibrous tissue, in a pattern that is inconsistent with benign mesothelial entrapment as part of a fibroinflammatory process. In addition, this biopsy showed no evidence of exudative inflammation. There is only minor cytological atypia.

biopsy tissue, taking into account that there is overlap in the cytologic abnormalities that occur in reactive mesothelial hyperplasias versus mesothelioma. However, [findings suggestive of a component of mesothelioma in situ] (especially in conjunction with effusion fluid cytology) may delineate "at risk" patients with "early" stage disease who require further investigation and follow-up. Because of the minimal and perhaps predominantly in situ tumor burden, the mesotheliomas may also be amenable to new modalities of therapy, and some of our "in situ" patients have had prolonged survivals.

Henderson et al.[119,490] also emphasized that in all of their cases,[489,679] biopsy or autopsy examination did

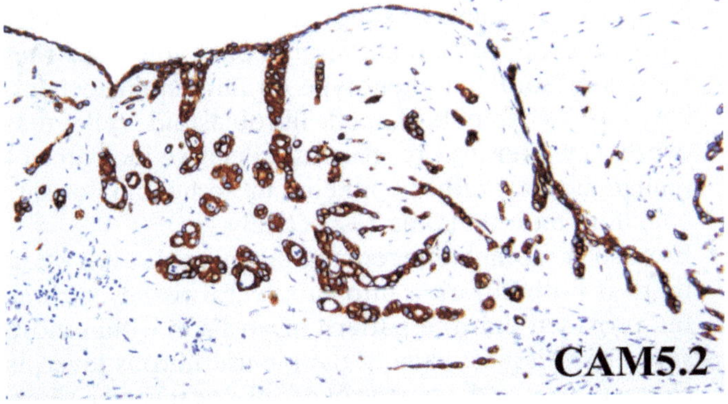

FIGURE 43.101. Same biopsy as illustrated in Figure 43.100, immunostained for low molecular weight cytokeratin (CAM5.2), illustrating the pattern of infiltration into the pleural fibrous layer.

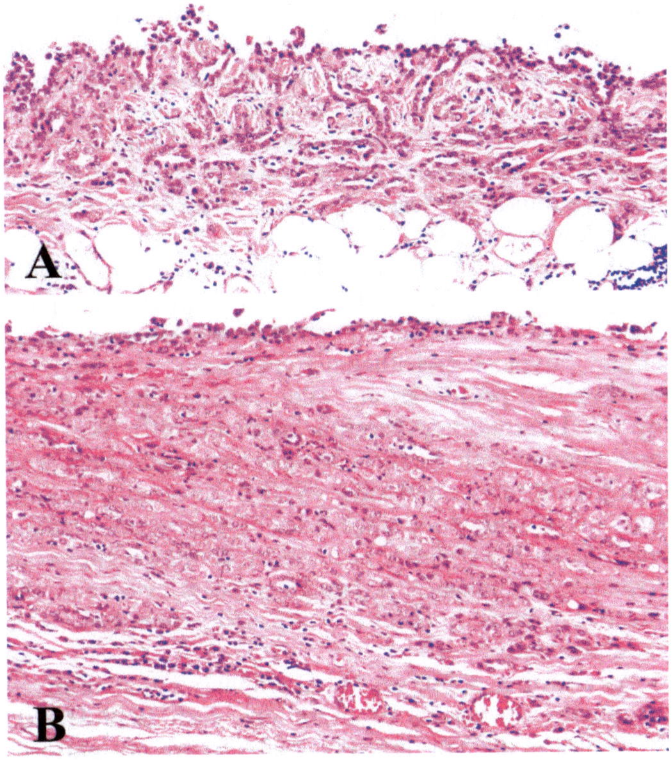

FIGURE 43.102. **(A,B)** Early-stage invasive malignant mesothelioma of epithelial type. Both of these figures are from the same case. The parietal pleural biopsy showed multiple foci of infiltration into the fibrous layer of the pleura, in the absence of exudative inflammation, with only equivocal and focal extension of a few mesothelial cells into the subjacent fat. The pattern of infiltration into the fibrous layer, with near-filling by linear and compressed tubular aggregates of mesothelial cells **(B)** is inconsistent with benign entrapment.

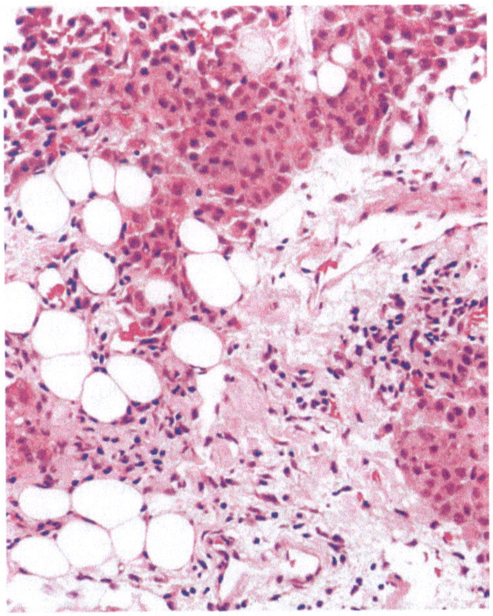

FIGURE 43.103. Area of invasion into subpleural adipose tissue, as a marker of malignancy for this mesothelial proliferation. The proliferation was noninvasive elsewhere in the biopsy.

confirm the development of invasive mesothelioma, but one patient was still alive at the time of writing[119] (with only a short period of follow-up). (Subsequently, Churg et al.[503] commented that in one instance in which Whitaker et al.[489] and Henderson et al.[119,679] "made a diagnosis of mesothelioma in situ without the presence of invasive tumor, the lesion appeared to have been benign on follow-up.")

Churg et al.[503] suggest that the term *mesothelioma in situ* not be used, and instead noninvasive atypical mesothelial proliferations should be designated as either "atypical mesothelial hyperplasia" or "atypical mesothelial proliferation" (the latter being favored by the International Mesothelioma Panel[37]). We have no argument with the term *atypical mesothelial proliferation* for entirely noninvasive atypical mesothelial lesions, but we would discourage use of the term *atypical mesothelial hyperplasia*, because by definition the word *hyperplasia* indicates a benign process, whereas the reactive versus neoplastic status for such lesions is indeterminate.

As a further point, we would emphasize that complex exophytic mesothelial proliferations, such as illustrated by Churg et al.[503] in their Fig. 4.23A,B, are not patterns usually or typically encountered with benign inflammation-induced mesothelial proliferations. Such appearances (Fig. 43.95A) raise a suspicion of MM where the invasive component (if present) has not been sampled by the biopsy. Such lesions should not be dismissed as benign; they are an indicator for close follow-up and further cytologic or biopsy investigation, as indicated by Churg et al. In other words, noninvasive atypical mesothelial proliferation in biopsy tissue does not correspond to a treatable disorder, but instead is a requirement for follow-up or further investigation.

It is sometimes stated that there is no proof that in situ mesothelial atypia in association with areas of invasive mesothelioma represents the same lesion.[503] However, Simon et al.[402] did report a single case of mesothelioma in situ in association with focal early-stage invasive mesothelioma. They investigated the lesion by laser microdissection and comparative genomic hybridization and found similar chromosomal alterations in both the areas of in situ mesothelial atypia and in the foci of early invasive mesothelioma. Accordingly, in the areas of mesothelioma in situ they recorded losses at 3p, 5q, 6q, 8p, 9p, 15q, 22q, and Y, with a gain on 7q; in the area of early invasive mesothelioma there were losses at 3p, 5pq, 6q, 8p, 9p, 15q, and 22q with no gain. In contrast, the advanced mesothelioma showed losses at 1p, 4pq, 6q, 9p, 13q, 14q, and 22q, with gains at 1q, 7pq, and 15q.

We still consider mesothelioma in situ to be a useful concept concerning the development of MM. In addition, by refocusing attention on the mesothelium itself as the target for neoplastic transformation, this concept points to the potential for diagnosis of noninvasive mesotheliomas, with the promise of more effective therapy in the future. We continue to believe that the term *mesothelioma in situ* represents a valid retrospective diagnosis in cases where at least early-stage invasive mesothelioma has been demonstrated.

As discussed above and illustrated in Figures 43.95B to 43.98, there can be substantial overlap in the degree of cytologic atypia encountered in proven atypical reactive mesothelial hyperplasias, versus proven invasive MMs of epithelial type. Although thick linear membrane-related labeling for EMA (using antibodies based upon the E29 clone) may sway the probability index toward a diagnosis of early-stage mesothelioma, this finding cannot be considered decisive or definitive, and at present there is no universally accepted immunohistologic or molecular marker for consistent discrimination between reactive mesothelial hyperplasia versus MM. This being so, histologic assessment of invasion is crucial to the diagnosis of MM and its discrimination from an atypical reactive mesothelial proliferation, in everyday diagnostic practice. We have found the following guidelines and caveats to be useful in the approach to differential diagnosis of mesothelial lesions where the discrimination between mesothelioma and hyperplasia is problematic:

- It is useful to correlate the histologic appearances with the findings on pleural effusion fluid cytology and with any abnormalities revealed by imaging studies, such as chest radiographs or CT scans. In this regard, the radiologic investigations can be regarded as a surrogate for gross anatomic findings. For example, radiologic demonstration of a confluent and nodular pleural lesion with encasement of the lung and contraction of the affected hemithorax together with an effusion (in which a florid atypical papillary mesothelial proliferation was found) can effectively substitute for the histologic detection of invasion, at a high order of confidence.
- Neoplastic invasion of subpleural adipose tissue (Fig. 43.103) or deeper structures by epithelioid cells that show a mesothelial phenotype on immunohistochemistry or by spindle-shaped fibroblastoid cells that express cytokeratins represents a decisive indicator of malignancy, for either epithelial mesothelioma or sarcomatoid mesothelioma respectively.
- Even so, mesothelioma remains diagnosable even when there is no infiltration into subpleural tissues such as fat, provided that the pattern of invasion within more superficial tissues, namely the pleural fibrous layer, is characteristic or diagnostic of neoplastic invasion (Figs. 43.99 to 43.102) as opposed to artifact or benign entrapment of mesothelial cells as part of an organizing fibroinflammatory process (see below).

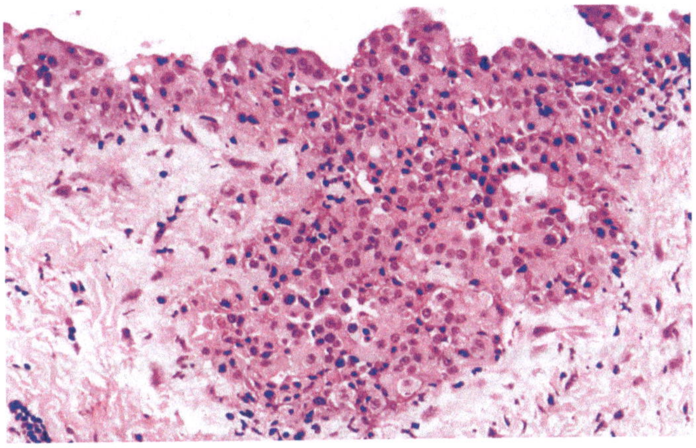

FIGURE 43.104. Pseudo-invasion in a case of benign reactive mesothelial hyperplasia, resulting from folding of the pleural membrane. (Same case as in Fig. 43.96.)

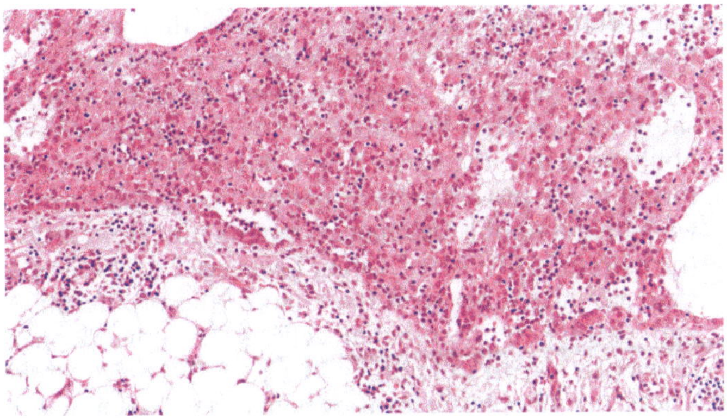

FIGURE 43.105. Prominent benign reactive mesothelial hyperplasia in a patient with proven tuberculous pleuritis. It is evident that the mesothelial proliferation is entirely noninvasive in character, and admixed with numerous inflammatory cells.

- We take great care to ensure that pleural biopsies are orientated correctly when subject to histologic sectioning, so that the tissue is embedded on edge, resulting in *en profile* as opposed to *en face* sections, because the latter can create problems concerning interpretation over what is, and what is not, acceptable evidence of invasion. When sufficient pleural membrane is available, we find it useful to prepare a *Swiss roll* from the biopsy and to fix the pleural tissue after the Swiss roll has been prepared, then taking a series of transverse sections, to facilitate correct orientation of the pleural membrane.
- It is necessary to discriminate between pseudo-invasion, for example, resulting from an *en face* plane of section through the biopsy or from folding of the pleural membrane (Fig. 43.104) versus genuine neoplastic infiltration of the submesothelial tissue. When there is doubt over whether the process represents pseudo-invasion versus genuine neoplastic invasion, we dismiss the appearances as inconclusive.
- Although most inflammation-driven reactive mesothelial hyperplasias are noninvasive (Fig. 43.105), some organizing serosal inflammatory reactions, especially in the pericardium in our experience, can result in the burying of hyperplastic mesothelial cells within the organizing and proliferative fibrous tissue, so that this well-recognized pattern of benign mesothelial entrapment requires distinction from genuine invasion (cf. Figs. 43.99 to 43.102 with Figs. 43.106 and 43.107). The presence of a florid fibrinous or neutrophilic inflammatory reaction should alert one to the likelihood of benign entrapment, but the authors have encountered cases of proven invasive mesothelioma with prominent associated inflammatory exudate. In such organizing inflammatory processes, the entrapment appears to be the result of burying of the site where the mesothelium is normally located, by a layer of inflammatory exudate that extends across the surface of the membrane, with subsequent organization. This process of entrapment of mesothelium is sometimes designated as mesothelial sequestration, but in many instances the lowermost level of the entrapped mesothelium seems actually to be situated at its original level. Instead, it is the surface of the pleura that has moved inward, into the lumen of

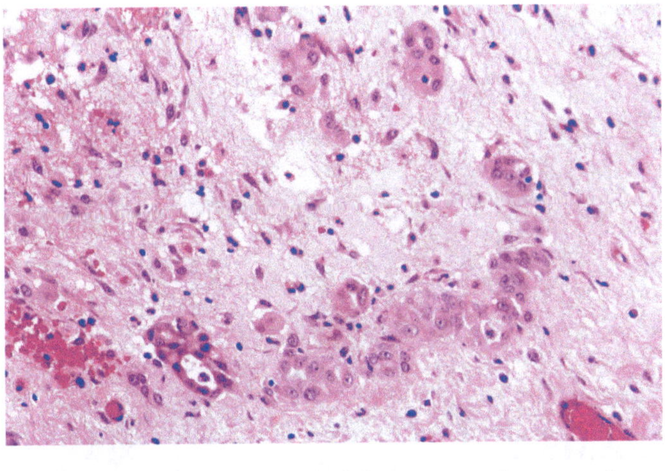

FIGURE 43.106. Benign mesothelial entrapment in a case of constrictive pericarditis, in a young man. Islands and tubules formed by mesothelial cells are evident within the fibrous tissue. There was prominent fibrinous inflammatory exudate near the surface of the pericardium (near the top left hand corner). In addition, the proliferative mesothelial cells in this biopsy showed scattered intracytoplasmic mucin-like droplets, stainable by the PAS-diastase stain. Follow-up for a period of over 5 years was entirely benign.

the pleura (or pericardium), a process that we sometimes liken to the shrinking of the Aral Sea and that we designate as the *Aral Sea effect*. In other words, ships marooned by the shrinkage of the Aral Sea have not moved into the surrounding desert, but rather the shoreline has moved away from the ships. In this regard, we find immunohistochemical staining for cytokeratins (or calretinin) to be of value, because it delineates a clear boundary between the zone of the proliferative and entrapped mesothelial cells, versus the deeper tissues, as shown in Figure 43.107.

- Therefore, neoplastic invasion remains the linchpin for diagnosis of early-stage mesotheliomas of epithelial type. When there is any doubt over whether genuine invasion is present or not, we prefer to err on the side of underdiagnosis of mesothelioma as opposed to inappropriate overdiagnosis. We base this approach on the principle that if the lesion is mesothelioma, it will declare itself as such soon enough, whereas inappropriate overdiagnosis of mesothelioma can lead to erroneous cytotoxic chemotherapy or even radical surgery, together with the anguish that a diagnosis of mesothelioma usually entails.
- Even when invasion cannot be found in a biopsy sample, there are several findings in combination that are suspicious of mesothelioma, although nondiagnostic by themselves. They include the extent of the mesothelial proliferation, the presence of a complex exophytic or papillary architecture at the surface of the pleura (in the absence of exudative inflammation), prominent cytologic atypia, focal necrosis within sheets of proliferative mesothelial cells in the pleura (Fig. 43.108), prominent intracytoplasmic vacuoles devoid of mucin-like content, and strong thick linear labeling for EMA (using antibodies based on the E29 clone). The presence of two or three or more such features is an indication for clinical follow-up or further investigation, to clarify the hyperplastic versus neoplastic properties of the mesothelial proliferation.

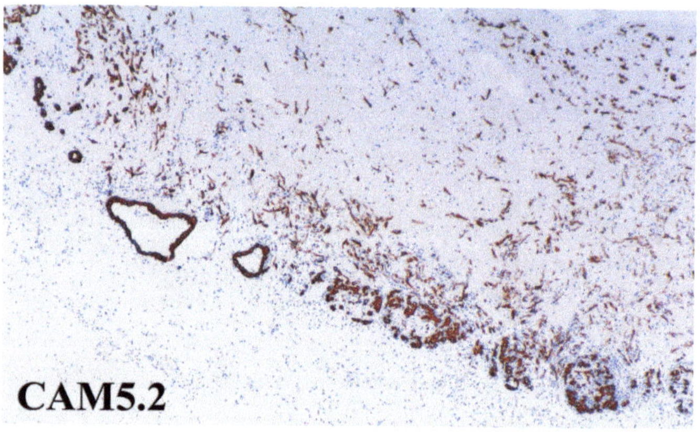

FIGURE 43.107. Same biopsy as illustrated in Figure 43.106, immunostained for low molecular weight cytokeratin (CAM5.2). Note the reasonably clear demarcation or boundary zone between the entrapped mesothelial cells and the deeper tissues, the appearances being unlike those of neoplastic invasion by a malignant mesothelioma, where the deep boundary of the lesion is less sharply demarcated and is infiltrative in character.

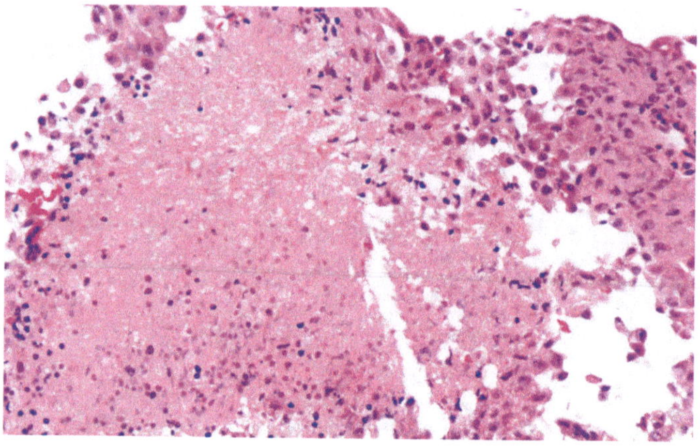

FIGURE 43.108. Focal tumor necrosis in an atypical mesothelial proliferation, as one indicator of malignant mesothelioma. Neoplastic invasion into subpleural adipose tissue was found in a different area of the same biopsy.

Small Cell Mesothelioma

In 1992, Mayall and Gibbs[772] drew attention to a small cell variant of MM, likely to be confused with small cell carcinoma of lung. In this regard, it is also worth emphasizing that Falconieri et al.[773] reported four cases of small cell carcinoma of lung with spread into the pleura, simulating pleural MM.

It is notable that most of the cases reported by Mayall and Gibbs[772] represented autopsy cases, with the potential for the small cell features being explicable at least in part by postmortem artifact. Krismann et al.[774] have expressed doubt about the existence of small cell mesothelioma, because the German Mesothelioma Registry, which contained more than 6000 mesothelioma cases as of 2004, did not contain a single example of small cell mesothelioma. Nonetheless, we have encountered extremely rare cases of mesothelioma with a small cell pattern (fewer than even lymphohistiocytoid mesothelioma). The following findings aid distinction of this form of mesothelioma from small cell carcinoma infiltrating pleura:

- In the cases of small cell mesothelioma the we have encountered, the tumor showed a transition from the small cell areas to other regions where the appearances were more characteristic of epithelioid mesothelioma.

- The nucleocytoplasmic features of small-cell mesothelioma differ subtly from those of small cell carcinoma (Figs. 43.30 and 43.31), so that the mesothelioma cells often possess greater amounts of cytoplasm, or alternatively, the nuclei are more open and vesicular in pattern with finely divided chromatin, in comparison to the "salt and pepper" nuclear chromatin pattern characteristic of small cell carcinomas, with nuclear molding.
- Immunohistochemical studies on these mesotheliomas reveal features characteristic of mesothelial differentiation, with no evidence of neuroendocrine differentiation as shown, for example, by immunostaining for synaptophysin or chromogranin.

Nonetheless, we have encountered extremely rare cases of mesothelioma where there was some focal evidence of neuroendocrine differentiation, but such cases appear not to have been described in any detail in the literature.

Deciduoid Mesothelioma

In 1994, Nascimento et al.[775] described three cases of peritoneal mesothelioma in young females, where the tumor cells possessed abundant eosinophilic cytoplasm and showed a resemblance to decidual cells, and such cases had no identifiable prior exposure to asbestos.[776] Reports of other cases of "deciduoid" mesothelioma followed.[776–780]

It is now recognized that deciduoid mesotheliomas (Fig. 43.25)[126,778,779,781–785] are confined neither to the peritoneum nor to young women, and they can arise in the pleura and in men.[786] Their natural history is akin to other epithelial mesotheliomas, although a few patients have had long survivals,[779] whereas the tumors comprising the original report[775] pursued an aggressive clinical course. Mesotheliomas that consist only of deciduoid tissue are rare, but it is not uncommon in biopsy tissue to see a transition from more usual patterns of epithelial mesothelioma to foci of deciduoid tissue. We do not consider deciduoid mesothelioma to represent a distinctive subtype, and instead we refer simply to these mesotheliomas as epithelioid mesotheliomas with focal deciduoid features. The immunophenotype of such "deciduoid" mesotheliomas is essentially the same as for other MMs of epithelioid type.[786]

Mucin-Positive Epithelial Mesotheliomas

Up to about 5% of epithelial mesotheliomas show focal staining with Mayer's mucicarmine, PAS-diastase, and Alcian blue/colloidal iron with hyaluronidase. We refer to these mesotheliomas as mucin-positive mesotheliomas.[505]

Ernst and Atkinson[787] reported seven of 18 epithelial mesotheliomas to be mucicarmine positive. They attributed the positive staining reaction to hyaluronic acid. The review article on MM by the U.S.–Canadian Mesothelioma Panel[788] illustrated a case of mucicarmine-positive mesothelioma and indicated this finding did not exclude the diagnosis of mesothelioma. Some mucin-positive epithelial mesotheliomas show staining of the cell membrane with mucin stains and are sensitive to hyaluronidase pre-digestion (Fig. 43.109). Others show intracellular droplet staining with Mayer's mucicarmine (Fig. 43.110), PAS-diastase (Fig. 43.111), and Alcian blue with and without hyaluronidase (Fig. 43.112). In our experience, these mucin-positive epithelial mesotheliomas are the ones that show crystalloid structures ultrastructurally (see Ultrastructural Features of Mesotheliomas, above).

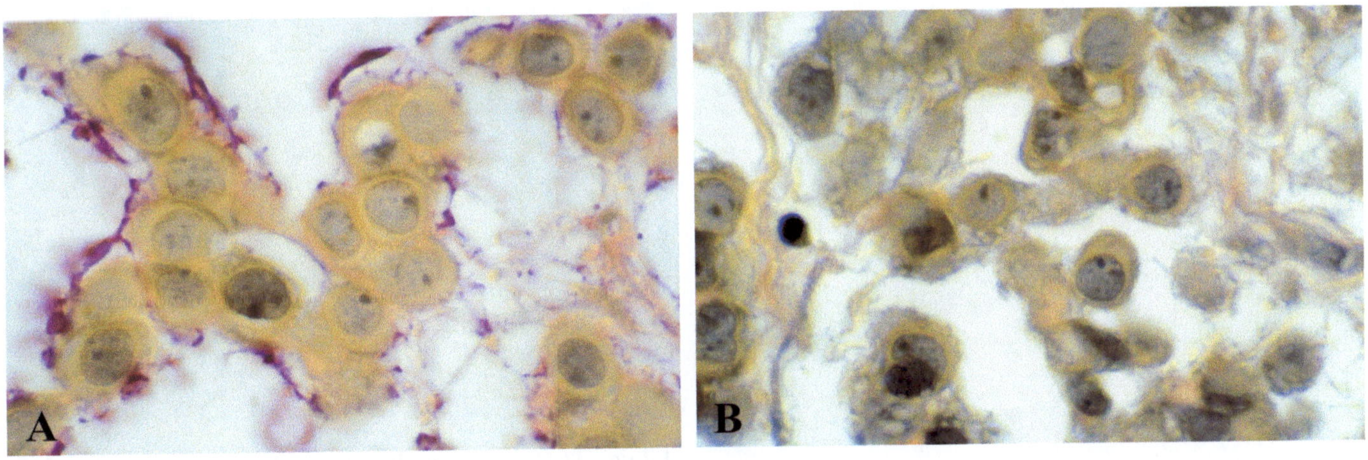

FIGURE 43.109. **(A)** This epithelial mesothelioma shows cell membrane staining for mucicarmine. **(B)** When pretreated with hyaluronidase, the mucicarmine staining does not occur, suggesting the mucicarmine staining is caused by hyaluronic acid.

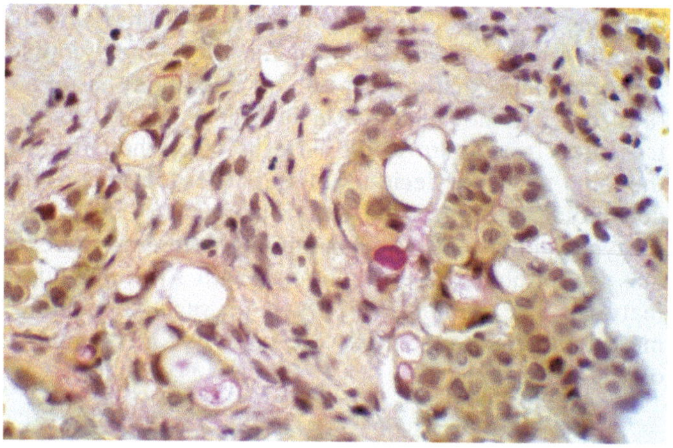

FIGURE 43.110. This epithelial mesothelioma shows intracellular droplet-like staining for mucicarmine that is resistant to hyaluronidase pre-digestion.

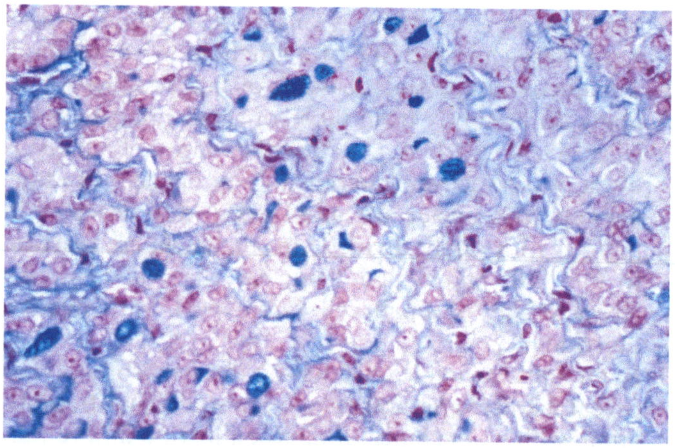

FIGURE 43.112. Alcian blue droplet-like staining is seen in this epithelial mesothelioma and is resistant to hyaluronidase pretreatment.

Benjamin and Ritchie[789] examined the staining results for glycogen and mucosubstance of 30 diffuse epithelial mesotheliomas. Tissue was fixed in formalin and processed using standard techniques. Tissue sections were stained with the WHO stain for mucin, PAS reagent with and without diastase, Hale's colloidal iron stain with and without hyaluronidase, potassium hydroxide–PAS technique, and Alcian blue at pH 1.0 and 2.5. They found that seven of the 30 mesotheliomas failed to stain by any method tested, and concluded the staining reactions of epithelial mesotheliomas with mucopolysaccharide stains were too inconsistent to be of much value in diagnosing epithelial mesotheliomas.

MacDougall et al.[539] reported a case of epithelial MM, the diagnosis documented by electron microscopy and immunohistochemistry, which was mucicarmine and PAS-D positive.

Gaucher Cell–Like Mesotheliomas

Gaucher cell–like mesotheliomas are one of the rarest, if not *the* rarest, epithelioid type of mesothelioma. These mesotheliomas are composed of large cells that are mostly round and contain intracytoplasmic inclusions and resemble Gaucher cells (Figs. 43.113 and 43.114). Ultrastructurally, these cells show some very unique crystalloid structures within the cisternae of the rough endoplasmic reticulum[211] (Fig. 43.115). We have seen this neoplastic pattern only in mesotheliomas and not in any other type of tumor.

Multicystic Mesothelioma

Multicystic mesotheliomas are well recognized in the peritoneal cavity,[790–807] mainly in women and less often in

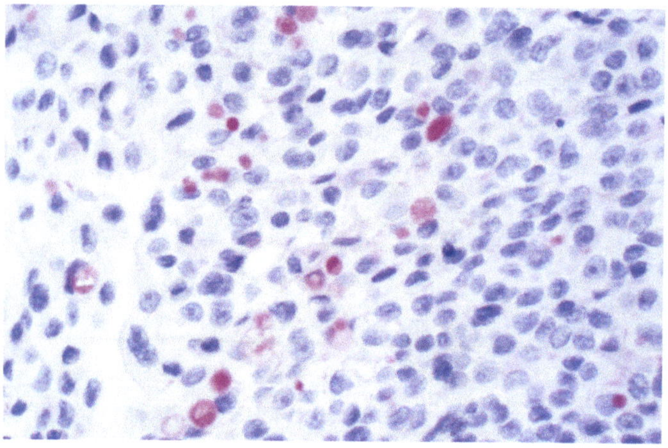

FIGURE 43.111. Intracellular PAS and PAS-diastase droplet-like staining is observed in this epithelial mesothelioma.

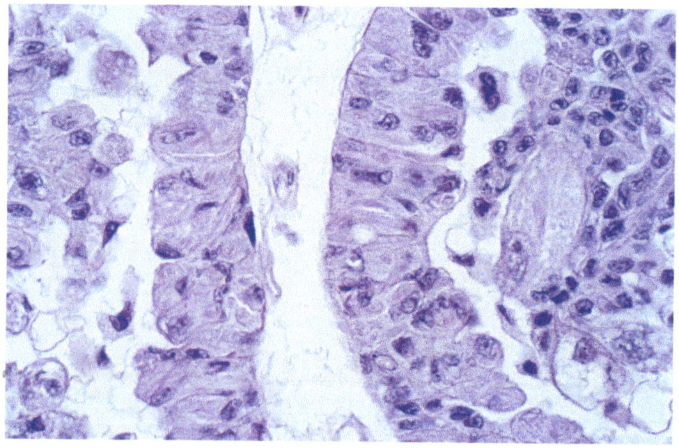

FIGURE 43.113. This epithelial mesothelioma is composed, in part, of numerous large cells with intracytoplasmic inclusions that resemble those seen in Gaucher cells.

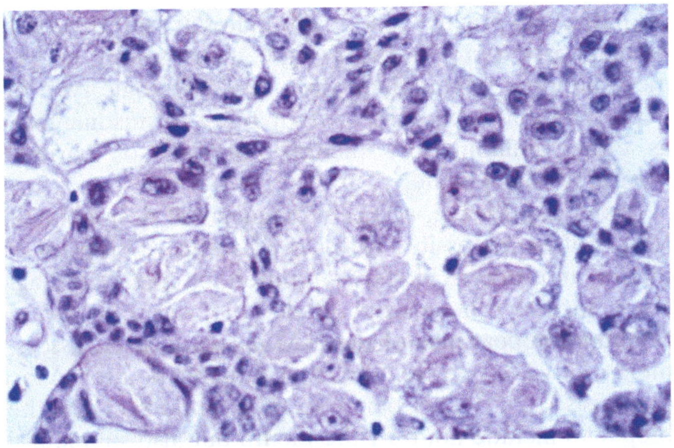

FIGURE 43.114. Gaucher-like cells with intracytoplasmic inclusions are a prominent component of this epithelial mesothelioma.

men.[808–813] In the peritoneal cavity, some lesions of this type appear to represent benign postinflammatory cystic lesions (for which an association with peritoneal inflammatory disorders, endometriosis, and antecedent surgical procedures has been recorded),[801,813–816] whereas other peritoneal multicystic mesotheliomas appear to represent indolent neoplasms of intermediate or low-grade malignant potential,[817] occasionally forming massive lesions that can recur locally[812,818,819] and require repeated surgical removal, although spread beyond the peritoneal cavity appears not to have been recorded.

We have encountered one case of a cystic mesothelioma of the peritoneum found during appendectomy in a man, with repeated local recurrences and with transition to a conventional malignant-appearing epithelial mesothelioma in late recurrences of the lesion. Gonzalez-Moreno et al.[820] also described malignant transformation of a peritoneal cystic mesothelioma in a 36-year-old woman.

Multicystic mesotheliomas most often affect young adults to middle-aged premenopausal women and they are found most often in the pelvic region, often localized to the pouch of Douglas. The patients may present with abdominal pain or abdominal swelling or a detectable mass lesion.

Characteristically, the cystic nature of this form of mesothelioma is evident on naked-eye inspection, and the cysts are lined by a single layer of flattened cells that express a mesothelial phenotype on immunohistochemistry, with fibrous tissue in the septa separating the individual cystic locules.

Multicystic mesotheliomas localized to the pleura are exceedingly rare. We know of only one report in the literature,[821] in a 37-year-old woman with a history of childhood exposure to asbestos (the size of the cystic locules was not specified). A single case of pleural cystic mesothelioma was also encountered in the Australian Mesothelioma Surveillance Program, in a young woman (the case being misdiagnosed initially as a cystic lymphangioma).[822] Again, the size of the cystic locules in that case is unknown, but the lesion did recur.

Multicystic mesotheliomas have no proven relationship to asbestos, and it seems likely that any association[821] is coincidental rather than causal. Given the extreme rarity of pleural multicystic mesothelioma, the following criteria are suggested for its diagnosis:

- The cystic character of the lesion should be evident on gross examination (either at thoracoscopy or thoracotomy, or on examination of a resected specimen).
- Throughout the entire lesion, the histologic appearances should be indistinguishable from those of a cystic mesothelioma of the peritoneum, with a requirement for it to be embedded in its entirety and sectioned.
- In particular, there should be no areas characteristic of conventional MM of epithelial type. Tumors showing areas of conventional mesothelioma we believe should be designated as MM with focal microcystic change. Nonetheless, adenomatoid areas are well recognized in conventional multicystic mesotheliomas.
- The mesothelial phenotype of the cells lining the cysts should be confirmed on immunohistochemistry or electron microscopy or both. In this regard, we reemphasize that cystic lymphangioma represents one differential diagnosis for these lesions, and that the antibody D2-40 labels both lymphatic endothelium and mesothelial cells,[632,753] as well as other cell types[605]; labeling of the

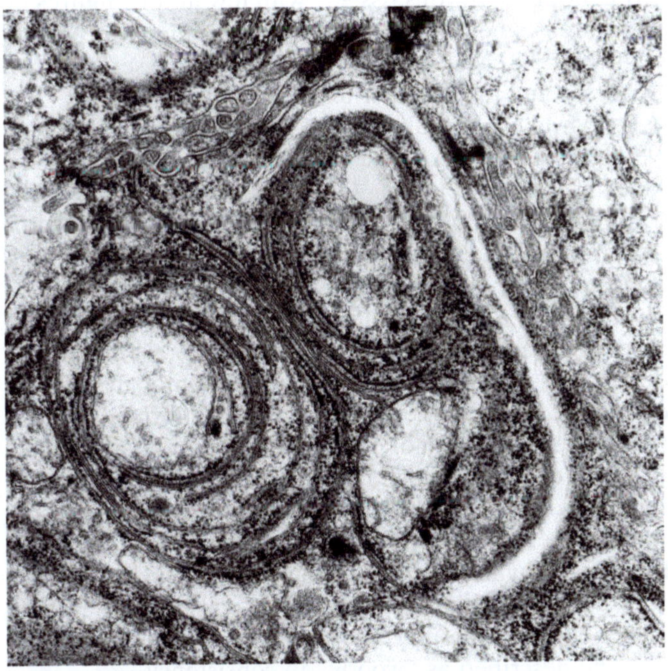

FIGURE 43.115. The cells with the inclusions show parallel arrays of membrane-like material within the cisterna.

relevant sections for cytokeratins or mesothelial markers such as calretinin facilitates the distinction.

Simple postinflammatory mesothelial cysts seen in the peritoneum do not seem to occur in relation to the pleura.

We have also seen several cases of peritoneal cystic mesothelioma where the patients had been informed that they had a (malignant) mesothelioma, and other cases where the patients were subjected to aggressive combination chemotherapy. Because of the distinct risk of clinical overreaction to these lesions, we prefer to designate most such lesions as peritoneal mesothelial inclusion cysts. If the term *cystic mesothelioma* is used in pathology reports, we consider it imperative to include a comment on the character of these lesions and their distinction from conventional MM.

Desmoplastic Sarcomatoid Mesothelioma of the Pleura and Its Distinction from Benign Fibrous Pleuritis

The first description of desmoplastic MM (DesMM) is usually attributed to Kannerstein and Churg[823] in 1980, and these lesions were further documented in 1982 by Cantin et al.,[824] but McCaughey[497] had emphasized the diagnostic problems imposed by "large amounts of hyaline collagen" in mesotheliomas as early as 1965. Much earlier, in their 1920 report of a case of pleural mesothelioma, Du Bray and Rosson[825] commented that much of the tumor showed a "marked desmoplastic reaction with the tumor cells scattered rather diffusely throughout the fibrous tissue," with few mitotic figures in those areas where the desmoplastic reaction was prominent. In 1998, Mangano et al.[826] reported a series of 31 DesMMs and proposed criteria for their diagnosis.

DesMMs are usually pleural in localization, although we have encountered uncommon cases of desmoplastic MM in the peritoneum. Of the 27 cases reported by Cantin et al.,[824] 26 were pleural in localization and only one was peritoneal; 19 represented sarcomatoid MMs, as opposed to six biphasic and two epithelial MMs.

About 2% to 10% of mesotheliomas can be described as desmoplastic,[37,119,507,823,827] and they are arbitrarily so designated when 50% or more of the tumor in an adequate biopsy represents hypocellular fibrous tissue[37] (when the proportion of paucicellular desmoplastic tissue is <50%, the authors simply designate the tumors as a sarcomatoid or other MM with desmoplastic features).

Characteristically, DesMMs comprise interweaving bundles of hyalinized fibrocollagenous tissue with variable numbers of intervening tumor cells, and the gross morphology is that of firm rubbery fibrous tissue that may even be described as "woody" in consistency.

Desmoplastic sarcomatoid MM is perhaps the most deceptive pattern of mesothelioma encountered in surgical pathology practice, and it stimulates greater diversity of diagnostic opinion and disagreement among expert mesothelioma panels than any other histologic type of mesothelioma,[788] because of its liability to misdiagnosis as either inflammatory pleural fibrosis[826] or parietal pleural fibrous plaque.

In our experience, accurate diagnosis of desmoplastic MM is often impossible with closed and core biopsies of pleura, and surgical biopsy is required for confident diagnosis, such as thoracoscopy-guided biopsies. Because of the bland appearance of the MM in many cases, assessment of invasion is often the most valuable pointer to the diagnosis.[119,503,822] This being so, it is important for the biopsy to include not only the pleura but also subpleural tissues for the assessment of invasion; the confidence index for a diagnosis of desmoplastic MM can be correlated directly with the extent of the biopsy and its depth. Even so, it is our experience that some cases of DesMM continue to be misdiagnosed histologically as benign fibrous pleuritis. As recorded by Mangano et al.[826] and in our experience,[119,822] several major features aid in the diagnosis of these deceptive lesions:

- *The architecture of the lesion and the presence or absence of "bland" necrosis.* Unlike the paucicellular laminated architecture of benign pleural fibrous plaques, DesMMs are usually characterized by interweaving areas of fibrocollagenous tissue, with a branched, whorled, micronodular, or storiform pattern, different from the architecture characteristic of benign pleural fibrous plaques or the more orderly stratified (zonal) pattern of benign fibrous pleuritis (cf. Figs. 43.116 and 43.117 with 43.118 to 43.120).

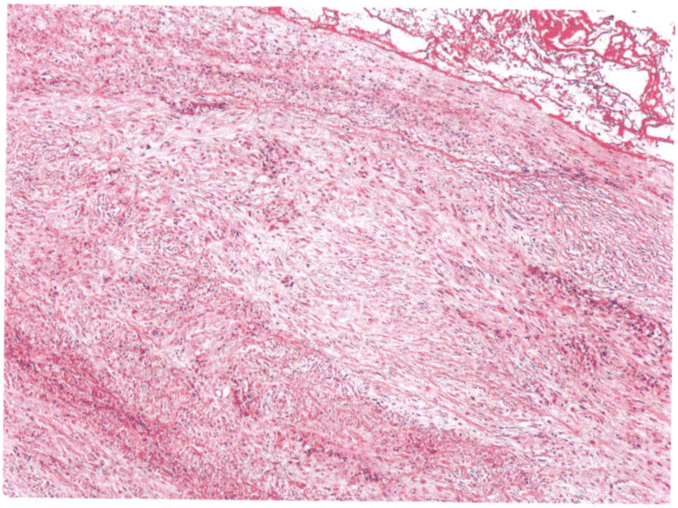

FIGURE 43.116. Desmoplastic sarcomatoid mesothelioma of pleura. At low magnification, the disordered architecture of the collagen-rich hypocellular tumor tissue is evident, especially in the lower left of this field.

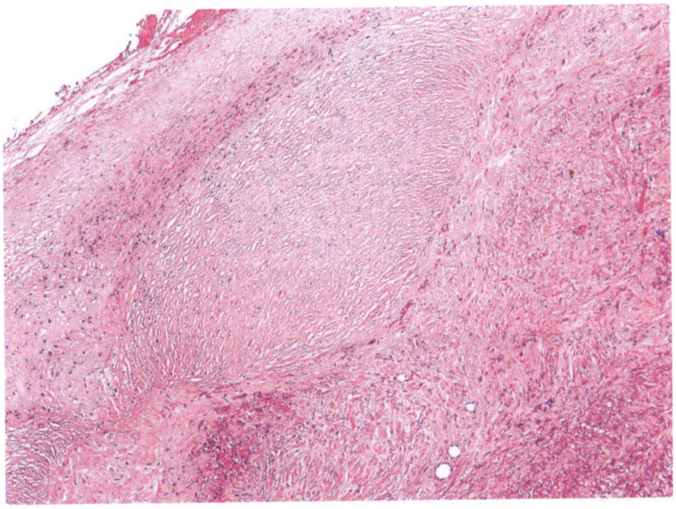

FIGURE 43.117. Pleural desmoplastic sarcomatoid mesothelioma. In addition to a disordered architecture of the desmoplastic tissue, this lesion shows a focal micronodular pattern, located near the center of the field. The desmoplastic tissue also shows greater cellularity in the deeper zone of the tumor (lower right field) than in the subsurface zone, a reversal of the zonation characteristic of a fibroinflammatory process affecting the pleura.

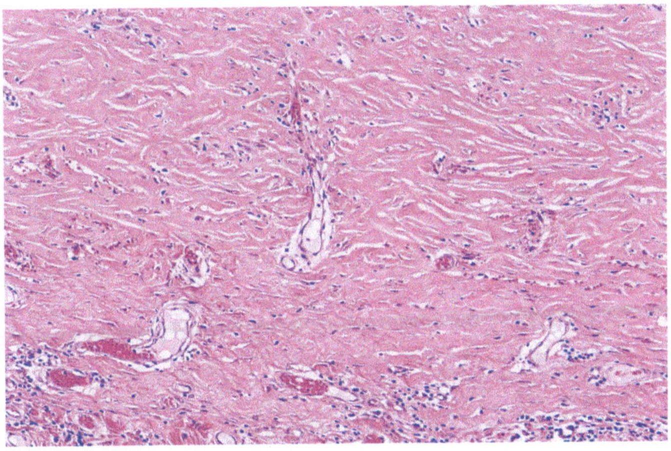

FIGURE 43.119. Benign fibrous pleuritis. This micrograph was taken close to the interface between the pleural fibrous tissue and subpleural adipose tissue and shows a reasonably orderly to laminated architecture, with no augmentation of cellularity in this zone. Small thin-walled blood vessels are evident within the fibrocollagenous tissue, one of which (center) extends almost vertically toward the pleural surface.

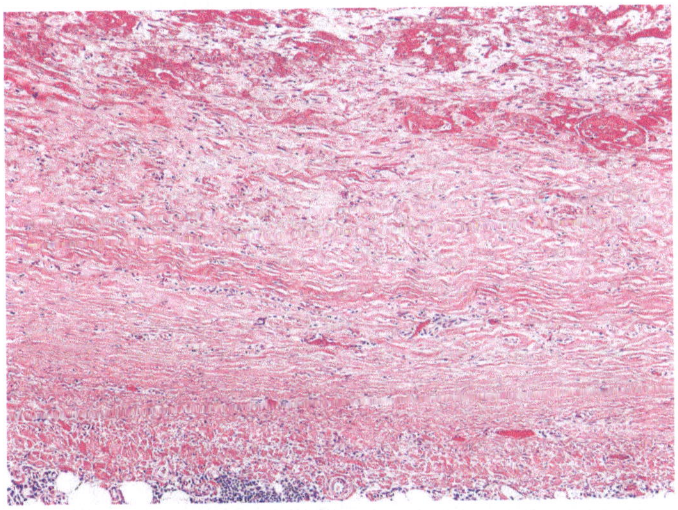

FIGURE 43.118. Benign fibrous pleuritis. Fibrinous exudate is evident near the upper zone of this field and the fibrous tissue shows no increase in cellularity, for example, near the interface between the pleural fibrous tissue and the subpleural fat, where there is a focal lymphocytic infiltrate, a feature often seen with benign fibrous pleuritis and also with pleural malignant mesotheliomas on occasions. The appearances of the fibrous pleuritis in this case are nonspecific, but the patient had a background of occupational exposure to asbestos with no clinical evidence of any alternative cause for pleuritis, so that the appearances were considered consistent with benign asbestos pleuritis with pleural fibrosis. Compare with Figures 43.116 and 43.117.

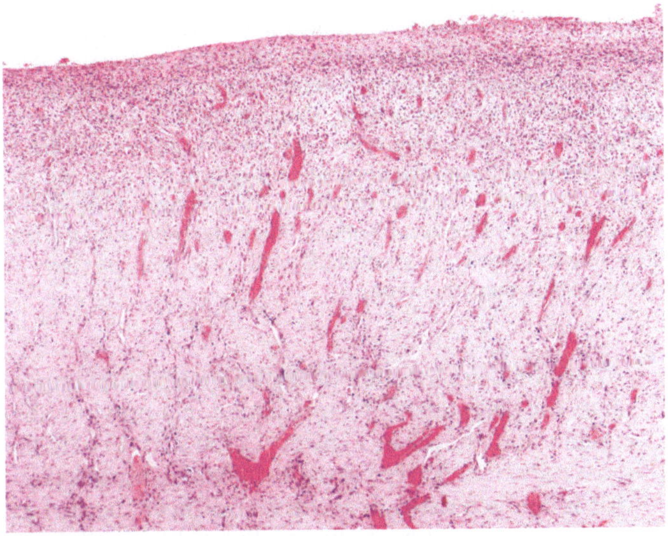

FIGURE 43.120. Benign fibrous pleuritis. In comparison to the desmoplastic mesothelioma illustrated in Figures 43.116 and 43.117, this benign inflammatory process shows a "top heavy" zonal pattern in terms of cellularity, whereby the most cellular tissue is located in the subsurface zone, with diminishing cellularity and increasing collagen deposition in the deeper zones of the thickened fibrous layer. In addition, there are multiple small and congested blood vessels that extend through most of the fibrous tissue illustrated, near-perpendicular to the free surface of the pleura and roughly parallel to each other. The overall architecture and zonation are characteristic of a benign fibroinflammatory process.

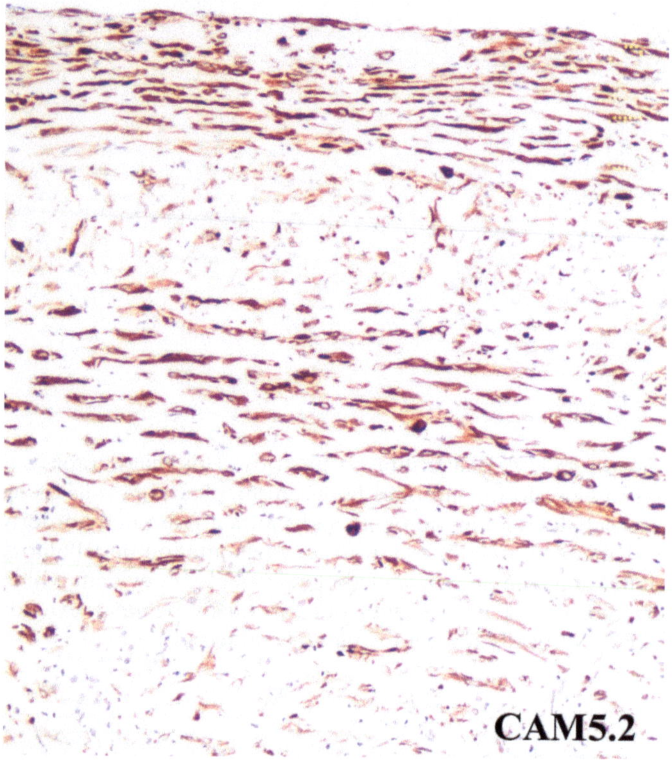

FIGURE 43.121. Benign fibrous pleuritis. The fibroblastoid cells in cases of benign fibrous pleuritis usually show positive expression of cytokeratins (CKs), illustrated here by staining for CK8/18 (CAM5.2). Again, the pattern of CK expression conforms to the zonal pattern of a benign fibroinflammatory disorder, whereby the most cellular tissue is located near the free surface, with diminishing cellularity toward the lower zone of this field. In addition, the fibroblastoid cells in this area are disposed with their long axes parallel to the surface of the pleura and roughly parallel to each other. This orderly pattern of zonation and cellularity is characteristically not seen in cases of desmoplastic mesothelioma.

The zonal architecture of the lesion is also of importance for diagnosis.[828] As mentioned in a previous discussion and shown in Figures 43.120 and 43.121, the most cellular and atypical tissue in benign fibrous pleuritis is characteristically located at or near the surface of the pleura, with gradually diminishing cellularity and increasing collagen deposition in the deeper zones of the fibrous tissue ("top heavy" cellularity[507]). In contrast, the most cellular and atypical tissue in DesMM is usually found near the deep boundary of the lesion (Fig. 43.117); in other words, DesMMs are characterized by reversal of the zonation typical of organizing pleural inflammation.

The architecture of the microvasculature within the fibrous tissue may be of diagnostic significance. In some instances, small blood vessels within benign fibrous pleuritis are arranged roughly in parallel and perpendicular or nearly so to the free surface of the pleura (Fig. 43.120), and they traverse almost the full thickness of the fibrotic tissue,[37,507] whereas this orderly and near-perpendicular vascular architecture is typically not seen in cases of DesMM.[507] Even so, two caveats are worth emphasis concerning this finding: (1) blood vessels with this pattern are not always or consistently evident in benign fibrous pleuritis, and (2) we have encountered rare cases of proven epithelial MM accompanied by a prominent fibroproliferative stromal reaction where there were parallel and near-perpendicular blood vessels of this type (Fig. 43.48 in biphasic mesothelioma section). Therefore, it seems that only the presence (not absence) of these blood vessels is of significance, and that they indicate that the fibrous tissue is benign in those areas where they are located.

When a disordered, storiform, or micronodular architecture is seen in combination with foci of so-called bland necrosis—defined as such by absence of a boundary inflammatory reaction (Fig. 43.122) and perhaps resulting from compression, invasion, or neoplastic outpacing of the stromal microvasculature—these two findings in combination can allow a diagnosis of desmoplastic sarcomatoid MM at a high order of confidence, even in the absence of overtly sarcomatoid tissue or in the absence of invasion (for example, when the biopsy is too superficial in character for this assessment).[826] Even so, laminated fibrocollagenous tissue that is essentially indistinguishable from pleural fibrous plaque tissue can be encountered in desmoplastic mesotheliomas,[822] and in such cases it is arguable as to whether such areas represent benign plaque tissue overgrown by the desmoplastic mesothelioma or whether the laminated paucicellular fibrocollagenous tissue is an integral part of the mesothelioma (as we consider it sometimes to be).

- *The cellularity and cytomorphology of the fibrocollagenous tissue.* Areas of overtly sarcomatoid tissue—defined as such by cellularity, cytologic atypia, and mitotic figures that are excessive for a benign fibrocollagenous lesion of the pleura such as benign fibrous pleuritis—are important markers of DesMM.[37,119,503,822,826] It is our impression that the most cellular and atypical tissue is sometimes found at the mediastinal aspect of the pleura, and in one of our cases a definitive diagnosis of DesMM could not be made on a surgical biopsy from the lateral parietal pleura, because of absence of overtly sarcomatoid tissue or invasion, but the diagnosis was suspected from the collagen pattern; because of this and the operative appearances, a further biopsy was taken from the mediastinal pleura and this revealed obvious sarcomatoid tissue.[822]
- *Clear evidence of invasion of chest wall structures or lung.* Invasion of subpleural adipose tissue (or even deeper chest wall structures) is one of the most impor-

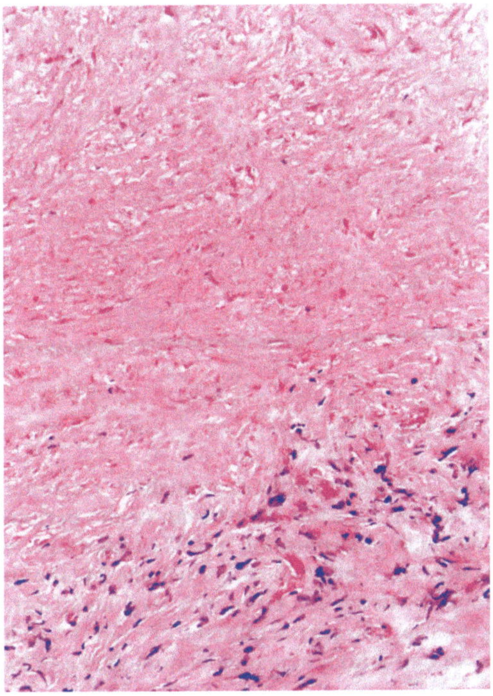

FIGURE 43.122. Desmoplastic sarcomatoid mesothelioma of pleura. An area of "bland" necrosis is illustrated, characterized by absence of an inflammatory reaction at the interface between the necrotic zone and the adjacent apparently viable desmoplastic sarcomatoid tissue.

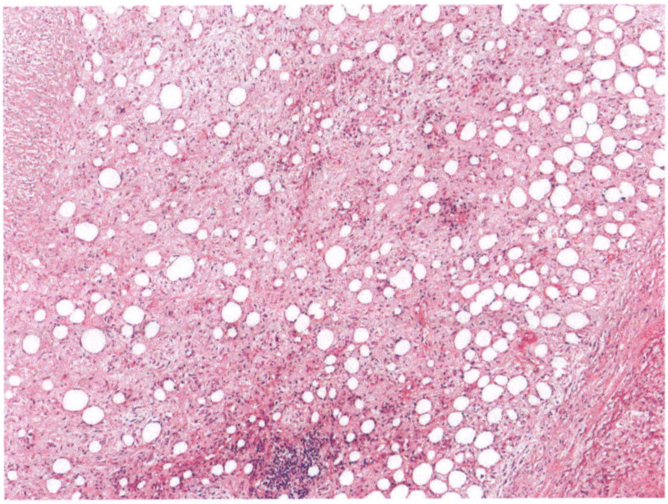

FIGURE 43.123. Desmoplastic sarcomatoid mesothelioma of pleura. The hypocellular tumor tissue shows a characteristic pattern of infiltration into the subpleural adipose tissue, whereby the neoplastic cells insinuate between individual adipocytes, splaying them apart and incorporating them into the advancing edge of the tumor, a pattern that we sometimes describe as Swiss cheese invasion.

tant markers for a diagnosis of desmoplastic sarcomatoid MM, and perhaps the most decisive. In particular, the demonstration of infiltration into subpleural tissue or deeper structures or into lung parenchyma by cytokeratin-positive spindle-shaped cells is perhaps the clearest indicator of sarcomatoid DesMM in surgical biopsy tissue (Figs. 43.123 to 43.127).[37,119,503,822,826] In this regard, it is our experience and that of others[503,515,829] that the great majority of sarcomatoid DesMMs show intense and widespread expression of cytokeratins (CKs), and the demonstration of invasion of subpleural tissues by CK-positive spindle cells represents a decisive indicator of MM[119] (Fig. 43.125). It is emphasized that the presence of CK-positive fibroblastoid cells is not of diagnostic importance by itself, because benign fibroinflammatory disorders of the pleura are usually characterized by CK expression by the reactive fibroblastoid cells (Fig. 43.121)[37]: instead, immunostaining for CKs is of value in this situation to facilitate assessment of invasion as a marker of malignancy (Fig. 43.125). In contrast, in our experience[119,822] and that of others,[37,515,829] infiltration of CK-positive fiboblastoid cells into subpleural adipose or other tissues is almost never seen with benign fibroinflammatory disorders (exceptions include rare examples of a biopsy of an antecedent biopsy site or needle track, with displaced mesothelial cells restricted to the zone of the wound).

Invasion into subpleural adipose tissue by the fibrocollagenous tissue comprising DesMM is often characterized by an insinuative pattern of invasion whereby the tumor cells extend between individual adipocytes, splaying them apart and incorporating them into the poorly delineated deep margin of the DesMM (Figs.

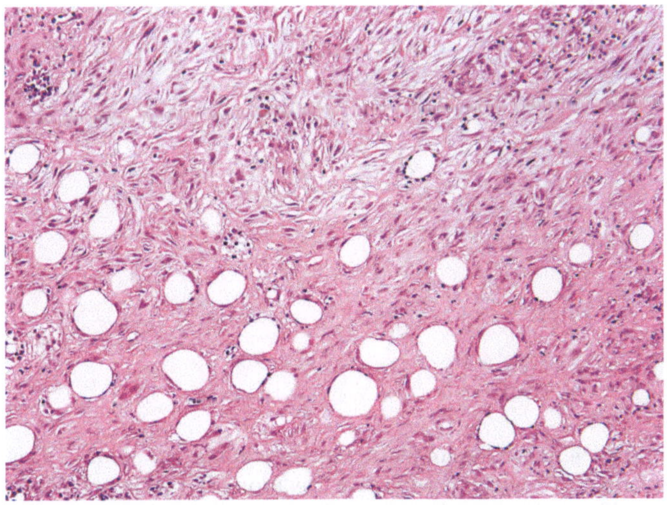

FIGURE 43.124. Desmoplastic sarcomatoid mesothelioma of pleura. This field illustrates the invasion at higher magnification, with splaying apart of the adipocytes by the hypocellular fibroblastoid tumor tissue.

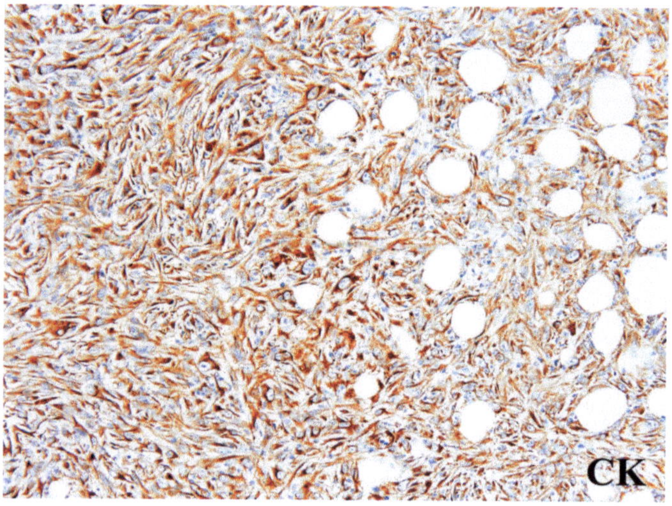

FIGURE 43.125. Pleural desmoplastic sarcomatoid mesothelioma. The demonstration of CK-positive fibroblastoid cells infiltrating into adipose tissue with separation of individual adipocytes is virtually diagnostic of malignancy in this context.

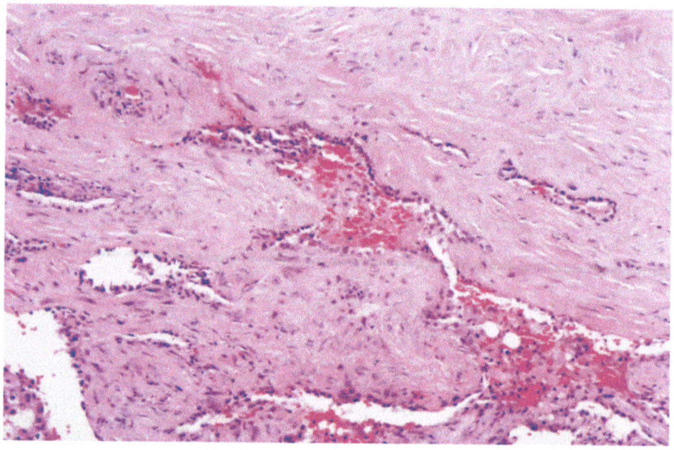

FIGURE 43.127. Desmoplastic sarcomatoid mesothelioma of pleura, infiltrating into the interstitium of the peripheral lung parenchyma, with incorporation into the tumor of remnants of alveolar spaces lined by alveolar epithelium. In other instances, the desmoplastic tissue can erupt into alveolar spaces, producing mimicry of organizing pneumonia, or even the architectural pattern of an epithelioid hemangioendothelioma of lung.

43.123 to 43.125). We often refer to this pattern of infiltration as *Swiss cheese* invasion. Although characteristic of DesMM, it is by no means diagnostic and can be found with other tumors, including non-Hodgkin's lymphomas.

When DesMM invades into lung parenchyma, it can infiltrate along the interstitium and interlobular septa, incorporating remnants of alveoli into the invasive margin of the mesothelioma (Fig. 43.127).

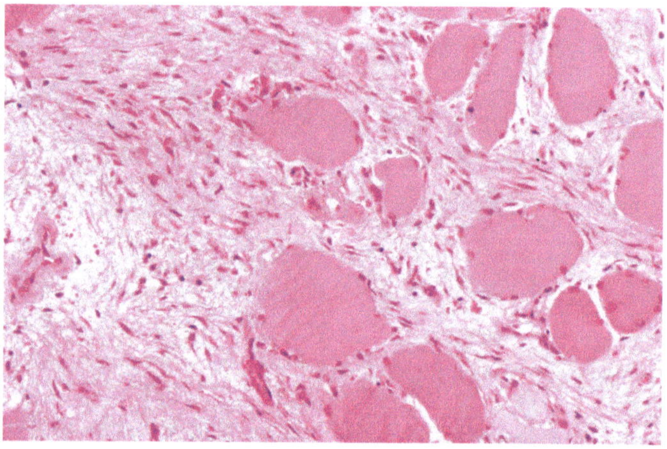

FIGURE 43.126. Desmoplastic mesothelioma of pleura. This micrograph depicts insinuative invasion of the hypocellular fibroblastoid tumor tissue into chest wall skeletal muscle, with separation of individual myocytes. The desmoplastic tumor tissue in this case extended almost to the perichondrium of a rib, where there was a CK-negative periosteal reaction with subperiosteal new (woven) bone formation.

The mesotheliomatous tissue may also burst into alveolar spaces, to mimic the histology of organizing pneumonia or even epithelioid hemangioendothelioma of lung.[37,503]

- *Rarely in surgical pathology, the identification of metastatic DesMM.* Wilson et al.[827] found evidence of metastatic spread in 14 of 16 cases of DesMM that came to autopsy. The contralateral lung was the site affected most commonly (75%), and on rare occasions an intrapulmonary metastatic deposit of DesMM may be found in biopsy tissue.[503] Other sites of metastasis recorded by Wilson et al. included liver, thyroid, kidney, adrenal gland, myocardium, and bone.

DesMM appears to have a propensity to metastasize to bone,[37,503,830] with the potential for misdiagnosis as a primary bone tumor if the antecedent medical history is unknown to the pathologist or if the metastatic deposit(s) represent the presenting manifestation of the DesMM. We have encountered several such cases (Figs. 43.128 and 43.129). In most cases, the bone metastasis presented as a pathologic fracture after diagnosis of the pleural DesMM, but one referral case presented as a fractured neck of femur in an elderly woman who had been diagnosed a short time beforehand with benign fibrous pleuritis. As in the other cases, the bone deposit was characterized by strong CK expression by the desmoplastic tissue, and was followed by reexamination of the original pleural biopsy and a revised diagnosis of pleural DesMM. The bone in such skeletal deposits is distinguishable from osseous differentiation within a DesMM[503] by (1) knowledge of the site whence the biopsy was taken; and (2) the presence of well-

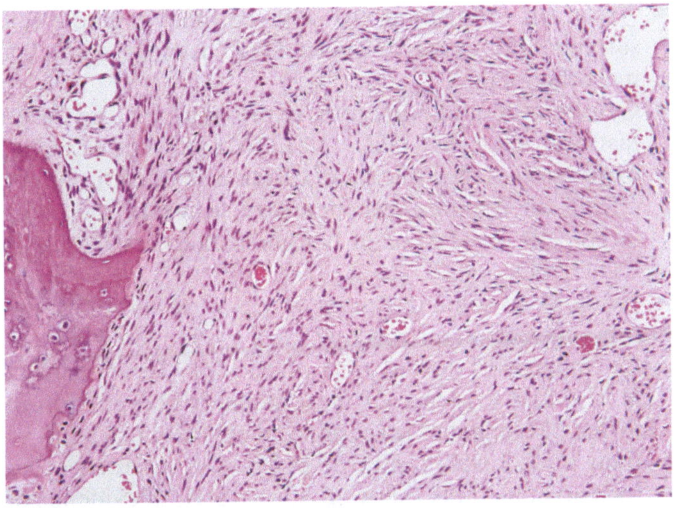

FIGURE 43.128. Metastatic deposit of desmoplastic sarcomatoid mesothelioma in bone, depicting the hypocellular tumor tissue.

developed trabeculae of lamellar bone, in addition to any woven bone related to a pathologic fracture.

Finally, it is worth emphasizing that although desmoplastic MMs lack many of the cytologic indicators of malignancy, these lesions represent a highly lethal form of pleural MM, with a mean survival of approximately 6 months following diagnosis,[824,827] in comparison to about 8 to 12 months following diagnosis of other forms of pleural MM.

Lymphohistiocytoid Mesothelioma

In 1988, Henderson et al.[831] described three cases of pleural MM with a striking lymphomatoid appearance in biopsy tissue, which they designated as lymphohistiocytoid mesothelioma (LHM). They considered this type of mesothelioma to represent a variant of predominantly sarcomatoid mesothelioma where the neoplastic cells were histiocytoid in appearance but were obscured by a prominent infiltrate of lymphocytes, accompanied by plasma cells and in one case eosinophils, imparting a histologic resemblance to either Hodgkin's or non-Hodgkin's lymphoma (Figs. 43.130 and 43.131); all three cases had been misdiagnosed at some stage as lymphoma.

The three cases represented 0.8% of all cases of pathologically proven mesotheliomas across Australia as accessioned in the Australian Mesothelioma Register as part of the Australian Mesothelioma Surveillance Program. Subsequently, additional cases have been reported by Khalidi et al.[832] and by Yao et al.[833] The cases reported by Yao et al. represented 3.3% of accessions, probably reflecting a referral bias for cases submitted to a reference center for ultrastructural pathology in the U.S. Galateau-Sallé et al.[37] reported a series of 22 cases reported by the MesoPath Group in France in 2003, representing less than 2% of their cases.

Of 12 cases of LHM described in detail in the literature,[831–835] 11 were pleural in location, and one was peritoneal (we have seen an additional case of peritoneal LHM (Fig. 43.131). The ages of the patients ranged from 31 to 74 years, with a mean of 59 years approximately, with a male-to-female ratio of 2:1.

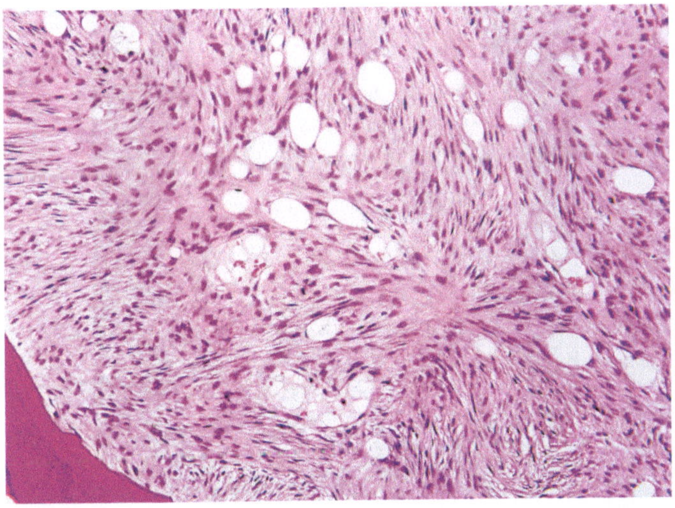

FIGURE 43.129. Metastatic deposit of desmoplastic sarcomatoid mesothelioma in bone. This was the most cellular area of the tissue in this biopsy specimen, showing a focal storiform architecture. The bone trabecula at the upper right of the field was predominantly lamellar in character.

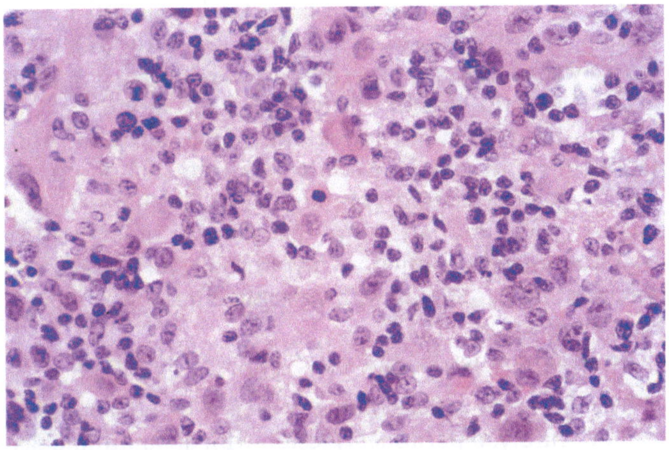

FIGURE 43.130. Pleural malignant mesothelioma, lymphohistiocytoid type. The tissue comprises an admixture of histiocytoid cells, with moderate amounts of pale eosinophilic cytoplasm, with numerous interspersed lymphocytes. (Case 3 from Henderson et al.[831])

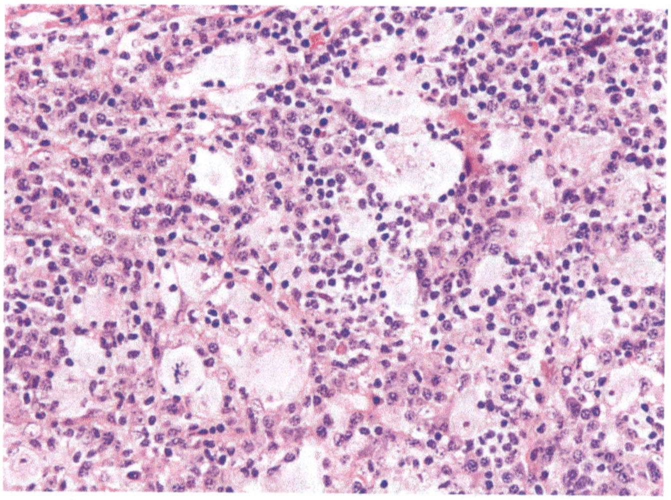

FIGURE 43.131. Peritoneal malignant mesothelioma of lymphohistiocytoid type. Among the background lymphocytes and plasma cells, there are larger pale neoplastic cells with multilobated nuclei, and one mitotic figure is evident. The large pale cells showed strong immunostaining for low molecular weight cytokeratins.

All three cases originally described by Henderson et al.[831] had a background of occupational exposure to asbestos, but no such history was recorded in the three cases reported by Khalidi et al.[832] and details of any asbestos exposure were unknown for three of the cases reported by Yao et al.,[833] whereas one of their cases had no history of exposure. There was a history of minor exposure to asbestos in the single case reported by Dorfmüller et al.[834] in 2004.

There was no evidence that the lymphohistiocytoid appearances of the cases conferred any major survival advantage. Three of the cases reported by Khalidi at al.[832] were alive with disease at 2, 3, and 72 months postdiagnosis, whereas the survival range for other cases averaged about 7 months, within a range of 2 to 20 months.

The differential diagnosis for LHM includes both Hodgkin's and non-Hodgkin's malignant lymphoma as well as lymphomatoid granulomatosis, primary or secondary thymoma affecting the pleura, inflammatory pseudotumor (inflammatory myofibroblastic tumor), and sarcomatoid carcinoma with a prominent stromal inflammatory reaction.[831–833,836]

Several findings facilitate the diagnosis of LHM:

- The presence of a confluent pleura-based (or, even more rarely, a peritoneal) lesion with an anatomic distribution indistinguishable from mesothelioma on imaging studies or at operation (Fig. 43.132).
- A lymphoma-like appearance on light microscopy, with scattered dispersed or indistinctly clustered atypical large histiocytoid cells (Figs. 43.130 and 43.131).
- Areas of transition to conventional spindle-cell sarcomatoid tissue, or even small foci of epithelial mesothelioma.
- Cytokeratin and vimentin expression by the large histiocytoid cells (Fig. 43.133) and, occasionally, expression of mesothelial markers such as calretinin or CK5/6 on immunohistochemistry, whereas the same large cells are devoid of lymphoid markers[503] such as CD45, CD3, or CD20.
- Evidence in some instances of mesothelial differentiation on electron microscopy, such as elongated serpentine microvilli devoid of a glycocalyx. Henderson et al.[831] found evidence of mesothelial differentiation in terms of elongated serpentine microvilli in two out of their three cases, and three of the four cases reported by Yao et al.[833] also showed ultrastructural evidence of mesothelial differentiation, whereas no electron microscopy findings were recorded in three cases described by Khalidi at al.[832]

Four further facets of LHM are worth emphasis:

- This variant of mesothelioma does not simply represent prominent lymphocytic infiltration in an epithelial mesothelioma.[837] Henderson et al.[831] considered LHM to be a variant of predominantly sarcomatoid mesothelioma, where there was an intimate admixture and intermingling of the background histiocytoid tumor

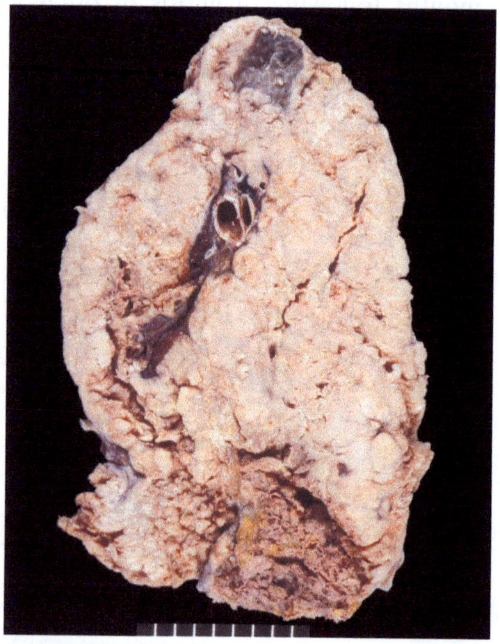

FIGURE 43.132. Pleural lymphohistiocytoid mesothelioma, gross appearances at autopsy. On histologic examination of the autopsy tissues, the lymphohistiocytoid features were depleted, and the tissue comprised mainly spindle-cell sarcomatoid tissue. (Case 3 from Henderson et al.[831])

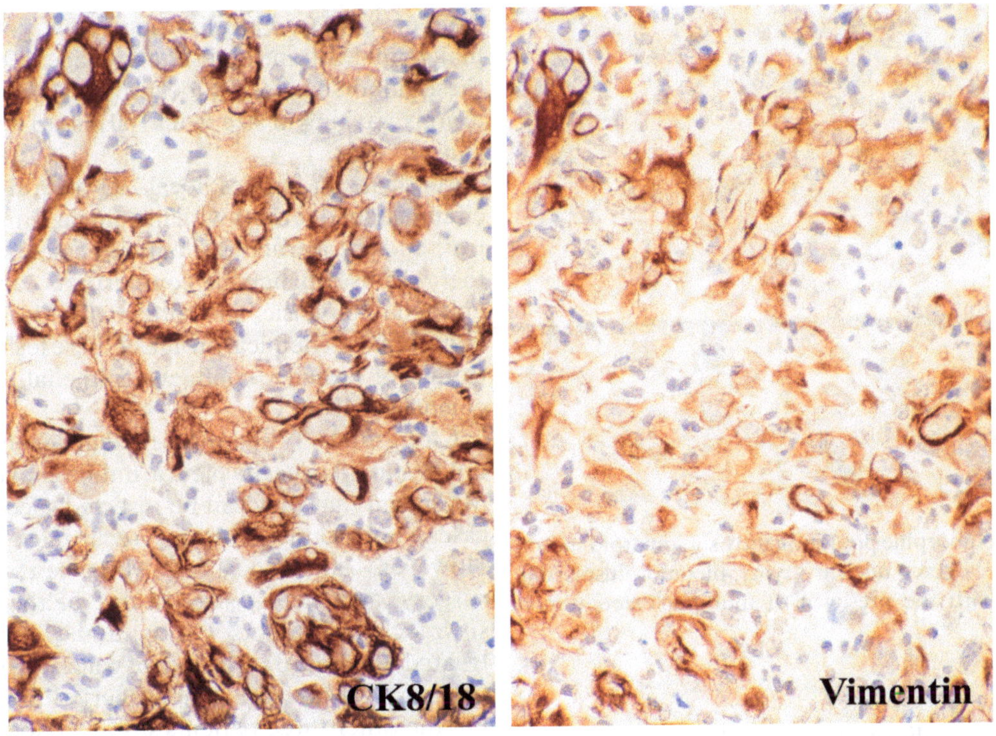

A B

FIGURE 43.133. **(A)** Pleural lymphohistiocytoid mesothelioma. The neoplastic cells show obvious expression of low molecular weight cytokeratins. (Case 3 from Henderson et al.[831]) **(B)** Coexpression of vimentin by the neoplastic cells.

cells with tumor-infiltrating lymphocytes, plasma cells, and in some areas, eosinophils.

- Focal lymphohistiocytoid features occur in otherwise conventional sarcomatoid mesothelioma, so that it is suggested—by analogy with desmoplastic mesothelioma—that at least 50% of the tissue in an adequate biopsy should be lymphohistiocytoid in appearance for a diagnosis of LHM.[37] When the proportion falls below 50%, we simply designate such cases as sarcomatoid mesotheliomas with focal lymphohistiocytoid features.
- The lymphohistiocytoid appearances presumably reflect an immunologic response on the part of the host to the mesothelioma itself. Henderson et al.[822] described the immunohistochemical findings in the tumor-infiltrating lymphocytes in 24 biopsies and autopsy tissue from 22 cases of mesothelioma (epithelial, biphasic, and sarcomatoid in type, including LHMs), and they found T-lymphocyte predominance in about 60% of cases, approximately equal representation of T and B cells in 20%, and B-lymphocyte predominance in the remaining 20%. In their cases, Khalidi et al.[832] found a predominance of T lymphocytes, but with the additional presence of B cells. Yao et al.[833] also recorded a predominance of T lymphocytes in all four cases, but with a minor component of CD20-positive B cells, accompanied by occasional eosinophils.
- The lymphohistiocytoid appearances may reflect a transient phase in the development of some sarcomatoid MMs. One of the three cases originally reported by Henderson et al.[831] had the histologic appearances of a conventional sarcomatoid mesothelioma at autopsy, suggesting depletion of immune-effector cells in the later stages of the mesothelioma. Robinson et al.[835] reported a single case of LHM in a woman who survived for 20 months. In contrast to the initial biopsy, no significant lymphoid infiltrate was detected at autopsy in her mesothelioma.

Pleomorphic Mesothelioma

Many epithelioid mesotheliomas show only low-grade cytologic atypia with minor nuclear pleomorphism and relatively little nuclear hyperchromasia, in comparison to the carcinomas from which they require distinction. Equally, although sarcomatoid MMs closely resemble equivalent soft tissue sarcomas, most notably fibrosarcoma and malignant fibrous histiocytoma (MFH), they may show only low-grade cytologic atypia and pleomorphism, especially desmoplastic mesotheliomas. However, rare mesotheliomas can show extreme cellularity, nuclear atypia, hyperchromasia, and pleomorphism, producing a close histologic resemblance to either an undifferentiated large cell carcinoma of lung or to the pleomorphic variant of MFH (Figs. 43.40, 43.41, and 43.134, respectively).

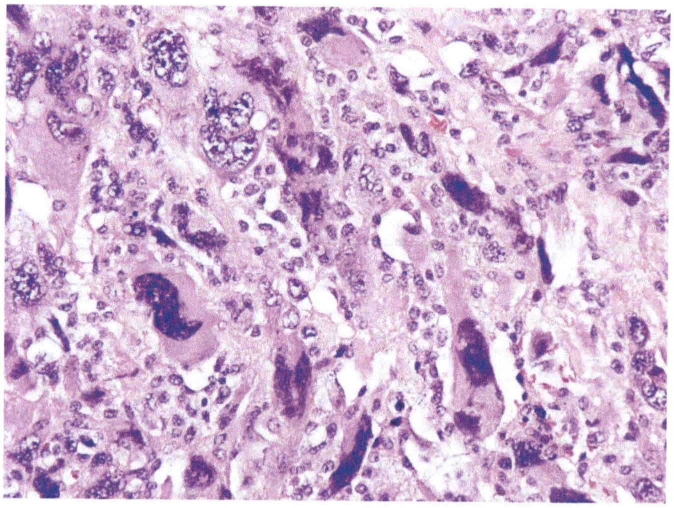

FIGURE 43.134. Pleomorphic predominantly sarcomatoid mesothelioma showing extreme nuclear atypia, pleomorphism, and hyperchromasia, with the presence of multinucleated tumor cells.

Accordingly, we believe that pleural tumors showing extreme pleomorphism should not be dismissed as large cell carcinoma or secondary sarcoma and that when they are pleura-based and have an anatomic distribution consistent with mesothelioma, they should be investigated accordingly.

The diagnosis of pleomorphic mesothelioma, whether epithelial or sarcomatoid, can be based on the following findings:

- A pleura-based tumor with an anatomic distribution that conforms to a diagnosis of mesothelioma, as revealed by imaging studies.
- A transition from the pleomorphic areas to other regions where the appearances are more characteristic of either epithelial or sarcomatoid MM.
- An immunohistochemical profile that conforms to a diagnosis of mesothelioma of either epithelial or sarcomatoid type, as opposed to secondary carcinoma or even secondary sarcoma (for example, when the neoplastic tissue shows strong positive labeling for cytokeratins throughout).
- Occasionally, ultrastructural evidence of mesothelial differentiation.

Localized Malignant Mesothelioma

In 1992, Henderson et al.[211] briefly referred to two cases of localized pleural MM, and further cases were subsequently described by Crotty et al.[838] and Allen et al.,[839] among others.[840–844] Localized pleural MM has been reported in men and women with about equal frequency, within an age range from the 40s to the 70s, although we have encountered localized and even polypoidal pleural malignant MMs in young adults of ages 20 to 30. Typically, these tumors represent localized sessile or pedunculated lesions, ranging in size from 100mm to a few centimeters (Fig. 43.135).

As the term implies, localized pleural MMs represent circumscribed tumors with histologic, immunohistochemical, and ultrastructural features essentially identical to their diffuse malignant counterparts, and they include epithelial, biphasic, and sarcomatoid lesions. Again, the immunohistochemical profile of these lesions corresponds to that of ordinary confluent epithelial, biphasic, or sarcomatoid MMs.

Churg et al.[503] commented that localized MMs tend not to spread over the pleura, unlike conventional pleural MMs, and that they can be resected successfully in some cases, apparently with no recurrence of the tumor. However, other localized MMs can recur following surgery, and metastasize. In one of the first reports of such localized tumors, Crotty et al.[838] recorded six cases treated by surgical resection, of which three had a disease-free survival for an extended period following excision, but the other three patients sustained local recurrence of the their disease and died within 2 years of initial resection. In one case mentioned by Henderson et al.[211]—a cytokeratin-positive sarcomatoid MM histologically resembling a malignant fibrous histiocytoma, located in an interlobar fissure and treated initially by surgical resection (bilobectomy)—the gross appearances of the recurrent tumor at autopsy were characteristic of mesothelioma.

When dealing with limited biopsy tissue, recognition of localized as opposed to diffuse MM requires information beyond that obtainable from the histologic sections alone. Some diffuse MMs can present with a dominant mass lesion, accompanied by other smaller tumor nodules, so that evidence of the purely localized character of the MM is needed for diagnosis of localized MM,[503] necessitating

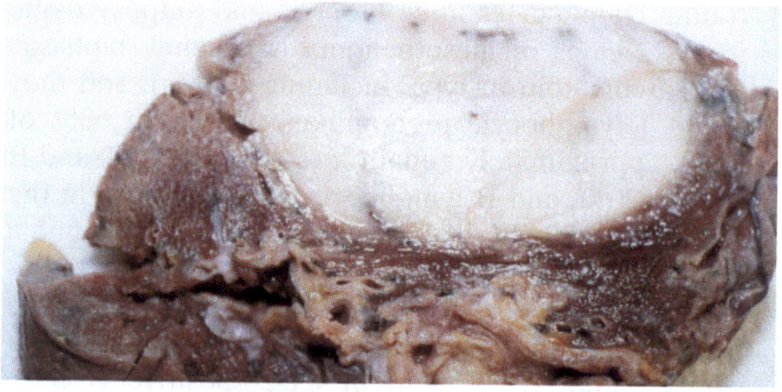

FIGURE 43.135. This localized pleural mesothelioma arose in the pleura and invaded lung parenchyma. It was diagnosed radiographically as a solitary pulmonary nodule.

integration of the histologic findings with organ-imaging studies or the gross appearances at operation.

It is sometimes claimed that the relationship between localized pleural MM and prior asbestos exposure is less well established than for diffuse pleural MMs. This may be so, perhaps explicable by the unusual gross and radiologic findings in such cases, so that an exhaustive exposure history may not be sought, and by the paucity of such localized cases reported to date; however, we have encountered such cases where there has been a clear history of antecedent asbestos exposure (including one case with childhood exposure). Therefore, on the basis of the prevailing evidence at this time, we believe that there is no compelling evidence to consider the relationship of such localized MMs to asbestos to be essentially different than for diffuse MMs.

Approach to Diagnosis/Differential Diagnosis

Our approach to the diagnosis of pleural neoplasms is to accurately classify a neoplasm according to its cytologic, histologic, immunohistochemical, and ultrastructural features. All types of specimens are potentially useful in making a specific diagnosis. In general, with respect to biopsy specimens, the larger the specimen, the more useful and potentially less difficult it is to make a specific diagnosis. Cytologic evaluation is also a potentially useful technique as described below.

The Cytology of Malignant Mesothelioma

The cytology specimens used for the investigation of a lesion suspicious of MM include effusion fluids and, less commonly, fine-needle aspiration biopsies (FNABs). As noted by some authors,[845] the difficulties that beset interpretation of effusion cytology specimens have "kept researchers and publishers in business over the last 20 years." Unfortunately, those difficulties can also lead to confusion among clinicians who may be uncertain over the interpretation of the cytopathology reports and assessment of the confidence index for a diagnosis. There are two main difficulties in pleural effusion cytology: (1) the distinction between MM and metastatic malignancy, and (2) the distinction between a reactive pleural effusion from MM. Nowadays, it is the second that is more problematic.

Numerous diagnostic criteria and ancillary investigations, such as immunohistochemical studies, electron microscopy,[846] flow cytometry,[847] atomic force microscopy,[848] and many more, have been proposed. Some techniques initially appeared to show promise in research laboratories, but that early promise was either not borne out in more extensive routine diagnostic testing, or the techniques were impractical for everyday diagnosis. There is currently no consensus concerning the optimal approach for difficult cytology specimens. There are several excellent textbooks and recent reviews on this subject[845,849–854] and it is not our aim to duplicate those comprehensive accounts. Rather, we highlight some of the problem areas and offer our approach to them (see also Mesothelioma in Chapter 45).

The main issues of importance in the cytologic diagnosis of pleural MM, as we see them, are as follows:

1. Some pathologists require the presence of invasion in a tissue specimen for a definitive diagnosis of MM, and consequently argue that a definitive diagnosis cannot be made from a cytology specimen alone.[854] Even when a combination of clinical and cytologic criteria is used, there is no consensus about the confidence index for a cytodiagnosis. Some authors believe that even distinction of MM in situ and invasive MM is possible in skilled hands.[849] However, the literature and, in particular, the criteria proposed for the diagnosis of MM in situ indicate that this specific diagnosis is almost impossible on cytology. Henderson et al.[490] recommended that invasive MM should be identified elsewhere in the same biopsy, a follow-up biopsy, or at autopsy as a requirement for the diagnosis of MM in situ. In our practice, we consider a biopsy-proven diagnosis to be optimal, but in many cases a confident diagnosis of mesothelioma can be reached from careful correlation of the cytologic findings with clinical-radiologic information, whereby the radiologic demonstration of a confluent pleura-based lesion with nodularity or other evidence of invasion can substitute for gross or histologic evidence of invasion. In particular, we require an atypical pleural mesothelial proliferation *plus* classic radiologic findings for a clear diagnosis of MM. Correlation with clinical and radiologic information can also avoid false-positive diagnosis.

These considerations also highlight the importance of clinicopathologic correlation in general; for example, if an FNAB is performed, the exact location of the biopsy (pleura-based lesion versus an intraparenchymal lung lesion impinging on pleura) must be recorded.

2. Different processing procedures can result in different appearances on the slide. It is important to be thoroughly familiar with the procedures employed in one's own laboratory.

3. Not all types of MM are equally amenable to diagnosis from effusion fluid cytology; MMs with an epithelial component (i.e., epithelial mesotheliomas and biphasic mesotheliomas) are far more likely to shed atypical and identifiable mesothelial cells into effusion fluids than sarcomatoid MMs, for which effusion fluids usually show low cellularity and a low frequency of atypical cells. It is our experience that desmoplastic sarcomatoid mesothelioma

is never diagnosable in practice on the basis of either effusion fluid cytology or FNAB.

4. Assessment of pleural effusion cytology (like assessment of biopsy tissue) is critically dependent on the adequacy of the specimen, the quality of specimen preparation, and the experience of the pathologist providing the service. The reported sensitivity and specificity of cytology on the diagnosis of MM varies greatly. In a 1989 review of 30 years of publications, sensitivity varied between 0% and 93%.[678] In later publications, sensitivity remained variable, between 32%[855] and 76%,[856] although the main problem appeared to be the adequacy of the specimen, rather than its assessment. Practicing cytopathologists seem now well aware of the problems in making the diagnosis, and we are not aware of any recent reports of false-positive diagnoses of MM based on cytologic specimens alone.

5. A dedicated service where the entire effusion fluid is received by the pathology laboratory and can be used for microscopy and ancillary studies is likely to give the greatest diagnostic yield. This is highlighted by Whitaker et al.[850] who, on reviewing slides for a published study that claimed low sensitivity of effusion fluid cytology for diagnosis of MM,[855] found that "poor samples were the cause of poor results." The use of immunohistochemical studies on cell-block sections can increase the sensitivity and specificity of cytologic assessment; in other words, a cell block is an essential adjunct to cytologic diagnosis.

There is no doubt that the interpretation of pleural effusion cytology is fraught with difficulty. We agree with Whitaker et al.[850] that "the cytological diagnosis of MMs can be a relatively straightforward exercise though it is often a challenge and occasionally, especially in desmoplastic cases, impossible."

The first step, the distinction of malignant cells, whether mesothelial or metastatic, from benign reactive mesothelial cells, can be problematic. Attention to cytologic detail and additional features in the specimen, such as background inflammation as well as relevant clinical-radiologic details, may all assist in cytodiagnosis. However, it is our approach to err on the side of underdiagnosis when there is uncertainty, on the basis that if the process is malignant (whether MM or secondary cancer), it will declare itself as such soon enough (the prognosis for any kind of pleural malignancy is poor and usually measured in months, with little available in terms of effective treatment options at the moment; see discussion of malignancy-associated pleural effusions in the section Secondary Malignant Neoplasms Affecting the Pleura).

Rapport with Clinician

Effective communication between the cytopathologist and the clinician can aid significantly in the assessment of specimens, and relevant radiologic information should be communicated. It is unfortunate that the current guidelines issued by the British Thoracic Society Pleural Disease Group state that "20 mL of pleural fluid is adequate for cytological examination," and although some of the recommendations regarding biochemical examination have been questioned, this statement seems not to have been challenged, despite the recommendation from some cytologists that the effusion fluid should be submitted in its entirety for optimal results.[850,857,858] No less unfortunate is the statement from the European Respiratory Society (ERS) on the management of malignant pleural effusions[859] that "monoclonal antibodies . . . cannot be relied on for diagnosis" and instead the ERS recommends that "identification of . . . aneuploidy by flow cytometry may add to routine cytology by detecting false negatives."

Macroscopic Appearance of Specimen and the Use of Tumor Markers

Useful information can be gained from observation of the volume, color, clarity, and viscosity of the effusion fluid. A massive effusion is more likely to be due to a malignant process than a small one, and exudative effusions are more likely to be malignant than transudates (see later discussion on malignancy-associated pleural effusions). Highly cellular fluids (as is typical of malignant effusions) may show a thick whitish layer at the bottom of the container if they have been allowed to stand for some time. High viscosity due to high levels of hyaluronic acid is characteristic of MM.[860–862] This finding is particularly useful when quantitative assessment of hyaluronic acid concentration is used in combination with cytologic criteria.[863] Sometimes the hyaluronic acid can be seen on the slides as flocculent background material.[851] Measurement of mesothelin levels in effusion fluid may also contribute to diagnosis[864] (see later discussion in this chapter). Other tumor markers have not been found to be particularly helpful, with the possible exception of CEA, which may be increased in malignant effusion related to secondary neoplasms but was not found to be elevated in any of the cases of MM investigated.[865]

Specimen Preparation

Cytology slides may be prepared as direct smears made from the pellet after centrifugation of the specimen, as smears of the clotted specimen, as direct cytospins of the whole effusion fluid, or as cytospin preparations after Ficol Hypaque gradient centrifugation. Finally, some laboratories also use the Thin-Prep technique originally developed for cervical smears. Each of these techniques has certain characteristics and advantages, but these technical variations may lead to variation in the appearances of the specimen. No significant advantage has been identified in the use of Thin-Prep preparations over cytospin slides,[866,867] in regard to background and the preservation of cytologic detail. Whenever sufficient material is available, a cell block should be prepared. Immunohistochemical studies are most reliable when performed on sections of cell blocks, as compared to cytospins or direct smears, with the least background staining (apparently due to the reduced proteinaceous background and the reduction of three-dimensional clusters of cells that may trap antibody, resulting in false-positive results[868]). Cell-block sections also allow for the best morphologic interpretation, approximating the results seen in surgical specimens except for invasion, and are the most economical of the techniques tested.

Not only is it important to have comprehensive knowledge of the preferred techniques used in one's own laboratory, but cytologists also need to be aware of these different types of specimen preparation when reviewing slides from other laboratories.

Specimen Adequacy

There is no quantitative rule for the minimal number of mesothelial cells on a slide to assess a specimen as adequate, but in general one can argue that the more cells the better. Our experience suggests that a reasonable assessment is generally possible on samples of 50 mL at least.

Although there is no doubt that specimens are best received fresh, it appears that storage at 4°C for up to 14 days does not significantly compromise assessment of effusion fluid specimens.[869] In particular, apart from increased numbers of cytoplasmic blebs and cytoplasmic vacuolation, morphologic detail remained sufficiently preserved for diagnosis, and immunocytochemistry performed on cell block material did not reveal significant loss of antigenicity. Even though the number of specimens examined was relatively small, the results nonetheless suggested that examination can be attempted with a good chance of obtaining a diagnosis on those specimens that reach the laboratory after considerable delay.

General Aspects of Specimen Assessment

The main differential diagnoses encompass a MM, an atypical but reactive mesothelial proliferation, and secondary neoplasia. The cytologic features that suggest mesothelial differentiation do not by themselves definitively distinguish between benign and malignant mesothelial processes, but a combination of features may be used to make the distinction. Ancillary techniques including immunocytochemistry may also be used, but some are somewhat controversial. In contrast, it is widely accepted that a distinction between a mesothelial process and a metastatic malignancy can usually be made with certainty using an appropriate immunocytochemical panel, discussed below.

Features Indicative of Mesothelial Differentiation, and Discrimination Between Benign Mesothelial Hyperplasia and Malignant Mesothelioma

Normal mesothelial cells may contain one or more round or oval nuclei with one or more nucleoli. There is uniform staining of nuclei and cytoplasm, and most nuclei are located centrally or slightly eccentrically within cells, but only rarely does the nucleus abut the cell border. The cells tend to form flat sheets, with obvious fenestrations between cells (Fig. 43.136), related to the presence of long microvilli between apposed cell membranes.[829] Single cells have finely microvillous (fuzzy) borders, again corresponding to the characteristic elongated and serpentine microvilli. Small three-dimensional balls may be present but usually comprise less than 20 cells. A central collagenous core may be noted. The background may contain erythrocytes, leukocytes, and necrotic debris.

Denser cytoplasm may be seen in reactive mesothelial cells, and larger three-dimensional cell balls containing

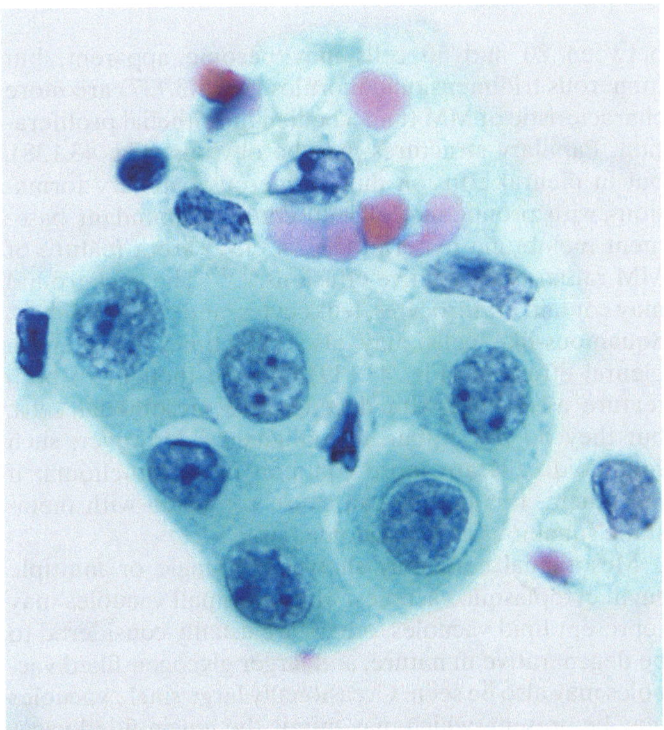

FIGURE 43.136. Atypical mesothelial cells in pleural effusion, thought to represent an atypical mesothelial hyperplasia. No biopsy was taken, but the patient was alive and well 4 years later. The cells are from a cytospin preparation, stained by the Papanicolaou (Pap) technique and show marked cytologic atypia with obvious fenestrations between cells.

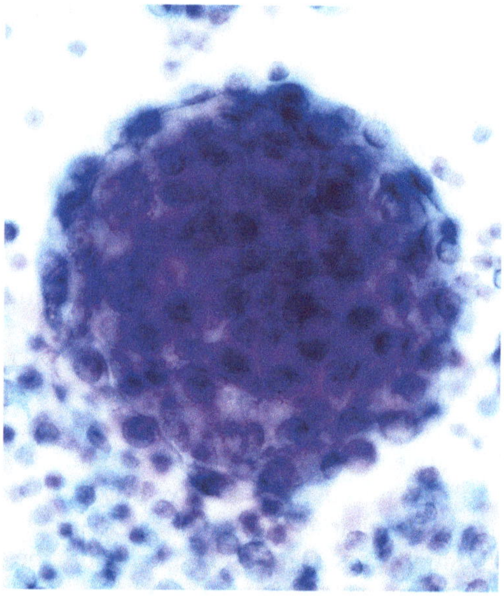

FIGURE 43.137. This Pap-stained cytospin preparation shows a large three-dimensional morule. There is some nuclear pleomorphism and some prominence of nucleoli. The nuclei remain central within most of the cells. This specimen of pleural effusion fluid came from a patient with biopsy-proven invasive MM of epithelial type.

between 20 and 50 cells may become apparent, but numerous tridimensional morules (Fig. 43.137) are more characteristic of MM than a benign mesothelial proliferation. Papillary structures may be obvious (Fig. 43.138), but in pleural effusion fluid numerous papillary formations with prominent collagen cores or abundant basement membrane material (Fig. 43.139) are a feature of MM rather than reactive effusions.[849,870] The background may contain erythrocytes, leukocytes, and cellular debris. Squamous-like cells may also sometimes be seen in pleural effusions (Fig. 43.139) and are thought to be a feature associated with degenerative mesothelial cells, but they do not equate to malignancy. However, such squamoid cells are more common in mesothelioma; if prominent, this finding can cause confusion with metastatic squamous cell carcinoma.[871]

Mesothelial cells may show large single or multiple small cytoplasmic vacuoles. Multiple small vacuoles may represent lipid vacuoles, others are usually considered to be degenerative in nature, and larger glycogen-filled vacuoles may also be seen. Occasionally large single vacuoles may be present, which may mimic the mucin-filled vacuoles seen in adenocarcinoma (Fig. 43.140). These are now thought to contain hyaluronic acid. However, adenocarcinoma cells may also contain different types of vacuoles, and all of these findings can be misleading. We routinely stain spare slides or cell-block sections with PAS and PAS-diastase stains.

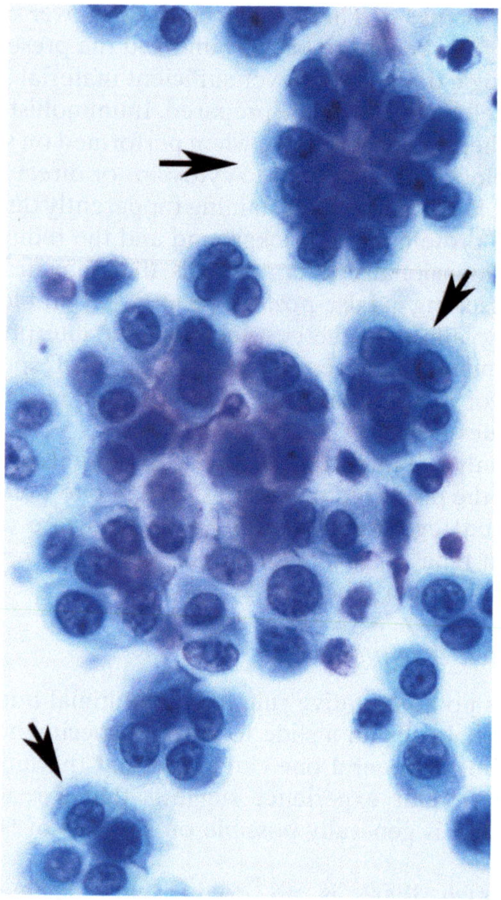

FIGURE 43.138. Atypical mesothelial proliferation. (Same case as in Figure 43.136.) This Pap-stained cytospin demonstrates papilla formation in a pleural effusion fluid (arrows).

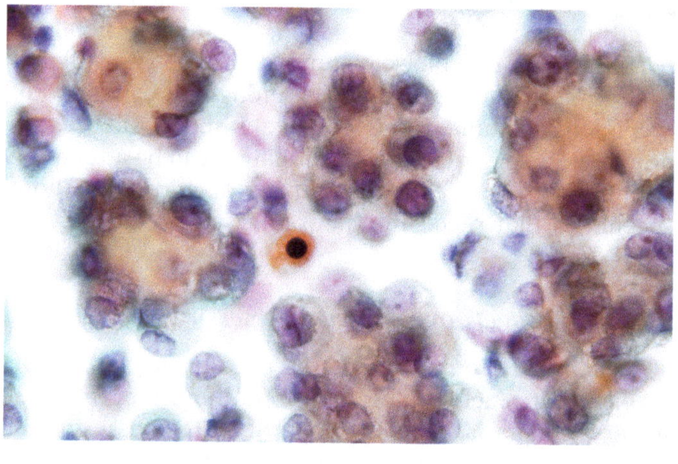

FIGURE 43.139. Mesothelial cells in pleural effusion, from a patient with biopsy-proven invasive MM of epithelial type, stained by the Pap technique. Thus micrograph depicts several papillary clusters of atypical mesothelial cells. The core in some of the papillae shows glassy orange staining, which correlated with the presence of PAS-positive basal laminal material. A small rounded squamoid cell with a pyknotic nucleus and intensely orangeophilic cytoplasm is also evident.

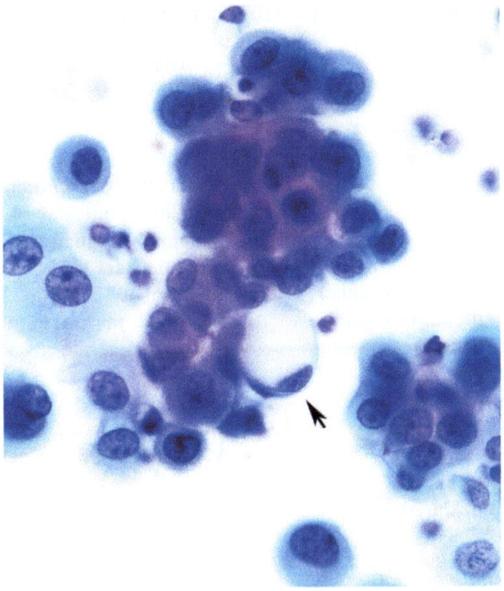

FIGURE 43.140. This Pap-stained cytospin preparation depicts a large intracytoplasmic vacuole in a mesothelial cell, with displacement of the nucleus to the periphery of the cell (arrow). For cells like this, the main differential diagnosis is adenocarcinoma. This patient had a biopsy-proven invasive MM, epithelial type.

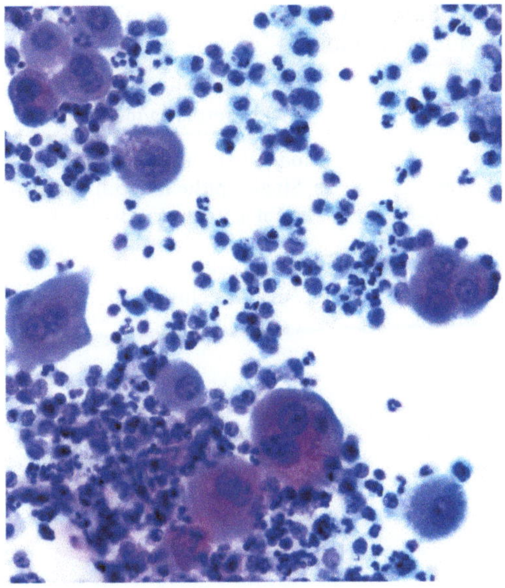

FIGURE 43.141. Multinucleation of cells may be seen in reactive processes as well as in MM. However, the presence of numerous multinucleated cells in virtually every high-power microscopic field examined supports a diagnosis of MM. This pleural fluid was taken from a patient with biopsy-proven invasive MM of epithelial type.

The cellularity of a specimen is important. In general, malignant effusions show greater cellularity than benign "reactive" effusions, but the cellularity seen on the slide may depend in part on the preparatory method used, and cellularity alone is insufficient for a diagnosis of malignancy. With increased cellularity, papillary structures can often be found in the effusion fluid; if found in significant numbers, they should suggest a malignant diagnosis (cf. Figs. 43.138 and 43.139). As mentioned previously, cytologic atypia alone is insufficient for a diagnosis of malignancy; MMs often do not show marked cytologic atypia and characteristically maintain a stable nuclear to cytoplasmic ratio, although a high nuclear-to-cytoplasmic ratio may occasionally be seen, and fenestrations may be evident between apposed cells (Fig. 43.136). Conversely, hyperplastic mesothelial cells can show substantial cytologic atypia, as well as nucleoli.

Although multinucleated mesothelial cells may be seen in reactive processes, the presence of numerous multinucleated cells—with multiple multinucleated cells in any given high-power microscopic field—has been found to correspond to MM (Fig. 43.141). The presence of cell-cell engulfment[872] or "cannibalism" in a pincer-like arrangement is also commonly seen in MM (Fig. 43.142) and may support a diagnosis of malignancy versus a reactive process. The presence of necrotic debris is a strong indicator of a malignant process.

The cytologic features that may aid in the differential diagnoses between a malignant pleural mesothelioma and a benign reactive mesothelial hyperplasia are summarized in Table 43.21, but a host of ancillary techniques has also been employed and these are discussed below.

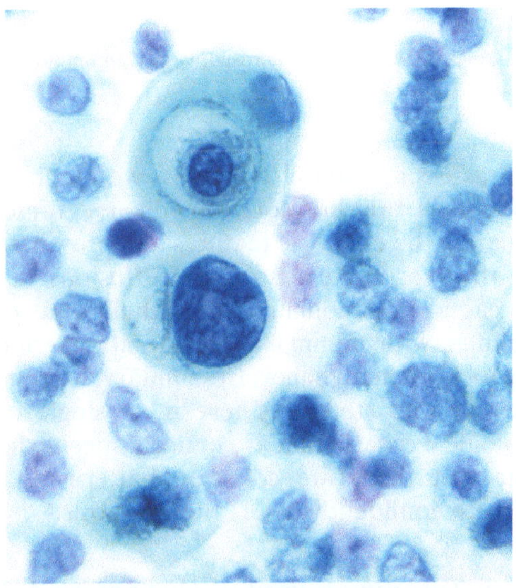

FIGURE 43.142. Cell-cell engulfment or "cannibalism" is considered to be a general feature of malignancy, but is common in MM. Shown here is the typical pincer-like cell-in-cell arrangement in a biopsy-proven case of invasive MM. The adjacent cell shows a high nuclear-to-cytoplasmic ratio.

TABLE 43.21. Summary of cytologic discriminants among reactive mesothelial hyperplasia, epithelial malignant mesothelioma, and secondary adenocarcinoma

Feature	Reactive mesothelial hyperplasia/mesotheliosis	Mesothelioma (epithelial, biphasic)	Metastatic adenocarcinoma
Low-power Cell population	Moderate to high cellularity • Single epithelioid cell population • ± Inflammatory cells	Cellular • Single epithelioid cell population	Cellular • Classically dual epithelioid cell population, but may be single malignant population
Cell disposition	• Single cells • Small 2D clusters/sheets and clumps (<20 cells)	• Single cells • Large 3D morules, (>50 cells) • Scalloped and complex outline of clusters • Papillary structures • Pseudoacini with collagen core	• Large clusters (>12 cells) smooth "cannonball" outline • Acini with peripheral nuclei • Cells in single-file row
Cytologic features	• Enlarged cells • Enlarged central nucleus	• Enlarged cells, N/C ratio same or less • Range of cell sizes • Many multinucleated cells, "cell-in-cell" • Giant mesothelial cells • Squamous-like cells	• Enlarged cells • Atypical and bizarre cells
Differentiating features	• Fenestrations between the cells in clusters/sheets • Central nuclei • Bi-tonal staining cytoplasm (dense orange around nucleus to green-blue at periphery in Pap stain, denser centrally in DQ) • Peripheral fringe • Cytoplasmic vacuoles may be present (no or only minimal PAS-diastase staining) • Atypia usually only moderate		• Mucin vacuoles indenting nucleus, PAS-diastase positive • Nuclei peripheral • Nuclei may be very atypical, often with coarse chromatin
IHC	• Calretinin (nuclear) • CK5/6 • WT1 (nuclear) • HBME-1 (linear membrane) • Thrombomodulin (linear membrane) • EMA: strong circumferential linear labeling more common in MM than reactive (clone E29), cytoplasmic labeling in adenocarcinoma		• CEA • B72.3, • CD15 • BG8 • Site specific markers, e.g., TTF-1, gross cystic disease fluid protein (GCDFP)
EM	Long slender serpentine microvilli; no glycocalyx		Short stubby microvilli; antennular glycocalyx

DQ, Diff Quick; EM, electron microscopy; IHC, immunohistochemistry; 2D, two-dimensional; 3D, three-dimensional.

When assessing pleural effusions, we emphasize that mesotheliomas are histologically diverse tumors, and consequently the cytologic features and presentation can also be diverse. For example, the effusions in biopsy-proven cases of sarcomatoid mesotheliomas are often paucicellular with minimal cytologic atypia, and hence not diagnostic of malignancy. In summary, we concur with Whitaker,[849] who stated, "There is no single or set of morphological criteria that are entirely specific for mesothelioma, yet there are common patterns that often permit us to confidently assert the diagnosis."

Ancillary Techniques used to Distinguish MM and Reactive Mesothelial Hyperplasia

Immunocytochemistry can be applied to Thin-Prep preparations and direct smears,[873] but we, like most others, prefer cell-block sections.[866,868] Labeling of cells in the typical linear distribution with antibodies against EMA[667] (clone E29) has also been found to be useful for the distinction between MM and reactive effusions,[662–664] because only MM showed strong and widespread (>10% of cells) membranous staining.[671] Although none of the reactive effusions showed staining in this pattern, only 75% of MMs tested showed this pattern of EMA labeling, with high specificity but low sensitivity. However, at the moment, this is the only ancillary technique available in most routine diagnostic laboratories to aid in the distinction between mesothelial hyperplasia and MM,[576] with the E29 clone being commercially available (Dako); we have found this to be a useful indicator of malignancy (Fig. 43.143).

In addition, immunohistochemical labeling for the one of the inhibitors of apoptosis proteins (IAPs), the X-linked-IAP (XIAP), has been found to be of value in distinguishing benign from malignant effusions, irrespec-

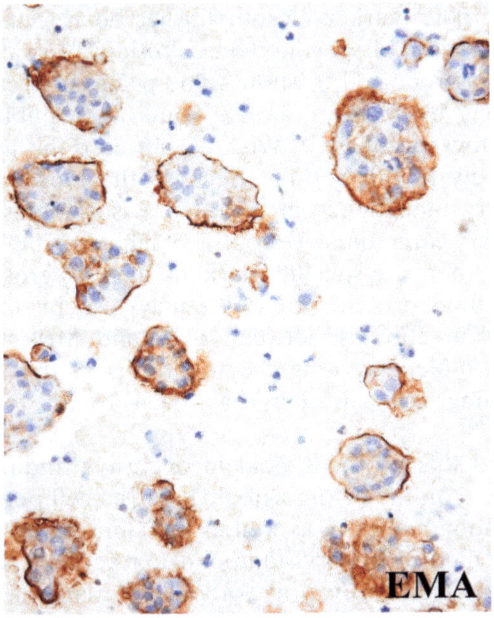

FIGURE 43.143. Immunocytochemical labeling of a cell-block section for EMA (clone E29) in a biopsy-proven case of MM reveals strong, circumferential membrane labeling of the cells and cell clusters, supporting a diagnosis of malignancy.

tive of the type of malignancy.[704] In the one study published to date, 80% of mesotheliomas showed positive labeling of mesothelial cells, whereas in reactive effusions positive labeling was limited to histiocytes in a minority of specimens (6%). This technique may prove to be useful, particularly in the distinction of reactive mesothelial hyperplasia and MM, but further validation of the results is required before routine use can be advocated, and identification of the type of malignant cells by other means (cytomorphology or immunohistochemistry) would still be necessary.

The use of immunohistochemistry for the distinction between MM and metastatic carcinoma is discussed in detail below.

Flow cytometry has been used to distinguish reactive and malignant mesothelial cell populations in pleural effusion fluids, based on the fact that malignant cells commonly show aneuploidy. Although high specificity has been reported in research laboratories, this approach appears at present to be too insensitive for routine diagnostic use.[874–876]

Image cytometry on de-stained Papanicolaou (Pap)-stained slides, which were then re-stained with the Feulgen stain, also assesses ploidy, and was found to be particularly helpful in the distinction of reactive mesothelial proliferations (all diploid) from MM (most aneuploid), but this technique is less useful for the distinction of MM from secondary adenocarcinoma, because both are mostly aneuploid.[876] Other studies found ploidy studies in isolation to be less useful, but suggested that prognostic information may be gained from ploidy studies on histologically confirmed MMs.[874,877]

Additional techniques that have been investigated include *silver nucleolar organizer region (AgNOR) staining*, which resulted in 95% sensitivity in small closed biopsies when combined with linear EMA labeling.[679] AgNOR testing appears to be fairly specific for malignant effusions and possibly more sensitive than ploidy studies by either fluorescence in-situ hybridization (FISH) or flow cytometry, but because of the high demands on either staff time or image analysis equipment, this technique has also not entered into routine diagnostic practice.[679,878,879]

Distinction Between Secondary Neoplasms Affecting the Pleura and Malignant Mesothelioma

The distinction between a malignant mesothelial process and a metastatic malignancy makes use of cytomorphology and ancillary techniques. On microscopic examination, the most obvious and important feature is the presence of a dual cell population (Fig. 43.144), although, rarely, a single population of metastatic malignant cells may be present and may mimic MM. The most common distinction is between MM and adenocarcinoma, with lung (for males) and breast (for females) being the most common primary sites (see Secondary Malignant Neoplasms Affecting the Pleura, below). However, other

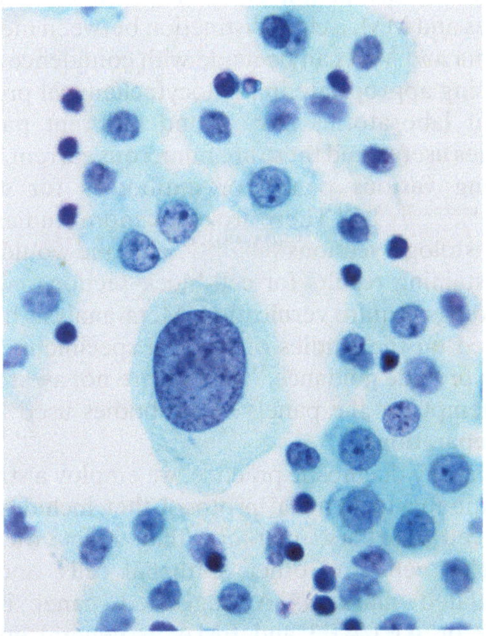

FIGURE 43.144. Pleural effusion fluid from a patient with documented disseminated breast carcinoma, showing a dual population of malignant cells. The large cell illustrated shows a high nuclear-to-cytoplasmic ratio.

types of malignancies, such as lymphoma or squamous cell carcinoma (SCC) may also enter the differential diagnosis. The exclusion of SCC is particularly important if the squamous-like cells sometimes seen in mesothelial proliferations are numerous. Lack of immunohistochemical labeling for calretinin in SCC is particularly useful in this situation.[637]

The effusions of metastatic adenocarcinoma are often very cellular, and may contain cell aggregates, but unlike the morules seen in MM, the cell aggregates in metastatic adenocarcinoma often have smooth contours. They may also show obvious acinar arrangements, with columnar cells featuring eccentric nuclei. Malignant mesothelial cells may be enlarged and even "giant," but classically the nuclear to cytoplasmic ratio is retained and frankly bizarre cells indicate a diagnosis of carcinoma.

Ancillary Techniques for the Distinction of Malignant Mesothelioma from Metastatic Neoplasms

Once a diagnosis of malignancy has been reached, and a distinction between MM and, for example, adenocarcinoma is required, ancillary techniques are particularly useful, and can be employed successfully by routine diagnostic laboratories. For example, mucin stains may distinguish intracytoplasmic mucin droplets of adenocarcinoma from prominent vacuoles in mesothelial cells. However, occasional mucin-producing mesotheliomas have been described.[505,539]

Unlike the distinction between reactive mesothelial processes and MM, a clear distinction between metastatic carcinoma and MM can be made with confidence in most cases, using appropriate immunocytochemical protocols. Different laboratories have found different panels of antibodies useful, and there are numerous current reviews suggesting various panels of antibodies for effusion fluids.[566,658,666,676,880–884] There are many more studies focusing on histologic sections[547,563,578–580] and one would expect similar staining results for cell-block sections, although such findings require verification. Meta-analysis has been attempted on the studies of surgical specimens, in an a effort to provide guidance,[547] but we are not aware of any such attempt for the panels of antibodies used in cytologic preparations.

In everyday diagnostic practice, we employ a standardized immunocytochemical protocol that includes mesothelial cell markers, markers that react with both mesothelial cells and other epithelial cells, and carcinoma-related markers. A suggested panel includes CAM5.2 or AE1/AE3 and EMA as general epithelial markers; CK5/6, calretinin, HBME-1, WT1, and thrombomodulin as mesothelial cell markers; and CEA, CD15, B72.3, and BG8 as carcinoma-related markers. Like many others, we have found calretinin to be particularly useful.[566] The marker mesothelin has been found to be less sensitive and specific than calretinin.[614] In contrast, D2-40 was reported to show some promise in cytologic specimens by some authors,[714] but other publications suggest low specificity.[605] We have not used this antibody extensively in this setting. Because the most common secondary malignancy in the pleura is a metastasis of pulmonary carcinoma, we routinely include TTF-1 in our panel. Other site-specific markers such as gross cystic disease fluid protein (GCDFP) may also be included. If the distinction is between SCC and MM, labeling for high-molecular weight cytokeratins in the absence of labeling for calretinin has been found to be of value.[632,637]

Should this protocol yield inconclusive findings, and depending on the cytomorphology of the cell population in the individual case, as well as the clinical background and past medical history, additional markers can be added (for example, further mesothelial, carcinoma-related markers and markers for endothelial and melanocyte differentiation and even lymphoid markers).[37,213] It also has been recommended that each laboratory should establish its own protocol that best meets its requirements and that yields consistent results, with high specificity and a high predictive value overall, keeping in mind that it is unlikely that a unique and reproducible immunoprofile will ever be established for a morphologically protean tumor such as MM.

Ancillary Techniques to Increase the Detection of Malignant cells in Effusion Fluids

To decrease the rate of false-positive fluids, the use of ancillary techniques has been suggested. However, immunocytology has not yielded convincing results in this regard. In one study there were only three of 26 cases of false-positive serous effusions where malignant cells could be detected using a panel of markers,[885] and similar results were seen in earlier studies.[639] This low cost-benefit ratio for such expensive and labor-intensive techniques has been considered as the main reason for the continued use of conventional cytology as first-line investigation.

Fine-Needle Aspiration in the Diagnosis of Malignant Mesothelioma

Fine-needle aspiration (FNA) has been performed with success on a range of pleural lesions, including MM, solitary fibrous tumors, synovial sarcoma, and unusual lesions such as myelolipoma.[886–892] The technique has also been found useful in the identification of local recurrence of MM.[893] In addition, primary diagnosis of MM based on an aspirate obtained from a supraclavicular lymph node has also been described.[894] The diagnostic considerations are similar to those associated with the assessment of pleural effusion fluid, in that clinicopathologic correlation is required. As for effusion fluids, a correct diagnosis of epithelial or biphasic MM may be possible based on the cellular findings in a sufficiently cellular specimen, but the diagnosis of sarcomatoid and, in particular, desmoplastic MM can be challenging or impossible. Ancillary techniques, in particular, immunohistochemistry and EM, may be extremely useful in reaching the correct diagnosis.

In addition, FNA has been employed in the diagnosis of metastatic MM, but there are only few reports available.[895–898] It appears that the cytomorphologic features of the metastatic tumors vary greatly, as might be expected in view of the morphologic variability of MM, and immunohistochemical techniques and clinical information, including knowledge of previous malignancy, play a major role in the diagnosis of these tumors.

Finally, percutaneous cutting needle biopsy under radiologic guidance, yielding a thin core of tissue, may be employed if insufficient material is sampled by FNA. This technique has a reported sensitivity of 86%, with 100% specificity,[899] and we have found this to be occasionally helpful in fibrous or desmoplastic lesions. The different techniques and lines of investigations available for diagnosis should be regarded as complementary.

Secondary Malignant Neoplasms Affecting the Pleura

Secondary neoplasms represent the most common pattern of malignancy affecting the pleura, and it has been estimated that malignant disease accounts for about 25% of all pleural effusions[900,901]—ranking after effusions related to congestive cardiac failure in the elderly and as a complication of pneumonia (parapneumonic effusion)[902]—and amounting to about 75% of exudative pleural effusions.[903] According to Matthay et al.,[902] among 1868 pleural effusions reported by different groups, 785 (42%) were linked to cancer, with a large increase in the percentage of malignancy-associated pleural effusions from the third and fourth decades with a further proportional rise in the seventh decade, followed by a fall in the eighth.

Because of its frequency and anatomic proximity to the pleura, carcinoma of the lung represents the most frequent cancer associated with malignant pleural disease—about 35% to 45% of pleural effusions related to cancer[900,902]—and it has been estimated that about 7% to 15% of lung cancer patients develop pleural effusion during the course of their disease.[903] Metastatic breast cancer accounts for about 25% of malignant pleural effusions,[900,902] followed by malignant lymphoma, including both Hodgkin's and non-Hodgkin's malignant lymphomas (about 10%).[900,902,903] In one series of cases,[904] women were almost twice as likely to develop metastasis to the pleura than men, related to the high frequency of pleural metastasis from breast cancer. These three categories of cancer account for about 75% of all malignancy-associated pleural effusions.[900] Metastatic carcinomas of ovarian or gastric origin, malignant melanoma, and sarcomas account for only a small percentage of cancer-associated pleural disease (about 5%).[900,902,903] In about 5% to 15% of cases with malignancy-associated pleural effusion, the primary site is unknown,[900,902,903] but it can often be identified using a panel of immunocytochemical markers.[905]

Adenocarcinoma represents the most frequent histologic type of lung cancer to result in a malignant pleural effusion—presumably because adenocarcinomas comprise a greater proportion of peripheral cancers than the other histologic types[903]—followed by squamous, small cell, and large cell undifferentiated carcinomas. As expected, adenocarcinomas represent the histologic type for cancers of breast, ovary, and stomach metastatic to the pleura.[902]

In some cases, malignancy-associated pleural effusions do not involve direct infiltration of the pleura by the cancer, and Sahn[903] designates such effusions as "paramalignant." As Sahn has emphasized, the lymphatic system of the parietal pleura, which joins the intercostal trunk vessels that drain predominantly toward the mediastinal lymph nodes, is the only pathway for clearance of fluid from the pleural cavities. Obstruction of this pathway at any point (for example, by mediastinal lymph node metastases) can result in a pleural effusion. Alternatively, a paramalignant effusion can result from obstructive pneumonitis as a consequence of lung cancer, or even from venous obstruction (for example, as part the superior vena cava syndrome).[902] In some instances, notably those resulting from lymphatic or venous obstruction, the effusion represents a transudate as opposed to a exudate. In contrast, effusions resulting directly from neoplastic infiltration of the pleura are characteristically exudative. Other causes of paramalignant pleural effusion include pulmonary embolism and low serum protein levels, or the effects of radiation or chemotherapy.[902] Depending on the anatomic site of the primary tumor, infiltration of the pleura can result from direct invasion of the visceral pleura by an underlying lung cancer or, alternatively, infiltration into the subpleural lymphatic plexus or from invasion of small branches of the pulmonary artery, with embolism of tumor cells to the periphery of the lung where they can then invade the visceral pleura. In the case of malignant pleural effusions resulting from subdiaphragmatic tumors, it has been suggested that the pleural involvement represents tertiary spread from hepatic metastases.[902,903]

Malignancy-associated pleural effusions need not be bilateral. Patients with lung cancer usually develop unilateral pleural effusion on the same side as the primary carcinoma, but occasionally the effusion is bilateral; an effusion restricted to the contralateral side is rare.[902] In contrast, with patients with breast cancer and subdiaphragmatic neoplasms (for example, stomach or ovary), there is no such predilection for the ipsilateral side.[902] It has been estimated that 50% of patients with disseminated breast cancer develop a pleural effusion during the course of their disease, on the same side as the original breast cancer in 60% of the patients, on the contralateral side in 25%, and bilaterally in about 15%.[902] In general, the interval between the diagnosis of the primary breast cancer and the subsequent development of an associated pleural effusion is about 2 years, but it can be as long as 20 years or more.[902]

The size of the pleural effusion in metastatic malignancy varies greatly. In about 75% of patients the effusion is moderate to large, within the range of about 500 to 2000mL; in about 10% the effusions are massive (with complete opacification of the affected hemithorax); and in a further 10%, approximately, the effusions are small (less than 500mL).[903] About 70% of patients with a massive effusion have an underlying cancer as the basis for the effusion.[903] Matthay et al.[902] referred to one series of 46 patients with massive pleural effusions from all causes: 31 (67%) had malignant pleural effusions, 27 as a consequence of metastatic carcinoma and one patient had a MM.

From an analysis of 500 documented cases of pleural effusion as a consequence of metastatic malignancy, Matthay et al.[902] found that the diagnostic yield from cytologic examination of pleural effusion fluid was 66%, versus 46% from pleural biopsy. Matthay et al. commented that pleural fluid cytologic examination is more sensitive for the diagnosis of metastatic cancer than pleural biopsy, and although cytology and biopsies are complementary to each other, pleural biopsy added little to cytologic examination. Matthay et al. commented further that the lower yield from pleural biopsy may represent operator technique or sampling error, the latter known to be a problem in that metastatic deposits can be widely scattered over the pleural membrane. They suggested that diagnostic yield can be increased by repeat cytology examinations and pleural biopsy. If a diagnosis is not obtained following repeat cytology examination and biopsy, thoracoscopy can be considered, and when multiple biopsies are taken at thoracoscopy, the diagnostic yield rises to about 80% to 97%.[902] Vargas and Teixeira[900] commented that pleural biopsies in cases of malignant pleural effusion establish the diagnosis in about 40% to 75%, but the combination of cytologic evaluation of the effusion fluid and a needle biopsy allows a diagnosis in about 80%. Medford and Maskell[906] commented that "blind" pleural biopsy increased the diagnostic yield over cytologic examination of effusion fluid by only 7% to 27%, and that at least four samples from one site are required to optimize the diagnostic return. These authors also set forth their perception that "blind" pleural biopsy no longer has a role in the investigation of malignant pleural disease and that it should be replaced by guided biopsies under imaging control.

In general, pleural metastatic deposits are a marker of advanced disease,[906] and survival of patients with pleural deposits from cancer of the lung, stomach, or ovary is usually measured in only a few months following diagnosis of the malignant pleural effusion.[902]

Although it is emphasized that lung and breast cancer and malignant lymphomas account for about 75% of malignancy-associated pleural effusions, almost any cancer with the capacity for metastasis to the lungs in particular also has the capacity for metastasis or spread to the pleura. Such unusual metastases can range from renal cell carcinomas to ependymomas arising in the central nervous system, among many others.

Pseudomesotheliomatous Tumors Affecting the Pleura Including Pseudomesotheliomatous Adenocarcinoma of Lung

By definition, pseudomesotheliomatous neoplasms affecting the pleura are characterized by diffuse infiltration of the pleura in a pattern essentially identical to, and indistinguishable from, pleural MM on gross examination or on radiologic studies, including CT scans.[907] In this regard, the neoplasm characteristically takes the form of multiple nodules, plaques, or a confluent rind of tumor, with an associated pleural effusion in many instances and with frequent obliteration of the pleural cavity in the later stages of the disease, sometimes with invasion into the chest wall, diaphragm, and pericardium, as seen at autopsy.

Most pseudomesotheliomatous neoplasms affecting the pleura are thought to originate from the lung,[908–923] but pseudomesotheliomatous metastases from carcinomas arising in other sites are well recorded, including the kidney,[918,924–926] thyroid gland,[497] larynx,[927] stomach,[918] and cutaneous malignant melanoma as well as various sarcomas, including malignant phyllodes tumor.[928]

In addition, with pseudomesotheliomatous carcinomas (PMCs) of the lung, adenocarcinoma is the most frequent histologic type, but other cell types can produce pseudomesotheliomatous spread, including SCC, small cell carcinoma,[773] large cell undifferentiated carcinoma, and carcinosarcoma.[532]

Pseudomesotheliomatous carcinomas of the lung were first described by Babolini and Blasi[929] in 1956, to emphasize that the symptoms in these patients were related predominantly to involvement of the pleura with recurrent exudative effusion, often accompanied by chest pain and dyspnea. Of five cases reported by Babolini and Blasi, two appear to have represented small cell carcinoma and the other three were adenocarcinomas. About

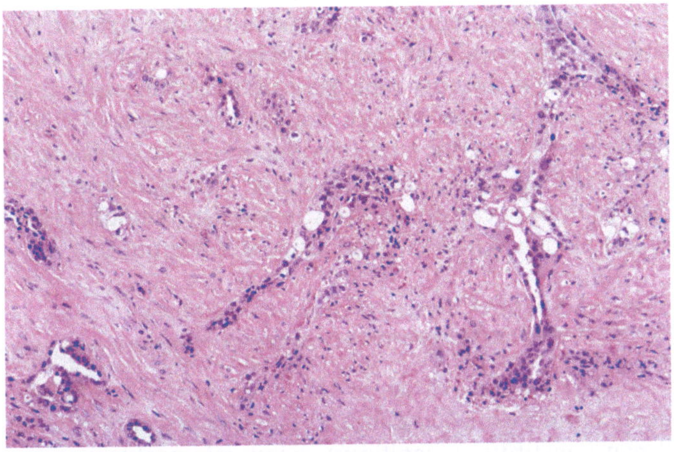

FIGURE 43.145. Pseudomesotheliomatous adenocarcinoma. Pleural biopsy from a 77-year-old man with a right pleural effusion. At thoracoscopy, the appearances were considered suggestive of a malignant mesothelioma. The neoplastic acini are embedded in a prominent fibrous stroma ("tubulo-desmoplastic adenocarcinoma").

20 years later, Harwood et al.[908] reported six cases of primary lung cancer with mimicry of mesothelioma in terms of the distribution of the carcinoma within the pleura, and they introduced the term *pseudomesotheliomatous carcinoma.* In two of their six cases there were small intraparenchymal nodules in the underlying lung parenchyma and all tumors were adenocarcinomas, with bronchioloalveolar features in five. The patients were all men of ages 50 to 76 years, and they had symptoms of dyspnea on exertion, chest pain, and weight loss. Koss et al.[916] also reported an underlying adenocarcinoma in the lung in seven out of 14 autopsy cases. Nonetheless, in some instances, pleural pseudomesotheliomatous adenocarcinomas show no evidence of an underlying intraparenchymal tumor, probably explicable by overgrowth of a small peripheral primary lung cancer by the predominant pleural extension.

In their review, Koss et al.[916] reviewed 15 previously published pseudomesotheliomatous adenocarcinomas of lung and added a further 15 examples from the files of the Armed Forces Institute of Pathology (AFIP) in Washington. Ninety percent of the patients were men with a median age of 61 years, and 17% had possible to definite occupational exposure to asbestos; one patient had proven asbestosis. The prognosis for pseudomesotheliomatous adenocarcinoma was similar to that of mesothelioma: the mean survival time in this series[916] was 4.7 months and the longest survival was 25 months.

Although PMCs are defined entirely by the gross anatomic distribution of the neoplasm (or on radiologic examination as a surrogate for gross examination), the acinar structures in pseudomesotheliomatous adenocarcinoma may or may not resemble an epithelial mesothelioma; that is, these tumors may comprise simplified or isolated glands in a fibrotic stroma, with appearances characteristic of adenocarcinoma; however, in some instances they can show a complex branching and anastomosing architecture producing a histologic resemblance to epithelial mesothelioma (Figs. 43.145 and 43.146). The acini, tubules, and nests of tumor cells in PMC are characteristically surrounded by thickened and fibrotic stromal tissue (Fig. 43.145), heightening the resemblance to mesothelioma (an appearance that Hammar and Dodson[907] have described as "tubulo-desmoplastic adenocarcinoma").

In the series reported by Koss et al.,[916] the main feature used for the diagnosis of pseudomesotheliomatous adenocarcinoma was the presence of PAS-diastase–positive mucin in gland lumina or as intracytoplasmic droplets (but "all of the AFIP surgical specimens . . . were selected on the basis of mucin-positivity within tumor cells"). The distinction between mesothelioma and pseudomesotheliomatous adenocarcinoma is usually straightforward on immunohistochemical staining, and the distinction is facilitated by use of a panel of mesothelial cell markers and generic carcinoma-related antibodies (Figs. 43.147 and 43.148), together with immunostaining for TTF-1.

A further issue that awaits clarification is whether a causal relationship between these tumors and asbestos exposure differs from other bronchopulmonary carcinomas. In our experience, a high proportion of pseudomesotheliomatous adenocarcinomas appear to have a background of occupational exposure to asbestos, but it is unclear whether this seemingly high proportion is

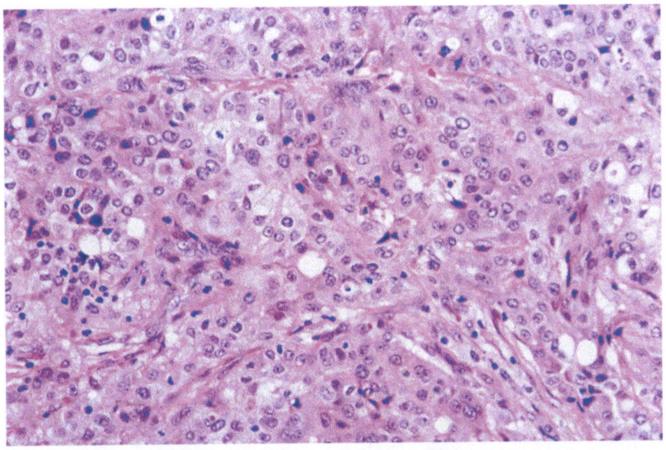

FIGURE 43.146. Pseudomesotheliomatous adenocarcinoma of pleura. This carcinoma is more cellular than the tumor illustrated in Figure 43.145, with a paucity of stromal tissue. The nuclei of the neoplastic cells are nonhyperchromatic and they show only moderate cytologic atypia. The appearances are similar to those seen in some epithelial mesotheliomas.

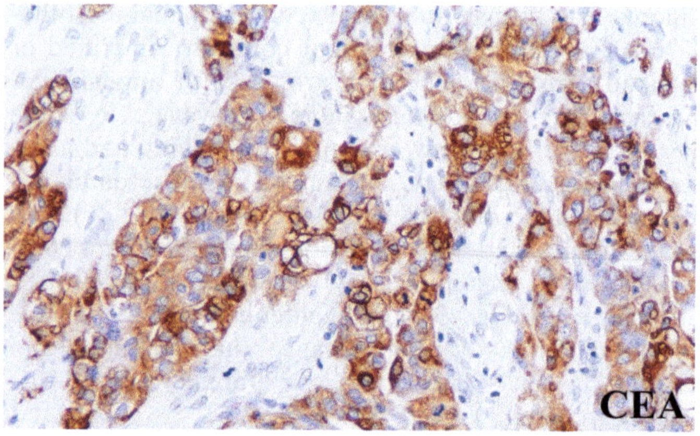

FIGURE 43.147. Pseudomesotheliomatous adenocarcinoma. (Same case as in Fig. 43.145.) The tumor shows positive staining for carcinoembryonic antigen (CEA).

explicable by (1) patterns of referral of cases for which mesothelioma is the differential diagnosis, or (2) whether the clinical and radiologic mimicry of mesotheliomas by these tumors stimulates a more detailed history concerning asbestos exposure than would be the case for conventional lung cancers (see also Chapter 27).

Spindle Cell Carcinoma and Carcinosarcoma of Lung

Although spindle cell (sarcomatoid) carcinomas of lung usually form localized intraparenchymal mass lesions, they can invade the pleura, with the potential for histologic mimicry of biphasic mesothelioma. In this regard, Mayall and Gibbs[532] reported two carcinosarcomas that presented as pleural tumors, with encasement of the lung in a pseudomesotheliomatous fashion in one patient. No site of origin within the lung could be identified for either tumor. These authors suggested that the following findings in such tumors militate against a diagnosis of mesothelioma: (1) neutral mucin production; (2) expression of CEA; (3) squamous differentiation, although squamous differentiation can occur rarely in MMs of epithelial type; or (4) evidence of neuroendocrine differentiation.

Serosal-Surface Serous Papillary Tumors

Because serous papillary adenocarcinomas arise predominantly from the ovaries or the peritoneal mesothelium itself, mimicry of *pleural* mesothelioma is exceptional, but it can constitute a significant diagnostic problem, especially because a high proportion of serous papillary carcinomas show no evidence of CEA expression on immunohistochemistry.[119,930–933] Even so, three patients with an underlying serous papillary adenocarcinoma of the peritoneum encountered by the authors[119] (Figs. 43.149 and 43.150) presented with unilateral pleural effusion, apparently related to spread from the underlying peritoneal tumor (in at least one of these cases, the primary peritoneal lesion was demonstrable only on CT imaging). The diagnosis in most instances can be made on detailed immunohistochemical studies, for example, including labeling with antibodies such as Ber-EP4 (Fig. 43.150), B72.3,[119,930,932,934] and BG8. In two cases in our files the diagnosis was established primarily by electron microscopy, which demonstrated short blunt microvilli with an antennular glycocalyx characteristic of carcinoma in one case, and by the presence of elongated branched microvilli in another case, where the microvilli lacked the sinuous and serpentine architecture characteristic of mesothelial microvilli.[119] The resemblance of such serous

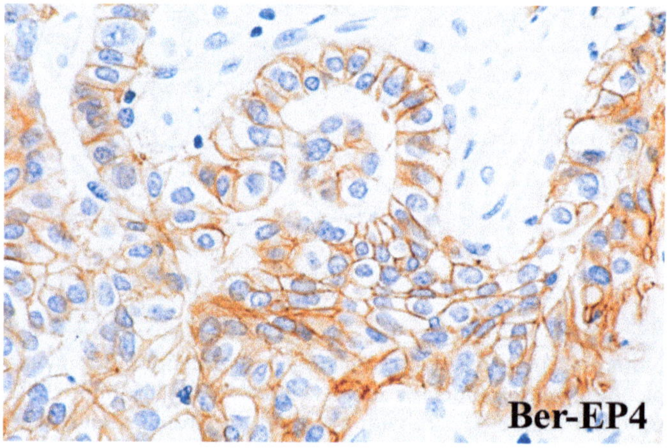

FIGURE 43.148. Pseudomesotheliomatous adenocarcinoma. Positive linear labeling of the neoplastic cells with Ber-EP4.

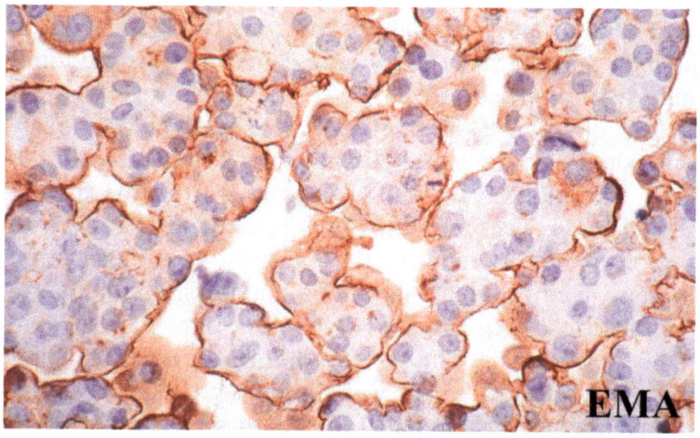

FIGURE 43.149. Pleural metastasis of a serous papillary adenocarcinoma of the peritoneum (cytology cell block section). Linear membrane-related staining for epithelial membrane antigen (EMA), essentially indistinguishable from labeling that characterizes epithelial mesotheliomas.

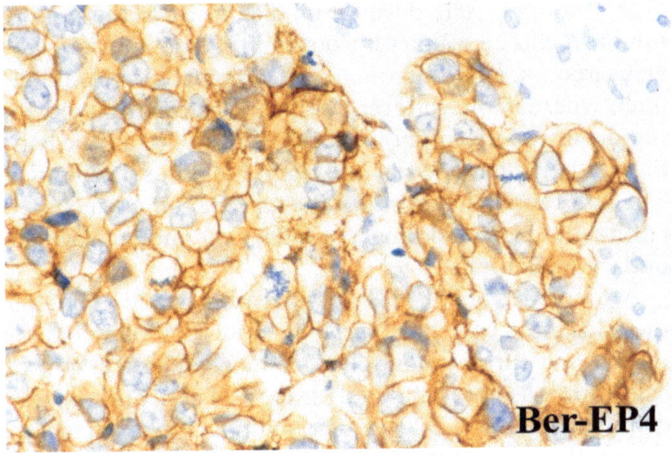

FIGURE 43.150. Pleural metastasis of a peritoneal serous papillary adenocarcinoma. (Same case as in Fig. 43.149.) positive linear labeling of the neoplastic cells with Ber-EP4 in a "chicken-wire" pattern.

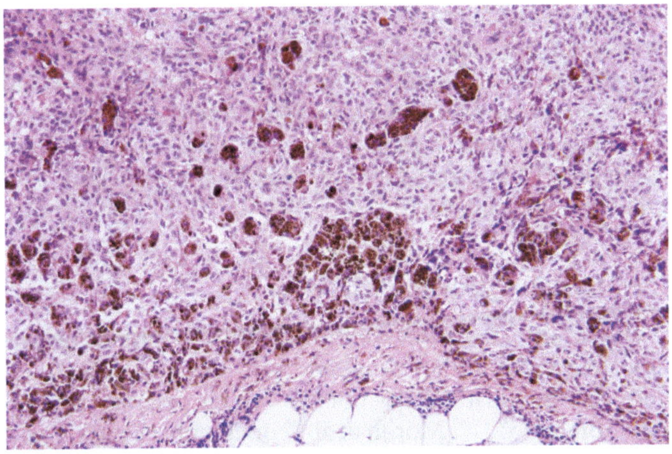

FIGURE 43.151. Pleural metastasis of malignant melanoma of unknown primary site, in an 83-year-old man with a recurrent blood-stained pleural effusion, thought on clinical grounds to be suspicious of mesothelioma. As illustrated, the melanoma showed confluent spread over the pleura. Plentiful melanin pigment is evident, mostly concentrated in stromal macrophages.

papillary carcinomas to mesothelioma is further enhanced by the pattern of EMA staining in some cases, with linear membrane-related labeling in some instances (Fig. 43.149).

Other Tumors that can Invade or Spread to the Pleura

We have also encountered cases of renal cell carcinoma and amelanotic malignant melanoma metastatic to the pleura[662] (Figs. 43.151 and 43.152), with mimicry of mesothelioma on rare occasions, and renal cell carcinomas with a spindle cell sarcomatoid pattern represent a potentially difficult differential diagnostic problem. In such instances, labeling of the tumor for renal cell carcinoma–related markers such as CD10 and renal cell carcinoma antigen may facilitate the diagnosis,[711] but whenever renal cell carcinoma enters into the differential diagnosis, we routinely recommend exclusion of an underlying renal tumor by noninvasive imaging procedures such as ultrasound or CT scanning.

Metastatic melanoma is distinguishable from mesothelioma by the absence or paucity of CK expression in most instances, and by positive labeling for S-100 proteins and other melanoma-related markers such as HMB-45[119,662] (Fig. 43.152) and melan-A.

We have also encountered rare cases of sarcoma metastatic to the pleura, with clinical and even histologic mimicry of mesothelioma on rare occasions, including one case of metastatic sclerosing epithelioid fibrosarcoma.[935,936] Such cases highlight the importance of comprehensive clinical data, including a history of any other neoplasm with the capacity for metastasis to the pleura, to avoid misdiagnosis of secondary sarcomas and other cancers as mesothelioma. At the same time, because mesotheliomas are most often encountered in patients over 55 years of age, many of our patients with proven pleural MM have had a history of antecedent cancer (for example, carcinoma of the prostate). When dealing with cases of this type it is crucial to compare the pleural lesion

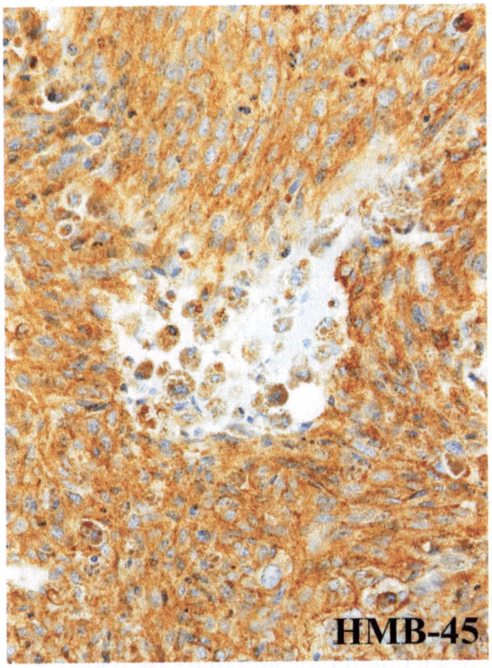

FIGURE 43.152. Positive staining of tumor cells with HMB-45. (Same case as in Fig. 43.151.) Immunostaining for cytokeratins was negative.

with any tissue available from the antecedent tumor whenever possible and to adjust the immunohistochemical protocol to encompass not only mesothelial cell and generic carcinoma markers but also more specific markers for the relevant carcinomas and other tumors (for example, TTF-1, prostate-specific antigen, prostatic acid phosphatase, and so forth).

Thymoma Affecting the Pleura

The literature contains several reports of thymoma affecting the pleura, either as spread into the pleura from an anterior mediastinal thymoma,[937] or as primary pleural thymomas.[836,938–941] Moran et al.[940] documented eight cases of thymoma that presented as pleural tumors requiring distinction from mesothelioma (most notably the lymphohistiocytoid variety). Six of their patients had diffuse pleural thickening, with encasement of the lung in four cases, and the tumor in one patient was obscured by a massive unilateral effusion. All of the cases comprising this series lacked radiographic evidence of a mediastinal tumor, but there was some uncertainty as to whether the thymomas were ectopic within the pleura or whether they represented spread from an underlying thymic tumor. More recently, the concept of primary pleural thymoma has become established,[836] but such pleural thymomas are distinctly rare and only about 25 to 30 cases have been reported in the literature to date.[836,938–941] They can present as localized masses or with diffuse pleural thickening.

The main histologic feature distinguishing lymphocyte-rich thymoma from lymphohistiocytoid mesothelioma is subdivision of the thymoma by bands of fibrocollagenous tissue, producing a lobulated architecture, and by a double cell population comprising epithelial cells and small lymphocytes only, the lymphocytes showing an immunohistochemical pattern of immature thymic lymphocytes. In other cases, the epithelial component predominates, with nesting, spindle-cell, and trabecular patterns, together with perivascular microcystic spaces.

Attanoos et al.[836,942] reported eight cases of pleural thymic epithelial tumors, four in males and four in females, with an age range of 19 to 75 years (median, 56 years). Three tumors occurred in the left hemithorax and four in the right, and the laterality was unknown in one case. In seven of the eight cases, the tumors were multinodular, with pleural thickening and partial encasement of the ipsilateral lung. In seven cases, low-magnification histologic examination showed a strikingly lobulated architecture, with fibrous septa subdividing cellular epithelial islands of tumor cells. In each case, there was a variable lymphoid cell population and one case had an extensively cystic appearance. The cases comprised WHO type A (medullary) thymic epithelial tumors, WHO type B1 (predominantly cortical) tumors, and WHO type B2 (cortical) tumors.[943] The differential diagnosis for the type A tumors included solitary fibrous tumor, monophasic synovial sarcoma, angiosarcoma, and sarcomatoid mesothelioma, whereas the differential diagnosis for the type B1 tumors included lymphohistiocytoid MM, metastatic lymphoepithelial carcinoma, and non-Hodgkin's lymphoma. The differential diagnosis for the type B2 tumors included epithelioid mesothelioma, secondary carcinoma, and secondary melanoma.

Attanoos et al.[836,942] also emphasized that thymic epithelial tumors can show variable expression of cytokeratin 5/6 and thrombomodulin, but nuclear expression of calretinin was not found in their cases. These authors also commented that CD20 expression in a cytokeratin-positive epithelial neoplasm and the presence of an immature lymphocyte population (demonstrable by immunostaining for CD1a, CD2, CD99, and terminal deoxynucleotidyl transferase [TdT]) indicates a thymic epithelial neoplasm, whereas nuclear expression of calretinin "favors MM."

Other Neoplasms Arising in the Pleura

Spindle Cell Neoplasms

Synovial Sarcoma of the Pleura

Both biphasic and monophasic synovial sarcomas (SSas) affecting somatic soft tissues and other sites have been extensively documented in the literature,[944–950] comprising up to about an estimated 5% to 14% of all sarcomas,[526,951] and characterized by a distinctive t(X;18) chromosomal translocation and the production of the resultant alternative fusion genes, *SYT-SSX1* or *SYT-SSX2*.[528–530] Most commonly, SSa affects the soft tissues of the extremities near—but only exceptionally in continuity with—large joints, and they have been described in most anatomic sites, including the head and neck region, the hypopharynx, abdominal wall, central nervous system, and prostate, among others.[951] They are now well recognized also as primary intrathoracic neoplasms in the mediastinum,[526,952,953] heart and pericardium,[954–957] lung,[526,958,959] and pleura[521–526,951,960–966] where the histologic appearances can potentially lead to confusion with either biphasic or sarcomatoid mesothelioma or carcinosarcoma (spindle cell carcinoma) of pulmonary or other origin, or biphasic pulmonary blastoma.

It is worth emphasizing that the term *synovial sarcoma* is quite inappropriate for these neoplasms, which have no phenotypic relationship to either synovial A or B cells (histiocytoid and fibroblastoid cells, respectively).[951,967–970] Instead, the epithelioid component of biphasic SSa shows clear evidence of epithelial differentiation as demonstrated by immunohistochemical studies and by electron microscopy (the term *carcinosarcoma* might be more correct for soft tissue SSas,[969] but *synovial sarcoma* is now standard, and terms such as *carcinosarcoma* for pleuropulmonary tumors would only invite confusion with carcinosarcoma of lung). For example, Ordóñez et al.[948] described the pathologic findings in 39 primary SSas of which 15 were biphasic and 24 monophasic, as well as 19 cases of metastatic SSa. The epithelial or spindle cells in each biphasic tumor, whether primary or metastatic, showed reactivity for cytokeratins and EMA, but only six primary tumors (five biphasic and one monophasic) showed detectable expression of CEA, which was confined to the epithelial component of the biphasic tumors. Of the monophasic SSas, 15 primary (63%) and four metastatic (25%) cases showed reactivity for cytokeratin, whereas seven primary and two metastatic SSas (29% and 13%, respectively) showed detectable expression of EMA. The same authors found that EM could facilitate the diagnosis when markers of epithelial differentiation were not expressed on immunohistochemical staining, and EM aided in differentiating monophasic SSas from other sarcomas with histologic similarities. (See also later discussion of the study reported by Miettinen et al.[527] concerning the immunohistochemical repertoire of biphasic, monophasic and poorly differentiated SSas, in comparison to mesothelioma.)

In 1989, Witkin et al.[952] reported four cases of primary mediastinal biphasic SSa, with a fifth case mentioned as an addendum to their report, and they also referred to another case, in a 5-year-old boy who had a localized pleural tumor with a histologic resemblance to SSa. Although the SSas described by Witkin et al. were frequently adherent to the pericardium or pleura, none appeared actually to arise from the mesothelial surface at either site.

Subsequently, Gaertner et al.[521] recorded five cases of pleural biphasic SSa. The average age of their patients was 25 years (significantly younger than the mean age of mesothelioma patients), and the tumors presented as a localized mass lesion, often surrounded by a pseudocapsule (Fig. 43.153).[119] Jawahar et al.[522] reported a further case of pleural biphasic SSa, and in the same year Kashima et al.[971] reported a case of peritoneal biphasic SSa that showed the characteristic t(X;18) translocation; in the following year, Langner et al.[955] described a pericardial SSa in a patient with occupational exposure to asbestos, thought initially to represent a pericardial mesothelioma.

Nicholson et al.[523] described three cases of pleural SSa, in a 28-year-old man and two 42-year-old men, with no known background of exposure to asbestos. Two of the tumors were monophasic in character and one was biphasic. All three tumors showed focal expression of either cytokeratins or EMA in the spindle-cell tissue, and they also showed positive staining for bcl-2 protein and CD99. Bégueret et al.[526] also reported a series of 40 t(X;18) cases of primary intrathoracic SSa, at least 19 of which represented lung tumors, whereas six affected the pleura. The others were designated as pleuropulmonary or they affected mediastinal structures, sometimes in apparent continuity with the pericardium or lung. In this series, only one SSa was biphasic. The remaining 39 were classified as monophasic (24 cases) or poorly differentiated SSas (15 cases). Aubry et al.[960] reported five cases of primary monophasic SSa of the pleura, confirmed by identification of the SYT-SSX fusion transcript. In the following year, Praet et al.[972] reported four cases of pleural SSa, three of which were monophasic. Molecular analysis revealed SYT-SSX transcripts in three of the four cases, with results pending for the remaining case.

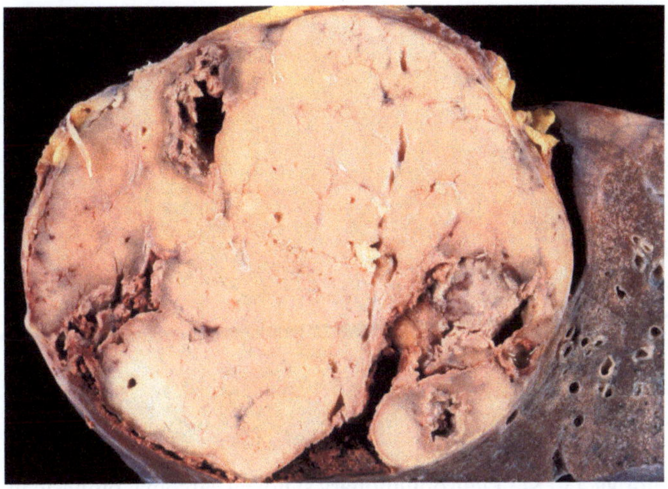

FIGURE 43.153. Gross appearances of a pleuropulmonary synovial sarcoma. Surgical resection specimen of upper lobe from an elderly woman. The tumor is well demarcated, and it indented the adjoining upper lobe. Yellow mediastinal fat is attached to the outer aspect of the tumor, in the upper part of this field. The tumor tissue itself is tan in color, with areas of necrosis and cystic degeneration. Other examples of pleural synovial sarcoma may take the form of pedunculated tumors or multinodular to confluent tumors that can mimic mesothelioma in their gross appearances.

Powers and Carbone[951] summarized the findings in 23 cases of primary SSa of the pleura reported in the literature.[419,521–523,961–965] The patients' ages ranged from 9 to 77 years (mean, 35.5 years, significantly less than the mean ages recorded for patients with pleural MM). There were 14 males and 9 females (M/F ratio = 1.56:1). Twelve of the SSas were monophasic, whereas 10 were biphasic, and the histologic type was unspecified for the remaining case.

In one of the largest studies reported to date, Miettinen et al.[527] described the immunohistochemical findings in 103 *extrapleural* SSas that included 41 biphasic tumors, 44 monophasic sarcomas, and 18 poorly differentiated SSas, in comparison to 23 epithelial and seven sarcomatoid mesotheliomas. They found that most biphasic SSas

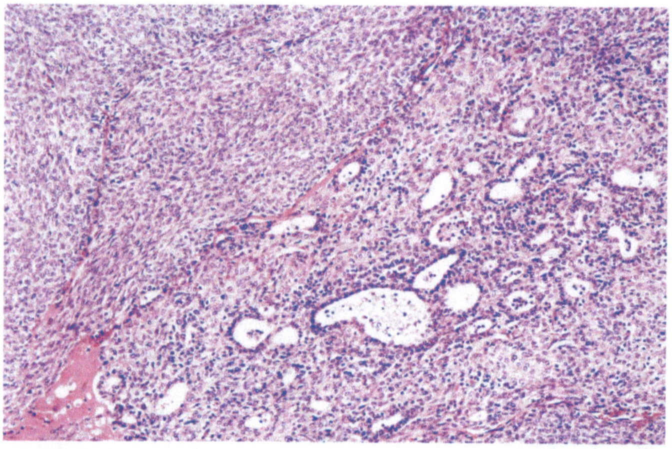

FIGURE 43.154. Pleuropulmonary synovial sarcoma, biphasic in type. The stromal component is illustrated in the upper left of this field, and the glandular component in the remainder of the field.

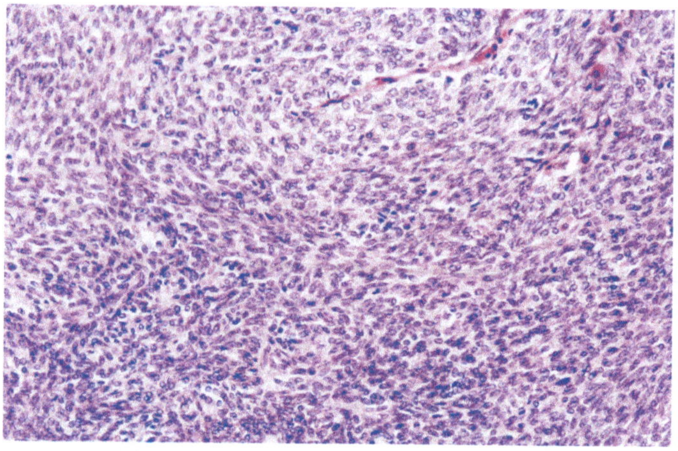

FIGURE 43.155. Stromal component of a pleuropulmonary synovial sarcoma. The stromal tissue is more cellular than the sarcomatoid tissue usually encountered in biphasic and sarcomatoid mesotheliomas, and typically the tumor cells tend to form curving poorly delineated fascicles as opposed to the storiform architecture often encountered in sarcomatoid and biphasic mesotheliomas.

(29/41; 71%) showed focal to extensive calretinin positivity, more often in the spindle-cell tissue (24/41 cases; 59%) than in the epithelial cells (14/41 cases; 34%), but only five of those cases showed calretinin positivity in ≥10% of the epithelial component; all of the biphasic SSas also stained with HBME-1. The monophasic and poorly differentiated SSas showed foci of calretinin positivity in 52% and 56% of cases, respectively. In comparison, all 23 epithelial mesotheliomas showed extensive calretinin positivity, and variable focal positive calretinin staining was seen in seven sarcomatoid mesotheliomas. They also found that two of 15 malignant peripheral nerve sheath tumors showed focal calretinin positivity, whereas there was no evidence of calretinin expression in epithelioid sarcomas, leiomyosarcomas, gastrointestinal stromal tumors (GISTs), or angiosarcomas. The biphasic SSas differed from mesothelioma by their more common Ber-EP4 positivity (90%), whereas focal Ber-EP4 staining was found in 13% of epithelial mesotheliomas. Expression of CD15 was rare in both mesotheliomas and SSas. Expression of Wilms' tumor antigen-1 (WT1) was not detected in any of the cases of SSa but was found in 12 out of 17 epithelial mesotheliomas. Miettinen et al. found that cytokeratins were present in the epithelial cells of both biphasic SSas and mesotheliomas (CK7 and CK19), but the expression was focal in both the monophasic and poorly differentiated SSas.

The findings of the International Mesothelioma Panel[37] and ours are useful for discrimination between biphasic/monophasic SSa and pleural MM:

- Typically, pleural SSas occur at a younger age (mean, 25–35 years) than pleural MM (mean, 65 years), although we have encountered some cases of SSa in the elderly.
- In terms of gross morphology, pleural SSa usually takes the form of a circumscribed mass lesion (Fig. 43.153), ranging from a few millimeters to 250 mm in diameter,[951] sometimes surrounded by a fibrous pseudocapsule and often accompanied by focal cystic degeneration[951] (Fig. 43.153), although diffuse pleural SSas can occur, mimicking MM in their anatomic distribution.
- There are significant histologic differences between either biphasic or monophasic SSa and biphasic/sarcomatoid MM (Figs. 43.154 to 43.156). The spindle-cell

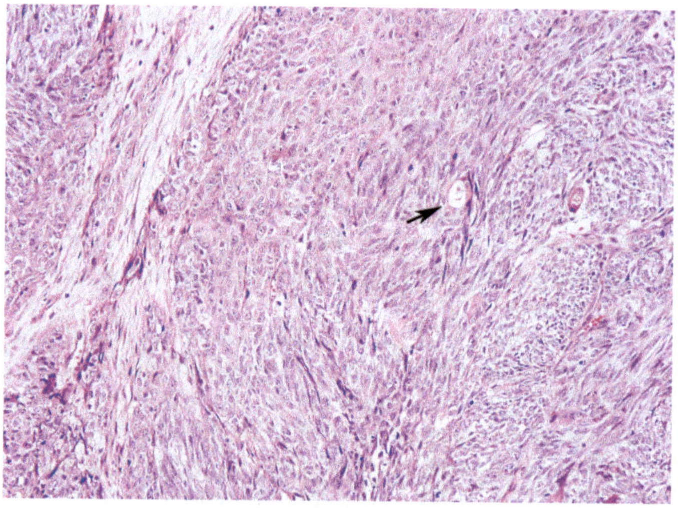

FIGURE 43.156. Localized pleural synovial sarcoma resected in a 67-year-old man. The fascicular architecture of the spindle-cell tissue is more obvious than in Figure 43.155. A rudimentary glandular structure can be seen (arrow).

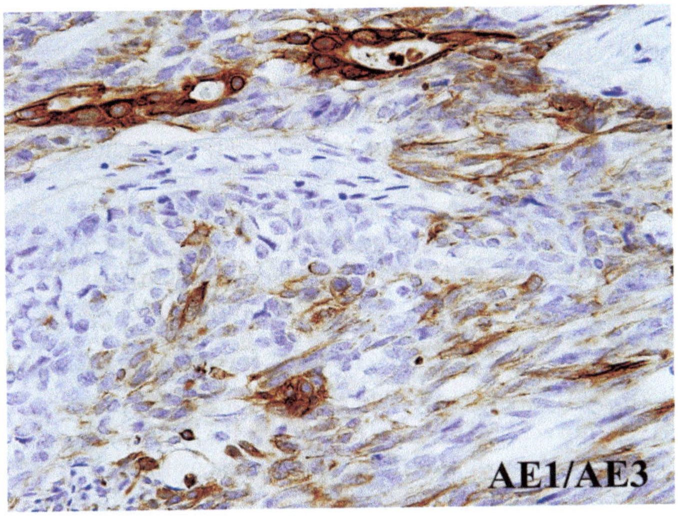

FIGURE 43.157. Biphasic synovial sarcoma of pleura, immunostained for pan-cytokeratins (AE1/AE3). Both the glandular component and the spindle-cell stromal tissue show expression of CKs, but labeling is more intense in the glandular tissue.

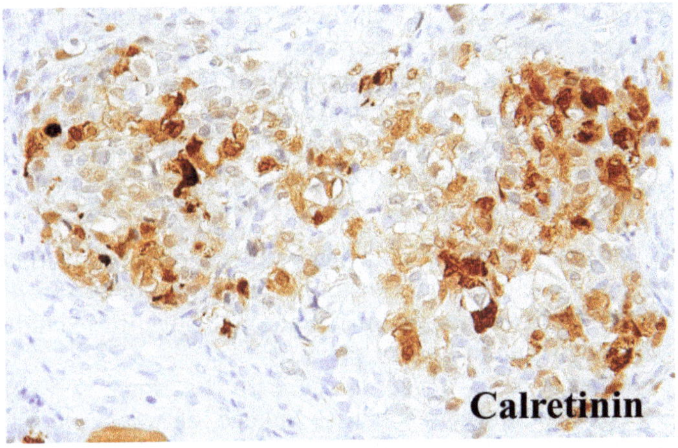

FIGURE 43.158. Pleural synovial sarcoma, biphasic type, showing focal staining for calretinin in both the cytoplasmic and nuclei of the tumor cells. (Same case as in Fig. 43.157.)

tissue in SSas is usually more cellular than the sarcomatoid component of mesotheliomas, and the cell size is smaller (Fig. 43.155). In addition, the spindle cells in SSa typically form interweaving fascicles (Figs. 43.155 and 43.156)—a "school of fish" pattern, a hemangiopericytic pattern, and foci of hyaline fibrosis (and even calcification[951]) are common in SSa but are not characteristic of mesothelioma. Frequent stromal mast cells are a characteristic finding in SSa, but not pleural mesothelioma.

- The glandular component of SSas (when present) frequently shows evidence of neutral mucin, whereas this finding typically does not occur in biphasic mesotheliomas, although mucin-positive mesotheliomas are well described.
- Powers and Carbone[951] considered that focal CK expression together with labeling for bcl-2, CD56, and CD99 in the context of undetectable staining for calretinin and WT1 suggests a diagnosis of SSa as opposed to pleural mesothelioma. In addition, expression of CKs by the stromal component of SSas is usually less intense and less extensive than in most cases of biphasic or sarcomatoid mesotheliomas (Fig. 43.157), and two cases of pleural monophasic SSa reported by Praet et al.[972] showed no detectable CK expression (the diagnosis in both was confirmed by detection of *SYT-SSX* transcripts).
- As indicated above, there is some overlap in calretinin expression between SSa and mesothelioma (Fig. 43.158), whereas nuclear staining for WT1 is frequent in mesothelioma but not in SSa.
- Both biphasic SSa and biphasic mesothelioma typically show positive staining for EMA, but whereas EMA expression in mesothelioma is typically linear and membrane-related in distribution, both membranous and cytoplasmic staining is found in biphasic SSa. Furthermore, expression of the epithelial markers, most notably Ber-EP4, CEA, or CD15 (Fig. 43.159) is not uncommon in biphasic SSa, but is substantially less frequent in mesotheliomas.
- By electron microscopy, the microvilli found on the epithelial cells of SSas are short and blunt,[946,947] and may even show structures resembling glycocalyceal bodies,[119] whereas the microvilli in mesothelioma are characteristically elongated, serpentine, and intertwining, with no evidence of a glycocalyx.

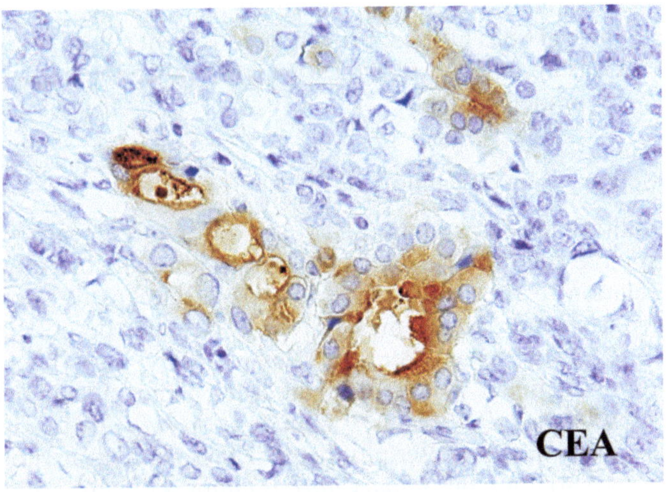

FIGURE 43.159. Biphasic synovial sarcoma of pleura, showing focal staining for carcinoembryonic antigen in the glandular component. (Same case as in Figs. 43.157 and 43.158.)

- Finally, the t(X;18) chromosomal translocation and expression of the resultant chimeric gene *SYT-SSX1* or *SYT-SXX2* are virtually diagnostic of SSa—both biphasic and monophasic—but are absent in mesotheliomas. Identification of this characteristic translocation is of particular value for the discrimination between poorly differentiated SSa and mesothelioma.[526]

Also, a diagnosis of primary pleuropulmonary SSa requires exclusion of a history of an antecedent SSa of somatic soft tissues or other anatomic sites, to exclude SSa metastatic to lung or pleura.[973]

In rare cases there appears to be some as yet unreported and unexplained linkage between pleural SSa and mesothelioma. We have encountered one case of a surgically resected pleural SSa that was followed about 1 year later by recurrent tumor in the same hemithorax, but the pathologic features of the recurrence were classical of mesothelioma and not SSa. In another referred case, biopsy of a confluent pleural tumor revealed features classical of epithelial mesothelioma, but the thoracic surgeon also identified a small and apparently separate polypoidal tumor in the same hemithorax, and biopsy of this lesion yielded findings characteristic of SSa.

The prognosis for pleural SSa, at least the localized tumors, appears to be somewhat more favorable than for patients with diffuse MM. About half of the 14 cases in the literature as tabulated by Aubry et al.[960] were alive without evidence of disease at 4 to 13 months postresection, and one patient was alive with disease at 8 years. However, diffuse pleural SSas and poorly differentiated SSas appear to represent highly aggressive lesions. The distinction of pleural SSa from pleural MM is also important, for two additional reasons:[951]

1. SSas may be responsive to ifosfamide-based chemotherapy, which is not the case for pleural MM.
2. Pleural SSas have no proven or consistent causal relationship to prior asbestos exposure, unlike the majority of pleural MMs.

Solitary Fibrous Tumors of Pleura

Solitary fibrous tumors (SFTs) are uncommon localized spindle-cell fibroblastoid neoplasms that usually occur in relation to the pleura, where they are thought to arise from submesothelial mesenchyme.[974–976] First described in 1931 by Klemperer and Rabin,[8] SFTs have been reported under a variety of different names, including *submesothelial fibroma*.[503] *Localized fibrous tumor* is arguably the best descriptor because these tumors are not always solitary, but *solitary fibrous tumor* is the preferred nomenclature at present.[503] The former designation *fibrous mesothelioma* is to be avoided, because the spindle cells comprising these lesions show no evidence of a mesothelial phenotype, and the term *fibrous mesothelioma* invites confusion with conventional mesothelial tumors.

Intrathoracic SFTs most often arise in relation to the visceral pleura (~80% of pleural SFTs[503])—where they frequently represent pedunculated lesions (Figs. 43.160 to 43.162)—or the parietal pleura,[974] but they can also arise within the mediastinum or as intraparenchymal lung tumors[977] (see Chapter 39 for complete discussion of intrapulmonary SFT), and in relation to the pericardium[978] and diaphragm.[979] Within the thorax, they can vary greatly in size (Figs. 43.160 and 43.161), ranging from 13 to 330 mm in greatest diameter in one series of cases.[980] Extrathoracic SFTs have been recorded with increasing frequency in a variety of sites,[981,982] such as the orbit,[983–986] nasal cavity,[981,987] paranasal sinuses[987] and nasopharynx,[988] soft tissues of the extremities,[981,989] retroperitoneum,[990] kidney, urinary bladder,[981,991] seminal vesicle and prostate,[981] spermatic cord, vagina,[992] parotid gland,[993] thyroid,[994] liver,[995] pancreas, omentum/mesentery,[996] and meninges.[985]

Solitary fibrous tumors have been recorded in patients of ages 5 to 87 years, but they are rare in patients under the age of 10 years, and the peak incidence is between the fourth and sixth decades of life. One review of 55 patients with pleural SFTs recorded an age range of 18 to 80 years, with a mean of 55 years.[997] A smaller series of 14 intrathoracic SFTs recorded an older age range of 44 to 73 years, with a mean of 60 years.[980] Both intrathoracic and extrathoracic SFTs have been recorded rarely during childhood, for example, in an 8-year-old boy (intrapulmonary)[998] and an 11-year-old girl (parotid gland).[993] In

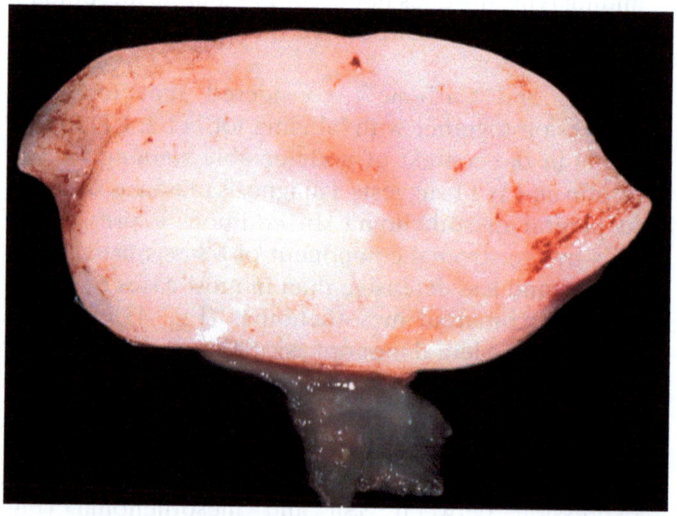

FIGURE 43.160. Small solitary fibrous tumor (SFT) from the visceral pleura. This lesion was pedunculated, and a portion of the pedicle can be seen in the lower center of this field, extending to the foot of the photograph.

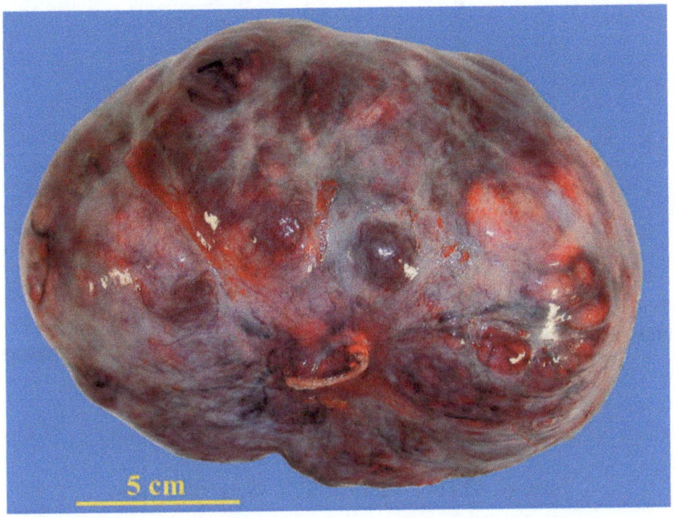

FIGURE 43.161. Pleural SFT. This lesion was resected from a 45-year-old woman, and required the use of obstetrics forceps to "deliver" the SFT through the thoracotomy incision. The lesion has a smooth if slightly bosselated surface, with areas of congested and hemorrhagic tumor tissue alternating with paler areas. The pedicle for this pedunculated tumor is shown near the lower center of this field. The scale at the foot of the photograph is in centimeters.

several series of intrathoracic SFTs, the tumors occurred more often in females than males, but one larger study had a male predominance (32 of 55 cases).[997] In a series of 27 consecutive intrathoracic SFTs from the files of one of the authors (D.W.H.), there were 13 male patients and 14 females, with an average age of 64 years; the tumors ranged in size from 16 to 224 mm (mean, 75 mm), as recorded for 16 cases.

Most commonly, SFTs are discovered incidentally on routine chest x-rays or CT scans in asymptomatic patients,[503,999] and the radiologic appearances may give some inkling of the diagnosis (for example, a smooth localized pleura-based tumor[503]), but definitive diagnosis requires histologic examination of either a biopsy or surgical resection specimen. When present, symptoms can be related to the size of the tumor and to compression of—or intrusion into—surrounding tissues.[999] In such circumstances, symptoms related to intrathoracic SFTs include systemic symptoms such as fatigue, fever, night sweats, and weight loss, whereas symptoms related to the intrathoracic location include cough, dyspnea, chest pain, digital clubbing, hypertrophic osteoarthropathy, and, less commonly, hypoglycemia related to production of insulin-like growth factor[1000] (Doege-Potter syndrome[503]). In one review of 79 cases of SFT[1001]—54 intrathoracic and 25 extrathoracic—89% of the intrathoracic lesions were asymptomatic, whereas 83% of the extrathoracic SFTs were associated with symptoms, which varied according to the range of sites in which the tumors arose.

The histologic appearances characteristically vary from one area to another within a single tumor and from one SFT to another, and they can range from the "patternless pattern" of Stout to "herringbone," cellular, short storiform, diffuse sclerosing, myxoid and hemangiopericytic or angiofibromatoid areas, and areas with neural-type palisading, and, in some instances SSa-like areas (Figs. 43.163 to 43.168).[503,974,976] The bipolar spindle-shaped cells resemble fibroblasts, and they often show a distinctive localization along and parallel to stromal collagen bundles (Fig. 43.164). Multinucleated giant cells occur in some cases, and calcification or ossification may be present (Fig. 43.169). Other changes include cystic degeneration, necrosis, and hemorrhage (Fig. 43.162). Varying degrees of nuclear atypia and pleomorphism, and mitotic activity can be found, and the mitotic index in particular appears to be a probability marker for a diagnosis of malignant SFT (see following discussion). Entrapped mesothelium may be present (or entrapped alveolar epithelium in the case of intrapulmonary SFTs)[503] (Figs. 43.170 and 43.171).

The differential diagnosis includes a variety of other spindle-cell fibroblastoid tumors that can arise in relation to the pleura, chest wall, mediastinum, and other sites where both intrathoracic and extrathoracic SFTs have

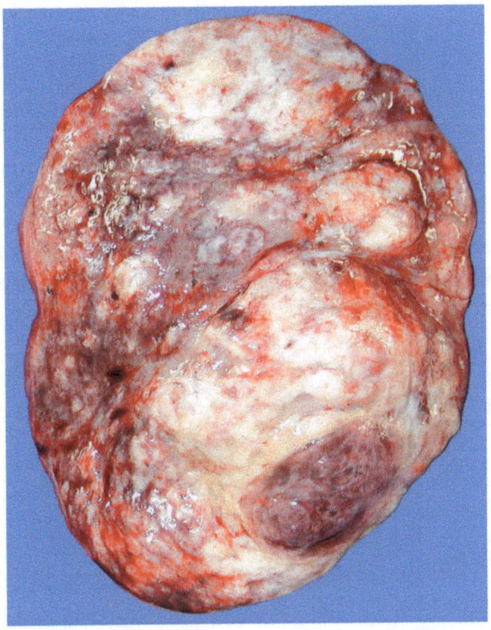

FIGURE 43.162. Pleural SFT. (Same case as in Fig. 43.161.) Areas of pale white tumor tissue alternate with hemorrhagic zones. Areas of necrosis were evident in this tumor, histologically resembling ischemic necrosis, so that the areas of hemorrhagic necrosis were thought probably to be related to partial torsion of the SFT around its pedicle. There were no histologic markers of malignancy, and the tumor tissue was uniform in appearance with only rare mitotic figures.

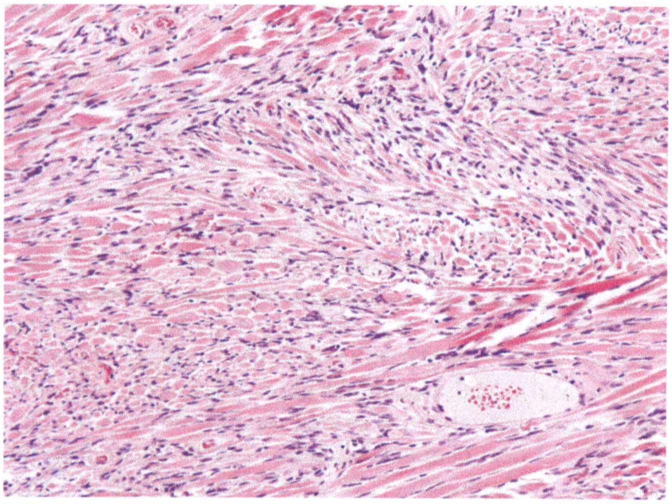

FIGURE 43.163. Pleural SFT. This field depicts intertwining fascicles of collagen bundles with intervening fibroblastoid cells, the appearances being characteristic of an SFT.

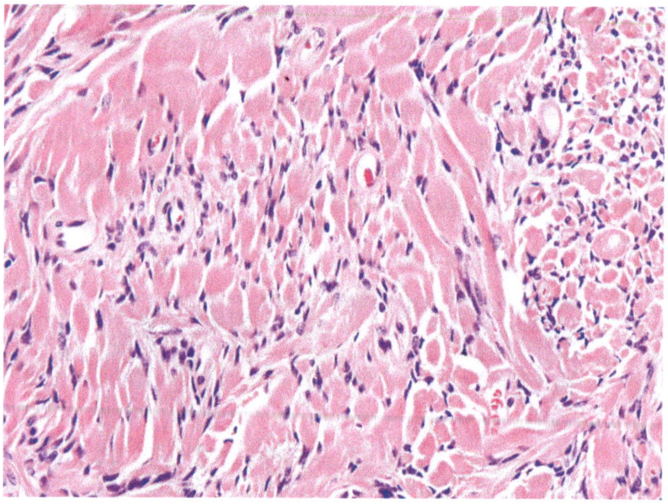

FIGURE 43.164. Pleural SFT. (Same case as in Fig. 43.163.) At higher magnification the collagen bundles and their intervening fibroblastoid cells are seen.

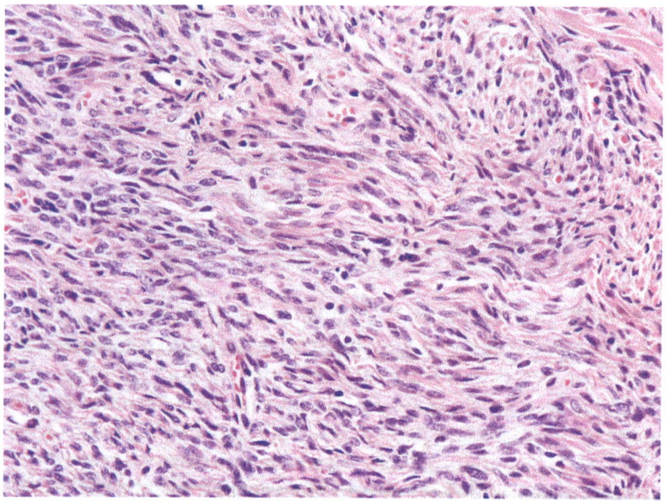

FIGURE 43.165. Pleural SFT. Area of cellular fibroblastoid tissue. This lesion showed no detectable expression of cytokeratins, but staining for CD34 was positive. The tumor cell nuclei are reasonably uniform, and mitotic figures were extremely rate in this case.

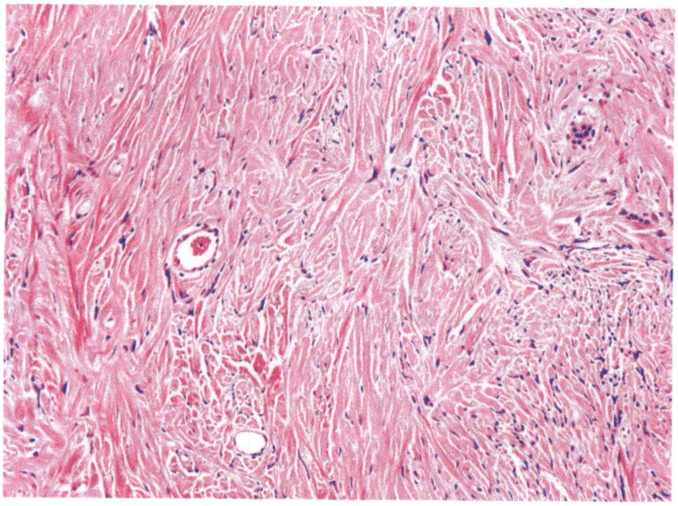

FIGURE 43.166. Pleural SFT. Sclerotic area.

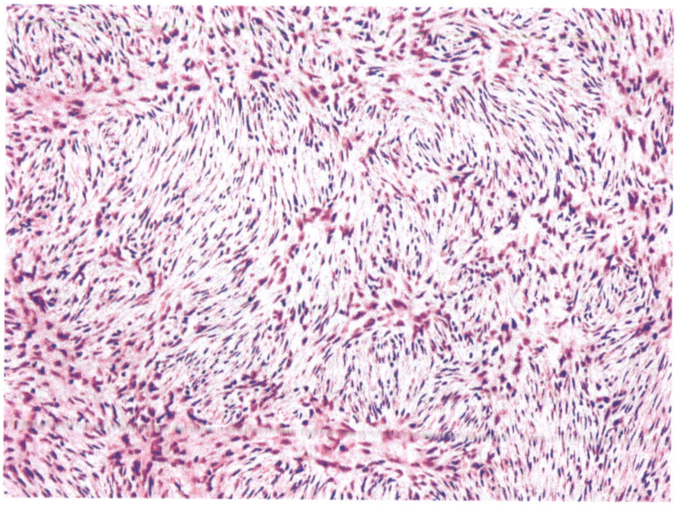

FIGURE 43.167. Pleural SFT that was considered to be malignant on the basis of invasion and areas of cytologically malignant tissue. The tumor has a prominent storiform architecture in this region.

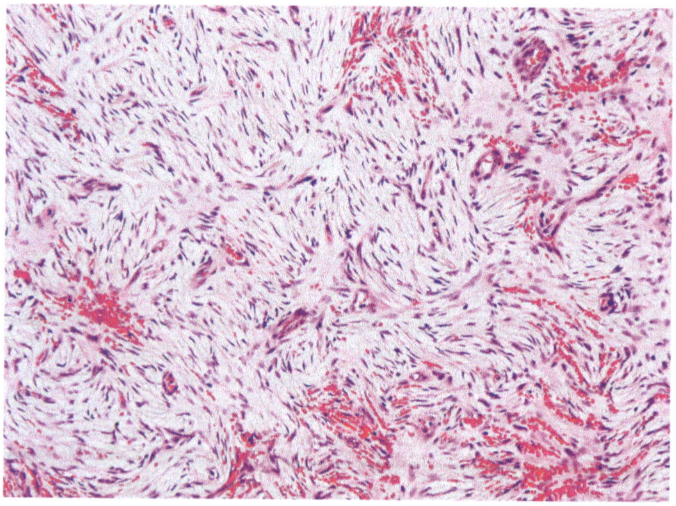

FIGURE 43.168. Pleural SFT, assessed as malignant on the basis of invasion and cytologic indicators of malignancy. An area of myxoid storiform tissue is shown.

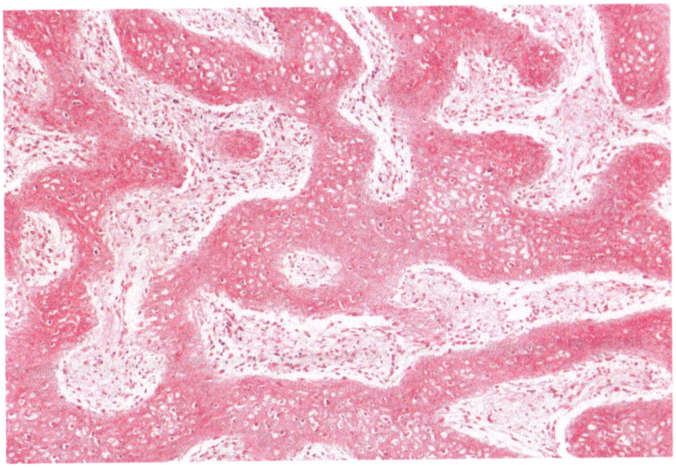

Figure 43.169. Area of bone formation in a solitary fibrous tumor of pleura that was malignant in terms of invasion but showed no cytologic markers of malignancy, with no identifiable mitotic figures.

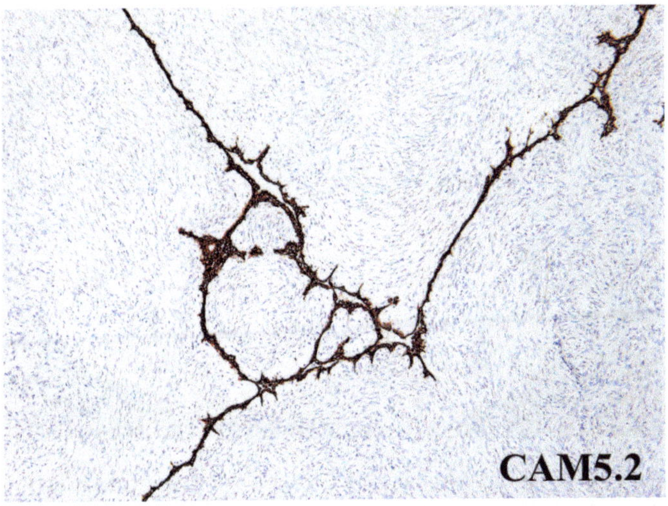

Figure 43.171. Malignant SFT of pleura, showing the multilobated pattern of tumor growth, with inclusion of linear formations of cytokeratin-positive mesothelium (CAM5.2).

been recorded, including extraintestinal gastrointestinal stromal tumors (EGISTs). In the case of pleural tumors, the major differential diagnoses include sarcomatoid and desmoplastic mesothelioma (which can occur as a localized tumor on occasions), fibroblastoid tumors arising in relation to the chest wall or ribs and including pleural desmoid tumors, monophasic SSa, schwannoma, inflammatory myofibroblastic tumor (inflammatory pseudotumor), calcifying fibrous (pseudo)tumor,[999] and perhaps a spindle cell carcinoma of lung with invasion of the pleura.

In most instances, the gross and histologic findings can discriminate between the differential diagnoses at a reasonable order of confidence, but immunohistochemical studies are crucial if there is doubt. Characteristically, the fibroblastoid cells comprising benign SFTs are devoid of CK expression (Fig. 43.171) in contrast to most sarcomatoid mesotheliomas, whether localized or not, and instead the cells show positive immunohistochemical staining for vimentin and CD34[503] (within a range of about 66% to 95%; Fig. 43.172), and less consistently for bcl-2[1002] and CD99.[971,985,1003,1004] However, in some malignant SFTs, the tumor may show depletion of CD34 expression either throughout the tumor or over extensive areas.[1005] In addition, malignant SFTs may show a lobulated growth pattern, with incorporation of linear arrays of hyperplastic mesothelial cells into the tumor, but the background fibroblastoid cells are still devoid of CK expression. The

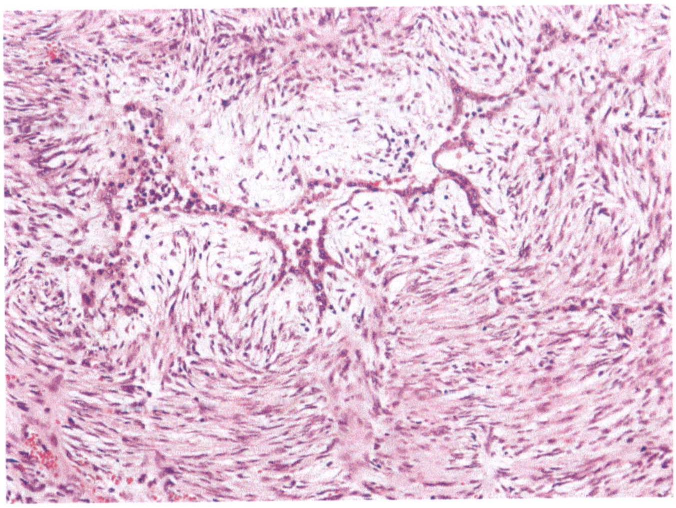

Figure 43.170. Malignant SFT of pleura, showing an area of incorporated mesothelium thought to have been enclosed by a multinodular pattern of tumor growth.

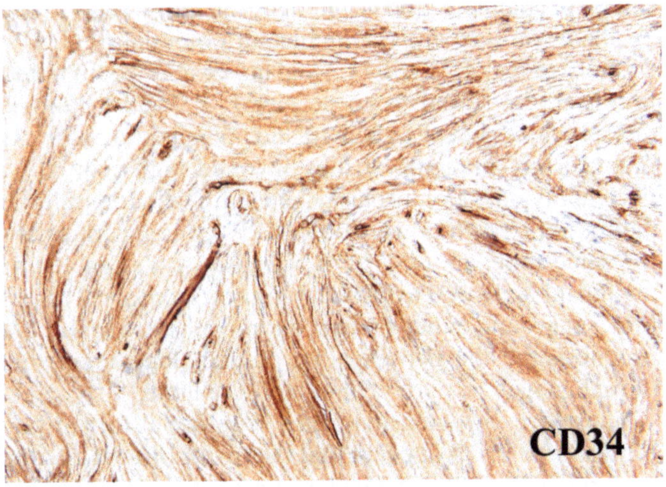

Figure 43.172. Pleural SFT. Expression of CD34.

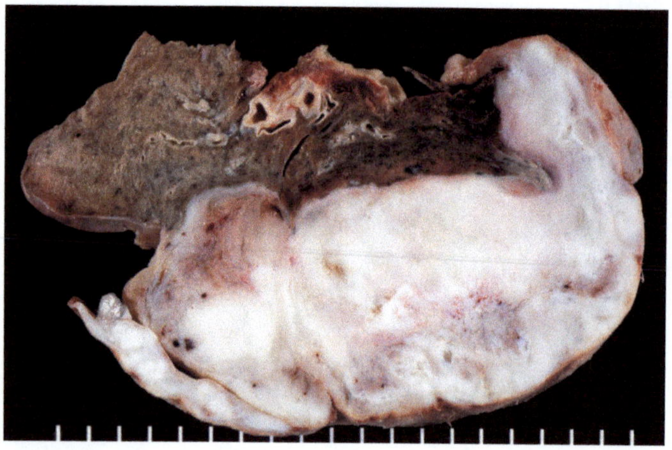

FIGURE 43.173. Malignant SFT of pleura (surgical resection specimen). The lesion forms a massive sessile tumor attached to the visceral pleura and lung, which measured almost 19 cm in vertical dimension (scale is in centimeters). The tumor tissue is pale and white, but there are no obvious areas of necrosis. Nonetheless, the lesion showed invasion into lung parenchyma, and there was also invasion along the parietal pleura. This tumor also showed focal osseous metaplasia (Fig. 43.169). The tumor tissue comprised uniform-appearing fibroblastoid cells throughout, with no mitotic figures identifiable on a protracted search of the sections; nonetheless, this lesion recurred rapidly within the same hemithorax, with a fatal outcome 10 months after the original presentation.

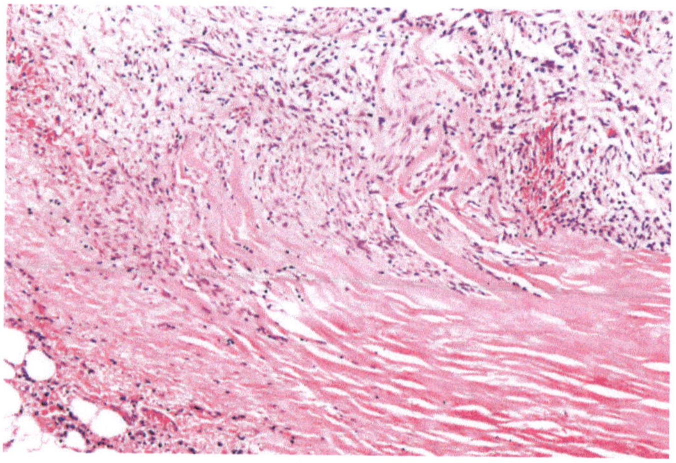

FIGURE 43.174. Malignant SFT of pleura. This patient had a background of occupational exposure to asbestos, with the presence of pleural plaques. Nonetheless, this lesion had histologic features and an immunoprofile characteristic of solitary fibrous tumor. In this field, the tumor is seen invading into pleural plaque, dissecting along and between the collagenous laminae making up the plaque.

EGISTs affecting the thorax (e.g., the mediastinum) can be excluded by the absence of staining for CD117 (c-kit); however, Miettinen et al.[1006] found that about 47% to 100% of GISTs showed positive staining for CD34, and others[1007] have reported positive staining of SFTs for CD117. Schwannomas can be excluded by labeling for S-100 proteins and other markers of schwannian differentiation.

Discrimination between benign and malignant SFTs can be problematic and is analogous in many ways to the problems of assessing the malignant potential of GISTs. In their series of 223 SFTs, England et al.[974] commented that there appeared to be no clearly defined histologic discriminators between benign and malignant tumors. As indicators of malignancy they invoked high cellularity, nuclear atypia, pleomorphism, and more than four mitotic figures per 10 high-power fields (HPFs), among others. At the same time, about 45% of the cases so designated as malignant appeared to have been cured by surgical resection, suggesting either that such tumors have a favorable prognosis or, alternatively, that the histologic indicators of malignancy were not consistently reliable.

Therefore, by extension of the criteria put forward by others,[503,842,974,976] it appears that the major discriminators, in perhaps the following order of rank, favor assessment of an SFT as malignant as opposed to benign, in biopsy tissue or a surgical resection specimen (Figs. 43.173 to 43.176):

- Invasion of adjacent structures (pleura, chest wall, lung (Figs. 43.173 and 43.174)
- Areas of overtly sarcomatous tissue within an SFT, and not resembling SFT (Fig. 43.176)
- Areas of tumor necrosis (as opposed to ischemic-type necrosis possibly related to partial torsion of the lesion; Fig. 43.175)
- More than four mitotic figures per 10 HPFs

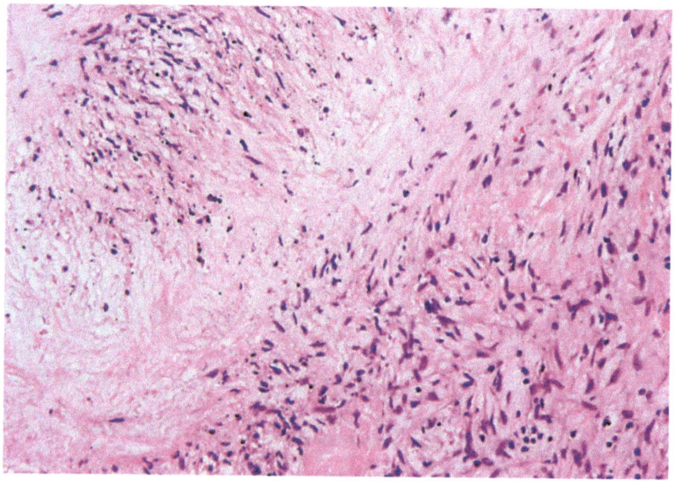

FIGURE 43.175. Malignant SFT of the pleura, showing an area of necrosis with a minor associated inflammatory infiltrate, accompanied by nuclear karyorrhexis.

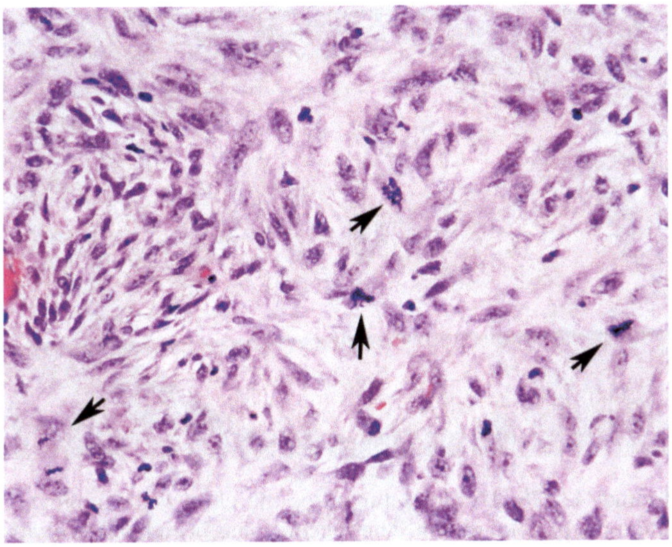

FIGURE 43.176. Malignant SFT of pleura. At least four mitotic figures are evident in this single high-power field (*arrows*). The tumor cells also show moderate nuclear atypia and pleomorphism.

- High cellularity, with prominent nuclear atypia and pleomorphism
- Occurrence on the parietal pleura
- Sessile tumor (Fig. 43.173)
- Large tumor size (>10cm; Fig. 43.173)
- Associated pleural effusion
- Local tumor recurrence following surgical resection (although otherwise benign SFTs can recur locally as multiple tumor nodules following incomplete resection)

With the exception of invasion (or metastasis), most of these markers may be regarded as probability indicators, and some are probably linked (nonindependent) variables. Assessment of the benign versus malignant status of an SFT is arguably best based on a combination of findings. Depending on the above combination of findings, we report SFTs as benign (no histologic evidence of malignancy), SFTs with features of malignancy (e.g., SFT with invasion), and SFTs of uncertain malignant potential. Accordingly, it seems that a small pedunculated tumor arising from the visceral pleura is likely to have a "benign" course following apparently complete surgical resection, irrespective of the cellularity and cytologic atypia seen focally within such a lesion. On the other hand, a large sessile tumor arising on parietal pleura, with areas of tumor necrosis and obvious invasion of the pleura is likely to pursue a "malignant" course, irrespective of the degree of nuclear pleomorphism and atypia. For example, we have encountered a case of a massive malignant SFT that arose as a sessile lesion in relation to the parietal pleura, with invasion of the pleura, chest wall, and lung, and which recurred with a fatal outcome within 10 months of incomplete surgical resection, although exhaustive histologic sampling of the tumor revealed no evidence of excessive cellularity, nuclear atypia, or pleomorphism, and no mitoses could be found (Fig. 43.173).

In the literature, benign SFTs appear to predominate within the thorax. In one study of 36 cases, only two recurred locally.[1008] Another series of 55 cases[997] revealed features of malignancy in four, but only one case showed aggressive behavior, with local recurrence. In another study, four of 14 cases were assessed as malignant[980]; the malignant tumors were larger in diameter (>20cm) and were soft and fleshy, and they showed high mitotic activity, with an average of about seven mitoses per 10 HPF. In a series of 92 extrathoracic SFTs reported by Vallat-Decouvelaere et al.,[1009] 10 recurred or had atypical histologic features (11%), with tumor relapse in eight cases and the development of metastases in five (in lung, liver, and bone). These authors concluded, "Nuclear atypia, hypercellularity, greater than 4 mitoses/10 HPFs, and necrosis . . . [occur] in up to 10% extrathoracic SFTs, and are associated with, but are not themselves predictive of, aggressive clinical behavior."

Wherever possible, management of SFT is by surgical resection.[503] It has been observed that incompletely resected pleural SFTs can recur locally, sometimes as multiple tumor nodules, even where there are no other indicators of malignancy. Therefore, we recommend that local resection of pleural SFTs should include a tumor-free margin of about 10mm around the base of the pedicle or base of the tumor, whenever feasible.

Calcifying Fibrous (Pseudo-)Tumor of the Pleura

Calcifying fibrous tumor (CFT) typically affects the subcutaneous and deeper soft tissues of the limbs, trunk, and neck of children, adolescents, and young adults,[503] but cases have been reported in relation to the pleura,[1010–1013] chest wall,[1014] mediastinum,[1015,1016] peritoneum,[1017] and mesentery.[1018] Pinkard et al.[1011] described three cases of pleural CFT in young adults, ages 23, 28, and 34 years. Typically, pleural CFTs are located in the inferior chest region, and they may represent either solitary mass lesions or multifocal tumor-like lesions, measuring about 30 to 120mm in greatest diameter.[503,1010] One case with multiple pleural lesions has been recorded in a 29-year-old woman who had no symptoms referable to the tumor.[1013]

On histologic examination, CFT comprises paucicellular fibrocollagenous tissue without a laminar (plaque-like) architecture, accompanied by a sparse lymphoplasmacytic infiltrate and with variable numbers of rounded calcified bodies of variable size, resembling psammoma bodies (Fig. 43.177). Points of distinction of CFT from either desmoplastic MM or solitary fibrous

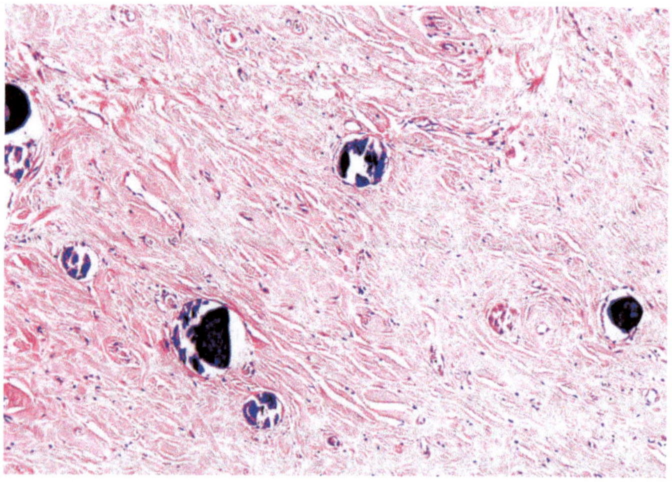

FIGURE 43.177. This calcifying fibrous (pseudo)tumor comprises paucicellular fibrocollagenous tissue with several rounded calcified bodies, some of which are partly shattered as a consequence of cutting the histologic section. (Courtesy of Dr. Goran Elmberger, Stockholm, Sweden.)

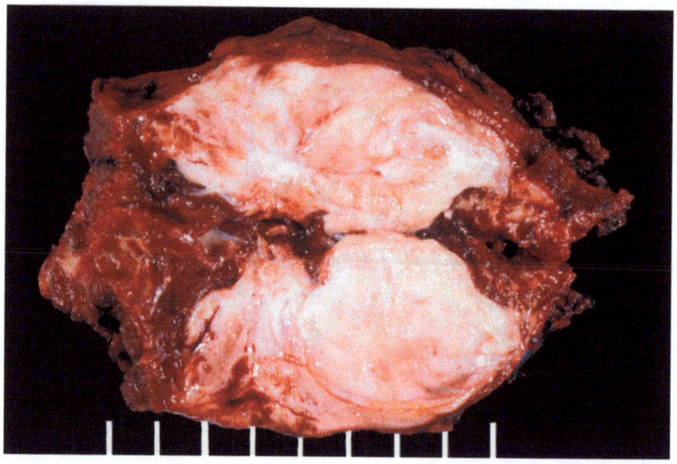

FIGURE 43.178. Desmoid tumor of the chest wall, impinging upon the parietal pleura. The specimen has been bivalved, with pleura at the top of the specimen as depicted, and at the bottom. The lesion is reasonably well localized, although obviously unencapsulated. It was clearly invasive on microscopy, and it had a firm rubbery white (slightly bosselated) cut surface. Scale is in centimeters.

tumor include negative reactions for both cytokeratins and CD34, whereas the fibroblastoid cells show positive staining for vimentin.[503] Pleural plaques are distinguishable by their paucicellular, laminated, and (frequently) hyalinized appearance; in addition, the pattern of psammoma-like calcification in CFTs differs from the finely punctate to sheet-like calcification seen in plaques.

A relationship to inflammatory myofibroblastic tumor has been debated,[1019–1021] but the pathogenesis of CFT remains obscure. These lesions are entirely benign in character and are usually treated successfully by surgical extirpation, but local recurrence has been recorded.[1022]

We have observed one case that occurred in a diffuse pleural distribution and was misdiagnosed as a desmoplastic mesothelioma.

Desmoid Tumors of the Pleura

Desmoid tumors in the region of the thorax, including the shoulder girdle region and chest wall, are well recognized in the literature; some chest wall lesions can impinge upon the parietal pleura (Fig. 43.178), but primary desmoid tumors of the pleura and lung are extremely rare. Pleural desmoid tumors carry the potential for misdiagnosis as an SFT in particular, as well as benign neurogenic tumors and even localized sarcomatoid mesotheliomas with desmoplastic features.

Wilson et al.[1023] reported four cases of pleural desmoid tumors, in two men and two women of ages 16 to 66 years (mean, 44 years). Three of the patients presented with chest pain and one had dyspnea. Three of the tumors affected the parietal pleura and one was located in the visceral pleura. The mean tumor size was 125 mm, and all showed a bosselated firm white cut surface (Fig. 43.178). The histologic appearances were essentially identical to those of desmoid tumors in extrapleural sites (Figs. 43.179 and 43.180). As with desmoid tumors in other locations, the lesions invariably showed invasive features, with

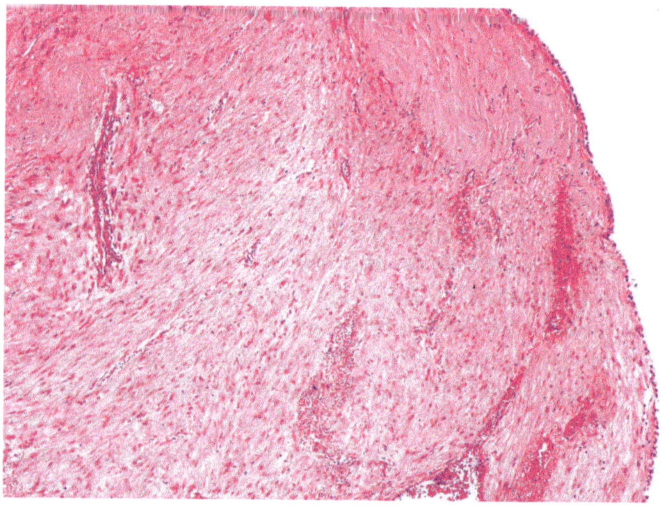

FIGURE 43.179. Pleural desmoid tumor from a 69-year-old man. This lesion was located near the apex of the pleura, with invasion of the thoracic inlet, so that complete surgical resection was impossible. A layer of cuboidalized mesothelium can be seen at the surface of the pleura, and the submesothelial tissues are expanded by a hypocellular collagen-producing spindle-cell lesion with histologic appearances and a pattern of invasion elsewhere that were characteristic of a desmoid tumor.

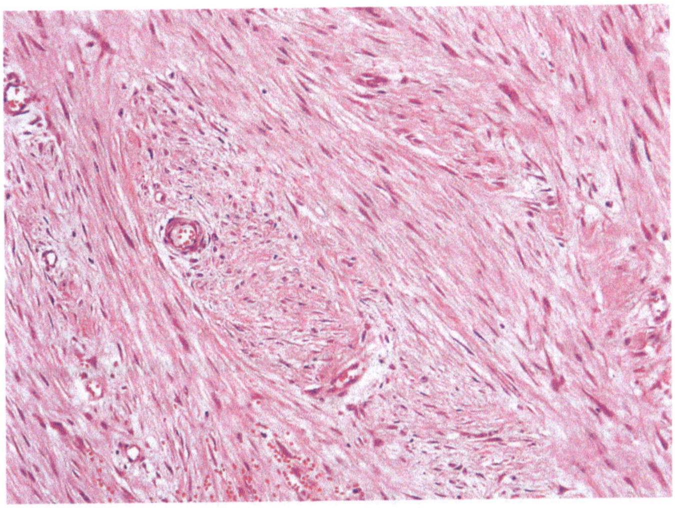

FIGURE 43.180. Detail of desmoid tumor of the pleura. The tumor comprises reasonably uniform spindle-shaped fibroblastoid cells separated by a collagenous matrix, with reasonably prominent blood vessels.

extension into fat or skeletal muscle. Wilson et al. found that the tumor cells showed immunoreactivity for vimentin, smooth muscle and muscle-specific actin, and desmin in three out of the four cases, and the lesions showed no evidence of S-100 protein immunoreactivity. The patients were treated by surgical resection, either complete or incomplete, and one case where resection was incomplete was managed further by radiation therapy and then complete surgical resection. Follow-up revealed stable residual disease at 12 months after treatment in one patient, and two of the patients had no evidence of residual disease at 12 and 96 months.

Subsequently, Andino et al.[1024] studied β-catenin expression and cyclin D-1 in a series of four thoracic desmoid tumors—one representing a pleural desmoid tumor, one intrapulmonary in location, and two affecting the pleura-chest wall—in comparison to five benign and six malignant SFTs of pleura. Diffuse, moderate to strong nuclear staining for β-catenin was found in all of the desmoid tumors, four out of five benign SFTs, and two of six malignant SFTs. Nuclear and cytoplasmic cyclin D-1 staining was seen in all groups. These authors also found that the distinction between desmoid tumors and SFTs was best made from CD34 expression (0/4 desmoid tumors versus 8/11 SFTs) and smooth muscle actin (found in all four desmoid tumors but in none of the 11 solitary fibrous tumors). Lack of S-100 protein expression also distinguishes pleural desmoid tumors from neurogenic lesions, and the distinction from a localized sarcomatoid mesothelioma with desmoplastic features can be made on the distinctive histologic appearances of desmoid tumors and the absence of cytokeratin expression (although, as mentioned elsewhere, cytokeratin-negative sarcomatoid mesotheliomas are well recognized).

Benign and Malignant Nerve Sheath Tumors

Neoplasms that have histologic and immunohistochemical features of nerve sheath tumors have been reported primary in the pleural cavity.[1025,1026] The benign growths typically show morphologic features of Verocay bodies with Antoni A and B areas, as well as hyaline vascular changes. They have features similar to nerve sheath tumors seen elsewhere. When malignant, these cells frequently do not show the typical benign features of nerve sheath tumors. Immunohistochemical staining with neural markers such as S-100 protein is helpful in confirming a neurogenic origin of these neoplasms.

Inflammatory Myofibroblastic Tumors

Inflammatory pseudotumors, also referred to as *plasma cell granulomas* and *inflammatory myofibroblastic tumors*, may occasionally involve the lung and rarely involve the pleura.[1027] These tumors have the histologic features of those neoplasms involving the lung and occurring elsewhere, typically made up of a proliferation of spindle cells with varying numbers of inflammatory cells, usually with an excess number of plasma cells. There has been a significant debate whether these tumors are true neoplasms or are reactive changes.[1028] (See Chapter 39).

Epithelioid Hemangioendothelioma and Angiosarcoma of the Pleura

Epithelioid hemangioendothelioma (EHE) is a distinctive malignant angioformative neoplasm in which the neoplastic endothelial cells are epithelioid and sometimes bland in appearance,[1029] often arranged as solid sheets or in a linear fashion, embedded in a hyaline or myxohyaline stroma.[237] These epithelioid endothelial neoplasms have been described in soft tissue,[1029] bone, liver, and lung; in the lung they were designated as intravascular bronchioloalveolar tumors (IVBATs) before their endothelial character was recognized.[533] The epithelioid appearances of the neoplastic cells stand in contrast to the angioformative and even papillary patterns of conventional angiosarcomas; EHEs in soft tissues are often considered to represent neoplasms intermediate in malignancy between conventional aggressive angiosarcomas and benign hemangiomas, but they have the potential for local recurrence and metastatic spread. The anatomic site where these tumors arise correlates with mortality, so that the mortality rate for EHEs of bone or liver is about double the mortality rate for those that arise within soft tissues.[503]

In 1993, Battifora[1030] recorded mimicry of mesothelioma by pleural EHE, and his report was followed in 1996 by the study carried out by Lin et al.[1031] on 14 cases of malignant vascular tumors of serous membranes producing mimicry of mesothelioma. The EHEs (epithelioid angiosarcomas) diffusely involved pleural, peritoneal, or pericardial cavities, producing a clinical picture that closely simulated mesothelioma. The patients ranged in age from 34 to 85 years at the time of diagnosis, with a mean age of 52 years. The patients included two women and one man with peritoneal EHE, eight men with pleural EHEs, and three men with pericardial tumors.

The histologic appearances took the form of a diffuse sheet-like and clustered pattern of tumor cells with variable degrees of vascular differentiation, and a tubulopapillary growth pattern was encountered in four cases. Nine cases showed varying numbers of spindle-shaped cells producing a focal biphasic architecture, heightening the resemblance to mesothelioma.

The initial diagnoses made on those cases included mesothelioma, secondary adenocarcinoma, and leiomyosarcoma. On immunohistochemical analysis, they were characterized by extensive strong vimentin staining (14/14 cases) in the face of weak (4/14) to moderate (2/14) immunostaining for CKs. The tumor cells expressed at least two of the four endothelial markers employed in the study (CD31, CD34, von Willebrand factor [factor VIII–related antigen; factor VIII–RAG], and *Ulex europaeus* agglutinin-1). Markers for mesothelial, epithelial, myoid, and neuronal differentiation were all negative. These serosal EHEs pursued a highly aggressive course; 12 of the patients presented with disseminated disease and most died within months of the initial presentation.

Subsequently, additional cases have been reported by Attanoos et al.,[1032] Crotty et al.,[1033] Zhang et al.,[519] Sporn et al.,[1034] and Al-Shraim et al.[1035] Zhang et al. found a total of 26 cases in the literature, to which they added five; 22 cases came from Western nations and nine from Japan. The patients were 22 to 79 years of age, with an average of 57 years, and with a male-to-female ratio of 9:1. A history of exposure to radiation or asbestos was noted in a few Western cases. The most common presentation took the form of pleural thickening accompanied by effusion, producing radiological mimicry of MM.

All three cases of pleural EHE reported by Attanoos et al.[1036] had a background of occupational exposure to asbestos, but ferruginous bodies were found in histologic sections from only one of the cases, and only in this patient was the asbestos fiber burden raised in comparison to the range of fiber counts for a nonexposed "background" population. The latent period between asbestos exposure and the diagnosis of the EHEs ranged from 18 to 60 years. These authors reported that no definitive conclusion concerning a relationship between asbestos and pleural EHE could be drawn from this small series of three cases, "but further investigation [was] warranted."

The six patients (five men and one woman) reported by Sporn et al.[1034] ranged in age from 55 to 80 years. All six presented with pleural thickening with or without an accompanying pleural effusion, and for the five for whom follow-up was available, all had died at periods ranging from 3 to 14 months. Oliveira and Carvalho[1037] reported a pleural EHE in a woman who survived for 29 months after diagnosis.

Not only do pleural EHEs essentially mimic mesothelioma in their presentation and the anatomic distribution of the pleural tumor as revealed, for example, by radiologic imaging studies, but the epithelioid appearances of the neoplastic cells can produce a pattern in H&E-stained sections that is virtually indistinguishable from mesothelioma. The neoplastic cells can closely resemble epithelioid cells in an MM, being disposed as sheets or as irregular clusters as shown in Figures 43.181 and 43.182. In some areas, abortive vascular differentiation may be found, and in many cases the neoplastic cells possess empty-appearing intracytoplasmic vacuoles that appear on electron microscopy examination to represent rudimentary vascular lumina (Figs. 43.181 and 43.183). The stroma of these tumors can vary from myxoid (Figs. 43.181 and 43.182) to hyaline, and there may be a spindle-cell sarcomatoid pattern producing mimicry of biphasic mesothelioma.

In 1984 three cases of angiosarcoma of serosal surfaces were described by McCaughey et al.[517] In general, the angiosarcomas are more pleomorphic and less epithelioid than the EHEs (Fig. 43.184).

Clues to the correct diagnosis of EHE include the following:

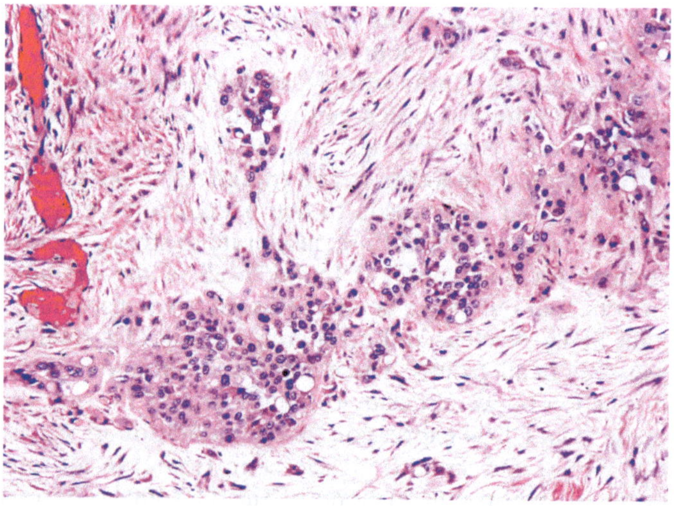

FIGURE 43.181. Pleural epithelioid hemangioendothelioma (EHE) in a middle-aged woman who presented with a unilateral pleural effusion. The tumor comprises an irregular ramifying collection of epithelioid cells embedded in a myxoid fibroproliferative matrix. Vacuoles are discernible in some of the neoplastic cells.

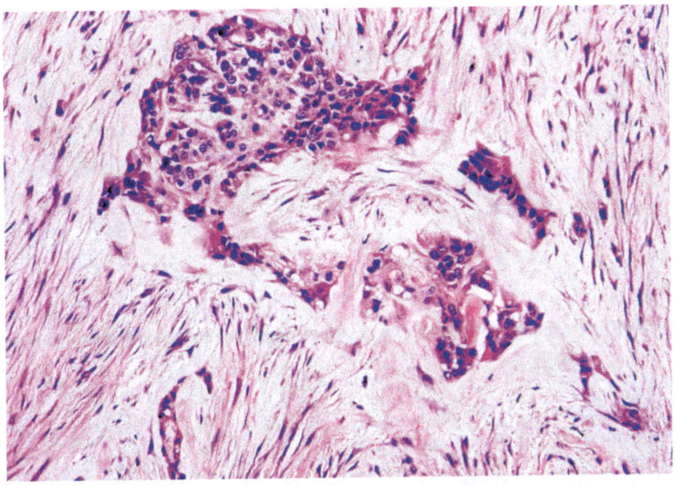

FIGURE 43.182. Pleural EHE. (Same case as in Fig. 43.181.) Collection of epithelioid tumor cells, surrounded by abundant myxoid matrix.

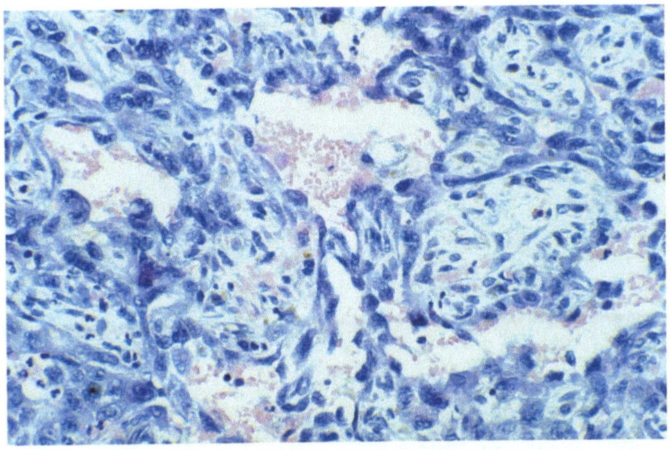

FIGURE 43.184. Histologically, angiosarcomas of the pleura are formed by pleomorphic cells showing vascular spaces

- Negative to weak or only moderate immunostaining for CKs, in comparison to disproportionately prominent reactivity for vimentin
- Absence of staining for mesothelial cell markers such as calretinin or with HBME-1 or for carcinoma-related markers
- Positive immunostaining for endothelial markers such as CD31, CD34 (Fig. 43.185) or factor VIII–RAG

For these reasons, we always include an endothelial marker as part of our immunohistochemical workup on cases of suspected mesothelioma, and we have encountered only two cases of proven mesothelioma that showed positive reactivity of the epithelioid cells for CD31.

On electron microscopy, these tumors show distinct features of endothelial differentiation, including the formation of rudimentary vascular structures, a surrounding basal lamina, and in some instances the presence of tubulated Weibel-Palade bodies in the cytoplasm (Figs. 43.186 and 43.187).

Desmoplastic Round Cell Tumors

Most desmoplastic round cell tumors occur in the pelvic cavity in young adults; rare cases have been reported in the pleura and thorax.[1038–1041]

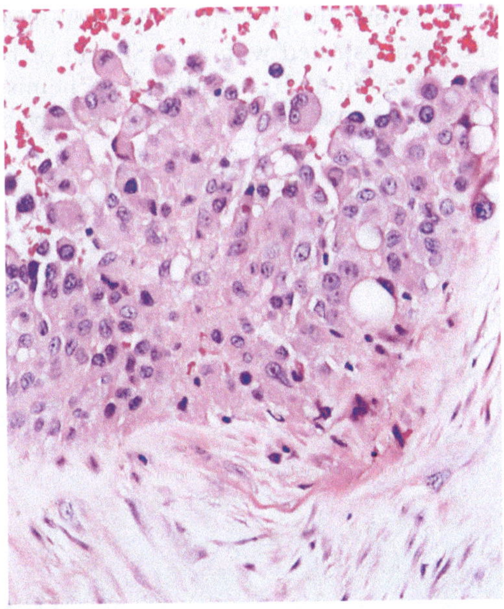

FIGURE 43.183. Pleural EHE. The epithelioid cells are depicted in greater detail, showing nuclear atypia and lucent intracytoplasmic vacuoles.

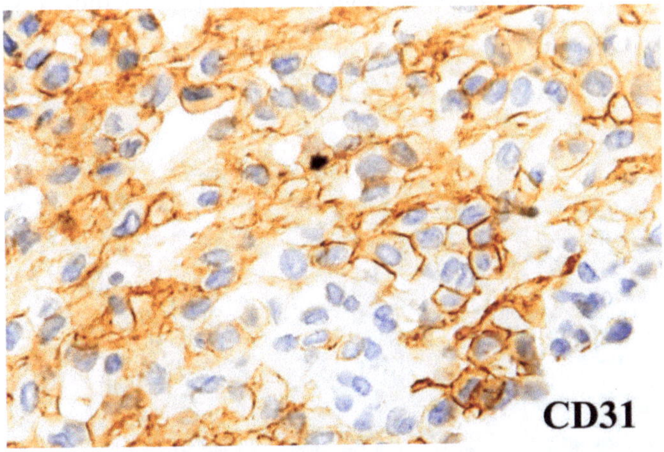

FIGURE 43.185. Pleural EHE. (Same case as in the preceding figures.) The immunoreactivity is seen on labeling for CD31. Identical labeling was seen for CD34. This case showed no detectable cytokeratin expression.

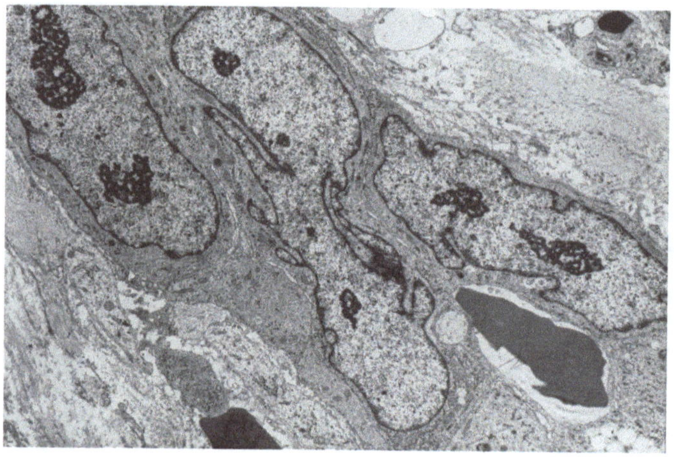

FIGURE 43.186. This electron micrograph shows elongated cells forming primitive vascular structures.

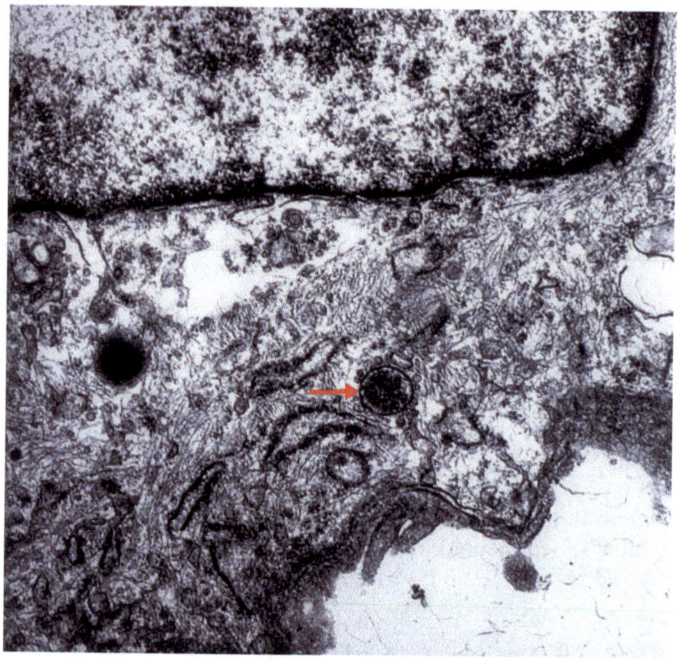

FIGURE 43.187. The structure (arrow) in the cytoplasm of the cell shown here is referred to as a Weibel-Palade body and is pathognomonic of an endothelial cell.

These neoplasms have the same morphology in the pleura as they do in the abdominal cavity, typically consisting of nests of small round cells with hyperchromatic nuclei and a dense fibrous or cellular spindle stroma (Fig. 43.188). The cytoplasm typically contains dot-like structures that correspond to intermediate filaments when examined ultrastructurally (Fig. 43.189). These neoplasms typically show immunostaining for cytokeratin and desmin, with the desmin being in a dot-like configuration (Fig. 43.188B) corresponding to the intermediate filaments seen ultrastructurally. In addition, these neoplasms typically show nuclear staining for WT1. Desmoplastic round cell tumors also characteristically show the translocation t(11;22)(p13;q12) by molecular analysis.[1042]

Primitive Neuroectodermal Tumor

Primitive neuroectodermal tumors (PNETs) are part of the spectrum of small round cell neoplasms that also includes Ewing's sarcoma. These tumors are also referred to as Askin tumors and are composed of sheets of small round cells with hyperchromatic nuclei that show areas of necrosis (Fig. 43.190).[1042] Rosette structures are common and cystic spaces are occasionally seen. The neoplastic cells have a high nuclear-cytoplasmic ratio, and the nuclei typically have vesicular, finely granular chromatin. Glycogen is frequently present in the neoplastic cells and can be demonstrated with a PAS stain or by ultrastructural examination. By immunohistochemistry, the neoplastic cells express CD99 and are usually negative

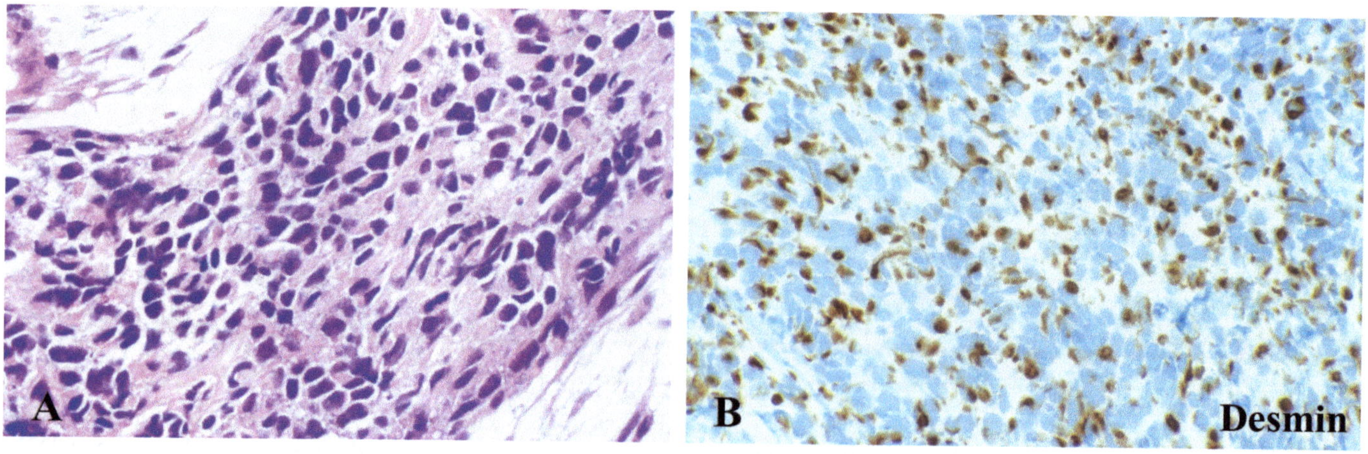

FIGURE 43.188. **(A)** This pleural tumor is composed of small round cells surrounded by cellular fibrous stroma. **(B)** Immunostain for desmin is positive in a dot-like pattern.

for keratin, although focal keratin positivity as well as chromogranin and synaptophysin immunostaining have been observed.[1043,1044] Histologically, these tumors can be confused with small cell mesotheliomas. Molecular analysis typically shows the characteristic translocation, t(11;22)(q24;q12), although this translocation is not specific (see Figs. 36.99 to 36.101 in Chapter 36, and Chapter 42).

Pleuropulmonary Blastoma

Pleuropulmonary blastomas are rare neoplasms that occur in the lung and pleura, predominantly in early childhood.[156,1045] Pleuropulmonary blastomas often have a hamartomatous appearance and frequently are associated with a family history. This neoplasm is different from the pulmonary blastoma that characteristically occurs in an adult. Pleuropulmonary blastoma is composed of primitive cells underneath an epithelium with a cambium layer-like appearance as seen in sarcoma botryoides. Rhabdomyoblasts may be found among the small cells. Occasional anaplastic sarcomatous elements, including embryonal rhabdomyosarcoma, fibrosarcoma, chondrosarcoma, and undifferentiated sarcoma (see Figs. 42.7 to 42.9 in Chapter 42) are observed.

Pleural Lymphomas

Primary pleural lymphomas are rare. The two lymphomas that are mentioned most frequently as involving the pleura are *primary effusion lymphoma (PEL)* and *pyothorax-associated lymphoma.*[1046,1047] Primary effusion lymphomas are composed of large B lymphoid cells (Fig. 43.191) and typically present as pleural effusions without detectable tumor masses elsewhere in the body. Primary effusion lymphomas are associated with human herpesvirus 8 and Kaposi's sarcoma, and typically occur in individuals with acquired immune deficiency syndrome (AIDS).[1046–1048] (See Chapter 32).

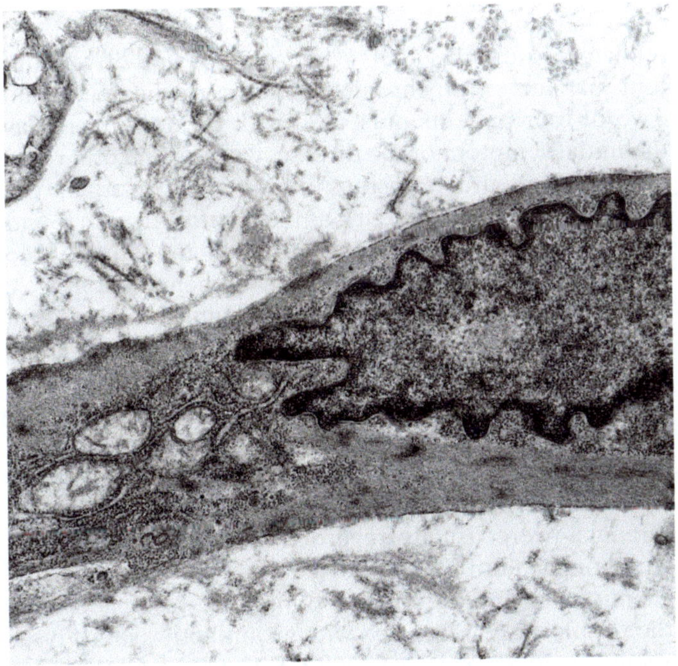

FIGURE 43.189. Ultrastructurally, the cells are round to spindle shaped and show intracytoplasmic intermediate filaments.

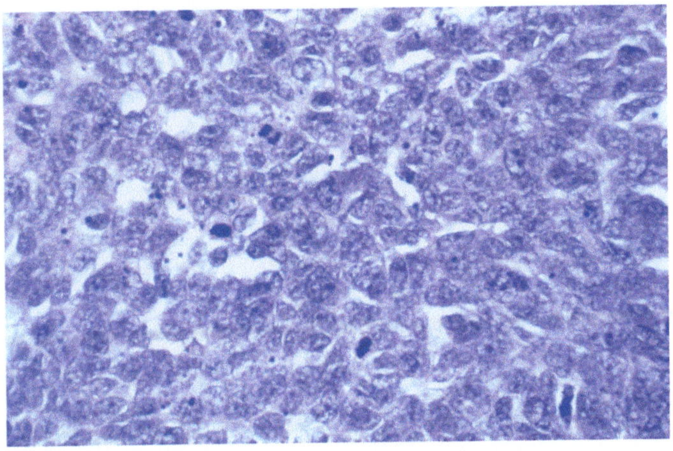

FIGURE 43.190. This small cell tumor involving the pleura has the histologic and immunohistochemical features of a primitive neuroectodermal tumor (PNET).

Pyothorax-associated lymphoma typically occurs in persons with a chronic pyothorax, often decades after the initial injury.[1049–1051] Pyothorax-associated lymphomas were first described in Japan and the largest series is from that country. Clinically, persons with pyothorax-associated lymphomas present with effusion, chest pain, weight loss, and dyspnea. Males are typically more frequently affected than females. Patients with pyothorax-associated lymphoma do not have a history of HIV infection or immunosuppression. The potential causes of pyothorax include tuberculosis and other inflammatory/infectious conditions. The pathogenesis is thought to be due to chronic antigen stimulation analogous to mucosa-associated lymphoid tissue (MALT) lymphomas of the stomach. Pyothorax-associated lymphomas typically are large (usually ≥10 cm) and are associated with pleural fibrosis. They often invade adjacent structures. Pyothorax-associated lymphomas are composed of large B lymphocytes with a smaller number of lymphoplasmacytoid cells. At the time of autopsy, over half the patients have disease limited to the thoracic region and the other half show extrathoracic extension. The neoplastic cells typically show expression of CD45, CD20, CD79, and occasionally CD138. The lymphoid cells are typically negative for CD3.

Diffuse large B-cell lymphomas have been reported to show pleuropulmonary involvement and typically are

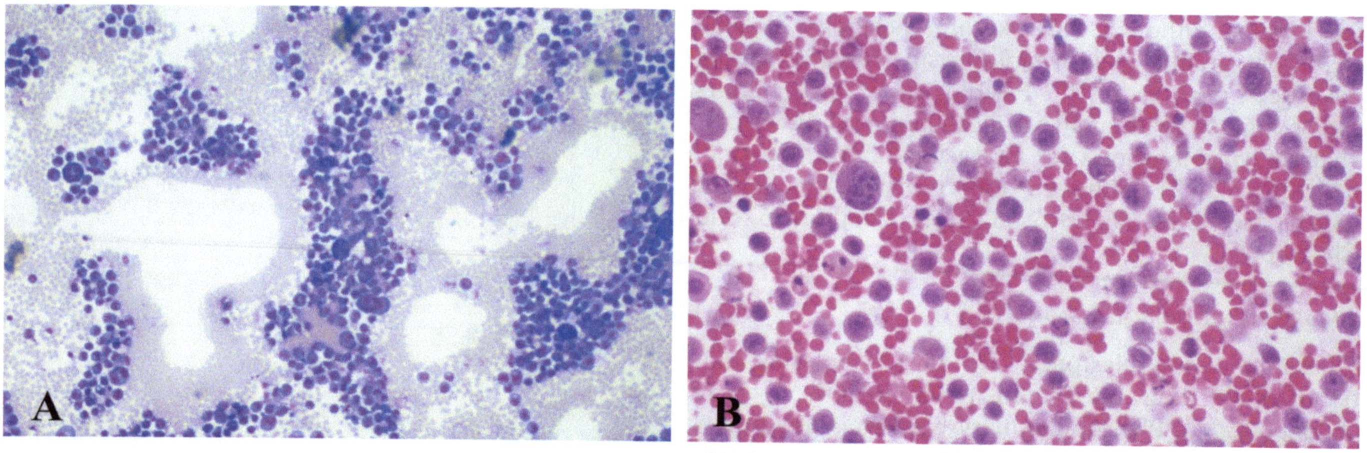

FIGURE 43.191. **(A,B)** The patient whose pleural fluid was evaluated was HIV positive. All cells in the fluid were CD20 positive and were diagnosed by flow cytometry as a large B cell lymphoma. There was no evidence of lymphoma elsewhere in the patient's body.

composed of cells that have immunoblastic features with plasmacytoid differentiation. These cells show frequent mitoses and have a high proliferative rate as demonstrated by MIB-1 evaluation. The cells also show immunostaining for CD45, CD79, and CD20 (see Chapter 32).

Primary sclerosing mediastinal B-cell lymphomas typically occur in young females and can show pleuropulmonary involvement. These lymphomas are thought to arise from perithymic B lymphocytes and typically show immunostaining for CD45, CD20, and CD30. They are CD15 negative.

Multiple myeloma has also been identified as primarily involving the pleura.[1052–1054]

The most recent report on lymphomas involving the pleura is by Vega et al.,[1055] who reviewed the clinicopathologic features of 34 patients with lymphoma involving the pleura proven by biopsy and classified these lymphomas according to the WHO classification. Nine (26.5%) patients had pleural involvement as the only site of disease, whereas 22 (64.7%) had other sites of involvement. Eighteen (56.3%) of 32 patients with adequate clinical data had a history of lymphoma, including three patients with pleural involvement as the only site of disease. According to the WHO classification, 17 (50%) were diffuse large B-cell lymphomas; five (14.7%) were follicular lymphomas, including a case with areas of diffuse large B-cell lymphoma; two (5.9%) were small lymphocytic lymphoma/chronic lymphocytic leukemia; two (5.9%) were precursor T-cell lymphoblastic lymphoma/leukemia; one (2.9%) was mantle cell lymphoma; one (2.9%) was posttransplant lymphoproliferative disorder; and one (2.9%) was a classical Hodgkin's lymphoma. The other five cases were B-cell lymphomas that could not be further classified. The authors concluded that most patients with lymphoma involving the pleura had simultaneous evidence of systemic involvement. The most frequent type was a diffuse large B-cell lymphoma followed by follicular lymphoma.

We have recently seen a mantle zone lymphoma proven by flow cytometry and immunohistochemistry primarily involving the pleura and associated with an epithelial mesothelioma.

Leukemic Involvement of the Pleura

The incidence of leukemic involvement of the pleura is difficult to determine. Relatively few cases have been reported. Bourantas et al.[1056] reported pleural effusion in four patients with chronic myelomonocytic leukemia. Two of four patients presented with pleural effusion as the initial symptom of the disease, whereas the other two developed pleural effusions during the course of the disease. In only one patient was the pleural effusion found to be due to leukemic infiltration. In the other three patients, it was considered a reactive phenomenon.

Schmitt-Graff et al.[1057] reported identification of focal leukemic infiltrates as the initial manifestation of acute myeloid leukemia. Eight patients had myelodysplastic syndrome, and over a 2-year period developed acute myelogenous leukemia. Focal leukemic infiltrates were localized in the skin, oral mucosa, lymph nodes, gastrointestinal tract, pleura, and retroperitoneum. These myelosarcomas were usually regarded as putative malignant lymphomas until further evaluation by immunohistochemistry or flow cytometry. By immunohistochemistry, the neoplastic cells reacted with an antibody against lysozyme, myeloperoxidase, CD68, CD43, CD56, CD117, and CD34. The authors stated that although bone marrow findings were inconclusive, a straightforward diagnosis was reached by considering the possibility of a myelosarcoma and performing the appropriate immunohistochemical/flow cytometric analyses.

Screening for Mesothelioma: Serum Levels of Soluble Mesothelin-Related Proteins and Osteopontin

Soluble Mesothelin-Related Proteins

A potentially significant recent development for the investigation of MM has been the retrospective demonstration[1058–1065] of elevated serum mesothelin-related protein (SMRP) levels in patients with mesothelioma; similar findings have also been reported in relation to osteopontin levels as a marker for MM.[1066,1067] Even so, these approaches are still at an investigational stage of development. The positive predictive value (PPV)[1068]* for an elevated blood level of SMRP or osteopontin (or both together) has yet to be established, as a precondition for the introduction of these tests into routine clinical practice for the screening or clinical investigation of individual patients for the prospective diagnosis of MM.

Mesothelin is a cell-surface glycoprotein present on normal mesothelial cells and is expressed in several cancers,[563,611,612] including mesotheliomas with an epithelioid component,[563,611,612,680] ovarian adenocarcinomas in particular,[563,864,1069,1070] squamous and large cell carcinomas and adenocarcinomas of lung,[583,680,1071] pancreatic adenocarcinomas,[615,1072] and some gastrointestinal cancers.[1069] The precursor protein product of the mesothelin gene occurs as a 69- to 71-kDa polypeptide with a glycosyl-phosphatidyl-inositol linkage that anchors it to the cell membrane.[1069,1073] This anchored precursor protein can be cleaved by a furin-like protease to yield a 31-kDa soluble protein called megakaryocyte potentiating factor (MPF)[1069,1073] and a 40-kDa cell membrane-bound protein called mesothelin. There is some evidence that mesothelin may be implicated in cell-cell adhesion,[1069] but knowledge of its normal biologic function is incomplete, and mice with a knockout of the mesothelin gene(s) have no obvious phenotypic abnormality.[1070] Although mesothelin is attached to the cell membrane, it can be shed like other cell membrane proteins, and some investigators, including Robinson's group,[1058–1062] have described a 42- to 44-kDa protein called soluble mesothelin/MPF-related (SMR) protein detectable in sera from patients with pleural MM and also ovarian carcinoma.

Antibodies to cell membrane-bound mesothelin were first prepared by inoculating BALB/c mice with the human ovarian carcinoma cell line OVCAR-3, generating the monoclonal antibody K-1,[615,1070] and K-1 has been used for some years for assessment of cancers by immunostaining of histologic sections.[611,612] However, we abandoned the use of antibodies against mesothelin for the immunohistochemical investigation of suspected MM because of its cross-reactivity with other cancers,[611,615,1070] and it appeared to have no particular advantage over other antibodies raised against mesothelial cells. Of course, detection of mesothelin by immunohistochemical analysis of histologic sections is an exercise different from quantitative estimates of blood SMRP levels.

The mechanisms whereby mesothelin is released from cell membranes are unclear as yet, but the release of SMRP might be due to an abnormal splicing event that unbinds or cleaves it from the cell surface.[1064] Robinson's group[1058,1062] detected SMRP using the OV569 monoclonal antibody, but Hassan et al.[1063] appear to have used a different approach to the generation of a mouse anti-mesothelin monoclonal antibody, making it difficult to compare their results with those of both Robinson's group[1058–1062] and Scherpereel et al.[1064] (the OV569 antibody appears to be the basis for the commercially-marketed Mesomark™ Fujirebio Diagnostics, Inc. Malvern, PA test[1065]). Testing for serum SMRP levels is determined by an enzyme-linked immunosorbent assay (ELISA) test using two monoclonal antibodies (e.g., OV569 and 4H3),[1062] which bind to different SMRP epitopes. Shiomi et al.[1074] found that the renal cell carcinoma gene *ERC*, which is expressed in a renal carcinoma model in Eker rats, which carry a mutation in the Tsc2 gene,[1073] is a homologue of the human mesothelin gene, and these investigators[1074] developed an ELISA system for the detection of mesothelin in the sera of mesothelioma patients, using specific antibodies prepared in the same laboratory against the 31-kDa N-terminal fragment of *ERC*.

Robinson et al.[1058] reported elevated blood SMRP levels in 37 of 44 patients previously diagnosed with MM (sensitivity = 84%) in contrast to one of 22 lung cancers (histologic types not specified) and seven of 40 asbestos-exposed control patients (three of whom developed MM 15 to 19 months after the SMRP sample had been taken). Robinson et al. reported their results in terms of the optical absorbance at 420 nm; in a more recent (2006) publication from the same laboratory, Creaney et al.[1062] reported the results as nanomoles (nM), with a mean value of 15.33 ± 20.48 nM in the mesothelioma group, in

---

*PPV is defined lucidly by Gigerenzer[1068] as "the proportion of p among all those who test positive who actually do have the disease (or condition); i.e. the true positives divided by the total number who test positive"; validity is the extent to which a test measures what it is intended to measure; reliability is the extent to which a test produces the same result when it is carried out at different times and by others using the same methodology. High reliability is necessary but does not guarantee high validity, and vice versa; both are required for a high PPV, among other factors. The sensitivity of a test can be defined as the proportion of patients with the disease in question who return a positive test for that disease.

comparison to a level of 0.925 ± 0.831 nM for healthy controls. Hassan et al.[1063] recorded elevated serum mesothelin levels in 40 of 56 mesothelioma patients (71%) and in 14 of 21 patients with ovarian cancer (67%); their results were expressed as nanograms per liter (ng/L).

Nonetheless, although a sensitivity of 84% and a claimed specificity of 100% as recorded by Robinson et al.[1058] may seem impressive at first sight, these figures do not necessarily translate to a PPV of the same order.

Beyer et al.[1065] investigated SMRP levels in the serum of 409 apparently healthy individuals, 177 patients with nonmalignant disorders, and 500 cancer patients who included 88 with pleural mesothelioma. The 99th percentile level for the reference group was 1.5 nM/L, whereas the mean level for the 88 mesothelioma patients was 7.5 nM/L (95% CI, 2.8–12.1). The SMRP levels were increased in 52% of the MM patients and 5% of asbestos-exposed individuals.

In another series, Scherpereel et al.[1064] reported blood SMRP levels in 74 mesothelioma patients, 35 patients with carcinomas metastatic to the pleura, and 28 cases of benign pleural lesions associated with asbestos exposure (BPLAE). They found that the serum SMRP levels were significantly higher for epithelioid MMs than for biphasic or sarcomatoid MMs. They also found that the median value for patients with pleural MM was 2.05 ± 2.5 nM/L, in comparison to a level of 1.02 ± 1.79 nM/L for the metastatic carcinoma group—there is significant overlap between these two values in term of the standard deviations (SDs)—and in BPLAE cases the level was 0.55 ± 0.59 nM/L.

In 2007, Creaney et al.[804] also reported mesothelin levels in effusion fluids from 52 patients with pleural MM, in comparison to 56 patients with malignancies other than mesothelioma and 84 with benign pleural effusions. Creaney et al. found significantly greater concentrations of mesothelin in pleural fluid from the MM patients than in the other two groups, with a specificity of 98% and a sensitivity of 67% for the mesothelioma group in comparison to those with nonneoplastic effusions. In seven of 10 cases, the mesothelin levels were elevated before the diagnosis of MM was made (by 0.75–10 months); four of eight such cases had elevated mesothelin concentrations in the effusion fluid but not in the serum. The highest mesothelin levels were found in peritoneal fluid in patients with ovarian carcinoma (exponentiated mean of log transformed data = 73.7 ± 0.77 nM); there were significant differences in the corresponding mean mesothelin values in pleural effusion fluid for epithelial (46.9 ± 1.1 nM), biphasic (30.1 ± 0.8), and sarcomatoid (4.5 ± 1.38) MMs, and for the cases designated "cytology only" the mesothelin level in pleural fluid was 39.2 ± 0.96 nM. For the pleural sarcomatoid MMs, the mesothelin concentrations did not differ significantly from patients with nonmalignant effusions. The median survival for MM patients with high concentrations of mesothelin in effusion fluid was 14 months, versus 8 months for those with low mesothelin levels, probably reflecting MMs with an epithelial component as opposed to sarcomatoid mesotheliomas.

Therefore, we draw the following conclusion:

1. Although blood SMRP levels are elevated in most cases of mesothelioma, nonmesothelial cancers can also be associated with significantly elevated serum SMRP concentrations, including lung and, in particular, ovarian cancers.[1063,1075]
2. Epithelial mesotheliomas are associated with higher mesothelin levels in serum and effusion fluid than biphasic or sarcomatoid mesotheliomas.
3. The diagnosis of MM remains an essentially pathologic exercise that employs routine light microscopy of cytology and biopsy specimens and autopsy tissue on occasion, together with mucin histochemistry, immunohistochemistry, and, in some cases, transmission electron microscopy.
4. At present, investigation of serum SMRP levels cannot replace cytologic or biopsy diagnosis of MM, except perhaps in extraordinary circumstances (e.g., an elderly patient whose poor physical condition precludes biopsy procedures or for whom past biopsies have been nondiagnostic, but who has high serum SMRP levels, such as levels >15 nM/L).
5. At present, it seems difficult or impossible to compare the SMRP results obtained by different laboratories, because of methodologic differences.
6. High serum SMRP levels (for example >7.5 or >15 nm/L) probably have a greater predictive value as a marker of MM, whereas levels in the range of ~2.0 nM/L are more problematic, and the PPVs for different blood levels of SMRP have yet to be evaluated.
7. Use of serum SMRP levels as a screening test for patients at high risk of MM should be approached with awareness of the limitations of the test and its potential ethical ramifications: (a) any test will produce occasional false-positive results, with a requirement to investigate further, and such further investigations for mesothelioma are necessarily invasive, with the potential for resultant morbidity; (b) a false-positive result can generate unnecessary anguish in the patient and family concerning a cancer well known to be highly aggressive; and (c) screening procedures are most cogently justifiable when there is an effective intervention or treatment for the disorder so detected, but there is no consistently curative or definitive treatment for mesothelioma at the present time.
8. High mesothelin levels in effusion fluid may prove useful as an adjunct to cytodiagnosis of such fluids when ovarian carcinoma is not an issue.
9. Apart from a role as a screening procedure or as an adjunct to pathologic diagnosis, assays of serum SMRP

levels may find a role as an indicator of prognosis (with the exception of sarcomatoid MMs) and as a means to assess the progress of the disease or its response to treatment.

Serum Osteopontin Levels

The significance of serum osteopontin (OPN) levels as a marker for mesothelioma is more problematic and open to greater doubt than testing for serum SMRP concentrations. OPN is an acidic glycoprotein normally synthesized by osteoblasts and—like the angiopoietin-1 (ANG-1) also produced by osteoblasts—OPN acts as a "constraining factor"[1076] on hemopoietic stem cell proliferation in the bone marrow. Although elevated blood OPN levels have been recorded in patients with mesothelioma,[1066] elevated levels have also been recorded in a variety of other disorders that include carcinomas of the head and neck region[1077,1078] and cervix,[1077] as well as ovarian,[1079] gastric,[1080] and hepatocellular carcinomas[1081]; elevated levels have also been found in patients with inflammatory bowel disease.[1082] Therefore, it appears that serum OPN levels have poor specificity for a diagnosis of mesothelioma, but serum OPN assays may find a role in assessment of the extent and prognosis of mesothelioma and its response to treatment.

Chemical Analysis of Pleural Fluid and Pleural Neoplasms for Hyaluronic Acid

The concentration of hyaluronic acid in pleural fluid and pleural neoplasms has been evaluated to determine if it is helpful in making a diagnosis of mesothelioma. The results have been variable. Friman et al.[1083] found an increased concentration of hyaluronic acid in pleural fluid in three cases of mesothelioma. Arai et al.[1084] reported a hyaluronic acid concentration of 7 μg/mL in a case of diffuse mesothelioma, 14 ± 8.6 μg/mL in four cases of tuberculous pleurisy, and 9.43 ± 5.13 μg/mL in seven cases of cancerous pleurisy. Other investigators[1085–1087] found similar variable results of hyaluronic acid concentration in pleural fluid. An anecdotal case report also noted increased pleural fluid hyaluronic acid in a patient with mesothelioma.[1088]

In 1988, Pettersson et al.[1089] reported their evaluation of hyaluronic acid concentration in pleural fluid from 85 patients with pleural effusions, including 15 with MM, 32 with other types of neoplasms, 31 with nonmalignant inflammatory disease, and seven with congestive heart failure. Eleven of 15 (73%) patients with MM and seven of 31 (23%) with nonmalignant inflammatory conditions had pleural fluid hyaluronic acid concentrations greater than 100 mg/L, whereas all 32 patients with other types of cancers and the seven patients with congestive heart failure had hyaluronic acid concentrations less than 100 mg/L. The authors also evaluated the usefulness of pleural fluid CEA concentrations in differentiating MM from other types of cancer. Four of 15 (27%) patients with MM and 12 of 32 (38%) patients with other malignant neoplasms had CEA concentrations greater than 10 μg/L. The authors concluded that, in pleural effusions associated with a malignant tumor, a high hyaluronic acid concentration and low CEA concentration in the pleural fluid suggested the diagnosis of MM as opposed to other malignant neoplasms. Using a cutoff of 100 μg/mL, Atagi et al.[860] also found that pleural fluid hyaluronic acid levels were higher in patients with mesothelioma versus metastatic carcinoma, and that the combination of elevated hyaluronic acid and low CEA levels possibly supported the diagnosis of mesothelioma.

In a somewhat similar study, Hillerdal et al.[1090] determined the hyaluronic acid concentration in serum and pleural fluid in 78 consecutive patients with pleural effusions. In three of nine (33%) patients with MM and five of 42 (12%) patients with metastatic malignant neoplasms, pleural fluid hyaluronic acid concentration was greater than 100 mg/L. In addition, in two of 11 (18%) patients with cardiac disease, three of four (75%) patients with viral infection, one patient with a postinfectious effusion, and two of two (100%) patients with benign asbestos-induced effusion had pleural fluid hyaluronic acid concentrations greater than 100 mg/L. The serum hyaluronic acid concentrations were lower than those found in the pleural fluid, and there was no correlation between pleural fluid hyaluronic acid concentrations and serum hyaluronic acid levels. In contrast to the conclusion of Pettersson et al.,[1089] Hillerdal et al. concluded that a high concentration of hyaluronic acid in pleural fluid was not specific for MM and could be found in other malignant conditions and in benign diseases. They also concluded that a low pleural fluid hyaluronic acid concentration did not exclude the diagnosis of MM. Soderblom et al.[1091] also concluded that elevated hyaluronic acid levels could be found not only in mesothelioma but also in patients with benign pleural effusions, especially those with rheumatoid arthritis. They speculated that hyaluronic acid was related to proinflammatory cytokines.

In tissue specimens, Arai and colleagues[1084] found at least 0.10 mg of hyaluronic acid per gram of dry tissue in four cases of mesothelioma, but only 0.02 to 0.03 mg of hyaluronic acid per gram of dry tissue in two cases of carcinomatous pleural tissue and in pleural tissue from two patients with asbestosis. Chiu et al.[1092] isolated glycosaminoglycans from 21 mesotheliomas, 34 primary lung carcinomas, 12 carcinomas from other sites, and four soft tissue sarcomas. Hyaluronic acid was identified qualitatively in 20 of 21 mesotheliomas, approximately half of the lung carcinomas, and all of the soft tissue sarcomas. Quantitatively, hyaluronic acid constituted 45% of the total glycosaminoglycan in mesotheliomas and 28% of the total in carcinomas of the lung. The mean value of hyaluronic acid in mesotheliomas was significantly higher (0.74 mg/g) than lung adenocarcinomas (0.08 mg/g), but was not significantly higher than in soft tissue sarcomas (2.01 mg/g) or ovarian serous carcinomas (0.92 mg/g). They concluded that a hyaluronic concentration of greater than 0.4 mg/g dry tissue extract supported the diagnosis of mesothelioma when the alternative diagnosis was primary pulmonary adenocarcinoma.

Nakano et al.[1093] also studied glycosaminoglycan concentration in five pleural mesotheliomas and contrasted it to that seen in one pulmonary adenocarcinoma. The average total amount of glycosaminoglycan was 7.9 times higher in the mesotheliomas than in the pulmonary adenocarcinoma, and hyaluronic acid and chondroitin sulfate were the main types of glycosaminoglycans found. They also found an increase in hyaluronic acid and chondroitin sulfate in pleural fluid from two patients with mesothelioma. Iozzo[1094] reviewed the subject of proteoglycans and their role in neoplasia in 1985, having previously reported[1095] that tissue extracts of mesotheliomas contain large amounts of chondroitin sulfate.

Afify et al.[1096] evaluated archival paraffin-embedded cell blocks of serous fluids from 28 cases of reactive mesothelial cells, 14 cases of MM, 20 cases of metastatic ovarian carcinomas, 17 cases of metastatic breast carcinomas, 12 cases of metastatic lung adenocarcinoma. and 12 cases of metastatic gastrointestinal adenocarcinoma by means of immunohistochemical staining for hyaluronic acid using a biotinylated hyaluronic acid binding protein (HABP) and CD44S. All MMs and 93% (26 of 28) of benign mesothelial cells were positive for intracytoplasmic hyaluronic acid versus none of the adenocarcinomas. CD44S was expressed in 100% of mesothelial hyperplasia cases and 86% (12 of 14) of MMs, 70% (14 of 20) ovarian carcinomas, 29% (five of 17) of breast carcinomas, 25% (three of 12) of gastrointestinal adenocarcinomas, and 8% (one of 12) of lung adenocarcinomas. The authors concluded immunostaining for hyaluronic acid was a reliable marker that could distinguish between cells of mesothelial origin (reactive mesothelial cells and MM) and adenocarcinoma. The authors also concluded that immunostaining for CD44S could be useful with other stains in the differential diagnosis of adenocarcinoma and mesothelioma.

Thylen et al.[1097] in a multivariate analysis confirmed that an elevated concentration of hyaluronan in pleural fluid was an independent predictor of longer survival in older patients and in patients receiving therapy for mesothelioma.

In summary, most mesotheliomas show reactivity for hyaluronic acid and manifest elevated concentrations of hyaluronic acid in pleural fluid, but the findings are neither specific nor sensitive enough to be used in a diagnostic setting.

Clinicopathologic Correlations

Patients with pleural mesothelioma usually present with nonspecific signs and symptoms consisting of chest pain, dyspnea on exertion, cough, weight loss, and a unilateral pleural effusion. Physical examination is usually nonspecific, but characteristically reveals dullness to percussion on the involved side and distant breath sounds by auscultation.

Approximately 10% to 20% of patients diagnosed with mesothelioma have "B" symptoms consisting of fever, night sweats, weight loss, and anorexia. About 20% to 30% of patients have anemia, typically a microcytic anemia. About 20% to 30% develop thrombocytosis, thought to be mediated by interleukin-6. We have seen four cases of individuals who have presented with spontaneous thrombosis of the subclavian vein with elevated platelet counts, the highest being over 1 million platelets per microliter, and other cases where a diagnosis of mesothelioma has been followed by thrombotic or thromboembolic complications related to thrombocytosis, such as cerebral infarction.

It is currently thought that the systemic manifestations of MM, including fever, cachexia, and thrombocytosis, may be related to the production of interleukin-6 by malignant cells.[1098]

Spread and Staging of Malignant Mesothelioma

The clinical course of MM is usually dominated by the primary tumor and its locoregional spread. Accordingly, pleural mesotheliomas typically compress and invade lung, mediastinum, and chest wall structures. On occasion, the neoplasm and its associated effusion may be so massive that it constitutes a tension effusion with tumor, with displacement of mediastinal structures to the contralateral side.[1099] Because mesothelioma can produce contraction of the affected hemithorax (Fig. 43.192), it can also displace mediastinal structures toward itself. Invasion of the mediastinum and pericardium may be complicated by the development of hemopericardium with tamponade, or by encasement of the great vessels or esophagus, sometimes with the development of dysphagia. Invasion of the chest wall is frequent,[211,190] especially along needle tracks, biopsy sites, or drainage wounds (Fig. 43.193),[211,503,716] with extension through the chest wall into the subcutaneous plane, sometimes complicated by ulceration.

Local invasion into lung parenchyma is also common, and when this occurs, unusual patterns of infiltration can develop, including a desquamative interstitial pneumonia (DIP)-like appearance whereby the invasive epithelial mesothelioma is accompanied by innumerable alveolar macrophages[1100] (Fig. 43.194); lepidic spread along preexisting alveolar walls can also occur, producing histologic

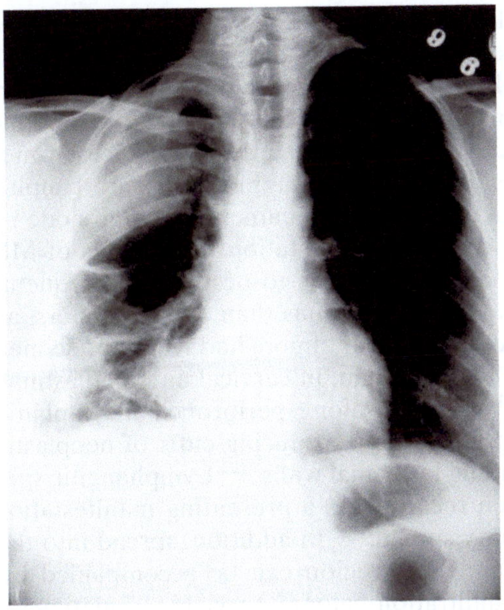

FIGURE 43.192. Right-sided pleural malignant mesothelioma in a young woman. Chest radiograph following aspiration of a massive pleural effusion. This was the first "environmental" mesothelioma from Wittenoom. The patient was 28 years old at the time of her presentation in 1975, with an abrupt onset of right pleuritic chest pain in the middle of the night. She had given birth to her third child a few weeks earlier and at first her pleural effusion was thought to be explicable by pulmonary thromboembolism. A pleural biopsy revealed a biphasic malignant mesothelioma with heterologous osseous differentiation (see Fig. 43.50). The patient had lived at Wittenoom for the first 12 years of her life, where her father was a miner (and subsequently developed asbestosis). Mine tailings were used to top-dress the lawn in the backyard of the family residence, and the patient frequently played in the tailings, looking for "fool's gold." She died from her mesothelioma about 6 months after presentation.

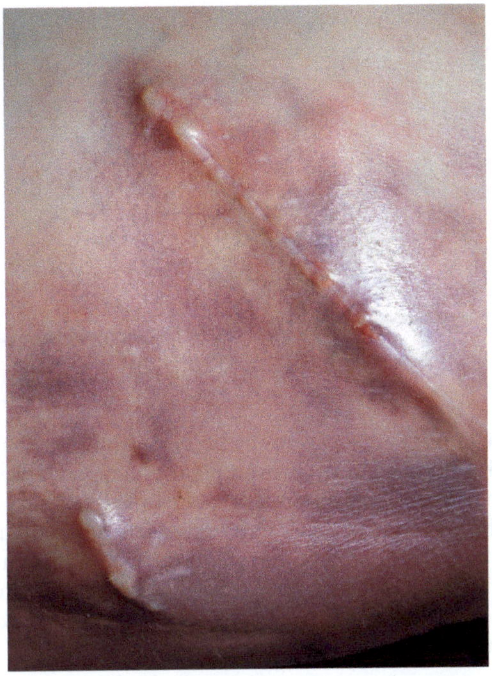

FIGURE 43.193. Pleural malignant mesothelioma with direct invasion into a thoracotomy scar and extension into the skin, which displays postmortem lividity. A similar pattern of chest wall invasion is also evident through the nearby drainage site. (Figure 4-5 from Churg A, Cagle PT, Roggli VL. Tumors of the Serosal Membranes, AFIP Atlas of Tumor Pathology, Fourth Series, American Registry of Pathology, Washington, DC 2006.)

mimicry of a bronchioloalveolar carcinoma.[1100,1101] When sarcomatoid and desmoplastic MMs invade into lung, they can infiltrate into and along the interstitium, and they can also erupt into alveolar spaces, producing histologic mimicry of either organizing pneumonia[37] or an intrapulmonary epithelioid hemangioendothelioma.[1100] Spread to the contralateral pleura or lung is also common in late-stage disease.[211]

Extension of mesothelioma through the diaphragm ("gravitational spread") can lead to seeding of the mesothelioma into the peritoneal cavity, complicated by the development of ascites[211] (Fig. 43.195). For right-sided pleural mesotheliomas, extension through the diaphragm may be accompanied by direct invasion into the liver. In some cases, ascites as a consequence of transdiaphragmatic spread dominates the clinical picture, and identification of the mesothelioma by cytologic examination of ascitic fluid or biopsy tissue from the abdomen can lead to misdiagnosis of the mesothelioma as a primary peritoneal lesion. Therefore, before diagnosis of a mesothelioma as a primary mesothelioma of the peritoneum (or pericardium or tunica vaginalis testis), we routinely recommend exclusion of an underlying pleural mesothelioma on the basis of the clinical and radiologic findings,

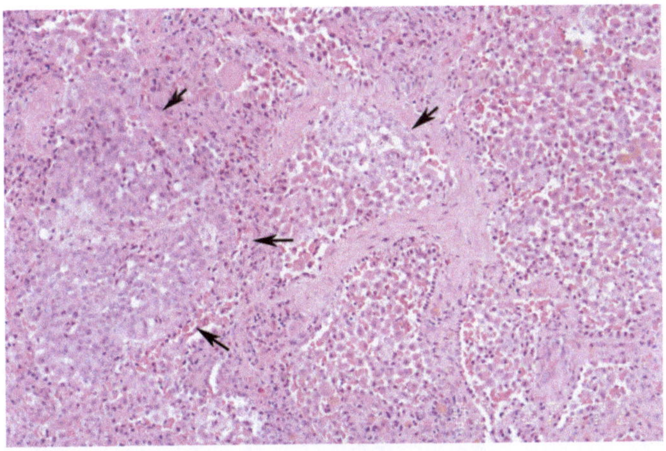

FIGURE 43.194. Invasion into lung parenchyma by a pleural malignant mesothelioma of epithelial type. The mesothelioma (arrows) extends into alveolar spaces where it blends with numerous alveolar macrophages, creating a histologic resemblance to desquamative interstitial pneumonia.

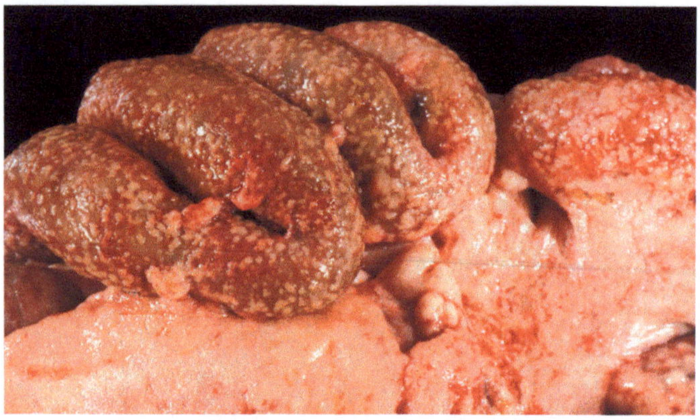

FIGURE 43.195. Transdiaphragmatic extension into the peritoneal cavity from a biopsy-proven pleural malignant mesothelioma. Apart from symptoms referable to the primary pleural tumor, the patient suffered from intractable ascites during the final few months of his life, as a consequence of this pattern of spread. Innumerable serosal nodular deposits of tumor are evident over the loops of small intestine, accompanied by a mesenteric "cake" of metastatic mesothelioma.

taking into account the fact that about 90% of all mesotheliomas arise in the pleura.[211] For example, a diagnosis of MM in one of our cases was established on an omental biopsy taken at an exploratory laparotomy for ascites. The primary pleural tumor was recognized in retrospect from abnormalities in the chest radiographs—contraction of one hemithorax plus a pleural effusion on the same side—which antedated the abdominal manifestations.[211] In another case, the diagnosis of mesothelioma was established from a resected vermiform appendix, in a patient suspected on radiologic grounds to have a pleural mesothelioma.[211]

In contrast to spread of mesothelioma from the pleura to the peritoneum, the reverse direction of spread is distinctly uncommon and seems to have occurred in only two cases accessioned into the Australian Mesothelioma Surveillance Program, as assessed from the clinical findings and the distribution of tumor at autopsy.[211]

Local invasion into and along lymphatic channels is often encountered (especially in pleuropneumonectomy specimens), accompanied in some instances by metastatic deposits in regional and more distant lymph nodes. Sussman and Rosai[746] documented lymph node metastasis as the initial manifestation in six cases of MM. This pattern of spread seems to occur more frequently with peritoneal mesotheliomas than pleural tumors, and four of the five peritoneal tumors had lymph node metastases above the diaphragm, in cervical and mediastinal lymph nodes.[746] Invasion along peribronchial lymphatic channels can also occur, producing cuffs of neoplastic tissue surrounding bronchial walls.[1102] Lymphangitic spread has also been recorded as a presenting manifestation,[1103] as has miliary spread.[1104] In addition, spread into the mediastinal and hilar region can be accompanied by retrograde infiltration along bronchi—sometimes within bronchial lymphatic vessels—with eruption of the tumor into the bronchial lumen, accounting for rare cases where mesothelioma is sampled by endoscopic bronchial biopsies (Fig. 43.196).

Autopsy studies have also shown that hematogenous metastases from mesothelioma often develop in sites such as lung, liver, adrenal glands, bone marrow, brain, and even kidney.[211] In this regard, such hematogenous spread can be encountered in three main circumstances:

1. *At autopsy:* In general, distant metastatic deposits from mesothelioma remain silent during life, so clinical evidence of extrathoracic spread is uncommon (about 10%).[190]

2. *Clinically apparent metastases in cases with antecedent biopsy-proven MM:* Such metastases include cerebral[1105–1111] and cutaneous[1112,1113] metastases. Brain metastases in three cases of mesothelioma in our files produced prominent clinical manifestations. In fact, MM has the capacity to metastasize to virtually any anatomic

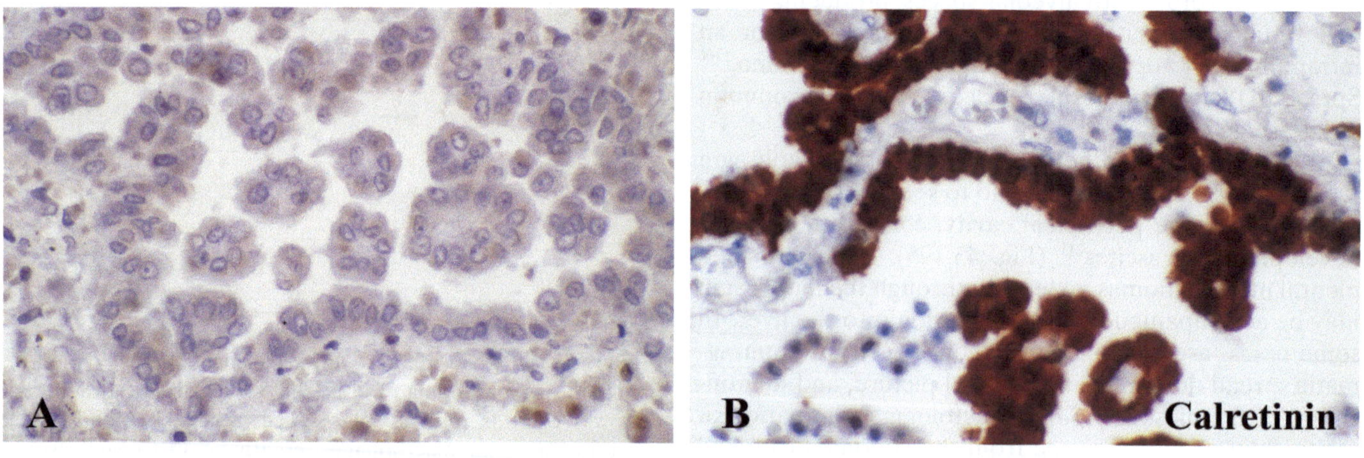

FIGURE 43.196. This transbronchial biopsy shows involvement by an epithelial neoplasm **(A)** that shows nuclear and cytoplasmic immunostaining for calretinin **(B)** and no immunostaining for CEA or TTF-1.

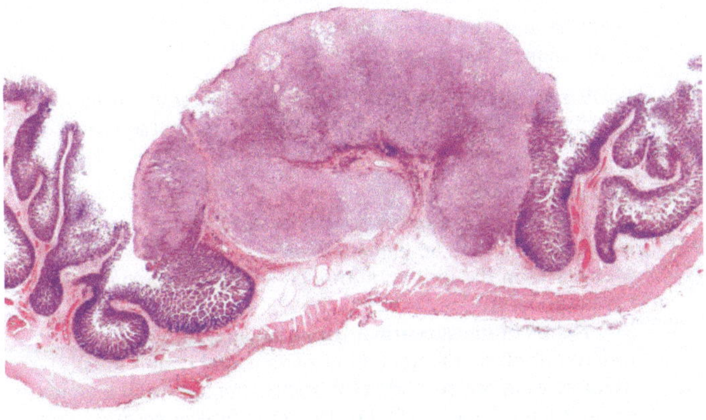

FIGURE 43.197. Metastasis of pleural malignant mesothelioma to small intestine. The patient was a 51-year-old man with a history of antecedent minor exposure to asbestos and who was found to have a pleural mass lesion. Fine-needle aspiration cytology and a core biopsy from the affected pleura yielded a diagnosis of highly probable to near-definite mesothelioma of epithelial type. About 2 years later, he developed intestinal obstruction and was found at laparotomy to have tumor nodules in the small intestine. Pathologic examination of the resected segment of small bowel revealed mucosal/submucosal deposits of metastatic mesothelioma, as shown in this figure. There is no evidence of extension into the muscularis externa and the serosa is unaffected.

site. Unusual other sites where metastases have been recorded on rare occasions include the orbit,[1114] tongue,[1115] intestine (Fig. 43.197), thyroid,[898,1116] and prostate,[1116] among others. As mentioned elsewhere in this chapter, desmoplastic mesotheliomas appear to have a propensity for metastasis to bone,[37,503,830] where they can be confused with primary fibroblastoid bone tumors.

3. *Rarely, metastases as the presenting manifestation of an underlying and hitherto undetected MM.*

Brenner et al.[85] reviewed 123 patients with pleural mesothelioma and found that the tumor was apparently confined to the thorax in all but nine at the time of diagnosis, but spread to the peritoneum or distant sites developed later in 33 of the remaining 114 patients (29%). "Distant" metastases were also recorded in 12 of 16 autopsy cases of pleural mesothelioma reported by Adams and Unni,[500] whereas Whitaker[495] recorded them in 45% of cases and Roberts[1117] in 47%. Huncharek and Muscat[1118] detected lymph node deposits in 19 of 42 autopsy cases (45%), whereas "distant" metastases were found in 32 cases (76%). Hulks et al.[1119] found autopsy evidence of metastatic disease in lymph nodes and distant sites on either side of the diaphragm, in 32 of 40 pleural MM patients from Western Glasgow (80%). In the last two series,[1118,1119] the histologic type of the mesothelioma did not appear to influence either the frequency of metastases or their distribution. In a later autopsy study of 22 cases of mesothelioma, King et al.[1120] found metastases in multiple sites that included omentum, stomach, intestine, mesentery, adrenal glands, ovary, pancreas, kidneys, liver, spleen, and vertebrae. Henderson et al.[211] recorded similar observations (Table 43.22), as did Hammar[289] in a tabular analysis of 11 different autopsy studies,[83,500,1117–1119,1121–1126] across which 58% of the cases had metastatic disease. Malignant mesothelioma has also been reported in other more unusual metastatic sites such as scalp, fingers, tonsil, and gluteal muscle.

TABLE 43.22. Spread of pleural malignant mesothelioma as found in 143 autopsy cases

Anatomic pattern of spread	Number of cases	Percentage
Direct/intrathoracic spread		
Contralateral pleura/lung	73	51
Pericardium	74	52
Myocardium/endocardium	17	12
Mediastinal/brachial great vessels	17	12
Esophagus	9	6
Transdiaphragmatic spread into peritoneal cavity	63	44
Lymph nodes: cervical, mediastinal, hilar, retroperitoneal	67	47
Distant metastases		
Axial bone marrow: sternum, ribs, vertebrae	23	16
Liver	36	25
Spleen	6	4
Kidney	19	13
Adrenal gland	20	14
Pancreas	4	3
Central nervous system: meninges, brain, spinal cord	5	4
Skin and subcutis	5	4
Other (muscle, thyroid, cecum)	11	8
Total with distant metastases	69	48

Source: Modified from Henderson DW, Shilkin KB, Whitaker D, Attwood HD, Constance TJ, Steele RH, Leppard PJ, The pathology of malignant mesothelioma, including immunohistology and ultrastructure. In: Henderson DW, Shilkin KB, Langlois SLeP, Whitaker D, eds. Malignant mesothelioma, pp. 69–139. Copyright 1992 by Hemisphere. Reproduced with permission of Informa Healthcare Books via Copyright Clearance Center.

TABLE 43.23. Staging of mesothelioma

DEFINITION OF TNM

IMIG Staging System for Diffuse Malignant Pleural Mesothelioma

Primary Tumor (T)

TX Primary tumor cannot be assessed
T0 No evidence of primary tumor
T1 Tumor involves ipsilateral parietal pleura, with or without focal involvement of visceral pleura
T1a Tumor involves ipsilateral parietal (mediastinal, diaphragmatic) pleura. No involvement of the visceral pleura
T1b Tumor involves ipsilateral parietal (mediastinal, diaphragmatic) pleura, with focal involvement of the visceral pleura
T2 Tumor involves any of the ipsilateral pleural surfaces with at least one of the following:
—confluent visceral pleural tumor (including fissure)
—invasion of diaphragmatic muscle
—invasion of lung parenchyma
T3* Tumor involves any of the ipsilateral pleural surfaces, with at least one of the following:
—invasion of the endothoracic fascia
—invasion into mediastinal fat
—solitary focus of tumor invading the soft tissues of the chest wall
—non-transmural involvement of the pericardium
T4** Tumor involves any of the ipsilateral pleural surfaces, with at least one of the following:
—diffuse or multifocal invasion of soft tissues of the chest wall
—any involvement of rib
—invasion through the diaphragm to the peritoneum
—invasion of any mediastinal organ(s)
—direct extension to the contralateral pleura
—invasion into the spine
—extension to the internal surface of the pericardium
—percardial effusion with positive cytology
—invasion of the myocardium
—invasion of the brachial plexus

*T3 describes locally advanced but potentially resectable tumor
**T4 describes locally advanced, technically unresectable tumor

Regional Lymph Nodes (N)

NX Regional lymph nodes cannot be assessed
N0 No regional lymph node metastases
N1 Metastases in the ipsilateral bronchopulmonary and/or hilar lymph node(s)
N2 Metastases in the subcarinal lymph node(s) and/or the ipsilateral internal mammary or mediastinal lymph node(s)
N3 Metastases in the contralateral mediastinal, internal mammary, or hilar lymph node(s) and/or the ipsilateral or contralateral supraclavicular or scalene lymph node(s)

Distant Metastasis (M)

MX Distant metastases cannot be assessed
M0 No distant metastasis
M1 Distant metastasis

STAGE GROUPING			
Stage I	T1	N0	M0
Stage IA	T1a	N0	M0
Stage IB	T1b	N0	M0
Stage II	T2	N0	M0
Stage III	T1, T2	N1	M0
	T1, T2	N2	M0
	T3	N0, N1, N2	M0
Stage IV	T4	Any N	M0
	Any T	N3	M0
	Any T	Any N	M1

Source: Used with the permission of the American Joint Committee on Cancer (AJCC), Chicago, Illinois. The original source for this material is the AJCC Cancer Staging Manual, Sixth Edition (2002) published by Springer Science and Business Media, LLC, www.springer.com.

Staging of Pleural Malignant Mesothelioma

The Butchart staging system[1127] for pleural MM has now been superseded by the tumor, node, metastases (TNM) staging system as developed by the International Mesothelioma Interest Group (IMIG)[37,1128] and as essentially set forth in the Cancer Staging Handbook from the American Joint Committee on Cancer (AJCC) (Table 43.23).[1116]

As previously stated, malignant pleural mesotheliomas not infrequently show diffuse spread to lung parenchyma when evaluated at autopsy. Radiographic diffuse metastases to lung parenchyma by pleural mesothelioma may show no abnormalities or a diffuse reticulonodular or variably nodular pattern. Ohishi et al.[1129] reported identifying mesothelial metastases by transbronchial biopsy. We have seen several cases of this phenomenon (Fig. 43.196).

Prognosis of Malignant Mesothelioma

Chailleux et al.[1130] evaluated 167 cases of pleural MM diagnosed between 1955 and 1985 in the St. Nazaire region of France; 135 mesotheliomas were epithelial, 25 biphasic, and seven sarcomatous; 131 (78%) were related to occupational exposure to asbestos. Eighty-eight patients were treated, including 14 by pleurectomy, 25 by partial pleurectomy, four by pleuropneumonectomy, 42 with chemotherapy (consisting of cisplatin alone, cisplastin, adriamycin and bleomycin, cyclophosphamide alone, and other combinations), 20 with talc pleurodesis and 1 with radiation plus chemotherapy. Survival from first symptoms was 54% at 1 year and 22% at 2 years with a median of 11 months. Survival from pathologic diagnosis was 39% at 1 year and 14% at 2 years with a median of 10 months. No patient was alive 4 years after diagnosis. Patients treated by chemotherapy, surgery, or talc poudrage had a longer survival, but there was no indication that one form of therapy was superior to another. One woman treated with cisplatin had a 15-month complete remission; no partial remissions were observed with chemotherapy. The histologic type of mesothelioma and a history of asbestos exposure had no predictive survival value. Patients younger than 60 years of age when the mesothelioma was diagnosed lived longer than those 60 years or older.

Antman et al.[1131] evaluated 180 patients with MM identified between 1965 and 1985, of which 136 were pleural, 37 peritoneal, five pericardial, and two testicular in origin. The median survival for those patients with pleural mesothelioma was 14 to 15 months. There was a significantly increased survival for those patients with a performance status between 0 and 1 (median, 31–32 months) versus those with a performance status >1 (median survival, 7 months), for those with epithelial histology (median survival, 17 months) versus sarcomatous histology (median survival, 7 months), for those with an absence of chest pain (median survival, 24 months) versus those with chest pain (median survival, 16 months), and those with an interval >6 months from the onset of symptoms (median survival, 16 months) versus those with an interval of ≤6 months from the onset of symptoms (median survival, 13 months), and possibly a better survival for those patients treated with chemotherapy or pleuropneumonectomy.

Alberts et al.[1132] evaluated survival rates and prognostic factors in 262 patients diagnosed between 1965 and 1985 with pleural MM who were treated with chemotherapy only, radiotherapy only, radiotherapy and chemotherapy, or with decortication combined with chemotherapy and radiotherapy. The median survival for all patients from the time of diagnosis was 9.6 months, which was the same for all treatment groups. In a univariate analysis, favorable prognostic factors included good performance status, duration of symptoms >6 months at the time of diagnosis, early stage of disease, white race, and female gender. In a multivariate analysis, good performance status, white race, duration of symptoms, and stage of disease were significant favorable prognostic factors. The authors found that the stepwise addition of treatment modalities did not increase survival.

Ruffie et al.[1126] performed a retrospective study of 332 patients diagnosed with pleural MM between 1965 and 1984. The median survival was 9 months. Using univariate analysis, three factors were found to have a significant effect on survival: (1) disease stage: stage 1, median survival 16.6 months, versus stage IV, 1.4 months; (2) weight loss: no weight loss, median survival, 10.5 months, versus weight loss, median survival, 4.8 months; and (3) histologic type: epithelial or mixed median survival of 9.9 and 9.2 months, respectively, versus sarcomatous median survival of 5.2 months. The authors found there were no drastic differences in survival among groups of patients subjected to different therapeutic measures. Radical surgery and radiotherapy were found to be ineffective; there was a low response rate to chemotherapeutic agents.

Harvey et al.[1133] also performed a retrospective analysis on 94 patients with pleural MM treated at one institution between 1965 and 1988. Group I patients ($n = 76$) received supportive care only, including pleurodesis as needed. Group II patients ($n = 9$) were managed with debulking procedures including decortication and pleurectomy. Group III patients ($n = 7$) were treated by extrapleural pneumonectomy. Median survival in group I patients was 231 days. Four patients in group I survived more than 2 years, and one patient who was treated with chemotherapy and tangential field external beam irradiation survived more than 5 years. Group II patients had a median survival of 360 days, and none were alive at the end of 2 years. Four of seven group III patients expired within 6 months after treatment, although one patient died 7 years after therapy and one 36-year-old man was alive 8 years after diagnosis. The authors concluded that selected patients (seven young patients) benefit from radical surgery and that debulking may also extend survival.

Ribak and Selikoff[1134] studied the clinical course of 457 consecutive fatal cases of pleural and peritoneal MM that occurred among 17,800 asbestos insulation workers observed prospectively from January 1967 to January 1987. In the pleural mesotheliomas, mean survival time was 11.4 months and median survival time 10 months. The mean survival time in peritoneal mesothelioma was 7.4 months. The median survival time from diagnosis to death for patients with pleural mesotheliomas was 5 months and for peritoneal mesothelioma 2 months. The authors found no differences for survival time between various treatment modalities or between treated and untreated patients. The authors concluded that survival time in MM was short, most patients die within 1 year from the onset of symptoms, and no effective therapy for MM was available.

Tammilehto[1135] prospectively studied 98 patients with histologically proven MM, 93 pleural and five peritoneal, diagnosed between 1981 and 1990. Treatment consisted of surgery ($n = 15$); surgery and chemotherapy ($n = 11$); surgery and radiotherapy ($n = 14$); surgery, chemotherapy, and radiotherapy ($n = 28$); chemotherapy ($n = 3$); chemotherapy and radiotherapy ($n = 9$); radiotherapy ($n = 8$); and no treatment ($n = 10$). The median survival for all 98 patients calculated from the date of histologic diagnosis was 9 months with a range of 0 to 81 months. Eighteen patients were alive 2 years after diagnosis and two patients 5 years after diagnosis. By univariate analysis, good prognostic factors included age ≤65 years (11 months median survival versus 6 months median survival for those >65), female gender (13 months median survival versus 8 months for males), epithelial histology (median survival 14 months versus 2 to 5 months for sarcomatous histology), performance status WHO ≤1 (13 months median survival versus 3 months for WHO >1), stage I to IIA (11.5 months versus 5 months for stage IIB, III, and IV), and a diagnostic delay of more than 6 months from first symptom to histologic diagnosis (14.5 months median survival versus 8 months for diagnostic delay of ≤6 months). Low S-phase fraction was associated with a better survival (16 months median survival) than a high S-phase fraction (median survival of 8 months), although DNA ploidy had no effect. Lung tissue fiber content of $<10^6$ fibers per gram of dry lung tissue was associated with a median survival of 26 months whereas a concentration $\geq 10^6$ fibers per gram of dry lung tissue showed a median survival of 13 months. Factors by multivariate analysis that were prognostically favorable included good performance status (WHO diagnostic delay of more than 6 months, epithelial histology, and clinical stage I or IIA). Although the patients who were treated with surgery, chemotherapy, or irradiation appeared to survive longer, this apparent increased survival was not significant when other factors were considered.

Sridhar et al.[1136] evaluated survival rates and prognostic factors in 49 patients with MM diagnosed between 1977 and 1991. The male-to-female ratio for patients with mesothelioma was 4:1, and the patients ranged in age between 36 and 77 years with a mean and median of 58 years. Asbestos exposure was identified in 75% of patients in whom a history was available. Most patients presented with Butchart stage 1 to 2 disease. Thirty-three patients were treated with a variety of combinations of chemotherapeutic agents, 14 were treated by various surgical modalities, and 10 patients received some type of radiation therapy. The median time from first symptom to diagnosis was 3 months. The median survival for pleural mesotheliomas was 13 months, and 15 months for peritoneal mesotheliomas from the onset of first symptom. Survival was longer in patients with earlier stage disease, a good performance status, a longer duration of symptoms, an absence of pain, and those who were treated with combined surgery and chemotherapy.

Pistolesi and Rusthoven[113] reviewed pleural MM, including current management and new therapeutic options. They stated that the stage of the disease was but one of the known variables that might influence survival. Two prognostic scoring systems were stated to have been developed for evaluating pleural MM on data collected from patients entered into large cooperative trials. Multivariate Cox analysis of a variety of variables (performance status, chest pain, dyspnea, platelet count greater than 400,000 per microliter, weight loss, serum lactate dehydrogenase level greater than 500 IU/L, pleural involvement, low hemoglobin level, high white blood cell count, and age greater than 75) demonstrated that pleural involvement, lactate dehydrogenase greater than 500 IU/L, poor performance status, chest pain, platelet count greater than 400,000 per microliter, nonepithelial histology, and age greater than 75 were independent predictors of reduced survival. Performance status was stated to have produced the most significant prognostic split. Six distinct prognostic subgroups were identified, with survival times ranging from 1.4 to 13.9 months. The best survival time was in patients less than 49 years of age with a performance status of 0 and a hemoglobin of 14.6 g/dL. The worst survival time was in patients with a performance status of 1 or 2 and a white blood cell count of greater than 15,600 per microliter. See Box 43.9 for a summary of prognostic factors.

Curran et al., of the European Organization for Research and Treatment of Cancer (EORTC)[1137] evaluated 13 factors via Cox proportional hazard regression model. Poor prognosis was stated to have been associated with a poor performance status, a high white blood cell count, a probable/possible histologic diagnosis of mesothelioma, male gender, and sarcomatoid histologic subtype. The EORTC classified patients into two prognostic groups: a good prognostic group (1-year survival of 40% having two or fewer poor prognostic factors) and a poor prognostic group (1-year survival of 12% having three or more poor prognostic factors).

Box 43.9. Prognostic Factors
(Expected Survival: 1.4 to 13.9 Months)

Independent predictors of reduced survival
(3 or more of the following)
Age 75 or older
Performance status 1 or 2
Nonepithelial histology or sarcomatoid subtype
Pleural involvement
Chest pain
Platelet count greater than 400,000 per microliter
WBC greater than 15,600 per microliter
Lactate dehydrogenase greater than 500 IU/L
Independent predictors of increased survival
Age 49 or younger
Performance status of 0
Hemoglobin of 14.6 g/dL

Among treatment modalities, radiation was stated to have been shown to have palliative benefit in reducing pain and symptoms of dyspnea. Surgical pleurodesis was stated to have reduced symptoms associated with recurrent or persistent pleural effusions. Chemotherapy was stated to have demonstrated palliative benefits in overall quality of life. Pistolesi and Rusthoven[113] concluded that treatment of pleural MM with more than palliative intent remained inadequate at all stages of presentation. Surgery, as a single modality, was stated to have failed to improve survival. Chemotherapy was stated to have generally failed to significantly impact survival.

Pistolesi and Rusthoven[113] discussed three procedures that are used in surgical management of pleural MM, including thoracoscopy with pleurodesis, pleurectomy/decortication, and extrapleural pneumonectomy. Thoracoscopy was stated to be useful not only for obtaining tissue for a diagnosis, but also for palliating recurrent symptomatic pleural effusions. Talc was stated to be the least expensive and could be administered via thoracoscope or instilled as a slurry through a chest tube. The authors stated that although often attempted with curative intent, neither extrapleural pneumonectomy nor pleurectomy/decortication appeared to offer a significant improvement in survival. The authors cited the Brigham and Women's Hospital Tri-Modality therapy. Those who survived surgery achieved a 2-year and 5-year survival rate of 38% and 15%, respectively.

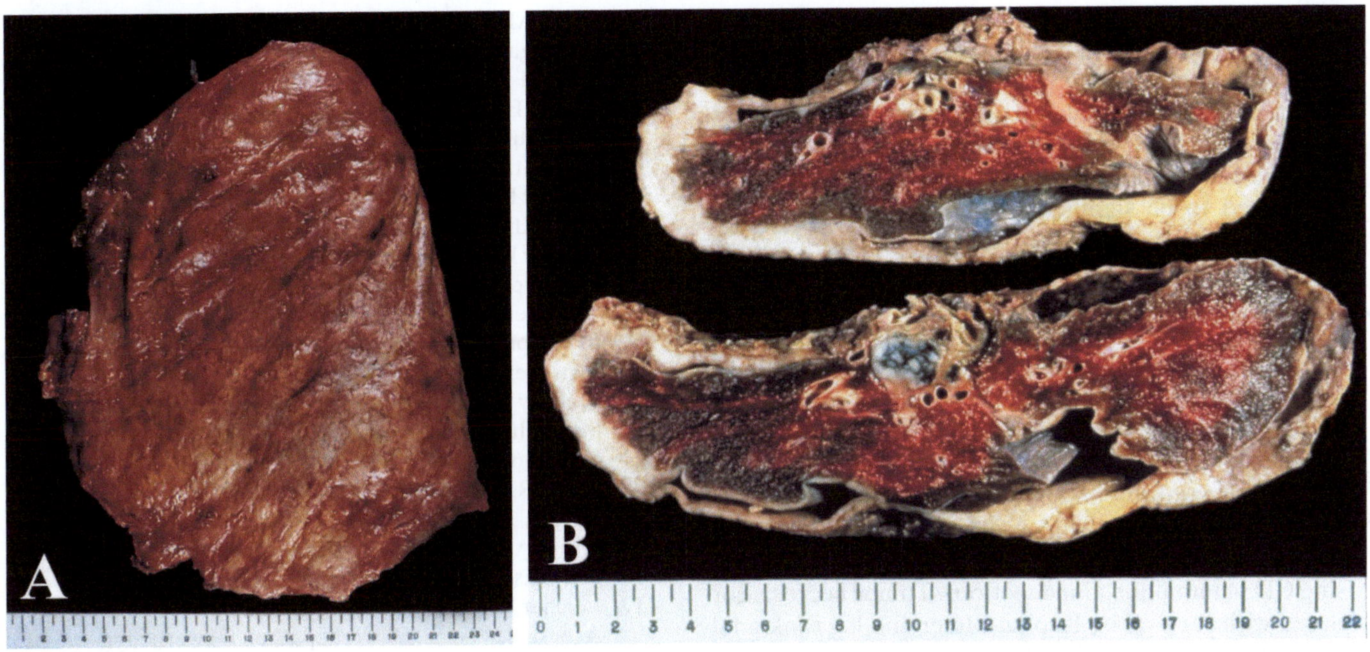

FIGURE 43.198. **(A)** Pleuropneumonectomy specimen resected from a patient with stage 1 epithelial mesothelioma. **(B)** Two cross-sectioned portions of lung and pleura are shown. Note the lack of complete encasement of the lung. Also note the whitish tissue within the hilar lymph node; this represents metastatic mesothelioma.

Reviews of radiation therapy were stated by Pistolesi and Rusthoven[113] to show no suggestion of a clear survival benefit for extensive radiation therapy. They stated that a report from the Joint Center for Radiation Therapy in Boston suggested a minimum effective dose of 40 Gy in order to achieve palliation.

With respect to chemotherapy, Pistolesi and Rusthoven[113] stated that most single agents that have been tested in malignant pleural mesothelioma have had response rates less than 20%, and survival benefit for single-agent chemotherapy has not been suggested in a single cohort study. A common combination of chemotherapy agents used at the present time is pemetrexed (Alimta®) and cisplatin. A response rate of about 42% has been reported.[113] Pistolesi and Rusthoven also discussed novel therapies for the treatment of mesothelioma. At this point in time, it is difficult to know whether these will be of any significance.

A more recent study from the Sugarbaker International Mesothelioma Group[1138] found a 5-year survival rate of 55% of those patients with anatomic stage 1 disease and epithelial histology. A typical pleuropneumonectomy specimen in shown in Figure 43.198. Note the extent of tumor and the rind of tumor that encases the lung. Also note that, in areas, the visceral and parietal pleura are not fused. Also note that in this case there is metastatic tumor in a hilar lymph node.

Takagi et al.[1139] reported on the surgical approach to diffuse pleural MM in Japan. They evaluated 189 surgical cases of diffuse MM between 1987 and 1996. The patients ranged between 18 and 80 years old and 154 were males, 33 were females and 2 were unspecified; 104 patients had an epithelial histology, 29 had a sarcomatous histology, and 46 had a biphasic histology. Pleuropneumonectomy was performed on 116 cases (61%) and limited resection was performed in 73 cases (39%). The goal of radical pleuropneumonectomy was stated to be radical resection of the tumor, which often required resection of adjacent structures. The tumor was stated to have been completely removed macroscopically in 84 cases (72%) of the 116 patients who underwent pleuropneumonectomy. Among those who had an epithelial mesothelioma that was completely removed by pleuropneumonectomy, the tumor recurred postoperatively in 43% of patients. Perioperative adjuvant therapy was performed in 83 of 116 patients who underwent pleuropneumonectomy. The 2-year and 5-year survival rates of those who underwent pleuropneumonectomy was 29.7% and 9.1%, respectively. The perioperative mortality was 6%.

Pass et al.[1140] analyzed the impact of preoperative and post-resection solid tumor volumes on the outcomes in 47 of 48 consecutive patients undergoing resection for pleural MM who were treated prospectively and randomized to photodynamic therapy or no photodynamic therapy. Forty-eight patients with pleural MM had cytoreductive debulking to 5 mm or less residual tumor by extrapleural pneumonectomy (n = 25) or pleurectomy/decortication (n = 23). Three-dimensional CT reconstructions of pre-resection and post-resection solid tumor were prospectively performed and the disease was staged postoperatively according to the new IMIG/AJCC staging. Median survival for all patients was 14.4 months (extrapleural pneumonectomy 11 months; pleurectomy/decortication 22 months). Median survival for preoperative volume less than 100cc was 22 months versus 11 months if 100cc or greater. Median survival for postoperative volume less than 9cc was 25 months versus 9 months if there were 9cc or greater. Tumor volumes associated with negative nodes were stated to be significantly smaller than those with positive nodes. The authors concluded that pre-resection tumor volume was representative of T status in pleural MM and could predict overall progression-free survival as well as postoperative stage. Large volumes were associated with nodal spread and post-resection residual tumor burden could predict outcome.

Edwards et al.[1141] evaluated the significance of tumor necrosis in cases of MM. They reviewed 171 routine formalin-fixed, paraffin-embedded, H&E-stained tumor sections by two independent observers. Angiogenesis was stated to have been assessed by microvessel count (MVC) using CD34 immunostained sections. Tumor necrosis correlated with survival by Kaplan-Meier and log rank analysis. Stepwise multivariate Cox models were used to compare tumor necrosis with angiogenesis and establish prognostic factors and prognostic scoring systems. Tumor necrosis was stated to have been identified in 39 cases (22.8%) and correlated with low hemoglobin level, thrombocytosis, and high microvessel counts, and was a poor prognostic factor in univariate analysis. Patients with tumor necrosis had a median survival of 5.3 months versus 8.3 months in cases without necrosis. Independent indicators of poor prognosis in multivariate analysis were nonepithelioid cell type, poor performance status, and increasing microvessel counts, but not tumor necrosis. Tumor necrosis contributed independently to prognosis according to the EORTC and to the Cancer and Leukemia Group B prognostic groups. Tumor necrosis correlated with angiogenesis and was stated to be a poor prognostic factor in MM.

References

1. Hillerdal G. Malignant mesothelioma: review of 4710 published cases. Br J Dis Chest 1983;77:321–343.
2. Hillerdal G. Mesothelioma: cases associated with non-occupational and low dose exposures. Occup Environ Med 1999;56:505–513.
3. Aisner J, Wiernick PH. Malignant mesothelioma. Current status and future prospects. Chest 1978;74:438–443.
4. Chahinian AP. Malignant mesothelioma. In: Holland JF, Frei E III, eds. Cancer medicine. Philadelphia: Lea & Febiger, 1982:1744–1751.
5. Wagner E. Das tuberkelahnliche lymphadenom. Arch Heilk 1870;11:495–525.
6. Robertson HE. "Endothelioma" of the pleura. Am J Cancer 1924;8:317–375.
7. Doll R. Mortality from lung cancer in asbestos workers. Br J Ind Med 1955;12:81–86.
8. Klemperer P, Rabin CB. Primary neoplasms of pleura: report of 5 cases. Arch Pathol 1931;11:385–412.
9. Stout AP, Murray MR. Localized pleural mesothelioma: investigation of its characteristics and histogenesis by the method of tissue culture. Arch Pathol 1942;34:951–964.
10. Foster EA, Ackerman LV. Localized mesotheliomas of the pleura: the pathologic evaluation of 18 cases. Am J Clin Pathol 1960;34:349–364.
11. Wedler HW. Uber den Lungenkrebs bei Asbestose. Dtsch Arch Klin Med 1943;191:189–209.
12. Wedler HW. Uber den Lungenkrebs bei Asbestose. Dtsch Med Wochenschr 1943;69:575–576.
13. Merewether ERA. Annual report of the chief inspector of factories for the year 1947. London: His Majesty's Stationery Office, 1949:78–81.
14. Mallory TB, Castleman B, Parris EE. Case records of the Massachusetts General Hospital #33111. N Engl J Med 1947;236:407–412.
15. Willis RA. Pathology of tumours, 4th ed. London: Butterworths, 1967.
16. Weiss A. Pleurakrebs bei Lungenasbestose, in vivo morphologisch Geishert. Medizienische 1953;3:93–94.
17. Leicher F. Primarer deckzellen Tumor des Bauchtells bei Asbestose. Arch Gewerbepathol Gewerbehyg 1954;13: 382–392.
18. Keal EE. Asbestosis and abdominal neoplasms. Lancet 1960;2:1211–1216.
19. Wagner JC, Sleggs CA, Marchand P. Diffuse pleural mesothelioma and asbestos exposure in North Western Cape Province. Br J Ind Med 1960;17:260–271.
20. Wagner JC. The discovery of the association between blue asbestos and mesotheliomas and the aftermath. Br J Ind Med 1991;48:399–403.
21. Wagner JC. Asbestos and mesothelioma: a personal reminiscence. In: Henderson DW, Shilkin KB, Langlois SLP, Whitaker D, eds. Malignant mesothelioma. New York: Hemisphere, 1992:xvii–xxv.
22. Roggli VL, Pratt PC, Brody AR. Asbestos fiber type in malignant mesothelioma: an analytical scanning microscopic study of 94 cases. Am J Ind Med 1993;23:605–614.
23. Dodson RF, O'Sullivan M, Corn CJ, et al. Analysis of asbestos fiber burden in lung tissue from mesothelioma patients. Ultrastruct Pathol 1997;21:321–336.
24. Smither WJ, Gilson JC, Wagner JC. Mesotheliomas and asbestos dust. Br Med J 1962;2:1194–1195.
25. McCaughey WTE, Wade OL, Elmes PC. Exposure to asbestos dust and diffuse pleural mesothelioma. Br Med J 1962;2:1397.
26. Wagner JC, Munday DE, Harington JS. Histochemical demonstration of hyaluronic acid in pleural mesotheliomas. J Pathol Bacteriol 1962;84:73–78.
27. Wagner JC. Experimental production of mesothelial tumours of the pleura by implantation of dusts in laboratory animals. Nature 1962;196:180–181.
28. Selikoff IJ, Churg J, Hammond EC. Relation between exposure to asbestos and mesothelioma. N Engl J Med 1965;272:560–565.
29. Selikoff IJ, Churg J, Hammond EC. Asbestos exposure and neoplasia. JAMA 1964;188:22–26.
30. Newhouse ML, Thompson H. Epidemiology of mesothelial tumors in the London area. Ann NY Acad Sci 1965; 132:579–588.

31. Newhouse ML, Thompson H. Mesothelioma of pleura and peritoneum following exposure to asbestos in the London area. Br J Ind Med 1965;22:261–269.
32. Goodwin MC. Diffuse mesotheliomas with comment on their relationship to localized fibrous mesotheliomas. Cancer 1967;10:298–319.
33. South Australian Cancer Registry. Epidemiology of cancer in South Australia: incidence, mortality and survival 1977 to 1999. Adelaide: Department of Human Services, 2000.
34. New South Wales Cancer Council (NSWCC). Cancer in New South Wales: incidence and mortality 1997. Sydney: NSWCC, 1999.
35. Ferlay J, Bray F, Pisani P, Parkin DM. Globocan 2000: cancer incidence, mortality and prevalence worldwide. Lyon: International Agency for Research on Cancer, 2001.
36. Leigh J, Hendrie L, Berry D. Malignant mesothelioma in Australia, 1945–2000. J Occup Health Safety Aust NZ 2001;17:453–470.
37. Galateau-Sallé F, ed. International Mesothelioma Panel: Brambilla E, Cagle PT, Churg AM, et al. Pathology of malignant mesothelioma. London: Springer, 2006.
38. Henderson DW, Rödelsperger K, Woitowitz H-J, Leigh J. After Helsinki: a multidisciplinary review of the relationship between asbestos exposure and lung cancer, with emphasis on studies published during 1997–2004. Pathology 2004;36:517–550.
39. Motley RL. The lid comes off. Trial 1980;15:21–24.
40. Brodeur P. Expendable Americans. New York: Viking, 1974.
41. Brodeur P. The asbestos industry on trial. I. A failure to warn. II. Discovery. III. Judgement. IV. Bankruptcy. New Yorker 1985;61:49–52+ (June 10); 45–48+ (June 17); 37–41+ (June 24); 36–38+ (July 1).
42. World Trade Organization (WTO) Dispute Settlement Report WT/DS135. European Communities—Measures Concerning Asbestos and Asbestos-Containing Products. Geneva: WTO, 2000. See also WTO Dispute Settlement Reports 2001;8:3303–4047 (DSR 2001: VIII). Cambridge: Cambridge University Press, 2004.
43. Leigh J, Robinson BWS. The history of mesothelioma in Australia 1945–2001. In: Robinson BWS, Chahinian AP, eds. Mesothelioma. London: Martin Dunitz, 2002: 55–86.
44. Health and Safety Executive (HSE). Mesothelioma occupation statistics: male and female deaths aged 16–74 in Great Britain 1980–2000 (excluding 1981). London: HSE, 2003.
45. Price B. Analysis of current trends in United States mesothelioma incidence. Am J Epidemiol 1997;145:211–218.
46. Teschke K, Morgan MS, Checkoway H, et al. Mesothelioma surveillance to locate sources of exposure to asbestos. Can J Public Health/Rev Can Santé Publique 1997; 88:163–168.
47. Tossavainen A. Asbestos, asbestosis and cancer: exposure criteria for clinical diagnosis. Asbestos, Asbestosis and Cancer. People and Work Research Reports 14. Helsinki: Finnish Institute of Occupational Health (FIOH), 1997; 14:8–27.
48. Tossavainen A, Takahashi K. Epidemiological trends for asbestos-related cancers. People and Work Research Reports 36. Helsinki: FIOH, 2000;36:26–30.
49. HSE. Mesothelioma. 2006: http://www.hse.gov.uk/statistics/causdis/meso.htm.
50. McDonald AD, Harper A, El Attar DA, McDonald JC. Epidemiology of primary malignant mesothelial tumors in Canada. Cancer 1970;26:914–919.
51. Theriault GP, Grand-Bois L. Mesothelioma and asbestos in the province of Quebec, 1969–1972. Arch Environ Health 1978;33:15–19.
52. Biava PM, Ferri R, Spacal B, et al. Cancro de lovora a Trieste: II mesothelioma della pleura. Sapere 1976;79: 41–45.
53. Greenberg M, Lloyd-Davies TA. Mesothelioma register 1967–1968. Br J Ind Med 1974;31:91–104.
54. McDonald All, McDonald JC. Malignant mesothelioma in North America. Cancer 1980;46:1650–1656.
55. Cutler SJ, Young JL. Third National Cancer Survey: incidence data. Natl Cancer Inst Monogr 1975;41:442.
56. Bruckman L, Rubino RA, Christine B. Asbestos and mesothelioma incidence in Connecticut. J Air Pollut Control Assoc 1977;27:121–126.
57. Churg A. Malignant mesothelioma in British Columbia in 1982. Cancer 1985;55:672–674.
58. Ferguson D. Malignant mesothelioma—the rising epidemic. Med J Austral 1989;150:233–235.
59. McDonald JC, McDonald AD. Epidemiology of mesothelioma from estimated incidence. Prev Med 1977;6: 426–446.
60. Hughes JM, Weill H. Asbestos exposure—quantitative assessment of risk. Am Rev Respir Dis 1986;133:5–13.
61. Selikoff IJ, Hammond EC, Seidman H. Mortality experience of insulation workers in the United States and Canada 1943–1976. Ann NY Acad Sci 1979;330: 91–116.
62. Huncharek M. Changing risk groups for malignant mesothelioma. Cancer 1992;69:2704–2711.
63. Environmental Working Group (EWG) Action Fund Report. The Asbestos Epidemic in America. 2004. http://wwwewgorg/reports/asbestos/facts/fact1php.
64. Price B. Analysis of current trends in the United States mesothelioma incidence. Am J Epidemiol 1997;145:211–218.
65. Connelly RR, Spirtas R, Myers MH, et al. Demographic patterns for mesothelioma in the United States. J Natl Cancer Inst 1987;78:1053–1060.
66. Peto J, Hodgson JT, Matthews FE, Jones JR. Continuing increase in mesothelioma mortality in Britain. Lancet 1995;345:535–539.
67. Hodgson JT, McElvenny DM, Darnton AJ, et al. The expected burden of mesothelioma mortality in Great Britian from 2002 to 2050. Br J Cancer 2005;92:587–593.
68. Health and Safety Executive Data. Cited in Kazan-Allen L. Asbestos and mesothelioma: worldwide trends. Lung Cancer 2005;49(suppl):S3–S8.
69. Treasure T, Waller D, Swift S, Peto J. Radical surgery for mesothelioma. BMJ 2004;328:237–238.
70. Roggli VL. Changing patterns of mesothelioma referral. Asbestos Med 2004;387–397.

71. Lemen RA. Epidemiology of asbestos-related diseases and the knowledge that led to what is known today. In: Dodson RF, Hammar SP, eds. Asbestos: risk assessment, epidemiology and health effects. Boca Raton: CRC Taylor Francis, 2006:217.
72. Wagner JC. Mesothelioma and mineral fibers. Cancer 1986;57:1905–1911.
73. Rom WM, Lockey JE. Diffuse malignant mesothelioma: a review. West J Med 1982;137:548–554.
74. Legha SS, Muggia FM. Pleural mesothelioma: clinical features and therapeutic implications. Ann Intern Med 1977;87:613–621.
75. Borow M, Conston A, Livornese L, Schalet N. Mesothelioma following exposure to asbestos: a review of 72 cases. Chest 1973;64:641–646.
76. Cochrane JC, Webster I. Mesothelioma in relation to asbestos fibre exposure. A review of 70 serial cases. S Afr Med J 1978;54:279–281.
77. Tagnon I, Blot WJ, Stroube RB, et al. Mesothelioma associated with the shipbuilding industry in coastal Virginia. Cancer Res 1980;40:3875–3879.
78. Whitwell F, Rawcliffe RM. Diffuse malignant pleural mesothelioma and asbestos exposure. Thorax 1971;26:6–22.
79. Hammar SP. Mesothelioma. In: Sheppard MN, ed. Practical pulmonary pathology. Boston: Little, Brown and Edward Arnold, 1995:264–288.
80. Taylor RA, Johnson LP. Mesothelioma: current perspectives. West J Med 1981;134:379–383.
81. Vogelzang NJ, Schultz SM, Iannucci AM, Kennedy BJ. Malignant mesothelioma: the University of Minnesota experience. Cancer 1984;53:377–383.
82. Peto J, Henderson BE, Pike MC. Trends in mesothelioma in the United States and the forecast epidemic due to asbestos exposure during World War II. In: Peto R, Schneiderman M, eds. Quantification of occupational cancer. Banbary Report 9. New York: Cold Spring Harbor Laboratory 1981:51–69.
83. Roggli VL, McGavran MH, Subach J, Sybers HD, Greenberg SD. Pulmonary asbestos body counts and electron probe analysis of asbestos body cores in patients with mesothelioma: a study of 25 cases. Cancer 1982; 50:2423–2432.
84. Oels HC, Harrison EG, Carr DT, Bernatz PE. Diffuse malignant mesothelioma of the pleura: a review of 37 cases. Chest 1971;60:564–470.
85. Brenner J, Sordillo PP, Magill GB, Golbey RB. Malignant mesothelioma of the pleura: review of 123 patients. Cancer 1982;49:2431–2435.
86. Ratzer ER, Pool JL, Melamed MR. Pleural mesotheliomas: clinical experiences with thirty-seven patients. Am J Radiol 1967;99:863–880.
87. Newhouse ML, Berry G. Patterns of mortality in asbestos factory workers in London. Ann NY Acad Sci 1979;330: 53–60.
88. Newhouse ML, Berry G. Predictions of mortality from mesothelial tumours in asbestos factory workers. Br J Ind Med 1976;33:147–151.
89. Epler GR, Gerlad MXF, Gaensler EA, Carrington CB. Asbestos-related disease from household exposure. Respiration 1980;39:229–240.
90. Chen W, Mottet NK. Malignant mesothelioma with minimal asbestos exposure. Hum Pathol 1978;9:253–258.
91. Iwatsubo Y, Pairon JC, Menard BO, et al. Pleural mesothelioma: dose-response relation at low levels of asbestos exposure in a French population-based case-controlled study. Am J Epidemiol 1998;148:133–142.
92. World Health Organization. Environmental Health Criteria 203. Chrysotile asbestos. Geneva: WHO, 1998.
93. Hodgson JT, Darnton A. The quantitative risks of mesothelioma and lung cancer in relation to asbestos exposure. Ann Occup Hyg 2000;44:565–601.
94. Rödelsperger K, Jockel H, Pohlabein H, Romer W, Woitowitz H. Asbestos and man-made vitreous fibers as risk factors for diffuse malignant mesothelioma: results from a German hospital-based case-control study. Am J Ind Med 2001;39:262–275.
95. Rolland P, Ducamp S, Gramond C, et al. Risk of pleural mesothelioma: a French population-based case-control study. Lung Cancer 2006;54(suppl):S9–S10.
96. Evaluation of EPA's analytical data from the El Dorado Hills Asbestos Evaluation Project. April 20, 2006:14.
97. Elimination of asbestos-related diseases. Policy paper. World Health Organization, 2006.
98. Anderson HA, Lils R, Daum SM, et al. Asbestosis among household contacts of asbestos factory workers. Ann NY Acad Sci 1979;330:387–399.
99. Vianna NJ, Polan AK. Non-occupational exposure to asbestos and malignant mesothelioma in females. Lancet 1978;1:1061–1063.
100. Kane MJ, Chahinian P, Holland JF. Malignant mesothelioma in young adults. Cancer 1990;65:1449–1455.
101. Cazzadori A, Malesani F, Romeo L. Malignant pleural mesothelioma caused by non-occupational childhood exposure to asbestos. Br J Ind Med 1992;49:599.
102. Dodoli D, Del Nevo M, Fiumalbi C, et al. Environmental household exposure to asbestos and occurrence of pleural mesothelioma. Am J Ind Med 1992;21:681–687.
103. Hammar SP, Roggli VL, Oury T. Malignant mesothelioma in women. Lung Cancer 1997;18(Suppl 1): 236.
104. Baris YI. Pleural mesotheliomas and asbestos pleurisies due to environmental asbestos exposure in Turkey: an analysis of 120 cases. Hacettepe Bull Med/Surg 1975;8: 165–185.
105. Baris YI, Sahin AA, Ozesmi M, et al. An outbreak of pleural mesothelioma and chronic fibrosing pleurisy in the village of Karain/Urgup in Anatolia. Thorax 1978;33: 181–192.
106. Artvinli M, Baris YI. Malignant mesotheliomas in a small village in the Anatolian region of Turkey: an epidemiologic study. J Natl Cancer Inst 1979;63:17–22.
107. Baris YI, Saracci R, Simonato L, Skidmore JW, Artvinli M. Malignant mesothelioma and radiological chest abnormalities in two villages in central Turkey. Lancet 1981; 1:984–987.
108. Artvinli M, Baris YL. Environmental fiber-induced pleuro-pulmonary diseases in an Anatolian village: an epidemiologic study. Arch Environ Health 1982;37: 177–181.
109. Lillis R. Fibrous zeolites and endemic mesothelioma in Cappadocia, Turkey. J Occup Med 1981;23:548–550.

110. Sebastien P, Gaudichet A, Bignon J, Baris YL. Zeolite bodies in human lungs from Turkey. Lab Invest 1981; 44:420–425.
111. Wagner JC, Skidmore JW, Hill RJ, Griffiths DM. Erionite exposure and mesotheliomas in rats. Br J Cancer 1985; 51:727–750.
112. Rohl AN, Langer AM, Moncure G, Selikoff IJ, Fischbein A. Endemic pleural disease associated with exposure to mixed fibrous dust in Turkey. Science 1982;216:518–520.
113. Pistolesi M, Rusthoven J. Malignant pleural mesothelioma. Update, current management, and newer therapeutic strategies. Chest 2004;126:1318–1329.
114. Roushady-Hammady I, Siegel J, Emri S, et al. Genetic susceptibility factor of malignant mesothelioma in the Cappadocian region of Turkey. Lancet 2001;357:444–445.
115. Hillerdal G, Berg J. Malignant mesothelioma secondary to chronic inflammation and old scars: two new cases and review of the literature. Cancer 1985;55:1968–1972.
116. Gentiloni N, Febbraro S, Barone C, et al. Peritoneal mesothelioma in recurrent familial peritonitis. J Clin Gastroenterol 1997;24:276–279.
117. Schneider J, Woitowitz H-J. Asbestos-related non-occupational malignant mesothelioma. In: Peters GA, Peters BJ, eds. Sourcebook on asbestos diseases. Charlottesville: Lexis, 1998;17:43–69.
118. Sakellariou K, Malamou-Mitsi V, Haritou A, et al. Malignant pleural mesothelioma from nonoccupational asbestos exposure in Metsovo (north-west Greece): slow end of an epidemic? Eur Respir J 1996;9:1206–1210.
119. Henderson DW, Comin CE, Hammar SP, et al. Malignant mesothelioma of the pleura: current surgical pathology. In: Corrin B, ed. Pathology of lung tumors. New York: Churchill Livingstone, 1997:241–280.
120. Kerrigan SA, Cagle P, Churg A. Malignant mesothelioma of the peritoneum presenting as an inflammatory lesion: a report of four cases. Am J Surg Pathol 2003;27:248–253.
121. Andersson M, Wallin H, Jonsson M, et al. Lung carcinoma and malignant mesothelioma in patients exposed to Thorotrast: incidence, histology and p53 status. Int J Cancer 1995;63:330–336.
122. de la Pena A, Lucas I. Malignant peritoneal mesothelioma as late complication of radiotherapy for Hodgkin's disease [letter; Spanish]. An Med Intern 1997;14:319.
123. Gold B, Kathren RL. Causes of death in a cohort of 260 plutonium workers. Health Phys 1998;75:236–240.
124. Van Kaick G, Dalheimer A, Hornik S, et al. The German thorotrast study: recent results and assessment of risks. Radiat Res 1999;152:S64–71.
125. Amin AM, Mason C, Rowe P. Diffuse malignant mesothelioma of the peritoneum following abdominal radiotherapy. Eur J Surg Oncol 2001;27:214–215.
126. Henley JD, Loehrer PJ Sr, Ulbright TM. Deciduoid mesothelioma of the pleura after radiation therapy for Hodgkin's disease presenting as a mediastinal mass. Am J Surg Pathol 2001;25:547–548.
127. Melato M, Rizzardi C. Malignant pleural mesothelioma following chemotherapy for breast cancer. Anticancer Res 2001;21:3093–3096.
128. Velissaris TJ, Tang AT, Millward-Sadler GH, et al. Pericardial mesothelioma following mantle field radiotherapy. J Cardiovasc Surg (Torino) 2001;42:425–427.
129. Travis LB, Fossa SD, Schonfeld SJ, et al. Second cancers among 40,576 testicular cancer patients: focus on long-term survivors. J Natl Cancer Inst 2005;97:1354–1365.
130. Neugut AI, Ahsan H, Antman KH. Incidence of malignant pleural mesothelioma after thoracic radiotherapy. Cancer 1997;80:948–950.
131. Austin MB, Fechner RE, Roggli VL. Pleural malignant mesothelioma following Wilms' tumor. Am J Clin Pathol 1986;86:227–230.
132. Anderson KA, Hurley WC, Hurley BT, Ohrt DW. Malignant pleural mesothelioma following radiotherapy in a 16-year-old boy. Cancer 1985;56:273–276.
133. Mizuki M, Yukishige K, Abe Y, Tsuda T. A case of malignant pleural mesothelioma following exposure to atomic radiation in Nagasaki. Respirology 1997;2:201–205.
134. da Silva Horta J, et al. Malignancy and late effects following administration of Thorotrast. Lancet 1965;2:201–205.
135. Maurer R, Egloff B. Malignant peritoneal mesothelioma after colangiography with Thorotrast. Cancer 1975;36: 1381–1385.
136. Babcock TL, et al. Radiation-induced peritoneal mesothelioma. J Surg Oncol 1976;8:369–372.
137. Stock RJ, Fu YS, Carter JR. Malignant peritoneal mesothelioma following radiotherapy for seminoma of the testis. Cancer 1979;44:914–919.
138. Brenner J, et al. Malignant mesothelioma of the pleura: review of 123 patients. Cancer 1982;49:2431–2435.
139. Antman KH, Corson JM, Li FP, et al. Malignant mesothelioma following radiation exposure. J Clin Oncol 1983;1: 695–700.
140. Antman KH, Ruxer RL, Aisner J, Vawter G. Mesothelioma following Wilms' tumor in childhood. Cancer 1984; 54:367–369.
141. Gilks B, et al. Malignant peritoneal mesothelioma after remote abdominal radiation. Cancer 1988;61:2019–2021.
142. Horie A, Hiraoka K, Yamamoto O, et al. An autopsy case of peritoneal malignant mesothelioma in a radiation technologist. Acta Pathol Jpn 1990;40:57–62.
143. Lerman Y, et al. Radiation-associated malignant pleural mesothelioma. Thorax 1991;46:463–464.
144. Hofmann J, et al. Malignant mesothelioma following radiation therapy. Am J Med 1994;97:379–382.
145. Shannon VR, Nesbitt JC, Libshitz HI. Malignant pleural mesothelioma after radiation therapy for breast cancer: a report of two additional patients. Cancer 1995;76: 437–441.
146. Cavazza A, Travis LB, Travis WD, et al. Post irradiation malignant mesothelioma. Cancer 1996;77:1379–1385.
147. Weissmann LB, et al. Malignant mesothelioma following treatment for Hodgkin's disease. J Clin Oncol 1996;14: 2098–2100.
148. Pappo AS, Santana VM, Furman WL, et al. Post irradiation malignant mesothelioma. Cancer 1997;79:192–193.
149. Tassile D, Roth AD, Kurt AM, et al. Colon cancer and peritoneal mesothelioma occurring 29 years after abdominal radiation for testicular seminoma: a case report and review of the literature. Oncol 1998;55:289–292.

150. Kramer G, et al. Long-term survival of a patient with malignant pleural mesothelioma as a late complication of radiotherapy for Hodgkin's disease treated with ^{90}yttrium-silicate. Lung Cancer 2000;27:205–208.
151. Teta MJ, et al. Therapeutic radiation for lymphoma: risk of malignant mesothelioma. Cancer 2007;109:1432–1438.
152. Talerman A, Montero JR, Chilcote RR, Okagaki T. Diffuse malignant peritoneal mesothelioma in a 13-year-old girl: report of a case and review of the literature. Am J Surg Pathol 1985;9:73–80.
153. Fraire AE, Cooper S, Greenberg SD, Buffler PA, Langston C. Mesothelioma of childhood. Lab Invest 1987;56:25A.
154. Fraire AE, Cooper S, Greenberg SD, Buffler P, Langston C. Mesothelioma of childhood. Cancer 1988;62:838–847.
155. Lin-Chu M, Lee Y, Ho MY. Malignant mesothelioma in infancy. Arch Pathol Lab Med 1989;113:409–411.
156. Priest JR, McDermott MB, Bhatia S, et al. Pleuropulmonary blastoma: a clinicopathologic study of 50 cases. Cancer 1997;80:147–161.
157. McDonald JC, McDonald A. Mesothelioma and asbestos exposure. In: Pass HI, Vogelzang NJ, Carbone M, eds. Malignant mesothelioma: advances in pathogenesis, diagnosis, and translational therapies. New York: Springer, 2005:267–292.
158. McDonald JC, McDonald AD. Mesothelioma: is there a background? In: Jaurand M-C, Bignon J, eds. The mesothelial cell and mesothelioma. New York: Marcel Dekker, 1994:37–45.
159. HSE. Health and Safety Statistics 1998/99. London: HSE Books, 1999.
160. Strickler HD, Goedert JJ, Devesa SS, et al. Trends in US pleural mesothelioma incidence rates following simian virus 40 contamination of early Poliovirus vaccines. J Natl Cancer Inst 2003;95:38–45.
161. Roggli VL, Oury TD, Moffatt EJ. Malignant mesothelioma in women. Anat Pathol 1997;2:147–163.
162. Roggli VL, Sharma A, Butnor KJ, et al. Malignant mesothelioma and occupational exposure to asbestos: a clinicopathological correlation of 1445 cases. Ultrastruct Pathol 2002;26:55–65.
163. Hillerdal G. Mesothelioma: cases associated with non-occupational and low dose exposures. Occup Environ Med 1999;56:505–513.
164. Di Maria GU, Comba P. Malignant pleural mesothelioma: the puzzling role of gene-environment interaction. Chest 2004;125:1604–1607.
165. Lynch HT, Katz D, Markvicka SE. Familial mesothelioma: review and family study. Cancer Genet Cytogenet 1985; 15:25–35.
166. Martensson G, Larsson S, Zettergren L. Malignant mesothelioma in two pairs of siblings: Is there a hereditary predisposing factor? Eur J Respir Dis 1984;65: 179–184.
167. Hammar S. Familial mesothelioma: a report of two families. Hum Pathol 1989;20:107–112.
168. Huncharek M, Kelsey K, Muscat J, Christiani D. Parental cancer and genetic predisposition in malignant pleural mesothelioma: a case-control study. Cancer Lett 1996;102: 205–208.
169. Heineman EF, Bernstein L, Stark AD, Spirtas R. Mesothelioma, asbestos, and reported history of cancer in first-degree relatives. Cancer 1996;77:549–554.
170. Ascoli V, Scalzo CC, Bruno C, Facciolo F, et al. Familial pleural malignant mesothelioma: clustering in three sisters and one cousin. Cancer Lett 1998;130:203–207.
171. Bianchi C, Brollo A, Ramani L, Bianchi T, Giarelli L. Familial mesothelioma of the pleura—a report of 40 cases. Ind Health 2004;42:235–239.
172. Ohar JA, Ampleford EJ, Howard SE, Sterling DA. Identification of a mesothelioma phenotype. Respir Med 2007;101:503–509.
173. Ascoli V, Aalto Y, Carnovale-Scalzo C, Nardi F, et al. DNA copy number changes in familial malignant mesothelioma. Cancer Genet Cytogenet 2001;127:80–82.
174. Musti M, Cavone D, Aalto Y, Scattone A, et al. A cluster of familial malignant mesothelioma with del(9p) as the sole chromosomal anomaly. Cancer Genet Cytogenet 2002;138:73–76173.
175. Bianchi AB, Mitsunaga SI, Cheng JQ, Klein WM, et al. High frequency of inactivating mutations in the neurofibromatosis type 2 gene (*NF2*) in primary malignant mesotheliomas. Proc Natl Acad Sci 1995;92:10854–10858.
176. Hemminki K, Li X. Familial risk of cancer by site and histopathology. Int J Cancer 2003;103:105–109.
177. Dawson A, Gibbs A, Browne K, et al. Familial mesothelioma: details of 17 cases with histopathologic findings and mineral analysis. Cancer 1992;70:1183–1187.
178. Serio G, Scattone A, Gentile M, et al. Familial pleural mesothelioma with environmental asbestos exposure: losses of DNA sequences by comparative genomic hybridization (CGH). Histopathology 2004;45:643–645.
179. Nelson HH, Christiani DC, Wiencke JK, et al. K-ras mutation and occupational asbestos exposure in lung adenocarcinoma: asbestos-related cancer without asbestosis. Cancer Res 1999;59:4570–4573.
180. Lynch HT, Anton-Culver H, Kurosaki T. Is there a genetic predisposition to malignant mesothelioma? In: Jaurand M-C, Bignon J, eds. The mesothelial cell and mesothelioma. New York: Marcel Dekker, 1994:47–69.
181. Pylkkänen L, Wolff H, Stjernvall T, et al. Reduced Fhit protein expression and loss of heterozygosity at FHIT gene in tumours from smoking and asbestos-exposed lung cancer patients. Int J Oncol 2002;20:285–290.
182. Pylkkänen L, Wolff H, Stjernvall T, et al. Reduced Fhit protein expression in human malignant mesothelioma. Virchows Arch 2004;444:43–48.
183. Hirvonen A, Saarikoski ST, Linnainmaa K, et al. Glutathione S-transferase and N-acetyltransferase genotypes and asbestos-associated pulmonary disorders. J Natl Cancer Inst 1996;88:1853–1856.
184. Puntoni R, Filiberti R, Cerrano PG, et al. Implementation of a molecular epidemiology approach to human pleural malignant mesothelioma. Mutat Res 2003;544:385–396.
185. Pott F. Asbestos use and carcinogenicity in Germany and a comparison with animal studies. Ann Occup Hyg 1994;38:589–600.
186. Klein G, Powers A, Croce C. Association of SV40 with human tumors. Oncogene 2002;21:1141–1149.

187. Immunization Safety Review Committee. Immunization Safety Review: SV40 Contamination of Polio Vaccine and Cancer. Washington, DC: National Academies Press, 2003.
188. Hubner R, Van ME. Reappraisal of the strong association between simian virus 40 and human malignant mesothelioma of the pleura (Belgium). Cancer Causes Control 2002;13:121–129.
189. British Thoracic Society Standards of Care Committee. Statement on malignant mesothelioma in the United Kingdom. Thorax 2001;56:250–265.
190. Lee YCG, de Klerk NH, Henderson DW, Musk AW. Malignant mesothelioma. In: Hendrick DJ, Burge PS, Beckett WS, Churg A, eds. Occupational disorders of the lung: recognition, management, and prevention. London: Saunders, 2002:359–379.
191. Lopez-Rios F, Illei PB, Rusch V, Ladanyi M. Evidence against a role for SV40 infection in human mesotheliomas and high risk of false-positive PCR results owing to presence of SV40 sequences in common laboratory plasmids. Lancet 2004;364:1157–1166.
192. Manfredi JJ, Dong J, Liu WJ, et al. Evidence against a role for SV40 in human mesothelioma. Cancer Res 2005; 65:2602–2609.
193. Leigh J, Driscoll T. Malignant mesothelioma in Australia, 1945–2002. Int J Occup Environ Health 2003;9:206–217.
194. Spirtas R, Heineman EF, Bernstein L, et al. Malignant mesothelioma: attributable risk of asbestos exposure. Occup Environ Med 1994;51:804–811.
195. Furuya S, Natori Y, Ikeda R. Asbestos in Japan. Int J Occup Environ Health 2003;9:260–265.
196. Albin M, Magnani C, Krstev S, et al. Asbestos and cancer: an overview of current trends in Europe. Environ Health Perspect 1999;107:289–298.
197. Miller A. Mesothelioma in household members of asbestos-exposed workers: 32 United States cases since 1990. Am J Ind Med 2005;47:458–462.
198. Schneider J, Straif K, Woitowitz HJ. Pleural mesothelioma and household asbestos exposure. Rev Environ Health 1996;11:65–70.
199. Browne K. Asbestos-related mesothelioma: epidemiological evidence for asbestos as a promoter. Arch Environ Health 1983;38:261–266.
200. Dupres JS, Mustard JF, Uffen RJ. Report of the Royal Commission on Matters of Health and Safety Arising from the Use of Asbestos in Ontario (2 vols). Toronto: Ontario Ministry of Government Services: Queen's Printer for Ontario, 1984.
201. Huncharek M, Capotorto JV, Muscat J. Domestic asbestos exposure, lung fibre burden, and pleural mesothelioma in a housewife. Br J Ind Med 1989;46:354–355.
202. Gibbs AR, Griffiths DM, Pooley FD, Jones JSP. Comparison of fibre types and size distributions in lung tissues of paraoccupational and occupational cases of malignant mesothelioma. Br J Ind Med 1990;47:621–626.
203. Anderson HA, Lilis R, Daum SM, Selikoff IJ. Asbestosis among household contacts of asbestos factory workers. Ann NY Acad Sci 1979;330:387–399.
204. Tweedale G. Magic mineral to killer dust: Turner & Newall and the asbestos hazard. Oxford: Oxford University Press, 2000.
205. Layman L. The blue asbestos industry at Wittenoom in Western Australia: a short history. In: Henderson DW, Shilkin KB, Langlois SL, Whitaker D, eds. Malignant mesothelioma. New York: Hemisphere, 1992:305–327.
206. Musk AW, de Klerk NH, Eccles JL, et al. Wittenoom, Western Australia: a modern industrial disaster. Am J Ind Med 1992;21:735–747.
207. Berry G, de Klerk NH, Reid A, et al. Malignant pleural and peritoneal mesotheliomas in former miners and millers of crocidolite at Wittenoom, Western Australia. Occup Environ Med 2004;61:e14.
208. Jones JSP, Smith PG, Pooley FD, et al. The consequences of exposure to asbestos dust in a wartime gas-mask factory. In: Wagner JC, ed. Biological effects of mineral fibres, vol. 2 IARC Scientific Publications no. 30. Lyon: IARC, 1980:637–653.
209. Brown SK. A review of occupational and environmental exposure to asbestos dust. Melbourne, Australia: CSIRO Division of Building Research, 1981.
210. Jarvholm B, Sanden A. Lung cancer and mesothelioma in the pleura and peritoneum among Swedish insulation workers. Occup Environ Med 1998;55:766–770.
211. Henderson DW, Shilkin KB, Whitaker D, et al. The pathology of mesothelioma, including immunohistology and ultrastructure. In: Henderson DW, Shilkin KB, Langlois SL, Whitaker D, eds. Malignant mesothelioma. New York: Hemisphere, 1992:69–139.
212. Hemminki K, Li X. Time trends and occupational risk factors for pleural mesothelioma in Sweden. J Occup Environ Med 2003;45:456–461.
213. Comin CE, de Klerk NH, Henderson DW. Malignant mesothelioma: current conundrums over risk estimates, and whither electron microscopy for diagnosis? Ultrastruct Pathol 1997;21:315–320.
214. Neumann V, Muller KM, Fischer M. Peritoneal mesothelioma—incidence and etiology [German]. Pathologe 1999;20:169–176.
215. Neumann V, Gunthe S, Muller KM, Fischer M. Malignant mesothelioma—German mesothelioma register 1987–1999. Int Arch Occup Environ Health 2001;74:383–395.
216. Rogers AJ, Leigh J, Berry G, et al. Relationship between lung asbestos fiber type and concentration and relative risk of mesothelioma: a case-control study. Cancer 1991; 67:1912–1920.
217. Hemminki K, Li X. Time trends and occupational risk factors for peritoneal mesothelioma in Sweden. J Occup Environ Med 2003;45:451–455.
218. Ferguson DA, Berry G, Jelihovsky T, et al. The Australian mesothelioma surveillance program 1979–1985. Med J Aust 1987;147:166–172.
219. Bianchi C, Brollo A, Ramani L, et al. Asbestos exposure in malignant mesothelioma of the pleura: a survey of 557 cases. Ind Health 2001;39:161–167.
220. Multiple authors. Consensus report: asbestos, asbestosis, and cancer: the Helsinki criteria for diagnosis and attribution. Scand J Work Environ Health 1997;23:311–316.
221. Craighead JE, Abraham JL, Churg A, et al. The pathology of asbestos-associated diseases of the lungs and pleural cavities: diagnostic criteria and proposed grading schema. Arch Pathol Lab Med 1982;106:544–596.

222. Henderson DW, Jones ML, DeKlerk N, et al. The diagnosis and attribution of asbestos-related diseases in an Australian cohort: report of the Adelaide Workshop on Asbestos-Related Diseases. October 6–7. Int J Occup Environ Health 2004;10:40–46.
223. Wagner JC, Pooley FD. Mineral fibres and mesothelioma. Thorax 1986;41:161–166.
224. Pott F. Problems in defining carcinogenic fibres. Ann Occup Hyg 1987;31:799–802.
225. Pott F, Huth F, Friedrichs KH. Tumorigenic effects of fibrous dusts in experimental animals. Environ Health Perspect 1974;9:313–315.
226. Pott F, Ziem U, Reiffer FJ, Huth F, Ernst H, Mohr U. Carcinogenicity studies on fibres, metal compounds and some other dusts in rats. Exp Pathol 1987;32:129–152.
227. Pott F, Roller M, Ziem U, et al. Carcinogenicity studies on natural and man-made fibres with the intraperitoneal test in rats. Symposium on Mineral Fibres in the Non-Occupational Environment, Lyon, September 8–9, 1987: 1–4.
228. Stanton MF, Wrench C. Mechanisms of mesothelioma including with asbestos and fibrous glass. J Natl Cancer Inst 1972;48:797–821.
229. Stanton MF, Layard M, Tegeris E, et al. Relation of particle dimension to carcinogenicity in amphibole asbestoses and other fibrous minerals. J Natl Cancer Inst 1981; 67:965–975.
230. Harington JS. Fiber carcinogenesis: epidemiologic observations and the Stanton hypothesis. J Natl Cancer Inst 1981;67:977–989.
231. Davis JMG, Jones AD. Comparisons of the pathogenicity of long and short fibres of chrysotile asbestos in rats. Br J Exp Pathol 1988;69:717–737.
232. Davis JMG, Addison J, Bolton RE, et al. The pathogenicity of long versus short fibre samples of amosite asbestos administered to rats by inhalation and intraperitoneal injection. Br J Exp Pathol 1986;67:415–430.
233. Donaldson K, Golyasnya G, Davis JMG. Long and short amosite asbestos samples: comparison of chromosome-damaging effects to cells in culture with in vivo pathogenicity. In: Davis JMG, Jaurand M-C, eds. Cellular and molecular effects of mineral and synthetic dusts and fibres. NATO ASI series, vol. H85. Berlin: Springer-Verlag, 1994.
234. Yegles M, Janson X, Dong HY, et al. Role of fibre characteristics on cytotoxicity and induction of anaphase/telophase aberrations in rat pleural mesothelial cells in vitro: correlations with in vivo animal findings. Carcinogenesis 1995;16:2751–2758.
235. Suzuki Y, Yuen SR. Asbestos tissue burden study on human malignant mesothelioma. Ind Health 2001;39: 150–160.
236. Dodson RF, Williams MG, Corn CJ, Brollo A, Bianchi C. Asbestos content of lung tissue, lymph nodes, and pleural plaques from former shipyard workers. Am Rev Respir Dis 1990;142:843–847.
237. Sebastien P, Janson X, Gaudicher A, Hirsh A, Bignon J. Asbestos retention in human respiratory tissues: Comparative measurements in lung parenchyma and in parietal pleura. In: Wagner JC, ed. Biological effects of mineral fibers. Lyon: IARC, 1980:237–246.
238. Suzuki Y, Yuen SR. Asbestos fibers contributing to the induction of human malignant mesothelioma. Ann NY Acad Sci 2002;982:160–176.
239. Dodson RF, O'Sullivan M, Huang J, Holiday DB, Hammar SP. Asbestos in extrapulmonary sites, omentum and mesentery. Chest 2000;117:486–493.
240. Boutin C, Dumortier P, Rey F, Viallat JR, DeVuyst P. Black spots concentrate oncogenic asbestos fibers in the parietal pleura: thoracoscopic and mineralogic study. Am J Respir Crit Care Med 1996;153:444–449.
241. Mitchev K, Dumortier P, DeVuyst P. "Black spots" and hyaline pleural plaques on parietal pleura of 150 urban necropsy cases. Am J Surg Pathol 2002;26:1196–1206.
242. Zeren EH, Gumurdulu D, Roggli VL, Tuncer I, Zorludemir S, Erikisi M. Environmental malignant mesothelioma in Southern Anatolia: a study of fifty cases. Environ Health Perspect 2000;108:1047–1050.
243. Selcuk ZT, Coplu L, Emri S, Kalyoncu AF, Sahin AA, Baris YI. Malignant pleural mesothelioma due to environmental mineral fiber exposure in Turkey. Chest 1992;102: 790–796.
244. Baris I, Simonato L, Artvinli M, et al. Epidemiological and environmental evidence of the health effects of exposure to erionite fibres: a four-year study in the Cappadocian region of Turkey. Int J Cancer 1987;39:10–17.
245. Johnson NF, Edwards RE, Munday DE, Rowe N, Wagner JC. Pluripotential nature of mesotheliomata induced by inhalation of erionite in rats. Br J Exp Pathol 1984;65: 377–388.
246. McDonald JC, Harris J, Armstrong B. Mortality in a cohort of vermiculite miners exposed to fibrous amphibole in Libby, Montana. Occup Environ Med 2004;61: 363–366.
247. Anderson BA, Dearwent SM, Durant JT, et al. Exposure pathway evaluations for sites that processed asbestos-contaminated vermiculite. Int J Hyg Environ Health 2005;208:55–65.
248. Churg A. The diagnosis of asbestosis. Hum Pathol 1981; 20:97–99.
249. Roggli VL, Pratt PC. Numbers of asbestos bodies on iron-stained tissue sections in relation to asbestos body counts in lung tissue digests. Hum Pathol 1983;14:355.
250. Dodson RF, O'Sullivan MF, Brooks DR, Bruce JR. Asbestos content of omentum and mesentery in non-occupationally exposed individuals. Toxicol Ind Health 2001;17:138–143.
251. Dodson RF, Greenberg SD, Williams MG, et al. Asbestos content in lungs of occupationally and nonoccupationally exposed individuals. JAMA 1984;252:68–71.
252. Breeding PH, Buss DH. Ferruginous (asbestos) bodies in the lungs of rural dwellers, urban dwellers, and patients with pulmonary neoplasms. South Med J 1976;69:401–404.
253. Roggli VL, Pratt PC, Brody AR. Asbestos content of lung tissue in asbestos associated diseases: a study of 110 cases. Br J Ind Med 1986;43:18–28.
254. Langer AM, Selikoff IJ, Sastre A. Chrysotile asbestos in the lungs from persons in New York City. Arch Environ Health 1971;22:348–361.

255. Dodson RF, Atkinson AL. Measurements of asbestos burden in tissues. Ann NY Acad Sci 2006;1076:281–291.
256. Roggli VL, McGavran MH, Subach J, Sybers HD, Greenberg SD. Pulmonary asbestos body counts and electron probe analysis of asbestos body cores in patients with mesothelioma: a study of 25 cases. Cancer 1982;50: 2423–2432.
257. Roggli VL. Human disease consequences of fiber exposures: a review of human pathology and fiber burden data. Environ Health Perspect 1990;88:295–303.
258. Srebro SH, Roggli VL. Asbestos-related disease associated with exposure to asbestiform tremolite. Am J Ind Med 1994;26:809–819.
259. Srebro SH, Roggli VL, Samsa GP. Malignant mesothelioma associated with low pulmonary tissue asbestos burdens: a light and scanning electron microscopic analysis of 18 cases. Mod Pathol 1995;8:614–621.
260. Roggli VL. The role of analytical SEM in the determination of causation in malignant mesothelioma. Ultrastruct Pathol 2006;30:31–35.
261. Dodson RF, Graef R, Shepherd S, O'Sullivan M, Levin J. Asbestos burden in cases of mesothelioma from individuals from various regions of the United States. Ultrastruct Pathol 2005;29:415–433.
262. Paoletti L, Batisti D, Bruno C, et al. Unusually high incidence of malignant pleural mesothelioma in a town of eastern Sicily: an epidemiological and environmental study. Arch Environ Health 2000;55:392–398.
263. Langer AM, Nolan RP, Constantopoulos SH, Moutsopoulos HM. Association of Metsovo lung and pleural mesothelioma with exposure to tremolite-containing whitewash. Lancet 1987;1:965–967.
264. Howel D, Gibbs A, Arblaster L, et al. Mineral fibre analysis and routes for exposure to asbestos in the development of mesothelioma in an English region. Occup Environ Med 1999;56:51–58.
265. Karjalainen A, Meurman LO, Pukkala E. Four cases of mesothelioma among Finnish anthophyllite miners. Occup Environ Med 1994;51:212–215.
266. Tuomi T, Segerberg-Konttinen M, Tammllehto L, et al. Mineral fiber concentration in lung tissue of mesothelioma patients in Finland. Am J Ind Med 1989;16: 247–254.
267. Andrion A, Bosia S, Paoletti L, et al. Malignant peritoneal mesothelioma in a 17-year-old boy with evidence of previous exposure to chrysotile and tremolite asbestos. Hum Pathol 1994;25:617–622.
268. Glickman LT, Domanski LM, Maguire TG, et al. Mesothelioma in pet dogs associated with exposure of their owners to asbestos. Environ Res 1983;32:305–313.
269. Frank AL, Dodson RF, Williams MG. Carcinogenic implications of the lack of tremolite in UICC reference chrysotile. Am J Ind Med 1998;34:314–317.
270. Davis JMG, Bolton RE, Miller BG, Niven K. Mesothelioma dose response following intraperitoneal injection of mineral fibres. Int J Exp Pathol 1991;72:263–274.
271. Egilman D, Fehnel C, Bohme SR. Exposing the "myth" of ABC, "anything but chrysotile." A critique of the Canadian asbestos mining industry and McGill University chrysotile studies. Am J Ind Med 2003;44:540–557.
272. De A. Petrology of dikes emplaced in the ultramafic rocks of South Eastern Quebec. PhD thesis, Princeton University, 1961.
273. Churg A. Chrysotile, tremolite, and malignant mesothelioma in man. Chest 1988;93:621–628.
274. Churg A, Wright JL, Vedal S. Fiber burden and patterns of asbestos-related disease in chrysotile miners and millers. Am Rev Respir Dis 1993;148:25–31.
275. Dufresne A, Begin R, Churg A, Masse S. Mineral fiber content of lungs in patients with mesothelioma seeking compensation in Quebec. Am J Respir Crit Care Med 1996;153:711–718.
276. Begin R, Gauthier J, Desmeules M, Ostiguy G. Work-related mesothelioma in Quebec, 1967–1990. Am J Ind Med 1992;22:531–542.
277. Langer AM, McCaughey WTE. Mesothelioma in a brake repair worker. Lancet 1982;1:1101–1103.
278. Nolan RP, Langer AM, Addison J. Lung content analysis of cases occupationally exposed to chrysotile asbestos. Environ Health Perspect 1994;102:245–250.
279. Churg A, Vedal S. Fiber burden and patterns of asbestos-related disease in workers with heavy mixed amosite and chrysotile exposure. Am J Respir Crit Care Med 1994; 150:663–669.
280. McDonald JC, Armstrong BG, Edwards CW, et al. Case-reference survey of young adults with mesothelioma: I. Lung fibre analysis. Br Occup Hyg Soc 2001;45:513–518.
281. Talcot J, Thurber W, Gaensler E, Antman K, Li FP. Mesothelioma in manufacturing of asbestos-containing cigarette filters. Lancet 1987;1:392.
282. Talcot JA, Thurber WA, Kantor AF, et al. Asbestos-associated diseases in a cohort of cigarette-filter workers. N Engl J Med 1989;321:1220–1223.
283. Dodson RF, Williams MG, Satterley JD. Asbestos burden in two cases of mesothelioma where the work history included manufacturing of cigarette filters. J Toxicol Environ Health 2002;65:1109–1102.
284. Dodson RF, Hammar SP. Pleural mesothelioma in a woman whose documented past exposure to asbestos was from smoking asbestos-containing filtered cigarettes: the comparative value of analytical transmission electron microscopic analysis of lung and lymph-node tissue. Inhal Toxicol 2006;18:679–684.
285. Levin JL, McLarty JW, Hurst GA, Smith AN, Frank AL. Tyler asbestos workers: mortality experiences in a cohort exposed to amosite. Occup Environ Med 1998;55:155–160.
286. Dodson RF, O'Sullivan M, Brooks DR, Hammar SP. Quantitative analysis of asbestos burden in women with mesothelioma. Am J Ind Med 2003;43:188–195.
287. Peto J, Decarli A, LaVecchia C, Levi, Negri E. The European mesothelioma epidemic. Br J Cancer 1999;79: 666–672.
288. De Klerk NH, Armstrong BK. The epidemiology of asbestos and mesothelioma. In: Henderson DW, Shilkin KB, Langlois SL, Whitaker D, eds. Malignant mesothelioma. New York: Hemisphere, 1992:223–250.
289. Hammar SP. Pleural diseases. In: Dail DH, Hammar SP, eds. Pulmonary pathology, 2nd ed. New York: Springer-Verlag, 1994:1463–1579.

290. Fattman CL, Chu CT, Oury TD. Experimental models of asbestos-related diseases. In: Roggli VL, Oury TD, Sporn TA, eds. Pathology of asbestos-associated diseases, 2nd ed. New York: Springer-Verlag, 2004:256–308.
291. Middleton AP, Beckett ST, Davis JM. Further observations on the short-term retention and clearance of asbestos by rats, using UICC reference samples. Ann Occup Hyg 1979;22:141–152.
292. Du Toit RS. An estimate of the rate at which crocidolite asbestos fibres are cleared from the lung. Ann Occup Hyg 1991;35:433–438.
293. De Klerk NH, Musk AW, Williams V, et al. Comparison of measures of exposure to asbestos in former crocidolite workers from Wittenoom Gorge, W. Australia. Am J Ind Med 1996;30:579–587.
294. Finkelstein MM, Dufresne A. Inferences on the kinetics of asbestos deposition and clearance among chrysotile miners and millers. Am J Ind Med 1999;35:401–412.
295. Rödelsperger K, Mándi A, Tossavainen A, et al. Inorganic fibres in the lung tissue of Hungarian and German lung cancer patients. Int Arch Occup Environ Health 2000; 74:133–138.
296. Peto J, Seidman H, Selikoff IJ. Mesothelioma mortality in asbestos workers: implications for models of carcinogenesis and risk assessment. Br J Cancer 1982;45:124–135.
297. Berry G. Models for mesothelioma incidence following exposure to fibers in terms of timing and duration of exposure and the biopersistence of the fibers. Inhal Toxicol 1999;11:111–130.
298. Bourdès V, Boffetta P, Pisani P. Environmental exposure to asbestos and risk of pleural mesothelioma: review and meta-analysis. Eur J Epidemiol 2000;16:411–417.
299. Magnani C, Agudo A, Gonzalez CA, et al. Multicentric study on malignant pleural mesothelioma and non occupational exposure to asbestos. Br J Cancer 2000;83: 104–111.
300. Magnani C, Dalmasso P, Biggeri A, et al. Increased risk of malignant mesothelioma of the pleura after residential or domestic exposure to asbestos: a case-control study in Casale Monferrato, Italy. Environ Health Perspect 2001; 109:915–919.
301. Rödelsperger K, Woitowitz HJ, Bruckel B, et al. Dose-response relationship between amphibole fiber lung burden and mesothelioma. Cancer Detect Prevent 1999; 23:183–193.
302. Pan X-I, Day HW, Wang W, et al. Residential proximity to naturally occurring asbestos and mesothelioma in California. Am J Respir Crit Care Med 2005;172:1019–1025.
303. Koskinen K, Pukkala E, Martikainen R, et al. Different measures of asbestos exposure in estimating risk of lung cancer and mesothelioma among construction workers. J Occup Environ Med 2002;44:1190–1196.
304. Industrial Injuries Advisory Council (UK). Asbestos-related diseases: report by the Industrial Injuries Advisory Council in Accordance with Section 171 of the Social Security Administration Act 1992 Reviewing the Prescription of the Asbestos-Related Diseases. London: HMSO, 2005.
305. Mossman BT. Mechanisms of asbestos carcinogenesis and toxicity: the amphibole hypothesis revisited. Br J Ind Med 1993;50:673–676.
306. Mossman BT, Gee JBL. Asbestos-related cancer and the amphibole hypothesis: 4: the hypothesis is still supported by scientists and scientific data. Am J Public Health 1997;87:689–690.
307. Cullen MR. The amphibole hypothesis of asbestos-related cancer—gone but not forgotten [editorial]. Am J Public Health 1996;86:158–159.
308. Stayner LT, Dankovic DA, Lemen RA. Occupational exposure to chrysotile asbestos and cancer risk: a review of the amphibole hypothesis. Am J Public Health 1996; 86:179–186.
309. Stayner LT, Dankovic DA, Lemen RA. Asbestos-related cancer and the amphibole hypothesis: 2: Stayner and colleagues respond. Am J Public Health 1997;87: 688.
310. Langer AMP, Nolan RPP. Asbestos-related cancer and the amphibole hypothesis: 3: The amphibole hypothesis: neither gone nor forgotten. Am J Public Health 1997;87: 688–689.
311. Cullen MR. Asbestos-related cancer and the amphibole hypothesis: 5: Cullen responds. Am J Public Health 1997; 87:690–691.
312. Stayner LT, Dankovic DA, Lemen RA. Asbestos-related cancer and the amphibole hypothesis: 6: Stayner and colleagues respond. Am J Public Health 1997;87:691.
313. McDonald AD, Case BW, Churg A, et al. Mesothelioma in Quebec chrysotile miners and millers: epidemiology and aetiology. Ann Occup Hyg 1997;41:707–719.
314. McDonald JC, McDonald AD. Chrysotile, tremolite and carcinogenicity. Ann Occup Hyg 1997;41:699–705.
315. Emri S, Demir A, Dogan M, et al. Lung diseases due to environmental exposures to erionite and asbestos in Turkey. Toxicol Lett 2002;127:251–257.
316. Coplu L, Dumortier P, Demir AU, et al. An epidemiological study in an Anatolian village in Turkey environmentally exposed to tremolite asbestos. J Environ Pathol Toxicol Oncol 1996;15:177–182.
317. Viallat JR, Boutin C, Steinbauer J, et al. Pleural effects of environmental asbestos pollution in Corsica. Ann NY Acad Sci 1991;643:438–443.
318. Goldberg P, Luce D, Billon-Galland MA, et al. Potential role of environmental and domestic exposure to tremolite in pleural cancer in New Caledonia [French]. Rev Epidemiol Santé Publique 1995;43:444–450.
319. Luce D, Bugel I, Goldberg P, et al. Environmental exposure to tremolite and respiratory cancer in New Caledonia: a case-control study. Am J Epidemiol 2000; 151:259–265.
320. McDonald JC, McDonald AD, Armstrong B, Sebastien P. Cohort study of mortality of vermiculite miners exposed to tremolite. Br J Ind Med 1986;43:436–444.
321. Amandus HE, Wheeler R. The morbidity and mortality of vermiculite miners and millers exposed to tremolite-actinolite: part ii: mortality. Am J Ind Med 1987;11: 15–26.
322. Case BW. Health effects of tremolite. Now and in the future. Ann NY Acad Sci 1991;643:491–504.

323. De Guire L, Labrèche F, Poulin M, Dionne M. The use of chrysotile asbestos in Quebec. Montreal, Quebec: Institut National de Santé Publique du Québec, 2005.
324. De Guire Le. The epidemiology of asbestos-related diseases in Quebec. Montreal, Québec: Institut National de Santé du Québec, 2004.
325. Yano E, Wang Z-M, Wang X-R, et al. Cancer mortality among workers exposed to amphibole-free chrysotile. Am J Epidemiol 2001;154:538–543.
326. Tossavainen A, Kovalevsky E, Vanhala E, Tuomi T. Pulmonary mineral fibers after occupational and environmental exposure to asbestos in the Russian chrysotile industry. Am J Ind Med 2000;37:327–333.
327. Tossavainen A, Kotilainen M, Takahashi K, et al. Amphibole fibres in Chinese chrysotile asbestos. Ann Occup Hyg 2001;45:145–152.
328. Williams-Jones AE, Normand C, Clark JR, et al. Controls of amphibole formation in chrysotile deposits: evidence from the Jeffrey Mine, Asbestos, Quebec. In: Nolan RP, Langer AM, Ross M, et al., eds. The health effects of chrysotile: contribution of science to risk-management decisions. Can Mineral 2001;spec publ 5:89–104.
329. Kashansky SV, Scherbakov SV, Kogan FM. Dust levels in workplace air (a retrospective view of "Uralasbest"). In: Peters GA, Peters BJ, eds. Sourcebook on asbestos diseases, vol. 15. Charlottesville: Lexis, 1997;15:337–354.
330. Scherbakov SV, Dommin SG, Kashansky SV. Dust levels in workplace air of the mines and mills of Uralasbest Company. In: Lehtinen S, Tossavainen A, Rantanen J, eds. Proceedings of the Asbestos Symposium for the Countries of Central and Eastern Europe, Budapest, December 1997. People and Work Research Reports 19. Helsinki: FIOH, 1998:104–108.
331. Kashansky SV. A 300-year history of the discovery of asbestos in the Urals. In: Peters GA, Peters BJ, eds. Sourcebook on asbestos diseases, vol. 20. Charlottesville: Lexis, 1999;20:129–144.
332. Kogan FM. Asbestos-related diseases in Russia. In: Banks DE, Parker JE, eds. Occupational lung disease: an international perspective. London: Chapman & Hall, 1998: 247–253.
333. Vudrag M, Krajnc K. Asbestos in the Republic of Slovenia. In: Lehtinen S, Tossavainen A, Rantanen J, eds. Proceedings of the Asbestos Symposium for the Countries of Central and Eastern Europe, Budapest, December 1997. People and Work Research Reports 19. Helsinki: FIOH, 1998;19:79–84.
334. Tcherneva-Jalova P, Lukanova R, Demirova M. Asbestos in Bulgaria. In: Lehtinen S, Tossavainen A, Rantanen J, eds. Proceedings of the Asbestos Symposium for the Countries of Central and Eastern Europe, Budapest, December 1997. People and Work Research Reports 19. Helsinki: FIOH, 1998;19:33–38.
335. Indulski J, Szeszenia-Dabrowska N. Asbestos in Poland. In: Lehtinen S, Tossavainen A, Rantanen J, eds. Proceedings of the Asbestos Symposium for the Countries of Central and Eastern Europe, Budapest, December 1997. People and Work Research Reports 19. Helsinki: FIOH, 1998;19:55–62.
336. Sturm W, Menze B, Krause J, Thriene B. Use of asbestos, health risks and induced occupational diseases in the former East Germany. Toxicol Lett 1994;72:317–324.
337. Sturm W, Menze B, Krause J, Thriene B. Asbestos-related diseases and asbestos types used in the former GDR. Exp Toxicol Pathol 1995;47:173–178.
338. Yano E, Wang ZM, Wang XR, et al. Does exposure to chrysotile asbestos without amphibole cause lung cancer? Epidemiology for Sustainable Health: The XV International Scientific Meeting of the International Epidemiological Association, 1999;209.
339. Dement JM, Brown DP, Okun A. Follow-up study of chrysotile asbestos textile workers: cohort mortality and case-control analyses. Am J Ind Med 1994;26:431–447.
340. Dement JM, Brown DP. Lung cancer mortality among asbestos textile workers: a review and update. Ann Occup Hyg 1994;38:525–532.
341. Morinaga K, Kohyama N, Yokoyama K, et al. Asbestos fibre content of lungs with mesotheliomas in Osaka, Japan: a preliminary report. IARC Sci Publ 1989:438–443.
342. Yarborough CM. Chrysotile as a cause of mesothelioma: an assessment based on epidemiology. Crit Rev Toxicol 2006;36:165–187.
343. Paustenbach DJ, Finley BL, Lu ET, Brorby GP. Environmental and occupational health hazards associated with the presence of asbestos in brake linings and pads (1900 to present): a "state-of"-the-art" review. J Toxicol Environ Health [B] 2004;7:25–80.
344. Lorimer WV, Rohl AN, Miller A, et al. Asbestos exposure of brake repair workers in the United States. Mt Sinai J Med 1976;43:207–218.
345. Rohl AN, Langer AM, Wolff MS, Weisman I. Asbestos exposure during brake lining maintenance and repair. Environ Res 1976;12:110–128.
346. Huncharek M, Muscat J, Capotorto JV. Pleural mesothelioma in a brake mechanic. Br J Ind Med 1989;46: 69–71.
347. Robinson C, Lemen R, Wagoner JK. Mortality patterns, 1940–1975, among workers employed in an asbestos textile friction and packing products manufacturing facility. In: Lemen R, Dement JM, eds. Dusts and diseases. Park Forest South, IL: Pathotox, 1979:131–143.
348. Berry G, Newhouse ML. Mortality of workers manufacturing friction materials using asbestos. Br J Ind Med 1983;40:1–7.
349. McDonald AD, Fry JS, Wooley AJ, Mcdonald JC. Dust exposure and mortality in an American chrysotile asbestos friction products plant. Br J Ind Med 1984;41: 151–157.
350. Newhouse ML, Sullivan KR. A mortality study of workers manufacturing friction materials: 1941–1986. Br J Ind Med 1989;46:176–179.
351. Yeung P, Patience K, Apthorpe L, Willcocks D. An Australian study to evaluate worker exposure to chrysotile in the automotive service industry. Appl Occup Environ Hyg 1999;14:448–457.
352. Kohyama N. Airborne asbestos levels in non-occupational environments in Japan. IARC Sci Publ 1989: 262–276.

353. Kauppinen T, Korhonen K. Exposure to asbestos during brake maintenance of automotive vehicles by different methods. Am Ind Hyg Assoc J 1987;48:499–504.
354. Weir FW, Tolar G, Meraz LB. Characterization of vehicular brake service personnel exposure to airborne asbestos and particulate. Appl Occup Environ Hyg 2001;16:1139–1146.
355. Rödelsperger K, Jahn H, Brückel B, et al. Asbestos dust exposure during brake repair. Am J Ind Med 1986;10: 63–72.
356. Butnor KJ, Sporn TA, Roggli VL. Exposure to brake dust and malignant mesothelioma: a study of 10 cases with mineral fiber analysis. Ann Occup Hyg 2003;47:325–330.
357. Dodson RF, Poye LW, Hammar SP. Asbestos burden in lung tissue from an individual with extensive exposure to brake dust. Submitted for publication 2007.
358. Goodman M, Teta MJ, Hessel PA, et al. Mesothelioma and lung cancer among motor vehicle mechanics: a meta-analysis. Ann Occup Hyg 2004;48:309–326.
359. Hessel PA, Teta MJ, Goodman M, Lau E. Mesothelioma among brake mechanics: an expanded analysis of a case-control study. Risk Analysis 2004;24:547–552.
360. Laden F, Stampfer MJ, Walker AM. Lung cancer and mesothelioma among male automobile mechanics. Rev Environ Health 2004;19:39–61.
361. Egilman DS, Billings MA. Abuse of epidemiology: automobile manufacturers manufacture a defense to asbestos liability. Int J Occup Environ Health 2005;11:360–371.
362. Egilman D, Bohme SR. Over a barrel: corporate corruption of science and its effects on workers and the environment. Int J Occup Environ Health 2005;11:331–337.
363. Gennaro V, Tomatis L. Business bias: how epidemiologic studies may underestimate or fail to detect increased risks of cancer and other diseases. Int J Occup Environ Health 2005;11:356–359.
364. Carel R, Boffetta P, Kauppinen T, et al. Exposure to asbestos and lung and pleural cancer mortality among pulp and paper industry workers. J Occup Environ Med 2002;44:579–584.
365. Henderson DW, de Klerk NH, Hammar SP, et al. Asbestos and lung cancer: is it attributable to asbestosis, or to asbestos fiber burden? In: Corrin B, ed. Pathology of lung tumors. New York: Churchill Livingstone, 1997:83–118.
366. Leigh J, Davidson P, Hendrie L, Berry D. Malignant mesothelioma in Australia, 1945–2000. Am J Ind Med 2002;41:188–201.
367. National Industrial Chemicals Notification and Assessment Scheme (NICNAS) (Australia). Full public report: chrysotile asbestos—priority existing chemical no. 9. NICNAS; National Occupational Health and Safety Commission (NOHSC). Sydney: Commonwealth of Australia, 1999.
368. Bradford Hill A. The environment and disease: association or causation? Proc R Soc Med 1965;58:295–300.
369. Popper K. The logic of scientific discovery. London: Routledge Classics (originally published as Logic der Forschung in Vienna: Verlag von Julius Springer 1935), 1959/2002.
370. Popper K. Conjectures and refutations: the growth of scientific knowledge. London: Routledge Classics, 1963/2002.
371. Kamp DW, Weitzman SA. The molecular basis of asbestos induced lung injury. Thorax 1999;54:638–652.
372. Bielefeldt-Ohlmann H, Jarnicki AG, Fitzpatrick DR. Molecular pathobiology and immunology of malignant mesothelioma. J Pathol 1996;178:369–378.
373. McLaren BR, Robinson BWS. The molecular pathogenesis of mesothelioma. In: Robinson BWS, Chahinian AP, eds. Mesothelioma. London: Martin Dunitz, 2002:307–323.
374. Ramos-Nino ME, Testa JR, Altomare DA, et al. Cellular and molecular parameters of mesothelioma. J Cell Biochem 2006;98:723–734.
375. Vogelstein B, Lane D, Levine AJ. Surfing the p53 network. Nature 2000;408:307–310.
376. Cugell DW, Kamp DW. Asbestos and the pleura: a review. Chest 2004;125:1103–1117.
377. Manning CB, Vallyathan V, Mossman BT. Diseases caused by asbestos: mechanisms of injury and disease development. Int Immunopharmacol 2002;2:191–200.
378. Schins RP. Mechanisms of genotoxicity of particles and fibers. Inhal Toxicol 2002;14:57–78.
379. Hesterberg TW, Barrett JC. Induction by asbestos fibers of anaphase abnormalities: mechanism for aneuploidy induction and possibly carcinogenesis. Carcinogenesis 1985;6:473–475.
380. Dopp E, Schiffmann D. Analysis of chromosomal alterations induced by asbestos and ceramic fibers. Toxicol Lett 1998;96–97:155–162.
381. Oloffson K, Mark J. Specificity of asbestos-induces chromosomal abnormalities in short term cultured human mesothelial cells. Cancer Genet Cytogenet 1989;41: 33–39.
382. Jaurand MC. Mechanisms of fiber-induced genotoxicity. Environ Health Perspect 1997;105:1073–1084.
383. Stanton MF, Layard M, Tegeris A, et al. Carcinogenicity of fibrous glass: pleural response in the rat in relation to fiber dimension. J Natl Cancer Inst 1977;58: 587–603.
384. Kamp DW, Greenberger MJ, Sbalchierro JS, et al. Cigarette smoke augments asbestos-induced alveolar epithelial cell injury: role of free radicals. Free Radic Biol Med 1998;25:728–739.
385. Unfried K, Schurkes C, Abel J. Distinct spectrum of mutations induced by crocidolite asbestos: clue for 8-hydroxydeoxyguanosine-dependent mutagenesis in vivo. Cancer Res 2002;62:99–104.
386. Fach E, Kristovich R, Long JF, et al. The effect of iron on the biological activities of erionite and mordenite. Environ Int 2003;29:451–458.
387. Ruotsalainen M, Hirvonen MR, Luoto K, Savolainen KM. Production of reactive oxygen species by man-made vitreous fibres in human polymorphonuclear leukocytes. Hum Exp Toxicol 1999;18:354–362.
388. Broaddus VC, Yang L, Scavo LM, et al. Crocidolite asbestos induces apoptosis of pleural mesothelial cells: role of reactive oxygen species and poly(ADP-ribosyl) polymerase. Environ Health Perspect 1997;105:1147–1152.
389. Kahlos K, Soini Y, Paakko P, et al. Proliferation, apoptosis, and manganese superoxide dismutase in malignant mesothelioma. Int J Cancer 2000;88:37–43.

390. Broaddus VC, Yang L, Scavo LM, et al. Asbestos induces apoptosis of human and rabbit pleural mesothelial cells via reactive oxygen species. J Clin Invest 1996;98:2050–2059.
391. Narasimhan SR, Yang L, Gerwin BI, Broaddus VC. Resistance of pleural mesothelioma cell lines to apoptosis: relation to expression of Bcl-2 and Bax. Am J Physiol 1998;275:L165–171.
392. Janssen Y, Marsh J, Quinlan T, et al. Activation of early cellular responses by asbestos: induction of c-FOS and c-JUN protooncogene expression in rat pleural mesothelial cells. In: Davis JMG, Jaurand M-C, eds. Cellular and molecular effects of mineral and synthetic dusts and fibres. NATO ASI Series, H85. Berlin: Springer-Verlag; 1994:205–213.
393. Vintman L, Nielsen S, Berner A, et al. Mitogen-activated protein kinase expression and activation does not differentiate benign from malignant mesothelial cells. Cancer 2005;103:2427–2433.
394. Appel JD, Fasy TM, Kohtz DS, et al. Asbestos fibers mediate transformation of monkey cells by exogenous plasmid DNA. Proc Natl Acad Sci USA 1988;85:7670–7674.
395. Tiainen M, Kere J, Tammilehto L, et al. Abnormalities of chromosomes 7 and 22 in human malignant pleural mesothelioma: correlation between Southern blot and cytogenetic analyses. Genes Chromosomes Cancer 1992;4:176–182.
396. Xio S, Li D, Vijg J, et al. Codeletion of p15 and p16 in primary malignant mesothelioma. Oncogene 1995;11:511–515.
397. Kivipensas P, Bjorkqvist AM, Karhu R, et al. Gains and losses of DNA sequences in malignant mesothelioma by comparative genomic hybridization. Cancer Genet Cytogenet 1996;89:7–13.
398. Cheng JQ, Jhanwar SC, Klein WM, et al. p16 alterations and deletion mapping of 9p21–p22 in malignant mesothelioma. Cancer Res 1994;54:5547–5551.
399. Both K, Turner DR, Henderson DW. Loss of heterozygosity in asbestos-induced mutations in a human mesothelioma cell line. Environ Mol Mutagen 1995;26:67–71.
400. Lee WC, Testa JR. Somatic genetic alterations in human malignant mesothelioma. Int J Oncol 1999;14:181–188.
401. Bjorkqvist AM, Wolf M, Nordling S, et al. Deletions at 14q in malignant mesothelioma detected by microsatellite marker analysis. Br J Cancer 1999;81:1111–1115.
402. Simon F, Johnen G, Krismann M, Muller KM. Chromosomal alterations in early stages of malignant mesotheliomas. Virchows Arch 2005;447:762–767.
403. Sekido Y, Pass HI, Bader S, et al. Neurofibromatosis type 2 (NF2) gene is somatically mutated in mesothelioma but not in lung cancer. Cancer Res 1995;55:1227–1231.
404. Deguen B, Goutebroze L, Giovannini M, et al. Heterogeneity of mesothelioma cell lines as defined by altered genomic structure and expression of the NF2 gene. Int J Cancer 1998;77:554–560.
405. Bianchi AB, Mitsunaga SI, Cheng JQ, et al. High frequency of inactivating mutations in the neurofibromatosis type 2 gene (NF2) in primary malignant mesotheliomas. Proc Natl Acad Sci USA 1995;92:10854–10858.
406. Kleymenova EV, Bianchi AA, Kley N, et al. Characterization of the rat neurofibromatosis 2 gene and its involvement in asbestos-induced mesothelioma. Mol Carcinog 1997;18:54–60.
407. Gusella JF, Ramesh V, MacCollin M, Jacoby LB. Merlin: the neurofibromatosis 2 tumor suppressor. Biochim Biophys Acta 1999;1423:M29–36.
408. Rihn B, Coulais C, Kauffer E, et al. Inhaled crocidolite mutagenicity in lung DNA. Environ Health Perspect 2000;108:341–346.
409. Papp T, Schipper H, Pemsel H, et al. Mutational analysis of N-ras, p53, p16INK4a, p14ARF and CDK4 genes in primary human malignant mesotheliomas. Int J Oncol 2001;18:425–433.
410. Ni Z, Liu Y, Keshava N, et al. Analysis of K-ras and p53 mutations in mesotheliomas from humans and rats exposed to asbestos. Mutat Res 2000;468:87–92.
411. Yang CT, You L, Lin YC, et al. A comparison analysis of anti-tumor efficacy of adenoviral gene replacement therapy (p14ARF and p16INK4A) in human mesothelioma cells. Anticancer Res 2003;23:33–38.
412. Yang CT, You L, Uematsu K, et al. P14(ARF) modulates the cytolytic effect of ONYX-015 in mesothelioma cells with wild-type p53. Cancer Res 2001;61:5959–5963.
413. Yang CT, You L, Yeh CC, et al. Adenovirus-mediated p14(ARF) gene transfer in human mesothelioma cells. J Natl Cancer Inst 2000;92:636–641.
414. Frizelle SP, Grim J, Zhou J, et al. Re-expression of p16INK4a in mesothelioma cells results in cell cycle arrest, cell death, tumor suppression and tumor regression. Oncogene 1998;16:3087–3095.
415. Ortega A, Malumbres M, Barbacid M. Cyclin D-dependent kinases, INK4 inhibitors and cancer. Biochim Biophys Acta 2002;1602:73–87.
416. Baldi A, Groeger AM, Esposito V, et al. Expression of p21 in SV40 large T antigen positive human pleural mesothelioma: relationship with survival. Thorax 2002;57:353–356.
417. Hirvonen A, Mattson K, Karjalainen A, et al. Simian virus 40 (SV40)-like DNA sequences not detectable in Finnish mesothelioma patients not exposed to SV40–contaminated polio vaccines. Mol Carcinog 1999;26:93–99.
418. Pilatte Y, Vivo C, Renier A, et al. Absence of SV40 large T-antigen expression in human mesothelioma cell lines. Am J Respir Cell Mol Biol 2000;23:788–793.
419. Carbone M, Rizzo P, Powers A, et al. Molecular analyses, morphology and immunohistochemistry together differentiate pleural synovial sarcomas from mesotheliomas: clinical implications. Anticancer Res 2002;22:3443–3448.
420. Carbone M, Rizzo P, Procopio A, et al. SV40–like sequences in human bone tumors. Oncogene 1996;13:527–535.
421. Butel JS, Lednicky JA, Stewart AR, et al. SV40 and human brain tumors. J Neurovirol 1997;1:S78–79.
422. Strickler HD, Rosenberg PS, Devesa SS, et al. Contamination of poliovirus vaccines with simian virus 40 (1955–1963) and subsequent cancer rates. JAMA 1998;279:292–295.
423. Olin P, Giesecke J. Potential exposure to SV40 in polio vaccines used in Sweden during 1957: no impact on cancer

incidence rates 1960 to 1993. Dev Biol Stand 1998;94: 227–233.
424. Shah KV. SV40 and human cancer: a review of recent data. Int J Cancer 2006;120:215–223.
425. Cicala C, Pompetti F, Carbone M. SV40 induces mesotheliomas in hamsters. Am J Pathol 1993;142:1524–1533.
426. Ke Y, Reddel RR, Gerwin BI, et al. Establishment of a human in vitro mesothelial cell model system for investigating mechanisms of asbestos-induced mesothelioma. Am J Pathol 1989;134:979–991.
427. Wang Y, Faux SP, Hallden G, et al. Interleukin-1beta and tumour necrosis factor-alpha promote the transformation of human immortalised mesothelial cells by erionite. Int J Oncol 2004;25:173–178.
428. Whitson BA, Kratzke RA. Molecular pathways in malignant pleural mesothelioma. Cancer Lett 2006;239: 183–189.
429. Strizzi L, Vianale G, Giuliano M, et al. SV40, JC and BK expression in tissue, urine and blood samples from patients with malignant and nonmalignant pleural disease. Anticancer Res 2000;20:885–889.
430. Catalano A, Romano M, Martinotti S, Procopio A. Enhanced expression of vascular endothelial growth factor (VEGF) plays a critical role in the tumor progression potential induced by simian virus 40 large T antigen. Oncogene 2002;21:2896–2900.
431. Mossman BT, Gruenert DC. SV40, growth factors, and mesothelioma: another piece of the puzzle. Am J Respir Cell Mol Biol 2002;26:167–170.
432. Strizzi L, Catalano A, Vianale G, et al. Vascular endothelial growth factor is an autocrine growth factor in human malignant mesothelioma. J Pathol 2001;193:468–475.
433. Kumar P, Kratzke RA. Molecular prognostic markers in malignant mesothelioma. Lung Cancer 2005;49: S53–60.
434. Kumar-Singh S, Weyler J, Martin MJ, et al. Angiogenic cytokines in mesothelioma: a study of VEGF, FGF-1 and -2, and TGF beta expression. J Pathol 1999;189:72–78.
435. Little M, Wells C. A clinical overview of WT1 gene mutations. Hum Mutat 1997;9:209–225.
436. Oates J, Edwards C. HBME-1, MOC-31, WT1 and calretinin: an assessment of recently described markers for mesothelioma and adenocarcinoma. Histopathology 2000;36:341–347.
437. Thorner P, Squire J, Plavsic N, et al. Expression of WT1 in pediatric small cell tumors: report of two cases with a possible mesothelial origin. Pediatr Dev Pathol 1999;2: 33–41.
438. Hoffmann R, Valencia A. A gene network for navigating the literature. Nature Genet 2004;36:664.
439. Maheswaran S, Park S, Bernard A, et al. Physical and functional interaction between Wt1 and p53 proteins. Proc Natl Acad Sci USA 1993;90:5100–5104.
440. Kumar-Singh S, Segers K, Rodeck U, et al. WT1 mutation in malignant mesothelioma and WT1 immunoreactivity in relation to p53 and growth factor receptor expression, cell-type transition, and prognosis. J Pathol 1997;181: 67–74.
441. Carbone M, Kratzke RA, Testa JR. The pathogenesis of mesothelioma. Semin Oncol 2002;29:2–17.
442. Xiao GH, Beeser A, Chernoff J, Testa JR. P21-activated kinase links Rac/Cdc42 signaling to merlin. J Biol Chem 2002;277:883–886.
443. Knudson A. Asbestos and mesothelioma: genetic lessons from a tragedy. Proc Natl Acad Sci USA 1995;92: 10819–10820.
444. Sozzi G, Sard L, De Gregorio L, et al. Association between cigarette smoking and FHIT gene alterations in lung cancer. Cancer Res 1997;57:2121–2123.
445. Nelson HH, Wiencke JK, Gunn L, et al. Chromosome 3p14 alterations in lung cancer: evidence that FHIT exon deletion is a target of tobacco carcinogens and asbestos. Cancer Res 1998;58:1804–1807.
446. Croce CM, Sozzi G, Huebner K. Role of FHIT in human cancer. J Clin Oncol 1999;17:1618–1624.
447. Cai YC, Roggli V, Mark E, et al. Transforming growth factor alpha and epidermal growth factor receptor in reactive and malignant mesothelial proliferations. Arch Pathol Lab Med 2004;128:68–70.
448. Destro A, Ceresoli GL, Falleni M, et al. EGFR overexpression in malignant pleural mesothelioma: an immunohistochemical and molecular study with clinicopathological correlations. Lung Cancer 2006;51:207–215.
449. Cesario A, Catassi A, Festi L, et al. Farnesyltransferase inhibitors and human malignant pleural mesothelioma: a first-step comparative translational study. Clin Cancer Res 2005;11:2026–2037.
450. Zanella CL, Posada J, Tritton TR, Mossman BT. Asbestos causes stimulation of the extracellular signal-regulated kinase 1 mitogen-activated protein kinase cascade after phosphorylation of the epidermal growth factor receptor. Cancer Res 1996;56:5334–5338.
451. Walker C, Everitt J, Ferriola PC, et al. Autocrine growth stimulation by transforming growth factor alpha in asbestos-transformed rat mesothelial cells. Cancer Res 1995;55:530–536.
452. Faux SP, Houghton CE, Hubbard A, Patrick G. Increased expression of epidermal growth factor receptor in rat pleural mesothelial cells correlates with carcinogenicity of mineral fibres. Carcinogenesis 2000;21:2275–2280.
453. Pache JC, Janssen YM, Walsh ES, et al. Increased epidermal growth factor-receptor protein in a human mesothelial cell line in response to long asbestos fibers. Am J Pathol 1998;152:333–340.
454. Janne PA, Taffaro ML, Salgia R, Johnson BE. Inhibition of epidermal growth factor receptor signaling in malignant pleural mesothelioma. Cancer Res 2002;62: 5242–5247.
455. Liu Z, Klominek J. Inhibition of proliferation, migration, and matrix metalloprotease production in malignant mesothelioma cells by tyrosine kinase inhibitors. Neoplasia 2004;6:705–712.
456. Mukohara T, Civiello G, Johnson BE, Janne PA. Therapeutic targeting of multiple signaling pathways in malignant pleural mesothelioma. Oncology 2005;68:500–510.
457. She Y, Lee F, Chen J, et al. The epidermal growth factor receptor tyrosine kinase inhibitor ZD1839 selectively potentiates radiation response of human tumors in nude mice, with a marked improvement in therapeutic index. Clin Cancer Res 2003;9:3773–3778.

458. Kari C, Chan TO, Rocha de Quadros M, Rodeck U. Targeting the epidermal growth factor receptor in cancer: apoptosis takes center stage. Cancer Res 2003;63:1–5.
459. Govindan R, Kratzke RA, Herndon JE, 2nd, et al. Gefitinib in patients with malignant mesothelioma: a phase II study by the Cancer and Leukemia Group B. Clin Cancer Res 2005;11:2300–2304.
460. Porta C, Mutti L, Tassi G. Negative results of an Italian Group for Mesothelioma (G.I.Me.) pilot study of single-agent imatinib mesylate in malignant pleural mesothelioma. Cancer Chemother Pharmacol 2007;59:149–150.
461. Baldi A, Santini D, Vasaturo F, et al. Prognostic significance of cyclooxygenase-2 (COX-2) and expression of cell cycle inhibitors p21 and p27 in human pleural malignant mesothelioma. Thorax 2004;59:428–433.
462. Cardillo I, Spugnini EP, Verdina A, et al. Cox and mesothelioma: an overview. Histol Histopathol 2004;20: 1267–1274.
463. Edwards JG, Faux SP, Plummer SM, et al. Cyclooxygenase-2 expression is a novel prognostic factor in malignant mesothelioma. Clin Cancer Res 2002;8:1857–1862.
464. O'Kane SL, Cawkwell L, Campbell A, Lind MJ. Cyclooxygenase-2 expression predicts survival in malignant pleural mesothelioma. Eur J Cancer 2005;41:1645–1648.
465. Edwards JG, Swinson DE, Jones JL, et al. EGFR expression: associations with outcome and clinicopathological variables in malignant pleural mesothelioma. Lung Cancer 2006;54:399–407.
466. Marrogi A, Pass HI, Khan M, et al. Human mesothelioma samples overexpress both cyclooxygenase-2 (COX-2) and inducible nitric oxide synthase (NOS2): in vitro antiproliferative effects of a COX-2 inhibitor. Cancer Res 2000;60:3696–3700.
467. Catalano A, Graciotti L, Rinaldi L, et al. Preclinical evaluation of the nonsteroidal anti-inflammatory agent celecoxib on malignant mesothelioma chemoprevention. Int J Cancer 2004;109:322–328.
468. Ohta Y, Shridhar V, Bright RK, et al. VEGF and VEGF type C play an important role in angiogenesis and lymphangiogenesis in human malignant mesothelioma tumours. Br J Cancer 1999;81:54–61.
469. Konig JE, Tolnay E, Wiethege T, Muller KM. Expression of vascular endothelial growth factor in diffuse malignant pleural mesothelioma. Virchows Archiv 1999;435:8–12.
470. Demirag F, Unsal E, Yilmaz A, Caglar A. Prognostic significance of vascular endothelial growth factor, tumor necrosis, and mitotic activity index in malignant pleural mesothelioma. Chest 2005;128:3382–3387.
471. Aoe K, Hiraki A, Tanaka T, et al. Expression of vascular endothelial growth factor in malignant mesothelioma. Anticancer Res 2006;26:4833–4836.
472. Konig J, Tolnay E, Wiethege T, Muller K. Co-expression of vascular endothelial growth factor and its receptor flt-1 in malignant pleural mesothelioma. Respiration 2000;67: 36–40.
473. Masood R, Kundra A, Zhu ST, et al. Malignant mesothelioma growth inhibition by agents that target the VEGF and VEGF-C autocrine loops. Int J Cancer 2003;104: 603–610.
474. Cacciotti P, Strizzi L, Vianale G, et al. The presence of simian-virus 40 sequences in mesothelioma and mesothelial cells is associated with high levels of vascular endothelial growth factor. Am J Respir Cell Mol Biol 2002;26:189–193.
475. Partanen R, Koskinen H, Hemminki K. Tumour necrosis factor-alpha (TNF-alpha) in patients who have asbestosis and develop cancer. Occup Environ Med 1995;52:316–319.
476. Yang H, Bocchetta M, Kroczynska B, et al. TNF-α inhibits asbestos-induced cytotoxicity via a NF-κB-dependent pathway, a possible mechanism for asbestos-induced oncogenesis. Proc Natl Acad Sci USA 2006;103:10397–10402.
477. Donaldson K, Li XY, Dogra S, et al. Asbestos-stimulated tumour necrosis factor release from alveolar macrophages depends on fibre length and opsonization. J Pathol 1992;168:243–248.
478. Falleni M, Pellegrini C, Marchetti A, et al. Quantitative evaluation of the apoptosis regulating genes Survivin, Bcl-2 and Bax in inflammatory and malignant pleural lesions. Lung Cancer 2005;48:211–216.
479. Gordon G, Mani M, Mukhopadhyay L, et al. Expression patterns of inhibitor of apoptosis proteins in malignant pleural mesothelioma. J Pathol 2007;211:447–454.
480. Gordon G, Mani M, Mukhopadhyay L, et al. Inhibitor of apoptosis proteins are regulated by tumour necrosis factor-alpha in malignant pleural mesothelioma. J Pathol 2007;211:439–446.
481. Liu Z, Ivanoff A, Klominek J. Expression and activity of matrix metalloproteases in human malignant mesothelioma cell lines. Int J Cancer 2001;91:638–643.
482. Zhong J, Gencay MM, Bubendorf L, et al. ERK1/2 and p38 MAP kinase control MMP-2, MT1–MMP, and TIMP action and affect cell migration: a comparison between mesothelioma and mesothelial cells. J Cell Physiol 2006; 207:540–552.
483. Hirano H, Tsuji M, Kizaki T, et al. Expression of matrix metalloproteinases, tissue inhibitors of metalloproteinase, collagens, and Ki67 antigen in pleural malignant mesothelioma: an immunohistochemical and electron microscopic study. Med Electron Microsc 2002;35:16–23.
484. Edwards JG, McLaren J, Jones JL, et al. Matrix metalloproteinases 2 and 9 (gelatinases A and B) expression in malignant mesothelioma and benign pleura. Br J Cancer 2003;88:1553–1559.
485. Liu Z, Klominek J. Regulation of matrix metalloprotease activity in malignant mesothelioma cell lines by growth factors. Thorax 2003;58:198–203.
486. Hoang CD, D'Cunha J, Kratzke MG, et al. Gene expression profiling identifies matriptase overexpression in malignant mesothelioma. Chest 2004;125:1843–1852.
487. Versnel MA, Hagemeijer A, Bouts MJ, et al. Expression of c-sis (PDGF B-chain) and PDGF A-chain genes in ten human malignant mesothelioma cells lines derived from primary and metastatic tumors. Oncogene 1988;2: 601–605.
488. Versnel MA, Claesson-Welch L, Hammacher A, et al. Human malignant mesothelioma cell lines express PDGF β-receptors whereas cultured normal mesothelial cells

express predominantly PDGF α-receptors. Oncogene 1991;6:2005–2011.
489. Whitaker D, Henderson DW, Shilkin KB. The concept of mesothelioma in situ: implications for diagnosis and histogenesis. Semin Diagn Pathol 1992;9:151–161.
490. Henderson DW, Shilkin KB, Whitaker D. Reactive mesothelial hyperplasia vs mesothelioma, including mesothelioma in situ: a brief review. Am J Clin Pathol 1998;110: 397–404.
491. Whitaker D, Papadimitriou JM, Walters MN-I. The mesothelium and its reactions: a review. CRC Crit Rev Toxicol 1982;10:81–144.
492. Whitaker D, Papadimitriou JM. Mesothelial healing: morphological and kinetic investigations. J Pathol 1985;145: 159–175.
493. Whitaker D, Manning LS, Robinson BW, Shilkin KB. The pathobiology of the mesothelium. In: Henderson DW, Shilkin KB, Langlois SL, Whitaker D, eds. Malignant mesothelioma. New York: Hemisphere, 1992:25–68.
494. Mutsaers SE, Whitaker D, Papadimitriou J. Stimulation of mesothelial healing by exudate macrophages enhances serosal wound healing in a murine model. Am J Pathol 2002;160:680–692.
495. Whitaker D. The mesothelium of the rat and its response to injury. Thesis, University of Western Australia, 1983.
496. Catalano A, Romano M, Robuffo I, et al. Methionine aminopeptidase-2 regulates human mesothelioma cell survival: role of Bcl-2 expression and telomerase activity. Am J Pathol 2001;159:721–731.
497. McCaughey WTE. Criteria for the diagnosis of diffuse mesothelial tumors. Ann NY Acad Sci 1965;132:603–613.
498. Kannerstein M, McCaughey WEE, Churg J, Selikoff IJ. A critique for the diagnosis of diffuse malignant mesothelioma. Mt Sinai J Med (NY) 1977;44:485–494.
499. Kannerstein M, Churg J, McCaughey WTE. Asbestos and mesothelioma: a review. Pathol Annu 1978:81–130.
500. Adams VI, Unni KK. Diffuse malignant mesothelioma of pleura: diagnostic criteria based on an autopsy study. Am J Clin Pathol 1984;82:15–23.
501. McCaughey WTE, Kannerstein M, Churg J. Tumors of the serous membranes. Washington, DC: Armed Forces Institute of Pathology, 1985.
502. Battifora H, McCaughey WTE. Tumors of the serosal membranes. Washington, DC: Armed Forces Institute of Pathology, 1994.
503. Churg A, Cagle PT, Roggli VL. Tumors of the Serosal Membranes. Washington DC: American Registry of Pathology/Armed Forces Institute of Pathology, 2006.
504. Hammar SP, et al. Round cell mesotheliomas with an emphasis on deciduoid mesothelioma. Submitted for publication.
505. Hammar SP, Bockus DE, Remington FL, Rohrbach KA. Mucin-positive epithelial mesotheliomas: a histochemical, immunohistochemical and ultrastructural comparison with mucin-producing pulmonary adenocarcinomas. Ultra Pathol 1996;20:293–325.
506. Ordóñez NG, Myhre M, Mackay B. Clear cell mesothelioma. Ultrastruct Pathol 1996;20:331–336.
507. Sporn TA, Roggli VL. Mesothelioma. In: Roggli VL, Oury TD, Sporn TA, eds. Pathology of asbestos-associated diseases, 2nd ed. New York: Springer, 2004:104–168.
508. Mayall FG, Goddard H, Gibbs AR. Intermediate filament expression in mesotheliomas: leiomyoid mesotheliomas are not uncommon. Histopathology 1992;21:453–457.
509. Battifora H. Leiomyoid mesotheliomas [letter]. Histopathology 1993;21:601.
510. Churg A, Roggli V, Galateau-Sallé F, et al. Mesothelioma. In: Travis WD, Brambilla E, Müller-Hermelink HK, Harris C, eds. Pathology and genetics of tumours of the lung, pleura, thymus and heart. Lyon: IARC, 2004:128–136.
511. Attanoos RL, Dojcinov SD, Webb R, Gibbs AR. Anti-mesothelial markers in sarcomatoid mesothelioma and other spindle cell neoplasms. Histopathology 2000; 37:224–231.
512. Hinterberger M, Reineke T, Storz M, et al. D2–40 and calretinin—a tissue microarray analysis of 341 malignant mesotheliomas with emphasis on sarcomatoid differentiation. Mod Pathol 2007;20:248–255.
513. Churg A, Colby TV, Cagle P, et al. The separation of benign and malignant mesothelial proliferations. Am J Surg Pathol 2000;24:1183–1200.
514. Montag AG, Pinkus GS, Corson JM. Keratin protein immunoreactivity of sarcomatoid and mixed types of diffuse malignant mesothelioma: an immunoperoxidase study of 30 cases. Hum Pathol 1988;19:336–342.
515. Battifora H. The pleura. In: Sternberg SS, ed. Diagnostic surgical pathology. New York: Raven Press, 1989:829–855.
516. Roggli VL, Kolbeck J, Sanfilippo F, Shelburne JD. Pathology of human mesothelioma: etiologic and diagnostic considerations. Pathol Annu 1987;22:91–131.
517. McCaughey WTE, Dardick I, Barr JR. Angiosarcoma of serous membranes. Arch Pathol Lab Med 1983;107: 304–307.
518. Falconieri G, Bussani R, Mirra M, Zanella M. Pseudomesotheliomatous angiosarcoma: a pleuropulmonary lesion simulating malignant pleural mesothelioma. Histopathology 1997;30:419–424.
519. Zhang PJ, Livolsi VA, Brooks JJ. Malignant epithelioid vascular tumors of the pleura: report of a series and literature review. Hum Pathol 2000;31:29–34.
520. Yousem SA, Hochholzer L. Malignant mesotheliomas with osseous and cartilaginous differentiation. Arch Pathol Lab Med 1987;111:62–66.
521. Gaertner E, Zeren EH, Fleming MV, et al. Biphasic synovial sarcomas arising in the pleural cavity: a clinicopathologic study of five cases. Am J Surg Pathol 1996;20: 36–45.
522. Jawahar DA, Vuletin JC, Gorecki P, et al. Primary biphasic synovial sarcoma of the pleura. Respir Med 1997;91: 568–570.
523. Nicholson AG, Goldstraw P, Fisher C. Synovial sarcoma of the pleura and its differentiation from other primary pleural tumours: a clinicopathological and immunohistochemical review of three cases. Histopathology 1998;33: 508–513.
524. Caliandro R, Terrier P, Regnard JF, et al. Primary biphasic synovial sarcoma of the pleura [Fr]. Rev Mal Respir 2000; 17:498–502.

525. Cappello F, Barnes L. Synovial sarcoma and malignant mesothelioma of the pleura: review, differential diagnosis and possible role of apoptosis. Pathology 2001;33:142–148.
526. Bégueret H, Galateau-Sallé F, Guillou L, et al. Primary intrathoracic synovial sarcoma: a clinicopathologic study of 40 t(X;18)-positive cases from the French Sarcoma Group and the Mesopath Group. Am J Surg Pathol 2005;29:339–346.
527. Miettinen M, Limon J, Niezabitowski A, Lasota J. Calretinin and other mesothelioma markers in synovial sarcoma: analysis of antigenic similarities and differences with malignant mesothelioma. Am J Surg Pathol 2001; 25:610–617.
528. Dos Santos NR, de Bruijn DR, Balemans M, et al. Nuclear localization of SYT, SSX and the synovial sarcoma-associated SYT-SSX fusion proteins. Hum Mol Genet 1997;6:1549–1558.
529. De Leeuw B, Balemans M, Olde Weghuis D, Geurts van Kessel A. Identification of two alternative fusion genes, SYT-SSX1 and SYT-SSX2, in t(X;18)(p11.2;q11.2)-positive synovial sarcomas. Hum Mol Genet 1995;4: 1097–1099.
530. Brett D, Whitehouse S, Antonson P, et al. The SYT protein involved in the t(X;18) synovial sarcoma translocation is a transcriptional activator localised in nuclear bodies. Hum Mol Genet 1997;6:1559–1564.
531. Argani P, Zakowski MF, Klimstra DS, et al. Detection of the SYT-SSX chimeric RNA of synovial sarcoma in paraffin-embedded tissue and its application in problematic cases. Mod Pathol 1998;11:65–71.
532. Mayall FG, Gibbs AR. "Pleural" and pulmonary carcinosarcomas. J Pathol 1992;167:305–311.
533. Colby TV, Koss MN, Travis WD. Tumors of the lower respiratory tract. Washington, DC: Armed Forces Institute of Pathology, 1995.
534. Travis WD, Colby TV, Corrin B. Histological typing of lung and pleural tumours, 3rd ed. Berlin: Springer, 1999.
535. Hansen T, Bittinger F, Kortsik C, et al. Expression of KIT (CD117) in biphasic pulmonary blastoma: novel data on histogenesis. Lung 2003;181:193–200.
536. Bolen JW, Hammar SP, McNutt MA. Reactive and neoplastic serosal tissue: a light-microscopic, ultrastructural and immunocytochemical study. Am J Surg Pathol 1986;10:34–47.
537. Dardick I, Al-Jabi M, McCaughey WTE, Srigley JR, van Nostrand AWP, Ritchie AC. Ultrastructure of poorly differentiated diffuse epithelial mesotheliomas. Ultrastruct Pathol 1984;7:151–160.
538. Cook HC. Carbohydrates. In: Bancroft JD, Stevens A, eds. Theory and practice of histological techniques. New York: Churchill Livingstone, 1982:180–216.
539. MacDougall DB, Wang SE, Zibar BL. Mucin-positive epithelial mesothelioma. Arch Pathol Lab Med 1992;116: 874–880.
540. Friedman HD, Litovsky SH, Abraham JL. Mucin-positive epithelial mesothelioma and pseudomesotheliomatous adenocarcinoma [letter; comment]. Arch Pathol Lab Med 1993;117:967.
541. Battifora H. Mesothelioma versus carcinoma: getting easier? Hum Pathol 2005;36:1153.
542. King JE, Galateau-Sallé F, Hasleton P. Histopathology of malignant pleural mesothelioma. In: O'Byrne K, Rusch V, eds. Malignant pleural mesothelioma. Oxford: Oxford University Press, 2006:61–103.
543. Bedrossian CWM, Bonsib S, Moran C. Differential diagnosis between mesothelioma and adenocarcinoma: a multimodal approach based on ultrastructure and immunocytochemistry. Semin Diagn Pathol 1992;9:124–140.
544. Betta P. Immunohistochemistry. In: Pass H, Vogelzang NJ, Carbone M, eds. Malignant mesothelioma. New York: Springer, 2005:490–507.
545. Coleman M, Henderson DW, Mukherjee TM. The ultrastructural pathology of malignant pleural mesothelioma. Pathol Annu 1989;24:303–353.
546. Lucas DR, Pass HI, Madan SK, et al. Sarcomatoid mesothelioma and its histologic mimics: a comparative immunohistochemical study. Histopathology 2003;42:270–279.
547. King JE, Thatcher N, Pickering CA, Hasleton PS. Sensitivity and specificity of immunohistochemical markers used in the diagnosis of epithelioid mesothelioma: a detailed systematic analysis using published data. Histopathology 2006;48:223–232.
548. Lumb PD, Suvarna SK. Metastasis in pleural mesothelioma: immunohistochemical markers for disseminated disease. Histopathology 2004;44:345–352.
549. Beer TW, Buchanan R, Matthews AW, et al. Prognosis in malignant mesothelioma related to MIB 1 proliferation index and histological subtype. Hum Pathol 1998;29: 246–251.
550. Comin CE, Anichini C, Boddi V, et al. MIB-1 proliferation index correlates with survival in pleural malignant mesothelioma. Histopathology 2000;36:26–31.
551. Leonardo E, Zanconati F, Bonifacio D, Bonito LD. Immunohistochemical MIB-1 and p27kip1 as prognostic factors in pleural mesothelioma. Pathol Res Pract 2001; 197:253–256.
552. Trupiano JK, Geisinger KR, Willingham MC, et al. Diffuse malignant mesothelioma of the peritoneum and pleura: analysis of markers. Mod Pathol 2004;17:476–481.
553. Bongiovanni M, Cassoni P, De Giuli P, et al. P27(kip1) immunoreactivity correlates with long-term survival in pleural malignant mesothelioma. Cancer 2001;92:1245–1250.
554. Beer TW, Shepherd P, Pullinger NC. P27 immunostaining is related to prognosis in malignant mesothelioma. Histopathology 2001;38:535–541.
555. Betta PG, Andrion A, Donna A, et al. Malignant mesothelioma of the pleura: the reproducibility of the immunohistological diagnosis. Pathol Res Pract 1997;193: 759–765.
556. Chang K, Pai HL, Batra J, et al. Characterization of the antigen (CAK1) recognized by monoclonal antibody K1 that is present on ovarian cancers and normal mesothelium. Cancer Res 1992;52:181–186.
557. Chang K, Pai LH, Pass H, et al. Monoclonal antibody K1 reacts with epithelial mesothelioma but not with lung adenocarcinoma. Am J Surg Pathol 1992;16:259–268.
558. O'Hara CJ, Corson JM, Pinkus GS, et al. ME1 a monoclonal antibody that distinguishes epithelial-type malignant mesothelioma from pulmonary adenocarcinoma

and extrapulmonary malignancies. Am J Pathol 1990; 136:421–428.
559. Abutaily AS, Addis BJ, Roche WR. Immunohistochemistry in the distinction between malignant mesothelioma and pulmonary adenocarcinoma: a critical evaluation of new antibodies. J Clin Pathol 2002;55:662–668.
560. Simsir A, Fetsch P, Mehta D, et al. E-cadherin, N-cadherin, and calretinin in pleural effusions: the good, the bad, the worthless. Diagn Cytopathol 1999;20:125–130.
561. Wieczorek TJ, Krane JF. Diagnostic utility of calretinin immunohistochemistry in cytologic cell block preparations. Cancer 2000;90:312–319.
562. Kitazume H, Kitamura K, Mukai K, et al. Cytologic differential diagnosis among reactive mesothelial cells, malignant mesothelioma, and adenocarcinoma: utility of combined E-cadherin and calretinin immunostaining. Cancer 2000;90:55–60.
563. Yaziji H, Battifora H, Barry TS, et al. Evaluation of 12 antibodies for distinguishing epithelioid mesothelioma from adenocarcinoma: identification of a three-antibody immunohistochemical panel with maximal sensitivity and specificity. Mod Pathol 2006;19:514–523.
564. Ordóñez NG. Role of immunohistochemistry in distinguishing epithelial peritoneal mesotheliomas from peritoneal and ovarian serous carcinomas. Am J Surg Pathol 1998;22:1203–1214.
565. Roberts F, McCall AE, Burnett RA. Malignant mesothelioma: a comparison of biopsy and postmortem material by light microscopy and immunohistochemistry. J Clin Pathol 2001;54:766–770.
566. Fetsch PA, Simsir A, Abati A. Comparison of antibodies to HBME-1 and calretinin for the detection of mesothelial cells in effusion cytology. Diagn Cytopathol 2001; 25:158–161.
567. Attanoos RL, Webb R, Dojcinov SD, Gibbs AR. Value of mesothelial and epithelial antibodies in distinguishing diffuse peritoneal mesothelioma in females from serous papillary carcinoma of the ovary and peritoneum. Histopathology 2002;40:237–244.
568. Ordóñez NG. The value of antibodies 44-3A6, SM3, HBME-1, and thrombomodulin in differentiating epithelial pleural mesothelioma from lung adenocarcinoma: a comparative study with other commonly used antibodies. Am J Surg Pathol 1997;21:1399–1408.
569. Riera JR, Astengo-Osuna C, Longmate JA, Battifora H. The immunohistochemical diagnostic panel for epithelial mesothelioma: a reevaluation after heat-induced epitope retrieval. Am J Surg Pathol 1997;21:1409–1419.
570. Wick MR. Immunophenotyping of malignant mesothelioma. Am J Surg Pathol 1997;21:1395–1398.
571. Zimmerman RL. There's madness in the methods. Diagn Cytopathol 2005;32:183–184.
572. Fetsch P, Simsir A, Abati A. There may be "madness in the methods" but the devil is in the detail. Diagn Cytopathol 2005;34:590–593.
573. Zimmerman RL. Response to Dr. Abati's letter to the editor. Diagn Cytopathol 2005;34:594–595.
574. Dejmek A, Hjerpe A. Immunohistochemical reactivity in mesothelioma and adenocarcinoma: a stepwise logistic regression analysis. APMIS 1994;102:255–264.
575. Brockstedt U, Gulyas M, Dobra K, et al. An optimized battery of eight antibodies that can distinguish most cases of epithelial mesothelioma from adenocarcinoma. Am J Clin Pathol 2000;114:203–209.
576. Dejmek A, Hjerpe A. Reactivity of six antibodies in effusions of mesothelioma, adenocarcinoma and mesotheliosis: stepwise logistic regression analysis. Cytopathology 2000;11:8–17.
577. Carella R, Deleonardi G, D'Errico A, et al. Immunohistochemical panels for differentiating epithelial malignant mesothelioma from lung adenocarcinoma: a study with logistic regression analysis. Am J Surg Pathol 2001;25: 43–50.
578. Ordóñez NG. The immunohistochemical diagnosis of epithelial mesothelioma. Hum Pathol 1999;30:313–323.
579. Ordóñez NG. The immunohistochemical diagnosis of mesothelioma: a comparative study of epithelioid mesothelioma and lung adenocarcinoma. Am J Surg Pathol 2003;27:1031–1051.
580. Ordóñez NG. Immunohistochemical diagnosis of epithelioid mesothelioma: an update. Arch Pathol Lab Med 2005;129:1407–1414.
581. Ordóñez NG. What are the current best immunohistochemical markers for the diagnosis of epithelioid mesothelioma? A review and update. Hum Pathol 2007;38:1–16.
582. Frisman DM. Immunoquery. 2006. http://www.ipox.org/login.cfm?IQMessage=1&RequestTimeout=200.
583. Butnor KJ, Sporn TA, Ordóñez NG. Recommendations for the reporting of pleural mesothelioma. Hum Pathol 2007;450:15–23.
584. Billing-Marczak K, Kuznicki J. Calretinin—sensor or buffer—function still unclear. Pol J Pharmacol 1999;51: 173–178.
585. Gotzos V, Vogt P, Celio MR. The calcium binding protein calretinin is a selective marker for malignant pleural mesotheliomas of the epithelial type [published erratum appears in Pathol Res Pract 1996;192:646]. Pathol Res Pract 1996;192:137–147.
586. Tos AP, Doglioni C. Calretinin: a novel tool for diagnostic immunohistochemistry. Adv Anat Pathol 1998;5:61–66.
587. Doglioni C, Tos AP, Laurino L, et al. Calretinin: a novel immunocytochemical marker for mesothelioma. Am J Surg Pathol 1996;20:1037–1046.
588. Comin CE, Novelli L, Boddi V, et al. Calretinin, thrombomodulin, CEA, and CD15: a useful combination of immunohistochemical markers for differentiating pleural epithelial mesothelioma from peripheral pulmonary adenocarcinoma. Hum Pathol 2001;32:529–536.
589. Ordóñez NG. Immunohistochemical diagnosis of epithelioid mesotheliomas: a critical review of old markers, new markers. Hum Pathol 2002;33:953–967.
590. Clover J, Oates J, Edwards C. Anti-cytokeratin 5/6: a positive marker for epithelioid mesothelioma. Histopathology 1997;31:140–143.
591. Ordóñez NG. Value of cytokeratin5/6 in distinguishing epithelial mesothelioma of pleura from lung adenocarcinoma. Am J Surg Pathol 1998;22:1215–1221.
592. Chu PG, Weiss LM. Expression of cytokeratin 5/6 in epithelial neoplasms: an immunohistochemical study of 509 cases. Mod Pathol 2002;15:6–10.

593. Bateman AC, Al-Talib RK, Newman T, et al. Immunohistochemical phenotype of malignant mesothelioma: predictive value of CA125 and HBME-1. Histopathology 1997;30:49–56.
594. Renshaw AA, Pinkus GS, Gorson JM. HBME-1 aids in distinguishing mesotheliomas and adenocarcinomas of the lung and breast. Mod Pathol 1995;8:152A.
595. Gonzalez-Lois C, Ballestin C, Sotelo MT, et al. Combined use of novel epithelial (MOC-31) and mesothelial (HBME-1) immunohistochemical markers for optimal first line diagnostic distinction between mesothelioma and metastatic carcinoma in pleura. Histopathology 2001;38:528–534.
596. Foster MR, Johnson JE, Olson SJ, Allred DC. Immunohistochemical analysis of nuclear versus cytoplasmic staining of WT1 in malignant mesotheliomas and primary pulmonary adenocarcinomas. Arch Pathol Lab Med 2001;125:1316–1320.
597. Gulyas M, Hjerpe A. Proteoglycans and WT1 as markers for distinguishing adenocarcinoma, epithelioid mesothelioma, and benign mesothelium. J Pathol 2003;199: 479–487.
598. Amin KM, Litzky LA, Smythe WR, et al. Wilms' tumor 1 susceptibility (WT1) gene products are selectively expressed in malignant mesothelioma. Am J Pathol 1995; 146:344–356.
599. Hecht JL, Lee BH, Pinkus JL, Pinkus GS. The value of Wilms tumor susceptibility gene 1 in cytologic preparations as a marker for malignant mesothelioma. Cancer 2002;96:105–109.
600. Ordóñez NG. The diagnostic utility of immunohistochemistry in distinguishing between mesothelioma and renal cell carcinoma: a comparative study. Hum Pathol 2004; 35:697–710.
601. Schacht V, Dadras SS, Johnson LA, et al. Up-regulation of the lymphatic marker podoplanin, a mucin-type transmembrane glycoprotein, in human squamous cell carcinomas and germ cell tumors. Am J Pathol 2005;166:913–921.
602. Chu AY, Litzky LA, Pasha TL, et al. Utility of D2–40, a novel mesothelial marker, in the diagnosis of malignant mesothelioma. Mod Pathol 2005;18:105–110.
603. Ordóñez NG. D2–40 and podoplanin are highly specific and sensitive immunohistochemical markers of epithelioid malignant mesothelioma. Hum Pathol 2005;36: 372–380.
604. Muller AM, Franke FE, Muller KM. D2–40: a reliable marker in the diagnosis of pleural mesothelioma. Pathobiology 2006;73:50–54.
605. Bassarova AV, Nesland JM, Davidson B. D2–40 is not a specific marker for cells of mesothelial origin in serous effusions. Am J Surg Pathol 2006;30:878–882.
606. Collins CL, Ordóñez NG, Schaefer R, et al. Thrombomodulin expression in malignant pleural mesothelioma and pulmonary adenocarcinoma. Am J Pathol 1992;141: 827–833.
607. Collins CL, Fink LM, Hsu S-M, et al. Thrombomodulin staining of mesothelioma cells [letter]. Hum Pathol 1992; 23:966.
608. Fink L, Collins CL, Schaefer R, et al. Thrombomodulin expression can be used to differentiate between mesotheliomas and adenocarcinomas. Lab Invest 1992;66: 113A.
609. Cury PM, Butcher DN, Fisher C, et al. Value of the mesothelium-associated antibodies thrombomodulin, cytokeratin 5/6, calretinin, and CD44H in distinguishing epithelioid pleural mesothelioma from adenocarcinoma metastatic to the pleura. Mod Pathol 2000;13:107–112.
610. Chang K, Pastan I, Willingham MC. Isolation and characterization of a monoclonal antibody, K1, reactive with ovarian cancers and normal mesothelium. Int J Cancer 1992;50:373–381.
611. Miettinen M, Sarlomo-Rikala M. Expression of calretinin, thrombomodulin, keratin 5, and mesothelin in lung carcinomas of different types: an immunohistochemical analysis of 596 tumors in comparison with epithelioid mesotheliomas of the pleura. Am J Surg Pathol 2003;27: 150–158.
612. Ordóñez NG. Value of mesothelin immunostaining in the diagnosis of mesothelioma. Mod Pathol 2003;16: 192–197.
613. Galloway ML, Murray D, Moffat DF. The use of the monoclonal antibody mesothelin in the diagnosis of malignant mesothelioma in pleural biopsies. Histopathology 2006;48:767–769.
614. Kachali C, Eltoum I, Horton D, Chhieng DC. Use of mesothelin as a marker for mesothelial cells in cytologic specimens. Semin Diagn Pathol 2006;23:20–24.
615. Hassan R, Laszik ZG, Lerner M, et al. Mesothelin is overexpressed in pancreatobiliary adenocarcinomas but not in normal pancreas and chronic pancreatitis. Am J Clin Pathol 2005;124:838–845.
616. Penno MB, Askin FB, Ma H, et al. High CD44 expression on human mesotheliomas mediates association with hyaluronan. Cancer J Sci Am 1995;1:196.
617. Roberts F, Harper CM, Downie I, Burnett RA. Immunohistochemical analysis still has a limited role in the diagnosis of malignant mesothelioma: a study of thirteen antibodies. Am J Clin Pathol 2001;116:253–262.
618. Battifora HA, Gown AM. Do we need two more mesothelial markers? Hum Pathol 2005;36:451–452.
619. Wang N-S, Huang S-N, Gold P. Absence of carcinoembryonic antigen-like material in mesothelioma: an immunohistochemical differentiation from other lung cancers. Cancer 1979;44:937–943.
620. Dejmek A, Hjerpe A. Carcinoembryonic antigen-like reactivity in malignant mesothelioma: a comparison between different commercially available antibodies. Cancer 1994;73:464–469.
621. Robb JA. Mesothelioma versus adenocarcinoma: false-positive CEA and Leu-M1 staining due to hyaluronic acid [letter]. Hum Pathol 1989;20:400.
622. Johnson BL, Lee I, Gould VE. Epidemiology, pathogenesis, and pathology. In: Kittle CF, ed. Mesothelioma: diagnosis and management. Chicago: Year Book Medical Publishers, 1987:1–29.
623. Sheibani K, Battifora H, Burke JS. Antigenic phenotype of malignant mesotheliomas and pulmonary adenocarcinomas: an immunohistologic analysis demonstrating the value of Leu M1 antigen. Am J Pathol 1986;123:212–219.

624. Sheibani K, Battifora H, Burke JS, Rappaport H. Leu-M1 antigen in human neoplasms: an immunohistologic study of 400 cases. Am J Surg Pathol 1986;10:227–236.
625. Leers MP, Aarts MM, Theunissen PH. E-cadherin and calretinin: a useful combination of immunochemical markers for differentiation between mesothelioma and metastatic adenocarcinoma. Histopathology 1998;32: 209–216.
626. Ordóñez NG. The immunohistochemical diagnosis of mesothelioma: differentiation of mesothelioma and lung adenocarcinoma. Am J Surg Pathol 1989;13:276–291.
627. Wick MR, Loy T, Mills SE, et al. Malignant epithelioid pleural mesothelioma versus peripheral pulmonary adenocarcinoma: a histochemical, ultrastructural, and immunohistologic study of 103 cases. Hum Pathol 1990;21: 759–766.
628. Attanoos RL, Goddard H, Thomas ND, et al. A comparative immunohistochemical study of malignant mesothelioma and renal cell carcinoma: the diagnostic utility of Leu-M1, Ber EP4, Tamm-Horsfall protein and thrombomodulin. Histopathology 1995;27:361–366.629.
629. Ordóñez NG. Mesothelioma with rhabdoid features: an ultrastructural and immunohistochemical study of 10 cases. Mod Pathol 2006;19:373–383.
630. Jordan DA, Jagirdar J, Kaneko M. Blood group antigens, Lewis^x and Lewis^y in the diagnostic discrimination of malignant mesothelioma versus adenocarcinoma. Am J Pathol 1989;135:931–938.
631. Ordóñez NG. Value of thyroid transcription factor-1, E-cadherin, BG8, WT1, and CD44H immunostaining in distinguishing epithelial pleural mesothelioma from pulmonary and nonpulmonary adenocarcinoma. Am J Surg Pathol 2000;24:598–606.
632. Ordóñez NG. The diagnostic utility of immunohistochemistry in distinguishing between epithelioid mesotheliomas and squamous carcinomas of the lung: a comparative study. Mod Pathol 2006;19:417–428.
633. Balzar M, Winter M, de Boer CJ, Litvinov SV. The biology of the 17–1A antigen (Ep-CAM). J Mol Med 1999;77: 699–712.
634. Winter MJ, Nagtegaal ID, van Krieken JH, Litvinov SV. The epithelial cell adhesion molecule (Ep-CAM) as a morphoregulatory molecule is a tool in surgical pathology. Am J Pathol 2003;63:2139–2148.
635. De Boer CJ, van Krieken JH, Janssen-van Rhijn CM, Litvinov SV. Expression of Ep-CAM in normal, regenerating, metaplastic, and neoplastic liver. J Pathol 1999; 188:201–206.
636. Osta WA, Chen Y, Mikhitarian K, et al. EpCAM is overexpressed in breast cancer and is a potential target for breast cancer gene therapy. Cancer Res 2004;64: 5818–5824.
637. Li Q, Bavikatty N, Michael CW. The role of immunohistochemistry in distinguishing squamous cell carcinoma from mesothelioma and adenocarcinoma in pleural effusion. Semin Diagn Pathol 2006;23:15–19.
638. Kortsik CS, Werner P, Freudenberg N, et al. Immunocytochemical characterization of malignant mesothelioma and carcinoma metastatic to the pleura: IOB3—a new tumor marker. Lung 1995;173:79–87.
639. Robinson RJ, Royston D. Comparison of monoclonal antibodies AUA1 and BER EP4 with anti-CEA for detecting carcinoma cells in serous effusions and distinguishing them from mesothelial cells. Cytopathology 1993;4:267–271.
640. Chenard-Neu MP, Kabou A, Mechine A, et al. Immunohistochemistry in the differential diagnosis of mesothelioma and adenocarcinoma: evaluation of 5 new antibodies and 6 traditional antibodies [Fr]. Ann Pathol 1998;18: 460–465.
641. Soosay GN, Griffiths M, Papadaki L, et al. The differential diagnosis of epithelial-type mesothelioma from adenocarcinoma and reactive mesothelial proliferation. J Pathol 1991;163:299–305.
642. Szpak CA, Johnston WW, Roggli V, et al. The diagnostic distinction between malignant mesothelioma of the pleura and adenocarcinoma of the lung as defined by a monoclonal antibody (B72.3). Am J Pathol 1986;122: 252–260.
643. Otis CN, Carter D, Cole S, Battifora H. Immunohistochemical evaluation of pleural mesothelioma and pulmonary adenocarcinoma: a bi-institutional study of 47 cases. Am J Surg Pathol 1987;11:445–456.
644. Ordóñez NG. Role of immunohistochemistry in differentiating epithelial mesothelioma from adenocarcinoma: review and update. Am J Clin Pathol 1999;112:75–89.
645. Skov BG, Lauritzen AF, Hirsch FR, et al. Differentiation of adenocarcinoma of the lung and malignant mesothelioma: predictive value and reproducibility of immunoreactive antibodies. Histopathology 1994;25:431–437.
646. Muller AM, Weichert A, Muller KM. E-cadherin, E-selectin and vascular cell adhesion molecule: immunohistochemical markers for differentiation between mesothelioma and metastatic pulmonary adenocarcinoma? Virchows Arch 2002;441:41–46.
647. Soler AP, Knudsen KA, Jaurand MC, et al. The differential expression of N-cadherin and E-cadherin distinguishes pleural mesotheliomas from lung adenocarcinomas. Hum Pathol 1995;26:1363–1369.
648. Bingle CD. Thyroid transcription factor-1. Int J Biochem Cell Biol 1997;29:1471–1473.
649. Minoo P, Hamdan H, Bu D, et al. TTF-1 regulates lung epithelial morphogenesis. Dev Biol 1995;172:694–698.
650. Lazzaro D, Price M, de Felice M, Di Lauro R. The transcription factor TTF-1 is expressed at the onset of thyroid and lung morphogenesis and in restricted regions of the foetal brain. Development 1991;113:1093–1104.
651. Stahlman MT, Gray ME, Whitsett JA. Expression of thyroid transcription factor-1 (TTF-1) in fetal and neonatal human lung. J Histochem Cytochem 1996;44:673–678.
652. Fabbro D, Di Loreto C, Stamerra O, et al. TTF-1 gene expression in human lung tumours. Eur J Cancer 1996; 32A:512–517.
653. Holzinger A, Dingle S, Bejarano PA, et al. Monoclonal antibody to thyroid transcription factor-1: production, characterization, and usefulness in tumor diagnosis. Hybridoma 1996;15:49–53.
654. Di Loreto C, Puglisi F, Di Lauro V, et al. TTF-1 protein expression in pleural malignant mesotheliomas and adenocarcinomas of the lung. Cancer Lett 1998;124:73–78.

655. Harlamert HA, Mira J, Bejarano PA, et al. Thyroid transcription factor-1 and cytokeratins 7 and 20 in pulmonary and breast carcinoma. Acta Cytol 1998;42:1382–1388.
656. Puglisi F, Barbone F, Damante G, et al. Prognostic value of thyroid transcription factor-1 in primary, resected, non-small cell lung carcinoma. Mod Pathol 1999;12:318–324.
657. Afify AM, al-Khafaji BM. Diagnostic utility of thyroid transcription factor-1 expression in adenocarcinomas presenting in serous fluids. Acta Cytol 2002;46:675–678.
658. Ng WK, Chow JC, Ng PK. Thyroid transcription factor-1 is highly sensitive and specific in differentiating metastatic pulmonary from extrapulmonary adenocarcinoma in effusion fluid cytology specimens. Cancer 2002;96: 43–48.
659. Zamecnik J, Kodet R. Value of thyroid transcription factor-1 and surfactant apoprotein A in the differential diagnosis of pulmonary carcinomas: a study of 109 cases. Virchows Arch 2002;440:353–361.
660. Rossi G, Marchioni A, Milani M, et al. TTF-1, cytokeratin 7, 34βE12, and CD56/NCAM immunostaining in the subclassification of large cell carcinomas of the lung. Am J Clin Pathol 2004;122:884–893.
661. Khoor A, Whitsett JA, Stahlman MT, et al. Utility of surfactant protein B precursor and thyroid transcription factor 1 in differentiating adenocarcinoma of the lung from malignant mesothelioma. Hum Pathol 1999;30: 695–700.
662. Henderson DW, Whitaker D, Shilkin KB. The differential diagnosis of mesothelioma: a practical approach to diagnosis during life. In: Henderson D, Shilkin K, Langlois SL, Whitaker D, eds. Malignant Mesothelioma. New York: Hemisphere, 1992:183–197.
663. Singh HK, Silvermann JF, Berns L, Haddad MG. The value of epithelial membrane antigen expression in separating benign mesothelial proliferation from malignant mesothelioma: a comparative study. Diagn Cytopathol 2005;32:156–159.
664. Esteban JM, Yokota S, Husain S, Battifora H. Immunocytochemical profile of benign and carcinomatous effusions: a practical approach to difficult diagnosis. Am J Clin Pathol 1990;94:698–705.
665. Cury PM, Butcher DN, Corrin B, Nicholson AG. The use of histological and immunohistochemical markers to distinguish pleural malignant mesothelioma and in situ mesothelioma from reactive mesothelial hyperplasia and reactive pleural fibrosis. J Pathol 1999;189:251–257.
666. Dejmek A, Hjerpe A. The combination of CEA, EMA, and BerEp4 and hyaluronan analysis specifically identifies 79% of all histologically verified mesotheliomas causing an effusion. Diagn Cytopathol 2005;32:160–166.
667. Leong AS-Y, Parkinson R, Milios J. "Thick" cell membranes revealed by immunocytochemical staining: a clue to the diagnosis of mesothelioma. Diagn Cytopathol 1990;6:9–13.
668. King JA, Tucker JA. Evaluation of membranous staining of mesothelioma. Cell Vis 1998;5:24–27.
669. Hammar SP, Bolen JW, Bockus D, et al. Ultrastructural and immunohistochemical features of common lung tumors: an overview. Ultrastruct Pathol 1985;9:283–318.
670. Krismann M, Thattamparambil P, Simon F, Johnen G. Differential diagnosis of preneoplastic lesions of the pleura and of early mesothelioma: immunohistochemical and morphological findings. Pathologe 2006;27:99–105.
671. Saad RS, Cho P, Yulin LL, Silverman JF. The value of epithelial membrane antigen expression in separating benign mesothelial proliferation from malignant mesothelioma: a comparative study. Diagn Cytopathol 2005; 32:156–159.
672. Whitaker D, Shilkin KB, Sterrett GF. Cytological appearances of malignant mesothelioma. In: Henderson DW, Shilkin KB, Langlois SL, Whitaker D, eds. Malignant mesothelioma. New York: Hemisphere, 1992:167–182.
673. Walts AE, Said JW, Shintaku IP. Epithelial membrane antigen in the cytodiagnosis of effusions and aspirates: immunocytochemical and ultrastructural localization in benign and malignant cells. Diagn Cytopathol 1987;3: 41–49.
674. Van der Kwast TH, Versnel MA, Delahaye M, et al. Expression of epithelial membrane antigen on malignant mesothelioma cells: an immunocytochemical and immunoelectron microscopic study. Acta Cytol 1988;32:169–174.
675. Lauritzen AF. Distinction between cells in serous effusions using a panel of antibodies. Virchows Arch A Path Anat Histopathol 1987;411:299–304.
676. Mason MR, Bedrossian CW, Fahey CA. Value of immunocytochemistry in the study of malignant effusions. Diagn Cytopathol 1987;3:215–221.
677. Silverman JF, Nance K, Phillips B, Norris HT. The use of immunoperoxidase panels for the cytologic diagnosis of malignancy in serous effusions. Diagn Cytopathol 1987; 3:134–140.
678. Whitaker D, Sterrett G, Shilkin K. Early diagnosis of malignant mesothelioma: the contribution of effusion and fine needle aspiration cytology and ancillary techniques. In: Peters GA, Peters BJ, eds. Asbestos disease update March 1989: a special supplement to the sourcebook on asbestos diseases: medical, legal, and engineering aspects. New York: Garland Law Publishing, 1989:73–112.
679. Wolanski KD, Whitaker D, Shilkin KB, Henderson DW. The use of epithelial membrane antigen and silver-stained nucleolar organizer regions testing in the differential diagnosis of mesothelioma from benign reactive mesothelioses. Cancer 1998;82:583–590.
680. Kushitani K, Takeshima Y, Amatya VJ, et al. Immunohistochemical marker panels for distinguishing between epithelioid mesothelioma and lung adenocarcinoma. Pathol Int 2007;57:190–199.
681. Zhu W, Michael CW. WT1, monoclonal CEA, TTF1, and CA125 antibodies in the differential diagnosis of lung, breast, and ovarian adenocarcinomas in serous effusions. Diagn Cytopathol 2007;35:370–375.
682. Hedman M, Arnberg H, Wernlund J, et al. Tissue polypeptide antigen (TPA), hyaluronan and CA 125 as serum markers in malignant mesothelioma. Anticancer Res 2003;23:531–536.
683. Kebapci M, Vardarell E, Adapinar B, Acikalin M. CT findings and serum CA 125 levels in malignant peritoneal mesothelioma: report of 11 new cases and review of the literature. Eur Radiol 2003;13:2620–2626.

684. Baratti D, Kusamura S, Martinetti A, et al. Circulating CA125 in patients with peritoneal mesothelioma treated with cytoreductive surgery and intraperitoneal hyperthermic perfusion. Ann Surg Oncol 2007;14:500–508.
685. Fleming MV, Guinee DG Jr, Chu WS, et al. Bcl-2 immunohistochemistry in a surgical series of non-small cell lung cancer patients. Hum Pathol 1998;29:60–64.
686. Navratil E, Gaulard P, Kanavaros P, et al. Expression of the bcl-2 protein in B cell lymphomas arising from mucosa associated lymphoid tissue. J Clin Pathol 1995;48:18–21.
687. Ben-Ezra JM, Kornstein MJ, Grimes MM, Krystal G. Small cell carcinomas of the lung express the Bcl-2 protein. Am J Pathol 1994;145:1036–1040.
688. Segers K, Ramael M, Singh SK, et al. Immunoreactivity for bcl-2 protein in malignant mesothelioma and non-neoplastic mesothelium. Virchows Arch 1994;424: 631–634.
689. Attanoos RL, Griffin A, Gibbs AR. The use of immunohistochemistry in distinguishing reactive from neoplastic mesothelium: a novel use for desmin and comparative evaluation with epithelial membrane antigen, p53, platelet-derived growth factor-receptor, P-glycoprotein and Bcl-2. Histopathology 2003;43:231–238.
690. King J, Thatcher N, Pickering C, Hasleton P. Sensitivity and specificity of immunohistochemical antibodies used to distinguish between benign and malignant pleural disease: a systematic review of published reports. Histopathology 2006;49:561–568.
691. Ramael M, Lemmens G, Eerdekens C, et al. Immunoreactivity for p53 protein in malignant mesothelioma and non-neoplastic mesothelium. J Pathol 1992;168:371–375.
692. Mayall FG, Goddard H, Gibbs AR. The frequency of p53 immunostaining in asbestos-associated mesotheliomas and non-asbestos-associated mesotheliomas. Histopathology 1993;22:383–386.
693. Mullick SS, Green LK, Ramzy I, et al. P53 gene product in pleural effusions: practical use in distinguishing benign from malignant cells. Acta Cytol 1996;40:855–860.
694. Cagle PT, Brown RW, Lebovitz RM. P53 immunostaining in the differentiation of reactive processes from malignancy in pleural biopsy specimens. Hum Pathol 1994;25: 443–448.
695. Esposito V, Baldi A, De Luca A, et al. p53 immunostaining in differential diagnosis of pleural mesothelial proliferations. Anticancer Res 1997;17:733–736.
696. Mayall F, Heryet A, Manga D, Kriegeskotten A. P53 immunostaining is a highly specific and moderately sensitive marker of malignancy in serous fluid cytology. Cytopathology 1997;8:9–12.
697. Schneider J, Presek P, Braun A, et al. p53 protein, EGF receptor, and anti-p53 antibodies in serum from patients with occupationally derived lung cancer. Br J Cancer 1999;80:1987–1994.
698. Isik R, Metintas M, Gibbs AR, et al. p53, p21 and metallothionein immunoreactivities in patients with malignant pleural mesothelioma: correlations with the epidemiological features and prognosis of mesotheliomas with environmental asbestos exposure. Respir Med 2001;95: 588–593.
699. Kettunen E, Nicholson AG, Nagy B, et al. L1CAM, INP10, P-cadherin, tPA and ITGB4 over-expression in malignant pleural mesotheliomas revealed by combined use of cDNA and tissue microarray. Carcinogenesis 2005;26: 17–25.
700. Lantuéjoul S, Laverriere MH, Sturm N, et al. NCAM (neural cell adhesion molecules) expression in malignant mesotheliomas. Hum Pathol 2000;31:415–421.
701. Ramaekers FCS, Haag D, Kant A, et al. Coexpression of keratin- and vimentin-type intermediate filaments in human metastatic carcinoma cells. Proc Natl Acad Sci USA 1983;80:2618–2622.
702. Scoones DJ, Richman PI. Expression of desmin and smooth muscle actin in mesothelial hyperplasia and mesothelioma. J Pathol 1993;169:166A.
703. Dai Y, Bedrossian CW, Michael CW. The expression pattern of β-catenin in mesothelial proliferative lesions and its diagnostic utilities. Diagn Cytopathol 2005;33: 320–324.
704. Wu M, Yuan S, Szporn AH, et al. Immunocytochemical detection of XIAP in body cavity effusions and washes. Mod Pathol 2005;18:1618–1622.
705. Soini Y, Jarvinen K, Kaarteenaho-Wiik R, Kinnula V. The expression of P-glycoprotein and multidrug resistance proteins 1 and 2 (MRP1 and MRP2) in human malignant mesothelioma. Ann Oncol 2001;12:1239–1245.
706. Ramael M, van den Bossche J, Buysse C, et al. Immunoreactivity for P-170 glycoprotein in malignant mesothelioma and in non-neoplastic mesothelium of the pleura using the murine monoclonal antibody JSB-1. J Pathol 1992;167:5–8.
707. Afify A, Zhou H, Howell L, Paulino AF. Diagnostic utility of GLUT-1 expression in the cytologic evaluation of serous fluids. Acta Cytol 2005;49:621–626.
708. Okamoto H, Matsuno Y, Noguchi M, et al. Malignant pleural mesothelioma producing chorionic gonadotropin: report of two cases. Am J Surg Pathol 1992;16:969–974.
709. McAuley P, Asa SL, Chiv B, et al. Parathyroid hormone-like peptide in normal and neoplastic mesothelial cells. Cancer 1990;66:1975–1979.
710. Chu P, Wu E, Weiss LM. Cytokeratin 7 and cytokeratin 20 expression in epithelial neoplasms: a survey of 435 cases. Mod Pathol 2000;13:962–972.
711. Butnor KJ, Nicholson AG, Allred DC, et al. Expression of renal cell carcinoma-associated markers erythropoietin, CD10, and renal cell carcinoma marker in diffuse malignant mesothelioma and metastatic renal cell carcinoma. Arch Pathol Lab Med 2006;130:823–827.
712. Tot T. The value of cytokeratins 20 and 7 in discriminating metastatic adenocarcinomas from pleural mesotheliomas. Cancer 2001;92:2727–2732.
713. Campbell F, Herrington CS. Application of cytokeratin 7 and 20 immunohistochemistry to diagnostic pathology. Curr Diagn Pathol 2001;7:113–122.
714. Saad RS, Lindner JL, Lin X, et al. The diagnostic utility of D2–40 for malignant mesothelioma versus pulmonary carcinoma with pleural involvement. Diagn Cytopathol 2006;34:801–806.
715. Kaufmann O, Fietze E, Mengs J, Dietel M. Value of p63 and cytokeratin 5/6 as immunohistochemical markers for

the differential diagnosis of poorly differentiated and undifferentiated carcinomas. Am J Clin Pathol 2001; 116:823–830.
716. Shieh S, Grassi M, Schwarz JK, Cheney RT. Pleural mesothelioma with cutaneous extension to chest wall scars. J Cutan Pathol 2004;31:497–501.
717. Ormsby AH, Snow JL, Su WP, Goellner JR. Diagnostic immunohistochemistry of cutaneous metastatic breast carcinoma: a statistical analysis of the utility of gross cystic disease fluid protein-15 and estrogen receptor protein. J Am Acad Dermatol 1995;32:711–716.
718. Barnetson RJ, Burnett RA, Downie I, et al. Immunohistochemical analysis of peritoneal mesothelioma and primary and secondary serous carcinoma of the peritoneum: antibodies to estrogen and progesterone receptors are useful. Am J Clin Pathol 2006;125:67–76.
719. Kafiri G, Thomas DM, Shepherd NA, et al. p53 expression is common in malignant mesothelioma. Histopathology 1992;21:331–334.
720. Suzuki Y, Churg J, Kannerstein M. Ultrastructure of human malignant diffuse mesothelioma. Am J Pathol 1976;85:241–262.
721. Klima M, Bossart MI. Sarcomatous type of malignant mesothelioma. Ultrastruct Pathol 1983;4:349–358.
722. d'Andiran G, Gabbiani G. A metastasizing sarcoma of the pleura composed of myofibroblasts. In: Fenoglio CM, Wolff M, eds. Progress in surgical pathology. New York: Mason, 1980:31–40.
723. Warhol MJ, Hickey WF, Corson JM. Malignant mesothelioma: ultrastructural distinction from adenocarcinoma. Am J Surg Pathol 1982;6:307–314.
724. Warhol MJ, Corson JM. An ultrastructural comparison of mesotheliomas with adenocarcinomas of the lung and breast. Hum Pathol 1985;16:50–55.
725. Burns TR, Greenberg SD, Mace ML, Johnson EH. Ultrastructural diagnosis of epithelial malignant mesothelioma. Cancer 1985;56:2036–2040.
726. Burns TRI, Johnson EH, Cartwright UR, Greenberg SD. Desmosomes of epithelial malignant mesothelioma. Ultra Pathol 1988;12:385–388.
727. Tiainen M, Tammilethol L, Rautonen J, Tumoi T, Mattson K, Knoutila S. Chromosomal abnormalities and their correlations with asbestos exposure and survival in patients with mesothelioma. Br J Cancer 1989;60: 618–626.
728. Hagemeijer A, Versnel MA, Van Drunen E, et al. Cytogenetic analysis of malignant mesothelioma. Cancer Genet Cytogenet 1990;47:1–28.
729. Hicks J. Biologic, cytogenetic, and molecular factors in mesothelial proliferations. Ultrastruct Pathol 2006;30: 19–30.
730. Davidson B, Holth A, Dong HP, et al. Chemokine receptors are rarely expressed on malignant or benign mesothelial cells. Lung Cancer 2006;54(S1):S14.
731. Jaurand MC. Asbestos, chromosomal deletions and tumor suppressor gene alterations in human malignant mesothelioma. Lung Cancer 2006;54(S1):S15.
732. Janne PA. Proteomic methods to identify novel therapeutic targets in malignant mesothelioma. Lung Cancer 2006;54(S1):S15.
733. Christensen JC, Marsit CJ, Nelson HH, et al. Asbestos burden, epigenetic silencing, and survival in malignant pleural mesothelioma. Lung Cancer 2006;54(S1):S21.
734. Rihn BH. Oxidative stress gene modulation in pleural mesothelioma as assessed by microarray in vitro, ex-vivo, and in-situ analysis. Lung Cancer 2006;54(S1):S21.
735. Bahnassy AA, Gaafar RM, Zekri AN, et al. Alterations of the G1 checkpoints in malignant pleural mesothelioma (MPM) in relation to pathogenesis and survival. Lung Cancer 2006;54(S1):S23.
736. Croonen AM, van der Valk P, Herman CJ, Lindeman J. Cytology, immunopathology and flow cytometry in the diagnosis of pleural and peritoneal effusions. Lab Invest 1988;58:725–732.
737. Hafiz MA, Becker RL Jr, Mikel UV, Bahr GF. Cytophotometric determination of DNA in mesotheliomas and reactive mesothelial cells. Anal Quant Cytol Histol 1988;58:120–126.
738. Frierson HF, Mills SE, Legier JF. Flow cytometric analysis of ploidy in immunohistochemically confirmed examples of malignant mesothelioma. Am J Clin Pathol 1988;90: 240–243.
739. Burmer GC, Rabinovitch PS, Kulander BG, Rusch V, McNutt MA. Flow cytometric analysis of malignant pleural mesothelioma: relationship to histology and survival. Hum Pathol 1989;20:777–783.
740. Dazzi H, Thatcher N, Hasleton PS, Chattlerjee AK, Lawson AM. DNA analysis by flow cytometry in malignant pleural mesothelioma: relationship to histology and survival. J Pathol 1990;162:51–55.
741. Tierney G, Wilkinson MJ, Jones JSP. The malignancy grading method is not a reliable assessment of malignancy in mesothelioma. J Pathol 1990;160:209–211.
742. El-Naggar AK, Ordone NG, Garnsey L, Batsakis JG. Epithelioid pleural mesotheliomas and pulmonary adenocarcinomas: a comparative DNA flow cytometric study. Hum Pathol 1991;22:972–978.
743. Esteban JM, Sheibani K. DNA ploidy analysis of pleural mesotheliomas: Its usefulness for their distinction from lung adenocarcinomas. Mod Pathol 1992;6:626–630.
744. Cakir C, Gulluoglu MG, Yilmazbayhan D. Cell proliferation rate and telomerase activity in the differential diagnosis between benign and malignant mesothelial proliferations. Pathology 2006;38:10–15.
745. Kim BS, Varkey B, Choi H. Diagnosis of malignant pleural mesothelioma by axillary lymph node biopsy. Chest 1987;91:278–81.
746. Sussman J, Rosai J. Lymph node metastasis as the initial manifestation of malignant mesothelioma: report of six cases. Am J Surg Pathol 1990;14:819–828.
747. Lloreta J, Serrano S. Pleural mesothelioma presenting as an axillary lymph node metastasis with anemonc cell appearance. Ultrastruct Pathol 1994;18:293–298.
748. Wills EJ. Pleural mesothelioma with initial presentation as cervical lymphadenopathy. Ultrastruct Pathol 1995;19: 389–394.
749. Colby TV. Benign mesothelial cells in lymph node. Adv Anat Pathol 1999;6:41–48.
750. Sion-Vardy N, Diomin V, Benharroch D. Hyperplastic mesothelial cells in subpleural lymph nodes mimicking

metastatic carcinoma. Ann Diagn Pathol 2004;8:373–374.
751. Walker AN, Mills SE. Surgical pathology of the tunica vaginalis testis and embryologically related mesothelium. Pathol Annu 1988;23;2:125–152.
752. Nogales FF, Isaac MA, Hardisson D, et al. Adenomatoid tumors of the uterus: an analysis of 60 cases. Int J Gynecol Pathol 2002;21:34–40.
753. Ordóñez NG. Podoplanin: a novel diagnostic immunohistochemical marker. Adv Anat Pathol 2006;13:83–88.
754. Kaplan MA, Tazelaar HD, Hayashi T, et al. Adenomatoid tumors of the pleura. Am J Surg Pathol 1996;20:1219–1223.
755. Handra-Luca A, Couvelard A, Abd Alsamad I, et al. Adenomatoid tumor of the pleura. Ann Pathol 2000;20:369–372.
756. Kannerstein M, Churg J, McCaughey WTE, Hill DP. Papillary tumors of the peritoneum in women: Mesothelioma or papillary carcinoma. Am J Obstet Gynecol 1977;127:306–314.
757. Goepel JR. Benign papillary mesothelioma of peritoneum: a histological, histochemical and ultrastructural study of six cases. Histopathology 1981;5:21–30.
758. Burrig KF, Pfitzer P, Hort W. Well-differentiated papillary mesothelioma of the peritoneum: a borderline mesothelioma: report of two cases and review of literature. Virchows Arch A Pathol Anat Histopathol 1990;417:443–447.
759. Daya D, McCaughey WT. Well-differentiated papillary mesothelioma of the peritoneum: a clinicopathologic study of 22 cases. Cancer 1990;65:292–296.
760. Lovell FA, Cranston PE. Well-differentiated papillary mesothelioma of the peritoneum. AJR Am J Roentgenol 1990;155:1245–1246.
761. Daya D, McCaughey WT. Pathology of the peritoneum: a review of selected topics. Semin Diagn Pathol 1991;8:277–289.
762. Lammer F, Scherrer C, Hacki WH. Well-differentiated papillary mesothelioma of the peritoneum: rare, but prognostically important differential diagnosis. Schweiz Med Wochenschr 1991;121:954–956.
763. Bouvier S, Baron O, Nomballais F, et al. Well-differentiated papillary mesothelioma of the peritoneum: an attenuated malignant tumor—review of the literature apropos of a case. Bull Cancer 1994;81:104–107.
764. Mangal R, Taskin O, Franklin R. An incidental diagnosis of well-differentiated papillary mesothelioma in a woman operated on for recurrent endometriosis. Fertil Steril 1995;63:196–197.
765. Hoekman K, Tognon G, Risse EK, et al. Well-differentiated papillary mesothelioma of the peritoneum: a separate entity. Eur J Cancer 1996;32A:255–258.
766. Shukunami K, Hirabuki S, Kaneshima M, et al. Well-differentiated papillary mesothelioma involving the peritoneal and pleural cavities: successful treatment by local and systemic administration of carboplatin. Tumori 2000;86:419–421.
767. Butnor KJ, Sporn TA, Hammar SP, Roggli VL. Well-differentiated papillary mesothelioma. Am J Surg Pathol 2001;25:1304–1309.
768. Chetty R. Well differentiated (benign) papillary mesothelioma of the tunica vaginalis. J Clin Pathol 1992;45:1029–1030.
769. Sane AC, Roggli VL. Curative resection of a well-differentiated papillary mesothelioma of the pericardium. Arch Pathol Lab Med 1995;119:266–267.
770. Galateau-Sallé F, Vignaud JM, Burke L, et al. Well-differentiated papillary mesothelioma of the pleura: a series of 24 cases. Am J Surg Pathol 2004;28:534–540.
771. Bolen JW, Hammar SP, McNutt MA. Serosal tissue: reactive tissue as a model for understanding mesotheliomas. Ultrastruct Pathol 1987;11:251–262.
772. Mayall FG, Gibbs AR. The histology and immunohistochemistry of small cell mesothelioma. Histopathology 1992;20:47–51.
773. Falconieri G, Zanconati F, Bussani R, Di Bonito L. Small cell carcinoma of lung simulating pleural mesothelioma: report of 4 cases with autopsy confirmation. Pathol Res Prac 1995;191:1147–1152.
774. Krismann M, Müller K-M, Jaworska M, Johnen G. Pathological anatomy and molecular pathology [of mesothelioma]. Lung Cancer 2004;45S:S29–S33.
775. Nascimento AG, Keeney GL, Fletcher CDM. Deciduoid peritoneal mesothelioma: an unusual phenotype affecting young females. Am J Surg Pathol 1994;18:439–445.
776. Gloeckner-Hofmann K, Zhu XZ, Bartels H, et al. Deciduoid pleural mesothelioma affecting a young female without prior asbestos exposure. Respiration 2000;67:456–458.
777. Okonkwo A, Musunuri S, Diaz L Jr, et al. Deciduoid mesothelioma: a rare, distinct entity with unusual features. Ann Diagn Pathol 2001;5:168–171.
778. Reis-Filho JS, Pope LZ, Milanezi F, et al. Primary epithelial malignant mesothelioma of the pericardium with deciduoid features: cytohistologic and immunohistochemical study. Diagn Cytopathol 2002;26:117–122.
779. Serio G, Scattone A, Pennella A, et al. Malignant deciduoid mesothelioma of the pleura: report of two cases with long survival. Histopathology 2002;40:348–352.
780. Gillespie FR, van der Walt JD, Derias N, Kenney A. Deciduoid peritoneal mesothelioma: a report of the cytological appearances. Cytopathology 2001;12:57–61.
781. Ordóñez NG. Epithelial mesothelioma with deciduoid features: report of four cases. Am J Surg Pathol 2000;24:816–823.
782. Puttagunta L, Vriend RA, Nguyen GK. Deciduoid epithelial mesothelioma of the pleura with focal rhabdoid change [letter]. Am J Surg Pathol 2000;24:1440–1443.
783. Shanks JH, Harris M, Banerjee SS, et al. Mesotheliomas with deciduoid morphology: a morphologic spectrum and a variant not confined to young females. Am J Surg Pathol 2000;24:285–294.
784. Talerman A. Deciduoid or pseudodecidual mesothelioma [letter; comment]. Am J Surg Pathol 2000;24:1179.
785. Monaghan H, Al-Nafussi A. Deciduoid pleural mesothelioma. Histopathology 2001;39:104–106.
786. Guinee DG, Travis WD. Pitfalls in the diagnosis of malignant mesothelioma. In: Pass HI, Vogelzang NJ, Carbone M, eds. Malignant mesothelioma: advances in pathogen-

esis, diagnosis, and translational therapies. New York: Springer, 2005:555–578.
787. Ernst CS, Atkinson BF. Mucicarmine positivity in malignant mesothelioma. Lab Invest 1980;42:113–114.
788. McCaughey WTE, Colby TV, Battifora H, et al. Diagnosis of diffuse malignant mesothelioma: experience of a US/Canadian mesothelioma panel. Mod Pathol 1991;4: 342–353.
789. Benjamin CJ, Ritchie AC. Histological staining for the diagnosis of mesothelioma. Am J Med Technol 1982; 48:905–908.
790. Mennemeyer R, Smith M. Multicystic, peritoneal mesothelioma: a report with electron microscopy of a case mimicking intra-abdominal cystic hygroma (lymphangioma). Cancer 1979;44:692–698.
791. Moore JH Jr, Crum CP, Chandler JG, Feldman PS. Benign cystic mesothelioma. Cancer 1980;45:2395–2399.
792. Blumberg NA, Murray JF. Multicystic peritoneal mesothelioma: a case report. S Afr Med J 1981;59:85–86.
793. Katsube Y, Mukai K, Silverberg SG. Cystic mesothelioma of the peritoneum: a report of five cases and review of the literature. Cancer 1982;50:1615–1622.
794. Schneider V, Partridge JR, Gutierrez F, et al. Benign cystic mesothelioma involving the female genital tract: report of four cases. Am J Obstet Gynecol 1983;145:355–359.
795. Nirodi NS, Lowry DS, Wallace RJ. Cystic mesothelioma of the pelvic peritoneum: two case reports. Br J Obstet Gynaecol 1984;91:201–204.
796. Philip G, Reilly AL. Benign cystic mesothelioma: case reports. Br J Obstet Gynaecol 1984;91:932–938.
797. Sienkowski K, Russell AJ, Dilly SA, Djazaeri B. Peritoneal cystic mesothelioma: an electron microscopic and immunohistochemical study of two male patients. J Clin Pathol 1986;39:440–445.
798. Weiss SW, Tavassoli FA. Multicystic mesothelioma: an analysis of pathologic findings and biologic behavior in 37 cases. Am J Surg Pathol 1988;12:737–746.
799. Santucci M, Biancalani M, Dini S. Multicystic peritoneal mesothelioma: a fine structure study with special reference to the spectrum of phenotypic differentiation exhibited by mesothelial cells. J Submicrosc Cytol Pathol 1989; 21:749–764.
800. Pollack CV Jr, Jorden RC. Benign cystic mesothelioma presenting as acute abdominal pain in a young woman. J Emerg Med 1991;9:21–25.
801. Scucchi L, Mingazzini P, Di Stefano D, et al. Two cases of "multicystic peritoneal mesothelioma": description and critical review of the literature. Anticancer Res 1994;14: 715–720.
802. Ozgen A, Akata D, Akhan O, et al. Giant benign cystic peritoneal mesothelioma: US, CT, and MRI findings. Abdominal Imaging 1998;23:502–504.
803. De Toma G, Nicolanti V, Plocco M, et al. Cystic peritoneal mesothelioma: report of a case. Surg Today 2000;30:98–100.
804. Moghe GM, Krishnamurthy SC. Multicystic mesothelioma of the peritoneum. Indian J Gastroenterol 2001; 20:202–203.
805. Omeroglu A, Husain A. Multilocular peritoneal inclusion cyst (benign cystic mesothelioma). Arch Pathol Lab Med 2001;125:1123–1124.
806. Petrou G, Macindoe R, Deane S. Benign cystic mesothelioma in a 60-year-old woman after cholecystectomy. ANZ J Surg 2001;71:615–618.
807. Bui-Mansfield LT, Kim-Ahn G, O'Bryant LK. Multicystic mesothelioma of the peritoneum. AJR 2002;178:402.
808. Ricci F, Borzellino G, Ghimenton C, Cordiano C. Benign cystic mesothelioma in a male patient: surgical treatment by the laparoscopic route. Surg Laparosc Endosc 1995; 5:157–160.
809. Kumar D, Dhar A, Jain R, et al. Benign cystic peritoneal mesothelioma in a man. Indian J Gastroenterol 1998; 17:156–157.
810. Colombat M, Carton S, Drouard F. Cystic mesothelioma of the peritoneum in a male. Ann Pathol 2000;20:59–61.
811. Ignjatovic M, Cerovic S, Cuk V. Mesothelial cyst and cystic mesothelioma of the greater omentum: case report and literature review. Acta Chir Iugosl 2001;48:77–83.
812. Hafner M, Novacek G, Herbst F, et al. Giant benign cystic mesothelioma: a case report and review of literature. Eur J Gastroenterol Hepatol 2002;14:77–80.
813. Vara-Thorbeck C, Toscano-Mendez R. Peritoneal cystic mesothelioma. Surg Endosc 2002;16:220.
814. Ross MJ, Welch WR, Scully RE. Multilocular peritoneal inclusion cysts (so-called cystic mesothelioma). Cancer 1989;64:1336–1346.
815. Groisman GM, Kerner H. Multicystic mesothelioma with endometriosis. Acta Obstet Gynecol Scand 1992;71: 642–644.
816. Drut R, Quijano G. Multilocular mesothelial inclusion cysts (so-called benign multicystic mesothelioma) of pericardium [letter]. Histopathology 1999;34:472–474.
817. Hutchinson R, Sokhi GS. Multicystic peritoneal mesothelioma: not a benign condition. Eur J Surg 1992;158: 451–453.
818. Miles JM, Hart WR, McMahon JT. Cystic mesothelioma of the peritoneum: report of a case with multiple recurrences and review of the literature. Cleve Clin Q 1986; 53:109–114.
819. Letterie GS, Yon JL. The antiestrogen tamoxifen in the treatment of recurrent benign cystic mesothelioma. Gynecol Oncol 1998;70:131–133.
820. Gonzalez-Moreno S, Yan H, Alcorn KW, Sugarbaker PH. Malignant transformation of "benign" cystic mesothelioma of the peritoneum. J Surg Oncol 2002;79:243–251.
821. Ball NJ, Urbanski SJ, Green FH, Kieser T. Pleural multicystic mesothelial proliferation: the so-called multicystic mesothelioma. Am J Surg Pathol 1990;14:375–378.
822. Henderson DW, Shilkin KB, Whitaker D, et al. Unusual histological types and anatomic sites of mesothelioma. In: Henderson DW, Shilkin KB, Langlois SL, Whitaker D, eds. Malignant mesothelioma. New York: Hemisphere, 1992:140–166.
823. Kannerstein M, Churg J. Desmoplastic diffuse malignant mesothelioma. In: Fenoglio CM, Wolff M, eds. Progress in surgical pathology. New York: Masson, 1980:19–29.
824. Cantin R, Al-Jabi M, McCaughey WT. Desmoplastic diffuse mesothelioma. Am J Surg Pathol 1982;6:215–222.
825. Du Bray ES, Rosson FB. Primary mesothelioma of the pleura: a clinical and pathologic contribution to pleural

malignancy, with report of a case. Arch Intern Med 1920;26:715–737.
826. Mangano WE, Cagle PT, Churg A, et al. The diagnosis of desmoplastic malignant mesothelioma and its distinction from fibrous pleurisy: a histologic and immunohistochemical analysis of 31 cases including p53 immunostaining. Am J Clin Pathol 1998;110:191–199.
827. Wilson GE, Hasleton PS, Chatterjee AK. Desmoplastic malignant mesothelioma: a review of 17 cases. J Clin Pathol 1992;45:295–298.
828. Churg A. Neoplastic asbestos-induced disease. In: Churg A, Green FHY, eds. Pathology of occupational lung disease, 2nd ed. Baltimore: Williams & Wilkins, 1998: 339–391.
829. Battifora H, McCaughey WTE. Tumors of the serosal membranes. Atlas of tumor pathology, 3rd series, fascicle 15. Washington, DC: Armed Forces Institute of Pathology, 1995.
830. Machin T, Mashiyama ET, Henderson JAM, McCaughey WTE. Bony metastases in desmoplastic pleural mesothelioma. Thorax 1988;43:155–156.
831. Henderson DW, Attwood HD, Constance TJ, et al. Lymphohistiocytoid mesothelioma: a rare lymphomatoid variant of predominantly sarcomatoid mesothelioma. Ultrastruct Pathol 1988;12:367–384.
832. Khalidi HS, Medeiros LJ, Battifora H. Lymphohistiocytoid mesothelioma: an often misdiagnosed variant of sarcomatoid mesothelioma. Am J Clin Pathol 2000;113: 649–654.
833. Yao DX, Shia J, Erlandson RA, Klimstra DS. Lymphohistiocytoid mesothelioma: a clinical, immunohistochemical and ultrastructural study of four cases and literature review. Ultrastruct Pathol 2004;28:213–228.
834. Dorfmüller P, Krismann M, Müller K-M. Mesotheliomas with leukocytic infiltration: aspects of differential diagnosis. Pathologe 2004;25:349–355.
835. Robinson BW, Robinson C, Lake RA. Localised spontaneous regression in mesothelioma—possible immunological mechanism. Lung Cancer 2001;32:197–201.
836. Attanoos RL, Galateau-Salle F, Gibbs AR, et al. Primary thymic epithelial tumours of the pleura mimicking malignant mesothelioma. Histopathology 2002;41:42–49.
837. Leigh RA, Webster I. Lymphocytic infiltration of pleural mesothelioma and its significance for survival. S Afr Med J 1982;61:1007–1009.
838. Crotty TB, Myers JL, Katzenstein AL, et al. Localized malignant mesothelioma: a clinicopathologic and flow cytometric study. Am J Surg Pathol 1994;18:357–363.
839. Allen TC, Cagle PT, Churg AM, et al. Localized malignant mesothelioma. Am J Surg Pathol 2005;29:866–873.
840. Myers J, Tazelaar H, Katzenstein AL, et al. Localized malignant epithelioid and biphasic mesothelioma of the pleura: clinicopathologic, immunohistochemical, and flow cytometric analysis of 3 cases. Lab Invest 1992;66: 115A.
841. Ojeda HF, Mech K Jr, Hicken WJ. Localized malignant mesothelioma: a case report. Am Surg 1998;64:881–885.
842. Churg AM. Localized pleural tumors. In: Cagle PT, ed. Diagnostic pulmonary pathology. New York: Marcel Dekker, 2000:719–735.
843. Okamura H, Kamei T, Mitsuno A, et al. Localized malignant mesothelioma of the pleura. Pathol Int 2001;51: 654–660.
844. Umezu H, Kuwata K, Ebe Y, et al. Microcystic variant of localized malignant mesothelioma accompanying an adenomatoid tumor-like lesion. Pathol Int 2002;52:416–422.
845. Zimmerman RL. Effusion cytology: keeping researchers and journals in business for the past 20 years—and it is not over yet. Current Diagn Pathol 2005;11:194–202.
846. Turbat-Herrera EA, Herrera GA. Electron microscopy renders the diagnostic capabilities of cytopathology more precise: an approach to everyday practice. Ultrastruct Pathol 2005;29:475–482.
847. Joseph MG, Banerjee D, Harris P, et al. Multiparameter flow cytometric DNA analysis of effusions: a prospective study of 36 cases compared with routine cytology and immunohistochemistry. Mod Pathol 1995;8: 686–693.
848. Ross B, Motherby H, Saurenbach F, et al. Atomic force microscopy in effusion cytology. Anal Quant Cytol Histol 1998;20:97–104.
849. Whitaker D. The cytology of malignant mesothelioma. Cytopathology 2000;11:139–151.
850. Whitaker D, Sterrett G, Shilkin KB. Mesotheliomas. In: Gray W, ed. Diagnostic cytopathology. Edinburgh: Churchill Livingstone, 1995:195–224.
851. DeMay RM. Cytology of malignant mesothelioma. In: Pass H, Vogelzang NJ, Carbone M, eds. Malignant mesothelioma. New York: Springer, 2005:481–489.
852. DeMay RM. The art and science of cytopathology. Chicago: ASCP Press, 1996.
853. Geisinger KR, Stanley MW, Raab SS, et al. Modern cytopathology. Philadelphia: Churchill Livingstone, 2003.
854. Pereira TC, Saad RS, Liu Y, Silverman JF. The diagnosis of malignancy in effusion cytology: a pattern recognition approach. Adv Anat Pathol 2006;13:174–184.
855. Renshaw AA, Dean BR, Antman KH, et al. The role of cytologic evaluation of pleural fluid in the diagnosis of malignant mesothelioma. Chest 1997;111:106–109.
856. DiBonito L, Falconieri G, Colautti I, et al. Cytopathology of malignant mesothelioma: a study of its patterns and histological bases. Diagn Cytopathol 1993;9:25–31.
857. Maskell NA, Butland RJ. BTS guidelines for the investigation of a unilateral pleural effusion in adults. Thorax 2003;58(suppl 2):8–17.
858. Tarn AC, Lapworth R. BTS guidelines for investigation of unilateral pleural effusion in adults. Thorax 2004;59:358–9; author reply 359.
859. Antony VB, Loddenkemper R, Astoul P, et al. Management of malignant pleural effusions. Eur Respir J 2001; 18:402–419.
860. Atagi S, Ogawara M, Kawahara M, et al. Utility of hyaluronic acid in pleural fluid for differential diagnosis of pleural effusions: likelihood ratios for malignant mesothelioma. Jpn J Clin Oncol 1997;27:293–297.
861. Boersma A, Degand P, Biserte G. Hyaluronic acid analysis and the diagnosis of pleural mesothelioma. Bull Eur Physiopathol Respir 1980;16:41–45.
862. Matzel W, Schubert G. Hyaluronic acid in pleural fluids: an additional parameter for clinical diagnosis on diffuse

mesotheliomas [German]. Arch Geschwulstforsch 1979; 49:146–154.
863. Welker L, Muller M, Holz O, et al. Cytological diagnosis of malignant mesothelioma-improvement by additional analysis of hyaluronic acid in pleural effusions. Virchows Arch 2007;450:455–461.
864. Creaney J, Yeoman D, Naumoff L, et al. Soluble mesothelin in effusions—a useful tool for the diagnosis of malignant mesothelioma. Thorax 2007;62:569–576.
865. Romero S, Fernandez C, Arriero JM, et al. CEA, CA 15–3 and CYFRA 21–1 in serum and pleural fluid of patients with pleural effusions. Eur Respir J 1996;9:17–23.
866. Fetsch PA, Simsir A, Brosky K, Abati A. Comparison of three commonly used cytologic preparations in effusion immunocytochemistry. Diagn Cytopathol 2002;26:61–66.
867. Ylagan LR, Zhai J. The value of ThinPrep and cytospin preparation in pleural effusion cytological diagnosis of mesothelioma and adenocarcinoma. Diagn Cytopathol 2005;32:137–144.
868. Gong Y, Sun X, Michael CW, et al. Immunocytochemistry of serous effusion specimens: a comparison of ThinPrep vs. cell block. Diagn Cytopathol 2003;28:1–5.
869. Manosca F, Schinstine M, Fetsch PA, et al. Diagnostic effects of prolonged storage on fresh effusion samples. Diagn Cytopathol 2007;35:6–11.
870. Whitaker D. Cell aggregates in malignant mesothelioma. Acta Cytol 1977;21:236–239.
871. Johnson JS, Edwards JM. Malignant mesothelioma mimicking squamous carcinoma in a pleural fluid aspirate. Cytopathology 2001;12:54–56.
872. Gupta K, Dey P. Cell cannibalism: diagnostic marker of malignancy. Diagn Cytopathol 2003;28:86–87.
873. Tickman RJ, Cohen C, Varma VA. Distinction between carcinoma cells and mesothelial cells in serous effusions: usefulness of immunohistochemistry. Acta Cytol 1990; 34:491–496.
874. Isobe H, Sridhar KS, Doria R, et al. Prognostic significance of DNA aneuploidy in diffuse malignant mesothelioma. Cytometry 1995:86–91.
875. Motherby H, Pomjanski N, Kube M, et al. Diagnostic DNA-flow- vs. -image-cytometry in effusion cytology. Anal Cell Pathol 2002;24(1):5–15.
876. Osterheld MC, Liette C, Anca M. Image cytometry: an aid for cytological diagnosis of pleural effusions. Diagn Cytopathol 2005;32:173–176.
877. Dejmek A, Stromberg C, Wikstrom B, Hjerpe A. Prognostic importance of the DNA ploidy pattern in malignant mesothelioma of the pleura. Anal Quant Cytol Histol 1992;14:217–221.
878. Jagirdar J, Levine Z, Gallo L, Lee T. Automated argyrophilic nucleolar organizer region (AgNOR) counts in the differential diagnosis of benign vs malignant mesothelial cells. Lab Invest 1992;66:114A.
879. Pomjanski N, Motherby H, Buckstegge B, et al. Early diagnosis of mesothelioma in serous effusions using AgNOR analysis. Anal Quant Cytol Histol 2001;23: 151–160.
880. Nagel H, Hemmerlein B, Ruschenburg I, et al. The value of anti-calretinin antibody in the differential diagnosis of normal and reactive mesothelial versus metastatic tumors in effusion cytology. Pathol Res Prac 1998;194:759–764.
881. Su XY, Li GD, Liu HB, Jiang LL. Significance of combining detection of E-cadherin, carcinoembryonic antigen, and calretinin in cytological differential diagnosis of serous effusion [Chin]. Ai Zheng 2004;23:1185–1189.
882. Ruitenbeek T, Gouw AS, Poppema S. Immunocytology of body cavity fluids: MOC-31, a monoclonal antibody discriminating between mesothelial and epithelial cells. Arch Pathol Lab Med 1994;118:265–269.
883. Lauritzen AF. Diagnostic value of monoclonal antibody B72.3 in detecting adenocarcinoma cells in serous effusions. APMIS 1989;97:761–766.
884. Ko EC, Jhala NC, Shultz JJ, Chhieng DC. Use of a panel of markers in the differential diagnosis of adenocarcinoma and reactive mesothelial cells in fluid cytology. Am J Clin Pathol 2001;116:709–715.
885. Nance KV, Silverman JF. Immunocytochemical panel for the identification of malignant cells in serous effusions. Am J Clin Pathol 1991;95:867–874.
886. Dusenbery D, Grimes MM, Frable WJ. Fine-needle aspiration cytology of localized fibrous tumor of pleura. Diagn Cytopathol 1992;8:444–450.
887. Sterrett GF, Whitaker D, Shilkin KB, Walters MN. Fine needle aspiration cytology of malignant mesothelioma. Acta Cytol 1987;31:185–193.
888. Nguyen GK, Akin MR, Villanueva RR, Slatnik J. Cytopathology of malignant mesothelioma of the pleura in fine-needle aspiration biopsy. Diagn Cytopathol 1999;21: 253–259.
889. Silverman JF, Berns LA, Holbrook CT, et al. Fine needle aspiration cytology of primitive neuroectodermal tumors: a report of these cases. Acta Cytol 1992;36:541–550.
890. Spanta R, Saleh HA, Khatib G. Fine needle aspiration diagnosis of extraadrenal myelolipoma presenting as a pleural mass: a case report. Acta Cytol 1999;43: 295–298.
891. Taylor CA, Barnhart A, Pettenati MJ, Geisinger KR. Primary pleuropulmonary synovial sarcoma diagnosed by fine needle aspiration with cytogenetic confirmation: a case report. Acta Cytol 2005;49:673–676.
892. Cho EY, Han JJ, Han J, Oh YL. Fine needle aspiration cytology of solitary fibrous tumours of the pleura. Cytopathology 2007;18:20–27.
893. Yu GH, Soma L, Hahn S, Friedberg JS. Changing clinical course of patients with malignant mesothelioma: implications for FNA cytology and utility of immunocytochemical staining. Diagn Cytopathol 2001;24:322–327.
894. Tafazzoli A, Raza A, Martin SE. Primary diagnosis of malignant mesothelioma by fine-needle aspiration of a supraclavicular lymph node. Diagn Cytopathol 2005;33: 122–125.
895. Yu GH, Baloch ZW, Gupta PK. Cytomorphology of metastatic mesothelioma in fine-needle aspiration specimens. Diagn Cytopathol 1999;20:328–332.
896. Cimbaluk D, Kasuganti D, Kluskens L, et al. Malignant biphasic pleural mesothelioma metastatic to the liver diagnosed by fine-needle aspiration. Diagn Cytopathol 2006;34:33–36.

897. Sneige N, Holder PD, Katz RL, et al. Fine-needle aspiration cytology of the male breast in a cancer center. Diagn Cytopathol 1993;9:691–697.
898. Schmid KW, Hittmair A, Ofner C, et al. Metastatic tumors in fine needle aspiration biopsy of the thyroid. Acta Cytol 1991;35:722–724.
899. Adams RF, Gray W, Davies RJ, Gleeson FV. Percutaneous image-guided cutting needle biopsy of the pleura in the diagnosis of malignant mesothelioma. Chest 2001;120: 1798–1802.
900. Vargas FS, Teixeira LR. Pleural malignancies. Curr Opin Pulm Med 1996;2:335–340.
901. Bonomo L, Feragalli B, Sacco R, et al. Malignant pleural disease. Eur J Radiol 2000;34:98–118.
902. Matthay RA, Coppage L, Shaw C, Filderman AE. Malignancies metastatic to the pleura. Invest Radiol 1990; 25:601–619.
903. Sahn SA. Malignancy metastatic to the pleura. Clin Chest Med 1998;19:351–361.
904. Chernow B, Sahn SA. Carcinomatous involvement of the pleura: an analysis of 96 patients. Am J Med 1977; 63:695–702.
905. Pomjanski N, Grote HJ, Doganay P, et al. Immunocytochemical identification of carcinomas of unknown primary in serous effusions. Diagn Cytopathol 2005;33:309–315.
906. Medford A, Maskell N. Pleural effusion. Postgrad Med J 2005;81:702–710.
907. Hammar SP, Dodson RF. Asbestos. In: Dail DH, Hammar SP, eds. Pulmonary pathology, 2nd ed. New York: Springer-Verlag, 1994:901–983.
908. Harwood TR, Gracey DR, Yokoo H. Pseudomesotheliomatous carcinoma of the lung: a variant of peripheral lung cancer. Am J Clin Pathol 1976;65:159–167.
909. Braganza JM, Butler EB, Fox H, et al. Ectopic production of salivary type amylase by a pseudomesotheliomatous carcinoma of the lung. Cancer 1978;41:1522–1525.
910. Broghamer WL Jr, Collins WM, Mojsejenko IK. The cytohistopathology of a pseudomesotheliomatous carcinoma of the lung. Acta Cytol 1978;22:239–242.
911. Tanaka I, Inoue M, Futonaka H, et al. An autopsy case of pseudomesotheliomatous lung cancer presenting as pneumothorax [Japanese]. Jap J Thorac Dis 1979;17: 582–587.
912. Lin JI, Tseng CH, Tsung SH. Pseudomesotheliomatous carcinoma of the lung. South Med J 1980;73:655–657.
913. Nishimoto Y, Ohno T, Saito K. Pseudomesotheliomatous carcinoma of the lung with histochemical and immunohistochemical study. Acta Pathol Jap 1983;33:415–423.
914. Simonsen J. Pseudomesotheliomatous carcinoma of the lung with asbestos exposure. Am J Forens Med Pathol 1986;7:49–51.
915. Dessy E, Pietra GG. Pseudomesotheliomatous carcinoma of the lung: an immunohistochemical and ultrastructural study of three cases. Cancer 1991;68:1747–1753.
916. Koss M, Travis W, Moran C, Hochholzer L. Pseudomesotheliomatous adenocarcinoma: a reappraisal. Semin Diagn Pathol 1992;9:117–123.
917. Moch H, Kiener S, Dalquen P, Gudat F. Pseudomesotheliomatous adenocarcinoma of the lung: immunohistochemical study with special reference to detection of blood group isoantigens and Ber-EP4 antigen [German]. Pathologe 1993;14:11–15.
918. Hartmann CA, Schütze H. Mesothelioma-like tumors of the pleura: a review of 72 autopsy cases. J Cancer Res Clin Oncol 1994;120:331–347.
919. Brunner-La Rocca HP, Schlossberg D, Vogt P. Pseudomesotheliomatous carcinoma in HIV infection [German]. Dtsch Med Wochenschr 1995;120:1312–1317.
920. Schreiner SR, Kirkpatrick BD, Askin FB. Pseudomesotheliomatous adenocarcinoma of the lung in a patient with HIV infection. Chest 1998;113:839–841.
921. Oka K, Otani S, Yoshimura T, et al. Mucin-negative pseudomesotheliomatous adenocarcinoma of the lung: report of three cases. Acta Oncol 1999;38:1119–1121.
922. Yuasa H, Tomoyasu M. Clinical comparison of diffuse malignant mesothelioma of the pleura and pseudomesotheliomatous carcinoma of the lung for each case [Japanese]. Jpn J Thorac Surg 1999;52:836–839.
923. Attanoos RL, Gibbs AR. "Pseudomesotheliomatous" carcinomas of the pleura: a 10-year analysis of cases from the Environmental Lung Disease Research Group, Cardiff. Histopathology 2003;43:444–452.
924. Taylor DR, Page W, Hughes D, Varghese G. Metastatic renal cell carcinoma mimicking pleural mesothelioma. Thorax 1987;42:901–902.
925. Ohgou T, Okahara M, Kishimoto T. Renal cell carcinoma with many transvenous pleural metastases [Japanese]. Nihon Kokyuki Gakkai Zasshi 1998;36:369–373.
926. Azuma T, Nishimatsu H, Nakagawa T, et al. Metastatic renal cell carcinoma mimicking pleural mesothelioma. Scand J Urol Nephrol 1999;33:140–141.
927. Huncharek M, Muscat J. Metastatic laryngeal carcinoma mimicking pleural mesothelioma. Respiration 1991;58: 204–206.
928. Hartmann CA, Minck C. Metastatic cystosarcoma phyllodes with pseudomesotheliomatous sarcomatosis of the contralateral pleura [German]. Pathologe 1988;9:119–123.
929. Babolini G, Blasi A. The pleural form of primary carcinoma of the lung. Dis Chest 1956;29:314–323.
930. Bollinger DJ, Wick MR, Dehner LP, al e. Peritoneal malignant mesothelioma versus serous papillary adenocarcinoma: a histochemical and immunohistochemical comparison. Am J Surg Pathol 1989;13:659–670.
931. Raju U, Fine G, Greenawald KA, Ohorodnik JM. Primary papillary serous neoplasia of the peritoneum: a clinicopathologic and ultrastructural study of eight cases. Hum Pathol 1989;20:426–436.
932. Wick MR, Mills SE, Dehner LP, et al. Serous papillary carcinomas arising from the peritoneum and ovaries: a clinicopathologic and immunohistochemical comparison. Int J Gynecol Pathol 1989;8:179–188.
933. Truong LD, Maccato ML, Awalt H, et al. Serous surface carcinoma of the peritoneum: a clinicopathologic study of 22 cases. Hum Pathol 1990;21:99–110.
934. Khoury N, Raju U, Crissman JD, et al. A comparative immunohistochemical study of peritoneal and ovarian serous tumors, and mesotheliomas. Hum Pathol 1990; 21:811–819.
935. Meis-Kindblom JM, Kindblom LG, Enzinger FM. Sclerosing epithelioid fibrosarcoma: a variant of fibrosarcoma

simulating carcinoma. Am J Surg Pathol 1995;19:979–993.
936. Antonescu CR, Rosenblum MK, Pereira P, et al. Sclerosing epithelioid fibrosarcoma: a study of 16 cases and confirmation of a clinicopathologically distinct tumor. Am J Surg Pathol 2001;25:699–709.
937. Rosai J, Gorich J. Pleural metastasis of malignant thymoma: a pitfall in the CT-diagnosis of pleural mesothelioma. Am J Surg Pathol 1990;14:819–828.
938. Payne CB, Jr,, Morningstar WA, Chester EH. Thymoma of the pleura masquerading as diffuse mesothelioma. Am Rev Respir Dis 1966;94:441–446.
939. Honma K, Shimada K. Metastasizing ectopic thymoma arising in the right thoracic cavity and mimicking diffuse pleural mesothelioma: an autopsy study of a case with review of the literature. Wien Klin Wochenschr 1986; 98:14–20.
940. Moran CA, Travis WD, Rosada-de-Christenson M, et al. Thymomas presenting as pleural tumors: report of eight cases. Am J Surg Pathol 1992;16:138–144.
941. Fushimi H, Tanio Y, Kotoh K. Ectopic thymoma mimicking diffuse pleural mesothelioma: a case report. Hum Pathol 1998;29:409–410.
942. Attanoos RL, Gibbs AR. Unusual “pseudomesotheliomatous” neoplasms: primary pleural thymic epithelial tumours. Histopathology 2002;41(suppl 2):170–173.
943. Travis WD, Brambilla E, Müller-Hermelink HK, Harris C, eds. Pathology and genetics of tumours of the lung, pleura, thymus and heart. Lyon: IARC, 2004:128–136.
944. Corson JM, Weiss LM, Banks-Schlegel SP, Pinkus G. Keratin proteins and carcinoembryonic antigen in synovial sarcomas: an immunohistochemical study of 24 cases. Hum Pathol 1984;15:615–621.
945. Nakamura T, Nakata K, Hata S, et al. Histochemical characterization of mucosubstances in synovial sarcoma. Am J Surg Pathol 1984;8:429–434.
946. Abenoza P, Manivel JC, Swanson PE, Wick MR. Synovial sarcoma: ultrastructural study and immunohistochemical analysis by a combined peroxidase-antiperoxidase/avidin-biotin-peroxidase complex procedure. Hum Pathol 1986;17:1107–1115.
947. Fisher C. Synovial sarcoma: ultrastructural and immunohistochemical features of epithelial differentiation in monophasic and biphasic tumors. Hum Pathol 1986;17: 996–1008.
948. Ordóñez NG, Mahfouz SM, Mackay B. Synovial sarcoma: an immunohistochemical and ultrastructural study. Hum Pathol 1990;21:733–749.
949. Dickersin GR. Synovial sarcoma: a review and update, with emphasis on the ultrastructural characterization of the nonglandular component. Ultrastruct Pathol 1991;15: 379–402.
950. Fisher C. Synovial sarcoma. Ann Diagn Pathol 1998;2: 401–421.
951. Powers A, Carbone M. Diagnosis of synovial sarcoma of the pleura and differentiation from malignant mesothelioma. In: Pass HI, Vogelzang NJ, Carbone M, eds. Malignant mesothelioma: advances in pathogenesis, diagnosis, and translational therapies. New York: Springer, 2005:543–554.
952. Witkin GB, Miettinen M, Rosai J. A biphasic tumor of the mediastinum with features of synovial sarcoma. A report of four cases. Am J Surg Pathol 1989;13:490–499.
953. Suster S, Moran CA. Primary synovial sarcomas of the mediastinum: a clinicopathologic, immunohistochemical and ultrastructural study of 15 cases. Am J Surg Pathol 2005;29:569–578.
954. Nicholson AG, Rigby M, Lincoln C, et al. Synovial sarcoma of the heart. Histopathology 1997;30:349–352.
955. Langner K, Schafer R, Muller KM, Goller T. Synovial sarcoma of the pericardium [German]. Pathologe 1998; 19:442–446.
956. Al-Rajhi N, Husain S, Coupland R, et al. Primary pericardial synovial sarcoma: a case report and literature review. J Surg Oncol 1999;70:194–198.
957. Vander Salm TJ. Unusual primary tumors of the heart. Semin Thorac Cardiovasc Surg 2000;12:89–100.
958. Hisaoka M, Hashimoto H, Iwamasa T, et al. Primary synovial sarcoma of the lung: report of two cases confirmed by molecular detection of SYT-SSX fusion gene transcripts. Histopathology 1999;34:205–210.
959. Keel SB, Bacha E, Mark EJ, et al. Primary pulmonary sarcoma: a clinicopathologic study of 26 cases. Mod Pathol 1999;12:1124–1131.
960. Aubry MC, Bridge JA, Wickert R, Tazelaar HD. Primary monophasic synovial sarcoma of the pleura: five cases confirmed by the presence of the SYT-SSX fusion transcript. Am J Surg Pathol 2001;25:776–781.
961. Colwell AS, D’Cunha J, Vargas SO, et al. Synovial sarcoma of the pleura: a clinical and pathologic study of three cases. J Thorac Cardiovasc Surg 2002;124:828–832.
962. Essary LR, Vargas SO, Fletcher CD. Primary pleuropulmonary synovial sarcoma: reappraisal of a recently described anatomic subset. Cancer 2002;94:459–469.
963. Hirano H, Kizaki T, Sashikata T, et al. Synovial sarcoma arising from the pleura: a case report with ultrastructural and immunohistochemical studies. Med Electron Microsc 2002;35:102–108.
964. Chan JA, McMenamin ME, Fletcher CDM. Synovial sarcoma in older patients: clinicopathologic analysis of 32 cases with emphasis on unusual histological features. Histopathology 2003;43:72–83.
965. Ng SB, Ahmed Q, Tien SL, et al. Primary pleural synovial sarcoma: a case report and review of the literature. Arch Pathol Lab Med 2003;127:85–90.
966. Vohra HA, Davies S, Vohra H, et al. Primary synovial sarcoma of the pleura: beware of misdiagnosis. Eur J Intern Med 2004;15:465–466.
967. Ghadially FN. Fine structure of synovial joints: a text and atlas of the ultrastructure of normal and pathological articular tissues. London: Butterworths, 1983.
968. Ghadially FN. Diagnostic electron microscopy of tumours, 2nd ed. London: Butterworths, 1985.
969. Henderson DW, Papadimitriou JM, Coleman M. Ultrastructural appearances of tumours. Diagnosis and classification of human neoplasia by electron microscopy, 2nd ed. Edinburgh: Churchill Livingstone, 1986.
970. Erlandson RA. Diagnostic transmission electron microscopy of tumors, with clinicopathological,

immunohistochemical, and cytogenetic correlations. New York: Raven Press, 1994.
971. Kashima T, Matsushita H, Kuroda M, et al. Biphasic synovial sarcoma of the peritoneal cavity with t(X;18) demonstrated by reverse transcriptase polymerase chain reaction. Pathol Int 1997;47:637–641.
972. Praet M, Forsyth R, Dhaene K, et al. Synovial sarcoma of the pleura: report of four cases. Histopathology 2002; 41:147–149.
973. Maruyama R, Mitsudomi T, Ishida T, et al. Aggressive pulmonary metastasectomies for synovial sarcoma. Respiration 1997;64:316–318.
974. England DM, Hochholzer L, McCarthy MJ. Localized benign and malignant fibrous tumors of the pleura: a clinicopathologic review of 223 cases. Am J Surg Pathol 1989;13:640–658.
975. Briselli M, Mark EJ, Dickersin GR. Solitary fibrous tumors of the pleura: eight new cases and review of 360 cases in the literature. Cancer 1981;47:2678–2689.
976. Moran CA, Suster S, Koss MN. The spectrum of histologic growth patterns in benign and malignant fibrous tumors of the pleura. Semin Diagn Pathol 1992;9:169–180.
977. Van de Rijn M, Lombard CM, Rouse RV. Expression of CD34 by solitary fibrous tumors of the pleura, mediastinum, and lung. Am J Surg Pathol 1994;18:814–820.
978. Segawa D, Yoshizu H, Haga Y, et al. Successful operation for solitary fibrous tumor of the epicardium. J Thorac Cardiovasc Surg 1995;109:1246–1248.
979. Kawashima K, Yokoi K, Matsuguma H, et al. Huge localized mesothelioma of the diaphragm in a 17-year-old female—a case report with calculated tumor volume doubling time. Nippon Kyobu Geka Gakkai Zasshi 1998; 46:225–230.
980. Chang YL, Lee YC, Wu CT. Thoracic solitary fibrous tumor: clinical and pathological diversity. Lung Cancer 1999;23:53–60.
981. Mentzel T, Bainbridge TC, Katenkamp D. Solitary fibrous tumour: clinicopathological, immunohistochemical, and ultrastructural analysis of 12 cases arising in soft tissues, nasal cavity and nasopharynx, urinary bladder and prostate. Virchows Arch 1997;430:445–453.
982. Fukunaga M, Naganuma H, Nikaido T, et al. Extrapleural solitary fibrous tumor: a report of seven cases. Mod Pathol 1997;10:443–450.
983. Segers K, Rodeck U, Backhovens H, et al. Solitary fibrous tumour of the orbit. J Pathol 1997;181:67–74.
984. Ing EB, Kennerdell JS, Olson PR, et al. Solitary fibrous tumor of the orbit. Ophthalmol Plast Reconstr Surg 1998;14:57–61.
985. Zamecnik M, Michal M. Solitary fibrous tumor (fibrous mesothelioma): report of 2 cases in an extraserous location. Cesk Patol 1998;34:58–62.
986. Festa S, Lee HJ, Langer P, Klein KM. Solitary fibrous tumor of the orbit: CT and pathologic correlation. Neuroradiology 1999;41:52–54.
987. Alobid I, Alos L, Blanch JL, et al. Solitary fibrous tumour of the nasal cavity and paranasal sinuses. Acta Otolaryngol 2003;123:71–74.
988. Ferrario F, Piantanida R, Spriano G, et al. Solitary fibrous tumor of the nasopharynx: apropos of a case. Ann Oto-Laryngol Chirurg Cervico-Faciale 1997;114:71–75.
989. Abe S, Imamura T, Tateishi A, et al. Intramuscular solitary fibrous tumor: a clinicopathological case study. J Comput Assist Tomogr 1999;23:458–462.
990. Piazza R, Blandamura S, Zattoni F, et al. Solitary fibrous tumour of the retroperitoneum mimicking a renal mass. Int Urol Nephrol 1996;28:751–754.
991. Leite KRM, Srougi M, Miotto A, Camara-Lopes LH. Solitary fibrous tumor in the bladder wall. Int Braz J Urol 2004;30:406–409.
992. Vadmal MS, Pellegrini AE. Solitary fibrous tumor of the vagina. Am J Dermatopathol 2000;22:83–86.
993. Thompson M, Cheng LHH, Stewart J, et al. A pediatric case of a solitary fibrous tumor of the parotid gland. Int J Pediatric Otorhinolaryngol 2004;68:481–487.
994. Kie JH, Kim JY, Park YN, et al. Solitary fibrous tumour of the thyroid. Histopathology 1997;30:365–368.
995. Levine TS, Rose DS. Solitary fibrous tumour of the liver. Histopathology 1997;30:396–397.
996. Hardisson D, Limeres MA, Jimenez-Heffernan JA, et al. Solitary fibrous tumor of the mesentery. Am J Gastroenterol 1996;91:810–811.
997. Cardillo G, Facciolo F, Cabazzana AO, et al. Localized (solitary) fibrous tumors of the pleura: an analysis of 55 patients. Ann Thorac Surg 2000;70:1808–812.
998. Kanamori Y, Hashizume K, Sugiyama M, et al. Intrapulmonary solitary fibrous tumor in an eight-year-old male. Pediatr Pulmonol 2005;40:262–264.
999. Henderson DW, Klebe S. Tumors, benign. In: Laurent GJ, Shapiro SD, eds. Encyclopedia of respiratory medicine, vol. 4. Oxford: Elsevier, 2006:312.
1000. Mori K, Ohtsuki Y, Hizuka N. Solitary fibrous tumor of the pleura with elevated high-molecular-weight insulin-like growth factor II and hypoglycemia. Nihon Kokyuki Gakkai Zasshi 1999;37:834–840.
1001. Gold JS, Antonescu CR, Hajdu C, et al. Clinicopathologic correlates of solitary fibrous tumors. Cancer 2002;94: 1057–1068.
1002. Chilosi M, Facchettti F, Dei Tos AP, et al. Bcl-2 expression in pleural and extrapleural solitary fibrous tumours. J Pathol 1997;181:362–367.
1003. Renshaw AA. O13 (CD99) in spindle cell tumors: reactivity with hemangiopericytoma, solitary fibrous tumors, synovial sarcoma, and meningioma, but rarely with sarcomatoid mesothelioma. Appl Immunohistochem 1995; 3:250–256.
1004. De Saint Aubain Somerhausen N, Rubin BP, Fletcher CD. Myxoid solitary fibrous tumor: a study of seven cases with emphasis on differential diagnosis. Mod Pathol 1999;12: 463–471.
1005. Yokoi T, Tsuzuki M, Yatabe Y, et al. Solitary fibrous tumor: significance of p53 and CD34 immunoreactivity in its malignant transformation. Histopathology 1998;32: 423–432.
1006. Miettinen M, Sobin LH, Sarlomo-Rikala M. Immunohistochemical spectrum of GISTs at different sites and their differential diagnosis with reference to CD117 (KIT). Mod Pathol 2000;13:1134–1142.

1007. Butnor KJ, Burchette JL, Sporn TA, et al. The spectrum of Kit (CD117) immunoreactivity in lung and pleural tumors: a study of 96 cases using a single-source antibody with a review of the literature. Arch Pathol Lab Med 2004;128:538–543.
1008. Kayser K, Trott J, Bohm G, et al. Localized fibrous tumors (LFT's) of the pleura: clinical data, asbestos burden, and syntactic structure analysis applied to newly defined angiogenic/growth-regulatory effectors. Pathol Res Pract 2005;201:791–801.
1009. Vallat-Decouvelaere AV, Dry SM, Fletcher CD. Atypical and malignant solitary fibrous tumors in extrathoracic locations: evidence of their comparability in intrathoracic tumors. Am J Surg Pathol 1998;22:1501–1511.
1010. Erasmus JJ, McAdams HP, Patz EFJ, et al. Calcifying fibrous pseudotumor of the pleura: radiologic features in three cases. J Comput Assist Tomogr 1996;20:63–65.
1011. Pinkard NB, Wilson RW, Lawless N, et al. Calcifying fibrous pseudotumor of pleura: a report of three cases of a newly described entity involving the pleura. Am J Clin Pathol 1996;105:189–194.
1012. Nascimento AE, Ruiz R, Hornick JL, Fletcher CD. Calcifying fibrous "pseudotumor": clinicopathologic study of 15 cases and analysis of its relationship to inflammatory myofibroblastic tumor. Int J Surg Pathol 2002;10:189–196.
1013. Hainaut P, Lesage V, Weynand B, et al. Calcifying fibrous pseudotumor (CFPT): a patient presenting with multiple pleural lesions. Acta Clin Belg 1999;54:162–164.
1014. Reed MK, Margraf LR, Nikaidoh H, Cleveland DC. Calcifying fibrous pseudotumor of the chest wall. Ann Thorac Surg 1996;62:873–874.
1015. Dumont P, de Muret A, Skrobala D, et al. Calcifying fibrous pseudotumor of the mediastinum. Ann Thorac Surg 1997;63:543–544.
1016. Jeong HS, Lee GK, Sung R, et al. Calcifying fibrous pseudotumor of mediastinum: a case report. J Korean Med Sci 1997;12:58–62.
1017. Kocova L, Michal M, Sulc M, et al. Calcifying fibrous pseudotumor of visceral peritoneum. Histopathology 1997;31:182–184.
1018. Ben-Izhak O, Czernobilsky B. Calcifying fibrous pseudotumor of the mesentery presenting with acute peritonitis: case report with immunohistochemical study and review of the literature. Int J Surg Pathol 2001;9:249–253.
1019. Van Dorpe J, Ectors N, Geboes K, et al. Is calcifying fibrous pseudotumor a late sclerosing stage of inflammatory myofibroblastic tumor? Am J Surg Pathol 1999;23: 329–335.
1020. Hill KA, Gonzalez-Crussi F, Chou PM. Calcifying fibrous pseudotumor versus inflammatory myofibroblastic tumor: a histological and immunohistochemical comparison. Mod Pathol 2001;14:784–790.
1021. Sigel JF, Smith TA, Reith JD, Goldblum JR. Immunohistochemical analysis of anaplastic lymphoma kinase expression in deep soft tissue calcifying fibrous pseudotumor: evidence of a late sclerotic phase of inflammatory myofibroblastic tumor? Ann Diagn Pathol 2001;5:10–14.
1022. Maeda A, Kawabata K, Kusuzaki K. Rapid recurrence of calcifying fibrous pseudotumor (a case report). Anticancer Res 2002;22:1795–1797.
1023. Wilson RW, Galateau-Sallé F, Moran CA. Desmoid tumors of the pleura: a clinicopathologic mimic of localized fibrous tumor. Mod Pathol 1999;12:9–14.
1024. Andino L, Cagle PT, Murer B, et al. Pleuropulmonary desmoids tumors: immunohistochemical comparison with solitary fibrous tumors and assessment of β-catenin and cyclin D1 expression. Arch Pathol Lab Med 2006;130: 1503–1509.
1025. Fletcher C, Krishman A, Mertens F. Tumor of soft tissue and bone. Lyon: WHO/IARC Press, 2002.
1026. Ordonez NG, Tornos C. Malignant peripheral nerve sheath tumor of the pleura with epithelial and rhabdomyoblastic differentiation: report of a case clinically simulating mesothelioma. Am J Surg Pathol 1997;21: 1515–1521.
1027. Galateau-Sallé F, ed. International Mesothelioma Panel: Brambilla E, Cagle PT, Churg AM, et al. Differential diagnosis: non-mesothelial tumors of serosal cavity: sarcomas. In: Pathology of malignant mesothelioma. London: Springer, 2006:169.
1028. Snyder CS, Dell-Aquila N, Munson P, et al. Clonal changes in inflammatory pseudotumor of lung. Cancer 1995;76: 1545–1549.
1029. Weiss SW, Enzinger FM. Epithelioid hemangioendothelioma: a vascular tumor often mistaken for carcinoma. Cancer 1882;50:970–981.
1030. Battifora H. Epithelioid hemangioendothelioma imitating mesothelioma. Appl Immunohistochem 1993;1:220–221.
1031. Lin BT-Y, Colby T, Gown AM, et al. Malignant vascular tumors of the serous membranes mimicking mesothelioma. Am J Surg Pathol 1996;20:1431–1439.
1032. Attanoos RL, Dallimore NS, Gibbs AR. Primary epithelioid haemangioendothelioma of the peritoneum: an unusual mimic of diffuse malignant mesothelioma. Histopathology 1997;30:375–377.
1033. Crotty EJ, McAdams HP, Erasmus JJ, et al. Epithelioid hemangioendothelioma of the pleura: clinical and radiologic features. AJR Am J Roentgenol 2000;175: 1545–1549.
1034. Sporn TA, Butnor KJ, Roggli VL. Epithelioid haemangioendothelioma of the pleura: an aggressive vascular malignancy and clinical mimic of malignant mesothelioma. Histopathology 2002;41:173–177.
1035. Al-Shraim M, Mahboub B, Neligan PC, et al. Primary pleural epithelioid haemangioendothelioma with metastases to the skin: a case report and literature review. J Clin Pathol 2005;58:107–109.
1036. Attanoos RL, Suvarna SK, Rhead E, et al. Malignant vascular tumours of the pleura in "asbestos" workers and endothelial differentiation in malignant mesothelioma. Thorax 2000;55:860–863.
1037. Oliveira A, Carvalho L. Epithelioid haemangioendothelioma of the pleura: 29 months survival. Rev Port Pneumol 2006;12:455–461.
1038. Parkash V, Gerald WL, Parma A, et al. Desmoplastic small round cell tumor of the pleura. Am J Surg Pathol 1995;19:659–665.
1039. Sapi Z, Szentirmay Z, Orosz Z. Desmoplastic small round cell tumor of the pleura: a case report with further

cytogenetic and ultrastructural evidence of mesothelial "blastemic" origin. Eur J Surg Oncol 1999;25:633–634.
1040. Venkateswaran L, Jenkins JJ, Kaste SC, et al. Disseminated intrathoracic desmoplastic small round-cell tumor: a case report. J Pediatr Hematol Oncol 1997;19:172–175.
1041. Liu J, Nau MM, Yeh JC, et al. Molecular heterogeneity and function of EWS-WT1 fusion transcripts in desmoplastic small round cell tumors. Clin Cancer Res 2000;6:3522–3529.
1042. Dehner LP. Primitive neuroectodermal tumor and Ewing's sarcoma. Am J Surg Pathol 1993;17:1–13.
1043. Perlman EJ, Dickman PS, Askin FB, et al. Ewing's sarcoma—routine diagnostic utilization of MIC2 analysis: a Pediatric Oncology Group/Children Cancer Group Intergroup Study. Hum Pathol 1994;25:304–307.
1044. Weidner N, Tjoe J. Immunohistochemical profile of monoclonal antibody O13: antibody that recognizes glycoprotein p30/32MIC2 and is useful in diagnosing Ewing's sarcoma and peripheral neuroepithelioma. Am J Surg Pathol 1994;18:486–494.
1045. Manivel JC, Priest JR, Watterson J, et al. Pleuropulmonary blastoma: the so-called pulmonary blastoma of childhood. Cancer 1988;62:1516–1526.
1046. Ansari MQ, Dawson DB, Nador R, et al. Primary body cavity-based AIDS-related lymphomas. Am J Clin Pathol 1996;105:221–229.
1047. Banks PM, Warnke RA. Primary effusion lymphoma. In: WHO classification of tumors of hematopoietic and lymphoid tissues. Lyon: IARC Press, 2001:179–180.
1048. Banks PM, Harris NL, Warnke RA. Primary effusion lymphoma. In: Travis WD, Brambilla E, eds. WHO classification of tumors of the lung, pleura and mediastinum. Lyon: IARC Press, 2004.
1049. Aozasa K, Ohsaw AM, Kanno H. Pyothorax-associated lymphoma: a distinctive type of lymphoma strongly associated with Epstein-Barr virus. Adv Anat Pathol 1997;4:58–63.
1050. Gaulard P, Harris NL. Pyothorax-associated lymphoma. In: Travis WD, Brambilla E, eds. WHO classification of tumors of the lung, pleura and mediastinum. Lyon: IARC Press, 2004.
1051. Ibuka T, Fukayama M, Hayashi Y, et al. Pyothorax-associated pleural lymphoma. Cancer 1994;73:738–744.
1052. Uluba G, Eynboglu FO, Simek A, Ozyilkan O. Multiple myeloma with pleural involvement: a case report. Am J Clin Oncol 2005;28:429–430.
1053. Giuliani N, Caramatti C, Roti G, et al. Hematologic malignancies with extramedullary spread of disease. Case 1. Multiple myeloma with extramedullary involvement of the pleura and testes. J Clin Oncol 2003;21:1887–1888.
1054. Quinquenel ML, Moualla M, Le Coz A, et al. Pleural involvement of myeloma. Apropos of two cases. Rev Mal Respir 1995;12:173–174.
1055. Vega F, Padula A, Valbuena JR, et al. Lymphomas involving the pleura: a clinicopathologic study of 34 cases diagnosed by pleural biopsy. Arch Pathol Lab Med 2006;130:1497–1502.
1056. Bourantas KL, Tsiara S, Pantel IA, et al. Pleural effusion in chronic myelomonocytic leukemia. Acta Hematol 1998;99:34–37.
1057. Schmitt-Graff A, Wickenhauser C, Kvasnicka HM, et al. Extramedullary initial manifestations of acute myeloid leukemia (AML). Pathologe 2002;23:397–404.
1058. Robinson BW, Creaney J, Lake R, et al. Mesothelin-family proteins and diagnosis of mesothelioma. Lancet 2003;362:1612–1616.
1059. Creaney J, Robinson BW. Detection of malignant mesothelioma in asbestos-exposed individuals: the potential role of soluble mesothelin-related protein. Hematol Oncol Clin North Am 2005;19:1025–1040.
1060. Robinson BW, Creaney J, Lake R, et al. Soluble mesothelin-related protein—a blood test for mesothelioma. Lung Cancer 2005;49:S109–S111.
1061. Robinson BWS, Musk A, Lake R. Malignant mesothelioma. Lancet 2005;366:397–408.
1062. Creaney J, Christansen H, Lake R, et al. Soluble mesothelin related protein in mesothelioma. J Thorac Oncol 2006;1:172–174.
1063. Hassan R, Remaley AT, Sampson ML, et al. Detection and quantitation of serum mesothelin, a tumor parker for patients with mesothelioma and ovarian cancer. Clin Cancer Res 2006;12:447–453.
1064. Scherpereel A, Grigoriu B, Conti M, et al. Soluble mesothelin-related protein in the diagnosis of malignant pleural mesothelioma. Am J Respir Crit Care Med ACJRCCM Articles in Press: e-publication 2006; doi:10.1164/rccm.200511–1789OC.
1065. Beyer HL, Geschwindt RD, Glover CL, et al. MESOMARK™: a potential test for malignant pleural mesothelioma. Clin Chem 2007;53:666–672.
1066. Pass HI, Lott D, Lonardo F, et al. Asbestos exposure, pleural mesothelioma, and serum osteopontin levels. N Engl J Med 2005;353:1564–1573.
1067. Cullen M. Serum osteopontin levels—is it time to screen asbestos-exposed workers for pleural mesothelioma? [editorial]. N Engl J Med 2005;353:1617–1618.
1068. Gigerenzer G. Calculated risks: how to know when numbers deceive you. New York: Simon & Schuster, 2002. Published in the United Kingdom as Reckoning with risk: learning to live with uncertainty. London: Allen Lane, 2002.
1069. Rump A, Morikawa Y, Tanaka M, et al. Binding of ovarian cancer antigen CA125/MUC16 to mesothelin mediates cell adhesion. J Biol Chem 2004;279:9190–9198.
1070. Yen MJ, Hsu C-Y, Mao T-L, et al. Diffuse mesothelin expression correlates with prolonged patient survival in ovarian serous carcinoma. Clin Cancer Res 2006;12:827–831.
1071. Ho M, Bera TK, Willingham MC, et al. Mesothelin expression in human lung cancer. Clin Cancer Res 2007;13:1571–1575.
1072. Baruch AC, Wang H, Staerkel GA, et al. Immunocytochemical study of the expression of mesothelin in fine-needle aspiration biopsy specimens of pancreatic adenocarcinoma. Diagn Cytopathol 2007;35:143–147.
1073. Maeda M, Hino O. Molecular tumor markers for asbestos-related mesothelioma: serum diagnostic markers. Pathol Int 2006;56:649–654.
1074. Shiomi K, Miyamoto H, Segawa T, et al. Novel ELISA system for detection of N-ERC mesothelin in the sera of mesothelioma patients. Cancer Sci 2006;97:928–932.

1075. Huang CY, Cheng WF, Lee CN, et al. Serum mesothelin in epithelial ovarian carcinoma: a new screening marker and prognostic factor. Anticancer Res 2006;26:4721–4728.
1076. Haylock DN, Nilsson SK. Osteopontin: a bridge between bone and blood. Br J Haematol 2006;134:467–474.
1077. Vordermark D, Said HM, Katzer A, et al. Plasma osteopontin levels in patients with head and neck cancer and cervix cancer are critically dependent on the choice of ELISA system. BMC Cancer 2006;6:207: doi:10.1186/471-2407-6-207.
1078. Teo M, Kodama S, Nomi N, et al. Clinical significance of elevated osteopontin levels in head and neck cancer patients. Auris Nasus Larynx 2007;34:343–346.
1079. Bao LH, Sakaguchi H, Fujimoto J, Tamaya T. Osteopontin in metastatic lesions as a prognostic marker in ovarian cancers. J Biomed Sci 2007;14:373–381.
1080. Wu CY, Wu MS, Chiang EP, et al. Elevated plasma osteopontin associated with gastric cancer development, invasion and survival. Gut 2007;56:782–789.
1081. Kim J, Ki SS, Lee SD, et al. Elevated levels of osteopontin levels in patients with hepatocellular carcinoma. Am J Gastroenterol 2006;101:2051–2059.
1082. Mishima R, Takeshima F, Sawai T, et al. High plasma osteopontin levels in patients with inflammatory bowel disease. J Clin Gastroenterol 2007;41:167–172.
1083. Friman C, Hellstrom PE, Juvani M, Riska H. Acid glycosaminoglycans (mucopolysaccharides) in the differential diagnosis of pleural effusion. Clin Chim Acta 1977;76:357–361.
1084. Arai H, Kang K, Sato H, et al. Significance of the quantification and demonstration of hyaluronic acid in tissue specimens for the diagnosis of pleural mesothelioma. Am Rev Respir Dis 1979;120:529–532.
1085. Castor CW, Naylor B. Acid mucopolysaccharide composition of serous effusions. Cancer 1967;20:462–466.
1086. Rasmussen KN, Faber V. Hyaluronic acid in 247 pleural fluids. Scand J Respir Dis 1967;48:366–371.
1087. Thompson ME, Bromberg PA, Amenta JS. Acid mucopolysaccharide determination: a useful adjunct for the diagnosis of malignant mesothelioma with effusion. Am J Clin Pathol 1969;52:335–339.
1088. Katayam N, Tokuda A, Nakatsumi Y, et al. A case of malignant mesothelioma presenting with recurrent pneumothorax. Nihon Kokyuki Gakkai Zasshi 2006;44:807–811.
1089. Pettersson T, Froseth B, Rista H, Klockars M. Concentration of hyaluronic acid in pleural fluid as a diagnostic aid for malignant mesothelioma. Chest 1988;94:1037–1039.
1090. Hillerdal G, Lindqvist U, Engstrom-Laurent A. Hyaluronan in pleural effusions and in serum. Cancer 1991;67:2410–2414.
1091. Soderblom T, Pettersson T, Nyberg P, et al. High pleural fluid hyaluronan concentrations in rheumatoid arthritis. Eur Respir J 1999;13:519–522.
1092. Chiu B, Churg A, Tengblad A, Pearce R, McCaughey WTE. Analysis of hyaluronic acid in the diagnosis of malignant mesothelioma. Cancer 1984;54:2195–2199.
1093. Nakano T, Fujii J, Tamura S, et al. Glycosaminoglycan in malignant pleural mesothelioma. Cancer 1986;57:106–110.
1094. Iozzo RV. Biology of disease. Proteoglycans: structure, function and role in neoplasia. Lab Invest 1985;53:373–396.
1095. Iozzo RV, Goldes JA, Chen W-J, Wight JN. Glycosaminoglycans of pleural mesothelioma: a possible biochemical variant containing chondroitin sulfate. Cancer 1981;48:89–97.
1096. Afify AM, Stern R, Michael CW. Differentiation of mesothelioma from adenocarcinoma in serous effusions: the role of hyaluronic acid and CD44 localization. Diagn Cytopathol 2005;32:145–150.
1097. Thylen A, Hjerpe A, Martensson G. Hyaluronan content in pleural fluid as a prognostic factor in patients with malignant mesothelioma. Cancer 2001;92:1224–1230.
1098. Monti G, Jaurand MC, Monnet I, et al. Intrapleural production of interleukin-6 during mesothelioma and its modulation by gamma interferon treatment. Cancer Res 1994;54:4419–4423.
1099. Langlois SL, Henderson DW. Radiological investigation of mesothelioma. In: Henderson DW, Shilkin KB, Langlois SL, Whitaker D, eds. Malignant mesothelioma. New York: Hemisphere, 1992:259–77.
1100. Nind NR, Attanoos RL, Gibbs AR. Unusual intraparenchymal growth patterns of malignant pleural mesothelioma. Histopathology 2003;42:150–155.
1101. Felner KJ, Wieczorek R, Kline M, et al. Malignant mesothelioma masquerading as a multinodular bronchioloalveolar cell adenocarcinoma with widespread pulmonary nodules. Int J Surg Pathol 2006;14:229–233.
1102. Jones JSP, ed. Pathology of the mesothelium. London: Springer-Verlag, 1987.
1103. Solomons K, Polakow R, Marchand P. Diffuse malignant mesothelioma presenting as bilateral malignant lymphangitis. Thorax 1985;40:682–683.
1104. Musk AW, Dewar J, Shilkin KB, Whitaker D. Miliary spread of malignant pleural mesothelioma without a clinically identifiable pleural tumour. Aust NZ J Med 1991;21:460–462.
1105. Kaye JA, Wang A-M, Joachim CL, et al. Malignant mesothelioma with brain metastases. Am J Med 1986;80:95–97.
1106. Asoh Y, Nakamura M, Maeda T, et al. Brain metastasis from primary pericardial mesothelioma: case report. Neurol Med Chir 1990;30:884–887.
1107. Bohn U, Gonzalez JL, Martin LM, et al. Meningeal and brain metastases in primary malignant pericardial mesothelioma [letter]. Ann Oncol 1994;5:660–661.
1108. Kitai R, Kabuto M, Kawano H, et al. Brain metastasis from malignant mesothelioma—case report. Neurol Med Chir 1995;35:172–174.
1109. Kawai A, Nagasaka Y, Muraki M, et al. Brain metastasis in malignant pleural mesothelioma. Intern Med 1997;36:591–594.
1110. Cheeseman SL, Ranson MR. Cerebral metastases in malignant mesothelioma: a case report. Eur J Cancer Care 1999;8:104–106.
1111. Kobayashi S, Ida M, Matsui O, et al. Lipomatous change in a brain metastasis from malignant pleural mesothelioma. Neuroradiology 2001;43:159–161.

1112. Dutt PL, Baxter JW, O'Malley FP, et al. Distant cutaneous metastasis of pleural malignant mesothelioma. J Cutan Pathol 1992;19:490–495.
1113. Prieto VG, Kenet BJ, Varghese M. Malignant mesothelioma metastatic to the skin, presenting as inflammatory carcinoma. Am J Dermatopathol 1997;19:261–265.
1114. Kubota K, Furuse K, Kawahara M, et al. A case of malignant pleural mesothelioma with metastasis to the orbit. Jpn J Clin Oncol 1996;26:469–471.
1115. Piattelli A, Fioroni M, Rubini C. Tongue metastasis from a malignant diffuse mesothelioma of the pleura: report of a case. J Oral Maxillofac Surg 1999;57:861–863.
1116. American Joint Committee on Cancer (AJCC). AJCC cancer staging handbook, 6th ed.: TNM classification of malignant tumors. New York: Springer, 2002.
1117. Roberts GH. Distal visceral metastases in pleural mesothelioma. Br J Dis Chest 1976;70:246–250.
1118. Huncharek M, Muscat J. Metastases in diffuse pleural mesothelioma: influence of histological type. Thorax 1987; 42:897–898.
1119. Hulks G, Thomas JSJ, Waclawski E. Malignant pleural mesothelioma in western Glasgow 1980–6. Thorax 1989; 44:496–500.
1120. King JA, Tucker JA, Wong SW. Mesothelioma: a study of 22 gases. South Med J 1997;90:199–205.
1121. Elmes PC, Simpson MJC. The clinical aspects of mesothelioma. Q J Med 1976;45:427–429.
1122. Doward AJ, Stack BHR. Diffuse malignant pleural mesothelioma in Glasgow. Br J Dis Chest 1981;75: 397–402.
1123. Chahinian AP, Pajak TF, Holand JF, et al. Diffuse malignant mesothelioma: prospective evaluation of 69 patients. Ann Intern Med 1982;96:746–755.
1124. Solomons K. Malignant mesothelioma—clinical and epidemiological features: a report of 80 cases. S Afr Med J 1984;66:407–412.
1125. Krumhaar D, Lange S, Hartman C, Anhuth D. Follow-up study of 100 malignant pleural mesotheliomas. Thorac Cardiovasc Surg 1985;33:272–275.
1126. Ruffie P, Feld R, Minkin S, et al. Diffuse malignant mesothelioma of the pleura in Ontario and Quebec: a retrospective study of 322 patients. J Clin Oncol 1989;7: 1157–1168.
1127. Butchart EG, Ashcroft T, Barnsley WC, Holden MP. Pleuropneumonectomy in the management of diffuse malignant mesothelioma of the pleura: experience with 29 patients. Thorax 1976;31:15–24.
1128. Rusch VW. A proposed new international TNM staging system for malignant pleural mesothelioma from the International Mesothelioma Interest Group. Lung Cancer 1996;14:1–12.
1129. Ohishi N, Oka T, Fukuhara T, et al. Extensive pulmonary metastases in malignant pleural mesothelioma: a rare clinical and radiographic presentation. Chest 1996;110: 296–298.
1130. Chailleux E, Dabouis G, Pioche D, et al. Prognostic factors in diffuse malignant pleural mesothelioma: a study of 167 patients. Chest 1988;93:159–162.
1131. Antman K, Shemin R, Ryan L, et al. Malignant mesothelioma: prognostic variables in a registry of 180 patients, the Dana-Farber Cancer Institute and Brigham and Women's Hospital experience over two decades, 1965–1985. J Clin Oncol 1988;6:147–153.
1132. Alberts AS, Falkson G, Goedhals L, Vorobiof DA, Van Dor Merwe CA. Malignant pleural mesotheliom: a disease unaffected by current therapeutic maneuvers. J Clin Oncol 1988;6:527–535.
1133. Harvey JC, Fleischman EH, Kagan AR, Streeter OE. Malignant pleural mesothelioma: a survival study. J Surg Oncol 1990;45:40–42.
1134. Ribak J, Selikoff IJ. Survival of asbestos insulation workers with mesothelioma. Br J Ind Med 1992;49:732–735.
1135. Tammilehto L. Malignant mesothelioma: Prognostic factors in a prospective study of 98 patients. Lung Cancer 1992;8:175–184.
1136. Sridhar KS, Doria R, Raub WA Jr, Thurer RJ, Saldana M. New strategies are needed in diffuse malignant mesothelioma. Cancer 1992;70:2969–2979.
1137. Curran D, Sahmoud T, Therasse P, et al. Prognostic factors in patients with pleural mesothelioma, the EORTC experience. J Clin Oncol 1998;16:145–152.
1138. Grondin SC, Sugarbaker DJ. Pleuropneumonectomy in the treatment of malignant pleural mesothelioma. Chest 1999;116:450S–454S.
1139. Takagi K, Tsuchy AR, Watanabi Y. Surgical approach to pleural diffuse mesothelioma in Japan. Lung Cancer 2001;31:57–65.
1140. Pass HI, Temeck BK, Kranda K, et al. Preoperative tumor volume is associated without common malignant pleural mesothelioma. J Thorac Cardiovasc Surg 1998;115:310–317.
1141. Edwards JG, Swinson DE, Jones JL, et al. Tumor necrosis correlates with angiogenesis and is a predictor of poor prognosis in malignant mesothelioma. Chest 2003;124: 1916–1923.

44
Metastases to and from the Lung

David H. Dail

Metastatic neoplasms to the lung are the most common category of tumor found in the lung. This chapter discusses general principles of metastases to lung, specific organ sources, and primary lung tumors and their own metastases. In autopsy studies, the lungs are involved with metastases in 20% to 54%[1–6] of cases of extrapulmonary malignancies, and in 15% to 25% the lung is the only site of such metastases.[1] Some selected excellent reviews of the basics of metastases,[7,8] their clinical, radiographic, and therapeutic details,[7,9–11] and their presence in the lung and pleura[7,9–13] are highly recommended for the interested reader.

The fact that the lungs are the organ system that acquires the most metastases of any system in the entire body is related to several unique features of the lungs: they receive the entire right-sided cardiac output continuously with every heartbeat, they have the densest capillary bed in the body, they are the first capillary plexus met by cells after most of the lymphatic drainage enters the venous system, and they consist of delicate membranes that may be beneficial for initially drawing on nearby oxygenated air for early sustenance. There are several other factors. In 1889, Stephen Paget[14] compared the apparent selectivity of hematogenously borne metastases to seeds needing to find the right soil, an idea that has become known as Paget's "seed and soil" theory. In 1928, James Ewing[15] proposed that metastases developed in the first organ to be exposed to drainage of tumor cell–bearing fluids such as lymph or blood. As nicely reviewed by Zetter in 1990,[8] both theories are partially correct; examples of direct flow carrying tumor cells, such as colon metastases to liver, and of selective implantation, such as the liver as a destination of choroidal melanomas, are well known.

Both primary and secondary pulmonary neoplasms are supplied by bronchial arteries whose circulation is high pressure, oxygenated, and part of the systemic supply. At the edge of growing tumor masses and in cases of bronchioloalveolar-type carcinomatous growth, most likely some sustenance is obtained from direct diffusion from adjacent alveoli or perfusion from adjacent pulmonary capillary venous or arterial blood, and the same sources may serve the establishment of early metastases.

Because of their overall frequency, carcinomas metastatic to the lung are the most common subgroup of malignancies, although lymphomas and sarcomas are also important and are also discussed. Virtually any malignancy may spread to the lungs. Most common sources, in approximate order of frequency, are breast, colon, stomach, pancreas, kidney, melanoma, prostate, liver, thyroid, adrenal glands, and male and female genital tracts. By absolute numbers, adenocarcinomas far outnumber the other extrathoracic solid tumors that metastasize to lung.

The pathologist is often challenged by whether a tumor in the lung is primary or metastatic. If known, a history of malignancy outside the lung is certainly helpful. The clinical and radiographic findings may favor one or the other in those with known tumor elsewhere. A comparison of pathology of the two tumors, or at times more than two tumors, should be conducted. General histology may give some clues. Even within the group of glandular-derived adenocarcinomas, "dirty necrosis" and tall hyperchromatic cells favor colon cancer; microacinar or cribriforming, relatively low-grade patterns favor prostate; and intracytoplasmic mucin droplets favor breast. Unique tumor characteristics such as with choriocarcinoma or differentiated sarcomas may be persuasive. A clear cell carcinoma in lung containing fat and sugar strongly favors metastatic renal carcinoma. Tumor in abundance in pulmonary artery branches is usually indicative of metastases (Fig. 44.1). A panel of immunoperoxidase markers, flow cytometry, hormone and other receptors, electron microscopy, or chromosomal aberrations may help make this distinction.

At times, however, there is no way to distinguish primary from secondary tumors with absolute certainty. Whether to treat a new lung lesion of identical cell type,

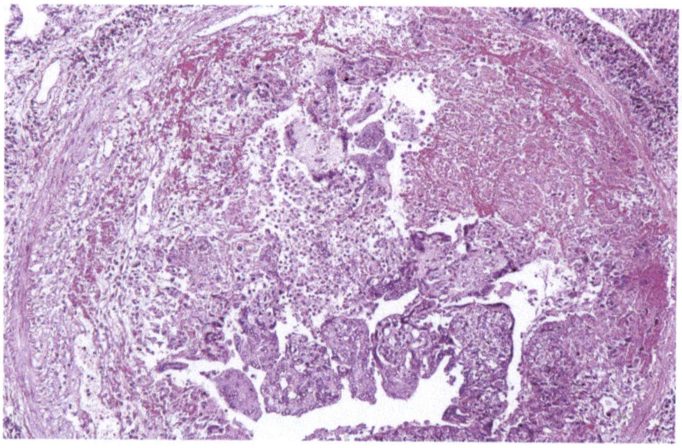

Figure 44.1. Metastatic choriocarcinoma in a smaller pulmonary artery. Note syncytiotrophoblasts.

without distinguishing markers, in a patient with known extrapulmonary malignancy as a metastatic or new primary lesion is a point often raised in tumor boards.

Immunohistochemistry has revolutionized anatomic pathology in our lifetime (see Special Situations in Metastases in Lung, below). Panels of antibodies are often necessary to correlate both positive and negative results. The typical history of a new "specific" antibody for an organ or tissue type is that it becomes less specific with broadening use but may still be helpful in the right setting within a panel.

There are rare cases of tumors, such as choriocarcinoma, melanoma, or synovial sarcoma,[16,17] which are generally metastatic, but when no primary can be found and when they are solitary, they may be considered primary in the lung. Caution is always necessary in cases such as choriocarcinomas or melanomas, for example, as sometimes they regress in their primary sites. Also salivary gland tumors or melanomas primary in lung are usually bronchus-associated, whereas metastases from elsewhere grow in more peripheral lung parenchyma.

Tumors may spread to the lung by different routes. Hematogenous spread is most important and includes varying sized tumor emboli. Tumor cells leaving their primary sites may gain access to venous blood by direct invasion or secondarily by lymphatic spread with lymph drainage eventually entering venous blood. Occasionally tumors spread by direct extension, such as surface spread within the lung, or through chest wall, mediastinum, or diaphragm, or via lymphatics permeating between these structures. Although direct extension to another organ is considered tumor spread, metastases usually imply discontinuous tumor deposits. Metastases in the lung may involve the lung parenchyma itself as nodules, either as solitary or multiple, either large or small, or may be more diffuse interstitial infiltrates, the latter often suggesting vascular spread. Tumors may likewise involve bronchi in a nodular or diffuse fashion, and may embolize to large and small blood vessels, lymphatics, pleura, or hilar-mediastinal or intraparenchymal lymph nodes. Even peritoneal-venous shunting of malignant ascites may deliver tumor cells to lungs.[18] Each of these situations is discussed separately here.

The most common situation for metastatic lung tumors is presentation in patients with known extrapulmonary neoplasm. Bilateral pulmonary nodules, often of somewhat different sizes, favor middle to lower peripheral lung fields, these areas being colonized presumably because of the volume of blood flow. The varying sized nodules may relate to different times when metastatic deposits were established in the lung, or the varying quality of the "soil," the growth rate of individual cells that establishes different nodules, or other factors. Similarly sized nodules (Fig. 44.2), when seen throughout the lungs bilaterally, may represent showers of tumor cells all of which originated about the same time.[9] The differential diagnosis of multinodular masses generally consists of various forms of vasculitis, synchronous or asynchronous primary tumors in the lung, or, if small, granulomatous

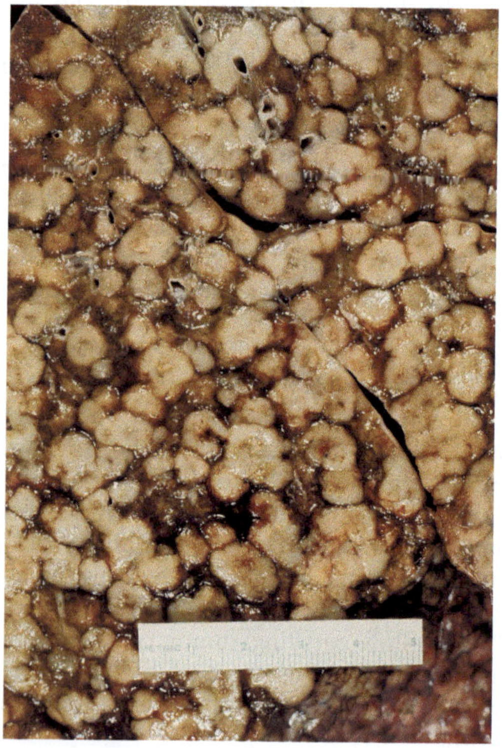

Figure 44.2. Metastatic cholangiocarcinoma. Multiple small nodules suggest "shower" of tumor cells perhaps occurring about the same time, in contrast to solitary or several larger or variably sized nodules of tumor, which may suggest different ages of metastases (see text).

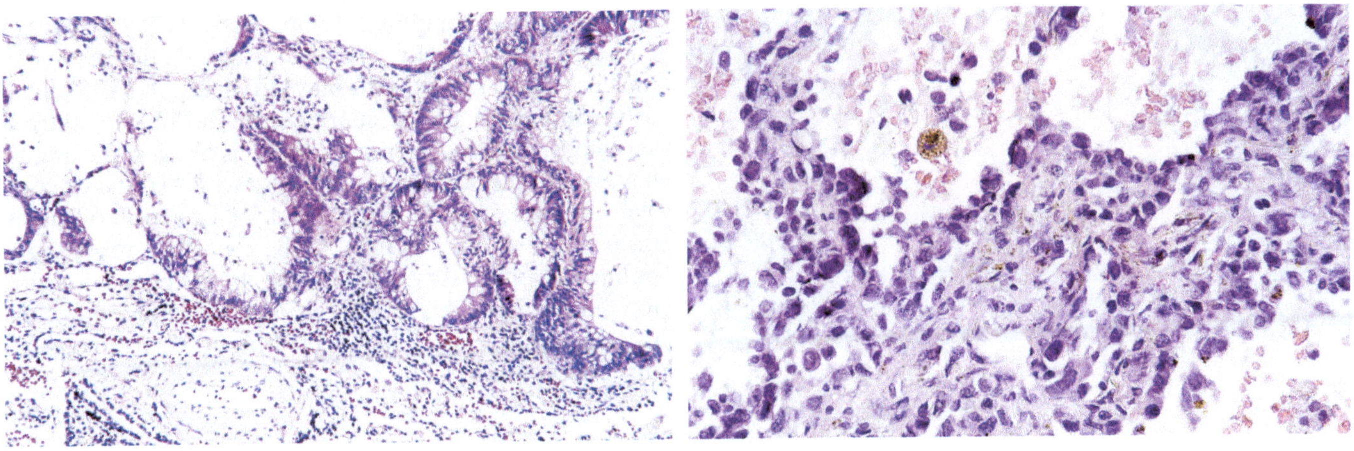

FIGURE 44.3. Simulating a bronchioloalveolar carcinoma (BAC). **(A)** Metastatic mucinous colon cancer simulating mucinous BAC. **(B)** An unusual case of metastatic melanoma focally lining alveoli simulating nonmucinous BAC.

disease or other inflammatory causes, or any combination of these.

Further generalizations concerning metastases are that they are usually smaller than lung primaries, often measuring less than 3cm in diameter; are more evenly contoured; grow more rapidly; are more peripherally located, and therefore may be less likely to be reached by the bronchoscope or biopsy forceps; or are less likely to have sloughed cells for cytology specimens. Exceptions to each of these generalizations occur. In-situ change may suggest a primary lung cancer, but is seen predominantly only in squamous carcinoma. More peripherally atypical adenomatous hyperplasia in lung parenchyma is thought a marker of more widespread glandular neoplasia, but each lesion is not necessarily destined to become cancer. See further discussion of this entity in Chapter 34. Metastatic cancers can invade bronchial mucosa and should not be mistaken for in-situ change. Some 3% to 7% of patients with primary lung cancers have independent primary malignancies at some other bodily location,[19] and the reverse is also detailed.

In one series from 1990, even before immunoperoxidase markers, up to 98% of the metastases were correctly identified as such.[20] However, atypical presentations of metastatic disease to the lung can cause confusion with primary lung cancer. This confusion occurs most often when metastases are solitary; have cavitation; are centrally placed, including in an endobronchial location; have hilar or mediastinal nodal involvement; are in an apical location invading the bronchial plexus, causing Pancoast syndrome; or have no distinguishing immunohistochemistry or other distinguishing characteristics. Further ambiguity can occur when any of these findings occur with cell types that can also be seen in primary lung carcinomas, or when no extrathoracic tumor is documented. Once tumor is in the lung, whether it arose there or arrived there secondarily, it may spread to the lung vessels, including the lymphatics and venous routes but also the arterial routes, or extend by direct continuity such as with endobronchial spread or through the pleura, or by surface spread, such as in bronchioloalveolar carcinoma or metastases simulating these carcinomas[21,22] (Fig. 44.3). At times the tumor will follow a combination of routes. A miliary pattern of small nodules is seen most often with medullary carcinoma of the thyroid,[23] melanoma,[24] renal cell carcinoma, and at times ovarian carcinoma.[25]

Solitary Metastases

Solitary metastases occur in 3% to 9% of cases of all metastases to the lung.[18,26,27] This situation occurs most often with metastases from the colon, which account for 30% to 40% of all cases,[26,27] breast, kidney (Fig. 44.4), urinary bladder, nonseminomatous testicular sources, nasopharyngeal sources, and sarcomas.[26,28–33] Large cannonball metastases, generally considered to be larger than 5cm, most often arise from neoplasms of breast, kidney, sarcomas, or melanomas.[7] Solitary metastases in the absence of a known primary in one series was reported in only 0.4% of cases.[26] As treatment and prognosis are so often different, an independent lung primary must always be considered and excluded as best as possible when evaluating a patient for metastatic disease.

At times primary lung tumors may be multiple and synchronous and may be of the same cell type or varying cell types. As summarized by Filderman et al.,[7] if a solitary lung nodule is detected in the face of extrathoracic malignancy, it is more likely to be a new primary than secondary deposits in cancers of the lung, breast, stomach, prostate, head, and neck,[33–35] is more often metastatic

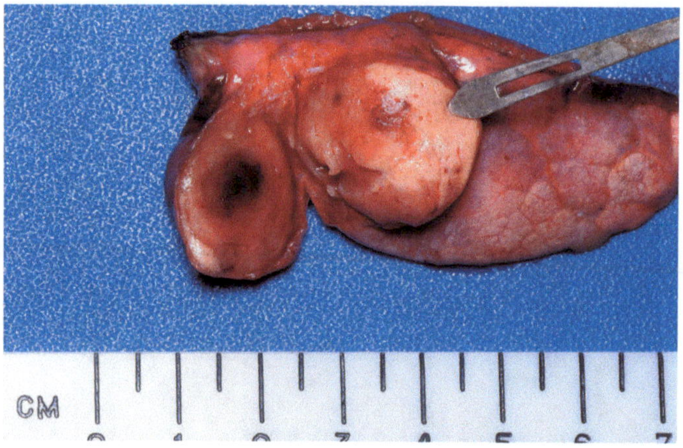

FIGURE 44.4. Solitary round evenly contoured metastasis from renal clear cell adenocarcinoma. Note focally yellow color. Lesion was soft.

than primary in melanomas and sarcomas,[26,36] and of about equal incidence in carcinomas of kidney, colon, or testes.[35,37] Certain malignancies that arise in lung are typically multifocal and bilateral without a dominant tumor mass and include bronchioloalveolar carcinoma and epithelioid hemangioendothelioma. At times what appears to be a solitary tumor on plain chest radiograph is shown to be multiple adjacent lesions using different procedures such as spiral computed tomography (CT),[38] positron emission tomography (PET), or magnetic resonance imaging (MRI) scans. This may still be treated effectively as a solitary nodule in many cases, and in one study of sarcomas, patients having as many as five lesions did not have a different survival from those with a solitary mass.[39] The term *metastasectomy* is used for resection of metastases. At least for sarcoma,[40] when feasible, resection of pulmonary metastases offers the best chance for prolonged survival. This is being studied for carcinomas.[41] An international registry has been formed to further study this procedure.[42]

Cavitation

Cavitation can occur in 4% of metastatic disease and 9% of primary lung cancers.[43] It is most often seen in squamous cell carcinoma in either situation. The most frequent sources of squamous carcinoma metastases are head and neck in men, the genitourinary tract in women,[43] and the esophagus and anus in either sex. Squamous carcinomas generally metastasize so rarely to the lung that finding such a lesion in the lung should be a good reason to suspect an independent primary cancer.[7] Other malignancies, such as sarcomas (Fig. 44.5) or adenocarcinomas, can form cavities, either in primary or secondary

A

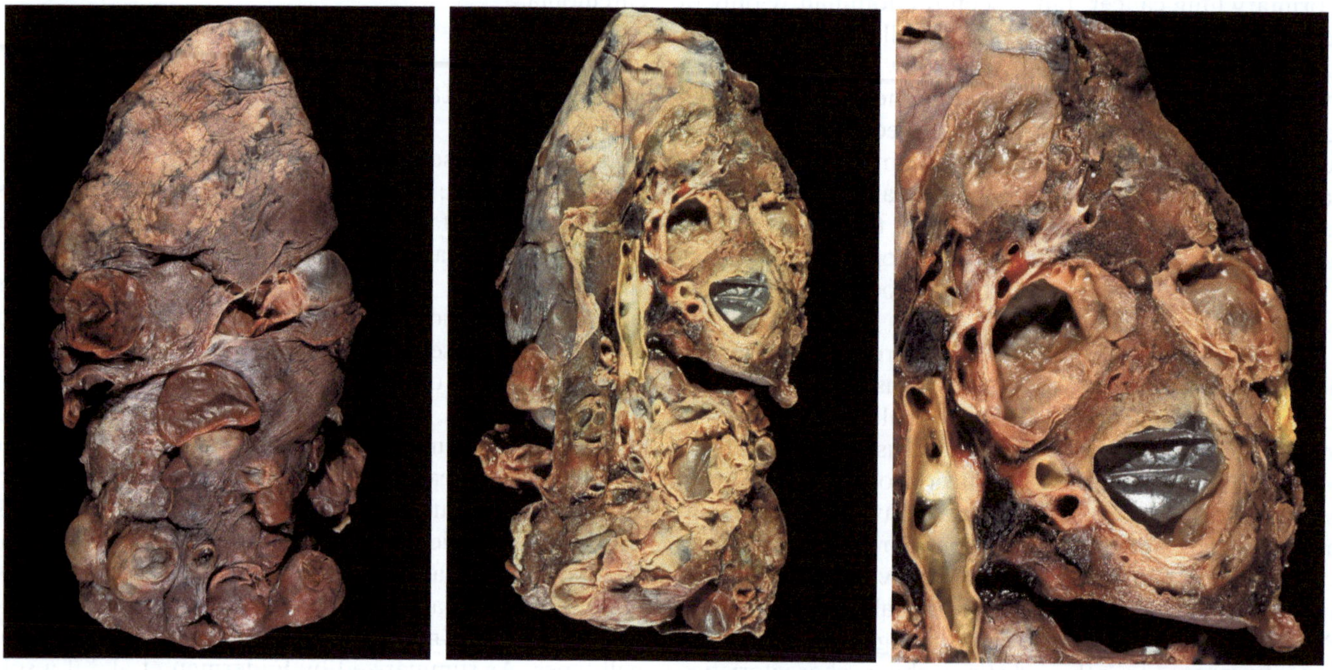

B,C

FIGURE 44.5. Metastatic low-grade uterine leiomyomasarcoma, documented at death 21 years after multiple uterine leiomyomas up to 12 cm were removed. Note variable size and extent of cyst formation and thin walls. **(A)** Surface view before sectioning. **(B)** Whole lung section showing multiple cystic metastases. **(C)** Close-up of gross cystic metastases. (Courtesy of A. A. Liebow Pulmonary Pathology Collection, original contributor Dr. B. Pocock.)

forms.[43–47] At times cavitation of tumor masses peripherally has a role in establishing bronchopleural fistula, as is described below.

Endobronchial Metastases

Because they can be confused with centrally placed primary lung carcinomas, endobronchial metastases may be a particular challenge in distinguishing metastatic from primary disease[48,49] (Fig. 44.6). This is true especially when the metastatic lesions are adenocarcinomas. True primary bronchial adenocarcinomas are rare and often derive from bronchial glands.[50,51] Most primary lung adenocarcinomas are peripheral, and consequently their typical classification as one of the major types of bronchogenic carcinomas is usually erroneous. Indeed the term *bronchogenic* is somewhat confusing, and some would translate this as making a bronchus instead of being derived from one; thus the term might be better replaced by *bronchocentric* or perhaps best discarded entirely. Pathologists rarely use this term, but all physicians learned it in medical school, and the term is carried forth for simplicity's sake especially among nonpulmonary physicians.

The incidence of endobronchial metastases varies; it was noted in 1.1% of bronchial tumor diagnoses by Bourke.[52] In the review by Braman and Whitcomb,[53] 2% to 5% of patients dying of extrathoracic solid tumors have easily identifiable, significant tumor spread to central bronchi. In another series it was 18%,[54] and when reviews are limited to only those specifying whether tumor was present or not in bronchi, or when microscopic spread is included, the percentage may be as high as 70%.[55] The most common sources for these tumors are breast[56,57] colon,[58] kidney,[59] rectum, melanoma, cervix, soft tissue, and sarcomas.[49,60] Other less frequent tumors include those from pancreas, prostate, choriocarcinoma, osteosarcoma, leiomyosarcoma, uterine cervix, ovary, skin, urinary bladder, penis, testes, stomach, larynx, or thyroid.[11,61–63] In one series,[60] sarcomas were found in 6 of 17 cases (35%). In another study by King and Castleman,[54] carcinomas and sarcomas had a relatively similar incidence of endobronchial spread once each tumor had established itself as metastatic in the lung. The trachea is a less common site of metastatic tumor involvement than the bronchus,[64] but metastases to this site have been noted coming from breast, colon, and other locations.[64–66] Whether proximal bronchial or tracheal in location, these tumors can often be biopsied through the bronchoscope.[52,67–69]

Possible mechanisms for endobronchial spread include hematogenous seeding, lymphatic spread, spread from immediately adjacent tumor in lung parenchyma, mediastinum, or nodes, or rarely by aerogenous routes.[53,54,57–60] It is possible a few metastases arise in the lung via spread from bronchial arteries, and perhaps a few rare ones in the central portions of nodes arise through nodal systemic arterial supply. Lymphangitic spread in bronchial walls can be detected with some regularity through the bronchoscope. As the tumor is "on the move" in this location, it may be a dilemma in the case of primary lung cancer whether to call a tumor in this site metastatic, with the possible misinterpretation as to whether the primary lesion, further out, is also interpreted as metastatic. In such instances the pathologist should be careful in describing the fact that tumor spreading in the bronchial wall may be related to a primary lung cancer.

As with primary lung cancers, symptoms of endobronchial tumor growth are cough, localized wheezing, dyspnea, or hemoptysis. Radiographically there may be separate lesions in lung parenchyma, postobstructive collapse, atelectasis, air-trapping, an obvious mass, or CT scan or bronchoscopy documentation of a lesion in the bronchus. Metastatic involvement of airways producing significant respiratory signs or symptoms or chest radiographic changes are reported to occur in less than 5% of those who die with solid extrapulmonary tumors.[53]

Vascular Metastases

This is an important route of spread, as most metastases arrive in the lung via the bloodstream (Figs. 44.1 and 44.7). As mentioned in the introduction, the lung is a particularly receptive organ because it receives the entire cardiac output, including most of the upstream lymph flow, and is a meshwork of delicate capillaries that easily entraps tumor cells and otherwise appears attractive to tumor growth. Tumors arising in whatever location, including the lung, may enter the circulation either directly through vascular penetration, or via the lymphatics, which then empty into the systemic venous circulation.

Most metastases in lung and other organs appear without associated identified endovascular tumor. This may be caused by tumor growing beyond the vessel lumen, not including the vessel of origin in the plane of sectioning, by obliteration of the vessel of origin by the neoplastic growth, or by origin from a small inapparent vessel, or perhaps spread by routes other than blood vessels. One might expect to see individual tumor cells in the blood circulating in the lung, and certainly some such cells are seen in smaller caliber vessels. Some malignancies do present with abundant loosely cohesive cells, sometimes with such a tumor cell burden that cancer cells are identified even on peripheral blood smears; this has been called carcinoma cell leukemia, or carcinocythemia.[70–74] In the peripheral circulation, small cell carcinomas from lung,[75–79] adenocarcinomas from breast,[80] and, less often, adenocarcinomas from intestine,[81]

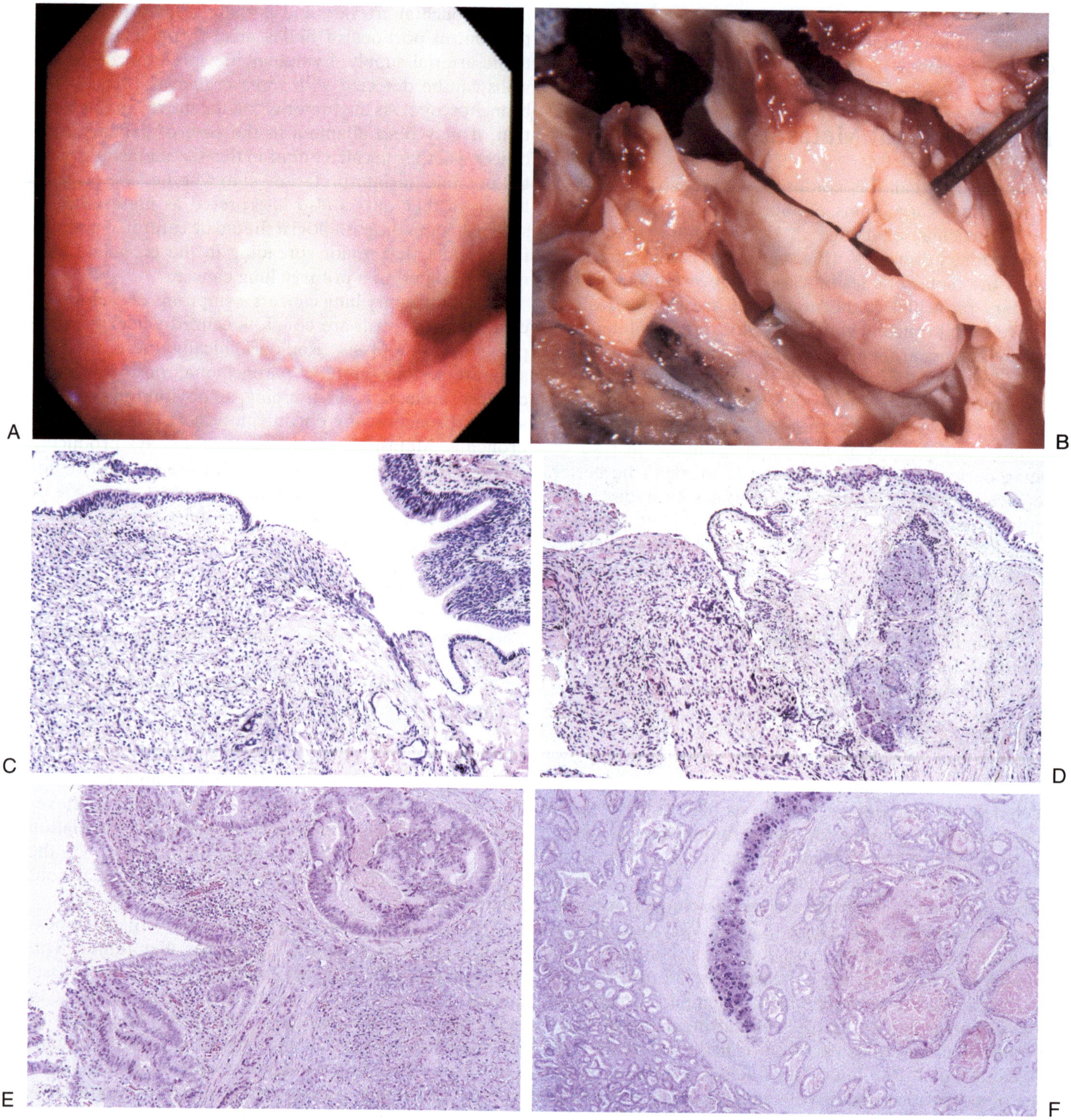

FIGURE 44.6. Endobronchial metastases. **(A)** Endoscopic view of nodule of metastatic esophageal adenocarcinoma. **(B)** Metastatic clear cell renal adenocarcinoma forms larger endobronchial mass. **(C)** Microscopic view of renal carcinoma in **B**. **(D)** Metastatic uterine leiomyosarcoma. **(E)** Metastatic colon cancer to larger bronchial wall. **(F)** Metastatic colon cancer filling smaller bronchial lumen and replacing bronchial lining. (**A:** Courtesy of Donald E. Low, M.D. Virginia Mason Thoracic Surgery, Seattle, WA.)

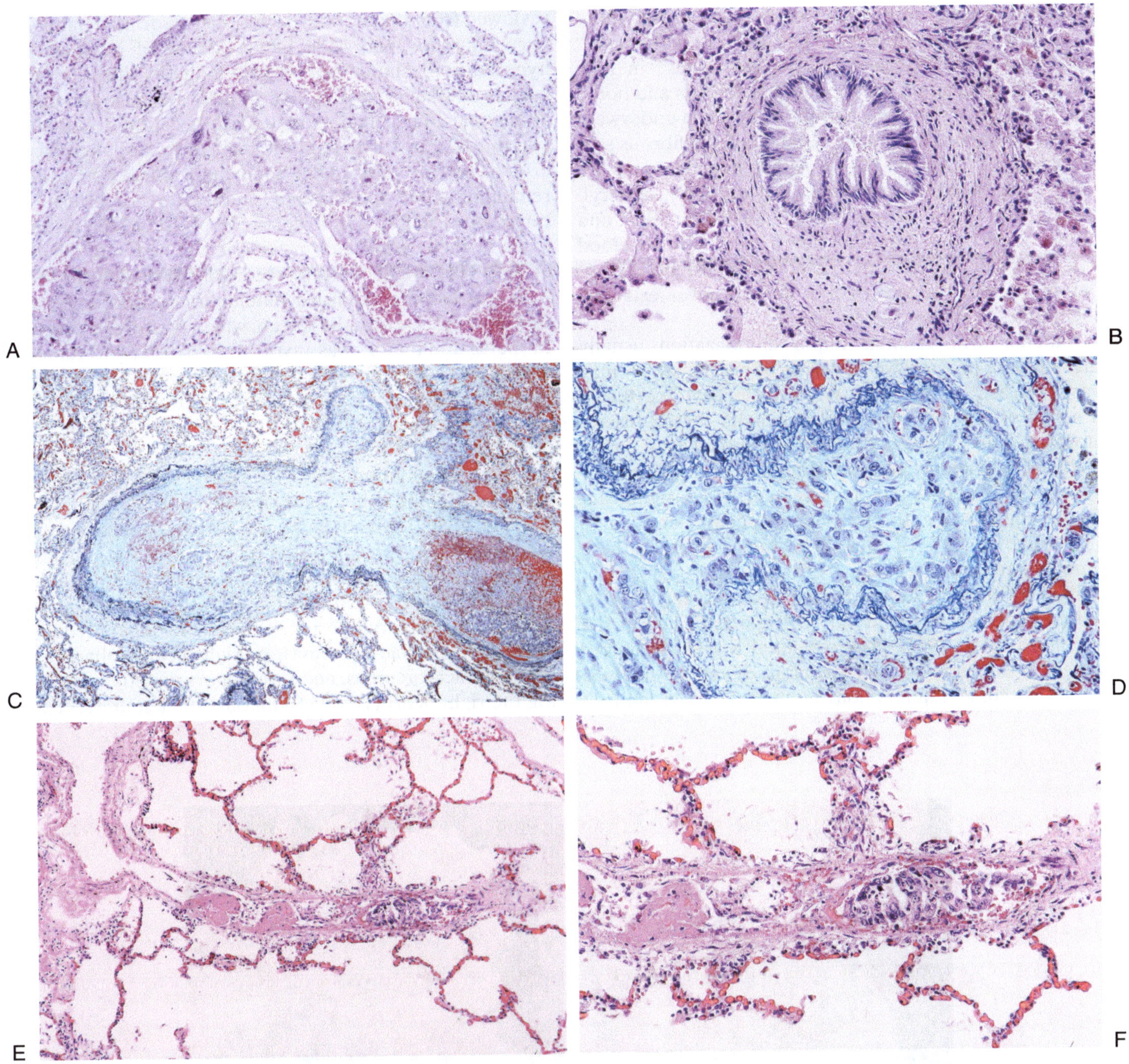

FIGURE 44.7. Endovascular metastases. **(A)** Metastatic pancreatic adenocarcinoma. **(B)** Metastatic well-differentiated colonic adenocarcinoma lining pulmonary artery lumen, simulating a bronchial structure at first glance. **(C)** Metastatic adenocarcinoma with fresher clot at right lower and older fibrous tumor plug in most of rest of vessel lumen. (Movat pentachrome stain.) **(D)** Higher power view top part of **C**. (Movat pentachrome stain.) **(E,F)** Fresher ovarian tumor emboli to smaller vessel with fibrin clots. **(E)** Lower power view. **(F)** Higher power view.

melanomas,[72] rhabdomyosarcomas,[82] or transitional cell carcinomas[72] have been thus identified.[70–72] Many leukemias and some lymphomas, also notorious for having leukemic phases, are seen both in the peripheral blood and in the blood circulating through the lung. (See following discussion.)

The interested reader is referred to the basics of tumor metastasis, as well reviewed by Filderman et al.,[7] and the many steps a tumor cell must go through to penetrate a blood vessel at its site of origin, live in the circulation, engraft, and grow to reestablish itself. Schmidt[83] in 1903 reviewed the nature of small emboli arriving in pulmonary vessels in humans and noted that blood and fibrin surround the tumor cells (Fig. 44.7E,F). Takahashi[84] and Iwasaki[85] in 1915 and Warren and Gates[86] in 1936 studied tumor emboli in experimental animals and noted that tumor cells that were entrapped by fibrin underwent degeneration and eventually became a focal fibrous scar in the intima[87] (Fig. 44.7C–F). Although carcinomas are most often involved, sarcomas can certainly undergo similar patterns of spread. Iwasaki, Willis[88] in 1934, and others[89] later pointed out that tumor cells in distant blood vessels should not be interpreted as metastatic disease per se, as many tumor emboli die and never establish themselves as metastases.

Patients with vascular tumor embolization usually present with progressive shortness of breath, which may vary from acute to subacute. Winterbauer et al.[89] reviewed a series of 366 patients with carcinoma of the breast, stomach, liver, kidney, or choriocarcinoma, and found 95 (26%) had some degree of tumorization of pulmonary vessels. In 30 (8%) this embolization was a significant factor contributing to the patient's death, and in 10 (3% of total, 10% of those with tumor emboli) these emboli were the direct cause of death. Although tumor emboli to lungs were first described in the early 1800s, Winterbauer et al. found only 30 reported cases in the literature up to 1967. They proposed a grading system based on the number and percentage of vessels involved on microscopic examination; in their 10 cases and 23 reviewed from the literature, 48% had associated pulmonary infarction and 45% had evidence of pulmonary hypertension. Tumor emboli may lodge in either larger vessels or smaller vessels, and in their series at autopsy, about one fourth had grossly identified tumor emboli, two thirds of which were in the main or lobar pulmonary artery and one third in the segmental arteries, and the remaining three fourths had small artery or arteriole tumor obstruction. The liver was involved in 36% of the cases in their series and in 50% in the series by Kane et al.[90] This might indicate secondary spread from the liver was feeding extensive pulmonary vascular spread. In Kane et al.'s series, the spleen, which is rarely receptive to metastatic tumor, was involved in 37.5%, and tumor emboli were present with dyspnea in some 50% of the cases. In other series, cough was present in 8% to 47%, pleuritic chest pain in 18% to 28%, and hemoptysis in 5% to 18%.[91–93]

Large vessel tumor embolization can lead to acute heart failure and other signs of a major acute embolus. Tumors giving rise to these are often connected with major systemic veins, with direct tumor extension into some part of this venous system; these most often include liver, kidney (Fig. 44.8), uterine smooth muscle tumors, and, rarely, primary inferior vena cava leiomyosarcoma, right-sided cardiac myxomas, or right heart pulmonary outflow tract sarcomas, and rare tumors directly infiltrating the right heart (Fig. 44.9) among other sources, such

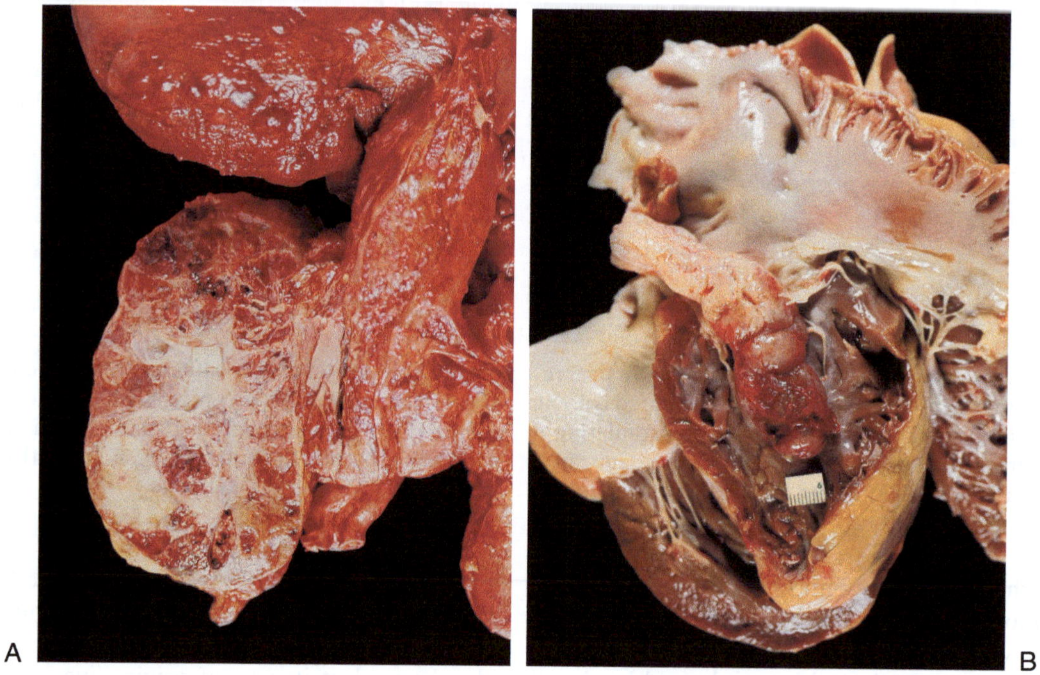

FIGURE 44.8. **(A)** Renal cell adenocarcinoma is replacing right kidney and distends and extends up inferior vena cava. **(B)** Tumor extends in continuity into right ventricle with its tip above ruler near apex. Patient had a strange heart murmur.

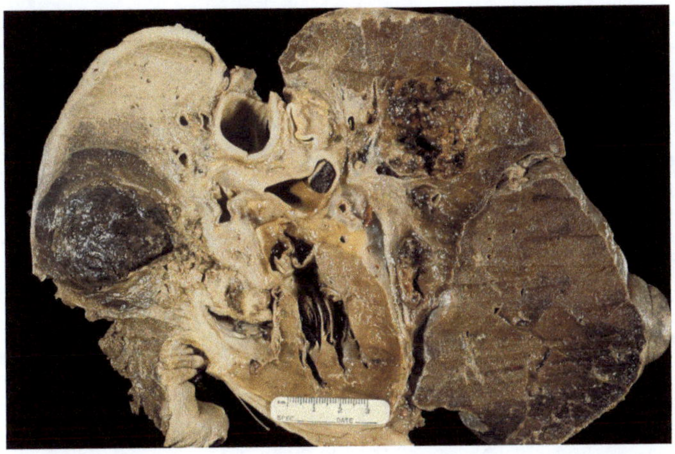

FIGURE 44.9. Large fibrosarcoma in right lung and right hilum directly invades right atrium. Tumor extension into left lung is perhaps through embolization from right heart.

as pancreas. In smaller caliber vessels, which have potential for collaterals and shunting to less involved vessels, heart failure is generally more subacute than it is acute, but acute heart failure has certainly been described in this situation along with pulmonary hypertension.[7,89–108] Vessels with tumor emboli of any size may undergo thrombosis or fibrous obliteration, sometimes causing a pulmonary infarct. At times, tumor emboli die leaving a thrombus, which may partially calcify (Fig. 44.10).

Tumors that spread to the smaller pulmonary vessels, generally those less than 2mm in diameter, including arterioles and capillaries, are most often seen in cancers from breast, stomach, colon, rectum, liver, pancreas, uterus, cervix, choriocarcinoma, ovarian tumors, prostate, urinary, and gallbladder origins.[90] In the series by Kane et al.,[90] vascular emboli were noted in 2.4% of 1085 consecutive autopsies for solid malignant neoplasms, and half of those involved had unexplained dyspnea; however, there was no significant difference in the mean percentage of small vessels involved within this group compared with those presenting without unexplained dyspnea. It is also interesting that there was no example of larger vessel tumor emboli in this large series. In the Soares et al.[105] series of 12 cases of tumor spread to pulmonary alveolar septal capillaries, including nine tumors with origin outside the chest, 11 (92%) had other pulmonary vascular compartments involved, those being lymphatics in nine, arterioles in seven, and veins in one; parenchymal tumor nodules were present in five of those nine that were metastatic to lung and presumably in all three arising in the lung. Only one of their cases had purely alveolar capillary spread, a case of squamous carcinoma of the cervix; this was compared to one other similar case reported by Abbondanzo et al.[99] in which the primary was in breast (Fig. 44.11A). This figure also illustrates several other examples of tumor emboli to small vessels and capillaries, including mesothelioma, melanoma, and intravascular lymphoma. Whether intravascular lymphoma, originally called malignant angioendotheliomatosis, is considered primary in any particular organ system is undetermined because it is considered primary in blood vessels themselves. It is in the differential diagnosis of intravascular malignancies, and may also be diagnosed by right-heart wedge catheterization[109] (Fig. 44.11F).

Pulmonary veins may also be involved with leukemia or tumors metastatic to lung as well as primary tumors arising there, and often represent one route for either tumor, once established in the lung, to move from that location. Venous spread is discussed more at the end of this chapter.

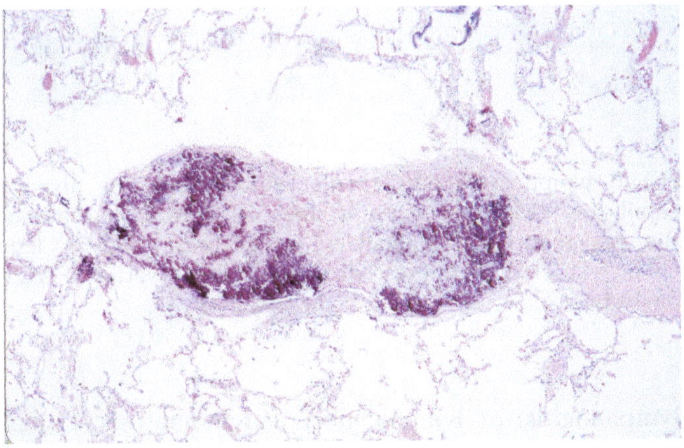

A

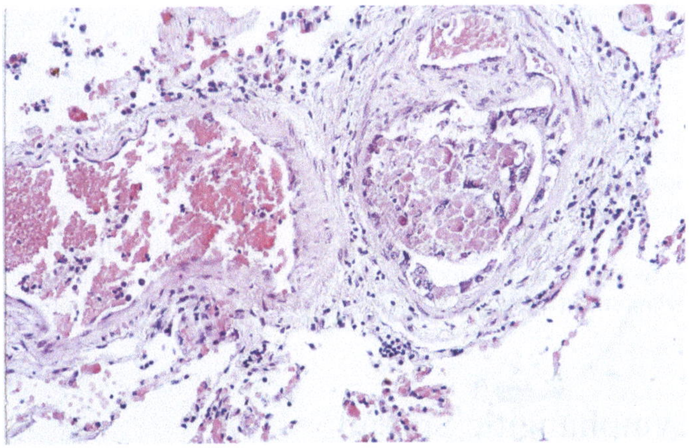

B

FIGURE 44.10. Metastatic ovarian carcinoma. **(A)** It has undergone calcification. No viable tumor cells are seen in this vessel. **(B)** Tumor in artery nearby with ring of adenocarcinoma, encircling more acute thrombus to right. Note also older septum with smaller partially recanalized patent vessel above and more patent vessel to left.

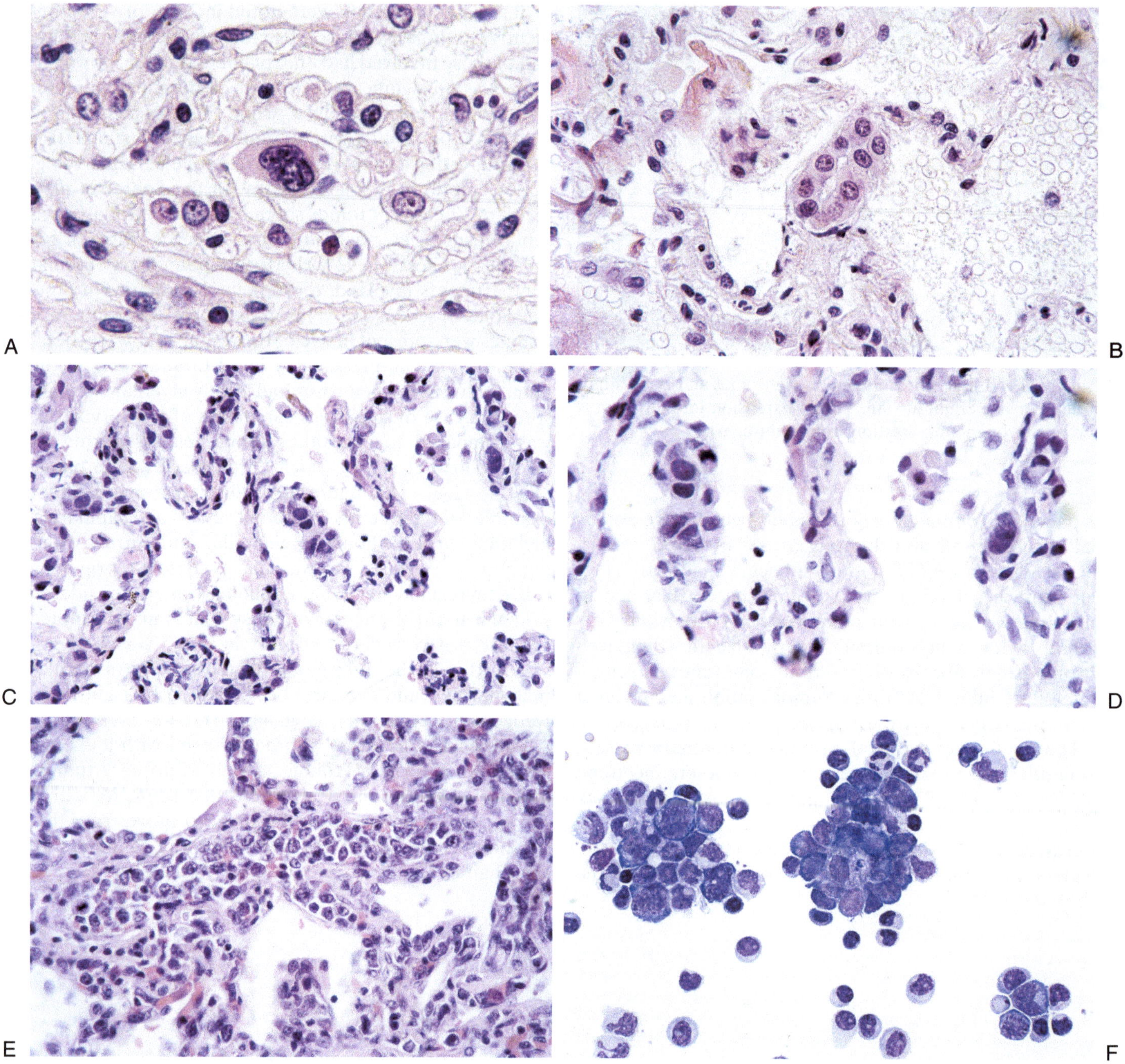

FIGURE 44.11. Tumor emboli in smaller vessels. **(A)** Breast cancer cell simulating a megakaryocyte. **(B)** One intracapillary gland of epithelioid mesothelioma in person with concurrent diagnosis of similar mesothelioma nearby. **(C,D)** Metastatic melanoma in two magnifications. **(E,F)** Intravascular lymphoma. **(E)** B lymphocytes plug smaller vessels including alveolar capillaries. **(F)** Right heart wedge catheterization retrieved the malignant B lymphocytes, which were lambda light chain restricted by fluorescence-activated cell sorter (FACS) analysis.

Lymphangitic Spread

It is generally accepted that about 6% to 8% of metastases to the lung appear as lymphangitic disease[110–112] (Figs. 44.12 and 44.13). This has also been called lymphangitic, lymphangitis, or lymphangiosis carcinomatosis. Others have noted higher incidences of lymphangitic spread, 24%[113] to 56%.[114] A summary of 275 cases reviewed from 1935 to 1971 by Yang and Lin[110] showed that 44% arose in the stomach, 23% in bronchus, 9% in breast, 5% in

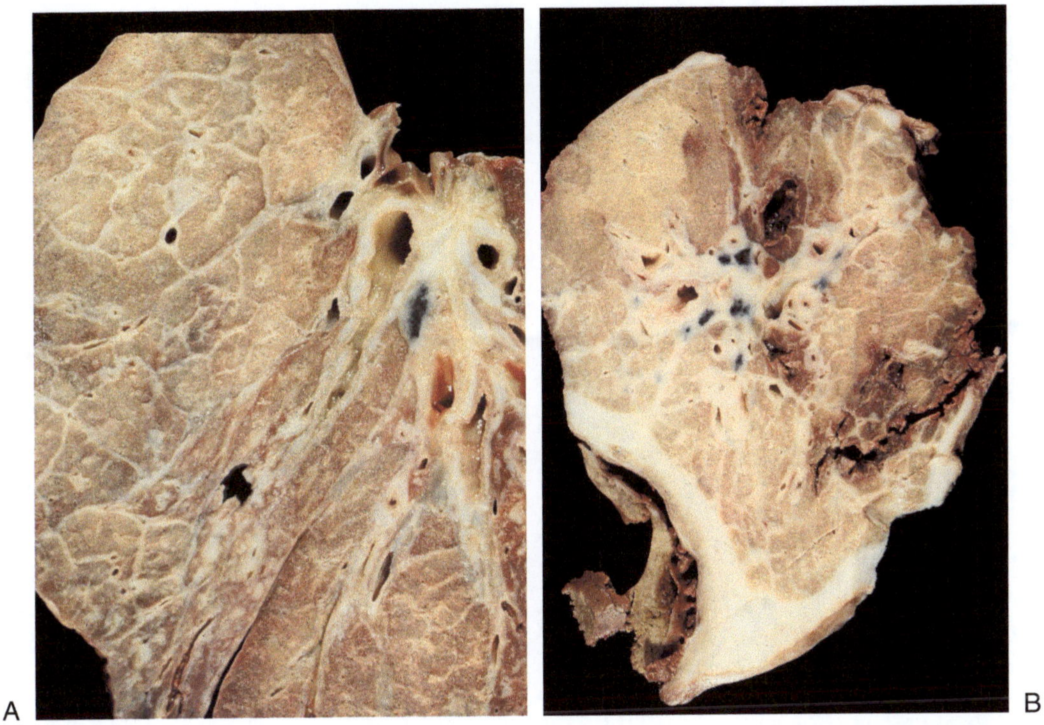

FIGURE 44.12. Lymphangitic breast adenocarcinoma. **(A)** Cancer cells thicken and highlight interlobular septal lymphatic spaces. Some bronchi are encased toward bottom of frame. **(B)** Same case as in **A**, where more dependent tumor thickens diaphragmatic pleura and peribronchial lymphatics are filled with tumor. Note sparing of tumor spread in more superior portion. Small tumor deposit is visible in at least one inferiorly placed node.

pancreas, and 4% each in uterus, colon-rectum, and prostate. The three series from the 1930s heavily favored the stomach.[110] In studying a single source, Goldsmith et al.[113] noted 24% of the patients with breast cancer had lymphangitic spread to the lungs, often with pleural effusion (see following). Breast cancer accounts for about half the cases now of lymphangitic spread in North America (Fig. 44.12), while gastric carcinoma is expected to account for a high percentage in Japan.[115] Other metastatic tumors proven to cause this pattern are from ovary, cervix, thyroid, liver, bladder, endometrium, nasopharynx, esophagus,[110,111,116] and malignant carcinoid arising in the abdomen.[117] Certainly primary lung cancers can spread frequently via lymphatics as do lymphomas (Fig. 44.13E).

As many as 50% of the cases of histologically proven pulmonary lymphatic carcinomatosis present with normal radiographs[113,118] and CT scans increase this sensitivity, often showing a beaded appearance.[119–122] Lymphangitic carcinomatosis causes more interstitial lymphatic septal thickening than lymphangitic lymphoma or lymphangitic sarcoidosis.[123] Perfusion scans may also highlight abnormalities in blood vessels.[103,124,125] Most cases are bilateral and diffuse but some are unilateral and focal, and these variations may depend on the source of the tumor and the route of spread in the lymphatics, as discussed later. About one third have associated hilar or mediastinal node enlargement, and two thirds have pleural disease.[110,116]

Lymphangitic tumor spread conveys a poor prognosis; about half the patients are dead within 3 months and 90% are dead within 6 months.[110] However, some rare cases have responded to treatment, including patients with breast,[126] prostate,[127] or ovarian carcinoma.[128]

The series by Yang and Lin[110] is of special note. They divided their 62 cases into four radiographic patterns. The first pattern showed progressive linear infiltrates bilaterally without hilar enlargement or tumor masses, and all these cases proved to be cancers spreading from gastric adenocarcinoma. The presumed route of spread with this pattern was anterograde through the diaphragm and pleural surfaces. The second group consisted of radiating linear lines from enlarged hilar masses, and this was found in association with gastric carcinoma in 25%, cervical carcinoma in 30%, breast carcinoma in 20%, and in fewer numbers, cancers from nasopharynx, prostate, pancreas, and thyroid. This pattern was presumed to be due to retrograde lymphangitic spread from bilateral hilar node metastases. The third pattern represented a focal lymphangitic spread from one portion of the lung, and this

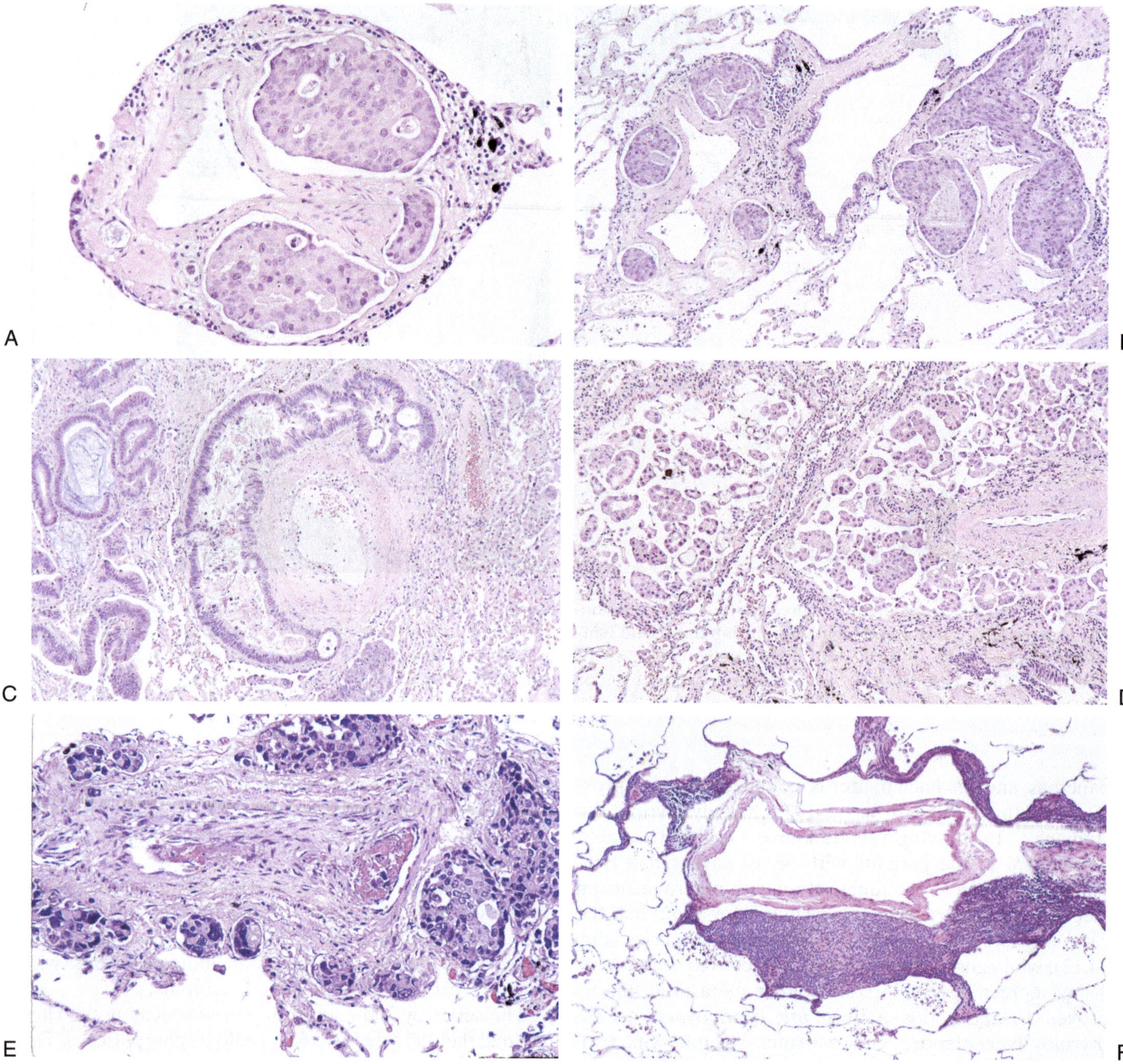

FIGURE 44.13. Lymphangitic spread of tumor. **(A)** A smaller muscular pulmonary artery is compressed by focally mucin-producing adenocarcinoma. **(B)** More extensive perivascular and peribronchiolar lymphangitic carcinoma with tumor necrosis. **(C)** Fanciful pattern of well-differentiated metastatic colon cancer in area strongly suggesting lymphangitic spread. Compare also with **B**. **(D)** Papillary adenocarcinoma distends spaces. **(E)** Metastatic adenocarcinoma in central vessel with clot, with surrounding lymphatic spread. **(F)** Small cell lymphoma in similar lymphatic pathway, here sometimes called lymphatic "tracking."

was typical of a centrally placed primary lung carcinoma, often involving bronchus. Their fourth pattern consisted of radiating tumor from a parenchymal primary lung tumor that was not centrally placed. They note that 91% of all of the cases were adenocarcinomas. Lymphatic spread has also been found in primary lung carcinomas (see following). In a study of unilateral yet fairly widespread lymphangitic carcinoma, Youngberg[129] found associated adenopathy in one third of cases and pleura disease in two thirds of cases. As already noted, nodes and pleura were also involved in similar frequencies in bilateral disease[110,116] and reflect lymphatic spread in both locations. (See following discussion on pleural spread.)

Three possible routes of lymphangitic spread have been described. The most likely one is via spread from adjacent blood vessels.[116,130] As noted in the first pattern of Yang and Lin,[110] direct lymphangitic invasion can also occur, particularly from gastric carcinoma and breast carcinoma (Fig. 44.12), and yet retrograde lymphatic spread also occurs. As a further example of retrograde spread, I have personally seen one case of two right-sided synchronous lung cancers, an adenocarcinoma in the right-middle lobe with lymphangitic and hilar node spread, and a right lower-lobe basilar compound tumor with a centrally placed large cell neuroendocrine carcinoma surrounded by a rim of keratinizing squamous carcinoma, with the surrounding lower lobe also showing lymphangitic spread of adenocarcinoma, presumably having occurred from retrograde spread. Adenocarcinomas in lymphatics may not form glands and may be more difficult to distinguish as adenocarcinoma, and may look more solid or squamoid in type (Fig. 44.13A). Some adenocarcinomas in lymphatics do, however, show a well-differentiated papillary (Fig. 44.13D) or glandular pattern (Fig. 44.13C), sometimes with psammomatous calcifications or mucin production giving a fanciful appearance.[9] Kaposi's sarcoma is characterized in the lung by lymphangitic spread, a fairly unique pattern of spread for sarcomas. At times, blood-filled vascular spaces where lymphatics are located are a clue to this disease (Fig. 44.14).

When tumor is confined to lymphatic spaces, there is little fibrin deposition, intraluminal fibrosis, or other evidence of organization.

Blood vessels are often coexistently involved with metastatic cancer when lymphatics are so involved (Fig. 44.13E). In the series by Janower and Blennerhassett,[116] arterial involvement was noted in 20 of 23 cases (87%) with lymphatic spread, and in the series by von Herbay et al.,[101] lymphatics were involved in 18 of 21 (86%) cases when blood vessels were so involved. In the first series,[116] nodes were radiographically enlarged in only five of 23 (22%) and histologically positive in only 11 (48%), while all cases had extensive hematogenous spread of metastases to other organs, which supports hematogenous arrival. The true incidence of both vascular and lymphatic spread is underestimated because histologic sampling of lung, even at autopsy, is limited.

Although the favored and most probable thesis for lymphangitic spread is invasion from peripheral arteries, such spread is hard to document histologically.[101] The reader should remember that there are no lymphatics in the alveoli themselves, but tumor cells that gain entrance to the free alveolar spaces may perhaps reenter the interstitium around the terminal bronchioles in a fashion similar to dust reentry in this location. In contrast, multifocal primary bronchioloalveolar carcinoma of lung is thought to spread to multiple sites, including bilateral lungs, principally by an aerogenous surface route without lymphatic invasion.

Some, and perhaps many, cases clinically thought to represent lymphangitic carcinomatosis may represent vascular tumor emboli.[103,125] The technique of peripheral pulmonary vascular sampling by right-heart catheterization, described in 1985 by Masson and Ruggieri,[131] with follow-up studies,[132] confirmed that with some experience and care, tumor cells can be identified. Although these patients are considered histologically as having lymphangitic carcinoma solely or predominantly, a high yield on withdrawing a small amount of arterial-capillary or venous blood must indicate tumor cells are inside the blood vessels, or, less likely, accessible via direct or traumatic access to lymphatic routes from the blood system.

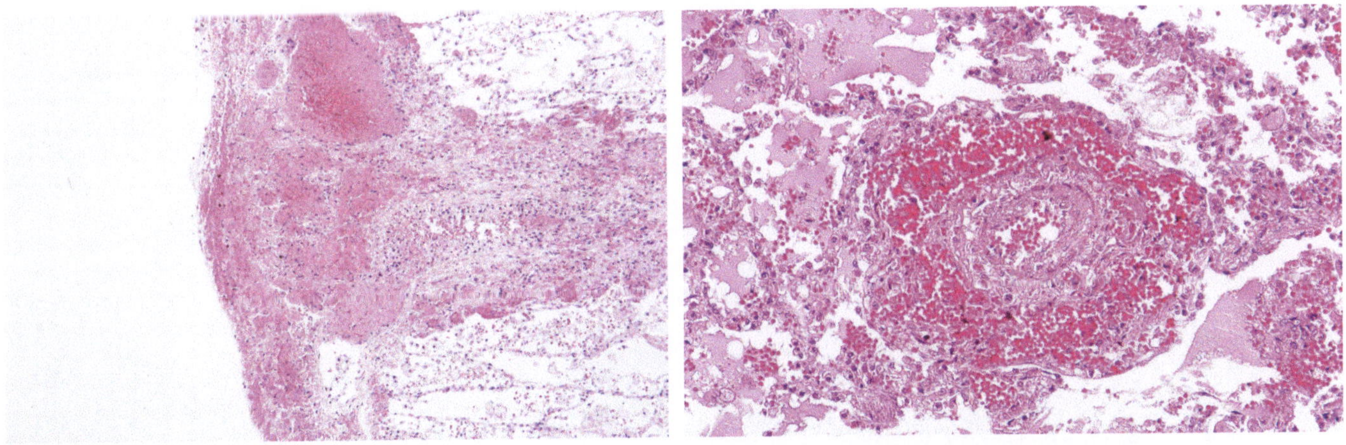

A B

FIGURE 44.14. Kaposi's sarcoma. Unique among lung sarcomas for degree of lymphangitic spread. **(A)** In pleura and in intersecting interlobular septum. **(B)** Sometimes a clue to Kaposi's sarcoma in lung is blood-filled spaces where lymphatics should be.

Megakaryocytes are sought in this procedure to prove peripheral vascular sampling. This cell is chosen because it is a normal component in capillaries of lung, and in fact the lung is the second richest source of megakaryocytes in the body after bone marrow.[133] In a study by Aabo and Hansen,[134] 365 consecutive hospital autopsies were compared with 21 forensic autopsies, the latter in previously healthy individuals who died suddenly. Intravascular megakaryocytes were found in 95% of the hospital series and 67% of the forensic series in an average number of lung samples reviewed. The average number of megakaryocytes was 37/cm^2 in the hospital series and 4/cm^2 in the forensic series. Therefore, the stresses of events preceding death in a hospital appear to increase the number of megakaryocytes. These authors used 25 megakaryocytes per cm^2 as the upper level of normal. This concentration is increased in myelofibrosis and may suggest extramedullary hematopoiesis in the lung, but it is also increased in intravascular coagulation, acute infections, bleeding, shock, cancer, and liver insufficiency, along with fever. An interesting companion study[135] of 55 cases of leukemia and 16 of multiple myeloma found an increased number of megakaryocytes in only one case in these diseases. A study by Soares,[136] noted increased pulmonary megakaryocytes with tumor metastases to lung. Megakaryocytes should not be mistaken for tumor cells (Fig. 44.11A), and appropriate immunostains will help distinguish these in problematic cases. (See Chapter 28, Fig. 28.38).

Intrathoracic Nodal Spread

It is logical that lymph nodes should be involved along with pleura when intraparenchymal pulmonary lymphatics are involved with tumor spread. As just discussed, nodal and pleural spread does not occur in as many cases as expected for the incidence of parenchymal lymphatic spread. Nodal spread may be either from a primary or secondary tumor, then representing secondary and tertiary metastases respectively.

Lymph node involvement in primary tumors is so valuable in cancer staging as to be one of the key findings here as elsewhere in the body. Certainly a unilateral lung mass with ipsilateral unilateral hilar nodal enlargement is considered cancer with nodal spread until proven otherwise. Looking at metastases to the chest from a nodal viewpoint, in a series of 1071 cases with various extrathoracic malignancies by McLoud et al.,[137] 25 patients (2.3%) showed nodal involvement on chest radiographs with 48% of these being from primary genitourinary malignancies, 32% from head and neck, 12% breast, and 8% melanomas. Tumor in nodes was accompanied by parenchymal involvement in 40% of this series, and the right paratracheal chain was involved most often (60%); unilateral hilar node involvement occurred in 32% and bilateral hilar node involvement in 28%. Subcarinal and posterior mediastinal lymph node involvement was uncommon, except in cases of testicular seminoma and, less often, other testicular neoplasms. Such posterior nodal spread is presumably in continuity along the periaortic nodes to account for this discrepancy.

The incidence of regional intrathoracic node involvement in metastatic lung neoplasia is 21%[138] to 28.6%[139] when regional nodes are histologically examined. Prognosis for this tertiary spread is worse than for only secondary pulmonary spread.[139] Hilar or mediastinal nodal spread may represent tertiary spread from intraparenchymal lung metastases, but also may represent secondary spread by alternate routes. Lymphatic drainage from the retroperitoneum continues directly into the mediastinum via the ductus lymphaticus and other collateral spaces. Lymphatic drainage into pleura may also occur via these routes with consequent movement of tumor cells via the pleural lymphatics to regional nodes.[140] The incidence of node involvement with metastatic melanoma to chest, similar to testis tumors, is unusually high (54%

A
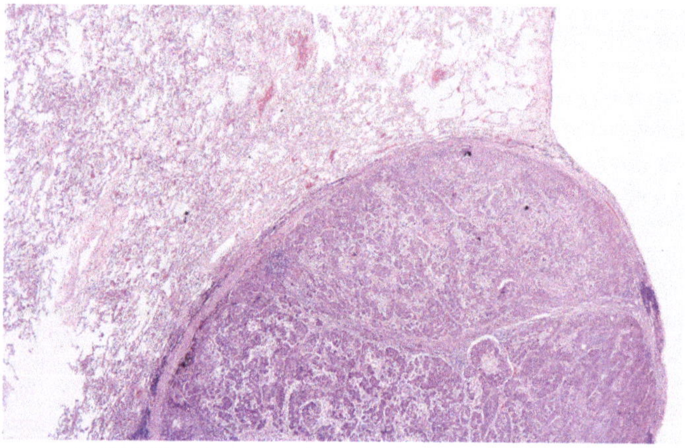
B
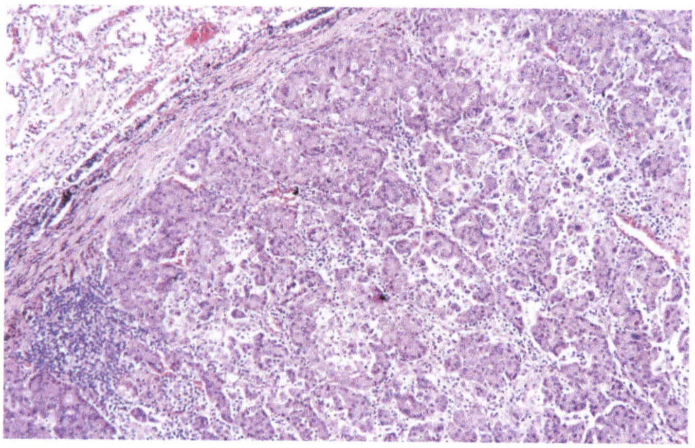

FIGURE 44.15. Metastatic hepatocellular carcinoma to intraparenchymal subpleural node. **(A)** Lower power. **(B)** Higher power.

to 55%).[141,142] In a study by Winterbauer et al.,[143] bilateral hilar adenopathy was found in 74 of 99 (74%) cases of sarcoid, 20 of 212 (9.4%) cases of lymphoma, four of 500 (0.8%) of primary lung cancer, and two of 1201 (0.2%) of extrathoracic malignancies. In this latter group of 1201 extrathoracic malignancies, 354 had pulmonary metastases, indicating an incidence of extrathoracic malignancies with pulmonary metastases and hilar adenopathy of two of 354 (0.6%). In the series by McLoud et al.,[137] 40% of the cases had evidence of pulmonary vascular lymphatic involvement with tumor spread to nodes occurring most often from head and neck, testes, kidney, breast, melanoma, gastrointestinal tract, and prostate primaries. Occasionally extrathoracic metastases are identified in intraparenchymal nodes (Fig. 44.15).

Pneumothorax and Bronchopleural Fistula in Malignancies

Whether primary or secondary tumors are involved, if the tumor nodule is peripheral, there is a chance of cavitation and erosion through the pleura, producing a bronchopleural fistula. This may also occur via direct tumor spread from aerated lung or bronchus to pleura, tumor cavitation, postobstructive pneumonia, or air-trapping, and is more common in skeleton-derived tumors in children[144] than it is in the adult population.[135] Metastatic bone tumors account for 70% of such cases in one pediatric series.[144] It has been described with cavitary metastases such as squamous carcinoma, adenocarcinoma, or angiosarcoma.[145] As 80% to 90% of bilateral multinodular metastases are peripheral and subpleural,[6,146] it is interesting that fistulas do not happen more often. In some cases metastatic tumor has been associated with bleb formation.[147]

Pleural Metastases

As has been noted, lymphatics run in pleura, and as with nodal spread it is not unusual to expect pleural spread with parenchymal lymphatic invasion (Fig. 44.12B). This may happen in an anterograde or retrograde fashion, the latter secondary to obstruction or other causes of high pressure. This topic has been well reviewed by Filderman et al.,[7] and the following discussion is drawn from this review.

Malignancy accounts for a significant percentage of pleural effusions, and this percentage increases with age. Chrétien and Jaubert[148] collected 1868 cases of pleural effusion from six series, including one of their own of 488 cases, in which there was an average rate of malignancy of 42% (range, 24–80%). Sahn[149] collected nine series, for a total of 1783 cases of malignant pleural effusion, and noted that 36% were from lung, 25% from breast, 10% from lymphoma, 5% from ovary, 2% from stomach, and 7% from unknown sources; similar findings were noted in another large review by Light.[150] Adenocarcinomas, whether from lung, breast, ovary, or stomach, lead the list of individual cell types, while other cell types are certainly included, including squamous carcinoma, small cell, or large cell undifferentiated cell types from lung.

Interesting work on pleural spread in both secondary and primary lung cancers has been done by Cantó et al.[151–153] In primary lung cancers,[152] 14 of 22 squamous carcinomas (64%), 21 of 24 adenocarcinomas (87.5%), and 26 of 29 small cell carcinomas (89.7%) have pleural spread. A contrasting study of 126 cases of metastatic breast carcinoma with malignant pleural effusion in 85 cases[153] showed the pleural space to be involved from the same side as the breast primary in 76.5% of cases and on the opposite side in 23.5%. When the contralateral side was involved, 80% represented spread from a left-sided chest wall primary to the right pleural space. These authors have shown that, whether primary lung cancer or metastatic lesions, the dependent portion of the pleural space is most subject to tumor studding, with the largest nodules most inferior, suggesting earliest arrival or implantation by settling in the most dependent locations (Fig. 44.12). Pleural fluid was positive for malignant cells in 43% of these histologically proven cases, of which 61% of the total were serous and 39% serosanguineous.

As also explained earlier, malignant cells may arrive in the pleural space from transdiaphragmatic chest wall or mediastinal lymphatics and from there be picked up by pleural lymphatics. Breast, gastric, and hepatic tumors are good examples of such spread. In several series, women have malignant pleural effusions more often than men because their incidence of breast cancer is greater.[154] Although this is partially compensated by men's increased incidence of lung cancer, the ratio for malignant pleural effusions is still two women for each man.[154] Malignant pleural effusions are usually moderate to large in volume, ranging from 500 to 2000 mL.[154,155] Not all pleural effusions in cancer patients are malignant, however, and the common pathway seems to be obstruction of the lymphatics, as mediastinal lymph nodes involved with malignancy have a high percentage of pleural effusions.[154,156] Pulmonary infiltrates were seen in 40%, and evidence of pulmonary metastases, either in lung or mediastinal lymphadenopathy, was present in an additional 31% in the series reported by Chernow and Sahn.[154] That lymphatic metastases of cancer appear to be an important mechanism in effusion formation is shown by the fact that sarcomas, even when they are in the pleura, excluding Kaposi's sarcoma, do not typically invade lymphatics[152] and do not usually have associated pleural effusion. Heart failure with chemotherapy and radiation treatment can affect lymph drainage in these cases. Of note, about 30%

of Hodgkin's disease cases have pleural effusion,[152] but in some cases this results from obstructive lymphatic drainage in the mediastinum. Spread to pleura could be through distal arterial-capillary vascular supply, lymphatics in the lung, or directly through chest wall via pleural space, such as noted in the case of breast, liver, and stomach. A 78% incidence of malignant pleural effusions occurred in one series of hepatic metastases,[156] and this is thought to be a contributing source for tertiary spread to pleura.[89,156]

Special Situations in Metastases in Lung

As reviewed by both Filderman et al.[7] and Fraser et al.,[9] there are some characteristics of specific organ system metastases to lung that are worthwhile emphasizing. What follows should be considered a summary and not comprehensive. Immunostains mentioned emphasize the most common types of tumors in each group. A tabular review of the essentials of immunostains for most carcinomas is given in Table 44.1.[157–160] A good general source for all tumors, including less common ones, is Dabbs.[158] This section begins with an immunostain review of lung cancer itself, as these tumors can spread within lung, and when comparing immunohistochemical characteristics, knowledge of primary organ site tumors is always critical.

Lung

The common distinction in deciding primary from secondary tumor in any organ is based on whether a tumor arises or "belongs" in that organ. Much progress has been made lately with the widespread use of immunohisto-

TABLE 44.1. Usual immunostain reactions in most frequent epithelial tumors

Tissue	CK7	CK20	BH11[a]	BE12[b]	Others
Lung					
Adenocarcinoma	+	(–)	+	(–)	TTF-1, EMA, B72-3, Leu M-1, BerEP-4, surfactant apoprotein, villin
Squamous	(–)	–	(–)[c]	+	CK5/6, p63
Large cell	(+)	–	+	(–)	
Small cell	(–)	–	+	–	TTF-1, neuroendocrine markers (synaptophysin, chromogranin A, others)
Mesothelioma	(+)	–	+	(+)	Vimentin, calretinin, CK5/6
Squamous (all sites)	(–)	–	(–)[c]	+	CK5/6, p63
Thyroid					
Papillary and follicular	+	–	+	(+)	TTF-1, thyroglobulin, HBME-1, CD57, CA19-9, ER, PR, vimentin, involucrin
Medullary	(+)	–	+	–	Calcitonin, chromogranin A, synaptophysin
Breast					
Ductal	+	–	+	(–)	ER, PR, GCDFP-15, E-cadherin, S-100
Lobular	+	–	+	(–)	ER, PR, GCDFP-15, (E-cadherin –)
Liver					
Hepatoma	(–)	–	+	–	HepPar1, other hepatocyte markers, CD34, (sinusoidal), CEA (canalicular)
Cholangiocarcinoma	+	(+)	+	(–)	CEA, villin
Gastrointestinal					
Stomach	(+)	(+)	+	–	CK17, CA19-9, CEA
Colon and rectum	–	+	+	(–)	CDX2, CA19-9, CK19
Pancreas	+	(+)	+	(–)	CK17, CEA, CA19-9, CA125
Adrenal	–	–	–	–	Melan A (A103), synaptophysin, inhibin A
Renal cell	(–)	–	+	–	RCC Ag, vimentin, CD10
Urothelial cell	+	(+)	+	(–)	Uroplakin, p63
Ovary					
Serous	+	(–)	+	(+)	WT-1, CK5/6, CA125, ER, PR
Mucinous	+	+	+	(+)	ER, PR, CEA
Endometrium	+	–	+	(+)	ER, PR, vimentin
Prostate	(–)	–	+	–	PSA, PAP, Amicar

[a]CAM 5.2 also.
[b]Also CK5/6 and p63.
[c]Negative in native squamous surface-derived tumors; often positive in those arising through glandular metaplasia to squamous cancer, or in lung.
CEA, carcinoembryonic antigen; EMA, epithelial membrane antigen; ER, estrogen receptor; GCDFP-15, gross cystic disease fluid protein fraction 15; PAP, prostatic acid phosphatase; PR, progesterone receptor; PSA, prostate-specific antigen; RCC, renal cell carcinoma; TTF-1, thyroid transcription factor-1; +, positive; (+), mostly positive; (–), mostly negative; –, negative.
Source: Data derived from Gown,[157] Dabbs,[159] and Chu et al.,[160] and a review by Dr. John Bolen, Virginia Mason Medical Center, Seattle, WA.

FIGURE 44.16. Comparison of incidence of common immunohistochemical markers in the most frequent non–small-cell lung cancers. (From Hammar.[161] Copyright 2002, with permission from Elsevier.)

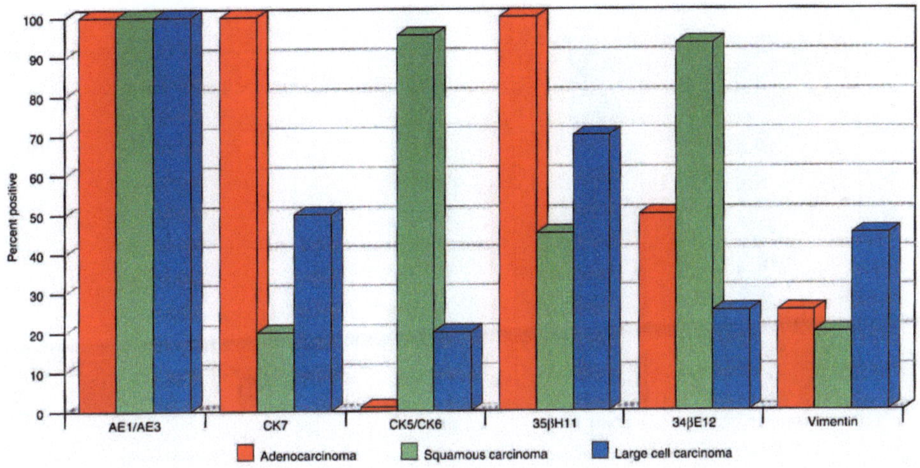

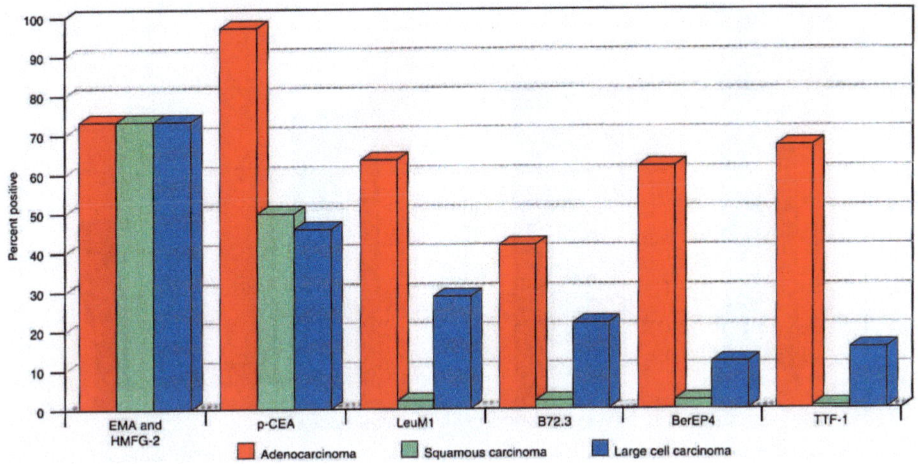

chemistry. Therefore, knowledge of primary lung tumors' characteristics is important, and a brief review is presented here. Much more extensive primary tumor immunocharacterization is available in each section dealing with each entity elsewhere in this book.

The battery of immunoperoxidase stains most characteristic of lung cancers is graphically illustrated by Dr. Samuel Hammar[161] and duplicated here as Figures 44.16 and 44.17. A basic panel may start with CK7, CK20, and thyroid transcription factor-1 (TTF-1), with the addition possibly of low and high molecular weight cytokeratin and vimentin. Panels often grow with additions of the other organs under consideration. Other organ-specific immunoperoxidase markers are summarized in Table 44.1 and are addressed more for each site to follow if not specifically mentioned in these tables.

Sarcomas

Sarcomas have a high incidence of spread to lung, especially after local recurrence. Clinically in life they have been detected in as many as 38% of cases[162,163] and at autopsy in up to 95% of cases.[163–166] Sarcomas are usually nodular and multiple and can become quite large,[167,168] may cavitate (Fig. 44.5) or have endobronchial spread (Fig. 44.6D),[169] may lead to spontaneous pneumothoraces,[170–175] present as thin-walled cysts,[176–178] or rarely have lymphatic spread as with Kaposi's sarcoma (Fig. 44.14). Especially pediatric bone-derived metastatic sarcomas to lung[144,145,179,180] have an especially high frequency of bronchopleural fistulas and pneumothorax. The spectrum of immunotyping of all sarcomas is broad, depending on the cell or tissue of origin.

Melanoma

The majority of disseminated metastatic melanoma patients have spread to lung.[181] In one series, 70% of 652 cases had pulmonary metastases, and in 7% the lungs were the only site of such metastases.[142] These metastases frequently have concurrent malignant pleural effusions and usually present as multiple nodules, being solitary in

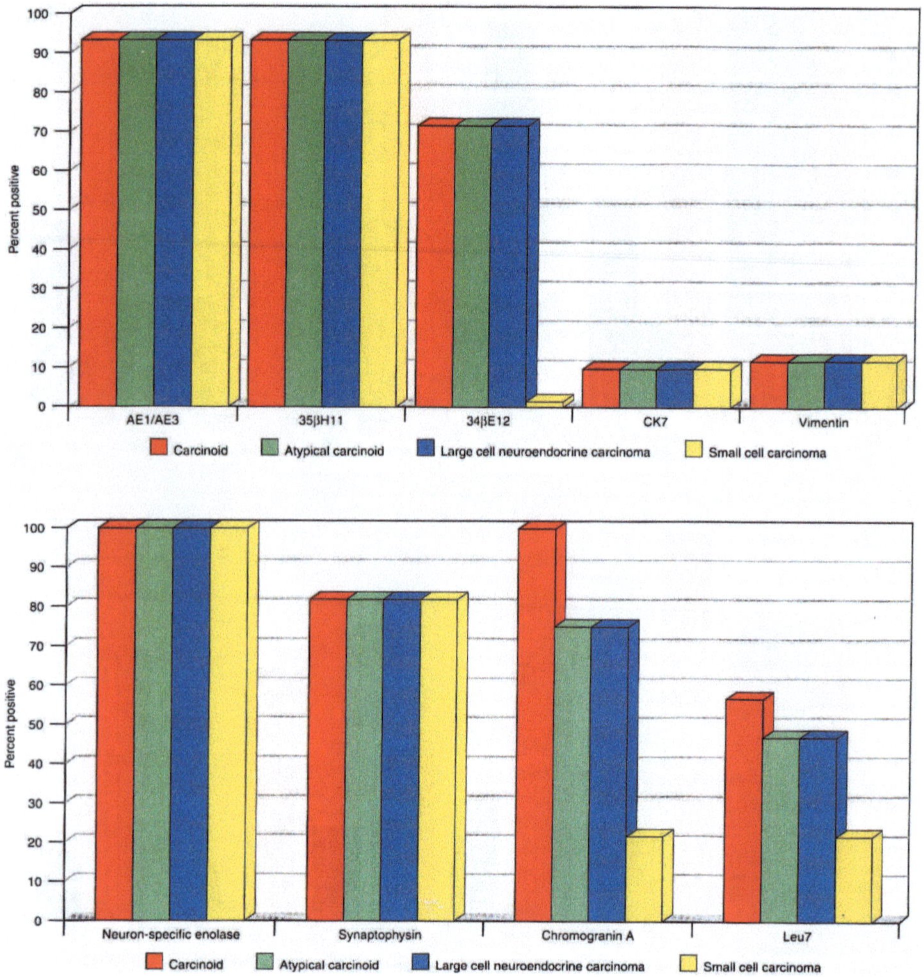

FIGURE 44.17. Comparison of common immunohistochemical markers for neuroendocrine carcinoma in lung. (From Hammar.[161] Copyright 2002, with permission from Elsevier.)

only 20% to 25% of those cases with thoracic metastases.[141,181,182] However, in a series of 200 melanomas with distant metastases, an asymptomatic pulmonary nodule was the first evidence of dissemination in 38% of cases.[183] A few are miliary, estimated to be 1.5% in one series[181] and 12% in another,[141] and lymphangitic spread occurred in some 8%. A rare case is illustrated in Figure 44.3B, which appears to be interstitial-alveolar and almost simulates an adenocarcinoma with a nonmucinous bronchioloalveolar component. I have seen several indisputable metastatic melanoma cases where in-situ severe melanocytic atypia replaces some bronchial or bronchiolar mucosa in the peripheral lung. This unfortunately has been one of the criteria used to suggest primary melanoma in lung! Balloon cell melanomas can be confused with finely vacuolated tumors of histiocytic or lipid-rich tumors of assorted types. Rarely individual cells or small cell clusters are seen circulating or trapped in lung capillaries (Figs. 44.11C,D). Some may be endobronchial[184] or rarely associated with diffuse pulmonary ossification.[185] Most metastatic melanomas to lung occur within 4 to 6 months of the diagnosis of the primary tumor, although exceptions to this generalization certainly occur. These are usually negative for assorted cytokeratins and positive for vimentin, HMB-45, Melan A (MART-1), S-100, and tyrosinase, among others.

Not all solitary lung nodules in melanoma patients are metastatic melanoma. In one series, 16 of 49 patients (33%) with pulmonary resections for suspected melanoma had benign disease.[186] In a series by Patel et al.,[187] another primary neoplasm somewhere in the body was present in 7.4% of patients with metastatic melanoma. At autopsy, melanoma is usually present in multiple metastatic sites, involving only one site in less than 1% of cases in another series.[182] A large single institution series of 945 cases of pulmonary metastatic melanoma is by Harpole and associates.[182]

Head and Neck

Squamous carcinomas, particularly those arising in the larynx, hypopharynx, tonsillar fossa, and nasopharynx, account for many of the cases from head and neck sources that become pulmonary metastases. The incidence ranges from 12.3% to 40.7%,[188–191] and cervical nodes are usually involved with metastases in 65% to 80% of cases[190,191] before lung lesions occur. The larynx and lung may have coexistent carcinomas, as was noted in one series[192] of 60 such cases. These concur because of common tobacco and other environmental pollutant exposure. In one study[193] of lung lesions with head and neck cancers, 28% were benign, 19% metastatic, and 53% were primary lung tumors, so it is important to evaluate a lung nodule as a possible separate primary malignancy. Some salivary gland tumors can recapitulate those arising in bronchial glands but usually metastasize to distal lung parenchyma and are not bronchus-associated as are primary tumors. Metastatic adenoid cystic carcinomas in lung may be among the very slowly growing metastatic tumors.[194] Squamous cell carcinomas arising in native squamous surfaces, versus arising through glandular to squamous metaplasia, are usually low molecular weight cytokeratin, CK7 and CK20 negative, and positive for high molecular weight cytokeratin markers, 34BE12, CK5, CK6, and P63.

Thyroid

Follicular and anaplastic thyroid carcinomas can spread hematogenously in the course of the disease and lodge in the lung.[195–198] Depending on cell type, it is estimated that 15% to 47% of thyroid carcinomas eventually spread to lung[195,196,199–202]; the papillary variant most often involves lymph nodes first, is more indolent, and may grow slowly in the lung once it arrives there.[195,203,204]

These metastases are often multiple but may be solitary or very small, and hilar and mediastinal nodes are involved in as many as 50% of the cases with lung metastases.[195] Thyroid carcinomas, especially the anaplastic ones but also some papillary and follicular types, can directly invade the trachea.[205] Young age and positive radionucleotide I^{131} uptake confer a better prognosis in tumors that have spread to lung.[206] Thyroid cancers usually stain for TTF-1, thyroglobulin, HBME-1, low and high molecular weight cytokeratin, and CK7, and are CK20 negative (Table 44.1). Vimentin is coexpressed in 50% of cases, becoming the dominant marker in anaplastic tumors. Neuroendocrine markers are most positive in medullary carcinomas.

Breast

Breast origin has been mentioned in many of the metastatic patterns discussed here. This is attributed to the high incidence of cancer in the breast, its ability to frequently metastasize, and its high frequency of being an adenocarcinoma, in addition to the proximity of the breast to the lung. Spread may be hematogenously or lymphatically, or by direct penetration of the chest wall, and then with lymphatic spread. About 50% of disseminated breast cancers have pleural effusions.[113,207] The sole manifestations of breast metastases were seen as lung metastases in 15% and as pleural metastases in 10%, in contrast to the high incidence of bone metastases as single-site metastases in 56%.[208] In another series, the lungs and pleura represented the initial sites of recurrence of breast cancer in 10% of cases.[209] Metastases are most often nodular, but they may also be lymphangitic, vascular (Fig. 44.11A), embolic, pleural with effusion, or endobronchial.[59,113,208–211] In one interesting series,[210] 3% of breast cancer patients had a solitary nodule in the lung at the time of diagnosis of the breast lesion, and of these 5% were benign, 43% represented metastatic breast cancer, and 52% represented new primary lung cancers. See Table 44.1 for immunoperoxidase characterization. Gross cystic disease fluid protein fraction 15 (GCDFP-15) is most helpful, especially in those tumors with apocrine differentiation. Common breast cancers may stain S-100 positive while being carcinoembryonic antigen (CEA) negative, but CEA is usually vividly positive in lung cancers.[212] ER, PR, and TTF-1 help distinguish these also.

Liver

The lungs represent the most common site of liver tumor metastases, which have been reported to occur in 37% to 70% of cases in autopsy series[213–215] but are less often clinically detected.[216] These present as nodules, often multiple, but pleural effusions are common; there is a tendency for more nodules to be in the right lower lobe, and a greater degree of effusion to occur in the lower[217] lobes, suggesting probable transdiaphragmatic spread. Occasionally they spread in a miliary pattern,[217] and occasionally they metastasize to intraparenchymal pulmonary nodes (Fig. 44.15). These tumors may also spread in continuity through the venous route directly, into the right heart as a large plug of tumor that may cause a major vessel embolus or as multiple smaller endovascular tumor emboli. The role of metastases in liver that then spread in a tertiary manner to the pleural space and pleural lymphatics has already been emphasized (Table 44.1). HepPar 1 and other hepatocyte markers are new helpful antigens. Fibrolamellar hepatocellular carcinomas are often CK7 positive. As noted in Table 44.1, CD34 often highlights sinusoidal lining cells and CEA canalicular structures in hepatocellular carcinomas.

Colon and Rectum

In general, 6% to 47% of colorectal carcinomas have pulmonary metastases,[218] which may be nodular, either

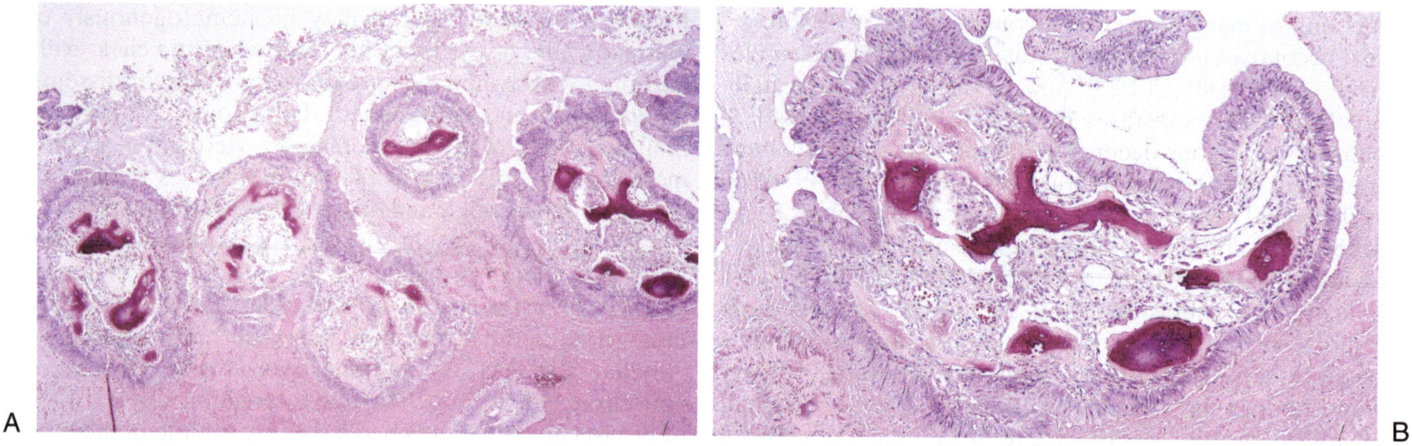

FIGURE 44.18. Metastatic colon cancer is the most frequent metastatic cancer in lung to undergo benign osseous metaplasia. **(A)** Lower power. **(B)** Higher power.

solitary or multiple, involve hilar, mediastinal, or intraparenchymal nodes (Fig. 44.15), and endobronchial (Fig. 44.6E,F) or endotracheal sites.[219] Of note, some 30% to 40% of all solitary metastases to lung are from the colon and rectum.[26,28] Many cancers arising in these sites go through the portal circulation and spread to the liver before the lungs. In a review of colorectal cancer metastases, 20% to 70% had liver spread and 10% to 20% lung spread.[220] Because collateral circulation from the left side of the colon avoids the liver, and because the original disease is often at an advanced stage at time of discovery, the rectum and, less often, the left colon have a higher incidence of pulmonary spread than the rest of the colon.[218,220–227] These metastases rarely ossify but ossification occurs in this group more often than with other tumor metastases[221] (Fig. 44.18 and Table 44.1). CDX2, although not totally specific,[228] is very helpful. It strongly stains a subset of primary adenocarcinomas of lung with goblet cell/colloid carcinoma morphology[229,230] but is not found in mucinous bronchioloalveolar carcinomas[231] or other primary lung tumors.

Pancreas

Pancreatic metastases usually involve nodes first and then liver, with spread to the lung thereafter. In an autopsy series of 104 patients, 62% had liver spread and 40% had lung spread.[232] Metastases may be nodular, both solitary and multiple, and incidence of lymphatic, pleural, and nodal spread is fairly high.[232] The nodular lesions can cavitate[232,233] or spread to endobronchus.[234] Tumors that arise in the tail of the pancreas more often have hilar and mediastinal node metastases than those that arise in the head and body.[232] The histology of these metastases, as with certain other poorly differentiated glandular primaries, is not always clear-cut adenocarcinoma (Fig. 44.7A). In addition to immunostains listed in Table 44.1, CDX2 has been useful in neuroendocrine neoplasms of gastrointestinal tract and pancreas.[235]

Renal Cell Carcinoma

Renal cell carcinoma spreads fairly frequently to the lung, perhaps because it frequently invades veins and then directly extends to (Fig. 44.8) or embolizes to lung as the next vascular network. It has been described in the lung in from 55% to 75% of series,[236–240] and all types of pulmonary spread have been described including nodules, occasionally quite large, both large and small vascular emboli, and endobronchial spread[241–246] is fairly common (Fig. 44.6B,C), as is lymphatic, hilar, and mediastinal node spread, occasionally with bilateral hilar adenopathy.[236,247–249] Of interest, 30% to 45% of patients with pulmonary spread have no symptoms referable to the primary kidney lesion.[237] Also, metastatic lesions in lung occasionally appear many years after the primary has been excised, sometimes up to 50 years later.[250] Immunohistochemical markers (Table 44.1) usually show low molecular weight cytokeratin, and, in about half, vimentin coexpression. CD10, epithelial membrane antigen (EMA), and renal cell carcinoma (RCC) antibodies are often positive. Uroplakin helps with urothelial cell–derived tumors. The main differential diagnosis in lung is with primary lung cancer with clear cell change and primary benign "sugar cell" tumors. Immunoperoxidase studies help sort this out, including lack of any cytokeratins and other renal markers and presence of HMB-45 and sometimes smooth muscle actin positivity in benign "sugar cell" tumors derived from the perivascular epithelioid cell (PEC). Of course, lipids and sugars, which are rich in renal cell and not primary lung carcinomas, both of which need special handling for documentation in routine histology. Renal cell adenocarcinoma is often the most frequent recipient and lung the most frequent donor of tumor to tumor metastases.[251]

Ovarian Cancer

As many as 50% of ovarian cancers have intrathoracic spread, including lung parenchyma and pleura.[252–254] This is the highest rate of intrathoracic spread of any gynecologic malignancy.[255,256] Pleural spread is most common, and is usually accompanied by malignant pleural effusion in up to 39% of all cases, being positive in 77% of those with thoracic metastases.[253] Parenchymal spread occurs in 7% to 39%[253,257,258] often in continuity with pleural tumor nodules.[258] Solitary lesions may occur in 7%, lymphatic spread in 6%, and nodal spread in 11%[242] with rare endobronchial spread.[259] Vascular spread also rarely occurs[260] (Figs. 44.7 and 44.10). Spread to the chest usually follows fairly extensive pelvic and peritoneal tumor,[253,254,258] and extensive small vessel tumor cell embolization to lung has sometimes been described with peritoneal-venous (LeVeen type) shunting for malignant ascites.[18,253] This has occasionally led to rapid death from respiratory failure with lung capillaries filled with tumor cells.[18,261–265] Common ovarian tumor groups are divided into serous and mucinous surface tumors (Table 44.1).

Uterus

The cervix, endometrium, and myometrium are considered here. Invasive carcinoma of the cervix has been reported as spreading to lung in 5.8%[266] to 33%[267] of cases, averaging about 10%.[268] In a study by Sostman and Matthay,[269] cervical adenocarcinomas spread with an incidence of 20% and were stage independent, while squamous carcinomas had an incidence of pulmonary spread of 4% and were stage dependent, supporting the vasoinvasiveness of adenocarcinomas. The lung may be the sole site of metastatic cervical carcinoma in 12%[268,272] to 25%[273] of cases. Multiple nodules are usual,[120,271,273,274] but in as many as one third of the cases they may be solitary[270–274] and sometimes are quite large "cannonballs." Cavitation[231,275] along with endobronchial spread[54,60,65,276,277] has been identified as well as lymphangitic spread.[110,278,279] At times hilar or mediastinal nodes are the only evidence of metastases,[280] and effusion may occur.[271] Endometrial cancers spread very rarely to lung, having occurred in only 2.3% of 470 cases in one series with a 2- to 12-year follow-up.[281] Pulmonary spread usually occurs late, often after disease is evident elsewhere. These are divided into endometrioid type and serous type. The high-grade serous carcinoma of endometrium usually stains vividly with p53 marker in 90% of cases compared to some staining in 20% of endometrioid carcinomas.[282] Ki-67 is usually very positive in these serous tumors.[282] Other immunostain characteristics are given in Table 44.1.

Uterine wall-derived smooth muscle tumors are frequent sources of spread to the lung. When a lower- or higher-grade smooth muscle nodule is found in the lung of a woman, the uterus frequently is the most likely source. The lower-grade ones are referred to as "benign" metastasizing leiomyomas[283–288] (Fig. 44.19, see also Figs. 39.21 and 39.22 in Chapter 39). Whether low or high grade, such nodules in lung are usually asymptomatic but rarely lead to respiratory failure and death.[178,283,286] Metastases are usually nodular and bilateral, occasionally cystic,[174,283] (Fig. 44.5) but micronodular[286,287] and miliary[289] patterns and endobronchial spread[290] (Fig. 44.6D) have been described. Some uterine-derived leiomyosarcomas or intravascular leiomyomas, as well as those primary in the inferior vena cava, extend up to and fill the inferior vena cava and may extend directly into the right heart, and even directly into pulmonary artery,[291] and they may break off as large tumor emboli (see Fig. 39.23 in Chapter 39).[292] Leiomyosarcomas are positive for smooth muscle actins and smooth muscle myosin, h-caldesmon, calponin, and to a lesser degree CD34 and CD30. Type IV collagen outlines individual tumor cells.

Endometrial stromal sarcomas when high grade often metastasize to lung. More recently, low-grade pulmonary metastases from these tumors have received attention[293–295] and occasionally show microcystic change or sex-cord–like differentiation,[295,296] even in their metastatic location (Fig. 44.19C,D). Occasionally they are grossly cystic and can be mistaken for lymphangioleiomyomatosis (LAM)[297] or account for some of those described as cystic mesenchymal hamartomas.[295,298] Some have pulmonary metastases up to 25 years after hysterectomy.[299] CD10 is positive in endometrial stromal sarcomas but not in leiomyosarcomas.

Female Gestational Choriocarcinomas

These tumors frequently present in the lung as nodules, either single or multiple,[300,301] and sometimes reach large size, or they can cause a diffuse miliary pattern[302–304] or vessel embolus (Fig. 44.1), again often large in size.[303,305–307] Cavitation[308] or pneumothorax[309] can occur. In one series, pulmonary metastases occurred in 87% of cases.[303] Spontaneous regression can occur but more often is induced by chemotherapy, with only focal fibrosis or dystrophic calcification remaining.[303,310,311] Occasionally, partially responding tumor can have unusual pathologic appearances,[312] and they rarely are mistaken for a primary large cell carcinoma of lung.[313] Some rare primary lung tumors show trophoblastic change with human chorionic gonadotropin (HCG) staining. I have seen one evolving out of a more routine adenocarcinoma. Immunostains show strong low molecular weight cytokeratin staining and frequent HCG,

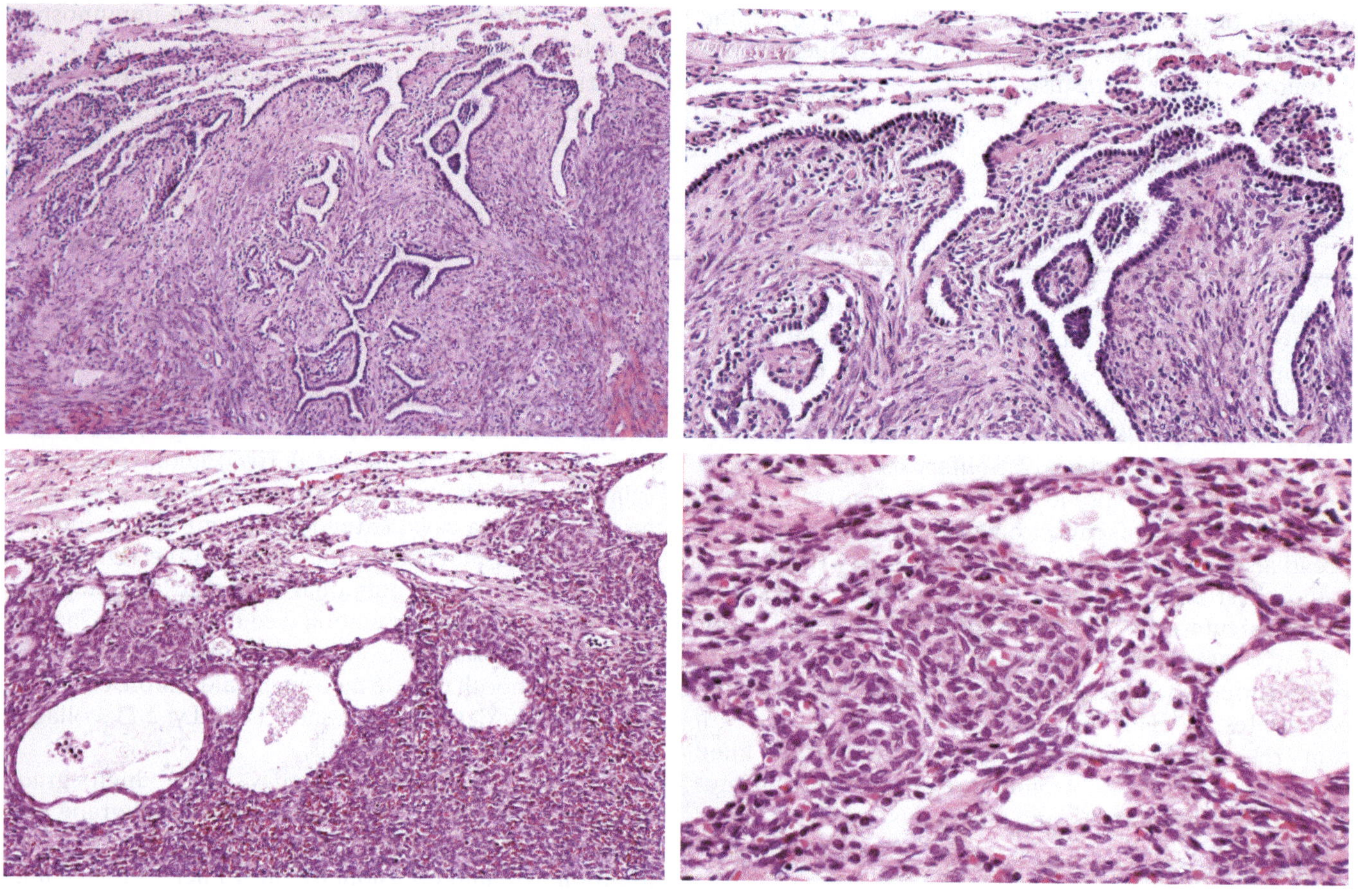

FIGURE 44.19. Myometrial stroma neoplasms in lung. **(A,B)** Benign metastasizing leiomyoma here stimulates benign metaplastic lining cells over edges of progressing low grade spindle cell tumor. **(A)** Lower power. **(B)** Higher power. **(C,D)** Metastatic low-grade endometrial stromal sarcoma. **(C)** Lower power. **(D)** Higher power. Note small cysts more at periphery in both. Note suggestion of sex-cord–like differentiation in **D**.

human placental lactogen (HPL), and placental alkaline phosphatase (PLAP) positivity. Mel-CAM (CD146) is under study to augment this panel.

Prostate

Prostatic adenocarcinoma most often extends regionally to lymphatics first, or frequently directly to bone, before extending to the lung.[314–316] Bone is almost invariably involved before lung,[317] but rare exceptions occur.[318,319] Retrograde venous spread from prostate to lower vertebral column may account for the higher incidence of tumor there than in lung.[316] Clinically only 5% to 15% of cases have lung metastases,[314,320,321] but autopsy series have noted more, 24%[320] to 38%.[321] These may be as solitary or multiple nodular metastases,[317] rarely with endobronchial,[63,322–325] lymphangitic,[326,327] or nodal spread.[328] Malignant pleural effusion has been noted in 14% of stage D prostate carcinomas.[328] Prostatic-specific antigen (PSA) and prostatic acid phosphatase (PAP) are helpful, although not exclusive here (Table 44.1).

Testes

Seminomas usually evolve slowly, and spread through nodes sequentially before pulmonary spread.[329] Nonseminomatous tumors, however, are more rapidly growing and spread to the lung early by both hematogenous and lymphatic routes.[329–331] Choriocarcinoma spreads via venous routes solely. Single or multiple nodules are seen most commonly[332] and may occasionally be large, and endobronchial spread[333,334] has been identified. Although lymphatic spread in lung is unusual,[332] direct spread up the periaortic node chain appears to account for mediastinal node involvement without lung involvement,[137,335] representing the most common manifestation of intrathoracic metastatic testis tumors.[336] Seminomas, embryonal carcinomas, and yolk sac tumors usually stain PLAP positive and choriocarcinomas HCG positive. (See above discussion for more on choriocarcinomas.) Up to 75% of nonseminomatous germ cell tumors are α-fetoprotein (AFP) positive. Some of the nonseminomatous germ cell neoplasms mature into teratomas either spontaneously or after chemotherapy,[337,338] and other testicular neoplasms respond to therapy and may leave only residual pulmonary cysts or lacunae.[339]

Metastases from the Lung

It is apparent from the extent of the foregoing discussion that metastases in the lung may be difficult to distinguish from primary pulmonary tumors, and, vice versa, primary tumors must in certain situations be distinguished from metastases and treated accordingly as independent primary cancer(s) in a patient with known malignancy elsewhere in the body. Some 3% to 7% of patients with lung cancer have metachronous tumors in another location.[19] Some general principles have been covered; central, solitary tumors with unilateral hilar node involvement are most often, but not always, primary carcinomas. Solitary metastases to lung do occur in some 3% to 9% of cases,[3,26,27] and endobronchial metastases add potential for further confusion. Primary lung cancers can be peripheral in the zone(s) of the lung most often involved with metastases.

Synchronous or metachronous multiple unilateral or bilateral primary lung cancers can occur as discussed in a review[9] and in two large single institutional series,[340,341] and were metachronous in two thirds of the series.[9,340] Either primary or secondary tumors that grow in the lung can metastasize from the lung, following similar routes. Primary tumors often spread through lymphatics, an important step in staging cancers. Regional nodes are most often involved followed by the upstream mediastinal nodes.

Primary lung cancer metastases favor liver, adrenal glands, and bone, although almost any site in the body can be involved. Of interest, early unilateral spread to adrenal glands is usually to the ipsilateral adrenal, suggesting this is transdiaphragmatic and probably lymphangitic. Later, when generalized hematogenous spread has occurred, this is not true.[342] Because lung tumors are prevalent, they can spread to unusual sites[343,344] such as the gastrointestinal tract, both male and female genital tracts including the placenta, the choroid coat of the eye, or the bones of hands and feet.

Some primary lung tumors, once they have gone throughout the lymphatics and venous exit pathways from their primary site, similarly can reenter the lung directly as secondary tumor or as tertiary metastases from secondary involvement of other sites such as liver. In one series,[345] the opposite lung was involved with metastatic small cell carcinoma in 8% of cases. Certainly lung cancers can primarily enter their own lymphatic spaces anterograde and drain to regional nodes, but such tumors can also spread back into other portions of lung in a retrograde fashion because of obstructed nodes (see foregoing discussion of lymphatic spread). Although primary lung tumors typically spread to unilateral hilar lymph nodes, they spread to bilateral hilar nodes in 0.8% of cases, which compares to secondary tumors with pulmonary involvement that show this spread in 0.6% of cases.[143] Primary lung cancers are also a significant cause of malignant pleural effusions, and in one series by Cantó et al.,[152] 14 of 22 squamous carcinomas (64%), 21 of 24 adenocarcinomas (87.5%), and 26 of 29 small cell carcinomas (89.7%) and all three primary lung tumors (100%) not otherwise specified had malignant spread to pleura. Spread of primary lung cancer to pleural space is important in staging, and usually indicates the lung cancer is incurable.[152]

In contrast, bronchioloalveolar carcinomas can spread aerogenously and despite their extensive and often bilateral spread, avoid the lymphatic pathways and regional nodes. As noted earlier, this tumor and epithelioid hemangioendotheliomas can present as multiple smaller nodules without a dominant tumor mass, and yet may still represent primary lung tumors. However, both tumors may also represent patterns of secondary spread.

Primary lung tumors can invade both pulmonary arteries and veins. Gonzalez-Vitale and Garcia-Bunuel[100] discussed pulmonary artery embolization from primary lung cancers, finding it present in 33 of 331 (10%) patients dying with non–small-cell primary lung cancers. In the same series, venous spread occurred in 79% and lymphangitic spread was noted in 84%. Adenocarcinoma showed this frequency in 16.5% of cases, compared to 5.8% for squamous carcinoma and 7.7% for large cell undifferentiated carcinomas. None of the classic bronchioloalveolar carcinomas did so. Coexistent lymphatic invasion occurred in 84% of the cases with vascular spread, focal in only 1%, and widespread or diffuse in the others. When focal, it was seen in the areas coexistent with tumor emboli in vessels. Tumor embolization within the lung may occur in the absence of widespread metastases and was present in 9% of the cases in one series.[96] In my and others[346] experience, primary adenocarcinoma of lung associated with scarring (so-called scar carcinomas) often shows thick-walled, compressed muscular arteries in the middle of the scar whose remnant collapsed luminal spaces contains tumor. The mechanism for this is unclear. Lung cancers are notorious for direct spread into adjacent structures, such as into the brachial plexus superiorly, producing Pancoast tumor and possibly Horner's syndrome, but also into other parts of the chest wall, the mediastinum, hilar structures, heart, pericardium, or diaphragm. Likewise, bony metastases from primary lung cancers are most often to ribs and vertebrae.

Massive malignant arterial emboli to systemic arteries are most often caused by lung cancer (Fig. 44.20), with only a rare case due to primary aortic cancer.[347,348] Of

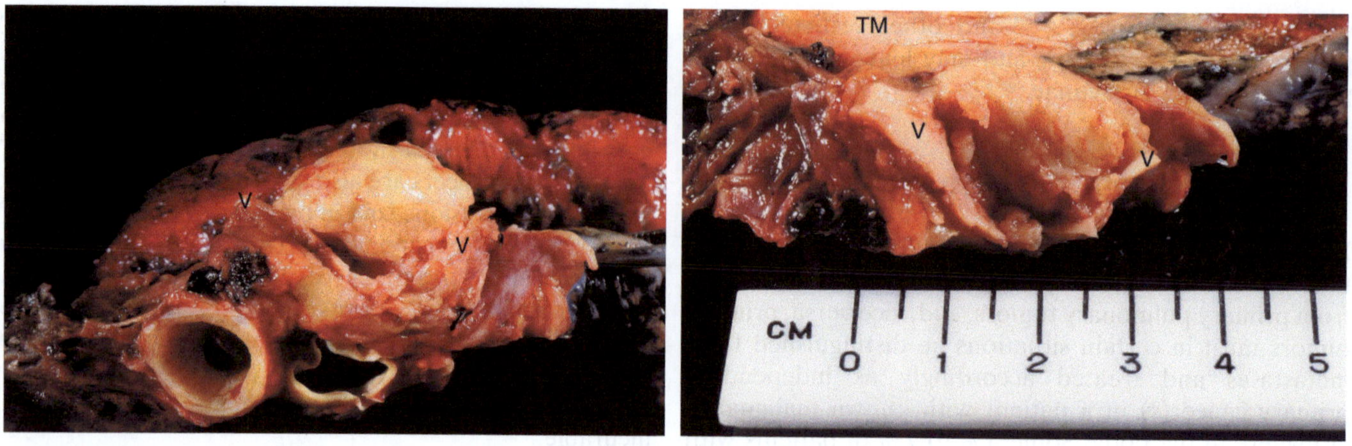

A B

FIGURE 44.20. Primary lung cancer grossly extends into pulmonary vein. **(A)** A 4.5-cm central primary pulmonary squamous carcinoma has invaded the central vein. Intact pneumonectomy specimen is viewed from hilum. Wall of vein (V) is noted around the tumor protruding into its lumen. Note main stem bronchus and main pulmonary artery below tumor. **(B)** On the cut surface of the lung above is seen a portion of the primary tumor (TM).

note, some of these tumor emboli from the lung come from metastatic lesions in the lung.[347] Occasionally a primary cardiac myxoma causes a massive embolus. Paradoxical tumor emboli passing through patent foramen ovale or interventricular septal defects may also present as systemic arterial emboli. Rarely, nonpulmonary malignancies directly penetrate the aortic wall and cause similar massive emboli to systemic vessels.[349]

References

1. Farrell JT Jr. Pulmonary metastasis: a pathologic, clinical, roentgenologic study based on 78 cases seen at necropsy. Radiology 1935;24:444–451.
2. Abrams HJ, Spiro R, Goldstein N. Metastases in carcinoma, analysis of 1000 autopsied cases. Cancer 1950;3: 74–85.
3. Rosenblatt MB, Lisa JR, Trinidad S. Pitfalls in the clinical and histological diagnosis of bronchogenic carcinoma. Dis Chest 1966;49:396–404.
4. Johnson RM, Lindskog GE. 100 cases of tumor metastatic to the lung and mediastinum. JAMA 1967;202:94–98.
5. Willis RA. The spread of tumours in the human body. London: Butterworths, 1973:167–174.
6. Crow J, Slavin G, Kreel L. Pulmonary metastasis: a pathologic and radiologic study. Cancer 1981;47:2595–2603.
7. Filderman AE, Coppage L, Shaw C, et al. Pulmonary and pleural manifestations of extrathoracic malignancies. Clin Chest Med 1989;10:747–807.
8. Zetter BR. The cellular basis of site specific tumor metastasis. N Engl J Med 1990;322:605–612.
9. Fraser RS, Müller NL, Colman N, et al. Diagnosis of diseases of the chest. 3rd ed. Philadelphia: WB Saunders, 1999:1381–1417.
10. Whitesell PL, Peters SG. Pulmonary manifestations of extrathoracic malignant lesions. Mayo Clin Proc 1993;68: 483–491.
11. Suster S, Moran CA. Unusual manifestations of metastatic tumors to the lungs. Semin Diagn Pathol 1995;12:193–206.
12. Luce JA. Metastatic malignant tumors. In: Murray JE, Nadel JA, Mason RJ, Boushey HA Jr, eds. Textbook of respiratory medicine. 3rd ed. Philadelphia: WB Saunders, 2000:1469–1476.
13. Cagle PT. Differential diagnosis between primary and metastatic carcinomas. Lung tumors: fundamental biology and clinical management. In: Brambilla C, Brambilla E, eds. Lung biology in health and disease, vol 124. New York: Marcel Dekker, 1999:127–137.
14. Paget S. The distribution of secondary growths in cancer of the breast. Lancet 1889;1:571–573.
15. Ewing J. A treatise on tumors. 3rd ed. Philadelphia: WB Saunders, 1928.
16. Zeren, H, Moran CA, Suster S, et al. Primary pulmonary synovial sarcomas with features of monophasic synovial sarcoma: a clinicopathologic, immunohistochemical, and ultrastructural study of 25 cases. Hum Pathol 1995;26: 474–480.
17. Okamoto S, Hisaoka M, Daa T, et al. Primary pulmonary synovial sarcoma: a clinicopathologic, immunohistochemical, and molecular study of 11 cases. Hum Pathol 2004;35: 850–856.
18. Fildes J, Narvaez GP, Baig KA, et al. Pulmonary tumor embolization after peritoneovenous shunting for malignant ascites. Cancer 1988;61:1973–1976.
19. Yesner R, Carter D. Pathology of carcinoma of the lung: changing patterns. Clin Chest Med 1982;3:257–289.
20. Muller KM, Respondek M. Pulmonary metastases: pathologic anatomy. Lung 1990;168(suppl):1137–1144.
21. Rosenblatt MB, Lisa JR, Collier F. Primary and metastatic broncho-alveolar carcinoma. Dis Chest 1967;52:147–152.
22. Wu H, Tino G, Gannon FH, et al. Lepidic intrapulmonary growth of malignant mesothelioma presenting as recurrent pneumothorax. Hum Pathol 1996;27:989–992.

23. Hie J, Stenwig AE, Kullman G, et al. Distant metastases in papillary thyroid cancer. Cancer 1988;61:1–6.
24. Dwyer AJ, Reichert CM, Woltering EA, et al. Diffuse pulmonary metastasis in melanoma: radiographic-pathologic correlation. AJR 1984;143:983–984.
25. Coppage L, Shaw C, Curtis AM. Metastatic disease to the chest in patients with extrathoracic malignancy. J Thorac Imaging 1987;2:24–37.
26. Steele JD. The solitary pulmonary nodule. J Thorac Cardiovasc Surg 1963;46:21–39.
27. Toomes H, Delphendahl A, Manke H, et al. The coin lesion of the lung: a review of 955 resected coin lesions. Cancer 1983;51:534–537.
28. Head JM. Surgery of pulmonary metastases. In: Choi WC, Grillo HC, eds. Thoracic Oncology. New York: Raven Press, 1983:359–365.
29. Clagett OT, Woolner LB. Surgical treatment of solitary metastatic pulmonary lesion. Med Clin North Am 1964;48: 939–943.
30. Paglicci A. Tumori metastatice del polmone: studio su 152 lasi (metastatic tumors of the lung: a study of 152 cases). Radiol Med (Tor) 1956;422:184–192.
31. Holmes EC, Ramming KP, Eiber FR. The surgical management of pulmonary metastases. Semin Oncol 1977;4:65–69.
32. Huth JF, Holmes EC, Vernon SE, et al. Pulmonary resection for metastatic carcinoma. Am J Surg 1980;140: 9–16.
33. Cahan WG, Castro EB. Significance of a solitary lung shadow in patients with breast cancer. Ann Surg 1975; 181:137–143.
34. Judson WF, Harbrecht PJ, Fry DE. Associated lung lesions in patients with primary head and neck carcinoma. Ann Surg 1973;178:703–705.
35. Saegesser F, Besson A, Kafai F. Pulmonary cold lesions and metastases. In: Saegesser F, Pettraral J, ed. Surgical oncology. Baltimore: Williams & Wilkins, 1970:539–610.
36. Cahan WG. Excision of melanoma metastases to lung: problems in diagnosis and management. Ann Surg 1973; 178:703–709.
37. Cahan WG, Castro EB, Hajdu SI. The significance of a solitary lung shadow in patients with colon carcinoma. Cancer 1974;33:414–421.
38. Herold CJ, Bankier AA, Fleischmann D. Lung metastases. Eur Radiol 1996;6:596–606.
39. Jablons D, Steinberg S, Roth J, et al. Metastasectomy for soft tissue sarcoma: further evidence for efficacy and prognostic mediators. J Thorac Cardiovasc Surg 1989;97: 695–704.
40. Billingsley KG, Burt ME, Jara E, et al. Pulmonary metastases from soft tissue sarcoma: analysis of patterns of diseases and postmetastasis survival. Ann Surg 1999;299: 602–610.
41. Monteiro A, Arce N, Bernardo J, et al. Surgical resection of lung metastases from epithelial tumors. Ann Thorac Surg 2004;77:431–437.
42. Anonymous. Long-term results of lung metastasectomy: prognostic analyses based on 5206 cases. The International Registry of Lung Metastases. J Thorac Cardiovasc Surg 1997;113:37–49.
43. Dodd GD, Boyle JJ. Excavating pulmonary metastases. AJR 1961;85:277–293.
44. Aronchick JM, Palevsky HI, Miller WT. Cavitary pulmonary metastases in angiosarcoma. Diagnosis by transthoracic needle aspiration. Am Rev Respir Dis 1989;139:252–253.
45. Gilman JK, Sievers DB, Thornsvard CT. Malignant fibrous histiocytoma manifesting as a cavitary lung metastasis. South Med J 1986;79:376–378.
46. Wright FW. Spontaneous pneumothorax and pulmonary malignant disease—a syndrome sometimes associated with cavitating tumors. Clin Radiol 1976;27:211–222.
47. Seo JB, Im JG, Goo JM, et al. Atypical pulmonary metastases: spectrum of radiologic findings. Radiographics 2001;21:403–417.
48. Trinidad S, Lisa JR, Rosenblatt MB. Bronchogenic carcinoma simulated by metastatic tumour. Cancer 1965;16: 1521–1529.
49. Sorenson JB. Endobronchial metastases from extrapulmonary solid tumors. Acta Oncol 2004;43:73–79.
50. Schnilla RA, Fazzini EP. Bronchial gland adenocarcinoma of the lung. Am Rev Respir Dis 1977;115(suppl):160 (abstr).
51. Hirata H, Noguchi M, Shimosato Y, et al. Clinicopathologic and immunohistochemical characteristics of bronchial gland cell type adenocarcinoma of the lung. Am J Clin Pathol 1990;93:20–25.
52. Bourke SA, Henderson AF, Stevenson RD, et al. Endobronchial metastases simulating primary carcinoma of the lung. Respir Med 1989;83:151-152.
53. Braman SS, Whitcomb ME. Endobronchial metastasis. Arch Intern Med 1975;135:543–547.
54. King DS, Castleman B. Bronchial involvement in metastatic pulmonary malignancy. J Thorac Surg 1943;12:305–315.
55. Seiler HH, Clagett T, McDonald JR. Pulmonary resection for metastatic malignant lesions. J Thorac Surg 1950;19: 655–679.
56. Albertini RE, Edberg NL. Endobronchial metastasis in breast cancer. Thorax 1980;35:435–440.
57. Schoenbaum S, Viamonte M. Subepithelial endobronchial metastases. Diagn Radiol 1971;101:63–69.
58. Furth J. Experiments on the spread of neoplastic cells through the respiratory passages. Am J Pathol 1946;22; 1101–1107.
59. Gerle R, Felson B. Metastatic endobronchial hypernephroma. Dis Chest 1963;44:225–233.
60. Fitzgerald RH. Endobronchial metastases. South Med J 1977;79:440–443.
61. Baumgartner WA, Mark JB. Metastatic malignancies from distant sites to the tracheobronchial tree. J Thorac Cardiovasc Surg 1980;79:499–503.
62. Shepherd MP. Endobronchial metastatic disease. Thorax 1982;37:362–365.
63. Lee DW, Ro JY, Sahin AA, et al. Mucinous adenocarcinoma of the prostate with endobronchial metastasis. Am J Clin Pathol 1990;94:641–645.
64. Garces M, Tsai E, Marsan RE. Endotracheal metastases. Chest 1974;65:350–351.
65. Coaker LA, Sobonya RE, David JR. Endobronchial metastases from uterine cervical squamous carcinoma. Arch Pathol Lab Med 1984;108:269–271.

66. Yeh TJ, Batayias G, Peters H, et al. Metastatic carcinoma to the trachea: report of a case of palliation by resection and marlex graft. J Thorac Cardiov Surg 1965;49:886–892.
67. Mohsenifar Z, Chopra SK, Simmons DH. Diagnostic value of fiberoptic bronchoscopy in metastatic pulmonary tumours. Chest 1978;74:369–371.
68. Chuang MT, Padilla ML, Teirstein AS. Flexible fiberoptic bronchoscopy in metastatic cancer to the lungs. Cancer 1983;52:1949–1951.
69. Poe RH, Ortiz C, Israel RH, et al. Sensitivity, specificity and predictive values of bronchoscopy in neoplasm metastatic to the lung. Chest 1985;88:84–88.
70. Carey RW, Taft PD, Bennett JM, et al. Carcinocythemia (carcinoma cell leukemia): an acute leukemia-like picture due to metastatic carcinoma cells. Am J Med 1976;60: 273–278.
71. Lugassy G, Vorst EJ, Varon D, et al. Carcinocythemia: report of two cases, one simulating a Burkitt lymphoma. Acta Cytol 1990;34:265–268.
72. Gallivan MV, Lokich JJ. Carcinocythemia (carcinoma cell leukemia): report of two cases with English literature review. Cancer 1984;53:1100–1102.
73. Seronie-Vivien S, Mery E, et al. Carcinocythemia as the single extension of breast cancer: report of a case and review of the literature. Ann Oncol 2001;12:1019–1022.
74. Rodriguez-Salas N, Jimenez-Gordo AM, Gonzalez E, et al. Circulating cancer cells in peripheral blood. A case report. Acta Cytol 2000;44:237–241.
75. Dannaher CI, Yam LT, McKeown JM. Metastatic carcinoma with carcinocythemia mimicking leukemia. South Med J 1979;72:622–624.
76. Ejeckam GC, Sogbeing SK, McLeish WA. Carcinocythemia due to metastatic oat cell carcinoma of the lung. Can Med Assoc J 1979;120:336–338.
77. Solanki DI, McCurdy PR. Oat cell carcinoma mimicking leukemia. Postgrad Med 1980;68:213–216.
78. Finkel GC, Tishkoff GH. Malignant cells in a peripheral blood smear. N Engl J Med. 1960;26:187–188.
79. Sile CC, Perry DJ, Nam L. Small cell carcinocythemia. Arch Pathol Lab Med 1999;123:426–428.
80. Myerowitz RD, Edwards PA, Sartiano GP. Carcinocythemia (carcinoma cell leukemia) due to metastatic carcinoma of the breast: report of a case. Cancer 1977;40: 3107–3111.
81. Rappaport H. Tumors of the hematopoietic system. Washington, DC: Armed Forces Institute of Pathology, 1966:418.
82. Krause JR. Rhabdomyosarcoma presenting as carcinocythemia. South Med J 1979;72:1007–1008.
83. Schmidt MB. Die verbreitungswege der karzinome und die beziehung generalisierter sarkome zu den leukämischen neubildungen. Jena: G Fisher, 1903, as quoted by Saphir.[87]
84. Takahashi M. An experimental study of metastasis. J Pathol Bacteriol 1915;20:1–13.
85. Iwasaki T. Histological and experimental observations on the destruction of tumor cells in the blood vessels. J Pathol Bacteriol 1915–16;20:85–105.
86. Warren S, Gates O. The fate of intravenously injected tumor cells. Am J Cancer 1936;27:485–492.
87. Saphir O. The fate of carcinoma emboli in the lung. Am J Pathol 1947;23:245–253.
88. Willis RA. The spread of tumours in the human body. London: Churchill, 1934.
89. Winterbauer RH, Elfenbein IB, Ball WC Jr. Incidence and clinical significance of tumor embolization to the lungs. Am J Med 1968;45:271–290.
90. Kane RD, Hawkins HK, Miller JA, et al. Microscopic pulmonary tumor emboli associated with dyspnea. Cancer 1975;36:1473–1482.
91. Shiner RW, Ryn JH, Edwards WD. Microscopic pulmonary tumor embolism causing subacute cor pulmonale: a difficult antemortem diagnosis. Mayo Clin Proc 1991;66: 143–148.
92. Goldhaber SZ, Dricker E, Buring JE, et al. Clinical suspicion of autopsy-proven thrombotic and tumor pulmonary embolism in cancer patients. Am Heart J 1987;114:1432–1435.
93. Chan CK, Hutcheon MA, Hyland RH, et al. Pulmonary tumor embolism: a critical review of clinical, imaging, and hemodynamic features. J Thorac Imaging 1987;2:4–14.
94. Fahrner RJ, McQueeney AJ, Mosley JM, et al. Trophoblastic pulmonary thrombosis with cor pulmonale. JAMA 1959;170:1898–1901.
95. Fanta CH, Compton CC. Microscopic tumour emboli to the lungs: a hidden cause of dyspnea and pulmonary hypertension. Thorax 1979;43:794–795.
96. Greenspan EB. Carcinomatous endarteritis of the pulmonary vessels resulting in failure of the right ventricle. Arch Intern Med 1934;54:625–644.
97. Marini JJ, Bilnoski W, Huseby JS. Acute cor pulmonale resulting from tumor microembolism. West J Med 1980; 132:77–80.
98. Storstein O. Circulatory failure in metastatic carcinoma of the lung. A physiologic and pathologic study of its pathogenesis. Circulation 1951;4:913–919.
99. Abbondanzo SL, Klappenbach RS, Tsou E. Tumor cell embolism to pulmonary alveolar capillaries. Arch Pathol Lab Med 1986;110:1197–1198.
100. Gonzalez-Vitale JC, Garcia-Bunuel R. Pulmonary tumor emboli and cor pulmonale in primary carcinoma of the lung. Cancer 1976;38:2105–2110.
101. von Herbay A, Illes A, Waldherr R, et al. Pulmonary tumor thrombotic microangiopathy with pulmonary hypertension. Cancer 1990;66:587–592.
102. Altemus LF, Lee RL. Carcinomatosis of the lung with pulmonary hypertension. Arch Intern Med 1967;119: 32–38.
103. Crane R, Rudd TG, Dail DH. Tumor microembolism: pulmonary perfusion pattern. J Nucl Med 1984;25:877–880.
104. Soares FA, Landell GAM, de Oliveira JAM. Pulmonary tumor embolism to alveolar septal capillaries: a prospective study of 12 cases. Arch Pathol Lab Med 1991;115:127–130.
105. Soares FA, Landell GAM, de Oliveira JAM. Pulmonary tumor embolism from squamous cell carcinoma of the vulva. Gynecol Oncol 1990;38:141–143.

106. Soares FA, Landell GAM, de Oliveira JAM. Pulmonary tumor embolism to alveolar septal capillaries. Arch Pathol Lab Med 1992;116:187–188.
107. Durham JR, Ashley PF, Dorencamp D. Cor pulmonale due to tumor emboli. JAMA 1961;175:107–110.
108. Kupari M, Laitinen L, Hekali P, et al. Cor pulmonale due to tumor cell embolization. Acta Med Scand 1981;210: 507–510.
109. Demirer T, Dail DH, Aboulafia DM. Four varied cases of intravascular lymphomatosis and a literature review. Cancer 1994;73:1738–1745.
110. Yang SP, Lin CC. Lymphangitic carcinomatosis of the lungs: the clinical significance of its roentgenologic classification. Chest 1972;62:179–187.
111. Harold JT. Lymphangitis carcinomatosa of the lungs. Q J Med 1952;21:353–360.
112. Minor GR. A clinical and radiologic study of metastatic pulmonary neoplasms. J Thorac Cardiovasc Surg 1950;20: 34–42.
113. Goldsmith HS, Bailey HD, Callahan EL, et al. Pulmonary lymphangitic metastases from breast cancer. Arch Surg 1967;94:483–488.
114. Fichera G, Hägerstrand I. The small lymph vessels of the lungs in lymphangiosis carcinomatosa. Acta Pathol Microbiol Scand 1965;65:505–513.
115. Thurlbeck WM. Neoplasia of the pulmonary vascular bed. In: Moser KM, ed. Pulmonary vascular disease. New York: Marcel Dekker, 1979;629–649.
116. Janower ML, Blennerhassett JB. Lymphangitic spread of metastatic cancer to the lung: a radiologic-pathologic classification. Radiology 1971;101:267–273.
117. Amundson DE, Weiss PJ. Hypoxemia in malignant carcinoid syndrome: a case attributed to occult lymphangitic metastatic involvement [letter]. Mayo Clin Proc 1991;66: 1178–1180.
118. Trapnell DH. The radiological appearance of lymphangitic carcinomatosa of the lung. Thorax 1964;19:251–260.
119. Johkoh T, Ikezoe J, Tomiyama N, et al. CT findings in lymphangitic carcinomatosis of the lungs: Correlation with histologic findings and pulmonary function tests. AJR 1992;158:1217–1222.
120. Stein MG, Mayo J, Müller N, et al. Pulmonary lymphangitic spread of carcinoma: appearance on ct scans. Radiology 1987;162:371–375.
121. Ren H, Hruban RH, Kuhlman JE, et al. Computed tomography of inflation-fixed lungs: the beaded septum sign of pulmonary metastases. J Comput Assist Tomogr 1989;13: 411–416.
122. Munk PL, Müller NL, Miller RR, et al. Pulmonary lymphangitic carcinomatosis: CT and pathologic findings. Radiology 1988;166(3):705–709.
123. Honda O, Johkoh T, Ichikado Y, et al. Comparison of high resolution CT findings of sarcoidosis, lymphoma and lymphangitic carcinoma: is there any difference of involved interstitium? J Comput Assist Tomogr 1999;23:374–379.
124. Sostman HD, Brown M, Toole A, et al. Perfusion scan in pulmonary vascular/lymphangitic carcinomatosis: the segmental contour pattern. AJR 1981;137:1072–1074.
125. Green N, Swanson L, Kern W. Lymphangitic carcinomatosis: lung scan abnormalities. J Nucl Med 1976;17:258–260.
126. Schimmel DH, Julien PJ, Gamsu G. Resolution of pulmonary lymphangitic carcinoma of the breast. Chest 1976; 69:106–108.
127. Heffner JE, Duffey DJ, Schwartz MI. Massive pleural effusions from prostatic lymphangitic carcinomatosis: resolution with endocrine therapy. Arch Intern Med 1982;142: 375–376.
128. Fernandez K, O'Hanlan KA, Rodriquez-Rodriquez L, et al. Respiratory failure due to interstitial lung metastases of ovarian carcinoma reversed by chemotherapy. Chest 1991;99:1533–1534.
129. Youngberg AS. Unilateral diffuse lung opacity. Radiology 1977;123:277–281.
130. Morgan D. The pathology of subacute cor pulmonale in diffuse carcinomatosis of the lungs. J Pathol Bacteriol 1959;61:75–84.
131. Masson RG, Ruggieri J. Pulmonary microvascular cytology: a new diagnostic application of the pulmonary artery catheter. Chest 1985;88:908–914.
132. Masson RG, Krikorian J, Lukl P, et al. Pulmonary microvascular cytology in the diagnosis of lymphangitic carcinomatosis. N Engl J Med 1989;321:71–76.
133. Scheinin TM, Koivuniemi AP. Megakaryocytes in the pulmonary circulation. Blood 1963;22:82–87.
134. Aabo K, Hansen KB. Megakaryocytes in pulmonary blood vessels. 1. Incidence at autopsy, clinicopathological relations especially to disseminated intravascular coagulation. Acta Path Microbiol Scand [A] 1978;86:285–291.
135. Hansen KB, Aabo K. Megakaryocytes in pulmonary blood vessels. 2. Relation to malignant hematological diseases especially leukemia. Acta Path Microbiol Scand [A] 1978;86:293–295.
136. Soares FA. Increased numbers of pulmonary megakaryocytes in patients with arterial pulmonary tumour embolism and with lung metastases seen at necropsy. J Clin Pathol 1992;45:140–142.
137. McLoud TC, Kalisher L, Stark P, et al. Intrathoracic lymph node metastases from extrathoracic neoplasms. AJR 1978;131:403–407.
138. Ercan S, Nichols FC 3rd, Trastek VF, et al. Prognostic significance of lymph node metastasis found during pulmonary metastasectomy for extrapulmonary carcinoma. Ann Thorac Surg 2004;77:1786–1791.
139. Faries MB, Bleicher RJ, Ye X, et al. Lymphatic mapping and sentinel lymphadenectomy for primary and metastatic pulmonary malignant neoplasms. Arch Surg 2004;139: 870–876.
140. Meyer KK. Direct lymphatic connections from the lower lobes of the lung to the abdomen. J Thorac Surg 1958; 35:726–733.
141. Webb WR, Gamsu G. Thoracic metastasis in malignant melanoma. Chest 1977;71:176–181.
142. Das Gupta T, Brasfield R. Metastatic melanoma: a clinicopathological study. Cancer 1964;17:1323–1339.
143. Winterbauer RH, Belic N, Moores KD. A clinical interpretation of bilateral hilar adenopathy. Ann Intern Med 1973;78:65–71.
144. D'Angio GJ, Lannaccone G. Spontaneous pneumothorax as a complication of pulmonary metastases in malignant tumors of childhood. Am J Roentgenol 1961;86:1092–1102.

145. Wright FW. Spontaneous pneumothorax and pulmonary malignant disease—a syndrome sometimes associated with cavitating tumors. Clin Radiol 1976;27:221–222.
146. Scholten ET, Kreel L. Distribution of lung metastases in the axial plane. Radiol Clin North Am 1977;46:248–265.
147. Samo RC, Carter BL. Bullous change by CT heralding metastatic sarcoma. Comput Radiol 1985;9:115–120.
148. Chrétien J, Jaubert F. Pleural responses in malignant metastatic tumors. In: Chrétien J, Bignon J, Hirsch A, eds. The pleura in health and disease. New York: Marcel Dekker, 1985:489–505.
149. Sahn SA. Malignant pleural effusion. In: Fishman AP, ed. Pulmonary diseases and disorders, 2nd ed. New York: McGraw-Hill, 1988:2159–2169.
150. Light RW. Tumors of the pleura. In: Murray JF, Nadel JA, eds. Textbook of respiratory medicine. Philadelphia: WB Saunders, 1988:1770–1780.
151. Cantó A, Rivas J, Saumench J, Morera R, et al. Points to consider when choosing a biopsy method in cases of pleurisy of unknown origin. Chest 1983;84:176–179.
152. Cantó A, Ferrer G, Romagosa V, Moya J, et al. Lung cancer and pleural effusion. Clinical significance and study of pleural metastatic locations. Chest 1985;87:649–652.
153. Cantó-Armengod A. Macroscopic characteristics of pleural metastases arising from the breast and observed by diagnostic thoracoscopy. Am Rev Respir Dis 1990;142: 616–618.
154. Chernow B, Sahn SA. Carcinomatous involvement of the pleura: an analysis of 96 patients. Am J Med 1977;63: 695–702.
155. Sahn SA. Malignant pleural effusions. Clin Chest Med 1985;6:113–125.
156. Meyer PC. Metastatic carcinoma of the pleura. Thorax 1966;21:437–443.
157. Gown AM. Clinical reference manual. 3rd ed. Seattle: PhenoPath Laboratories, 2001:11–15.
158. Dabbs DJ, ed. Diagnostic immunohistochemistry. New York: Churchill-Livingstone, 2002.
159. Dabbs DJ. Carcinomatous differentiation and metastatic carcinoma of unknown primary. In: Dabbs DJ, ed. Diagnostic immunohistochemistry. New York: Churchill-Livingstone, 2002:163–196.
160. Chu P, Wu E, Weiss LM. Cytokeratin 7 and cytokeratin 20 expression in epithelial neoplasms: a survey of 435 cases. Med Pathol 2000;13:953–972.
161. Hammar SP. Lung and pleural neoplasms. In: Dabbs DJ, ed. Diagnostic immunohistochemistry. New York: Churchill-Livingstone, 2002:267–312.
162. Cantin J, McNeer GP, Chu FC, et al. The problem of local recurrence after treatment of soft tissue sarcoma. Ann Surg 1968;168:47–53.
163. Jeffree GM, Price CH, Sissons HA. The metastatic patterns of osteosarcoma. Br J Cancer 1975;32:87–107.
164. Marcove RC, Mike V, Hajek JV, et al. Osteogenic sarcoma under the age of twenty-one. J Bone Joint Surg [Am] 1970; 52:411–423.
165. Scranton PE, DeCicco FA, Totten RS, et al. Prognostic factors in osteosarcoma. A review of 20 years' experience at the University of Pittsburgh Health Center Hospitals. Cancer (Philadelphia) 1975;36:2179–2191.
166. Vezeridis MP, Moore R, Karakousis CP. Metastatic patterns in soft-tissue sarcomas. Arch Surg 1983;118:915–918.
167. Aronchick JM, Palevsky HI, Miller WT. Cavitary pulmonary metastases in angiosarcoma. Diagnosis by transthoracic needle aspiration. Am Rev Respir Dis 1989;139:252–253.
168. Gilman JK, Sievers DB, Thorsvard CT. Malignant fibrous histiocytoma manifesting as a cavitary lung metastasis. South Med J 1986;79:376–378.
169. Flynn KJ, Kim HS. Endobronchial metastasis of uterine leiomyosarcoma. JAMA 1978;240:2080.
170. Hinton AA, Sandler MP, Shaff MI, et al. Pulmonary nodules and spontaneous pneumothorax in an adolescent female. Invest Radiol 1984;19:479–483.
171. Lodmell EA, Capps SC. Spontaneous pneumothorax associated with metastatic sarcoma. Radiology 1949;52:88–93.
172. Thornton TF, Bigelow RR. Pneumothorax due to metastatic sarcoma. Arch Pathol 1944;37:334–336.
173. Shaw AB. Spontaneous pneumothorax from secondary sarcoma of lung. Br Med J 1951;1:278–280.
174. Sherman RS, Birant EE. An x-ray of spontaneous pneumothorax due to cancer metastases to the lungs. Chest 1954;26:328–337.
175. Dines DE, Cortese DA, Brennan MD, et al. Malignant pulmonary neoplasms predisposing to spontaneous pneumothorax. Mayo Clin Proc 1973;48:541–544.
176. Crow NE, Brogdon BG. Cystic lung lesions from metastatic sarcoma. Am J Roentgenol Radium Ther Nucl Med 1959;81:303–304.
177. Traweek ST, Rotter AJ, Swartz Azumi N. Cystic pulmonary metastatic sarcoma. Cancer 1990;65:1805–1811.
178. Pocock B, Craig JR, Bullock WK. Metastatic uterine leiomyoma. A case report. Cancer 1976;38:2090–2100.
179. Spittle MF, Heal J, Harmer C, et al. The association of spontaneous pneumothorax with pulmonary metastases in bone tumours of children. Clin Radiol 1968;19:400–403.
180. Janetos GP, Ochsner SF. Bilateral pneumothorax in metastatic osteogenic sarcoma. Am Rev Respir Dis 1963;88: 73–76.
181. Chen JTT, Dahrnash NS, Ravin CE, et al. Metastatic melanoma to the thorax: report of 130 patients. AJR 1981; 137:293–298.
182. Harpole DH Jr, Johnson CM, Wolfe WG, et al. Analysis of 945 cases of pulmonary metastatic melanoma. J Thorac Cardiovasc Surg 1992;103:743–750.
183. Balch CM, Soong SJ, Murad TM, et al. A multifactorial analysis of melanoma: prognostic factors in 200 melanoma patients with distant metastases. J Clin Oncol 1983;1: 126–134.
184. Sutton FS, Jr., Vestal RE, Creagh CE. Varied presentations of metastatic pulmonary melanoma. Chest 1974;65:415–419.
185. Kayser K, Stute H, Tuengerthal S. Diffuse pulmonary ossification associated with metastatic melanoma of the lung. Respiration 1987;52:221–227.
186. Pogrebniak HW, Stovroff M, Roth JA, et al. Resection of pulmonary metastases from malignant melanoma: results of a 16-year experience. Ann Thorac Surg 1988;46:20–23.
187. Patel JK, Didolkar MS, Pickren JW, et al. Metastatic pattern of malignant melanoma: a study of 216 autopsy cases. Am J Surg 1978;135:807–810.

188. Demington ML, Carter DR, Meyers AD. Distant metastases in head and neck epidermoid carcinoma. Laryngoscope 1980;90:196–201.
189. O'Brien PH, Carlson R, Steubner BA, et al. Distant metastases in epidermoid cell carcinoma of the head and neck. Cancer 1971;27:304–307.
190. Papec R. Distant metastases from head and neck cancer. Cancer 1984;53:342–345.
191. Probert JC, Thompson RW, Bagshaw MA. Patterns of distant metastases in head and neck cancer. Cancer 1974; 33:128–133.
192. Cahan WG, Montemayor PB. Cancer of the larynx and lung in the same patient. J Thorac Cardiovasc Surg 1962; 44:309–320.
193. Malefetto JP, Kasimis BS, Moran EM, et al. The clinical significance of radiographically detected pulmonary neoplastic lesions in patients with head and neck cancer. J Clin Oncol 1984;2:625–630.
194. Lampe JL, Zatzkin H. Metastases of pseudoadenomatous basal cell carcinoma. Radiology 1948;53:379–385.
195. Massin J-P, Savoie J-C, Gamier H, et al. Pulmonary metastases in differentiated thyroid carcinoma. Study of 58 cases with implications for the primary tumor treatment. Cancer 1984;53:982–992.
196. Samaan NA, Schultz PN, Haynie TP, et al. Pulmonary metastasis of differentiated thyroid carcinoma: treatment results in 101 patients. J Clin Endocrinol Metab 1985;60: 376–380.
197. Franssila KG. Prognosis in thyroid carcinoma. Cancer 1975;36:1138–1146.
198. McKenzie AD. The natural history of thyroid cancer. A report of 102 cases analyzed 10 to 15 years after diagnosis. Arch Surg 1971;102:274–277.
199. Rasmusson B. Carcinoma of the thyroid. Acta Radiol 1978;17:177–188.
200. Nemec J, Pohunková D, Zamrazil V, et al. Pulmonary metastases of thyroid carcinoma. Czech Med 1979;2:78–83.
201. Hoie J, Stenwig AE, Kullmann G, et al. Distant metastases in papillary thyroid cancer: a review of 91 patients. Cancer 1988;61:1–6.
202. Venkatesh YS, Ordonez NG, Schultz PN, et al. Anaplastic carcinoma of the thyroid. A clinicopathologic study of 121 cases. Cancer 1990;66:321–330.
203. McGee AR, Warren R. Carcinoma metastatic from the thyroid to the lungs. Radiology 1966;87:516–517.
204. Chariot P, Feliz A, Monnet I. Miliary opacities diagnosed as lung metastases of a thyroid carcinoma after 13 years of stability. Chest 1993;104:981–982.
205. Tsumori T, Nakao K, Miyata M, et al. Clinicopathologic study of thyroid carcinoma infiltrating the trachea. Cancer 1985;56:2843–2848.
206. Ronga G, Filesi M, Montesano T, et al. Lung metastases from differentiated thyroid carcinoma. A 40 years' experience. Q J Nucl Med 2004;48:12–19.
207. Fracchia AA, Knapper WH, Carey JT, et al. Intrapleural chemotherapy for effusion from metastatic breast carcinoma. Cancer 1970;26:626–629.
208. Cutler SJ, Asire AJ, Taylor SG. Classification of patients with disseminated cancer of the breast. Cancer 1969;24: 861–869.
209. Winchester DP, Sener SF, Khandekar JD, et al. Symptomatology as an indicator of recurrent or metastatic breast cancer. Cancer 1979;43:956–960.
210. Casey JJ, Stempel BG, Scanlon EF, et al. The solitary pulmonary nodule in the patient with breast cancer. Surgery 1984;96:801–805.
211. DeBeer RA, Garcia RL, Alexander SC. Endobronchial metastasis from cancer of the breast. Chest 1978;73: 94–96.
212. Raab SS, Berg LC, Swanson PE, et al. Adenocarcinoma in the lung in patients with breast cancer. A prospective analysis of the discriminatory value of immunohistochemistry. Am J Clin Pathol 1993;100:27–35.
213. Eppstein S. Primary carcinoma of the liver. Am J Med Sci 1964;247:43–50.
214. MacDonald RA. Primary carcinoma of the liver. A clinicopathologic study of one hundred eight cases. Arch Intern Med 1957;99:266–279.
215. Patton RB, Horn RC. Primary liver carcinoma. Autopsy study of 60 cases. Cancer 1964;17:757–768.
216. Levy JI, Geddes EW, Kew MC. The chest radiograph in primary liver cancer. An analysis of 449 cases. S Afr Med J 1976;50:1323–1326.
217. Tsai GL, Liu JD, Siauw CP, et al. Thoracic roentgenologic manifestations in primary carcinoma of the liver. Chest 1984;86:430–434.
218. August DA, Ottow RT, Sugarbaker PH. Clinical perspective of human colorectal cancer metastasis. Cancer Metastasis Rev 1984;5:303–324.
219. Berg HK, Petrelli NJ, Herrera L, et al. Endobronchial metastasis from colorectal carcinoma. Dis Colon Rectum 1984;27:745–748.
220. Penna C, Nordlinger B. Colorectal metastasis (liver and lung). Surg Clin North Am 2002;82:1075–1090.
221. Birzele J, Schmitz I, Muller KM. Ossification in lung metastases of primary colorectal adenocarcinomas [in German]. Pathologe 2003;24:66–69.
222. Dionne L. The pattern of bloodborne metastasis from carcinoma of rectum. Cancer 1965;18:775–781.
223. Langer B. Colorectal cancer: managing distant metastases. Can J Surg 1985;28:419–421.
224. Russell AH, Tong D, Dawson LE, et al. Adenocarcinoma of the proximal colon. Sites of initial dissemination and patterns of recurrence following surgery alone. Cancer 1984;53:360–367.
225. Taylor FW. Cancer of the colon and rectum: a study of routes of metastases and death. Surgery 1962;52:305–308.
226. McCormack PM, Attiyeh FF. Resected pulmonary metastases from colorectal cancer. Dis Colon Rectum 1979; 22:553–556.
227. Pihl E, Hughes ES, McDermott FT, et al. Lung recurrence after curative surgery for colorectal cancer. Dis Colon Rectum 1987;30:417–419.
228. Li MK, Folpe AL. CDX-2, a new marker for adenocarcinoma of gastrointestinal origin. Adv Anat Pathol 2004;11: 101–105.
229. Rossi G, Murer B, Cavazza A, et al. Primary mucinous (so-called colloid) carcinomas of the lung: a clinicopathological and immunohistochemical study with special reference

to CDX-2 homeobox gene and MUC2 expression. Am J Surg Pathol 2004;28:442–452.
230. Yatabe Y, Koga T, Mitsudomi T, et al. CK20 expression, CDX2 expression K-ras mutation and goblet cell morphology in a subset of lung adenocarcinomas. J Pathol 2004; 203:645–652.
231. Saad RS, Cho P, Silverman JF, et al. Usefulness of CDX2 in separating mucinous bronchioloalveolar adenocarcinoma of the lung from metastatic mucinous colorectal adenocarcinoma. Am J Clin Pathol 2004;122:421–427.
232. Lisa JR, Trinidad S, Rosenblatt MB. Pulmonary manifestations of carcinoma of the pancreas. Cancer 1964;17: 395–401.
233. Bunker SR. Klein DL. Multiple cavitated pulmonary metastases in pancreatic adenocarcinoma. Br J Radiol 1982;55:455–456.
234. Cassiere SG, McLain DA, Emory WB, et al. Metastatic carcinoma of the pancreas simulating primary bronchogenic carcinoma. Cancer 1980;46:2319–2321.
235. Barbareschi M, Roldo C, Zamboni G, et al. CDX2 homeobox gene product expression in neuroendocrine tumors: its role as a marker of intestinal neuroendocrine tumors. Am J Surg Pathol 2004;28:1169–1176.
236. Greenberg BE, Young JM. Pulmonary metastasis from occult primary sites resembling bronchogenic carcinoma. Dis Chest 1958;33:496–505.
237. Latour A, Shulman HS. Thoracic manifestations of renal cell carcinoma. Radiology 1976;121:43–48.
238. Mountain CF. Pulmonary metastatic disease—progress in a neglected area. Int J Radiat Oncol Biol Phys 1976;1: 755–757.
239. Bennington JL, Beckwith JB. Tumors of the kidney, renal pelvis, and ureter. Atlas of tumor pathology. Second Series, vol 12. Washington, DC: Armed Forces Institute of Pathology, 1975:168.
240. Saitoh H. Distant metastasis of renal adenocarcinoma in patients with a tumor thrombus in the renal vein and/or vena cava. J Urol 1982;127:652–653.
241. Amer B, Guy J, Vaze B. Endobronchial metastasis from renal adenocarcinoma simulating a foreign body. Thorax 1981;36:183–184.
242. Gerle R, Felson B. Metastatic endobronchial hypernephroma. Dis Chest 1963;44:225–233.
243. Jariwalla AG, Seaton A, McCormack RJ, et al. Intrabronchial metastases from renal carcinoma with recurrent tumor expectoration. Thorax 1981;36:179–182.
244. Merine D, Fishman EK. Mediastinal adenopathy and endobronchial involvement in metastatic renal cell carcinoma. J Comput Tomogr 1988;12:216–.219.
245. Themelin D, Duchatelet P, Boudaka W, et al. Endoscopic resection of an endobronchial hypernephroma metastasis using a polypectomy snare. Eur Respir J 1990;3:732–736.
246. Noy S, Michowitz M, Lazebnik N, et al. Endobronchial metastasis of renal cell carcinoma. J Surg Oncol 1986;31: 268–270.
247. Reinke RT, Higgins CB, Niwayama G, et al. Bilateral pulmonary hilar lymphadenopathy. Radiology 1976;121:49–53.
248. King TE, Fisher J, Schwarz MI, et al. Bilateral hilar adenopathy: an unusual presentation of renal cell carcinoma. Thorax 1982;37:317–318.
249. Kutty K, Varkey B. Metastatic renal cell carcinoma simulating sarcoidosis: analysis of 12 patients with bilateral hilar lymphadenopathy. Chest 1984;85:533–536.
250. Katzenstein A-LA, Purvis RW Jr, Gmelich JT, et al. Pulmonary resection for metastatic renal adenocarcinoma. Cancer 1978;41:712–723.
251. Sella A, Ro JY. Renal cell cancer: Best recipient of tumor-to-tumor metastasis. Urology 1987;30:35–38.
252. Kerr V. Pulmonary metastases and ovarian cancer. Conn Med 1984;48:770–776.
253. Kerr VE, Cadman E. Pulmonary metastases in ovarian cancer. Cancer 1985;56:1209–1213.
254. Piatkowski Z. Distant metastases in cases of primary ovarian carcinoma. Pol Med J 1972;11:147–151.
255. Bernstein P. Tumors of the ovary. A study of 1,101 cases of operations for ovarian tumor. Am J Obstet Gynecol 1936; 32:1023–1039.
256. Meigs JV. Cancer of the ovary. Surg Gynecol Obstet 1940; 71:44–53.
257. Dauplat J, Hackner NF, Nieberg RK, et al. Distant metastases in epithelial ovarian carcinoma. Cancer 1987;60: 1561–1566.
258. Dvoretsky PM, Richards KA, Angel C, et al. Distribution of disease at autopsy in 100 women with ovarian cancer. Hum Pathol 1988;19:57–63.
259. Merrill CR, Hopkirk JAC. Late endobronchial metastasis from ovarian tumour. Br J Dis Chest 1982;76:253–254.
260. Smith JP, Day TG Jr. Review of ovarian cancer at the University of Texas Systems Cancer Center, MD Anderson Hospital and Tumor Institute. Am J Obstet Gynecol 1979; 135:984–993.
261. Chew SY, Stemmerman GN. Fatal pulmonary tumor microembolism complicating peritoneovenous shunt. Hawaii Med J 1981;40:130–134.
262. Lokich J, Reinhold R, Silverman M, et al. Complications of peritoneovenous shunting for malignant ascites. Cancer Treat Rep 1980;64:305–309.
263. Matt B, Oosterlee J, Spoos JA, et al. Dissemination of tumor cells via LeVeen shunt. Lancet 1979;1:988.
264. Oosterlee J. Peritoneovenous shunting for ascites in cancer patients. Br J Surg 1980;67:663–666.
265. Smith RL, Steinberg SS, Paglia MA, et al. Fatal pulmonary tumor embolization following peritoneovenous shunting for malignant ascites. J Surg Oncol 1981;16:27–35.
266. Carlson V, Delclos L, Fletcher GH. Distant metastases in squamous cell carcinoma of the uterine cervix. Radiology 1967;88:961–966.
267. Badib AO, Kurohara SS, Webster JH, et al. Metastasis to organs in carcinoma of the uterine cervix. Cancer 1968; 21:434–439.
268. Tellis CJ, Beechler CR. Pulmonary metastasis of carcinoma of the cervix: a retrospective study. Cancer 1982;59:1705–1709.
269. Sostman HD, Matthay RA. Thoracic metastases from cervical carcinoma: current status. Invest Radiol 1980;15:113–119.
270. Braude S, Thompson PJ. Solitary pulmonary metastases in carcinoma of the cervix. Thorax 1983;38:953–954.
271. D'Orsi CJ, Bruckman J, Mauch P, et al. Lung metastases in cervical and endometrial carcinoma. AJR 1979;133: 719–722.

272. Bouras D, Papadakis K, Siafakas N, et al. Patterns of pulmonary metastasis from uterine cancer. Oncology 1996;53:360–363.
273. Seaman WB, Arneson AN. Solitary pulmonary metastases in carcinoma of the cervix. Obstet Gynecol 1953;1: 165–176.
274. Omenn GS. Pancoast syndrome due to metastatic carcinoma from the uterine cervix. Chest 1971;60:268–270.
275. Kirubakaran MG, Pulimood BM, Ray D. Excavating pulmonary metastases in carcinoma of the cervix. Postgrad Med J 1975;51:243–245.
276. Kennedy PS, Stockman G, Smith FE. Endobronchial metastasis from cervical cancer: a case report. Gynecol Oncol 1976;4:340–344.
277. King TE Jr, Neff TA, Ziporin P. Endobronchial metastasis from the uterine cervix: presentation as primary lung abscess. JAMA 1979;242:1651–1652.
278. Buchsbaum HJ. Lymphangitis carcinomatosis secondary to carcinoma of cervix. Obstet Gynecol 1970;36:850–860.
279. Kennedy KE, Christopherson WA, Buchsbaum HJ. Pulmonary lymphangitic carcinomatosis secondary to cervical carcinoma: a case report. Gynecol Oncol 1989;32: 253–256.
280. Scott I, Bergin CJ, Muller NL. Mediastinal and hilar lymphadenopathy as the only manifestation of metastatic carcinoma of the cervix. J Can Assoc Radiol 1986;37:52–53.
281. Ballon SC, Donaldson RC, Growdon WA, et al. Pulmonary metastases in endometrial carcinoma. In: Weiss L, Gilbet HA, eds. Pulmonary metastasis. Boston: GK Hall, 1978:182.
282. Soslow RA, Isacson C. Diagnostic immunohistochemistry of the female genital tract: In: Dabbs DJ, ed. Diagnostic immunohistochemistry. New York: Churchill Livingstone, 2002:486–516.
283. Wolff M, Kaye G, Silva F. Pulmonary metastases (with admixed epithelial elements) from smooth muscle neoplasms. Am J Surg Pathol 1979;3:325–342.
284. Gal AA, Brooks JSJ, Pietra GG. Leiomyomatous neoplasms of the lung: a clinical, histologic and immunohistochemical study. Mod Pathol 1989;2:209–216.
285. Cho KR, Woodruff JD, Epstein JI. Leiomyoma of the uterus with multiple extrauterine smooth muscle tumors: a case report suggesting multifocal origin. Hum Pathol 1989;20:80–83.
286. Kaplan C, Katoh A, Shamoto M, et al. Multiple leiomyomas of the lung: benign or malignant. Am Rev Respir Dis 1973;108:656–659.
287. Boyce CR, Buddhdev HN. Pregnancy complicated by metastasizing leiomyomas of the uterus. J Obstet Gynecol 1973;42:252–258.
288. Barnes HM, Richardson PJ. Benign metastasizing fibroleiomyoma. A case report. J Obstet Gynaecol Br Commonw 1973;80:569–573.
289. Lipton JH, Fong TC, Burgess KR. Miliary pattern as presentation of leiomyomatosis of the lung. Chest 1987;91: 781–782.
290. Flynn KJ, Kim H-S. Endobronchial metastasis of uterine leiomyosarcoma. JAMA 1978;240:2080.
291. Akatsuka N, Tokunaga K, Isshiki T, et al. Intravenous leiomyomatosis of uterus with continuous extension into the pulmonary artery. Jpn Heart J 1984;25:651–659.
292. Norris HJ, Parmley T. Mesenchymal tumors of the uterus. V: Intravenous leiomyomatosis. A clinical and pathologic study of 14 cases. Cancer 1975;36:2164–2178.
293. Dail DH. Pulmonary metastases of uterine stromal sarcoma: unique histologic appearance suggesting their source. Lab Invest 1980;42:110a(abstr).
294. Abrams J, Talcott J, Corson JM. Pulmonary metastases in patients with low-grade endometrial stromal sarcoma: clinicopathologic findings with immunohistochemical characterization. Am J Surg Pathol 1989;13:133–140.
295. Aubry M-C, Meyers JL, Colby TV, et al. Endometrial stromal sarcoma metastatic to the lung: a detailed analysis of 16 patients. Am J Surg Pathol 2002;26:440–449.
296. Clement PB, Scully RE. Uterine tumors resembling ovarian sex-cord tumors. Am J Clin Pathol 1976;66:512–525.
297. Itoh T, Mochizuki M, Kumazaki S, et al. Cystic pulmonary metastases of endometrial stromal sarcoma of the uterus, mimicking lymphangioleiomyomatosis: a case report with immunohistochemistry of HMB45. Pathol Int 1997;47: 725–729.
298. Mark E. Mesenchymal cystic hamartoma of the lung. N Engl J Med 1986;315:1255–1259.
299. Inayama Y, Shoji A, Odagiri S, et al. Detection of pulmonary metastasis of low-grade endometrial stromal sarcoma 25 years after hysterectomy. Pathol Res Pract 2000;196: 129–134.
300. Hendin AS. Gestational trophoblastic tumors metastatic to the lungs. Cancer 1984;53:58–61.
301. Kumar J, Ilancheran A, Ratnam SS. Pulmonary metastases in gestational trophoblastic disease: a review of 97 cases. Br J Obstet Gynecol 1988;95:70–74.
302. Tsao M-S, Schraufnagel D, Wang N-S. Pulmonary metastasis of choriocarcinoma with a miliary radiographic pattern. Arch Pathol Lab Med 1981;105:557–558.
303. Bagshawe KD, Noble MIM. Cardiorespiratory aspects of trophoblastic tumours. Q J Med 1966;35:39–54.
304. Burton RM. A case of chorion-epithelioma with pulmonary complications. Tubercle 1963;44:487–490.
305. Bagshawe KD, Garnett ES. Radiological changes in the lungs of patients with trophoblastic tumours. Br J Radiol 1963;36:673–679.
306. Carlson JA Jr, Day TG Jr, Kuhns JG, et al. Endoarterial pulmonary metastasis of malignant trophoblast associated with a term intrauterine pregnancy. Gynecol Oncol 1984; 17:241–248.
307. Bagshawe KD, Brooks WDW. Subacute pulmonary hypertension due to chorioepithelioma. Lancet 1959;1:653–658.
308. Evans KT, Cockshott WP, de V Hendrickse JP. Pulmonary changes in malignant trophoblastic disease. Br J Radiol 1965;38:161–167.
309. Santhosh-Kumar CR, Vijayaraghauan R, Harakati MS, et al. Spontaneous pneumothorax in metastatic choriocarcinoma. Respir Med 1991;85:81–83.
310. Cockshott WP, de V Hendrickse JP. Pulmonary calcification at the site of trophoblastic metastases. Br J Radiol 1969;42:17–20.
311. Xu LT, Sun CF, Wang YE, et al. Resection of pulmonary metastatic choriocarcinoma in 43 drug-resistant patients. Ann Thorac Surg 1985;39:257–259.

312. Mazur MT. Metastatic gestational choriocarcinoma: unusual pathologic variant following therapy. Cancer 1989; 63:1370–1377.
313. Hatch KD, Shingleton HM, Gore H, et al. Human chorionic gonadotropin-secreting large cell carcinoma of the lung detected during follow-up of a patient previously treated for gestational trophoblastic disease. Gynecol Oncol 1980;10:98–104.
314. Bumpus HC. Carcinoma of the prostate: a clinical study of one thousand cases. Surg Gynecol Obstet 1926;43: 150–154.
315. Ware JL. Prostate tumor progression and metastasis. Biochim Biophys Acta 1987;907:279–298.
316. Bubendorf L, Schopfer A, Wagner U, et al. Metastatic patterns of prostate cancer: an autopsy study of 1,589 patients. Hum Pathol 2000;31:578–583.
317. Varkarakis MJ, Winterberger AR, Gaeta J, et al. Lung metastases in prostatic carcinoma: clinical significance. Urology 1974;3:447–452.
318. Petras AD, Wollett FC. Metastatic prostatic pulmonary nodules with normal bone image. J Nucl Med 1983;24: 1026–1027.
319. Saitoh H, Hida M, Shimbo T, et al. Metastatic patterns of prostatic cancer: correlation between sites and number of organs involved. Cancer 1984;54:3078–3084.
320. Mintz ER, Smith GG. Autopsy finding in 100 cases of prostatic cancer. N Engl J Med 1934;211:479–487.
321. Elkin M, Mueller HP. Metastases from cancer of the prostate: autopsy and roentgenological findings. Cancer 1954; 7:1246–1248.
322. Scoggins WG, Witten JA, Texter JH, et al. Endobronchial metastasis from prostatic cancer in patients with renal cell carcinoma. Urology 1978;12:207–209.
323. Lali C, Gogia H, Raju L. Multiple endobronchial metastases from carcinoma of prostate. Urology 1983;21:164–165.
324. Scherz H, Schmidt JD. Endobronchial metastasis from prostate carcinoma. Prostate 1986;8:319–324.
325. Kenny JN, Smith WL, Brawer MK. Endobronchial metastases from prostatic carcinoma. Ann Thorac Surg 1988; 45:223–224.
326. Legge DA, Good CA, Ludwig J. Roentgenologic features of pulmonary carcinomatosis from carcinoma of the prostate. AJR 1971;11:360–364.
327. Mestitz H, Pierce RJ, Holmes PW. Intrathoracic manifestations of disseminated prostate adenocarcinoma. Respir Med 1989;83:161–166.
328. Apple JS, Paulson DF, Baber C, et al. Advanced prostatic carcinoma: pulmonary manifestations. Radiology 1985;54: 601–604.
329. Skinner DG, Scardino PT, Daniels JR. Testicular cancer. Annu Rev Med 1981;32:543–557.
330. Bosl GJ, Geller NL, Cirrincione C, et al. Multivariate analysis of prognostic variables in patients with metastatic testicular cancer. Cancer Res 1983;43:3403–3407.
331. Prognostic factors in advanced non-seminomatous germ-cell testicular tumours: results of a multicentre study. Report from the medical council working party on testicular tumours. Lancet 1985;1:8–11.
332. Bergman SM, Lippert M, Javapour N. The value of whole lung tomography in the early detection of metastatic disease in patients with renal cell carcinoma and testicular tumors. J Urol 1980;124:860–862.
333. Varkey B, Heckman MG. Diagnosis of a case of embryonal carcinoma by bronchial biopsy. Chest 1972;62: 758–760.
334. Toner GC, Geller NL, Lin SY, et al. Extragonadal and poor risk nonseminomatous germ cell tumors. Survival and prognostic features. Cancer 1991;67:2049–2057.
335. Wood A, Robson N, Tung K, et al. Patterns of supradiaphragmatic metastases in testicular germ cell tumours. Clin Radiol 1996;51:273–276.
336. Williams MP, Husband JE, Heron CW. Intrathoracic manifestations of metastatic testicular seminoma: a comparison of chest radiographic and CT findings. AJR 1987; 149:473–475.
337. Mandelbaum I, Williams SD, Einhorn LH. Aggressive surgical management of testicular carcinoma metastatic to lungs and mediastinum. Ann Thorac Surg 1980;30: 224–229.
338. Vogelzang NJ, Stenlund R. Residual pulmonary nodules after combination chemotherapy of testicular cancer. Radiology 1983;146:195–197.
339. Charig MJ, Williams MP. Pulmonary lacunae: sequelae of metastases following chemotherapy. Clin Radiol 1990;42: 93–96.
340. Deschamps C, Pairolero PC, Trastek VF, et al. Multiple primary lung cancers: results of surgical treatment. J Thorac Cardiovasc Surg 1990;99:769–778.
341. Rosengart TK, Martini N, Ghosn P, et al. Multiple primary lung carcinoma: prognosis and treatment. Ann Thorac Surg 1991;52:773–779.
342. Karolyi P. Do adrenal metastases from lung cancer develop by lymphogenous or hematogenous route? J Surg Oncol 1990;43:154–156.
343. Matthews MJ. Problems in morphology and behavior of bronchopulmonary malignant disease. In: Israel L, Chahanian P, eds. Lung cancer: natural history, prognosis and therapy. New York: Academic Press, 1976:23–62.
344. Auerbach O, Garfinkel L, Parks UR. Histologic type of lung cancer in relation to smoking habits, year of diagnosis and sites of metastases. Chest 1975;67:382–387.
345. Hirsch FR. Histopathologic classification and metastatic pattern of small cell carcinoma of the lung. Copenhagen: Munksgaard, 1983.
346. Kolin A, Koutoulakis T. Role of arterial occlusion in pulmonary scar cancers. Hum Pathol 1988;19:1161–1167.
347. Prioleau PG, Katzenstein A-LA. Major peripheral arterial occlusion due to malignant tumor embolism: histologic recognition and surgical management. Cancer 1978;42: 2009–2014.
348. Heitmiller RF. Prognostic significance of massive bronchogenic tumor embolus. Ann Thorac Surg 1992;53:153–155.
349. Van Way CW III, Lawler MR. Osteogenic sarcomatous emboli to the femoral arteries. Am J Surg 1969;117: 745–747.

45
Cytopathology of Pulmonary Neoplasia

N. Paul Ohori and Elise R. Hoff

Cytopathologic techniques have the potential to provide useful diagnostic information from specimens obtained through minimally invasive procedures including expectorated sputum, washings, lavages, brushings, and aspiration procedures. These procedures provide access to almost any site within the thorax. Given optimal conditions, many neoplasms can be diagnosed by cytology procedures. However, it is important to understand the strengths and limitations of cytopathologic evaluation. While pulmonary neoplastic classification is relatively stable, recent histopathologic, immunohistochemical, and molecular studies underscore the complexity of neoplasms. Cytologic sampling may be representative of the entire tumor or may represent the "tip of the iceberg." An understanding of biologic complexity of pulmonary neoplasms helps to avoid overdiagnosing an entity. To provide an ideal cytopathologic diagnosis and report that accurately reflect the entire process, the pathologist should take a number of steps.

First, the sampling must be ample for the diagnosis of neoplastic processes since certain diagnoses require ancillary studies for complete or precise characterization. For example, a peripheral lung lesion is often an adenocarcinoma that represents a primary or metastatic neoplasm. This type of lesion is best approached by computer tomography guided needle aspiration/biopsy procedure combined with immediate cytologic evaluation for the best probability of attaining an adequate sample. Second, the staining and cytologic processing methods must be optimized for each procedure taken. Third, the diagnostic categorization must be compatible with that used for surgical pathology.

In this chapter, we use the 2004 World Health Organization/International Agency for Research on Cancer (WHO/IARC) classification of pulmonary neoplasia.[1] Although the adenocarcinoma, squamous cell carcinoma, large cell undifferentiated carcinoma, and small cell carcinoma comprise approximately 95% of primary pulmonary malignancies, almost any type of primary or metastatic cancer may be seen in the lung. To make a pathologic diagnosis, multiple parameters are often evaluated and some of these parameters may be beyond cytologic observation. The diagnosis of bronchioloalveolar carcinoma requires that the neoplastic cells strictly grow along alveolar septa without invading into the underlying stroma. Therefore, this diagnosis cannot be made by cytologic evaluation alone. Furthermore, many neoplasms are complex and exhibit tumor heterogeneity.

Cytologic sampling may not be representative of the entire process. As stated above, the strengths and limitations of cytologic evaluation must be appreciated. Even under the best of conditions, there are times when the cytomorphology and ancillary studies cannot discriminate between a reactive process and a neoplastic lesion. These cases are placed in one of the indeterminate categories (atypical, suspicious). At our institution, the "atypical" diagnosis has a lower positive predictive value than a "suspicious" diagnosis. Other institutions combine all indeterminate diagnoses into one category. Whatever the system, it is important to perform cytohistologic correlation exercises and follow-up studies to attain an understanding of the degree of suspicion. While an indeterminate diagnosis is not precise, it provides impetus for the clinician to perform the next diagnostic procedure for a more definitive diagnosis. An understanding of the current and evolving management algorithms for pulmonary malignancies is helpful in preparing an insightful cytopathology report.

In this chapter, we take a practical approach to the diagnosis of pulmonary neoplasms by cytologic procedures. Pattern recognition, differential diagnoses, and specific cytologic diagnostic issues are emphasized. Cytologic sampling has great potential in obtaining valuable information from minimally invasive procedures. It is important for pathologists handling pulmonary cytology specimens to understand the potentials and limitations of cytopathology practice. The primary goal is to place a neoplasm in one of the categories in Table 45.1. If

TABLE 45.1. Major diagnostic categories for malignant pulmonary neoplasms

Small cell carcinoma
Small cell carcinoma
Combined small cell carcinoma
Non–small-cell carcinoma
Adenocarcinoma
Squamous cell carcinoma
Large cell undifferentiated carcinoma
Carcinoma with pleomorphic, sarcomatoid, and sarcomatous elements
Neuroendocrine neoplasm
Typical carcinoid tumor
Atypical carcinoid tumor
Large cell neuroendocrine carcinoma
Mesothelioma
Epithelioid
Sarcomatoid
Biphasic
Sarcoma
Epithelioid hemangioendothelioma
Pleuropulmonary blastoma
Inflammatory myofibroblastic tumor
Pulmonary vein sarcoma
Pulmonary artery sarcoma
Synovial sarcoma
Lymphoma
Extranodal marginal zone B-cell lymphoma (MALT lymphoma)
Diffuse large B-cell lymphoma
Lymphomatoid granulomatosis
Other non-Hodgkin's lymphoma
Hodgkin's disease

possible, a specific diagnosis is made. Otherwise, a comment on a list of differential diagnoses would be clinically useful. Pathologists act as consultants to clinicians in recommending the most effective procedures and rendering the best diagnostic, prognostic, and treatment information necessary for optimal patient care.

Respiratory Cytology Specimens: Acquisition Procedure, Collection, Processing, and Slide Preparation

Sputum

Sputum sampling represents spontaneously exfoliated cells and secretions from all levels of the respiratory tract from the oropharynx to the alveoli. It is an inexpensive and easily collected specimen that is useful for detection of centrally located malignant tumors and premalignant lesions. Due to the noninvasive nature of the collection procedure, sputum samples are considered to be the method of choice for screening of patients who are at high risk for developing lung cancer. The sample represents a wide area of the pulmonary parenchyma and is not localized to a specific site. Furthermore, sputum cytology is not effective in sampling tumors covered by intact epithelium (submucosal tumors) that do not communicate with the airways, or peripheral tumors.

Specimen Procurement and Collection

Early morning spontaneously produced deep cough specimens provide the best material for cytologic examination rather than samples collected at other times of the day (for best yield and better cell preservation).[2] Otherwise, specimens may be induced by inhalation of a nebulized hypertonic solution.[3] Maximum diagnostic yield is obtained with three to five consecutive early morning specimens.[4,5] Ideally, samples should be submitted immediately to the cytology lab in the fresh state, as delays lead to cellular degeneration that can render a sample unsatisfactory for evaluation. If delay is expected, samples should be either refrigerated or submitted in a fixative, such as Saccomanno fixative (2% polyethylene glycol and 50% ethyl alcohol). Any samples that are pooled should be submitted in Saccomanno fixative. Specimens should not be submitted in 50% alcohol, as this will cause cellular clumping and hardening of the sample, making smear preparation difficult.[6]

Specimen Processing

The two main techniques used to process sputum are the pick and smear technique (used for fresh samples) and the Saccomanno technique (used for sputum fixed in Saccomanno fluid). The pick and smear technique for fresh samples involves picking out any potentially diagnostic material from the sample, placing it on two glass slides, and smearing it between two other clean slides. Material to be picked out includes any white-streaked or blood-tinged particles or threads. The amount of material placed on each slide should be less than 1 cm in diameter. The slides are fixed in alcohol before staining. Watery specimens may be centrifuged and smears are made from the sediment.[6]

The Saccomanno technique is used for specimens submitted in Saccomanno fixative.[7] The alcohol in Saccomanno fluid acts as a fixative for the cells, and the 2% polyethylene glycol is a wax (Carbowax) that protects cells from air-drying once they are smeared onto slides. As this fixative contains alcohol, some clumping and hardening of the sputum will occur, requiring mechanical force (i.e., emulsification with a blender or with vigorous shaking) to break apart any clumps. The emulsified specimen is centrifuged for 10 minutes and the button is resuspended in an equal amount of supernatant. Drops of the resuspended button can then be either smeared directly onto slides or put into wells for cytospin preparations. Then, prior to staining, the slides are dipped into alcohol to remove the Carbowax, so that the Papanicolaou stain can penetrate the cells. Often, sputum contains abundant mucus, which makes slide smearing and preparation difficult. Mucolytic agents, such as DL-dithiothreitol (DDT) may be added to break up the mucus. It has been used at our institution for this purpose, as it has been found to be a very effective mucolytic agent.

Bronchial Washings

Bronchial washings represent mechanically exfoliated epithelial cells from the endobronchial surface. They consist of saline fluid that has been instilled onto and over an area of interest in a bronchus. This method facilitates better localization of lesions than sputum samples and is suited for the detection of airway-associated and mucosal-based lesions, such as squamous cell carcinoma, bronchogenic adenocarcinoma, and small cell carcinoma. Washings sample an area larger than that sampled by bronchial brushings.

Specimen Procurement and Collection

Washings are obtained by wedging a flexible bronchoscope into the bronchus of interest, followed by instilling and aspirating sequential aliquots (approximately 5 to 10 mL each) of warm saline until approximately 25 to 30 mL of fluid is collected. This fluid is sent to the cytology laboratory either in the fresh state or in Saccomanno fixative.

Specimen Processing

Bronchial washes may be covered with a layer of mucoid froth, which can be removed, fixed in 50% alcohol, and used for cell-block preparations.[6] The remainder of the specimen can be processed in a fashion similar to that for sputum samples. Pieces of interest (i.e., white-streaked or blood-tinged particles or flecks) can be removed from the original sample, placed into another conical tube, mixed with mucolytic agents if necessary, and centrifuged. For bloody specimens, red blood cell lysing agents (e.g., Cytorich Red, Thermo Electron Corp., Pittsburgh, PA) can also be mixed with the original sample prior to centrifuging. If the sample size is small, the whole sample is centrifuged. These slides may be coverslipped or the centrifuged pellet may be resuspended and smeared.

Bronchial Brushings

Bronchial brushing specimens represent surface epithelial cells and elements that have been mechanically removed from the surface of a bronchus by a small brush attached to a flexible bronchoscope. This method is useful for localizing and accurately sampling tumors that are present on the surface epithelium of the main airways. Such tumors include squamous cell carcinoma, small cell carcinoma, bronchogenic adenocarcinoma, and others. Submucosal tumors (e.g., carcinoid tumors) are not well sampled by the brushing technique.

Specimen Procurement and Collection

A flexible bronchoscope with a channel containing a retractable small circular stiff-bristle brush is inserted into the airway of interest. The area of interest is brushed and the brush and scope are removed. Care must be taken to avoid scraping the diagnostic material off the brush when retracting the brush into the channel. Direct smears are made by rolling the brush on frosted slides and fixing the smears immediately in 95% alcohol. Alternatively, the brush may be cut off from its shaft and placed in Saccomanno fixative or balanced saline.[7]

Specimen Processing

Slides are prepared from the balanced saline rinse solution into which the brush is placed. To optimize cellular yield, the brush is either vigorously agitated in the rinse, or the brush is scraped, to dislodge any attached material into the rinse. Subsequently, the sample is then centrifuged to produce a cytocentrifugation slide specimen or a cell block from the cell enriched material. Otherwise, slides may be produced from one of the monolayer methods. The combination of bronchial washing and brushing specimens results in a diagnostic sensitivity of approximately 90%.[6,7]

Bronchoalveolar Lavage

Bronchoalveolar lavage (BAL) samples the terminal air spaces and is most useful for the evaluation of diffuse disease processes, particularly identification of fungal organisms such as *Aspergillus*, *Mucor*, *Candida*, and *Pneumocystis*, and viral inclusions. Peripheral or diffuse malignancies with alveolar involvement, such as some peripheral adenocarcinomas and lymphomas, can also be identified with BAL specimens. The presence of alveolar macrophages indicates alveolar sampling. To be considered satisfactory, abundant alveolar macrophages without a significant number of inflammatory cells, ciliated bronchial cells. or superficial squamous cells should be present. Quantitatively, a total of 2×10^6 cells is considered a minimum requirement. Furthermore, more than 10 macrophages should be present in a high-powered microscopic field and degenerative changes should cover less than 20% of the specimen area on the slide. If the number of squamous epithelial cells, bronchial cells, red blood cells, or inflammatory cells exceeds that of macrophages, the specimen is considered unsatisfactory.[8–10]

Specimen Procurement and Collection

The BAL specimens are obtained by wedging the end of a flexible bronchoscope into the lobar, segmental, or subsegmental bronchus. Warmed saline in sequential aliquots of 20mL is instilled into the air spaces, aspirated, and collected in a container. A total of 100 to 200ml of collected lavage fluid is sent fresh to the cytology laboratory.

Specimen Processing

If the BAL specimen requires only a cytologic evaluation, it can be processed in a fashion similar to that for bronchial washes. Portions of the original sample are mixed with mucolytic or red blood cell lysing agents if necessary, and then centrifuged. The pellet is resuspended in enough liquid (which can be a fixative solution, with or without additional mucolytic or red blood cell lysing agents) to achieve sufficient turbidity to yield a monolayer on cytospin preparations. Air-dried slides are stained with the Wright-Giemsa or Diff-Quik stain and alcohol fixed slides with Papanicolaou stain.[11] Cell counts can be performed by use of an automated particle counter, hemocytometer, or manual counting of a set number of cells on a smear without a hemocytometer.

Transbronchial Fine-Needle Aspirates

The primary indication for any fine-needle aspirate of the lung is the evaluation of a localized mass or nodule that cannot be diagnosed by exfoliative cytology. Transbronchial aspirates in particular are useful for identification of centrally located masses that are covered by intact epithelium or other tissue (e.g., granulation tissue). The procedure is performed by a pulmonologist who inserts a flexible bronchoscope into the patient's airway and targets the lesion with a needle, which is threaded through the bronchoscope. Mediastinal and hilar lymph nodes and masses are also amenable to sampling with this technique, which makes transbronchial fine-needle aspiration (FNA) useful in staging known pulmonary carcinomas. This method is not useful for identification of very small or peripheral nodules or lesions located far from the main airways.

To be considered to represent the bronchial area, a transbronchial FNA should contain at least respiratory bronchial epithelial cells. However, determination of adequacy requires clinical and radiologic correlation. This depends on the index of clinical suspicion and often requires the presence of abnormal or lesional cells for a specimen to be considered adequate.

Specimen Procurement and Collection

Transbronchial aspirates are obtained with a needle that is attached to a flexible bronchoscope, which is inserted (under radiologic guidance) through a bronchial wall into a mass or lymph node. Material is aspirated and may be used for a variety of purposes, including smear preparation, microbiologic cultures, flow cytometric immunophenotypic analysis, and cell block preparation.

Specimen Processing

The aspirated material is first expelled onto labeled slides that are smeared, then either air-dried or fixed immediately into 95% alcohol, depending on the type of stain. Air-dried slides are stained with the Diff-Quick stain and alcohol-fixed slides are stained with either Papanicolaou stain or hematoxylin and eosin stain. The needle used for aspiration is placed into a fixative solution of 50% alcohol and rinsed well by repeated aspiration and expulsion. The rinsed material is centrifuged and the pelleted material may be placed on slides or embedded as cell block material.

Transthoracic Fine-Needle Aspirates

This technique targets peripheral lesions and those not associated with main airways. The procedure is performed by a radiologist who localizes the needle into the lesion by using computed tomographic guidance. If immediate adequacy evaluation is requested, the cytopathologist stains representative air-dried slides with Diff-Quik stain and provides feedback to the radiologist regarding presence or absence of diagnostic material. Transthoracic FNA is capable of making the diagnosis of primary neoplasms (benign and malignant), metastatic malignancies, and nonneoplastic processes that may mimic malignancies. Due to the minimally invasive nature, transthoracic FNA is suitable for patients who cannot tolerate more extensive procedures. Pneumothorax is the main complication, encountered in approximately 30% to 40% of cases. Respiratory epithelial cells or macrophages should be present to state that a transthoracic FNA represents the lung parenchyma. To be diagnostic, lesional cells must be present in addition.

Specimen Procurement and Collection

The aspirated material is collected as smears (air-dried or alcohol fixed), needle rinse fluid in 50% ethanol (for cytocentrifugation), and fragments in buffered formalin (for cell block preparation).

Specimen Processing

Material from transthoracic aspirates is used and processed in the same way as that from transbronchial aspirates.

Pleural Fluid

Pleural fluid specimens are examined for documenting the presence of neoplasia, infection, inflammation, and other reactive processes. Approximately 50% of pleural effusions are due to a malignant process. One of the most common diagnostic problems evolves around the differential diagnosis of metastatic carcinoma and reactive mesothelial cells. Cytomorphologic features distinguishing these processes have been detailed.[12,13] While many cases are diagnosed by morphologic examination alone, occasional cases are difficult to classify. For such cases, ancillary studies on cell-block material are helpful.

Specimen Procurement and Collection

Pleural fluid specimens are collected by thoracentesis procedure, in the operating room during thoracic surgery or from chest tube drainage. Depending on the clinical indication, the specimen is triaged and submitted to the clinical chemistry laboratory, microbiology laboratory, or cytopathology laboratory. For cytopathologic evaluation, the specimen may be collected fresh or fixed in an equal volume of 50% ethanol.

Specimen Processing

The amount of pleural fluid specimen submitted to the cytopathology laboratory ranges from a few milliliters to volumes greater than a liter. Any clotted or solid material should be removed and processed as a cell block (see below). In general, the entire specimen or a representative sample of the fluid is placed in a capped tube and centrifuged at 2000 revolutions per minute for 10 minutes. The supernatant is decanted and the cell button is smeared to create an even monolayer. For specimens that are less cellular, several drops of pleural fluid may be placed in a cytofunnel for centrifugation of the fluid specimen onto a slide (cytocentrifugation). If immediate processing of the specimen is not possible, it may be placed in the refrigerator at 4°C.

Cell Block Preparation

Cell blocks are prepared from fragments of tissue obtained from aspirated material or fluid specimens. The tissue fragments are collected in buffered formalin or 50% ethanol and by the use of forceps, placed in cassettes with sponges on both sides of the specimen to prevent loss during processing. When the amount of material is scant, the cellular component may be captured in a gel-type material such as Histogel™ (Richard–Allan Scientific, Kalamazoo, MI). By this procedure, the fluid with scant material is centrifuged to produce a cell button. Histogel is heated to liquify. The supernatant is decanted and the cellular material is resuspended in liquified Histogel and allowed to solidify at room temperature. The solidified gel material is removed from the bottom of the centrifugation tube and placed in a histology cassette and processed as a cell block.

Preparation of a cell block is encouraged since it allows for additional studies that may not be performed on cytologic slides (smears and cytocentrifuged slides) alone. Using cell blocks, ancillary studies such as histochemical and immunohistochemical stains are performed in the same manner as they are performed for routine paraffin-embedded blocks. Known histology tissue blocks are used for positive and negative controls. Immunohistochemical stains may be performed on cytology smears and cytocentrifuged slides. However, the interpretation of staining results may be treacherous since the reliability of "positive" staining is uncertain. Unless there is a protocol for routinely collecting and preserving unstained cytologic slides of various cell and tissue types, adequate controls are difficult to obtain on a regular and reliable basis. For this reason, immunohistochemical stains are best performed on cell-block material.

Practical Classification of Pulmonary Neoplasms for Cytopathology

Malignant Neoplasms

Non–Small-Cell Carcinoma

Adenocarcinoma

By definition, pulmonary adenocarcinoma is a malignant epithelial neoplasm with evidence of glandular differentiation or mucin production. The tumor cells show acinar, papillary, bronchioloalveolar, or solid growth patterns. Pulmonary adenocarcinomas are often complex and may exhibit a mixture of these patterns. Furthermore, the degree of differentiation ranges from well to poorly differentiated. The combination and permutation of the patterns and differentiation are reflected in the wide spectrum of appearances on cytology preparations. While well-differentiated adenocarcinoma is relatively uniform in appearance, adenocarcinomas of higher grades are more variable. The neoplastic cells may be round to oval, small to large, and have poorly defined cell borders (in contrast to squamous cell carcinoma) with a nuclear to cytoplasmic (N/C) ratio that may be low in some tumors (Fig. 45.1). Architectural patterns appreciated on cytologic specimens include acinar clusters, glands, and papillary fragments. The nucleus is often enlarged when compared to benign reactive bronchial epithelial cells. The individual cells may be columnar, cuboidal, or round with or without vacuolization, reflecting mucin production. The cytoplasm of cells without mucin production is pale to dense. The nuclei range from those with round, smooth nuclear contours and fine granular chromatin pattern to those with nuclear membrane irregularities,

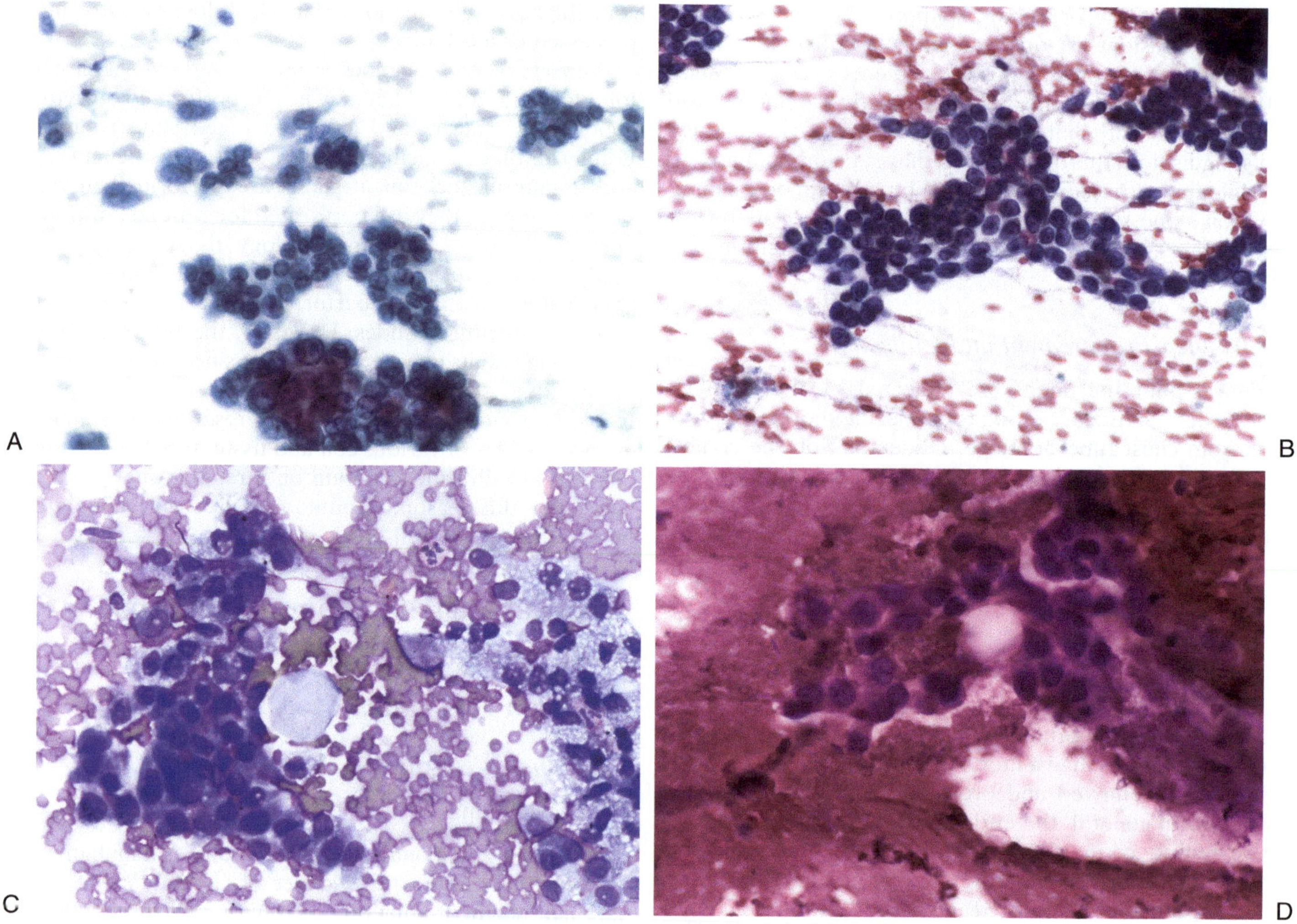

FIGURE 45.1. **(A)** Moderate to poorly differentiated adenocarcinoma is composed of neoplastic cells with enlarged nuclei, elevated nuclear to cytoplasmic (N/C) ratio, and variability in appearance from cluster to cluster. Cell borders are ill-defined. Crowding and nuclear overlapping are noted. (Papanicolaou stain.) **(B)** Adenocarcinoma with micropapillary fragment. The individual intermediate size cells are crowded and show monomorphism. The nuclei are hyperchromatic and nucleoli are inconspicuous. (Papanicolaou stain.) **(C)** The cytoplasm of these adenocarcinoma cells shows varying degrees of vacuolization. (Diff-Quik stain.) **(D)** The background is bloody and the neoplastic cells show gland formation with intraluminal mucin.

prominent nucleoli, and coarse chromatin pattern. The number of nucleoli, which are conspicuous, range from none to multiple. Intranuclear pseudo-inclusions, representing surfactant apoprotein, may also be identified.

Ancillary studies, which help confirm the diagnosis of adenocarcinoma, include the histochemical and immunohistochemical studies discussed in Chapter 35. Histochemical and immunohistochemical stains are best performed on cell-block material since routine paraffin-embedded tissue may be used as positive controls. In principle, the approach to workup should be similar to that in evaluating small biopsy specimens. Histochemical and immunohistochemical stains should be ordered as a panel and include markers that are expected to be positive as well as negative. By evaluating the cytomorphology and clinical presentation, a list of differential diagnoses is created. Markers selected are ideally specific for entities listed in the differential diagnosis.

Diastase-digested periodic acid-Schiff (PAS-D) stain and mucicarmine stain positivity help confirm the presence of cellular mucin production by the neoplastic cells in the absence of convincing gland formation. The cytokeratin 7–positive/cytokeratin 20–negative profile (CK7+/CK20–) is expected in approximately 80% to 90% of primary pulmonary adenocarcinomas. Likewise, thyroid transcription factor-1 (TTF-l) is also positive in 72% of pulmonary adenocarcinomas (Fig. 45.2).[14] Of notable exception is the mucinous type bronchioloalveolar carci-

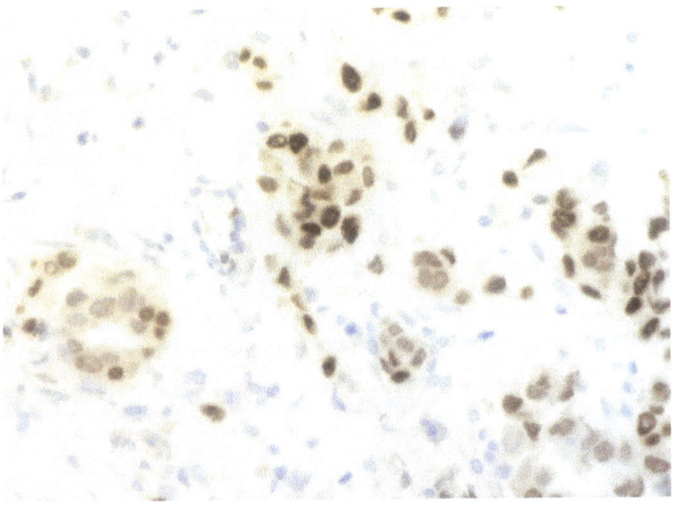

FIGURE 45.2. Thyroid transcription factor-1 (TTF-1) is helpful in identifying adenocarcinoma of pulmonary origin. Distinct nuclear staining is required for a positive stain interpretation. (Immunocytochemical stain for TTF-1 on cell block.)

noma, which is often negative with TTF-1 and may not demonstrate the classic CK7+/CK20– immunostaining profile.[15]

Pulmonary adenocarcinomas are usually peripheral lesions, and therefore, sputum cytology, bronchial washing, and endobronchial brushing have low sensitivity (49%, 48%, and 59%, respectively) in obtaining a diagnostic sample.[16] Methods with higher sensitivity for diagnosing adenocarcinoma include transbronchial fine-needle aspirate (66.6%), transthoracic fine-needle aspirate (85%), and transbronchial biopsy (82%).[17] The combination of multiple transbronchial and transthoracic procedures increases the diagnostic sensitivity to 92%.[18]

In addition to sensitivity, the accuracy for making the specific diagnosis of adenocarcinoma on cytology specimens ranged from 67.8% to 91.6%.[19] These values vary due to the type of procedure used to obtain the cytologic specimen. The most accurate diagnoses are made by the use of FNA specimens.[20] Furthermore, even if the cytology specimen shows unequivocal evidence of adenocarcinoma, there is a possibility that another type of neoplasm is present in the lesion. Pulmonary neoplasms are potentially heterogeneous; from area to area they may differ in grade and in the type of differentiation. The presence of "gland formation" may be mimicked by other neoplasms (e.g., carcinoid tumor) demonstrating similar structures. Therefore, the presence of intracytoplasmic mucin is a more reliable criterion. However, it should be noted that squamous cell carcinoma and other non–small-cell carcinomas may have rare foci of mucin production occupying up to 10% of the neoplasm. In other words, the diagnosis of adenosquamous carcinoma requires at least 10% of the neoplasm to show glandular differentiation. If gland formation or mucin production is only focal or not convincing, it is judicious to make the diagnosis of non–small-cell carcinoma and discuss the findings in a comment.

The diagnosis of the bronchioloalveolar carcinoma (BAC) subtype of adenocarcinoma has attracted much attention in the cytopathology and surgical pathology literature. There have been a number of studies stating that a cytologic diagnosis of BAC is possible through the application of a number of morphologic criteria.[21–27] Cytologic features such as clean background, fine granular chromatin, nuclear grooves, flat sheets, orderly arrangement of mucinous or nonmucinous cells with round uniform nuclei, absence of nuclear overlap, and absence of irregular nuclear membranes have been reported as characteristic findings in BAC. However, it is important to understand that the diagnosis of BAC has evolved over the past four decades. Under the current WHO/IARC 2004 classification, these neoplasms are in-situ neoplastic proliferations that grow along the alveolar septal framework without evidence of invasion. The prospective cytopathologic diagnosis of this entity is not possible since the cytologic features representing the in-situ proliferation or the bronchioloalveolar pattern (listed above) are also observed in mixed adenocarcinoma and BAC, and in papillary adenocarcinoma[28] (Fig. 45.3). Due to the lack of specificity for the bronchioloalveolar growth pattern, an unequivocal cytopathologic diagnosis should not be made. Nonetheless, the recognition of the bronchioloalveolar pattern is important since it implies the possibility of aerogenous spread and multifocal disease. Furthermore, there are cytologic patterns that overlap with the bronchioloalveolar pattern described above. Micropapillary clusters are defined as small, three-dimensional clusters consisting of greater than three but less than 20 neoplastic cells. The presence of these micropapillary clusters in cytology specimens correlates with micropapillary pattern in adenocarcinoma and suggests a poorer prognosis than that associated with localized BAC.[29]

The cytologic distinction between BAC and atypical adenomatous hyperplasia (AAH) is not possible since AAH is a small lesion (usually 5 mm or less) that is usually incidentally discovered in a resection specimen. These lesions would not be expected to exfoliate and yield cellular samples by bronchial washings or sputum specimens. Bronchial brushing procedures would not reach the peripheral air spaces where these lesions are located. Radiologically guided FNA procedures are able to localize lesions less than 1 cm. However, there is overlap in the cytologic features of AAH, reactive bronchial proliferations, and small BACs. If columnar or cuboidal cells with elevated N/C ratio, slight pleomorphism, and nuclear atypia are noted on a cytology sample, the diagnosis of

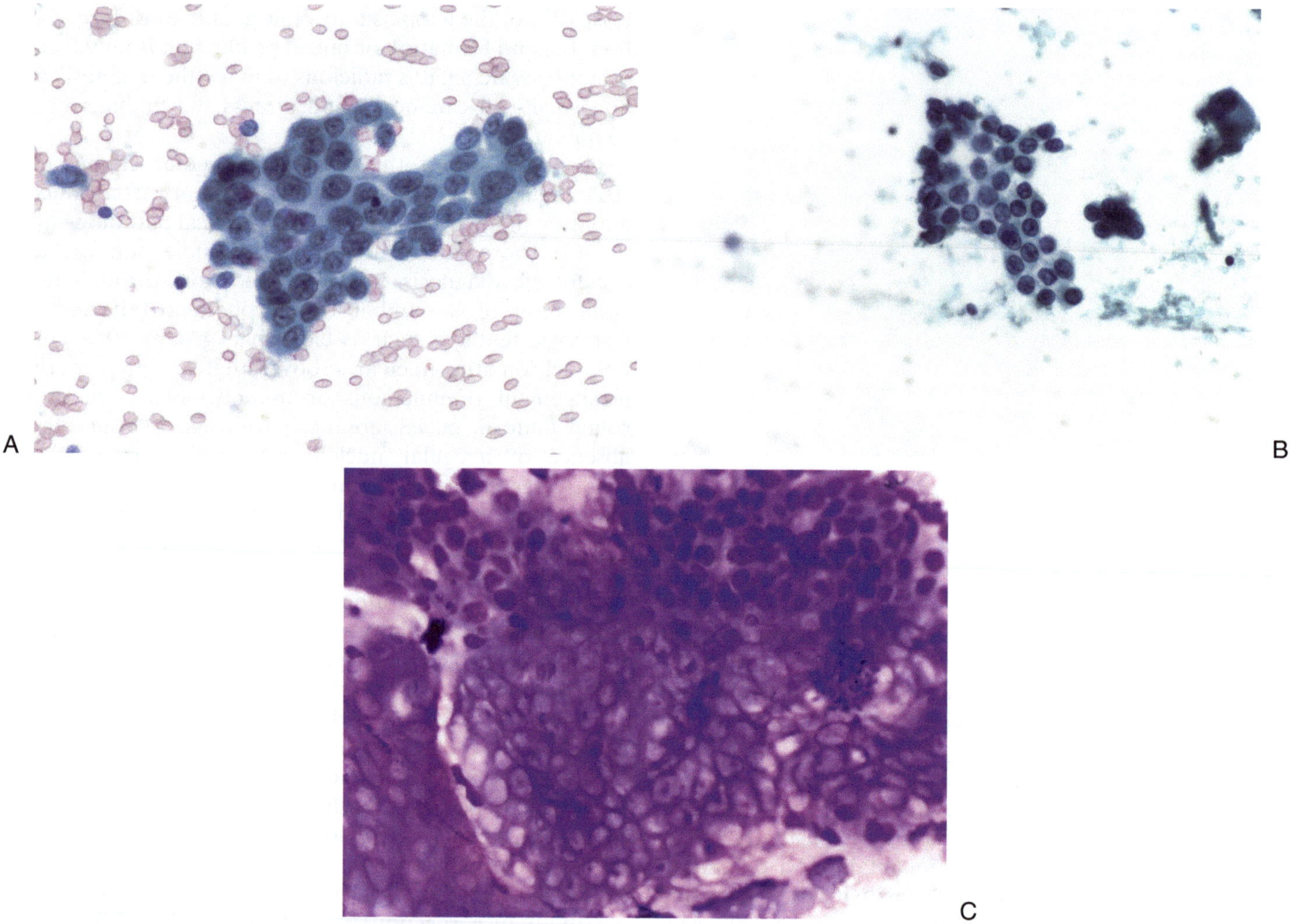

FIGURE 45.3. **(A)** Invasive adenocarcinoma with peripheral bronchioloalveolar (BA) growth pattern. The cytologic BA pattern is noted in adenocarcinomas that have a peripheral lepidic growth pattern. This pattern is not specific for bronchioloalveolar carcinoma and is observed also in mixed adenocarcinoma and papillary adenocarcinoma. (Papanicolaou stain.) **(B)** Bronchioloalveolar carcinoma (BAC), nonmucinous type. A small cluster from BAC shows a uniform monomorphic cell population with even spacing of cells and nuclei. The architecture appears micropapillary; however, this pattern is common to both BA and papillary growth patterns. (Papanicolaou stain.) **(C)** Bronchioloalveolar carcinoma, mucinous type. Numerous columnar epithelial cells with cytoplasmic mucin arranged in a honeycomb pattern are noted. The nuclei are relatively small round and regular. These cell clusters were abundant in this specimen. (Diff-Quik stain.)

"atypical cells" with a comment on the differential diagnosis would be appropriate.

Metastatic adenocarcinoma may mimic pulmonary adenocarcinoma. Most notably, ductal carcinomas of breast and pancreatico-biliary area are capable of producing metastases that are cytologically very similar if not identical to pulmonary adenocarcinoma (Fig. 45.4). Metastatic adenocarcinoma may also spread along alveolar septal structures, and therefore, present cytologically with a bronchioloalveolar growth pattern. Immunohistochemical studies including TTF-1, surfactant apoprotein, cytokeratin 7, cytokeratin 20, gross cystic disease fluid protein, thyroglobulin, prostate-specific antigen, and CDX2 on cell block material are potentially useful in determining the origin of the adenocarcinoma (see Chapter 44). Furthermore, adenocarcinoma cells are usually positive for monoclonal carcinoembryonic antigen (mCEA), BER-EP4, B72.3, and Leu-M1. In addition to the cytomorphologic features of adenocarcinoma cells, these markers along with mesothelial cell markers including calretinin and WT-1 are useful in distinguishing adenocarcinoma from mesothelioma.

The distinction from reactive pneumocytes is also potentially challenging. In most instances, reactive cells

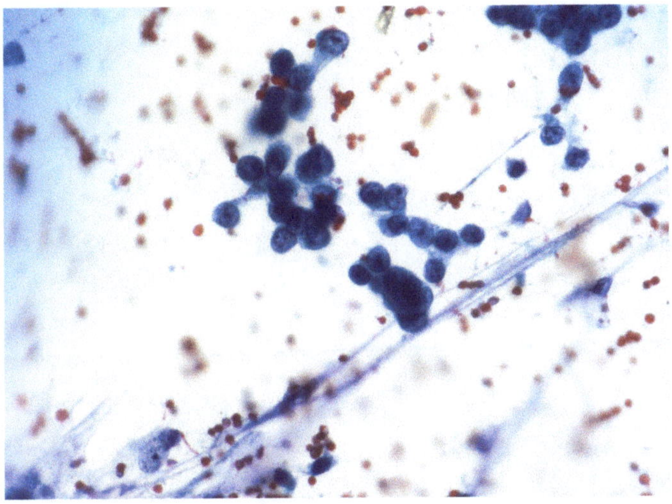

FIGURE 45.4. Metastatic ductal carcinoma from breast shows neoplastic cells that are similar to those of pulmonary adenocarcinoma. The neoplastic cells show disorganization, high N/C ratio, and prominent nucleoli. Immunocytochemical stains are helpful in determining the site of origin. (Papanicolaou stain.)

show variability in size and shapes of cells and nuclei (Fig. 45.5). Ironically, well-differentiated adenocarcinoma, including BAC, shows less nuclear pleomorphism than some reactive proliferations. The presence of cilia or terminal bars is helpful in determining the benign nature of the cell population. In areas with ulceration and inflammation, epithelial cells demonstrate a repair-type reaction with pavementing of cells, vesicular nuclei, and prominent nucleoli. These cells are present in flat sheets and the nuclear membranes are relatively homogeneous.

Squamous Cell Carcinoma

Squamous cell carcinoma (SCC) is a malignant epithelial tumor showing keratinization or intercellular bridges. The cytologic features are quite varied, with cases ranging from well to moderate to poorly differentiated. The variants include papillary, clear cell, small cell, and basaloid subtypes. Many of the patterns overlap with features of other non–small-cell carcinomas. For practical purposes, the cytologic diagnosis of non–small-cell carcinoma is made when criteria for the diagnosis of small cell carcinoma are not fulfilled (see below). Cytologically, SCC presents with irregular cell fragments, loosely cohesive groups, syncytial tissue fragments, and single cells (Fig. 45.6). The individual cells are round, polygonal, spindled, or multinucleated with giant cell forms. The cytoplasmic cell borders are generally well defined. The nuclear chromatin is fine to coarse with parachromatin clearing in many cases. Single micro- or macronucleoli are present. Keratinization manifests as orangeophilic, cyanophilic, or yellow hyaline globules. Intercellular bridges are not readily apparent on cytologic samples.

Ancillary studies are often used to distinguish SCC from adenocarcinoma. In contrast to adenocarcinoma, the PAS-D and mucicarmine stains are generally negative (although up to 10% of the neoplastic cells of SCC may show mucin positivity). Thyroid transcription factor-1 is demonstrable in only approximately 5% of SCC cases. In contrast, p63 and p16 (INK4A) are positive in the majority of SCC.[30] The CK7/CK20 profile is variable, in contrast

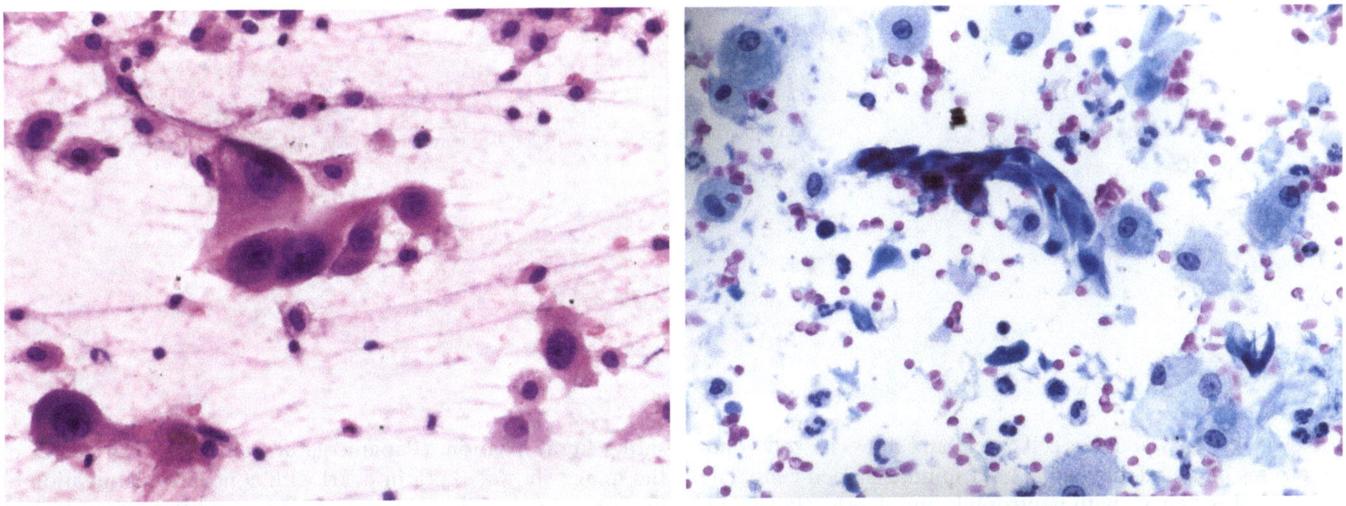

A B

FIGURE 45.5. **(A)** Reactive pneumocytes from diffuse alveolar damage shows markedly pleomorphic cells with coarse chromatin and prominent nucleoli. However, in contrast to malignant neoplastic cells, these cells are displayed in a flat sheet, have relatively low N/C ratio, and the nuclear membranes are smooth and even. **(B)** Repair reaction with a flat sheet of slender epithelial cells. The nuclei are enlarged and hyperchromatic. However, the N/C ratio is low. (Papanicolaou stain.)

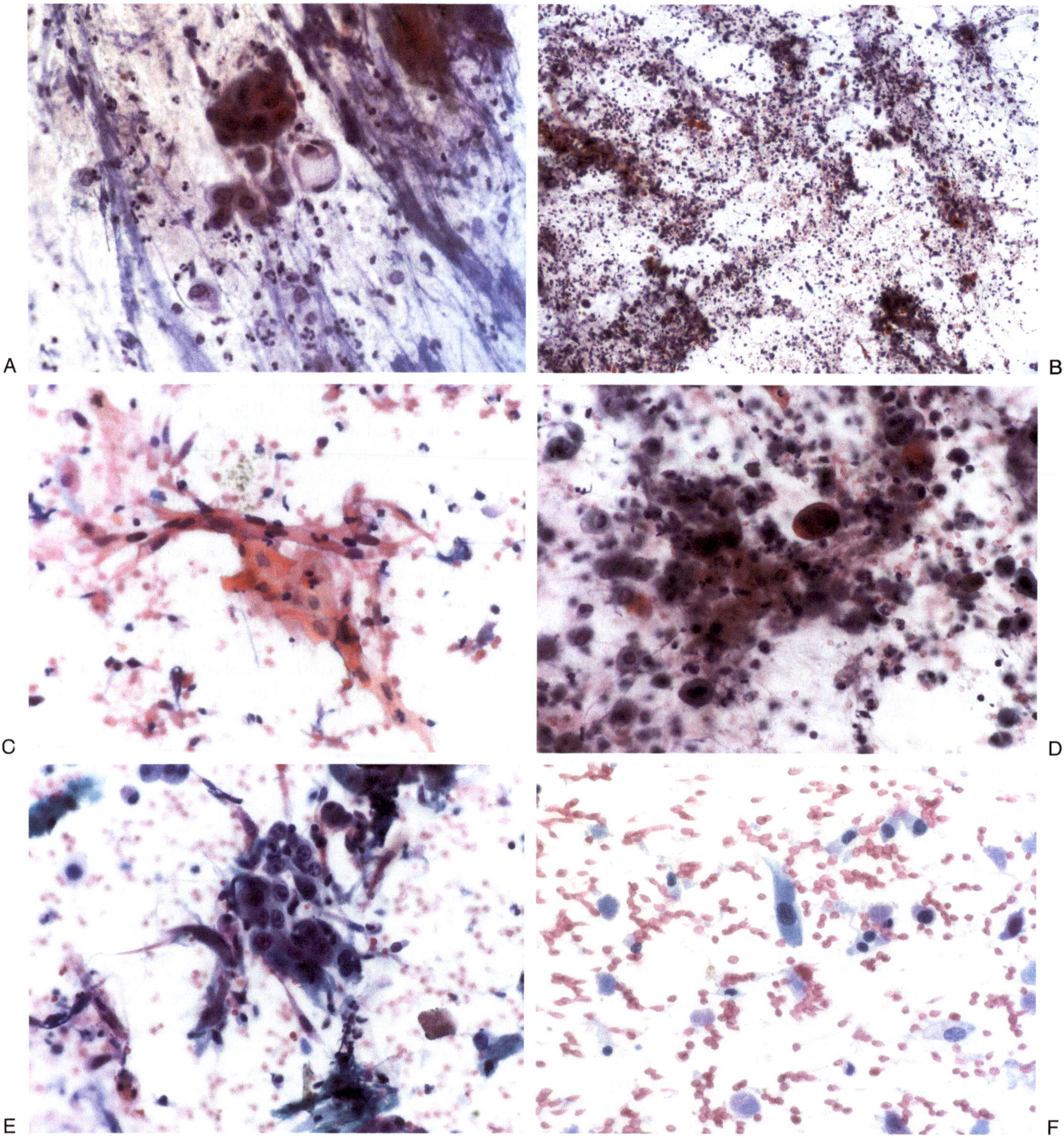

FIGURE 45.6. **(A)** Squamous cell carcinoma shows loosely cohesive groups of round, polygonal, and spindle-shaped cells. The background is "dirty" with neutrophils and debris. (Papanicolaou stain.) **(B)** Low-power image of the dirty background of squamous cell carcinoma shows cell aggregates and degenerated debris. (Papanicolaou stain.) **(C)** High-power magnification of a well-differentiated squamous cell carcinoma shows slightly enlarged and hyperchromatic nuclei. The N/C ratio is not markedly elevated while the cytoplasm of the spindle-shaped cells shows keratinization. (Papanicolaou stain.) **(D)** The center of the image shows a keratin pearl with concentric lamination of keratin. (Papanicolaou stain.) **(E)** Poorly differentiated squamous cell carcinoma shows spindle cells but lack of overt keratinization. (Papanicolaou stain.) **(F)** Mildly dysplastic cells from the bronchial mucosa cytomorphologically overlap with reactive cells. There is slight nuclear enlargement and hyperchromasia. (Papanicolaou stain.)

G

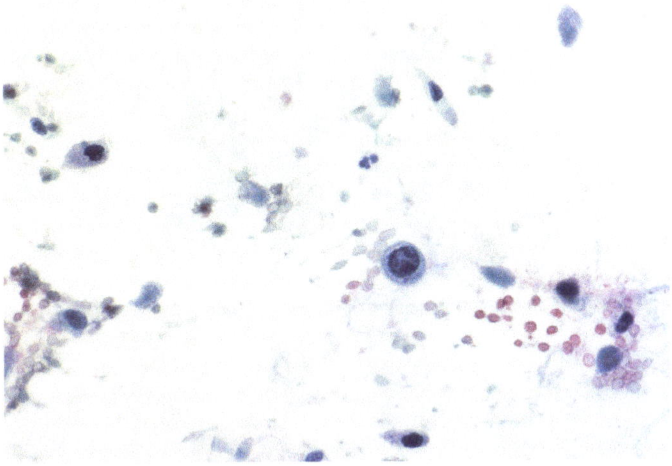

FIGURE 45.6. **(G)** Severely dysplastic cells show marked elevation of N/C ratio, nuclear hyperchromasia, and nuclear membrane thickening. (Papanicolaou stain.)

to adenocarcinoma which shows a CK7+/CK20– profile in the majority of cases.

Since SCCs are most often centrally located lesions, bronchial washing, bronchial brushing, transbronchial FNA, transthoracic FNA, and sputum cytology specimens have good diagnostic sensitivity. For patients with SCC, a diagnosis of malignancy is made in 88% of cases, and in 75% of cases the correct preoperative typing of SCC is made.[31] The degree of interobserver variability for SCC is intermediate (80%) when compared to other major lung carcinomas such as adenocarcinoma (75%) and small cell carcinoma (95%).[32]

Squamous cell carcinoma develops through sequential changes in the bronchial epithelium from benign columnar bronchial epithelium to metaplastic squamous epithelium to dysplastic squamous epithelium and carcinoma in situ (see Chapter 34). The cytomorphology of high-grade dysplasia and carcinoma in situ overlaps with invasive SCC. Therefore, such distinction between these in situ processes and invasive carcinoma cannot be made from cytology specimens alone. In contrast to adenocarcinoma that is positive for TTF-1, the majority of SCC cases do not express an analogous organ-specific marker. By current methods, distinction between primary pulmonary and metastatic SCC is best evaluated by clinical parameters.

Since SCC is often a centrally located neoplasm, diagnostic specimens may be obtained from sputum cytology, bronchial brushing, bronchial washing, or fine-needle aspirates. As for adenocarcinoma, obtaining multiple specimens increases diagnostic yield due to sampling variability. Once an adequate sample is obtained, the diagnosis of a primary pulmonary SCC is established through four steps. First, the determination of non–small-cell carcinoma is made. If the neoplasm is not clearly a carcinoma, a cytokeratin immunostain (e.g., AE1/AE3) will help support the epithelial nature. Some other tumors such as malignant melanoma, mesothelioma, thymic carcinoma, and sarcoma are notorious for mimicking non–small-cell carcinoma. Second, the presence of squamoid features in the specimen is confirmed. By the WHO/IARC 2004 criteria, SCC demonstrates keratinization or intercellular bridges. On cytologic specimens, keratinization manifests as orangeophilic cytoplasm or keratin pearls. Characteristically, SCC has well-defined cell borders. However, other tumors may also have this feature, and therefore the presence of well-defined cell borders alone may be misleading (Fig. 45.7). While the presence of intercellular bridges is a diagnostic criterion, this feature is present only in well-preserved tissue fragments and is not represented on many cytologic specimens of SCC. Third, the specimen is evaluated for other types of differentiation. The most common consideration will be for the differentiation seen in other pulmonary neoplasms such as adenocarcinoma, small cell carcinoma, other neuroendocrine tumors, and sarcomatous neoplasms. If significant portions of the cytologic sample show divergent differentiation, the possibility of a combined neoplasm should be considered. The WHO/IARC 2004 criteria defines a combined neoplasm as one in which the secondary component occupies at least 10% of the entire neoplasm. From cytologic sampling, the estimation of the secondary component is not possible. Therefore, when divergent differentiation is identified, the cytologic features are best described in a comment. Fourth, determine if the squamous cell carcinoma is clinically consistent with a primary pulmonary neoplasm.

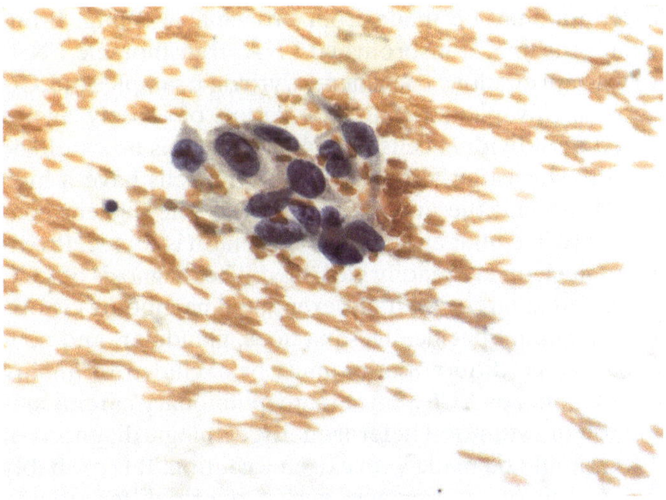

FIGURE 45.7. Some adenocarcinomas have areas mimicking squamous cell carcinoma with well-defined cell borders and spindled cells. (Papanicolaou stain.)

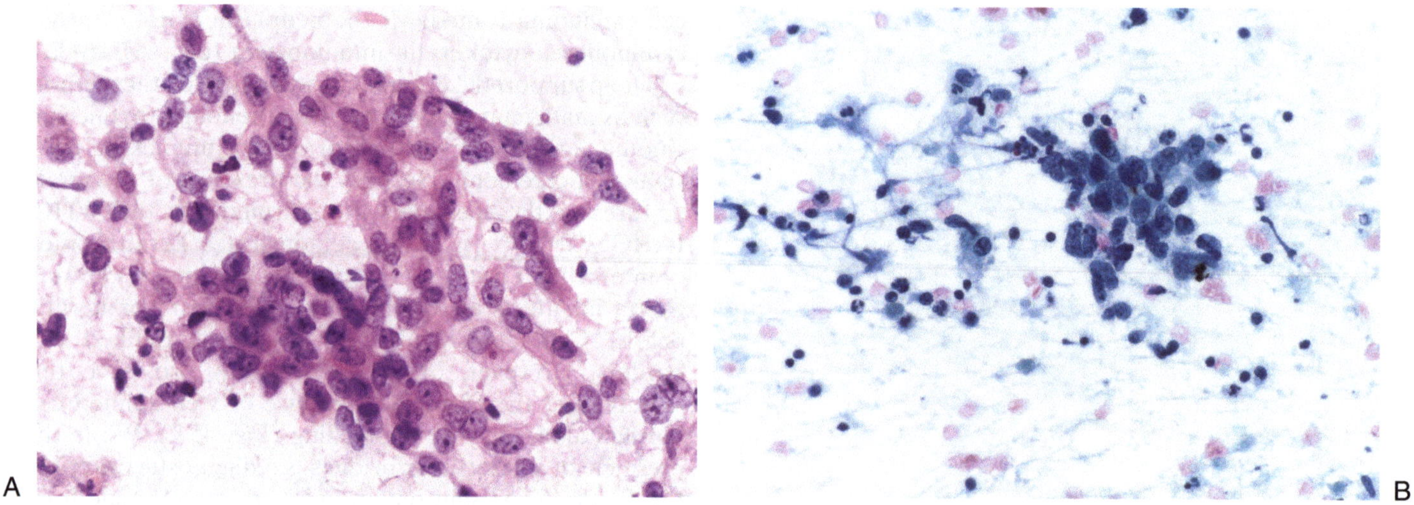

FIGURE 45.8. **(A)** Large cell carcinoma is a diagnosis of exclusion. Squamous, glandular, and neuroendocrine features are not observed. This diagnosis is difficult to make from cytologic specimens since areas of differentiation may not be sampled. **(B)** A subtype of large cell carcinoma, lymphoepithelioma-like carcinoma shows clusters of poorly differentiated carcinoma cells with lymphocytes in the background. (Papanicolaou stain.)

As stated above, there is no organ-specific marker (e.g., TTF-1) for primary pulmonary SCC. Therefore, the determination of whether a neoplasm is primary in the lung or not is best determined by clinical parameters. However, for some cases, even after thorough clinical and pathologic evaluation, the site of origin may not be established with certainty.

Large Cell Carcinoma

Like adenocarcinoma, large cell carcinoma (LCC) is often a peripheral neoplasm. It tends to be large, so an endobronchial component is often present. Therefore, the diagnosis may be made from bronchial washing, bronchial brushing, transbronchial FNA, transthoracic FNA, or sputum cytology specimens. Cytologic samples of LCC show highly pleomorphic population of loosely aggregated or individual cells (Fig. 45.8). There is no cytologic feature suggesting differentiation. The cells have a high N/C ratio and the cytoplasm is dense. The nuclear contours are irregular and nuclear chromatin is coarse. Prominent nucleoli are readily identified. The diagnosis of LCC (also called large cell undifferentiated carcinoma) is one of exclusion. Specifically, squamous, glandular, and neuroendocrine differentiation must be excluded to qualify a carcinoma as LCC. Since many pulmonary carcinomas exhibit intratumoral heterogeneity, cytologic diagnosis of LCC should be made with extreme caution. It is probably more judicious to diagnose such a poorly differentiated carcinoma as non–small-cell carcinoma.

The broader category of large cell carcinoma in the current WHO/IARC 2004 classification includes large cell neuroendocrine carcinoma, basaloid carcinoma, lymphoepithelioma-like carcinoma, clear cell carcinoma, and large cell carcinoma with rhabdoid phenotype. Large cell neuroendocrine carcinoma is discussed below (see Other Neuroendocrine Neoplasms). Basaloid carcinoma is listed as a large cell carcinoma, although, ironically, the neoplastic cells may superficially resemble small cell carcinoma. In contrast to small cell carcinoma, basaloid carcinoma does not exhibit as much nuclear molding or as fine chromatin pattern (Fig. 45.9).[33] However, such

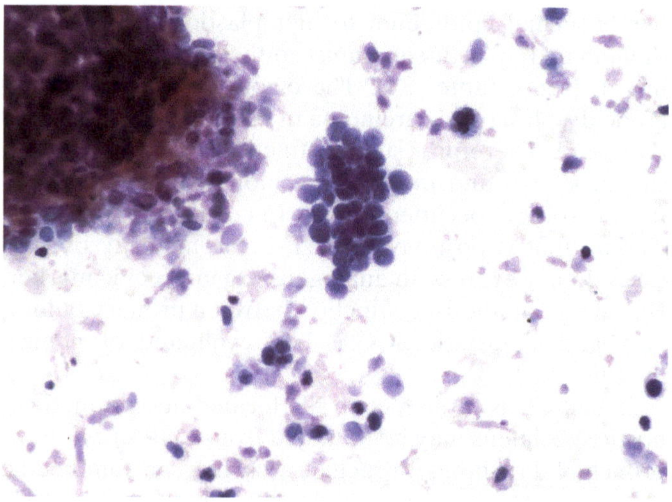

FIGURE 45.9. Basaloid carcinoma may appear similar to small cell carcinoma. Crowded cellular groups with occasional "molding" can be observed. However, the chromatin pattern is not a fine as in small cell carcinoma.

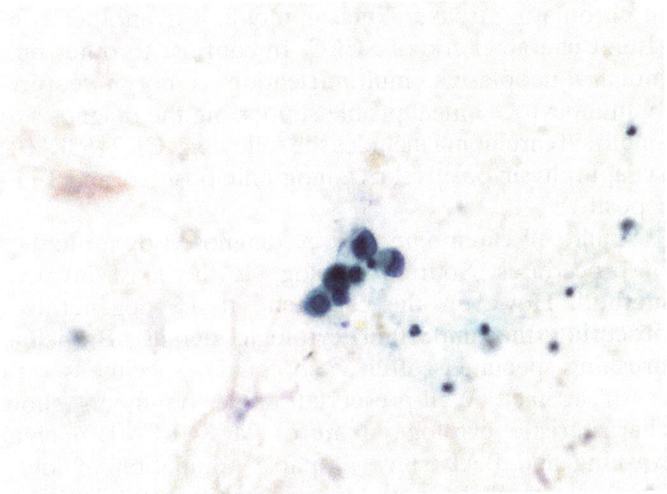

FIGURE 45.10. Clear cell carcinoma. Clear cell change is seen in variety of carcinomas and is not specific for clear cell carcinoma. The differential diagnosis includes metastatic renal cell carcinoma, hepatocellular carcinoma with clear cell change, melanoma, myoepithelioma, and other clear cell neoplasms. (Papanicolaou stain.)

distinction may be difficult to make on cytologic samples, and immunocytochemical staining with neuroendocrine markers may be beneficial. When employing immunocytochemical stains, one should be aware that small cell carcinoma has a tendency to have weak or focal neuroendocrine marker (e.g., chromogranin or synaptophysin) positivity. Therefore, a negative result must be interpreted with caution. Another useful marker is TTF-1, which is positive in the majority of small cell carcinomas but rarely expressed in basaloid carcinoma. Lymphoepithelioma-like carcinoma is similar to its nasopharyngeal counterpart. Due to the heavy lymphocytic background, other types of carcinoma (e.g., metastasis), melanoma, and lymphoid neoplasms (e.g., Hodgkin's disease) need to be considered in the differential diagnosis (Fig. 45.8B).[34] The diagnosis of clear cell carcinoma is also one of exclusion (Fig. 45.10). Since clear cell differentiation is seen in a variety of neoplasms (e.g., adenocarcinoma, squamous cell carcinoma, malignant melanoma, metastatic renal cell carcinoma), it is best to describe the clear cell feature of the neoplastic cell population and provide a list of differential diagnoses in the comment. Large cell carcinoma with rhabdoid phenotype is rarely encountered in cytologic specimens and insufficiently reported in the cytology literature.

Sarcomatoid Carcinoma

These neoplasms appear anaplastic and show sarcoma or sarcoma-like elements. Spindle cells and giant cells are a common feature of these tumors.[35] In general, adequate samples tend to be quite cellular, with the neoplastic cells manifesting as single cells, clusters, or syncytial fragments. The neoplastic cells are large with large nuclei and nucleoli. However, the N/C ratio may be variable, and the shapes of the cells range from round to polygonal to spindle shaped (Fig. 45.11). The category of sarcomatoid carcinoma is further subdivided into pleomorphic carcinoma, spindle cell carcinoma, giant cell carcinoma, carcinosarcoma, and pulmonary blastoma. Precise cytologic diagnosis of these tumors is extremely difficult since marked intratumoral heterogeneity is noted in many. Even on resected specimens, extensive sampling is

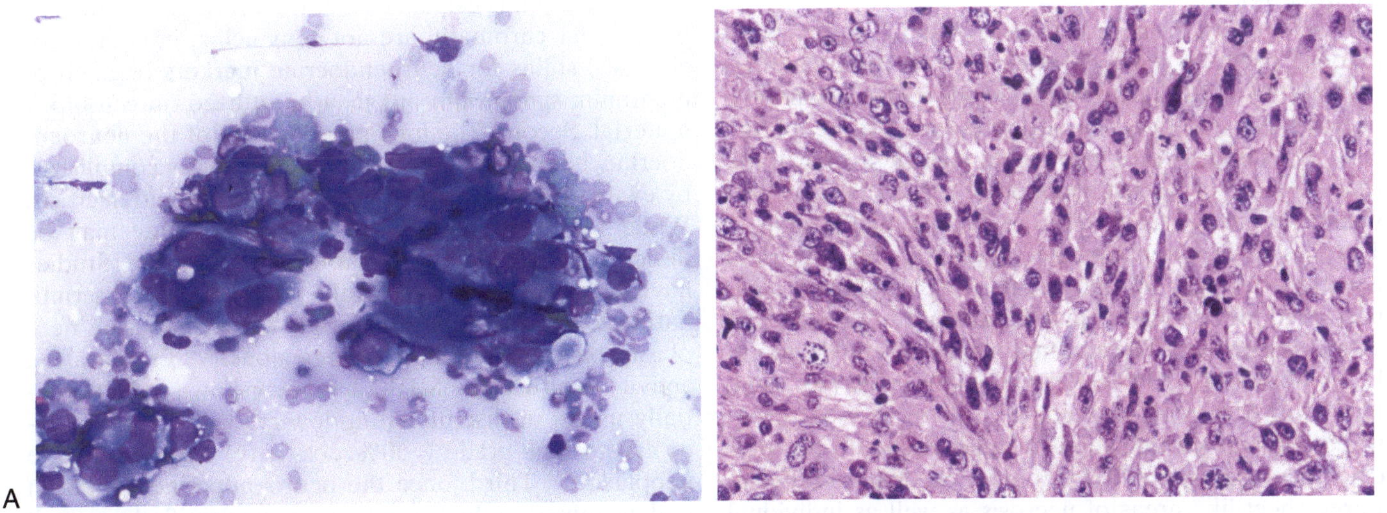

FIGURE 45.11. Sarcomatoid carcinoma often shows pleomorphic epithelioid areas (**A**, Diff-Quik stain) and spindled cell areas (**B**, hematoxylin and eosin [H&E]). Biphasic neoplasms are not necessarily carcinosarcomas, and therefore careful evaluation with clinical correlation and ancillary studies are important.

required as the carcinomatous component may be elusive. Therefore, on cytology specimens, overtly pleomorphic pulmonary neoplasms are best approached judiciously. The differential diagnosis includes reactive processes, primary and metastatic sarcoma, melanoma, mesothelioma, and other metastases. Immunocytochemical stains for a variety of cytokeratin markers and epithelial membrane antigen (EMA) on a cytology sample may be negative in sarcomatoid carcinoma (since the expression may be focal and present in an unsampled area). Thus, a cytokeratin-negative spindle cell malignant neoplasm on a cytologic sample does not necessarily represent a mesenchymal neoplasm.

It is important not to overstate the cytologic diagnosis. For example, carcinosarcoma is a subset of sarcomatoid carcinoma and requires the demonstration of heterologous elements such as malignant cartilage, bone, or skeletal muscle for diagnosis. The mere presence of a "sarcomatoid" spindle cell population is not sufficient for the diagnosis of carcinosarcoma. In addition, cytokeratin positivity in a spindle cell population must be interpreted with caution since some sarcomas (e.g., synovial sarcoma) are cytokeratin positive.

Small Cell Carcinoma

Small cell carcinoma (SCLC) is a high-grade malignant epithelial neoplasm consisting of small cells with high N/C ratio and demonstrating neuroendocrine differentiation. With adequate sampling, the cytologic diagnosis of SCLC is highly accurate.[36–40] This diagnosis is important since confirmatory tissue biopsies may not be performed and the diagnosis leads to medical-oncologic management. Unlike SCC and adenocarcinoma, the precursor lesion of SCLC has not yet been recognized (see Chapter 34).

Cytologically, the neoplastic cells of SCLC are arranged in loose, irregular cell aggregates, or syncytial tissue fragments (Fig. 45.12). Individual single cells, often in a necrotic background, are also present. The neoplastic cells are small to intermediate in size (less than three times the size of resting lymphocyte). The shape of individual cells varies from round to oval to spindle shaped. There is scant cytoplasm, and therefore the N/C ratio is extremely high. Mitotic count is high, although well-preserved mitotic figures may be difficult to identify in a cytology specimen. The chromatin pattern is finely granular in most cells, and nucleoli are usually small or absent. However, occasional prominent nucleoli may be recognized and the identification of nucleoli should not preclude the diagnosis of SCLC if other criteria are fulfilled. Large sheet-like areas of necrosis as well as individual cell necrosis/degeneration and apoptosis are common. Necrotic and degenerated cells demonstrate pyknotic nuclei with lack of chromatin detail. Crush artifact results in chromatin streaks. Nuclear molding is another consistent characteristic of SCLC. In contrast to other pulmonary neoplasms, multinucleation is not a feature. Immunocytochemical profile supporting the diagnosis of small cell carcinoma includes the following: CK7+/CK20–, synaptophysin positive, chromogranin positive, and TTF-1 positive.

Small cell carcinoma may be diagnosed by a number of procedures. Sputum cytology is the least invasive method. However, the cells tend to be degenerated, obscuring the important cytologic details. Bronchial brushing specimens often yield cellular specimens with crush artifact. Well-preserved tissue fragments show characteristic cytologic features of SCLC. Bronchial washing and BAL show a sparse population of loose aggregates of SCLC with less crush artifact. While SCLC is susceptible to crush artifact, FNA specimens generally yield preserved tissue fragments.

The differential diagnosis of SCLC includes stripped bronchial epithelial cells, lymphocytes, lymphoma, typical carcinoid tumor, atypical carcinoid tumor, large cell neuroendocrine carcinoma, basaloid and small cell variant of SCC, poorly differentiated adenocarcinoma, salivary gland carcinoma (e.g., adenoid cystic carcinoma), thymoma, metastatic carcinoma, and melanoma. Nuclear molding, cell size, finely granular or salt and pepper chromatin, and scant, delicate cytoplasm are cited as the most useful criteria in discriminating SCLC from other neoplasms.[39,41] These features yield sensitivity and specificity of greater than 90%. Accuracy of cytologic diagnosis of SCLC approaches 98%.[36] Generally, the diagnosis is in agreement with surgical pathology specimens except when the SCLC is combined with other neoplasms.[42]

The approach to the diagnosis of SCLC involves three steps. First, the neuroendocrine nature of the neoplastic cell population is established. If the cytologic features of the nuclear chromatin are not convincing, immunocytochemical stains for neuroendocrine markers (e.g., chromogranin, synaptophysin) may be utilized on cell-block material. Second, the high-grade nature of the neuroendocrine neoplasm is determined. This is accomplished by evaluating the degree of mitotic activity and necrosis. While these parameters are reasonable, they may be difficult to evaluate on cytologic specimens. Studies have demonstrated the difficulty in consistently discriminating low-grade from high-grade neuroendocrine neoplasms based on cytomorphology alone.[43,44] Proliferation activity measured by MIB-1 has been shown to be potentially useful in discriminating low-grade (<25% positivity) from high-grade (>50% positivity) neuroendocrine neoplasms.[44] Third, once the neuroendocrine neoplasm is determined as high grade, it is subclassified as small or large cell type. By definition, neoplastic cells of SCLC are smaller than three small round lymphocytes. However, some cells of SCLC demonstrate intratumoral

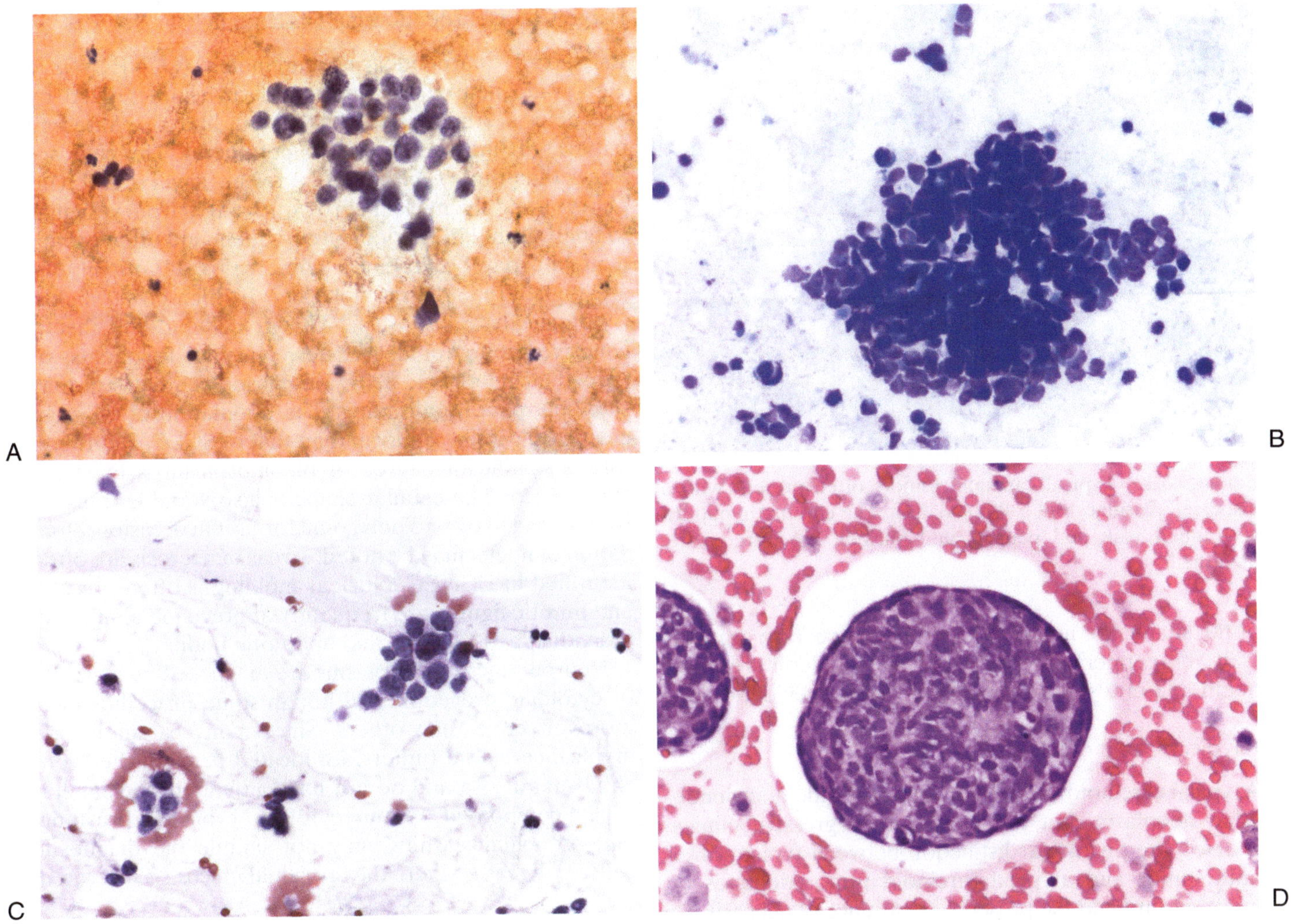

Figure 45.12. **(A)** Small cell carcinoma shows fine stippled chromatin pattern, characteristic of neuroendocrine neoplasms. (Papanicolaou stain.) **(B)** On Diff-Quik stain, the nuclear chromatin is not as clearly detailed. Nuclear crowding and molding are appreciated. (Diff-Quik stain.) **(C)** When the sampling of the neoplasm is sparse and the diagnostic features are not all present, the diagnosis should be approached with caution. There are other neoplasms with "small" cells. These include poorly differentiated squamous cell carcinoma, basaloid carcinoma, carcinoid tumor, melanoma, and a variety of metastatic tumors. (Papanicolaou stain.) **(D)** Small cell carcinoma in pleural fluid may form "balls" with some cells becoming elongated.

heterogeneity and occasional neoplastic cells may be large. Such findings are focal in the majority of SCLC. Nonetheless, in some cases, the distinction between SCLC and large cell neuroendocrine carcinoma (LCNEC) may be difficult. Furthermore, in fluid samples (e.g., pleural effusion), SCLC may show altered cytomorphology with neoplastic cells in rows and layers.[45,46]

Other Neuroendocrine Neoplasms

Typical Carcinoid Tumor

Typical carcinoid tumor is a low-grade neuroendocrine neoplasm that is located centrally, beneath the bronchial mucosa, or peripherally within the lung parenchyma. Peripheral carcinoid tumors are usually not adherent to the visceral pleura as is often the case with peripheral adenocarcinoma. By definition, carcinoid tumor is a neuroendocrine neoplasm characterized by organoid, trabecular, insular, palisading, acinar, ribbon or rosette-like patterns. Cytologically, the neoplastic cells present as clusters or dispersed individual cells. The clusters may aggregate in a nested, acinar, sheet-like, or trabecular pattern. On occasion, gland-like or papillary structures, mimicking adenocarcinoma, are identified.[47,48] The cells are uniform with a moderate amount of finely granular cytoplasm, which may be amphophilic or eosinophilic. The shapes of the individual cells range from round to oval to spindle. Nuclei are round to oval with smooth nuclear membranes and may be eccentrically placed, giving a plasmacytoid appearance (Fig. 45.13). Regardless

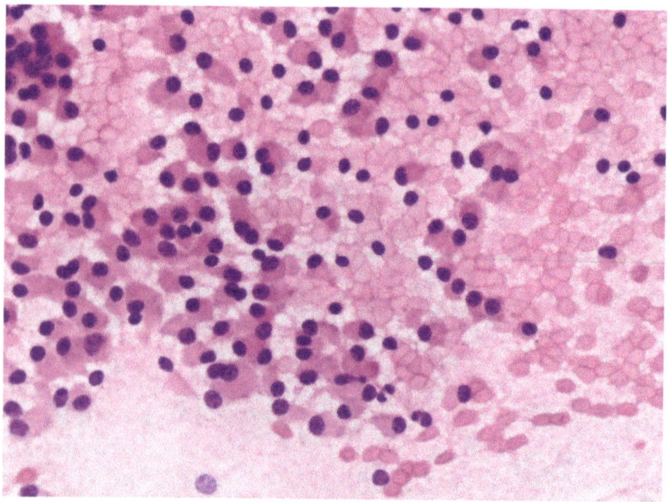

FIGURE 45.13. Typical carcinoid tumors often present with a dispersed plasmacytoid cell population. The chromatin pattern is granular (salt and pepper) and nucleoli are infrequently identified.

of the shape, the nuclei have a relatively coarse granular (salt and pepper) chromatin pattern. Nucleoli are infrequent and mitoses are rare. No necrosis is evident.

Atypical Carcinoid Tumor

Atypical carcinoid tumor is also a low-grade neuroendocrine neoplasm, but it has a more aggressive clinical course. The histologic distinction between typical carcinoid tumor and atypical carcinoid tumor depends on mitotic count and the presence or absence of necrosis. By histologic criteria, neoplasms with a mitotic count between two and 10 per 10 high-power fields or necrosis are designated as atypical carcinoid tumors. Other more subjective criteria include cytologic atypia, lymphatic invasion, prominent nucleoli, increased cellularity, and disorganized architecture. The cytologic distinction between typical carcinoid and atypical carcinoid tumor is more challenging since counting mitotic figures on cytology specimens is not as reliable as on histologic sections (Fig. 45.14). Furthermore, the presence or absence of punctate necrosis (characteristic of atypical carcinoid tumor) may not be present on cytology specimens due to sampling. At the other end of the spectrum, the distinction between atypical carcinoid and LCNEC or SCLC can be difficult also. As stated above in the discussion on SCLC, proliferation marker studies (e.g., Ki-67, MIB-1) have been utilized in the grading of neuroendocrine tumors including carcinoid tumors. Proliferation activity measured by MIB-1 may discriminate low-grade (<25% positivity) from high-grade (>50% positivity) neuroendocrine neoplasms.[44] However, its application to the distinction between typical and atypical carcinoid tumors requires further investigation.

Large Cell Neuroendocrine Carcinoma

Large cell neuroendocrine carcinoma (LCNEC) is a high-grade neuroendocrine neoplasm characterized by organoid, nesting, trabecular, rosette-like, or palisading patterns. It may be central or peripheral. The cells are larger than three times that of a resting small round lymphocyte, and the nuclear chromatin ranges from vesicular to finely granular. Nucleoli are frequent and often prominent but may be absent in some cases. Mitotic counts are higher than 11 or more per 10 high-power fields. Cytologically, cases of LCNEC are cellular with sheets, cohesive groups or aggregates, syncytial fragments, or individual neoplastic cells. Neoplastic cell clusters may show peripheral palisading. The population of the neoplastic cells is less uniform than that of SCLC, and therefore a significant degree of pleomorphism is expected (Fig. 45.15). The cellular shape is also variable, ranging from round to oval to polygonal forms. On occasion, elongation of nuclei may be noted. Areas of necrosis are often identified in LCNEC. Nuclear molding is often present, and mitotic figures are frequently appreciated along with individual cell necrosis and apoptotic bodies.[49]

Neuroendocrine neoplasms are diagnosed by a variety of cytologic procedures, although some procedures are more effective than others. Since many carcinoid and atypical carcinoid tumors are located beneath the bronchial submucosa and do not have an endobronchial epithelial component, sputum cytology, bronchial brushing, and bronchial washing may not sample the diagnostic cells.[50,51] In cases where the bronchial mucosa is ulcerated,

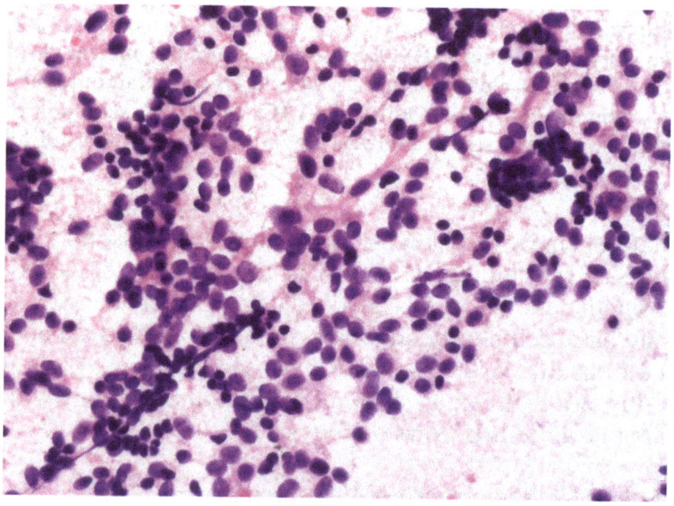

FIGURE 45.14. Atypical carcinoid tumors may show slightly increased pleomorphism in comparison to typical carcinoid tumors. However, pleomorphism is not a reliable criterion. The most useful distinguishing features—mitotic counts and punctate necrosis—are often not reliably identified on cytology specimens due to sampling.

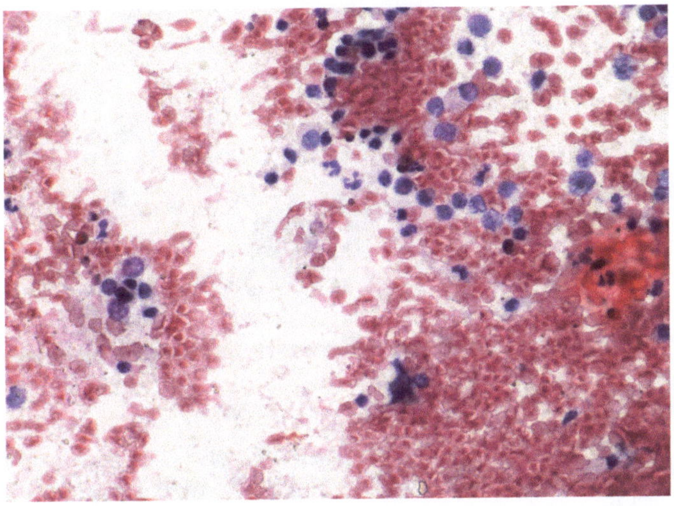

FIGURE 45.15. Large cell neuroendocrine carcinoma is composed of a pleomorphic population neoplastic cells. The differential diagnosis includes small cell carcinoma and other non–small-cell carcinomas.

the neoplastic cells may be obtained by these methods. However, mucosal hemorrhage could result in dilution of the neoplastic cell population. Otherwise, transbronchial or transthoracic FNA are often successful in acquiring the diagnostic cells of interest. Since centrally located LCNECs often show endobronchial invasion and mucosal ulceration, they may be diagnosed by bronchial brushing or FNA procedures.[52,53] The location and radiographic images of the neoplasm are important in selecting the most effective diagnostic procedures.

The precise classification and grading of neuroendocrine neoplasms by cytologic procedures may be possible on only a subset of cases and requires the understanding of the limitations of cytopathology. In a study by Nicholson and Ryan,[54] fewer than half of the cases of neuroendocrine neoplasms were classified correctly. In the remainder that were initially interpreted as either non–small-cell carcinoma, carcinoma not otherwise specified, or atypical-indeterminate for malignancy, the vast majority of them were found to show neuroendocrine features on reevaluation. In particular, neuroendocrine neoplasms with acinar or rosette-like arrangement may be mistaken for adenocarcinoma or other types of non–small-cell carcinoma. Although typical carcinoid tumor, atypical carcinoid tumor, and LCNEC are neuroendocrine carcinomas that are distinct from SCLC, it is best not to classify these neoplasms as non–small-cell carcinomas since the clinical management is often different from that for adenocarcinoma, SCC, and large cell undifferentiated carcinoma. Appreciation of the neuroendocrine (salt and pepper) chromatin pattern in the neoplastic cells found in well-preserved area helps avoid this pitfall. If cell-block material is available, application of histochemical studies for mucin (mucicarmine or PAS-D) or immunohistochemical studies for neuroendocrine markers (chromogranin, synaptophysin) are useful in this differential diagnosis.

The cytologic distinction between SCLC and LCNEC also may be challenging since the neoplastic cells of SmCC may show some pleomorphism and an occasional larger cell surpassing the "three lymphocyte" size criterion may be found. Furthermore, some LCNECs have a finely granular chromatin pattern similar to that of SCLC, and some SCLC cells have prominent nucleoli. In such cases, the cytologic diagnosis of high-grade neuroendocrine carcinoma is appropriate, and the final diagnosis should be deferred to another procedure such as a biopsy. Finally, neuroendocrine carcinoma (e.g., LCNEC) may be combined with a non–small-cell carcinoma or SCLC. Unless the components are well represented, these neoplasms are difficult to diagnose by cytologic procedures alone. A rare focus of divergent differentiation does not necessarily indicate a combined or mixed neoplasm since the secondary component must comprise at least 10% of the entire neoplasm. The value of good sampling and processing of cytologic specimens cannot be overemphasized. Misclassifications are often made on specimens that retrospectively are deemed suboptimal.

Mesothelioma

In pleural fluid specimens, the neoplastic cells of mesothelioma are arranged in sheets, clusters, or individual cells. Some of the clusters demonstrate papillary configuration. Between cells, a clear space ("window") is noted. Cellular engulfment or clasping is also a common feature. In comparison to reactive mesothelial cells, the clusters tend to be larger. The individual neoplastic cells are round, polygonal, or spindle shaped. The cytoplasm is generally dense and may show peripheral vacuolization. The nuclear appearance is variable, with some neoplastic cells showing very bland features while others demonstrate marked pleomorphism. Correspondingly, the chromatin pattern ranges from fine, granular, and homogeneous to coarse and clumped. Nucleoli may be prominent and mitoses are observed (Fig. 45.16).

The cytologic diagnosis of malignant mesothelioma involves two main issues: (1) distinction from adenocarcinoma and other malignancies, and (2) distinction from benign reactive mesothelial cells. These issues mainly stem from the protean manifestation of mesothelial cells. The major histologic subtypes of mesothelioma are the epithelioid, sarcomatoid, and biphasic types. Accordingly, a number of different cytologic patterns, including tubular, acinar, papillary, and solid patterns, are recognized. Cytologically, the epithelioid type predominantly presents with round to polygonal cells, whereas the

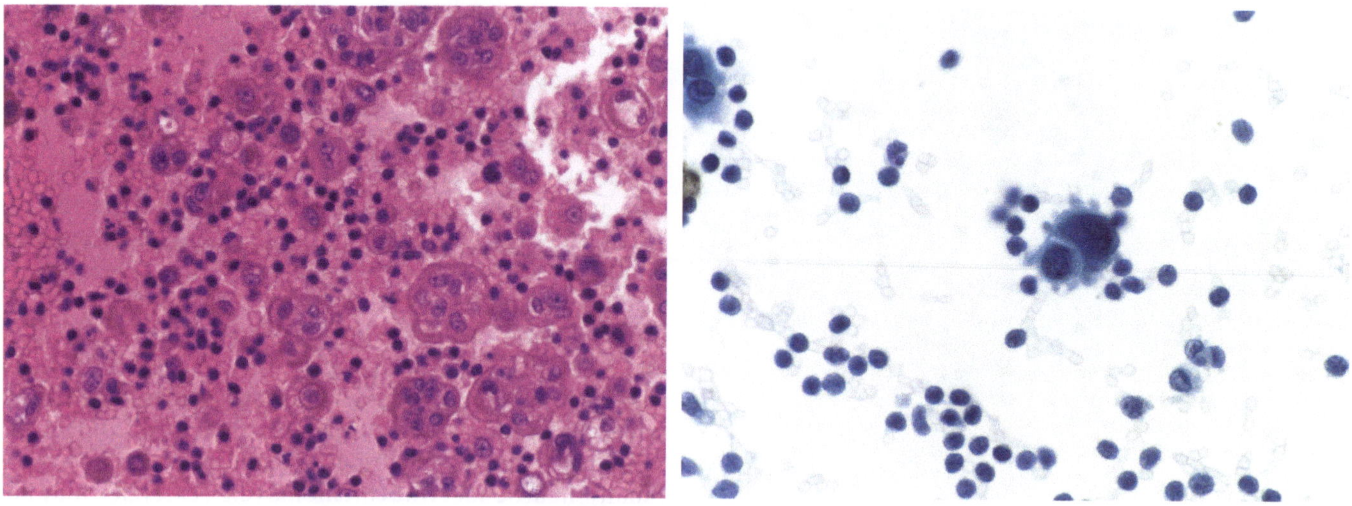

A B

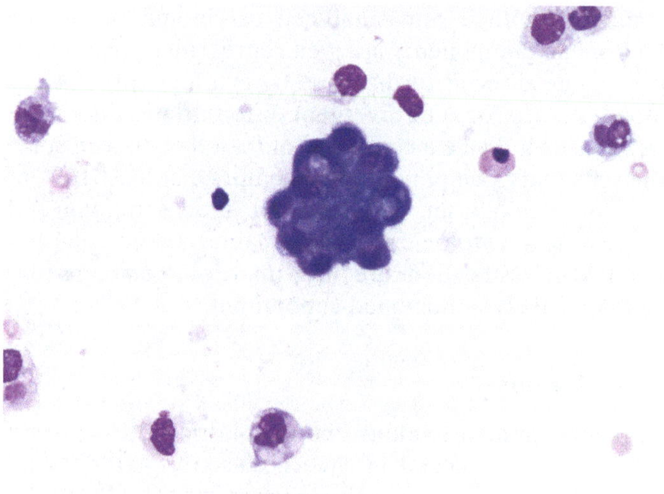

C

FIGURE 45.16. **(A)** The cytologic diagnosis of mesothelioma is challenging. For well-differentiated mesotheliomas, clusters of neoplastic cells demonstrate little pleomorphism and the chromatin shows some areas of clearing. **(B)** Cytoplasmic "window" is noted between these two neoplastic mesothelial cells. (Papanicolaou stain.) **(C)** Knobby cell contour of mesothelioma is characteristic. In contrast, adenocarcinoma cell clusters have smooth borders. (Diff-Quik stain.)

sarcomatoid types are for the most part spindled in cellular morphology. The sarcomatoid subtype may also show heterologous elements including chondroid, osteoblastic, rhabdomyoblastic, or neurogenic differentiation.

Pleural fluid specimens from thoracentesis procedures should be searched for clots to obtain cell-block material. If clots are not present, cytocentrifugation and use of Histogel (PERK Scientific, Inc., Devon, PA) may capture cells for ancillary studies. Cytologic samples tend to be cellular and usually yield material for a cell block. Cytologically, epithelioid mesotheliomas typically show large clusters of cells that are solid or hollow in the center, giving a "lacunar" appearance. The periphery of these clusters is knobby in contrast to adenocarcinoma that shows smooth contours. The cellular features of mesothelioma are related to the degree of differentiation. The well-differentiated mesothelioma shows cytoplasmic characteristics that are common to all mesothelial cells (dense cytoplasm, peripheral vacuoles, cytoplasmic blebs, central or eccentric nuclei, conspicuous nucleoli, variable N/C ratio, intercellular "windows"). The distinction from metastatic adenocarcinoma is difficult when the mesothelial cells demonstrate papillary, glandular, or acinar patterns. Furthermore, some mesotheliomas show cytoplasmic vacuolization mimicking signet ring adenocarcinoma. The identification of a separate and distinct cell population has been traditionally cited as the key to making the diagnosis of metastatic adenocarcinoma. However, this distinction may be difficult at times. Occasionally, adenocarcinoma may simulate the appearance of mesothelioma by demonstrating intercellular windows, cytoplasmic blebs, and knobby borders.

Immunohistochemical and histochemical studies on cell-block material are particularly useful by providing phenotypic information that distinguishes mesothelial cells from carcinoma cells. Immunohistochemical stains that mark for mesothelial cells include calretinin and Wilms' tumor marker (WT-1). Markers for adenocarcinoma include monoclonal carcinoembryonic antigen (CEA), B72.3, Leu-M1, Ber-EP4, and PAS-D.[55] In addition, site-specific adenocarcinoma markers including TTF-1 for lung, gross cystic disease fluid protein (GCDFP) for breast, CDX2 for gastrointestinal tract, and PSA are useful (see Chapters 43 and 44).

Other malignant neoplasms may also involve the pleural cavity, although the frequency is less than that of adenocarcinoma. These include SCC, SCLC, urothelial cell carcinoma, malignant melanoma, lymphoma, multiple myeloma, leukemia, and sarcoma. A detailed clinical history and prudent use of ancillary studies are important in determining the origin of the malignant neoplasm. For these neoplasms, the cytomorphologic appearances may be sufficiently distinctive to differentiate them from malignant mesothelioma. For cases in which the cells of interest are sparse or lacking in morphologic specificity, ancillary studies may assist in the diagnosis. Relatively specific immunohistochemical markers include p63 (for SCC), S-100, HMB-45, and Melan-A (for melanoma), and CD3, CD20 (L26), CD138, and CD43 and other hematolymphoid markers (for lymphoma, myeloma, and leukemia). On cytologic specimens, the distinction between sarcoma and sarcomatoid mesothelioma is difficult (see Fig. 45.22, below). In some cases, the cellularity of the neoplastic spindle cell population may be sparse. Furthermore, there is marked overlap in the cytomorphologic features, so ancillary studies are useful. If the neoplastic spindle cell population marks positively with a broad-spectrum cytokeratin marker (e.g., pan-keratin, AE1/AE3), the diagnosis of mesothelioma is favored. However, some sarcomas (e.g., malignant fibrous histiocytoma) may show aberrant cytokeratin and calretinin positivity in a minority of cases.

Differential diagnosis between reactive mesothelial cells and malignant mesothelioma is more challenging. In general, malignant mesothelial cells present as uniformly enlarged cells aggregating in larger clusters, in comparison to reactive mesothelial cells. However, this morphologic distinction is more easily stated than applied in practice. As expected, the cytologic diagnosis of well-differentiated mesotheliomas is particularly difficult. Currently, there is no reliable immunohistochemical marker differentiating benign from malignant mesothelial cells. Techniques evaluating molecular and cytogenetic changes hold promise. For this differential diagnosis, fluorescence in-situ hybridization evaluating deletion of CDKN2A, p16INK4a, and NF2, and polysomy of chromosomes 7 and 9 have been studied.[56,57] (See also Chapter 43 for further discussion of cytology of mesothelioma).

Lymphoma

Primary lymphoma arising in the lung is uncommon, comprising only 0.5% of primary lung cancer and approximately 3% to 4% of extranodal lymphomas. In contrast, secondary involvement of lymphoma in the lung is seen in 38% of Hodgkin disease and 24% of non-Hodgkin lymphomas.[58] Both primary and secondary lymphoma may present in a variety of gross and histologic patterns including peribronchial, vascular, nodular, alveolar, interstitial, or pleural distribution (see Chapter 32). The cytologic diagnosis of pulmonary lymphoma depends on the pattern and extent of involvement and the techniques (cytomorphology, flow cytometric immunophenotypic studies, and molecular analysis) utilized.

Over 80% of the primary pulmonary lymphomas are of the low-grade type, predominantly consisting of extranodal marginal zone B-cell lymphoma. The remainder is composed of other types including follicular center cell lymphoma, diffuse large B-cell lymphoma, lymphomatoid granulomatosis, and Hodgkin disease. The types of lymphoma that secondarily involve the lung include diffuse large B-cell lymphoma, small lymphocytic lymphoma/chronic lymphocytic leukemia, follicular lymphoma, Burkitt's lymphoma, and mantle cell lymphoma. Clinical history and radiologic information are important in arriving at the correct diagnosis. As a general rule, the lymphoid neoplasm consists of a cytologically monomorphic population of neoplastic lymphoid cells. These lymphoid cells may be broadly characterized into large, intermediate, and small cell types. Many lymphomas are associated with a reactive lymphoid cell component. If these areas are sampled along with the neoplastic cell population, the cytologic pattern may be difficult to discern (Fig. 45.17). For extranodal marginal zone B-cell lymphoma, the lymphoid cell population consists of intermediate-size cells with occasional small round

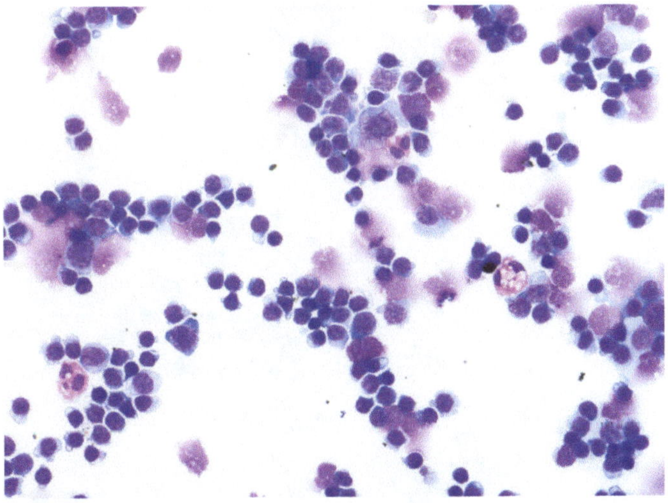

FIGURE 45.17. Extranodal marginal zone B-cell lymphoma shows a lymphoid cell population consisting of intermediate sized neoplastic cells and small round lymphocytes. Plasmacytoid morphology is observed in some of the intermediate-size cells. (Diff-Quik stain.)

lymphocytes and transformed cells in the background.[59] The intermediate-size cells have a moderate amount of cytoplasm, and the nuclear membranes are slightly irregular. Nucleoli are inconspicuous. In some cases, the intermediate cells demonstrate plasmacytoid morphology. Flow cytometric immunophenotypic studies show a predominance of B cells with light chain restriction. Coexpression of CD19/CD5 and expression of CD10 are not observed.

The distinction between extranodal marginal zone B-cell lymphoma and reactive lymphoid proliferation is potentially difficult. Characteristically, reactive lymphoid proliferations demonstrate a spectrum of reactive lymphoid cells ranging from small round lymphocytes to intermediate-size lymphocytes to occasional blastic type large lymphocytes. Proportionately, the small round lymphocytes predominate and the intermediate and larger cells comprise a minority population. With extranodal marginal zone B-cell lymphoma, the neoplastic cell population is slightly larger than small round lymphocytes and is characteristically intermediate in size with slightly more cytoplasm than small round lymphocytes. The key to the diagnosis is in the recognition and distinction of the intermediate-size lymphoid cell population with slight nuclear membrane irregularity and inconspicuous nucleoli from small round lymphocytes. The recognition of the plasmacytoid appearance of the neoplastic cells in this context is a helpful feature also.

Diffuse large B-cell lymphoma involves the lung on rare occasion.[60] Cytologic specimens show a cellular population of large noncleaved or immunoblastic cells. The nuclear membrane is irregular and the nuclear chromatin is coarse, clumped, and granular with areas of clearing (Fig. 45.18). The nucleoli are variable in size. Areas of necrosis and occasional granulomas may be found. The neoplastic cells are readily recognized as cytologically malignant; however, on some occasions, the distinction from nonlymphoid malignancies may be difficult. The differential diagnosis includes poorly differentiated carcinoma, melanoma, and sarcoma. Ancillary immuno-

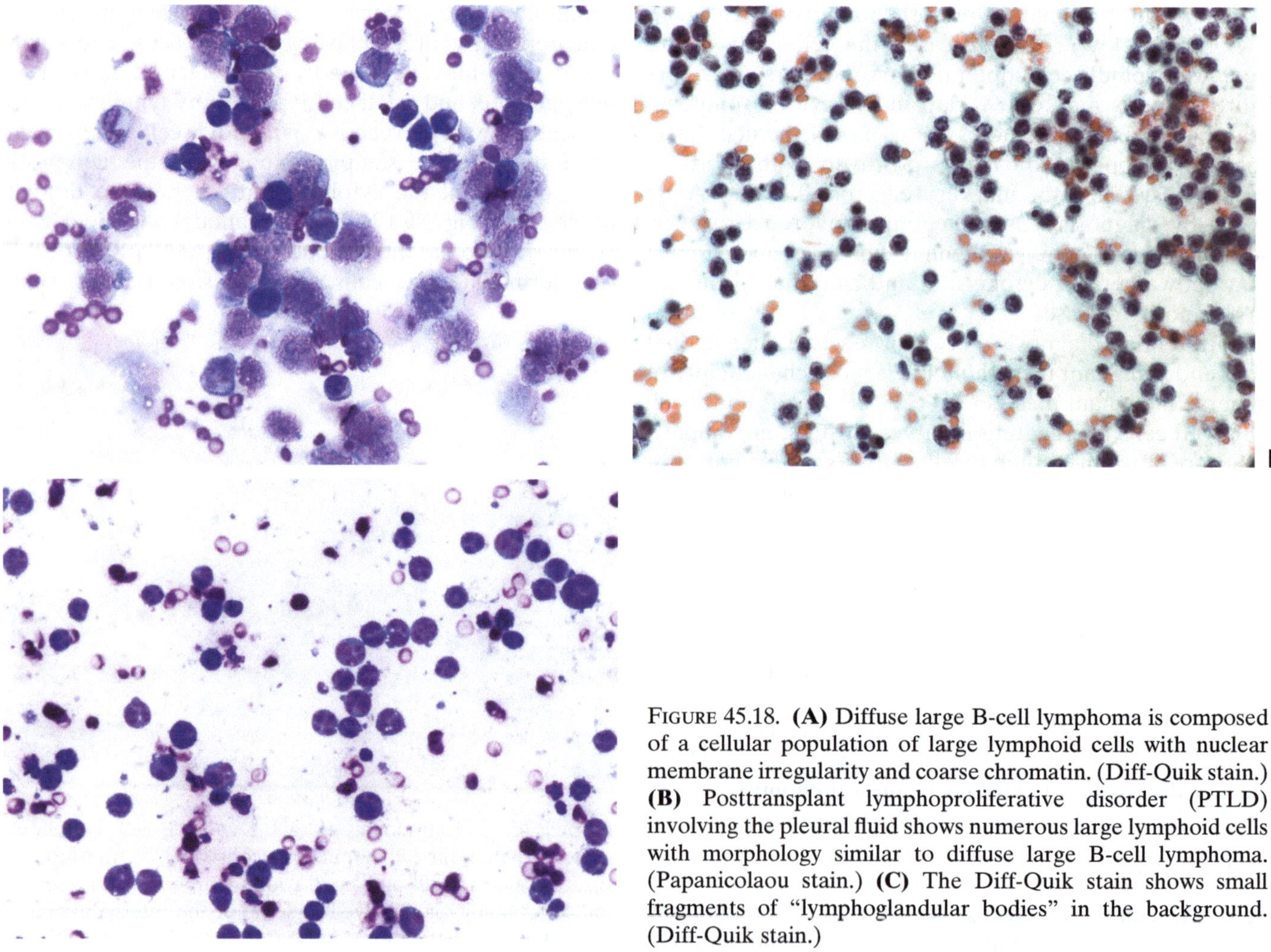

A B C

FIGURE 45.18. **(A)** Diffuse large B-cell lymphoma is composed of a cellular population of large lymphoid cells with nuclear membrane irregularity and coarse chromatin. (Diff-Quik stain.) **(B)** Posttransplant lymphoproliferative disorder (PTLD) involving the pleural fluid shows numerous large lymphoid cells with morphology similar to diffuse large B-cell lymphoma. (Papanicolaou stain.) **(C)** The Diff-Quik stain shows small fragments of "lymphoglandular bodies" in the background. (Diff-Quik stain.)

cytochemical or flow cytometric immunophenotypic studies demonstrating a CD20-positive population of lymphoid cells with light chain restriction are useful in establishing the diagnosis. Furthermore, the distinction of diffuse large B-cell lymphoma from a high-grade follicular lymphoma may be difficult by cytologic evaluation. Lymphomas may secondarily involve the pleural cavity or may present as a primary effusion lymphoma (PEL). Identification of human herpesvirus-8 is possible by polymerase chain reaction on direct smears or cell-block material.[61]

In addition to cytologic and immunophenotypic analysis, clinical correlation with the patient's immunologic status is especially important. Patients with autoimmune conditions are prone to developing lymphoid hyperplasias, which may mimic neoplastic lymphoid proliferations. Transplant patients not infrequently develop posttransplant lymphoproliferative disorder (PTLD), which may be morphologically identical to lymphoma but biologically is considered to be a potentially reversible disorder (treated by reduction of immunosuppression) (Fig. 45.18B).[62] Posttransplant lymphoproliferative disorder is classified as polymorphous (with mature lymphocytes, immature lymphocytes, plasma cells, and macrophages) or monomorphous (with a diffuse population of large lymphoid cells; see Chapter 32). Lymphoglandular bodies are identified in the background (Fig. 45.18C). Most PTLDs are B-cell proliferations associated with Epstein-Barr virus (EBV). These features are useful diagnostically. Demonstration of a predominantly B-cell population with EBV positivity (by immunocytochemistry or in-situ hybridization) provides support for the diagnosis of PTLD. Like high-grade lymphomas, PTLD may secondarily involve the pleural cavity or may present as a primary effusion PTLD.[63] Patients with human immunodeficiency virus infections are also susceptible to developing lymphoid proliferations, many of which are high grade in nature.

While the evaluation of the lymphoproliferative conditions by cytologic procedures has advanced over the last decades, there are limitations that must be understood. In general, sputum cytology is not yielding in determining the diagnosis of lymphoma. Bronchoalveolar lavage and bronchial washings may be useful for lymphomas that have alveolar patterns of involvement. However, the lymphoid cell population may be diluted by the instilled saline, and material may not be available for flow cytometric immunophenotypic studies. Bronchial brushing specimens may obtain the diagnostic lymphoid cell population in a situation where the lymphoma involves the peribronchial and bronchial areas. Unless planned in advance, material for flow cytometric immunophenotypic studies is difficult to obtain. Fine-needle aspiration procedures are ideal for nodular, pleural, and other localized processes. They provide the best chance for obtaining a cellular sample that could be divided for morphologic, immunocytochemical, and flow cytometric studies.

While the characteristic pathologic findings of common lymphoproliferative disorders have been described in the lung. The primary diagnosis of lymphoma in the lung may be difficult to establish by cytologic procedures alone. Lymphomas are notorious for demonstrating intratumoral heterogeneity and complexity. The extent to which such complexity is clinically relevant is an issue of further investigation.

If aberrant features are identified on cytologic evaluation, the final diagnosis of primary lymphoma is best reserved for evaluation on resected tissue samples.

Sarcoma

Primary pulmonary sarcomas are extremely rare and account for approximately 0.2% of primary lung cancers. Due to the presence of pluripotential tissue in the lung, virtually all morphologic types of primary pulmonary sarcoma have been reported (see Chapters 39 and 40). Sarcomas may manifest as spindle cells or a mixture of spindle cells and epithelioid cells. These cells are arranged in clusters, loose aggregates, and fascicles. Primary spindle cell pulmonary sarcomas include leiomyosarcoma, rhabdomyosarcoma, malignant fibrous histiocytoma, malignant peripheral nerve sheath tumor, fibrosarcoma, osteosarcoma, chondrosarcoma, liposarcoma, and angiosarcoma. The primary sarcomas of epithelioid types include rhabdomyosarcoma, extraosseous Ewing's sarcoma/peripheral neuroectodermal tumor (Askin tumor), neuroblastoma, granulocytic sarcoma, synovial sarcoma, and epithelioid hemangioendothelioma. The diagnostic criteria for these entities are identical to those of primary sarcomas of soft tissue. The cytologic and architectural patterns of the cell population provide clues for the differentiation of sarcomas. Cytologic diagnosis is challenging due to the possibility of localized sampling of a potentially complex neoplasm and the amount of material available for ancillary studies. Nonetheless, characteristic findings have been documented.

Leiomyosarcoma is characterized by single and cohesive groups of spindle cells with dense homogeneous cytoplasm. The nuclear shapes range from oval to fusiform and the chromatin tends to be finely granular (Fig. 45.19). The identification of mitotic figures and necrosis is variable.[64–66] Rhabdomyosarcoma (RMS) shows a population of pleomorphic neoplastic cells with ill-defined cell borders and granular cytoplasm with occasional globular material. Muscle striation, which is a characteristic feature of RMS, is only found occasionally in cytology samples. The nuclei are elongated with chromatin clumping and prominent nucleoli.[67] Synovial sarcomas are monophasic or biphasic. The monophasic type

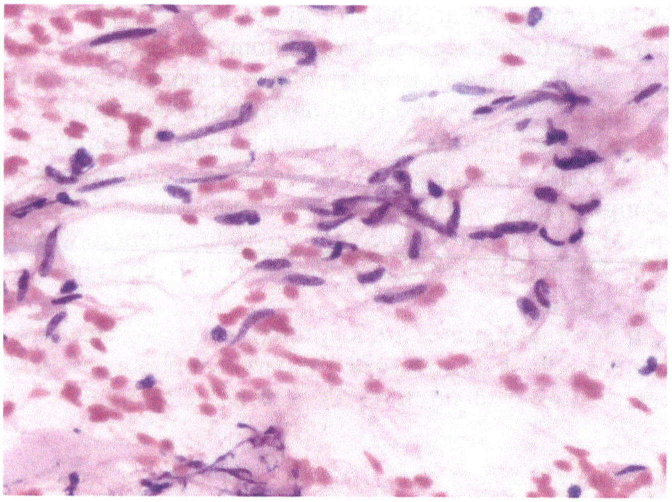

FIGURE 45.19. Neoplastic spindle cell population from leiomyosarcoma shows dense cytoplasm and cigar-shaped nuclei.

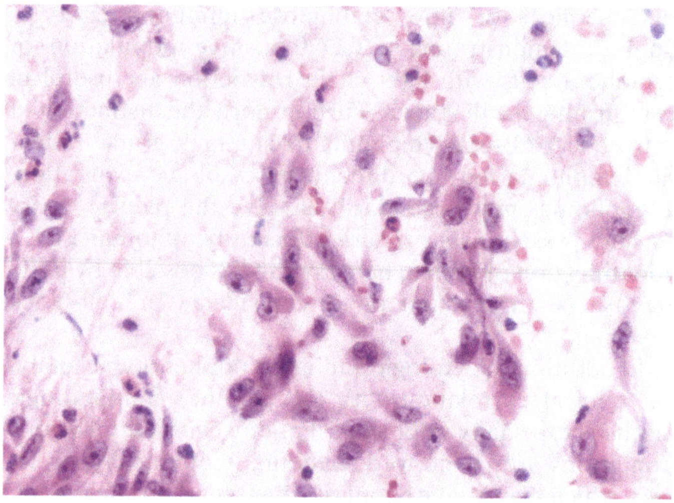

FIGURE 45.20. Like other pleomorphic neoplasms, malignant fibrous histiocytoma (MFH) is a diagnosis of exclusion. Clinical correlation and ancillary studies excluding specific differentiation are valuable.

is characterized by relatively uniform spindle cells with oval to elongated nuclei, fine granular chromatin, and inconspicuous nucleoli. Cytologically, these cells can be difficult to differentiate from those of other spindle cell sarcomas, epithelioid sarcoma (e.g., primitive neuroectodermal tumor), or carcinoma. The biphasic pattern of synovial sarcoma includes an element of epithelioid cells that can show ill-defined rosette formation or nuclear molding. In isolation, the epithelioid cell population on cytologic specimens mimics carcinoma. Identification of X:18 translocation by cytogenetic studies is useful in adding support to the diagnosis.[68]

Fine-needle aspiration specimens from malignant fibrous histiocytoma (MFH) demonstrate a cellular population of highly pleomorphic cells that vary from round, oval, and polygonal to spindle shapes. There may be single or multiple nuclei with small or conspicuous nucleoli. The chromatin pattern tends to be coarse and clumped (Fig. 45.20). Mitoses and areas of necrosis are identified in a typical representative sample. While a malignant diagnosis is reached easily, the final diagnosis of MFH requires thorough clinicopathologic correlation since MFH is a diagnosis of exclusion.[69] In general, ancillary studies are highly valuable in evaluating sarcomas, especially since many sarcomas require the demonstration of specific immunophenotypic expression as part of their diagnostic criteria.

There are three main issues regarding the diagnosis of primary pulmonary sarcoma. First, a bland spindle cell population from a pulmonary specimen is more likely to be benign, representing a reactive or neoplastic condition that is benign or low grade in malignant potential (Fig. 45.21). These include granuloma, organizing pneumonia, hamartoma, neurilemoma, solitary fibrous tumor, and inflammatory myofibroblastic tumor.[70] While most of these are composed of a relatively uniform spindle cell population, the degree of pleomorphism in some of these processes may be misleading. Second, a malignant-appearing spindle cell population is more likely to be a spindle cell population from a primary pulmonary carcinoma, carcinoid tumor, or mesothelioma than a sarcoma. The actual carcinoma may be a poorly differentiated SCC, adenocarcinoma, large cell undifferentiated carcinoma, pleomorphic carcinoma, or spindle cell carcinoma. Perhaps the most important diagnosis to exclude prior to

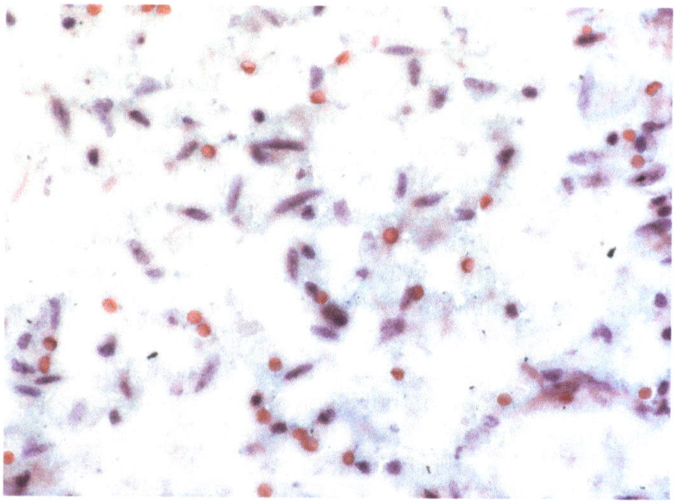

FIGURE 45.21. These bland spindled cells are derived from a neurilemoma. The nuclei and cytoplasm are tapered at the ends. The background shows degeneration. (Papanicolaou stain.)

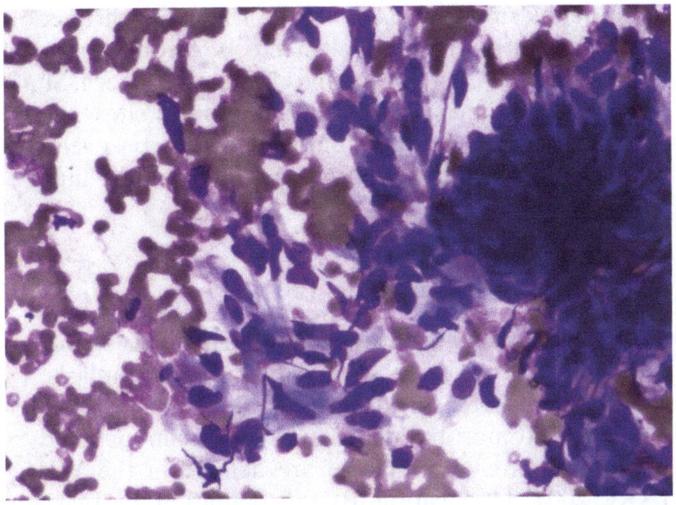

FIGURE 45.22. Sarcomatoid mesothelioma with malignant spindled cells mimics sarcoma. (Diff-Quik stain.)

considering the diagnosis of a primary pulmonary sarcoma is the possibility of a carcinoma with spindle cell morphology or sarcomatoid mesothelioma (Fig. 45.22). Clinical correlation and immunohistochemical studies with keratin and mesothelial cell markers are useful in evaluating these possibilities. One should note that many pleomorphic carcinomas might be focally negative with keratin markers. Furthermore, some sarcomas may have focal keratin positivity. Therefore, the presence or absence of keratin does not necessarily prove or discount the possibility of carcinoma versus sarcoma. Third, the possibility of metastasis should also be considered. Metastatic carcinoma, sarcoma, and melanoma may all present with a pleomorphic spindle cell population on cytology specimens (Fig. 45.23). When a sarcoma is encountered in the lung, it more likely represents a metastasis from another primary site. Clinical history is particularly important in considering this possibility since virtually any type of sarcoma may metastasize to the lung. Overall, a specific cytopathologic diagnosis on a spindle cell neoplasm is rendered in approximately 85% of cases.[70] While this figure is encouraging, cytopathologic evaluation may misclassify a neoplasm occasionally. In particular, synovial sarcoma and melanoma are potential mimickers of other types of tumor.[71,72]

Endobronchial Carcinoma (Salivary Gland Type)

Endobronchial carcinomas are rare and most arise from the submucosal salivary gland tissue (see Chapter 38). Therefore, the morphology of these neoplasms is similar to the salivary gland counterparts in the head and neck area. In this section, we discuss two neoplasms that can be encountered by cytologic sampling (bronchial washing, bronchial brushing, and FNA).

Mucoepidermoid carcinoma (MEC) is exophytic and polypoid with solid and cystic areas, grossly. The size may vary from a few millimeters to a few centimeters in diameter, and the larger ones obstruct the airways. Histologically, MEC is composed of three cell types—mucinous, intermediate, and squamous cells. The proportion of these cells varies depending on the grade of the neoplasm. The more common low-grade MEC is predominantly composed of mucinous cells and intermediate cells forming cystic and glandular structures. On the other hand, high-grade MEC shows more solid areas with squamous and intermediate cells showing significant pleomorphism, areas of necrosis, and frequent mitotic figures. Cytologic samples of MEC showing the low-grade component are predominated by mucinous and intermediate cells (Fig. 45.24).[73–75] The distinction from mucinous adenocarcinoma may be difficult, especially if the intermediate cells are not well represented. These intermediate cells are small and polygonal with amphophilic cytoplasm and round and bland nuclei. No significant pleomorphism, areas of necrosis, or elevated mitotic count is noted. At the other end of the spectrum, high-grade MEC is predominated by pleomorphic squamous cells and intermediate cells. While the squamous cells do not show keratinization, the cytologic distinction from SCC may not be possible. When both low- and high-grade components are present, the distinction of MEC from adenosquamous carcinoma is extremely challenging.

Adenoid cystic carcinoma (ACC) arises in the major bronchi, producing a polypoid mass or infiltrating along the bronchial wall. Histologically, cribriform, tubular, and solid patterns are encountered. Of these, the cribriform pattern is most characteristic. The neoplastic cells of ACC

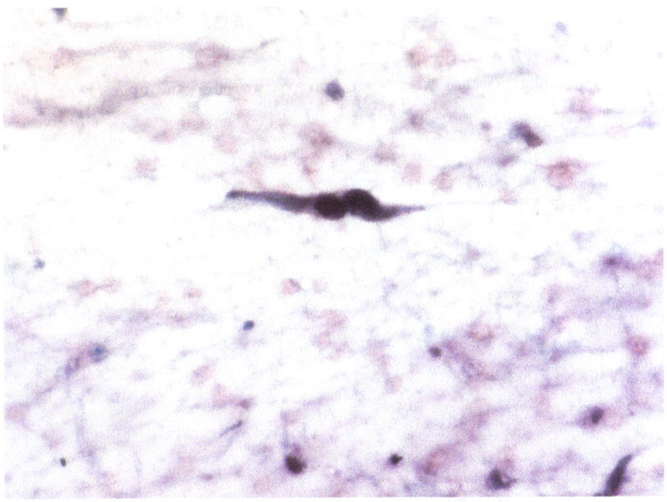

FIGURE 45.23. A rare atypical spindled cell was later shown to represent metastatic sarcoma on a biopsy specimen. (Papanicolaou stain.)

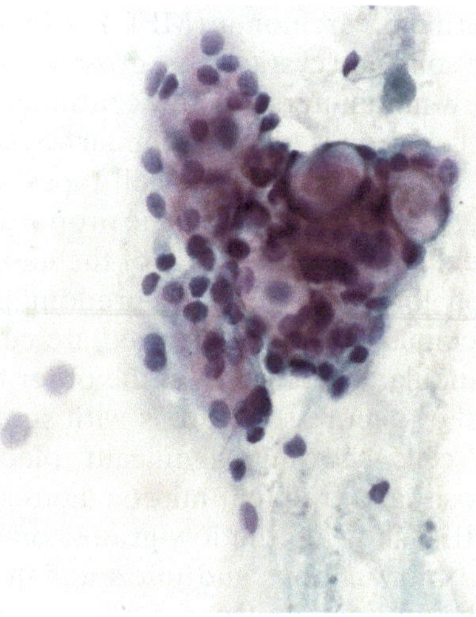

FIGURE 45.24. A well-differentiated mucoepidermoid carcinoma shows vacuolated mucinous cells and smaller "intermediate" cells that resemble transitional cells. These intermediate cells demonstrate well-defined cell borders, high N/C ratio, and a low degree of pleomorphism. (Papanicolaou stain.)

are small with relatively scant cytoplasm and line cystic and cylindrical spaces that are filled with basophilic basement membrane material. Cytologically, cases that are diagnostic show the acellular basement membrane material surrounded by small cuboidal/polygonal cells with bland nuclei (Fig. 45.25). Mitotic figures are not readily encountered and necrosis is not seen in most cases.[76–78] The small cells of ACC are relatively bland cytologically. However, with sparse sampling they may be mistaken for other neoplasms, especially SCLC. The major distinction is the lack of individual cell necrosis, frequent mitotic figures, and the neuroendocrine chromatin pattern. Since MEC and ACC may arise in extrapulmonary sites, metastasis to the lung is a possibility that must be excluded before reporting the neoplasm as primary to the lung.

Premalignant Lesion: Squamous Cell Dysplasia

Like other mucosa, the bronchus gives rise to SCC through a stepwise progression from squamous metaplasia to changes with increasing degrees of dysplasia (see Chapter 34). The histomorphologic features of squamous cell dysplasia and carcinoma in situ are defined in the WHO/IARC 2004 classification. By this definition, dysplasia is categorized as mild, moderate, or severe. Severe dysplasia is further distinguished from carcinoma in situ.

There are a few issues regarding the cytologic diagnosis of bronchial squamous dysplasia, especially at the ends of the spectrum. Cytologically, metaplastic squamous cells are present in small clusters or as single cells. They are round with dense cyanophilic cytoplasm on Papanicolaou-stained slides. The N/C ratio is low, and the nuclei are round with smooth even nuclear membranes. The chromatin pattern is homogeneous and the nucleoli are small or inconspicuous.

The distinction between mild dysplasia and reactive atypia is difficult. Squamous cells with mild dysplasia show a slight increase in N/C ratio, mild nuclear pleomorphism and variability, some nuclear membrane thickening and irregularity, and hyperchromasia. Nucleoli are

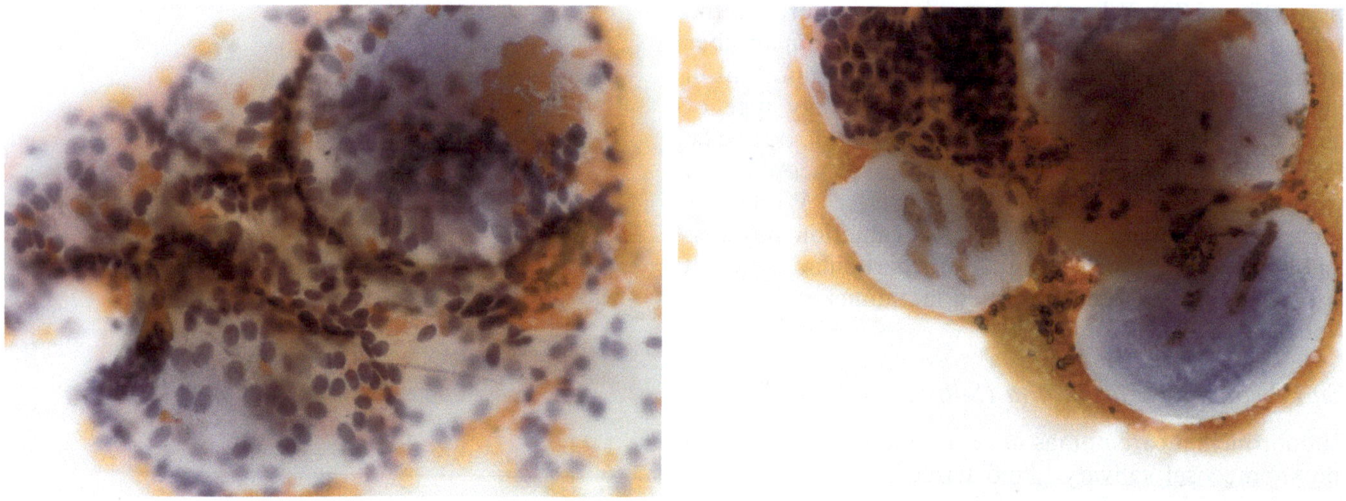

A B

FIGURE 45.25. **(A,B)** The cytologic diagnosis of adenoid cystic carcinoma depends on the identification of the characteristic hyaline globules surrounded by small pyknotic cells with high N/C ratio. This cytomorphologic presentation correlates with the cribriform pattern on histologic sections. The other patterns of adenoid cystic carcinoma—tubular and solid are not as characteristic on cytology specimens. (Papanicolaou stain.)

small and inconspicuous. These features overlap with other benign inflammatory and reactive conditions including changes from lung injury, infection, and radiation/chemotherapy (Fig. 45.6F). For cells with moderate dysplasia, the nuclei and N/C ratio are increased to a greater degree. The nuclear chromatin is coarser and the cytoplasm may be dyskeratotic. Severe dysplasia is characterized cytologically by small to large pleomorphic cells with elevated N/C ratio, single or loose clusters of cells, nuclear enlargement, hyperchromasia, irregular nuclear membranes, and prominent nucleoli (Fig. 45.6G). Severely dysplastic cells have dyskeratotic or dense cytoplasm with hyperchromatic or pyknotic nuclei that may only be slightly enlarged. Therefore, the N/C ratio may not be very high. Like low-grade dysplasia, a variety of nonneoplastic reactive conditions secondary to cell injury and inflammation are in the differential diagnosis of high-grade dysplasia. In particular, reactive changes secondary to diffuse alveolar damage produce markedly abnormal cytologic features. Inflammatory changes in the background would favor a reactive process. Furthermore, the cytologic distinction between high-grade dysplasia and carcinoma in situ is another problem area. Despite these borderline issues, the cytologic identification of severe squamous cell dysplasia is associated with an underlying carcinoma in approximately half of the patients. Therefore, such finding warrants close follow-up.[79]

On biopsy specimens, the expression of p63 immunoreactivity has been shown to correlate with the progression from preneoplastic and preinvasive lesions to invasive SCC.[80] The application of this marker to cytopathologic specimens may provide useful information for diagnosis. Due to these issues, the diagnosis of squamous cell dysplasia on pulmonary cytology samples is best approached carefully with thorough clinical and histologic correlation. The atypia identified in squamous cells in these specimens may not necessarily represent dysplasia.

Atypical adenomatous hyperplasia and diffuse neuroendocrine cell hyperplasia are also preinvasive lesions (see Chapter 34). Due to the fact that these lesions are small and clinically and radiologically difficult to localize, cytologic correlates have not been defined. By chance, should these cells be found on cytology specimens, they would most likely be mixed with other benign and nonlesional cellular components. Given the likely sparse representation of the lesional cells, prospective diagnosis is difficult to achieve. Atypical columnar/cuboidal type cells may be found under a variety of reactive and inflammatory processes as well as at the periphery of adenocarcinomas where the neoplastic cells grow along the preexisting alveolar framework. Likewise, neuroendocrine (Kulchitsky) cells are prevalent throughout the bronchi and bronchioles. Rare representation of these cells on cytologic specimens may not necessarily indicate diffuse neuroendocrine cell hyperplasia.

Benign Lesions

Cytologic evaluation of benign pulmonary neoplasms is relatively uncommon. The important issue regarding the cytologic diagnosis of benign neoplasms is not to overinterpret them as malignant neoplasms. Determination of benignity depends on cytologic appearance as well as the differentiation of the neoplastic cells. Furthermore, recognition of the clinical presentation is important in avoiding misdiagnosis. Particularly, radiographic formation detailing the precise location and the gross characteristics of the lesion are important. Two important benign lesions that may be encountered in cytologic specimens are hamartoma and sclerosing hemangioma.

Pulmonary Hamartoma

The radiographic appearance of a pulmonary nodule with "popcorn" calcification is characteristic of this lesion. The majority of hamartomas are now thought to be benign mesenchymal neoplasms, often with a prominent chondromyxoid component, with entrapped epithelial cells. For this reason, the term *mesenchymoma* is preferred, although *pulmonary hamartoma* is entrenched in the literature. The cytologic diagnosis is based on the identification of the fibromyxoid and chondroid elements admixed with epithelial cells. The fibromyxoid material is composed of fibrillary fragments with elongated fibroblast nuclei embedded in the matrix material (Fig. 45.26). Mature cartilage is present in a minority of cases.[81,82] The main difficulty in providing a cytologic diagnosis rests on the identification of the fibromyxoid fragments that may be mimicked by fibrous tissue, mucus, and clusters of

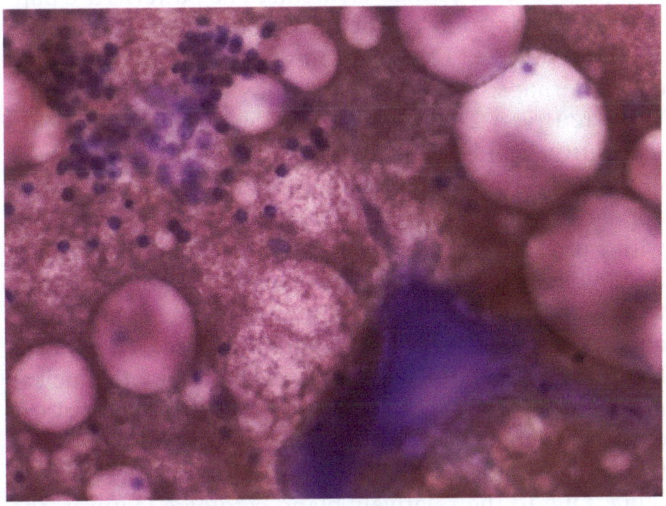

FIGURE 45.26. Pulmonary hamartoma shows bland epithelial cells in the upper left and chondroid matrix in the lower right. The chondroid cells that are the proliferating neoplastic cell population are often not sampled.

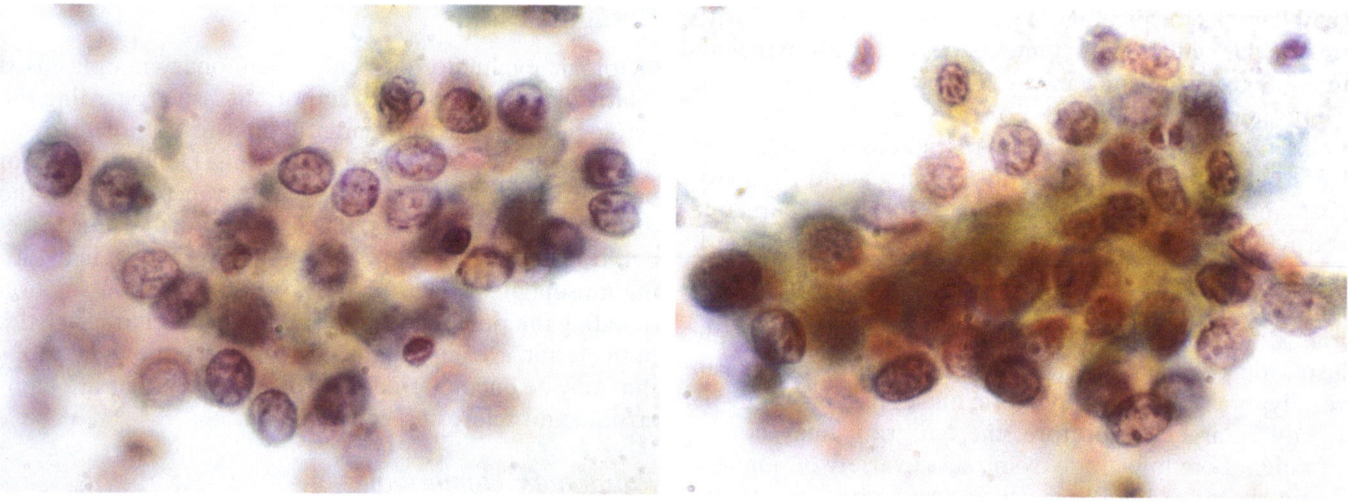

A B

FIGURE 45.27. **(A,B)** The cytologic diagnosis of sclerosing hemangioma is challenging. The characteristic cells are the bland polygonal "inverted" pneumocytes. These cells have abundant homogeneous cytoplasm, fine nuclear chromatin pattern, smooth nuclear membranes, and occasional grooves. (Papanicolaou stain.) (Courtesy of Dr. Anthony Gal, Emory University, Department of Pathology, Atlanta, GA.)

macrophages. Furthermore, fibromyxoid material may be found in a number of lesions. The most common differential diagnoses include chondroma, chondrosarcoma, pleomorphic adenoma, and other neoplasms with a chondroid element.

Sclerosing Hemangioma

Sclerosing hemangioma exhibits architectural heterogeneity and diverse cellular elements. The patterns are papillary, sclerotic, solid, and hemorrhagic. The neoplastic cell elements are the "round" stromal cells and the epithelial cells. Perhaps, one of the synonyms for this entity, "inverted type 2 pneumocytoma" more aptly describes this entity. Cytologically, the round cells that are embedded in the stroma are characteristic of this lesion; they appear in sheets with evenly spaced small, round cells with round to oval nuclei (Fig. 45.27). There is abundant homogeneous cytoplasm. The chromatin pattern is coarser than that of epithelial cells. The epithelial cells are larger and round, polygonal or spindled shaped. These cells have fine chromatin pattern, even and smooth nuclear membranes, and occasional grooves.[83,84] The cytologic diagnosis depends on the identification of these two cells types. This could be challenging depending on the sampling. Due to the relatively bland cytologic features, the differential diagnosis includes bronchioloalveolar carcinoma, papillary carcinoma, carcinoid tumor, and other low-grade neoplasms.

References

1. Travis WD, Brambilla E, Müller-Hermelink HK, Harris CC. Tumours of the lung, pleura, thymus, and heart. Lyon: IARC Press, 2004.
2. Johnston WW, Frable WJ. The cytopathology of respiratory tract: a review. Am J Pathol 1976;84:372–414.
3. Sproul EE, Huvos A, Brisch C. A two-year follow up study of 261 patients examined by use of superheated aerosol induced sputum. Acta Cytol 1962;6:409–412.
4. Koss LG, Melamed MR, Goodner JT. Pulmonary cytology: a brief survey of diagnostic results from July 1st, 1952 until December 31st, 1960. Acta Cytol 1964;8:104–113.
5. Boecking A, Biesterfeld S, Chatelain R, Gien-Gerlach G, Esser E. Diagnosis of bronchial carcinoma on secretions of paraffin-embedded sputum. Sensitivity and specificity of an alteration to routine cytology. Acta Cytol 1992; 36–47.
6. Greenstreet P, Purslow MJ, Kini SR. Respiratory specimen types for cytologic diagnoses, specimen procurement, collection methods, specimen submission, cytopreparation, and staining. In: Kini SR. Color atlas of pulmonary cytopathology. New York: Springer-Verlag, 2002:6–26.
7. Papanicolaou Society of Cytopathology Task Force on Standards of Practice. Guidelines of the Papanicolaou Society of Cytopathology for the examination of cytologic specimens obtained from the respiratory tract. Diagn Cytopathol 1999;21:61–69.
8. Rankin JA, Naegel GP, Reynolds HY. Use of a central laboratory for analysis of bronchoalveolar lavage fluid. Am Rev Respir Dis 1986;133:186–190.

9. Chamberlain DW, Braude AC, Rebuck AS. A critical evaluation of bronchoalveolar lavage: criteria for identifying unsatisfactory specimens. Acta Cytol 1987;31:599–605.
10. Taskinen EI, Tukiainen PS, Alitalo RL, Turunen J-P. Bronchoalveolar lavage: cytological techniques and interpretation of the cellular profiles. Pathol Annu 1994;29 (pt 2):121–155.
11. Robinson-Smith TM, Saad A, Baughman RP. Interpretation of the Wright-Giemsa stained bronchoalveolar lavage specimen. Lab Med 2004;35:553–557.
12. Bedrossian CW. Diagnostic problems in serous effusions. Diagn Cytopathol 1998;19:131–137.
13. Bottles K, Reznicek MJ, Holly EA, et al. Cytologic criteria to diagnose adenocarcinoma in pleural effusions. Mod Pathol 1991;4:677–681.
14. Yatabe Y, Mitsudomi T, Takahashi T. TTF-1 expression in pulmonary adenocarcinomas. Am J Surg Pathol 2002;26: 767–773.
15. Shah RN, Badve S, Papreddy D, Schindler S, Laskin WB, Yeldandi AV. Expression of cytokeratin 20 in mucinous bronchioloalveolar carcinoma. Hum Pathol 2002;33:915–920.
16. Schreiber G, McCrory DC. Performance characteristics of different modalities for diagnosis of suspected lung cancer: summary of published evidence. Chest 2003;123: 115S–128S.
17. Baba M, Iyoda A, Yasufuku K, et al. Preoperative cytodiagnosis of very small-sized peripheral-type primary lung cancer. Lung Cancer 2002;37:277–280.
18. Lachman MF, Schofield K, Cellura K. Bronchoscopic diagnosis of malignancy in the lower airway. A cytologic review. Acta Cytol 1995;39:1148–1151.
19. Barbazza R, Toniolo L, Pinarello A, et al. Accuracy of bronchial aspiration cytology in typing operable (stage I-II) pulmonary carcinomas. Diagn Cytopathol 1992;8:3–7.
20. Dahlstrom JE, Langdale-Smith GM, James DT. Fine needle aspiration cytology of pulmonary lesions: a reliable test. Pathology 2001;33:13–16.
21. Roger V, Nasiell M, Linden M, Enstad I. Cytologic differential diagnosis of bronchiolo-alveolar carcinoma and bronchogenic adenocarcinoma. Acta Cytol 1976;20:303–307.
22. Silverman JF, Finley JL, Park HK, Strausbauch P, Unverferth M, Carney M. Fine needle aspiration cytology of bronchioloalveolar-cell carcinoma of the lung. Acta Cytol 1985;29:887–894.
23. Tao LC, Weisbrod GL, Pearson FG, Sanders DE, Donat EE, Filipetto L. Cytologic diagnosis of bronchioloalveolar carcinoma by fine-needle aspiration biopsy. Cancer 1986;57: 1565–1570.
24. Lozowski W, Hajdu SI. Cytology and immunocytochemistry of bronchioloalveolar carcinoma. Acta Cytol 1987;31: 717–725.
25. Auger M, Katz RL, Johnston DA. Differentiating cytological features of bronchioloalveolar carcinoma from adenocarcinoma of the lung in fine-needle aspirations: a statistical analysis of 27 cases. Diagn Cytopathol 1997;16: 253–257.
26. Zaman SS, van Hoeven KH, Slott S, Gupta PK. Distinction between bronchioloalveolar carcinoma and hyperplastic pulmonary proliferations: a cytologic and morphometric analysis. Diagn Cytopathol 1997;16:396–401.
27. MacDonald LL, Yazdi HM. Fine-needle aspiration biopsy of bronchioloalveolar carcinoma. Cancer 2001;93:29–34.
28. Ohori NP, Santa Maria. Cytopathologic diagnosis of bronchioloalveolar carcinoma. Does it correlate with the 1999 World Health Organization definition? Am J Clin Pathol 2004;122:44–50.
29. Hoshi R, Tsuzuku M, Horai T, et al. Micropapillary clusters in early-stage lung adenocarcinomas. A distinct cytologic sign of significantly poor prognosis. Cancer Cytopathol 2004;102:81–86.
30. Zhang H, Liu J, Cagle PT, et al. Distinction of pulmonary small cell carcinoma from poorly differentiated squamous cell carcinoma: an immunohistochemical approach. Mod Pathol 2005;18:111–118.
31. Edwards SL, Robert C, McKean ME, et al. Preoperative histological classification of primary lung cancer: accuracy of diagnosis and use of the non-small cell category. J Clin Pathol 2000;53:537–540.
32. Evans DM, Shelley G. Respiratory cytodiagnosis: study in observer variation and its relation to quality of material. Thorax 1982;37:259–263.
33. Dugan JM. Cytologic diagnosis of basal cell (basaloid) carcinoma of the lung. A report of two cases. Acta Cytol 1995;39:539–542.
34. Chow LT, Chow WH, Tsui WM, et al. Fine needle aspiration cytologic diagnosis of lymphoepithelioma-like carcinoma of the lung. Report of two cases with immunohistochemical study. Am J Clin Pathol 1995;103:35–40.
35. Hummel P, Cangiarella JF, Cohen J-M, et al. Transthoracic fine-needle aspiration biopsy of pulmonary spindle cell and mesenchymal lesions. A study of 61 cases. Cancer Cytopathol 2001;93:187–198.
36. Roggli VL, Vollmer RT, Greenberg SD, et al. Lung cancer heterogeneity: a blinded and randomized study of 100 consecutive cases. Hum Pathol 1985;16:569–579.
37. Caya JG, Wollenberg NJ, Clowry LJ, Tieu TM. The diagnosis of pulmonary small-cell anaplastic carcinoma by cytologic means: a 13-year experience. Diagn Cytopathol 1988;4: 202–205.
38. Delgado PI, Jorda M, Ganjar-Azar P. Small cell carcinoma versus other lung malignancies: diagnosis by fine-needle aspiration cytology. Cancer Cytopathol 2000;90:279–285.
39. Sturgis CD, Nassar DL, D'Antonio JA, Raab SS. Cytologic features useful for distinguishing small cell from non-small cell carcinoma in bronchial brush and wash specimens. Am J Clin Pathol 2000;114:197–202.
40. Bavikatty NR, Michael CW. Cytologic features of small-cell carcinoma on ThinPrep. Diagn Cytopathol 2003;29: 8–12.
41. Arora VK, Singh N, Chaturvedi S, Bhatia A. Significance of cytologic criteria in distinguishing small cell from non-small cell carcinoma of lung. Acta Cytol 2003;47:216–220.
42. Zaharopoulos P, Wong JY, Stewart GD. Cytomorphology of the variants of small-cell carcinoma of the lung. Acta Cytol 1982;26:800–808.
43. Szyfelbein WM, Ross JS. Carcinoids, atypical carcinoids, and small-cell carcinoma of the lung: differential diagnosis of

fine-needle aspiration biopsy specimens. Diagn Cytopathol 1988;4:1–8.
44. Lin O, Olgac S, Green I, et al. Immunohistochemical staining of cytologic smears with MIB-1 helps distinguish low-grade from high-grade neuroendocrine neoplasms. Am J Clin Pathol 2003;120:209–216.
45. Salhadin A, Nasiell M, Nasiell K, et al. The unique cytologic picture of oat cell carcinoma in effusions. Acta Cytol 1976;20:298–302.
46. Chhieng DC, Ko EC, Yee HT, et al. Malignant pleural effusions due to small-cell lung carcinoma: a cytologic and immunohistochemical study. Diagn Cytopathol 2001;25: 356–360.
47. Pilotti S, Rilke F, Lombardi L. Pulmonary carcinoid with glandular features. Report of two cases with positive fine needle aspiration biopsy cytology. Acta Cytol 1983;27: 511–514.
48. Evans H, Blaney R. Pulmonary carcinoid with papillary structure: report of a case with fine-needle aspiration cytology. Diagn Cytopathol 1994;11:178–181.
49. Wiatrowska BA, Krol J, Zakowski MF. Large-cell neuroendocrine carcinoma of the lung: proposed criteria for cytologic diagnosis. Diagn Cytopathol 2001;24:58–64.
50. Nguyen GK. Cytopathology of pulmonary carcinoid tumor in sputum and bronchial brushing. Acta Cytol 1995;39: 1152–1160.
51. Aron M, Kapila K, Verma K. Carcinoid tumors of the lung: a diagnostic challenge in bronchial washings. Diagn Cytopathol 2004;30:62–66.
52. Kakinuma H, Mikami T, Iwabuchi K, et al. Diagnostic findings of bronchial brush cytology for pulmonary large cell neuroendocrine carcinomas: comparison with poorly differentiated adenocarcinomas, squamous cell carcinomas, and small cell carcinomas. Cancer Cytopathol 2003;99: 247–254.
53. Yang YJ, Steele CT, Ou XL, et al. Diagnosis of high-grade pulmonary neuroendocrine carcinoma by fine-needle aspiration biopsy: nonsmall-cell or small-cell type? Diagn Cytopathol 2001;25:292–300.
54. Nicholson SA, Ryan MR. A review of cytologic findings in neuroendocrine carcinomas including carcinoid tumors with histologic correlation. Cancer Cytopathol 2000;90: 148–161.
55. Ordonez NG. The immunohistochemical diagnosis of mesothelioma: a comparative study of epithelioid mesothelioma and lung adenocarcinoma. Am J Surg Pathol 2003;27: 1031–1051.
56. Illei PB, Ladanyi M, Rusch VW, Zakowski MF. The use of CDKN2A deletion as a diagnostic marker for malignant mesothelioma in body cavity effusions. Cancer Cytopathol 2003;99:51–56.
57. Shin HJ, Shin DM, Tarco E, Sneige N. Detection of numerical aberrations of chromosome 7 and 9 in cytologic specimens of pleural malignant mesothelioma. Cancer Cytopathol 2003;99:233–239.
58. Costa MBG, Siqueira SA, Saldiva PH, et al. Histologic patterns of lung infiltration of B-cell, T-cell, and Hodgkin lymphomas. Am J Clin Pathol 2004;121:718–726.
59. Crapanzano JP, Lin O. Cytologic findings of marginal zone lymphoma. Cancer Cytopathol 2003;99:301–309.
60. Orucevic A, Reddy VB, Selvaggi SM, et al. Fine-needle aspiration of extranodal and extramedullary hematopoietic malignancies. Diagn Cytopathol 2000;23:318–321.
61. Wakely PE, Menezes G, Nuovo GJ. Primary effusion lymphoma: cytopathologic diagnosis using in situ molecular genetic analysis for human herpesvirus 8. Mod Pathol 2002;15:944–950.
62. Dusenbery D, Nalesnik MA, Locker J, Swerdlow SH. Cytologic features of post-transplant lymphoproliferative disorder. Diagn Cytopathol 1997;16:489–496.
63. Ohori NP, Whisnant RE, Nalesnik MA, Swerdlow SH. Primary pleural effusion posttransplant lymphoproliferative disorder: distinction from secondary involvement and effusion lymphoma. Diagn Cytopathol 2001;25:50–53.
64. Cordes BG, Collins BT, McDonald JW, et al. Fine needle aspiration biopsy of primary leiomyosarcoma arising from pulmonary vein. Acta Cytol 1999;43:523–526.
65. Lazure T, Essamet W, Palazzo L, et al. Cytological findings of a primary mediastino-pulmonary leiomyosarcoma. Report of a case diagnosed by endoscopic ultrasonography-guided fine needle aspiration. Cytopathology 2001;12: 410–413.
66. Yamaguchi T, Imamura Y, Nakayama K, et al. Primary pulmonary leiomyosarcoma. Report of a case diagnosed by fine needle aspiration cytology. Acta Cytol 2002;46: 912–916.
67. Gray J, Ngyugen G. Primary pulmonary Rhabdomyosarcoma diagnosed by fine-needle aspiration cytology. Diagn Cytopathol 2003;29:181–182.
68. Hummel P, Yang GCH, Kumar A, et al. PNET-like features of synovial sarcoma of the lung: a pitfall in the cytologic diagnosis of soft-tissue tumors. Diagn Cytopathol 2001;24: 283–288.
69. Hsiu JG, Kreuger JK, D'Amato NA, Morris JR. Primary malignant fibrous histiocytoma of the lung. Fine needle aspiration cytologic features. Acta Cytol 1987;31: 345–350.
70. Hummel P, Cangiarella JF, Cohen J. Transthoracic fine-needle aspiration biopsy of pulmonary spindle cell and mesenchymal lesions. Cancer Cytopathol 2001;93:187–188.
71. Ryan MR, Stasny JF, Wakely PE. The cytopathology of synovial sarcoma. A study of six cases, with emphasis on architecture and histopathologic correlation. Cancer Cytopathol 1998;84:42–49.
72. Slagel DD, Raab SS, Silverman JF. Fine needle biopsy of metastatic malignant melanoma with "rhabdoid" features. Frequency, cytologic features, pitfalls, and ancillary studies. Acta Cytol 1997;41:1426–1430.
73. Tao LC, Robertson DI. Cytologic diagnosis of bronchial mucoepidermoid carcinoma by fine needle aspiration. Acta Cytol 1978;22:221–224.
74. Brooks B, Baandrup U. Peripheral low-grade mucoepidermoid carcinoma of the lung. Fine needle aspiration cytologic diagnosis and histology. Cytopathology 1992;3: 259–265.
75. Segletes LA, Steffee CH, Geisinger KR. Cytology of primary pulmonary mucoepidermoid and adenoid cystic carcinoma. A report of four cases. Acta Cytol 1999;43:1091–1097.
76. Anderson RJ, Johnston WW, Szpak CA. Fine needle aspiration of adenoid cystic carcinoma metastatic to the lung.

Cytologic features and differential diagnosis. Acta Cytol 1985;29:527–532.
77. Smith RC, Amy RW. Adenoid cystic carcinoma metastatic to the lung: report of a case diagnosed by fine needle aspiration biopsy. Acta Cytol 1985;29:533–534.
78. Radhika S, Dey P, Rajwanshi A, et al. Adenoid cystic carcinoma in a bronchial washing: a case report. Acta Cytol 1993;37:97–99.
79. Risse EK, Vooijs GP, van't Hof MA. Diagnostic significance of "severe dysplasia" in sputum cytology. Acta Cytol 1988; 32:629–634.
80. Pelosi G, Pasini F, Olsen Stenholm C, et al. p63 immunoreactivity in lung cancer: yet another player in the development of squamous cell carcinoma? J Pathol 2002;198:100–109.
81. Dunbar F, Leiman G. The aspiration cytology of pulmonary hamartomas. Diagn Cytopathol 1989;5:174–180.
82. Hughes JH, Young NA, Wilbur DC, et al. Fine-needle aspiration of pulmonary hamartoma. A common source of false-positive diagnoses in the College of American Pathologists interlaboratory comparison program in non-gynecologic cytology. Arch Pathol Lab Med 2005;129: 19–22.
83. Chow LT, Chan SK, Chow WH, Tsui MS. Pulmonary sclerosing hemangioma. Report of a case with diagnosis by fine needle aspiration. Acta Cytol 1992;36:287–292.
84. Gal AA, Nassar VH, Miller JI. Cytopathologic diagnosis of pulmonary sclerosing hemangioma. Diagn Cytopathol 2002; 26:163–166.

Index

G

H

M

N

MIX
Papier aus verantwortungsvollen Quellen
Paper from responsible sources
FSC® C105338

If you have any concerns about our products,
you can contact us on
ProductSafety@springernature.com

In case Publisher is established outside the EU,
the EU authorized representative is:
Springer Nature Customer Service Center GmbH
Europaplatz 3, 69115 Heidelberg, Germany

Printed by Libri Plureos GmbH
in Hamburg, Germany